P9-CKO-656

Allergy and Allergic Diseases

To my mentors
John Crofton, Robin Coombs
and Frank Austen

Allergy and Allergic Diseases

Edited by A.B. Kay FRSE
PhD DSc FRCP FRCPath
Head, Allergy and Clinical Immunology
Imperial College School of Medicine at the
National Heart and Lung Institute
and Honorary Consultant Physician
Royal Brompton Hospital, London

Foreword by R.R.A. Coombs FRS

IN TWO VOLUMES
VOLUME 1

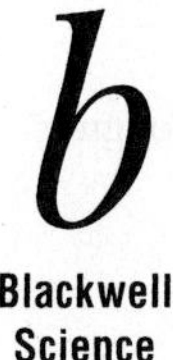

Blackwell
Science

Editorial Offices:
Osney Mead, Oxford OX2 0EL
25 John Street, London WC1N 2BL
23 Ainslie Place, Edinburgh EH3 6AJ
350 Main Street, Malden
MA 01248-5018, USA
54 University Street, Carlton
Victoria 3053, Australia

Other Editorial Offices:
Blackwell Wissenschafts-Verlag GmbH
Kurfürstendamm 57
10707 Berlin, Germany

Zehetnergasse 6
A-1140 Wien
Austria

Set by Excel Typesetters, Hong Kong
Printed and bound in Italy
by Rotolito Lombarda S.p.A., Milan

The Blackwell Science logo is a trade mark of Blackwell Science Ltd, registered at the United Kingdom Trade Marks Registry

First published 1997

A catalogue record for this title
is available from the British Library

ISBN 0-86542-867-0

Library of Congress
Cataloging-in-publication Data

Allergy and allergic diseases / edited by
A.B. Kay.
p. cm.
Includes bibliographical references
and index.
ISBN 0-86542-867-0
1. Allergy–Pathophysiology.
2. Asthma–Pathophysiology.
I. Kay, A.B.
[DNLM:
1. Hypersensitivity–immunology.
2. Asthma–immunology.
3. Allergens–immunology.
4. Immunotherapy. WD 300
A4326 1997]
RC585.A445 1997
616.97–dc20
DNLM/DLC
for Library of Congress 96-13727
CIP

DISTRIBUTORS

Marston Book Services Ltd
PO Box 269
Abingdon
Oxon OX14 4YN
(*Orders*: Tel: 01235 465500
Fax: 01235 46555)

USA
Blackwell Science, Inc.
Commerce Place
350 Main Street
Malden, MA 02148-5018
(*Orders*: Tel: 800 759 6102
617 388 8250
Fax: 617 388 8255)

Canada
Copp Clark Professional
200 Adelaide Street West, 3rd Floor
Toronto, Ontario M5H1W7
(*Orders*: Tel: 416 597-1616
800 815-9417
Fax: 416 597-1617)

Australia
Blackwell Science Pty Ltd
54 University Street
Carlton, Victoria 3053
(*Orders*: Tel: 03 9347 0300
Fax: 03 9347 5001)

Contents

List of Contributors, x

Foreword, xvii

Preface, xx

VOLUME 1

Part 1: Immunological Basis of the Allergic Response

1 A Short History of Allergological Diseases and Concepts, 3
AL de Weck

2 Concepts of Allergy and Hypersensitivity, 23
AB Kay

3 T and B Lymphocytes and the Development of Allergic Reactions, 36
CJ Corrigan

4 Immunoglobulin Structure, Synthesis and Genetics, 58
AR Venkitaraman

5 IgE and IgE Receptors, 81
BJ Sutton & HJ Gould

6 Regulation of IgE Synthesis, 96
S Romagnani

7 Antigen Processing and Presentation, 113
JM Austyn

8 Immunological Tolerance and T-cell Anergy, 131
GF Hoyne, C Hetzel & JR Lamb

Part 2: Inflammatory Cells and Mediators

9 Human Mast Cells and Basophils, 149
MK Church, P Bradding, AF Walls & Y Okayama

10 Eosinophils and the Allergic Inflammatory Response, 171
AJ Wardlaw, RM Moqbel & AB Kay

11 The Neutrophil, 198
C Haslett & ER Chilvers

12 Platelets, 214
CM Herd & CP Page

13 Macrophages and Dendritic Cells in Allergic Reactions, 228
PG Holt

14 Leucocyte Adhesion in Allergic Inflammation, 244
AJ Wardlaw

15 Airway Epithelium in Asthma, 263
LA Cohn, BM Fischer, TM Krunkosky, DT Wright & KB Adler

16 Endothelial Cells in Allergy, 284
A-B Tonnel, D Jeannin, S Molet, P Gosset, Y Delneste, B Wallaert & M Joseph

17 Fibroblasts and Bronchial Asthma, 298
WR Roche

18 Complement and Antigen–Antibody Complexes, 307
WJ Schwaeble & K Whaley

19 Intrinsic Coagulation/Bradykinin-Forming Cascade, 324
AP Kaplan, M Silverberg & S Reddigari

20 Cytokines (Interleukins), 340
CJ Corrigan

21 Role of IL-5, IL-3 and GM-CSF in the Pathophysiology of Asthma and Allergy, 354
AB Kay

22 Chemokines, 365
CA Dahinden

23 Lipid Mediators—Leukotrienes, Prostanoids and Platelet-Activating Factor, 380
SMS Nasser & TH Lee

Part 3: Pharmacology

24 Histamine and Antihistamines, 421
FER Simons

25 Vascular Permeability and Plasma Exudation, 439
CGA Persson

26 Neuropeptides, 447
MG Belvisi & AJ Fox

27 The Autonomic Nervous System in Asthma and Rhinitis, 481
SJ Smart & TB Casale

28 Neuropharmacology, 505
AD Watkins

29 Endothelin and Nitric Oxide, 518
DR Springall & JM Polak

30 Theophylline and Isoenzyme-Selective Phosphodiesterase Inhibitors, 531
MA Giembycz, G Dent & JE Souness

31 Adrenergic Agonists and Antagonists, 568
TR Bai

32 Nedocromil Sodium and Sodium Cromoglycate: Pharmacology and Putative Modes of Action, 584
RP Eady & AA Norris

33 Cholinergic Antagonists, 596
NJ Gross

34 Potassium Channel Openers as Anti-Asthma Drugs, 609
RC Small & RW Foster

35 Glucocorticosteriods, 619
PJ Barnes

36 Immunosuppressants (Drugs and Monoclonal Antibodies), 642
CA Bonham & AW Thomson

Part 4: Physiology

37 Physiological Aspects of Airway, Pulmonary and Respiratory Muscle Function in Asthma, 667
NB Pride

38 Bronchial Hyperresponsiveness, 682
R Pauwels

39 Exercise-Induced Asthma, 692
SD Anderson

40 Mucus and Mucociliary Clearance, 712
PJ Wills & PJ Cole

41 New Approaches in Aerosol Drug Delivery for the Treatment of Asthma, 730
V Knight & JC Waldrep

42 Airway Smooth Muscle, 742
IW Rodger

Part 5: Cellular and Molecular Techniques in the Study of Allergic Disease

43 T-Cell Cloning, 755
RE O'Hehir, BA Askonas & JR Lamb

44 *In Situ* Hybridization, 766
Q Hamid

45 Immunocytochemistry, 775
Q Hamid

46 Polymerase Chain Reaction, 784
CJ Corrigan
Appendix, Ai

VOLUME 2

Part 6: Allergens

47 Biochemistry of Allergens, 797
O Cromwell

48 Molecular Cloning of Allergens, 811
WR Thomas

49 Allergen Extracts and Standardization, 825
S Klysner & H Løwenstein

50 Grass, Tree and Weed Pollens, 835
JC Emberlin

51 Fungi and Actinomycetes as Allergens, 858
J Lacey

52 Dust Mites and Asthma, 888
TAE Platts-Mills & JA Woodfolk

53 Animal Allergens, 900
C Schou

54 Allergens in the Workplace, 909
RD Tee

55 Allergens from Stinging Insects, 927
TJ Lintner, WMW Guralnick & H Løwenstein

56 Cockroach Allergens and their Role in Asthma, 942
MD Chapman, LD Vailes, ML Hayden, TAE Platts-Mills & LK Arruda

57 Chironomidae, 952
V Liebers & X Baur

58 Food Allergens, 961
SB Lehrer, SL Taylor, SL Hefle & RK Bush

59 Latex Allergy, 981
JE Slater

Part 7: Diagnostic Methods and the Assessment of Allergic Diseases

60 Principles and Interpretation of Laboratory Tests for Allergy, 997
RMR Barnes

61 Skin Tests, 1007
AJ Frew

62 Quantification of IgE both as Total Immunoglobulin and as Allergen-Specific Antibody, 1012
TG Merrett

Part 8: Major Animal Models of Asthma and Hyperresponsiveness

63 Primate Models of Allergic Asthma, 1037
RH Gundel

64 Sheep Models of Allergic Bronchoconstriction, 1045
WM Abraham

65 Murine Models of Allergy, Asthma and Hyperresponsiveness, 1056
GP Geba & PW Askenase

66 The Allergic Response in Rats, 1068
KF Chung

67 The Rabbit as an Animal Model of Allergy, Asthma and Airway Hyperresponsiveness, 1079
CM Herd & CP Page

68 The Sensitized Guinea Pig as a Model of Allergic Asthma, 1093
E Minshall & S Sanjar

69 Canine Models of Asthma and Hyperresponsiveness, 1103
C Emala & CA Hirshman

Part 9: Human Models of Allergic Inflammation (Late-Phase Reactions)

70 Human Late Asthmatic Responses, 1113
AM Bentley, AB Kay & SR Durham

71 Late-Phase Skin Reactions, 1131
AJ Frew

72 Late-Phase Reactions in the Nose, 1139
RS Peebles & A Togias

Part 10: General Principles of the Allergic Response in Humans

73 Allergy and Helminthic Parasites: are Atopics Protected against Infection?, 1163
RM Moqbel & DI Pritchard

74 Familial Inheritance of Asthma and Allergy, 1177
B Sibbald

75 Genetics of Atopy, 1187
JM Hopkin

76 Genetics of Allergy and Asthma, 1196
ER Bleecker & DA Meyers

77 Epidemiology of Atopy and Atopic Disease, 1208
D Jarvis & P Burney

Part 11: Allergen Injection Immunotherapy

78 Mechanisms, 1227
SR Durham & VA Varney

79 Indications for Specific Immunotherapy, 1234
J Bousquet, A Des Roches, L Paradis, J Knani, H Dhivert & F-B Michel

80 Practical Immunotherapy, 1243
H-J Malling

Part 12: The Practice of Allergology

81 Allergology as a Medical Specialty or Sub-Specialty, 1261
AB Kay

82 Principles and Practice of Diagnosis and Treatment of Allergic Disease, 1271
AB Kay

Part 13: Seasonal and Perennial Rhinitis

83 The Classification and Diagnosis of Rhinitis, 1293
IS Mackay & SR Durham

84 Structure and Function of the Upper Airways, 1300
N Mygind & H Jacobi

85 Seasonal and Perennial Allergic Rhinitis, 1311
PH Howarth

86 Treatment and Management of Allergic Rhinitis, 1327
MA Calderón-Zapata & RJ Davies

Part 14: Asthma

87 Definition, Clinical Features, Investigations and Differential Diagnosis of Asthma, 1347
LM Fabbri, G Caramori & P Maestrelli

88 Post-Mortem Pathology in Asthma, 1360
JC Hogg

89 Aetiology and Pathogenesis of Asthma, 1366
ST Holgate

90 The T-Cell Hypothesis of Chronic Asthma, 1379
AB Kay, AJ Frew, CJ Corrigan & DS Robinson

91 Air Pollution and Allergic Disease, 1395
AJ Wardlaw

92 Pathology of Asthma, 1412
PK Jeffery

93 Treatment of Chronic Asthma in Adults, 1429
PJ Barnes

94 Delivery Systems, 1440
GK Crompton

95 Childhood Asthma, 1451
JO Warner

96 Occupational Asthma, 1464
P Cullinan & AJ Newman-Taylor

Part 15: Other Allergic Diseases

97 Extrinsic Allergic Alveolitis, 1489
P Cullinan & AJ Newman-Taylor

98 Pulmonary Eosinophilia, 1502
MW Elliott & AJ Newman-Taylor

99 Food Allergy, 1517
HA Sampson

100 Anaphylaxis, 1550
SJ Lane & TH Lee

101 Atopic Dermatitis, 1573
CAFM Bruijnzeel-Koomen, GC Mudde & A Kapp

102 Urticaria and Angioedema, 1586
A Kobza Black & MW Greaves

103 Contact Dermatitis, 1608
JD Wilkinson & S Shaw

104 Otitis Media, 1632
P Fireman

105 Ocular Allergy, 1645
M Hingorani & S Lightman

106 Drug Reactions, 1671
M Pradal & D Vervloet

107 Insect-Sting Allergy, 1693
PW Ewan

Part 16: Prevention of Allergic Disease and Future Trends

108 Prevention of Allergic Diseases and Sensitization, 1709
R Dahl & S Halken

109 Prevention of Allergy in the Fetus and Newborn, 1715
D Hide & JA Warner*

110 New Treatment Drugs for Asthma, 1726
OM Kon & NC Barnes

Index, i

List of Contributors

W.M. Abraham, Mount Sinai Medical Center, 4300 Alton Road, Miami Beach, Florida 33140, USA

K.B. Adler, Department of Anatomy, Physiological Sciences and Radiology, College of Veterinary Medicine, North Carolina State University, 4700 Hillsborough Street, Raleigh, North Carolina 27545, USA

S.D. Anderson, Department of Respiratory Medicine, Royal Prince Alfred Hospital, Missenden Road, Camperdown, NSW Australia 2050

L.K. Arruda, Asthma and Allergic Diseases Center, Departments of Internal Medicine and Microbiology, University of Virginia, Charlottesville, Virginia, USA

P.W. Askenase, Yale University School of Medicine, 904 LC1, P.O.Box 208013, New Haven, Connecticut 06520-8013, USA

B.A. Askonas, Infection and Immunity Section, Department of Biology, Imperial College of Science, Technology and Medicine, Prince Consort Road, London SW2 7BB, UK

J.M. Austyn, Nuffield Department of Surgery, University of Oxford, John Radcliffe Hospital, Headington, Oxford, OX3 9DU, UK

T.R. Bai, Respiratory Division, University of British Columbia, Pulmonary Research Laboratory, St Paul's Hospital, 1081 Burrard Street, Vancouver BC, Canada V6Z 1Y6

N.C. Barnes, Thoracic Medicine, London Chest Hospital, Bonner Road, London, E1 9JX, UK

P.J. Barnes, Thoracic Medicine, Imperial College School of Medicine at The National Heart and Lung Institute, Dovehouse Street, London, SW3 6LY, UK

R.M.R. Barnes, Department of Immunology, Royal Liverpool University Hospital, Liverpool, UK

X. Baur, BGFA, Institut an der Ruhr-Universität Bochum, Burkle-de-la-Camp-Platz 1, D-44789 Bochum, Germany

M.G. Belvisi, Thoracic Medicine, Imperial College School of Medicine at The National Heart and Lung Institute, Dovehouse Street, London, SW3 6LY, UK

A.M. Bentley, Osler Chest Unit, Churchill Hospital, Headington, Oxford, OX3 7LJ, UK

E.R. Bleecker, University of Maryland at Baltimore, School of Medicine, Division of Pulmonary and Critical Care Medicine, University Center, Baltimore, Maryland 21201, USA

C.A. Bonham, Department of Surgery, University of Pittsburgh Medical Center, W154OC Biomedical Science Tower, 200 Lothrop Street, Pittsburgh, Pennsylvania 15213, USA

J. Bousquet, CHU Montpellier, Service des Maladies Respiratoires, Hôpital Arnaud de Villeneuve, 371 Avenue du Doyen G. Giraud, 34295 Montpellier, Cedex 5, France

P. Bradding, Immunopharmacology Group, Centre Block, Southampton General Hospital, Tremona Road, Southampton, SO16 6YD, UK

C.A.F.M. Bruijnzeel-Koomen, Department of Dermatology, University Hospital Utrecht, P.O. Box 85500, 3508 GA Utrecht, The Netherlands

P. Burney, United Medical and Dental Schools, Division of Public Health Services, Block 8, St Thomas's Hospital, Lambeth Palace Road, London, SE1 7EH, UK

R.K. Bush, Department of Medicine, Allergy and Clinical Immunology Section, University of Wisconsin, Madison, Wisconsin, USA; Wm.S.Middleton Memorial VA Hospital, Madison, Wisconsin, USA

M.A. Calderón-Zapata, Academic Department of Respiratory Medicine, St Bartholomew's, London Chest Hospital, Bonner Road, London, E2 9JX, UK

G. Caramori, Institute of Respiratory and Infectious Diseases, Via Fossato di Mortara, 64/B, 44100 Ferrara, University of Ferrara, Italy

T.B. Casale, Nebraska Medical Research Institute, 401 East Gold Coast Road, Suite 326, Papillon, Nebraska 68128-4796, USA

M.D. Chapman, Asthma and Allergic Diseases Center, Departments of Internal Medicine and Microbiology, University of Virginia, Charlottesville, Virginia, USA

E.R. Chilvers, Respiratory Medicine Unit, Department of Medicine, University of Edinburgh, Royal Infirmary, Lauriston Place, Edinburgh, EH3 9YW, UK

K.F. Chung, Thoracic Medicine, Imperial College School of Medicine at The National Heart and Lung Institute and Royal Brompton Hospital, London, SW3, UK

M.K. Church, Immunopharmacology Group, Centre Block, Southampton General Hospital, Tremona Road, Southampton, SO16 6YD, UK

L.A. Cohn, University of Missouri, College of Veterinary Medicine, Veterinary Teaching Hospital, 374 Clydesdale Hall, Columbia, Missouri 65211, USA

P.J. Cole, Host Defence Unit, Imperial College School of Medicine at The National Heart and Lung Institute, Emmanuel Kaye Building, Manresa Road, London, SW3 6LR, UK

C.J. Corrigan, Department of Medicine, Charing Cross and Westminster Medical School (University of London), Charing Cross Hospital, Fulham Palace Road, London, W6 8RF, UK

G.K. Crompton, Respiratory Unit, Western General Hospitals NHS Trust, Crewe Road, Edinburgh, EH4 2XU, UK

O. Cromwell, Allergopharma Joachim Ganzer KG, Hermann-Körner Strasse 52, 21465 Reinbek, Hamburg, Germany

P. Cullinan, Occupational and Environmental Medicine, Imperial College School of Medicine at The National Heart and Lung Institute, Emmanuel Kaye Building, Manresa Road, London, SW3 6LR, UK

C.A. Dahinden, Institute of Immunology and Allergology, University Hospital, Inselspital, CH 3010 Bern, Switzerland

R. Dahl, Department of Respiratory Disease, University Hospital of Aarhus, DK-8000 Aarhus C., Denmark

R.J. Davies, Academic Depertment of Respiratory Medicine, St Bartholomew's and the Royal London School of Medicine and Dentistry, The London Chest Hospital, Bonner Road, London, E2 9JX, UK

Y. Delneste, INSERM U 416, Institut Pasteur, P.O. Box 245, F-59019 Lille, France

G. Dent, Krankenhaus Großhansdorf, Zentrum für Pneumologie und Thoraxchirurgie, LVA Hamburg, Wöhrendamm, D-22927, Großhansdorf, Germany

A. Des Roches, CHU Montpellier, Service des Maladies Respiratoires, Hôpital Arnaud de Villeneuve, 371 Avenue du Doyen G. Giraud, 34295 Montpellier, Cedex 5, France

H. Dhivert, CHU Montpellier, Service des Maladies Respiratoires, Hôpital Arnaud de Villeneuve, 371 Avenue du Doyen G. Giraud, 34295 Montpellier, Cedex 5, France

S.R. Durham, Nose Clinic, Royal Brompton Hospital, Allergy and Clinical Immunology, Imperial College School of Medicine at The National Heart and Lung Institute, Dovehouse Street, London, SW3 6LY, UK

R.P. Eady, Astra Charnwood, Bakewell Road, Loughborough, Leicestershire, LE11 5RH, UK

M.W. Elliott, Consultant Chest Physician, St James's Respiratory Unit, St James's University Hospital, Beckett Street, Leeds, LS9 7TF, UK

C. Emala, The Johns Hopkins School of Hygiene and Public Health, Room 7006, 615 N. Wolfe Street, Baltimore, Maryland 21205, USA

J.C. Emberlin, Pollen Research Unit, Worcester College of Higher Education, Henwick Grove, Worcester, WR2 6AJ, UK

P.W. Ewan, Molecular Immunopathology Unit, Medical Research Council Centre, and Allergy Clinic, Addenbrooke's Hospital NHS Trust, Hills Road, Cambridge, CB2 2QH, UK

L.M. Fabbri, Institute of Respiratory and Infectious Diseases, Via Fossato di Mortara, 64/B, 44100 Ferrara, University of Ferrara, Italy

P. Fireman, Division of Immunology and Rheumatology, University of Pittsburgh School of Medicine, Children's Hospital of Pittsburgh, One Children's Place, 3705 Fifth Avenue at DeSoto Street, Pittsburgh, Pennsylvania 15213-2583, USA

B.M. Fischer, Department of Anatomy, Physical Sciences and Radiology, College of Veterinary Medicine, North Carolina State University, 4700 Hillsborough Street, Raleigh, NC 27606, USA

A.J. Frew, University Medicine, Level D, Centre Block, Southampton General Hospital, Tremona Road, Southampton, SO16 6YD, UK

R.W. Foster, Smooth Muscle Pharmacology Research Group, School of Biological Sciences, University of Manchester, Oxford Road, Manchester, M13 9PT, UK

A.J. Fox, Thoracic Medicine, Imperial College School of Medicine at The National Heart and Lung Institute, Dovehouse Street, London, SW3 6LY, UK

G.P. Geba, Sections of Pulmonary and Critical Care and Allergy and Immunology, Department of Medicine, Yale University School of Medicine, 333 Cedar Street, New Haven, Connecticut 06520, USA

M.A. Giembycz, Thoracic Medicine, Imperial College School of Medicine at The National Heart and Lung Institute, Dovehouse Street, London, SW3 6LY, UK

P. Gosset, INSERM U 416, Institut Pasteur, P.O. Box 245, F-59019 Lille, France

H.J. Gould, The Randall Institute, King's College London, 26 Drury Lane, London, WC2B 5RL, UK

M.W. Greaves, St Johns Institute of Dermatology, St Thomas's Hospital, London, SE1 7EH, UK

N.J. Gross, Departments of Medicine and Molecular Biochemistry, Division of Pulmonary and Critical Care Medicine, Edward Hines Jr. Hospital, P.O. Box 1430, Hines, Illinois 60141

R.H. Gundel, Pharmacology Department, Biotechnology, Bayer Corporation, Berkeley, California, 94701-1986, USA

W.M.W. Guralnick, Vespa Laboratories, Inc., R.D. NBR1, Spring Mills, Pennsylvania, 16875, USA

S. Halken, Department of Pediatrics, Soenderborg Hospital, DK-6400 Soenderborg, Denmark

Q. Hamid, Departments of Medicine and Pathology, Meakins-Christie Laboratories, McGill University, 3626 St Urbain Street, Montreal, Quebec H2X 2P2, Canada

C. Haslett, Respiratory Medicine Unit, Department of Medicine (RIE), University of Edinburgh, Royal Infirmary, Lauriston Place, Edinburgh, EH3 9YW, UK

M.L. Hayden, Asthma and Allergic Diseases Center, Departments of Internal Medicine and Microbiology, University of Virginia, Charlottesville, Virginia, USA

S.L. Hefle, University of Nebraska, Department of Food Science and Technology, Lincoln, Nebraska, USA

C.M. Herd, Biomedical Sciences Division, Pharmacology Group, King's College, University of London, Manresa Road, London, SW3 6LX, UK

C. Hetzel, Infection and Immunity Section, Department of Biology, Imperial College of Science, Technology and Medicine, Prince Consort Road, London SW7 2BB, UK

D. Hide (*deceased) Former Consultant in Clinical Allergy/Senior Lecturer in Child Health

M. Hingorani, Institute of Ophthalmology and Department of Clinical Ophthalmology, Moorfield's Eye Hospital, London, UK

C.A. Hirshman, The Johns Hopkins School of Hygiene and Public Health, Room 7006, 615 N. Wolfe Street, Baltimore, Maryland 21205, USA

J.C. Hogg, UBC Pulmonary Research Laboratory, St Paul's Hospital, 1081 Burrard Street, Vancouver, BC V6Z1Y6, Canada

S.T. Holgate, University Medicine, Level D, Centre Block, Southampton General Hospital, Tremona Road, Southampton, SO16 6YD, UK

P.G. Holt, Institute for Child Health Research, PO Box 855, West Perth, Western Australia 6872

J.M. Hopkin, Osler Chest Unit, Churchill Hospital, Oxford, OX3 7LJ, UK

P.H. Howarth, University Medicine, Southampton General Hospital, Tremona Road, Southampton, SO16 6YD, UK

G.F. Hoyne, Infection and Immunity Section, Department of Biology, Imperial College of Science, Technology and Medicine, Prince Consort Road, London, SW7 2BB, UK

H. Jacobi, Allergy Clinic, Department of Internal Medicine TTA, Rigshospitalet, DK-2100 Copenhagen, Denmark

D. Jarvis, United Medical and Dental Schools, Division of Public Health Services, Block 8, St Thomas's Hospital, Lambeth Palace Road, London, SE1 7EH, UK

P. Jeannin, INSERM U 416, Institut Pasteur, P.O. Box 245, F-59019 Lille, France

P.K. Jeffery, Lung Pathology Unit, Department of Histopathology, Royal Brompton/National Heart and Lung Institute, Sydney Street, London, SW3 6LY, UK

M. Joseph, INSERM U 416, Institut Pasteur, P.O. Box 245, F-59019 Lille, France

A.P. Kaplan, Division of Allergy, Rheumatology and Clinical Immunology, Department of Medicine, SUNY—Stony Brook, Health Sciences Center, Stony Brook, New York 11794, USA

A. Kapp, Department of Dermatology, University of Hanover, Hanover, Germany

A.B. Kay, Allergy and Clinical Immunology, Imperial College School of Medicine at The National Heart and Lung Institute, Dovehouse Street, London, SW3 6LY, UK

S. Klysner, Research ALK Laboratories, P.O. Box 408, Bøge Alle, 10–12, DK-2970, Hørsholm, Denmark

J. Knani, CHU Montpellier, Service des Maladies Respiratoires, Hôpital Arnaud de Villeneuve, 371 Avenue du Doyen G. Giraud, 34295 Montpellier Cedex 5, France

V. Knight, Department of Molecular Physiology and Biophysics, Baylor College of Medicine, One Baylor Plaza, Houston, Texas 77030, USA

A. Kobza Black, St Johns Institute of Dermatology, St Thomas's Hospital, London, SE1 7EH, UK

O.M. Kon, Department of Clinical Immunology, Imperial College School of Medicine at The National Heart and Lung Institute, Dovehouse Street, London, UK

T.M. Krunkosky, Department of Anatomy, Physiological Sciences and Radiology, College of Veterinary Medicine, North Carolina State University, 4700 Hillsborough St, Raleigh, North Carolina 27606, USA

J. Lacey, Crop and Disease Management Department, IACR-Rothamstead, Harpenden, Hertfordshire, AL5 2JQ, UK

J.R. Lamb, Infection and Immunity Section, Department of Biology, Imperial College of Science, Technology and Medicine, Prince Consort Road, London, SW7 2BB, UK

S.J. Lane, Department of Respiratory Medicine, 4th Floor Hunt's House, Guy's Hospital, London, SE1 9RT, UK

T.H. Lee, Department of Respiratory Medicine, 4th Floor Hunt's House, Guy's Hospital, London, SE1 9RT, UK

S.B. Lehrer, Tulane University School of Medicine, Department of Medicine, Section of Allergy and Immunology, New Orleans, Louisiana, USA

V. Liebers, BGFA, Institut an der Ruhr Universität Bochum, Bürkle-de-la-Camp-Platz 1, 44789 Bochum, Germany

S. Lightman, Institute of Ophthalmology and Department of Clinical Ophthalmology, Moorfield's Eye Hospital, City Road, London, EC1V 2PD, UK

T.J. Lintner, Vespa Laboratories, Inc., R.D. NBR1, Spring Mills, Pennsylvania 16875, USA

H. Løwenstein, Research, ALK Laboratories, P.O. Box 408, Bøge Alle 10-12, DK-2970 Hørsholm, Denmark

I.S. Mackay, Nose Clinic, Royal Brompton Hospital, Sydney Street, London, SW3 6NP, UK

P. Maestrelli, Institute of Occupational Diseases, University of Padova Via Facciolati 71, 35127, Padova, Italy

H.-J. Malling, Allergy Unit 7551, National University Hospital, Tagensvej 20, DK-2200 Copenhagen N, Denmark

T.G. Merrett, Allergy Analysis Centre Ltd., Glyn Rhonwy, Llanberis, Caernarfon, Gwynedd, LL55 4EL, UK

D.A. Meyers, Johns Hopkins University School of Medicine, Meyer 4-139, Baltimore, Maryland 21205, USA

F.-B. Michel, CHU Montpellier, Service des Maladies Respiratoires, Hôpital Arnaud de Villeneuve, 371 Avenue du Doyen G. Giraud, 34295-Montpellier, Cedex 5, France

E. Minshall, Meakins-Christie Laboratories, McGill University, 3626 St Urbain Street Montreal, Quebec H2X 2P2, Canada

S. Molet, INSERM U 416, Institut Pasteur, P.O. Box 245, F-59019 Lille, France

R.M. Moqbel, Department of Medicine, Pulmonary Research Group, 574 Heritage Medical Research Centre, University of Alberta, Edmonton, Alberta, Canada T6G 2S2

G.C. Mudde, Sandoz Research Institut, 1235 Vienna, Austria

N. Mygind, Department of Lung Diseases, Århus Kommunehospital, Nørrebrogade 44, DK 8000 Århus, Denmark

S.M.S. Nasser, Department of Allergy and Clinical Immunology, Addenbrooke's NHS Trust, Hills Road, Cambridge, CB2 2QQ, UK

A.J. Newman-Taylor, Occupational and Environmental Medicine, Imperial College School of Medicine at The National Heart and Lung Institute, Emmanuel Kaye Building, Manresa Road, London, SW3 6LR, UK

A.A. Norris, Rhône-Poulenc Rover, Respiratory Development, Summerpool Road, Loughborough, Leicestershire, LE11 5DY, UK

R.E. O'Hehir, Department of Allergy and Clinical Immunology, Alfred Hospital Group, Commercial Road, Prahan, Melbourne, Victoria 3181, Australia

Y. Okayama, Immunopharmacology Group, Centre Block, Southampton General Hospital, Tremona Road, Southampton, SO16 6YD, UK

C.P. Page, Biomedical Sciences Division, Pharmacology Group, King's College London, Manresa Road, London, SW3 6LX, UK

L. Paradis, CHU Montpellier, Service des Maladies Respiratoires, Hôpital Arnaud de Villeneuve, 371 Avenue du Doyen G. Giraud, 34295-Montpellier, Cedex 5, France

R. Pauwels, Department of Respiratory Diseases, University Hospital, De Pintelaan 185, B9000 Ghent, Belgium

R.S. Peebles, Center for Lung Research, T-1217 MCN Vanderbilt University Medical Center, Nashville, Tennessee 37232-2650, USA

C.G.A. Persson, Department of Clinical Pharmacology, University Hospital, S22185 Lund, Sweden

T.A.E. Platts-Mills, Asthma and Allergic Diseases Center, Departments of Internal Medicine and Microbiology, University of Virginia, Charlottesville, Virginia, USA

J.M. Polak, Department of Histochemistry, Royal Postgraduate Medical School, Hammersmith Hospital, Du Cane Road, London, W12 0HS, UK

M. Pradal, Allergy Division, Chest Diseases Department, Hôpital Sainte-Marguerite, Marseille, France

N.B. Pride, Department of Medicine (Respiratory Division), Royal Postgraduate Medical School, Hammersmith Hospital, Du Cane Road, London, W12 0HS, UK

D.I. Pritchard, Department of Life Sciences, University of Nottingham, Nottingham, NG7 2RD, UK

S. Reddigari, Division of Allergy, Rheumatology and Clinical Immunology, Department of Medicine, SUNY—Stony Brook, Health Sciences Center, Stony Brook, New York 11794, USA

D.S. Robinson, Allergy and Clinical Immunology, Imperial College School of Medicine at The National Heart and Lung Institute, Dovehouse Street, London, SW3 6LY, UK

W.R. Roche, Pathology, University of Southampton, Southampton General Hospital, Tremona Road, Southampton, SO16 6YD, UK

I.W. Rodger, Merck Frosst Centre for Therapeutic Research, P.O. Box 1005, Pointe Claire-Dorval, Quebec, Canada, H9R 4P8

S. Romagnani, Clinical Immunology and Allergology, Instituto di Medica Interna and Immuno-Allergologia, Policlinico di Careggi, 50134 Florence, Italy

H.A. Sampson, Pediatric Clinical Research Center, Johns Hopkins University School of Medicine, Johns Hopkins Hospital, 600 N. Wolfe Street, Baltimore, Maryland 21287-3923, USA

S. Sanjar, Respiratory Diseases Unit, Glaxo-Wellcome Research and Development, Medicines Research Centre, Gunnels Wood Road, Stevenage, Hertfordshire SG1 2NY, UK

C. Schou, Research Department, ALK-Abello Group, Postbox 408, Boge Alle 10-12, DK-2970 Hørsholm, Denmark

W.J. Schwaeble, Department of Microbiology and Immunology, University of Leicester, Leicester, LE1 9RH, UK

S. Shaw, Amersham General Hospital, Whielden Street, Amersham, Buckinghamshire, HP7 0JD, UK

B. Sibbald, National Primary Care Research and Development Centre, Williamson Building, The University of Manchester, Oxford Road, Manchester, M13 9PL, UK

M. Silverberg, Division of Allergy, Rheumatology and Clinical Immunology, Department of Medicine, SUNY—Stony Brook, Health Sciences Center, Stony Brook, New York 11794, USA

F.E.R. Simons, Department of Pediatrics and Child Health, Head, Section of Allergy and Clinical Immunology, Faculty of Medicine, University of Manitoba, Winnipeg, Manitoba, Canada R3A 1S1

J.E. Slater, Center for Molecular Mechanisms of Disease, Children's Research Institute; Department of Asthma, Allergy and Pulmonary Medicine, Children's National Medical Center; Department of Pediatrics, George Washington University Medical Center, USA

R.C. Small, Smooth Muscle Pharmacology Research Group, School of Biological Sciences, University of Manchester, Oxford Road, Manchester, M13 9PT, UK

S.J. Smart, Department of Allergy and Immunology, Wilford Hall Medical Center, Lackland AFB, TX 78236, USA

J.E. Souness, Discovery Biology, Rhône-Poulenc Rover Ltd., Rainham Road South, Dagenham, Essex, RM10 7XS, UK

D.R. Springall, Department of Histochemistry, Royal Postgraduate Medical School, Hammersmith Hospital, Du Cane Road, London, W12 0HS, UK

B.J. Sutton, The Randall Institute, King's College London, 26 Drury Lane, London, WC2B 5RL, UK

S.L. Taylor, University of Nebraska, Department of Food Science and Technology, Lincoln, Nebraska, USA

R.D. Tee, Occupational and Environmental Medicine, Imperial School of Medicine at the National Heart and Lung Institute, Manresa Road, London, SW3 6LR, UK

W.R. Thomas, TVW Telethon Institute for Child Health Research, P.O. Box 855, West Perth, Western Australia 6872

A.W. Thomson, Molecular Genetics and Biochemistry, University of Pittsburgh Medical Center, W1544 Biomedical Science Tower, 200 Lothrop Street, Pittsburgh, Pennsylvania 15213, USA

A. Togias, Johns Hopkins Asthma and Allergy Center, Allergy and Clinical Immunology Division, 5501 Hopkins Bayview Circle, Baltimore, Maryland 21224-6801, USA

A.-B. Tonnel, INSERM U 416, Institut Pasteur, P.O. Box 245, F-59019 Lille, France

L.D. Vailes, Asthma and Allergic Diseases Center, Departments of Internal Medicine and Microbiology, University of Virginia, Charlottesville, Virginia, USA

V.A. Varney, Nose Clinic, Royal Brompton Hospital, Allergy and Clinical Immunology, Imperial School of Medicine at the National Heart and Lung Institute, Dovehouse Street, London, SW3 6LY, UK

A.R. Venkitaraman, Medical Research Council, Laboratory of Molecular Biology, Hills Road, Cambridge, CB2 2QH, UK

D. Vervloet, Department des Maladies Respiratories, Hôpital Sainte-Marguerite, BP 29, 13274 Marseille Cedex 9, France

J.C. Waldrep, Department of Molecular Physiology and Biophysics, Baylor College of Medicine, One Baylor Plaza, Houston, Texas 77030, USA

B. Wallaert, INSERM U 416, Institut Pasteur, P.O. Box 245, F-59019 Lille, France

A.F. Walls, Immunopharmacology Group, Centre Block, Southampton General Hospital, Tremona Road, Southampton, SO16 6YD, UK

A.J. Wardlaw, Department of Respiratory Medicine, Leicester University Medical School, Glenfield Hospital, Groby Road, Leicester, LE3 9QP, UK

J.O. Warner, Department of Child Health, University of Southampton, Southampton General Hospital, Tremona Road, Southampton, SO16 6YD, UK

J.A. Warner, Department of Child Health, Southampton General Hospital, Tremona Road, Southampton, SO16 6YD, UK

A.D. Watkins, University Medicine, Level D, Centre Block, Tremona Road, Southampton, SO16 6YD, UK

A.L. de Weck, Allergy Research Laboratory, Gerimm Foundation, 16 Grands Places 16, CH 1700 Fribourg, Switzerland

K. Whaley, Department of Immunology, Leicester Royal Infirmary, Leicester, LE1 5WW, UK

J.D. Wilkinson, Amersham General Hospital, Whielden Street, Amersham, Buckinghamshire, HP7 0JD, UK

P.J. Wills, Host Defence Unit, Imperial College School of Medicine at The National Heart and Lung Institute, Emmanuel Kaye Building, Manresa Road, London, SW3 6LY, UK

J.A. Woodfolk, Asthma and Allergic Disease Center, Departments of Internal Medicine and Microbiology, University of Virginia Charlottesville, Virginia, USA

D.T. Wright, NJC Enterprises Ltd., P.O. Box 14145, Research Triangle Park, North Carolina 27709, USA

Foreword

I was touched when Professor Kay asked whether I would write a Foreword for this book: for after completing his medical training he embarked on research on his PhD degree on *Eosinophil Leucocytes and Allergic Tissue Reactions* in my laboratory. I was, at first, hesitant in accepting this invitation, having always been a general immunologist. Also it is now already 7 years since I retired from my University Chair at Cambridge. However, when I saw a draft of the book — its extensive coverage, with exciting new developments, and its presentation—I was full of enthusiasm and enrolled forthwith.

This book is unquestionably a substantial treatise in 110 chapters written by world authorities. It deals firstly with the basic allergic responses to allergens (antigens) and then focuses mainly on the allergic reactions underlying perennial allergic rhinitis and asthma at the cellular and molecular levels. Asthma is now a much more complex and intractable disease than earlier supposed. To describe and cover the relevant pharmacology today receives 12 chapters. In another section there are three strictly physiological chapters which I consider extremely helpful for scientists who did their physiology many years ago or may have had no training at all in physiology. Other very important chapters in this section deal with exercise-induced asthma, airway hyperresponsiveness and aerosol-drug delivery.

I am very pleased that Professor Kay includes a section with seven chapters on experimental animal models for asthma research. In many allergic diseases, where complex inflammatory processes are involved, animal experimentation is essential. However, the pattern of allergic reactivity differs so much from one animal species to another, that considerable knowledge is required in selecting the most appropriate model.

A section with 13 chapters chronicles the latest position in the extraction, identification, purification and biochemical structure of some of the major allergens in the environment with clinical significance. I found especially helpful the chapters describing, in simple language, certain new cellular and molecular technologies, e.g. molecular cloning of allergens, T cell cloning, *in situ* hybridization and the polymerase chain reaction. The prevalence, assessment and treatment of perennial rhinitis and asthma in all age groups is covered in 35 chapters. There is special emphasis on what is now referred to as the allergen-induced 'late-phase reaction' in asthma and how this relates to airway hyperresponsiveness and inflammation. These mechanisms are steadily being elucidated and the chapters dealing with these issues are most revealing. Also covered in the text is allergen-injection immunotherapy and the prevention of atopic allergic diseases. There are also comprehensive chapters on extrinsic allergic alveolitis, food allergy and anaphylaxis, as well as atopic and contact dermatitis.

Professor Kay and his team deserve considerable credit for establishing the importance of T lymphocytes and their products in the pathogenesis of asthma and atopic allergic disease. Their work (reviewed in Chapters 21 and 90) has focused extensively on the role of type 2 cytokines, particularly interleukin-4 and interleukin-5, and has led to the evaluation of 'anti-T cell agents' such as cyclosporin A in the treatment of severe corticosteroid-dependent asthma. The importance of chronically-activated T lymphocytes in the airways of asthmatics has now been established and biotechnology companies and other commercial organizations are developing selective 'immunosuppressive agents' as therapeutic alternatives for the severe forms of this disease (see Chapters 36 and 110).

Immunology and allergology are frequently criticized over their terminologies which are found to be inconsistent and confusing. The tangled history of the various discoveries accounts for much of this, but some is due to laxity and disregard of literate discipline. With regard to allergology and the word 'allergy' itself, difficulties have arisen because, although the word coined by von Pirquet in 1906 was generally adopted, it was not (as noted in Chapter 2) used in the meaning or sense intended. von Pirquet had foreseen that, with the discoveries of the tissue-damaging so-called 'paradoxical reactions' such as anaphylaxis, Arthus reactions and serum sickness etc.—all involving antigens and antibodies, it would be quite inconsistent to call these 'immune responses' and 'immune reactions'. And so a new word was needed and the word he suggested was 'allergy'. He intended it to cover the (primary biological) responses of an individual to allergen or antigen, but the word was to remain *uncommitted* as to whether the effects were to be prophylactic (leading to protection or immunity) or antiphylactic (new word)—harmful. Over the years the word allergy (and its adjectival form allergic) has been used as if synonymous with the antiphylactic reactions only. This is quite contrary to what von Pirquet had in mind and so this particular confusion in terminology has continued. I especially want to commend the efforts Professor Kay has made in his book to set this right and to build on the suggestion and teaching of von Pirquet, one of the original and greatest pioneers of Allergology.

If I may, I would like to take this opportunity to proffer further illustrations of such inappropriate and confusing terminology in Immunology in general. (1) An immunogen is not any antigen: it is an antigen (usually of a micro-organism) which produces *protective* antibodies concerned with immunity. There are many antigens on or within a micro-organism which produce antibodies but which are quite irrelevant in establishing immunity: these are not immunogens. The term should not be used for any indiscriminate antigen. Researchers concerned with production of vaccines are rightly sensitive about this thoughtless usage. (2) One does not immunize, say a rabbit, by injecting antigens such as egg albumin or bovine serum albumin: the question of immunity is not involved. If anything, it could lead to a hypersensitivity reaction. One can raise antibodies to egg albumin by injecting this antigen—not by immunizing. (3) The commonly used word 'auto-immunity' is very ill-conceived. A very distinguished physician and medical writer asked so sensibly 'How can you develop immunity to yourself?' In fact, when you produce auto-antibodies you may become allergic to youself or rather to antigens of your tissues or cells. The correct word should be 'auto-allergy' and likewise the disease, e.g. auto-allergic thyroiditis, auto-allergic haemolytic anaemia. There is no immunity or protection implied—in fact just the opposite. By convention most people still refer, correctly, to auto-allergic encephalomyelitis! (4) It is not immune responses that give rise to the allergic or hypersensitivity reactions: this is contradictory. It is the allergic responses (uncommitted) that give rise to either immunity or the hypersensitivity reactions. (5) And lastly, as a further illustration of such paradoxes, I have recently read in a medical journal '... post-transfusion purpura is a rare serious adverse transfusion reaction. It affects mainly women beyond the age of 50 who have been *pre-immunized* (my italics) by pregnancies and/or blood transfusions'. These women have not been immunized—just the opposite; they have been pre-sensitized or, quite acceptably, pre-allergized.

In the introduction to many textbooks on allergy there is often an apologia, as it were, on the confused terminology of the subject. However, if we fail to take note of von Pirquet's foresight and fail to act on it, this terminological confusion will continue. Even the *Journal of Allergy*, when it started publication in 1929, had difficulties. I will quote from the statement on the frontispiece of the first issue—'In view of the differences of opinion of how the word 'allergy' should be used we believe it evident that it does not possess an established meaning in scientific usage. However, the term is generally employed by clinicians, who apply it, to conditions of specific hypersensitiveness, exclusive of anaphylaxis in lower animals. Its sense in the title of this journal corresponds to its current medical usage'. This was quite contrary to what von Pirquet intended — and what a prejudice they had against the lower species! I sincerely hope Professor Kay's book will help in establishing the proper usage.

In the excellent clinical and scientific book *'Allergy'* (1944) by Erich Aubach (the then Chief of Allergy Service, Jewish Hospital, Philadelphia, USA) he discusses at some length the considerable difficulties with terminology. He does actually talk of 'allergized cells' and 'allergized tissues' in the sense of sensitization—a usage I like very much. In 1968 we note Wagner reiterating the real need that Immunology had for this new word 'allergy' being uncommitted or partial to either immunity or hypersensitivity, but embracing both. Richard Wagner, a some-time clinical assistant to von Pirquet and subsequently Senior Paediatrician, New England Center Hospitals, USA, wrote a most readable and learned medical biography of von Pirquet.

Phillip Gell and myself, as the editors of the first three editions of *'Clinical Aspects of Immunology'* (1963, 1968 and 1975) based the terminology, as far as we were able, on the teaching of von Pirquet. We were most gladdened that

Carl Prausnitz, who was then living in England, agreed to write the Foreword for our book. Prausnitz had also served at one time (probably 1910–1912) as a clinical assistant to von Pirquet and was also, of course, another one of the great pioneers in the field of allergy, having developed the so-called PK reaction (1921) which was the first means of measuring reagin (IgE antibody). He was so delighted that we had taken this stand on terminology. Unfortunately the editors of the subsequent editions let this lapse. It was then such a pleasant surprise when I first went through the draft chapters of '*Allergy and Allergic Diseases*' to find that Professor Kay had also set his presentation in line with the thoughts of von Pirquet, which makes such good sense. Like Phillip Gell and myself he has included a translation of von Pirquet's original article as an Appendix.

It is gratifying that the types I to IV classification of adverse allergic reactions introduced in the first edition (1963) of *Clinical Aspects of Immunology* (with minor modifications in the third edition in 1975) has stood the test of time. Professor Kay's enlargement of the scheme, based on a similar modification originally proposed by Janeway & Travers (1995), is a logical extension of our earlier concepts. In particular, the suggestion that the type II and type IV reactions could be subdivided on the basis of important differences in the initiating events and their subsequent outcomes does, I believe, provide greater clarification and adequately incorporates the newer scientific concepts on the pathogenesis of allergic disease.

The comprehensiveness of the book with entries of so much up-to-date research in almost all fields makes this, for me, a very exciting book. I have no doubt that it will be likewise greatly appreciated by scientists in their laboratories and on the clinical side not only by clinical allergists but also by other clinicians in closely allied specialities. I wish the book all the success it deserves.

ROBIN COOMBS

References

Coombs, R.R.A. & Gell, P.G.H. (1975) The classification of allergic reactions responsible for clinical hypersensitivity and disease. In: *Clinical Aspects of Immunology* (eds P.G.H. Gell, R.R.A. Coombs & P.J. Lachmann), 3rd edn, pp. 761–81. Oxford: Blackwell Scientific Publications.

Janeway, C. & Travers, P. (1995) *Immunobiology*, 2nd edn. London: Garland Press, Chapter 11.

Prausnitz, C. & Küstner, H. (1921) Studies on supersensitivity. *Centralbl. f. Bakteriol. 1. Abt. Orig.*, **86**, 160–9. Translated from the German original by Prausnitz, C. In: *Clinical Aspects of Immunology* (eds P.G.H. Gell & R.R.A. Coombs) (1963), 1st edn. Oxford: Blackwell Scientific Publications.

Urbach, E. (1944) *Allergy*. London: William Heinemann Ltd.

Wagner, R. (1968) *Clements von Pirquet. His Life and Work*. Baltimore: The Johns Hopkins Press.

von Pirquet (1906) Allergie. *Münch. med. Wochenschr.*, **30**, 1457. (Translated from the German by Prausnitz, C. In: P.G.H. Gell & R.R.A. Coombs (eds) (1963) *Clinical Aspects of Immunology*. Blackwell Scientific Publications, Oxford.)

Preface

The primary aim of this book is to provide a detailed source of information on the rapidly growing subject of Allergy and Allergic Diseases. There have of course been other textbooks in this field, many from the USA. However, these two volumes have a distinctly European flavour, particularly in regard to concepts of mechanisms and approaches to the diagnosis and treatment of allergic diseases. In this sense it fulfils an unmet need since there has been no fully comprehensive text on this topic from this side of the Atlantic in recent years.

Producing a book of this size has been an enormous task but I have been very fortunate in having critical comments from many colleagues on various aspects of the individual chapters submitted. Several authors have also acted as reviewers of other contributors' chapters and for this I am most grateful. However, I owe a special debt of thanks to members of my own department (both past and present), and others, for painstakingly going through many of the chapters in detail. In particular, I would like to thank Dr Andrew Alexander, Dr Luis Barata, Professor Jean Bousquet, Dr Sherwood Burge, Professor Martin Church, Professor Tim Clark, Dr Christopher Corrigan, Dr William Frankland, Dr Tony Frew, Professor Hannah Gould, Dr Robert Gundel, Professor Patrick Holt, Dr Marc Humbert, Dr Onn Min Kon, Dr Mark Larché, Professor Tak Lee, Dr Douglas Robinson, Dr David Springall, Professor Ron Thompson and Dr Andrew Wardlaw.

I am also most grateful to Professor Robin Coombs FRS, for dignifying this book with a Foreword. He has been fully supportive of my attempts, where possible, to adhere to the original and correct 'von Pirquet terminology'. Furthermore, he has taken a great interest in this ambitious project and spent many hours and days reading, and in many instances re-reading, several chapters of the book. I am most appreciative of his sound advice and for his invaluable help at many stages of the editorial process.

Blackwell Science have given constant help and reassurance throughout these proceedings and for this I would like to thank Dr Stuart Taylor (Senior Editor) and Ms Jody Ball (Senior Production Editor) for their skill, management and attention to detail. Above all, I am indebted to my Editorial Assistant, Miss Jennifer Mitchell, without whom the publication of this book would not have taken place. She has nursed *Allergy and Allergic Diseases* from its inception through to its gestation. The editorial aspects of this work have been truly monumental and no praise can be high enough for Jennifer's untiring efforts in seeing this volume through to a successful conclusion.

A.B. KAY

PART 1
Immunological Basis of the Allergic Response

CHAPTER 1

A Short History of Allergological Diseases and Concepts

A.L. de Weck

Introduction

The history of allergy and allergic diseases mingles in part with the history of immunology but also has a number of picturesque aspects of its own. In fact, an accurate recording of major and minor events and concepts which have contributed to our present knowledge of allergic diseases has become as complex as the disciplines of allergy and immunology themselves.

This may explain why many young allergologists and immunologists nowadays seem to possess only a relatively poor idea of their own intellectual background and little curiosity for the lives, ideas and achievments of those scientists who have preceded them in the field. This, of course, is not a phenomenon particular to young scientists and physicians. Nor are the more or less bitter criticisms proferred by elders about frequent disinterest of the young in history a new phenomenon particular to the present generation. It is, in fact, quite physiological and natural that young incoming physicians and scientists will be more interested in the present and the future than in the past.

It seems, however, that in the medical and biomedical professions at the verge of the 21st century, the knowledge and interest of young scientists for their own past has become even more dim than it was 50 years ago, at a time when the second golden age of immunology and allergology started. Those of us who had the good fortune to live through a most exciting period of discoveries since the end of World War II will recall that, at the time, a thorough knowledge about the previous 100 years of immunology and allergology and about the scientists who had provided the milestones was a prerequisite for further progress and new experiments. Immunology and allergology were taught in medical and biological courses and textbooks in historical perspectives. Particularly in the French and German medical literature, newly described diseases, discoveries and concepts were often attributable and attributed to the name of a single, more or less famous scientist and physician, thereby enticing the student to get better acquainted with the scientist and with the circumstances of their discovery.

During the last half-century, a number of circumstances have contributed to make younger generations less aware of their past, which I had the opportunity to follow during 40 years in teaching (de Weck, 1994). The accelerated pace to acquire new scientific information, the explosion of published papers and results and the intense pressure for scientists and physicians to keep abreast with the newest information leaves no time for contemplation or reflection on the past. Teaching of allergology and immunology has so many current concepts and facts to communicate that there is usually no time to look behind and to assess not only where we stand and where we want to go but also how we got there!

Modern computer technology, which, on the one hand, favours acquisition and retrieval of new data (and may possibly make the task of future historians easier!), on the other hand, makes it less palatable for many of us in a hurry to go back to the old books buried in some dusty archives. It has become customary for many of us to limit literature search to the last 5 years, in the mistaken belief that anything older is so out of date that it no longer contributes to research and progress. This may be true for technical details but is seldom the case for concepts, ideas and imaginative prescient visions, which, indeed, form the young mind to recognize new unexpected observations and which are the basis of new discoveries. It has become much easier and faster to retrieve the medical literature by electronic means but there is also some danger that younger generations will believe that medical science started in earnest in 1966, the first year recorded in full on a CD-ROM disk. If doing so, much time, effort, money and false pride may be wasted in reinventing the wheel, albeit under another name.

Another sign of the ambivalent attitude of scientists and physicians towards the history of biomedical science is that strictly historical books on allergy or immunology are not bestsellers and will not so easily find a publisher. In fact, some of the most informative and delightful books on history of allergy which have appeared during the past decade are all 'private prints' in limited edition sponsored by some donor (Samter, 1969; Avenberg & Harper, 1980; Cohen & Samter, 1992), which leaves them out of reach for the younger generation.

Some of us older witnesses, sorting out events we have thoroughly read about or through which we lived, are left with a difficult responsibility, namely to point out and highlight the really significant events in the field, in the hope that 'scientific culture' will still, in the long run, make the difference between leaders and mere robots or executors. It is therefore to be welcomed that a treatise on allergic dieases should start with a chapter on history of allergy.

However, how to find here the right way? What should the reader of such a treatise expect to learn about history? Particularly during the past years, a number of books (Samter, 1969; Avenberg & Harper, 1980; Cohen & Samter, 1992; Simons, 1994) and reviews (Humphrey & White, 1970; Klein, 1982; Silverstein, 1982), including some extensive treatises (Schadewaldt, 1979–82), have appeared which in a readable and sometimes humorous manner provide a great deal of information and a number of anecdotes about earlier observations and the historical development of allergy and immunology as biomedical disciplines. To produce, as an introductory chapter, a condensed version of these books, which all follow a chronological historical perspective, is not particularly exciting and probably also not particularly useful. This is why I have chosen another approach, which may be more palatable to the reader in a hurry, namely to order historical events and discoveries in a topic-orientated manner rather than in a merely chronological pot-pourri approach. I have also limited myself to mere statements without describing in detail the historical and anecdotal circumstances which the statements are based on. A critical evaluation of history of allergy and of the evolution of its various pathophysiological concepts in view of current knowledge and perspectives, as recently performed for asthma (Emanuel & Howarth, 1995), would indeed be of great interest but might become a treatise in itself. I hope that the approach chosen here will allow young allergologists to acquire at least a minimal historical varnish and the curiosity to look at the sources given for more information about the scientists, their times and the unabated drive for knowledge.

The concept of immunity and the origins of immunology

The term 'immune' derives from the Latin word *immunis* which at the time meant 'free of obligations', such as taxes or military service, regardless of whether they were imposed by the emperor or by the law. *Immunis* was then originally a legal term. This is not to be interpreted, as pointed out by an old teacher of immunology at the start of his course, that immunologists endeavour to teach tax evasion and dodging military duties.

In a medical sense, immunity refers to the defense of the organism against pathogenic external and internal agents, and, in a broader sense, to protection against disease. We are not quite clear about the first conscious use of the word *immunis* in its medical sense: in any case, it is recorded in the description of Colley as immunity acquired during a plague epidemic, described in his paper '*Equibus deigracidego immunis evast*'.

In Greek mythology, the concept of immunity found its most prominent subject in the semi-god Achilles, who was said to have become invulnerable to war wounds, with the exception of his famous weak heel, after having been held by the heels in early infancy and immersed head down first in the holy river Styga. The heels were therefore not rendered tolerant or immune to wounds like the rest of the body and this eventually led to his death during the Trojan war.

During what may be called the empirical period of immunology (Silverstein, 1982), which in fact lasted from mythological times until about the middle of the 19th century, a number of recorded events and writings point to immunological phenomena and even therapies. However, and even if many facts and observations became known, the immunological mechanisms underlying them were not recognized. Empirical immunology has left its traces not only in the western world, where records may be better available, but also in various other civilizations, particularly in China, India and Central America. During its long history, many theories bordering on theology, magics and physico-medical approaches were debated but these are beyond the scope of this chapter.

The most well known events and descriptions relating

to basic concepts of immunology and immune reactions are:

3000 (?) BC	Achilles	Early acquisition of 'immunity' (to wounds) by early 'preventive' treatment.
431–4 BC	Thukidides	First decription of lifelong immunity in patients having survived plague.
132–63 BC	Mithridates	King of Pontus, known for induction of oral tolerance to plant poisons.

During the middle ages and from the 16th century onwards, a number of authors described various diseases of an immunological nature, such as hay fever and asthma (see the corresponding sections), but a relationship between natural immunity occurring in a number of infectious diseases and adverse reactions to external elements was not established.

1717	Lady Mary Montague	First introduction of variolation against smallpox to England, based on her observations among Turks. Variolation practised in China for over 5000 years.

19th century: immunology emerges as a biomedical science

The experiments performed by Jenner on vaccination with cowpox, certainly in the western world, represent a turning point and the start of experimental immunology. Almost 70 years had to elapse, however, before the microbiological era of immunology was introduced by the brilliant works of Louis Pasteur and Robert Koch. Soon this was followed by a first golden era of immunology, in which both humoral and cellular immune mechanisms were recognized and put to work in the prevention of major infectious diseases, such as diphtheria, tetanus and rabies.

Milestones and major discoveries: microbiological era and first pathophysiological concepts

1798	Edward Jenner	First vaccination against smallpox with cowpox pustule fluid. Description of accelerated secondary local inflammatory response in smallpox-immune patient.
1885	Louis Pasteur	First vaccinations against fowl cholera, sheep anthrax, swine erysipelas, rabies in dog and humans. Partial heat sterilization.
1886	Theobald Smith	Protection of pigeons from cholera infections by heat-killed cultures of chicken cholera bacilli.
1888	Pierre Roux Alexandre Yersin	Discovery of diphtheria exotoxin.
1882	Robert Koch	Discovery of tuberculosis bacillus, tuberculin and *Vibrio cholerae*. Altered reaction of infected animals to reinfection ('Koch's Grundversuch').
1893	Elie Metchnikoff	Description of phagocytosis of bacteria by leucocytes and role of cells in immunity.
1890	Emil von Behring	Production of diphtheria antitoxin and vaccination.
1894	Shibasaburo Kitasato	Discovery of tetanus bacillus, production of tetanus toxin, antitoxin and vaccination.
1894	Pierre Roux	Cure of diphtheria by serum from immunized horses.
1894	Richard Pfeiffer	Discovery of killing effect *in vitro* on cholera bacillus by serum from animals immunized against *Vibrio cholerae*. Requirement for guinea pig serum.
1898	Richard Pfeiffer	Formation of antibodies mainly in spleen, bone marrow, lymph nodes and lungs.
1894	Hans Büchner	Loss of bacteria killing ability when antiserum is heated at 56°C: discovery of 'alexin'.
1895	Jules Bordet	Description of complement, a

		thermolabile component of serum required to act with antibody for killing *Vibrio cholerae in vitro*.
1903	Almroth Wright	Concept of 'opsonization': killing by macrophages of bacilli coated with antibodies—a compromise view between humoral and cellular immunity.
1917	O.T. Avery	Serological differentiation of pneumococci.

Molecular immunology and immunochemistry

Based on the immense progress of organic chemistry in the second half of the 19th century, the biological phenomena observed by early immunologists were soon interpreted in chemical terms. Most important in this development were the contributions of Paul Ehrlich and Karl Landsteiner, who established immunology and immunochemsitry as a truly molecular science.

1897	Paul Ehrlich	Theory of chemical nature of antigen–antibody interaction and side-chain concept.
1900	Karl Landsteiner	Discovery of ABO blood group antigens.
1917–40	Karl Landsteiner	Studies on fine specificity of antibodies by immunization with haptens.
1926	Lloyd D. Felton	Antibodies recognized as proteins.
1928	Edward Dienes	Induction of cellular delayed hypersensitivity by protein antigens.
1934	John Marrack	Development of the lattice hypothesis of antigen–antibody interaction.
1932	Felix Haurowitz	Template theory of antibody formation.
1942	Merrill W. Chase	Transfer of tuberculin sensitivity by cells from immunized animals.
1945	Merrill W. Chase	Transfer of contact dermatitis to simple chemicals by sensitized leucocytes.

Biomolecular immunology: the second golden age

Following World War II and based on the development of interdisciplinary medical research, fast progress occurred in immunology: this was a most exciting time (Sela, 1987; de Weck, 1994). Immunology also yielded practical dividends, such as vaccination against poliomyelitis, treatment of immunodeficiency diseases, organ transplantation, immunosuppression in the treatment of autoimmune (or autoallergic — see Chapter 2) diseases and better understanding and management of allergic disorders. Between 1945 and 1970 the main characteristic of immunology and immunologists was that the scientists involved had very different scientific backgrounds, thus bringing in a variety of points of view and technical skills. Immunology developed on a multicentric basis and, in most countries, only started to become institutionalized around 1970.

Since 1970, various departments and institutes of immunology throughout the world took over teaching and core research in the field. Immunology became recognized in medical and biological schools as an independent discipline, which steadily started to produce immunologists with some common education and background. Once again, however, fertilization has come also from the outside, with a great influence from cellular biology, genetics and molecular biology in the last decade. In fact, the limits and identity of immunology have again started to become somewhat blurred, the more as immunological phenomena and/or techniques are now affecting all domains of medicine and biological sciences.

Important milestones that have contributed to modern immunology include those in the following list.

1945	Ray D. Owen	Description of natural immunological tolerance to blood group antigens in dizygotic cattle sharing the same placenta (acquired immunological tolerance).
1948	Astrid Fagraeus	Synthesis of immunoglobulins by plasma cells.
1949	MacFarlane Burnet	Theory of acquired immunological tolerance.
1952	Peter Medawar	Discovery of acquired immunological tolerance to skin grafts by neonatal injection of lymphoid cells.

1958 1962	Jean Dausset Jan van Rood	Description of anti-leucocyte antibodies directed against human leucocyte antigen (HLA) histocompatibility antigens.
1956	Bruce Glick	Role of the bursa of Fabricius in antibody formation in chicken.
1955	Niels K. Jerne	Natural selection theory of antibody formation.
1956	Jacques Oudin	Discovery of immunoglobulin allotypes.
1957	Alick Isaacs Jean Lindenmann	Discovery of interferon as anti-viral lymphokine.
1957	David W. Talmage	Clonal selection theory.
1957	MacFarlane Burnet	Clonal selection theory of antibody production.
1959	Rodney R. Porter	Chemical structure of immunoglobulins, recognition of Fc and Fab fragments.
1959	Michael Sela	Synthetic antigen polymers and antigen structure, synthetic vaccines.
1961	Gerald M. Edelman	Recognition of immunoglobulin heavy and light chains.
1961	Jacques Miller	Role of thymus and T cells in control of antibody production.
1962–68	Baruj Benacerraf Hugh O. McDevitt	Identification of immune response genes (Ir) as linked to major histocompatibility antigens.
1963	Jacques Oudin	Discovery of immunoglobulin idiotypes.
1963	Henry Kunkel	Antinuclear and anti-idiotypic antibodies in autoimmune diseases.
1965	Thomas B. Tomasi	Role of IgA in secretory immunity.
1966	Henry N. Claman	Cooperation of T and B lymphocytes in antibody production.
1966	Barry R. Bloom John R. David	Description of lymphokine-induced cell interaction: macrophage migration inhibitory factor (MIF).
1970	Richard K. Gershon	Demonstration of suppressor T cells as cause of immunological tolerance.
1973	Peter C. Doherty Rolf Zinkernagel	T-cell restriction determined by HLA complex.
1974	Niels K. Jerne	Network theory of idiotypic regulation.
1976	Susumu Tonegawa	Generation of antibody diversity by rearrangement of *V* and *C* immunglobulin genes.

Natural and experimental allergic and immune deficiency diseases

Description and interpretation of diseases as due to 'immunological' phenomena and reactions has fostered the creation of a new medical specialty: clinical immunology. Some of the milestones in this respect were as follows.

1837	Johann Schoenlein	First description of rheumatic purpura.
1882	Eduard Henoch	Second description of rheumatic purpura.
1872	Heinrich Quincke	First description of angioneurotic oedema.
1905	Bela Schick	First description of serum disease.
1915	Warfield T. Longcope	Experimental lesions in organs from animals repeatedly injected with foreign proteins.
1934	Mataso Masugi	Experimental glomerulonephritis with anti-kidney antiserum.
1932 1948	Wilhelm Löffler André Essellier	Description of evanescent eosinophilic pulmonary infiltrations associated with *Ascaris* infection.
1941	Joseph Harkavy	Bronchial asthma with recurrent pulmonary eosinophilic infiltration and polyserositis.
1948	Malcolm H. Hargraves	Description of the neutrophil leucocyte phagocytosing nuclear material, characteristic

		of autoimmune/ autoallergic diseases with antinuclear antibodies (lupus erythematosus).
1956	Robert A. Good	Hypo- and agammaglobulinaemia syndromes, role of thymus in immunodeficiencies.
1957	Ernest Witebsky	Experimental autoallergic thyroiditis; pathology and criteria of autoimmune diseases.
1963	Frank J. Dixon	Role of antigen–antibody complexes in disease.

Milestones in acute, adverse allergic reactions

Untoward allergic reactions were already reported in ancient times. However, and particularly when considering diseases with a relatively clear-cut clinical pattern, such as a hayfever and asthma attack, it is remarkable that reports were not in fact more frequent or would not have been an important part of medicine.

This may be due to the fact that allergic diseases were in fact, until the 20th century, relatively rare (Sela, 1987).

The origins of the first reported adverse allergic reactions to external agents

2641 BC	Menes	Egyptian pharaoh reported to have died from a wasp ('kehb') sting (first report of an anaphylactic shock?). However, interpretation of hieroglyph controversial (Avenberg & Harper, 1980).
b.375 BC	Hippocrates	Description of asthma, eczema and allergy to goats' milk and cheese.
AD b.41	Britannicus	Reported as afflicted by acute allergic reactions to horses.
b.1478	Thomas Moore	Report on acute skin eruption of King Richard III due to ingestion of strawberries (Shakespeare!).
c. 1584	Johann Schenk	Coins the term 'idiosyncrasy'.

Early reports of general anaphylactic reactions

Although sudden deaths after bee or wasp stings are the first examples of natural anaphylactic reactions, the beginning of an understanding that the immune response, so helpful in defense against bacteria, may also cause harmful reactions dawned on us from the discovery of experimental anaphylaxis. The discovery of anaphylaxis therefore, is for allergy what the beginning of vaccination is for immunology: the first experimental evidence and reproduction of a major natural biological phenomenon.

1839	François Magendie	Description of sudden death of dogs repeatedly injected with egg albumin.
1894	Samuel Flexner	Experimental 'toxic death' whilst injecting dog serum into rabbits.
1902	Charles Richet Paul Portier	Discovery of experimental anaphylaxis in dogs (Fig. 1.1).
1903	Theobald Smith	Observations of anaphylactic reactions of guinea pigs to horse serum.

Pathophysiological concepts in the allergic diseases

Studies on anaphylactic and similar reactions proceeded rather slowly. After it was first realized, at the start of this century, that ana- or anti-phylactic reactions provided a major new concept for explaining a number of diseases, diagnostic and therapeutic attempts remained rather empirical for several decades. Retrospectively, it is obvious that the main reason for this state of affairs is that the tools and techniques which had provided so many insights into bacterial immunology were inappropriate for the study of allergic diseases. Only with the development of suitable technology, which led first to the identification of IgE in 1967, did the era of modern and scientific allergology really begin.

In that sense, and despite the many insights gained more or less empirically by pioneers, allergology is still a relatively young branch of science. Some of the main milestones in the development of allergy science are as follows.

1877	Paul Ehrlich	Description and staining of mast cells (1877) and eosinophils (1879) (Fig. 1.2).

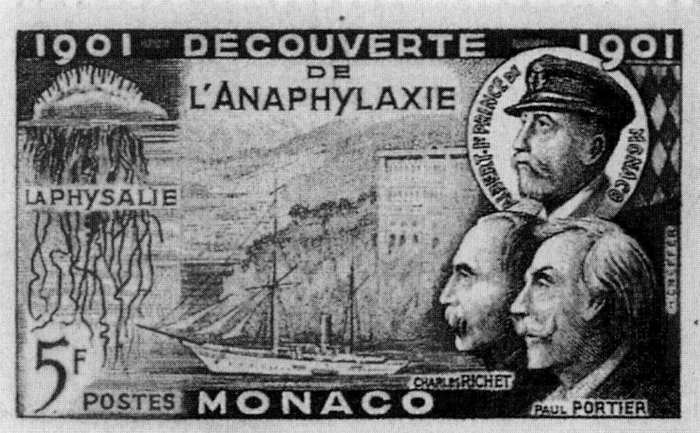

Fig. 1.1 *Charles R. Richet* (1850–1935) and *Paul J. Portier* (1866–1962). Discovered anaphylaxis. The story behind this commemorative postage stamp is provided by Richet (Richet, C. (1913) *Anaphylaxis* (translated by J.M. Bligh). Liverpool University Press; Constable, London).

> During a cruise on Prince Albert of Monaco's yacht, the Prince suggested to Portier and myself a study of the toxin production of *Physalia* (the jelly-fish known as Portuguese Man-of-War) found in the South Seas. On board the Prince's yacht, experiments were carried out proving that an aqueous glycerine extract of the filaments of *Physalia* is extremely toxic to ducks and rabbits. On returning to France, I could not obtain *Physalia* and decided to study comparatively the tentacles of *Actinaria* (sea anemone). . . . While endeavouring to determine the toxic dose (of extracts), we soon discovered that some days must elapse before fixing it; for several dogs did not die until the fourth or fifth day after administration or even later. We kept those that had been given insufficient to kill, in order to carry out a second investigation upon these when they had recovered. At this point an unforeseen event occurred. The dogs which had recovered were intensely sensitive and died a few minutes after the administration of small doses. The most typical experiment, that in which the result was indisputable, was carried out on a particularly healthy dog. It was given at first 0.1 ml of the glycerin extract without becoming ill; 22 days later, as it was in perfect health, I gave it a second injection of the same amount. In a few seconds it was extremely ill; breathing became distressful and panting; it could scarcely drag itself along, lay on its side, was seized with diarrhoea, vomited blood and died in 25 minutes.

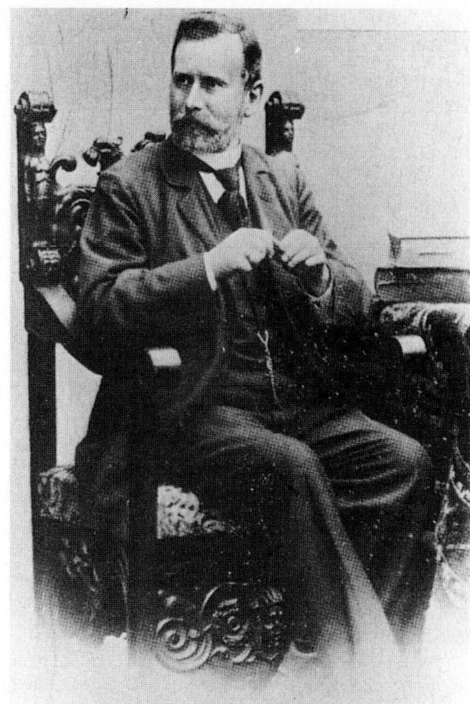

Fig. 1.2 *Paul Ehrlich (1854–1915).* An exceptionally creative bioscientist who, along with many other accomplishments, described the side-chain theory of antibody formation and discovered the mast cell and the eosinophil. (From Mahmoud & Austen, 1980.)

1903	Maurice Arthus	Experimental localized acute necrotizing vasculitis, first described as local anaphylaxis (Fig. 1.3).
1905	Clemens von Pirquet	Studies on serum sickness, coined the term 'allergy' (Fig. 1.4).

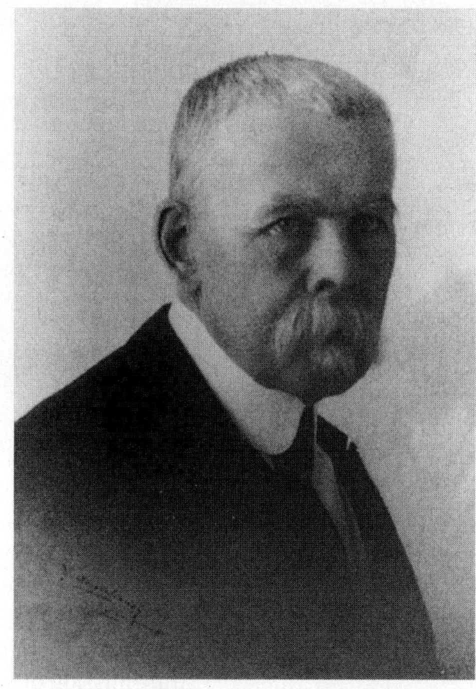

Fig. 1.3 *Nicholas-Maurice Arthus (1862–1945).* The 'Arthus reaction' is an experimental localized acute necrotizing vasculitis first described as local anaphylaxis. (From Cohen & Samter, 1992.)

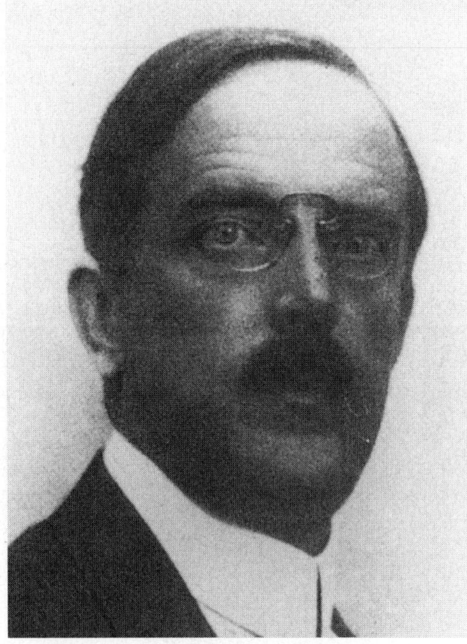

Fig. 1.4 *Clemens von Pirquet (1874–1929).* von Pirquet conceived the term 'allergy' (see Appendix). He meant it to include any situation where there was 'changed reactivity' irrespective of whether this resulted in immunity or hypersensitivity (see Chapter 2). He also introduced tuberculin skin tests in diagnosis. (From Cohen & Samter, 1992.)

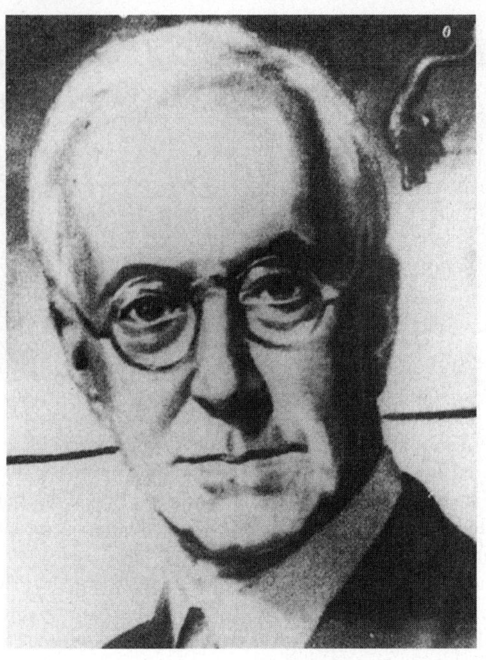

Fig. 1.5 *Sir Henry H. Dale (1875–1968).* Established the role of histamine in anaphylaxis and demonstrated chemical transmission of nerve impulses. (From Cohen & Samter, 1992.)

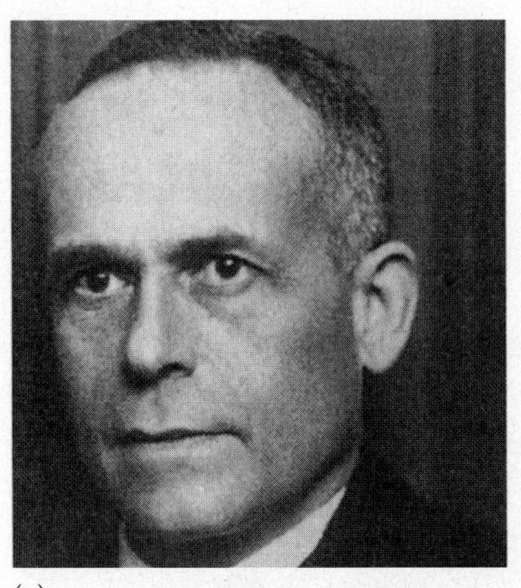

(a)

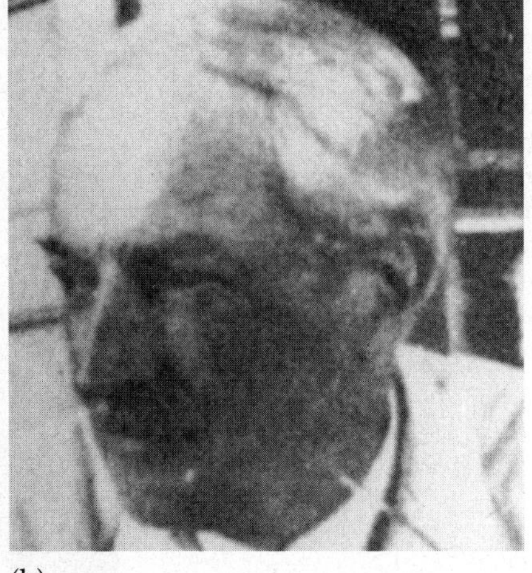

(b)

Fig. 1.6 (a) *Otto Carl W. Prausnitz (Giles) (1876–1963).* (b) *Heinz Küstner (1897–1963).* The passive transfer of immediate skin reactivity by interdermal injection of serum from an allergic patient ('reagin') is called the Prausnitz–Küstner (or P–K) test. (From Cohen & Samter, 1992.)

1911	Henry Dale	Role of histamine in anaphylaxis and studies on chemical transmission of nerve impulses (Fig. 1.5).
1919	M.A. Ramirez	Horse dander asthma following blood transfusion.
1921	Carl Prausnitz Heinz Küstner	Passive transfer of immediate skin reactivity of fish allergen by intradermal injection of serum from allergic patient ('reagins') (Fig. 1.6).

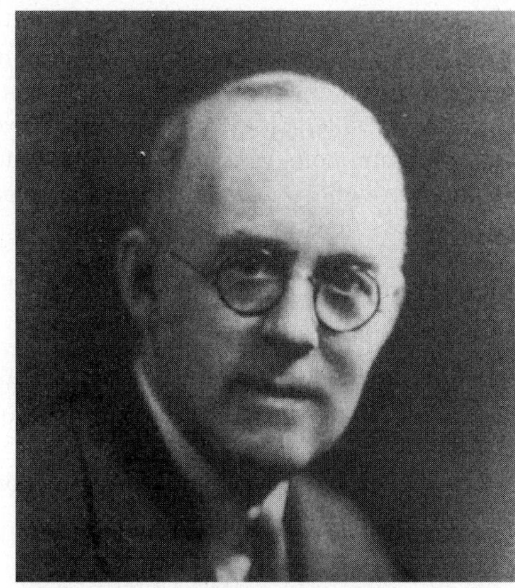

Fig. 1.7 *Arthur Fernandez Coca (1875–1959).* Coca introduced the term 'atopy' (now recognized as IgE-mediated hypersensitivity). (From Cohen & Samter, 1992.)

1921	Arent de Besche	Passive transfer of serum from horse asthmatics sensitized to horse proteins by injection of diphtheria vaccine.
1923	Arthur Coca	Coined the term 'atopy' (Fig. 1.7).
1927	Thomas Lewis	Description of similarities between urticaria and skin vascular reactions to histamine (vasodilatation, flare and local oedema as triple response).

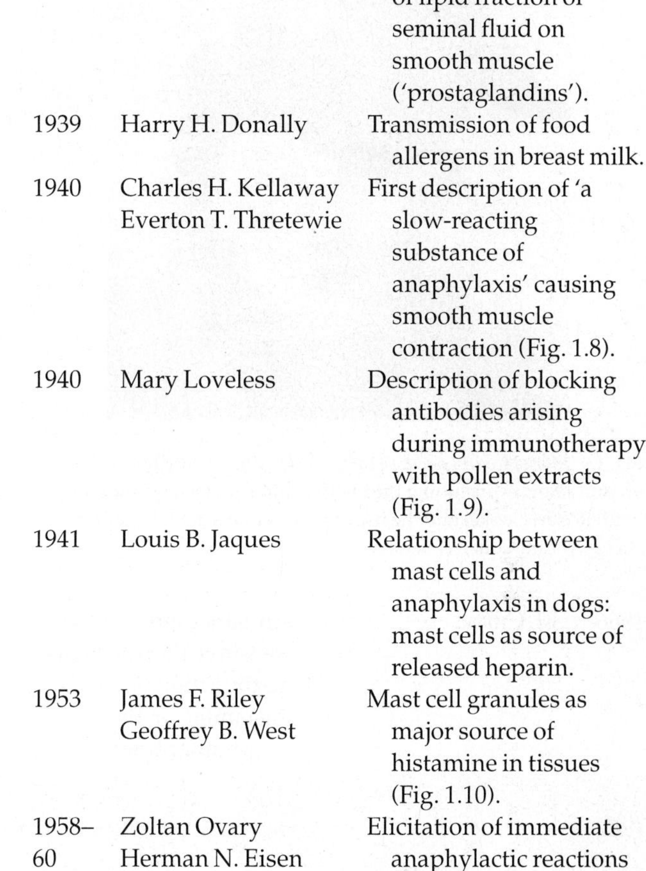

1927	Bret Ratner	Experiments on allergic sensitization *in utero.*
1935	Ulf von Euler	Discovery of the activity of lipid fraction of seminal fluid on smooth muscle ('prostaglandins').
1939	Harry H. Donally	Transmission of food allergens in breast milk.
1940	Charles H. Kellaway Everton T. Thretewie	First description of 'a slow-reacting substance of anaphylaxis' causing smooth muscle contraction (Fig. 1.8).
1940	Mary Loveless	Description of blocking antibodies arising during immunotherapy with pollen extracts (Fig. 1.9).
1941	Louis B. Jaques	Relationship between mast cells and anaphylaxis in dogs: mast cells as source of released heparin.
1953	James F. Riley Geoffrey B. West	Mast cell granules as major source of histamine in tissues (Fig. 1.10).
1958–60	Zoltan Ovary Herman N. Eisen	Elicitation of immediate anaphylactic reactions requires bridging of antibody molecules by bi- or multivalent allergen.

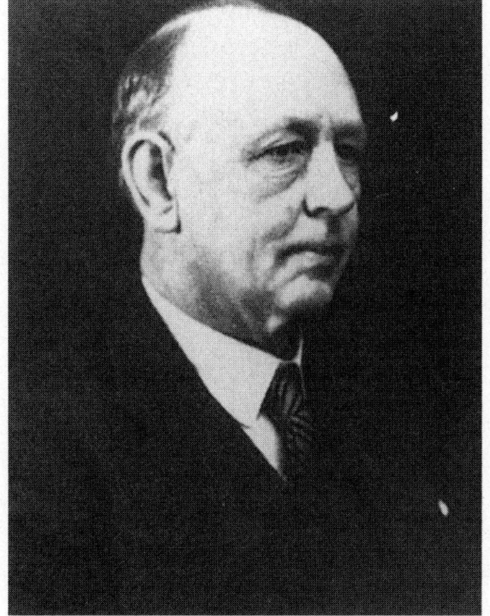

(a)

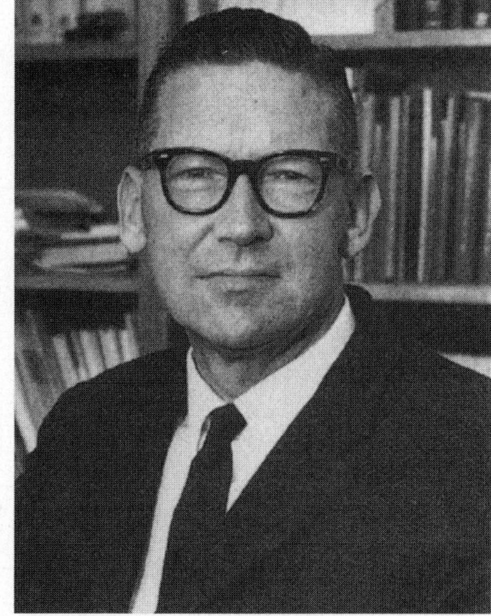

(b)

Fig. 1.8 (a) *Charles H. Kellaway (1889–1952).* (b) *Everton R. Trethewie (1913–84).* First description of a 'slow-reacting substance of anaphylaxis' causing smooth muscle contraction. (From Cohen & Samter, 1992.)

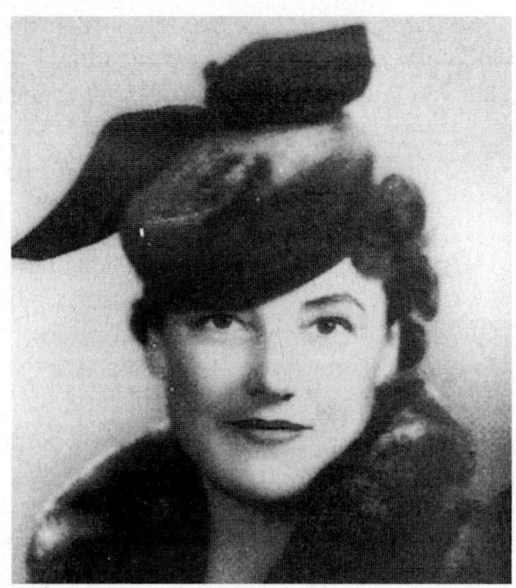

Fig. 1.9 *Mary Hewitt Loveless (1899–1991).* Major contributions to immunotherapy including the identification of blocking antibody (with Robert Cooke) and the use of pure venoms in hymenoptera allergy. (From Cohen & Samter, 1992.)

1966	J.J. Curry	Asthmatics more sensitive than normals to the action of histamine on the respiratory tract.

IgE

The discovery of IgE as a new immunoglobulin class responsible for some of the major manifestations of allergy really inaugurated a modern era and a deeper understanding of allergic phenomena. Combined with cellular, genetic and molecular approaches originating mainly from basic immunology, various impulses have contributed to make allergology one of the most exciting fields of applied immunology. A comprehensive history of the numerous discoveries and contributions of the past 25 years is still to be written.

1963	K. Frank Austen	Biochemistry of mast cell mediator release (Fig. 1.11).
1967	Kimishige Ishizaka Teruko Ishizaka	Characterization of reagins as IgE immunoglobulins (Fig. 1.12).
1967	Hans Bennich Gunnar Johansson	Identification of myeloma ND as IgE immunoglobulin (Fig. 1.13).
1981	K. Frank Austen	Biological properties of leukotrienes.
1983	Bengt I. Samuelson	Identification of leukotrienes as slow-reacting substance of anaphylaxis, role in allergic diseases (Fig. 1.14).

Hayfever—allergic rhinitis

Hayfever or allergic rhinitis is certainly the most prevalent allergic disease in most parts of the world today. There is much indirect, and some direct, evidence that this was not always so (Emanuel, 1988). In fact, and somewhat paradoxically, hayfever, despite being due primarily to contact

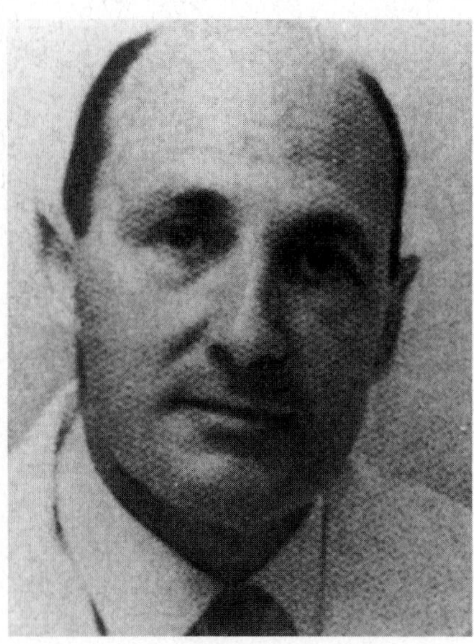

(a)

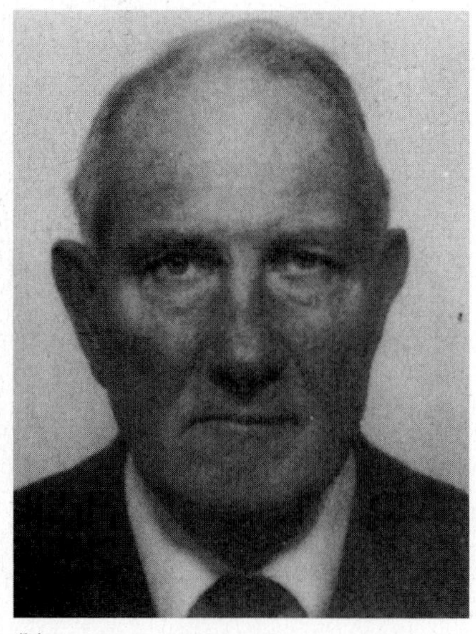

(b)

Fig. 1.10 (a) *James F. Riley (1912–85).* (b) *Geoffrey B. West (1916–).* Riley and West discovered that the mast cell granule was the major source of histamine in tissues. (From Cohen & Samter, 1992.)

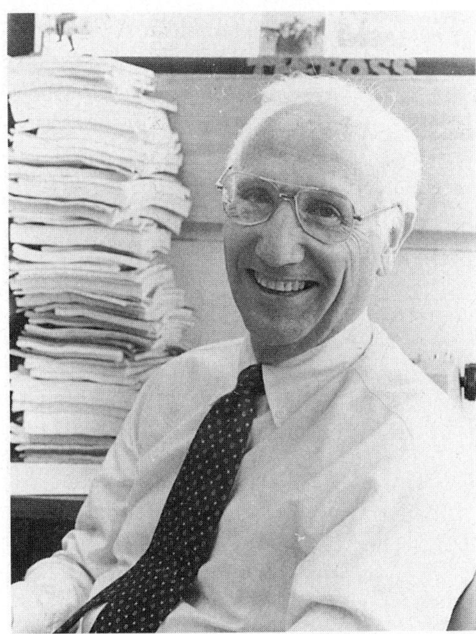

Fig. 1.11 *K. Frank Austen (1928–).* Pioneered the biochemistry of mast cell mediator release and the biological properties of leukotrienes.

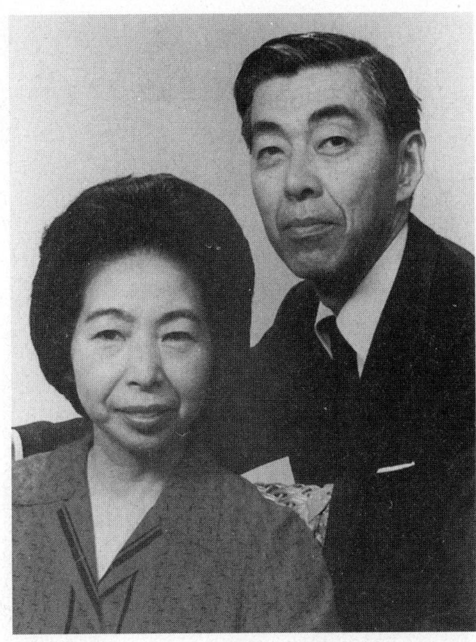

Fig. 1.12 (Left) *Kimshige Ishizaka (1925–).* (Right) *Teruko Ishizaka (1926–).* Characterized reaginic antibody as IgE.

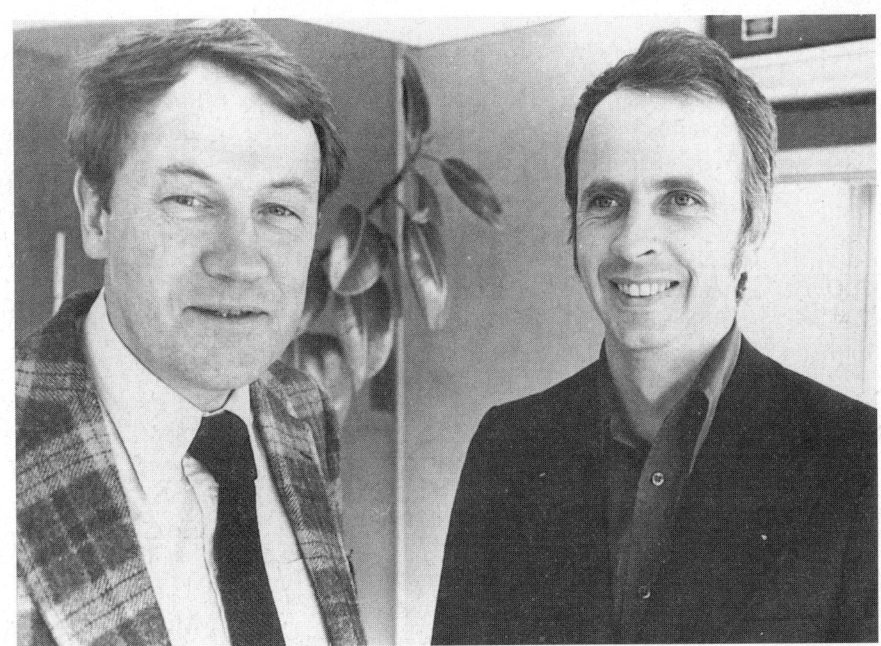

Fig. 1.13 (Left) *Hans Bennich (1930–).* (Right) *Gunnar Johansson (1938–).* Identification of IgND as IgE immunoglobulin and with L. Wide developed the Radio-AllergoSorbent Technique (RAST). (Courtesy of Pharmacia, Uppsala, Sweden.)

with agricultural 'products', seems to have flourished with the advent of the industrial revolution in the middle of the 19th century and to have taken a real 'turn for the worst' since about 1970 (Emanuel, 1988). Although still debated, the increase in hayfever prevalence does not appear to be due to better recognition of the disease by physicians or the public; this may have been the case 100 years ago, when the origin and mechanisms of hayfever attacks were not yet well known, but it is certainly not the case today.

Early descriptions and theories

AD b.865	Rhazes	Description of seasonal catarrh due to roses in Persia.

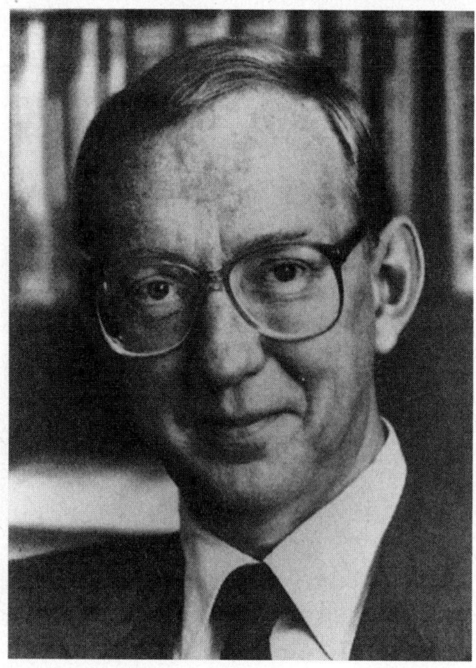

Fig. 1.14 *Bengt I. Samuelsson (1934–).* Identification and chemical characterization of the SRS-A leukotrienes. (From Cohen & Samter, 1992.)

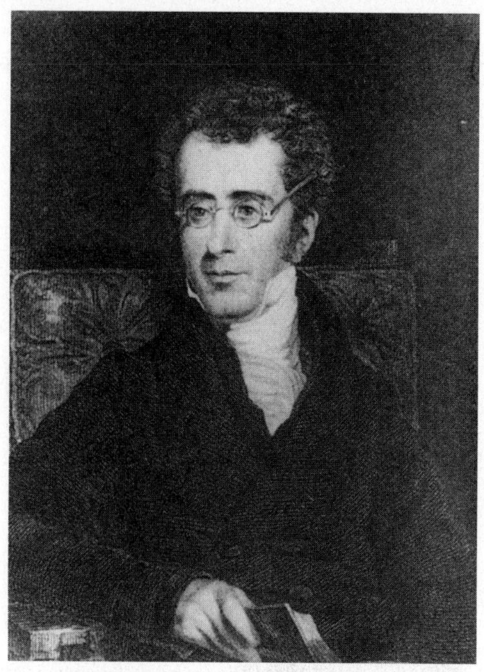

Fig. 1.15 *John Bostock (1773–1846).* Described 'catarrhus aestivus', later recognized as summer hayfever. (From Cohen & Samter, 1992.)

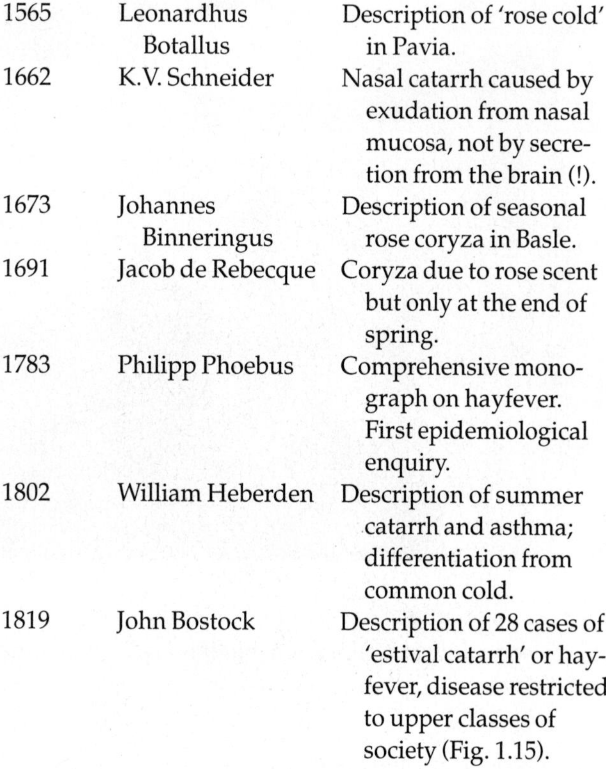

1565	Leonardhus Botallus	Description of 'rose cold' in Pavia.
1662	K.V. Schneider	Nasal catarrh caused by exudation from nasal mucosa, not by secretion from the brain (!).
1673	Johannes Binneringus	Description of seasonal rose coryza in Basle.
1691	Jacob de Rebecque	Coryza due to rose scent but only at the end of spring.
1783	Philipp Phoebus	Comprehensive monograph on hayfever. First epidemiological enquiry.
1802	William Heberden	Description of summer catarrh and asthma; differentiation from common cold.
1819	John Bostock	Description of 28 cases of 'estival catarrh' or hayfever, disease restricted to upper classes of society (Fig. 1.15).

Identification of causes of hayfever

In earlier times, roses were singled out as the main culprit for seasonal catarrh and it was only around 1873 that pollens were definitely shown to be a major cause.

1872	Morrill Wyman	Description of autumnal catarrh in USA and identification of ragweed pollen as cause.
1873–80	Charles Blackley	Experimental demonstration of role of grass pollens in hayfever, first pollen counts (Fig. 1.16).
1906	A. Wolff-Eisner	Relationship of human hayfever and urticaria to experimental anaphylaxis.

Milestones in asthma

Asthma has a history closely mingled with that of hayfever and has certainly been observed in China since the oldest recorded times. Theories on the pathogenesis of asthma have, however, gone through many historical cycles, sometimes emphasizing nervous and psychosomatic causes, sometimes IgE and anaphylactic reactions, sometimes T lymphocytes, cellular immunity, bacterial allergy, and so on (Emanuel & Howarch, 1995). The continued discussions and controversies probably reflect the fact that asthma is a heterogeneous syndrome.

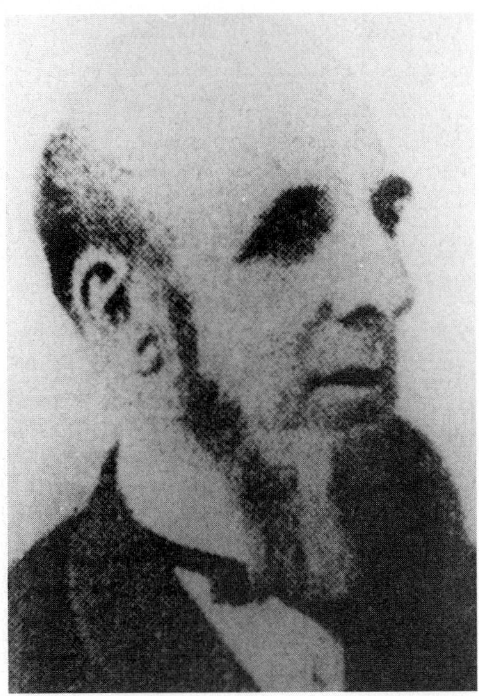

Fig. 1.16 *Charles H. Blackley (1820–1900).* Identified pollen as a cause of hayfever and devised methods for pollen counts and clinical challenge tests. (From Cohen & Samter, 1992.)

Early descriptions and theories on the pathophysiology of asthma

2698 BC	Huang Ti	First decription of asthma ('noisy breathing') in the Nei Ching, oldest treatise of internal medicine.
460–375 BC	Hippocrates	Description of asthma and eczema.
25 BC–AD 40	Aulus Celsus	Thorough description of dyspnoea, asthma and orthopnoea in treatise 'De medica'.
120–AD 180	Aretaeus of Cappadocia	First detailed description and coining of the word asthma.
1135–1204	Moses Maimonides	Author of famous 'Treatise on Asthma'. Physician of Sultan Saladin (Fig. 1.17).
1603	Felix Platter	Asthma due to obstruction of small pulmonary arteries or to nerve disturbances.
1680	Thomas Willis	Studies of asthma as bronchial disease and role of bronchial innervation; asthma as nervous disease (Fig. 1.18).

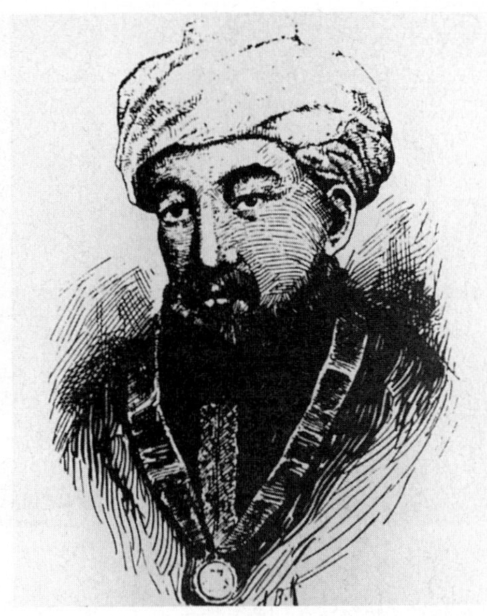

Fig. 1.17 *Moses Maimonides (1135–1204).* A prolific writer and author of a famous 'Treatise on Asthma'. (From Cohen & Samter, 1992.)

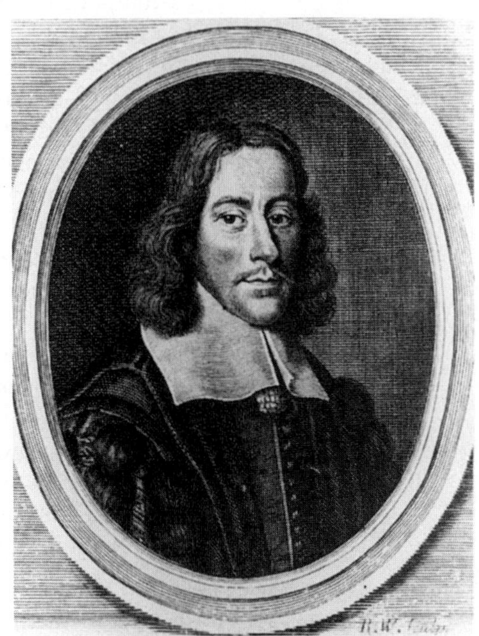

Fig. 1.18 *Thomas E. Willis (1621–75).* Recognized the importance of bronchial innervation in asthma; asthma as a 'nervous disease'. (From Cohen & Samter, 1992.)

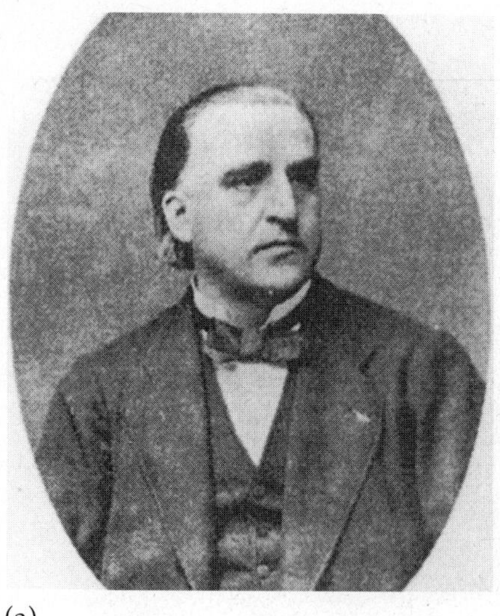

(a)

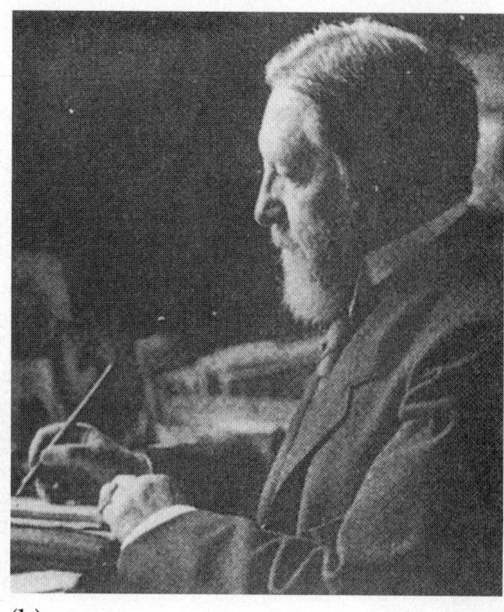

(b)

Fig. 1.19 (a) *Jean Martin Charcot (1825–93).* (b) *Ernst V. von Leyden (1832–1910).* The needle-like (eosinophil-derived) crystals characteristic of asthmatic sputum are named after Charcot and Leyden. (From Cohen & Samter, 1992.)

1682	Joan van Helmont	Description of seasonal asthma with itching skin eruption (atopic dermatitis?) and of psychosomatic asthma.
1816	Henri Laennec	Invents stethoscope. Identifies bronchospasm as important component of asthma.
1853 1886	Jean Martin Charcot Ernst van Leyden	Description of Charcot–Leyden crystals in sputum of asthmatics: asthma is not just a 'nervous disease' (Fig. 1.19).
1909	William B. Osler	Asthma associated with neurotic disease.
1910	S. Meltzer	Bronchial asthma as a phenomenon of anaphylaxis.
1918	Francis Rackemann	Description of intrinsic and extrinsic asthma: asthma is not always of allergic origin (Fig. 1.20).

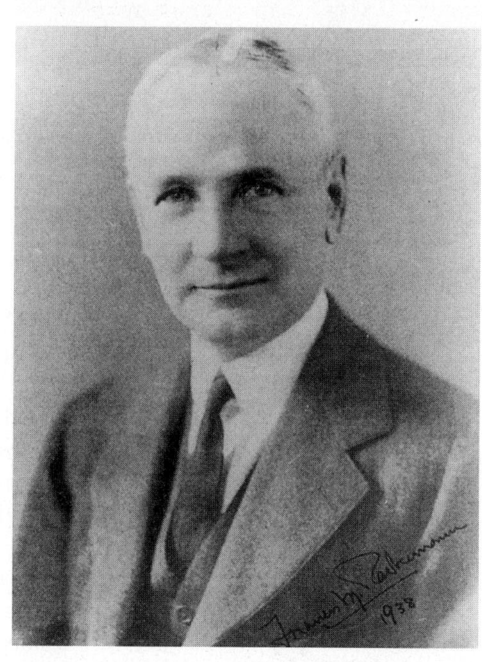

Fig. 1.20 *Francis M. Rackemann (1887–1973).* Introduced the term 'intrinsic asthma'. (From Cohen & Samter, 1992.)

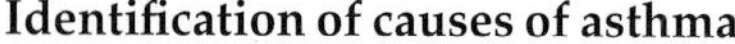

Identification of causes of asthma

Retrospectively, the deleterious effect of the 'scent' provided by various classical inhalation allergens has been recognized empirically since the Middle Ages. More on this topic may be found by assessing the historical records for various types of allergens (see below).

1552	Jerome Cardan	Cures asthma of Archbishop Hamilton of St Andrew by elimination of bedding feather pillows.

c. 1630	Sanctorius	Description of asthma to cat hair.
1656	Pierre Borel	Weakness, fainting and asthma upon contact with cats, mice, dogs and horses (particularly in Germans?).
1698	John Floyer	Description of asthma causes (tobacco smoke, dust, foods, exercise, emotions, environmental factors). First description of heredity in asthma (Fig. 1.21).
1713	Bernardino Ramazzini	First systematic description of occupational diseases, in particular baker's asthma (Fig. 1.22).
1868	Henry Hide Salter	Description of asthma with various causes (animal emanations, foods, hayfever), intrinsic asthma, cells in sputum (later identified as eosinophils) (Fig. 1.23).

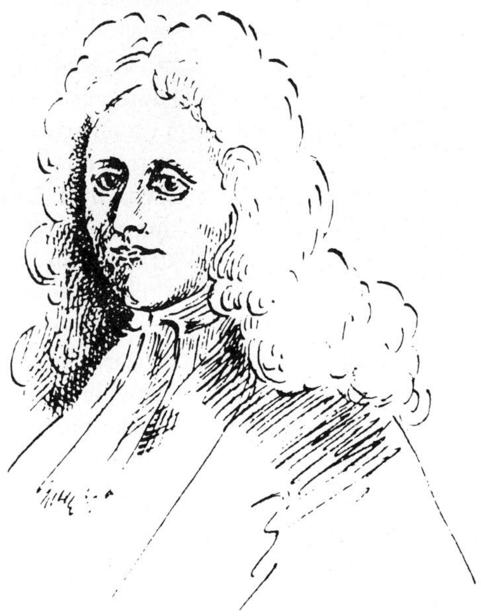

Fig. 1.21 *Sir John Floyer (1649–1734).* Recognition of asthma as a multifactorial disease with many triggers (e.g. tobacco smoke, dust, foods, exercise, emotions, environmental factors). First description of heredity in asthma. (From Cohen & Samter, 1992.)

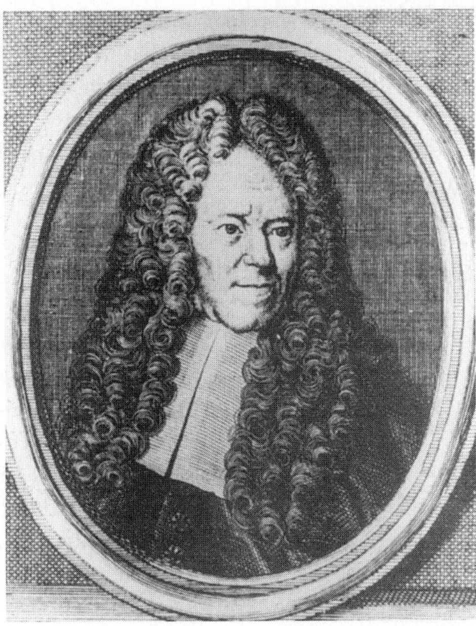

Fig. 1.22 *Bernardino Ramazzini (1633–1714).* First description of occupational diseases, in particular baker's asthma. (From Cohen & Samter, 1992.)

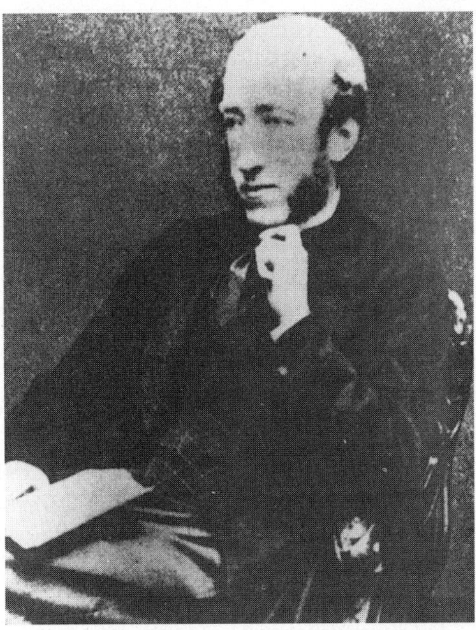

Fig. 1.23 *Henry Hyde Salter (1823–71).* Description of the various causes of asthma and of cells (now known as eosinophils) in sputum. (From Cohen & Samter, 1992.)

Identification of major allergen sources

From mere empirical observations, the causative role of allergens in the induction of allergic reactions was in general proven by provocation and, later, by skin testing.

With the advent of IgE serology and of refined immunological techniques, it became possible to identify major allergens as single proteins and finally to produce them as recombinant proteins. A detailed history of the evolution of knowledge about major allergens over the past 20 years has yet to be written.

Pollens and other inhalant allergens

AD b.41	Britannicus	Reported as afflicted by acute allergic reactions to horses.
AD *c.* 40	Marcus Terrentius Varro	'Very small animals invisible to the eye, floating in the air, growing in damp places, inhaled and giving rise to serious diseases' (mites ?).
1552	Jerome Cardan	Asthma due to bedding feather pillows.
1570	Pietro Mattioli	First reported challenge of a cat allergic patient by stay in a room containing a concealed cat.
c. 1630	Sanctorius	Description of asthma to cat hair.
c. 1680	Nehemiah Green	First micrcopic studies of pollen grains.
1913	William Dunbar	Methodology for pollen extraction, identification of allergenic protein.
1924	F.T. Codham	First description of mould allergy.
1928	Storm van Leeuwen	Inhalation allergy to house dust.
1963	Jack Pepys	Identification of moulds and anti-*Thermosopora* IgG antibodies as cause of farmer's lung (Fig. 1.24).
1967	Reindert Voorhorst Frederick Spieksma	Identification of *Dermatophagoides* mites as major allergen source in house dust.

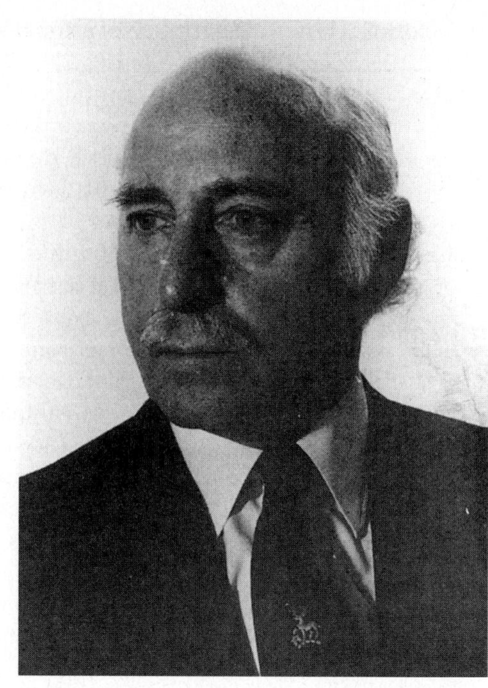

Fig. 1.24 *Jack Pepys (1914–96).* Identified thermophilic actinomycetes as a cause of farmer's lung. Major contributions to our understanding of the aetiology and pathogenesis of allergic alveolitis, occupational asthma and allergic bronchopulmonary aspergillosis. (From Cohen & Samter, 1992.)

Food allergies

The fact that some foods may cause allergic reactions, particularly skin urticaria, has been known for a very long time, and some of the classical food allergens are still with us.

b.460 BC	Hippocrates	Description of allergy to goats' cheese.
AD b.131	Galen	Description of untoward reactions to various milks (goat, cow, ewe, camel, ass): allergy?
1530	Thomas Moore	Report on acute skin eruption of King Richard III due to ingestion of strawberries (Shakespeare!).
1665	Philipp Jacob Sachs	Description of a case of urticaria caused by strawberries and of shock upon ingestion of fish.
1675	Theophile Bonet	Idiosyncrasies to bread, strawberries and wine.
1775	William Cullen	Hereditary idiosyncrasy to eggs in 'Historia de Materia Medica'.
1778	Stolpertus	Description of acute angioneurotic oedema following ingestion of eggs.

1783	Friedrich Schademantal	Allergic urticaria due to ingestion of fresh pork meat.

Insect allergies

2641 BC	Menes	Egyptian pharaoh reported to have died from a wasp ('kehb') sting (first report of an anaphylactic shock?). However, interpretation of hyeroglyph controversial.
1765	Debrest	Description of sudden death by bee sting in Montpellier.
1914	A.T. Waterhouse	Anaphylactic reactions of beekeepers to stings.

Drug allergies

A number of natural substances and plants used as drugs were described or known to cause allergies. With the advent of chemical drugs around the end of the 19th century, however, a vast 'can of worms' was opened and is still with us today, although the main culprits change with time and therapeutic habits. For example, adverse allergic reactions to salvarsan, the antisyphilitic drug created by Paul Ehrlich and which dominated syphylis therapy for 40 years, have disappeared. They were to some extent replaced, in terms of frequency, by reactions towards β-lactam antibiotics.

1648 1776	Thomas Dover Johann Murray	Introduction of ipecacuanha root (emetine), causes asthma attacks in pharmacists.
1895	Josef Jadassohn	Description of various types of drug reactions in the skin.
1916	Robert A. Cooke	Description of allergic drug reactions (Fig. 1.25).
1922	Fernand Widal	Nasal polyps and asthma due to aspirin intolerance, haemolytic anaemia, leukopenia in anaphylaxis.
1960	Bernard. B. Levine Alain L. de Weck	Identification of major and minor antigenic determinants in penicillin allergy.
1967	Bernard Halpern	Lymphocyte stimulation test in drug allergy.

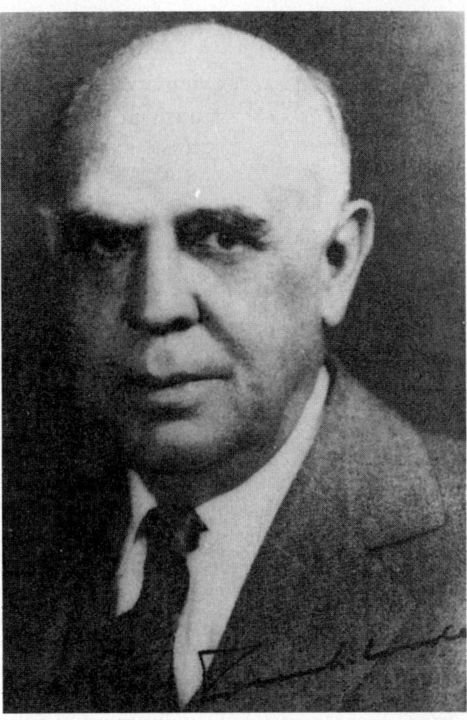

Fig. 1.25 *Robert A. Cooke (1880–1960).* Introduced the protein nitrogen unit (PNU) for standardization of allergen extracts, realized the role of hereditary factors in hayfever and described allergic drug reactions. Cooke also discovered 'blocking antibody' with Mary Loveless. (From Cohen & Samter, 1992.)

Milestones in immunological techniques

Although concepts and theories are important, as the motors of experimentation, practical results and confirmation may only be obtained as a result of the discovery and development of new tools and methods. In fact, in immunology, the discovery of such tools has been, most of the time, the decisive event which permitted progress. Modern immunology really started with the serological techniques developed by microbiologists around 1880–90.

1889	Albert Charrin Georges Roger	Detection of anti-*Pseudomonas pyocyanea* antibodies by agglutination.
1896	Max von Gruber	Description of microbial agglutinin reactions.
1896	Georges Widal	Application of the agglutination reaction to clinical diagnosis of enteric fever.
1897	Rudolf Kraus	Precipitation between serum of immunized animal and bacterial

		culture filtrate: discovery of precipitins.
1929	Michael Heidelberger	Quantitative aspects of antigen–antibody reactions (preciptin curve), basic immunochemistry.
1939	Arne Tiselius Elvin A. Kabat	Identification of antibodies as gammaglobulins by electrophoresis.
1941	Albert H. Coons	Identification of immunoglobulins in tissues with fluorescent-labelled antibodies (immunocytochemistry).
1942	Jules Freund	Adjuvant oil emulsions and production of experimental autoimmune disorders.
1945	Robin A. Coombs	Antiglobulin passive haemaglutination techniques (Fig. 1.26).
1948	Orjan Ouchterlony	Development of gel double-diffusion techniques.
1948	Jacques Oudin	Development of gel immunodiffusion techniques.
1952	Zoltan Ovary	Development of passive cutaneous anaphylaxis (PCA) for quantitation of anaphylactic antibodies.
1955	Pierre Grabar	Development of immunoelectrophoresis.
1960	Rosalyn S. Yalow Solomon A. Berson	Development of radioimmunoassay.
1962	Niels K. Jerne	Plaque assay for cellular antibody formation.

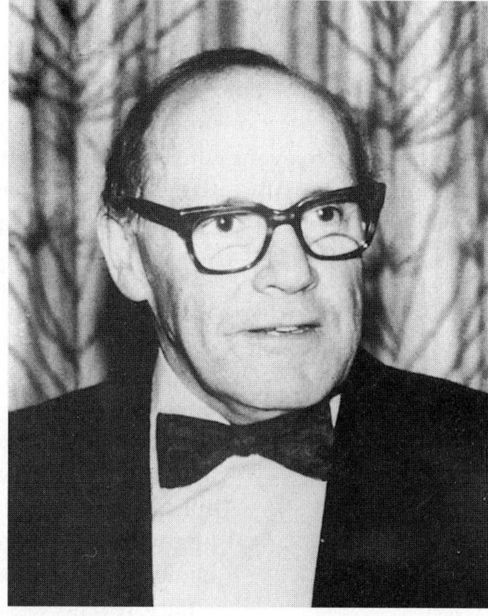

Fig. 1.26 *Robin A. Coombs (1921–).* Described the antiglobulin ('Coombs') test and, with Philip Gell, classified the hypersensitivity reactions (see Chapter 2).

Milestones in allergological diagnostic techniques

Like immunology, progress in clinical allergy has been dependent upon the availability of investigational tools. Most of them are still with us.

1570	Pietro Mattioli	First reported challenge of a cat allergic patient by stay in a room containing a concealed cat.
1656	Pierre Borel	Blister upon applying egg on skin of hypersensitive patient (first skin test?).
b.1603	Kenelm Digby	Blister to rose petal applied on cheek of English court lady hypersensitive to roses (first patch test?).
1895	Josef Jadassohn	Establishment of patch tests in contact dermatitis.
1905	Bela Schick	Skin test for susceptibility to diphtheria.
1905	Clemens von Pirquet	Introduced tuberculin skin test in diagnosis.
1909	William Schultz	Detection of anaphylaxis by contraction of isolated smooth muscle *in vitro*.
1911	Tomaso Casoni	Skin test in patients infected with *Echinococcus*.
1912	Oscar M. Schloss	Use of scratch test in allergy to foods.
1916	Robert A. Cooke	Standardization of allergen extracts—protein nitroger unit (PNU), role of hereditary factors in hayfever, description

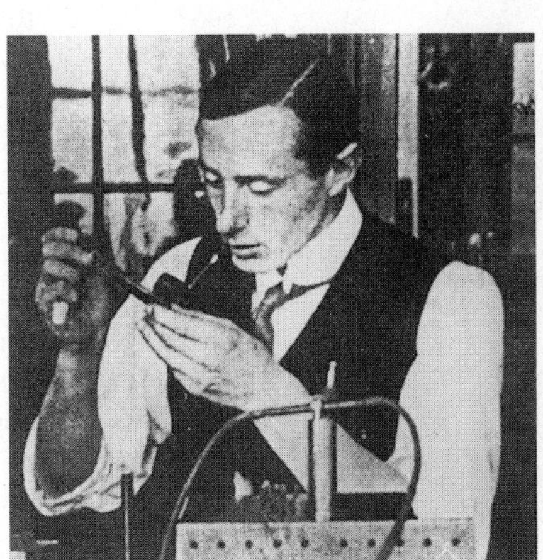

(a)

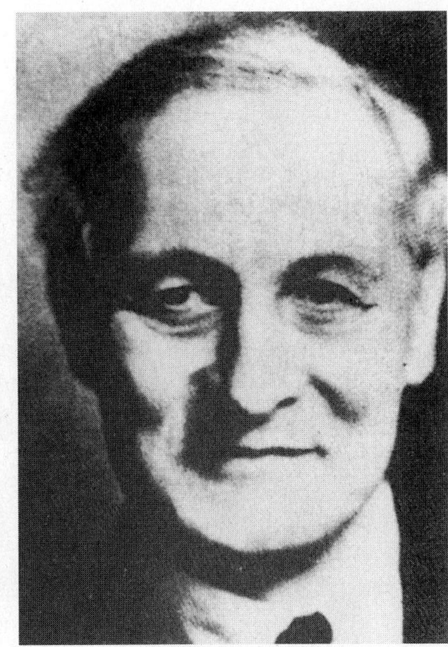

(b)

Fig. 1.27 (a) *Leonard Noon (1877–1913)*. (b) *John Freeman (1877–1962)*. Noon and Freeman introduced the treatment of hayfever by immunization with pollen extracts. (From Cohen & Samter, 1992.)

		of allergic drug reactions (Fig. 1.25).
1923	Arthur Coca	Reagent for allergen extraction (Fig. 1.7).
1962	Alain L. de Weck Charles W. Parker	Diagnostic skin testing for penicillin allergy with synthetic penicilloyl-polylysine polymers.
1964	Lawrence M. Lichtenstein Abraham G. Osler	Development of allergen-specific histamine release test.
1964	T.E. King	Identification of major allergen in ragweed.
1966	David Marsh	Identification of major grass allergens.
1967	L. Wide Gunnar Johannsson	Development of a RAdioSorbent Test (RAST) for detection of allergen-specific IgE.

Milestones in allergy therapy

The major therapeutic weapons of the allergologists are still nowadays identification and avoidance of the allergen(s) responsible, allergen-specific immunotherapy and symptomatic treatment with a variety of anti-allergic drugs. A real causal treatment and definite cure for allergic sensitization is still out of our reach, even if some such claims are periodically made, praising one or the other of the alternative methods.

Allergen avoidance

1552	Jerome Cardan	Elimination of feather bedding pillows.

Allergen-specific immunotherapy

1910	William Dunbar	Methodology for pollen extraction first approaches to pollen immunotherapy.
1911	Leonard Noon John Freeman	Wide use of immunotherapy with pollen extracts in hayfever patients (Fig. 1.27).
1940	Mary Loveless	Use of pure venoms in immunotherapy for hymenoptera allergy (Fig. 1.9).
1954	William Frankland Rosa Augustin	First placebo-controlled clinical trial of desensitization (allergen-injection immunotherapy).

Anti-allergic drugs

28th cent. BC	Shen Nung	First reference to an anti-asthmatic plant ('ma-huang'), shown later to contain ephedrine, in the first herbal

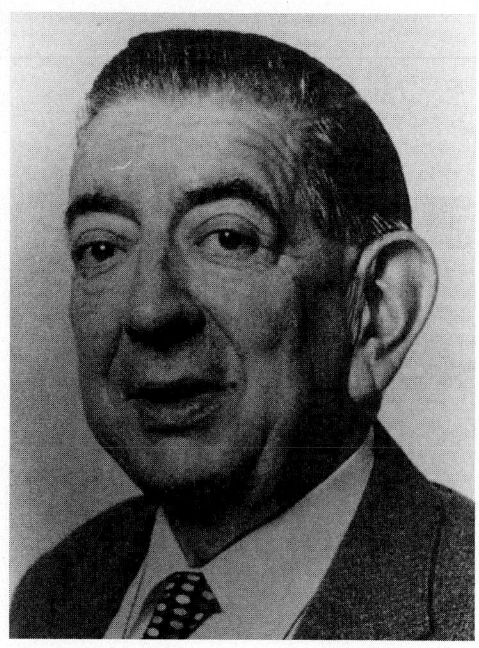

Fig. 1.28 *Roger E.C. Altounyan (1922–87).* Discovered sodium cromoglycate. (From Cohen & Samter, 1992.)

		compendium Pen Ts'ao.
AD *c.* 60	Pedanius Dioscorides	Remedies for asthma in classical pharmacology treatise 'De Materia Medica'.
b.1306	John of Arderne	Prescription of a syrup for the asthmatic.
1900	Solomon Solis-Cohen	Role of autonomic imbalance in allergic diseases. Use of adrenal substance in hayfever and asthma.
1924	Ko Kuei Shen Carl F. Schmidt	Systematic investigations of pharmacological actions of ephedrine, the active component of 'ma-huang'.
1937	Daniel Bovet	First synthesis of antihistaminic drugs.
1949	Philip S. Hench Edward C. Kendall	Isolation of cortisone from adrenals for therapy of rheumatoid arthritis.
1967	Roger Altounyan	Discovery of sodium cromoglycate as anti-asthmatic drug (Fig. 1.28).

Conclusion

The portraits of many individuals who have had a major impact on our understanding of allergic diseases including asthma are contained in Figs 1.1–1.28.

The history of the allergic diseases and their relationship to basic immunology is truly fascinating and knowledge of it helps considerably in the acquisition of an overview of the whole discipline. It is only in evaluating and reflecting upon the past that we shall advance with a sure footing towards the future.

References

Avenberg, K.M. & Harper, S.D. (1980) *Footnotes on Allergy*. Pharmacia, Uppsala.

Cohen, S.G. & Samter, M. (1992) *Excerpts from Classics in Allergy*, 2nd edn. Symposia Foundation (Oceanside Publications), Providence, Rhode Island.

Emanuel, M.B. (1988) Hay fever, a post industrial revolution epidemic: a history of its growth during the 19th century. *Clin. Allergy*, **18**, 295–304.

Emanuel, B. & Howarth, P.H. (1995) Asthma and anaphylaxis: a relevant model for chronic disease? An historical analysis of directions of asthma research. *Clin. Exp. Allergy*, **25**, 73–9.

Humphrey, J. & White, R.G. (1970) *Immunology for Students of Medicine*, 3rd edn. Blackwell Scientific Publications, Oxford.

Klein, J. (1982) History of immunology. In: *Immunology*. John Wiley, Chichester.

Mahmoud, A.A.F. & Austen, K.F. (eds) (1980) *The Eosinophil and Health and Disease*, p. 5. Grune & Stratton, New York.

Samter, M. (1969) *Excerpts from Classics in Allergy*. Ross Laboratories.

Schadewaldt, H. (1979–82) *Geschichte der Allergie*, Bd 1–4. Dustri, München.

Sela, M. (1987) A peripatetic and personal view of molecular immunology for one third of the century. *Ann. Rev. Immunol.*, **5**, 1.

Silverstein, A.M. (1982) History of immunology. Development of the concept of immunologic specificity II. *Cell. Immunol.*, **71**, 183–95.

Simons, E.E. (1994) *Ancestors of Allergy*. Global Medical Communications, New York.

de Weck, A.L. (1994) Farewell address. 40 years allergo-immunology: from the nipple unto milk. *Clin. Exp. Allergy*, **24**, 490–6.

CHAPTER 2

Concepts of Allergy and Hypersensitivity

A.B. Kay

Problems of terminology

With the passage of time the word 'allergy' has become corrupted. It is frequently used synonymously with immunoglobulin E (IgE)-mediated hypersensitivity. This restricted meaning was not originally intended. von Pirquet (1906)* who introduced the term allergy, used it to describe the situation of 'changed reactivity' (to antigenic stimulation) irrespective of whether this resulted in immunity (protection) or hypersensitivity. Hypersensitivity (or supersensitivity) was, and still is, a general term used to describe an adverse clinical reaction to an antigen (or allergen). Such an antigen could be bacteria-derived, as in a classic delayed-type hypersensitivity reaction to tuberculo-protein, or an allergen such as pollen giving rise to IgE-mediated hypersensitivity.

Today, the terms 'allergy' and 'hypersensitivity' mistakenly tend to be used interchangeably to describe any exaggerated response of the 'immune system' to external antigenic, or allergenic substances. This is unsatisfactory as, by definition, the role of the so-called 'immune system' is to effect immunity. For example, hypersensitivity states may occur in response to autoantigens, as in 'autoimmune thyroiditis — better and properly called autoallergic thyroiditis (in the same way that experimental allergic encephelomyelitis is not referred to as 'immune' encephalomyelitis). Most of the difficulty is removed if instead of 'allergy' we refer to 'allergic diseases' and confine the word allergy (as von Pirquet originally intended) to the 'uncommitted' biological response (Fig. 2.1). In the individual, this uncommitted response may lead either to immunity (which is beneficial), or allergic disease (which is harmful). Therefore, the allergic response—in producing antibodies and specifically reacting lymphocytes — supplies the common armaments for both the reactions of immunity and those of hypersensitivity (allergic disease).

This teaching, stemming from von Pirquet, affords a satisfactory layout for this volume (*Allergy and Allergic Diseases*)—'*Allergy*' covers (i) the allergic responses—the first section, and (ii) mechanisms and clinical aspects of '*Allergic Diseases*'—the rest of the book.

Some examples of hypersensitivity reactions fall outside the scope of this work, e.g. antigen/antibody (Ag/Ab) (or so-called 'immune complex-mediated') reactions such as erythema nodosum leprosum, Ag/Ab complex glomerulonephritis and haemolytic disease of the newborn. For reasons which are somewhat arbitrary these areas will not be covered in this text. Instead, the volume is concerned with allergic diseases elicited by external ('foreign'), non-infectious substances which are inhaled, ingested or injected, or which come into contact with a mucosal surface. Hypersensitivity states caused by infectious agents, or by self- or autoantigens, will not be addressed.

The restricted usage of the term allergy to 'allergic disease' is reflected in the practice of clinical allergy ('allergology') where physicians diagnose and treat only selected examples of hypersensitivity states, rather than the wide spectrum of immunological disorders (see Fig. 2.1). In many countries (see Chapter 81) clinical allergists manage only the IgE-mediated ('atopic') diseases, e.g. summer hayfever, perennial rhinitis, allergic asthma,

*This article, translated from the German original by Carl Prausnitz, appears as an Appendix to this volume.

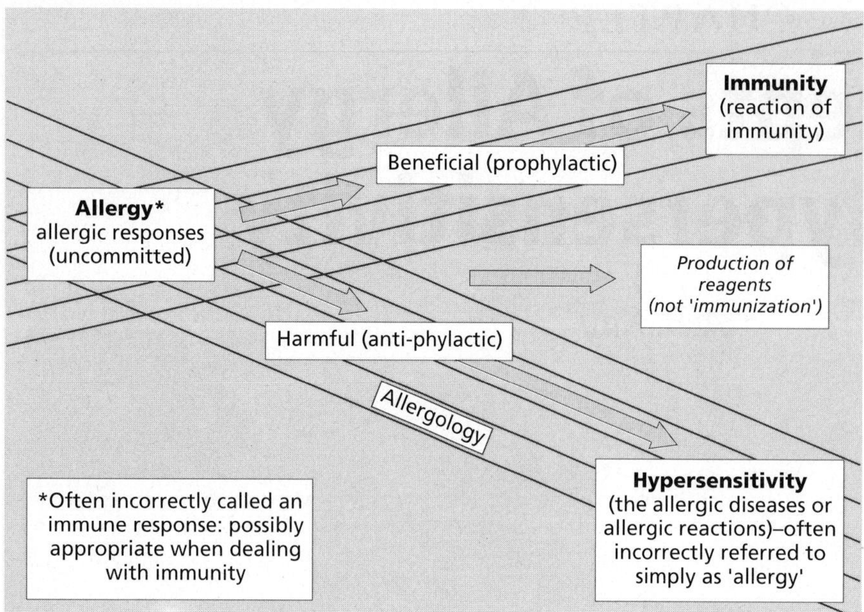

Fig. 2.1 A paradigm for reinstating the word 'allergy' to the original meaning intended by von Pirquet. The diagram illustrates how the biological expression of allergy can be protective as in *immunity* or harmful as in the *allergic diseases* (*'allergology'*). A further inconsistency in terminology is also mentioned. The scientist does not 'immunize' a rabbit to produce a reagent such as, for example, specific antibody to egg albumin. The actual procedure is *injecting antigen*; the animal is not rendered 'immune' to egg albumin.

allergy to stinging insects, food anaphylaxis and atopic dermatitis (see below for a definition of 'atopy'). Other 'hypersensitivity diseases', such as coeliac disease and contact dermatitis, are usually treated by the relevant organ-based specialist. Furthermore, the clinical allergist often deals with patients whose signs and symptoms mimic those of true allergic disease, i.e. where there is evidence of local or generalized release of histamine and other pharmacological reagents but where a proven allergic abnormality cannot be identified. Such reactions are sometimes called 'pseudo-allergy' and can occur in certain susceptible individuals following exposure to certain foods, food additives, radiocontrast media and various drugs. They are believed to involve the direct release of pharmacological agents from target mediator-containing cells. An overview of the principles and practice of diagnosis and management of allergic disease is given in Chapter 82.

Classification of the hypersensitivity reactions

A distinction should be made between a *classification of mechanisms of hypersensitivity*, which may play a role in certain allergic conditions, and a *classification of the allergic diseases* themselves. In considering mechanisms it is useful to reappraise briefly the classic work of Coombs and Gell (1963) who described a '. . . classification of allergic reactions which may be deleterious to the tissues and harmful to the host'. This still remains extremely useful to practising physicians, scientists and students because it relates mechanisms to disease entities. The authors predicted correctly that in any one disease it was likely that more than one kind of allergic process was involved. They also emphasized the fact that their classification was primarily one of *initiating mechanisms* and not of the *subsequent events* or the diseases themselves.

The types I to IV hypersensitivity reactions of Coombs and Gell were as shown in Fig. 2.2. The *type I reaction* was initiated by allergen or antigen reacting with tissue cells passively sensitized by antibody produced elsewhere, leading to the release of pharmacologically active substances. These *anaphylactic reactions* included both general anaphylaxis in humans and other animals and local manifestations of anaphylaxis, such as that observed in the skin following diagnostic skin-prick tests, as well as local responses in the respiratory and gastrointestinal tracts. A further example was instances of sudden death in infancy in which anaphylactic hypersensitivity to cows' milk proteins was a proposed mechanism (Parish *et al.*, 1960).

Type II reactions (cytolytic or cytotoxic) were initiated by antibody reacting either with an antigenic component of a tissue cell, or with an antigen or hapten intimately associated with these cells. Complement was usually, but not always, necessary to effect the cellular damage. Examples include drug-induced haemolytic anaemia in association with chlorpromazine or phenacetin and thrombocytopenic purpura caused by the now obsolete sedative, Sedormid. There are many examples of type II reactions outside the province of the 'clinical allergist'. These include incompatible blood transfusion reactions, Rhesus incompatibility and autoallergic (autoimmune) haemolytic anaemia.

In some instances antibodies against cell surface receptors have cell stimulatory (agonist) effects without necessarily being cytotoxic. An example is Graves' disease (hyperthyroidism, autoallergic thyroiditis) in which IgG antibodies directed against the thyroid-stimulating hormone (TSH)-receptor is produced. These have agonist

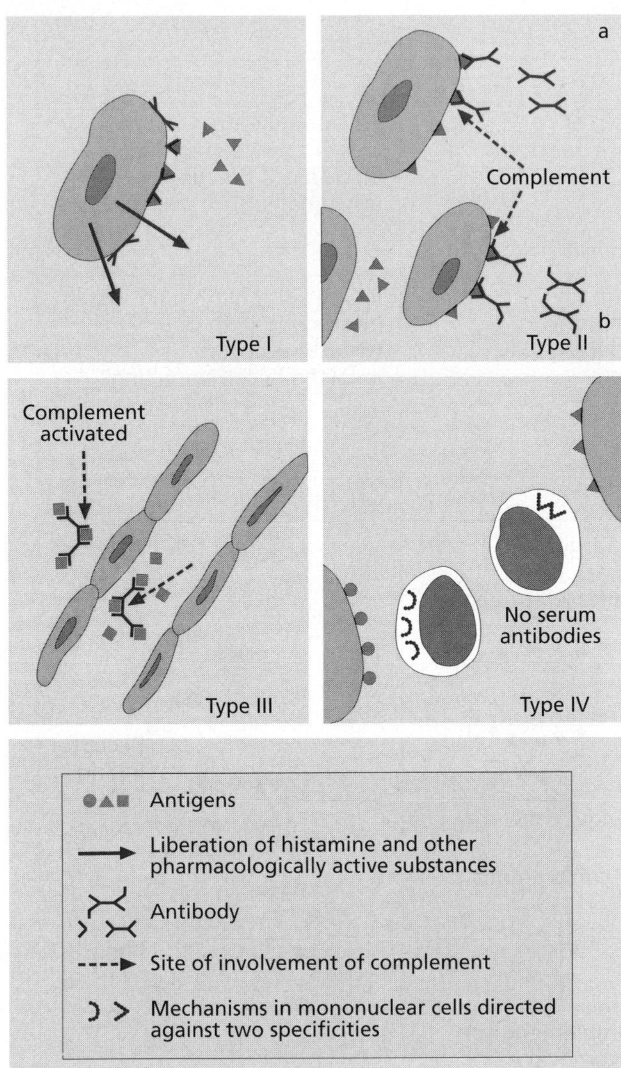

Fig. 2.2 The original Coombs and Gell classification of 'hypersensitivity reactions which may be deleterious to the tissues and harmful to the host'. The initiating events in the various types is as follows. *Type I*, free antigen reacting with antibody passively sensitizing cell surface; *type II*, antibody reacting with (a) cell surface or (b) with antigen or hapten which becomes attached to cell surface —complement plays a major destructive role; *type III*, antigen and antibody reacting in antigen excess forming complexes which, possibly with the aid of complement, are toxic to cells; *type IV*, specifically modified nononuclear cells reacting with allergen or antigen deposited at a local site. (From Coombs & Gell, 1963.)

effects by stimulating thyroid hormone production with subsequent thyrotoxicosis and goitre formation. Similarly, some patients with chronic urticaria have histamine-releasing IgG autoantibodies against the α subunit of the high-affinity IgE receptor (FcεRIα) (Hide *et al.*, 1993). The antibody is believed to activate normal mast cell function by receptor cross-linking and in this sense is cytostimulating, rather than cytolytic (in which there is destruction of the cells with liberation of pre-formed histamine). In myasthenia gravis, on the other hand, autoantibodies directed against acetylcholine receptors have been identified. These have antagonist properties leading to a failure to sustain a maintained or repeated contraction of striated muscle. Although, in both situations, the initiating event is IgG bound to cell-surface antigen, the outcome is quite different, giving on the one hand, cytolytic or cytotoxic reactions, and on the other a cyto-stimulating hypersensitivity reaction in which there is altered cell function (or cell signalling) with IgG antibody acting either as an agonist or an antagonist. For these reasons, Janeway and Travers (1995) proposed that the classic Coombs and Gell type II cytotoxic or cell-stimulatory reaction is subdivided into type IIa (cytotoxic) and type IIb (cell-stimulating) responses (Fig. 2.3) (Gell & Coombs, 1975).

Type III reactions (Arthus reactions and 'immune complex' or toxic complex syndrome) occur when antigen and antibody, reacting in antigen excess, form complexes which, possibly with the aid of complement, are toxic to cells. Examples include farmer's lung (and other forms of extrinsic allergic alveolitis), erythema nodosum leprosum, serum sickness, Ag/Ab complex glomerulonephritis and deposition of Ag/Ab complexes at other sites such as the skin as in certain vasculitic skin rashes.

For many years the Arthus-type reaction (i.e. the Coombs and Gell type III response) was considered to be the major mechanism operative in tissue damage in extrinsic allergic alveolitis. The concept was that inhaled antigen interacting with IgG ('precipitating') antibody formed toxic Ag/Ab complexes in and around the alveolar capillaries. The classic works of Pepys (1969) and Pepys *et al.* (1963) described serum precipitating antibody in association with hypersensitivity responses to inhaled fungal, microbial and animal-derived antigens. In particular, they demonstrated the aetiological role of thermophilic actinomycetes in the pathogenesis of farmer's lung indicating that, in this disease, inhalation of the spores of *Thermopolyspora polyspora* and *Micropolyspora vulgaris* and possibly other antigen-producing thermophilic actinomycetes were the major antigens. This, in turn, led to the development of a diagnostic precipitation test. Subsequently there was interest in the role of cell-mediated responses in extrinsic allergic alveolitis with identification of sensitized T cells which respond in proliferation assays to the allergen in question (Fink *et al.*, 1975). Thus, there may be an additional type IV component to the clinical expression of extrinsic allergic alveolitis.

Type IV reactions refer to situations where specifically sensitized T cells react with allergen or antigen deposited at the local site, as in delayed- or tuberculin-type hypersensitivity. Classical delayed-type hypersensitivity involves predominantly CD4+ T cells with antigen presented in a major histocompatibility complex (MHC) class II restricted fashion. These reactions are characterized by infiltration of T lymphocytes with a restricted cytokine

	Type I	Type II	
		a	b
Descriptive term	Immediate-type (IgE-dependent, or anaphylactic) hypersensitivity	Cytolytic, or cytotoxic, reactions	Cell-stimulating reactions involving altered cell function (or signalling)
Initiating event	Antigen (allergen) interacting with mast cells or basophils passively sensitized by IgE	IgG antibody interacting with cell surface antigen	IgG cell-stimulating antibody interacting with cell surface receptors involved in cell signalling
Antigen	Soluble	Cell-associated	Cell-associated
Simplified scheme of the proposed mechanism	Mast cell/basophil 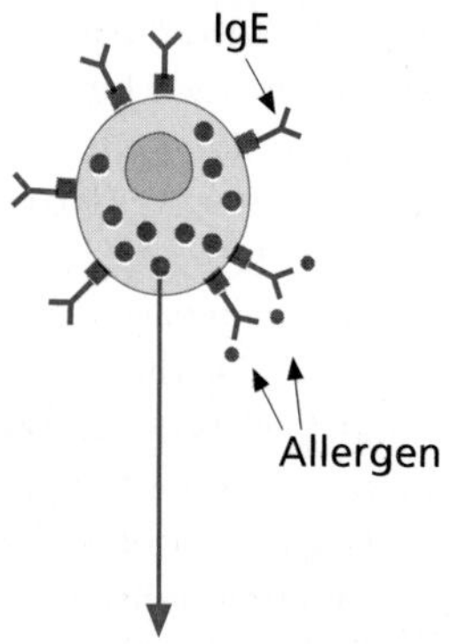 IgE Allergen Release of granule-associated mediators (e.g. histamine) and membrane-derived lipid mediators of hypersensitivity	Target cell 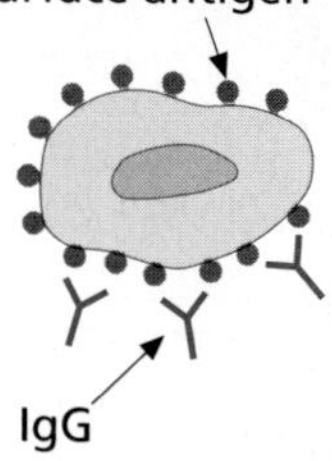 Cell surface antigen IgG +/– complement Complement lysis or removal by the RE system	Target cell 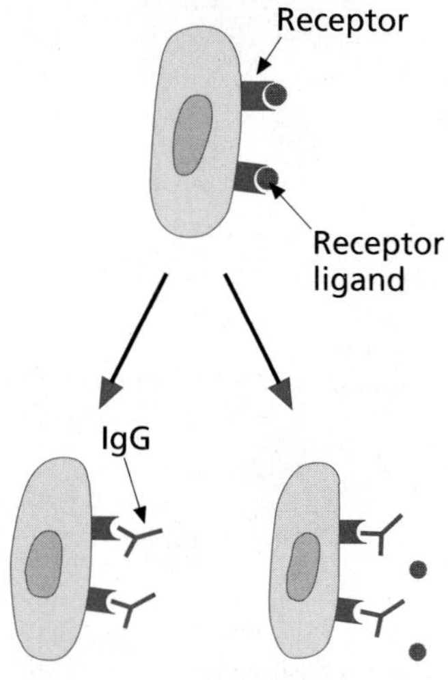 Receptor Receptor ligand IgG Agonist Antagonist
Examples in humans	• Acute symptoms of allergic rhinitis • General and local anaphylaxis • Early-phase allergic reactions (in experimental models of atopic allergic disease)	• Certain allergic drug reactions (e.g. penicillin) • Incompatible transfusion reactions • Autoallergic ('autoimmune') haemolytic anaemia	• Chronic urticaria (Anti-FcεRIα antibody – agonist) • Graves disease (Thyroid stimulating antibody – agonist) • Myasthenia gravis (Anti-acetylcholine receptor antibody – antagonist)

Fig. 2.3 (*Above and opposite.*) A modification to the Coombs and Gell classification (1963) of hypersensitivity reactions based on more recent knowledge of the initiating events but restricted to human allergic disease. Immediate-type (type I) reactions involve soluble antigen interacting with cell-bound IgE. As explained in the text, the role of non-IgG homocytotropic antibodies in human allergic disease has not been clarified. Type I reaction involves IgE antibodies bound to high-affinity (FcεRI) IgE receptors on mast cells or basophils (and possibly macrophages or even eosinophils). Antigen (allergen) induces the release of granule-associated and membrane lipid-derived mediators of hypersensitivity as well as several cytokines including IL-5, IL-3 and GM-CSF (see Fig. 2.4). Type II reactions are subdivided into type IIa, cytolytic or cytotoxic reactions originally described by Coombs and Gell, in which antibody-sensitized cells are destroyed by complement lysis or removed by the reticuloendothelial (RE) system, and type IIb, those in which

Type III	Type IV	Type IV	Type IV
	a_1	a_2	b
Arthus type (or antigen-antibody complex) – often called 'immune complex' – hypersensitivity reaction	Classical delayed-type hypersensitivity	Cell-mediated eosinophilic hypersensitivity *or* chronic allergic inflammation	Tissue injury by cytotoxic T lymphocytes
Antigen-antibody complexes, in and around the micro-vasculature, which activate complement	Antigen presentation to sensitized CD4+ type 1 T lymphocytes (also called T helper (Th) type 1 cells)	Antigen presentation to sensitized CD4+ type 2 T lymphocytes. *Sensitized CD8+ type 2 T lymphocytes (also called T cytotoxic (Tc) type 2 cells) may also participate*	Cytotoxic CD8+ T lymphocytes recognise fragments of antigen on the surface of target cells
Soluble	Soluble	Soluble	Cell-associated
Microvasculature; Antigen-antibody complexes + complement; Neutrophil-rich inflammatory response	T Lymphocyte; CD4+ type 1; TCR; AF; MHC Class II; APC; Type 1 cytokines; Macrophage-rich inflammatory response	T Lymphocyte; CD4+ type 2; MHC Class II; APC; Type 2 cytokines; Eosinophil- (and possibly basophil-) rich inflammatory response	T Lymphocyte; CD8+ cytotoxic; MHC Class I; Target cell; Cytotoxicity (apoptosis)
• Serum sickness • Extrinsic allergic alveolitis • Antigen-antibody complex ('immune complex') glomerulonephritis	• Tuberculin reaction • Contact dermatitis • Rheumatoid arthritis	• Chronic asthma • Chronic allergic rhinitis • Atopic eczema • Late-phase allergic reactions (in experimental models of atopic allergic disease)	• Early-onset, insulin-dependent diabetes • Graft rejection

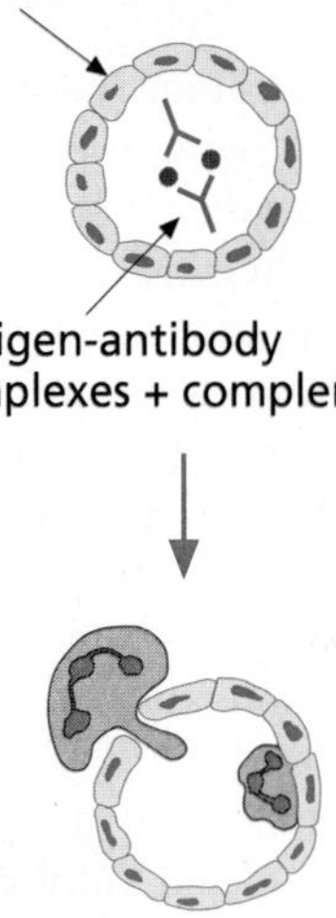

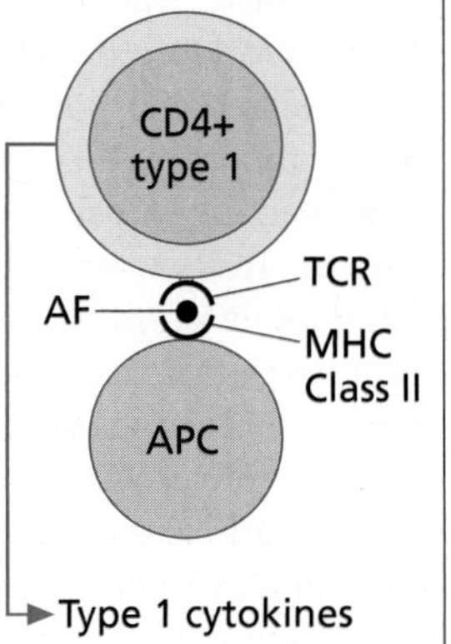

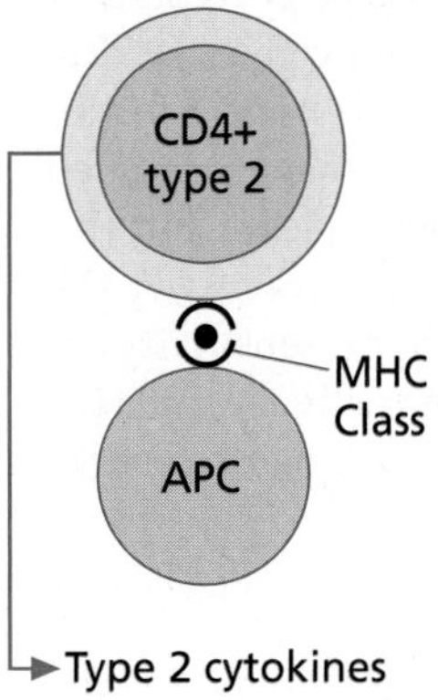

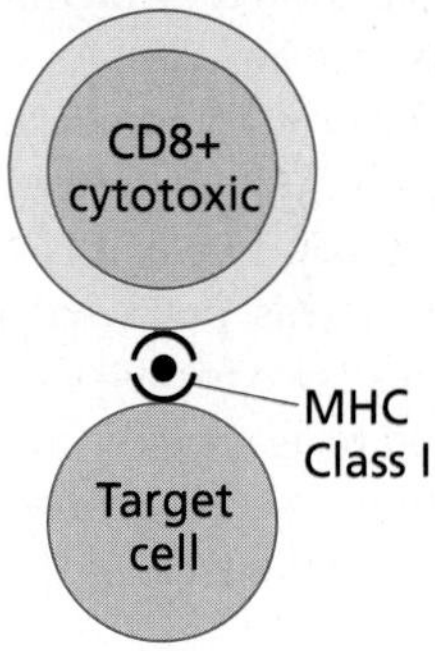

antibodies directed against cell-surface receptors cause altered cell function or signalling. In type IIb, antibody is cell-stimulating (cyto-stimulatory) and acts as either an agonist or antagonist. The type III Arthus-type, or Ag/Ab-complex reaction (mostly called immune-complex reaction) is mediated by soluble antigen and involves IgG, complement and an inflammatory reaction which initially is neutrophil-rich. Type IV reactions are subdivided into (i) classical delayed-type hypersensitivity initiated by CD4+ Th1-type lymphocytes (type IVa_1), (ii) cell-mediated eosinophilic hypersensitivity *or* chronic allergic reactions involving CD4+ (and sometimes CD8+) Th2-type cells (type IVa_2). Basophils may also be involved in type IVa_2 reactions, and (iii) reactions in which tissue damage is evoked by CD8+ cytotoxic T lymphocytes (type IVb). (From Janeway & Travers, 1995.)

profile. As described below, and in detail elsewhere, these cells preferentially produce interferon-γ (IFN-γ) and interleukin-2 (IL-2), as opposed to IL-4 and IL-5, and are therefore characteristic of the T helper (Th) type 1 lymphocyte* (Cher & Mosmann, 1987; Tsicopoulos *et al.*, 1992). Contact dermatitis, an important allergic disease, is another example of a type IV reaction with a prominent Th1-type cytokine response (Kapsenberg *et al.*, 1992). Some T lymphocyte-mediated hypersensitivity reactions, of which early onset (insulin-dependent) diabetes is an example, involves CD8+ cytotoxic T cells. These recognize cell-surface antigen presented to T cells in a MHC class I restricted fashion. After cell–cell contact, programmed cell death (apoptosis) of the target is initiated. Although, in the healthy body, cytotoxic T cells provide a basic 'immune' mechanism for dealing with viruses and other insoluble antigens, in the context of insulin-dependent diabetes and graft rejection they mediate a variant of type IV hypersensitivity (see Fig. 2.3). As stated, the effector cell in classical delayed-type hypersensitivity is the CD4+ type 1 (or Th type 1) lymphocyte whereas in tissue damage mediated by cytotoxic T cells it is the CD8+ T lymphocyte. For this reason it was proposed by Janeway and Travers (1995) that these two forms of cell-mediated hypersensitivity are referred to as type IVa and type IVb respectively, since the initiating event involves T lymphocytes with distinct characteristics (see Fig. 2.3).

Mechanisms in type I reactions

The basic mechanisms involved in immediate type I hypersensitivity are still the subject of intense investigation although, over the years, considerable advances have been made. Very shortly after the publication of the Coombs and Gell classification, passive tissue-sensitizing, or 'homocytotropic', antibody was identified as IgE (Ishizaka & Ishizaka, 1967, 1968). Coombs and Gell had speculated that 'non-atopic antibodies', i.e. the equivalent of the heat-stable antibodies found in lower animals, would also initiate type I reactions in humans. This possibility remains unresolved. Whereas IgG1 binds to macrophages (LoBuglio *et al.*, 1967) and basophils (Ishizaka *et al.*, 1979), the functional, and in turn the clinical, significance of these interactions is still uncertain.

The discovery and characterization of the high- (FcεRI) (Ishizaka *et al.*, 1970; Kulczycki & Metzger, 1974) and low- (FcεRII) (Lawrence *et al.*, 1975; Conrad & Peterson, 1984) affinity IgE receptors and their distribution on various cell types has added further to the complexity of the type I reaction. Cell surface high-affinity IgE receptors have been identified on mast cells (Ishizaka *et al.*, 1972), basophils (Kulczycki *et al.*, 1974) and Langerhans' cells (Wang *et al.*, 1992) and at a much lower density on eosinophils (Soussi Gounni *et al.*, 1994; Sihra *et al.*, 1996a) and monocytes (Maurer *et al.*, 1994; Sihra *et al.*, 1996a). Low-affinity FcεRII receptors (CD23) are found predominantly on cells of the monocyte/macrophage series (Melewicz *et al.*, 1982) as well as B cells (Yukawa *et al.*, 1987) and a subset of T cells (Suemura *et al.*, 1986). FcεRII appears to be functionally significant since cells of the monocyte/macrophage series can initiate CD23-dependent mediator release following interaction with IgE Ag/Ab complexes (Rouzer *et al.*, 1982; Borish *et al.*, 1991). High-affinity IgE receptors appear to be essential for the development of the anaphylactic reaction since, in mice, disruption of the α-chain of FcεRI abolishes this response (Dombrowicz *et al.*, 1993).

Early work on the pharmacological mediators released from isolated cells and tissues following type I reactions related almost exclusively to histamine (or serotonin) and 'slow-reacting substance of anaphylaxis' (SRS-A) (Kellaway & Trethewie, 1940). It was then established that histamine is prepackaged within mast cell and basophil granules in close association with the glycosaminoglycan core (see Chapter 9). Mast cell granules also contain neutral proteases, acid hydrolases and numerous cytokines. In addition, mast cells, basophils and eosinophils (Moqbel *et al.*, 1994) synthesize, store and release a wide array of cytokines.

In the 1970s, SRS-A was identified as a membrane-derived newly-generated mediator and fully characterized and synthesized as the sulphidopeptide leukotrienes LTC_4 and LTD_4 (Samuelsson, 1983). Other membrane-derived products released by IgE-dependent mechanisms by various cell types include LTB_4, cyclo-oxygenase products, and platelet-activating factor (PAF) (see Chapter 23).

For many years it was convenient to consider type I reactions as the principal mechanism in diseases such as hayfever and asthma. Although these conditions clearly have an immediate-type hypersensitivity component, asthmatics undergoing inhalational challenge with specific allergen (i.e. experimental, provoked asthma under controlled conditions in the clinical laboratory) frequently developed an additional delayed-in-time *late-phase response* (LPR) (Herxheimer, 1952). The LPR is used extensively as a model of chronic allergic inflammation, especially as mucosal inflammation is recognized as an integral feature of ongoing perennial atopic diseases such as asthma and allergic rhinitis. There has been considerable debate as to whether the LPR is the result of a prolonged effect of mast cell-derived mediators such as LTC_4/D_4 and PAF, or to Ag/Ab complexes interacting

* The reader approaching the subject for the first time could be understandably confused by, on the one hand, the terms 'type I and type II hypersensitivity reactions', and on the other 'T helper type 1 and type 2 lymphocytes'.

with complement, or a form of cell-mediated hypersensitivity. Biopsies of allergen-induced LPR elicited in the skin of atopic subjects revealed a strong inflammatory component with eosinophils and CD4+ T cells being prominent (Frew & Kay, 1988). Allergen-induced LPR in several organs and tissues, including the bronchi and nose as well as skin, all had the appearance of an 'eosinophilic cell-mediated hypersensitivity' response with a preponderance of cells which are messenger ribonucleic acid positive (mRNA+) for Th2-type cytokines (Kay *et al.*, 1991; Durham *et al.*, 1992; Robinson *et al.*, 1992). These features have also been observed in biopsies from ongoing chronic allergic asthma (Azzawi *et al.*, 1990; Bradley *et al.*, 1991; Hamid *et al.*, 1991; Ying *et al.*, 1993) as well as atopic dermatitis. For these reasons, it is proposed that classical delayed-type hypersensitivity, originally termed type IV hypersensitivity by Coombs and Gell (1963) and type IVa by Janeway and Travers (1995) should now be designated type IVa_1 and that chronic allergic inflammatory tissue reaction (or 'cell-mediated eosinophilic hypersensitivity') is referred to as type IVa_2. Thus the initiating cells in type IVa_1 and type IVa_2 are the CD4+ type 1 (or Th1 type) and CD4+ type 2 (or Th2 type) lymphocyte, respectively (Fig. 2.3). Present evidence suggests that the LPR may have both a type IVa_2 (Sihra, 1996b) *and* a type I hypersensitivity component since the reaction can be elicited *in vivo* by challenge with anti-IgE antibody (Solley *et al.*, 1976). This suggests that the allergen-induced LPR has both a mast cell- and a T-cell component.

The mechanisms by which eosinophils accumulate in allergic tissue reactions are discussed elsewhere (see Chapter 10) although these can be summarized briefly, as follows. Terminal differentiation of the eosinophil precursor and mobilization from the bone marrow (Collins *et al.*, 1995) is largely under the control of IL-5. IL-5, together with granulocyte macrophage colony-stimulating factor (GM-CSF) and IL-3, promote hyperadherence of eosinophils to vascular endothelium (Walsh *et al.*, 1990). The C-C chemokines, e.g. RANTES, MCP-3, MIP-1α and the newly discovered eotaxin (Jose *et al.*, 1990; Ponath *et al.*, 1996) promote selective directional migration of eosinophils across the vessel wall. IL-5, GM-CSF and IL-3 also contribute to local eosinophil accumulation by acting as survival factors (in which apoptosis is delayed (Stern *et al.*, 1992)). Eosinophils produce tissue damage, particularly at mucosal surfaces, through the release of basic proteins and lipid mediators (reviewed in Wardlaw *et al.*, 1995; Chapter 10).

Basophils are also prominent cells in various models of chronic allergic inflammation and there is evidence that, in humans, basophils and eosinophils are derived from the same precursor cell (Denburg *et al.*, 1985). Thus, basophils appear together with eosinophils in allergen-induced LPR in the nose (Bascom *et al.*, 1988) and skin (Charlesworth *et al.*, 1989). These observations are reminiscent of the phenomenon known as cutaneous basophil hypersensitivity (CBH), first described in the guinea pig (Dvorak *et al.*, 1970) and in which large numbers of basophils, together with eosinophils, were observed 6–24 hours after injection of soluble allergen into the skin of sensitized animals. The time-course of CBH (peaking at 12–24 hours) was more typical of an allergen-induced LPR (type IVa_2) than classical delayed-type hypersensitivity (type IVa_1) which is usually maximal at 48–72 hours. It is of considerable interest that, on one hand, the basophil contains histamine which, as in mast cells, is released by allergen cross-linking of IgE bound to FcεRI (as in a type I reaction). On the other hand it is recruited, along with eosinophils, in certain chronic allergic cell-mediated inflammatory reactions (type IVa_2).

The concept of acute and chronic allergic tissue reactions being a combination of type I and type IVa_2 reaction is diagrammatically illustrated in Fig. 2.4.

T-cell dichotomy and the allergic response

It is now widely believed that IgE synthesis, the accumulation of eosinophils and basophils and the increase in mast cell numbers associated with the inflammatory component of the allergic response, are all dependent on the production of cytokines from Th2-type cells. These comprise IL-4, IL-5, IL-10 and IL-13 in mice, and IL-4, IL-5 and IL-13 in humans (see Chapter 6). The concept of a subdivision of helper (CD4) T cells based on their cytokine profile was first proposed by Mosmann and Coffman (1987). Th2-type cells preferentially transcribe and translate RNA (mRNA) for IL-4 and IL-5 and predominate in inflammatory responses associated with atopic allergy and helminthic parasitic infections. IL-4 is an essential cofactor for the production of IgE by B cells, a property also shared by IL-13. IL-5, together with GM-CSF and IL-3, promote eosinophil maturation from CD34+ precursor cells, as well as eosinophil activation and survival (see Chapter 10). The counterpart of the Th2-type cell is the Th1-type cell. Through the elaboration of IFN-γ and IL-2 (but not IL-4 and IL-5), Th-type 1 cells regulate classical delayed-type (type IVa) hypersensitivity reactions and other effector functions usually associated with macrophage activation and T-cell-mediated immunity.

Although this dichotomy of T cells is firmly established in mice, there was initial scepticism about the existence of a human counterpart of type 1 and type 2 CD4+ cells. It was found, however, that allergen-specific T-cell clones derived from the peripheral blood of atopic donors secreted cytokines according to a Th2-type pattern, whereas bacterial antigen-specific clones secreted cytokines according to a Th1-type pattern (Parronchi *et al.*,

1991). Furthermore, as described above, skin biopsy (Kay *et al.*, 1991), nasal biopsy (Durham *et al.*, 1992), bronchoalveolar lavage (BAL) (Robinson *et al.*, 1992) and bronchial biopsy (Ying *et al.*, 1995) specimens obtained from atopic donors challenged with a specific allergen contained an inflammatory infiltrate rich in cells expressing mRNA encoding predominantly IL-4 and IL-5, rather than IL-2 and IFN-γ.

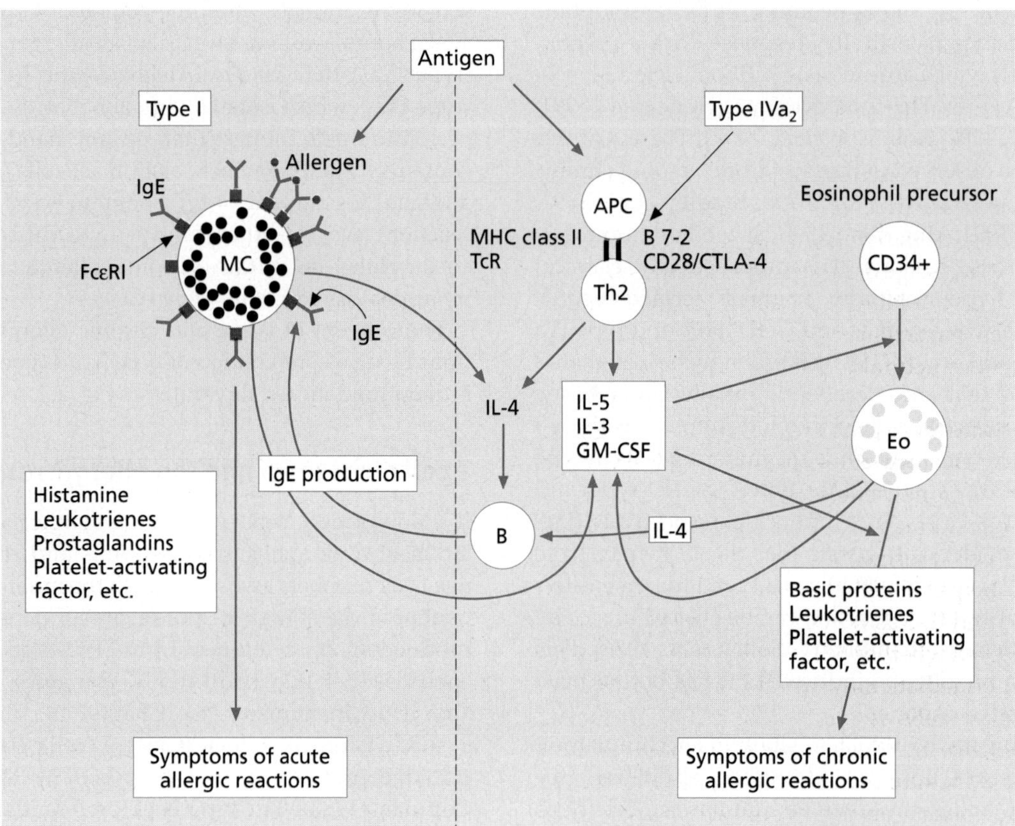

Fig. 2.4 Acute and chronic atopic allergic tissue reactions as a combination of type I and type IVa_2 hypersensitivity responses. The left-hand side represents the classic type I hypersensitivity reaction with mast cells (MC) sensitized with IgE via high-affinity IgE receptors (FcεRI). Antigen (Ag)—in this situation a soluble allergen—induces the non-cytotoxic energy-dependent release of preformed granule-associated mediators such as histamine, as well as membrane-derived lipid mediators, e.g. leukotrienes (LT), prostaglandins (PG) and platelet-activating factor (PAF). These reactions occur within minutes and are believed to produce the symptoms of the acute allergic response. Histamine is the principal mediator. Lipid mediators such as PG, LT and PAF have a more prolonged effect and may in part explain the oedematous component of the allergen-induced late-phase response (LPR). MC also synthesize, store and secrete cytokines such as IL-5, IL-3 and GM-CSF. In this way MCs may also contribute to chronic allergic reactions. The right hand side of the diagram represents a scheme for chronic allergic reactions (type IVa_2 reaction (see Fig. 2.3)). This mechanism may also be operative in the LPR but is more characteristic of the changes which occur after chronic antigen/allergen exposure (i.e., cell-mediated eosinophilic hypersensitivity) as occurs in diseases such as ongoing perennial allergic asthma and allergic rhinitis. Interleukin-4 (IL-4) is an essential co-factor for IgE synthesis by B cells and is derived from Th2-type T lymphocytes as well as MC, basophils (not shown) and eosinophils. The relative amounts of IL-4 produced by these various cell types is unknown. IL-4 contributes not only to IgE production but creates a microenvironment which favours the Th2 phenotype. Antigen (or allergen) is presented to Th2-type CD4+ helper lymphocytes by antigen-presenting cells (APC) i.e. the type IVa_2 reaction. Preference for B7-2 co-stimulatory molecules in reactions involving Th2-type cells has been suggested. The Th2-type cytokines include IL-4 and IL-5. IL-5, together with IL-3 and granulocyte macrophage colony-stimulating factor (GM-CSF), are referred to as eosinophil-survival or eosinophil-activating cytokines. Eosinophils themselves synthesize, store and secrete several cytokines including IL-5, IL-3 and GM-CSF. Eosinophil recruitment may result from local release of C-C chemokines such as eotaxin, RANTES and MCP-3 (not shown). IL-5, IL-3 and GM-CSF are involved in eosinophil maturation, mobilization (from the bone marrow), activation, recruitment and survival. Eosinophils are derived from CD34+ haematopoetic progenitor cells with the initial maturation/commitment being under the influence of IL-3 and GM-CSF. IL-5 promotes terminal differentiation of the committed eosinophil precursor. Activated eosinophils are believed to cause allergic tissue damage through the release of basic proteins from the crystalloid granule as well as membrane-derived lipids such as leukotrienes (particularly LTC_4) and PAF.

Conceptual difficulties regarding the control and differentiation of the Th1- and Th2-type T-cell subgroups remain (Kay, 1994). One problem is how Th cells differentiate between bacterial and allergen antigens, since there is no evidence that such antigens have specific structural features that Th cells might recognize. In some diseases, such as leprosy and human immunodeficiency virus (HIV) infection, Th1- or Th-2 type responses may predominate in different persons at different stages of the disease, although the Th cells presumably recognize the same array of foreign antigens. Since the antigen specificity of a Th cell is established apparently randomly in the thymus, it is difficult to conceptualize how Th cells recognizing a particular antigen could be preprogrammed at this stage of development to secrete a particular pattern of cytokines in a subsequent encounter with this antigen, particularly since this ability may result from permanent structural alterations in the genome of the Th cell.

To accommodate these problems, it has been suggested that, at any inflammatory site, Th1- and Th2-type helper T cells differentiate from a common antigen-specific post-thymic precursor termed 'Thp' that produces IL-2 (see Chapter 6). A cell intermediate between Thp and Th1- and Th2-type helper T cells that produces both sets of cytokines (IL-4 and IL-5 as well as IL-2 and IFN-γ) has also been described, but whether this cell type (termed 'Th0') is an essential intermediate in the development of Thp into Th1- or Th2-type cells is still unclear. Several factors appear to influence the development of Th1- and Th2-type cells. These include the nature and concentration of antigen, the type of antigen-presenting cell (APC), and the presence or absence of cytokines secreted by other cells in the microenvironment.

One view is that even a committed Th1 cell can convert to a Th2 cell and vice versa. Under such conditions the addition of IL-4 to Th1-type T cell clones proliferating in response to specific antigen alters the profile of secreted cytokines away from a Th1-type and towards a Th2-type profile. Furthermore, IL-4 promotes the differentiation of Th2 cells in the early stages of an antigen-specific response of Th cells and together with IL-10 inhibits the secretion of cytokines by Th1-type cells. Conversely, as described in Chapter 6, IFN-γ promotes the differentiation of Th1-type cells and inhibits the responses of Th2-type cells. IFN-γ production is regulated by IL-12 with the balance between IL-12 and IL-4 determining the Th-type 1 or 2 response.

The alternative view is that the pattern of cytokine secretion by two subtypes is immutable and already established in Th cells before clonal expansion. In this case, the changes brought about by treatments with such cytokines as IL-4, IFN-γ and IL-12 may reflect population shifts in mixtures of irreversibly committed Th cells, rather than changes in differentiation at the clonal level. In either case there is the question of whether these alterations are somehow imprinted on the genotype or phenotype of Th cells that proliferate at localized inflammatory sites so that they can be passed on to progeny memory Th cells and, if so, how could this be accomplished in molecular terms?

There is now increasing evidence for the existence of Th2-like CD8+ T lymphocytes in humans and mice (Mosmann & Sad, 1996). These have been referred to as Tc1 and Tc2 to denote T cytotoxic type 1 and T cytotoxic type 2 cells, respectively. Chronic asthma is associated with viral infections, a situation where Tc2 cells (i.e. CD8+ cells secreting the type 2 cytokines, IL-4 and IL-5) may be operative. In mice, lymphocytic choriomeningitis virus (LCMV)-specific CD8+ T cells secreting IL-5 have been shown to be associated with airway eosinophilia (Coyle *et al.*, 1995). The existence of Tc2-type cell in humans is supported by the work of Till *et al.* (1995) who described CD8+ IL-5-secreting T-cell lines from BAL cells from asthmatic subjects. Type 1 and type 2 T-helper and T-cytotoxic cells together with the hypersensitivity reactions in which they may feature are listed in Table 2.1.

With regard to the role of APC in this process, it has been shown that Th1 and Th2 pathways are differentially activated by two costimulatory molecules, B7-1 (CD80) and B7-2 (CD86), expressed on APC (Kuchroo *et al.*, 1995;

Table 2.1 Th-type 1 and 2 and T cytotoxic cells.

Cell type	Abbreviation	Hypersensitivity response in which they feature	Classification
T helper type 1 CD4+ lymphocyte	Th1-type	Classical delayed-type hypersensitivity	Type IVa_1
T helper type 2 CD4+ lymphocyte	Th2-type	Cell-mediated eosinophilic hypersensitivity (chronic allergic inflammation) in association with atopy	Type IVa_2
T cytotoxic type 1 CD8+ lymphocyte	Tc1-type	Tissue injury by cytotoxic T cells	Type IVb
T cytotoxic type 2 CD8+ lymphocyte	Tc2-type	Cell-mediated eosinophilic hypersensitivity (chronic allergic inflammation) in association with viral mucosal infection	Type IVa_2

Thompson, 1995). Anti-B7-1 reduced the incidence of experimental allergic encephalomyelitis (EAE) while anti-B7-2 increased disease severity. Thus, interaction of B7-1 and B7-2 with their shared counter-receptors, CD28 and CTLA-4, may result in very different outcomes in clinical disease by influencing commitment of precursors to a Th1 or Th2 lineage.

Atopy

The term 'atopy' was first used by Coca to describe a tendency to develop immediate-type hypersensitivity reactions to common allergens (Coca & Cooke, 1923). The word is derived from the Greek *atopia* (strangeness).* The predisposition to atopy was present in certain susceptible individuals but not in others and was partly hereditary. Atopy was known to be associated with large amounts of tissue-sensitizing antibody, now recognized as IgE, but originally referred to as atopic or 'reaginic' antibody.

There is a lack of general agreement as to the precise definition of atopy and how the atopic individual can be identified. Most UK physicians use the term to describe all individuals who develop a positive weal-and-flare reaction after skin-prick tests to extracts of common aeroallergens, irrespective of whether or not they have symptomatology. Others believe that atopic individuals should be defined as those who have clear manifestations of atopic disease (allergic rhinitis, asthma or atopic dermatitis). Some patients with these diseases may have negative skin-prick tests and serum concentrations of IgE antibody within the normal range (e.g. intrinsic asthma) while in others, the presence of specific IgE antibody may not relate clearly to the disease process (e.g. atopic dermatitis). In any event, all individuals presumably have the capacity to produce antigen-specific IgE following helminthic parasitic infections. Also, many patients with IgE-mediated anaphylactic reactions to bee and wasp venom are non-atopic, i.e. skin-test negative to extracts of common environmental allergens.

It is clear that the genetic basis of atopy is critical to a clear understanding of the expression of the IgE response. Population, family and twin studies support the view that the propensity of individuals to secrete elevated serum concentrations of IgE is genetically controlled, although the mode of inheritance remains unclear (see Chapter 74). Somewhat different results have been obtained using either nuclear family studies or extended family studies. It has been suggested that 'high serum IgE' is inherited as an autosomal recessive trait in nuclear family studies whereas there is evidence of genetic heterogeneity in extended family studies (see Chapter 74). The complexities of the subject are further compounded by the association between atopy and asthma. Many asthmatics, but not all, are atopic and asthma also runs in families. There is clearly a close association of asthma with atopic status as shown by the relationship between serum IgE and the incidence of asthma-like symptoms in population studies (Burrows *et al.*, 1989). Nevertheless, there is considerable controversy over the mode of inheritance of asthma, probably because multiple genes are involved and environmental factors also play an important role (see Chapters 74–77). Cookson *et al.* (1989) have suggested that atopy, as defined by elevated IgE synthesis, is inherited as an autosomal dominant trait and that an abnormal locus exists on the short arm of chromosome 11 close to the centromere (11q13). Sandford *et al.* (1993) have identified a locus on chromosome 11q within the encoding region of the β-chain of FcεRI and found that the linkage of atopy to this locus was stronger when the abnormal gene was inherited through the mother. The specific abnormality on the intramembrane portion of the β-chain of FcεRI was identified as two specific amino acid substitutions at positions 181 and 183 (isoleucine to leucine; valine to leucine, respectively). When inherited maternally, Leu-181/Leu-183 identified a genetic risk factor for atopy and bronchial hyperresponsiveness (Hill *et al.*, 1995). Marsh *et al.* (1994) have evidence of linkage of atopy to a locus on chromosome 5 close to the gene encoding IL-4, whereas Meyers *et al.* (1994) have shown linkage between markers close to both the IL-4 gene cluster and β_2-adrenoreceptors and indices of atopy (IgE) and asthma. Of particular interest is a study showing that a trait for elevated total serum IgE levels is co-inherited with a trait for bronchial hyperresponsiveness and that a gene governing bronchial hyperresponsiveness is located near a major locus that regulates serum IgE levels on chromosome 5q (Postma *et al.*, 1995).

There are also important associations between IgE responsiveness to specific allergens and the human leucocyte antigen (HLA) system. Thus, in addition to the regulatory loci, significant associations between HLA class II DR and DP phenotypes and allergic IgE and IgG responses to environmental allergens (including ragweed, pollen, ryegrass and house dust mite) have been identified (Young *et al.*, 1994). Furthermore, a linkage has been observed between specific sequences on the α-chain of the T-cell receptor encoded on chromosome 14 and the allergic phenotype which increases the complexity of the genetics of atopy and asthma (Moffat *et al.*, 1994).

*The term was coined in consultation with Edward Delevan Perry (1854–1938), Professor of Greek and Sanskrit at Columbia University (Cohen & Samter, 1992).

Summary and conclusions

The word allergy, if used correctly (as 'changed, or altered, reactivity'), encompasses the whole of the science of immunology. However, over the years, the term has become restricted perversely to a description of the IgE-mediated diseases, i.e. atopy, as well as certain non-IgE-mediated conditions such as farmer's lung, contact dermatitis and coeliac disease. The Coombs and Gell classification of the *hypersensitivity reactions* with updated modifications remains conceptually useful as it provides a fundamental basis for understanding the range of adverse reactions mediated by antibody or specifically sensitized T cells, including hypersensitivity reactions to autoantigens as well as those directed against bacterial and helminthic antigens.

There have been exciting advances in our understanding of molecular and cellular mechanisms of the hypersensitivity reactions. These include the structure of IgE and its receptors, the characterization of leukotrienes and other lipid mediators, and the concept of a subdivision of T lymphocytes into atopy-associated (Th-type 2 cells) and classical delayed-type hypersensitivity-associated (Th-type 1 cells), based on their cytokine profile. There has also been a growth of information on the genetics and mode of inheritance of allergic diseases.

References

Azzawi, M., Bradley, B., Jaffery, P.K. *et al.* (1990) Identification of activated T lymphocytes and eosinophils in bronchial biopsies in stable atopic asthma. *Am. Rev. Resp. Dis.*, **142**, 1407–13.

Bascom, R., Wachs, M., Naclerio, R.M. *et al.* (1988) Basophil influx occurs after nasal antigen challenge: effects of topical corticosteroid pre-treatment. *J. Allergy Clin. Immunol.*, **81**, 580–9.

Borish, L., Mascali, J.J. & Rosenwasser, L.J. (1991) IgE-dependent cytokine production by human peripheral blood mononuclear phagocytes. *J. Immunol.*, **146**, 63–7.

Bradley, B.L., Azzawi, M., Jacobson, M. *et al.* (1991) Eosinophils, T-lymphocytes, mast cells, neutrophils and macrophages in bronchial biopsies from atopic asthmatics: comparison with atopic non-asthma and normal controls and relationship to bronchial hyperresponsiveness. *J. Allergy Clin. Immunol.*, **88**, 661–74.

Burrows, B., Martinez, F.D., Halonen, M., Barbee, R.A. & Cline, M.G. (1989) Association of asthma with serum IgE levels and skin-test reactivity to allergens. *New Engl. J. Med.*, **320**, 271–7.

Charlesworth, E.N., Hood, A.F., Soter, N.A. *et al.* (1989) Cutaneous late-phase response to allergen. Mediator release and inflammatory cell infiltration. *J. Clin. Invest.*, **83**, 1519–26.

Cher, D.I. & Mosmann, T.R. (1987) Two types of murine helper T cell clones. II. Delayed-type hypersensitivity is mediated by Th1 clones. *J. Immunol.*, **138**, 3688–94.

Coca, A.F. & Cooke, R.A. (1923) On the classification of the phenomenon of hypersensitiveness. *J. Immunol.*, **8**, 163.

Cohen, S.G. & Samter, M. (eds) (1992) *Excerpts from Classics in Allergy*, 2nd edn. Symposia Foundation/Oceanside Publications, Providence, Rhode Island, p. 94.

Collins, P.D., Marleau, S., Griffith-Johnson, D.A., Jose, P.J. & Williams, T.J. (1995) Cooperation between interleukin-5 and the chemokine eotaxin to induce eosinophil accumulation *in vivo*. *J. Exp. Med.*, **182**, 1169–74.

Conrad, D.H. & Peterson, L.H. (1984) The murine lymphocyte receptor for IgE. I. Isolation and characterization of the murine B cell Fc epsilon receptor and comparison with Fc epsilon receptors from rat and human. *J. Immunol.*, **132**, 796–803.

Cookson, W.O.C.M., Sharp, P.A., Faux, P.A. & Hopkin, J.M. (1989) Linkage between immunoglobulin E responses underlying asthma and rhinitis and chromosome 11q. *Lancet*, **i**, 1292–5.

Coombs, R.R.A. & Gell, P.G.H. (1963) The classification of allergic reactions underlying disease. In: Gell P.G.H. & Coombs R.R.A. (eds) *Clinical Aspects of Immunology*. Blackwell Scientific Publications: Oxford, 317–37.

Coyle, A.J., Erard, F., Bertrand, C., Walti, S., Pircher, H. & Le Gros, G. (1995) Virus-specific CD8+ cells can switch to interleukin 5 production and induce airway eosinophilia. *J. Exp. Med.*, **181**, 1229–33.

Denburg, J.A., Telizyn, S., Messner, H. *et al.* (1985) Heterogeneity of human peripheral blood eosinophil-type colonies: evidence for a common basophil-eosinophil progenitor. *Blood*, **66**, 312–18.

Dombrowicz, D., Flamand, V., Brigman, K.K., Koller, B.V. & Kinet, J.-P. (1993) Abolition of anaphylaxis by targeted disruption of the high affinity immunoglobulin E receptor α chain gene. *Cell*, **75**, 969–76.

Durham, S.R., Ying, S., Varney, V.A. *et al.* (1992) Cytokine messenger RNA expression for IL-3, IL-4, IL-5 and GM-CSF in the nasal mucosa after local allergen provocation: relationship to tissue eosinophilia. *J. Immunol.*, **148**, 2390–4.

Dvorak, H.F., Dvorak, A.M., Simpson, B.A. *et al.* (1970) Cutaneous basophil hypersensitivity. II. A light and electron microscopic description. *J. Exp. Med.*, **132**, 558–82.

Fink, J.N., Moore, V.L. & Barboriak, J.J. (1975) Cell-mediated hypersensitivity in pigeon breeders. *Int. Arch. Allergy Appl. Immunol.*, **49**, 831–6.

Frew, A.J. & Kay, A.B. (1988) The relationship between infiltrating CD4+ lymphocytes, activated eosinophils and the magnitude of the allergen-induced late phase cutaneous reaction in man. *J. Immunol.*, **141**, 4159–64.

Gell, P.G.H., Coombs, R.R.A. & Lachman, M. (eds) (1975) *Clinical Aspects of Immunology*, 3rd edn. Blackwell Scientific Publications, Oxford.

Hamid, Q., Azzawi, M., Ying, S. *et al.* (1991) Expression of mRNA for interleukin-5 in mucosal bronchial biopsies from asthma. *J. Clin. Invest.*, **87**, 1541–6.

Herxheimer, H. (1952) The late bronchial reaction in induced asthma. *Int. Arch. Allergy Appl. Immunol.*, **3**, 323–8.

Hide, M., Francis, D.M., Grattan, C.E.H., Hakimi, J., Kochan, J.P. & Greaves, M.W. (1993) Autoantibodies against the high-affinity IgE receptor as a cause of histamine release in chronic urticaria. *New Engl. J. Med.*, **328**, 1599–1604.

Hill, M.R., James, A.L., Faux, J.A. *et al.* (1995). FcεRI-β polymorphism and risk of atopy in a general population sample. *Brit. Med. J.*, **311**, 776–9.

Ishizaka, K. & Ishizaka, T. (1967) Identification of gamma-E antibodies as a carrier of reaginic activity. *J. Immunol.*, **99**, 1187–98.

Ishizaka, K. & Ishizaka, T. (1968) Human reaginic antibodies and immunoglobulin E. *J. Allergy*, **42**, 330–63.

Ishizaka, T., Ishizaka, K. & Tomioka, H. (1972) Release of histamine and slow reacting substance of anaphylaxis (SRS-A) by IgE–anti-IgE reactions on monkey mast cells. *J. Immunol.*, **108**, 513–20.

Ishizaka, T., Sterk, A.R. & Ishizaka, K. (1979) Demonstration of Fc-γ receptors on human basophil granulocytes. *J. Immunol.*, **123**, 578–83.

Ishizaka, T., Tomioka, H. & Ishizaka, K. (1970) Mechanisms of passive sensitization. I. Presence of IgE and IgG molecules on human leukocytes. *J. Immunol.*, **105**, 1459–67.

Janeway, C. & Travers, P. (1995) *Immunobiology*, 2nd edn. Garland Press, London, Chapter 11.

Jose, P.J., Griffiths-Johnson, D.A., Collins, P.D. *et al.* (1994) Eotaxin: a potent eosinophil chemoattractant-cytokine detected in a guinea pig model of allergic airways inflammation. *J. Exp. Med.*, **179**, 881–2.

Kapsenberg, M.L., Wierenga, E.A., Stiekema, F.E.M., Tiggelman, A.M.B.C. & Bos, J.D. (1992) TH1 lymphokine production profiles of nickel-specific CD4+ T lymphocyte clones from nickel contact allergic and non-allergic individuals. *J. Invest. Dermatol.*, **98**, 59–63.

Kay, A.B. (1994) Editorial. Origin of type 2 helper T cells. *New Engl. J. Med.*, **330**, 567–9.

Kay, A.B., Ying, S., Varney, V. *et al.* (1991) Messenger RNA expression of the cytokine gene cluster, IL-3, IL-4, IL-5 and GM-CSF in allergen-induced late-phase cutaneous reactions in atopic subjects. *J. Exp. Med.*, **173**, 775–8.

Kellaway, C. & Trethewie, E. (1940) The liberation of slow reacting smooth muscle stimulating substance in anaphylaxis. *Q. J. Med.*, **30**, 121–45.

Kuchroo, V.K., Das, M.P., Brown, J.A. *et al.* (1995) B7-1 and B7-2 costimulatory molecules activate differentially the Th1/Th2 developmental pathways: application to autoimmune disease therapy. *Cell*, **80**, 707–18.

Kulcyzcki, A. Jr., Isersky, C. & Metzger, H. (1974) The interaction of IgE with rat basophilic leukemia cells. I. Evidence for specific binding of IgE. *J. Exp. Med.*, **139**, 600–16.

Kulcyzcki, A. Jr. & Metzger, H. (1974) The interaction of IgE with rat basophilic leukemia cells. II. Quantitative aspects of the binding reaction. *J. Exp. Med.*, **140**, 1676–95.

Lawrence, D.A., Weigle, W.O. & Spiegelberg, H.L. (1975) Immunoglobulins cytophilic for human lymphocytes, monocytes, and neutrophils. *J. Clin. Invest.*, **55**, 368–87.

LoBuglio, A.F., Cotran, R.S. & Jandl, J.H. (1967) Red cells coated with immunoglobulin G: binding sphering by mononuclear cells in man. *Science*, **158**, 1582–5.

Maurer, D., Fiebiger, E., Reininger, B. *et al.* (1994) Expression of functional high affinity immunoglobulin E receptors (FcεRI) on monocytes of atopic individuals. *J. Exp. Med.*, **179**, 745–50.

Melewicz, F.M., Kline, L.E., Cohen, A.B. & Spiegelberg, H.L. (1982) Characterization of Fc receptors for IgE on human alveolar macrophages. *Clin. Exp. Immunol.*, **49**, 364–70.

Meyers, D.A., Postma, D.S., Panhuysen, C.I.M. *et al.* (1994) Evidence for a locus regulating total serum IgE levels mapping to chromosome 5. *Genomics*, **23**, 464–70.

Moffatt, M.F., Hill, M.R., Cornelis, F. *et al.* (1994) Genetic linkage of T-cell receptor α/δ complex to specific IgE responses. *Lancet*, **343**, 1597–600.

Moqbel, R., Levi-Schaffer, F. & Kay, A.B. (1994) Cytokine generation by eosinophils. *J. Allergy Clin. Immunol.*, **94** (Suppl.), 1183–8.

Mosmann, T.R. & Coffman, R.L. (1987) Two types of mouse helper T cell clone: implications for immune regulation. *Immunol. Today*, **8**, 223–7.

Mosmann, T.R. & Sad, S. (1966) The expanding universe of T-cell subsets: Th1, Th2 and more. *Immunol. Today*, **17**, 138–46.

Parish, W.E., Barrett, A.M., Coombs, R.R.A., Gunther, M. & Camps, F.E. (1960) Hypersensitivity to milk and sudden death in infancy. *Lancet*, **ii**, 1106–10.

Parronchi, P., Macchia, D., Piccinni, M.P. *et al.* (1991) Allergen- and bacterial antigen-specific T lymphocyte clones established from atopic donors show a different profile of cytokine production. *Proc. Nat. Acad. Sci. USA*, **88**, 4538–42.

Pepys, J. (1969) Hypersensitivity disease of the lungs due to fungi and other organic dusts. *Monogr. Allergy*, **4**, 44.

Pepys, J., Jenkins, P.A., Festenstein, G.N., Gregory, P.H., Lacey M. & Skinner, F.A. (1963) Farmer's lung: thermophilic actinomycetes as a source of farmer's lung hay antigen. *Lancet*, **2**, 607–11.

von Pirquet, C. (1906). Allergie. *Münch. med. Wochenschr.*, **30**, 1457. (Translated from the German by Prausnitz, C. In: Gell, P.G.H. & Coombs, R.R.A. (eds) (1963) *Clinical Aspects of Immunology*. Blackwell Scientific Publications, Oxford.)

Ponath, P.D., Qiu, S., Ringler, D.J. *et al.* (1996) Cloning of the human eosinophil chemoattractant, eotaxin. Expression, receptor binding and functional properties provide a mechanism for the selective recruitment of eosinophils. *J. Clin. Invest.*, **97**, 604–12.

Postma, D.S., Bleecker, E.R., Amelung, P.J. *et al.* (1995) Genetic susceptibility to asthma — bronchial hyperresponsiveness co-inherited with a major gene for atopy. *New Engl. J. Med.*, **333**, 894–900.

Robinson, D.S., Hamid, Q., Ying, S. *et al.* (1992). Predominant TH2-like bronchoalveolar T-lymphocyte population in atopic asthma. *New Engl. J. Med.*, **326**, 298–304.

Rouzer, C.A., Scott, W.A., Hamill, A.L., Liu, F.-D., Katz, D.H. & Cohn, Z.A. (1982) Secretion of leukotriene C and other arachidonic metabolites by macrophages challenged with immunoglobulin E immune complexes. *J. Exp. Med.*, **156**, 1077.

Samuelsson, B. (1983) Leukotrienes: mediators of hypersensitivity reactions and inflammation. *Science*, **220**, 568–75.

Sandford, A.J., Shirakawa, T., Moffatt, M.F. *et al.* (1993) Localisation of atopy and the β subunit of the high affinity IgE receptor (FcεRI) on chromosome 11q. *Lancet*, **341**, 332–4.

Sihra, B.S., Durham, S.R., Walker, S., Kon, O.M., Barnes, N.C. & Kay, A.B. (1996a) Inihibition of the allergen-induced late asthmatic responses by cyclosporin A. Submitted.

Sihra, B.S., Kon, O.M., Grant, J.A. & Kay, A.B. (1996b) Expression of the high affinity IgE receptor (FcεRI) on peripheral blood basophils, monocytes and eosinophils in atopic and non-atopic subjects: relationship to total serum immunoglobulin (IgE) concentrations. *J. Allergy Clin. Immunol.* (in press).

Solley, G.O., Gleich, G.J., Jordan, R.E. & Schroeter, A.L. (1976) Late phase of the immediate wheal and flare skin reactions: its dependence on IgE antibodies. *J. Clin. Invest.*, **58**, 408–20.

Soussi Gounni, A.S., Lamkhioued, B., Ochiai, K. *et al.* (1994) High-affinity IgE receptor on eosinophils is involved in defence against parasites. *Nature*, **367**, 183–6 (erratum *Nature*, **368**, 473).

Stern, M., Meagher, L., Savill, J. & Haslett, C. (1992) Apoptosis in human eosinophils: programmed cell death in the eosinophil leads to phagocytosis by macrophages and is modulated by IL-5. *J. Immunol.*, **148**, 3543–9.

Suemura, M., Kikutani, H., Barsumian, E.L. *et al.* (1986) Monoclonal anti-Fcε receptor antibodies with different specificities and studies on the expression of Fcε receptors on human B and T cells. *J. Immunol.*, **137**, 1214–20.

Thompson, C.B. (1995) Distinct roles for the costimulatory ligands B7-1 and B7-2 in T helper cell differentiation? *Cell*, **81**, 979–82.

Till, S.J., Li, B., Durham, S. *et al.* (1995) Secretion of the eosinophil-active cytokines interleukin-5, granulocyte/macrophage colony-stimulating factor and interleukin-3 by bronchoalveolar lavage CD4+ and CD8+ T cell lines in atopic asthmatics, and atopic and non-atopic controls. *Eur. J. Immunol.*, **25**, 2727–31.

Tsicopoulos, A., Hamid, Q., Varney, V. *et al.* (1992) Preferential mRNA expression of Th1-type cells (IFNγ^+, IL-2$^+$), in classical delayed-type (tuberculin) hypersensitivity reactions in human skin. *J. Immunol.*, **148**, 2058–61.

Walsh, G.M., Hartnell, A., Wardlaw, A.J., Kurihara, K., Sanderson, C.J. & Kay, A.B. (1990) IL-5 enhances the *in vitro* adhesion of human eosinophils, but not neutrophils, in a leucocyte integrin (CD 11/18)-dependent manner. *Immunology*, **71**, 258–65.

Wang, B., Rieger, A., Kilgus, O. *et al.* (1992) Epidermal Langerhans cells from normal human skin bind monomeric IgE via FcεRI. *J. Exp. Med.*, **175**, 1353–65.

Wardlaw, A.J., Moqbel, R. & Kay, A.B. (1995) Eosinophils: biology and role in disease. *Adv. Immunol.*, **60**, 151–266.

Ying, S., Durham, S.R., Corrigan, C.J., Hamid, O. & Kay, A.B. (1995) Phenotype of cells expressing mRNA for TH2-type (interleukin-4 and interleukin-5) and TH1-type (interleukin-2 and interferon-gamma) cytokines in bronchoalveolar lavage and bronchial biopsies from atopic asthmatics and normal control subjects. *Am. J. Resp. Cell. Mol. Biol.*, **12**, 477–87.

Young, R.P., Dekker, J.W., Wordsworth, B.P. *et al.* (1994) HLA-DR and HLA-DP genotypes and immunoglobulin E responses to common major allergens. *Clin. Exp. Allergy*, **24**, 431–9.

Yukawa, K., Kikutani, H., Owaki, H. *et al.* (1987) A B cell-specific differentiation antigen, CD23, is a receptor for IgE (FcεR) on lymphocytes. *J. Immunol.*, **138**, 2576–80.

CHAPTER 3

T and B Lymphocytes and the Development of Allergic Reactions

C.J. Corrigan

Introduction

T lymphocytes play a fundamental role in the initiation and regulation of inflammatory responses. Through their specific antigen receptors, they are capable of recognizing invading foreign antigens and initiating appropriate immune responses, which may be characterized predominantly by 'cell-mediated' reactions, in which effector immune cells play a major role, or 'humoral' reactions, in which antibody responses are more prominent. Although immature B lymphocytes express surface IgM with low binding affinity for foreign antigens, these cells are largely dependent on T lymphocytes for their subsequent activation and proliferation, and for antibody affinity maturation. There is now abundant evidence that T lymphocytes orchestrate both the initiation and the propagation of allergic reactions largely through the secretion of cytokines, and that the particular combination of cytokines secreted during the course of these inflammatory responses is responsible for the type of hypersensitivity reaction which ensues, including whether the reaction is predominantly cellular or humoral in nature. It is the purpose of this chapter to describe the fundamental properties of T lymphocytes and the factors which govern their secretion of cytokines in various inflammatory conditions, particularly in allergic inflammation and asthma, and how these cytokines influence immunoglobulin (Ig) synthesis, particularly that of IgE, by B lymphocytes. Finally, it will be shown how the secretion of various patterns of cytokines can influence the course and nature of the ensuing inflammatory response.

The atopic diathesis, allergic diseases and asthma

It is now widely accepted that chronic inflammation of the relevant mucosal surface plays a fundamental role in the genesis of the clinical features of asthma and atopic diseases such as allergic rhinitis. The most striking feature of this inflammation is the intense infiltration of the mucosa with eosinophils and lymphocytes (Houston *et al.*, 1953; Dunnill, 1960; Dunnill *et al.*, 1969). In fact, these diseases have many of the histopathological features of a chronic, cell-mediated hypersensitivity reaction. Later in this chapter, it will be seen how cytokine and chemokine products of activated T lymphocytes have the propensity to bring about selective eosinophil accumulation and activation at mucosal surfaces. The eosinophil appears to be a key cell in producing injury to mucosal surfaces, particularly the asthmatic bronchial mucosa (Filley *et al.*, 1982). This injury is in turn believed to result, ultimately, in the *chronic* clinical features of asthma and allergic diseases, although the precise mechanisms through which mucosal damage causes these clinical features remain unclear.

Atopy refers to the genetic predisposition of certain individuals to synthesize, inappropriately, IgE specific for protein components of inhaled aeroallergens such as grass pollen. Cells with high- and low-affinity IgE Fc receptors bind to allergen-specific IgE, thus sensitizing them. Further allergen exposure then brings about the release of inflammatory agents from these sensitized cells. One principal feature of this process is its *immediacy*, which has resulted in the term 'immediate hypersensitivity'. IgE-mediated mechanisms are assumed to play a fundamental role in the pathogenesis of allergic diseases such as rhinitis, since many of the symptoms of these diseases occur immediately in relation to aeroallergen exposure, and they can be alleviated, at least partly, by mediator antagonists such as antihistamines. Furthermore, with very few exceptions, these diseases are seen only in sensitized, atopic individuals, although not all atopic subjects develop them.

Asthma is often, although not invariably, associated with atopy. Some atopic asthmatics sensitized to environmental aeroallergens experience an exacerbation of their disease on exposure to these allergens. Such patients have traditionally been referred to as 'extrinsic' asthmatics, reflecting the clear relationship of their disease to external environmental factors (although unlike rhinitics these patients do not respond to antihistamines). Non-atopic asthmatics, who are not apparently sensitized to a wide range of environmental allergens (although it is impossible to make this list exhaustive), and in whom IgE-mediated mechanisms do not obviously operate, have been labelled 'intrinsic'. Following Rackemann's initial description of intrinsic asthma (Rackemann, 1940, 1947), it is now generally accepted that this term is used to describe a group of asthmatics who are skin-prick-test negative in response to extracts of common aeroallergens, and have serum total IgE concentrations within the normal range. As a group, these patients tend to develop symptoms for the first time in adulthood (although some child asthmatics are non-atopic), and their disease is often relatively difficult to control. In addition, some patients develop asthma after exposure to specific proteins or small-molecular-weight chemicals at work; these 'occupational' asthmatics form a third clinical category. An IgE response specific for the sensitizing agent can sometimes, but not always, be demonstrated in these patients.

The relative roles of IgE-mediated mechanisms and chronic inflammation of mucosal surfaces brought about by interactions of activated T lymphocytes with eosinophils in asthma and allergic diseases therefore remain unclear. Perhaps 'rhinitis without asthma' and 'intrinsic asthma' represent the two ends of a continuous spectrum of the relative prominence of these processes. It will be argued later in this chapter that activated T lymphocytes may drive asthmatic inflammation independently of IgE-mediated mechanisms, although the nature of the antigen(s) involved in this activation process remains a subject for speculation. The concept that there are indeed fundamental pathogenetic differences between 'extrinsic' and 'intrinsic' asthma has also been challenged by epidemiological studies showing that, irrespective of atopic status as defined by skin-prick tests, the prevalence of self-reported asthma in individuals relates closely to their serum concentrations of IgE corrected for age and sex (Burrows *et al.*, 1989). This suggests that IgE-mediated mechanisms may play at least some role in the pathogenesis of asthma in all patients. Whatever the case, it is clear that IgE-mediated mechanisms are certainly not sufficient for the development of asthma and allergic diseases, since not all atopic subjects develop these diseases. It is possible to speculate that, as has been proposed for many other diseases, asthma and allergic disease develop following environmental influences on individuals with an inherited predisposition (see below).

In summary, while IgE-mediated mechanisms may clearly be important in allergen-induced short-term *exacerbations* of disease in atopic individuals, their role in the *pathogenesis* of chronic disease, particularly asthma, is less certain. Despite these observations, many studies on the 'pathogenesis' of asthma and allergic disease address changes in cell numbers and activation after experimental allergen challenge of atopic patients with rhinitis and asthma.

T-lymphocyte antigen recognition

T lymphocytes recognize antigens through specific cell-surface receptors composed of a pair of polypeptide chains (either α/β or γ/δ). Unlike antibodies, which recognize the *shape* of antigens, T-cell receptors specifically recognize the *sequence* of small peptide fragments ('epitopes') derived from the intact antigen. These fragments are presented to T lymphocytes after partial hydrolysis, or 'denaturation' of the antigen by antigen-presenting cells (APC). Antigenic epitopes cannot be recognized in isolation, but must be 'presented' to T lymphocytes bound to major histocompatibility complex (MHC) molecules on the surface of APC (MHC class I molecules in the case of CD8 T-lymphocytes and class II molecules in the case of CD4 cells). As with immunoglubulins, the presence of multiple germ-line gene segments encoding 'hypervariable' regions in those parts of the T-lymphocyte receptor proteins which contact both the epitope and its associated MHC molecules accounts for variable specificity of epitope binding. Again analagously with immunoglobulins, the T-lymphocyte receptor gene rearrangements which take place during maturation of individual T lymphocytes from their precursors is fixed during ontogeny, so that each mature T cell can recognize only a limited range of epitopes. The potential variability of these gene rearrangements is more than enough, however, to ensure that T cells recognizing any particular epitope will be generated during maturation of T cells in the thymus.

Epitopes derived from both 'self' and 'non-self' proteins can associate with MHC molecules. Indeed, self peptides are processed as efficiently as those derived from foreign proteins (Adorini *et al.*, 1988), and so mechanisms must exist whereby the potential ability of T lymphocytes to recognize and respond to self epitopes is eliminated. Experimental data from several systems (McDuffie *et al.*,

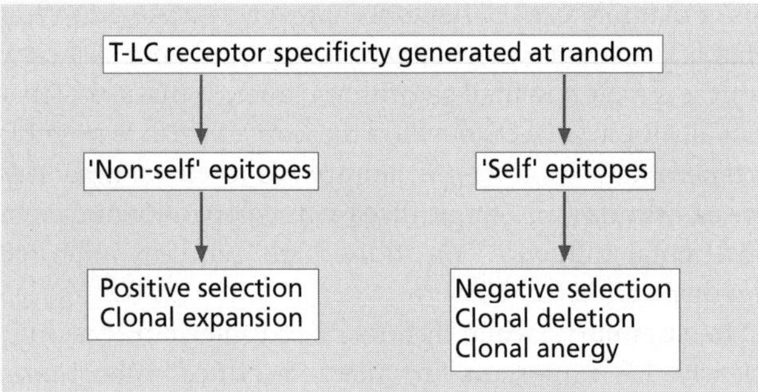

Fig. 3.1 Clonal selection in the thymus. T-lymphocyte (T-LC) epitope specificity is generated at random during thymic development. 'Non-self' reactive cells are positively selected for expansion in the periphery. 'Self' reactive cells are negatively selected by deletion (death) or induction of anergy.

1987; Kappler *et al.*, 1988; Kisielow *et al.*, 1988; MacDonald *et al.*, 1988) provide strong evidence that the majority of self-reactive T lymphocytes are removed either by clonal deletion or the induction of clonal 'anergy', during their development in the thymus. The majority of cells leaving the thymus possess receptors which are capable of recognizing non-self or 'foreign' antigenic peptides in association with self-MHC molecules, but not self peptides associated with self-MHC molecules (Fig. 3.1). T cells expressing autoreactive antigen specificities either die in the thymus or are functionally inactivated, probably by encountering their specific epitopes under conditions incompatible with cell activation (McDuffie *et al.*, 1987; Kisielow *et al.*, 1988; MacDonald *et al.*, 1988; Blackman *et al.*, 1990).

What signals, other than presentation of specific antigenic peptides on appropriate MHC molecules, are then required for T-lymphocyte activation? One important signal is interleukin-1 (IL-1) secreted by the APC (Durum *et al.*, 1985). In addition, cell contact between the APC and the antigen-specific T lymphocyte is required (Fig. 3.2). This conclusion is supported by the observation that antigen-pulsed APC fixed with agents such as ethyl carbo-diimide (ECDI) fail to stimulate antigen-specific T lymphocytes and, furthermore, induce a state of non-responsiveness (Mueller *et al.*, 1989). If the APC are activated prior to fixation, tolerance is not induced, suggesting that one or more cell-surface molecules, whose expression is increased during activation, are responsible for this 'second signal'. The ability of allogeneic, unfixed APC to rescue T-lymphocyte activation in mixing experiments with fixed, syngeneic antigen-pulsed APC supports this conclusion.

There is now considerable evidence implicating the homologous glycoproteins CD28 and CTLA-4, expressed on the surface of T lymphocytes, as costimulator molecules responsible for this requirement for contact with APC during T-lymphocyte activation (Fig. 3.2). Cellular signals induced by engagement of these molecules synergize with signals arising from the engaged T-lymphocyte antigen receptor to induce T-lymphocyte proliferation (Harding *et al.*, 1992). Both CD28 and CTLA-4 interact with the same ligands on APC, namely CD80 (also known as B7) and the more recently described B70 (or B7-2) (Linsley *et al.*, 1991; Lanier *et al.*, 1995). These molecules are highly homologous and are expressed on most activated APC including B lymphocytes and also, interestingly, on activated T cells and natural killer (NK) cells. Currently available evidence suggests that successful T-lymphocyte activation requires up-regulation of both CD28/CTLA-4 and CD80/B70.

Evidence that CD28 is a costimulatory molecule for T lymphocytes has been provided by the finding that non-stimulatory anti-CD28 antibody Fab fragments completely inhibit the provision of costimulation to T lymphocytes by activated B lymphocytes (Harding *et al.*, 1992). CD28 cross-linking in the presence of phorbol ester results in IL-2 production by T lymphocytes which is resistant to inhibition by cyclosporin A (June *et al.*, 1990), suggesting that CD28 signals by a biochemical pathway distinct from that used by the T-lymphocyte antigen receptor.

The CD28 ligand CD80 (B7) is a heavily glycosylated

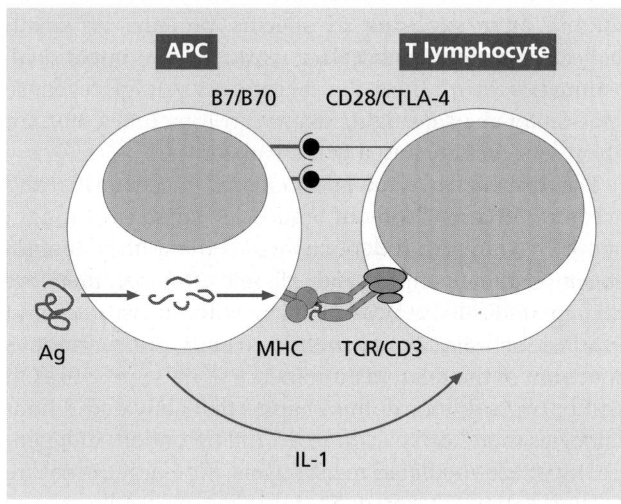

Fig. 3.2 Role of accessory molecules in T-lymphocyte activation/anergy. Antigen (Ag) processed by antigen-presenting cells (APC) is presented as small peptides to T cells on major histocompatibility complex (MHC) molecules. Additional cytokine signals such as interleukin-1 (IL-1) are important for T-cell activation. In addition, engagement of the T-cell ligands CD28/CTLA-4 and their counter-receptors B7/B70 on APC are also essential. If these signals are not provided then the T cell is rendered non-responsive or 'anergic' to the particular epitope. This may represent at least one mechanism for physiological anergy.

membrane glycoprotein. As might be expected for a co-stimulatory ligand, CD80 is constitutively expressed on dendritic cells, is induced on activated B lymphocytes and monocytes, and is not expressed on resting T lymphocytes. Expression of CD80 on B lymphocytes is induced by cross-linking of their surface immunoglobulin or MHC class II molecules (Nabavi *et al.*, 1992; Schwartz, 1992), as may occur during presentation of antigen to T lymphocytes. Anti-CD80 antibodies or a fusion protein composed of the extracellular domain of CTLA-4 fused to the human IgG_1 Fc region (CTLA-4-Ig) blocked the proliferation of T lymphocytes in response to antigen presented by a variety of CD80 expressing accessory cells (Jenkins *et al.*, 1991).

T lymphocytes, B lymphocytes and IgE synthesis

Primary antibody responses are mounted by antibodies of the IgM class. Since these antibodies generally express germ-line-determined variable region genes that have not yet been modified by somatic mutation, they bind antigen only with low affinity. This is partially compensated for by their 10 antigen-binding sites, which enables avid binding to multimeric antigens. IgM antibodies can destroy or opsonize target cells through their very efficient fixation of complement. Nevertheless, the low affinity of IgM antibody, its pentameric structure which limits its diffusion capacity and its short half-life *in vivo* suggest that IgM antibodies are probably less well adapted than IgG antibodies to protect the host against repeated infections by pathogens.

Antibodies of the IgG, IgA and IgE classes are made later than IgM during a primary immune response, but account for most of the antibody that is made during a memory response. Although isotype switching and affinity maturation are independent processes, they usually occur simultaneously (Fish *et al.*, 1989), so that the increased affinity of bivalent antibodies of isotypes other than IgM is rapidly enhanced. IgG antibody is the predominant isotype in plasma and lymph, while IgA antibody predominates at mucosal surfaces and in secretions from these surfaces.

The regulation of IgE synthesis in humans is covered in some detail in Chapter 6. It is relevant here, however, to briefly emphasize the important role which T-lymphocyte-derived cytokines play in this process.

The antigen-binding specificity of an immunoglobulin molecule is determined by the amino termini of its heavy and light chains, which are highly variable in structure. By contrast, the carboxy terminus of the heavy chain has a constant sequence which determines the effector functions of the immunoglobulin molecule, such as binding to particular Fc receptors. The variable region of immunoglobubin is encoded by multiple germ-line elements which are assembled into complete V(D)J variable regions during B-lymphocyte differentiation by a common enzymatic activity termed recombinase. These variable region genes are then juxtaposed to germ-line constant region (C_H) region genes which determine the isotype, and thus the functional porperties of, the immunoglobulin. During an immune response, a B- lymphocyte can express different heavy-chain isotypes sharing the same V(D)J region. This phenomenon, known as class switching, allows a single B-lymphocyte clone to secrete antibodies of the same antigen specificity in association with different C_H region genes. Intervening sequences, including previously expressed C_H region genes, are deleted. Class switching involves characteristic repetitive sequences (S regions), composed of short tandem repeats, located upstream of the Cμ gene, and corresponding regions located immediately upstream of each C_H gene except for Cδ. In B lymphocytes predisposed to undergo class switching to a particular isotype such as ε, the C_H locus to which switching is directed is transcribed before switching into a 'germ-line' transcript (Fig. 3.3). These transcripts initiate approximately 2 kb upstream of the S region involved in switch recombination and are processed to an mRNA in which an exon (designated I exon) located 100–500 bp upstream of the relevant C_H exon, and the C_H exon itself, are spliced directly together. The resulting 'germ-line' transcripts do not appear to be capable of encoding for protein products, since the I exon contains stop codons in all three reading frames. The I exon is 200–300 bp shorter than the V(D)J region present in

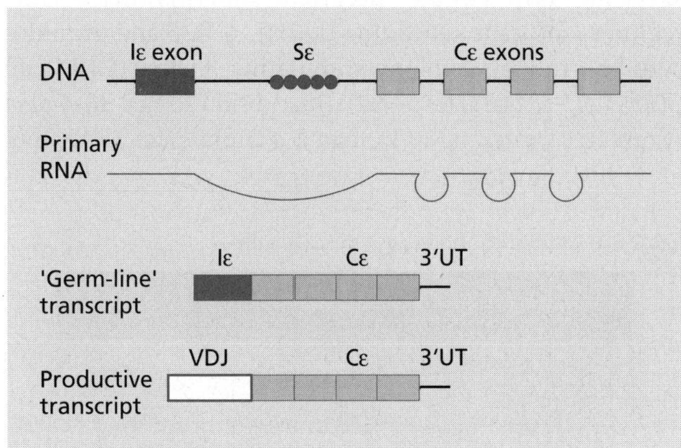

Fig. 3.3 Switching to IgE synthesis in B lymphocytes. During switching, Cε exons encoding the constant region of the IgE heavy chain are juxtaposed to the variable (V(D)J) region genes by looping out of intervening DNA sequences at the adjacent switch recombinase site (Sε). During the switching process, the Cε exons are brought near to the Iε exon, the transcription of which product results after RNA processing in a 'germ-line' transcript. Later, the Cε exons are juxtaposed to the V(D)J regions, the transcription of which product results in a productive IgE heavy chain transcript.

mature transcripts, so that germ-line transcripts are also correspondingly shorter (Fig. 3.3). The precise significance of germ-line transcripts remains to be defined, but they appear in the course of switching in B lymphocytes and are a useful marker of switching when studying the effects of cytokines on this process.

The role of cytokines in regulating IgE synthesis

Cytokines play an important role in the control of switching of antibody isotypes in humans away from IgM during the evolution of the immune response, and also in regulating the amounts of antibody which are secreted through their growth-regulating effects on B lymphocytes. In the case of IgE, cytokines which play a role in this process may be classified as follows (Table 3.1).

1 *Cytokines which specifically induce IgE switching in B lymphocytes.* These cytokines have in common the ability to induce the transcription of germ-line C_H transcripts, as described above. IL-4 induces switching to IgE synthesis in human B lymphocytes, which is preceded by the synthesis of germ-line Cε transcripts (Gauchat *et al.*, 1990). Until recently, it was thought that no other cytokine could substitute for IL-4 in this process; it is now clear, however, that IL-13 can also cause Cε germ-line transcript expression and IgE switching in human B lymphocytes (Punnonen *et al.*, 1993). Although IL-13 and IL-4 show limited (30%) structural homology, all the residues contributing to the hydrophobic central core of IL-4 are conserved or have conservative replacements in IL-13 (Zurawski *et al.*, 1993). There is some evidence that IL-13 competes with IL-4 for binding to its receptor (Zurawski *et al.*, 1993). The gene encoding IL-13 is located in chromosome 5q31 in the same region as the genes encoding IL-3, IL-4, IL-5 and granulocyte macrophage colony-stimulating factor (GM-CSF) (Zurawski & De Vries, 1994). In addition to IgE, IL-4 also stimulates switching of human B lymphocytes to synthesis of IgG4, although IgG4 is detectable earlier, consistent with the interpretation that the switch from IgM to IgE typically involves an initial switch to an IgG4 and then a second switch to IgE (Gascan *et al.*, 1991).

2 *Cytokines which influence IgE production by B lymphocytes through effects other than the induction of switching.* Some of these cytokines are generally facilitatory or inhibitory to B-lymphocyte activation and clonal expansion. Thus, interferon-α (IFN-α), IFN-γ, TGF-β, IL-8 and IL-12 inhibit IL-4-induced IgE synthesis, whereas IL-2, IL-5, IL-6 and TNF-α enhance it (Pene *et al.*, 1988a,b; Vercelli *et al.*, 1989; Miyajima *et al.*, 1991; Gauchat *et al.*, 1992; Kimata *et al.*, 1992; Kinawa *et al.*, 1992). Endogenous IL-6 is crucially involved in IL-4-dependent IgE induction *in vitro*, since anti-IL-6 antibodies strongly inhibit IgE synthesis (Vercelli *et al.*, 1989).

Table 3.1 Cytokines and IgE synthesis *in vitro*.

Cytokine group	Function
1 IL-4 IL-13	Induce IgE switching in human B cells
2 IFN-γ IFN-α TGF-β IL-8 IL-12	Inhibit IgE synthesis by switched B cells
3 IL-2 IL-5 IL-6 TNF-α	Enhance IgE synthesis by switched B cells

A second B-lymphocyte activating signal is required for IgE synthesis

The cytokines IL-4 and IL-13 are necessary, but not sufficient, for the induction of IgE synthesis by B lymphocytes. A variety of second IgE-inducing signals have been described which are necessary for IgE secretion and which synergize with IL-4/13 in this process (Fig. 3.4). Allergen-specific CD4 T lymphocytes are activated when processed fragments of allergen are presented to their T-cell recep-

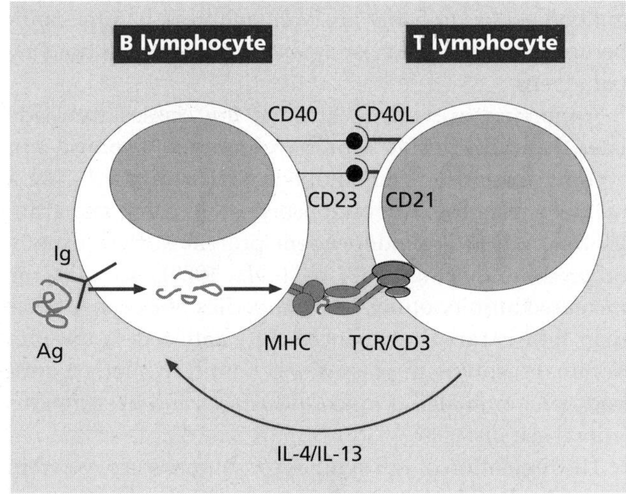

Fig. 3.4 Signals essential for IgE switching in B lymphocytes. B lymphocytes internalize specific antigen (Ag) bound to surface immunoglobulin (Ig) and process it into fragments ('epitopes') which are then presented to T lymphocytes on class II major histocompatibility complex (MHC) molecules. The antigen-specific T lymphocytes will support IgE synthesis if they secrete interleukin-4 (IL-4) or IL-13. In addition, T/B-cell contact through the molecules CD40 and CD23, and their respective ligands CD40L and CD21 (and perhaps other surface molecules), is essential for B-lymphocyte IgE switching.

tor/CD3 complex by APC on MHC class II molecules (see above). B lymphocytes process and present antigen in this way. Following presentation, the activated, allergen-specific T lymphocytes secrete cytokines, including IL-4 and IL-13. In addition to these 'cognate' interactions between allergen-specific T lymphocytes and B lymphocytes, additional signals are provided to B lymphocytes through T-lymphocyte contact which along with IL-4/13 are essential for subsequent secretion of allergen-specific IgE. At least two signals are important in this respect.

1 *CD40/CD40 ligand interaction*. CD40 is a surface glycoprotein expressed on immature and mature B lymphocytes as well as thymic epithelial cells and dendritic cells (Clark & Leadbetter, 1994). The importance of this interaction was first inferred when it was discovered that anti-CD40 monoclonal antibodies could replace contact with activated T lymphocytes in induction of IgE synthesis (Jabara *et al.*, 1990; Gascan *et al.*, 1991). These experiments conversely suggested the presence of a ligand for CD40 (CD40L) on T lymphocytes. Recently, CD40L has been cloned from cDNA libraries constructed from activated T lymphocytes (Hollenbaugh *et al.*, 1992). In contrast to activated CD4 T lymphocytes, resting cells do not express CD40L. Interestingly, human mast cells have also been shown to express CD40L, which was functional in the sense that mast cells could induce IgE synthesis by human B lymphocytes in the presence of IL-4 (Gauchat *et al.*, 1993).

2 *CD21/CD23 interaction*. CD23 is the low-affinity receptor for IgE present on many cells including B lymphocytes, monocytes and a subset of T lymphocytes, whereas CD21, identified as the Epstein–Barr virus and C3 desArg receptor on B lymphocytes, is also found on some T lymphocytes as well as follicular dendritic cells. It was shown recently (Aubry *et al.*, 1992) that triggering of CD21, either with anti-CD21 antibody or recombinant soluble CD23, increased IL-4-induced IgE production by B lymphocytes.

Interactions between these ligand pairs may explain why non-cognate interactions between T lymphocytes and B lymphocytes may result in IgE synthesis in the presence of exogenous IL-4 (Parronchi *et al.*, 1990). Hydrocortisone also induces IL-4-dependent IgE synthesis by normal unfractionated mononuclear cells (Sarfati *et al.*, 1989). The mechanism of this phenomenon is unknown.

In summary, it is clear that the T-lymphocyte-derived cytokines IL-4 and IL-13 play an indispensable role in the initiation and propagation of IgE synthesis by B lymphocytes. The need for both cytokines and cellular contact mediated by specific receptor/ligand interactions in this process bears many similarities to the requirements for T-lymphocyte activation by APC (see above). Conversely, B lymphocytes may themselves influence local cytokine synthesis by T lymphocytes, for example by their differential capacity to present soluble antigen to Th1- and Th2-like T cells (see above).

Cytokines and eosinophil recruitment

The pro-inflammatory properties of eosinophils and a summary of the evidence implicating them in the pathogenesis of asthma and allergic inflammation will be found in Chapter 10 of this volume. It is relevant here, however, to consider the role of T-lymphocyte-derived cytokines in the genesis of the marked and specific infiltration of eosinophils into the relevant mucosal surfaces, which is the hallmark of these diseases.

Eosinophils are non-dividing, granular cells which arise principally in the bone marrow. Eosinophil differentiation, like that of all leucocytes, is influenced by cytokines. Of the cytokines secreted by activated T lymphocytes, IL-3, IL-5 and GM-CSF promote maturation, activation and prolonged survival of the eosinophil (Lopez *et al.*, 1986; Rothenberg *et al.*, 1988, 1989). IL-5 is unique in that, unlike IL-3 and GM-CSF, it acts specifically on eosinophils when undergoing activation, hyperadhesion and terminal differentiation of the eosinophil precursor (Lopez *et al.*, 1988; Walsh *et al.*, 1990). IL-5 may be the most important cytokine for eosinophil differentiation since it is released principally by T lymphocytes, and eosinophilia associated with parasitic infections is T-lymphocyte dependent (Basten & Beeson, 1970). This hypothesis is further supported by the observation that transgenic mice constitutively expressing the gene for IL-5 show a marked, specific expansion of blood and tissue eosinophils (Dent *et al.*, 1990).

One fundamental problem with asthma pathogenesis is the mechanism by which eosinophils preferentially accumulate in the inflamed mucosa. Established eosinophil chemoattractants such as platelet activating factor, while highly potent (Wardlaw *et al.*, 1986), are non-specific in the sense that they also attract neutrophils. Local expression of eosinophil-specific cytokines such as IL-5 may partly account for this phenomenon by selectively enhancing eosinophil differentiation and survival, although these cytokines exhibit only weak eosinophil chemotactic activity *in vitro*. Chemoattractants may also play a role. Cytokines such as IL-5, IL-3 and GM-CSF have been shown to prime eosinophils for an enhanced chemotactic response to other chemoattractants, including chemokines such as IL-8 (Warringa *et al.*, 1991; Sehmi *et al.*, 1992). The T-lymphocyte-derived cytokines, lymphocyte chemoattractant factor (LCF) and IL-2 are also relatively potent eosinophil chemoattractants (Rand *et al.*, 1991a,b). The LCF protein exerts its activity by binding to CD4 molecules, so that in addition to affecting lymphocytes it also specifically acts on eosinophils as compared with other granulocytes, since only eosinophil granulocytes express

CD4 (Rand *et al.*, 1991a). An exciting recent observation has been that the chemokines eotaxin and MCP-4 (see Chapter 10), as well as RANTES, MCP-3 and, to a lesser extent, MIP-1α are all powerful and selective chemoattractants for eosinophils and basophils *in vitro* (Baggiolini & Dahinden, 1994). An investigation of whether these proteins are generated in the bronchial mucosa of asthmatic patients is now urgently required.

Another revealing field of study has been the role of adhesion molecules in selective eosinophil migration. Three major families of adhesion molecules have been defined as being involved in leucocyte migration: (i) the immunoglobulin superfamily, including intercellular cell adhesion molecule (ICAM)-1/2 and vascular cell adhesion molecule (VCAM)-1; (ii) the integrins, including β1-integrins such as VLA1-6 and the β2-integrins such as LFA-1 and Mac-1; (iii) the selectins, including E-selectin, P-selectin and L-selectin. Leucocyte migration is initiated by an interaction between receptors on the cell surface with their ligands on the surface of vascular endothelial cells. Selectins mediate the initial weak tethering of leucocytes to the endothelial wall. Eosinophils can bind to endothelium using all three selectins, with no apparent differences between these cells and neutrophils. Both eosinophils and neutrophils exhibit surface shedding of L-selectin on activation, which may facilitate endothelial transmigration (Smith *et al.*, 1992). Other leucocyte surface β2-integrins, such as LFA-1 and Mac-1, mediate firm adhesion and transmigration by binding to immunoglobulin-like molecules, such as ICAM-1 and VCAM-1, on the endothelium (Kyan-Aung *et al.*, 1991; Bochner *et al.*, 1993). Eosinophils appear to be unique, however, in that IL-3 and IL-5 up-regulate eosinophil, but not neutrophil, adhesion to unstimulated endothelial cells (Walsh *et al.*, 1990). Furthermore, eosinophils, but not neutrophils, express the β1-integrin VLA-4, which is a ligand for VCAM-1 on the surface of stimulated endothelial cells (Walsh *et al.*, 1991). The expression of VCAM-1 on endothelial cells is increased by exposure to IL-4, which enhanced VLA-4/VCAM-1-dependent adherence of eosinophils, but not neutrophils, to endothelium (Schleimer *et al.*, 1992). Bronchial mucosal endothelial cells do not express VCAM-1, at least in mild atopic asthmatics, but this molecule does appear following allergen bronchial challenge (Bentley *et al.*, 1993a). Eosinophils may also use VLA-4 for binding to tissue fibronectin (Elices *et al.*, 1990), which prolongs their survival *in vitro*, possibly by inducing autocrine secretion of IL-3 (Anwar *et al.*, 1993). Such mechanisms offer further possible explanations for the selective recruitment and activation of eosinophils observed in asthmatic inflammation. The important role of cytokines in this process is self-evident.

Table 3.2 Functional properties of subsets of human T lymphocytes.

Cytokine secretion	Th0	Th1	Th2
Cytokine secretion			
IL-2	+++	+++	−
IFN-γ	+++	+++	−
TNF-β	+	+++	−
TNF-α	++	+++	+
IL-3	+	+	++
IL-10	+	±	++
GM-CSF	++	+	++
IL-4	+	−	+++
IL-5	+	−	+++
IL-6	+	+	++
IL-13	+	+	+++
IL-9		−	++
Cytolytic activity	++	+++	±
Help for IgE synthesis	±	−	+++
Help for IgG/A/M synthesis			
Low T/B-cell ratios	++	++	++
High T/B-cell ratios	±	+++	

Typical functions and profiles of cytokine secretion of Th0-, Th1- and Th2-type T-lymphocytes. +++, characteristically of this subset; ++, considerable but not unique to this subset; +, trivial and not unique to this subset; ±, not always seen; −, characteristically not of this subset.

Functional heterogeneity of T lymphocytes

In recent years it has become clear that the nature of the allergic response initiated by CD4 T lymphocytes is at least partly dependent on the 'selection' or preferential activation of particular subsets of CD4 T lymphocytes which secrete defined patterns of cytokines (Table 3.2). These patterns of cytokine release result in the initiation and propagation of distinct immune effector mechanisms. Initial studies of mouse CD4 T-lymphocyte clones revealed that these could be divided into two basic functional subsets termed Th1 and Th2. Th1 T lymphocytes were characterized by the predominant secretion of IL-2, IFN-γ and tumour necrosis factor-β (TNF-β) while Th2 cells characteristically predominantly secreted IL-4, IL-5, IL-6 and IL-10. Other cytokines, such as TNF-α, IL-3 and GM-CSF, were produced by both Th1 and Th2 cell subsets (Mosmann *et al.*, 1986; Mosmann & Moore, 1991). These differing patterns of cytokine secretion by CD4 T lymphocytes result in distinct effector functions (Mosmann & Coffman, 1989). Broadly, Th1 cells participate in delayed-type hypersensitivity reactions (Cher & Mosmann, 1987), but also provide help for B-lymphocyte immunoglobulin synthesis under certain circumstances. Th2 cells, on the other hand, by their pattern of secretion of B-lymphocyte costimulatory cytokines, enhance the synthesis of all immunoglobulins, including IgE, in immune responses (see 'The role of cytokines in regulating IgE synthesis' above). In the centre of this spectrum, T-lymphocyte clones secreting cytokines characteristic of both Th1 and Th2 cells, termed Th0 cells, were also described (Firestein *et al.*, 1989). It is still not clear whether these Th0 cells represent distinct functional subsets or precursor cells in the process of differentiating into Th1 or Th2 cells.

Initial studies on mitogen-stimulated or alloreactive human T-lymphocyte clones raised from the peripheral blood of normal donors suggested that only a few CD4 T-lymphocyte clones showed clear-cut Th1 or Th2 phenotypes, while the majority resembled Th0 cells (Paliard *et al.*, 1988). A different picture emerged when human T-lymphocyte clones specific for particular antigens were raised, particularly when these antigens were implicated in prototype immunological mechanisms such as delayed-type hypersensitivity to mycobacterial antigens or nickel on the one hand, and IgE-mediated responses to helminth allergens on the other. For example, study of a large series of T-lymphocyte clones raised from the peripheral blood of healthy individuals specific for purified protein derivative (PPD) of *Mycobacterium tuberculosis* or the excretory/secretory antigens of *Toxocara canis* (TES) revealed that the majority of the PPD-specific clones showed a Th1-like cytokine profile, with excess secretion of IL-2 and IFN-γ, whereas the TES-specific clones showed a Th2-like profile, with excess IL-4 and IL-5 secretion (Del Prete *et al.*, 1991a). Similarly, many T-lymphocyte clones specific for intracellular bacteria such as *Borrelia burgdorferi* showed a Th1-like pattern of cytokine secretion (Yssel *et al.*, 1991). In patients with atopic dermatitis, T-lymphocyte clones specific for house dust mite (*Dermatophagoides pteronyssinus*) allergen raised from the peripheral blood secreted IL-4 and not IFN-γ, whereas all clones specific for *Candida albicans* or tetanus toxoid raised from the same donors secreted an excess of IFN-γ and relatively little IL-4 (Parronchi *et al.*, 1991). CD8 T lymphocytes also appear to exhibit functional heterogeneity in terms of their cytokine secretion profile. For example, CD8 T-cell clones specific for *Mycobacterium leprae* antigens showed patterns of cytokine secretion consistent with both Th1- and Th2-like phenotypes (Salgame *et al.*, 1991).

There is some evidence for mutual cross-inhibition of proliferation and cytokine secretion by Th1 and Th2 T lymphocytes, which is mediated by particular cytokines (Fig. 3.5). For example, exogenous IL-4 favours the growth and proliferation of Th2 T lymphocytes, whereas Th2 clones are exquisitely sensitive to inhibition by IFN-γ. IL-2 is a growth factor for both Th1 and Th2 cells. Whereas in mice IL-10 significantly inhibits the proliferation and cytokine secretion of Th1 cells (Fiorentino *et al.*, 1989), human IL-10 significantly inhibits proliferation of, and cytokine secretion by, both Th1- and Th2-like clones responding to specific antigen or lectin, and is itself a product of both Th1- and Th2-like clones (Del Prete *et al.*, 1993a).

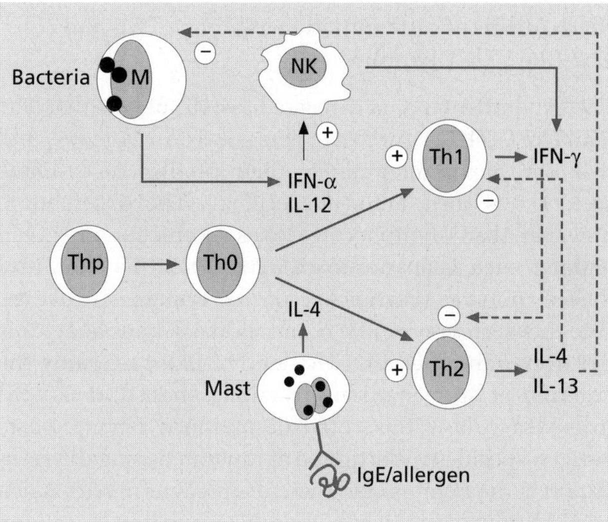

Fig. 3.5 Factors thought to influence development of Th1- and Th2-like T lymphocytes. Although it is suggested in this figure that both Th1- and Th2-like T cells arise from precursor (Thp) and Th0-like cells, this is by no means certain. Intracellular infection of monocytes (M) by organisms such as bacteria and viruses results in secretion of IFN-α and IL-12, which promote Th1-like development of T cells and activate NK (NK) cells to secrete IFN-γ, which is inhibitory to Th2-like cell development. It is not known precisely what favours Th2-like T-cell development *in vivo*, although local IL-4 released, for example, from allergen-triggered mast cells (Mast) may play a role. Once established, Th2-like T cells inhibit Th1-like development through the synthesis of IL-4 and IL-13, which also inhibit the activation of monocytes.

Human Th1 and Th2 cells also differ in the nature of their help for immunoglobulin synthesis by autologous B lymphocytes and in their cytolytic potential (Table 3.2). In the presence of specific antigen, Th2-like clones were able to induce the synthesis of IgM, IgG, IgA and IgE by autologous B lymphocytes (Del Prete *et al.*, 1991b). Under the same conditions, Th1-like clones induced synthesis of IgM, IgG and IgA, but not IgE, with a peak response at a T-cell/B-cell ratio of 1:1. At higher T-cell/B-cell ratios, immunoglobulin synthesis was reduced, possibly reflecting the cytolytic activity of the Th1-like clones against autologous B lymphocytes at higher T-cell/B-cell ratios. This inhibition of immunoglobulin synthesis by Th1-like cells may represent an important mechanism whereby the production of antibodies other than IgE in immune responses is self-regulated. In contrast, the failure of such an intrinsic regulatory mechanism in the case of Th2 cells may explain, at least partly, why IgE antibody responses may persist despite the cessation of antigen exposure.

Mechanisms of differentiation of human Th1- and Th2-like CD4 T lymphocytes

The experimental data discussed above suggest that Th1 and Th2 CD4 T-lymphocyte clones exist in humans, and that one factor determining their profiles of cytokine secretion is their antigen specificity. The observation, however, that T-lymphocyte clones specific for any given antigen, such as tetanus toxoid, can exhibit Th1, Th2 and Th0 phenotypes (Parronchi *et al.*, 1991) suggests that the cytokine secretion profile of individual T lymphocytes is not irrevocably 'set' in a Th1- or Th2-like pattern by the criterion of antigen specificity alone. Indeed, it is hard to envisage how this could occur, since T-lymphocyte antigen specificity is acquired at random during differentiation in the thymus, and therefore predetermination of a particular cytokine secretion profile according to antigen specificity would have to invoke some mechanism to 'imprint' such a profile on a T lymphocyte before it has encountered its specific antigen, which is not impossible but seems unlikely.

In order to address this problem, it has been suggested that, at least in mice, Th1 and Th2 cells may represent memory cells that have matured into different functional phenotypes in the face of repeated stimulation by specific antigen. This hypothesis invokes the putative existence of antigen-naive precursor T lymphocytes (Thp) which secrete principally IL-2 and develop into early memory Th0 effector cells after first encounter with specific antigen (Fig. 3.5) (Swain *et al.*, 1990). These cells then terminally differentiate into Th1 or Th2 cells following repetitive antigen stimulation.

The concept that Th0, Th1 and Th2 effector cells differentiate from a common pool of precursor cells raises the question of which factors influence the differentiation of a T lymphocyte to the Th1- or Th2-like phenotype. There is some evidence that exogenous cytokines may play a role in this differentiation process. For example, early addition of IL-4 to uncloned peripheral blood mononuclear cells stimulated with PPD shifted the subsequent differentiation of PPD-specific T lymphocytes from a Th1-like towards a Th0- or Th2-like phenotype. Conversely, in similar cultures, early addition of both IFN-γ and anti-IL-4 antibody induced many allergen- or TES-specific T-lymphocyte clones to differentiate into Th0- and Th1-like, instead of Th2-like clones (Maggi *et al.*, 1992). These data suggest that the presence or absence of exogenous IL-4 or IFN-γ at the time of antigen stimulation of resting T cells may influence their subsequent development into Th1- or Th2-like clones, regardless of any pre-existing functional bias. In addition, the cytokines IFN-α and IL-12 (both activators of natural killer (NK) cells which induce IFN-γ synthesis) were also found to promote the differentiation of allergen- or TES-specific T-lymphocyte clones towards a Th0- or Th1-like phenotype instead of the usual Th2-like phenotype, whereas neutralization of endogenous IL-12 by specific antibody promoted the differentiation of PPD-specific T lymphocytes towards a Th0- or Th2-like phenotype instead of the typical Th1-like phenotype (Romagnani, 1992). These observations have led to the hypothesis (Romagnani, 1992) that infection of cells such as macrophages with viruses and intracellular bacteria may favour a Th1-like response through local release of IFN-α and IL-12, which might in turn activate NK cells resulting in local release of IFN-γ (Fig. 3.5). It is less clear what could favour the differentiation of Th2-like effector T-lymphocytes from precursors *in vivo*, although it is possible to speculate that allergens or helminth-derived antigens, in contrast to intracellular parasites, might envoke relatively little IL-12 release from monocytes and therefore low local concentrations of IFN-γ. This, coupled with the presence of local IL-4 released from IgE-sensitized mast cells in patients with atopic disease or helminthic infections, might favour the local differentiation of Th2-like effector T lymphocytes. In addition, IL-13, like IL-4, inhibits secretion of IFN-α and IL-12 by monocytes (De Waal-Malefyt *et al.*, 1993). The local emergence of Th2-like T lymphocytes, themselves a rich source of IL-4 and IL-13 (Zurawski & De Vries, 1994), might therefore be expected to encourage the further development of Th2-like T lymphocytes and discourage the development of Th1-like cells.

The nature of the APC which activate antigen-naive T lymphocytes may also play a role in their subsequent development towards a Th1- or Th2-like phenotype. For example, at sites where the dominant APC are dendritic cells, which constitutively express CD80 (see above), both Th1- and Th2-like responses might be initiated. On the other hand, soluble antigen present at low concentrations in the periphery, such as at a mucosal surface, might be preferentially taken up and presented by resting B lymphocytes expressing antigen-specific surface immunoglobulin. When CD80-negative resting B lymphocytes serve as APC, however, Th1-like T lymphocytes fail to become activated and, furthermore, are rendered unresponsive (Gilbert & Weigle, 1992). In contrast, it is difficult to induce unresponsiveness in Th2-like T lymphocytes (Williams *et al.*, 1992), which can be activated, at least in mice, by resting B lymphocytes (Gajewski *et al.*, 1991), suggesting that the CD28/CD80 interaction may not always be essential for activation of Th2-like T lymphocytes. The cytokines IL-4 and IL-10 secreted by activated Th2-like T lymphocytes might then inhibit macrophage co-stimulation. This, coupled with the lack of secretion of IFN-γ, which is required for the induction of B7 expression on resting macrophages, might further down-regulate Th1-like responses in the presence of low concentrations of antigen.

Roles of Th1 and Th2 T lymphocytes in immune responses

The existence of CD4 and CD8 T lymphocytes which secrete defined combinations of cytokines in response to various antigenic stimuli, and a consideration of the properties of these cytokines, allows the view that particular patterns of cytokine release during inflammatory responses play an important role in determining the type of immune effector mechanism that a foreign antigen may elicit. Thus, Th1-like cells, through their predominant secretion of IL-2 and IFN-γ, might be expected to promote the development of cytotoxic T lymphocytes, enhance the bactericidal activity of macrophages and stimulate the activity of NK and LAK cells. These effector mechanisms would be particularly effective for the elimination of viruses and other intracellular pathogens. On the other hand, the secretion of cytokines such as IL-4, IL-6 and IL-10 by Th2-like T lymphocytes would be expected to inhibit local activation of macrophages and dendritic cells but would favour the synthesis and release of specific antibody, including IgE, by activated B lymphocytes. Such humoral responses have a well-defined role in the elimination of invading extracellular micro-organisms such as bacteria and their secreted products.

There is some evidence that secretion of Th2 cytokines may be detrimental to the host, in addition to their possible role in eliminating certain infections. In several infectious diseases of humans, a Th1-like pattern of cytokine secretion is associated with resistance to infection, whereas a Th2-like pattern may be associated with progressive, uncontrolled infection. The Th2 cytokines IL-4, IL-10 and IL-13 (Minty *et al.*, 1993), although enhancing antibody production, may suppress cell-mediated immune responses. For example, IL-4 blocks the IL-2-dependent proliferation of Th1-like T lymphocytes through down-regulation of IL-2 receptors (Martinez *et al.*, 1990), and abrogates the antimicrobial activity of monocytes activated by IFN-γ (Lehn *et al.*, 1989). IL-10 inhibits antigen-specific T-lymphocyte responses by interfering with antigen presentation by monocytes and macrophages and by down-regulation of their MHC class II molecule expression (De Waal-Malefyt *et al.*, 1991a). IL-10 also inhibits the release from macrophages of cytokines with antimicrobial functional properties (De Waal-Malefyt *et al.*, 1991b). A good example of how Th2-like cytokines might impair host responses to infection is provided by leprosy, which presents as a clinical and immunological spectrum of disease — on the one hand, patients with tuberculoid leprosy exemplify the resistant response restricting growth of the pathogen, on the other hand, patients with lepromatous leprosy suffer from uncontrolled proliferation of the *Mycobacterium leprae* organism despite demonstrating a marked humoral response to the pathogen. These clinical patterns of disease are associated with distinct cytokine patterns in skin lesions of patients with leprosy (Yamamura *et al.*, 1992), with elevated concentrations of mRNA encoding IL-2 and IFN-γ in tuberculoid lesions and elevated concentrations of mRNA encoding IL-4, IL-5 and IL-10 in lepromatous lesions. Spontaneous 'conversion' of the disease from the lepromatous to the tuberculoid form was associated with an alteration in the corresponding cytokine pattern observed in skin lesions. These differences in cytokine profiles have been confirmed in both CD4 and CD8 T lymphocytes at the clonal level (Salgame *et al.*, 1991). In addition to providing further evidence for the existence of Th1 and Th2 CD4 and CD8 T lymphocytes, these studies also implicate Th2 cytokines in suppressing cell-mediated immunity to such an extent that infection is allowed to proceed unabated.

In summary, these experimental data provide convincing evidence for specific patterns of cytokine release by both CD4 and CD8 T-lymphocyte clones in the course of immune responses to invading micro-organisms and in various immunopathological diseases. However, some of the most convincing evidence for a role for Th1- and Th2-like cytokines in orchestrating distinct inflammatory responses *in vivo* has come from studies of allergic inflammation and asthma, as described in detail below.

Evidence for mucosal inflammation in asthma and allergic diseases

Most recent studies on the histopathology of asthma have compared mild asthmatic and normal volunteers, utilizing the techniques of bronchoalveolar lavage (BAL) and bronchial biopsy. Elevated numbers of eosinophils, both in the bronchial mucosa and in BAL fluid, were constant features of mild asthma (Kirby *et al.*, 1987; Wardlaw *et al.*, 1988; Azzawi *et al.*, 1990). Similarly, increased numbers of activated lymphocytes, identified either as irregular, atypical lymphocytes by transmission electron microscopy (Jeffery *et al.*, 1989) or as CD25+ cells as shown by immunocytochemistry were also invariably seen. Most of the CD25-expressing cells in these biopsies were shown to be T lymphocytes (Hamid *et al.*, 1992a). The numbers of activated, 'memory' T lymphocytes were also increased in the BAL fluid of mild, atopic asthmatics as compared with controls (Robinson *et al.*, 1993a). There is evidence that activation of T lymphocytes and subsequent eosinophil recruitment and secretion may contribute both to epithelial damage and to bronchial hyperresponsiveness (Salvato, 1968; Laitinen *et al.*, 1985; Beasley *et al.*, 1989). In contrast, these studies demonstrated no significant changes in the numbers of mast cells and their sub-types or neutrophils in the bronchial mucosa (Fabbri *et al.*, 1988; Beasley *et al.*, 1989; Jeffery *et al.*, 1989, 1992; Bradley *et al.*,

1991; Bentley *et al.*, 1992b,c). Cell numbers do not, however, necessarily correlate with function: it was shown, for example, that spontaneous release of mediators from mast cells is elevated in asthmatic patients (Wardlaw *et al.*, 1988).

The present clinical classification of asthma discussed above (intrinsic, extrinsic and occupational) implies possible variability in its pathogenesis. Are such distinctions apparent in histopathological terms? Preliminary studies addressing this question would suggest that they are not: an autopsy study of the bronchial mucosa of a patient who had died with severe occupational asthma showed histological changes similar to those seen in fatal non-occupational asthma (Fabbri *et al.*, 1988), while immunocytochemical studies (Bentley *et al.*, 1992b,c) comparing bronchial biopsies from extrinsic, intrinsic and occupational asthmatics, showed marked similarities in terms of their inflammatory cell infiltrate. Examination of BAL fluid obtained from a group of intrinsic asthmatics (Mattoli *et al.*, 1991) showed increased numbers of activated T lymphocytes, eosinophils and neutrophils when compared with normal controls. These observations suggest that the bronchial response in patients with asthma has similar characteristics regardless of the nature of identifiable provoking agents, and regardless of the prominence of IgE-mediated mechanisms.

Atopic rhinitis is also associated with chronic inflammation of the nasal mucosa. The nature of this inflammation bears many similarities to that seen in the bronchial mucosa in asthma (Bentley *et al.*, 1992a; Varney *et al.*, 1992). There is infiltration of activated T lymphocytes as well as a marked, specific eosinophil infiltrate.

CD4 T lymphocytes and the pathogenesis of asthma and rhinitis

CD4 T lymphocytes and eosinophils

CD4 T lymphocytes are clearly an important source of the cytokines IL-5, IL-3 and GM-CSF, and may be an important source of chemokines such as regulated on activation normal T expressed and secreted (RANTES), macrophage inflammatory protein (MIP-1α) and monocyte chemotactic protein (MCP-3). The possible roles of these agents in enhancing eosinophil survival, maturation, activation and local accumulation have been discussed above (see above). These observations emphasize the fact that cytokines and other products of activated CD4 T lymphocytes have the propensity to bring about *selective* accumulation and activation of eosinophils in tissues, and that this need not involve immunological processes dependent on the presence of antibodies, including IgE.

Cytokine secretion by cells other than T lymphocytes

In addition to T lymphocytes, it is clear that many other cells which are normally present in the bronchial and nasal mucosa, or which migrate into it in association with allergic inflammation, are potential sources of cytokines and chemokines. For example, eosinophils have the capacity to elaborate cytokines and chemokines, including transforming growth factor-α (TGF-α), TGF-β, TNF-α, MIP-1α, IL-1, IL-3, IL-5, IL-6, IL-8 and GM-CSF (Wong *et al.*, 1990; Kita *et al.*, 1991; Moqbel *et al.*, 1991; Broide *et al.*, 1992b; Hamid *et al.*, 1992b; Braun *et al.*, 1993; Costa *et al.*, 1993; Weller *et al.*, 1993; Moqbel *et al.*, 1995). The secretion of such mediators by eosinophils may enable them to participate in the propagation of asthmatic inflammation through autocrine and juxtacrine effects. It is also clear that mast cells and basophils can store a number of cytokines, including IL-4, IL-5, IL-6 and TNF-α (Ohkawara *et al.*, 1992; Arock *et al.*, 1993; Bradding *et al.*, 1994), probably in their intracytoplasmic granules. In a study comparing bronchial biopsies from mild atopic asthmatics and non-atopic normal controls (Bradding *et al.*, 1994), serial thin glycol methacrylate sections were used to define the cellular provenance of IL-4, IL-5, IL-6 and TNF-α using immunocytochemistry with monoclonal antibodies directed against these cytokines and cellular phenotypic markers. Both asthmatic and normal bronchial mucosae contained numerous cells staining positively for all four cytokines, with the majority identified as mast cells owing to their tryptase content. The total numbers of mucosal mast cells were similar in the asthmatics and the controls, as has been observed in other studies (Beasley *et al.*, 1989; Bradley *et al.*, 1991; Bentley *et al.*, 1992b,c). The numbers of mast cells staining positively with antibodies against IL-4 and TNF-α were elevated in the asthmatics compared with the controls, whereas the numbers of cells staining with IL-5 and IL-6 antibodies were similar in both groups. This study suggests that mast cells have a potential role in the initiation and propagation of asthmatic mucosal inflammation, at least in atopic subjects. In particular, mast cell-derived IL-4 and IL-5 may play a role in eosinophil recruitment (see above), while IL-4 may direct T-lymphocyte maturation towards a Th2-like phenotype during the initiation of mucosal inflammation (see above). Interestingly, the authors were unable to demonstrate cytokine staining of T lymphocytes in this study (Bradding *et al.*, 1994), whereas T lymphocytes were shown to be the predominant source of IL-4 and IL-5 mRNA in BAL fluid cells from atopic asthmatics and the nasal mucosa of patients with atopic rhinitis (Ying *et al.*, 1993, 1995), with a smaller but significant contribution from mast cells and eosinophils. Aside from an idiosyncracy of the staining technique in these heavily fixed sections, these observations suggest the possibilities that secretion and storage of cytokine proteins in leucocytes may not be synchronous with transcription of their mRNA, and that T lymphocytes may secrete cytokines rapidly, without storage, following synthesis, such that intracytoplasmic cytokines are not detectable by immunocytochemistry. The resolution of these important questions, and the relative contributions of individual inflammatory cells to local cytokine release, must await futher studies. Nevertheless, T lymphocytes are unique amongst inflammatory cells in the sense that they can recognize and respond to processed antigens directly, and may play a pivotal role in initiating and sustaining immunologically driven chronic asthma, particularly in situations where the IgE response is absent or minimal.

T lymphocytes and asthmatic inflammation

Immunohistochemical studies of bronchial biopsies taken from patients with asthma (Jeffery *et al.*, 1989; Azzawi *et al.*, 1990; Bradley *et al.*, 1991; Bentley *et al.*, 1992b,c) have shown that activated (CD25+) T lymphocytes can be detected in the bronchial mucosa, and that their numbers can be correlated both with the numbers of local activated eosinophils and with disease severity. Activated (CD25+, HLA-DR+) CD4, but not CD8, T lymphocytes were also detected in the peripheral blood of patients with severe asthma (Corrigan *et al.*, 1988; Corrigan & Kay, 1990; Corrigan *et al.*, 1993), and their numbers were reduced following glucocorticoid therapy to a degree which correlated with the degree of clinical improvement. Similarly, activated CD4 and CD8 T lymphocytes were observed in the peripheral blood of child asthmatics (Gemou-Engesaeth *et al.*, 1994), and the numbers of activated CD4 cells correlated with both disease severity and the numbers of peripheral blood eosinophils. In one of these studies (Corrigan *et al.*, 1993), elevated serum concentrations of IL-5 were also detected in a proportion of the asthmatics, but not in non-asthmatic controls, and again concentrations were reduced in association with glucocorticoid therapy. Elevated serum concentrations of IL-5 were also seen in a proportion of patients with severe, glucocorticoid-dependent asthma (Alexander *et al.*, 1994). As shown (Doi *et al.*, 1994) by semiquantitative polymerase chain amplification of reverse transcribed cytokine-specific mRNA, peripheral blood T lymphocytes from both atopic and non-atopic severe asthmatics contained elevated quantities (relative to β-actin) of mRNA encoding IL-5 when compared with controls. The quantities of IL-5 mRNA were reduced in association with oral glucocorticoid therapy of the asthmatics and clinical improvement. Peripheral blood T lymphocytes from asthmatics clinically resistant to glucocorticoid therapy were shown to express activation markers *in vivo* (Corrigan *et al.*, 1991a) and to be refractory to the inhibitory effects of glucocorticoids *in vitro* (Corrigan *et al.*, 1991b; Haczku *et al.*, 1994). These studies suggest that glucocorticoids exert their anti-asthma effect at least partly by inhibiting the release of cytokines from activated T lymphocytes.

Some (Graham *et al.*, 1985), but not all (Wardlaw *et al.*, 1988) studies have demonstrated increased numbers of lymphocytes in the BAL fluid of patients with mild asthma, and preferential activation of memory CD4 T lymphocytes in the BAL fluid of mild atopic asthmatics was observed to correlated with asthma symptoms and bronchial hyperresponsiveness (Robinson *et al.*, 1993a). In another study of intrinsic and extrinsic asthmatics (Walker *et al.*, 1991), it was shown that while both CD4 and CD8 T lymphocytes in BAL fluid expressed activation markers, only the numbers of activated CD4 cells correlated with the numbers of BAL eosinophils and disease severity.

Measurement of cytokines *in vivo* is problematical because of their low concentrations, rapid metabolism and unquantifiable degree of dilution. Furthermore, 'physiological' concentrations of cytokines have in general not been defined, and so it is often unknown whether a specific assay, such as enzyme-linked immunosorbent assay (ELISA), is sufficiently sensitive. This problem is illustrated by a recent study of BAL fluid from mild asthmatics (Broide *et al.*, 1992a), where cytokines were detectable only after considerable concentration of the BAL fluid. Clearly, such a procedure might result in variable loss of specific proteins. One alternative to the direct measurement of cytokines is the detection of their mRNA using the technique of *in situ* hybridization with cytokine-specific cRNA probes or riboprobes. Although this is not a strictly quantitative technique, and with the proviso that mRNA synthesis does not necessarily equate with secretion of the corresponding protein, it does have the advantage that it can localize the secretion of cytokines within cells and tissues. Using this technique it was demonstrated that IL-5 mRNA was elaborated by cells in bronchial biopsies from a majority of mild asthmatics but not normal controls (Hamid *et al.*, 1991). The numbers of IL-5 mRNA signals correlated broadly with the numbers of activated T lymphocytes and eosinophils in biopsies from the same subjects. In another study (Robinson *et al.*, 1992), it was shown that significantly elevated percentages of BAL cells expressed mRNA encoding IL-2, IL-3, IL-4, IL-5 and GM-CSF but not IFN-γ in mild atopic asthmatics when compared with non-atopic normal controls. Separation of CD2+ T lymphocytes from the remainder of the BAL cells showed that the majority (<90%) of the cells expressing IL-5 and IL-4 mRNA were T lymphocytes. Over a broad range of asthma severity, the percentages of BAL fluid cells from atopic asthmatics expressing mRNA encoding IL-5, IL-4, IL-3 and GM-CSF, but not IL-2 and IFN-γ, could be correlated with the severity of asthma symptoms and bronchial hyperresponsiveness (Robinson *et al.*, 1993b). Elevated percentages of peripheral blood CD4, but not CD8, T lymphocytes from patients with exacerbation of asthma expressed mRNA encoding IL-3, IL-4, IL-5 and GM-CSF but not IL-2 and IFN-γ when compared with controls (Corrigan *et al.*, 1995). Elevated spontaneous secretion of IL-3, IL-5 and GM-CSF was also shown in these patients using an eosinophil survival-prolonging assay. Again, the percentages of CD4 T lymphocytes expressing mRNA encoding IL-3, IL-5 and GM-CSF, as well as spontaneous secretion of these cytokines by the CD4 T lymphocytes, were reduced in association with glucocorticoid therapy and clinical improvement. In a double-blind, parallel group study, therapy of mild atopic asthmatics with oral prednisolone, but not placebo, resulted in clinical impovement associated with a reduction in the percentages of BAL fluid cells expressing IL-5 and IL-4 and an increase in those expressing IFN-γ (Robinson *et al.*, 1993c). Conversely, artificial exacerbation of asthma by allergen bronchial challenge of sensitized atopic asthmatics was associated with increased numbers of activated T lymphocytes and eosinophils and increased expression of mRNA encoding IL-5 and GM-CSF in the bronchial mucosa (Bentley *et al.*, 1993b).

The chronic mucosal inflammatory processes associated with allergic rhinitis are very similar to those seen in asthma. Studies on nasal biopsies from grass pollen-sensitive patients with seasonal rhinitis showed accumulation of CD4 T lymphocytes and eosinophils, and preferential expression of Th2-like cytokines (IL-4 and IL-5) at the level of mRNA synthesis in the nasal mucosa in association with both local allergen challenge and natural seasonal exposure (Bentley *et al.*, 1992a; Durham *et al.*, 1992; Varney *et al.*, 1992). Using sequential immunocytochemistry and *in situ* hybridization, it was demonstrated that the principal source of mRNA encoding IL-4 and IL-5 (approximately 80% of the positive signals) in these nasal mucosal biopsies was the T lymphocyte, with a smaller, but significant contribution from mast cells and eosinophils (Sun Ying *et al.*, 1994, 1995). In patients with hayfever, topical glucocorticoid therapy inhibited both the early- and late-phase responses following local nasal allergen challenge (Masuyama *et al.*, 1994). This was associated with a reduction in T-lymphocyte and eosinophil infiltration in the nasal mucosa, and a marked decrease in the numbers of cells expressing mRNA encoding IL-4.

Taken together, these studies provide persuasive evidence in support of the general hypothesis that, in both asthmatic and allergic inflammation, activated CD4 T lymphocytes secrete cytokines which are relevant to the accumulation and activation of eosinophils in the relevant mucosa, and that glucocorticoids exert their therapeutic effect, at least partly, by reducing the synthesis of cytokines by these cells (see Chapter 90). They also suggest that the properties of CD4 T lymphocytes in the peripheral blood of asthmatics closely resemble those of T lymphocytes in the bronchial mucosa and BAL fluid, owing perhaps to a 'spill-over' effect of these cells from the mucosa into the peripheral blood. Thus, there seems considerable scope for examining the properties of asthmatic T lymphocytes at the level of the peripheral blood, obviating the problem of performing fibreoptic bronchoscopy in patients with severe disease.

Are asthmatic CD4 T lymphocytes 'Th2-like'?

Some of the most convincing evidence for a role for Th1- and Th2-like cytokines in orchestrating distinct inflammatory responses *in vivo* has come from studies of cytokine mRNA expression in asthma and rhinitis, as described above. In other studies employing *in situ* hybridization, the cutaneous inflammatory responses to challenge with allergen in atopic subjects and tuberculin in non-atopic subjects were compared (Kay *et al.*, 1991; Tsicopoulos *et al.*, 1992). Both types of response (late-phase allergic and delayed-type hypersensitivity (DTH)) were associated with an influx of activated CD4 T lymphocytes, but whereas mRNA molecules encoding IL-2 and IFN-γ were abundant within the tuberculin reactions, very little mRNA encoding these cytokines was observed in the late-phase allergic reactions. Conversely, mRNA encoding IL-4 and IL-5 was abundant in the late-phase allergic but not the tuberculin reactions. Furthermore, the relative numbers and types of granulocytes infiltrating these reactions reflected these different patterns of cytokine release (Gaga *et al.*, 1991). Similar differences were observed in the mRNA profiles of BAL T lymphocytes from patients with atopic asthma and pulmonary tuberculosis (Robinson *et al.*, 1994). These observations provide direct evidence in support of the hypothesis that activated T lymphocytes, through their patterns of cytokine secretion, regulate the types of granulocyte which participate in inflammatory reactions. Furthermore, they demonstrate that Th1- and Th2-like CD4 T-cell responses can be detected in humans under physiological conditions, and that the antigen specificity of the T cell might be one factor which determines which type of response is initiated. Taken together, they provide a considerable body of evidence for the existence of Th1- and Th2-like *patterns* of cytokine secretion *in vivo* in human asthma, although it cannot be ascertained from such studies whether or not these cytokines originate from the same cells. Further information in this regard must arise from a closer scrutiny of patterns of cytokine secretion by T-lymphocyte lines or clones isolated from the relevant mucosal surface in patients with asthma and allergic disease. Some data concerning patterns of cytokine secretion in atopic diseases are already available. For example, following mitogen stimulation, the majority of T lymphocytes derived from the conjunctival infiltrates of patients with vernal conjunctivitis developed into Th2-like clones (Maggi *et al.*, 1991). Similarly, high proportions of Th2-like clones were obtained from the skin lesions of patients with atopic dermatitis (Van der Heijden *et al.*, 1991; Ramb-Lindhauer *et al.*, 1991). A proportion of these skin-derived T-lymphocyte clones were specific for house dust mite or grass pollen allergens. T-lymphocyte clones obtained from nasal and bronchial biopsies of atopic patients with grass pollen-induced asthma or rhinitis 48 hours after allergen challenge were enriched for allergen-specific T lymphocytes, exhibited a Th2-like profile of cytokine secretion and induced IgE synthesis by autologous B lymphocytes. In contrast, clones derived from sites challenged with diluent control in the same patients yielded few allergen-specific cells and few clones showing a clear Th2-like cytokine profile (Del Prete *et al.*, 1993b). These studies directly implicate Th2-like, allergen-specific T lymphocytes in the pathogenesis of asthma, at least in atopic subjects.

The 'cause' of asthma and allergic disease

The studies described above have provided considerable insight into the role of Th2-like T lymphocytes in the pathogenesis of the chronic eosinophil-rich mucosal infiltration seen in asthma and rhinitis and in the regulation of IgE synthesis. They do not, however, explain why only some individuals develop allergen-specific IgE antibodies, atopic disease and/or asthma.

The phenomenon of atopy, defined in its broadest sense as the inappropriate synthesis of allergen-specific IgE, and without reference to the development of disease, shows a strong heritable tendency. Indeed, there is now good evidence that 'atopy' defined in this way is closely linked to a locus on chromosome 11q13 (Sandford *et al.*, 1993). One candidate gene at this locus is that encoding the β-subunit of the high-affinity IgE receptor; a common allelic variant of this gene (Ile-Leu substitution at amino acid 181) has been demonstrated in unrelated nuclear families with extrinsic asthmatic probands (Shirakawa *et al.*, 1994). How precisely this might predispose to the development of atopy is not clear, although dysregulation of the expression of IgE receptors on inflammatory effector cells or dysregulation of the expression of cytokines such as IL-4 which enhance IgE synthesis (possibilities for which there is as yet little good evidence) may play a role.

It is clear from many of the studies discussed above that both atopic and non-atopic adults have T lymphocytes in the peripheral blood which recognize epitopes derived from inhalant allergens. In atopic individuals, however, these T lymphocytes are more likely to be Th2-like, whereas in non-atopics they are more likely to be Th1-like. There is increasing interest in the so-called 'window of susceptibility' to atopy in infancy and early childhood, during which persistent IgE responses to both inhaled and dietary allergens may or may not be initiated. One view expounded by Holt (1994) is that exposure of mucosal surfaces to potential allergens, whether inhaled or consumed, results in active immunological recognition comprising cross-competing Th1-like and Th2-like allergen-specific T-lymphocyte clones. During repeated rounds of normal environmental restimulation, either a Th1-like or a Th2-like response eventually becomes dominant, resulting in a reservoir of memory T lymphocytes which directs the nature of the response to these allergens throughout later life. Supporting evidence shows that most children develop transient serum IgE antibody responses against common food allergens during the first year of life, the magnitude and duration of which reflects the incidence of atopy in their parents (Hattevig *et al.*, 1987). A similar pattern is seen with inhalant allergens (Hattevig *et al.*, 1993), although the IgE responses commence later and persist longer. It is possible that, in those children who go on to develop atopic disease, this transient Th2-like response persists, rather than being 'overwhelmed' by Th1-like responses. In addition to genetic predisposition, environmental factors which are known to influence the risk of sensitization to allergens (Holt *et al.*, 1990) may play a role in 'tipping the balance' of the Th1/Th2-like responses.

Both atopic and non-atopic subjects may develop asthma, and here even less is known about the key factors which influence this process. The heritability of asthma is more complex than that of atopy, and no single pattern of inheritance has emerged. Perhaps the clearest evidence that asthma may be initiated in previously disease-free subjects by exposure to novel, inhaled antigens comes from occupational asthma. Interestingly, in these subjects there is again a 'window of susceptibility' to asthma and allergic disease, in the sense that most subjects who are going to develop these diseases as a consequence of occupational exposure do so within about 3 years of the initiation of this exposure. The influences of environmental factors, such as cigarette smoking and genetic predisposition to atopy, are also apparent. Sensitizing antigen-specific IgE and Th2-like T-lymphocyte responses can be detected with varying prominence, according to the nature of the sensitizing agent. Nevertheless, of those subjects who develop these responses *de novo*, not all develop asthma. Clearly, further critical factors, be they environmental, immunological, physiological or heritable, need to be taken into account before the true 'cause' of asthma can be defined.

New therapeutic strategies in asthma and allergic disease

Peptide immunotherapy

The evidence discussed above suggests that Th2-like T lymphocytes, at least some of which are specific for aeroallergens, play a fundamental role in the pathogenesis of allergic diseases and asthma through the secretion of cytokines which both promote IgE synthesis (IL-4, IL-13) (see 'T lymphocytes, B lymphocytes and IgE synthesis') and orchestrate this specific accumulation of eosinophils at mucosal surfaces (IL-3, IL-5, GM-CSF) (see 'Cytokines and eosinophil recruitment' above). Since, as described above, the activation of CD4 T lymphocytes depends on the recognition of peptide fragments of allergen bound to MHC class II molecules, considerable interest has been generated in the use of immunotherapy with allergen-derived T-lymphocyte epitopes to modulate the function of allergen-specific Th2-like T cells. Therapeutically beneficial alterations in T-lymphocyte function might include failure to provide help for B-lymphocyte IgE synthesis, failure to undergo clonal expansion, failure to secrete Th2-like cytokines or an altered pattern (Th2-like to Th1-like) of cytokine secretion upon re-exposure to allergen. The mechanisms of this allergen-specific T-lymphocyte unresponsiveness are not completely understood, although current evidence suggests that allergen-derived peptide immunotherapy 'tolerizes' allergen-specific T lymphocytes. A lack of appropriate costimulation of T lymphocytes at the point of T-cell/peptide interaction appears to be critical for this process (see above). This may reflect the properties of particular APC at differing sites of antigen delivery, since studies in animals suggest that the route of administration is critical for determining the outcome of tolerance induction (Briner *et al.*, 1993; Hoyne *et al.*, 1993). The advantages of using allergen-derived peptides, compared with intact allergens for immunotherapy, include the potential for enhanced specificity of modulation of the T-cell response, and the removal of the risk of anaphylaxis associated with injection of sensitized subjects with intact allergen.

Two essential steps in this process are to identify those epitopes of particular allergens which appear to be critical for the activation of allergen-specific T cells (the so-called 'immunodominant' epitopes), and to define the specificity of HLA class II molecules (HLA-DP, -DQ and -DR) which restrict T-cell recognition of these epitopes. The identification of 'immunodominant' epitopes in allergen molecules is not always straightforward. For example, analysis of the immunodominant peptides of both group I (*Der p* I) and group II (*Der p* II) allergens of the house dust mite (*Dermatophagoides pteronyssinus*) has shown that, while particular epitopes are more frequently recognized, there is qualitative and quantitative variability in responses between individuals (Higgins *et al.*, 1992; Yssel *et al.*, 1992; O'Hehir *et al.*, 1993; Verhoef *et al.*, 1993). Also, the HLA class II restriction of T-lymphocyte recognition of house dust mite allergens is heterogeneous, involving HLA-DP, -DQ and -DR molecules of different specificities (Table 3.3). Furthermore, within an individual a single T-cell epitope may bind to more than one HLA class II molecule (O'Hehir *et al.*, 1990, 1991; Verhoef *et al.*, 1993). These observations would make the design of a 'universal' epitope vaccine, effective in all individuals, very difficult. More success has been claimed with immunodominant epitopes of the major cat dander allergen *Fel d* I, where in a majority of individuals the T-cell response is specific for two epitopes within one of the two *Fel d* I polypeptide chains (Briner *et al.*, 1993). Mice immunized with *Fel d* I chain 1 generate T-cell responses to these two epitopes. If, however, the animals are subsequently challenged subcutaneously with a mixture of the two dominant peptides, T-cell responses to the entire protein are abrogated, despite the presence of other potential, minor T-cell epitopes (a phenomenon referred to as 'determinant spreading'). It remains to be seen whether these epitopes are effective for immunotherapy of cat-allergic subjects at the population level.

Table 3.3 Human leucocyte antigen (HLA) class II restriction specificities of T-cell responses to house dust mite allergens. (After O'Hehir *et al.*, 1990, 1991; Verhoef *et al.* 1993.)

HLA-D region genes
DRB1 (DR1; DR2; DR5; DR8)
DRB3 (DR52 Dw25)
DRB4 (DR53)
DRB5 (DR2 Dw2; –Dw12; –Dw21)
DPB1 (DP4.1; DP4.2)
DQB1 (DQ7(3))

Allergen-specific T-lymphocyte clones may also be rendered unresponsive to further allergen exposure *in vitro* by incubation with supra-optimal concentrations of peptide epitopes regardless of the presence or absence of APC (Lamb *et al.*, 1983). This 'anergy' may be reversed by the addition of exogenous IL-2 and, indeed, is characterized by an inability of anergized T cells to secrete IL-2. 'Anergized' T cells fail to proliferate or to provide help to B lymphocytes for IgE synthesis. The loss of functional activity is accompanied by complex phenotypic changes, including down-regulation of the surface expression of the T-cell receptor/CD3 complex and the costimulatory receptor CD28 (see above), and up-regulation of CD25, the IL-2 receptor (Table 3.4). During the induction phase of anergy, cytokine-specific intracellular mRNA concentra-

Table 3.4 Effects of peptide-mediated 'anergy' on expression of T-cell surface membrane protein molecules.

Elevated	Diminished	Unaltered
CD2	TCR/CD3	CD71
CDIIa/18	CD4*	MHC class II
CD25	CD5*	
CD44	CD28	
CD54	CD29	
MHC class I*	CD43	

* Not seen in all anergized T-cell clones.

tions are enhanced; after re-stimulation with allergen, however, the cells failed to secrete IL-4 and IL-5, although IFN-γ secretion remained unaltered (Schall *et al.*, 1992). This would be expected to antagonize IgE synthesis and allergic inflammation. Whether or not this *in vitro* phenomenon is relevant to the genesis of allergen-specific T-lymphocyte unresponsiveness *in vivo* is not yet clear.

Conventional allergen immunotherapy

Conventional injection immunotherapy with intact allergen molecules has a proven role in the therapy of selected patients with severe grass pollen hayfever refractory to topical glucocorticoid therapy (Varney *et al.*, 1991), although its possible role in asthma therapy remains controversial. Immunotherapy of sensitized patients was associated with a marked inhibition of specific allergen-induced late-phase cutaneous responses (Varney *et al.*, 1993). Biopsies of these responses showed equivalent infiltration of cells expressing mRNA encoding IL-4 and IL-5, 24 hours following allergen challenge in both placebo- and immunotherapy-treated patients (despite the fact that in the latter patients the late response was markedly inhibited). In contrast, significant increases in cells expressing mRNA encoding IL-2 and IFN-γ were observed only in the immunotherapy-treated patients. These data are compatible with the hypothesis that immunotherapy promotes the development of allergen-specific Th1-like T lymphocytes whose products are effective in inhibiting the clinical response of sensitized atopic patients to allergen exposure. The possible mechanisms for this are not yet clear. While increased activation of Th1-like allergen-specific cells may inhibit allergen-specific IgE synthesis, most studies of immunotherapy do not show that this is associated with clinically significant reductions in serum concentrations of allergen-specific IgE. *Local* modulation of allergen-specific IgE synthesis within the inflamed mucosa may be more important in this regard. The production of allergen-specific antibodies of classes other than IgE may play a role in 'blocking' IgE-mediated responses. Again, it is not clear how the promotion of Th1-like allergen-specific cells might inhibit the pro-inflammatory effects of *established* Th2-like responses. The answers to these questions must await further studies.

Drug therapy

Data from many of the studies discussed above are consistent with the hypothesis that glucocorticoids ameliorate asthma and allergic disease at least partly by inhibiting the local synthesis of Th2-like cytokines in the inflamed mucosa. This raises the possibility that other drugs which inhibit activated CD4 T lymphocytes or their cytokine products may also be useful for the therapy of asthma and rhinitis. While glucocorticoids form the mainstay of anti-asthma therapy for a majority of patients, the rising mortality and morbidity from this disease attest to the possibility that not all asthmatics respond well to this therapy. It has recently been shown that cyclosporin A, an anti-T-lymphocyte drug which also has inhibitory effects on granulocytes such as eosinophils and basophils, was effective in improving disease severity in a proportion of chronic, severe, glucocorticoid-dependent asthmatics (Alexander *et al.*, 1992). Other possible novel approaches to drug therapy include cytokine antagonists, adhesion molecule antagonists and therapy with antibodies which neutralize CD4 T lymphocytes or cytokines.

Conclusion

There now exists considerable support for the hypothesis that asthma and allergic disease represent a specialized form of cell-mediated hypersensitivity (type IVc) reactions (see Chapter 2), in which cytokines and possibly other mediators secreted by activated T lymphocytes bring about the specific accumulation and activation of eosinophils in the bronchial and nasal mucosa. These cytokines are secreted in the context of a Th2-type pattern and putatively reflect a locally directed T-lymphocyte response against mucosal antigens, including aeroallergens. IgE-mediated mechanisms, the presence or absence of which are also highly influenced by Th2-like cytokines, are also likely to play a significant role in the pathogenesis of asthma and allergic diseases, although the relative contributions of these when compared with those mediated directly by T lymphocytes is not always clear, and may vary with the clinical presentation of the disease (Fig. 3.6). Inhibition of activated T lymphocytes, either by immunotherapy in the case of allergic disease or by drugs in allergic diseases and asthma, is likely to continue to form part of the fundamental basis for the therapy of these diseases.

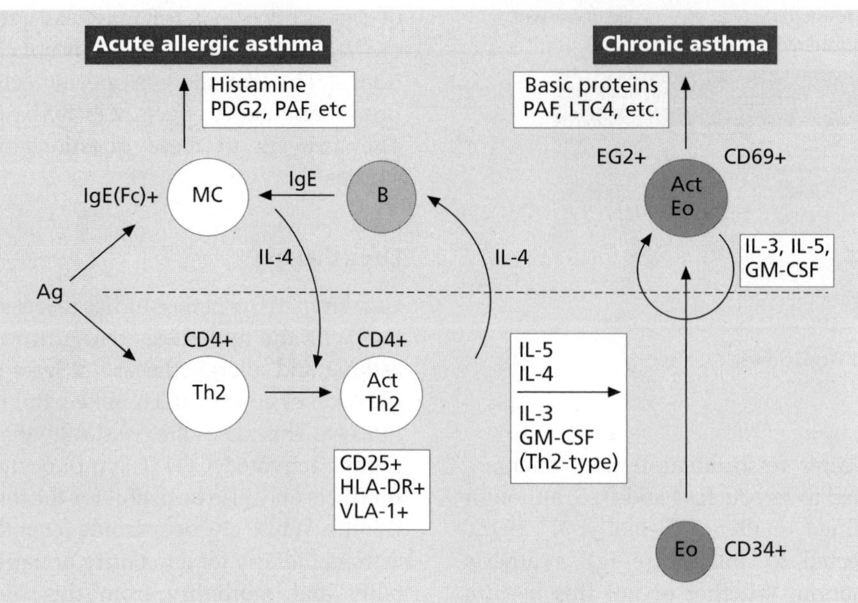

Fig. 3.6 Inflammatory mechanisms in asthma and allergic inflammation. Activation of Th2-like CD4+ T cells (TH) by specific antigen (Ag) results in the secretion of cytokines, particular IL-5, IL-4, IL-3 and GM-CSF, which influence eosinophil survival, differentiation, activation and adherence (Eo, Act Eo), and are implicated in orchestrating the specific eosinophil infiltration which characterizes mucosal inflammation in allergic disease and asthma. In parallel, allergens may trigger inflammatory processes through the cross-linking of surface IgE on mast cells (MC), resulting in the release of mediators such as histamine and leukotrienes. The relative importance of these processes in asthmatic and allergic inflammation in different clinical settings remains to be determined. The two systems are interdependent, in the sense that IL-4 derived from Th2-like TH cells is essential for IgE switching by B lymphocytes (B), and thus mast cell sensitization, whereas IL-4 release from IgE-triggered mast cells may further promote Th2-like T-lymphocyte development.

References

Adorini, L., Muller, S., Cardinaux, F., Lehmann, P.V., Falcioni, F. & Nagy, Z.A. (1988) *In vivo* competition between self peptides and foreign antigens in T-cell activation. *Nature*, **334**, 623–5.

Alexander, A.G., Barkans, J., Moqbel, R., Barnes, N.C., Kay, A.B. & Corrigan, C.J. (1994) Serum interleukin-5 concentrations in atopic and non-atopic patients with glucocorticoid-dependent chronic severe asthma. *Thorax*, **49**, 1231–3.

Alexander, A.G., Barnes, N.C. & Kay, A.B. (1992) Trial of cyclosporin A in corticosteroid-dependent chronic severe asthma. *Lancet*, **339**, 324–8.

Anwar, A.R.E., Moqbel, R., Walsh, G.M., Kay, A.B. & Wardlaw, A.J. (1993) Adhesion to fibronectin prolongs eosinophil survival. *J. Exp. Med.*, **177**, 819–24.

Arock, M., Merle-Beral, H., Dugas, B. *et al.* (1993) IL-4 release by human leukemic and activated normal basophils. *J. Immunol.*, **151**, 1441–7.

Aubry, J.-P., Pochon, S., Graber, P., Jansen, K.U. & Bonnefoy, J.-Y. (1992) CD21 is a ligand for CD23 and regulates IgE production. *Nature*, **358**, 505–7.

Azzawi, M., Bradley, B., Jeffery, P.K. *et al.* (1990) Identification of activated T lymphocytes and eosinophils in bronchial biopsies in stable atopic asthma. *Am. Rev. Resp. Dis.*, **142**, 1410–13.

Baggiolini, M. & Dahinden, C.A. (1994) CC chemokines in allergic inflammation. *Immunol. Today*, **15**, 127–33.

Basten, A. & Beeson, P.B. (1970) Mechanism of eosinophilia. II: Role of the lymphocyte. *J. Exp. Med.*, **131**, 1288–305.

Beasley, R., Roche, W., Roberts, J.A. & Holgate, S.T. (1989) Cellular events in the bronchi in mild asthma and after bronchial provocation. *Am. Rev. Resp. Dis.*, **139**, 806–17.

Bentley, A.M., Jacobson, M.R., Cumberworth, V. *et al.* (1992a) Immunohistology of the nasal mucosa in seasonal allergic rhinitis: increases in activated eosinophils and epithelial mast cells. *J. Allergy Clin. Immunol.*, **89**, 821–9.

Bentley, A.M., Maestrelli, P., Saetta, M. *et al.* (1992b) Activated T-lymphocytes and eosinophils in the bronchial mucosa in isocyanate-induced asthma. *J. Allergy Clin. Immunol.*, **89**, 821–9.

Bentley, A.M., Menz, G., Storz, C. *et al.* (1992c) Identification of T-lymphocytes, macrophages and activated eosinophils in the bronchial mucosa in intrinsic asthma: relationship to symptoms and bronchial responsiveness. *Am. Rev. Resp. Dis.*, **146**, 500–6.

Bentley, A.M., Durham, S.R., Robinson, D.S. *et al.* (1993a) Expression of the endothelial and leucocyte adhesion molecules ICAM-1, E-selectin and VCAM-1 in the bronchial mucosa in steady state and allergen-induced asthma. *J. Allergy Clin. Immunol.*, **92**, 857–68.

Bentley, A.M., Qiu Meng, Robinson, D.S., Hamid, Q., Kay, A.B. & Durham, S.R. (1993b) Increases in activated T-lymphocytes, eosinophils and cytokine messenger RNA for IL-5 and GM-CSF in bronchial biopsies after allergen inhalation challenge in atopic asthmatics. *Am. J. Resp. Cell Mol. Biol.*, **8**, 35–42.

Blackman, M., Kappler, J. & Marrack, P. (1990) The role of the T-cell receptor in positive and negative selection of developing T-cells.

Science, **248**, 1335–41.

Bochner, B.S., Luscinskas, F.W, Gimbrone, M.A.J. *et al.* (1993) Adhesion of human basophils, eosinophils and neutrophils to IL-1 activated human vascular endothlial cells: contributions of endothelial cell adhesion molecules. *J. Exp. Med.*, **173**, 1553–7.

Bradding, P., Roberts, J.A., Britten, K.M. *et al.* (1994) Interleukin-4, -5, -6 and tumor necrosis factor-α in normal and asthmatic airways: evidence for the human mast cells as a source of these cytokines. *Am. J. Respir. Cell Mol. Biol.*, **10**, 471–80.

Bradley, B.L., Azzawi, M., Assoufi, B. *et al.* (1991) Eosinophils, T-lymphocytes, mast cells, neutrophils and macrophages in bronchial biopsies from atopic asthmatics: comparison with atopic non-asthma and normal controls and relationship to bronchial hyperresponsiveness. *J. Allergy Clin. Immunol.*, **88**, 661–74.

Braun, R.K., Franchini, M., Erard, F. *et al.* (1993) Human peripheral blood eosinophils produce and release interleukin-8 on stimulation with calcium ionophore. *Eur. J. Immunol.*, **23**, 956–90.

Briner, T.J., Kuo, M.C., Keating, K.M., Rogers, B.L. & Greenstein, J.L. (1993) Peripheral T-cell tolerance induced in naive and primed mice by subcutaneous injection of peptides from the major cat allergen *Fel dI*. *Proc. Nat. Acad. Sci. USA*, **90**, 7608–12.

Broide, D.H., Lotz, M., Cuomo, A.J., Cobum, D.A., Federman, E.C. & Wasserman, S.I. (1992a) Cytokines in symptomatic asthma airways. *J. Allergy Clin. Immunol.*, **89**, 958–67.

Broide, D.H., Paine, M.M. & Firestein, G.S. (1992b) Eosinophils express interleukin-5 and granulocyte/macrophage colony-stimulating factor mRNA at sites of allergic inflammation in asthmatics. *J. Clin. Invest.*, **90**, 1414–24.

Burrows, B., Martinez, F.D., Halonen, M., Barbee, R.A. & Cline, M.G. (1989) Association of asthma with serum IgE levels and skin-test reactivity to allergens. *New Engl. J. Med.*, **320**, 271–7.

Cher, D.J. & Mosmann, T.R. (1987) Two types of murine helper T cell clone. II: Delayed-type hypersensitivity is mediated by Th1 clones. *J. Immunol.*, **138**, 3688–94.

Clark, E.A. & Leadbetter, J.A. (1994) How B- and T-cells talk to each other. *Nature*, **367**, 425–8.

Corrigan, C.J., Brown, P.H., Barnes, N.C., Tsai, J.J. & Kay, A.B. (1991a) Glucocorticoid resistance in chronic asthma: peripheral blood T-lymphocyte activation and a comparison of the T-lymphocyte inhibitory effects of glucocorticoids and cyclosporin A. *Am. Rev. Resp. Dis.*, **144**, 1026–32.

Corrigan, C.J., Brown, P.H., Barnes, N.C., Tsai, J.J. & Kay, A.B. (1991b) Glucocorticoid resistance in chronic asthma: glucocorticoid pharmacokinetics, glucocorticoid receptor characteristics and inhibition of peripheral blood T-cell proliferation by glucocorticoids *in vitro*. *Am. Rev. Resp. Dis.*, **144**, 1016–25.

Corrigan, C.J., Haczku, A., Gemou-Engesaeth, V. *et al.* (1993) CD4 T-lymphocyte activation in asthma is accompanied by increased concentrations of interleukin-5: effect of glucocorticoid therapy. *Am. Rev. Resp. Dis.*, **147**, 540–7.

Corrigan, C.J., Hamid, Q., North, J. *et al.* (1995) Peripheral blood CD4, but not CD8 T-lymphocytes in patients with exacerbation of asthma transcribe and translate messenger RNA encoding cytokines which prolong eosinophil survival in the context of a TH2-type pattern: effect of glucocorticoid therapy. *Am. J. Respir. Cell Mol. Biol.*, **12**, 567–78.

Corrigan, C.J., Hartnell, A. & Kay, A.B. (1988) T-lymphocyte activation in acute severe asthma. *Lancet*, **i**, 1129–31.

Corrigan, C.J. & Kay, A.B. (1990) CD4 T-lymphocyte activation in acute severe asthma. Relationship to disease severity and atopic status. *Am. Rev. Resp. Dis.*, **141**, 970–7.

Costa, J.J., Matossian, K., Resnick, M.B. *et al.* (1993) Human eosinophils can express the cytokines tumour necrosis factor-alpha and macrophage inflammatory protein-1 alpha. *J. Clin. Invest.*, **91**, 2673–84.

De Waal-Malefyt, R., Abrams, J., Bennett, B., Figdor, C.G. & De Vries, J.E. (1991a) Interleukin-10 (IL-10) inhibits cytokine synthesis by human monocytes: an autoregulatory role of IL-10 produced by monocytes. *J. Exp. Med.*, **174**, 1209–20.

De Waal-Malefyt, R., Haanen, J., Spits, H. *et al.* (1991b) Interleukin-10 (IL-10) and viral IL-10 strongly reduce antigen-specific human T-cell proliferation by diminishing the antigen presenting capacity of monocytes via down-regulation of class II major histocompatibility complex expression. *J. Exp. Med.*, **174**, 915–24.

De Waal-Malefyt, R., Figdor, C.G., Huijbens, R. *et al.* (1993) Effects of IL-13 on phenotype, cytokine production and cytotoxic function of human monocytes. *J. Immunol.*, **191**, 6370–81.

Del Prete, G.F., De Carli, M., Mastromauro, C. *et al.* (1991a) Purified protein derivative of *Mycobacterium tuberculosis* and excretory-secretory antigen(s) of *Toxocara canis* expand *in vitro* human T cells with stable and opposite (type 1 T helper or type 2 T helper) profile of cytokine production. *J. Clin. Invest.*, **88**, 346–50.

Del Prete, G.F., De Carli, M., Ricci, M. & Romagnani, S. (1991b) Helper activity for immunoglobulin synthesis of Th1 and Th2 human T cell clones. The help of Th1 clones is limited by their cytolytic capacity. *J. Exp. Med.*, **174**, 809–13.

Del Prete, G.F., De Carli, M., Almerigogna, F., Giudizi, M.G., Biagiotti, R. & Romagnani, S. (1993a) Human IL-10 is produced by both type 1 helper (Th1) and type 2 helper (Th2) T cell clones and inhibits their antigen-specific proliferation and cytokine production. *J. Immunol.*, **150**, 353–60.

Del Prete, G.F., De Carli, M., D'Elios, M.M. *et al.* (1993b) Allergen exposure induces the activation of allergen-specific Th2 cells in the airway mucosa of patients with allergic respiratory disorders. *Eur. J. Immunol.*, **23**, 1445–9.

Dent, L.A., Strath, M., Mellor, A.L. & Sanderson, C.J. (1990) Eosinophilia in transgenic mice expressing interleukin-5. *J. Exp. Med.*, **172**, 1425–31.

Doi, S., Gemou-Engesaeth, V., Kay, A.B. & Corrigan, C.J. (1994) Polymerase chain reaction quantification of cytokine messenger RNA expression in peripheral blood mononuclear cells of patients with severe asthma: effect of glucocorticoid therapy. *Clin. Exp. Allergy*, **24**, 854–67.

Dunnill, M.S. (1960) The pathology of asthma with special reference to changes in the bronchial mucosa. *J. Clin. Pathol.*, **13**, 27–33.

Dunnill, M.S., Massarella, G.R. & Anderson, J.A. (1969) A comparison of the quantitative anatomy of the bronchi in normal subjects, in status asthmaticus, in chronic bronchitis and in emphysema. *Thorax*, **24**, 176–9.

Durham, S.R., Sun Ying, Varney, V.A. *et al.* (1992) Cytokine messenger RNA expression for IL-3, IL-4, IL-5 and GM-CSF in the nasal mucosa after local allergen provocation: relationship to tissue eosinophilia. *J. Immunol.*, **148**, 2390–4.

Durum, S.K., Schmidt, J.A. & Oppenheim, J.J. (1985) Interleukin 1: an immunological perspective. *Ann. Rev. Immunol.*, **3**, 263–82.

Elices, M.J., Osborn, L., Takada, Y. *et al.* (1990) VCAM-1 on activated endothelium interacts with the leucocyte integrin VLA-4 at a site distinct from the VLA-4/fibronectin binding site. *Cell*, **60**, 577–84.

Fabbri, L.M., Danielli, D., Crescioli, S. *et al.* (1988) Fatal asthma in a subject sensitised to toluene disocyanate. *Am. Rev. Resp. Dis.*, **137**, 1494–8.

Filley, W.V., Holley, K.E., Kephart, G.M. & Gleich, G.J. (1982) Identification by immunofluorescence of eosinophil granule major basic protein in lung tissues of patients with bronchial asthma. *Lancet*, **ii**, 11–16.

Fiorentino, D.F., Bond, M.W. & Mossmann, T.R. (1989) Two types of mouse T helper cells. IV. Th2 clones secrete a factor that inhibits cytokine production by Th1 clones. *J. Exp. Med.*, **170**, 2081–95.

Firestein, G.S., Roeder, W.D., Laxer, J.A. *et al.* (1989) A new murine CD4+ T cell subset with an unrestricted cytokine profile. *J. Immunol.*, **143**, 518–25.

Fish, S., Zenowich, E., Fleming, M. & Manser, T. (1989) Molecular analysis of original antigenic sin. I. Clonal selection, somatic mutation and isotype switching during a memory B cell response. *J. Exp. Med.*, **170**, 1191–209.

Gaga, M., Frew, A.J., Varney, V.A. & Kay, A.B. (1991) Eosinophil activation and T-lymphocyte infiltration in allergen-induced late phase skin reactions and classical delayed-type hypersensitivity. *J. Immunol.*, **147**, 816–22.

Gajewski, T.F., Pinnas, M., Wong, T. & Fitch, F.W. (1991) Murine Th1 and Th2 clones proliferate optimally in response to distinct antigen-presenting cell populations. *J. Immunol.*, **146**, 1750–8.

Gascan, H., Gauchat, J-F., Aversa, G., Van Vlasselaer, P. & De Vries, J.E. (1991) Anti-CD40 monoclonal antibodies or CD4+ T cell clones induce IgG4 and IgE switching in purified human B cells via different signalling pathways. *J. Immunol.*, **147**, 8–13.

Gauchat, J.-F., Henchoz, S., Mazzei G. *et al.* (1993) Induction of human IgE synthesis by mast cells and basophils. *Nature*, **365**, 340–3.

Gauchat, J.-F., Aversa, G.G., Gascan, H. & De Vries, J.E. (1992) modulation of IL-4 induced germline ε mRNA synthesis in human B-cells by tumor necrosis factor-α, anti-CD40 monoclonal antibodies or transforming growth factor-β correlates with levels of IgE production. *Int. Immunol.*, **4**, 397–406.

Gauchat, J-F., Lebman, D.A., Coffman, R.L., Gascan, H. & De Vries, J.E. (1990) Structure and expression of germline ε transcripts in human B cells induced by IL-4 to switch to IgE production. *J. Exp. Med.*, **172**, 463–73.

Gemou-Engesaeth, V., Kay, A.B., Bush, A. & Corrigan, C.J. (1994) Activated peripheral blood CD4 and CD8 T-lymphocytes in childhood asthma: correlation with eosinophilia and disease severity. *Ped. Allergy Immunol.*, **5**, 170–7.

Gilbert, K.M. & Weigle, W.O. (1992) B cell presentation of a tolerogenic signal to Th clones. *Cell. Immunol.*, **139**, 58–71.

Graham, D.R., Luksza, A.R. & Evans, C.C. (1985) Bronchoalveolar lavage in asthma. *Thorax*, **40**, 717.

Haczku, A., Alexander, A., Brown, P., Kay, A.B. & Corrigan, C.J. (1994) The effect of dexamethasone, cyclosporin A and rapamycin on T-lymphocyte proliferation *in vitro*: comparison of cells from corticosteroid sensitive and corticosteroid resistant chronic asthmatics. *J. Allergy Clin. Immunol.*, **93**, 510–19.

Hamid, Q., Azzawi, M., Ying, S. *et al.* (1991) Expression of mRNA for interleukin-5 in mucosal bronchial biopsies from asthma. *J. Clin. Invest.*, **87**, 1541–6.

Hamid, Q., Barkans, J., Abrams, J.S. *et al.* (1992b) Human eosinophils synthesize and secrete interleukin-6 *in vitro*. *Blood*, **80**, 1496–501.

Hamid, Q., Barkans, J., Robinson, D.S., Durham, S.R. & Kay, A.B. (1992a) Co-expression of CD25 and CD3 in atopic allergy and asthma. *Immunology*, **75**, 659–63.

Harding, F.A., McArthur, J.G., Gross, J.A., Raulet, D.H. & Allison, H.P. (1992) CD28-mediated signalling co-stimulates murine T-cells and prevents induction of anergy in T-cell clones. *Nature*, **356**, 607–9.

Hattevig, G., Kjellman, B. & Bjorksten, B. (1987) Clinical symptoms and IgE responses to common proteins and inhalants in the first 7 years of life. *Clin. Allergy*, **17**, 571–8.

Hattevig, G., Kjellman, B. & Bjorksten, B. (1993) Appearance of IgE antibodies to ingested and inhaled allergens during the first 12 years of life in atopic and non-atopic children. *Ped. Allergy Immunol.*, **4**, 182–6.

Higgins, J.A., Lamb, J.R., Marsh, S.G.E. *et al.* (1992) Peptide-induced non-responsiveness of HLA-DP restricted human T-cells reactive with *Dermatophagoides* spp. (house dust mite). *J. Allergy Clin. Immunol.*, **90**, 749–56.

Hollenbaugh, D., Grosmaire, L.S., Kullas, C.D. *et al.* (1992) The human T cell antigen gp39, a member of the TNF gene family, is a ligand for the CD40 receptor: expression of a soluble form of gp39 with B cell co-stimulatory activity. *EMBO J.*, **11**, 4313–21.

Holt, P.G. (1994) A potential vaccine strategy for asthma and allied atopic diseases during early childhood. *Lancet*, **344**, 456–8.

Holt, P.G., McMenamin, C. & Nelson, D. (1990) Primary sensitisation to inhalant allergens during infancy. *Ped. Allergy Immunol.*, **1**, 3–13.

Houston, J.C., De Navasquez, S. & Trounce, J.R. (1953) A clinical and pathological study of fatal cases of status asthmaticus. *Thorax*, **8**, 207–13.

Hoyne, G.F., O'Hehir, R.E., Wraith, D.C., Thomas, W.R. & Lamb, J.R. (1993) Inhibition of T-cell antibody responses to house dust mite allegen by inhalation of the dominant T-cell epitope in naive and sensitised mice. *J. Exp. Med.*, **178**, 1783–8.

Jabara, H.H., Fu, S.M., Geha, R.S. & Vercelli, D. (1990) CD40 and IgE: synergism between anti-CD40 monoclonal antibody and IL-4 in the induction of IgE synthesis by highly purified human B cells. *J. Exp. Med.*, **172**, 1861–4.

Jeffery, P.K., Godfrey, R.W., Adelroth, E., Nelson, F., Rogers, A. & Johansson, S.-A. (1992) Effects of treatment on airway inflammation and thickening of reticular collagen in asthma: a quantitative light and electron microscopic study. *Am. Rev. Resp. Dis.*, **145**, 890–9.

Jeffery, P.K., Wardlaw, A.J., Nelson, F.C., Collins, J.V. & Kay, A.B. (1989) Bronchial biopsies in asthma: an ultrastructural, quantitative study and correlation with hyperreactivity. *Am. Rev. Resp. Dis.*, **140**, 1745–53.

Jenkins, M.K., Taylor, P.S., Norton, S.D. & Urdhal, K.B. (1991) CD28 delivers a co-stimulatory signal involved in antigen-specific IL-2 production by human T cells. *J. Immunol.*, 147, 2461–6.

June, C.H., Ledbetter, J.A., Linsley, P.S. & Thompson, C.B. (1990) Role of the CD28 receptor in T cell activation. *Immunol. Today*, **11**, 211–16.

Kappler, J.W., Staerz, U., White, J. & Marrack, P.C. (1988) Self tolerance eliminates T-cells specific for Mls-modified products of the major histocompatibility complex. *Nature*, **332**, 35–40.

Kay, A.B., Ying, S., Varney, V. *et al.* (1991) Messenger RNA expression of the cytokine gene cluster IL-3, IL-4, IL-5 and GM-CSF in allergen-induced late phase cutaneous reactions in atopic subjects. *J. Exp. Med.*, **173**, 775–8.

Kimata, H., Yoshida, A., Ishioka, C., Lindley, L. & Mikawa, H. (1992) Interleukin-8 selectively inhibits immunoglobulin E production induced by IL-4 in human B-cells. *J. Exp. Med.*, **176**, 1227–31.

Kinawa, M., Gately, M., Gabler, V., Chizzonite, R., Fargeas, C. & Delespesse, G. (1992) Recombinant interleukin-12 suppresses the synthesis of IgE by interleukin-4-stimulated human lymphocytes. *J. Clin. Invest.*, **90**, 262–9.

Kirby, J.G., Hargreave, F.E., Gleich, G.J. & O'Byrne, P.M. (1987) Bronchoalveolar cell profiles of asthmatic and non-asthmatic subjects. *Am. Rev. Resp. Dis.*, **136**, 379–83.

Kisielow, P., Bluthmann, H., Staerz, U.D., Steinmetz, M. & Von Boehmer, H. (1988) Tolerance in T-cell receptor transgenic mice involves deletion of non-mature CD4+ and CD8+ T-lymphocytes. *Nature*, **333**, 742–6.

Kita, H., Ohnishi, T., Okubo, Y., Wiler, D., Abrams, J.S. & Gleich, G.J. (1991) GM-CSF and interleukin-3 release from human peripheral blood eosinophils and neutrophils. *J. Exp. Med.*, **174**, 743–8.

Kyan-Aung, U., Haskard, D.O., Poston, R.N., Thornhill, M.H. & Lee, T.H. (1991) Endothelial leukocyte adhesion molecule 1 and intercellular adhesion molecule 1 mediate adhesion of eosinophils to endothelial cells *in vitro* and are expressed by endothelium in allergic cutaneous inflammation *in vivo*. *J. Immunol.*, **146**, 521–8.

Laitinen, L.A., Heino, M., Laitinen, A., Kava, T. & Haahtela, T. (1985) Damage of airway epithelium and bronchial reactivity in patients with asthma. *Am. Rev. Resp. Dis.*, **131**, 599–606.

Lamb, J.R., Skidmore, B.J., Green, N., Chiller, J.M. & Feldmann, M. (1983) Induction of tolerance in influenza virus-immune T-lymphocyte clones with synthetic peptides of influenza hemagglutinin. *J. Exp. Med.*, **157**, 1434–40.

Lanier, L.L., O'Fallon, S., Somoza, C. *et al.* (1995) CD80 (B7) and CD86 (B70) provide similar costimulatory signals for T-cell proliferation cytokine production, and generation of CTL. *J. Immunol.*, **154**, 97–105.

Lehn, M., Weiser, W.Y., Engelharn, S.J., Gillis, S. & Remold, H.G. (1989) IL-4 inhibits H_2O_2 production and anti-leishmanial capacity of human cultured monocytes mediated by IFN-γ. *J. Immunol.*, **143**, 3020–4.

Linsley, P.S., Brady, W., Urnes, M., Grosmaire, L.S., Damle, N.K. & Ledbetter, J.A. (1991) CTLA-4 is a second receptor for the B-cell activation antigen B7. *J. Exp. Med.*, **174**, 561–9.

Lopez, A.F., Williamson, D.J., Gamble, J.R. *et al.* (1986) Recombinant human granulocyte-macrophage colony stimulating factor stimulates *in vitro* mature human eosinophil and neutrophil function, surface receptor expression and survival. *J. Clin. Invest.*, **78**, 1220–8.

Lopez, A.F., Sanderson, C.J., Gamble, J.R., Campbell, H.D., Young, I.G. & Vadas, M.A. (1988) Recombinant human interleukin-5 is a selective activator of eosinophil function. *J. Exp. Med.*, **167**, 219–24.

MacDonald, H.R., Pedrazzini, T., Schneider, R., Louis, J.A. & Zinkernagel, R.M. (1988) Intrathymic elimination of Mlsa-reactive (V(beta6)+) cells during neonatal tolerance induction to Mlsa-encoded antigens. *J. Exp. Med.*, **167**, 2005–10.

McDuffie, M., Roehm, N., Born W., Marrack, P. & Kappler, J.W. (1987) T-cell receptor/MHC interactions in the thymus and the shaping of the T-cell repertoire. *Transpl. Proc.*, **19**(S7), 111–16.

Maggi, E., Biswas, P., Del Prete, G. *et al.* (1991) Accumulation of Th2-like helper T cells in the conjunctiva of patients with vernal conjunctivitis. *J. Immunol.*, **146**, 1169–174.

Maggi, E., Parronchi, P., Manetti, R. *et al.* (1992) Reciprocal regulatory role of IFN-γ and IL-4 on the *in vitro* development of human Th1 and Th2 clones. *J. Immunol.*, **148**, 2142–7.

Martinez, O.M., Gibbons, R.S., Gavoroy, M.R. & Aronson, F.R. (1990) IL-4 inhibits IL-2 receptor expression and IL-2-dependent proliferation of human T cells. *J. Immunol.*, **144**, 2211–15.

Masuyama, K., Jacobosn, M.R., Rak, S. *et al.* (1994) Topical glucocorticosteroid (fluticasone propionate) inhibits cytokine mRNA expression for interleukin-4 (IL-4) in the nasal mucosa in allergic rhinitis. *Immunology*, **82**, 192–9.

Mattoli, S., Mattoso, V.L., Soloperto, M., Allegra, L. & Fasoli, A. (1991) Cellular and biochemical characteristics of bronchoalveolar lavage fluid in symptomatic nonallergic asthma. *J. Allergy Clin. Immunol.*, **87**, 794–802.

Minty, A., Chalon, P., Derocq, J.-M. *et al.* (1993) Interleukin-13 is a new human lymphokine regulating inflammatory and immune responses. *Nature*, **362**, 248–50.

Miyajima, H., Hirano, T., Hirose, S., Karasuyama, H., Okumara, K. & Ovary, Z. (1991) Suppression by IL-2 of IgE production by B cells stimulated by IL-4. *J. Immunol.*, **146**, 457–62.

Moqbel, R., Ying, S., Barkans, J. *et al.* (1995) Identification of mRNA for interleukin-4 in human eosinophils with granule localization and release of the translated product. *J. Immunol.*, **155**, 4939–47.

Moqbel, R., Hamid, Q., Sun Ying *et al.* (1991) Expression of mRNA and immunoreactivity for the granulocyte/macrophage colony stimulating factor (GM-CSF) in activated human eosinophils. *J. Exp. Med.*, **174**, 749–52.

Mosmann, T.R., Cherwinski, H., Bond, M.W., Gedlin, M.A. & Coffman, R.L. (1986) Two types of murine helper T-cell clones. I. Definition according to profiles of lymphokine activities and secreted proteins. *J. Immunol.*, **136**, 2348–57.

Mosmann, T.R. & Coffman, R.L. (1989) Th1 and Th2 cells: different patterns of lymphokine secretion lead to different functional properties. *Ann. Rev. Immunol.*, **7**, 145–73.

Mosmann, T.R. & Moore, K.W. (1991) The role of IL-10 in cross-regulation of Th1 and Th2 responses. *Immunoparasitol. Today*, **12**, 49–53.

Mueller, D.L., Jenkins, M.K. & Schwartz, R.H. (1989) Clonal expansion versus functional clonal inactivation: a costimulatory signalling pathway determines the outcome of T-cell receptor occupancy. *Ann. Rev. Immunol.*, **7**, 445–63.

Nabavi, N., Freeman, G.J., Gault, A. *et al.* (1992) Signalling through the MHC class II cytoplasmic domain is required for antigen presentation and induces B7 expression. *Nature*, **360**, 266–8.

O'Hehir, R.E., Aguilar, B.A., Schmidt, T.J., Gollnick, S.O. & Lamb, J.R. (1991) Functional activation of *Dermatophagoides* spp. (house dust mite) reactive human T-cell clones. *Clin. Exp. Allergy*, **21**, 209–15.

O'Hehir, R.E., Mach, B., Berte, C. *et al.* (1990) Direct evidence for a functional role of HLA-DRB1 and -DRB3 gene products in the recognition of *Dermatophagoides* spp. (house dust mite) by helper T-lymphocytes. *Int. Immunol.*, **2**, 885–92.

O'Hehir, R.E., Verhoef, A., Panagiotopoulou, E. *et al.* (1993) Analysis of human T-cell responses to the group II allergen of *Dermatophagoides* species: localisation of major antigenic sites. *J. Allergy Clin. Immunol.*, **92**, 105–13.

Ohkawara, Y., Yamauchi, K., Tanno, Y. *et al.* (1992) Human lung mast cells and pulmonary macrophages produce tumor necrosis factor-α in sensitised lung tissue after IgE receptor triggering. *Am. J. Respir. Cell Mol. Biol.*, **7**, 385–92.

Paliard, X., De Waal Malefyt, R., Yssel, H. *et al.* (1988) Simultaneous production of IL-2, IL-4 and interferon-gamma by activated human CD4+ and CD8+ T-cell clones. *J. Immunol.*, **141**, 849–55.

Parronchi, P., Tiri, A., Macchia, D. *et al.* (1990) Noncognate contact-dependent B-cell activation can promote IL-4-dependent *in vitro* human IgE synthesis. *J. Immunol.*, **144**, 2102–6.

Parronchi, P., Macchia, D., Piccinni, M.P. *et al.* (1991) Allergen and bacterial antigen-specific T-cell clones established from atopic donors show a different profile of cytokine production. *Proc. Nat. Acad. Sci. USA*, **88**, 4538–42.

Pene, J., Rousset, F., Briere, F. *et al.* (1988a) IgE regulation by normal human lymphocytes is induced by interleukin-4 and suppressed by interferons γ and α and prostaglandin E_2. *Proc. Nat. Acad. Sci. USA*, **85**, 6880–4.

Pene, J., Rousset, F., Briere, F. *et al.* (1988b) Interleukin-5 enhances interleukin-4-induced IgE production by normal human B-cells. The role of soluble CD23 antigen. *Eur. J. Immunol.*, **18**, 929–35.

Punnonen, J., Aversa, G., Cocks, B.G. *et al.* (1993) Interleukin-13 induces interleukin-4-independent IgG4 and IgE synthesis and CD23 expression by human B-cells. *Proc. Nat. Acad. Sci. USA*, **90**, 3730–4.

Rackemann, F.M. (1940) Intrinsic asthma. *J. Allergy*, **11**, 147–62.

Rackemann, F.M. (1947) A working classification of asthma. *Am. J. Med.*, **3**, 601–6.

Ramb-Lindhauer, C., Feldmann, A., Rotte, M. & Neumann, C. (1991) Characterization of grass pollen reactive T cell lines derived from lesional atopic skin. *Arch. Dermatol. Res.*, **283**, 71–6.

Rand, T.H., Cruikshank, W.W., Center, D.M. & Weller, P.F. (1991a) CD4-mediated stimulation of human eosinophils: lymphocyte chemoattractant factor and other CD4-binding ligands elicit eosinophil migration. *J. Exp. Med.*, **173**, 1521–8.

Rand, T.H., Silberstein, D.S., Kornfeld, H. & Weller, P.F. (1991b) Human eosinophils express functional IL-2 receptors. *J. Clin. Invest.*, **88**, 825–32.

Robinson, D.S., Hamid, Q., Ying, S. *et al.* (1992) Evidence for a predominant 'Th2-type' bronchoalveolar lavage T-lymphocyte population in atopic asthma. *New Engl. J. Med.*, **326**, 298–304.

Robinson, D.S., Ying, S., Bentley, A.M. *et al.* (1993b) Relationships among numbers of bronchoalveolar lavage cells expressing messenger ribonucleic acid for cytokines, asthma symptoms, and airway methacholine responsiveness in atopic asthma. *J. Allergy Clin. Immunol.*, **92**, 397–403.

Robinson, D.S., Hamid, Q., Ying, S. *et al.* (1993c) Prednisolone treatment in asthma is associated with modulation of bronchoalveolar lavage cell interleukin-4, interleukin-5 and interferon-gamma cytokine gene expression. *Am. Rev. Resp. Dis.*, **148**, 420–6.

Robinson, D.S., Ying, S., Taylor, I.K. *et al.* (1994) Evidence for a Th1-like bronchoalveolar T cell subset and predominance of IFN-gamma gene activation in pulmonary tuberculosis. *Am. J. Resp. Crit. Care Med.*, **149**, 989–93.

Robinson, D.S., Bentley, A.M., Hartnell, A., Kay, A.B. & Durham, S.R. (1993a) Activated memory T helper cells in broncoalveolar lavage from atopic asthmatics. Relationship to asthma symptoms, lung function and bronchial responsiveness. *Thorax*, **48**, 26–32.

Romagnani, S. (1992) Induction of Th1 and Th2 response: a key role for the 'natural' immune response? *Immunol. Today*, **13**, 379–81.

Rothenberg, M.E., Owen, W.F., Silberstein, D.S. *et al.* (1988) Human eosinophils have prolonged survival, enhanced functional properties and become hypodense when exposed to human interleukin-3. *J. Clin. Invest.*, **81**, 1986–92.

Rothenberg, M.E., Petersen, J., Stevens, R.L. *et al.* (1989) IL-5 dependent conversion of normodense human eosinophils to the hypodense phenotype uses 3T3 fibroblasts for enhanced viability, accelerated hypodensity and sustained antibody-depedent cytotoxicity. *J. Immunol.*, **143**, 2311–16.

Salgame, P., Abrams, J.S., Clayberger, C. *et al.* (1991) Differing cytokine profiles of functional subsets of human CD4 and CD8 T cell clones. *Science*, **254**, 279–82.

Salvato, G. (1968) Some histological changes in chronic bronchitis and asthma. *Thorax*, **23**, 168–72.

Sandford, A.J., Shirakawa, T., Moffatt, M.F. *et al.* (1993) Localisation of atopy and β subunit of high-affinity IgE receptor (FcεRI) on chromosome 11q. *Lancet*, **341**, 332–4.

Sarfati, M., Luo, H. & Delespesse, G. (1989) IgE synthesis by chronic lymphocytic leukaemia cells. *J. Exp. Med.*, **170**, 1775–80.

Schall, T.J., O'Hehir, R.E., Goeddel, D.V. & Lamb, J.R. (1992) Uncoupling of cytokine mRNA expression and protein secretion during the induction phase of T-cell anergy. *J. Immunol.*, **148**, 381–7.

Schleimer, R.P., Sterbinsky, S.A., Kaiser, J. *et al.* (1992) IL-4 induces adherence of human eosinophils and basophils but not neutrophils to endothelium: association with expression of VCAM-1. *J. Immunol.*, **148**, 1086–92.

Schwartz, R.H. (1992) Co-stimulation of T lymphocytes: the role of CD28, CTLA-4 and B7/BB1 in IL-2 production and immunotherapy. *Cell*, **71**, 1065–8.

Sehmi, R., Wardlaw, A.J., Cromwell, O., Kurihara, K., Waltmann, P. & Kay, A.B. (1992) IL-5 selectively enhances the chemotactic response of eosinophils obtained from normal but not eosinophilic subjects. *Blood*, **79**, 2952–9.

Shirakawa, T., Li, A., Dubowitz, M. *et al.* (1994) Association between atopy and variants of the β-subunit of the high-affinity immunoglobulin E receptor. *Nature Genet.*, **7**, 125–30.

Smith, J.B., Kunjummen, R.D., Kishimoto, T.K. & Anderson, D.C. (1992) Expression and regulation of L-selectin on eosinophils from human adults and neonates. *Ped. Res.*, **32**, 465–71.

Ying, S., Durham S.R., Barkans J. *et al.* (1993) T cells are the principal source of interleukin-5 mRNA in allergen-induced rhinitis. *Am. J. Respir. Cell Mol. Biol.*, **9**, 356–60.

Ying, S., Durham, S.R., Jacobson M.R. *et al.* (1994) T lymphocytes and mast cells express messenger RNA for interleukin-4 in the nasal mucosa in allergen-induced rhinitis. *Immunology*, **82**, 200–6.

Ying, S., Durham, S.R., Corrigan, C.J., Hamid, Q. & Kay, A.B. (1995) Phenotype of cells expressing mRNA for Th2-type (interleukin-4 and interleukin-5) and Th1-type (interleukin-2 and interferon-gamma) cytokines in bronchoalveolar lavage and bronchial biopsies from atopic asthmatics and normal control subjects. *Am. J. Respir. Cell Mol. Biol.*, **12**, 477–87.

Swain, S.L., Weinberg, A.D. & English, M. (1990) CD4+ T cell subsets: lymphokine secretion of memory cells and efector cells which develop from precursors *in vitro*. *J. Immunol.*, **144**, 1788–98.

Tsicopoulos, A., Hamid, Q., Varney, V. *et al.* (1992) Preferential messenger RNA expression of Th1-type cells (IFN-γ+, IL-2+) in classical delayed-type (tuberculin) hypersensitivity reactions in human skin. *J. Immunol.*, **148**, 2058–61.

Van der Heijden, F.L., Wierenga, E.A., Bos, J.D. & Kapsenberg, M.L. (1991) High frequency of IL-4 producing CD4+ allergen-specific T lymphocytes in atopic dermatitis leisonal skin. *J. Invest. Dermatol.*, **97**, 389–94.

Varney, V.A., Jacobson, M.R., Sudderick, R.M. *et al.* (1992) Immunohistology of the nasal mucosa following allergen-induced rhinitis. Indentification of activated T-lymphocytes, eosinophils and neutrophils. *Am. Rev. Resp. Dis.*, **145**, 170–6.

Varney, V.A., Hamid, Q.A., Gaga, M. *et al.* (1993) Influence of grass pollen immunotherapy on cellular infiltration and cytokine mRNA expression during allergen-induced late-phase cutaneous responses. *J. Clin. Invest.*, **92**, 644–51.

Varney, V., Gaga, M., Frew, A.J., Aber, V.A., Kay, A.B. & Durham, S.R. (1991) Usefulness of immunotherapy in patients with severe summer hayfever uncontrolled by anti-allergic drugs. *Brit. Med. J.*, **302**, 265–9.

Vercelli, D., Jabara, H.H., Arai, K.-I., Yokota, T. & Geha, R.S. (1989) Endogenous IL-6 plays an obligatory role in IL-4-induced human IgE synthesis. *Eur. J. Immunol.*, **19**, 1419–24.

Verhoef, A., Higgins, J.A., Thorpe, C.J. *et al.* (1993) Clonal analysis of the atopic immune response to the group 2 allergen of *Dermatophagoides* spp. Identification of HLA-DR and -DQ restricted T-cell epitopes. *Int. Immunol.*, **5**, 1589–97.

Walker, C., Kaegi, M.K., Braun, M.D. & Blaser, K. (1991) Activated T cells and eosinophils in bronchoalveolar lavages from subjects with asthma correlated with disease severity. *J. Allergy Clin. Immunol.*, **88**, 935–42.

Walsh, G.M., Hartnell, A., Mermod, J-J., Kay, A.B. & Wardlaw, A.J.

(1991) Human eosinophil, but not neutrophil adherence to IL-1 stimulated HUVEC is α4β1 (VLA-4) dependent. *J. Immunol.*, **146**, 3419–23.

Walsh, G.M., Hartnell, A., Wardlaw, A.J., Kurihara, K., Sanderson, C.J. & Kay, A.B. (1990) IL-5 enhances the *in vitro* adhesion of human esoinophils, but not neutrophils, in a leucocyte integrin (CD11/CD18)-dependent manner. *Immunology*, **71**, 258–65.

Wardlaw, A.J., Moqbel, R., Cromwell, O. & Kay, A.B. (1986) Platelet activating factor: a potent chemotactic and chemokinetic factor for human eosinophils. *J. Clin. Invest.*, **78**, 1701–6.

Wardlaw, A.J., Dunnette, S., Gleich, G.J., Collins, J.V. & Kay, A.B. (1988) Eosinophils and mast cells in bronchoalveolar lavage in mild asthma: relationship to bronchial hyperreactivity. *Am. Rev. Resp. Dis.*, **137**, 62–9.

Warringa, R.A., Koenderman, L., Kok, P.T., Kreukniet, J. & Bruijnzeel, P.L. (1991) Modulation and induction of eosinophil chemotaxis by granulocyte/macrophage colony stimulating factor and IL-3. *Blood*, **77**, 2694–700.

Weller, P.F., Rand, T.H., Barrett, T., Elovic, A., Wong, D.T.W. & Finberg, R.W. (1993) Accessory cell function of human eosinophils: HLA-DR dependent, MHC-restricted antigen presentation and interleukin-1α formation. *J. Immunol.*, **150**, 2554–62.

Williams, M.E., Shea, C.M., Lichtman, A.H. & Abbas, A.K. (1992) Antigen receptor-mediated anergy in resting lymphocytes and T cell clones. *J. Immunol.*, **149**, 1921–6.

Wong, D.T., Weller, P.F., Galli, S.J. *et al.* (1990) Human eosinophils express transforming growth factor alpha. *J. Exp. Med.*, 172, 673–81.

Yamamura, M., Wagn, X.-H., Ohmen, J.D. *et al.* (1992) Cytokine patterns of immunologically mediated tissue damage. *J. Immunol.*, **149**, 1470–5.

Yssel, H., Johnson, K.E., Schneider, P.V. *et al.* (1992) T-cell activation-inducing epitopes of the house dust mite allergen *Der p I*: proliferation and lymphokine production patterns by *Der p I*-specific CD4+ T-cell clones. *J. Immunol.*, **148**, 738–45.

Yssel, H., Shanafelt, M.C., Soderberg, C., Schneider, P.V., Anzola, J. & Peitz, G. (1991) *Borrelia burgdorferi* activates a T helper type 1-like T cell subset in lyme arthritis. *J. Exp. Med.*, **174**, 593–601.

Zurawski, G. & De Vries, J.E. (1994) Interleukin-13, an interleukin-4-like cytokine that acts on monocytes and B-cells, but not on T-cells. *Immunol. Today*, **15**, 19–26.

Zurawski, S.M., Vega, F., Huyghe, G. & Zurawski, G. (1993) Receptors for interleukin-13 and interleukin-4 are complex and share a novel component that functions in signal transduction. *EMBO J.*, **12**, 2663–70.

CHAPTER 4

Immunoglobulin Structure, Synthesis and Genetics

A.R. Venkitaraman

Introduction

Antibody or immunoglobulin (Ig) molecules were first recognized by Boehringer and Kitasato in the late 19th century as humoral factors mediating the specific response to immunizing agents such as bacteria or their toxins. The identification of these factors as proteins (Heidelberger & Kendall, 1929), their purification from patients (Edelman & Gall, 1962) or animals (Potter, 1972) with multiple myeloma, and their structural characterization (Hilschmann & Craig, 1965; Edelman, 1973; Porter, 1973) laid the foundations for the modern field of molecular immunology.

It has by now become apparent that Ig molecules perform two distinct but complementary roles in the immune system (Fig. 4.1). Historically, the role of *secreted* Ig molecules was the first to be defined. These molecules are the primary mediators of humoral immunity or hypersensitivity, triggering effector mechanisms such as cytotoxicity, phagocytosis or the complement system when bound to antigen. More recently, it has been demonstrated that *membrane-bound* Ig molecules serve as antigen receptors on the surface of B lymphocytes and enable the antigen-specific clonal activation or silencing, expansion or deletion that is the basis of immune system function. The structure of Ig molecules and the genes that encode them is very highly adapted to these two functional roles. This chapter will review the present knowledge of the manner in which the structure, synthesis and genetics of Ig molecules underlies their function.

Ig structure

Ig classes

Ig molecules consist of pairs of polypeptide chains (Edelman, 1973; Porter, 1973), termed the *heavy* (H) and *light* (L) chains (Fig. 4.2). A complete Ig molecule is a tetramer of two H and two L chains held together by disulphide bonds. In humans and mice, five different *isotypes* or *classes* of Ig molecules (IgM, IgD, IgG, IgE and IgA) exist and are determined by the presence of H chains corresponding to each class (μ, δ, γ, ε and α) (Heidelberger & Pedersen, 1937; Deutsch *et al.*, 1956; Rowe & Fahey, 1965; Tomasi *et al.*, 1965; Ishikaza & Ishikaza, 1966). In addition, there are two classes of L chains (κ and λ) (Korngold & Lipari, 1956) and each may associate with any of the five H-chain isotypes to form complete Ig tetramers. It must be noted that the two H chains within any Ig tetramer are identical to one another, as are the two L chains. Thus, for example, an IgM molecule may have a $\mu 2\kappa 2$ or $\mu 2\lambda 2$ composition.

H chains of the γ and α classes may be further split into numbered subclasses (Table 4.1). Membrane-bound and secretory forms of each H-chain class are distinguished by the presence of a hydrophobic transmembrane anchor sequence and cytoplasmic tail in the membrane-bound form (Fig. 4.2(b)). These are replaced by a short segment of hydrophilic amino acids (the secretory tailpiece) in the secretory form, which may vary in length between different classes (Table 4.1). The genetic events which account for the production of these alternative forms of Ig H chains are discussed on p. 72.

The ratio in which the two L-chain classes are used in Ig

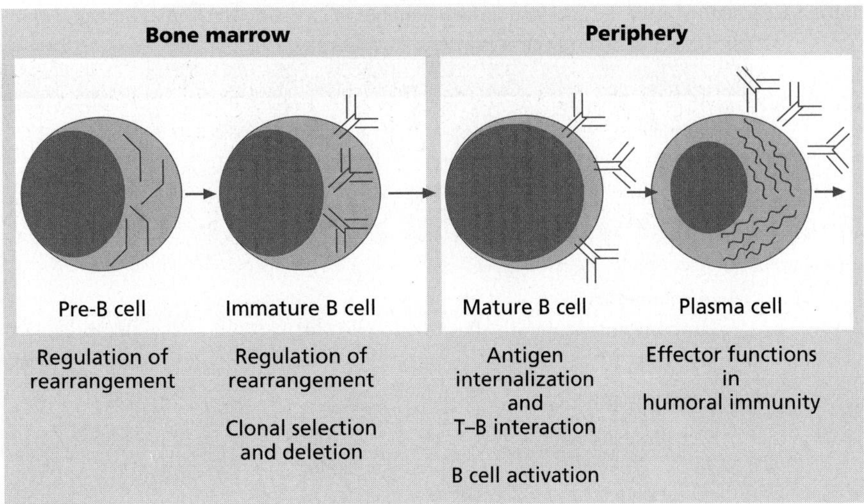

Fig. 4.1 Expression and function of Ig molecules during B-lymphocyte differentiation.

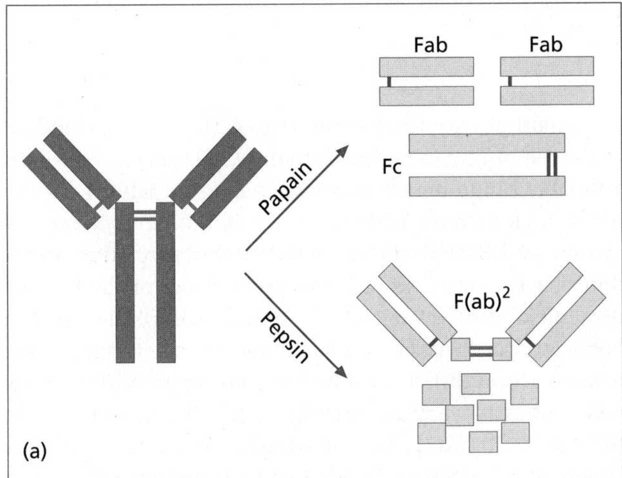

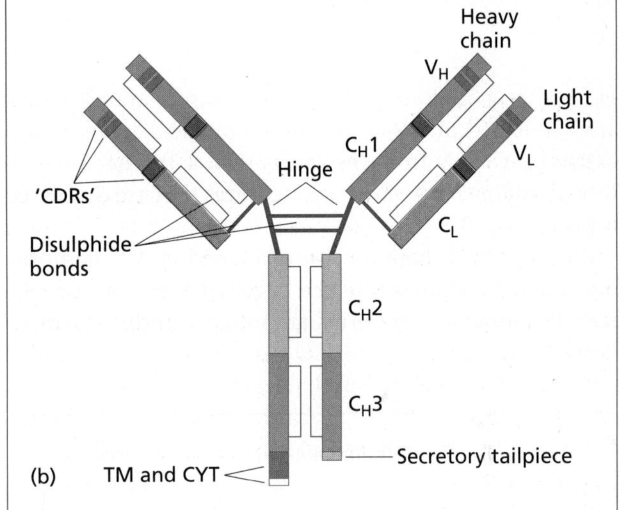

Fig. 4.2 Structure of Ig molecules. (a) Proteolytic fragments of IgG generated by digestion with pepsin and papain are denoted Fab, F(ab)2 (monovalent and divalent antigen binding fragments) and Fc (crystallizable fragment). (b) The general features of an IgG molecule are depicted. One membrane-bound and one secretory H chain are shown for convenience, but such an association does not occur naturally. CDR, complementarity determining region; TM, transmembrane segment; CYT, cytoplasmic tail. Glycosylation sites are not shown. (Modified from Venkitaraman, 1994.)

molecules varies from species to species for as yet unknown reasons. Human antibodies have a κ : λ ratio of roughly 60 : 40, whereas in murine antibodies the ratio is 95 : 5.

Domain structure of the H and L chains

The individual polypeptide chains of Ig molecules are subdivided into amino-terminal variable (V) and carboxyl-terminal constant (C) regions. The C region determines the class to which the chain belongs. In contrast, the V regions, which are involved in antigen binding, exhibit great amino-acid sequence diversity even amongst chains belonging to the same class.

Each chain is modular in its organization, the basic module (termed the immunoglobulin superfamily or *IgSF* domain) comprising approximately 110 amino-acid residues (Williams & Barclay, 1988). Whilst the Ig L chains contain two IgSF domains each, Ig H chains may contain either four or five. Individual IgSF domains in a chain are connected by short polypeptide strands which permit them to rotate relative to one another. Each IgSF domain assumes a three-dimensional structure consisting of two β-pleated sheets about 90–100 nm (9–10Å) apart, approximately parallel to one another and held together by a disulphide bond (Davies *et al.*, 1975; Amzel & Poljak, 1979; Davies & Metzeger, 1983). In C region IgSF domains, one

Table 4.1 Structure of murine (Mo) and human (Hu) heavy chains. (After Venkitaraman, 1994.)

	μ	δ	γ	ε	α
C_H domains	C_H1–4	C_H1 and C_H3 (Mo) C_H1–3 (Hu)	C_H1–3	C_H1–4	C_H1–3
Subclasses	—	—	γ1, γ2a/b, γ3 (Mo) γ1–4 (Hu)	—	α1,2 (Hu)
Size in amino acids					
Hinge region	0	35 (Mo) 70 (Hu)	13, 16, 22, 17 (Mo) 15, 12, 62, 20 (Hu)	0	14 (Mo) 10, 24 (Hu)
Cytoplasmic tail	3	3	28	28	14
Secretory tailpiece	20	22 (Mo) 8 (Hu)	2	8	20
M_r (kDa)	72	63	51–56	72	57

of the sheets has four, and the second three, strands which are connected at either end by amino-acid loops which extend outwards from the sheets (Fig. 4.3). The V region IgSF domains have additional features that are discussed below.

A typical Ig H chain consists of a V region (V_H) comprising one IgSF domain, which together with the first C-region domain (C_H1) forms an antigen binding 'arm' in combination with the L chain (Fig. 4.2). The arm is linked to the remaining C-region domains C_H2 and C_H3 through a flexible hinge region of variable length (Table 4.1). The hinge regions have little sequence homology between H chains of different classes, except for the relative abundance of Pro and Cys residues accounting for their structural flexibility (Kabat *et al.*, 1991). Disulphide bridges between the two H chains in an H_2/L_2 tetramer are formed through Cys residues in the hinge regions (Fig. 4.2), and may vary in number from one (in δ) to 11 (in human γ3). In μ and ε H chains the hinge region is replaced by an entire, additional IgSF domain (numbered C_H2) and so these two H chains include a total of four rather than three C-region domains (Kabat *et al.*, 1991).

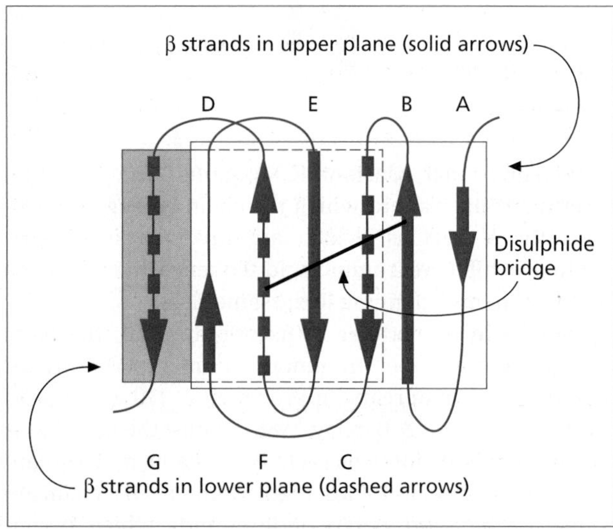

Fig. 4.3 Structure of a C-region IgSF domain. A side view is shown. Beta strands are designated by letters, those in the upper plane are thick lines and those in the lower plane are broken lines. The loops connecting the strands are thin lines, as is the disulphide bridge between strands B and F. (Modified from Venkitaraman, 1994.)

All IgH chains bear N-linked glycosylation sites. They vary in number from one in the C_H2 domain of γ-chains to five and six respectively in μ- and ε-chains. The function of glycosylation is not fully understood. It has been postulated to contribute to the stability of H_2/L_2 tetramers.

Each L chain comprises a single V_L domain linked to a constant Cκ or Cλ domain (Fig. 4.2(b)). Although subclasses of L chain C regions exist (e.g. there are at least nine Cλ subclasses and a single Cκ class in humans), there is very little difference between their amino-acid sequences.

Antigen binding

The antigen binding site of Ig molecules is formed by the paired V-region domains contributed by the Ig H/L chains (Davies *et al.*, 1975; Amzel & Poljak, 1979; Davies

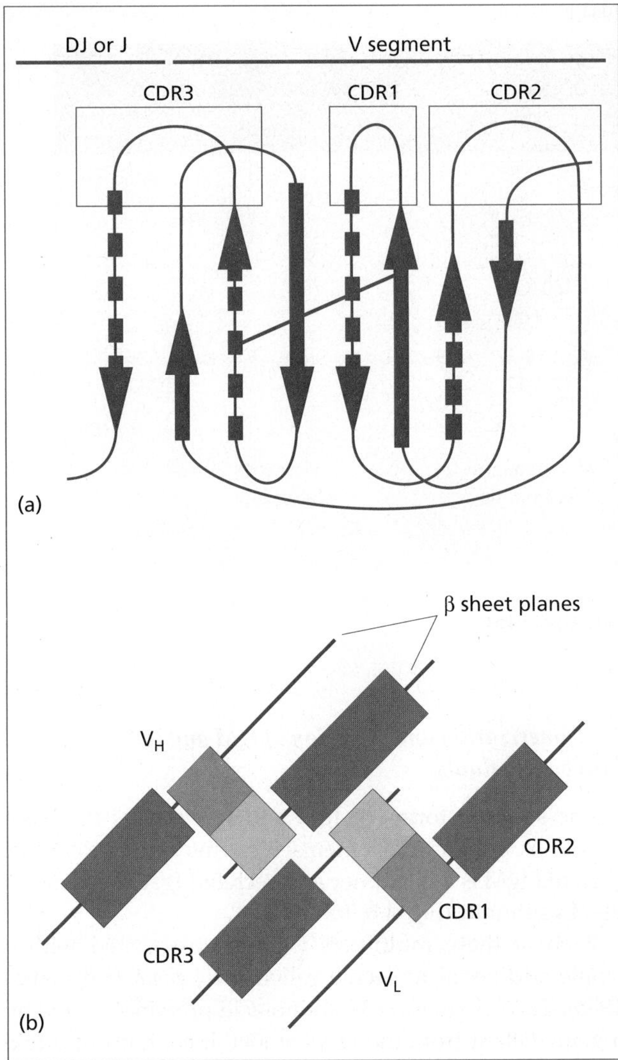

Fig. 4.4 The antigen binding site. (a) A V-region IgSF domain in side view (cf. Fig. 4.3). The portions of the polypeptide encoded by the *V*, *D*, and *J* segments are marked, as are the CDR loops. (b) The antigen binding site in top view. The CDR loops depicted as rectangles surmount the planes of the β-sheets shown in (a) and extend outwards and upwards from the page. (Modified from Venkitaraman, 1994.)

& Metzeger, 1983). Each V-region domain (Fig. 4.4(a)) assumes a structure similar to the C-region IgSF domains depicted in Fig. 4.3, except that there is an extra strand in the lower β-pleated sheet. Alignment of the amino-acid sequences of multiple V-region domains reveals four regions with little variability (the 'framework' regions FR1-4), surrounding three highly variable regions (the 'hypervariable' or 'complementarity determining' regions CDR1-3) (Wu & Kabat, 1970). X-ray crystallographic studies (Amit *et al.*, 1986) show that the CDR are loops extending out from the β-pleated sheets formed by the frameworks (FR) (Fig. 4.3); the CDR loops of the paired V domains together shape the antigen combining site (Fig. 4.4(b)), which may range from a flat surface to a deep pocket. Thus, it has been possible in at least a few examples to transfer the specificity of antigen binding simply by 'grafting' appropriate CDR upon an irrelevant FR (Jones *et al.*, 1986). However, this result is far from general, as discussed below.

Although in theory each CDR loop could assume a large number of possible conformations, analysis of solved structures suggests that in fact only a relatively small number of *canonical* CDR conformations exists (Chothia *et al.*, 1989). However, differences in the FR regions (which alter the relative positions of the CDR loops), as well as sequence differences in a few critical residues near the centre of the antigen combining site, conspire to enable specific binding to diverse antigens. It is therefore important to note that in many instances FR residues distant from the actual antigen contact sites may have dramatic effects upon binding.

Ig allotypes and idiotypes

As discussed previously, differences in the C regions of the murine and human Ig chains generate the five H-chain and two L-chain isotypes or classes which are found in all members of these species. In addition, there are allelic differences (termed *allotypes*) in the C regions of the H and L chains which give rise to differences between individuals of the same species (Natvig & Kunkel, 1973 and references therein; Kabat *et al.*, 1991). For example, allelic variants of the γ1–4 and α2 H chains and the κ L chain (termed the Gm, Am and Km allotypes, respectively) are found in humans.

The V region of each Ig molecule is distinct, and therefore distinguishes it from other Ig molecules in the same individual (Natvig & Kunkel, 1973, and references therein; Kabat *et al.*, 1991). These variations give rise to *idiotypic* differences, some of which are unique to a specific Ig molecule (private idiotypes), while others may be shared between a small group (public idiotypes).

Class-specific differences in structure and function

Although Ig H chains of all the five classes are remarkably similar in their overall structure, small but highly conserved differences between them give rise to class-specific differences in Ig function (Morgan & Weigle, 1987; Burton & Woof, 1992). The most striking differences are in the capacity of secreted Ig molecules of different classes to bind to and activate components of the complement cascade, and to bind to specific Fc receptors at the cell

Table 4.2 Properties of human secreted Ig molecules. (After Venkitaraman, 1994.)

			IgG					IgA	
	IgM	IgD	G1	G2	G3	G4	IgE	A1/2	sec
Composition									
H_2/L_2 units	5	1		1			1	1	2
Assoc. chains	J	—		—			—	—	J, SC
Approx M_r (kDa)	950	175		160 (G3) 150 (other)			190	160	415
Serum conc.* (per cent of serum Ig)	1 (5–10)	0.03 (0.5)		15 (70–85)			trace —		2 (5–15)
Complement activation†	++	–	+	±	+	–	–		–
Distribution of Fc receptors	—	—		Macrophages Neutrophils			Mast cells Basophils		—
Placental transfer	–	–	+	–	+	±	–		–

* Average serum concentration in adults (mg/ml).
† Classical pathway activation is shown. IgG4 and IgA also activate the alternative pathway.

surface. These differences in protein binding can generally be ascribed to amino-acid variations in the hinge, C_H2 and C_H3 domains (reviewed in Morgan & Weigle, 1987; Burton & Woof, 1992). For example, receptors for the Fc portion of IgG (FcγRI) bind to the distal hinge region, whilst the first component of complement binds to the C_H2 domain. Table 4.2 summarizes the differences between isotypes; two specific examples are considered in greater detail below. It must be noted that the transmembrane and cytoplasmic segments of membrane-bound Ig H chains also differ from class to class (Kabat *et al.*, 1991; see Table 4.1), although the functional role of these differences is not yet understood.

Binding of IgE to Fc receptors

The binding of serum IgE to Fc receptors on mast cells and basophils is a critical event in the initiation of many allergic reactions. The high-affinity Fc receptor for IgE (FcεRI) is a four-chain complex consisting of one α- and one β-chain with a disulphide-linked γ-chain dimer (Blank *et al.*, 1989). Each FcεRI complex binds a single IgE molecule with an affinity of about $10^{-10}\,M^{-1}$, but does not bind Ig molecules of other classes. Binding occurs through the α-chain of FcεRI, with which a short region at the Cε2–Cε3 junction in the ε H chain interacts (Helm *et al.*, 1988). Mast cells and basophils are activated when bound IgE is cross-linked by multivalent antigen. The γ-chain of FcεRI, also shared by Fc receptors for IgG (Kurosaki *et al.*, 1992), is strikingly homologous to the ξ component of the T-cell receptor and plays an important role in activation (Orloff *et al.*, 1990; Takai *et al.*, 1994).

Multimerization and secretion of IgM and IgA into bodily fluids

In the secreted forms of IgM and IgA classes the basic H_2/L_2 subunits may themselves multimerize. Thus, secreted IgM is a pentamer and secreted IgA is a dimer of H_2/L_2 subunits (Fig. 4.5, Table 4.2).

Each of these multimers is found associated with a single additional molecule called the *J chain* (Koshland, 1985). The J chain is a 137-amino-acid protein encoded by a gene distant from the Ig gene loci. It contains multiple Cys residues which form intrachain disulphide bonds, as well as linkages to the associated Ig H chains.

Secretory IgM contains a region in its carboxyl terminus (Davis *et al.*, 1989; Sitia *et al.*, 1990) which binds the endoplasmic reticulum resident protein BiP (binding protein, discussed further on p. 73). Thus, monomeric forms are retained intracellularly whilst pentamer formation displaces BiP and allows secretion.

Dimeric IgA/J chain is particularly abundant in fluids such as saliva, breast milk and the secretions of the respiratory, gastrointestinal and genitourinary tracts. In these secretions the IgA/J-chain complex is associated with secretory component (SC) (Brandtzaeg & Prydz, 1984), a protein consisting of five IgSF domains. SC is the extracellular portion of a receptor for polymeric Ig found on the surface of epithelial cells (Mostov *et al.*, 1980; Crago *et al.*, 1989). This receptor binds to circulating IgA/J chain and transports the complex to the luminal surface of the epithelial cell, whereupon it is cleaved and free IgA/J chain is released into the secretions bound to the extracellular portion of the receptor (Fig. 4.5).

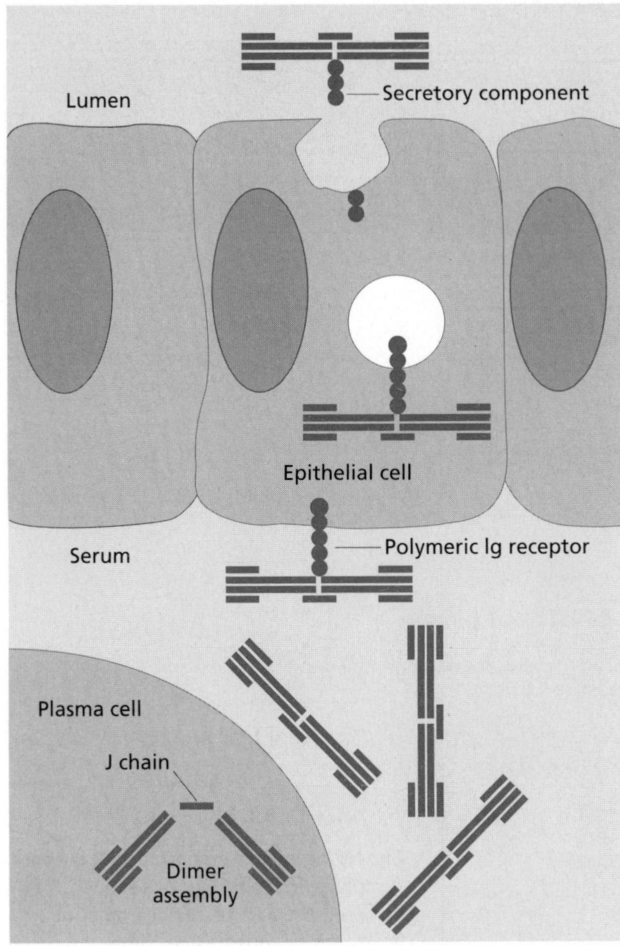

Fig. 4.5 Secretion and transepithelial transport of IgA. Dimer assembly with J chain occurs in plasma cells, and follows the intracellular pathway detailed in Fig. 4.13. The polymeric Ig receptor on epithelial cells lining the gastrointestinal, respiratory and genitourinary tracts mediates transepithelial transport. Assembly, secretion and transport of pentameric IgM/J-chain complexes is similar.

Monoclonal antibodies and antibody engineering: exploitation of structure–function relationships in Ig molecules

Immunization of animals with antigens results in a *polyclonal* response: that is, a variety of distinct Ig molecules of different classes, with differing affinities of antigen binding and with different specificities, are found in the serum. A method was described in 1975 for making immortalized rodent plasma cell lines ('hybridomas') that secrete an unlimited quantity of a single (*monoclonal*), predetermined species of Ig molecule (Köhler & Milstein, 1975; Milstein, 1980). A wide range of different monoclonal antibodies has since been developed that have a number of applications in diagnosis and therapy, although the vast majority are of rodent rather than human origin.

Newer approaches to the synthesis of monoclonal antibodies have taken advantage of the known relationships between the structure and functional properties of Ig molecules (reviewed in Winter & Milstein, 1991). For example, the C regions of the H chains determine how well particular Ig isotypes bind to and activate the complement cascade. 'Grafting' of the C regions from different human IgG subclasses onto the same antigen binding V region using the techniques of genetic engineering has shown that the $\gamma1$ subclass is the most effective at mediating complement-dependent lysis, whilst the $\gamma4$ subclass is the least. These techniques thereby enable the production of 'chimeric' antibodies containing human C regions with the desired effector properties, and murine V regions with the desired antigen binding specificity (Reichmann *et al.*, 1988), which are likely to be less immunogenic when used for therapy in humans.

The techniques of genetic engineering have also been used to synthesize artifical Ig molecules entirely *in vitro* without the need for animal immunization. It has proven possible to use *Escherichia coli*-based expression systems with phage lambda vectors (Huse *et al.*, 1989) or single-stranded filamentous phage particles (McCafferty *et al.*, 1990) to isolate antigen-binding Ig molecules or fragments thereof, which can, if required, be 'grafted' onto C regions or other molecules such as toxins with the desired effector properties. These techniques have since been greatly refined to enable the rapid isolation of antibody fragments with high affinity for virtually any desired antigen (Winter *et al.*, 1994, and references therein).

Organization of Ig genes

Ig molecules are required to mediate the recognition of an enormous number of diverse antigens. Given the impossibility of encoding each specificity as a discrete gene, it was recognized as early as 1965 (Dreyer & Bennett, 1965) that the Ig genes must have a specialized organization to fulfil the biological imperative to generate great diversity starting from a limited amount of genetic information. This prediction was confirmed with the demonstration that a series of somatic DNA rearrangements is required to generate a functional Ig gene (Hozumi & Tonegawa, 1976; Brack *et al.*, 1978; Early *et al.*, 1980).

The Ig genes are unique in their segmental organization in the chromosome (Leder, 1982; Ellison & Hood, 1983; Tonegawa, 1983) in that the antigen binding V-region domains are encoded by two or three distinct gene segments (*V*, variable; *D*, diversity; *J*, joining, see Fig. 4.6), which are separated in the germ-line and brought together by a series of DNA rearrangements during lymphocyte development. The number of distinct *V* segments

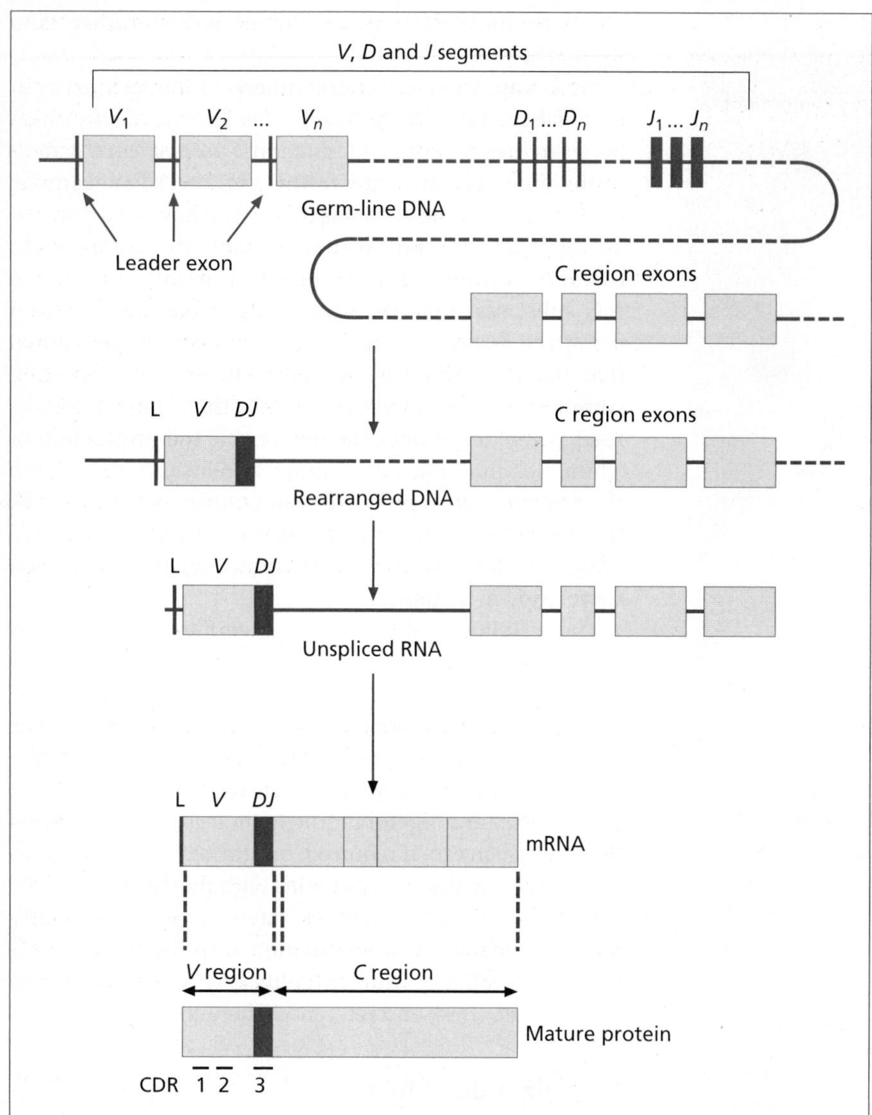

Fig. 4.6 Segmental organization of Ig genes. A prototypic H-chain locus is shown. *V*, *D* and *J* segments and *C*-region exons are boxes, and introns are lines; large gaps in the DNA strand are indicated by broken lines. The correspondence of regions of the mature IgH protein to the mRNA encoding it is shown at the bottom. Note that the leader peptide is cleaved from the mature protein post-translationally.

may run into the hundreds, and when combined with tens of *D* and *J* segments, a very large pool of receptor specificities can be generated combinatorially.

Not all Ig chains make use of *D* segments. The antigen binding V-region domains of the κ and λ L chains of Ig are encoded by rearranged *V–J* (and not *V–D–J*) segments.

Each rearranged *V–D–J* or *V–J* segment may be linked to constant region exons, permitting Ig molecules of a given *C*-region class to assume virtually any specificity of antigen binding. Furthermore, in the case of Ig H chains, a given *V–D–J* segment may be linked to *C*-region exons of each of the five classes at different stages in the life history of a single B cell. Thus, antibody molecules of different classes may have identical V-region domains and assume identical specificities of recognition.

The *V*, *D*, *J* gene segments and *C*-region exons encoding each of the Ig chains are clustered together in loci (Fig. 4.6). Varying numbers of these segments (as well as some *C* regions) are pseudogenes which are incapable of encoding functional polypeptide chains. In general within each locus the clusters encoding *V* segments are 5′ to the *D* and *J* clusters, which are in turn upstream to the *C*-region exons (Fig. 4.6). However, this 5′ to 3′ order need not always apply.

The chromosomal locations of the Ig loci and the estimated numbers of *V*, *D* and *J* segments are presented in Table 4.3. The nucleotide and amino-acid sequences of the coding regions of all known murine and human Ig H and L genes have been compiled, as have those of a number of different *V*, *D* and *J* segments (Kabat *et al.*, 1991).

Table 4.3 Features of the Ig loci.

	Chromosomal location	Estimated numbers (pseudogenes in brackets) *V*	*D*	*J*
IgH				
Murine	12	~128 (?)	12	4
Human	14	~95 (30–40)	~30 (?)	6 (3)
Igκ				
Murine	6	~160 (?)	–	5
Human	2	~76 (30)	–	5
Igλ				
Murine	16	2	–	4
Human	22	~50 (?)	–	>9 (~3)

The Ig H-chain locus

The discussion which follows is based upon the well-characterized human and murine IgH loci.

C_H *genes*

The eight murine C_H genes (Shimizu *et al.*, 1981; Honjo, 1983), separated by long intervening sequences, are contained within a 200-kb fragment of genomic DNA (Fig. 4.7). Each gene consists of multiple exons, three or four of which encode the C_H protein domains and one, the hinge region (where present). The C_H exons are flanked by introns of 100–300 bp, but are separated by a much longer intron from the two exons encoding the transmembrane segment and short cytoplasmic tail of the membrane-bound forms of the H chains. Two polyadenylation (polyA) sites are present, one is distal to the secretory tail-piece and the second, to the transmembrane exons. The Cμ gene is shown in Fig. 4.7.

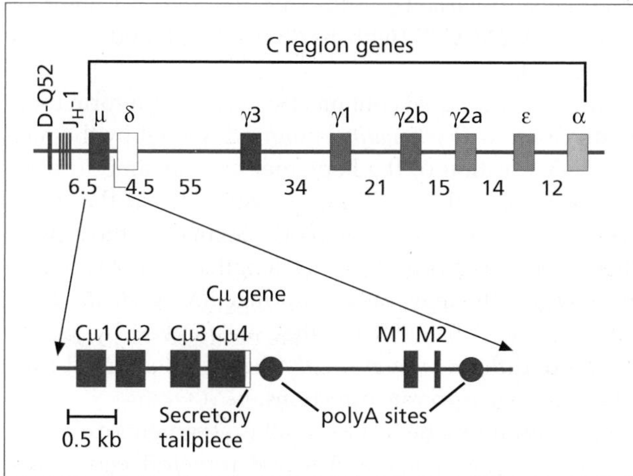

Fig. 4.7 The Ig H-chain gene locus. The murine Ig H gene locus is shown in the top half of the figure, with intergenic distances between the J_H cluster and *C*-region genes in kb (not to scale). The exon/intron structure of the murine *C*μ gene is shown below. Exons are shown as boxes, and introns as lines; M1 and M2 denote the two membrane exons; polyadenylation (polyA) sites are circles. (Modified from Venkitaraman, 1994.)

In humans, the 350-kb C_H locus contains nine genes and three pseudogenes (prefixed with a ψ) in the following 5′ to 3′ order (Ravetch *et al.*, 1981; Ellison & Hood, 1982; Flanagan & Rabbitts, 1982; Walter *et al.*, 1990): J_H–9 kb–μ–8 kb–δ–60 kb–γ3–26 kb–γ1–19 kb–ψε1–13 kb–α1–35 kb–ψγ–25 kb–γ2–19 kb–γ4–23 kb–ε–10 kb–α2. Thus, a gene duplication event has given rise to two copies of the γ–γ–ε–α set at the 3′ end.

In humans additional C_H pseudogenes may be found outside the IgH locus. A second ε pseudogene—ψε2—is located on chromosome 9, and there is evidence for the existence of at least one more ψγ.

D *and* J *segment clusters*

The D_H and J_H segments together encode between 17 and 38 amino acids at the carboxyl-terminal end of the V-region domain corresponding to CDR3 (Figs 4.4(a) & 4.6). D_H segments vary between three and 40 nucleotides in length, and J_H segments, between 45 and 60.

In the mouse, 11 D_H segments grouped into two families (*D*-SP2 with nine members and *D*-FL16 with two) map within a 60-kb DNA fragment (Kurosawa & Tonegawa, 1982; Wood & Tonegawa, 1983) located 20 kb upstream to the J_H cluster which contains four segments (J_H1–4) (Sakano *et al.*, 1980; Honjo, 1983). An additional single D_H segment (*D*-Q52) lies just 700 bp upstream of J_H1 (Fig. 4.7).

The human J_H cluster of about 3 kb contains six segments (J_H1–6) and three pseudogenes (ψJ_H1–3), and lies 9 kb upstream to Cμ (Ravetch *et al.*, 1981; Walter *et al.*, 1990). A single *D* segment homologous to the murine *D*-Q52 is contained within the J_H cluster between the 5′-most pseudogene ψJ_H1 and the first functional segment J_H1. The number and organization of the remaining D_H segments has not yet been established, but they may be dispersed within the locus on chromosme 14 (Buluwela *et al.*, 1988; Matsuda *et al.*, 1988) and may also be found on chromosomes 15 and 16. At least four D_H segments lie in a 33-kb region upstream of the J_H cluster, and may even be upstream of at least some V_H segments.

V_H *genes*

Each V_H segment consists of a 5′ exon of about 80 bp encoding the leader sequence of the mature Ig H-chain polypeptide. It is separated by a short intron from the V_H

exon of 300 bp that encodes the first 100 amino acids of the V-region protein domain, including CDR 1 and 2 (Figs 4.4(a) & 4.6).

Approximately 128 murine V_H segments are grouped into 14 families containing from one to 60 members each (Kabat *et al.*, 1991). Within each family, nucleotide sequence homologies are of the order of 80%. Members of each V_H family cluster together on the chromosome (Brodeur & Riblet, 1984; Rathbun *et al.*, 1987; Krawinkel *et al.*, 1989).

A recently completed physical map of the human V_H locus (Matsuda *et al.*, 1993; Cook *et al.*, 1994) reveals 95 V_H segments in a region extending some 1100 kb upstream of the J_H cluster on chromosome 14. Of these, about 30 represent pseudogenes, and 14 have not yet been detected in functional rearrangements (Tomlinson *et al.*, 1992). The exact number of functional V_H segments (roughly 50) varies from individual to individual depending on the haplotype. They fall into seven families (V_H1–7), which, in contrast to their murine counterparts, are interspersed in their chromosomal localization. It should be noted that additional human V_H segments on chromosomes 15 and 16 are located distant from the Ig H-chain locus; however, not all have associated D_H and J_H segments and so their functional importance is uncertain.

The Ig L-chain gene loci

One V_L and one J_L segment rearrange to encode the V-region protein domains of both κ and λ L chains, whilst the C_L domain is encoded by a single exon.

The murine κ locus (Max *et al.*, 1981) includes five *J*κ segments located 3 kb 5′ to a single *C*κ exon. An estimated 160 murine *V*κ segments, each similar in its structure to a V_H segment, are currently grouped into 19 families. The human κ locus differs somewhat in its organization (Zachau, 1993). Seventy-six *V*κ segments have been mapped; about 40 are proximal and 36 distal to the *J*κ cluster containing four *J*κ segments. Human *V*κ segments are grouped into seven families, of which the first three families include the most members. A strong but unexplained bias is observed in the repertoire of *V*κ segments expressed in human antibodies (Cox *et al.*, 1994): the *V*κ segments that are distal to *J*κ are highly under-represented.

In mice, the λ locus (Selsing *et al.*, 1989) contains two repeats of a *V*λ–*J*λ–*C*λ–*J*λ–*C*λ unit, making a total of two *V*λ segments, and four *C*λ segments each with a *J*λ just 5′. The distance between the two repeats is not known. The restricted repertoire of *V* and *J* segments may be related to the fact that only 5% of murine antibodies use a λ L chain. In contrast, nearly half of human antibodies use a λ L chain and the human λ gene locus is correspondingly more diverse. At least 36 *V*λ segments exist (Williams & Winter, 1993), grouped into nine families (Chuchana *et al.*, 1990; Kabat *et al.*, 1991). Nine *C*λ genes, each with an adjacent *J*λ segment, have been identified, and six are linked in a 50-kb fragment (Hieter *et al.*, 1981).

Ig gene rearrangement

Genetic studies on the segmental organization of the Ig genes in the germ-line discussed in the preceding section demonstrated that functional Ig genes must be assembled during B lymphopoiesis by gene rearrangement. It quickly became apparent that the process of rearrangement is highly ordered and stringently controlled at different stages of B-cell differentiation (Alt *et al.*, 1981, 1984). Current knowledge of the underlying principles that govern the operation of the complex rearrangement machinery will be outlined here.

Joining signals and the 12/23 rule

For gene rearrangement to work, its enzymatic machinery must in some way recognize the segments that are available for rearrangement. Comparison of the nucleotide sequences of unrearranged and rearranged Ig gene segments has revealed these 'joining signals', which consist of conserved heptamer and nonamer sequences separated by a degenerate spacer element of either 12 or 23 base pairs (Max *et al.*, 1979; Sakano *et al.*, 1979, 1980). The joining signals, which may take the form 5′-hepatamer–spacer–nonamer-3′ (or its complement), flank each *V*, *D* or *J* segment on either side. The consensus heptamer sequence is 5′-CACAGTG-3′ (with the first four bases essentially invariant), and that of the nonamer is 5′-ACAAAAACC-3′ (with positions 2, 5, 6 and 7 highly conserved).

Each joining signal contains two pieces of information. Firstly, it has a *directionality* conferred upon it by the relative 5′–3′ position of the heptamer and nonamer (in this discussion it will be arbitrarily assumed that the signal points 'towards' the nonamer). Secondly, the spacer element assumes one of two set lengths: 12 or 23 bp. Two gene segments may only rearrange (Max *et al.*, 1979; Sakano *et al.*, 1979, 1980) if they are flanked by joining signals of different *spacer length* (the so-called 12/23 rule) which point in opposite directions.

For example, in the IgH locus all V_H segments carry a 5′-heptamer–23 bp–nonamer-3′ signal at their 3′ end, whilst D_H segments are flanked on both sides by signals of 12-bp spacer length that point outwards (Fig. 4.8). Since J_H segments have a 5′-nonamer–23 bp–heptamer signal at their 5′ end, it will be seen that *V-D-J* rearrangement will only occur in that order, and *V-V*, *D-D*, *J-J* or *V-J* joins cannot usually occur, although rare exceptions have been reported (Meek, *et al.*, 1989). Thus, the nucleotide

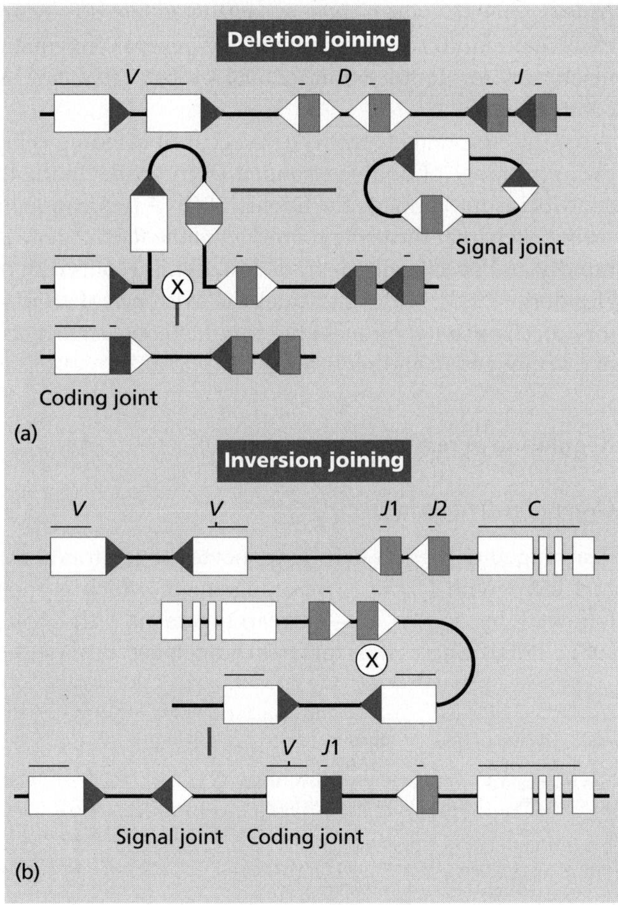

Fig. 4.8 Mechanisms of joining. Joining signals are depicted by triangles, with filled triangles denoting signals containing a 23-bp spacer and open triangles, those with a 12-bp spacer. Triangles point 'towards' the nonamer sequence. Transcriptional orientation of *V*, *D* and *J* segments is shown by arrows. Note that inversion joining (b) occurs between segments in the opposite orientation. (Modified from Venkitaraman, 1994.)

sequence of joining signals flanking particular types of gene segments governs the 5′–3′ order of rearrangement within the locus.

Mechanisms of joining

Two general mechanisms (Alt & Baltimore, 1982; Reth & LeClerq, 1987; Schatz *et al.*, 1992, and references therein) account for the types of join which have been detected in rearranged Ig genes (Fig. 4.8). The first mechanism, *deletion joining*, occurs between segments in the same 5′–3′ transcriptional orientation and results in the production of rearranged segments (the 'coding joint') and a DNA circle containing the fused joining signals (the 'signal joint'). The second mechanism, *inversion joining*, occurs between segments that are in opposite transcriptional orientations. In this case the signal joint is left linked to the rearranged segments on the same DNA strand. Rarely, rearrangements may occur between gene segments on different chromosomes by sister chromatid exchange.

Imprecision and nucleotide addition at coding joints

An important property of the rearrangement machinery is that the formation of coding joints (but not signal joints) is very imprecise (Alt & Baltimore, 1982; Reth & LeClerq, 1987), with nucleotide deletions and additions of between one and 12 bases. The imprecision inherent in this process contributes greatly to the diversity of antigen receptor repertoires, since the junctional regions encode a part of CDR3 (Fig. 4.3).

Nucleotide additions in coding joints fall into two classes. *N regions* consist of nucleotides added by the enzyme terminal deoxynucleotide transferase (TdT) to the ends of segments (Alt & Baltimore, 1982; Landau *et al.*, 1987); G and C additions are preferred (Lieber *et al.*, 1988). The role of TdT in *N*-region addition has been confirmed in mutant mice carrying a disrupted TdT gene on both alleles: rearranged Ig genes recovered from these animals contain no *N* regions (Gilfillan *et al.*, 1993). *P regions* are not random, but consist of between one and three base additions which are exactly complementary to the last few nucleotides of the segments to which they are added (Schatz *et al.*, 1992, and references therein). The enzyme(s) responsible for *P*-region additions have not yet been identified.

Genetic analysis of the rearrangement machinery

It is clear that rearrangement must involve several distinct modifications of DNA, beginning with the recognition of joining signals, double-stranded DNA cutting, nucleotide losses and additions at the segment boundaries, and, finally, DNA repair. The enzymatic machinery which mediates these steps is not yet clear, although it has been shown to be the same in both B and T cells. Genetic analyses have revealed the identity of a number of components of the rearrangement machinery in addition to terminal deoxynucleotide transferase.

A pair of genes (the recombination activating genes *RAG-1* and *RAG-2*) have recently been isolated whose products are necessary and sufficient to cause rearrangement in cells *in vitro*, although their enzymatic properties are not yet understood (Oettinger *et al.*, 1990; van Ghent *et al.*, 1995). *RAG-1* and *RAG-2* are expressed primarily in lymphoid cells (Oettinger *et al.*, 1990; Schatz *et al.*, 1992), and their pattern of expression coincides with the onset of rearrangement. Moreover, targetted disruption of either gene in the mouse germ-line results in an animal lacking mature lymphocytes because of an inability to initiate rearrangement (Mombaerts *et al.*, 1992; Shinkai *et al.*, 1992).

Transfection of *RAG-1* and *RAG-2* into non-lymphoid cells is sufficient to allow rearrangement of substrates containing heptamer–nonamer signals (Oettinger *et al.*, 1990). This suggests that most of the other components of the rearrangement machinery are ubiquitous. Indeed, the naturally occurring murine mutation *scid* (which induces a failure to form coding but not signal joints in T and B cells) also exhibits a general defect in double-stranded DNA break repair (Lieber *et al.*, 1988; Fulop & Phillips, 1990). Conversely, many mutations giving rise to defects in double-stranded DNA break repair also have defective *V–D–J* rearrangement. Complementation analysis has recently led to the identification of the double-stranded DNA binding protein Ku80—a target of autoantibodies in several autoimmune diseases—as one such ubiquitous component of the rearrangement machinery (Taccioli *et al.*, 1994). This molecule forms part of a DNA-dependent protein kinase complex rendered defective by the murine *scid* mutation (Blunt *et al.*, 1995). Thus, Ig gene rearrangement, which begins with site-specific DNA cleavage, requires components of the general enzymatic machinery for double-stranded DNA break repair for its completion.

If *V-D-J* rearrangement were to occur in dividing cells, the appearance of double-stranded DNA breaks in the Ig gene loci would impede the fidelity of DNA replication. It seems likely that the protein product of the *RAG-2* gene is rapidly and specifically degraded in dividing cells (Lin & Desiderio, 1993), which indicates the existence of regulatory mechanisms to prevent the simultaneous occurrence of rearrangement and replication.

Regulation of rearrangement (Fig. 4.9)

Order of rearrangement

Rearrangement begins in B-lymphocyte progenitors at the IgH locus with D_H to J_H rearrangement, which is then followed by V_H to D_H–J_H rearrangement (Alt *et al.*, 1981, 1984). Successful IgH rearrangement allows the

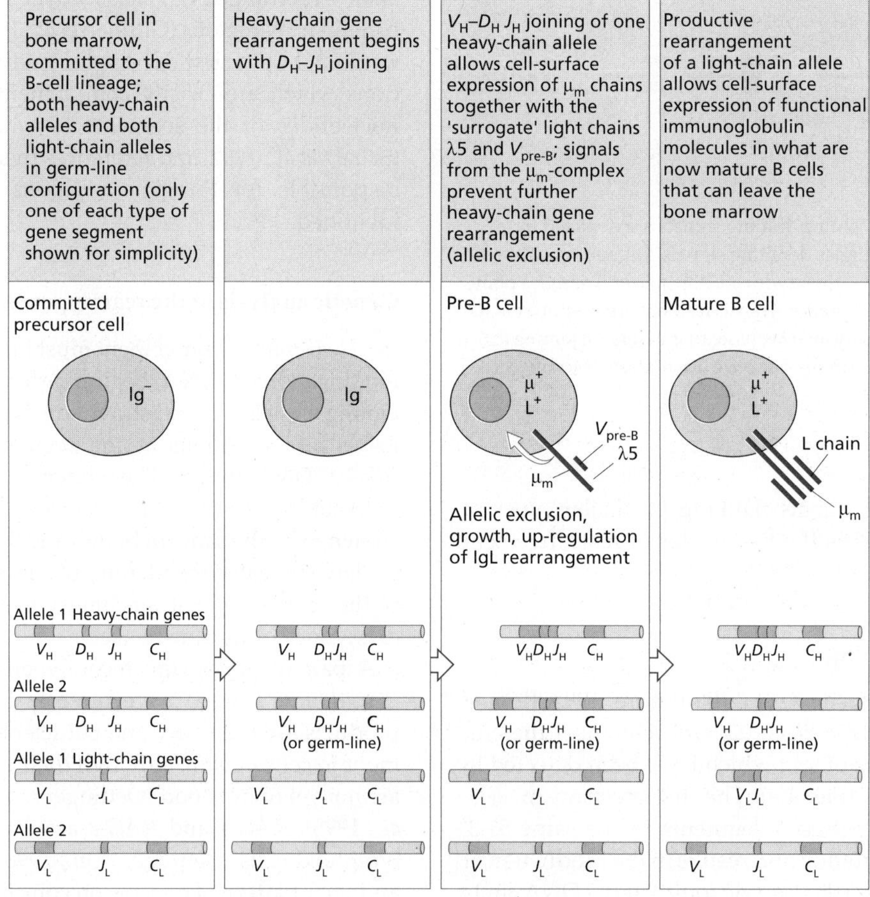

Fig. 4.9 Regulation of Ig rearrangement and allelic exclusion. The role of surrogate L chains V pre-B and λ5 in allowing cell surface expression of the μ H chain prior to L-chain rearrangement and in the postulated mechanism of allelic exclusion is depicted. (From Venkitaraman, 1992.)

rearrangement of the Ig L-chain genes to proceed (Reth *et al.*, 1987; Kitamura & Rajewsky, 1992).

The order of rearrangement in the L-chain loci remains unclear. The choice between κ and λ rearrangement appears to be made stochastically in humans, where the κ and λ loci are equally large. In the mouse, the κ locus is likely to be the first to rearrange with *V*κ to *J*κ joining. Multiple *V*κ to Jκ joins may occur, ensuring that most murine B cells carry a functionally rearranged κ L chain. However, in some cells, a *V*κ segment joins to a heptamer–nonamer joining signal located about 20 kb distal to the Cκ gene (the κ deleting element), resulting in deletion of the κ locus (Durdik *et al.*, 1984). Cells which have undergone κ deletion in this way may then proceed to initiate *V*λ to *J*λ rearrangement in their λ gene loci. However, λ rearrangements occur normally even in mice where the κ locus has been ablated by gene targetting (Zou *et al.*, 1993), which suggests that the order of rearrangement may be determined stochastically, just as in humans.

Cell-type specificity of rearrangement

Rearrangement of Ig genes normally occurs only in B lymphocytes. Although *D* to *J* rearrangements may be somewhat promiscuous, *V* to *D–J* rearrangements in the IgH locus and *V–J* rearrangements in the IgL loci are very strictly regulated. Sterile transcription of unrearranged *V* segments precedes their rearrangement (Yancopoulos & Alt, 1985; Schlissl & Baltimore, 1989), suggesting that cell-type specificity and timing are regulated through the control of 'accessibility' of the rearranging loci to nuclear enzymes.

Allelic exclusion

It is essential that each lymphocyte bears antigen receptors of only a single specificity, or the selective clonal expansion and elimination of lymphocytes which characterizes the immune system would be impossible. However the imprecision inherent in the rearrangement process means that two out of every three coding joints are likely to be non-functional because they contain shifts in the translational reading frame. Therefore, gene rearrangements occur in both alleles of any given gene locus to maximize the chances of a productive rearrangement. It follows that once a productive *V–D–J* or *V–J* rearrangement is made on any one allele, further rearrangement in that locus must be stopped (reviewed in Venkitaraman, 1992). This process is termed *allelic exclusion*.

During B-lymphocyte development in the bone marrow, successful rearrangement of the IgH locus on any one allele first results in the synthesis of a membrane-bound H-chain protein of the μ class (Fig. 4.9), with the Cμ gene being closest in position to the rearranged *V–D–J* segments. Thus, allelic exclusion at the IgH locus must hinge upon the ability to detect this protein.

The mechanism by which this occurs is not completely understood. Transmission of a transmembrane signal must play a role, because introduction of a transgene encoding a fully rearranged secretory Ig H chain into the mouse germ-line does not induce allelic exclusion of endogenous genes, whereas the membrane-bound form of the same molecule does (Nussenzweig *et al.*, 1987). Moreover, targetted disruption of the transmembrane exons of the Cμ gene in the mouse germ-line results in an animal that makes secretory IgM but fails to undergo allelic exclusion (Kitamura & Rajewsky, 1992).

Since μ H chains are not transported to the cell surface in the absence of L chains (see Fig. 4.13), it has been difficult to understand how H-chain allelic exclusion could occur prior to L-chain gene rearrangement. It has recently been shown that during IgH rearrangement, B-lymphocyte progenitors express two non-rearranging genes, *V* pre-B and λ5 (located together on murine chromosome 16 or human chromosome 22), which are important for allelic exclusion to occur (Melchers *et al.*, 1994 and references therein). The *V* pre-B gene encodes a single IgSF domain similar in structure to V_L, and the λ5 protein is somewhat larger than, but similar to, a C_L domain. The V pre-B and λ5 proteins together form a 'surrogate' L chain which can associate with the newly synthesized membrane-bound μ H chain and as yet unidentified proteins to form a μ-surrogate L-chain complex. It is believed that complex formation induces IgH allelic exclusion (Kitamura *et al.*, 1992) via a signal transmitted by the Ig-associated protein CD79b (see p. 73) (Papavasiliou *et al.*, 1995), whereupon the cell proceeds to IgL rearrangement which culminates in the synthesis of a κ or λ L-chain protein (Fig. 4.9). Association of membrane-bound μ with κ or λ could then signal for IgL allelic exclusion in a similar manner. Cells which fail to make both H- and L-chain gene rearrangements successfully are induced by an unknown mechanism to undergo programmed cell death or apoptosis. Several genes that may regulate apoptosis in developing B cells have been identified (Boise *et al.*, 1993; Li *et al.*, 1993).

Generation of diversity

It has been estimated that Ig molecules must recognize in the order of 10^9–10^{11} antigenic specificities. Several features contribute to the generation of this vast repertoire.

Combinatorial and junctional diversity

Much of the diversity of Ig specificities arises as a result of the gene rearrangement mechanism (Leder, 1982; Tonegawa, 1983; Alt *et al.*, 1987). Firstly, there is the *combinator-*

Table 4.4 Potential repertoires of Ig specificities. (After Venkitaraman, 1994.)

	IgH/κ
Combinations of *V* segment pairing between chains	2×10^4 (human) to 250×10^4 (murine)
Diversity in *D–J* junctional regions*	10^{11}

* Including the contributions of: *D*/*J* segment usage, nucleotide additions at junctions, differences in translational reading frame at junctions.

ial diversity generated by the rearrangement of hundreds of distinct *V* segments with tens of *J* (and sometimes *D*) segments. Secondly, *junctional diversity* is generated by the addition or deletion of nucleotides at the ends of the rearranging segments with resultant changes in the encoded protein. Finally, the random pairing of Ig H and L chains, each of which contributes to antigen specificity, multiplies the number of specificities that can potentially be recognized.

Estimates of the potential repertoire of the Ig genes based on known numbers of *V*, *D* and *J* segments and observed junctional diversity are presented in Table 4.4.

Allelic variation is another feature of Ig loci (Rathbun *et al.*, 1987; Matsuda *et al.*, 1993; Cook *et al.*, 1994; Cox *et al.*, 1994). Many human and murine *V* segments occur in different allelic forms which vary from individual to individual, or strain to strain. Inbred mouse strains may also carry genomic deletions which encompass the *V* segment clusters; similar deletions have also been reported in humans.

Affinity maturation and somatic hypermutation of Ig genes

Further mechanisms enlarge the diversity of the Ig repertoire in secondary immune responses. Antibodies that are produced during a secondary immune response (i.e. after re-challenge with a foreign antigen) have in general a higher affinity for antigen than those in a primary response, and also display more rapid kinetics of binding (Foote & Milstein, 1991). Two processes account for the improvement in binding. Firstly, the *V* segments used in secondary antibodies are often completely different to those used in a primary response (reviewed in Berek & Milstein, 1987; Nossal, 1992). Secondly, amino-acid sequence analysis reveals mutations which are clustered in and around the CDR of the H and L chains; at the nucleotide sequence level these mutations predominantly take the form of base substitutions in the rearranged *V–D–J* or *V–J* segments. This latter phenomenon is termed 'somatic hypermutation' (Crews *et al.*, 1981; Heinrich *et al.*, 1984).

Somatic hypermutation has several characteristic features (Berek & Milstein, 1987). The observed frequency of hypermutation is of the order of 10^{-3}/nucleotide/cell division, which is about 10^4–10^5 times greater than the frequency of random mutation in chromosomal DNA. Mutations are specifically targeted to rearranged *V–D–J* or *V–J* segments; with the caveat that the frequency of mutation in germ-line *V* segments is difficult to measure. Mutations cluster at so-called 'hotspots' in and around the regions encoding CDR 1–3, and exhibit a distinct predilection for certain types of base substitution.

The mechanism of somatic hypermutation is poorly understood, but it is now known that non-coding DNA sequences in the Ig gene loci, including known Ig transcriptional enhancers (Fig. 4.10), are responsible for the

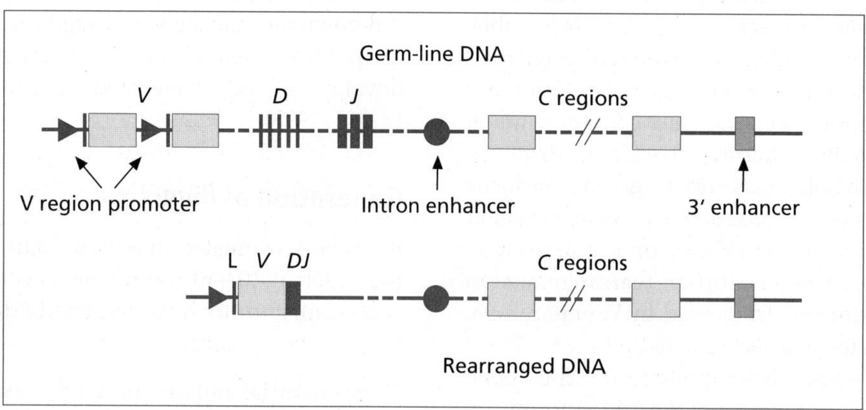

Fig. 4.10 Ig gene promoters and enhancers. The location of known promoter and enhancer sequences in a typical H-chain gene locus is shown schematically in germ-line (top) and rearranged (bottom) configurations. Note that their location ensures that these sequences are not disturbed by Ig rearrangement or class switching (bottom).

'targetting' of somatic mutation (Betz *et al.*, 1994), and that the *V* segment itself is not required (Yelamos *et al.*, 1995).

Ig synthesis and its regulation

The expression of rearranged Ig genes is tightly regulated at many levels. The specificity of gene transcription ensures that the genes are expressed only in cells belonging to the appropriate lineage. In the Ig H-chain gene loci, another type of DNA rearrangement enables expression of H chains of the five different isotypes. Finally, post-transcriptional mechanisms account for the changes in expression of the membrane-bound and secretory forms of each isotype.

Transcriptional regulation

Cis-acting DNA sequence elements which are responsible for the cell-type specificity of Ig gene transcription (reviewed in Calame & Ghosh, 1995) have been identified (Fig. 4.10). Each V_H and V_L segment in the germ-line carries its own promoter element just 5′ to the leader exon, containing a well-conserved octanucleotide sequence which is essential for its function. The long intron between the J_H cluster and the Cμ gene (Fig. 4.10) contains a strong, B-lineage-specific, transcriptional enhancer element (the IgH intron enhancer) of about 400 bp (Ephrussi *et al.*, 1985). The intron enhancer contains at least four short sequence motifs which serve as binding sites for transcription factors, as well as a copy of the octanucleotide sequence. A similar intron enhancer is found between the *J*κ cluster and *C*κ. Additionally, all three Ig loci contain a second strong enhancer element at their far 3′ end. In the IgH locus the 3′ enhancer is distal to the *C*α gene (Pettersson *et al.*, 1990), and in the κ locus, to *C*κ. The λ locus contains several 3′ enhancer elements downstream of the multiple *C*λ genes.

It is important to note that the location of the promoter and enhancer elements within the Ig gene loci ensures that they remain intact after gene rearrangement (Fig. 4.10).

Many nuclear factors which interact with the Ig gene promoters and enhancers have been identified (Calame & Ghosh, 1995). One of the first to be cloned and characterized was the factor NF-κB, which binds to the sequence GGGGACTTTCC in the κ and IgH intron enhancers. Several other proteins have been characterized more recently (Nelsen *et al.*, 1993; Strubin *et al.*, 1995). Surprisingly, like NF-κB, not many of these proteins display strict lineage restriction in their expression patterns, which has led to the proposal that transcriptional specificity is determined in a combinatorial manner by the interactions of multiple proteins with multiple *cis*-acting sequence elements.

The up- or down-regulation of Ig gene transcription during B-cell differentiation and activation is determined, at least in part, by regulation of these nuclear factors in response to receptor-mediated signals. For example, NF-κB is normally dormant in the cytoplasm in complex with an inhibitor I-κB which prevents its nuclear translocation (Sen & Baltimore, 1986). Receptor-mediated signals induce phosphorylation of I-κB on serine and threonine residues, resulting in NF-κB release and nuclear transport.

Class switching in IgH genes

Once a successful *V–D–J* rearrangement has taken place in the IgH locus, the V-region domain encoded by that rearrangement may be expressed in linkage with a C region encoded by any of the different H-chain isotypes. Mature B cells initially co-express IgM and IgD, and upon secondary antigenic challenge may switch to the expression of IgG, IgE or IgA.

Co-expression of IgM and IgD

While definitive proof is lacking, there is much evidence that B cells which co-express IgM and IgD produce separate transcripts by differential splicing of a single long precursor mRNA (Fig. 4.11). Thus, the same rearranged *V–D–J* could be spliced in-frame to the first exon of *C*μ or, alternatively, to the first exon of *C*δ with consequent splicing out of *C*μ. The mechanism governing the choice of splice site is not understood, but clearly it must be regulated to allow variations in the relative levels of IgM versus IgD.

When B cells co-expressing IgM and IgD first encounter antigen, they differentiate into antibody-secreting plasma cells. In these cells, IgM secretion predominates (although some IgD is also synthesized), and it is for this reason that IgM is the major circulating isotype in a primary immune response. The choice between IgM and IgD synthesis may be exerted at an additional level in plasma cells, in which most IgH gene transcription terminates at the distal end of the *C*μ gene without proceeding into *C*δ.

Switch recombination

Primary antigenic challenge of IgM/IgD co-expressing B lymphocytes induces differentiation not only into plasma cells but also into long-lived memory cells, in which the process of somatic hypermutation occurs. Secondary antigenic challenge of memory B cells includes class switching to other isotypes. Unlike the IgM/IgD switch, this involves a process of DNA rearrangement in the C_H genes.

Upstream to the *C*μ gene and each of the other C_H genes apart from *C*δ are regions ranging from 2 to 10 kb in length (Nikaido *et al.*, 1981), consisting of multiple repeats of short conserved sequence motifs called the switch regions

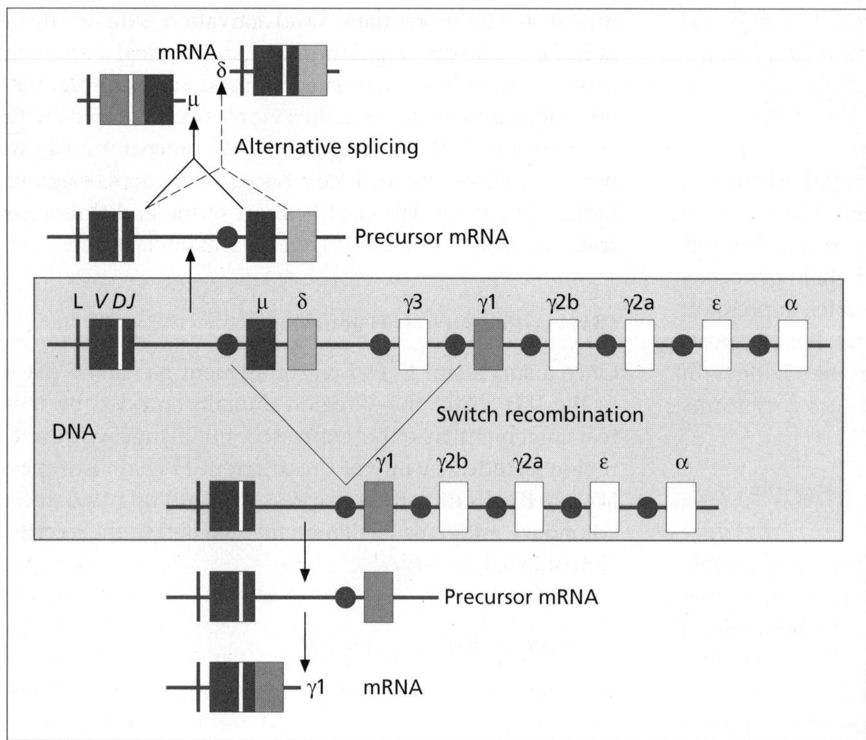

Fig. 4.11 Ig H-chain isotype switching. The central panel shows the murine IgH locus (not to scale), with a rearranged leader (*L*)-*VDJ* segment 5′ to the *C*-region genes. Switch regions are marked by circles. Class switching mediated by RNA processing is shown in the top part of the figure; the bottom part depicts class switch recombination. (Modified from Venkitaraman, 1994.)

(termed *S*μ, *S*γ, etc.). Switch recombination occurs at these regions. During switch recombination, a rearranged *V–D–J* segment is moved from its location 5′ of Cμ to a new location 5′ of another C_H gene (Fig. 4.11). Interventing sequences between *S*μ and the switch region to which recombination takes place are deleted. For example, once switch recombination from *S*μ to *S*α occurs, expression of intervening isotypes such as IgG and IgE is no longer possible.

Mechanism of directed switch recombination to IgE

The predominant class of Ig secreted by activated B lymphocytes varies in a predictable way, depending upon the antigenic stimulus. For example, serum IgE levels are elevated in parasitic infestations and allergic reactions. Whilst the exact mechanism underlying directed switch recombination is not yet understood, it is clear that cytokines secreted by T cells play a critical role (Coffman *et al*., 1993). Interleukin-4 (IL-4) has emerged as the critical factor directing switch recombination to IgE, although the related molecule IL-13 is also likely to be involved. Indeed, total serum IgE levels in humans exhibit a genetic linkage to the IL-4 gene on chromosome 5 (Marsh *et al*., 1994). Overexpression of IL-4 in transgenic mice results in vastly elevated serum IgE, and certain manifestations of allergy. Conversely, targetted disruption of the IL-4 gene results in the ablation of the IgE response to parasitic infestation (Kuhn *et al*., 1991).

Directed class switch recombination, just like *V–D–J* recombination, is preceded by germ-line transcription of the targetted gene. The effect of IL-4 is due at least in part to the induction of germ-line transcripts originating from a 179-bp DNA sequence 5′ of the *S*ε region (Bottaro *et al*., 1994; Schindler *et al*., 1994). The level of germ-line transcription *per se* determines the frequency but not the efficiency of the switch recombination process and so additional factors are likely to be involved.

Synthesis of membrane-bound and secreted forms of Ig H chains

H chains of each of the five Ig isotypes exist in two forms—one is membrane bound and the other is secreted. B lymphocytes synthesize the membrane-bound form upon activation by antigen, differentiate into plasma cells which secrete Ig (Fig. 4.1). Production of membrane-bound and secreted Ig molecules is regulated primarily at the level of mRNA processing.

Regulation has been studied most extensively at the murine Cμ gene (reviewed in Cook *et al*., 1987). Appended to the 3′ end of the exon encoding the Cμ4 domain are 20 codons which encode the secretory tailpiece (Fig. 4.7 & Table 4.1), distal to which are two exons M1 (of roughly 120 bp) and M2 (of just 6 bp) which encode the transmembrane segment and cytoplasmic tail of membrane-bound μ H chains. The M1 exon is separated from Cμ4 by a long intron of about 2 kb.

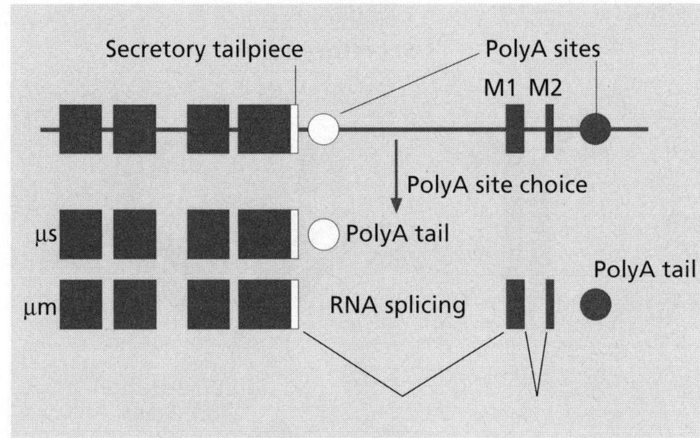

Fig. 4.12 Origin of secretory and membrane-bound Ig H-chain transcripts. Splice junctions between the exons are shown, as are the two mechanisms (polyA site choice and RNA splicing) regulating the production of the two forms of transcript. (Modified from Venkitaraman, 1994.)

Two polyadenylation sites are found. The first is in the Cμ4-M1 intron, and the second is 3′ to the M2 exon. Thus, use of the first polyadenylation site produces a secretory transcript, whereas use of the second site, together with splicing out of the secretory tailpiece codons, produces a membrane-bound transcript (Fig. 4.12).

A similar mechanism has been invoked to explain the production of membrane-bound and secretory forms of the γ, ε and α isotypes, in which the C_H genes have a similar organization to Cμ. In Cδ the secretory tailpiece is encoded in a separate exon located between Cδ3 and M1 and so, unlike the other isotypes, regulation occurs exclusively by differential mRNA splicing.

B lymphocytes synthesize slightly more of the membrane-bound than the secretory transcript, whilst plasma cells contain a vast excess of the secretory transcript. However, both cell types produce both forms of transcript, implying that further layers of regulation (at the translational and post-translational levels) must exist to explain why plasma cells lack membrane-bound Ig at the cell surface (see p. 74).

Intracellular transport of secreted Ig molecules

Once synthesized in plasma cells, secreted Ig H chains of all five isotypes do not exit the endoplasmic reticulum (ER) prior to L-chain association. ER retention is mediated by the binding of the ER resident protein BiP to a region of the C_H1 domain (Haas & Wabl, 1983; Hendershot *et al.*, 1990); L-chain association displaces BiP (Fig. 4.13). In pre-B cells (which have not rearranged their L-chain genes) a similar function may be served by the surrogate L-chain proteins V pre-B and λ5.

Secreted IgM molecules must be further assembled into pentamers before they are exported, or else they too are retained in the ER (Sitia *et al.*, 1990). A conserved Cys residue in the secreted tailpiece of the μ H chain may enable disulphide bridging between the μ_2L_2 subunits of the pentamer (Sitia *et al.*, 1990); prior to pentamerization this residue mediates intracellular retention by BiP binding. IgA molecules are secreted as dimers and it is of note that α H chains also contain an analogous Cys residue.

Structure and synthesis of membrane Ig (the B-cell antigen receptor)

Antigen receptors expressed at the surface of B lymphocytes are multimeric complexes which include several transmembrane glycoproteins in addition to the membrane-bound Ig H_2/L_2 tetramer. Whereas the Ig molecules function in specific antigen recognition, the associated proteins are essential for receptor transport and signal transduction. The assembly of membrane Ig complexes is tightly regulated to prevent the expression of incomplete, and therefore non-functional, complexes at the cell surface.

Components of the B-cell antigen receptor

Membrane-bound Ig molecules of all five isotypes are expressed at the cell surface in complex with at least two transmembrane proteins (Venkitaraman *et al.*, 1991; Reth, 1992, and references therein) which bear sequence homology to the CD3 chains of the T-cell receptor (Fig. 4.13). These proteins have been termed the Igα (CD79a) and Igβ (CD79b) subunits, and are the products of the *mb-1* and *B29* genes, respectively. The stoichiometry of subunit associations has not been precisely determined.

The Igα and Igβ proteins contain a single extracellular IgSF domain with multiple N-glycosylation sites. Variable glycosylation of Igα is observed, depending on the isotype of Ig with which it is associated (Venkitaraman *et al.*, 1991). Thus, membrane-bound IgM receptor complexes in murine cells contain a 32-kDa Igα subunit, and IgD complexes contain a 34-kDa Igα subunit. The human Igα protein is extensively glycosylated and larger in molecular weight (40–45 kDa) than murine Igα, whilst both human and murine Igβ proteins are 36–38 kDa.

Given the structural and presumed functional heterogeneity of the five classes of membrane-bound H chains, it is somewhat surprising that they all form the same canonical membrane complex with Igα/β. There is recent evidence (Kim *et al.*, 1994) to suggest that there are differences in the cytosolic proteins associated with membrane Ig complexes of different classes, but at this time the significance of the data is unclear.

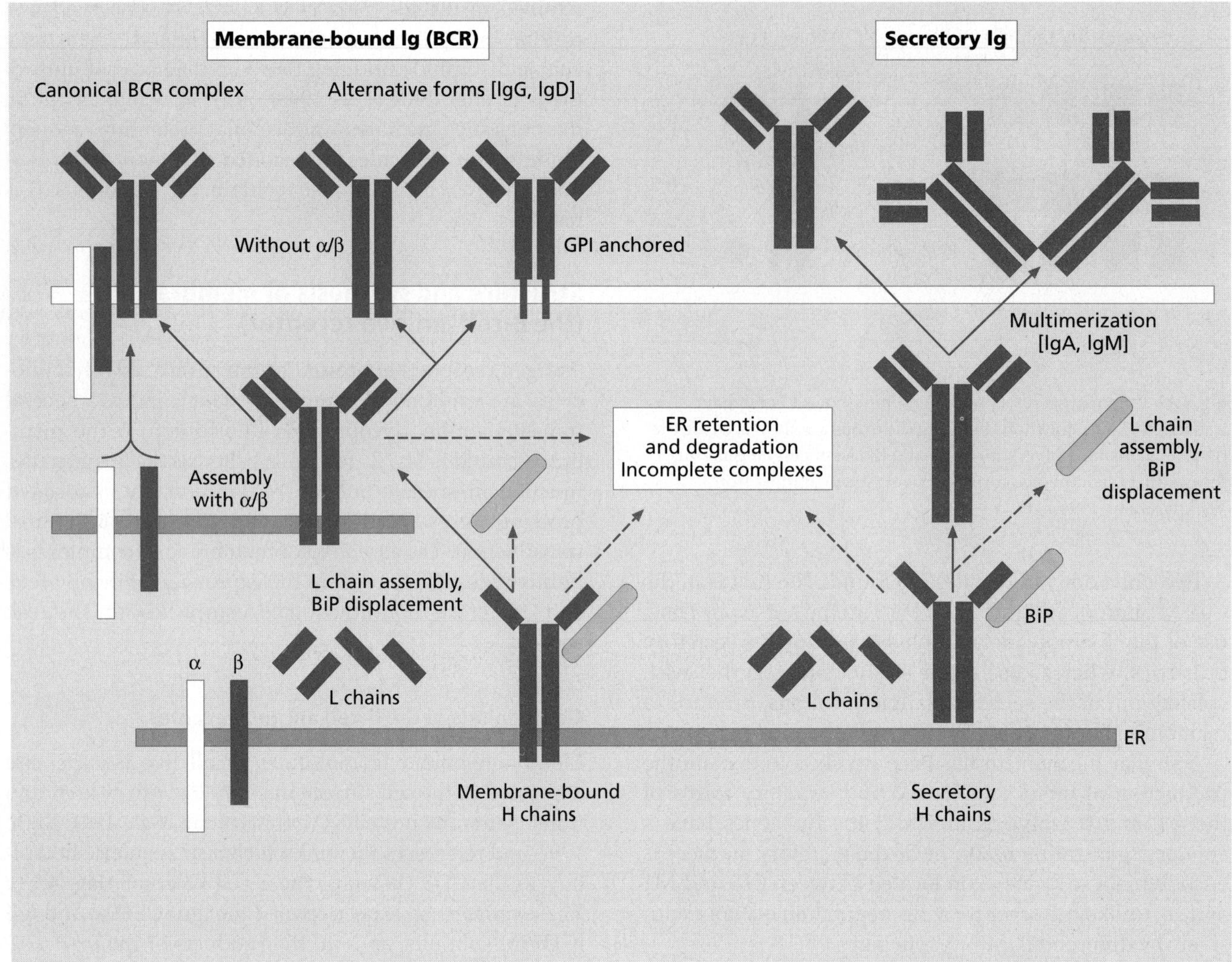

Fig. 4.13 Assembly and intracellular transport of the membrane-bound Ig complex and secretory Ig. Pathways of intracellular transport of membrane-bound and secreted Ig are shown on the left and right halves, respectively. Multimerization of secretory IgA and IgM with J chain is not shown—refer to the text for details. The composition of the canonical membrane-bound Ig complex (B-cell receptor, or BCR) of all five Ig isotypes is shown at the top, as are the alternative forms of membrane-bound IgD and IgG. Only IgD occurs in the glycophosphatidylinositol (GPI) linked form. Note that: (a) the stoichiometry of Igα/β subunit associations in the membrane Ig complex and (b) the relative chronological order of L-chain association versus Igα/β subunit association with the H chains have not been determined. Both are arbitrarily depicted. The Ig H-chain binding protein (BiP) is a shaded oval.

Assembly and surface transport of the B-cell antigen receptor

Membrane-bound IgM, IgE and IgA molecules fail to reach the cell surface in the absence of the Igα and Igβ subunits, and are retained and degraded in the ER. Interestingly, membrane-bound IgD and IgG2b molecules may not require Igα/β association for surface transport (Venkitaraman *et al.*, 1991), although they can associate with Igα/β when present. Membrane IgD in the absence of Igα/β may also be inserted into the cell membrane (Wienands & Reth, 1992) by a glycosyl-phosphatidylinositol (GPI) anchor (Fig. 4.13).

Whilst Igβ is expressed at all stages of B-cell differentiation, Igα is found only in pre-B and B cells. Thus, murine plasma cells, which lack Igα, do not transport membrane-bound Ig to the cell surface and it is retained in the ER. Retention in the absence of α/β is mediated by polar residues in the transmembrane segment of membrane-bound H chains (Williams *et al.*, 1990).

Functions of membrane-bound Ig (Fig. 4.14)

Transmembrane signalling

Antigen-specific activation of B cells is mediated by the transmission of a transmembrane signal through the B-cell antigen receptor (BCR) following its engagement by

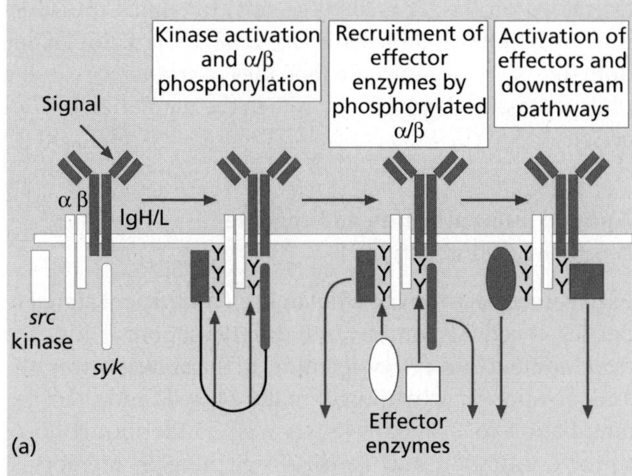

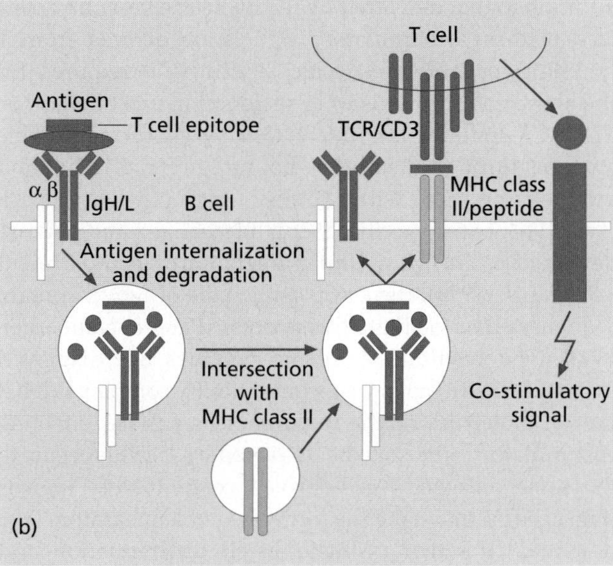

Fig. 4.14 Functions of the BCR. (a) Early biochemical events in transmembrane signalling by the BCR. Inactive kinases of the *src* family, and the *syk* kinase are shown as open boxes. BCR engagement results in kinase activation (filled boxes) and phosphorylation of the Igα/β subunits on Tyr residues (marked *Y*), although this cannot, as yet, be ascribed to one particular species of kinase. Effector enzymes are then recruited to the BCR by phosphotyrosine-*src* homology-2 subunit interactions. *Src* kinases, *syk* kinase and the activated effector enzymes may all contribute to downstream signalling pathways (indicated by arrows). (b) The mechanism of antigen internalization by the BCR and its role in cognate T-cell–B-cell interactions. Intracellular degradation of internalized antigen, its intersection with MHC class II molecules and recycling of peptide-loaded MHC and empty Ig to the cell surface are shown schematically. Note that the costimulatory signal from T cells may be delivered via a soluble mediator (as shown) or via an interaction between membrane-bound molecules.

antigen. The cytoplasmic tails of the membrane-bound Ig H chains are very short, and therefore unlikely to be solely responsible for transmembrane signal transduction. This function is performed by the associated Igα/β polypeptides and accessory molecules.

Antigen receptor signalling motif (ITAM or ARAM)

Consistent with this role, the juxtamembrane portion of the cytoplasmic tails of the Igα/β chains contains a short conserved motif consisting of precisely spaced Tyr and Leu residues in a context of about 26 amino acids (Reth, 1989). This motif, D/E-X(7)-D/E-X-X-*Y*-*X*-*X*-*L*-X(7)-*Y*-*X*-*X*-*L*/*I* (where X is any amino acid), is also found in the cytoplasmic tails of the Fc receptors for IgE and in the CD3 γ, δ, ε, ζ chains of the T-cell receptor. The motif is sufficient to confer antigen receptor signalling function when transferred to a heterologous protein. In particular, the integrity of the *Y*-*X*-*X*-*L* sequence may be essential.

Biochemical events following B-cell antigen receptor ligation

Tyrosine phosphorylation of cellular proteins is a prominent and early consequence of BCR ligation (Gold *et al*., 1990); indeed Igα/β chains are themselves tyrosine phosphorylated. Since none of the subunits of the B-cell antigen receptor complex contains kinase catalytic domains, this must be the result of activation of one or more non-receptor protein tyrosine kinases (PTK).

Non-receptor PTKs belonging to the *src* family of proto-oncogenes may be important in signal transduction by the BCR. Association of the cytoplasmic tails of Igα/β with *src* family members (Fig. 4.14(a)) is readily detected (Yamanishi *et al*., 1991; Clark *et al*., 1992). For example, $p59^{fyn}$, $p53/56^{lyn}$ and $p55^{blk}$ associate with Igα, and are activated upon receptor ligation. A novel, non-*src* PTK (PTK 72 or *syk*), which associates with the membrane-bound Ig complex, has also been identified. Despite the functional redundancy in the recruitment of tyrosine kinases by the BCR, there is recent evidence to suggest that *syk* (Cheng *et al*., 1995; Turner *et al*., 1995) and *lyn* (Hibbs *et al*., 1995) are of particular importance in signalling. Tyrosine phosphorylation following antigen receptor ligation results in the activation of phospholipase C (PLC)γ (in particular the γ2 isoform), an enzyme which catalyses the formation of the second messengers diacylglycerol (DAG) and inositol triphosphate (IP_3) from membrane phospholipids (Bjisterboch *et al*., 1985; Carter *et al*., 1991). DAG activates protein kinase C (PKC), whereas IP_3 causes the mobilization of Ca^{2+} from intracellular stores. The tyrosine kinase *syk* may couple the BCR directly or indirectly to this pathway, since

PLCγ is not phosphorylated in *syk*-deficient cells (Takata *et al.*, 1994). In addition, IP_3-independent mechanisms which are not impaired by *syk* deficiency also contribute to the observed Ca^{2+} mobilization.

Other second messenger systems have also been implicated in antigen receptor signal transduction (reviewed in Moller, 1993). There is evidence that a trimeric G protein couples to the BCR, although it has not yet been identified. BCR ligation also results in the recruitment and activation (Fig. 4.14(a)) of a number of other cytosolic enzymes (such as, for example, the proto-oncogene *vav*, phosphatidylinositol 3-kinase, *ras*-GAP and MAP kinases) to the α/β chains, but their role in BCR signalling remains to be clarified. Some, but not all, of these interactions occur when the phosphotyrosine binding *src* homology 2 domains in intracellular enzymes bind to phosphorylated Tyr residues in the antigen receptor signalling motifs in the cytoplasmic tails of α/β.

Accessory molecules associated with the BCR

Accessory molecules that associate with the BCR may augment or diminish transmembrane signals transmitted through the antigen receptor, and thereby serve to fine-tune the B-cell response. For example, the BCR is associated with the accessory molecules CD19, CD21, CD35 and TAPA-1 (Matsumoto *et al.*, 1993). The CD21 molecule is a 145-kDa receptor for the complement component C3d, and independently binds to CD35 (a receptor for C3b and C4b) and CD19. Little is known about the functions of TAPA-1 and CD19. CD19 has a large cytoplasmic domain which is tyrosine phosphorylated upon antigen receptor ligation, and contains conserved motifs which may serve as substrates for the binding of enzymes such as phosphatidylinositol 3-kinase involved in signal transduction. Co-cross-linking of CD19 with membrane-bound Ig greatly augments B-cell activation, and so it has been proposed that one function of the CD19/CD35/CD21 structure is to aid B-cell activation by circulating antigen–antibody–complement aggregates (Carter & Fearon, 1992). Analogously, an independent ligand for CD19 may exist but it has not yet been identified.

Signalling may be regulated in a different manner by the accessory molecule CD22, which is associated with the BCR and exerts an inhibitory effect upon it through the action of a protein tyrosine phosphatase PTP-1C bound to the cytoplasmic tail of CD22. This inhibitory effect is terminated when CD22 engagement by ligands expressed on other lymphocytes prevents its association with the BCR (Doody *et al.*, 1995). Autoimmunity is a feature of mutations in PTP-1C, which suggests that this interaction may play a role in the silencing of autoreactive B lymphocytes (Cyster & Goodenow, 1995).

The glycoprotein CD45, the B220 isoform of which is expressed on B cells, is also essential for signal transduction in B cells (Kishihara *et al.*, 1993). The cytoplasmic domain of this molecule encodes a protein tyrosine phosphatase and may play a role in the regulation of PTK activity.

Antigen internalization and cognate B-cell–T-cell interactions

Engagement of the BCR is not in itself a sufficient signal to permit B-cell activation and differentiation. Thus, the development of B-cell progenitors in the bone marrow, the antigen-specific activation of mature B cells and their differentiation to plasma cells, as well as the induction of somatic mutation and Ig class switching in memory B cells, all require some form of costimulatory signal in addition to that delivered by the BCR. The best characterized of these costimulatory signals are derived from T lymphocytes; antigen-specific T-cell help is required for the activation of B cells to Ig secretion in most instances. The BCR initiates this interaction by capturing soluble antigens through membrane-bound Ig (Fig. 4.14(b)), and internalizing them with extremely high efficiency (Rock *et al.*, 1984; Lanzavecchia, 1985). Internalized antigens are delivered to an intracellular degradative compartment (West *et al.*, 1994); the cytoplasmic tails of Igα/β contain sequences that facilitate this process (Patel & Neuberger, 1993). The resulting antigenic peptides are displayed in complex with major histocompatibility complex (MHC) class II molecules on the B-lymphocyte surface, enabling costimulatory signals to be delivered by T cells specific to the same antigen. T-cell-derived costimulatory signals (Fig. 4.14(b)) may take the form of soluble mediators (e.g. IL-4 and IL-5 that promote B-cell differentiation and mediate Ig class switching) or membrane-bound molecules that interact with ligands on the B-cell surface (e.g. T cell expressed *gp39* that interacts with the CD40 molecule on B cells). The pivotal role of the cognate B-cell–T-cell interaction is demonstrated by defective formation of germinal centres in secondary lymphoid tissue and subsequent humoral immune responses in humans or mice deficient in CD40 or its ligand (reviewed in Banchereau *et al.*, 1994).

Summary

There has been a remarkable increase in knowledge of the structure, genetics and cell biology of Ig molecules in the past 15 years. These advances have been due primarily to the application of recombinant DNA techniques and the ability to isolate lymphocytes producing monoclonal antibodies. Quite apart from their relevance to immunology, studies on Ig have proven to be remarkably fertile in yielding insights into the fundamental processes that regulate the development and function of mammalian cells. Thus, they have had important general implications for many areas of biology and medical science. Recent advances have been of particular relevance to clinical medicine. Detailed understanding of the structural basis of antigen recognition, when combined with the techniques of molecular biology, has now created a wealth of possibilities for the use of genetically engineered Ig molecules in the diagnosis and treatment of human disease.

References

Alt, F.W. & Baltimore, D. (1982) Joining of immunoglobulin heavy chain gene segments: implications from a chromosome with three D-JH fusions. *Proc. Nat. Acad. Sci. USA*, **79**, 4118–22.

Alt, F.W., Blackwell, T.K. & Yancopoulos, G.D. (1987) Development of the primary antibody repertoire. *Science*, **238**, 1079–87.

Alt, F.W., Rosenberg, N., Lewis, S., Thomas, E. & Baltimore, D. (1981) Organization and reorganization of immunoglobulin genes in A-MuLV transformed cells: rearrangement of heavy but not light chain genes. *Cell*, **27**, 381–90.

Alt, F.W., Yancopoulos, G.D., Blackwell, T.K. *et al.* (1984) Ordered rearrangement of immunoglobulin heavy-chain variable region gene segments. *Eur. Mol. Biol. Organ. J.*, **3**, 1209–19.

Amit, A., Mariuzza, R., Phillips, S. & Poljak, R.J. (1986) Three-dimensional structure of an antigen–antibody complex at 2.8 Å resolution. *Science*, **233**, 747–53.

Amzel, L.M. & Poljak, R.J. (1979) Three-dimensional structure of antibody molecules. *Ann. Rev. Biochem.*, **48**, 961–97.

Banchereau, J., Bazan, F., Blanchard, D. *et al.* (1994) The CD40 antigen and its ligand. *Ann. Rev. Immunol.*, **12**, 881–922.

Berek, C. & Milstein, C. (1987) Mutation drift and repertoire shift in the maturation of the immune response. *Immunol. Rev.*, **96**, 23–41.

Betz, A.G., Milstein, C., Gonzalez-Fernandez, A., Pannell, R., Larson, T. & Neuberger, M.S. (1994) Elements regulating somatic hypermutation of an immunoglobulin κ gene: critical role for the intron enhancer/matrix attachment region. *Cell*, **77**, 239–48.

Bjisterboch, M.K., Meade, C.J., Turner, G.A. & Klaus, G.G.B. (1985) B lymphocyte receptors and phosphoinositide degradation. *Cell*, **41**, 999–1006.

Blank, U., Ra, C., Miller, L., White, K., Metzeger, H. & Kinet, J.-P. (1989) Complete structure and expression in transfected cells of the high-affinity receptor for IgE. *Nature*, **337**, 187–9.

Blunt, T., Finnie, N.J., Taccioli, G.E. *et al.* (1995) Defective DNA-dependent protein kinase activity is linked to V(D)J recombination and DNA repair defects associated with the murine *scid* mutation. *Cell*, **80**, 813–23.

Boise, L.H., Gonzalez-Garcia, M., Postema, C.E. *et al.* (1993) *bcl-x*, a *bcl-2* related gene that functions as a dominant regulator of apoptotic cell death. *Cell*, **74**, 597–608.

Bottaro, A., Lansford, R., Xu, L., Zhang, J., Rothman, P. & Alt, F.W. (1994) S region transcription *per se* promotes basal IgE class switch recombination but additional factors regulate the efficiency of the process. *Eur. Mol. Biol. Organ. J.*, **13**, 665–74.

Brack, C.M., Hirama, M., Schuller, R. & Tonegawa, S. (1978) A complete Ig gene is created by somatic recombination. *Cell*, **15**, 1–14.

Brandtzaeg, P. & Prydz, H. (1984) Direct evidence for an integrated function of J chain and secretory component in epithelial transport. *Nature*, **311**, 71–4.

Brodeur, P.H. & Riblet, R. (1984) The immunoglobulin heavy chain variable region locus in the mouse. I. One hundred Igh-V genes comprise seven families of homologous genes. *Eur. J. Immunol.*, **14**, 922–30.

Buluwela, L., Albertson, D.G., Sherrington, P., Rabbitts, P.H., Spurr, N. & Rabbitts, T.H. (1988) The use of chromosomal translocations to study human immunoglobulin gene organization: mapping DH segments within 35 kb of the Cμ gene and the identification of a new DH locus. *Eur. Mol. Biol. Organ. J.*, **7**, 2003–10.

Burton, D.R. & Woof, J.M. (1992) Human antibody effector function. *Adv. Immunol.*, **51**, 1–84.

Calame, K. & Ghosh, S. (1995) Regulation of immunoglobulin gene transcription. In: *Immunoglobulin Genes* (eds T. Honjo & F.W. Alt), p. 387. Academic, London.

Carter, R.H. & Fearon, D.T. (1992) Lowering the threshold for antigen receptor stimulation of B lymphocytes. *Science*, **256**, 105–7.

Carter, R.H., Park, D.J., Rhee, S.G. & Fearon, D.T. (1991) Tyrosine phosphorylation of phospholipase C induced by membrane immunoglobulin in B lymphocytes. *Proc. Nat. Acad. Sci. USA*, **88**, 2745–9.

Cheng, A.M., Rowley, B., Pao, W., Hayday, A., Bolen, J.B. & Pawson, T. (1995) The Syk tyrosine kinase is required for mouse viability and B cell development. *Nature*, **378**, 303–6.

Chothia, C., Lesk, A., Tramontano, A. *et al.* (1989) Conformations of immunoglobulin hypervariable regions. *Nature*, **342**, 877–83.

Chuchana, P., Blancher, A., Brockly, F., Alexandre, D., LeFranc, G. & LeFranc, M.-P. (1990) Definition of the human immunoglobulin variable lambda (IGLV) gene subgroups. *Eur. J. Immunol.*, **20**, 1317–25.

Clark, M.R., Campbell, K.S., Kazlaukas, A. *et al.* (1992) The B cell antigen receptor complex: association of Igα and Igβ with distinct cytoplasmic effectors. *Science*, **258**, 123–6.

Coffman, R.L., Lebman, D.A. & Rothman, P. (1993) The mechanism and regulation of immunoglobulin isotype switching. *Adv. Immunol.*, **54**, 229–49.

Cook, G.P., Tomlinson, I.M., Walter, G. *et al.* (1994) A map of the human immunoglobulin VH locus completed by analysis of the telomeric region of chromosome 14q. *Nature Genet.*, **7**, 162–8.

Cook, G.P., Mason, J.O. & Neuberger, M.S. (1987) Immunoglobulin gene expression. In: *Molecular Genetics of Immunoglobulin* (eds F. Calabi & M.S. Neuberger), p. 153. Elsevier Science, Amsterdam.

Cox, J.P.L., Tomlinson, I.M. & Winter, G. (1994) A directory of human germ-line Vκ segments reveals a strong bias in their usage. *Eur. J. Immunol.*, **24**, 827–36.

Crago, S.S., Word, C. & Tomasi, T.B. (1989) Antisera to secretory component recognize the murine Fc receptor for IgA. *J. Immunol.*, **142**, 3909–14.

Crews, S., Griffin, J., Huang, H., Calame, K.L. & Hood, L.E. (1981) A single VH gene segment encodes the immune response to phosphorylcholine: somatic mutation is correlated with the class of antibody. *Cell*, **25**, 59–66.

Cyster, J.G. & Goodenow, C.C. (1995) Protein tyrosine phosphatase 1C negatively regulates antigen receptor signalling in B lymphocytes and determines thresholds for negative selection. *Immunity*, **2**, 13–24.

Davies, D.R. & Metzeger, H. (1983) Structural basis of antibody function. *Ann. Rev. Immunol.*, **1**, 87–118.

Davies, D.R., Padlan, E.A. & Segel, D.M. (1975) Three-dimensional structure of immunoglobulins. *Ann. Rev. Biochem.*, **44**, 639–67.

Davis, A.C., Collins, C., Yoshimura, Y.I., D'Agostaro, G. & Shulman, M.J. (1989) Mutations of the mouse μ H chain which prevent polymer assembly. *J. Immunol.*, **143**, 1352–9.

Deutsch, H.F., Morton, J.I. & Kratochvil, C.H. (1956) Antigenic identity of hyperglobulinemic serum components with proteins of normal serum. *J. Biol. Chem.*, **222**, 39–51.

Doody, G.M., Justement, L.B., Delibrias, C. *et al.* (1995) A role in B cell activation for CD22 and the protein tyrosine phosphatase SHP. *Science*, **269**, 242–4.

Dreyer, W.J. & Bennett, J.C. (1965) The molecular basis of antibody formation: a paradox. *Proc. Nat. Acad. Sci. USA*, **54**, 864–9.

Durdik, J., Morre, M.W. & Selsing, E. (1984) Novel κ light chain gene rearrangements in mouse lambda light chain producing B lymphocytes. *Nature*, **307**, 749–52.

Early, P., Huang, H., Davis, M.M., Calame, K. & Hood, L.E. (1980) An immunoglobulin heavy-chain gene is generated from three segments of DNA: *VH, D* and *JH*. *Cell*, **19**, 981–92.

Edelman, G.M. (1973) Antibody structure and molecular immunology. *Science*, **180**, 830–40.

Edelman, G.M. & Gally, J. (1962) The nature of Bence-Jones proteins: chemical similarities to polypeptide chains of myeloma globulins and normal γ-globulins. *J. Exp. Med.*, **116**, 207–29.

Ellison, J. & Hood, L.E. (1982) Linkage and sequence homology of two human immunoglobulin γ heavy chain constant regions. *Proc. Nat. Acad. Sci. USA*, **79**, 1984–8.

Ellison, J.W. & Hood, L.E. (1983) Human antibody genes: evolutionary and molecular genetic perspectives. *Adv. Hum. Genet.*, **13**, 113.

Ephrussi, A., Church, G.M., Tonegawa, S. & Gilbert, W. (1985) B lineage-specific interactions of an immunoglobulin enhancer with cellular factors *in vivo*. *Science*, **227**, 134–40.

Flanagan, J.G. & Rabbitts, T.H. (1982) Arrangement of human immunoglobulin heavy chain constant region genes implies evolutionary duplication of a segment containing gamma, epsilon and alpha genes. *Nature*, **300**, 709–13.

Foote, J. & Milstein, C. (1991) Kinetic maturation of an immune response. *Nature*, **352**, 530–2.

Fulop, G.M. & Phillips, R.A. (1990) The *scid* mutation causes a general defect in DNA repair in the mouse. *Nature*, **347**, 479–82.

Gilfillan, S., Dierich, A., Lemeur, M., Benoist, C. & Mathis, D. (1993) Mice lacking TdT: mature animals with an immature lymphocyte repertoire. *Science*, **261**(5125), 1175–8.

Gold, M.R., Law, D.A. & DeFranco, A.L. (1990) Stimulation of protein tyrosine phosphorylation by the B lymphocyte antigen receptor. *Nature*, **345**, 810–12.

Haas, I.G. & Wabl, M. (1983) Immunoglobulin heavy chain binding protein. *Nature*, **306**, 387–9.

Heidelberger, M. & Kendall, F. (1929) A quantitative study of the precipitant reaction between type III pneumococcus polysaccharide and purified homologous antibody. *J. Exp. Med.*, **50**, 809–19.

Heidelberger, M. & Pedersen, K.O. (1937) The molecular weight of antibodies. *J. Exp. Med.*, **65**, 393–414.

Heinrich, G., Traunecker, A. & Tonegawa, S. (1984) Somatic mutation creates diversity in the major group of mouse immunoglobulin k light chains. *J. Exp. Med.*, **159**, 417–35.

Helm, B., Marsh, P., Vercelli, D., Padlan, E., Gould, H. & Geha, R. (1988) The mast cell binding site on human immunoglobulin E. *Nature*, **331**, 180–3.

Hendershot, L.M. (1990) Immunoglobulin heavy chain and binding protein complexes are dissociated *in vivo* by light chain addition. *J. Cell Biol.*, **111**, 829–37.

Hibbs, M.L., Tarlinton, D.M., Armes, J. *et al.* (1995) Multiple defects in the immune system of Lyn-deficient mice, culminating in autoimmune disease. *Cell*, **83**, 310–21.

Hieter, P.A., Hollis, G.F., Korsmeyer, S.J., Waldmann, T.A. & Leder, P. (1981) Clustered arrangement of immunoglobulin lambda constant regions in man. *Nature*, **294**, 536–40.

Hilschmann, N. & Craig, L.C. (1965) Amino acid sequence studies with Bence-Jones proteins. *Proc. Nat. Acad. Sci. USA*, **53**, 1403–9.

Honjo, T. (1983) Immunoglobulin genes. *Ann. Rev. Immunol.*, **1**, 499–528.

Hozumi, N. & Tonegawa, S. (1976) Evidence for somatic rearrangement of immunoglobulin genes coding for variable and constant regions. *Proc. Nat. Acad. Sci. USA*, **73**, 3628–33.

Huse, W., Sastry, L., Iverson, S.A. *et al.* (1989) Generation of a large combinatorial library of the immunoglobulin repertoire in phage lambda. *Science*, **246**, 1275–81.

Ishikaza, K. & Ishikaza, T. (1966) Physiochemical properties of reaginic antibody. I. Association of reaginic activity with an immunoglobulin other than γA or γG globulin. *J. Allergy*, **37**, 169.

Jones, P.T., Dear, P.H., Foote, J., Neuberger, M.S. & Winter, G. (1986) Replacing the complementarity determining regions in a human antibody with those from a mouse. *Nature*, **321**, 522–5.

Kabat, E.A., Wu, T.T., Perry, H.M., Gottesman, K.S. & Foeller, C. (1991) *Sequences of Proteins of Immunological Interest.* US Department of Health and Human Services, Public Health Service, National Institutes of Health, Bethesda.

Kim, K.M., Adachi, T., Nielson, P.J. *et al.* (1994) Two new proteins preferentially associated with membrane immunoglobulin D. *Eur. Mol. Biol. Organ. J.*, **13**, 3793–800.

Kishihara, K., Penninger, J., Wallace, V.A. *et al.* (1993) Normal B lymphocyte development but impaired T cell maturation in CD45-exon 6 protein tyrosine phosphatase deficient mice. *Cell*, **74**, 143–56.

Kitamura, D., Kudo, A., Schaal, S., Müller, W., Melchers, F. & Rajewsky, K. (1992) A critical role of the λ5 protein in B cell development. *Cell*, **69**, 823–31.

Kitamura, D. & Rajewsky, K. (1992) Targeted disruption of the μ chain membrane exon causes loss of heavy chain allelic exclusion. *Nature*, **356**, 154–6.

Köhler, G. & Milstein, C. (1975) Continuous cultures of fused cells secreting antibody of predefined specificity. *Nature*, **256**, 52–3.

Korngold, L. & Lipari, R. (1956) The antigenic relationship of Bence-Jones proteins to normal gamma globulin and multiple myeloma serum proteins. *Cancer*, **9**, 262.

Koshland, M.E. (1985) The coming of age of immunoglobulin J chain. *Ann. Rev. Immunol.*, **3**, 425–53.

Krawinkel, K., Christoph, T. & Blankenstein, T. (1989) Organisation of the Ig V_H region in mice and humans. *Immunol. Today*, **10**, 339–44.

Kuhn, R., Rajewsky, K. & Muller, W. (1991) Generation and analysis of interleukin-4 deficient mice. *Science*, **254**, 707–10.

Kurosaki, T., Gander, I., Wirthmueller, U. & Ravetch, J.V. (1992) The beta subunit of the Fc epsilon RI is associated with the Fc gamma RIII on mast cells. *J. Exp. Med.*, **175**, 447–51.

Kurosawa, Y. & Tonegawa, S. (1982) Organization, structure and assembly of immunoglobulin heavy-chain diversity DNA segments. *J. Exp. Med.*, **155**, 201–18.

Landau, N.R., Schatz, D.G., Rosa, M. & Baltimore, D. (1987) Increased frequency of *N*-regional insertion in a murine pre-B cell line infected with a TdT retroviral expression vector. *Mol. Cell. Biol.*, **7**, 3237–43.

Lanzavecchia, A. (1985) Antigen-specific interaction between T and B cells. *Nature*, **314**, 538–9.

Leder, P. (1982) The genetics of antibody diversity. *Sci. Am.*, **246**, 102.

Li, Y.S., Hayakawa, K. & Hardy, R.R. (1993) The regulated expression of B lineage associated genes during B cell differentiation in bone marrow and fetal liver. *J. Exp. Med.*, **178**, 951–60.

Lieber, M.R., Hesse, J.E., Lewis, S. *et al.* (1988) The defect in murine severe combined immunodeficiency: joining of signal sequences but not coding segments in *V(D)J* recombination. *Cell*, **55**, 7–16.

Lin, W. & Desiderio, S. (1993) Regulation of *V(D)J* recombination activator protein RAG-2 by phosphorylation. *Science*, **260**, 953–9.

Marsh, D.G., Neely, J.D., Breazeale, D.R. *et al.* (1994) Linkage analysis of IL4 and other chromosome 5q31.1 markers and total serum immunoglobulin E concentrations. *Science*, **264**(5162), 1152–6.

Matsuda, F., Lee, K.H., Nakai, S. *et al.* (1988) Dispersed localization of *D* segments within the human immunoglobulin heavy-chain locus. *Eur. Mol. Biol. Organ. J.*, **7**, 1047–51.

Matsuda, F., Shin, E.K., Nagaoka, H. *et al.* (1993) Structure and physical map of 64 variable segments in the 3′ 0.8 Mb region of the human immunoglobulin heavy-chain locus. *Nature Genet.*, **3**, 88–94.

Matsumoto, A.K., Martin, D.R., Carter, R.H., Klickstein, L.B., Ahearn, J.M. & Fearon, D.T. (1993) Functional dissection of the CD21/CD19/TAPA-1/Leu-13 complex of B lymphocytes. *J. Exp. Med.*, **178**, 1407–17.

Max, E.E., Maizel, J.V. & Leder, P. (1981) The nucleotide sequence of a 5.5 kb DNA segment containing the mouse kappa Ig *J* and C region genes. *J. Biol. Chem.*, **256**, 5116–20.

Max, E.E., Seidman, J.G. & Leder, P. (1979) Sequences of five potential recombination sites encoded close to an immunoglobulin κ constant region gene. *Proc. Nat. Acad. Sci. USA*, **76**, 3450–4.

McCafferty, J., Griffiths, A.D., Winter, G. & Chiswell, D. (1990) Phage antibodies: filamentous phage displaying antibody variable domains. *Nature*, **348**, 552–4.

Meek, K.D., Hasemann, C.A. & Capra, J.D. (1989) Novel rearrangements at the immunoglobulin D locus. Inversions and fusions add to IgH somatic diversity. *J. Exp. Med.*, **170**, 39–57.

Melchers, F., Haasner, D., Grawunder, U. *et al.* (1994) Role of IgH and L chains and of surrogate L chains in the development of the B lymphocyte lineage. *Ann. Rev. Immunol.*, **12**, 209–21.

Milstein, C. (1980) Monoclonal antibodies. *Sci. Am.*, **243**(4), 66.

Moller, G. (1993) *The B Cell Antigen Receptor Complex*. Immunol. Reviews, vol. 132. Munksgaard, Copenhagen.

Mombaerts, P., Iocamini, J., Johnson, R.S., Herrup, K., Tonegawa, S. & Papaicannou, V.E. (1992) Rag-1 deficient mice have no mature B and T lymphocytes. *Cell*, **68**, 869–77.

Morgan, E.L. & Weigle, W.O. (1987) Biological activities residing in the Fc region of immunoglobulin. *Adv. Immunol.*, **40**, 61–134.

Mostov, K.E., Krahenbuhl, J.-P. & Blobel, G. (1980) Receptor-mediated transcellular transport of immunoglobulin: synthesis of secretory component as multiple and larger transmembrane forms. *Proc. Nat. Acad. Sci. USA*, **77**, 7257–61.

Natvig, J.B. & Kunkel, H.G. (1973) Human immunoglobulins: classes, subclasses, genetice variants and idiotypes. *Adv. Immunol.*, **16**, 1.

Nelsen, B., Tian, G., Erman, B. *et al.* (1993) Regulation of lymphoid-specific immunoglobulin mu heavy chain gene enhancer by ETS-domain proteins. *Science*, **261**, 82–6.

Nikaido, T., Nakai, S. & Honjo, T. (1981) Switch region of Ig Cμ gene is composed of simple tandem repetitive sequences. *Nature*, **292**, 845–9.

Nossal, G.J.V. (1992) The molecular and cellular basis of affinity maturation in the antibody response. *Cell*, **68**, 1–2.

Nussenzweig, M.C., Shaw, A.C., Sinn, E. *et al.* (1987) Allelic exclusion in transgenic mice that express the membrane form of immunoglobulin M. *Science*, **236**, 816–9.

Oettinger, M.A., Schatz, D.G., Gorka, C. & Baltimore, D. (1990) RAG-1 and RAG-2, adjacent genes that synergistically activate *V(D)J* recombination. *Science*, **248**, 1517–23.

Orloff, D.G., Ra, C., Frank, S.J., Klausner, R.D. & Kinet, J.-P. (1990) The zeta and eta chains of the T cell and the gamma chain of Fc receptors form a family of disulphide-linked dimers. *Nature*, **347**, 189–91.

Papavasiliou, F., Misulovin, Z., Suh, H. & Nussenzweig, M.C. (1995) The role of Ig beta in precursor B cell transition and allelic exclusion. *Science*, **268**(5209), 408–11.

Patel, K.J. & Neuberger, M.S. (1993) Antigen presentation by the B cell antigen receptor is driven by the a/b sheath and occurs independently of its cytoplasmic tyrosines. *Cell*, **74**, 939–46.

Pettersson, S., Cook, G.P., Brüggeman, M., Williams, G.T. & Neuberger, M.S. (1990) A second B cell specific enhancer sequence 3′ of the immunoglobulin heavy chain locus. *Nature*, **344**, 165–8.

Porter, R.R. (1973) Structural studies of immunoglobulins. *Science*, **180**, 713–6.

Potter, M. (1972) Immunoglobulin-producing tumours and myeloma proteins of mice. *Physiol. Rev.*, **52**, 631–719.

Rathbun, G.A., Capra, J.D. & Tucker, P.W. (1987) Organization of the murine immunoglobulin VH complex in the inbred strains. *Eur. Mol. Biol. Organ. J.*, **6**, 2931–7.

Ravetch, J.V., Siebenlist, U., Korsemeyer, S., Waldmann, T. & Leder, P. (1981) Structure of the human immunoglobulin μ locus: characterization of embryonic and rearranged *J* and *D* segments. *Cell*, **27**, 583–91.

Reichmann, L., Clark, M., Waldmann, H. & Winter, G. (1988) Reshaping human antibodies for therapy. *Nature*, **332**, 323–27.

Reth, M. (1989) Antigen receptor tail clue. *Nature*, **338**, 383.

Reth, M. (1992) The B cell antigen receptor. *Ann. Rev. Immunol.*, **10**, 97–121.

Reth, M. & LeClerq, L. (1987) Assembly of immunoglobulin variable region gene segments. In: *Molecular Genetics of Immunoglobulin* (eds F. Calabi & M.S. Neuberger), p. 111. Elsevier Science Publishers, Amsterdam.

Reth, M., Petrac, E., Wiese, P., Lobel, L. & Alt, F.W. (1987) Activation of Vκ rearrangement in pre-B cells follows the expression of membrane-bound immunoglobulin heavy chains. *Eur. Mol. Biol. Organ. J.*, **6**, 3299–305.

Rock, K.L., Benacerraf, B. & Abbas, A.K. (1984) Antigen presentation by hapten-specific B lymphocytes. I. Role of surface immunoglobulin receptors. *J. Exp. Med.*, **160**, 1102.

Rowe, D.S. & Fahey, J.L. (1965) A new class of human immunoglobulins. I. A unique myeloma protein. II. Normal serum IgD. *J. Exp. Med.*, **121**, 171–99.

Sakano, H., Hüppi, K., Heinrich, G. & Tonegawa, S. (1979) Sequences at the somatic recombination sites of immunoglobulin light-chain genes. *Nature*, **280**, 288–94.

Sakano, H., Maki, R., Kurosawa, Y., Roeder, W. & Tonegawa, S. (1980) Two types of somatic recombination are necessary for the generation of complete immunoglobulin heavy-chain genes. *Nature*, **286**, 676–83.

Schatz, D.G., Oettinger, M.A. & Schlissl, M.S. (1992) *V(D)J* recombination: molecular biology and regulation. *Ann. Rev. Immunol.*, **10**, 359–83.

Schindler, C., Kashleva, H., Pernis, A., Pine, R. & Rothman, P. (1994) STF-IL-4: a novel IL-4-induced signal transducing factor. *EMBO J.*, **13**, 1350–6.

Schlissl, M.S. & Baltimore, D. (1989) Activation of immunoglobulin kappa rearrangement correlates with induction of germline kappa gene transcription. *Cell*, **58**, 1001–7.

Selsing, E., Durdik, J., Moore, M.W. & Persani, D.M. (1989) Immunoglobulin λ genes. In: *Immunoglobulin Genes* (eds T. Honjo, F.W. Alt & T.H. Rabbitts), p. 111. Academic, London.

Sen, R. & Baltimore, D. (1986) Inducibility of kappa Ig enhancer binding protein NF kappa B by a post-translational mechanism. *Cell*, **46**, 921–8.

Shinkai, Y., Rathbun, G., Lam, K.P. *et al.* (1992) Rag-2 deficient mice lack mature lymphocytes owing to inability to initiate *V(D)J* recombination. *Cell*, **68**, 855–67.

Shimizu, A., Takahashi, N., Yamakawi-Kataoka, Y., Nishida, Y., Kataoka, T. & Honjo, T. (1981) Ordering of mouse immunoglobulin heavy-chain genes by molecular cloning. *Nature*, **289**, 149–53.

Sitia, R., Neuberger, M., Alberini, C. *et al.* (1990) Developmental regulation of IgM secretion: the role of the carboxy-terminal cysteine. *Cell*, **60**, 781–90.

Strubin, M., Newell, J.W. & Matthias, P. (1995) OBF-1, a novel B cell-specific coactivator that stimulates immunoglobulin promoter activity through association with octamer-binding proteins. *Cell*, **80**, 497–506.

Taccioli, G.E., Gottleib, T.M., Blunt, T. *et al.* (1994) Ku80: product of the *XRC5* gene and its role in DNA repair and *V(D)J* recombination. *Science*, **265**, 1442–5.

Takai, T., Li, M., Sylvestre, D., Clynes, R. & Ravetch, J.V. (1994) FcR gamma chain deletion results in pleitrophic effector cell defects. *Cell*, **76**, 519–29.

Takata, M., Sabe, H., Hata, A. *et al.* (1994) Tyrosine kinases Lyn and Syk regulate B cell receptor coupled Ca^{2+} mobilization through distinct pathways. *Eur. Mol. Biol. Organ. J.*, **13**, 1341–9.

Tomasi, T., Tan, E., Solomon, A. & Prendergast, R. (1965) Characteristics of an immunoglobulin common to certain external secretions. *J. Exp. Med.*, **121**, 101–24.

Tomlinson, I.M., Walter, G., Marks, J.D., Llewelyn, M.B. & Winter, G. (1992) The repertoire of human germline VH sequences reveals about fifty groups of VH segments with different hypervariable loops. *J. Mol. Biol.*, **227**, 776–98.

Tonegawa, S. (1983) Somatic generation of antibody diversity. *Nature*, **302**, 575–81.

Turner, M., Mee, P.J., Costello, P.S. *et al.* (1995) Perinatal lethality and blocked B cell development in mice lacking the tyrosine kinase Syk. *Nature*, **378**, 298–302.

van Ghent, D.C., McBlane, J.F., Ramsden, D., Sadofsky, M., Hesse, J. & Gellert, M. (1995) Initiation of *V(D)J* recombination in a cell-free system. *Cell*, **81**, 925–34.

Venkitaraman, A.R. (1992) Light chain surrogacy. *Curr. Biol.*, **10**, 559.

Venkitaraman, A.R. (1994) Antigen receptors. In: *Cellular Immunology LabFax* (ed. P.J. Delves), p. 155. BIOS Scientific, Oxford.

Venkitaraman, A.R., Williams, G.T., Dariavach, P. & Neuberger, M.S. (1991) The B cell antigen receptory of the five immunoglobulin classes. *Nature*, **352**, 777–81.

Walter, M.A., Surti, U., Hofker, M.H. & Cox, D.W. (1990) The physical organization of the human immunoglobulin heavy chain gene complex. *Eur. Mol. Biol. Organ. J.*, **9**, 3303–13.

West, M.A., Lucocq, J.M. & Watts, C. (1994) Antigen processing and class II MHC peptide-loading compartments in human B-lymphoblastoid cells. *Nature*, **369**(6476), 147–51.

Wienands, J. & Reth, M. (1992) Glycosylphosphatidylinositol linkage as a mechanism for the cell surface expression of IgD. *Nature*, **356**, 246–8.

Williams, A.F. & Barclay, A.N. (1988) The immunoglobulin superfamily: domains for cell surface recognition. *Ann. Rev. Immunol.*, **6**, 381–405.

Williams, G.T., Venkitaraman, A.R., Gilmore, D. & Neuberger, M.S. (1990) The sequence of the μm transmembrane segment determines the tissue specificity of the transport of immunoglobulin M to the cell surface. *J. Exp. Med.*, **171**, 947–52.

Williams, S.C. & Winter, G. (1993) Cloning and sequencing of human immunoglobulin Vλ segments. *Eur. J. Immunol.*, **23**, 1456–61.

Winter, G., Griffiths, A.D., Hawkins, R.E. & Hoogenboom, H.R. (1994) Making antibodies by phage display technology. *Ann. Rev. Immunol.*, **12**, 433–55.

Winter, G. & Milstein, C. (1991) Man-made antibodies. *Nature*, **349**, 293–9.

Wood, C. & Tonegawa, S. (1983) Diversity and joining segments of mouse immunoglobulin heavy chain genes are closely linked and in the same orientation: implications for the joining mechanism. *Proc. Nat. Acad. Sci. USA*, **80**, 3030–4.

Wu, T.T. & Kabat, E.A. (1970) An analysis of the sequences of the variable regions of Bence Jones proteins and myeloma light chains and their implications for antibody complementarity. *J. Exp. Med.*, **132**, 211–50.

Yamanishi, Y., Kakiuchi, T., Mizuguchi, J., Yamamoto, T. & Toyoshima, K. (1991) Association of B cell antigen receptor with protein tyrosine kinase Lyn. *Science*, **251**, 192–4.

Yancopoulos, G. & Alt, F.W. (1985) Developmentally controlled and tissue-specific expression of unrearranged VH gene segments. *Cell*, **40**, 271–81.

Yelamos, J., Klix, N., Goyenechea, B. *et al.* (1995) Targeting of non-Ig sequences in place of the *V* segment by somatic hypermutation. *Nature*, **376**, 225–9.

Zachau, H.G. (1993) The immunoglobulin kappa locus — or — what has been learned from looking closely at one-tenth of a percent of the human genome. *Gene*, **135**, 167–73.

Zou, Y., Takeda, S. & Rajewsky, K. (1993) Gene targeting in the Ig k locus: efficient generation of lambda chain expressing B cells independent of Ig k gene rearrangements. *Eur. Mol. Biol. Organ. J.*, **12**, 811–20.

CHAPTER 5

IgE and IgE Receptors

B.J. Sutton & H.J. Gould

Introduction

Antibody molecules of the class known as immunoglobulin E (IgE) play a crucial role in allergy and allergic diseases. The existence of a blood factor that could transfer sensitivity to allergens was first demonstrated by Prausnitz and Küstner (1921), but only much later was this identified as a novel class of antibody (Ishizaka & Ishizaka, 1967), and named IgE after the erythema that results from allergenic challenge in the skin of sensitized individuals. More recently, two cell-surface receptors for IgE have been identified. The first, found principally on mast cells and basophils, binds IgE with an affinity ($K_a \approx 10^{10}\,M^{-1}$) that is higher than that of any other rceptor for an antibody (Metzger, 1992a). It is termed FcεRI, since it binds to the Fc region of the ε-chain of IgE (as described below), and is responsible for the release of histamine and other inflammatory mediators in hypersensitivity reactions when the receptors are cross-linked by allergen–IgE complexes.

The second receptor also binds to the Fc region of IgE, but with a lower affinity ($K_a \approx 10^{8}\,M^{-1}$), and is known as FcεRII. It was first identifed on B cells, and is identical to the surface antigen CD23 by which name it is also known. However, it is also found on a variety of inflammatory cells (macrophages, eosinophils) as well as follicular dendritic cells (FDC), Langerhans cells and T cells, and has been implicated in a number of functions including IgE-dependent antigen presentation by B cells to T cells, IgE-dependent phagocytosis, cell adhesion between B and T cells, and B-cell homing in germinal centres (Delespesse *et al.*, 1992; Gordon, 1993; Conrad *et al.*, 1994). A further feature of this receptor is that soluble fragments (sFcεRII) are released from the cell membrane and display various cytokine activities (Delespesse *et al.*, 1992) including the ability to stimulate B-cell proliferation and specifically up-regulate IgE synthesis (Aubry *et al.*, 1992). Since it has also been demonstrated that IgE and IgE–antigen complexes can down-regulate IgE levels by means of their interaction with FcεRII (Sherr *et al.*, 1989), it is clear that this 'low-affinity receptor' plays an important role in the control of IgE responses. This was subsequently confirmed *in vivo* with antibodies to FcεRII (Flores-Romo *et al.*, 1993), and is strongly suggested by the results of gene 'knock-out' experiments in mice (Fujiwara *et al.*, 1994; Yu *et al.*, 1994).

This functional diversity of FcεRII, together with the fact that it belongs to the C-type lectin superfamily (see below) and yet does not recognize the carbohydrate moities of IgE (Vercelli *et al.*, 1989), had led to the suspicion that a counter-molecule for FcεRII must exist in addition to IgE. This was finally confirmed in 1992 by Bonnefoy, who identified the glycosylated cell-surface molecule known variously as CR2 (complement receptor 2), CD21 and the EBV (Epstein–Barr virus) receptor, as a counter-structure for FcεRII (Aubry *et al.*, 1992). CR2 is expressed on B cells, FDCs, some T cells and also on basophils, and the pairing of FcεRII and CR2 may enhance B-cell–T-cell adhesion and thus contribute to the up-regulation of IgE (Bonnefoy *et al.*, 1993b). The interaction between these two proteins also constitutes a direct link between the IgE antibody and complement systems. The importance of complement in the generation of antibody responses has long been recognized (Erdei *et al.*, 1991), and CR2 plays a role in B-cell proliferation in its own right as receptor for the complement fragments (such as C3dg) generated by antibody-dependent or antibody-independent complement activation by antigen (Matsumoto *et al.*, 1991).

In 1995 FcεRII was discovered to have a link with yet another family of proteins, namely the integrin receptors (Lecoanet-Henchoz *et al.*, 1995). FcεRII binds to the CD11b and CD11c components of integrin receptor complexes CD11b/CD18 (Mac-1) and CD11c/CD18, and this interaction accounts for the ability of FcεRII to modulate monocyte activation and enhance the release of pro-inflammatory agents. Other counter-structures of FcεRII may well exist.

While FcεRI is clearly involved in immediate allergic responses, and FcεRII in IgE regulation, IgE-dependent antigen presentation and phagocytosis, a closer relationship between the two receptors recently emerged with the discovery that FcεRI was also present on Langerhans cells (Wang *et al.*, 1992) and on eosinophils (Gounni *et al.*, 1994). FcεRI may therefore also contribute locally to antigen presentation, and to defence against parasites (Bieber, 1994). To complete this apparent reversal of roles, sFcεRII has been found to enhance histamine release from normal blood basophils, by interacting with the CR2 molecules which these cells express on their surface (Bacon *et al.*, 1993). There may therefore be significant functional overlap between these two receptors.

Functional diversification among the receptors may also extend to the cells which bear them. The two signals required for switching B cells to produce IgE are IL-4 and CD40 ligand (CD40L), a T-cell surface counter-molecule for CD40. In the lymph nodes, T cells supply these two signals. However, mast cells and basophils not only release IL-4, but also express CD40L on their surface, and thus all the requirements for induction of IgE synthesis are available locally at the site of allergenic challenge (Gauchat *et al.*, 1993). IgE switching may therefore occur in the periphery (in lung and skin etc.), not only in the lymph nodes, and the whole network of molecular interactions that control the IgE response may thus operate locally as well as systemically.

In addition to the molecular components discussed so far (IgE, FcεRI, FcεRII, CR2 and CD11b/CD11c), there is a class of proteins termed IgE-binding or ε-binding proteins (εBP) with the potential to modulate the allergic response by binding to IgE and/or FcεRI (Liu, 1993). Their role is less well defined at present, but they belong to the S-type lectin (or galectin) family, and their presence underlines the importance of both protein–carbohydrate and protein–protein interactions in the regulation of the IgE network.

Each molecular component of this network, which is summarized in Fig. 5.1, will now be considered in turn. Our aim is to rationalize their functional properties in terms of their three-dimensional structures and capacities for interaction with each other. By understanding these interactions at the molecular level it may be possible to design agents to intervene in this network and control allergic responses. Indeed, it is already true that as a result of recent advances in our knowledge of these molecules, new approaches for therapeutic intervention, and targets for structure-based drug design, have been identified and are being pursued.

The IgE molecule

The basic architecture of the IgE molecule, with two identical heavy chains (ε class) and two identical light chains (κ or λ type), is very similar to that of antibodies of other classes. These polypeptide chains fold into tandemly arranged domains of 110 amino-acid residues, each with an intradomain disulphide bond and the characteristic 'immunoglobulin fold' structure, as seen in crystal structures of IgG molecules and their fragments and in other members of the immunoglobulin superfamily (Williams & Barclay, 1988). This arrangement of polypeptide chains, their inter- and intrachain disulphide bridges, and the nomenclature of the variable (V) and constant (C) domains, are shown on the left in Fig. 5.2. On the right, the expected quaternary structural arrangement of the domains is illustrated schematically although no crystal structure of any IgE fragment has yet been determined. Like IgG, IgE can be cleaved proteolytically into antigen-binding Fab fragments, and a constant Fc fragment, which contains the sites of antibody receptor binding. However, in contrast to IgG which has a flexible 'hinge' segment in each heavy chain between the Fab and Fc regions, IgE has an additional constant domain (Cε2) which has been shown to pair as in Fig. 5.2 (Helm *et al.*, 1991). The Fc of IgE thus consists of a disulphide-linked dimer of the Cε2, Cε3 and Cε4 domains.

In the absence of a crystal structure for IgE-Fc, three-dimensional atomic models have been generated (Padlan & Davies, 1986; Helm *et al.*, 1991) based upon its homology with IgG-Fc. The Cε3 and Cε4 domains are expected to adopt a structure similar to the Cγ2 and Cγ3 domains of the IgG–Fc crystal structure (Deisenhofer, 1981), including the *N*-linked glycosylation site at Asn 394 in each Cε3 domain, which is homologous to Asn 297 in Cγ2 and is conserved across antibodies of other classes. (In addition to this conserved glycosylation site, there are two ε-chain specific *N*-linked sites, Asn 265 in Cε2 and Asn 371 in Cε3, as shown in Fig. 5.2.) There is no homologue for the Cε2 domains, however, and although a paired arrangement is expected and can be modelled, the disposition of the $(C\varepsilon2)_2$ pair relative to the rest of the Fc structure cannot be predicted. As we shall see later, the structure of this region between Cε2 and Cε3 is critically important for receptor binding.

The IgE molecule is depicted in Fig. 5.2 as a planar Y-

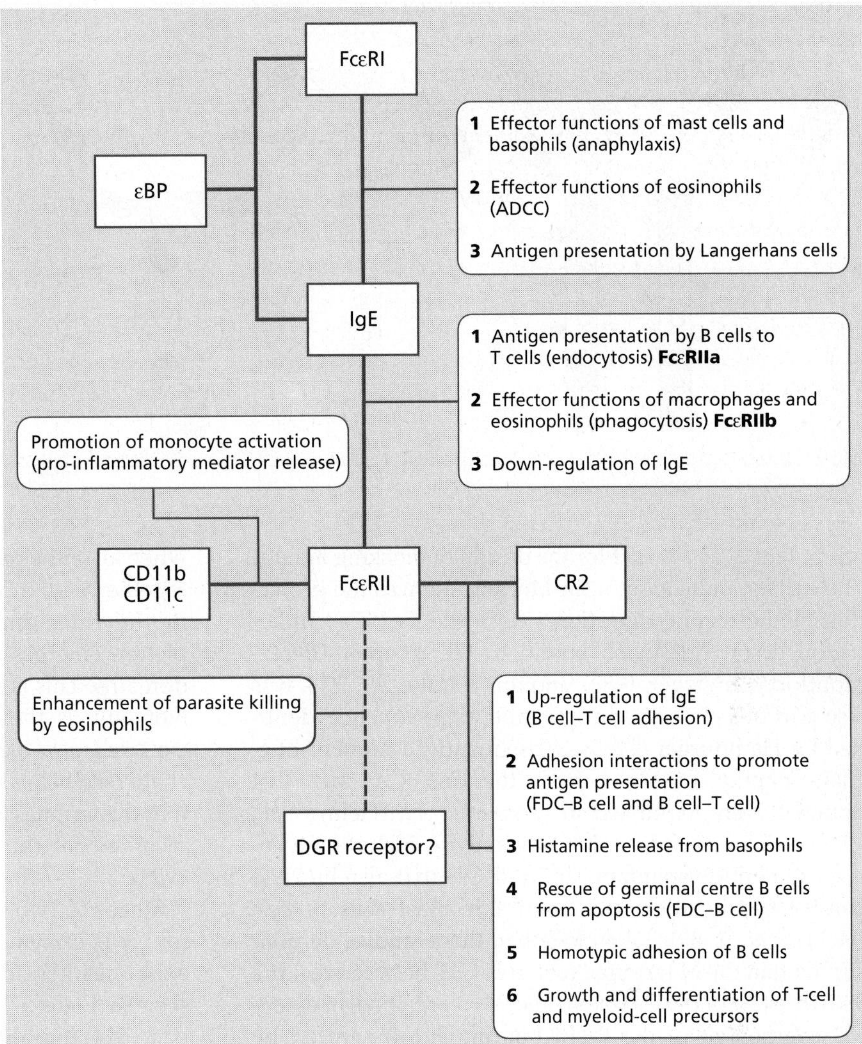

Fig. 5.1 Components of the IgE network and their functional interactions. See text for definition of abbreviations.

shaped structure, but spectroscopic studies in solution, in which the distance between chromophores attached to the extremities of the molecule is measured by resonance energy transfer (Zheng *et al.*, 1991), reveal that in fact it has a compact, bent structure. Whereas the distance between the antigen binding sites and the C termini of the Cε4 domains is expected to be 17.5 nm in a planar structure, it is in fact 6.9 nm. This bent structure was found not only for free IgE, but also when bound to FcεRI (Zheng *et al.*, 1991), and thus a more realistic image of the molecule is that shown in Fig. 5.4. This compact structure is also consistent with early solution X-ray scattering data (Davis *et al.*, 1990), and has been confirmed by more recent X-ray and neutron scattering studies (Beavil *et al.*, 1995a).

One consequence of this asymmetrical structure is that it can help to rationalize the observed stoichiometry of binding between IgE and FcεRI, which is 1 : 1 (Robertson, 1993), rather than the ratio of 1 : 2 which might have been expected for a structurally two-fold symmetrical IgE molecule. Clearly IgE must not be capable of binding two receptors, since this could lead to receptor cross-linkng and cell activation in the absence of allergen. The IgE–Fc, however, also has a stoichimetry of binding of 1 : 1 to the soluble IgE-binding α-chain of FcεRI (Keown *et al.*, 1995), suggesting that the Fc region itself is bent, and this has been confirmed by X-ray and neutron scattering studies which also show that the bend most likely occurs between the Cε2 and Cε3 domains (Beavil *et al.*, 1995a). This structure may be visualized by remodelling the extended linker region between the Cε2 and Cε3 domains of the earlier model (Helm *et al.*, 1991), to generate a compact, bent IgE–Fc structure. This can be seen in Plate 5.1 opposite page 524, and will now be used to discuss the location of the receptor binding sites.

Identification of the binding site for FcεRI in IgE has been a major focus of attention for many years, as it clearly

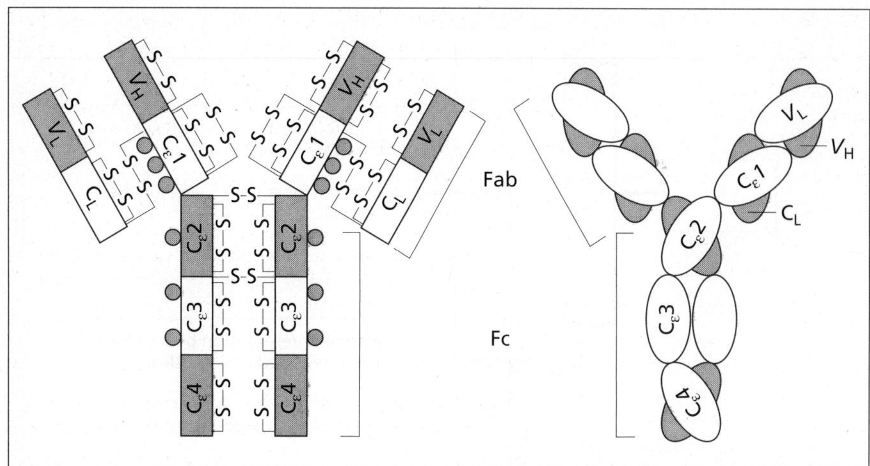

Fig. 5.2 Polypeptide and domain structure of the IgE molecule. Interchain and intradomain disulphide bridges are shown, and filled circles represent the *N*-linked glycosylation sites.

has potential as a target for the design of blocking agents. The earliest indication of the binding site was the protection of the tryptic digestion site in the Cε2/Cε3 linker region of rat IgE when bound to the receptor (Perez-Montfort & Metzger, 1982), and this residue, Arg 334, was also part of a class-specific pentapeptide sequence identified by Hamburger (1975). Subsequently, a number of ε-chain peptides derived from the Cε2, Cε3 and Cε4 domains were expressed in *Escherichia coli* (Helm *et al.*, 1988) and assayed for inhibitory activity, including a 76-residue peptide spanning Cε2 and Cε3 that also blocked passive sensitization of human skin mast cells *in vivo* (Helm *et al.*, 1989). Taken together, these studies demonstrated that the N-terminal region of Cε3, between residue 330 (the start of the Cε3 exon) and 361, contained an essential component of the FcεRI binding site (reviewed by Gould, 1992). A synthetic peptide consisting of residues 345–52 was also found to inhibit passive sensitization of human basophils at high concentration (Nio *et al.*, 1993). In an alternative approach to mapping the site, chimeric IgE molecules were generated with individual domains substituted either by mouse IgE or IgG sequences (Weetall *et al.*, 1990; Nissim *et al.*, 1993). These experiments confirmed the involvement of the Cε3 domain, but the final proof that this domain alone is sufficient has come from the production of a Cε3–Cε4 fragment (Basu *et al.*, 1993) and a Cε3 domain peptide with FcεRI binding activity (A.J. Henry, B.J. Sutton & H.J. Gould, unpublished data).

The most detailed mapping of the site has come from site-directed mutagenesis experiments. In a very comprehensive study investigating almost the whole surface of Cε3 (Presta *et al.*, 1994), a number of residues were identified, including a patch located distant from the N-terminal region of the domain. Yet mutagenesis of Pro 333 and Arg 334 in the N-terminal region has also demonstrated the involvement of these residues (Beavil *et al.*, 1993; Henry, Sutton & Could unpublished data). However, when all of the residues identified by Presta *et al.* are taken together with those in the N-terminal region, and located in the three-dimensional structure of IgE-Fc, a clear picture emerges of an extensive site spanning both Cε3 domains. This is shown in Plate 5.1(a), opposite page 524. Not only is the extent of the site consistent with that expected of a high-affinity interaction with the FcεRI α-chain (see below), but the compact shape of the complex that this implies is in agreement with hydrodynamic data recorded for the IgE–Fc/FcεRIα complex (Keown *et al.*, 1995).

Since the two Cε3 domains are related by a local two-fold axis of symmetry in the IgE–Fc structure, two sites exist on either side of the molecule. These two sites can be seen in Plate 5.1(b) (coloured red and green), opposite page 524, revealing the striking fact that their location is such that in the bent IgE–Fc, one site is occluded while the other is exposed. The extent of the bend between Cε2 and Cε3 is uncertain, but even as depicted in Plate 5.1(b), opposite page 524, the effect upon the two sites is clear. Thus, the asymmetrical, bent structure of IgE and its Fc fragment may account for the observed 1 : 1 stoichiometry.

Another interesting feature of this site is its structural homology to the receptor binding sites that have been identified in IgG. The first IgG residues to be implicated in FcγRI, II and III binding by mutagenesis studies were in the vicinity of Leu 235 in the N-terminal region of the Cγ2 domain (Duncan *et al.*, 1988; Jefferis *et al.*, 1990); the structural homologue of this residue is Pro 333 in the N-terminal region of Cε3, one of the residues depicted in Plate 5.1(a & b), opposite page 524. Other adjacent regions of IgG have since been implicated, in particular residues in the loop between β-strands F and G of the Cγ2 domain (Canfield & Morrison, 1991), and these are structurally homologous to IgE residues identified in FcεRI binding (Presta *et al.*, 1994) and shown in Plate 5.1(a & b), opposite page 524. This comparison with IgG–Fcγ receptor interactions may also shed light on the uniquely high affinity of the IgE–FcεRI interaction, which is two orders of magnitude higher than that of IgG for any of its receptors (Ravetch & Kinet, 1991). The relative affinities of the different subclasses of human IgG for each receptor (IgG1 ≈ IgG3 > IgG2 ≈ IgG4) approximately mirrors the relative hinge lengths in these subclasses, suggesting that antibody flexibility and accessibility to the receptor binding site (located as it is, close to the hinge) is a determinant of affinity. In contrast to the flexible IgG, a rigidly bent IgE (for spectroscopic studies not only indicate a bent, but also an inflexible molecule relative to IgG (Zheng *et al.*, 1992)), and a fully exposed site may contribute to the high affinity.

The binding site for the lower-affinity receptor FcεRII is not so well defined, but various approaches, including inhibition by monoclonal antibody binding (Chrétien *et al.*, 1988; Vercelli *et al.*, 1989), peptide inhibition (Ghaderi & Stanworth, 1993) and generation of chimeric antibodies (Nissim *et al.*, 1993), have been employed. It is clear, however, that this site also lies within the Cε3 domain. The results of these studies are illustrated in Plate 5.1(c), which probably overestimates the region of interaction since precise definition of the site has yet to be achieved. Nevertheless, it can be seen that the two symmetry-related sites are well separated from each other, and that bending of the IgE–Fc has no effect upon the accessibility of either FcεRII binding site (Plate 5.1(d)). It might be predicted, therefore, that the stoichiometry of binding between FcεRII and IgE–Fc is 2 : 1, and this has been confirmed by analytical ultracentrifugation (R. Ghirlando, B.J. Sutton & H.J. Gould unpublished data).

The FcεRI and FcεRII receptor binding sites in IgE are therefore clearly distinct, although there may be some degree of overlap. In particular they appear to be located strategically in regions of the IgE–Fc that lead to different stoichiometries of binding to their receptors which, as we shall see, has important functional implications.

The high-affinity receptor FcεRI

FcεRI consists of four polypeptide chains, $\alpha\beta\gamma_2$, which together form an integral membrane protein complex with seven transmembrane segments, as depicted schematically in Fig. 5.3. The β-chain and the two disulphide-linked γ-chains act synergistically to promote signal transduction, and each contains the sequence motif DxxYxxLxxxxxxxYxxL, which is known as the immunotyrosine activation motif (ITAM; Cambier, 1995). This motif, which is also found in the accessory molecules of other receptors such as the α- and β-chains of the mIgM antigen receptor, and the ξ-chain of the T-cell receptor, becomes phosphorylated at the tyrosine (Y) residues and then interacts with tyrosine kinases to initiate a cascade of reactions leading to cell activation. Tyrosine kinase *lyn* is associated with the unactivated FcεRIβ chain, and upon receptor aggregation phosphorylates the β- and γ-chains of an adjacent receptor (*trans*-phosphorylation; Pribluda *et al.*, 1994). This induces association with the kinase *syk*, activation of which initiates the cascade (Jouvin *et al.*, 1994; Wilson *et al.*, 1995). The trigger for activation is therefore receptor cross-linking in the presence of multivalent antigen (Metzger, 1992b), which is mediated by the principally extracellular and IgE-binding α-chain (Metzger, 1992a).

The extracellular sequence of the α-chain contains two domains that belong to the immunoglobulin superfamily. These domains, labelled α(1) and α(2) in Fig. 5.3, have been modelled upon immunoglobulin C domain crystal structures (Padlan & Helm, 1992), and upon the domain structures found in cell-surface antigens such as CD2 and CD4 (Beavil *et al.*, 1993; McDonnell *et al.*, 1996), which are

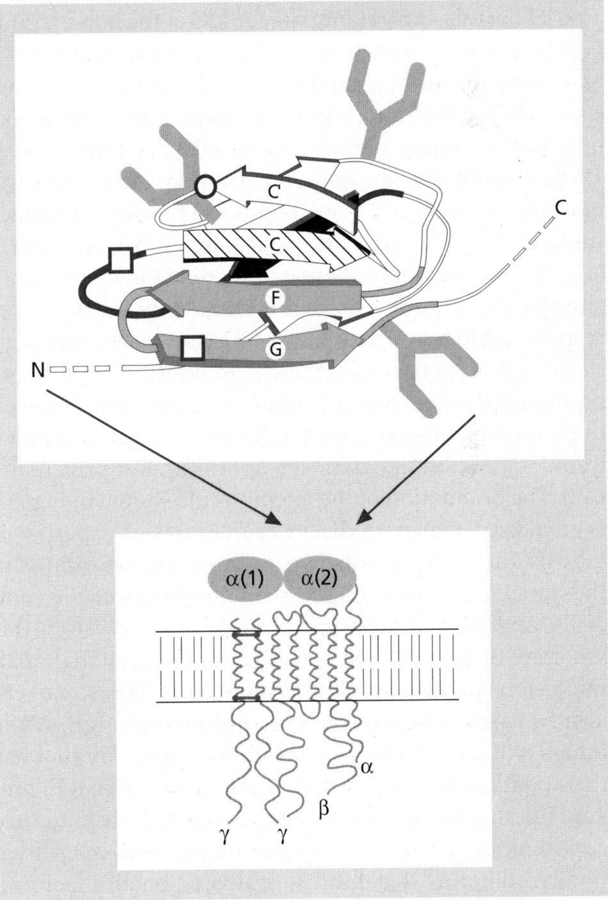

Fig. 5.3 Schematic illustration of the arrangement of polypeptide chains within FcεRI, and the predicted fold of the second, IgE-binding domain of the α-chain. The broad arrows represent β-strands, and the hatched, shaded and black segments, and residue positions (circle and squares), which implicate the C'CFG face in IgE binding, are discussed in the text. The three potential *N*-glycosylation sites are also shown.

intermediate in structure between the V and C domain types and are known as C2 (Williams & Barclay, 1988). The IgE-binding site has been shown to lie principally in α(2), by phage display of individual domains (Robertson, 1993; Scarselli *et al.*, 1993), and expression of chimeric α-chain (Mallamaci *et al.*, 1993), but maximal affinity is observed only when both domains are present. The schematic arrangement of β-strands within α(2) is shown in Fig. 5.3 and it is the C′CFG face of this domain which appears, from a number of lines of evidence, to be the region which interacts with IgE.

Firstly, this face is not glycosylated, and glycosylation does not interfere with IgE binding (Blank *et al.*, 1991; Letourneur *et al.*, 1995). Secondly, a stretch of seven residues conserved between human and rat FcεRI, but not FcγR sequences, corresponds to strand C (cross-hatched in Fig. 5.3). Thirdly, an antibody to the peptide corresponding to strand B (covered by carbohydrate) and the BC loop (shown black in Fig. 5.3) blocks IgE binding (Riske *et al.*, 1991). Fourthly, the binding site for IgG in the homologous FcγRII has been shown to involve residues in strands F and G and the intervening loop (F and G in Fig. 5.3; Hulett *et al.*, 1993, 1994), and a parallel study with FcγRIII also implicates residues in the CC′ and EF loops (Hibbs *et al.*, 1994). Finally, polymorphic substitutions that affect IgE binding to the homologous FcγRII are found on this face (indicated by the circle and squares in Fig. 5.3; Hogarth *et al.*, 1992). In addition, there is now direct evidence from site-specific mutagenesis, and inhibition by peptides corresponding to this face of α(2) (McDonnell *et al.*, 1996).

The topology of binding of IgE to FcεRI may therefore be depicted as in Fig. 5.4, with an interaction between the Cε3 domains of a bent IgE molecule, and the two immunoglobulin-like domains of FcεRIα, but principally α(2). The orientation of the IgE molecule shown in Fig. 5.4 is also consistent with distances determined experimentally by energy transfer between chromophores located in the antigen combining sites, the C terminus of the molecule, and the cell membrane (Zheng *et al.*, 1991). In this structure of the complex it may readily be seen that of all monoclonal antibodies that recognize free IgE, some will also be capable of binding to receptor-bound IgE, while others will not. It is this second class of antibody that has therapeutic potential, since they can remove free IgE, prevent binding to the receptor, and yet are unable to induce cross-linking of the IgE–receptor complex and cell activation. Antibodies that bind to epitopes on the 'convex' surface of the free IgE molecule would be expected to fall into this class, since these epitopes are hidden by the receptor on one side of the molecule, and occluded by the Fab regions on the other. Such antibodies are under development for the treatment of allergy and asthma (Davis *et al.*, 1993; Kolbinger *et al.*, 1993; Saban *et al.*, 1994).

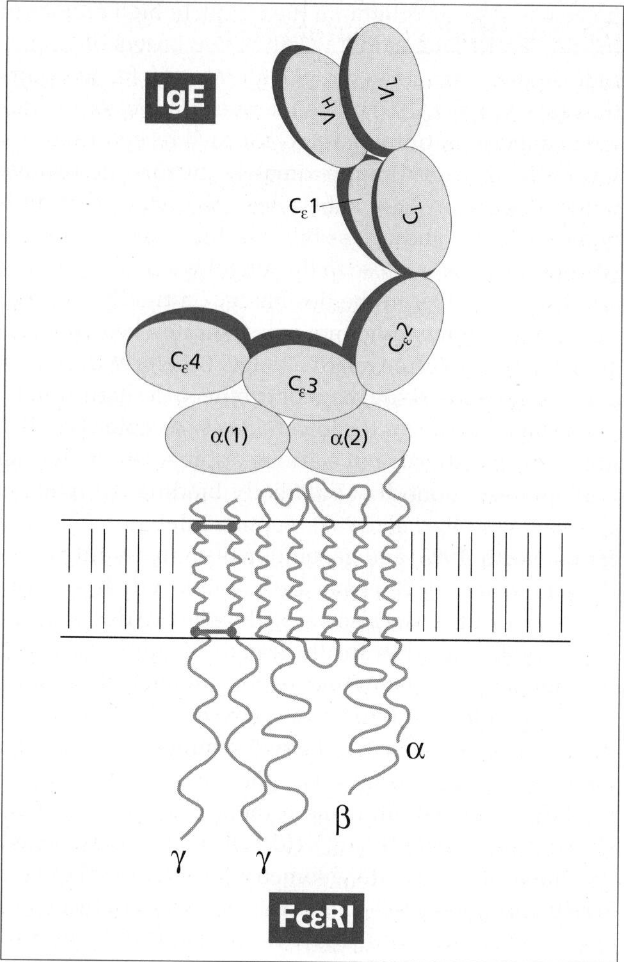

Fig. 5.4 Schematic representation of the complex formed between IgE and FcεRI. The bent structure of IgE is consistent with experimental data (refer to text), and the IgE binds principally to the α(2) domain of the receptor, through a site (shown in Plate 5.1(a) & (b), opposite p. 524) which spans both Cε3 domains on the convex side of the IgE molecule.

While the IgE–FcεRI interaction is clearly one target for therapeutic intervention, little is known about the way in which the four polypeptides of the receptor interact and function as a unit. Knowledge of the overall architecture of the receptor might open up alternative strategies. The discovery of an association between sequence variants of the FcεRIβ chain and atopy (Shirakawa *et al.*, 1994), in particular at position 181 within the fourth transmembrane segment of the chain, suggests that subtle changes in the spatial arrangement of the chains may indeed influence activity. Furthermore, spectroscopic studies of IgE binding to the cell-bound, intact receptor suggest that there may be a change in the conformational state of the receptor upon ligand binding (Ortega *et al.*, 1991). Much remains to be learned about the structure and function of FcεRI *in situ*.

The low-affinity receptor FcεRII

This molecule stands alone among the immunoglobulin receptors as the only one which is not a member of the immunoglobulin superfamily. It is a type II integral membrane protein (i.e. it has an intracellular N terminus), with an extracellular domain that is homolgous to the C-type (Ca^{2+}-dependent) lectins (Fig. 5.5), a family which includes cell-surface molecules such as the asialoglycoprotein receptor (AsgpR) and the selectins (Drickamer & Taylor, 1993). Another distinctive feature of this receptor is that various soluble fragments (sFcεRII) of different sizes are released from the cell membrane by proteolysis, apparently with their own functional activities. All sFcεRII forms contain the lectin domain, but subtle structural differences may be responsible for their characteristic functional properties.

Between the lectin domain and the single transmembrane segment lies an extensive region of the sequence in which a repeating pattern of amino-acid residues has been observed. Not only is this region coded by a tandem array of homologous exons (three in human, four in murine FcεRII), presumably the result of gene duplication, but also the sequence exhibits a periodicity in the nature of the amino-acid residues throughout the whole of this region. A heptad repeat of hydrophobic residues, characteristic of that found in α-helical coiled-coil proteins such as tropomyosin, can be identified (Beavil *et al.*, 1992), and is shown schematically in Fig. 5.5. Hydrophobic residues predominate at the first and fourth positions of the heptad (on the left in Fig. 5.5), and indeed in the middle of this region, a series of leucine residues spaced seven residues apart, a 'leucine zipper' motif, can be seen. This sequence implies the existence of an α-helical coiled-coil structure (Beavil *et al.*, 1992), and thus an oligomeric receptor. The sequence is compatible with either a two- or three-stranded structure, but the existence of trimers of murine FcεRII, and also trimers of membrane-bound FcεRII, was subsequently confirmed experimentally by chemical cross-linking studies (Dierks *et al.*, 1993; Beavil *et al.*, 1995b).

The intracellular region of the sequence exists in two forms, a and b, which differ in their first six or seven residues (Fig. 5.5). These two forms of the receptor result from separate first exons spliced to a common mRNA sequence, and are differentially expressed: FcεRIIa is found only on antigen-activated B cells before differentiation into antibody-secreting plasma cells, and FcεRIIb expression is induced by IL-4 on a variety of inflammatory cells as well as B cells (Yokota *et al.*, 1988). The two forms have also been shown to mediate distinct activities: endocytosis in FcεRIIa-expressing cells, and IgE-dependent phagocytosis in FcεRIIb-expressing cells. Critical residues responsible for these functional differences have been

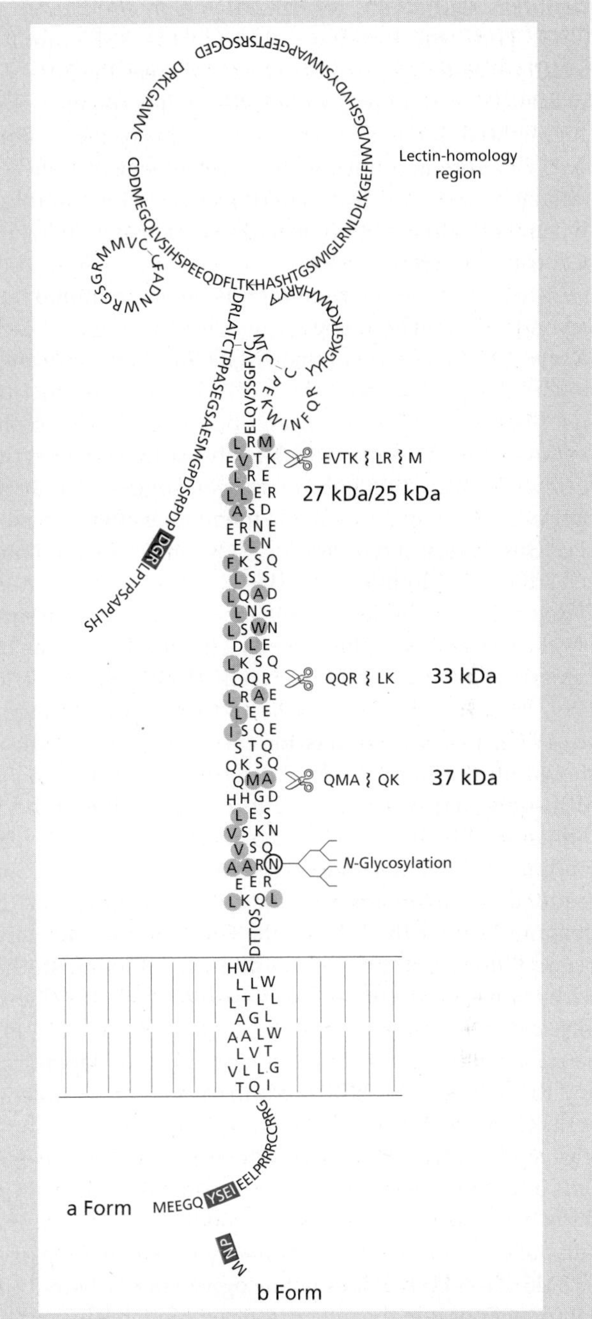

Fig. 5.5 The sequence and schematic structure of human FcεRII indicating: the functional motifs (YSEI and NP) within the N-terminal regions of the two alternative forms of the receptor; the single transmembrane segment; the region of heptad repeats, with hydrophobic residues circled; the sites of proteolytic cleavage and molecular weights of the soluble fragments released; the site of *N*-glycosylation; the C-type lectin homology region with conserved disulphide bridges; the C-terminal tail containing the potential adhesion motif (DGR).

identified within the N-terminal region (Yokota *et al.*, 1992). Thus, the tyrosine residue in the YSEI motif in FcεRIIa is essential for endocytosis, whereas the NP motif in FcεRIIb is required for IgE-dependent phagocytosis (highlighted in Fig. 5.5). These two forms of the receptor may therefore account for the involvement of FcεRII in antigen presentation by B cells (Pirron *et al.*, 1990) and IgE-dependent cytotoxicity of macrophages against parasites (Capron *et al.*, 1986).

At the other end of the molecule, in a C-terminal 'tail' beyond the lectin homology region, lies the sequence DGR (a reverse of the more common RGD, Arg-Gly-Asp), and a potential adhesion motif (Fig. 5.5). No counter-structure, nor function has yet been ascribed definitively to this region of the molecule (which is absent from the murine form of FcεRII), although it has been suggested that the part of FcεRII remaining in the membrane after release of sFcεRII serves as a receptor for FcεRII in FcεRII-mediated cell adhesion (Moulder *et al.*, 1993).

Returning to the lectin domain, the crystal structures of other members of the C-type lectin family, such as the trimeric mannose binding protein (MBP; Sheriff *et al.*, 1994; Weis & Drickamer, 1994) and E-selectin (Graves *et al.*, 1994), provide models for this region of FcεRII, as shown on the right in Fig. 5.6. Of the two Ca^{2+} sites in MBP, only that shown as Ca2 in Fig. 5.6 is conserved in human FcεRII, but it is known that both IgE and CR2 binding is Ca^{2+} dependent. The Ca^{2+} ion is probably required to maintain the structural integrity of the domain. Neither the IgE nor the CR2 binding sites have been located within this lectin domain, although studies with chimeric FcεRII molecules (Bettler *et al.*, 1992) have implicated several regions in IgE binding (shaded in Fig. 5.6). The interation with CR2 is carbohydrate dependent, and the homologous MBP binds to carbohydrate moieties at the Ca^{2+} site (Weis *et al.*, 1992), and so this may define at least a part of the CR2 binding site in FcεRII. The two sites thus appear to be in a region of the domain distant from the α-helical coiled-coil structure and the DGR-containing tail, but it is not known to what extent they overlap, if at all. Although FcεRII does not recognize the carbohydrate component of IgE, the interaction is inhibitable by certain sugars (Delespesse *et al.*, 1992), implying that the two sites may overlap at the carbohydrate binding site.

The overall architecture of the FcεRII molecule in the cell membrane is also shown in Fig. 5.6. The trimeric structure disposes the three lectin heads for interaction with their protein ligands at the top of a triple α-helical coiled-coil 'stalk' of length 15 nm (18 nm in murine FcεRII). A model for this trimeric disposition of lectin heads is provided by the crystal structures of the MBP trimer, which includes a short region of triple α-helical coiled-coil (Sheriff *et al.*, 1994; Weis & Drickamer, 1994). The 'stalk' of the soluble MBP consists principally of a collagen triple

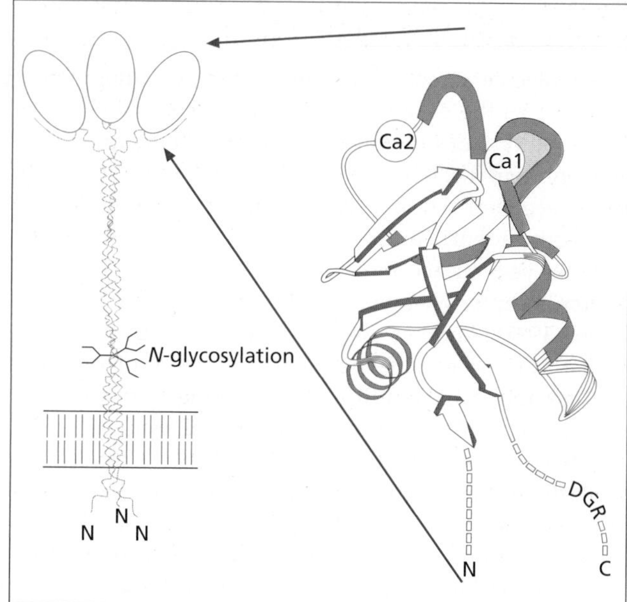

Fig. 5.6 Schematic representation of trimeric human FcεRII showing the triple α-helical coiled-coil stalk region, and the three lectin heads. The single *N*-linked glycosylation site is shown at the base of the stalk, and the molecule and membrane are drawn to scale. The fold of the polypeptide chain within the lectin domain is also shown, based upon the crystal structure of mannose binding protein (MBP, refer to text). Of the two Ca^{2+} sites in MBP, that marked Ca2 is conserved in human FcεRII. Regions implicated in IgE binding are shaded.

helix however, which places this protein in the family of 'collectins' (collagenous C-type lectins; Holmskov *et al.*, 1994). FcεRII belongs to a family of trimeric cell-surface receptor molecules with predicted α-helical coiled-coil stalks of different lengths (including AsgpR, 7.5 nm; and Kupffer cell receptor, 45 nm; Beavil *et al.*, 1992), but a common feature of all of these molecules is the enhanced effective affinity (avidity) for their ligands that results from the multipoint attachment afforded by their oligomeric structure. Indeed, there is a striking similarity between the endocytotic role of AsgpR in glycoprotein clearance, and the internalization of soluble IgE–antigen complexes by FcεRII for antigen presentation.

The stalk region not only acts as a spacer between the lectin domains and the membrane, but also contains the sites of cleavage that release the sFcεRII fragments. The principal sites are indicated in Fig. 5.5, together with the sizes of corresponding fragments. Figure 5.5 also shows that there is an *N*-glycosylation near the base of the stalk, and it is close to this site that the first cleavage occurs to produce a 37-kDa fragment; it may be significant that this cleavage site occurs in a region where the heptad repeat pattern appears to break down. Subsequent cleavage generates a 33-kDa fragment and a relatively stable 25-kDa fragment which has no stalk region. A 16-kDa fragment has also been identified that lacks the C-terminal tail and consists only of the lectin domain. All of these fragments retain IgE binding activity, but differ with respect to their cytokine activities; thus, while the larger fragments promote IgE synthesis (Delespesse *et al.*, 1992), the 16-kDa fragment inhibits this activity (Sarfati *et al.*, 1992). It is clear from Fig. 5.6, however, that while the larger fragments that include regions of the stalk may remain oligomeric in solution, the smaller fragments must be monomeric, and this may account for their functional differences.

It has been suggested that FcεRII possesses autoproteolytic activity (Letellier *et al.*, 1990), perhaps initiated by the action of an external protease, but this has yet to be clarified. Certainly FcεRII is a potential target for exogenous proteases, and it is possible that the potency of many common allergens derives in part from their protease activity and a direct effect upon FcεRII (Hewitt *et al.*, 1995; Schultz *et al.*, 1995).

A possible mode of binding between two lectin 'heads' of FcεRII and the two accessible sites on either side of the IgE Fc in the Cε3 domains (Plate 5.1(c & d)) is depicted in Fig. 5.7(a). The engagement and cross-linking of FcεRII on B cells by IgE immune complexes suppresses B-cell proliferation (Luo *et al.*, 1991) and IgE synthesis (Sherr *et al.*, 1989), but in addition to this down-regulatory signal, the binding of IgE and IgE complexes is known to inhibit the release of soluble fragments from FcεRII (Lee *et al.*, 1987). Inhibition of sFcεRII formation will block the potentially up-regulatory effects of these fragments on B-cell proliferation and IgE synthesis, and thus IgE and IgE immune complexes exert their negative effect in two ways. It is clear from the relative dimensions of these molecules and the location of the primary site of proteolysis at the base of the stalk, that this inhibition of FcεRII proteolysis at the membrane by IgE cannot be via a steric mechanism. Rather, an allosteric mechanism, perhaps involving stabilization of the trimeric structure, must be envisaged (Gould *et al.*, 1991).

In contrast to these down-regulatory effects upon IgE synthesis, the up-regulatory function of FcεRII and its soluble fragments depends upon its interaction with CR2, and this will be discussed below.

The counter-receptor for FcεRII: CR2

CR2 (CD21) is a glycosylated membrane protein that consists of a tandem array of homologous domains known as short consensus repeats (SCR), a constituent domain of many complement-related proteins. The SCR unit consists principally of a β-sheet structure (Norman *et al.*, 1991), and CR2 is an extended flexible molecule approximately 40 nm long (Moore *et al.*, 1989). It is shown in Fig. 5.7(b), together with the locations of its *N*-linked glycosylation sites, and the signal transduction molecule CD19 with which it is associated in the membrane. (CR2/CD19 in fact form part of a larger signal transduction complex on B cells; Tedder *et al.*, 1994.) The binding site in CR2 for fragments of the complement component C3 have been mapped with monoclonal antibodies to the two N-terminal domains and do not involve carbohydrate (Lowell *et al.*, 1989), but FcεRII binding has been localized to domains 5–8 and shown to involve the recognition of carbohydrate chains attached to domains 5 and 6 (Aubry *et al.*, 1994; see Fig. 5.7(b)). FcεRII is also known to exhibit a specificity for galactose residues (Kijimoto-Ochiai *et al.*, 1994). Indeed, FcεRII only appears to recognize certain glycoforms of CR2 (Aubry *et al.*, 1992), and this may be functionally important since differences exist in the pattern of glycosylation across the population. In addition to a direct role in IgE up-regulation, FcεRII is reported to degranulate basophils by cross-linking CR2 (Bacon *et al.*, 1993), and this may also indirectly enhance IgE production via the release of IL-4.

FcεRII and CR2 may thus form an adhesion pair as shown in Fig. 5.7(b), mediating interactions between B and T cells and contributing to IgE synthesis (Bonnefoy *et al.*, 1993b). This same molecular pairing may be involved in the rescue of germinal centre B cells from apoptosis (Bonnefoy *et al.*, 1993a), and perhaps also antigen presentation, since FDC express both FcεRII and CR2. Homotypic aggregation of B cells has also been shown to be mediated by FcεRII–CR2 interactions (Björck *et al.*, 1993). However, in addition to purely adhesion interactions between cells, FcεRII or oligomeric forms of sFcεRII could also cross-link CR2 and deliver a growth signal to a B cell (as do anti-CR2 antibodies), as shown in Fig. 5.7(c). For other CR2 ligands such as C3 fragments, only multivalent forms cause B-cell proliferation, whereas monovalent foms inhibit (Esparza *et al.*, 1991), and it may be that the same is true for FcεRII, thus accounting for the differential effects of the various sFcεRII species as B-cell growth or inhibition factors (Delespesse *et al.*, 1992). Furthermore, the potential of sFcεRII to interact with both IgE *and* CR2 provides a mechanism for the specific up-regulation of IgE; B cells committed to IgE synthesis will express both mIgE and CR2 and thus, as shown in Fig. 5.7(d), oligomeric sFcεRII may cross-link these molecules at the cell surface.

The discovery of CR2 as a counter-structure for FcεRII placed the 'low-affinity receptor for IgE' in an entirely new light, and at last provided a mechanism for some of the multifarious activities of this molecule, both IgE dependent and IgE independent. On account of its role in the regulation of IgE levels, FcεRII is clearly a potential target for intervention in allergy therapy, but much more needs to be learned about its interaction with CR2 before this becomes a feasible proposition.

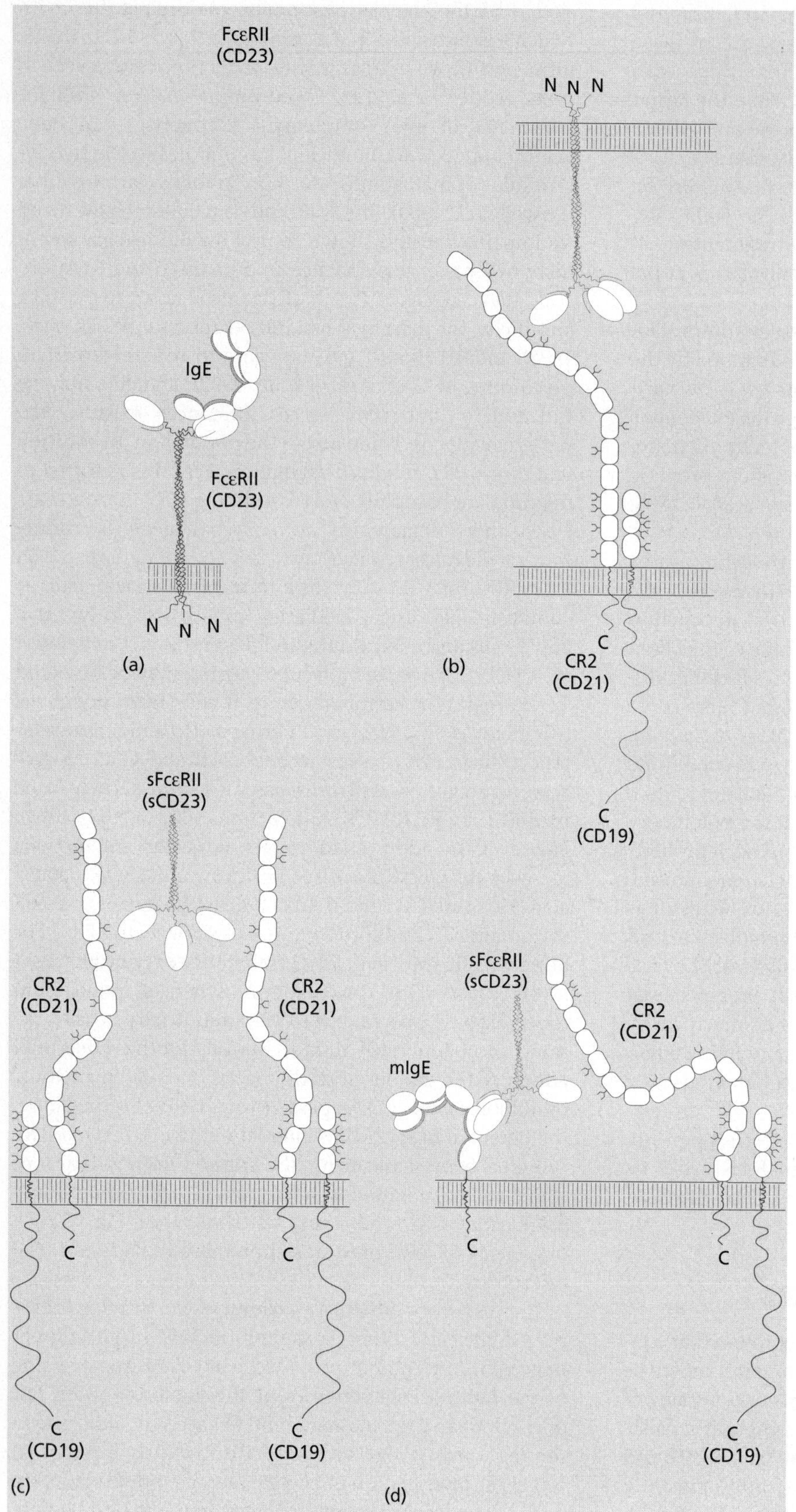

Fig. 5.7 Potential interactions between IgE, FcεRII and CR2. (All molecules and membrane are drawn to scale.) (a) IgE may bind to two lectin domains of FcεRII, through the sites (shown in Plate 5.1c & d, opposite page 524) on each of the two Cε3 domains. (b) Cell-surface FcεRII and CR2 may form an adhesion pair between various cell types (B cell–T cell, B cell–FDC, as described in the text). Glycosylation sites in CR2 and CD19 are indicated. (c) Oligomeric soluble forms of FcεRII may cross-link CR2 and lead to cell activation. (d) Oligomeric soluble forms of FcεRII may cross-link membrane-bound IgE and CR2 on the surface of B cells committed to IgE synthesis, and thereby provide a mechanism for specific activation of IgE synthesis.

Other counter-receptors for FcεRII: CD11b and CD11c

Despite the identification of two counter-structures for FcεRII, other functional properties implied the existence of yet futher ligands. Increased levels of FcεRII have been reported in a variety of inflammatory conditions such as rheumatoid arthritis, and this observation led to the discovery of a specific interaction between FcεRII and the CD11b and CD11c components of the integrin adhesion molecule complexes CD11b/CD18 (also known as Mac-1) and CD11c/CD18 on human blood monocytes (Lecoanet-Henchoz *et al.*, 1995). These integrins are involved in various well-documented cell adhesion interactions (Springer, 1990). The interaction of FcεRII with these molecules, however, is Ca^{2+} dependent, involves carbohydrate, and is partially inhibited by IgE (Lecoanet-Henchoz *et al.*, 1995); FcεRII thus behaves as a C-type lectin, as in its interaction with CR2. The functional effect of this interaction is the release of pro-inflammatory mediators such as nitric oxide and cytokines (Lecoanet-Henchoz *et al.*, 1995), and thus FcεRII appears to have a role in the regulation of monocyte activation. Inhibition of this interaction may provide a way to control inflammation, and anti-FcεRII antibodies have been shown to have such an effect in a mouse model for human rheumatoid arthritis (Plater-Zyberk & Bonnefoy, 1995).

In common with IgE and CR2, the binding of CD11b and CD11c does not appear to involve the reverse RGD sequence in the C-terminal tail of FcεRII (Lecoanet-Henchoz *et al.*, 1995; Fig. 5.5), despite the fact that a number of integrins do recognize RGD motifs. There is therefore still no counter-structure identified for this region of the molecule. However, the inhibition of IgE-dependent cytotoxicity against parasites by pre-incubation of eosinophils with this peptide sequence, or anti-peptide antibodies (Grangette *et al.*, 1989), implies that an adhesion interaction between this motif and a fourth, as yet unidentified, counter-receptor may exist (Fig. 5.1), and influence FcεRII activity on these cells.

ε-binding proteins

ε-binding protein (εBP), also known as Mac-2 and CBP35, is a soluble protein found associated with the cell surface of both mast cells and macrophages, with the ability to bind to both IgE and FcεRI. Its expression is enhanced when mast cells are activated by IgE complexes. It contains a tandemly repeated proline-rich N-terminal region which may mediate dimerization, and an S-type lectin (now termed galectin) C-terminal domain with specificity for galactose, through which it recognizes the carbohydrate moieties of IgE and FcεRI (Liu, 1993). (In the new terminology, εBP is now also known as galectin-3; Barondes *et al.*, 1994.) It thus has the capability to enhance the cross-linking of these molecules at the mast cell surface and, since it selectively recognizes particular glycoforms of these proteins (Robertson & Liu, 1991), has the potential to explain the variation between individual susceptibility to mast cell activation. In particular, the interaction with IgE is known to be prevented by sialylation of the *N*-linked oligosaccharide chains (Robertson & Liu, 1991), which blocks otherwise exposed terminal galactose residues. εBP has also been detected on neutrophils, and the binding of IgE complexes to cell-surface-associated εBP promotes activation of these cells (Truong *et al.*, 1993) which may therefore play a role in IgE-associated diseases. In a similar way, εBP has been found associated with Langerhans cells (which express both FcεRI and FcεRII), where it enhances the binding of IgE molecules that display terminal galactose residues (Wollenberg *et al.*, 1993).

εBP clearly has the ability to enhance allergic inflammatory responses, and more must be learned about the functional properties of this molecule, in particular its interactions with IgE and FcεRI and affinities for different glycoforms of these molecules. The crystal structures of two homologous mammalian S-type lectins (galectin-1 and galectin 2) have been determined (Barondes *et al.*, 1994) and found, remarkably, to have the same three-dimensional structure as plant lectins such as concanavalin A, despite the lack of any sequence homology with this latter family. The structure consists of a five-stranded and a six-stranded β-sheet, and all the residues of galectin-1 and galectin-2 that interact with carbohydrate in the crystal structures are conserved in εBP (galectin-3). Furthermore, a crystal structure of the dimeric galectin-1 cross-linked by biantennary carbohydrate chains of the complex type found on IgE and FcεRI (Bourne *et al.*, 1994) provides a model for the way in the which εBP may interact with glycoprotein carbohydrate chains that terminate in galactose. While εBP (galectin-3) contains only a single carbohydrate binding domain, the proline-rich repeating domain may facilitate dimerization, and hence IgE and/or FcεRI cross-linking.

A related protein with homology to the galectins, the Charcot–Leyden crystal protein (lysophospholipase), is a major constituent of eosinophils and basophils and is found in secretions from sites of inflammation in asthma and other allergic diseases (Ackerman *et al.*, 1993). While its IgE and receptor binding properties have yet to be established, it clearly has structural similarity to εBP (Leonidas *et al.*, 1995) and thus the potential to interact with glycoprotein components of the IgE network.

The existence of other factors that are characterized by their ability to release histamine from basophils and mast cells in an IgE-dependent manner, and which therefore may bind to IgE, has been suspected for many years. One such protein has now been identified and sequenced (MacDonald *et al.*, 1995), and appears to recognize a heterogeneity in IgE which may be a function of its glycosylation. This histamine-releasing factor appears to be linked to the severity of the late phase of the allergic reaction, and understanding the nature of its interaction with IgE may suggest why only certain individuals experience such a reponse, and how it might be controlled.

The IgE network and prospects for therapeutic intervention

Since the original discovery of IgE, a network of interacting proteins has been uncovered. No doubt more components of this system have yet to be identified. In contrast to IgG and its family of receptors, the IgE network encompasses at least five major superfamilies of proteins (Fig. 5.1): the immunoglobulin-like family (IgE, FcεRI), the C-type lectins (FcεRII), the S-type lectins or galectins (εBP), the integrins (CD11b, CD11c), and the family of proteins with complement SCR modules (CR2). FcεRII, in particular, appears to be engaged in an unprecedented array of interactions and functional activities, compounded by the fact that not only does it exist in two membrane-bound forms (FcεRIIa and FcεRIIb), but also in a variety of soluble forms with different oligomeric states. This receptor appears to play an important role in the regulation of IgE levels, and possible mechanisms for its role in both up-regulation (via CR2) and down-regulation (via IgE) have been mentioned above. Nevertheless, the overall picture of how these positive- and negative-feedback loops operate among the various cell populations that carry these receptors is still evolving (Sutton & Gould, 1993), and the ability to experiment with the intact system through the gene 'knockout' approach will no doubt enhance our understanding of the network as a whole.

Knowledge of the structures of the principal components and the nature of their interactions has, however, opened up a number of possibilities for therapeutic intervention. Blocking the binding of IgE to FcεRI to control the immediate hypersensitivity reaction has been approached by generating humanized anti-IgE antibodies (e.g. Davis *et al.*, 1993; Saban *et al.*, 1994), developing peptide inhibitors (Gould, 1992; McDonnell *et al.*, 1996) or by a vaccine strategy based upon IgE-derived peptides (Stanworth *et al.*, 1990) or whole domains, targetting the anti-IgE antibodies to the receptor binding region (Hellman, 1994). Indeed, it has been shown *in vitro* that naturally occurring IgG anti-IgE antibodies can either up-regulate or down-regulate the release of histamine from mast cells and basophils, depending upon their epitope specificity (Shakib *et al.*, 1995). These autoantibodies may also modulate IgE synthesis via their effect upon IgE binding to FcεRII (Shakib *et al.*, 1995), and an anti-IgE antibody has been shown to suppress a specific IgE response *in vivo*, by inhibiting FcεRII expression (Haak-Frendscho *et al.*, 1994). Inoculation of whole IgE into neonatal mice has been found to elicit an anti-IgE response and long-term suppression of IgE synthesis (Haba & Nisonoff, 1994). In contrast, the potentially harmful properties of anti-IgE and anti-FcεRI antibodies as histamine-releasing agents are exemplified by the demonstration of their important role in the pathogenesis of the allergic condition of chronic urticaria (Grattan *et al.*, 1991).

The FcεRI α-chain has also been considered as a target, either for the development of antireceptor antibodies (Riske *et al.*, 1991), or the soluble receptor itself (e.g. Ra *et al.*, 1993), which has been shown to inhibit allergic reactions *in vivo* (Naito *et al.*, 1995). Anti-FcεRII antibodies are known to inhibit the IgE response *in vivo* (Flores-Romo *et al.*, 1993), and soluble chimeric proteins containing the extracellular regions of CR2 have been found to suppress the immune response (Hebell *et al.*, 1991). A variety of molecular targets and strategies are thus being persued. The recent discovery that the two signals required to switch B cells to IgE synthesis, namely IL-4 and CD40L, may be supplied locally at sites of allergenic challenge, suggests that these earlier events may also be promising targets for therapeutic intervention in the future.

Acknowledgements

The authors wish to thank Dr Rebecca Beavil for the preparation of the figures, and the Medical Research Council, The Wellcome Trust and the National Asthma Campaign for supporting their work in this field.

References

Ackerman, S.J., Corrette, S.E., Rosenberg, H.F. *et al.* (1993) Molecular cloning and characterisation of human eosinophil Charcot–Leyden crystal protein (lysophospholipase). *J. Immunol.*, **150**, 456–68.

Aubry, J.-P., Pochon, S., Gauchat, J.-F. *et al.* (1994) CD23 interacts with a new functional extracytoplasmic domain involving N-linked oligosaccharides on CD21. *J. Immunol.*, **152**, 5806–13.

Aubry, J.-P., Pochon, S., Graber, P., Jansen, K.U. & Bonnefoy, J.-Y. (1992) CD21 is a ligand for CD23 and regulates IgE production. *Nature*, **358**, 505–7.

Bacon, K., Gauchat, J.-F., Aubry, J.-P. *et al.* (1993) CD21 expressed on basophilic cells is involved in histamine release triggered by CD23 and anti-CD23 antibodies. *Eur. J. Immunol.*, **23**, 2721–4.

Barondes, S.H., Cooper, D.N.W., Gitt, M.A. & Leffler, H. (1994) Galectins: structure and function of a large family of animal lectins. *J. Biol. Chem.*, **269**, 20807–10.

Basu, M., Hakimi, J., Dharm, E. *et al.* (1993) Purification and characterization of human recombinant IgE-Fc fragments that bind to the human high affinity IgE receptor. *J. Biol. Chem.*, **296**, 13118–27.

Beavil, A.J., Beavil, R.L., Chan, C.M.W. *et al.* (1993) Structural basis of the IgE–FcεRI interaction. *Biochem. Soc. Trans.*, **21**, 968–72.

Beavil, A.J., Edmeades, R.L., Gould, H.J. & Sutton, B.J. (1992) α-Helical coiled-coil stalks in the low-affinity receptor for IgE (FcεRII/CD23) and related C-type lectins. *Proc. Nat. Acad. Sci. USA*, **89**, 753–7.

Beavil, A.J., Young, R.J., Sutton, B.J. & Perkins, S.J. (1995a) Bent domain structure of recombinant human IgE-Fc in solution by X-ray and neutron scattering in conjunction with an automated curve fitting procedure. *Biochemistry*, **34**, 14449–61.

Beavil, R.L., Graber, P., Aubonney, N., Bonnefoy, J.-Y. & Gould, H.J. (1995b) CD23/FcεRII and its soluble fragments can form oligomers on the cell surface and in solution. *Immunology*, **84**, 202–6.

Bettler, B., Texido, G., Raggini, S., Rüegg, D. & Hofstetter, H. (1992) Immunoglobulin E-binding site in Fcε receptor (FcεRII/CD23) identified by homolog-scanning mutagenesis. *J. Biol. Chem.*, **267**, 185–91.

Bieber, T. (1994) FcεRI on human Langerhans cells: a receptor in search of new functions. *Immunol. Today*, **15**, 52–3.

Björck, P., Elenström-Magnusson, C., Rosén, A., Severinson, E. & Paulie, S. (1993) CD23 and CD21 function as adhesion molecules in homotypic aggregation of human B lymphocytes. *Eur. J. Immunol.*, **23**, 1771–5.

Blank, U., Ra, C. & Kinet, J.-P. (1991) Characterization of truncated α chain products from human, rat and mouse high affinity receptor for IgE. *J. Biol. Chem.*, **266**, 2639–46.

Bonnefoy, J.-Y., Henchoz, S., Hardie, D., Holder, M.J. & Cordon, J. (1993a) A subset of anti-CD21 antibodies promote the rescue of germinal center B cells from apoptosis. *Eur. J. Immunol.*, **23**, 969–72.

Bonnefoy, J.-Y., Pochon, S., Aubry, J.-P. *et al.* (1993b) A new pair of surface molecules involved in human IgE regulation. *Immunol. Today*, **14**, 1–2.

Bourne, Y., Bolgianor, B., Liao, D.-I. *et al.* (1994) Crosslinking of mammalian lectin (galectin-1) by complex biantennary saccharides. *Nature Struct. Biol.*, **1**, 863–70.

Cambier, J.C. (1995) New nomenclature for the Reth motif (or ARH1/TAM/ARAM/YXXL). *Immunol. Today*, **16**, 110.

Canfield, S.M. & Morrison, S.L. (1991) The binding affinity of human IgG for its high affinity Fc receptor is determined by multiple amino acids in the C_H2 domain and is modulated by the hinge region. *J. Exp. Med.*, **173**, 1483–91.

Capron, A., Dessaint, J.P., Capron, M., Joseph, M., Ameisen, J.C. & Tonnel, A.B. (1986) From parasites to allergy a second receptor for IgE. *Immunol. Today*, **7**, 15–18.

Chrétien, I., Helm, B.A., Marsh, P.J., Padlan, E.A., Wijdenes, J. & Banchereau, J. (1988) A monoclonal antibody anti-IgE antibody against an epitope (aminoacids 367–376) in the CH3 domain inhibits IgE binding to the low affinity IgE receptor (CD23). *J. Immunol.*, **141**, 3128–34.

Conrad, D.H., Campbell, K.A., Bartlett, W.C., Squire, C.M. & Dierks, S.E. (1994) Structure and function of the low affinity IgE receptor. *Adv. Exp. Med. Biol.*, **347**, 17–30.

Davis, F.M., Gossett, L.A., Pinkston, K.L. *et al.* (1993) Can anti-IgE be used to treat allergy? *Springer Semin. Immunopathol.*, **15**, 51–73.

Davis, K.G., Glennie, M., Harding, S. & Burton, D.R. (1990) A model for the solution conformation of rat IgE. *Biochem. Soc. Trans.*, **18**, 935–6.

Deisenhofer, J. (1981) Crystallographic refinement and atomic models of a human Fc fragment and its complex with fragment B of protein A from *Staphylococcus aureus* at 2.9 and 2.8 Å resolution. *Biochemistry*, **20**, 2361–70.

Delespesse, G., Sarfati, M., Wu, C.Y., Fournier S. & Letellier, M. (1992) The low-affinity receptor for IgE. *Immunol. Rev.*, **125**, 77–97.

Dierks, S.E., Bartlett, W.C., Edmeades, R.L., Gould, H.J., Roa M. & Conrad, D.H. (1993) The oligomeric nature of the murine FcεRII/CD23. *J. Immunol.*, **150**, 2372–82.

Drickamer, K. & Taylor, M.E. (1993) Biology of animal lectins. *Ann. Rev. Cell Biol.*, **9**, 237–64.

Duncan, A.R., Woof, J.M., Partridge, L.J., Burton, D.R. & Winter, G. (1988) Localization of the binding site for the human high-affinity Fc receptor on IgG. *Nature*, **332**, 563–4.

Erdei, A., Füst, G. & Gergely, J. (1991) The role of C3 in the immune response. *Immunol. Today*, **12**, 332–7.

Esparza, I., Becherer, J.D., Alsenz, J. *et al.* (1991) Evidence for multiple sites of interaction in C3 for complement receptor type 2 (C3d/EBV receptor, CD21). *Eur. J. Immunol.*, **21**, 2829–38.

Flores-Romo, L., Shields, J., Humbert, Y. *et al.* (1993) Inhibition of an *in vivo* antigen-specific IgE response by antibodies to CD23. *Science*, **261**, 1038–41.

Fujiwara, H., Kikutani, H., Suematsu, S. *et al.* (1994) The absence of IgE antibody-mediated augmentation of immune responses in CD23-deficient mice. *Proc. Nat. Acad. Sci. USA*, **91**, 6835–9.

Gauchat, J.-F., Henchoz S., Mazzei G. *et al.* (1993) Induction of human IgE synthesis in B cells by mast cells and basophils. *Nature*, **365**, 340–3.

Ghaderi, A.A. & Stanworth, D.R. (1993) Epitope mapping of the site(s) of binding of FcεRII/CD23 within human IgE. *Mol. Immunol.*, **30**, 1655–63.

Gordon, J. (1993) CD23 and CD72: C-type lectins and B-lymphocyte regulation. *Adv. Mol. Cell. Immunol.*, **1A**, 71–96.

Gould, H.J. (1992) The interaction between immunoglobulin E and its high-affinity receptor. In: *Genetics of Asthma* (eds S.T. Holgate & M.K. Church), pp. 293–304. Gower, London.

Gould, H.J., Sutton, B.J., Edmeades, R.L. & Beavil, A.J. (1991) CD23/FcεRII: C-type lectin membrane protein with a split personality? *Monogr. Allergy*, **29**, 28–49.

Gounni, A.S., Lamkhioued, B., Ochiai, K. *et al.* (1994) High-affinity IgE receptor on eosinophils is involved in defence against parasites. *Nature*, **367**, 183–6.

Grangette, C., Gruart, V., Ouaissi, M.A. *et al.* (1989) IgE receptor on human eosinophils (FcεRII). Comparison with B cell CD23 and association with an adhesion molecule. *J. Immunol.*, **143**, 3580–8.

Grattan, C.E.H., Francis, D.M., Hide, M. & Greaves, M.W. (1991) Detection of circulating histamine releasing autoantibodies with functional properties of anti-IgE in chronic urticaria. *Clin. Exp. Allergy*, **21**, 695–704.

Graves, B.J., Crowther, R.L., Chandran, C. *et al.* (1994) Insight into E-selectin/ligand interaction from the crystal structure and mutagenesis of the lec/EGF domains. *Nature*, **367**, 532–8.

Haak-Frendscho, M., Robbins, K., Lyon, R. *et al.* (1994) Administration of an anti-IgE antibody inhibits CD23 expression and IgE production *in vivo*. *Immunology*, **82**, 306–13.

Haba, S. & Nisonoff, A. (1994) Effects of syngeneic anti-IgE antibodies on the development of IgE memory and on the secondary IgE response. *J. Immunol.*, **152**, 51–7.

Hamburger, R.N. (1975) Peptide inhibition of the Prausnitz–Küstner reaction. *Science*, **189**, 389–90.

Hebell, T., Ahearn, J.M. & Fearon, D.T. (1991) Suppression of the immune response by a soluble complement receptor of B lymphocytes. *Science*, **254**, 102–5.

Hellman, L. (1994) Profound reduction in allergen sensitivity following treatment with a novel allergy vaccine. *Eur. J. Immunol.*, **24**, 415–20.

Helm, B.A., Kebo, D., Vercelli, D. *et al.* (1989) Blocking of passive sensitization of human mast cells and basophil granulocytes with IgE antibodies by a recombinant human ε-chain fragment of 76 amino acids. *Proc. Nat. Acad. Sci. USA*, **88**, 9465–9.

Helm, B.A., Ling, Y., Teale, C., Padlan, E.A. & Brüggemann, M. (1991) The nature and importance of the inter-ε chain disulfide bonds in human IgE. *Eur. J. Immunol.*, **21**, 1543–8.

Helm, B.A., Marsh, P., Vercelli, D., Padlan, E., Gould, H.J. & Geha, R. (1988) The mast cell binding site on human immunoglobulin E. *Nature*, **331**, 180–3.

Hewitt, C.R.A., Brown, A.P., Hart, B.J. & Pritchard, D.I. (1995) A major house dust allergen disrupts the IgE network by selectively cleaving CD23: innate protection by antiproteases. *J. Exp. Med.*, **182**, 1537–44.

Hibbs, M.L., Tolvanen, M. & Carpén, O. (1994) Membrane-proximal Ig-like domain of FcγRIII (CD16) contains residues critical for ligand binding. *J. Immunol.*, **152**, 4466–74.

Hogarth, P.M., Hulett, M.D., Ierino, F.L., Tate, B., Powell, M.S. & Brinkworth, R.I. (1992) Identification of the immunoglobulin binding regions (IBR) of FcγRII and FcεRI. *Immunol. Rev.*, **125**, 21–35.

Holmskov, U., Malhotra, R., Sim, R.B. & Jensenius, J.C. (1994) Collectins: collagenous C-type lectins of the innate immune defense system. *Immunol. Today*, **15**, 67–74.

Hulett, M.D., McKenzie, I.F.C. & Hogarth, P.M. (1993) Chimeric Fc receptors identify immunoglobulin-binding regions in human FcγRII and FcεRI. *Eur. J. Immunol.*, **23**, 640–5.

Hulett, M.D., Witort, E., Brinkworth, R.I., McKenzie, I.F.C. & Hogarth, P.M. (1994) Identification of the IgG binding site of the human low affinity receptor for IgG FcγRII. *J. Biol. Chem.*, **269**, 15287–93.

Ishizaka, K. & Ishizaka, T. (1967) Identification of γE-antibodies as a carrier of reaginic activity. *J. Immunol.*, **99**, 1187–98.

Jefferis, R., Lund, J. & Pound, J. (1990) Molecular definition of interaction sites on human IgG for Fc receptors (huFcγR). *Mol. Immunol.*, **27**, 1237–40.

Jouvin, M.-H.E., Adamczewski, M., Numerof, R., Letourneur, O., Vallé & Kinet, J.-P. (1994) Differential control of the tyrosine kinases Lyn and Syk by the two signaling chains of the high affinity immunoglobulin E receptor. *J. Biol. Chem.*, **269**, 5918–25.

Keown, M.B., Ghirlando, R., Young, R.J. *et al.* (1995) Hydrodynamic studies of a complex between the Fc fragment of human IgE and a soluble fragment of the FcεRI α chain. *Proc. Nat. Acad. Sci. USA*, **92**, 1841–5.

Kijimoto-Ochiai, S., Horimoto, E. & Uede, T. (1994) Demonstration of the interaction between the CD23 molecule and the galactose residue of glycoproteins. *Immunol. Letts.*, **40**, 49–53.

Kolbinger, F., Saldanha, J., Hardman, N. & Bendig, M. (1993) Humanization of a mouse anti-human IgE antibody: a potential therapeutic for IgE-mediated allergies. *Protein Eng.*, **6**, 971–80.

Lecoanet-Henchoz, S., Gauchat, J.-F., Aubry, J-P. *et al.* (1995) CD23 regulates monocyte activation through a novel interaction with the adhesion molecules CD11b–CD18 and CD11c–CD18. *Immunity*, **3**, 119–25.

Lee, W.T., Rao, M. & Conrad, D.H. (1987) The murine lymphocyte receptor for IgE. IV. The mechanism of ligand-specific receptor upregulation on B cells. *J. Immunol.*, **139**, 1191–8.

Letellier, M., Nakajima, T., Pulido-Cejudo, G., Hofstetter, H. & Delespesse, G. (1990) Mechanism of formation of human IgE-binding factors (soluble CD23): III. Evidence for a receptor (FcεRII)-associated proteolytic activity. *J. Exp. Med.*, **172**, 693–700.

Letourneur, O., Sechi, S., Willette-Brown, J., Robertson, M.W. & Kinet, J.-P. (1995) Glycosylation of human truncated FcεRI α chain is necessary for efficient folding in the endoplasmic reticulum. *J. Biol. Chem.*, **270**, 8249–56.

Liu, F.T. (1993) S-type mammalian lectins in allergic inflammation. *Immunol. Today*, **14**, 486–90.

Lowell, C.A., Klickstein, L.B., Carter, R.H., Mitchell, J.A., Fearon, D.T. & Ahearn, J.M. (1989) Mapping of the Epstein–Barr virus and C3dg binding sites to a common domain on complement receptor type 2. *J. Exp. Med.*, **170**, 1931–46.

Luo, H., Hofstetter, H., Banchereau, J. & Delespesse, G. (1991) Cross-linking of CD23 antigen by its natural ligand (IgE) or by anti-CD23 antibody prevents B lymphocyte proliferation and differentiation. *J. Immunol.*, **146**, 2122–9.

MacDonald, S.M., Rafnar, T., Langdon, J. & Lichtenstein, L.M. (1995) Molecular identification of an IgE-dependent histamine-releasing factor. *Science*, **269**, 688–90.

McDonnell, J.M., Beavil, A.J., Mackay, G.A. *et al.*, (1996) Structure based design and characterization of peptides that inhibit IgE binding to its high-affinity receptor. *Nature Struct. Biol.*, **3**, 419–26.

Mallamaci, M.A., Chizzonite, R., Griffin, M. *et al.* (1993) Identification of sites on the human FcεRIα subunit which are involved in binding human and rat IgE. *J. Biol. Chem.*, **268**, 22076–83.

Matsumoto, A.K., Kopicky-Burd, J., Carter, R.H., Tuveson, D.A., Tedder, T.F. & Fearon, D.T. (1991) Intersection of the complement and immune systems: a signal transduction complex of the B lymphocyte containing complement receptor type 2 and CD19. *J. Exp. Med.*, **173**, 55–64.

Metzger, H. (1992a) The receptor with high affinity for IgE. *Immunol. Rev.*, **125**, 37–48.

Metzger, H. (1992b) Transmembrane signalling: the joy of aggregation (A.A.I. Presidential address). *J. Immunol.*, **149**, 1477–87.

Moore, M.D., DiScipio, R.G., Cooper, N.R. & Nemerov, G.R. (1989) Hydrodynamic, electron microscopic, and ligand-binding analysis of the Epstein–Barr virus/C3dg receptor (CR2). *J. Biol. Chem.*, **264**, 20576–82.

Moulder, K., Barton, A. & Weston, B. (1993) CD23-mediated homotypic cell adhesion: the role of proteolysis. *Eur. J. Immunol.*, **23**, 2066–71.

Naito, K., Hirama, M., Okumura, K. & Ra, C. (1995) Soluble form of the human high-affinity receptor for IgE inhibits recurrent allergic reaction in a novel mouse model of type I allergy. *Eur. J. Immunol.*, **25**, 1631–7.

Nio, N., Seguro, K., Ariyoshi, Y. *et al.* (1993) Inhibition of passive sensitization of human peripheral basophils by synthetic human immunoglobulin E peptide fragments. *FEBS Letts.*, **319**, 225–8.

Nissim, A., Schwarzbaum, S., Siraganian, R. & Eshhar, Z. (1993) Fine specificity of the IgE interaction with the low and high affinity Fc receptor. *J. Immunol.*, **150**, 1365–74.

Norman, D.G., Barlow, P.N., Baron, M., Day, A.J., Sim, R.B. & Campbell, I.D. (1991) Three-dimensional structure of a complement control protein module in solution. *J. Mol. Biol.*, **219**, 717–25.

Ortega, E., Schweitzer-Stenner, R. & Pecht, I. (1991) Kinetics of ligand binding to the type I Fcε receptor on mast cells. *Biochemistry*, **30**, 3473–83.

Padlan, E.A. & Davies, D.R. (1986) A model of the Fc of immunoglobulin E. *Mol. Immunol.*, **23**, 1063–75.

Padlan, E.A. & Helm, B.A. (1992) A modelling study of the α-subunit of human high-affinity receptor for immunoglobulin E. *Receptor*, **2**, 129–42.

Perez-Montfort, R. & Metzger, H. (1982) Proteolysis of soluble IgE-receptor complexes: localization of sites on IgE which interact with the Fc receptor. *Mol. Immunol.*, **19**, 1113–25.

Pirron, U., Schlunck, T., Prinz, J.C. & Rieber, E.P. (1990) IgE-dependent antigen focusing by B lymphocytes is mediated by the low-affinity receptor for IgE. *Eur. J. Immunol.*, **20**, 1547–51.

Plater-Zyberk, C. & Bonnefoy, J.-Y. (1995) Marked amelioration of established collagen-induced arthritis by treatment with antibodies to CD23 *in vivo*. *Nature Med.*, **1**, 781–5.

Prausnitz, C. & Küstner, H. (1921) Stüdien uber die Ueberempfindlichkeit. *Zentralbl. Bakteriol. Parasit. Infektion. Hygiene*, **86**, 160–9.

Presta, L., Shields, R., O'Connell, L. *et al.* (1994) The binding site on human immunoglobulin E for its high affinity receptor. *J. Biol. Chem.*, **269**, 26368–73.

Pribluda, V.S., Pribluda, C. & Metzger, H. (1994) Transphosphorylation as the mechanism by which the high-affinity receptor for IgE is phosphorylated upon aggregation. *Proc. Nat. Acad. Sci. USA*, **91**, 11246–50.

Ra, C., Kuromitsu, S., Hirose, T. *et al.* (1993) Soluble human high-affinity receptor for IgE abrogates the IgE-mediated allergic reaction. *Int. Immunol.*, **5**, 47–54.

Ravetch, J.V. & Kinet, J.-P. (1991) Fc receptors. *Ann. Rev. Immunol.*, **9**, 457–92.

Riske, F., Hakimi, J., Mallamaci, M. *et al.* (1991) High affinity human IgE receptor (FcεRI). Analysis of functional domains of the α-subunit with monoclonal antibodies. *J. Biol. Chem.*, **266**, 11245–51.

Robertson, M.W. (1993) Phage and *Escherichia coli* expression of the human high affinity immunoglobulin E receptor α-subunit ectodomain. *J. Biol. Chem.*, **268**, 12736–43.

Robertson, M.W. & Liu, F.-T. (1991) Heterogeneous IgE glycoforms characterized by differential recognition of an endogenous lectin (IgE-binding protein). *J. Immunol.*, **147**, 3024–30.

Saban, R., Haak-Frendscho, M., Zine, M. *et al.* (1994) Human FcεRI-IgG and humanized anti-IgE monoclonal antibody MaE11 block passive sensitization of human and rhesus monkey lung. *J. Allergy Clin. Immunol.*, **94**, 863–43.

Sarfati, M., Bettler, B., Letellier, M. *et al.* (1992) Native and recombinant soluble CD23 fragments with IgE suppressive activity. *Immunology*, **76**, 662–7.

Scarselli, E., Esposito, G. & Traboni, C. (1993) Display of functional domains of the human high affinity IgE receptor on the M13 phage surface. *FEBS Letts.*, **329**, 223–6.

Schultz, O., Laing, P., Sewell, H.F. & Shakib, F. (1995) *Der p* 1, a major allergen of the house dust mite, proteolytically cleaves the lower affinity receptor for human IgE (CD23). *Eur. J. Immunol.*, **25**, 3191–4.

Shakib, F., Smith, S.J. & Pritchard, D.I. (1995) Do autoantibodies to IgE play a role in IgE-mediated events? *Immunol. Cell Biol.*, **73**, 109–12.

Sheriff, S., Chang, C.Y. & Ezekowitz, R.A.B. (1994) Human mannose-binding protein carbohydrate recognition domain trimerizes through a triple α-helical coiled-coil. *Nature Struct. Biol.*, **1**, 789–94.

Sherr, E., Macy, E., Kimata, H., Gilly, M. & Saxon, A. (1989) Binding the low affinity FcεR on B cells suppresses ongoing human IgE synthesis. *J. Immunol.*, **142**, 481–9.

Shirakawa, T., Li, A., Dubowitz, M., Dekker, J.W. *et al.* (1994) Association between atopy and variants of the β subunit of the high-affinity immunoglobulin E receptor. *Nature Genet.*, **7**, 125–30.

Springer, T.A. (1990) Adhesion receptors in the immune system. *Nature*, **346**, 425–34.

Stanworth, D.R., Jones, V.M., Lewin, I.V. & Nayyar, S. (1990) Allergy treatment with a peptide vaccine. *Lancet*, **336**, 1279–81.

Sutton, B.J. & Gould, H.J. (1993) The human IgE network. *Nature*, **366**, 421–8.

Tedder, T.F., Zhou, L.-J. & Engel, P. (1994) The CD19/CD21 signal transduction complex of B lymphocytes. *Immunol. Today*, **15**, 437–42.

Truong, M.-J., Gruart, V., Kusnierz, J.-P. *et al.* (1993) Human neutrophils express immunoglobulin E (IgE)-binding proteins (Mac-2/εBP) of the S-type lectin family: role in IgE-dependent activation. *J. Exp. Med.*, **177**, 243–8.

Vercelli, D., Helm, B.A., Marsh, P., Padlan, E., Geha, R.S. & Gould, H. (1989) The B-cell binding site on human immunoglobulin E. *Nature*, **338**, 649–51.

Wang B., Rieger, A., Kilgus, O. *et al.* (1992) Epidermal Langerhans cells from normal human skin bind monomeric IgE via FcεRI. *J. Exp. Med.*, **175**, 1353–8.

Weetall, M., Shopes, B., Holowka, D. & Baird, B. (1990) Mapping the site of interaction between murine IgE and its high affinity receptor with chimeric Ig. *J. Immunol.*, **145**, 3849–54.

Weis, W.I. & Drickamer, K. (1994) Trimeric structure of a C-type mannose-binding protein. *Structure*, **2**, 1227–40.

Weis, W.I., Drickamer, K. & Hendrickson, W.A. (1992) Structure of a C-type mannose-binding protein complexed with an oligosaccharide. *Nature*, **360**, 127–34.

Williams, A.F. & Barclay, A.N. (1988) The immunoglobulin superfamily — domains for cell surface recognition. *Ann. Rev. Immunol.*, **6**, 381–405.

Wilson, B.S., Kapp, N., Lee, R.J. *et al.* (1995) Distinct functions of the FcεRI γ and β subunits in the control of FcεRI-mediated tyrosine kinase activation and signaling responses in RBL-2H3 mast cells. *J. Biol. Chem.*, **270**, 4013–22.

Wollenberg, A., de la Salle, H., Hanau, D., Liu, F.-T. & Bieber, T. (1993) Human keratinocytes release the endogenous β-galactoside-binding soluble lectin immunoglobulin E (IgE)-binding protein which binds to Langerhans cells where it modulates their binding capacity for IgE glycoforms. *J. Exp. Med.*, **178**, 777–85.

Yokota, A., Kikutani, H., Tanaka, T. *et al.* (1988) Two species of human Fcε receptor II (FcεRII/CD23): tissue-specific and IL-4-specific regulation of gene expression. *Cell*, **55**, 611–18.

Yokota, A., Yukawa, K., Yamamoto, A. *et al.* (1992) Two forms of the low-affinity Fc receptor for IgE differentially mediate endocytosis and phagocytosis: identification of the critical cytoplasmic domains. *Proc. Nat. Acad. Sci. USA*, **89**, 5030–4.

Yu, P., Kosco-Vilbois, M., Richards, M., Köhler, G. & Lamers, M.C. (1994) Negative feedback regulation of IgE synthesis by murine CD23. *Nature*, **369**, 753–6.

Zheng, Y., Shopes, B., Holowka, D. & Baird, B. (1991) Conformations of IgE bound to its receptor FcεRI and in solution. *Biochemistry*, **30**, 9125–32.

Zheng, Y., Shopes, B., Holowka, D. & Baird, B. (1992) Dynamic conformations compared for IgE and IgG1 in solution and bound to receptors. *Biochemistry*, **31**, 7446–56.

CHAPTER 6

Regulation of IgE Synthesis

S. Romagnani

Introduction

Atopic allergy is a genetically determined disorder characterized by an enhanced ability of B lymphocytes to produce immunoglobulin E (IgE) antibodies in response to certain groups of ubiquitous antigens that can activate the immune system after inhalation, ingestion, and perhaps after penetration through the skin (allergens). The evidence that IgE is important in atopic disease states comes from both epidemiological association and animal models (Ishizaka & Ishizaka, 1978). IgE antibodies are capable of binding to high-affinity (type I) Fcε receptors (FcεRI) on the surface of mast cells/basophils and allergen-induced FcεRI cross-linking triggers the release of vasoactive mediators, chemotactic factors and cytokines that are responsible for the allergic cascade (Siraganian, 1993). In addition to IgE-producing B cells and IgE-binding mast cells/basophils, eosinophils are also consistently involved in the pathogenesis of allergic reactions, inasmuch as these cells usually accumulate in the sites of allergic inflammation and the toxic products they release significantly contribute to the induction of tissue damage (Sur *et al.*, 1993).

In the past few years, the cellular basis of IgE regulation has been actively investigated to gain insights into the pathogenesis of a condition which affects a considerable proportion of the population. The investigation of molecular events underlying IgE synthesis has provided an interesting model to identify and characterize the signals involved in isotype-specific regulation of Ig synthesis in humans. More importantly, intense study of the functional properties of T helper (Th) cells that collaborate with B cells for Ig synthesis has clarified the mechanisms accounting for the joint involvement of IgE-producing B cells, mast cells/basophils and eosinophils in the pathogenesis of allergic reactions.

This chapter gives a brief account of the molecular mechanisms underlying Ig synthesis. Following this, the regulatory mechanisms of IgE synthesis in humans are focused on. Finally, the mechanisms that regulate the development of type 2 Th cells (Th2), which are responsible for both the synthesis of IgE by B cells and the recruitment and activation of the other cell types involved in the allergic reactions, are discussed.

Ig class switching

The antigen specificity of an Ig molecule is determined by the highly variable regions of their heavy (V_H) and light (V_L) chains (idiotypic heterogeneity). By contrast, the effector functions of the Ig molecule (isotype heterogeneity) are related to the constant amino-acid sequence of the heavy chain (C_H). The variable region of Ig is encoded by multiple germ-line elements that are assembled into complete V(D)J variable regions during B-cell differentiation by a common enzymatic activity (recombinase), which is encoded by the *RAG* genes (Schatz *et al.*, 1989). Ig isotypes (IgM, IgD, IgG, IgA, IgE) are encoded by constant heavy genes that are aligned in tandem in the same transcriptional orientation, downstream to the V_HDJ_H gene complex, which encodes specificity for antigen. Human C_H genes are located on chromosome 14 with a 300-kb region in the following order: μ, δ, γ3, γ1, ψε, α1, γ2, γ4, ε and α2 (Fig. 6.1). In addition to the Ig heavy-chain complex, some repetitive sequences (S or switch regions) located upstream to each C_H gene have been demon-

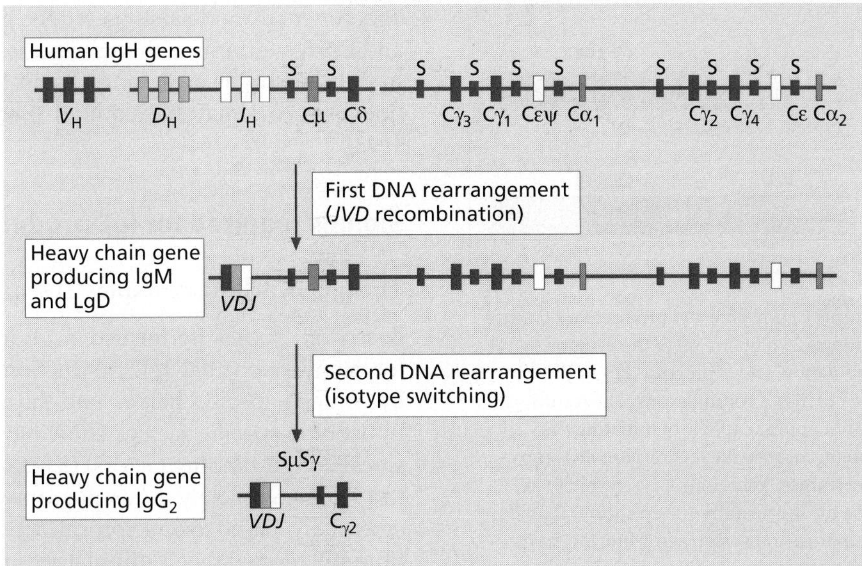

Fig. 6.1 A schematic representation of the human gene-line heavy-chain locus and of its rearrangement during B-cell life. The first DNA rearrangement occurring during B-cell ontogeny assembles three regions (variable or V_H, diversity or D_H, and joining or J_H) into the variable portion of the Ig molecule, resulting in the expression of an IgM (and IgD) with a given antigen specificity. The second DNA rearrangement, occurring following the recognition by the B cell of specific antigen and its interaction with the corresponding Th cell, involves the homologous switch sites (S) that precede each constant (C_H) gene. This results in a more distal constant gene, such as C2, moving next to the rearranged *V(D)J*, as in an IgG2-producing cell (isotype switch). (Modified from Vercelli & Geha, 1993.)

strated. S regions are 2–10 kb in length and their sequence consists of short tandem repeats (GAGCT, GGGCT). During an immune response, the same B lymphocyte can express different C_H region genes in association with the same V(D)J region. This phenomenon that allows a single B-cell clone to produce antibodies that retain antigen specificity in association with a different effector function is known as heavy-chain class (or isotype) switching (Snapper & Finkelman, 1993).

Recombinational mechanisms

Isotype switching is thought to result generally from a non-homologous recombination event between two sites on the same DNA segment within one chromosome, but more rarely it may occur betwen two different chromosomes. Unlike the V(D)J recombination occurring during ontogenesis that is a stochastic process (Fig. 6.1), recombination responsible for the isotype switching is a directed (non-random) process that can be regulated by mitogens, lymphokines, and probably other signals as well. Recombination juxtaposes a downstream C_H gene to the expressed *V(D)J* gene (Fig. 6.1). Intervening sequences, including the previously expressed C_H genes, are looped out and deleted (Matsuoka *et al.*, 1990). S regions play an essential role in heavy-chain class switching, by both facilitating and directing non-homologous recombination. Although looping out and deletion are well-established mechanisms of Ig isotype switching, it is likewise clear that switching to a given C_H gene does not always occur from Cμ but may occur through sequential deletional events. For example, B cells that have switched from IgM to IgG1 may later be able to undergo a second switch event to IgE. The type of stimulus appears to be critical in favouring direct switching from IgM to IgE rather than to IgE through IgG1. It is presumed that at least one DNA recombinase must be involved in deletional isotype switching, but the recombinase has yet to be identified and it remains to be determined whether a single recombinase (or set of recombinases) mediates switching to all isotypes. Finally, non-deletional mechanisms of isotype switching have also been demonstrated. However, the frequency with which they occur in normal cells and their biological importance relative to deletional switching are still being debated and investigated (Snapper & Finkelman, 1993).

Molecular requirements

At least two different processes are required for the induction of Ig isotype switching: (i) expression of germ-line RNA for the C_H gene to which switching will occur, and (ii) DNA synthesis (i.e. B-cell proliferation). The C_H gene that encodes the specific Ig isotype to which a given B cell

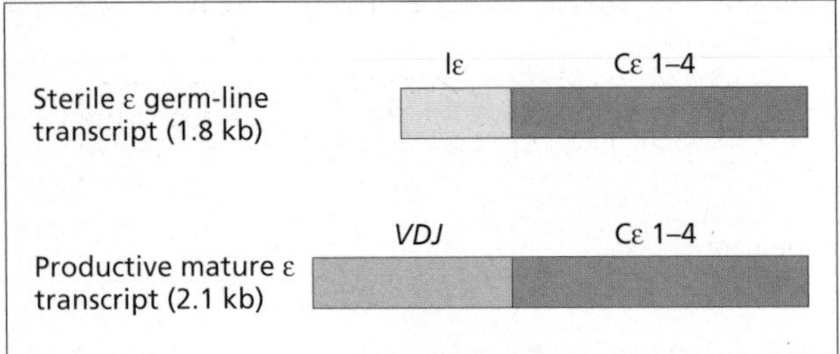

Fig. 6.2 Comparison of sterile ε germ-line and productive ε mature mRNA. The transcript initiates 2 kb upstream of the *S* region involved in switch recombination, and is processed to an RNA in which the *Iε* exon is spliced to the Cε coding exons. The resulting germ-line transcript does not appear capable of initiating the synthesis of a mature protein, because the *Iε* exon contains stop codons in all three reading frames. Therefore, it is referred to as 'sterile' transcript. Because the *Iε* is usually 300 bp shorter than the *V(D)J* exon present in the mature transcript, germ-line transcript is 0.3 kb smaller than mature transcript. (Modified from Vercelli & Geha, 1993.)

would switch is transcriptionally active and is transcribed in their germ-line configuration. Germ-line C_H RNA differs from mRNA encoded by a rearranged C_H gene, in that it lacks the exon that encodes V_HDJ_H ('truncated' RNA transcript) (Fig. 6.2). Therefore, this germ-line C_HRNA fails to initiate the synthesis of a mature Ig protein, and since it is not translated this RNA transcript is also referred to as 'sterile'. The exact role of germ-line transcripts in isotype switching is not completely clear. All germ-line transcripts initiate 5′ of the switch region, suggesting the possibility that transcription through a targetted region may favour accessibility for the action of a recombinase ('accessibility model') (Stavnezer-Nordgren & Sirlin, 1986; Yancopoulos *et al.*, 1986). The accessibility model predicts that an increase in steady-state levels of germ-line C_HRNA results from an increase in transcriptional rate of the C_H gene. Cytokines, such as interleukin-4 (IL-4), interferon-γ (IFN-γ) and transforming growth factor (TGF-β), have been shown to increase the steady-state levels of germ-line γ1 and ε, γ2a and γ3, and γ2b and α, respectively (see later). Alternatively, germ-line transcripts may favour the switching process by some direct enzymatic activity that participates in recombination, by stabilizing the open DNA configuration, by encoding a regulatory protein, or by splicing to a VDJ-CμRNA, which would then allow for non-deletional expression of a new Ig class. On the other hand, it cannot be excluded that germ-line transcripts do not play an active role in the switch event, but rather represent non-functional byproducts of activation of the switch mechanism. In addition to germ-line C_H gene expression, isotype switching requires DNA synthesis by the B cell. Indeed, DNA synthesis inhibitors selectively inhibit IgG, as opposed to IgM production, by mitogen-stimulated B cells. Finally, some experimental models suggest that germ-line expression and DNA synthesis, although necessary, are not sufficient to induce isotype switching. An additional, as yet undefined, process may be required (Snapper & Finkelman, 1993).

Signals required for IgE production

The IgE-switching cytokines: IL-4 and IL-13

Based on studies performed in rodents, it was thought for many years that IgE production could be regulated by antigen-specific helper and suppressor T cells, and by isotype-specific factors showing affinity for IgE (the so-called IgE-binding factors) (Ishizaka & Ishizaka, 1978). In 1986, a completely different pathway of IgE regulation, essentially based on reciprocal activity of IL-4 (at that time still termed B-cell stimulatory factor-1, or BSF-1) and IFN-γ, was discovered in mice. BSF-1 was indeed found to be able to induce production of IgE and IgG_1 by murine B cells stimulated *in vitro* with lipopolysaccharide (LPS), and its activity was strongly inhibited by IFN-γ (Coffman & Carty, 1986). The crucial role of IL-4 in the induction of murine IgE synthesis has also been confirmed *in vivo*. Suppression of *in vivo* polyclonal IgE responses was obtained by injection of a monoclonal anti-IL-4 antibody. More importantly, no IgE synthesis was detectable in an IL-4-deficient mouse mutant obtained by gene targetting in murine embryonic stem cells (Kuhn *et al.*, 1991). In murine B cells, stimulation with IL-4 and LPS induces the appearance of a 1.7–1.9 kb Cε germ-line transcript, that occurs at the transcriptional level. This transcript contains an Iε exon, located 2 kb upstream to Sε, spliced to the Cε1–Cε4 exons (Fig. 6.2). Two different proteins are induced by IL-4 that can bind to the transcriptional initiation site of Iε (Rothman *et al.*, 1991).

The crucial role of IL-4 in the induction of human IgE synthesis was demonstrated in 1988 by an *in vitro* model based on the use of T-cell clones (Del Prete *et al.*, 1988; Pene *et al.*, 1988a). PHA- or anti-CD3 antibody-stimulated T-cell clones, as well as their supernatants, were found to be able to provide helper activity for IgE synthesis. When the ability of PHA-induced T-cell clones (or their supernatants) to induce IgE synthesis was compared with their ability to produce (or to contain) IL-2, IL-4 and IFN-γ, a significant positive correlation between helper function for IgE and production of IL-4 was found. In contrast, there was a significant inverse correlation between the IgE helper activity of T-cell clones (or supernatants derived from them) and their ability to produce IFN-γ (Del Prete *et al.*, 1988). This opposite regulatory role for IL-4 and IFN-γ in the synthesis of human IgE was confirmed by the observations that: (i) human recombinant IL-4 can induce the synthesis of IgE in peripheral blood mononuclear cells

(Del Prete *et al.*, 1988; Pene *et al.*, 1988a), and (ii) this effect is inhibited by addition of recombinant IFN-γ (Del Prete *et al.*, 1988; Pene *et al.*, 1988a). More importantly, an anti-IL-4 antibody markedly suppressed the IgE synthesis induced by all active T-cell clones or their supernatants tested, whereas it had little, if any, inhibitory activity on the synthesis of IgM and IgG. IL-4 was also found to be able to induce the production of IgG_4, the human equivalent of murine IgG_1 (Gascam *et al.*, 1991).

As in the mouse, IL-4 induces transcription through the Sε region, resulting in the synthesis of germ-line ε transcript (Gauchat *et al.*, 1990). The structure of germ-line ε transcript by human B cells has recently been characterized. It consists of an approximately 134-bp Iε exon located approximately 3.5 kb upstream from Cε. The Iε exon is directly spliced to Cε by removal of the intervening sequences from the primary transcript (Vercelli & Geha, 1993). The germ-line transcript contains all four Cε exons, as well as the 3′ untranslated region. The human Iε does not contain an initiation codon in frame with the Cε region, and stop codons are present in all three reading frames, suggesting that no protein is encoded by these transcripts. Germ-line ε transcripts can be induced by IL-4 in resting B cells, indicating that no previous *in vivo* activation is required for expression of germ-line ε transcripts in response to IL-4 stimulation (Vercelli & Geha, 1993).

More recently IL-13, a second cytokine showing poor homology with IL-4 (about 30%) but possessing similar IgE-switching activity, was discovered (Punnonen *et al.*, 1993a). Mouse and human IL-13 are not active on T cells, have similar effects on macrophages, but different effects on B cells (Table 6.1). Mouse IL-13 is inactive on B cells, whereas human IL-13 has IL-4-like effects, being able to induce both B-cell proliferation and switching to IgE and IgG_4 production. Like IL-4, IL-13 also induces germ-line ε mRNA expression in highly purified B cells, supporting the notion that it is able to direct switching to the IgE isotype. IL-13, which generally is two- to fivefold less potent than IL-4 in inducing IgE production, has no additive or synergistic effects with IL-4 on induction of IgE or IgG_4. This favours the possibility that IL-4 and IL-13 use common signalling pathways for the induction of these Ig isotypes. Indeed, it has recently been shown that receptors for IL-4 and IL-13 are distinct but share a common subunit (γ-chain) (Zurawski & de Vries, 1994). As human IL-4, human IL-13 is produced by activated T cells, but its kinetics of production is markedly different from that of induction of IL-4. IL-13 mRNA expression peaks approximately 2 hours after activation, but considerable steady levels of IL-13 mRNA are still observed after 72 hours. In contrast, IL-4 mRNA peaks after 4–6 hours and its levels are minimal or undetectable after 24 hours. Based on this observation, it was inferred that IL-13 may play an important role in the regulation of enhanced IgE synthesis in allergic patients (Zurawski & de Vries, 1994).

Table 6.1 Comparison of the major biological activities of human IL-4 and IL-13.

Cell type	IL-4	IL-13
Monocytes/macrophages		
MHC class II	Up	Up
Fcγ receptors	Down	Down
CD23	Up	Up
Proinflammatory cytokines	Down	Down
Chemokines	Down	Down
IL-1ra	Up	Up
APC function	Up	Up
ADCC activity	Down	Down
B cells		
CD23, CD71, CD72, MHC class II	Up	Up
Proliferation	+	+
Differentiation (Ig switching)	Up	Up
T cells		
Proliferation	+	–
CD8α induction	+	–
Induction of Th2 development	+	–

See text for definition of abbreviations.

T–B cell-to-cell contact-mediated signals

Although both IL-4 and IL-13 are by themselves sufficient for the initiation of germ-line transcription through the ε locus, additional signals are necessary for the expression of mature ε mRNA transcripts and for the production of IgE protein. Both IL-4 and IL-13 are ineffective in inducing IgE synthesis in highly purified B cells, but the IL-4-dependent IgE synthesis can be restored by re-addition of appropriate concentrations of autologous or allogeneic T cells, and the inclusion of monocytes potentiates this response (Romagnani, 1990). In contrast, IgE synthesis by highly purified B cells was not restored by using mixtures of optimal concentrations of T-cell- and monocyte-derived cytokines, suggesting that a physical interaction between T and B cells is required for IL-4- (and IL-13-) dependent IgE synthesis. More direct evidence was provided by assaying IgE synthesis in a double-chamber system. When T and B cells are cultured in different chambers separated by a millipore membrane, permeable to molecules but not to cells, IL-4 cannot induce the synthesis of IgE. IgE synthesis occurs only when T and B cells are cultured in the same chamber (Vercelli *et al.*, 1989b; Parronchi *et al.*, 1990). This observation led us (Romagnani, 1990), and others (Vercelli & Geha, 1991), to propose a two-signal model for the induction of human IgE synthesis (Fig. 6.3). Our

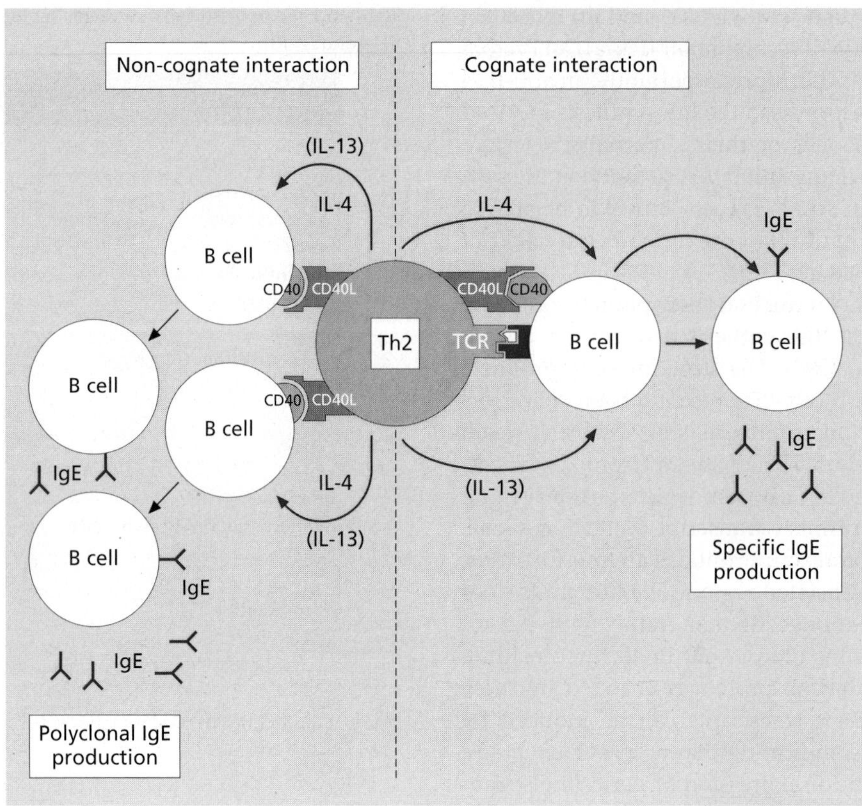

Fig. 6.3 A simplified view of the 'two-signal' model for the induction of human IgE synthesis. MHC class II-restricted interaction between a B cell and a Th2-type CD4+ T-cell specific for the same antigen (cognate interaction) results in the production of IL-4 (and/or IL-13) and expression of CD40L by the activated Th2 cell. IL-4 (and/or IL-13) induces the expression of ε germ-line transcript by the B cell (first signal). Interaction between CD40L and CD40 provides the second signal required for the expression of mature ε transcript, which results in the production of specific IgE antibody (right part). In some circumstances (i.e. helminthic infestations, acute transplant rejection), activated Th2 cells producing IL-4 (and/or IL-13) and expressing CD40L may also stimulate IgE production by B cells specific for different antigens, thus resulting in polyclonal IgE production (left part). (Modified from Romagnani, 1990.)

hypothesis was that cognate T–B cell-to-cell interaction was required to induce the release of IL-4 (or IL-13) by the activated T cell, but the molecules involved in the contact-mediated signalling were independent of the TCR-CD3/MHC (major histocompatibility complex) class II (Romagnani, 1990). Indeed, PHA-induced T-cell clones, both CD4+ and CD8+, were found to be able to induce IgE synthesis by B cells from randomly selected donors if large amounts of exogenous IL-4 were added to the cultures. Additional evidence for the role of a non-cognate interaction in the induction of IgE synthesis was provided by assaying the activity of an alloreactive Th2-like T-cell clone (TR46). This clone could induce the synthesis of IgE when cultured with B cells possessing the appropriate alloantigen (DR4). When the DR4-positive B cells were irradiated, IgE synthesis did not occur, but it could be restored by the addition of DR4-negative unirradiated B cells. More importantly, in the presence of exogenously added IL-4, TR46 enabled B cells from all donors tested to produce IgE, irrespective of whether they possessed the DR4 alloantigen (Parronchi *et al.*, 1990). Finally, mouse EL-4 thymoma cells potently induce IgE synthesis by human B cells if both PMA and exogenous IL-4 are added (Romagnani, 1990).

CD40/CD40L-mediated signal

The nature of the molecule(s) involved in the contact-mediated non-cognate signalling required for IgE production has recently been clarified. Different couples of molecules may be operating in T-cell/B-cell interaction; however, the most critical signalling is provided by the interaction of CD40 present on the B cell with its ligand (CD40L) expressed by the activated T cell (Armitage *et al.*, 1992). CD40 is a 50-*K*Da surface glycoprotein expressed on all human B lymphocytes, but not by T cells and monocytes. It is a member of the tumour necrosis factor receptor (TNF-R) superfamily which includes, in addition to CD40, both forms of TNF-R (types I and II); the nerve growth factor receptor; and CD27, CD30, and the Fas antigen (Smith *et al.*, 1990). Studies using monoclonal antibodies (mAb) to CD40 have indicated that a diverse array of biological activities occurs as a result of signalling through CD40. These include proliferation of anti-IgM cross-linked B cells and rescue of germinal centrocytes from apoptosis. Moreover, anti-CD40 mAb were shown to replace activated T cells in induction of IgE synthesis by IL-4 (Armitage *et al.*, 1992). The ability of anti-CD40 mAb to replace T cells in induction of IgE synthesis suggested the presence of the CD40L on activated T cells. CD40L has indeed been cloned from cDNA libraries constructed from activated T cells (Armitage *et al.*, 1992). This cDNA encodes a 33-kDa type II glycoprotein with significant homology to TNF-α and TNF-β. In contrast to activated CD4+ T cells, resting Th cells, which cannot assist B-cell differentiation, do not express CD40L. Transfectants expressing CD40L induced B-cell proliferation and differentiation into IgE-secreting cells in the presence of IL-4, indicating that all signals required for IgE switching can be delivered by CD40L and IL-4 (Spriggs *et al.*, 1992). More importantly, the gene encoding CD40L was mapped on the X-chromosomal location q26.3–q27.1, the same region in which a gene defect in patients with X-linked hyper-IgM syndrome was identified. Patients with hyper-IgM syndrome, who have minimal levels of IgG, IgA and IgE in their sera, have mutations in their CD40L gene, resulting in defective expression of CD40L and impaired isotype switching *in vivo* (Arrufo *et al.*, 1993). Also, T cells from a subset of patients suffering from common variable immunodeficiency were found to express suboptimal levels of CD40L, further supporting an essential role for CD40/C40L interactions in productive T-cell/B-cell collaboration (Farrington *et al.*, 1994).

The effect of CD40 triggering on Cε transcription was analysed in B cells stimulated with anti-CD40 mAb and IL-4. As expected, Cε germ-line transcript, but not mature ε mRNA, were detected in B cells stimulated with IL-4 alone. Anti-CD40 mAb by itself did not induce either germ-line transcript or mature Cε transcripts, but synergized with IL-4 to enhance ε germ-line transcript accumulation (an approximately sevenfold increase). A mature mRNA was observed only in B cells stimulated with both IL-4 and anti-CD40 mAb for 10 days (Vercelli & Geha, 1995). These results indicate that the CD40 signal induced isotype switching and the production of mature ε mRNA. The effects of CD40 engagement were totally dependent on the presence of IL-4. These findings are consistent with the hypothesis that the induction of germ-line transcripts may result in increased accessibility of the downstream S region for deletional switch recombination with Sμ ('accessibility model') (see above). Interestingly, it has recently been shown that the CD40-mediated generation of Sμ/Sε switch fragment in B cells treated with IL-4 was completely inhibited by disodiumcromoglycate (Loh *et al.*, 1994).

Other T/B-cell contact-mediated signals

When B cells are stimulated with anti-CD40 mAb in the presence of activated CD4+ T cells and optimal concentrations of IL-4, a synergistic effect on IgE synthesis is observed. This suggests that membrane-bound molecules other than CD40L may also be involved in the events leading to B-cell activation, proliferation and differentiation. Indeed, the 26-kDa membrane form of TNF-α (mTNF-α), expressed on CD4+ T cells after activation, is another molecule associated with productive T-cell–B-cell interactions. mAb specific for TNF-α strongly inhibit IgE synthesis induced by activated CD4+ T-cell clones or their membranes (Aversa *et al.*, 1993), as well as Ig production induced by human immunodeficiency virus (HIV)- or herpes virus saimiri (HVS)-infected CD4+ T-cell clones (Macchia *et al.*, 1993; Del Prete *et al.*, 1994). Likewise, the ligation of B-cell CD58 (LFA-3) by CD2, its natural ligand on T cells, or by anti-CD58 mAb, in concert with IL-4-stimulated ε germ-line transcription, induced the appearence of productive ε-transcripts and IgE production (Diaz-Sanchez *et al.*, 1994). Interestingly, mAb specific for CD58 also inhibited Ig production by HVS-infected CD4+ T-cell clones (Del Prete *et al.*, 1994). More recently, another member of the TNF superfamily, the CD30 ligand (CD30L), was cloned (Smith *et al.*, 1993), and found to be very active in inducing CD40L-independent IgE secretion (Shanebeck *et al.*, 1995). Thus, although CD40/CD40L interactions appear to be essential for B-cell differentiation and Ig isotype switching, other molecules, including mTNF-α, CD2 and CD30L can modulate the isotype switching events during T-cell–B-cell interactions.

T-cell-independent models of IL-4-dependent IgE synthesis

Apart from the above-mentioned model of IgE synthesis induced in highly purified B cells by stimulation with IL-4 and anti-CD40 mAb (that mimics the activity of CD40L expressed on activated T cells), other T-cell-independent systems of IgE synthesis have been described (Vercelli & Geha, 1995).

Epstein–Barr virus (EBV)

Stimulation with IL-4 and EBV induces T-cell-independent IgE synthesis in human B cells (Thyphronitis *et al.*, 1989). IgE production is likely to result from *de novo* induction of isotype switching, rather than from expansion of a committed surface-IgE-positive (sIgE+) B-cell subset, which has undergone Cε switching *in vivo*, because sIgE⁻ B cells could produce IgE in response to EBV and IL-4. A small fraction of B cells which have undergone EBV transformation (<2%) are responsible for IgE synthesis induced by EBV and IL-4; however, virtually all IgE-producing cells expressed *EBNA-1* and *EBNA-2*, two viral genes which are known to be present in all cells immortalized by EBV (Vercelli & Geha, 1995). The respective roles played by IL-4 and EBV in the induction of IgE synthesis are not completely clear. IL-4 itself is able to induce ε germ-line transcription by normal B cells. By contrast, mature ε transcripts were detected only after stimulation with both IL-4 and EBV, supporting the concept of the two-signal model for isotype switching to IgE. No signal was detected in RNA from EBV B cells which were not treated with IL-4 and secreted Ig isotypes other than IgE. These results suggest that IgE-secreting B cells obtained by activation with EBV and IL-4 contain both mature and germ-line Cε transcripts. Interestingly, when IL-4 was added to IgM- or IgG-secreting EBV B-cell lines which had been maintained in culture for over 3 months, induction of germ-line, but not mature, Cε transcripts was observed. Thus, in established EBV B-cell lines stimulated with IL-4, there is a dissociation between germ-line Cε transcription and isotype switching to IgE expression. The nature of the EBV-mediated signal favouring the transcription of mature Cε transcripts is at present unknown. However, it does not simply result from engagement of the EBV receptor/CD21/complement receptor 2 (CR2). Indeed, mAb to different CD21 epitopes could not synergize with IL-4 in IgE induction. EBV infection results in the expression of a variety of viral genes in B cells, one of which may facilitate recombination indirectly, through effects on transcription or cell proliferation (Vercelli & Geha, 1995).

Hydrocortisone

IgE synthesis can be induced in human CD5+ leukaemic B cells by a combination of IL-4 and hydrocortisone (Sarfati *et al.*, 1989). Normal polyclonal IgE⁻ B cells isolated by cell sorting are also inducible to IgE synthesis by hydrocortisone and IL-4, in the absence of both T cells and monocytes. The nature of the hydrocortisone-derived signal is unknown. Analysis of the effects of hydrocortisone on ε germ-line transcription showed that hydrocortisone by itself did not induce ε germ-line transcripts, but modestly enhanced their accumulation (an approximately twofold increase versus a sevenfold increase induced by CD40 engagement). Since both hydrocortisone and CD40 engagement induced vigorous IgE synthesis in the presence of IL-4, it is likely that IgE synthesis induced by hydrocortisone also reflects effect(s) on step(s) other than ε germ-line transcription (Jabara *et al.*, 1991).

Mast cells and basophils

Recently, the ability of mast and basophilic cell lines to increase IgG and to induce IgE synthesis in purified B cells stimulated with IL-4 in the absence of T cells has been reported. IgE production was preceded by a marked increase in IL-4-induced ε germ-line RNA. The induction of IgE and the increase in IgG synthesis brought about by mast and basophilic cells in the presence of IL-4 was inhibited by competion with a chimeric recombinant fusion protein, consisting of the extracellular domain of human CD40 fused to a murine IgG constant region (CD40-Fc) (Gauchat *et al.*, 1993). These results suggest that mast or basophilic cell lines can replace T cells to provide the contact-mediated signal that is required, in conjunction with IL-4, for the induction of IgE production. Inhibition of this production by CD40-Fc indicates involvement of CD40L. Normal purified lung mast cells and blood basophils were also found to be able to support IgE production by B cells in the absence of T cells (Gauchat *et al.*, 1993). In contrast to mast cells, basophils were able to induce IgE synthesis even in the absence of exogenous IL-4. This may be consistent with the observation that basophils are able to release IL-4 (Brunner *et al.*, 1993), whereas the ability of normal mast cells to release IL-4 (Bradding *et al.*, 1992) is more controversial. Based on these findings, it has been suggested that mast cells and basophils may play a role in the regulation of IgE synthesis *in vivo* and that Ig isotype switching may occur outside the germinal centres in peripheral organs such as the lung or the skin (Gauchat *et al.*, 1993). However, the *in vivo* relevance of this *in vitro* model is doubt. Indeed, it would be somewhat surprising that mast cells are capable of inducing IgE synthesis *in vivo*, because no antigen-specific receptor molecules on mast cells have been identified, and the means of controlling the specificity of the mast cell-induced IgE synthesis is not known.

Modulation of IgE synthesis

IgE-enhancing factors

It is well known that T-cell/IL-4-dependent IgE synthesis can be modulated by lymphokines other than IL-4. IL-2, IL-5, IL-6, TNF-α (Punnonen *et al.*, 1994) and IL-9 (Dugas *et al.*, 1993) enhance IL-4-induced IgE synthesis (Table 6.2). IL-5 and IL-6 have been shown to up-regulate the IgE production induced by IL-4 in unfractionated mononuclear cells. IgE up-regulation by IL-5 could be observed only when suboptimal IL-4 concentrations were used (Pene *et al.*, 1988b), whereas IL-6 could up-regulate IgE synthesis even in the presence of high concentrations of IL-4 (Vercelli *et al.*, 1989a). IL-6 is known to act at a late stage in B-cell differentiation with no isotype preference. IL-6

Table 6.2 Regulatory factors of human IgE synthesis.

Positive regulatory factors		
T–B cell-to-cell interaction (CD40L-CD40; others ?)	Inducing factors	Enhancing factors
Anti-CD40 antibody	+	IL-6
EBV infection	IL-4	TNF-α
Corticosteroids	or	IL-5
	IL-13	IL-9
Negative regulatory factors		
1 Acting on T cells		
IFN-γ		
IFN-α		
PGE_2		
IL-10		
IL-12		
2 Acting on B cells		
TGF-β		
IL-8		
PAF-acether		
CD23		

See text for definition of abbreviations.

induces the secretion of IgG1 by co-ordinated transcriptional activation, selective accumulation of mRNA for the secreted form of IgG, and possibly differential mRNA stabilization. Thus, IL-6 may amplify IgE secretion by similar mechanisms. However, no direct evidence is available (Punnonen *et al.*, 1994). The mechanisms responsible for the enhancing effect of IL-2 and TNF-α on IgE synthesis are not completely clear. Both cytokines are indeed active in the proliferation of both T and B lymphocytes, as well as in the differentiation of B cells into antibody-producing cells. However, the effects of IL-2 and TNF-α on IgE production induced in the presence of T cells or in their absence (stimulation of purified B cells with anti-CD40 antibody or soluble CD40L) have not been compared. Interestingly, in the T-cell-dependent model, IL-2 was found to exert opposite effects on IgE helper activity by naive and memory T cells. IgE helper activity by naive T cells was inhibited, whereas in the presence of IL-2 the IgE helper activity of memory T cells was enhanced (van Kooten *et al.*, 1992). However, the finding that IL-2 was able to potentiate T-cell-/IL-4-dependent IgE synthesis, even when T cells had been treated with mitomycin C, suggests that the enhancing effect of IL-2 on IgE synthesis is due not merely to its activity of T-cell growth factor (Maggi *et al.*, 1989).

IgE-inhibitory factors

Other cytokines or mediators, such as IFN-α, IFN-γ (Del Prete *et al.*, 1988; Pene *et al.*, 1988a), TGF-β (Gauchat *et al.*, 1992), IL-8 (Kimata *et al.*, 1992), IL-10 (Punnonen *et al.*, 1993b), IL-12 (Kiniwa *et al.*, 1992), platelet-activating factor (PAF)-acether (Deryckx *et al.*, 1992) and prostaglandin E_2 (Pene *et al.*, 1988a), have been shown to down-regulate IgE synthesis (Punnonen *et al.*, 1994). IFN-α and IFN-γ have been reported to inhibit IL-4-dependent IgE synthesis in both mice and humans (Coffman & Carty, 1986; Del Prete *et al.*, 1988; Pene *et al.*,1988a). The mechanisms by which IFNs inhibit IgE synthesis are not well defined. IFN-γ profoundly suppressed the expression of ε germ-line transcripts in murine B cells stimulated with LPS and IL-4. By contrast, no inhibition was observed when IFN-γ was added to highly purified human B cells stimulated with IL-4, suggesting that activation of ε germ-line transcription and switch recombination may not necessarily be coupled. Unlike IFN-γ, TGF-β and PAF-acether suppress both ε germ-line transcription and IgE synthesis in human B cells stimulated with IL-4. IL-8 also suppresses IgE synthesis by purified B cells stimulated with IL-4 and anti-CD40 mAb, but the inhibitory mechanism has not been investigated. More recently, IL-8 has also been found to block spontaneous IgE synthesis, and such an effect appeared to be mediated by its ability to decrease the production of IL-6 and TNF-α (Kimata *et al.*, 1995). On the other hand, IL-10 blocks IgE synthesis by peripheral blood mononuclear cells by inhibiting the accessory cell function of monocytes (Punnonen *et al.*, 1993b), but it also directly stimulates B cells cultured in the presence of IL-4 and anti-CD40 mAb cross-linked to CD32 (FcγRII) on murine L cells (Rousset *et al.*, 1992). The mechanism responsible for the inhibitory activity of IL-12 on IgE synthesis is unknown. However, its activity may be mediated by IFN-γ, since IL-12 is a powerful inducer of IFN-γ release by both T cells and natural killer (NK) cells (Chehimi & Trinchieri, 1994).

CD23

The issue of the effects on human IgE production of signals delivered via CD23 deserves separate discussion. CD23 is the low-affinity receptor for IgE. It shows no homology to the high-affinity IgE receptor (FcεRI) expressed on mast cells and basophils. Two forms of CD23, FcεRIIa and FcRIIb, which differ only in their N-terminal cytoplasmic portions, are generated through the use of different transcription sites and alternative RNA splicing (Yokota *et al.*, 1988). FcεRIIa is expressed exclusively by B cells, but FcεRIIb is also expressed by monocytes and Langheran's cells after activation by IL-4. CD23 is a labile protein, in that a soluble fragment is released from the carboxy-terminal extracellular portion of the molecule, giving rise to soluble CD23 (sCD23). Studies on the role of sCD23 in the regulation of IgE synthesis have resulted in somewhat contradictory results. Supernatants of CD23+ B-cell lines or purified forms of sCD23 were shown to enhance IgE synthesis (Sarfati & Delespesse, 1988; Scherr *et al.*, 1989), and mAb specific for CD23 inhibited B-cell proliferation and differentiation (Luo *et al.*, 1991). By contrast, other studies suggest that recombinant sCD23 does not have any B-cell growth-promoting activity *in vitro* (Uchibayashi *et al.*, 1989). Recently, it was shown that administration of mAb specific for CD23 to mice strongly inhibits antigen-specific IgE synthesis (Bonnefoy *et al.*, 1990), suggesting a role for the CD23 molecule in the regulation of IgE production *in vivo*. In addition, CD21 was shown to be another ligand for CD23 and to be able to regulate IgE production (Aubry *et al.*, 1992). More recent experiments performed in both CD23 gene-tragetted and CD23 transgenic mice suggest that membrane CD23 certainly plays a feedback regulatory role in IgE synthesis (Fujiwara *et al.*, 1994; Texido *et al.*, 1994; Yu *et al.*, 1994). Such a regulatory effect is probably mediated by a negative signal delivered by the interaction of IgE-containing immune complexes with CD23 expressed on the B-cell surface (Yu *et al.*, 1994). In contrast, the role of sCD23 in the regulation of IgE synthesis, at least in these very reliable experimental models, does not seem to be noteworthy.

Modulation of Th2 development

The Th1/Th2 dichotomy

The role of Th cells and Th-cell-derived cytokines in the induction of IgE synthesis was further emphasized and clarified by the demonstration that functionally distinct subsets of CD4+ Th cells reminiscent of those already described in mice (Mosmann *et al.*, 1986) do exist in humans as well (Romagnani, 1991). So far, two polarized forms of the specific Th cell-mediated response, based on their distinct and mutually exclusive pattern of cytokine secretion, have been described. Th1, but not Th2 cells, produce IFN-γ and TNF-β, whereas Th2, but not Th1, produce IL-4 and IL-5. Production of other cytokines, such as IL-2, IL-10 and IL-13, is less restricted than in mice, although IL-2 is mainly released by Th1 cells, whereas IL-10 and IL-13 are mainly released by Th2 cells (Table 6.3). Different cytokine patterns imply distinct effector functions (Table 6.3). Th1 cells, which trigger both cell-mediated immunity and production of opsonizing antibodies, mediate phagocyte-dependent defence in response to intracellular infectious agents (Romagnani, 1994a). In contrast, Th2 cells, which are responsible for IgE and IgG4 antibody production, differentiation and activation of mast cells and eosinophils, and inhibition of some macrophage functions, are mainly involved in the phagocyte-independent defence against large extracellular parasites (Romagnani, 1994a) (Fig. 6.4). In addition to cells that fit into the Th1- or Th2-polarized phenotypes, CD4+ Th cells have been identified (Th0 cells), that show a composite profile, including production of both Th1- and Th2-type cytokines, and mediate effects that depend on the ratio of cytokines produced (Romagnani, 1994a). More recently, human T-cell clones producing Th2-type cytokines were found to differ from those producing Th1-type cytokines for the ability to express CD30 (Del Prete *et al.*, 1995), a member of the TNF-R superfamily (Smith *et al.*, 1990), and to release the soluble form of CD30 (sCD30) (Manetti *et al.*, 1994; Del Prete *et al.*, 1995).

Table 6.3 Main properties of human Th1 and Th2 cells.

Property	Th1	Th2
Cytokine secretion		
IFN-γ	+++	–
TNF-β	+++	–
IL-2	+++	+
TNF-α	+++	+
GM-CSF	++	++
IL-3	++	+++
IL-10	+	+++
IL-13	+	+++
IL-4	–	+++
IL-5	–	+++
Cytolytic potential	+++	–
B-cell help for Ig synthesis		
IgE	–	+++
IgM, IgG, IgA		
At low T : B cell ratios	+++	++
At high T : B cell ratios	–	+++
Macrophage activation		
Induction of PCA	+++	–
TF production	+++	–
CD30 expression and release	±	+++

–, no activity; ±, exceptional; +, low; ++, mean; +++, strong.

Role of allergen-specific Th2 cells in the pathogenesis of allergy

The discovery that IL-4 was essential for IgE production and had mast cell-growth factor activity, together with the observation that IL-5 was the critical factor for the differentiation and activation of eosinophils, allowed speculation that allergen-specific Th2-like cells may have an important role in the pathogenesis of allergic (atopic) disorders. Indeed, the allergen-specific Th2 cell represents an excellent candidate for an explanation of why the mast cell/eosinophil/IgE-producing B-cell triad is involved in atopy (Romagnani, 1994b).

The analysis of cytokine production by T-cell clones specific for different antigens has clearly shown that, in

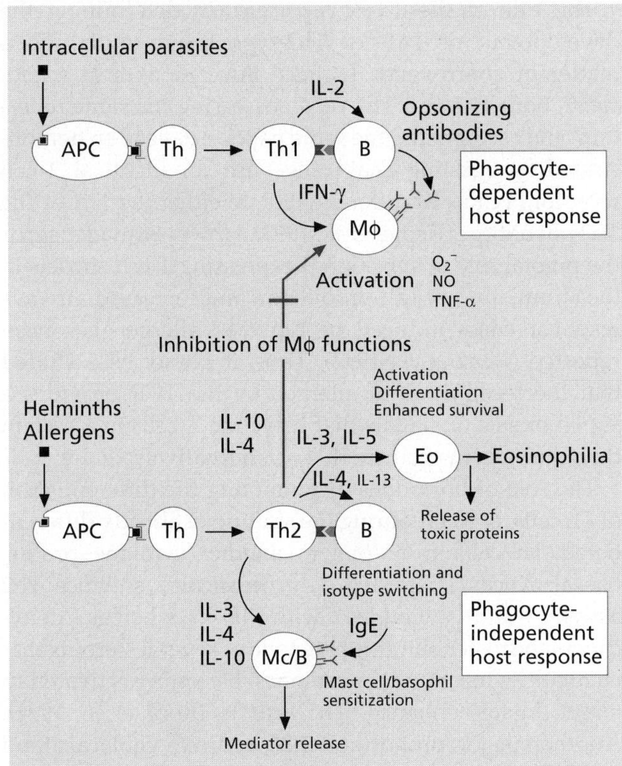

Fig. 6.4 Th1 and Th2 cells as polarized forms of Th-cell response. Th1 cells mainly develop in response to infections by intracellular parasites (i.e. mycobacteria and *Leishmania tropica major*). Th1 cells are responsible for the activation of macrophages (via IFN-γ), which are involved in delayed-type hypersensitivity (DTH), and for the production of opsonizing antibodies which collaborate with phagocytes (phagocyte-dependent host response). Th2 cells mainly develop in response to helminthic infestations and (in atopic people) in response to common environmental allergens. Th2-cell activation results in the growth of mast cells and basophils, differentiation and activation of eosinophils and production of Ig of different classes, including IgE. Some cytokines produced by Th2 cells, such as IL-4 and IL-10, inhibit different macrophage functions (phagocyte-independent host response). (Modified from Romagnani *et al.*, 1994.)

contrast to clones specific for bacterial antigens that show a prevalent Th1/Th0 phenotype, the great majority of allergen-specific T-cell clones generated from peripheral blood lymphocytes of atopic donors express a Th0/Th2 phenotype, with high production of IL-4 and IL-5, and no or low production of IFN-γ (Wierenga *et al.*, 1990; Parronchi *et al.*, 1991). Evidence suggesting that Th2-like cells accumulate at the level of target organs in different allergic disorders has been provided by using either cloning techniques or *in situ* hybridization. Upon mitogen stimulation, the majority of T-cell clones generated from the conjunctival infiltrates of patients with vernal conjunctivitis (a disease in which an allergic pathogenesis is suspected but not proved) were found to develop into Th2 clones (Maggi *et al.*, 1991). Using *in situ* hybridization, cells showing mRNA for Th2, but not Th1, cytokines were detected at the site of late-phase skin reactions in skin biopsies from atopic patients, in mucosal bronchial biopsies or bronchoalveolar lavage (BAL) from patients with asthma (Hamid *et al.*, 1991; Kay *et al.*, 1991; Robinson *et al.*, 1992) and after local allergen challenge in nasal mucosa of patients with allergen-induced rhinitis (Bradding *et al.*, 1993). Likewise, increased levels of IL-4 and IL-5 were measured in the BAL of allergic asthmatics, whereas in non-allergic asthmatics IL-2 and IL-5 predominated (Walker *et al.*, 1992). Finally, proportions ranging from 14 to 22% of T-cell clones, generated from airway mucosae of grass-allergic patients following inhalation challenge with grass pollen, appeared to be specific for grass allergens and most of them exhibited a definite Th2 profile (Del Prete *et al.*, 1993). Accordingly, high proportions of *Dermatophagoides pteronyssimus* (DP)-specific Th2-like CD4+ T-cell clones were generated from intact skin of patients with atopic dermatitis (AD) taken after contact challenge with DP (van Rejisen *et al.*, 1992). Very recently, it has been shown that CD30, a member of the TNF-R superfamily (Smith *et al.*, 1993), is preferentially expressed by T-cell clones able to produce Th2-type cytokines (Del Prete *et al.*, 1995). CD30 expression was therefore evaluated in circulating CD4+ T cells from six grass pollen-sensitive patients and six non-atopic controls before and during the seasonal exposure to grass pollens. No CD4+CD30+ cells were detected in any of the non-atopic donors or the atopic patients examined before the grass pollination season, whereas four out of six grass-sensitive donors examined during the season, when they were suffering from allergic symptoms, showed small proportions of circulating CD4+CD30+ cells (from 0.08 to 0.3%). Circulating CD4+ T cells from these patients were fractionated into CD30+ and CD30– cells by sorting with an anti-CD30 mAb, the two cell fractions expanded by culturing in IL-2, and then assessed for their ability to produce type 1 (IFN-β and TNF-β) or type 2 (IL-4 and IL-5) cytokines and to proliferate in response to *Lolium perenne* group I (Lol p I) allergen. Only CD30+ cells proliferated in response to Lol p I and exhibited the ability to produce IL-4 and IL-5, whereas production of both IFN-γ and TNF-β was prevalent in the CD30– cell fractions (Del Prete *et al.*, 1995). These findings clearly demonstrate that grass allergen-reactive CD4+ CD30+ T cells, inducible to the production of Th2 cytokines, can circulate in the peripheral blood of grass-sensitive patients during *in vivo* natural exposure to grass pollen allergens. The ligand for CD30 (CD30L) has been found to be expressed by both activated T cells and macrophages (Smith *et al.*, 1993).

Additional evidence for the role of Th2-like cells in the pathogenesis of allergic disorders was provided by two recent studies, devoted to investigation of the effect of allergen-specific immunotherapy on the cytokine profile of T cells. Grass pollen immunotherapy did not affect the expression of Th2-type cytokine pattern in response to allergen exposure at the level of allergen-induced late-phase cutaneous reactions, but expression of mRNA for Th1-type cytokines was enhanced in many patients showing clinical improvement (Varney *et al.*, 1993). In another study, successful immunotherapy was found to reduce IL-4 production by allergen-specific CD4+ T cells to levels observed with T cells from non-allergic subjects, whereas production of IFN-γ was not affected (Secrist *et al.*, 1993). Finally, both decreased production of IL-4 and increased production of IFN-γ was observed in bee venom-sensitized patients treated with specific immunotherapy (Jutel *et al.*, 1995; McHugh *et al.*, 1995). Although these reports are partially discordant, probably because of the different experimental approaches used, they all support the concept that cytokine profiles of allergen-specific memory CD4+ T cells are mutable and can be manipulated by *in vivo* therapies. This possibility is also supported by studies in mice injected with chemically modified allergen (Gieni *et al.*, 1993) or infected with *Leishmania tropica major* and treated with IL-12 and Pentostam (Nabors *et al.*, 1995).

Regulatory mechanisms of Th2 development

The mechanisms responsible for the preferential development of allergen-reactive Th2 cells in atopic subjects have not yet been completely clarified. Attention has been focused on the possible role of antigen-presenting cells (APC), the T-cell repertoire and soluble factors present in the microenvironment at the time of allergen presentation. It is highly probable that Langerhans cells (LC) present in the skin, as well as dendritic cells (DC) that are localized in the respiratory mucosa, represent the primary point of contact between the immune system and allergens coming into contact with the skin or the respiratory airways, respectively. Skin LC and mucosal DC are probably involved in allergen transport to regional lymph nodes where allergen presentation to allergen-specific CD4+ T cells occurs. Some data suggest that atopic patients with asthma may have higher numbers of intra-epithelial DC than non-asthmatic subjects, and that, in the presence of allergen molecules, these cells can induce T-cell activation and release of IL-4 and IL-5 (Schon-Hegrad *et al.*, 1991). However, the actual role played by APC in driving the development of allergen-reactive Th2-like cells remains to be elucidated. It will be of interest to establish whether alterations of CD30L expression and/or activity may play some role in the develepment of allergen-specific Th2 responses in atopic individuals. In preliminary experiments, it has been shown that blocking of CD30L on APC may shift the *in vitro* differentiation of allergen-specific T cells from the Th0/Th2 to the Th0/Th1 phenotype.

The role of the T-cell repertoire in determining the development of Th1- or Th2-type responses is still a matter of controversy. In mice infected with *L. tropica major*, both Th1 and Th2 cells possessing the same repertoire and recognizing the same peptide have been demonstrated, suggesting that cells with an identical T-cell receptor (TCR) can differentiate into either the Th1 or the Th2 phenotype (Reiner *et al.*, 1993). However, evidence for the pivotal role of specific Vβ-expressing T-cell subsets in the stimulation of IgE production and increased airways responsiveness induced by ragweed allergen has been reported (Renz *et al.*, 1993). Thus, it cannot be excluded that the recognition of allergen by the TCR provides a signal or sets of signals that drive the T cells in a certain direction, e.g. to produce IL-4 or, alternatively, IFN-γ.

The role of hormones in promoting the differentiation of Th cells, or in favouring the shifting of already differentiated Th cells from one to another cytokine profile, has also been suggested. Glucocorticoids enhance Th2 activity, and synergize with IL-4, whereas dehydroepiandrostenone sulphate (one of several steroids that circulate as inactive prohormones, becoming activated in target organs) enhances Th1 activity (Rook *et al.*, 1994). Another major prohormone, 25-hydroxy cholecalciferol (25(OH)-vitamin D3), may have a reverse effect on the Th1/Th2 balance. There is intense conversion of 25(OH)-vitamin D3 to 1,25$(OH)_2$-vitamin D3 (calcitriol), which is able to decrease output of IL-2 and IFN-γ and, when administered peripherally with antigen, evokes a Th2 pattern of response localized to mucosal surfaces. More importantly, calcitriol analogues can rival cyclosporin A in their ability to prolong the survival of skin grafts by inhibiting Th1 activity (Rook *et al.*, 1994). Finally, progesterone favours the *in vitro* development of human Th cells producing Th2-type cytokines and promotes both IL-4 production and membrane CD30 expression in established human Th1 clones (Romagnani, 1994b). This may represent one of the mechanisms involved in the Th1/Th2 switch which has been hypothesized to occur at the maternal–fetal interface, in order to improve fetal survival and promote successful pregnancy (Wegmann *et al.*, 1993). Thus, increasing evidence is accumulating to suggest that hormones and peripherally activated prohormones may regulate the Th1/Th2 balance.

So far, however, the clearest examples of factors affecting the differentiation pathways of both murine and human Th cells appear to be cytokines released by APC and/or other cell types at the time of antigen presentation (Fig. 6.5). Thus, IFN-α, IL-12 and TGF-β produced by macrophages and B cells, particularly in response to intracellular bacteria, have been shown to play an important role in the induction of Th1 expansion in various systems (Romagnani, 1992). IFN-γ, which is produced mainly by T cells and NK cells, also promotes the differentiation of

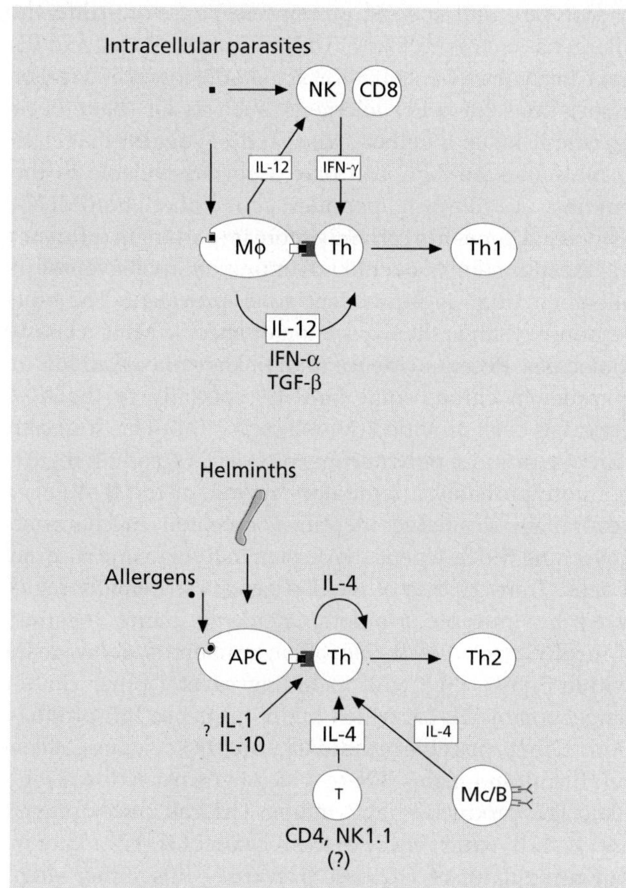

Fig. 6.5 Role for cells of the 'natural' immunity in the differentiation of Th cells into the Th1 or the Th2 profile. Intracellular parasites stimulate the production of IL-12 by macrophages. IL-12, either directly or indirectly via the induction of IFN-γ by NK cells and T cells, creates a microenvironment at the level of the antigen-presentation triad (APC/antigen/Th cell) which favours the development of the Th cell into a Th1 cell. Production of IFN-γ and TGF-β in the same site can also contribute to the Th1 development. Early production of IL-4 at the antigen-presentation level is required for the development of Th2 cells, which occurs in response to helminths and (in atopic people) to allergens. It is not yet clear whether early IL-4 production is due to cells of the mast cell/basophil lineage activated through FcR-independent mechanisms to a subset of memory T cells showing an unusual phenotype (CD4+NK1.1+) (Yashimoto & Paul, 1994) or to the mice Th cell itself. Early production of IL-1 and IL-10 can play an ancillary role in the Th2 development. (Modified from Romagnani, 1992.)

Th1 cells (Maggi *et al.*, 1992). Likewise, IL-12, which is a powerful IFN-γ inducer (Chehimi & Trinchieri, 1994), appears to be the most important natural initiator of Th1 responses by acting either directly or indirectly via the induction of IFN-γ production (Hsieh *et al.*, 1993; Manetti *et al.*, 1993).

The effect of cytokines produced by macrophages and/or B cells on the development of Th2 cells seems to be less critical. IL-10 has been shown to favour the development of Th2 cells both in mouse and humans. IL-1 is a selective co-factor for the growth of some murine Th2 clones, and can favour the *in vitro* development of human Th2-like clones (Romagnani, 1994b). However, most striking is the requirement for IL-4 for maturation of Th cells into Th2 cells (Fig. 6.5). In both murine and human systems, IL-4 appears to be the most dominant factor in determining the likelihood for Th2 polarization in cultured cells (Maggi *et al.*, 1992; Swain, 1993). Accordingly, IL-4-gene-targetted mice fail to generate mature Th2 cells *in vivo* and to produce IgE antibodies (Kopf *et al.*, 1993), suggesting that early IL-4 production by another cell type must be involved. Possible candidates include a peculiar CD4+NK1.1+ T-CD1-restricted cell subset (Yashimoto & Paul, 1994), as well as mast cells and basophils, which have been shown to release stored IL-4 in response to FcεR triggering (Bradding *et al.*, 1992; Brunner *et al.*, 1993). However, parasites or allergens should be able to activate CD4+NK1.1+ T cells or they would be able to cross-link FcεR receptors on mast cells/basophils prior to a specific immune response that had produced parasite-specific IgG and IgE antibodies. On the other hand, mast cell-deficient mice develop normal Th2 responses (Wershil *et al.*, 1994). Finally, in IL-4-deficient mice only those mice which are reconstituted with IL-4-producing T (but not with IL-4-producing non-T) cells produce antigen-specific IgE (Schmitz *et al.*, 1994). Thus, IL-4 production by mast cells triggered by antigen–IgE antibody immune complexes may play a role in amplifying secondary responses to parasites, but cannot account for the Th2 development in primary immune responses.

An alternative explanation is that some proteolytic enzymes, which are produced in large quantity by many helminth parasites, or anaphylotoxins formed via the alternative complement pathway, trigger mast cells to release IL-4 and other cytokines that induce a Th2 differentiation in the primary response. In this regard, it is of note that some environmental allergens are proteases. In addition, injection of papain in BALB/c mice resulted in 10–30-fold increases in IL-4 and IL-5 but not IFN-γ or IL-2 in draining lymph nodes, whereas inactivated papain was much less potent (Finkelman & Urban, 1992). However, many allergens are not enzymes. Thus, a more likely possibility is that the source of IL-4 in the primary response is the naive Th cells themselves. Indeed, low-intensity signalling of TCR, such as that mediated by low peptide doses or by mutant peptides, led to secretion of low levels of IL-4 by murine naive T cells (Pfeiffer *et al.*, 1995). Moreover, human naive T cells were found to develop into IL-4-producing cells in the absence of any pre-existing source of IL-4, and in spite of the presence of anti-IL-4 antibodies (Kalinski *et al.*, 1995). Thus, the fact that allergens induce Th2-type responses only in selected people suggests that atopic individuals would have genetic disregulation in the production of IL-4 (and/or of cytokines exerting regulatory effects on the development and/or function of Th2 cells) at the level of T cells. Recently, the role of IFN-γ released by MHC class I-restricted CD8+ T cells in preventing the development of Th2-like cells in response to non-replicating antigens presented at mucosal surfaces has been suggested (Kemeny & Diaz-Sanchez, 1993; McMenamin & Holt, 1993). Furthermore, nebulized but not parenteral IFN-γ decreased IgE production and normalized airways function in a murine model of allergen sensitization (Lack *et al.*, 1993), suggesting that the immediate allergic response to allergen sensitization via the airways may be immunomodulated by locally produced cytokines (and possibly by hormones, as well).

Possible alterations favouring Th2-type responses in atopic subjects

Traditionally, the immunogenetic mechanisms underlying heightened IgE responsiveness seen in the atopic diseases may be divided into two types, antigen specific and non-antigen specific (Marsh *et al.*, 1994). The former is strongly influenced by human leucocyte antigen (HLA)-D-encoded MHC class II genes and involves cognate T-cell/B-cell interaction. The latter, non-cognate regulation of IgE, could involve primarily mast cells, basophils, and possibly other FcεRI+ cells, and obviously Th2 cells.

The possible role of MHC class II molecules has been extensively investigated by both genetic and molecular approaches. Significant associations between certain HLA haplotypes, and specific immune responses to different allergens, such as Amb a V, Amb a VI and Lol p I, II and III, have been observed (Marsh *et al.*, 1994). However, weaker associations for other allergens, such as DP, have been reported. Taken together, these studies suggest that class II molecules on APC can play a permissive role in the binding of allergen peptides, but other non-MHC-associated genes are certainly more important in influencing the induction of overall IgE immune responsiveness to allergens (that is equivalent to a prevalent Th2-type response) than is the expression of specific MHC class II molecules. Recent evidence for a linkage of overall IgE to markers in chromosome 5q31.1, especially to the IL-4 gene, has been provided (Marsh *et al.*, 1994). This suggests that one or more polymorphisms exist in a coding region or, more probably, a regulatory region, of the IL-4 gene. Several studies have identified potential mechanisms governing the IL-4 gene expression in human and murine T cells. Transcription of the IL-4 gene is stringently regulated by multiple promoter elements acting together (Murphy *et al.*, 1993). However, numerous genes map within 5q31.1 (Fig. 6.6), including several other candidates, notably IL-13, which might influence IgE production. Other possible candidates are *IRF1*, whose gene product up-regulates IFN-α, which in turn can down-regulate IgE production and inhibit Th2 cell development and IL-12B, which encodes the β-chain of IL-12, a known down-regulator of Th2 cells (Fig. 6.6). Thus, either alterations of molecular mechanisms directly involved in the regulation of IL-4 gene expression, or deficient regulatory

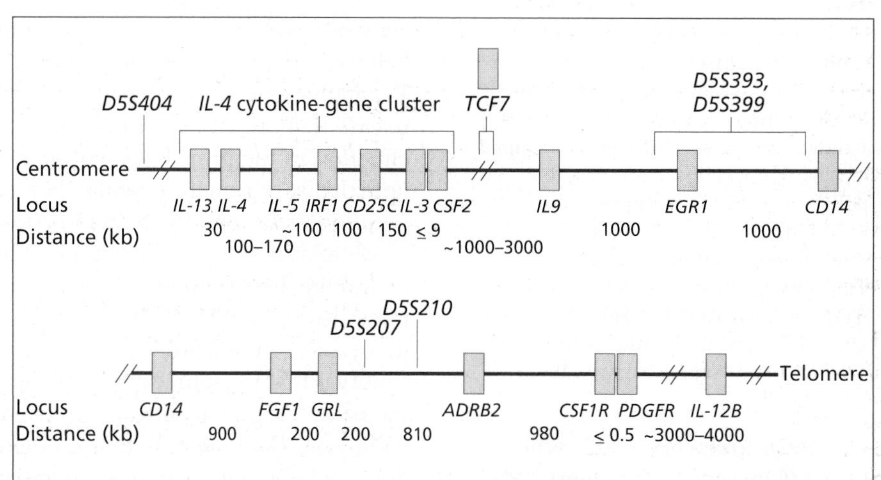

Fig. 6.6 A map showing genes of known physical location and certain polymorphic microsatellite markers in and around human chromosome 5q31.1–q33. Besides various interleukin genes (IL-3, IL-4, IL-5, IL-9, IL-12 β-chain, IL-13), the map includes the following: genes: *IRF*, IFN-regulatory factor-1, which encodes a transcription activator of IFN-α and IFN-β and other IFN-inducible genes; CDC25C, cell division cycle; CSF2, granulocyte macrophage colony-stimulatory factor (GM-CSF); TCF7, T-cell-specific transcription factor-7; EGR1, early growth factor response-1; CD14, cell antigen 14; GFG-1, fibroblast growth factor-1; GRL, lymphocyte-specific glucocorticoid receptor; ADRB2, the β_2-adrenergic receptor; CSF1-R, colony-stimulatory factor-1 receptor; PDGF-R, platelet-derived growth factor receptor. (Modified from Marsh *et al.*, 1994.)

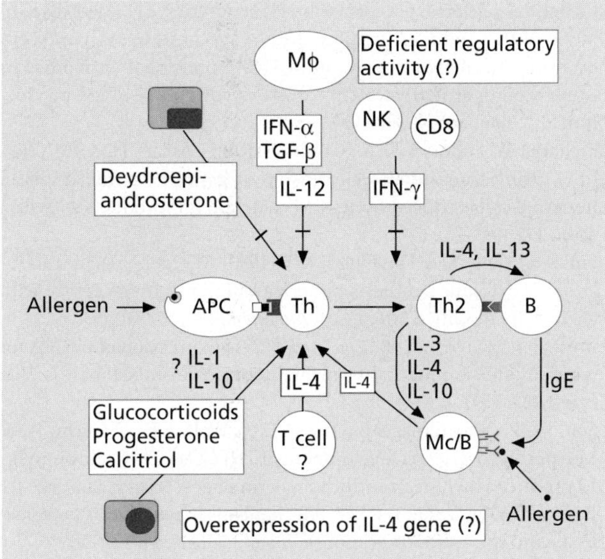

Fig. 6.7 A hypothetical scheme of cellular, hormonal and cytokine interactions leading to allergen-specific Th2 responses. Possible overexpression of IL-4 gene and/or deficient activity of genes encoding for cytokines showing Th2-regulatory activity cells may be responsible for the preferential development of allergen-specific Th2 cells in atopic individuals. (From Romagnani, 1994b.)

activity of cytokines responsible for inhibition of Th2-cell development (such as IFN-α and IL-12), or both, may account for the the preferential Th2-type response towards environmental allergens in atopic people (Fig. 6.7). An overexpression of other cytokine genes (IL-3, IL-5, GM-CSF and IL-9) located together with IL-4 and IL-13 within the same cluster of chromosome 5 may also co-exist (Fig. 6.7). The overexpression of the above genes can account for the preferential development of Th2 cells in resonse to allergens, as well as for the production by Th2 cells, and even by other cell types of the cytokines involved in the allergic inflammation, and therefore explain the persistent histological, pathophysiological and clinical aspects of allergic disorders.

Concluding remarks and summary

The mechanisms accounting for the joint involvement of IgE-producing B cells, mast cells/basophils and eosinophils in the pathogenesis of allergic reactions have remained unclear until the existence of distinct subsets of CD4+ Th cells, based on their profile of cytokine secretion, was discovered. So far, at least three different subsets of Th cells have been described in both mice and humans: Th1 cells that produce IL-2, IFN-γ and TNF-β; Th2 cells that produce IL-4, IL-5 and IL-10; Th0 cells that produce both Th1- and Th2-type cytokines. IL-3, GM-CSF and TNF-α are variably produced by all Th subsets. It is of note that IL-3, IL-4 and IL-10 are growth factors for mast cells and IL-5 is a selective activating and differentiating factor for eosinophils. Finally, it has clearly been shown that IgE synthesis results from the collaboration between Th2 cells and B cells. To this end, Th2 cells provide B cells with at least two signals. One signal is delivered by IL-4, the other is represented by a T-cell/B-cell physical interaction, occurring between the CD40 molecule constitutively expressed on the B cell and the CD40L expressed on the activated Th cell. The Th2-cell-derived IL-4 induces germ-line ε expression on the B cell, whereas the CD40L/CD40 interaction is required for the expression of productive mRNA and for the synthesis of IgE protein. Recently, it has been demonstrated that another cytokine, IL-13, is also able to induce germ-line ε expression, but its role in the pathogenesis of allergic reaction is still unclear. On the other hand, Th1 cells that produce IFN-γ but not IL-4, as well as Th0 cells that produce high concentrations of IFN-γ in addition to IL-4 and/or IL-13, are unable to support, or rather they suppress, the IL-4-dependent IgE synthesis. Other soluble factors produced by both T cells and non-T cells have also been shown to exert, at least *in vitro*, positive (IL-5, IL-6, TNF-α) or negative (IFN-α, TGF-β, IL-8, IL-10, IL-12) regulatory effects on human IgE synthesis.

The question of how and why common environmental allergens preferentially evoke Th2 responses, even though in a minority of the population, is still obscure. The recent demonstration that one or more polymorphisms exist in a coding region or, more probably, in a regulatory region of the IL-4 gene suggests that alterations of molecular mechanisms involved in the regulation of IL-4 gene expression is involved. An overexpression of other cytokine genes, such as IL-13 and IL-5, located together with IL-4 within the same cluster of chromosome 5 (5q31.1), may also occur. In this respect, of note is that IL-4 not only acts as the main IgE switching cytokine, but also represents the critical factor required for the differentiation of both naive and memory Th cells into the Th2-type functional subset. On the other hand, the possible role of a deficient regulatory activity of cytokines, such as IL-12, IFN-α and IFN-γ, exerting inhibitory activity on both IgE synthesis and development of Th2 cells, cannot be excluded.

References

Armitage, R., Fanslow, W., Strockbine, L. *et al.* (1992) Molecular and biological characterization of a murine ligand for CD40. *Nature*, **357**, 80–2.

Aruffo, A., Farrington, M., Hollenbaugh, D. *et al.* (1993) The CD40 ligand, gp39, is defective in activated T cells from patients with X-linked hyper IgM syndrome. *Cell*, **72**, 291–300.

Aubry, J.-P., Pochon, S., Graber, P., Jansen, K.U. & Bonnefoy, J.-Y. (1992) CD21 is a ligand for CD23 and regulates IgE production. *Nature*, **358**, 505–7.

Aversa, G., Punnonen, J. & de Vries, J.E. (1993) The 26-kD transmembrane form of tumor necrosis factor α on activated CD4+ T cell clones provides a co-stimulatory signal for human B-cell activation. *J. Exp. Med.*, **177**, 1575–85.

Bonnefoy, J.-Y., Shields, J. & Mermod, J.-J. (1990) Inhibition of human interleukin-4-induced IgE synthesis by a subset of anti-CD23/FcεRII monoclonal antibodies. *Eur. J. Immunol.*, **20**, 139–44.

Bradding, P., Feather, I.H., Howarth, P.H. *et al.* (1992) Interleukin 4 is localized and released by human mast cells. *J. Exp. Med.*, **76**, 1381–6.

Bradding, P., Feather, I.H., Wilson, S. *et al.* (1993) Immunolocalization of cytokines in nasal mucosa of normal and perennial rhinitic subjects. *J. Immunol.*, **151**, 3853–65.

Brunner, T., Heusser, C.H. & Dahinden, C.A. (1993) Human peripheral blood basophils primed by interleukin 3 (IL-3) produce IL-4 in response to immunoglobulin E receptor stimulation. *J. Exp. Med.*, **177**, 605–11.

Chehimi, J. & Trinchieri, G. (1994) Interleukin-12: a bridge between innate resistance and adaptive immunity with a role in infection and acquired immunodeficiency. *J. Clin. Immunol.*, **14**, 149–61.

Coffman, R.L. & Carty, J. (1986) A T cell activity that enhances polyclonal IgE production and its inhibition by interferon. *J. Immunol.*, **136**, 949–54.

Del Prete, G.F., Maggi, E., Parronchi, P. *et al.* (1988) IL-4 is an essential factor for the IgE synthesis induced *in vitro* by human T cell clones and their supernatants. *J. Immunol.*, **140**, 4193–8.

Del Prete, G.F., De Carli, M., D'Elios, M.M. *et al.* (1993) Allergen exposure induces the activation of allergen-specific Th2 cells in the airway mucosa of patients with allergic respiratory disorders. *Eur. J. Immunol.*, **23**, 1445–9.

Del Prete, G.-F., De Carli, M., D'Elios, M.M. *et al.* (1994) Polyclonal B cell activation induced by Herpesvirus saimiri-transformed human CD4+ T cell clones: role for membrane TNF-α/TNF-α receptors and CD2/CD58 interactions. *J. Immunol.*, **153**, 4872–9.

Del Prete, G.F., De Carli, M., Almerigogna, F. *et al.* (1995) Preferential expression of CD30 by human CD4+ T cells producing Th2-type cytokines. *FASEB J.*, **9**, 81–6.

Deryckx, S., de Waal Malefyt, R., Gauchat, J.-F., Vivier, E., Thomas Y. & de Vries, J.E. (1992) Immunoregulatory functions of paf-acether. VIII. Inhibition of IL-4-induced human IgE synthesis. *J. Immunol.*, **148**, 1465–70.

Diaz-Sanchez, D., Chegini, S., Zhang, K. & Saxon, A. (1994) CD58 (LFA-3) stimulation provides a signal for human isotype switching and IgE production distinct from CD40. *J. Immunol.*, **153**, 10–20.

Dugas, B., Renauld, J.C., Péne, J. *et al.* (1993) Interleukin-9 potentiates the interleukin-4-induced immunoglobulin (IgG, IgM and IgE) production by normal human B lymphocytes. *Eur. J. Immunol.*, **23**, 1687–92.

Farrington, M., Grosmaire, L.S., Nonoyama, S. *et al.* (1994) CD40 ligand is defective in a subset of patients with common variable immunodeficiency. *Proc. Nat. Acad. Sci. USA*, **91**, 1099–103.

Finkelman, F.D. & Urban, J.F. (1992) Cytokines: making the right choice. *Parasitol. Today*, **8**, 311–4.

Fujiwara, H., Kikutani, H., Suematsu, S. *et al.* (1994) The absence of IgE antibody-mediated augmentation of immune responses in CD23-deficient mice. *Proc. Nat. Acad. Sci. USA*, **91**, 6835–9.

Gascan, H., Gauchat, J.F., Aversa, G.G., van Vlasselaer P., de Vries, J.E. (1991) Anti-CD40 monoclonal antibodies or CD40+ T cell clones and IL-4 induce IgG4 and IgE switching in purified human B cells via different signalling pathways. *J. Immunol.*, **147**, 8–13.

Gauchat, J.-F., Henchoz, S., Mazzei, G. *et al.* (1993) Induction of human IgE synthesis in B cells by mast cells and basophils. *Nature*, **365**, 340–3.

Gauchat, J.-F., Aversa, G.C., Gascan, H. & de Vries, J.E. (1992) Modulation of IL-4-induced germline ε RNA synthesis in human B cells by tumor necrosis factor-α, anti-CD40 monoclonal antibodies or transforming growth factor-β correlates with levels of IgE production. *Int. Immunol.*, **4**, 397–406.

Gauchat, J.-F., Lebman, D.A., Coffman, R.L., Gascan, H. & de Vries, J.E. (1990) Structure and expression of germline ε transcripts in human B cells induced by IL-4 to switch to IgE production. *J. Exp. Med.*, **172**, 463–73.

Gieni, R.S., Yang, X. & HayGlass, K.T. (1993) Allergen-specific modulation of cytokine synthesis pattern and IgE responses *in vivo* with chemically modified allergen. *J. Immunol.*, **150**, 302–10.

Hamid, Q., Azzawi, M., Ying, S. *et al.* (1991) Expression of mRNA for interleukin-5 in mucosal bronchial biopsies from asthma. *J. Clin. Invest.*, **87**, 1541–6.

Hsieh, C.-S., Macatonia, S.E., Tripp, C.S., Wolf, S.F., O'Garra, A. & Murphy, K.M. (1993) Development of Th1 CD4+ T cells through IL-12 produced by *Listeria*-induced macrophages. *Science*, **260**, 547–9.

Ishizaka, K. & Ishizaka, T. (1978) Mechanisms of reaginic hypersensitivity and IgE antibody response. *Immunol. Rev.*, **41**, 122–48.

Jabara, H.H., Ahern, D.J., Vercelli, D. & Geha, R.S. (1991) Hydrocortisone and IL-4 induce IgE isotype switching in human B cells. *J. Immunol.*, **147**, 1557–60.

Jutel, M., Pichler, W.J., Skrbic, D., Urwyler, A., Dahinden, C. & Muller, U.R. (1995) Bee venom immunotherapy results in decrease of IL-4 and IL-5 and increase of IFN-γ secretion in specific allergen-stimulated T cell cultures. *J. Immunol.*, **154**, 4187–94.

Kalinski, P., Hilkens, G.M.U., Wierenga, E.A. *et al.* (1995) Functional maturation of human naive T helper cells in the absence of accessory cells. Generation of IL-4-producing T helper cells does not require exogenous IL-4. *J. Immunol.*, **154**, 3753–60.

Kay, A.B., Ying, S., Varney, V. *et al.* (1991) Messenger RNA expression of the cytokine gene cluster, interleukin 3 (IL-3), IL-4, IL-5, and granulocyte/macrophage colony-stimulating factor, in allergen-induced late-phase cutaneous reactions in atopic subjects. *J. Exp. Med.*, **173**, 775–8.

Kemeny, D.M. & Diaz-Sanchez, D. (1993) The role of CD8+ T cells in the regulation of IgE. *Clin. Exp. Allergy*, **23**, 466–70.

Kimata, H., Lindley, I. & Furusho, K. (1995) Selective inhibition of spontaneous IgE and IgG4 production by interleukin-8 in atopic patients. *Blood*, **85**, 3191–8.

Kimata, H., Yoshida, A., Ishioka, C., Lindley, I. & Mikawa, H. (1992) Interleukin 8 (IL-8) selectively inhibits immunoglobulin E production induced by IL-4 in human B cells. *J. Exp. Med.*, **176**, 1227–31.

Kiniwa, M., Gately, M., Gubler, U., Chizzonite, R., Fargeas, C. & Delespesse, G. (1992) Recombinant interleukin-12 suppresses the synthesis of immunoglobulin E by interleukin-4 stimulated human lymphocytes. *J. Clin. Invest.*, **90**, 262–6.

Kopf, M., Le Gros, G., Bachmann, M., Lamers, M.C., Bluthmann, H. & Kohler, G. (1993) Disruption of the murine IL-4 gene blocks Th2 cytokine responses. *Nature*, **362**, 245–8.

Kuhn, R., Rajewski, K. & Muller, W. (1991) Generation and analysis of IL-4-deficient mice. *Science*, **254**, 707–10.

Lack, G., Renz, H., Saloga, J. *et al.* (1993) Nebulized but not parenteral IFN-γ decreases IgE production and normalizes airways function in a murine model of allergen sensitization. *J. Immunol.*, **152**, 2546–54.

Loh, R.K.S., Jabara, H.H. & Geha, R.S. (1994) Disodium cromoglycate inhibits S S deletional switch recombination and IgE synthesis in human B cells. *J. Exp. Med.*, **180**, 663–71.

Luo, H., Hofstetter, H., Banchereau, J. & Delespesse, G. (1991) Cross-linking of CD23 antigen by its natural ligand (IgE) or by anti-CD23 antibody prevents B lymphocyte proliferation and differentiation. *J. Immunol.*, **146**, 2122–9.

Macchia, D., Almerigogna, F., Parronchi, P., Ravina, A., Maggi, E. & Romagnani, S. (1993) Membrane tumor necrosis factor-α is involved in the polyclonal B-cell activation induced by HIV-infected human T cells. *Nature*, **363**, 464–6.

McHugh, S.M., Deighton, J., Stewart, A.G., Lachmann, P.J. & Ewan, P.W. (1995) Bee venom immunotherapy induces a shift in cytokine responses from a Th2 to a Th1 dominant pattern: comparison of rush and conventional immunotherapy. *Clin. Exp. Allergy*, **25**, 828–38.

McMenamin, C. & Holt, P.G. (1993) The natural immune response to inhaled soluble protein antigens involved Major Histocompatibility Complex (MHC) Class I-restricted CD8+ T cell-dependent immune deviation resulting in selective suppression of immunoglobulin E production. *J. Exp. Med.*, **178**, 889–99.

Maggi, E., Del Prete, G.F., Parronchi, P. *et al.* (1989) Role for T cells, IL-2 and IL-6 in the IL-4-dependent *in vitro* human IgE synthesis. *Immunology*, **68**, 300–6.

Maggi, E., Biswas, P., Del Prete, G.F. *et al.* (1991) Accumulation of Th2-like helper T cells in the conjunctiva of patients with vernal conjunctivitis. *J. Immunol.*, **146**, 1169–74.

Maggi, E., Parrochi, P., Manetti, R. *et al.* (1992) Reciprocal regulatory role of IFN- and IL-4 on the *in vitro* development of human Th1 and Th2 clones. *J. Immunol.*, **148**, 2142–8.

Manetti, R., Annunziato, F., Biagiotti, R. *et al.* (1984) CD30 expression by CD8+ T cells producing type 2 helper cytokines. Evidence for large numbers of CD8+CD30+ T cell clones in human immunodeficiency virus infection. *J. Exp. Med.*, **180**, 2407–12.

Manetti, R., Parrochi, P., Giudizi, M.-G. *et al.* (1993) Natural killer cell stimulatory factor (interleukin 12) induces T helper type 1 (Th1)-specific immune responses and inhibits the development of IL-4-producing Th cells. *J. Exp. Med.*, **177**, 1199–204.

Marsh, D.G., Neely, J.D., Breazeale, D.R. *et al.* (1994) Linkage analysis of IL-4 and other chromosome 5q31.1 markers and total serum immunoglobulin E concentration. *Science*, **264**, 1152–6.

Matsuoka, M., Yoshida, K., Maeda, T., Usuda, S. & Sakano, H. (1990) Switch circular DNA formed in cytokine-treated mouse splenocytes: evidence for intramolecular DNA deletion in immunglobulin class switching. *Cell*, **148**, 3830–6.

Mosmann, T.R., Cherwinski, H., Bond, M.W., Giedlin, M.A. & Coffman, R.L. (1986) Two types of murine helper T-cell clone. I. Definition according to profiles of lymphokine activities and secreted proteins. *J. Immunol.*, **136**, 2348–56.

Murphy, K.M., Murphy, T.L., Gold, J.S. & Szabo, S.J. (1993) Current understanding of IL-4 gene regulation in T cells. *Res. Immun.*, **144**, 575–8.

Nabors, G.S., Afonso, L.C.C., Farrell, J.P., Scott, P. (1995) Switch from a type 2 to a type 1 T helper cell response and cure of established *Leishmania major* infection in mice is induced by combined therapy with interleukin 12 and pentostam. *Proc. Nat. Acad. Sci. USA*, **91**, 3142–6.

Parronchi, P., Tiri, A., Macchia, D. *et al.* (1990) Noncognate contact-dependent B cell activation can promote IL-4-dependent *in vitro* human IgE synthesis. *J. Immunol.*, **44**, 2102–8.

Parronchi, P., Macchia, D., Piccinni, M.-P. *et al.* (1991) Allergen- and bacterial antigen-specific T-cell clones established from atopic donors show a different profile of cytokine production. *Proc. Nat. Acad. Sci. USA*, **88**, 4538–42.

Pene, J., Rousset, F., Briere F. *et al.* (1988a) IgE production by normal human B cells is induced by interleukin 4 and suppressed by interferon γ and α and prostaglandin E2. *Proc. Nat. Acad. Sci. USA*, **85**, 6880–4.

Pene, J., Rousset, F., Briere, F. *et al.* (1988b) Interleukin 5 enhances interleukin-4-induced IgE production by normal human B cells. The role of soluble CD23 antigen. *Eur. J. Immunol.*, **18**, 929–35.

Pfeiffer, C., Stein, J., Southwood, S., Ketelaar, H., Sette, A. & Bottomly, K. (1995) Altered peptide ligands can control CD4 T lymphocyte differentiation *in vivo*. *J. Exp. Med.*, **181**, 1569–74.

Punnonen, J., Aversa, G., Cocks, B.G. *et al.* (1993a) Interleukin 13 induces interleukin 4-independent IgG4 and IgE synthesis and CD23 expression by human B cells. *Proc. Nat. Acad. Sci. USA*, **90**, 3730–4.

Punnonen, J., Aversa, G., Cocks, B.G. & de Vries, J.E. (1994) Role of interleukin-4 and interleukin-13 in synthesis of IgE and expression of CD23 by human B cells. *Allergy*, **49**, 576–86.

Punnonen, J., de Waat Malefyt, R., van Vlasselaer, P., Gauchat, J-F. & de Vries, J.E. (1993b) IL-10 and viral IL-10 prevent IL-4-induced IgE synthesis by inhibiting the accessory cell function of monocytes. *J. Immunol.*, **151**, 1280–9.

Reiner, S.L., Wang, Z.-E., Hatam, F., Scott, P. & Locksley, R.M. (1993) Th1 and Th2 cell antigen receptors in experimental leishmaniasis. *Science*, **259**, 1457–60.

Renz, H., Saloga, J., Bradley, K.L. *et al.* (1993) Specific Vβ T cell subsets mediate the immediate hypersensitivity response to ragweed allergen. *J. Immunol.*, **151**, 1907–17.

Robinson, D.S., Hamid, Q., Ying, S. *et al.* (1992) Predominant Th2-like bronchoalveolar T-lymphocyte population in atopic asthma. *New Engl. J. Med.*, **326**, 295–304.

Romagnani, S. (1990) Regulation and deregulation of human IgE synthesis. *Immunol. Today*, **11**, 316–21.

Romagnani, S. (1991) Human Th1 and Th2: doubt no more. *Immunol. Today*, **12**, 256–8.

Romagnani, S. (1992) Induction of Th1 and Th2 responses: a key role for the 'natural' immune response? *Immunol. Today*, **13**, 379–80.

Romagnani, S. (1994a) Lymphokine production by human T cells in disease states. *Annu. Rev. Immunol.*, **12**, 227–57.

Romagnani, S. (1994b) Regulation of Th2 development in allergy. *Curr. Opin. Immunol.*, **6**, 838–46.

Romagnani, S., Maggi, E. & Del Prete, G.-F. (1994) An alternative view of the Th1/Th2 switch hypothesis in HIV infection. *AIDS Res. Hum. Retrovir.*, **10**, 3–9.

Rook, G.A.W., Hernandez-Pando, R. & Lightman, S.L. (1994) Hormones, peripherally activated prohormones and regulation of the Th1-Th2 balance. *Immunol. Today*, **15**, 301–3.

Rothman, P., Li, S.C., Gorham, B., Glimcher, L., Alt, F. & Boothby, M. (1991) Identification of a conserved lipopolysaccharide-plus-intereukin-4 responsive element located at the promoter of germ line ε transcripts. *Mol. Cell. Biol.*, **11**, 5551–61.

Rousset, F., Garcia, E., DeFrance, T. *et al.* (1992) Interleukin-10 is a potent growth and differentiation factor for activated human B lymphocytes. *Proc. Nat. Acad. Sci. USA*, **89**, 1890–4.

Sarfati, M. & Delespesse, G. (1988) Possible role of human lymphocyte receptor for IgE (CD23) or its soluble fragments in the *in vitro* synthesis of human IgE. *J. Immunol.*, **141**, 2195–9.

Sarfati, M., Luo, H. & Delespesse, G. (1989) IgE synthesis by chronic lymphocytic leukemia cells. *J. Exp. Med.*, **170**, 1775–80.

Schatz, D.G., Oettinger, M.A. & Baltimore, D. (1989) The V(D)J recombination activating gene, RAG-1. *Cell*, **59**, 1035–48.

Scherr, E., Macy, E., Kimata, H., Gilly, M. & Saxon, A. (1989) Binding the low affinity FcR on B cells suppresses ongoing human IgE synthesis. *J. Immunol.*, **142**, 481–9.

Schmitz, J., Thiel, A., Khun, R. *et al.* (1994) Induction of interleukin-4 (IL-4) expression in T helper (Th) cells is not dependent on IL-4 from non-T cells. *J. Exp. Med.*, **179**, 1349–53.

Schon-Hegrad, M.A., Oliver, J., McMenamin, P.G. & Holt, P.G. (1991) Studies on the density, distribution and surface phenotype of intraepithelial Class II MHC (Ia) antigen-bearing dendritic cells in the conductive airways. *J. Exp. Med.*, **173**, 1345–56.

Secrist, H., Chelen, C.J., Wen, Y., Marshall, J.D. & Umetsu, D.T. (1993) Allergen immunotherapy decreases interleukin 4 production in CD4+ T cells from allergic individuals. *J. Exp. Med.*, **178**, 2123–30.

Shanebeck, K.D., Maliszewski, C.R., Kennedy, M.K. *et al.* (1995) Regulation of murine B cell growth and differentiation by CD30 ligand. *Eur. J. Immunol.*, **25**, 2147–53.

Siraganian, R.P. (1993) Mechanism of IgE-mediated hypersensitivity. In: *Allergy. Principles and Practice.* (ed E. Middleton), pp. 105–34. Mosby, St Louis.

Smith, C.A., Davis, T., Anderson, D. *et al.* (1990) A receptor for tumor necrosis factor defines an unusual family of cellular and viral proteins. *Science*, **248**, 1019–23.

Smith, C.A., Gruss, H.-J., Davis, T. *et al.* (1993) CD30 antigen, a marker for Hodgkin's lymphoma, is a receptor whose ligand defines an emerging family of cytokines with homology to TNF. *Cell*, **273**, 1349–60.

Snapper, C.M. & Finkelman, F.D. (1993) Immunoglobulin class switching. In: *Fundamental Immunology* (ed. W. Paul), pp. 837–63. Raven, New York.

Spriggs, M.K., Armitage, R.J., Strockbine, L. *et al.* (1992) Recombinant human CD40 ligand stimulates B cell proliferation and immunoglobulin E secretion. *J. Exp. Med.*, **176**, 1543–50.

Stavnezer-Norgren, J. & Sirlins, S. (1986) Specificity of immunoglobulin heavy chain switch correlates with activity of germline heavy chain genes prior to switching. *EMBO J.*, **5**, 95–102.

Sur, S., Adolphson, C.R. & Gleich, G.J. (1993) Eosinophils. Biochemical and cellular aspects. In: *Allergy. Principles and Practice* (ed E. Middleton), pp. 169–200. Mosby, St Louis.

Swain, S.L. (1993) IL-4 dictates T-cell differentiation. *Res. Immunol.*, **144**, 616–20.

Texido, G., Eibel, H., Le Gros, G. & van der Putten, H. (1994) Transgene CD23 expression on lymphoid cells modulates IgE and IgG1 responses. *J. Immunol.*, **153**, 3028–42.

Thyphronitis, G., Tsokos, G.C., June, C.H., Levine, A.D. & Finkelman, F.D. (1989) IgE secretion by Epstein–Barr virus-infected purified human B lymphocytes is stimulated by interleukin 4 and suppressed by interferon γ. *Proc. Nat. Acad. Sci. USA*, **86**, 5580–4.

Uchibayashi, N., Kikutani, H., Barsumian, E. *et al.* (1989) Recombinat soluble Fcε receptor II (FcεRII/CD23) has IgE binding activity but no B cell growth promoting activity. *J. Immunol.*, **142**, 3901–8.

van Kooten, C., van der Pouw Kraan, T., Rensink, I., van Oers, R. & Arden, L. (1992) Both naive and memory T cells can provide help for human IgE production, but with different cytokine requirements. *Eur. Cytokine Netw.*, **3**, 289–97.

van Reijsen, F.C., Bruijnzeel-Koomen, C.A.F.M., Kalthoff, F.S. *et al.* (1992) Skin-derived aeroallergen-specific T-cell clones of Th2 phenotype in patients with atopic dermatitis. *J. Allergy Clin. Immunol.*, **90**, 184–92.

Varney, V.A., Hamid, Q., Gaga, M. *et al.* (1993) Influence of grass pollen immunotherapy on cellular infiltration and cytokine mRNA expression during allergen-induced late-phase cutaneous responses. *J. Clin. Invest.*, **92**, 644–51.

Vercelli, D. & Geha, R.S. (1991) Regulation of IgE synthesis in humans: a tale of two signals. *J. Allergy Clin. Immunol.*, **8**, 285–95.

Vercelli, D. & Geha, R.S. (1993) Control of IgE synthesis. In: *Allergy. Principles and Practice* (eds E. Middleton *et al.*), pp. 93–104. Mosby, St Louis.

Vercelli, D. & Geha, R.S. (1995) Regulation of immunoglobulin E synthesis. In: *Asthma and Rhinitis* (eds W.W. Busse & S.T. Holgate), pp. 437–49. Blackwell Science, Boston.

Vercelli, D., Jabara, H.H., Arai, K., Yokota, T. & Geha, R.S. (1989a) Endogenous IL-6 plays an obligatory role in IL-4-induced human IgE synthesis. *Eur. J. Immunol.*, **19**, 1419–24.

Vercelli, D., Jabara, H.H., Arai, K. & Geha, R.S. (1989b) Induction of human IgE synthesis requires interleukin-4 and T/B cell interactions involving the T cell receptor/CD3 complex and MHC class II antigens. *J. Exp. Med.*, **169**, 1295–307.

Walker, C., Bode, E., Boer, L., Hansel, T.T., Blaser, K. & Virchow, J.-C. (1992) Allergic and nonallergic asthmatics have distinct patterns of T-cell activation and cytokine production in peripheral blood and bronchoalveolar lavage. *Am. Rev. Resp. Dis.*, **146**, 109–15.

Wegmann, T.G., Lin, H., Guilbert, L. & Mosmann, T.R. (1993) Bidirectional cytokine interactions in the maternal–fetal relationship: is successful pregnancy a Th2 phenomenon? *Immunol. Today*, **14**, 353–6.

Wershil, B.K., Theodos, C.M., Galli, S.J. & Titus, R.G. (1994) Mast cells augment lesion size and persistence during experimental *Leishmania major* infection in the mouse. *J. Immunol.*, **152**, 4563–71.

Wierenga, E.A., Snoek, M., de Groot, C. *et al.* (1990) Evidence for compartmentalization of functional subsets of CD4+ T lymphocytes in atopic patients. *J. Immunol.*, **144**, 4651–6.

Yancopoulos, G.D., DePinho, R.A., Zimmerman, K.A., Lutzker, S.G., Rosenberg, N. & Alt, F.W. (1986) Secondary genomic rearrangement events in pre-B cells: VHDJH replacement by a LINE-1 sequence and directed class switching. *EMBO J.*, **5**, 3259–66.

Yashimoto, T. & Paul, W.E. (1994) CD4^{pos}, NK1.1^{pos} T cells promptly produce interleukin 4 in response to *in vivo* challenge with anti-CD3. *J. Exp. Med.*, **179**, 1285–95.

Yokota, A., Kikutani, H., Tanaka, T. *et al.* (1988) Two species of human Fc epsilon receptor II (Fc epsilon RII/CD23): tissue-specific and IL-4-specific regulation of gene expression. *Cell*, **55**, 611–8.

Yu, P., Kosco-Vilbois, M., Richards, M., Kholer, G. & Lamers, M.C. (1994) Negative feedback regulation of IgE synthesis by murine CD23. *Nature*, **369**, 753–6.

Zurawski, G. & de Vries, J.E. (1994) Interleukin 13, an interleukin 4-like cytokine that acts on monocytes and B cells, but not on T cells. *Immunol. Today*, **15**, 19–26.

CHAPTER 7

Antigen Processing and Presentation

J.M. Austyn

Introduction

Antigen processing and presentation are central events for most adaptive (lymphocyte-mediated) immune responses, and T-cell responses in particular. T cells survey cell surfaces for the presence of foreign antigens in the form of peptide–MHC (major histocompatibility complex) complexes (Owen & Lamb, 1988). The terms antigen processing and presentation refer respectively to the collective mechanisms by which antigens are modified to 'processed' forms that can bind to MHC molecules, and to the subsequent display of these complexes at cell surfaces for recognition by T-cell receptors (TcR). Cells expressing peptide–MHC complexes that can be recognized by T cells are termed antigen-presenting cells (APC) (Austyn, 1989). Whereas T cells survey cell membranes for processed antigens presented by APC, B cells monitor the fluid phase for soluble or particulate antigens, frequently in their native conformations, recognition being mediated by membrane-bound antibodies (immunoglobulins, Ig; membrane Ig, mIg) (Klaus, 1990). Before T cells and B cells can function in immune responses, they need to recognize the respective forms of antigen (via TcR or mIg, respectively) and become activated from small lymphocytes in their resting state to large lymphoblasts with the capacity to synthesize a variety of different molecules that ultimately contribute to the removal of antigen. It is therefore appropriate to distinguish between the *afferent* or initiation phase of adaptive immune responses, during which antigen-specific lymphocytes are activated or sensitized, and the *efferent* or effector phase, when sensitized lymphoblasts elicit a number of different mechanisms that bring about or effect the removal of antigen. Antigen processing and presentation are central to both afferent and efferent phases of most T-cell and B-cell responses.

Different subsets of T cells (and B cells (Klaus, 1990)) have been identified. In the case of T lymphocytes, it is usual to distinguish between T cells with cytotoxic, helper and suppressive functions. Cytotoxic T lymphocytes (Tc) are responsible for killing the APC they recognize, often termed target cells, through the secretion of a variety of toxic molecules termed *cytolysins* (Berke, 1994). In contrast, when helper T cells (Th) recognize APC they secrete a variety of molecules termed *cytokines* (Romagnani, 1994; Seder & Paul, 1994) that act on the APC being recognized, and other cells, to modify their biological and immunological functions.

Depending on the precise spectrum of cytokines secreted by helper cells, it is possible to define Th1 and Th2 cells as polarized extremes, with Th0 cells having an intermediate pattern of cytokine secretion. However, subsets of cytotoxic cells that secrete distinct patterns of cytokines have also been identified, so the distinction between Th and Tc is not absolute. Moreover, while cytokines can exert positive or stimulatory effects on immune responses, many have negative or inhibitory functions. In the latter case, T cells secreting these cytokines could be considered to be suppressor T cells (Ts), so the distinction between Th and Ts also becomes blurred. Thus, the concept of distinct functional subsets of T cells (Tc, Th, Ts) may be an oversimplification, but it serves as a useful generalization. This applies perhaps particularly to T cells bearing αβ TcR, on which this article focuses; T cells expressing structurally related, but distinct, γδ TcR will be considered only in passing.

Under normal circumstances, the immune system

mounts an appropriate response to a foreign antigen and ultimately leads to its elimination. However, in some circumstances, inappropriate or exaggerated responses to a foreign antigen are induced, and these can result in tissue damage and immunopathology. Such responses are termed hypersensitivity reactions, of which four, or perhaps five, broad groups have been categorized. Modifications to this classification are suggested in Chapter 2. Of these, the type I or immediate hypersensitivity reactions mediated by IgE are known as atopic allergic responses (Ishizaka & Ishizaka, 1989; de Vries, 1994). Examples include atopic dermatitis, asthma and rhinitis, depending on whether the pathological responses are manifested within the skin, or the airways of the lung or nose, respectively. (Originally, the terms allergy and atopy meant 'altered reactivity' and 'out of place'.) The antigens that elicit such responses are termed allergens. One of the earliest of the many immunological events that occur, from the time of an individual's first encounter with an allergen to the development of atopic allergy, is processing of the allergen and its presentation to T cells. This chapter reviews antigen processing and presentation at the molecular level and the cellular level, in the context of immune responses in general. These are put briefly into the context of atopic allergic responses in the section on allergy. Throughout, the emphasis will be on the initiation, or afferent phase, of these responses.

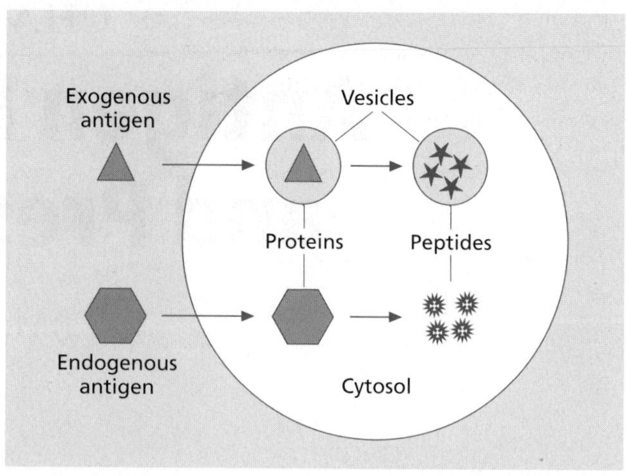

Fig. 7.1 Exogenous and endogenous antigens. Exogenous antigens are soluble molecules or particulates that are internalized by cells and degraded to peptides within endosomal/lysosomal compartments. Endogenous antigens gain direct access to the cytoplasm, and are degraded to peptides within the cytosol. The term antigen processing refers to the cellular mechanisms involved in degradation of protein-containing antigens prior to antigen presentation to T cells.

Molecular aspects of antigen processing and presentation, and T-cell-mediated immune responses

Exogenous and endogenous antigens

A foreign, or non-self, antigen can be defined as anything not normally produced within an individual that can be recognized by antigen-specific receptors of lymphocytes (i.e. TcR or mIg). Antigens that can be recognized by T cells can be classified into two types: *exogenous* and *endogenous* antigens (Fig. 7.1). Exogenous antigens are taken up by cells from their extracellular environment and are retained in membrane-bound compartments within the cell; in this sense they can be viewed as being in a topologically external milieu. Examples of exogenous foreign antigens are soluble molecules, such as bacterial toxins, that are internalized by cells through the process of pinocytosis, and particulates, such as bacteria and yeasts, that are internalized by phagocytosis. Most if not all allergens are exogenous antigens. In contrast, endogenous antigens gain direct access to the cytoplasm. Typical endogenous foreign antigens are viruses that have infected cells.

Most cells are capable of pinocytosis, the process by which soluble molecules are taken up in the bulk fluid phase or after binding to cellular receptors. In many cases, pinocytosed molecules are utilized for normal cellular processes; for example, in the case of iron that is complexed to transferrin and taken up via transferrin receptors. Phagocytosis, on the other hand, is a property of more specialized cell types such as macrophages which play an important scavenging role in taking up dead and dying cells and micro-organisms, thus clearing them from the body. In other cases, endocytosis, a term often used to cover both pinocytosis and phagocytosis, is a first step in the initiation of immune responses. In these situations internalized protein-containing antigens, and antigens within the cytosol, are degraded intracellularly to peptides, by mechanisms collectively termed antigen processing, prior to their binding to MHC molecules and the subsequent presentation of cell-surface foreign peptide–MHC complexes to T cells. MHC molecules can thus be considered as receptors for peptides, that allow the immune system to recognize intracellular contents at the cell surface.

MHC molecules

The MHC of mice is termed H-2, while that of humans is designated HLA (human leucocyte antigen) (Fig. 7.2); a nomenclature related to the latter is used for the MHC of other species (Guillemot *et al.*, 1988). MHC genes encode a number of molecules; some comprise, or contribute to, the formation of two different though structurally and functionally related heterodimers, termed class I and class II MHC molecules (Fig. 7.3). Class I molecules are composed of an MHC-encoded α-chain associated with β_2-microglobulin, which is encoded elsewhere in the genome. Both the α- and β-chains of class II molecules are encoded within the MHC, and these molecules can associate with a third chain, the invariant chain, which is encoded elsewhere. Some class I molecules are expressed or inducible on essentially all cell types, whereas class II molecules can only be expressed by a more limited number of cell types.

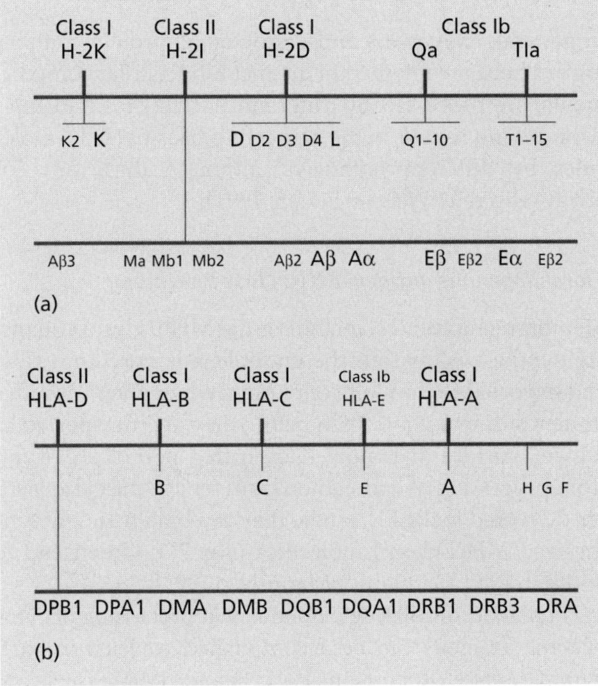

Fig. 7.2 Highly simplified genetic maps of the MHC in mice (H-2) and humans (HLA). The principal MHC class I and class II loci that encode classical MHC molecules involved in conventional antigen presentation to T cells are indicated.

Of the 30–40 class I and class I-related loci that have been identified within the mouse MHC, only two or three encode the α-chains of so-called 'classical' class I molecules that are generally involved in conventional antigen presentation to T cells. In the mouse, these are designated H-2K and H-2D (and H-2L if present); the equivalent loci in humans are designated HLA-A, HLA-B and HLA-C (Guillemot *et al.*, 1988). The majority of class I loci of the mouse encode non-classical class I molecules, which include the Qa and Tla molecules (Shawat *et al.*, 1994). These loci are considerably less polymorphic than the classical class I genes, and their products are expressed at detectable levels only by a limited number of cell types, may be anchored to the cell surface by phosphatidylinositol linkages rather than via transmembrane portions, and their function is not clearly established. Homologues of mouse Qa and Tla loci have not yet been detected in the human, although several non-classical class I loci have been identified.

The class II region of the mouse MHC is designated H-2I, and contains loci encoding the α- and β-chains of IA and IE molecules which are involved in conventional antigen presentation to T cells; the corresponding loci in humans encode the heterodimeric HLA-DP, DQ and DR molecules (Guillemot *et al.*, 1988). In both species the class II regions also contain loci encoding class II-related molecules that have been implicated in processing and/or

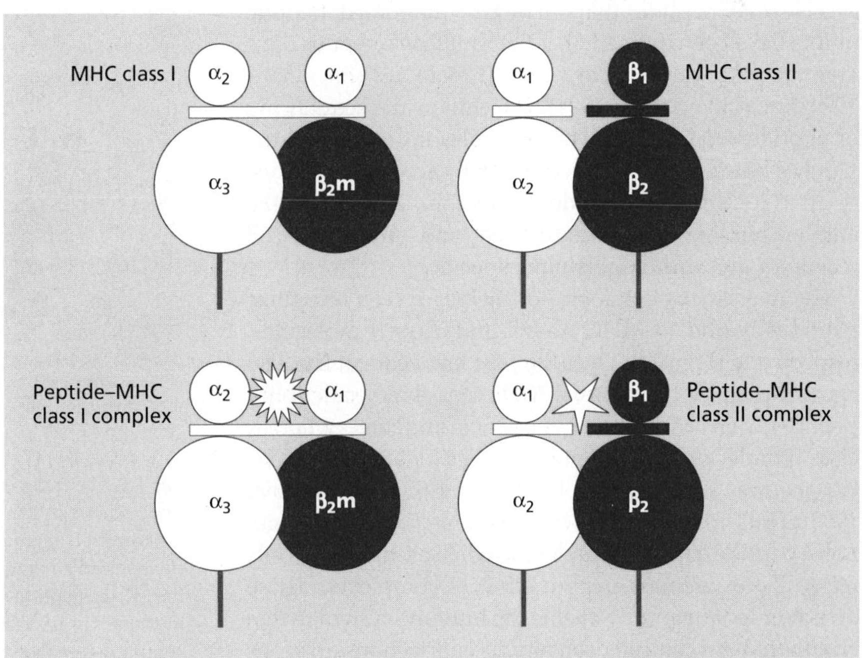

Fig. 7.3 MHC class I and class II molecules. MHC class I α-chains contain three Ig-like domains, and are associated with β_2-microglobulin to form heterodimers; MHC class II molecules are heterodimers of α1 and β-chains, each containing two Ig-like domains (top). Both MHC class I and class II molecules contain peptide-binding grooves that can accomodate peptides derived from antigen processing (bottom).

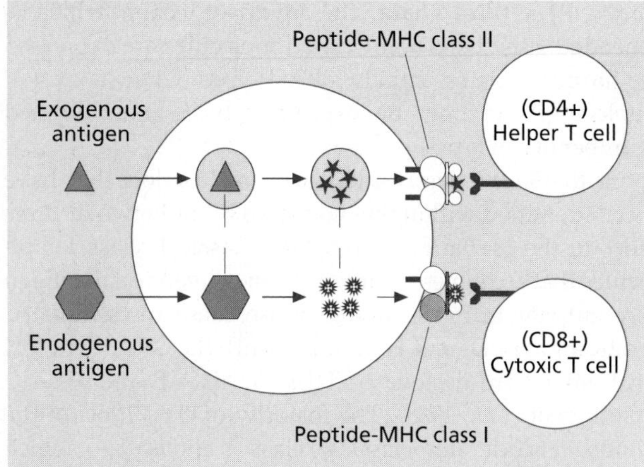

Fig. 7.4 Antigen-processing and presentation pathways. Peptides derived from exogenous antigens tend to associate with MHC class II molecules, for recognition primarily by helper T cells. Peptides derived from endogenous antigen tend to associate with MHC class I molecules, for recognition primarily by cytotoxic T cells. Cells expressing peptide–MHC complexes that can be recognized by (i.e. presented to) T cells are termed antigen-presenting cells.

presentation of exogenous antigens (see below), and loci encoding class II molecules with a limited tissue or cell distribution and unclear function (Karisson *et al.*, 1991).

Peptides from foreign antigens bind within the so-called peptide-binding groove of MHC molecules which, for several class I and class II alleles, have been visualized by X-ray crystallography (Fig. 7.3) (Bjorkman *et al.*, 1987; Stern *et al.*, 1994). Many polymorphic residues (amino acids) are located within the peptide-binding groove, determining its topography and thereby controlling the precise set of peptides that can be accommodated. Peptide motifs have been defined, that determine whether or not a given peptide can bind to an MHC molecule (Engelhard 1994; Rotzschke & Falk, 1994). The elution and sequencing of peptides bound to class I molecules indicates that the peptide-binding groove can potentially accommodate one of up to 10^7 different peptides at any time. In contrast, the antigen binding sites of antibodies, and probably T-cell receptors, are considerably more specific.

The majority of cytotoxic and helper T cells recognize peptides bound to MHC class I and class II molecules, respectively (Fig. 7.4). Over the past few years, it has also become clear that, in general, MHC class I molecules bind peptides derived from endogenous antigens, whereas class II molecules bind peptides from exogenous antigens (see below; Townsend & Bodmer, 1989; Lanzavecchia, 1990). Thus, many cytotoxic T cells can recognize endogenous peptide–class I complexes, whereas helper T cells recognize exogenous peptide–class II complexes. These dichotomies apparently enable the immune system to discriminate between cells containing endogenous antigens (e.g. viruses within the cytoplasm) that need to be killed, and cells that have internalized antigens whose effector functions can be induced or potentiated after recognition by helper T cells.

Antigen processing and peptide–MHC association

In general, exogenous and endogenous protein-containing antigens are retained in distinct intracellular compartments, are processed by different mechanisms and their peptides are routed to the respective class of MHC molecules by different pathways, although these are not always discrete (Weiss & Bogen, 1991).

The endogenous antigen–MHC class I pathway

Membrane molecules, including the MHC glycoproteins, are synthesized within the endoplasmic reticulum (ER) and exported to the Golgi apparatus where their carbohydrate residues are modified before they are transported to the cell surface. It is now known that peptides derived from processing of endogenous antigens in the cytoplasm are delivered to the ER, where they can bind to newly synthesized MHC class I molecules (Fig. 7.5) (Townsend & Bodmer, 1989; Germain & Margulies, 1993).

There is accumulating evidence that processing of cytoplasmic antigens can be accomplished, at least in part, by *proteasomes* (Robertson, 1991; Peters, 1994). These are highly conserved, large, multisubunit, macromolecular structures within the cytoplasm and nucleus of eukaryotic cells (and related structures are even present in archaebac-

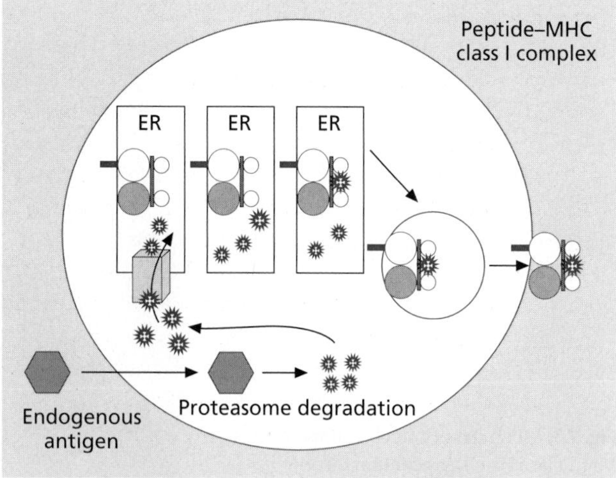

Fig. 7.5 The endogenous antigen–MHC class I pathway. Endogenous antigens are processed within the cytosol, at least in part through degradation by proteasomes. Peptides are then transported into the lumen of the ER by peptide transporters. Within the ER, the peptides bind to newly synthesized MHC class I molecules in association with β_2-microglobulin. Peptide–MHC complexes are then transported to the cell surface.

teria) that function as endopeptidases. They are readily visualized by electron microscopy and are essentially cylindrical, consisting of a stack of four rings, each of which appears to contain about six to eight subunits. Proteasomes catalyse the non-lysosomal, adenosine triphosphate (ATP)-dependent proteolysis of proteins that generally, but not always, first need to be ubiquitinated. As such they are associated with the *ubiquitin* system, a normal intracellular pathway by which aberrant or incorrectly folded proteins are modified by the addition of the protein ubiquitin and degraded by ubiquitin-dependent proteases (Hershko, 1988). Two proteasome subunits, LMP2 and LMP7, are encoded within the MHC class II region. Interferon-γ (IFN-γ) treatment increases expression of these and perhaps other subunits, but decreases expression of two or more different subunits (Tanaka, 1994). This appears to alter the proteolytic specificity of the proteasome, and may potentiate processing and presentation of endogenous foreign antigens. However, much remains to be learnt about the precise functions of these structures and their relative importance to the class I antigen-processing pathway compared with other mechanisms.

Once peptides have been generated within the cytoplasm, they are delivered into the lumen of the ER. Two genes have been identified within the MHC of mice, rats and humans that have a striking homology to the so-called ATP binding cassette (ABC) proteins which are expressed in micro-organisms and are known to be involved in peptide transport across cell membranes. The products of these genes, known as TAP1 and TAP2, appear to associate to form a functional *peptide transporter* protein in mammalian cells which is responsible for transport of peptides from the cytoplasm into the lumen of the ER (Howard, 1995). Here, peptide–MHC class Iα-chain–β_2-microglobulin complexes are formed. It was originally suggested that peptides can associate with MHC class Iα chains soon after or during their biosynthesis, and thereby induce a conformational change in the α-chain that permits the association of β_2-microglobulin and subsequent transport of the peptide–MHC class I complex to the cell surface (Townsend & Bodmer, 1989). Subsequently, however, evidence was presented that class Iα-chain–β_2-microglobulin dimerization occurs *before* peptide binding (Neefjes *et al.*, 1993). Further, it has been suggested that class Iα–β_2-microglobulin dimers first bind to TAP molecules to facilitate their association with TAP-transported peptides (Howard, 1995). (There is also evidence that a small proportion of class I molecules lacking bound peptides, so-called empty MHC molecules, can reach the cell surface, as can some class Iα-chains not associated with β_2-microglobulin (Ljunggren *et al.*, 1990).) Thus, the precise order of peptide binding to class I molecules within the ER has yet to be settled at the time of writing.

Peptides have been eluted from purified MHC class I molecules and found to be quite homogeneous in size, the majority of these 'naturally processed' peptides being nine amino acids in length (Engelhard, 1994). The reasons for this are not yet clear but they could, for example, relate to properties of the cytoplasmic proteases involved in processing or of the peptide transporter proteins, or could result from trimming of peptides to the appropriate size by proteases located within the ER. It is, however, quite clear that MHC class I molecules select peptides according to certain binding motifs (Rammensee, 1995), and that limited polymorphisms in the *TAP* genes can contribute to the spectrum of peptides that is transported into the ER (Momberg *et al.*, 1994a,b).

The exogenous antigen–MHC class II pathway

In contrast to the endogenous antigen–class I pathway outlined above, exogenous antigens are processed within membrane-bound vesicles, and peptides encounter MHC class II molecules only after their biosynthesis and export from the ER and Golgi apparatus (Fig. 7.6) (Lanzavecchia, 1990; Germain & Margulies, 1993).

After uptake by cells, endocytosed molecules and par-

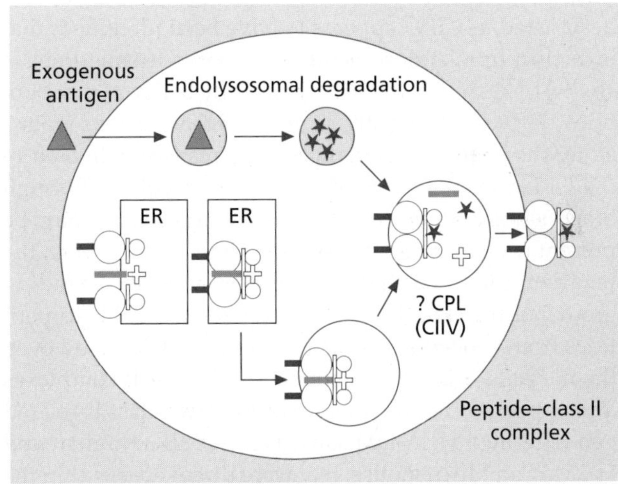

Fig. 7.6 The exogenous antigen–MHC class II pathway. Exogenous antigens are processed within endosomal/lysosomal compartments, at least in part through the action of acid proteases. They are then thought to be transported into specialized 'compartments for peptide loading'. MHC class II molecules and invariant chain molecules are synthesized within the ER and the complexes are thought to be also exported to the specialized 'compartments for peptide loading'. Here, or in earlier compartments, the invariant chain is degraded, and the final degradation product (CLIP peptide) is removed by a mechanism that seems to involve the DM molecule (not shown). Consequently, the peptide-binding groove is made available for peptide binding. Peptide–MHC complexes are then transported to the cell surface.

ticulates are contained within vesicles that are collectively termed early *endosomes*. These compartments are progressively acidified and their contents become susceptible to degradation by acid proteases, particularly in endolysosomes which are generated by fusion of late endosomes with other vesicles termed lysosomes containing these enzymes. Classical studies utilizing lysosomotropic agents which prevent acidification of endosomes, such as chloroquine, ammonium chloride and monensin, have demonstrated the importance of acidic proteases in class II-restricted antigen presentation by cells such as macrophages.

Peptides are prevented from binding to newly synthesized MHC class II molecules within the lumen of the ER, because these molecules are associated with a third chain, the *invariant chain* (Sant & Miller, 1994). Trimers containing an MHC class IIα-chain, a β-chain and an invariant chain are assembled within the ER, and these trimerize to form nine-subunit structures which are exported to and through the Golgi apparatus (Roche *et al.*, 1991). The presence of the invariant chain blocks the peptide-binding groove of class II heterodimers, so that peptides are prevented from binding to class II molecules within the ER, and this molecule contains sequences that route the class II molecules to the appropriate intracellular compartments.

A specialized *compartment for peptide loading* (CPL, also designated as CIIV) appears to have been identified, that is distinct from endosomes and lysosomes (Amigorena *et al.*, 1994; West *et al.*, 1994). It is currently believed that peptides derived from antigen processed at various points along the endo(lyso)somal pathway may be delivered to the CPL, along with MHC class II molecules (although other studies indicate that class II molecules may be present even in early endosomes). Here, or elsewhere, the invariant chain is degraded to render the peptide-binding groove of the class II αβ heterodimers accessible to peptides from exogenous antigens within the CPL. However, the normal assembly of peptide–MHC class II complexes also appears to require the products of two class II-related genes, termed HLA-DMA and HLA-DMB in human and H-2Ma and Mb in mouse, that were discovered within the MHC (Cho *et al.*, 1991; Kelly *et al.*, 1991; Fling *et al.*, 1994). These molecules are located intracellularly, perhaps being expressed primarily in endosomal compartments and/or the CPL, although their precise function is presently unclear. The peptides that can bind to class II molecules are generally longer and more heterogeneous than those bound to class I molecules (Rotzschke & Falk, 1994; Rammensee, 1995).

Self and non-self peptide complexes

Up to this point, only foreign or non-self antigens have been considered. However, most MHC molecules expressed at the surface of normal cells are probably occupied by peptides derived from self proteins. For example, many peptides eluted from the HLA-B27 class I molecule were derived from abundant cytosolic and nuclear proteins (Engelhard, 1994). Thus, it seems likely that a representative set of endogenous peptides from proteins normally synthesized within a cell can bind to MHC molecules, presumably via the class I pathway. Likewise, a representative set of exogenous peptides from internalized self proteins, such as normal serum components, may be directed into the class II pathway. Normally, of course, immune responses are not generated to these self peptide–MHC complexes. Self–non-self discrimination within the immune system occurs primarily at the level of T cells. These cells are usually unable to respond to self peptide–MHC complexes because they are rendered tolerant, through the process of negative selection. This involves at least two mechanisms, clonal deletion and clonal anergy or functional inactivation, which act on developing thymocytes within the thymus and/or mature T cells in the periphery (Fowlkes & Pardoll, 1989; Mueller *et al.*, 1989). The end result of negative selection is the development of a T-cell repertoire that responds only to foreign peptide–MHC complexes, except in cases of autoimmunity.

Molecules for T-cell antigen recognition and responses

T cells recognize peptide–MHC complexes via TcR (Owen & Lamb, 1988; Terhorst *et al.*, 1988). These heterodimers are of two types, composed of αβ- or γδ-chains. In the mouse, αβ TcR+ T cells predominate in secondary lymphoid tissues of the adult, whereas γδ TcR+ T cells are localized to skin epithelium and other topologically external tissues such as the gut and airways (Haas *et al.*, 1993). In the human, the distribution of these two types of T cell is more equal, but αβ TcR+ T cells are quantitatively more frequent. Conventional MHC-restricted antigen recognition is a function of αβ TcR+ T cells. The function of γδ TcR+ T cells is less clear, although some of these cells may have cytotoxic activity. They may recognize peptides associated with the non-classical class I MHC molecules, Qa and Tla, or with the class I-related family of molecules, CD1, the peptides in some cases perhaps being derived from heat-shock proteins (Haas *et al.*, 1993). γδ TcR+ T cells are not considered further in this chapter.

TcR are associated with a group of molecules, the CD3 complex, which is involved in signal transduction after T-cell antigen recognition (Chan *et al.*, 1994). These signals initiate a variety of intracellular biochemical events that may lead ultimately to new gene transcription and T-cell activation. One chain of the CD3 complex is also associated with other signal-transducing receptors, particularly membrane-bound antibodies of B cells and some Fc receptors (Irving & Weiss, 1991). However, the signals required for T-cell activation are many and varied, and other molecules are involved in T-cell responses. Two such molecules are CD4 and CD8 (Bierer *et al.*, 1989).

In general, T cells that recognize peptide–MHC class I complexes express CD8, whereas class II-restricted T cells express CD4, irrespective of the function of the T cells (Fig. 7.4). The majority of Tc and Th cells express CD8 or CD4, respectively, but there are also smaller subsets of CD4+ Tc cells (Ottenhoff & Mutis, 1990) and CD8+ Th cells. CD4 and CD8 bind the respective class of MHC molecule, can increase the overall avidity of a T cell for its antigen (e.g. if the TcR has a low affinity for a particular peptide–MHC complex), and deliver intracellular signals that can result in the activation of adhesion mechanisms, such as those mediated by CD11b/CD18 (LFA-1) (see below). Both CD4 and CD8 are associated with a cytoplasmic tyrosine kinase, $p56^{lck}$, which is responsible for phosphorylation of the cytoplasmic portions of certain membrane molecules, an important biochemical event in T-cell responses; TcR are associated with the tyrosine kinase $p59^{fyn}$ (Bierer *et al.*, 1989; Collins *et al.*, 1994). Phosphorylation by kinases can be regulated in turn by molecules such as CD45, the leucocyte common antigen (LCA), which has intrinsic protein tyrosine phosphatase activity and can therefore dephosphorylate intracellular components (Trowbridge & Thomas, 1994). This molecule is expressed by all leucocytes but different isoforms are produced by differential gene transcription and are variably expressed by different leucocytes, and by T cells in different stages of development or activation.

Although the TcR–CD3 complex is required for peptide–MHC recognition and subsequent T-cell responses, there are additional or alternative pathways for T-cell activation. For example, CD2, the ligand for which is CD58 (LFA-3), provides an alternative pathway for T-cell activation which is linked to the intracellular signalling cascade mediated via the TcR–CD3 complex (Bierer *et al.*, 1989; Makgoba *et al.*, 1989). A separate cascade is activated by ligation of CD28, and perhaps CTLA-4, which are expressed by many Tc and Th cells (Linsley *et al.*, 1991; Linsley & Ledbelter, 1993; Allison, 1994). The ligands for these molecules are members of the B7 family designated B7-1 (CD80), B7-2 (CD86), and possibly B7-3 that can be expressed by dendritic cells, activated B cells, and some other cell types (Larsen *et al.*, 1994). Signal transduction via CD28 regulates cytokine production by T cells at both transcriptional (DNA) and post-transcriptional (RNA) levels.

Other membrane molecules of T cells are required for their adhesion to endothelial cells and subsequent entry to tissues from the blood (T-cell trafficking), and for interactions with the extracellular matrix and with APC within tissues (Dustin & Springer, 1991). For entry of a T cell (and other types of leucocyte) from the blood to the tissues, at least three sets of adhesive interactions are required. Firstly, the T cell rolls along the endothelium, its attachment being mediated by transient interactions between *selectins* (Dustin & Springer, 1991; McEver, 1994) and their carbohydrate ligands. For example, L-selectin is expressed by T cells. It is an example of a 'homing receptor' that facilitates the attachment of T cells to high endothelial venules in lymph nodes and at certain inflammatory sites and their recirculation through blood and lymph; the complementary ligands expressed by endothelial cells have been termed 'vascular addressins'. Secondly, in the presence of an appropriate stimulus (e.g. a chemoattractant), the cell becomes partially activated and adheres more firmly to the endothelium. This attachment is mediated particularly by certain *integrins* (Dustin & Springer, 1991; Collins *et al.*, 1994; Picker, 1994), a superfamily of heterodimeric molecules that can be subdivided into three subfamilies, the β1, β2 and β3 integrins, which are categorized according to the particular shared beta subunit common to each. One such molecule is CD11a/CD18 (LFA-1), a β2 integrin, the ligands for which are ICAM-1 (CD54), ICAM-2 and ICAM-3. The avidity of CD11a/CD18 for CD54 is transiently increased when the T cell is activated. Thirdly, the T cell crawls along the endothelium, passes between the endothelial cells, and enters the tissue. Here it interacts with the extracellular matrix, via molecules such as some of the β1 and β3 integrins. Some of these molecules can also deliver costimulatory signals to the T cell, i.e. they synergize with other membrane molecules in inducing a T-cell response (Hemler, 1990). It is only after these (and other) complex cellular and molecular events that T cells can interact with APC within the tissue, and antigen presentation can occur.

Cellular aspects of antigen processing and presentation, and T-cell-mediated immune responses

Afferent, efferent and memory phases of immune responses: resting, activated and memory T cells

Resting T cells are functionally inert, small lymphocytes. These T cells predominate in secondary lymphoid tissues such as spleen and lymph nodes. Most are localized in T-cell areas (e.g. central white pulp of spleen and interfollicular areas of lymph nodes) where they are intimately associated with interdigitating cells (IDC), members of the dendritic cell (DC) family (see below).

In the afferent phase of immune responses, resting T cells develop into activated T cells (Fig. 7.7); responses of previously unsensitized T cells are termed primary responses. Activated T cells express increased levels of a

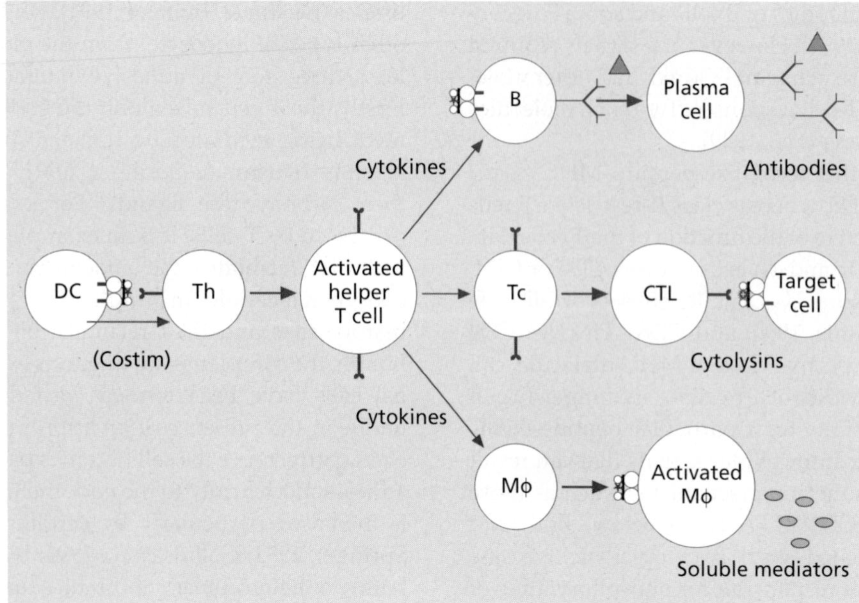

Fig. 7.7 A simplified overview of the afferent and efferent phases of adaptive immune responses. In the afferent phase, dendritic cells present foreign peptide–MHC complexes to resting helper T cells (Th) and deliver costimulatory signals for T-cell activation. Activated Th cells can then secrete cytokines that act on various cell types, including B cells, cytotoxic T cells (Tc) and macrophages (Mϕ). In the efferent phase, plasma cells secrete antibodies, cytotoxic T lymphocytes (CTL) secrete cytolysins, and activated macrophages secrete a wide variety of soluble mediators, all of which are involved in bringing about or effecting the removal of antigen.

variety of surface components including adhesion molecules, and new activation antigens such as receptors for transferrin and cytokines, e.g. high-affinity interleukin-2 (IL-2) receptors. T lymphoblasts enter the blood and migrate into sites of inflammation and infection in non-lymphoid tissues. Here they can recognize specific antigens on APC, proliferate, and secrete cytokines or cytolysins which contribute to the effector phase of immune responses.

During or after the efferent phase, some T cells develop into memory cells (Vitetta *et al.*, 1991). These small lymphocytes no longer express activation antigens, but do express higher levels of certain membrane molecules, and they may secrete a different spectrum of cytokines on re-stimulation than resting T cells (Ehlers & Smith, 1991; Vitetta *et al.*, 1991). Memory T cells recirculate between blood and lymph, largely due to their capacity to adhere to and cross high endothelial venules of lymph nodes. Immunological memory, the more rapid and efficient response elicited by antigens to which the cells were previously sensitized, is a consequence of the increased frequency of antigen-specific lymphocytes, due to their clonal expansion during primary responses, and possibly the greater ease with which they can be activated.

A critical difference between resting, activated and memory T cells is their requirement for interactions with different types of APC. Sensitization of resting T cells requires interaction with dendritic cells that present the requisite foreign peptide–MHC complexes and deliver essential costimulatory signals for T-cell activation (Inaba & Steinman, 1984; Steinman, 1991). Activated T cells no longer seem to require these specialized signals, and may respond to any APC presenting the relevant peptide–MHC complexes for which they are specific.

DC and the initiation of immune responses

The family of DC is distributed throughout lymphoid and most non-lymphoid tissues (Fig. 7.8). These cells are present in epithelia such as the skin, lung and airways, and gut, and in the interstitial spaces of solid organs such as heart and kidney (Steinman, 1991; Austyn, 1992). DC have a distinctive phenotype, can express high levels of MHC class I and class II molecules, and play a central role in the initiation of T-dependent immune responses. These cells are generated within the bone marrow as MHC class II-negative *progenitors* (Inaba *et al.*, 1992; Sallusto & Lanzavecchia, 1994). They enter the blood and migrate into non-lymphoid tissues where they apparently develop into *immature* MHC class II-positive DC.

Immature DC can endocytose and process protein-containing antigens but they have little or no capacity to activate resting T cells (Steinman, 1991; Austyn, 1992). Perhaps under the influence of inflammatory cytokines,

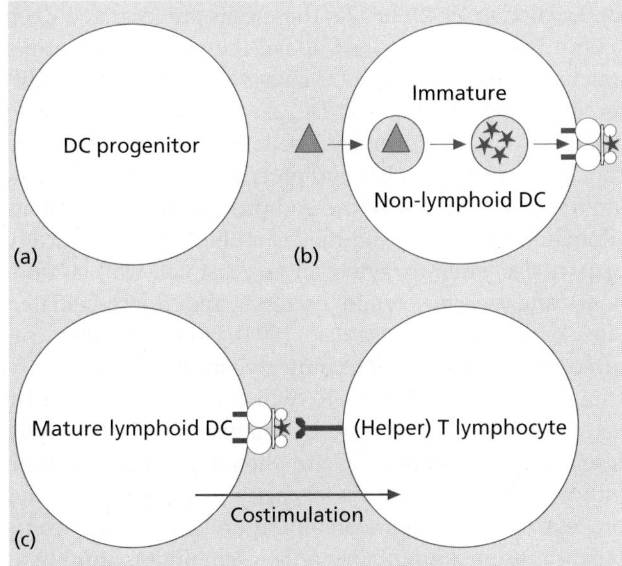

Fig. 7.8 An outline of dendritic cell (DC) development and maturation. DC progenitors are generated within the bone marrow and travel in the blood to non-lymphoid tissues. Here they develop into MHC class II-positive 'immature' DC which have optimal antigen uptake and processing capabilities but little or no costimulatory activity. Under the influence of various cytokines, these cells begin to mature and migrate into lymphoid tissues. Here, the 'mature' DC present foreign peptide–MHC complexes to resting T cells and deliver newly acquired costimulatory signals for T-cell activation.

produced in non-lymphoid tissues prior to the initiation of antigen-specific lymphocyte (adaptive) responses, these cells begin to mature and enter the lymph or blood, from where they migrate into lymph nodes or spleen, respectively (see below). Within secondary lymphoid tissues, the *mature* DC can present foreign peptide–MHC complexes to resting T cells, and have acquired the capacity to deliver costimulatory signals for T-cell activation (Metlay *et al.*, 1989; Steinman, 1991). The maturation and migration pathways of DC thus determine how, when and where T-cell-mediated immune responses are initiated (Austyn, 1992).

Lymphoid dendritic cells

DC isolated from lymphoid tissues are termed lymphoid DC. They can be identified on the basis of both phenotype, since they do not express a variety of lymphoid and myeloid cell markers but do express several DC-restricted markers in the mouse, and through their specialized functional properties. In particular, they have the specialized capacity to trigger primary T-cell responses *in vitro* (also termed immunostimulation, or T-cell sensitization) (Metlay *et al.*, 1989; Steinman, 1991). One of the first responses to be studied in this context was the allogeneic mixed leucocyte response (MLR), a large T-cell proliferative response that occurs when T cells are cultured with allogeneic DC. This response is largely due to the proliferation of Th cells, but mature cytotoxic T lymphocytes (CTL) also develop and proliferate in these cultures. While the development of CTL from their precursors frequently requires cytokines produced by activated Th cells, it is possible that DC can activate both subsets directly since they can induce CD8+ CTL even in the absence of CD4+ T cells (although the participation of a small subset of CD8+ Th cells has not been excluded).

Lymphoid DC can also stimulate primary antigen-specific lymphocyte responses *in vitro*, such as T-dependent antibody formation by B cells and antiviral CTL responses, as well as polyclonal T-cell proliferative responses, e.g. oxidative mitogenesis. Using these assays, rigorously purified populations of other leucocytes, such as splenic macrophages and small B cells, have been found to be unable to initiate primary T-cell responses, and depletion of DC from heterogeneous lymphoid cell populations ablates their stimulatory capacity. Activated B cells can also express costimulatory activities (Metlay *et al.*, 1989), but it is difficult to envisage how these cells could contribute to the initiation of primary immune responses, since in many cases B-cell activation requires the participation of DC-sensitized Th cells.

The importance of DC in the afferent phase of immune responses is also evident from the capacity of antigen-bearing DC to induce antigen-specific T-cell sensitization after administration *in vivo* (Steinman, 1991; Austyn, 1992). For example, DC were isolated from lymph nodes draining sites of skin to which contact sensitizers were applied, or from the lung after administration of antigens in aerosol form, or from pseudoafferent lymph-draining regions of gut into which antigens were injected, or isolated DC were pulsed with antigens *in vitro*. They were then transferred to naive recipients, which became sensitized to the respective antigens.

A close physical association of DC and T cells, or clustering, is essential for the initiation of *in vitro* responses, and this is likely to involve antigen-independent adhesion systems that function prior to antigen recognition by T cells (see above). Clustering is a prerequisite for subsequent antigen presentation to T cells, i.e. TcR recognition of specific peptide–MHC complexes expressed by DC, after which adhesion between the two cell types may be strengthened (e.g. via integrins). Almost certainly, these and other intermolecular interactions then lead to further intracellular signalling, such as occurs via CD28 and/or CTLA-4 following ligation of B7 molecules on DC, and through the interaction of CD40 ligand with CD40 which is also expressed by DC (Caux, 1994; Larsen *et al.*, 1994). Additionally, clustering is likely to facilitate the delivery of cytokines in a bidirectional manner. For example, DC can elaborate IL-12 (G. Schuler, personal communication), which plays an important role in the development of Th1 cells (see below), and IFN-γ produced by T cells can modulate DC expression of B7 molecules.

There is evidence that MHC class II-positive DC are situated in at least two distinct subcompartments of mouse spleen, and similar populations may also be present in other lymphoid tissues (Austyn, 1992). In the central white pulp, in intimate association with the bulk of resting T cells, are found IDC. In mouse, these cells express the NLDC145 (DEC 205) and J11d antigens, but do not appear to express the 33D1 marker. Within splenic marginal zones, where T cells enter the spleen from the blood, there is another population of DC that was first identified by the anti-CD11c/CD18 antibody N418 and which expresses 33D1, but not NLDC145 or J11d. The latter population seems to predominate in lymphoid DC isolated by techniques involving mechanical disruption of spleens, whereas IDC may be liberated in significant numbers only after collagenase digestion. Despite this clear phenotypic heterogeneity, possible functional differences between these DC subsets remain to be defined. Similar studies have not as yet been carried out in such detail with lymph node DC.

DC isolated from the thymus are also heterogeneous, although the relative proportion of the subsets usually obtained from this tissue is the converse of that from spleen. Within the thymus, DC are localized within the medulla (IDC) and at the corticomedullary junction. In contrast to their role in secondary lymphoid tissues—the initiation of responses of mature T cells to foreign peptide–MHC complexes—there is evidence that thymic DC are involved in the induction of tolerance of developing thymocytes to self peptide–MHC complexes (Fairchild & Austyn, 1990). Nevertheless, isolated thymic DC are similar to other lymphoid DC in their capacity to stimulate primary T-cell responses *in vitro*.

Non-lymphoid DC

A number of studies have documented the presence of MHC class II-positive leucocytes, often with dendritic profiles, in most non-lymphoid tissues. In some cases, functional criteria have confirmed that these cell are members of the DC system. Because of the importance of the skin and mucosal epithelia of the airways in atopic allergic responses, this section will focus particularly on properties of DC from these sites.

Langerhans cells

Perhaps the best characterized DC from non-lymphoid tissues are Langerhans cells (LC) from skin (Steinman, 1991; Austyn, 1992). *In situ*, these cells are localized deep within the epidermis, just above the epidermal–dermal junction. Freshly isolated LC have a phenotype that is different to that of lymphoid DC, and relatively little or no capacity to initiate primary T-cell responses *in vitro*. They can, however, internalize and process antigens. In particular, fresh LC can pinocytose and process protein antigens (Romani *et al.*, 1989), and they can phagocytose a variety of particles, such as zymosan (a yeast cell-wall component) and yeasts, certain bacteria, and fluoresceinated latex beads (Reis e Sousa *et al.*, 1993). However, when cultured in the presence of granuloctye macrophage colony-stimulating factor (GM-CSF), which can be produced by keratinocytes for example, LC mature into cells closely resembling lymphoid DC in phenotype and function. Importantly, they lose the capacity to phagocytose and process native protein-containing antigens, but become potent immunostimulatory cells resembling mature lymphoid DC (see above).

The loss of antigen-processing activity during culture of LC correlates with several intracellular changes. Biosynthesis of MHC class II molecules and the invariant chain (which is highly sialylated in these cells) is very high immediately after isolation, but virtually undetectable after culture in the presence of GM-CSF (Pure *et al.*, 1990). The cells also lose a number of acidic organelles normally associated with the capacity to process exogenous antigens, particularly early endosomes, as well as Birbeck granules (LC-specific organelles present in some species that may be endocytic in origin) (Stossel *et al.*, 1990). Nevertheless, cultured LC show increased expression of cell-surface MHC class II molecules, and for several days they can retain antigens acquired at an earlier stage in an immunogenic form, presumably as peptide–MHC complexes (Romani *et al.*, 1989). In culture they also acquire the capacity for antigen-independent clustering with T cells, which most likely contributes to their newly acquired immunostimulatory function.

DC in lung

MHC class II-positive leucocytes have also been identified in rodent and human lung and airways (Holt *et al.*, 1987; Rochester *et al.*, 1988; Nicod *et al.*, 1989a,b; Holt *et al.*, 1990, 1993; Pollard & Lipscomb, 1990). *In situ*, these cells are localized both within alveolar septae, and within and beneath the airway epithelium (see Chapter 13). Their distribution resembles that of LC in skin although, unlike the latter, they are juxtaposed to macrophages along the airway (Holt *et al.*, 1987). DC can be obtained by enzyme digestion of the lung parenchyma, whereas macrophages are typically obtained by lavage (Nicod *et al.*, 1989a). In the mouse, many isolated lung DC express CD25 (IL-2 receptor p50 chain), CD32 (FcγRII), NLDC145 and J11d, and the cultured DC but not macrophages from the same tissue can stimulate the allogeneic MLR (Pollard & Lipscomb, 1990). In the rat, the isolated DC can also present protein antigens, previously delivered to the lungs in aerosol form, to T-cell clones, whereas macrophages are suppressive (Holt *et al.*, 1987, 1993). It is not known to what extent the cells *in situ* resemble immature rather than mature DC. A reasonable hypothesis is that these cells are relatively immature, meaning that they have the capacity to endocytose and process antigens but that their full immunostimulatory capacity only develops after an inflammatory stimulus or after they have begun to migrate from these tissues into lymphoid tissues (see below).

Other non-lymphoid DC

As outlined above, DC in the lung and airways tend to be localized immediately below the epithelial cells lining these tissues, as in skin; the same is generally true for other topologically external sites, such as the gut and genitourinary tract. DC are also present in a subendothelial location in blood vessels. These cells therefore seem to be ideally situated to acquire antigens, such as pathogens, that may have breached this first line of defence, after which they may migrate primarily via the lymph into lymph nodes for the initiation of T-cell responses (see below). Within solid organs such as kidney and heart, similar cells are situated within the interstitial spaces, and have been termed interstitial DC (Hart & McKenzie, 1990). These cells have been isolated from various solid non-lymphoid tissues, and their functions have been studied in culture (Klinkert *et al.*, 1982). In most cases the cultured cells can stimulate primary T-cell responses, particularly the allogeneic mixed lymphocyte response (MLR), whereas other leucocytes, such as macrophages isolated from the same tissues, lack this function. However, DC purified from mouse heart and kidneys are unable to stimulate the allogeneic MLR or oxidative mitogenesis, unless they are cultured overnight (Austyn *et al.*, 1994). In this respect the cells resemble immature DC (cf. fresh LC), and the immunostimulatory function reported for DC isolated from these and other non-lymphoid organs seems likely to be a consequence of maturation in culture.

Migration pathways of DC

The behaviour of DC during both skin grafting and heart transplantation has been studied in mice. These studies have revealed the remarkable migratory properties of DC, and strongly suggest that migration of DC from non-lymphoid into lymphoid tissues is a critical event for the initiation of primary immune responses (Austyn & Larsen, 1990). To date there have been no similar systematic studies on the migration of DC from other tissues such as lung and airways or gut, but similar behaviour to LC of skin might be anticipated, because of the topological relationship between these tissues. In outline, it appears that DC from topologically external, epithelial tissues migrate primarily via afferent lymph to lymph nodes, whereas DC from solid, internal organs migrate both via this route and via blood to the spleen. Within these lymphoid tissues, it seems probable that the DC can then present peptide–MHC complexes (derived from foreign antigens acquired in the periphery) to specific T cells, and initiate immune responses.

Skin transplantation

Soon after skin grafting or in organ culture, a very rapid (within 4 hours) increase in MHC class II expression and size of epidermal LC was noted (Larsen *et al.*, 1990). The cells then left the epidermis, appeared in the dermis, and by 3–4 days they entered structures resembling dermal lymphatics. In organ culture, the cells migrated out of the skin and accumulated in the culture vessels, presumably mimicking events prior to their entry into lymphatics and migration to draining lymph nodes *in vivo* (where it is likely that skin-graft rejection is initiated). Studies on the migratory cells revealed changes in phenotype and function, compared to freshly isolated LC, characteristic of maturation. Direct visualization of the migration of LC into lymph nodes has been achieved after fluorochrome labelling of LC isolated from epidermal sheets, instillation into subcutaneous skin pockets in mice, and subsequent detection of labelled cells within the draining lymph nodes (M.I. Liddington, personal communication).

It has been suggested that changes in LC seen after grafting (i.e. the commencement of maturation and migration) are induced by inflammatory mediators because some of these events occurred within 4 hours, well before induction of an adaptive immune response (Larsen *et al.*, 1990). These mediators seem to be locally produced (e.g. by keratinocytes) and independent of the host, since similar changes were observed for isografts, allografts and in organ culture. This view is consistent with other reports (Enk *et al.*, 1993; Cumberbatch *et al.*, 1994), and is strengthened by the data from studies of migration of non-lymphoid DC in response to systemically administered endotoxin or cytokines (see below).

Heart transplantation

Using a fully vascularized, heterotopic cardiac allograft model in mice, DC were observed to migrate rapidly out of the transplants into recipient spleens (Larsen *et al.*, 1990). These (MHC class II+ CD45+ CD44+ CD3– CD4– CD8– Ig–) cells homed to the peripheral white pulp (B areas) and associated with CD4+ T cells. These cells migrated via the blood, a pathway demonstrated in earlier studies (Austyn *et al.*, 1988; Kupiec-Weglinski *et al.*, 1988), since the spleen lacks an afferent lymphatic supply and because DC from heart-cell suspensions are unable to enter spleens from the peritoneal cavity, the site of allografting. Similar observations have been made in a rat limb transplant model (Codner *et al.*, 1990).

In skin grafts (see above), various cytokine mediators produced in the transplanted heart, for example as a consequence of surgical trauma or ischaemia, may promote the maturation and migration of DC from this organ. In keeping with this view, in subsequent experiments it was found that systemic administration of bacterial lipopolysaccharide (LPS; endotoxin) to mice promoted a profound loss of DC from heart and kidney, apparently because the elicited cytokines induced DC migration (presumably into lymphoid tissues); qualitatively similar effects were observed following administration of tumour necrosis factor-α (TNF-α) and/or IL1-α (Roake *et al.*, 1996a). At the same time, systemic LPS lead to recruitment of MHC class II-negative DC progenitors (as well as monocyte/macrophages and neutrophils) into these tissues (Roake *et al.*, 1996b), perhaps to repeat the cycle—development of the progenitors into immature DC within the tissue, followed by maturation and migration to lymphoid tissues. Although these findings were made in transplant organs, it seems most likely that DC would behave similarly in antigen-specific responses. Thus, entry of antigen into a non-lymphoid tissue (e.g. an epithelium), accompanied by inflammation, may promote antigen uptake and processing by the immature DC, their migration to lymphoid tissues, and antigen presentation by the mature DC with newly acquired costimulatory activities.

APC and the efferent phase of immune responses

Activated T cells are essential for the efferent phase of adaptive immune responses, and their interactions with different types of APC are of paramount importance. Only a very brief overview will be provided here.

Interactions between activated Th cells and APC

When activated Th cells recognize foreign peptide–MHC complexes on APC they secrete cytokines that can act directly on the APC being recognized (during so-called cognate interactions) and induce or up-regulate their effector functions. For example, some cytokines activate macrophages into potent microbicidal cells that can secrete a variety of toxic molecules (e.g. proteases and reactive oxygen and nitrogen intermediates), that mediate their effector functions and lead to the elimination of extracellular and intracellular organisms (Nathan, 1987). Such molecules could, presumably, also contribute to the tissue damage seen in atopic allergy.

B cells also function as APC for activated Th cells (Metlay *et al.*, 1989; Klaus, 1990; Lanzavecchia, 1990). After binding to membrane Ig molecules, native antigens are internalized and processed intracellularly, and their peptide–MHC class II complexes can subsequently be recognized by activated Th cells. These T cells then produce the requisite cytokines for B-cell activation, their development into plasma cells, and the secretion of antibodies which mediate the effector functions of B cells. Cognate interactions presumably also occur between activated Th cells and cells that do not normally express MHC class II molecules, but on which they are induced in the course of immune responses, and some cytokines may act at a distance on cells that never express detectable class II.

The precise course of the efferent phase of immune responses is determined to a large extent by the spectrum of cytokines secreted by Th cells. Different subsets of CD4+ T cells, Th1 and Th2 cells, can produce different cytokines (see below) (Romagnani, 1994; Seder & Paul, 1994). Although there is some evidence that Th2 cells are derived from Th1 cells, perhaps as different stages of development or activation, there is conflicting evidence on this point and T cells secreting intermediate patterns of cytokines have also been identified (Th0 cells). The relevance of these subsets to atopic allergy is considered below.

Interactions between activated Tc cells and APC

Cytokines produced by activated Th cells are often required for the development of CTL. Although DC may activate Tc cells directly, it is possible that recognition of foreign peptide–class I complexes on other APC by precursor Tc cells is sufficient to induce responsiveness to Th-cell-derived cytokines (i.e. priming), which, if and when produced, may promote their final development into effector cells. Of these, IL-4 seems primarily to be required for development of full cytolytic activity, while IL-2 drives proliferation of the cells.

Recognition of foreign peptide–MHC class I complexes on cell membranes by CTL results in the secretion of a variety of toxic molecules collectively termed cytolysins (Berke, 1994). These molecules mediate the effector mechanism of CTL, i.e. cellular cytotoxicity, and can be divided into two groups, depending on whether or not they lead to the appearance of characteristic pores in target cell membranes. These are composed of pore-forming proteins called perforins, which polymerize into polyperforins. In many respects these pores resemble those generated by the C6–C9 components of complement, to which perforin has structural homology (Tschopp & Nabholz, 1990). Candidate non-pore-forming molecules of CTL include a family of serine esterases or granzymes, TNF-α, TNF-β and related molecules (e.g. leukalexins). Some of these, like perforins, are contained within granules of CTL and are secreted after recognition of the target cell (Peters *et al.*, 1991). One important difference between the cytotoxic mechanisms mediated by complement and CTL is that complement induces necrosis by damaging cell membranes, whereas CTL can also induce apoptosis, an important characteristic of the latter being early degradation of nuclear DNA before any changes in the cell membrane are evident. Apoptosis can be triggered by membrane molecular interactions between Fas, on the target cell, and Fas ligand, expressed by activated T cells (Lowin *et al.*, 1994).

Allergy

The antigens that give rise to atopic allergic reactions are termed allergens (Ishizaka & Ishizaka, 1989; de Vries, 1994). Most are soluble proteins or glycoproteins of molecular weight 5–50 kDa. It is unclear why they preferentially induce IgE rather than other classes of antibody.

There are clear MHC associations in allergy. For example, allergic responses to the Amb a 5 and Amb a 4 allergens of short ragweed pollen are more common in individuals expressing the DR2/Dw2 and DR5 HLA class II molecules, respectively, and those to rye grass pollen Lol p 1 and Lol p 2 components are associated with DR3/Dw3 genotypes. It is most likely that these responses are controlled in part by the MHC class II molecules themselves, by virtue of the polymorphisms that determine the binding of a particular peptide or set of peptides for presentation to T cells. However, in some cases, MHC associations may indicate the function of closely linked genes. Either way, it is highly likely that other genes also contribute to the atopic state; for example, general immune hyperresponsiveness is associated with HLA-B8 and DRW3, a non-MHC-linked autosomal dominant gene controls low IgE levels and, conversely, the enhanced IgE production in atopy is linked to chromosome 5q31.1 (see below).

For the induction of atopic allergic reactions, it is likely that the allergen is taken up and processed by APC at mucosal surfaces. Presentation to Th cells leads to the production of cytokines that help B cells secrete IgE. The IgE then binds to Fc receptors on mast cells and basophils which become sensitized. Subsequent exposure to the allergen cross-links the specific IgE bound to these receptors and causes degranulation and mediator release, which gives rise to the pathology recognized as the atopic allergic state. These stages are briefly considered below.

DC–resting T-cell interactions in allergy

Given the central role of DC in the induction of immune responses, it seems most likely that the primary response to the allergen follows uptake and processing by these cells in mucosal sites, for example by (immature) DC of the lung and skin for inhaled and topically encountered allergens, respectively. Subsequently, these cells would migrate into lymphoid tissues, where (as mature DC) they could present the relevant peptide–MHC complexes to Th cells and deliver costimulatory signals for T-cell activation. This scheme is consistent with the capacity of immature (non-lymphoid) DC to internalize particles by phagocytosis (or soluble molecules by endocytosis), with their optimal antigen-processing capabilities at this stage, with their migration pathways, and with the specialized costimulatory functions of mature (lymphoid) DC (Steinman, 1991; Austyn, 1992).

It is well established that DC can express Fc receptors, particularly FcγR for IgG by immature (non-lymphoid) DC, and there is accumulating evidence that, at least at some stage, they can also express FcεR for IgE (see below). The functions of Fc receptors on DC are unknown. Following the very first exposure to the allergen, it seems most unlikely that these Fc receptors could be involved in the subsequent response, since specific Ig would not yet be formed. However, once IgG or IgE had been produced against the allergen, and on subsequent encounter with it, it is conceivable that these classes of antibody could bind to the respective FcR on DC and either mediate uptake of the allergen by the cells and/or modulate DC function. Therefore, DC could play a very important role, not only in initiating the immune response to allergens, but also in determining the direction of the subsequent response, particularly the induction of Th2 versus Th1 cells (see below).

Activated T-cell–APC interactions in allergy

Having been activated by DC, T cells can then recognize other APC. Central to atopic allergy must be T-cell/B-cell interactions, which ultimately lead to IgE responses. The vast majority of B-cell responses to protein antigens (e.g. allergens) require T-cell help. For these, activated T cells need to recognize the same peptide–MHC class II complexes to which they were first sensitized. Although B cells are not phagocytic, it is clear that soluble antigens can be internalized by B cells after binding to membrane Ig. Subsequently, these antigens can be processed within the cell, and the peptides loaded onto class II molecules. Expression of membrane peptide–MHC complexes then permits recognition by specific T cells. Cognate interactions between T cells and B cells permit membrane–molecular interactions that result in intracellular signalling to the B cell, and the production of cytokines by the T cell that may also act on B cells at a distance.

T-cell-derived cytokines can act upon B cells in a number of ways. Firstly, some cytokines, such as IL-4, can directly activate resting B cells, which enter the cell cycle; B-cell activation can also be triggered by other routes, for example following antigen binding to and cross-linking of mIg and the delivery of intracellular signals for B-cell activation. Secondly, particular cytokines can induce class switching in B cells, i.e. the production of a different class of antibody with the same antigen specificity which is then expressed at the cell surface; it is generally believed that naive, unstimulated B cells express both IgM and IgG, but that expression of other classes such as IgE normally requires the action of T-cell-derived cytokines. Thirdly, certain cytokines promote production of the secretory (vs. membrane-anchored) form of the Ig, and induce antibody secretion by the plasma cell. This series of events can therefore result in a B cell that recognizes a given native antigen via its mIg, becoming a plasma cell that secretes a different class of antibody specific for the same antigen.

It seems likely that the T cells responsible for triggering B-cell responses must first be activated by DC, due to the specialized costimulatory functions of the latter. In culture in the presence of antigen, DC form tight aggregates with resting T cells and B cells during the induction of T-dependent antibody responses. However, there is accumulating evidence that activated B cells can express similar costimulatory functions to DC. For example, it has been shown that antigen binding to mIg on resting B cells can induce B-cell activation, development into lymphoblasts, and expression of costimulatory molecules such as CD40 and B7; such B cells can subsequently activate resting T cells. This pathway may result in the activation of more antigen-specific T cells, that in turn can activate additional B cells, thereby amplifying the response. Nevertheless, the cytokines secreted by the T cells play a central role in controlling whether or not an allergic state is subsequently induced (see below).

In addition to IgE-secreting B cells, mast cells and eosinophils are centrally involved in atopic allergic reactions. Both cell types can express MHC class II molecules, and could therefore interact with activated Th cells. In addition, mast cells can phagocytose bacteria and antibody-coated (opsonized) erythrocytes, so that particulate antigens could, in principle, be internalized and directed into the class II pathway. However, much remains to be learnt about these processes, particularly in the context of atopic allergic disease.

Cytokines and allergy

Clones of CD4+ T cells secreting polarized patterns of cytokines have been identified, as noted above (Fig. 7.9). Th1 cells secrete IL-2, IFN-γ and TNF-β, whereas Th2 cells secrete IL-4, IL-5 and IL-10 and perhaps IL-9 and IL-13; both subsets can produce IL-3, TNF-α and GM-CSF. Rather than representing discrete CD4+ T-cell subsets, it appears that Th1 and Th2 cells both develop from Th0 cells which secrete an intermediate pattern of cytokines. Their development into Th1 or Th2 cells is most likely determined by the precise spectrum of cytokines encountered during activation; thus, for example, IL-12 preferentially induces Th1 cells, and IL-4 induces Th2 cells (Seder

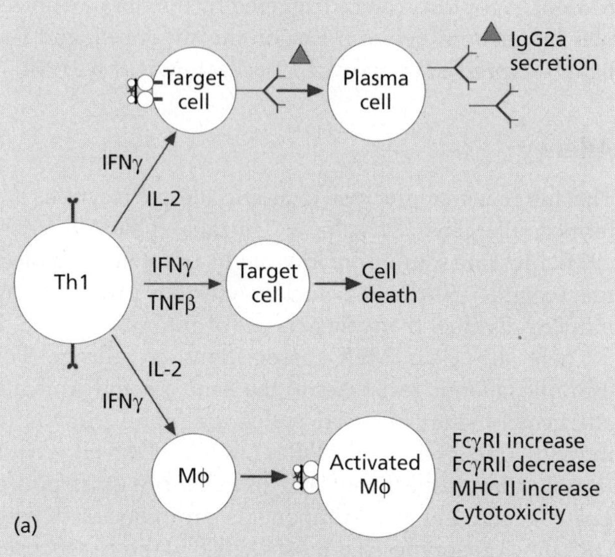

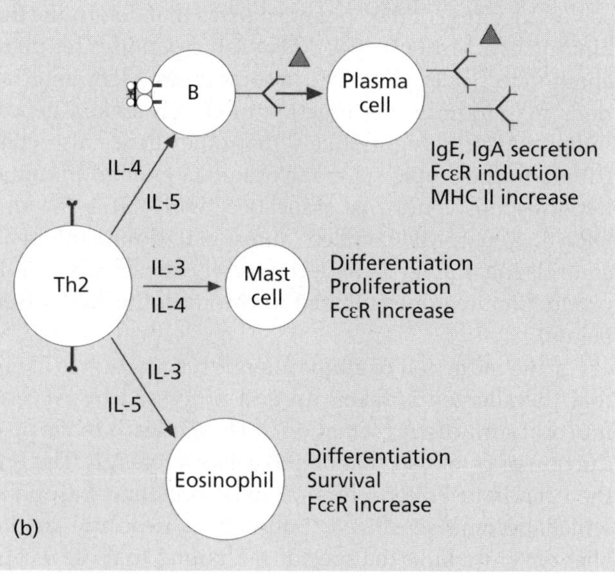

Fig. 7.9 Actions of Th1 and Th2 cells. A few examples of the cytokines secreted by CD4+ T cells and some of their actions. The cytokines secreted by Th1 cells tend to promote delayed-type hypersensitivity reactions, whereas those secreted by Th2 cells are involved in immediate-type hypersensitivity reactions such as allergy. There is evidence that similar polarized extremes also exist for CD8+ T cells.

& Paul, 1994). A detailed consideration of the factors controlling the induction of Th1 vs. Th2 cells, the various functions of these subsets, and detailed actions of the respective cytokines, is beyond the scope of this chapter. However, as a general rule, these subsets are involved in different pathological, as well as normal immunological, conditions (Romagnani, 1994). In particular, Th2 responses are responsible for triggering allergic or atopic conditions; these cells also preferentially develop during helminthic infections. In contrast, Th1 cells tend to be involved in type IV or delayed-type hypersensitivity reactions and in certain autoimmune conditions; these cells also predominate during infections by bacteria, protozoa and viruses. It should be noted that CD8+ T cells can also produce polarized patterns of cytokines.

The importance of Th2 cells in allergy is illustrated by the fact that most allergen-specific CD4+ T-cell clones from atopic donors have been found to secrete a Th2/Th0 pattern of cytokines, with high IL-4 but little or no IFN-γ, whereas clones derived from non-atopic donors exhibit a Th1/Th0 phenotype (Romagnani, 1994). Different, but polarized, patterns of cytokine production are also seen for CD8+ T cells from allergic donors. For example, there are reports that CD8+ T-cell clones specific for inhaled toluene diisocyanate, obtained by bronchial asthma biopsy, tend to produce IL-5 and IFN-γ but not IL-4. A question unanswered is why different individuals appear to respond differently to the same antigen. The genetic linkage of atopy to chromosome 5q31.1 is intriguing, given that this region contains the *IL-4* and *IL-13* genes (together with *IL-3*, *IL-5*, *IL-9* and *GM-CSF*); conceivably, this linkage could indicate a cytokine gene regulation defect in atopic individuals.

The precise spectrum of cytokines produced by T cells determines the nature of the subsequent immune response, as illustrated by the following examples. In the case of Th2 cells, IL-4 and also IL-13 can induce isotype switching of B cells to IgE expression; combinations of IL-3, IL-4 and IL-10 stimulate the production and proliferation of mucosal mast cells; IL-5 stimulates colony formation, differentiation and survival of eosinophils, and combinations of IL-4, IL-5 and IL-13 promote eosinophilia; and IL-4 and/or IL-5 induce the expression of FcεR (CD23) on mast cells and eosinophils as well as B cells (note that binding of IgE complexes to CD23 on B cells has been shown to increase B-cell antigen processing and presentation; see above). All these events are likely to contribute to the development of immediate-type (type I) hypersensitivity reactions, i.e. allergic atopic disorders. In contrast, IL-2 produced by Th1 cells promotes IgG2a secretion by B cells; IFN-γ induces macrophage expression of FcγRI, which is specific for monomeric IgG2a and mediates antibody-dependent cellular cytotoxicity, but down-regulates expression of FcγRII (specific for complexed or aggregated IgG2b); and IL-2 also increases macrophage cytotoxicity. These events are therefore more likely to result in delayed-type (type IV) hypersensitivity reactions. Th1 and Th2 cells cross-regulate their responses: for example, IL-10 produced by Th2 cells inhibits cytokine production by Th1 cells, and IFN-γ produced by Th1 cells can counteract many of the effects of IL-4 produced by Th2 cells. This knowledge suggests obvious strategies that are being explored to inhibit or prevent atopic allergy.

Mediators in allergy

A central event in atopic allergic reactions is binding of allergen-specific IgE to mast cells and basophils via FcεR, which mediate release of mediators on subsequent binding of allergen (Ishizaka & Ishizaka, 1989). Two classes of membrane-bound FcεR have been identified: the high-affinity FcεRI and low-affinity FcεRII or CD23. FcεRI is expressed by mast cells, basophils and Langerhans cells (Wang *et al.*, 1992; Bieber, 1994). It comprises an α-chain, composed of two Ig-like C2 domains, associated with a β-chain and a disulphide-linked γ-chain dimer (which is identical to the human CD16 FcγRIII γ-chain, and may mediate signal transduction). FcεRII (CD23) is structurally unrelated to FcεRI and contains a C-type lectin domain. Human CD23 is expressed in alternatively spliced forms, IIa and IIb, differing in seven amino acids at the N-terminal, cytoplasmic portion. The IIa form is expressed by mature B cells, whereas the IIb form is expressed by a variety of cells including eosinophils, monocytes and IL-4-activated macrophages. There are indications that CD23 may also be expressed by Langerhans cells (Buckley *et al.*, 1993). Proteolysis of membrane CD23 generates a number of fragments, some of which can also bind IgE. Mouse CD23 is homologous to the human IIa form, and is present on mature B cells.

Ligation of the FcεR receptors on eosinophils, mast cells, basophils and macrophages leads to the production of a wide variety of mediators, the precise spectrum of which depends on the particular receptor, cell type and response involved. However, in allergic atopic conditions, the key mediators of mast cells and basophils are spasmogens, activators and chemoattractants. Some are stored within granules and are released during the explosive degranulation that occurs after receptor ligation. One such example is histamine from human mast cells. Other mediators of mast cells are newly synthesized, such as the arachidonic acid metabolites, including prostaglandins and leukotrienes, platelet activating factor and a wide variety of cytokines. Likewise, eosinophils produce major basic protein, eosinophil peroxidase and eosinophil cationic protein. Acting in concert, these mediators produce the early and late phases of atopic allergic reactions and result in the tissue damage that is, for example, recognized clinically as atopic asthma, rhinitis or dermatitis. Further knowledge of the processing and presentation of allergens may lead to strategies to overcome atopic allergic conditions, by manipulation of the afferent phase of these responses.

Acknowledgements

The sections on molecular aspects and cellular aspects of antigen processing and presentation are based on Austyn (1993), with appropriate updating and modification.

References

Allison, J.P. (1994) CD28-B7 interactions in T-cell activation. *Curr. Opin. Immunol.*, **6**, 414–19.

Amigorena, S., Drake, J.R., Webster, P. & Mellman, I. (1994) Transient accumulation of new class II MHC molecules in a novel endocytic compartment in B lymphocytes. *Nature*, **369**, 113–20.

Austyn, J.M. (1989) *Antigen-Presenting Cells*. In: *Focus Series* (ed. D. Male). IRL Press, Oxford.

Austyn, J.M. & Larsen, C.P. (1990) Migration patterns of dendritic leukocytes. Implications for transplantation. *Transplantation*, **49**, 1–17.

Austyn, J.M. (1992) Antigen uptake and presentation by dendritic leukocytes. In: *Antigen Trapping and Presentation in vivo. Seminars in Immunology* (ed. J.G. Tew). WB Saunders, London.

Austyn, J.M. (1993) The initiation of immune responses and allograft rejection. In: *Immunology of Heart and Lung Transplantation* (eds M.L. Rose & M.H. Yacoub), pp. 22–41. Edward Arnold, London.

Austyn, J.M., Hankins, D.F., Larsen, C.P., Morris, P.J., Rao, A.S. & Roake, J.A. (1994) Isolation and characterization of dendritic cells from mouse heart and kidney. *J. Immunol.*, **152**, 2401–10.

Austyn, J.M., Kupiec-Weglinski, J.W., Hankins, D.F. & Morris, P.J. (1988) Migration patterns of dendritic cells in the mouse. Homing to T cell-dependent areas of spleen, and binding within marginal zone. *J. Exp. Med.*, **167**, 646–51.

Berke, G. (1994) The binding and lysis of target cells by cytotoxic lymphocytes: molecular and cellular aspects. *Ann. Rev. Immunol.*, **12**, 735–73.

Bieber, T. (1994) Fc epsilon RI on human Langerhans cells: a new receptor in search of new functions. *Immunol. Today*, **15**, 52–3.

Bierer, B.E., Sleckman, B.P., Ratnofsky, S.E. & Burakoff, S.J. (1989) The biologic roles of CD2, CD4, and CD8 in T-cell activation. *Ann. Rev. Immunol.*, **7**, 579–99.

Bjorkman, P.J., Saper, M.A., Samaroui, B., Bennett, W.S., Strominger, J.L. & Wiley, D.C. (1987) The foreign antigen binding site and T cell recognition regions of class I histocompatibility antigens. *Nature*, **329**, 512–18.

Buckley, C., Ivison, C., Poulter, L.W. & Rustin, M.H. (1993) CD23/Fc epsilon RII expression in contact sensitivity reactions: a comparison between aeroallergen patch test reactions in atopic dermatitis and the nickel patch test reaction in non-atopic individuals. *Clin. Exp. Immunol.*, **91**, 357–61.

Caux, C., Massacrier, C., Vanbervliet, B. *et al.* (1994) Activation of human dendritic cells through CD40 cross-linking. *J. Exp. Med.*, **179**, 1263–72.

Chan, A.C., Desai, D.M. & Weiss, A. (1994) The role of protein tyrosine kinases and protein tyrosine phosphatases in T cell antigen receptor signal transduction *Ann. Rev. Immunol.*, **12**, 555–92.

Cho, S., Attaya, M. & Monaco, J.J. (1991) New class II-like genes in the murine MHC. *Nature*, **353**, 573–6.

Codner, M.A., Shuster, B.A., Steinman, R.M., Harper, A.D., LaTrenta, G.S. & Hoffman, L.A. (1990) Migration of donor leukocytes from limb allografts into host lymphoid tissues. *Ann. Plast. Surg.*, **25**, 353–9.

Collins, T.L., Kassner, P.D., Bierer, B.E. & Burakoff, S.J. (1994) Adhesion receptors in lymphocyte activation. *Curr. Opin. Immunol.*, **6**, 385–93.

Cumberbatch, M., Fielding, I. & Kimber, I. (1994) Modulation of epidermal Langerhans' cell frequency by tumour necrosis factor-alpha. *Immunology*, **81**, 395.

Dustin, M.L. & Springer, T.A. (1991) Role of lymphocyte adhesion receptors in transient interactions and cell locomotion. *Ann. Rev. Immunol.*, **9**, 27–66.

Ehlers, S. & Smith, K.A. (1991) Differentiation of T cell lymphokine gene expression: the *in vitro* acquisition of T cell memory. *J. Exp. Med.*, **173**, 25–36.

Engelhard, V.H. (1994) Structure of peptides associated with class I molecules. *Curr. Opin. Immunol.*, **6**, 13–23.

Enk, A.H., Angeloni, V.L., Udey, M.C. & Katz, S.I. (1993) An essential role for Langerhans cell-derived IL-1 beta in the initiation of primary immune responses in skin. *J. Immunol.*, **150**, 3689.

Fairchild, P.J. & Austyn, J.M. (1990) Thymic dendritic cells: phenotype and function. *Int. Rev. Immunol.*, **6**, 187–96.

Fling, S.P., Arp, B. & Pious, D. (1994) HLA-DMA and -DMB genes are both required for MHC class II/peptide complex formation in antigen-presenting cells. *Nature*, **368**, 554–8.

Fowlkes, B.J. & Pardoll, D.M. (1989) Molecular and cellular events of T cell development. *Adv. Immunol.*, **44**, 207–64.

Germain, R.N. & Margulies, D.H. (1993) The biochemistry and cell biology of antigen processing and presentation. *Ann. Rev. Immunol.*, **11**, 403–50.

Guillemot, F., Auffray, C., Orr, H.T. & Strominger, J. (1988) MHC antigen genes. In: *Molecular Immunology* (eds B.D. Homes & D.M. Glover), pp. 81–143. IRL Press, Oxford.

Haas, S., Pereira, P. & Tonegawa, S. (1993) Gamma/delta cells. *Ann. Rev. Immunol.*, **11**, 637–85.

Hart, D.N.J. & McKenzie, J.L. (1990) Interstitial dendritic cells. *Int. Rev. Immunol.*, **6**, 128–49.

Hemler, M.E. (1990) VLA proteins in the integrin family: structures, functions, and their role on leukocytes. *Ann. Rev. Immunol.*, **8**, 365–400.

Hershko, A. (1988) Ubiquitin-mediated protein degradation. *J. Biol. Chem.*, **263**, 15237–40.

Holt, P.G., Oliver, J., Bilyk, N. *et al.* (1993) Downregulation of the antigen presenting cell function(s) of pulmonary dendritic cells *in vivo* by resident alveolar macrophages. *J. Exp. Med.*, **177**, 397–407.

Holt, P.G., Schon-Hegrad, M.A. & McMenamin, P.G. (1990) Dendritic cells in the respiratory tract. *Int. Rev. Immunol.*, **6**, 139–49.

Holt, P.G., Schon-Hegrad, M.A. & Oliver, J. (1987) MHC class II antigen-bearing dendritic cells in pulmonary tissues of the rat. Regulation of antigen presentation activity by endogenous macrophage populations. *J. Exp. Med.*, **167**, 262–74.

Howard, J.C. (1995) Supply and transport of peptides presented by class I MHC molecules. *Curr. Opin. Immunol.*, **7**, 69–76.

Inaba, K. & Steinman, R.M. (1984) Resting and sensitized T lymphocytes exhibit distinct stimulatory (antigen presenting cell) requirements for growth and lymphokine release. *J. Exp. Med.*, **160**, 1717–35.

Inaba, K., Inaba, M., Romani, N. *et al.* (1992) Generation of large numbers of dendritic cells from mouse bone marrow cultures supplemented with granulocyte/macrophage colony-stimulating factor. *J. Exp. Med.*, **176**, 1693–72.

Irving, B.A. & Weiss, A. (1991) The cytoplasmic domain of the T cell receptor zeta chain is sufficient to couple to receptor-associated signal transduction pathways. *Cell*, **64**, 891–901.

Ishizaka, K. & Ishizaka, T. (1989) Allergy. In: *Fundamental Immunology* (ed. W.E. Paul), 2nd edn, pp. 867–88. Raven, New York.

Karisson, L., Surh, C.D., Sprent, J. & Peterson, P.A. (1991) A novel class II MHC molecule with unusual tissue distribution. *Nature*, **351**, 485–8.

Kelly, A.P., Monaco, J.J., Cho, S. & Trowsdale, J. (1991) A new human HLA class II-related locus, DM. *Nature*, **353**, 571–73.

Klaus, G. (1990) B lymphocytes. In: *Focus Series* (ed. D. Male). IRL Press, Oxford.

Klinkert, W.E.F., Labadie, J.H. & Bowers, W.E. (1982) Accessory and stimulating properties of dendritic cells and macrophages isolated from various rat tissues. *J. Exp. Med.*, **156**, 1–19.

Kupiec-Weglinski, J.W., Austyn, J.M. & Morris, P.J. (1988) Migration patterns of dendritic cells in the mouse. Traffic from the blood, and T-cell-dependent and -independent entry to lymphoid tissues. *J. Exp. Med.*, **167**, 632–45.

Lanzavecchia, A. (1990) Receptor-mediated antigen uptake and its effect on antigen presentation to class II-restricted T lymphocytes. *Ann. Rev. Immunol.*, **8**, 773–93.

Larsen, C.P., Morris, P.J. & Austyn, J.M. (1990) Migration of dendritic leukocytes from cardiac allografts into host spleens: a novel pathway for initiation of rejection. *J. Exp. Med.*, **171**, 370–14.

Larsen, C.P., Ritchie, S.C., Hendrix, R. *et al.* (1994) Regulation of immunostimulatory function and costimulatory molecule (B7-1 and B7-2) expression on murine dendritic cells. *J. Immunol.*, **152**, 5208–19.

Larsen, C.P., Steinman, R.M., Witmer-Pack, M., Hankins, D.F., Morris, P.J. & Austyn, J.M. (1990) Migration and maturation of Langerhans cells in skin transplants and explants. *J. Exp. Med.*, **172**, 1483–93.

Linsley, P.S. & Ledbetter, J.A. (1993) The role of the CD28 receptor during T cell responses to antigen. *Ann. Rev. Immunol.*, **11**, 191–212.

Linsley, P.S., Brady, W., Urnes, M., Grosmaire, L., Damle, N.K. & Ledbetter, J.A. (1991) CTLA-4 is a second receptor for the B cell activation antigen B7. *J. Exp. Med.*, **173**, 721–30.

Ljunggren, H-G., Stam, N.J., Ohlen, C. *et al.* (1990) Empty MHC class I molecules come out in the cold. *Nature*, **346**, 476–80.

Lowin, B., Hahne, M., Mattmann, C. & Tschoop, J. (1994) Cytolytic T-cell cytotoxicity is mediated through perforin and Fas lytic pathways. *Nature*, **370**, 650–2.

Makgoba, M.W., Sanders, M.E. & Shaw, S. (1989) The CD2-LFA-3 and LFA-1-ICAM pathways: relevance to T-cell recognition. *Immunol. Today*, **10**, 417–22.

McEver, R.P. (1994) Selectins. *Curr. Opin. Immunol.*, **6**, 75–84.

Metlay, J.P., Pure, E. & Steinman, R.M. (1989) Control of the immune response at the level of antigen-presenting cells: a comparison of the function of dendritic cells and B lymphocytes. *Adv. Immunol.*, **47**, 45–116.

Momburg, F., Roelse, J., Howard, J.C., Butcher, G.W., Hammerling, G.J. & Neefjes, J.J. (1994a) Selectivity of MHC-encoded peptide transporters from human, mouse and rat. *Nature*, **367**, 648–51.

Momburg, F., Roelse, J., Hammerling, G.J. & Neefjes, J.J. (1994b) Peptide size selection by the major histocompatibility complex-encoded peptide transporter. *J. Exp. Med.*, **179**, 1613–23.

Mueller, D.L., Jenkins, M.K. & Schwartz, R.H. (1989) Clonal expansion versus functional clonal inactivation: a costimulatory signalling pathway determines the outcome of T cell antigen receptor occupancy. *Ann. Rev. Immunol.*, **7**, 445–80.

Nathan, C.F. (1987) Secretory products of macrophages. *J. Clin. Invest.*, **79**, 319–26.

Neefjes, J.J., Hammerling, G.J. & Momburg, F. (1993) Folding and assembly of major histocompatibility complex class I heterodimers in the endoplasmic reticulum of intact cells precedes the binding of peptide. *J. Exp. Med.*, **178**, 1971–80.

Nicod, L.P., Lipscomb, M.F., Weissler, J.C., Lyons, C.R., Alberton, J. & Toews, G.B. (1989a) Mononuclear cells in human lung paren chyma: characterization of a potent accessory cell not obtained by bronchoalveolar lavage. *Am. Rev. Resp. Dis.*, **136**, 818–23.

Nicod, L.P., Lipscomb, M.F., Weissler, J.C., & Toews, G.B. (1989b) Mononuclear cells from human lung parenchyma support antigen-induced T lymphocyte proliferation. *J. Leuk. Biol.*, **45**, 336–44.

Ottenhoff, T.H. & Mutis, T. (1990) Specific killing of cytotoxic T cells and antigen-presenting cells by CD4+ cytotoxic T cell clones. A novel potentially immunoregulatory T–T interaction in man. *J. Exp. Med.*, **171**, 2011–24.

Owen, M.J. & Lamb, J.R. (1988) Immune recognition. In: *Focus Series* (ed. D. Male). IRL Press, Oxford.

Peters, J.M. (1994) Proteasomes: protein degradation machines of the cell. *Trends Biochem. Sci.*, **19**, 377–82.

Peters, P.J., Borst, J., Oorschot, V. *et al.* (1991) Cytotoxic T lymphocyte granules are secretory lysosomes, containing both perforin and granzymes. *J. Exp. Med.*, **173**, 1099–109.

Picker, L.J. (1994) Control of lymphocyte homing. *Curr. Opin. Immunol.*, **6**, 394–406.

Pollard, A.M. & Lipscomb, M.F. (1990) Characterization of murine lung dendritic cells: similarities to Langerhans cells and thymic dendritic cells. *J. Exp. Med.*, **172**, 159–68.

Pure, E., Inaba, K., Crowley, M.T. *et al.* (1990) Antigen processing by epidermal Langerhans cells correlates with the level of biosynthesis of major histocompatibility complex class II molecules and expression of invariant chain. *J. Exp. Med.*, **172**, 1459–70.

Rammensee, H.-G. (1995) Chemistry of peptides associated with MHC class I and class II molecules. *Curr. Opin. Immunol.*, **7**, 85–96.

Reis e Sousa, C., Stahl, P.D. & Austyn, J.M. (1993) Phagocytosis of antigens by Langerhans cells *in vitro*. *J. Exp. Med.*, **178**, 509–19.

Roake, J.A., Rao, A.S., Morris, P.J., Larsen, C.P., Hankins, D.F. & Austyn, J.M. (1996a) Dendritic cell loss from non-lymphoid tissues following systemic administration of lipopolysaccharide, tumour necrosis factor, and interleukin-1. *J. Exp. Med.* (in press).

Roake, J.A., Rao, A.S., Morris, P.J., Larsen, C.P., Hankins, D.F. & Austyn, J.M. (1996b) Systemic lipopolysaccharide recruits dendritic cell progenitors to non-lymphoid tissues. *Transplantation* (in press).

Robertson, M. (1991) Antigen processing. Proteosomes in the pathway. *Nature*, **353**, 300–1.

Roche, P., Marks, M. & Cresswell, P. (1991) Formation of a nine subunit complex by HLA class II glycoproteins and the invariant chain. *Nature*, **354**, 392–394.

Rochester, C.L., Goodell, E.M., Stoltenborg, J.K. & Bowers, W.E. (1988) Dendritic cells from rat lung are potent accessory cells. *Am. Rev. Resp. Dis.*, **138**, 121–8.

Romagnani, S. (1994) Lymphokine production by human T cells in disease states. *Ann. Rev. Immunol.*, **12**, 227–57.

Romani, N., Koide, S., Crowley, M. *et al.* (1989) Presentation of exogenous protein antigens by dendritic cells to T cell clones. Intact protein is presented best by immature, epidermal Langerhans cells. *J. Exp. Med.*, **169**, 1169–78.

Rotzschke, O. & Falk, K. (1994) Origin, structure and motifs of naturally processed MHC class II ligands. *Curr. Opin. Immunol.*, **6**, 45–51.

Sallusto, F. & Lanzavecchia, A. (1994) Efficient presentation of soluble antigen by cultured human dendritic cells is maintained by granulocyte/macrophage colony stimulating factor plus interleukin 4 and down regulated by tumor necrosis factor alpha. *J. Exp. Med.*, **179**, 1109–18.

Sant, A.J. & Miller, J. (1994) MHC class II antigen processing: biology of invariant chain. *Curr. Opin. Immunol.*, **6**, 57–63.

Seder, R.A. & Paul, W.E. (1994) Acquisition of lymphokine-producing phenotype by CD4+ T cells. *Ann. Rev. Immunol.*, **12**, 635–73.

Shawar, S.M., Vyas, J.M., Rodgers, J.R. & Rich, R.R. (1994) Antigen presentation by major histocompatibility complex class I-B molecules. *Ann. Rev. Immunol.*, **12**, 839–80.

Steinman, R.M. (1991) The dendritic cell system and its role in immunogenicity. *Ann. Rev. Immunol.*, **9**, 271–96.

Stern, L.J., Brown, J.H., Jardetzky, T.S. *et al.* (1994) Crystal structure of the human class II MHC protein HLA-DR1 complexes with an influenza virus peptide. *Nature*, **368**, 215–21.

Stossel, H., Koch, F., Kampgen, E. *et al.* (1990) Disappearance of certain acidic organelles (endosomes and Langerhans cell granules) accompanies loss of antigen processing capacity upon culture of epidermal Langerhans cells. *J. Exp. Med.*, **172**, 1471–82.

Tanaka, K. (1994) Role of proteasomes modified by interferon-gamma in antigen processing. *J. Leuk. Biol.*, **56**, 571–5.

Terhorst, C., Alarcon, B., de Vries, J. & Spits, H. (1988) T lymphocyte recognition and activation. In: *Molecular Immunology* (eds B.D. Homes & D.M. Glover). IRL Press, Oxfrod.

Townsend, A. & Bodmer, H. (1989) Antigen recognition by class I-restricted T lymphocytes. *Ann. Rev. Immunol.*, **7**, 601–24.

Trowbridge, I.S. & Thomas, M.L. (1994) CD45: an emerging role as a protein tyrosine phosphatase required for lymphocyte activation and development. *Ann. Rev. Immunol.*, **12**, 85–116.

Tschopp, J. & Nabholz, M. (1990) Perforin-mediated target cell lysis by cytolytic T lymphocytes. *Ann. Rev. Immunol.*, **8**, 279–302.

Vitetta, E.S., Berton, M.T., Burger, C., Kepron, M., Lee, W.T. & Xin, X.M. (1991) Memory B cells and T cells. *Ann. Rev. Immunol.*, **9**, 193–218.

de Vries, J. (ed.) (1994) Atopic allergy and other hypersensitivities. *Curr. Opin. Immunol.*, **6**, 835–73.

Wang, B., Rieger, A., Kilgus, O. *et al.* (1992) Epidermal Langerhans cells from normal human skin bind monomeric IgE via Fc epsilon RI. *J. Exp. Med.*, **175**, 1353–65.

Weiss, S. & Bogen, B. (1991) MHC class II-restricted presentation of intracellular antigen. *Cell*, **64**, 767–76.

West, M.A., Lucocq, J.M. & Watts, C. (1994) Antigen processing and class II MHC peptide-loading compartments in human B-lymphoblastoid cells. *Nature*, **369**, 147–51.

CHAPTER 8

Immunological Tolerance and T-Cell Anergy

G.F. Hoyne, C. Hetzel & J.R. Lamb

During development, T and B cells express an antigen-specific receptor on their surface. If the rearranged receptor displays a high affinity for a self antigen, the maturation of that cell is terminated. Thus, mature T and B cells present in the peripheral circulation are selected to express antigen receptors that specifically respond to foreign antigens and ignore self proteins. A failure to control the development of self-reactive lymphocytes could lead to the development of autoimmune (or autoallergic — see Chapter 2) diseases. This review will mainly focus on the mechanisms for controlling T-cell development in the thymus and in the periphery, but where appropriate we shall see how similar mechanisms operate to control the fate of self-reactive B cells.

Unlike the foreign antigen receptor on B cells (the immunoglobulin (Ig) molecule) which recognizes a tertiary conformation on a foreign protein, antigen-specific receptors (TcR) expressed on the surface of all T cells cannot bind to intact proteins. Instead the TcR recognizes processed peptide presented in association with a self major histocompatibility complex (MHC) molecule on the surface of a target cell or antigen-presenting cell (APC). For the majority of circulating peripheral T cells, the TcR is a heterodimeric protein composed of α- and β-chains (Davis & Bjorkman, 1988; Matis, 1988). A second type of TcR has recently been defined, consisting of γ- and δ-chains. T cells expressing this latter class of receptor are highly tropic for mucosal sites such as the skin and gut (Goodman & Lefrancois, 1989; Havran *et al.*, 1989a,b; Lefrancois & Goodman, 1989; Lefrancois *et al.*, 1990). However, this chapter will focus exclusively on the function of T cells expressing the αβ TcR, since they have been most extensively studied.

T cells can be divided into two functionally distinct groups, based on whether the TcR recognizes antigen in association with class I or class II MHC molecules. The TcR on CD8+ cytotoxic T cells (Tc) recognizes antigen derived from intracellular biosynthesis (e.g. virus-infected cells or autologous proteins) presented on class I MHC molecules, while CD4+ T helper cells (Th) respond to exogenously derived antigen presented in association with class II MHC. Class I and class II MHC molecules therefore sample peptides derived from different intracellular compartments, and after peptide loading they are transported to the cell surface where they can be surveyed by passing T cells. Class I MHC molecules are expressed on all somatic cells, while the expression of class II MHC molecules is restricted to specialized cells (APC), which include dendritic cells, macrophages and B cells. Because of the limitations of this review, it is impossible to cover the area of antigen presentation in depth, but readers are referred to Chapter 7 and other reviews which have been written on this topic (Jenkins & Schwartz, 1987; Brodsky & Guargliardi, 1991). The recognition of a foreign antigen requires that a T cell must come into contact with an APC, and this involves a large number of different molecules. Some of these molecules have been identified in recent years and are shown in Fig. 8.1. When a T cell and APC first come together, the association between the cells is weak and is mediated by adhesion molecules (e.g. LFA-1, CD2, LFA-3, ICAM-1). This allows the TcR to scan the surface of the APC for appropriate ligands to which it can bind. If such ligands are found, then the adhesion between the T cell and APC is greatly increased and this allows for TcR to become cross-linked. T cells form clusters around an APC and these clusters can last for several hours,

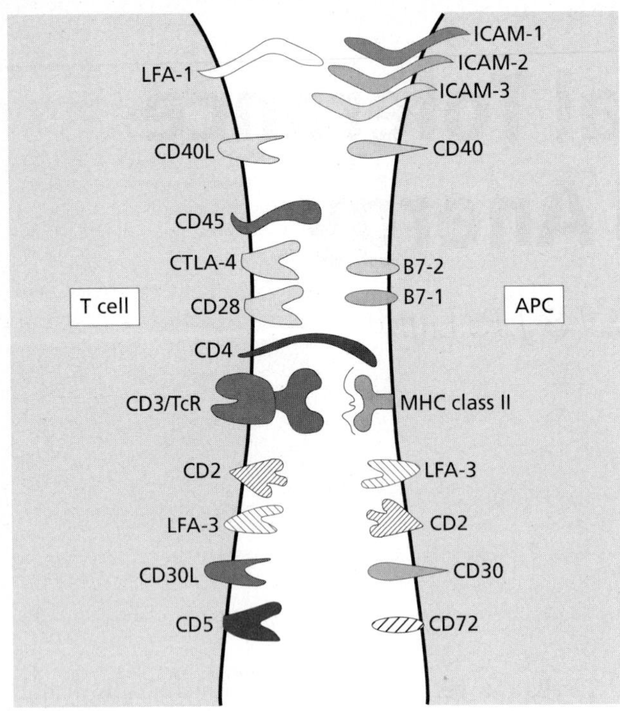

Fig. 8.1 Antigen-dependent and -independent interactions between a T cell and APC. The various molecules which play an important role in T-cell recognition of a foreign antigen are shown.

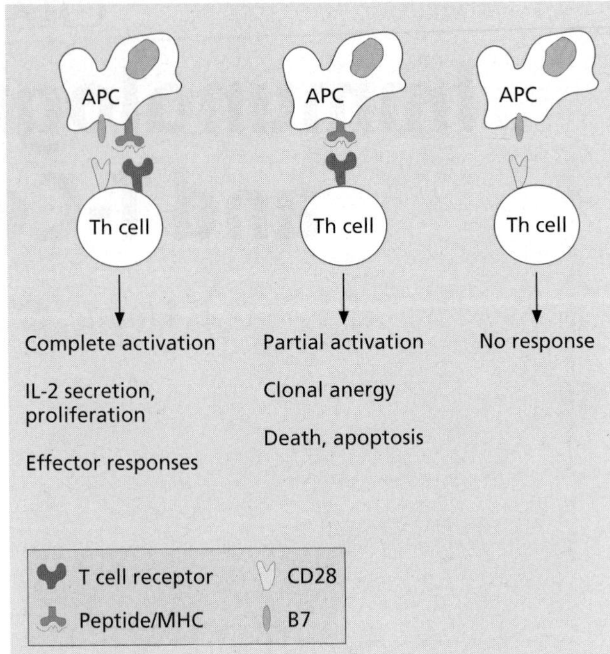

Fig. 8.2 Potential outcomes following T-cell recognition of antigen on the surface of an APC. To achieve complete activation, a T cell must recognize a peptide–MHC complex in association with a second non-specific signal. Th B7-1 and B7-2 ligands are expressed on the surface of professional APC and interact with the CD28 and CTLA-4 antigens on the surface of the T cell. The signals delivered through CD28 synergize with those transduced through the TcR, and induce maximal activation of the IL-2 gene and IL-2 receptor gene expression. When a T cell responds to a peptide–MHC complex alone this delivers only a partial signal to the T cell and will render it refractory to further stimulation. The state of non-responsiveness which develops has been termed clonal anergy. Finally, the binding of the CD28 molecule to B7-1 or B7-2 alone, in the absence of TcR-derived signals, is insufficient to induce T-cell activation.

allowing for maximal stimulation of the T cell. Eventually the T cell will move away from the APC, and it will then begin to proliferate and secrete lymphokines.

Signals involved in T-cell activation

T-cell activation requires the delivery of two separate signals (Fig. 8.2). Signal one is delivered through the TcR upon recognition of a peptide–MHC complex. Signal two is a non-specific signal delivered by the APC and is mediated through the CD28 receptor on T cells. Recent studies have identified that the surface molecules B7-1 and B7-2 present on professional APC are the natural ligands for the CD28 molecule, and the signals they deliver can synergize with those derived from the TcR to give rise to complete activation of the T cell (Jenkins & Schwartz, 1987; Linsley *et al.*, 1991a; Harding *et al.*, 1992). A second molecule expressed on activated T cells, referred to as CTLA-4, was originally identified by Linsley and coworkers and was also shown to be important in T-cell activation. The CTLA-4 molecule has a 20-fold higher affinity for B7-1 and B7-2 than CD28 (Linsley *et al.*, 1991b), and a fusion protein containing the extracellular portion of the CTLA-4 molecules fused to the Fc portion of a human IgG molecule, called CTLA-4Ig, can effectively block the signals delivered by the B7 molecules at the time of antigen recognition and thus can inhibit T-cell activation (Linsley *et al.*, 1992). Using murine T-cell clones it was shown that TcR recognition of the peptide–MHC complex alone on an APC delivers only a partial signal, and the T cell becomes refractory to further signalling through its receptor (Schwartz, 1990). The state of non-responsiveness that develops has been termed clonal anergy and is characterized by a failure of T cells to proliferate and secrete interleukin-2 (IL-2) when re-stimulated *in vitro* (Jenkins *et al.*, 1988; Schwartz, 1990). Anergy can also be induced in T cells by the addition of CTLA-4Ig into cultures at the time of antigen recognition, supporting the notion that the signals delivered by B7-1 and B7-2 are involved in costimulating T cells (Tan *et al.*, 1993).

Human T-cell clones can also be rendered anergic *in vitro*, by treatment with either supra-optimal concentrations of peptide or with superantigens (Lamb *et al.*, 1983; O'Hehir *et al.*, 1991). Human T cells normally display phenotypic changes after the induction of anergy, which includes down-modulation of TcR, CD3 and CD28 and a concomitant increase in expression of CD2 and CD25 (IL-2Rα) (O'Hehir *et al.*, 1991). Anergic T cells normally show heightened proliferative responses to exogenous IL-2 *in vitro*, due most likely to the up-regulation of CD25 expression (O'Hehir *et al.*, 1991). Anergy is normally induced by signalling T cells through their receptor in the absence of costimulation, and thus agents such as soluble anti-TcR, anti-CD3 monoclonal antibodies (mAb) (Go & Miller, 1992) or Con A (Kang *et al.*, 1992) are all effective in inducing anergy. Also T cells can be rendered anergic by treatment with ionophore alone (Schwartz, 1990). The induction of T-cell anergy can be abrogated either by the addition of IL-2 (Schwartz, 1990) or by cross-linking the CD28 molecule on the surface of T cells (Harding *et al.*, 1992). More recently, it has been shown that anergy can be abrogated by signalling T cells through the IL-2Rγc chain (Boussiotis *et al.*, 1994). The IL-2Rγc chain is also shared by other cytokine receptors, such as IL-4 and IL-7, and thus treatment of T cells during the induction phase of anergy with either IL-4 or IL-7 can also successfully abrogate the induction of anergy (Boussiotis *et al.*, 1994).

Intrathymic self-tolerance

A major problem that has hampered studies on lymphocyte development in the past, was the low frequency of antigen-specific T or B cells in the peripheral circulation, in the order of $1:10^5$ cells. However, this problem has been technically overcome by the development of molecular techniques that have enabled the transgenic expression of T-cell receptor α- and β-chains specific for a particular antigen. In TcR transgenic mice, as many as 90% of peripheral T cells can express the TcR of interest. Thus, the fate of such antigen-reactive cells can be followed *in vivo*, using mAb directed against specific α or β TcR chains; in some cases mAb against the whole TcR complex, referred to as the clonotype, have been developed (von Boehmer, 1990; Miller & Morahan, 1992). B-cell receptor transgenic mice, that overexpress the heavy and light chain genes from an antibody molecule specific for a particular antigen, have also been developed. These mice have proven to be valuable tools in dissecting the mechanisms determining the fate of self-reactive B cells (Goodnow, 1992).

To ensure T cells leaving the thymus recognize antigen in an MHC-restricted fashion, only immature thymocytes whose TcR have sufficient binding affinity for peptide–MHC complexes expressed on thymic stromal cells will be given the signal to differentiate further (Lo & Spent, 1986; Kisielow *et al.*, 1988). This process is known as positive selection. Early studies with TcR transgenic mice demonstrated that engagement of the TcR on class I MHC molecules allows differentiation to the CD4– CD8+ T-cell lineage, whereas, recognition of peptide–class II MHC complexes leads to differentiation to the CD4+ CD8– T-cell lineage (Teh *et al.*, 1988). If thymocytes express a TcR with high affinity for peptide–self MHC complexes, there are two well-defined mechanisms by which these self-reactive cells can be controlled—clonal deletion and clonal anergy. A significant proportion of the deletion of immature thymocytes has been shown to occur by a process called activation-induced programmed cell death (PCD), or apoptosis (Smith *et al.*, 1989; Suth & Sprent, 1994). Typically, thymocytes undergoing PCD show cytoplasmic changes, including membrane blebbing, chromatin condensation and nucleosome length DNA fragmentation (Wyllie, 1980). Although clonal deletion is the main way of inducing tolerance in the thymus, clonal anergy can also occur. This may be important as a back-up mechanism to prevent autoreactive cells that avoid negative selection from reaching the periphery. Two independent research groups, using bone marrow chimeras, showed the important role for clonal anergy in the induction of central tolerance in the thymus (Ramsdell *et al.*, 1989; Roberts *et al.*, 1990). They found that T cells bearing certain self-reactive V_β sequences were not deleted in the thymus, but rather when these cells were cultured with the self antigen (*Mls*^{1a}) they did not proliferate *in vitro* with F1 APC or with TcR-specific anti-V_β antibodies.

Only a small percentage (≈ 10%) of thymocytes are ever positively selected, thus ensuring that the majority of potentially autoreactive T cells never reach the periphery. Thymic APC are unlikely to be able to present the whole myriad of potential self peptides to thymocytes, and so a substantial number of T cells probably enter the peripheral circulation with the potential for autoreactivity (Guerder *et al.*, 1994). Therefore, there must be mechanisms in place in the periphery to prevent activation of these self-reactive T cells, since a failure to control them could give rise to an autoimmune/autoallergic disease. The mechanisms that have been identified will be reviewed below. In addition, the way in which the immune system regulates responses to innocuous antigens that pose no significant threat to the body will be examined. The generation of an aberrant response against dietary or inhaled antigens could result in the development of allergic disease and thus be detrimental to the host.

Mechanisms of peripheral T-cell tolerance to self and foreign antigens

Peripheral T-cell deletion

Although the thymus is recognized as the primary site for T-cell deletion, recent experiments suggest that mature self-reactive T cells can also undergo deletion in the periphery upon recognition of self antigen. Female mice which expressed a transgenic TcR specific for the male H-Y antigen, were injected with male (H-Y+) lymph node cells and it was noticed that within 7 days there was a decline in the number of T cells expressing the transgenic receptor which lasted for over 2 months. The decrease was not due to natural attrition of TcR+ cells or to cells being anatomically sequestered. Rather, the decrease was due to deletion, since there was a decrease in the absolute number of T cells in the periphery (Zhang *et al.*, 1992). In support of this, TcR transgenic T cells were observed to be undergoing PCD 4 days after injection of male H-Y+ lymph node cells (Carlow *et al.*, 1992). Peripheral T-cell deletion was also observed in transgenic mice which expressed the L^d antigen on pancreatic acinar cells and a TcR specific for the L^d molecule. Thymocyte development proceeded normally in these double transgenic mice, but a large depletion in TcR+ cells was seen in the periphery (Fields & Loh, 1992).

Sprent and colleagues demonstrated that tolerance to the minor histocompatibility antigen, *Mls*^{1a}, can involve clonal deletion. In these experiments recipient mice were thymectomized in order to monitor the fate of the *Mls*-reactive T cells *in vivo*. Mice were injected with *Mls* disparate splenocytes intravenously and the induction of tolerance was found to coincide with an initial expansion of $V_\beta6$+ T cells over the first 4 days, followed by deletion of $V_\beta6$+ T cells by day 14 (Webb *et al.*, 1990). In another study, T cells from a female mouse expressing a transgenic receptor specific for the male-specific antigen H-Y were injected into recipient male nude mice. Over the first 5 days, the $V_\beta5$+ H-Y TcR+ T-cell population expanded in number and then rapidly disappeared from the peripheral circulation within 9 days (Rocha & von Boehmer, 1991). In both of these studies, deletion of self-reactive T cells is likely to be mediated by apoptosis. Another mechanism to eliminate self-reactive T cells from the peripheral circulation has been identified through the effect of veto cells. Here specific lymphoid cells can kill T cells whose TcR recognize antigen on the veto cell itself. Veto cells, however, have only been shown to kill class I-restricted T cells (Rammensee, 1989).

Partial deletion

Some studies have identified that tolerance to extrathymic antigens can result from partial deletion of self-reactive T cells. In these studies, autoreactive T cells with high affinity for the self antigen were deleted, leaving behind only low-affinity clones in the peripheral circulation. It has been demonstrated that an APC must present a critical number of peptide–MHC complexes in order to elicit a T-cell response (Harding & Unanue, 1990). Therefore low-affinity T cells would require a high concentration of self antigen in order to be activated, and it is unlikely that this level would be achieved in the periphery (Jones-Youngblood *et al.*, 1990; Whiteley *et al.*, 1990; Wieties *et al.*, 1990; Yui *et al.*, 1990, 1992; Poindexter *et al.*, 1992).

Clonal anergy of self-reactive peripheral T cells

Perhaps one of the best studied disease models in experimental animals is for the development of diabetes. The equivalent disease in humans is insulin-independent diabetes mellitus (IDDM). Autoimmune Autoimmune/autoallergic diabetes involves lymphocytic destruction of the pancreatic islets due to infiltrating CD4+ and CD8+ T cells which are activated by recognition of islet-specific antigens. The identity of some of these potential target autoantigens has been identified in recent years in both rodents and humans (Kaufman *et al.*, 1993; Tisch *et al.*, 1993). Experimental models of autoimmunity/autoallergy have been developed, using either single or double transgenic mice. Single transgenic mice display tissue-specific expression of either an allo-MHC molecule or foreign antigen (e.g. influenza haemagglutinin (HA) protein, Fig. 8.3). Under both conditions the transgenic protein is treated as a self protein by the animal, and thus the development of tolerance to the transgenic proteins can be studied. To generate a double transgenic animal, mice with tissue-specific expression of the target antigen (e.g. HA on pancreatic islet β-cells) are cross-bred with mice expressing a TcR specific for the target antigen (Fig. 8.3). Examples of the different transgenic model systems that have been used to study autoimmune diseases are listed in Table 8.1.

One of the first studies to be reported used an I-E– strain of mouse and introduced the I-E^k gene under an insulin promoter, therefore directing expression of I-E^k to the pancreatic islet β-cells. Mice expressing the transgenic I-E^k did not develop insulinitis, indicating that self-reactive T cells were tolerant to the I-E molecule, and this was confirmed by a failure of peripheral T cells and thymocytes from these mice to proliferate *in vitro* in the presence of I-E^k-expressing splenocytes (Lo *et al.*, 1988). Expressing I-E^k under the elastase promoter on pancreatic acinar cells achieved the same result and the animals did not develop diabetes. Again, both peripheral T cells and thymocytes were unresponsive to I-E^k-expressing splenocytes *in vitro*. In both these studies, tolerance to the I-E^k molecule did not involve clonal deletion of Vβ5$^+$- or Vβ17$^+$-expressing T cells but was due to the induction of clonal anergy (Burkly *et al.*, 1989; Lo *et al.*, 1989). This was confirmed by the fact that peripheral T cells from I-E^k-expressing mice were unresponsive to anti-Vβ5 or anti-Vβ17 antibodies. When pancreatic β-cells expressing the I-E^k transgene were used to present antigen to a T-cell clone *in vitro*, it was noticed the T cell was rendered anergic, suggesting that pancreatic

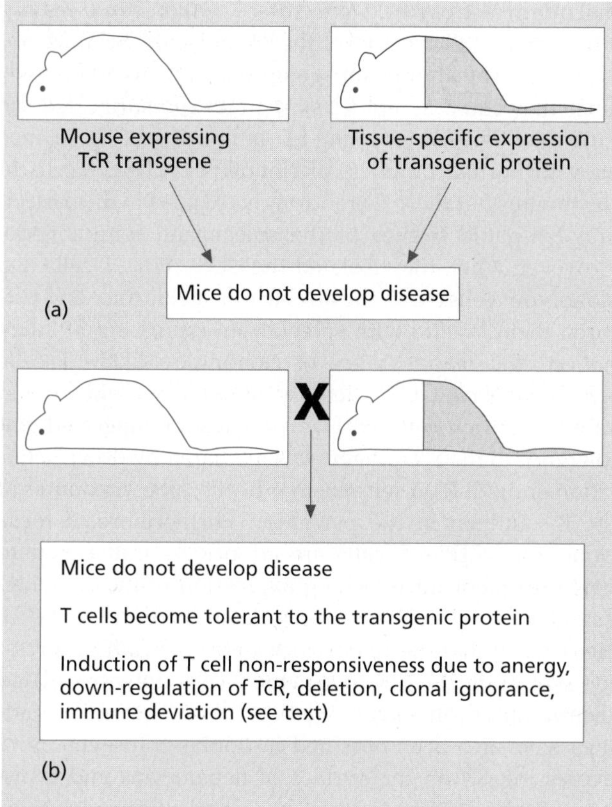

Fig. 8.3 T-cell tolerance in transgenic mice. Mice which express either a transgenic TcR or display tissue-specific expression of a transgenic protein do not normally develop autoimmune disease. When the two strains of mice are bred together the double transgenic mice do not develop disease either, and studies have shown that this may be due to the induction of clonal anergy, deletion, TcR down-regulation, clonal ignorance or immune deviation (see text).

β-cells lack expression of the molecules required to costimulate T-cell function (Markmann *et al.*, 1988). Similar findings were also observed in another study, where expression of the K^b molecule was directed to pancreatic β-cells and these K^b-expressing mice were then bred with mice carrying a TcR transgene specific for the K^b molecule. The double transgenic mice did not develop diabetes, accepted K^b skin grafts and their peripheral T cells did not display cytotoxic T lymphocyte (CTL) activity to K^b-bearing target cells *in vitro*. The number of TcR clonotype+ cells did not diminish in these double transgenic animals, suggesting that self-reactive T cells were anergic (Morahan *et al.*, 1989).

If the induction of anergy in the model systems described above was due to TcR recognition of self antigen–MHC complexes on tissue APC in the absence of costimulation, the prediction would be that by supplying these tissue APC with the necessary costimulatory molecules it should be possible to induce an autoimmune autoallergic disease, since they should be able to activate self-reactive T cells normally present in the periphery. This question was recently addressed in an elegant experiment, in which mice expressing the I-E^k molecule on pancreatic acinar cells were crossed with mice displaying transgenic expression of the B7-1 costimulatory molecule under the insulin promoter which directs its expression to the surface of pancreatic β-cells (Guerder *et al.*, 1994). Transgenic mice that express either I-E^k alone or B7-1 alone do not develop spontaneous diabetes (Guerder *et al.*, 1994). However, double transgenic mice co-expressing I-E^k and B7-1 do develop diabetes, with lymphocytic infiltrates that eventually destroy the pancreatic islet β-cells (Guerder *et al.*, 1994). These findings support the previous

Table 8.1 Transgenic models for studying peripheral T-cell tolerance.

Antigen	Site of tissue expression	TcR specificity	T-cell tolerance *in vitro*	T-cell tolerance *in vivo*	Mechanism of tolerance	Reference
L^d	Acinar cells	L^d CD8+ TcR	ND	Yes	Deletion	Fields & Loh, 1992
I-E^k	Islet β-cells, acinar cells		Yes	Yes	Anergy*	Lo *et al.*, 1988, 1989
K^b	Islet β-cells	K^b CD8+ TcR	Yes	Yes	Anergy	Morahan *et al.*, 1989
LCMV GP	Islet β-cells	LCMV-CD8+ TcR	No	Yes	Ignorance	Olhashi *et al.*, 1991
LCMV GP, NP	Islet β-cells	K^b CD8+ TcR	No	Yes	Ignorance	Oldstone *et al.*, 1991
K^b	Neuroectoderm		No	Yes	TcR down-regulation	Schonrich *et al.*, 1991a
K^b	Hepatocytes	K^b CD8+ TcR	No	Yes	Anergy	Schonrich *et al.*, 1991b
Flu HA†	Islet β-cells	HA- CD4+ TcR	No	Yes	Immune deviation	Scott *et al.*, 1994

*Stimulated T cells *in vitro* with α-Vβ5 or α-Vβ 17 mAb.
† Flu HA, influenza haemagglutinin protein.
ND, not tested.

in vitro observations made by Markmann *et al.* (1988), that tissue APC induce anergy because they are unable to costimulate potentially autoreactive T cells.

Clonal ignorance

Tolerance to some extrathymic self antigens is thought to arise because the protein is expressed in an immunologically privileged site and is thus inaccessible to self-reactive T cells. Therefore, a situation could exist where potentially autoreactive T cells could circulate in the periphery, but would not be activated because either the T cells cannot gain access to the particular tissue or, alternatively, tissue APC may be unable to provide adequate co-stimulation to the T cell. To demonstrate this *in vivo,* transgenic mice expressing the glycoprotein from the lymphocytic choriomeningitis virus (LCMV) on pancreatic β-cells (Ohashi *et al.*, 1991) were crossed with transgenic mice expressing a CD8+ TcR specific for the epitope 32–42 on the LCMV antigen presented in association with H-$2D^b$. The double transgenic mice did not develop spontaneous diabetes, although they had circulating T cells in the periphery which could lyse D^b-bearing target cells *in vitro,* and the absolute number of TcR+ T cells were unaltered when compared with numbers obtained in single TcR transgenic mice (Ohashi *et al.*, 1991). Therefore, tolerance was not due to deletion or clonal anergy. If the double transgenic mice were infected with the LCMV virus, they developed diabetes, indicated by a rise in blood glucose and destruction of the β-cell islets by a CD8+ T-cell infiltrate (Ohashi *et al.*, 1991). A similar study employed transgenic mice which expressed either the LCMV nuclear protein (NP) or glycoprotein (GP) on the surface of pancreatic β-cells, and under normal conditions the NP- or GP-transgenic mice did not develop spontaneous diabetes, but only did so after infection with the wild-type LCMV virus (Oldstone *et al.*, 1991). The results obtained from these two independent studies might suggest that the potentially autoreactive T cells did not induce disease, because they were not given the appropriate activation signals by tissue APC. Alternatively, the T cells may not be able to gain access into the tissue where the target antigen is expressed. Thus, it was only after the viral infection through the release of inflammatory cytokines which may have altered either the vascular permeability and/or the migration properties of lymphocytes that have allowed access of the viral-specific CD8+ T cells into the target tissue.

T-cell receptor down-regulation

A further method for inhibiting the function of self-reactive T cells in the periphery has emerged. Transgenic mice expressing the H-$2K^b$ molecule on cells of neuroectodermal origin (astrocytes) were crossed with mice expressing a transgenic TcR specific for the K^b molecule (Schonrich *et al.*, 1991a). The double transgenic mice were tolerant to K^b, since they could accept K^b skin grafts and supported the growth of the K^b-expressing EL-4 tumour cell. These mice showed normal numbers of clonotype+ CD8+ T cells in the thymus but these were strongly reduced in the peripheral lymphoid tissues of the spleen and lymph node. However, when they isolated the CD8– TcR– T cells (i.e. clonotype⁻ cells) from the double transgenic mice and cultured them *in vitro* with splenocytes expressing K^b, they noticed the reappearance of clonotype+ CD8+ T cells which displayed CTL activity on K^b-expressing target cells (Schonrich *et al.*, 1991a). These results suggested that tolerance to the K^b antigen was mediated by down-regulation of the TcR on self-reactive T cells, after encounter of the K^b antigen in the periphery. Furthermore, if these clonotype⁻ CD8– T cells are adoptively transferred to naive recipient mice lacking expression of the K^b molecule, TcR expression was up-regulated (Ferber *et al.*, 1994). However, if these recipient mice were given a K^b-expressing skin graft, the TcR transgenic T cells down-regulated their receptors once again (Ferber *et al.*, 1994). Similar findings have also been obtained in double transgenic mice expressing K^b on the surface of hepatocytes and transgenic T cells specific for the K^b molecule (Schonrich *et al.*, 1991b), except that the down-regulation of CD8 and TcR expression was not reversible in culture with K^b-expressing splenocytes (Schonrich *et al.*, 1991b). It remains to be determined why recognition of K^b molecules on these different tissue APC does not induce anergy, as has previously been observed with expression of target antigens on pancreatic β-cells (Lo *et al.*, 1988; Morahan *et al.*, 1989). Tissue APC from various sites may express different levels of peptide–MHC complexes on the surface, or they may utilize different accessory or costimulatory molecules; therefore, depending on the tissue microenvironment, TcR occupancy may have distinct outcomes.

Immune deviation

Studies on long-term murine CD4+ T-cell clones demonstrated that Th cells could be divided into two subsets called Th1 or Th2, based on the patterns of lymphokine secretion (Mosmann & Coffman, 1989). The concept of Th1/Th2 differentiation (Fig. 8.4) has been substantiated *in vivo* in different animal models of infection (Seder & Paul, 1994). Resistance or susceptibility to disease in various mouse strains has been shown to correlate with the type of lymphokines produced *in vivo* by antigen-specific Th cells. Th1 cells secrete IL-2, interferon-γ (IFN-γ), tumour necrosis factor-α (TNF-α) and usually provide minimal B-cell help (i.e. by promoting IgG2a synthesis) (Seder & Paul, 1994). Th1 cells are more commonly

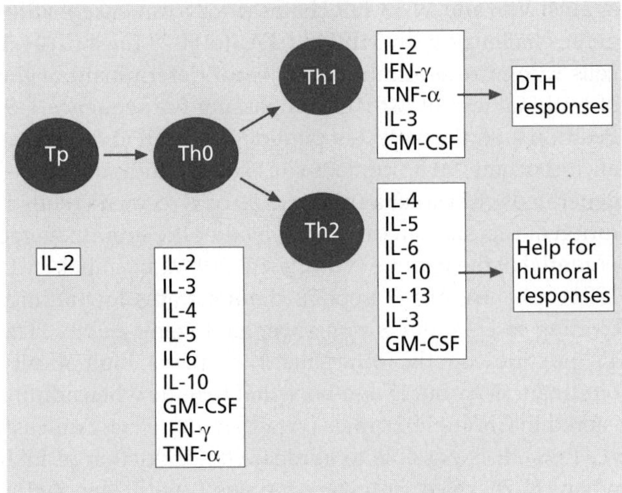

Fig. 8.4 Development of Th cells. Naive T cells which first enter the peripheral circulation have a minimal potential to secrete lymphokines and are referred to as proliferative T cells (Tp). Upon antigen recognition, the T cells have the capacity to secrete a large number of lymphokines and are termed Th0 cells. Depending on the previous encounter with antigen, the Th0 cell may terminally differentiate to become either a Th1 or Th2 cell.

involved in eliciting delayed-type hypersensitivity (DTH) reactions, and thus are especially effective in controlling responses to parasitic infection. Th2 cells, on the other hand, are more efficient in inducing humoral responses to foreign antigens, and when activated can secrete IL-4, IL-5, IL-6, IL-10 and IL-13. IL-4 and IL-6 are growth factors for B cells, with IL-4 being especially important for promoting isotype switching to IgE. In addition, Th2 cells promote the production of isotypes IgG1, IgG2b and IgA (Seder & Paul, 1994). Human Th2-like cells also support the production of isotypes IgG3 and IgG4. It is now well established that the lymphokines secreted by Th1 and Th2 cells are mutually antagonistic. For instance, IFN-γ secreted by Th1 cells can inhibit the growth of Th2 cells. Alternatively, IL-4 and IL-10 have mutually antagonistic activities, and can inhibit the activation and growth of Th1 cells. Such are the reciprocal effects of these lymphokines that it provides great potential for polarization of the immune response to an antigen (Seder & Paul, 1994).

Recently it has been shown that tolerance to a self antigen may involve non-MHC gene effects that may be explained in terms of immune deviation. In one study, transgenic mice expressed the influenza virus HA protein on pancreatic β-cells and were bred with mice expressing a transgenic TcR specific for an epitope on the HA protein that is recognized by CD4+ T cells. The double transgenic mice that were first generated were F1 hybrids on an H-2^{bxd} background and did not develop spontaneous diabetes (Scott *et al.*, 1994). These mice had normal numbers of TcR+ T cells in the thymus and peripheral lymphoid tissues compared with single TcR transgenic mice, and they showed normal levels of surface expression of the TcR chains. Peripheral T cells from double transgenic mice were not anergic, since they proliferated strongly to HA antigen *in vitro*. Also, these mice did not develop diabetes when they were infected with whole influenza virus (Scott *et al.*, 1994). However, it was identified that the incidence of spontaneous diabetes dramatically increased in offspring, as mice were bred to homozygosity on the H-2^d background. Mice that were bred to the H-2^b background did not develop disease. When T cells were obtained from mice from the third-generation backcross from the H-2^d background vs. the H-2^b background, it was noticed that the former group had T cells that produced high levels of IFN-γ and IL-4 when stimulated *in vitro*, whereas T cells from the H-2^b background mice secreted IFN-γ and only very low levels of IL-4 (Scott *et al.*, 1994). Therefore resistance to diabetes correlated with the induction of a Th2-like response to the self antigen *in vivo*. This was the first reported example where non-MHC genes, e.g. lymphokine genes, have been shown to determine susceptibility to an autoimmune disease (Scott *et al.*, 1994).

Tolerance in B lymphocytes

In mammals the maturation of B cells does not occur in a defined organ, unlike T-cell development which occurs in the thymus. Immature B cells leave the bone marrow and undergo several stages of maturation in the peripheral circulation. Studies on B-cell tolerance to self antigens have identified that clonal anergy, clonal deletion and clonal ignorance can all function to control the development of autoreactive B cells (Nossal, 1983; Goodnow, 1992). As discussed above, thymocytes which express a TcR with high affinity for self-MHC will be deleted, and the same fate is followed by B cells whose rearranged Ig receptor has high affinity for self antigens (Nossal, 1983; Goodnow, 1992). However, another novel mechanism has recently been identified that can lead to the deletion of self-reactive B cells, which involves competition between antigen-reactive B cells and self-reactive B cells at the level of entry into follicular compartments in lymphoid tissues (Cyster *et al.*, 1994). Upon activation with antigen, specific B cells enter germinal centres of lymphoid follicles where they receive signals to survive and their Ig genes can undergo somatic hypermutation to generate higher affinity antibodies and isotype switching (MacLennan *et al.*, 1991). In a very elegant series of experiments using transgenic mice, it was demonstrated that self-reactive B cells, although they could enter lymphoid tissues, were denied access into lymphoid follicles (Cyster *et al.*, 1994). Thus, self-reactive B cells would accumulate at the marginal zone of the follicle and eventually die. Self-reactive B cells that overexpressed the *Bcl-2* gene displayed increased survival, but they were still denied access into the lymphoid follicle (Cyster *et al.*, 1994). Thus, these studies highlight important differences between self-reactive B cells and antigen-specific B cells that have not previously been appreciated. It is not clear at this stage if the self-reactive B cells die because they are unable to respond to a growth factor released by stromal cells in the follicle, or whether they lack expression of a specific adhesion molecule that would normally allow them to migrate into the germinal centre.

Manipulation of the peripheral immune response to self antigens

T cells play an important role in the development of a number of different autoimmune diseases in humans. The induction of an autoimmune response leads to inflammation of the target tissue and in some cases to its eventual destruction. There has been much interest in recent years in trying to develop specific forms of immunotherapy for autoimmune diseases. The main aim of these therapies is to inactivate or delete self-reactive T cells from the peripheral circulation. A number of animal models of autoimmune disease have been studied experimentally, and often the clinical symptoms displayed by affected animals have an immunopathology similar to the equivalent disease state in humans. Some of these animal models are listed in Table 8.2.

Experimental allergic encephalomyelitis (EAE) is a demyelinating disease of rodents which is thought to be equivalent to multiple sclerosis in humans (Zamvil & Steinman, 1990). The disease is mediated by CD4+ T cells reactive to myelin basic protein (MBP) (Yui *et al.*, 1990). The murine disease is characterized by an oligoclonal T-cell response, and the TcR of autoreactive T cells displays restricted usage of *V*β gene sequences (Acha-Orbea *et al.*, 1988). Thus, it is possible to prevent the induction of EAE in mice of the H-2^u haplotype by treating them with mAb against Vβ8 and Vβ13 TcR chains prior to an encephalitogenic challenge with MBP in CFA. In H-2^u mice CD4+ T cells recognize an immunodominant determinant at the N-terminal end of MBP encompassing the sequence 1–9. Position 4 on the MBP 1–9 peptide has been identified as an important MHC contact site, and peptide analogues generated with either an alanine (A) or tyrosine (Y) substitution at this site can dramatically alter the immunogenic potential of the peptide (Wraith *et al.*, 1989a,b; Smilek *et al.*, 1991). The 4A Ac1–9 peptide demonstrates low-affinity binding to I-A^u and is non-encephalitogenic *in vivo*. The 4Y peptide, on the other hand, displays high-affinity binding to I-A^u but is non-encephalitogenic when administered in CFA to H-2^u mice (Wraith *et al.*, 1989a; Smilek *et al.*, 1991). It is possible to abrogate the induction of EAE when H-2^u mice are co-immunized with the Ac1–9 peptide plus the 4A analogue in CFA (Wraith *et al.*, 1989a; Smilek *et al.*, 1991). It is still unknown how the 4A peptide analogue prevents EAE, but possibilities such as antigenic competition for binding to I-A^u and the induction of anergy in MBP-specific T cells have been ruled out.

Immunotherapy of autoallergic disease

It is well established that administering proteins or peptides through mucosal surfaces can inhibit the response of antigen-specific CD4+ T cells *in vivo* (Mowat, 1987; Weiner *et al.*, 1994). Studies with animals have established that feeding antigens results in oral tolerance, which affects both the humoral and cellular arms of the immune response. Depending on the dose of antigen administered, inhibition of T-cell responses can result from the induction of clonal anergy or active suppression mediated by regulatory T cells that secrete inhibitory cytokines (Weiner *et al.*, 1994). Oral tolerance has been shown to be effective in preventing autoimmune disease in a number of different animal models. Also, inhalation of retinal antigens can prevent the induction of the autoallergic disease experimental allergic uveoretinitis in rats (Dick *et al.*, 1993).

Table 8.2 Animal models of autoallergy.

Disease	Animal	Target organ	Target antigen	T-cell effector	Human disease equivalent
EAE	Mouse/rat	Nervous system	MBP, PLP	CD4+ T cell	Multiple sclerosis
EAU	Mouse/rat	Retina (eye)	S retinal antigen	CD4+ T cell	Retinitis
CIA	Mouse/rat	Limb joints	Collagen	CD4+ T cell	Rheumatoid arthritis
AIA	Mouse/rat	Limb joints	Collagen	CD4+ T cell	Arthritis
Diabetes	Mouse*/rat	Pancreas	GAD	CD4+ T cell	IDDM

EAE, experimental allergic encephalomyelitis; EAU, experimental allergic uveoretinitis; CIA, collagen-induced arthitis; AIA, adjuvant-induced arthritis; GAD, glutamic acid decarboxylase; IDDM, insulin-independent diabetes mellitis; PLP, proteolipid protein.

* The most studied murine model of diabetes is the NOD mouse, non-obese diabetic mouse. The NOD gene defect has been bred onto various H-2 backgrounds.

Similar success has been reported with the intranasal administration of an immunodominant peptide derived from collagen type II, in the prevention of a rat model of collagen-induced arthritis (Staines *et al.*, 1994). The success obtained with some of the preclinical trials has allowed doctors to begin human clinical trials based on similar forms of therapy (see review in Weiner *et al.*, 1994). These involve patients being fed with homogenized extracts of tissues containing the appropriate self antigen. The therapy trials in progress include those for patients suffering with multiple sclerosis, rheumatoid arthritis and uveoretinitis (summarized in Weiner *et al.*, 1994).

Peptide-based immunotherapy has also been studied in experimental systems. Recently, Metzler & Wraith (1993) showed that inhalation of a high dose of the Ac1–9 peptide in naive H-2^u mice could prevent the induction of EAE. In addition, intranasal peptide treatment could prevent EAE following immunization with whole-spinal-cord homogenate (Metzler & Wraith, 1993). The immunological mechanisms underlying the control of T-cell function in this sytem remain to be defined. It has also been possible to prevent the induction of EAE in H-2^u mice following intraperitoneal injection of the Ac1–9 peptide in IFA (Gaur *et al.*, 1992). This route of administration has previously been shown to effective in inhibiting T-cell responses to whole-protein antigens *in vivo* (Ria *et al.*, 1990). The loss of T-cell responsiveness to MBP in this system was shown to be due to the induction of anergy in peptide-specific T cells (Gaur *et al.*, 1992).

Administering antigenic peptides intravenously can inhibit T-cell responses to protein antigens *in vivo* as a result of clonal anergy (Gammon & Sercarz, 1989). Recently, it was shown that intravenous administration of peptide could inhibit the development of diabetes in the LCMV transgenic model described above (Ohashi *et al.*, 1991). Aichele *et al.* (1994) showed that intravenous injection of 300 μg of the 32–42 LCMV peptide is thought to bring about clonal anergy in peptide-specific CD8+ T cells, thus rendering animals non-responsive to challenge with the native LCMV virus.

Antagonism and partial agonism of the TcR

The activation of CD4+ T cells can be blocked either *in vitro* or *in vivo* by mixing an antigenic peptide with a non-stimulatory MHC binding peptide (Adorini *et al.*, 1988, 1989). This strategy is referred to as MHC blockade, and it has been proposed that it could be useful in immunotherapy of autoimmune autoallergic diseases (Adorini *et al.*, 1990). However, the main drawbacks with this approach are that it lacks specificity and that the MHC blocking peptides are likely to have a short half-life in the peripheral circulation (Ishioka *et al.*, 1994). However, in recent years another novel strategy has emerged that may provide a more effective way of regulating T-cell responses *in vivo*. This approach is based on the use of synthetic peptide analogues that carry amino-acid substitutions at critical TcR contact sites. De Magistris *et al.* (1992) first showed that peptide analogues of the influenza haemagglutinin epitope recognized by CD4+ T cells, HA 307–319, could interact with the TcR but did not activate the T cell, such that they failed to secrete IL-2 or proliferate and did not mobilize intracellular calcium when re-stimulated *in vitro* (Ruppert *et al.*, 1993). The HA analogues did not induce anergy, but instead are thought to act as TcR antagonists and mediate their effects in an antigen-specific manner (De Magistris *et al.*, 1992). Thus, recent findings suggest that the function of TcR to distinguish between antigenic peptides and antagonistic peptides lies in the junctional regions of the TcR (Ostrov *et al.*, 1993). TcR antagonists or altered peptide ligands (APL) have now been identified for both CD4+ and CD8+ T cells (Evavold & Allen, 1991; Evavold *et al.*, 1993; Jameson *et al.*, 1993; Racioppi *et al.*, 1993). A characteristic pattern is emerging, however, as more APL are being identified. The general consensus from these studies suggests that T-cell recognition of an APL alters at least one of the possible effector responses of that T cell. For example, Evavold and Allen demonstrated that recognition of a myoglobin peptide analogue abrogated proliferation but did not affect IL-4 production by a Th2 cell (Evavold & Allen, 1991). Other studies have identified uncoupling of cytolysis from proliferation in CD8+ and CD4+ T-cell clones, respectively (Evavold *et al.*, 1993; Jameson *et al.*, 1993). Racciopi *et al.* (1993) have identified that TcR recognition of an APL on a mutant class II could give rise to receptor antagonism. T cells that responded to the APL secreted normal levels of IL-3, showed up-regulation of IL-2R expression but did not secrete IL-2. More recently, APL have been shown to be able to induce clonal anergy in both Th1 and Th2 clones *in vitro* (Sloan-Lancaster *et al.*, 1993, 1994a). Unlike previous studies, where clonal anergy was induced in murine Th1 clones by recognition of antigen on fixed APC (Jenkins & Schwartz, 1987; Jenkins *et al.*, 1988; Schwartz, 1990; Linsley *et al.*, 1991a,b, 1992; Harding *et al.*, 1992), or by blocking B7 derived co-stimulatory signals (Chen & Nabavi, 1994), APL could induce anergy on live APC (Sloan-Lancaster *et al.*, 1993, 1994a). The induction of anergy in both Th1 and Th2 cells appeared to be long lived. The induction of anergy induced by an APL has been shown to generate a unique pattern of tyrosine phosphorylation, characterized by a lack of ξ-chain phosphorylation and a failure of the Zap70 tyrosine kinase to associate with the TcR (Sloan-Lancaster *et al.*, 1994b).

The mechanisms regulating TcR antagonism are still largely unknown. Some studies suggest that APL may fail to induce appropriate T-cell–APC clustering, and therefore this may not allow T cells to receive adequate costimulation (Ruppert *et al.*, 1993). Alternatively, recognition of the APL may only elicit a low-affinity interaction between the TcR and peptide–MHC complex, and this could affect the nature of the signals transduced through the TcR (Ruppert *et al.*, 1993). Thus, the studies on APL have further highlighted the complexity of TcR–peptide–MHC interactions. It would appear that there exists a continuum of interactions between TcR and peptide–MHC, ranging from full agonism to complete antagonism (reviewed in Kuchroo *et al.*, 1994). A number of peptides have been identified that contain a mixture of agonist/antagonist properties and which elicit a subset of responses when recognized by T cells.

Since APL can uncouple T-cell effector responses *in vitro*, it has been proposed that they may one day be applied clinically in the therapy of immunologically based diseases. Early results are now emerging from experimental studies which demonstrate that an APL derived from a T-cell epitope on myelin proteolipid protein can act *in vivo* as a TcR antagonist and can prevent the induction of EAE (Kuchroo *et al.*, 1994). Similarly, the generation of allergen-specific APL with the capacity to inhibit IL-4 synthesis in CD4+ T cells may be useful in allergen injection immunotherapy. However, it is still to be determined if APL turn out to be effective in modulating T-cell responses *in vivo* in other experimental systems.

Regulating immune responses to dietary and inhaled protein antigens

The lung and the gastrointestinal tract are two sites of the body which are under constant antigenic exposure, and therefore the mucosal immune system present in these organs faces the task of discriminating between harmless antigens and those associated with pathogenic microorganisms. A failure to do so could lead to a potentially deleterious response, and thus result in allergic sensitization to a common dietary antigen or an inoffensive aeroallergen. The body has available a number of innate immune mechanisms that essentially act as barriers to prevent access of antigens into the peripheral circulation, and these have been recently reviewed by Holt (Holt & McMenamin, 1989; Holt *et al.*, 1990). As illustrated above, animal models have provided an excellent insight into the mechanisms which regulate T-cell tolerance to self antigen. In addition, animal models have also been valuable in aiding our understanding of how allergic responses to environmental antigens are regulated.

It was originally demonstrated in 1911 by Wells that feeding proteins to guinea pigs made them refractory to a further immunogenic challenge with the same antigen. The phenomenon of oral tolerance has mainly been studied in experimental animals (Thomas *et al.*, 1979; Challacombe & Tomasl, 1980; Mowat & Ferguson, 1981, 1982a,b; Mowat *et al.*, 1982; Mowat & Parrot, 1983; Mowat, 1985; Strobel & Ferguson, 1985; Bitmar & Whitacre, 1988; MacLennan *et al.*, 1991; Miller *et al.*, 1991, 1994; Whitacre *et al.*, 1991; Hoyne *et al.*, 1993, 1994; McMenamin & Holt, 1993; Metzler & Wraith, 1993), but a recent paper has also demonstrated that oral tolerance operates in human volunteers fed keyhole limpet haemocyanin (KLH) (Husby *et al.*, 1994). Early studies presented evidence for a role of CD8+ T suppressor (Ts) cells in mediating oral tolerance, but more recent studies have not supported earlier findings. It appears that feeding antigens to experimental animals elicits a strong CD4+ T-cell response (Hoyne *et al.*, 1993) that eventually leads to the induction of anergy (Whitacre *et al.*, 1991; Melamed & Friedman, 1993; Garside *et al.*, 1994). Hoyne *et al.* (1993) recently showed that in OVA-fed mice, CD4+ T cells from the mesenteric lymph node (MLN), Peyer's patch and spleen were able to secrete IFN-γ, granulocyte macrophage colony-stimulating factor (GM-CSF) but no IL-2 or IL-4, and did not proliferate when stimulated with antigen *in vitro*. Also, after OVA feeding, CD4+ T-cell responses to the I-A^d restricted epitope OVA323–339 were abrogated, whereas under conditions which lead to intragastric priming of CD4+ T cells to OVA, T-cell responses to this epitope were unaffected (Hoyne *et al.*, 1994).

The development of oral tolerance to MBP in rats has led to conflicting mechanisms being suggested for the control of T-cell function (Bitmar & Whitacre, 1988; Miller *et al.*, 1991, 1994). Recent studies have provided a reason for this conflict, and have shown that distinct mechanisms can be induced that are dependent on the dose of antigen fed. Feeding high doses of antigen will lead to the development of clonal anergy in CD4+ T cells (Whitacre *et al.*, 1991; Weiner *et al.*, 1994), whereas feeding low doses of MBP can lead to the activation of CD8+ Ts cells (Miller *et al.*, 1991) which mediate their suppressive effects on CD4+ T cells by secreting transforming growth factor-β1 (TGF-β1), which in turn can profoundly inhibit their proliferative response. More recently, Chen *et al.* isolated MBP-reactive CD4+ T-cell clones from the MLN from MBP-fed mice (Chen *et al.*, 1994). These cells predominantly secrete IL-4, IL-10 and TGF-β1. The authors suggest that feeding may therefore preferentially activate CD4+ T cells that secrete regulatory cytokines, and these cells will limit the effector response being elicited to the fed antigen. Another study has also reported that feeding tends to preferentially activate CD4+ T cells with the capacity to secrete IL-4, by examining the T-cell responses elicited in orally sensitized mice (Xu-Amano *et al.*, 1993).

Holt and coworkers originally showed that nebulizing low doses of protein antigens to mice or rats can elicit a transient IgE response that is down-regulated over time (Holt *et al.*, 1981; Holt & Leivers, 1982; Sedgwick & Holt, 1983, 1984, 1985). Recent studies indicate that early after antigen exposure, CD4+ T cells become sensitized to the inhaled protein and secrete IL-4 and IL-2. This CD4+ T-cell (Th2-like) response is short-lived, however, and is replaced by a Th-1-like response dominated by the secretion of IFN-γ by antigen-specific CD8+ T cells (McMenamin & Holt, 1993). Furthermore, these CD8+ T cells can inhibit the function of antigen-specific CD4+ T cells when adoptively transferred to a naive recipient (McMenamin *et al.*, 1991). It has recently been discovered that these regulatory CD8+ T cells express the γδ TcR, and need only be present in low numbers to mediate their suppressive effects *in vivo* (McMenamin *et al.*, 1994). This is the first demonstration that γδ+ T cells can directly inhibit the function of CD4+ αβ+ T cells. Thus, further studies are required to elucidate how these CD8+ γδ T cells become activated following presentation of an exogenous protein *in vivo*, and moreover, to identify the mechanism by which the suppression is mediated, i.e. by inhibitory cytokines or direct cell–cell interactions.

In a similar model, mice which are nebulized daily with the soluble protein ovalbumin become sensitized to the protein, produce IgE against the inhaled protein and develop airways hyperresponsiveness (Renz *et al.*, 1992). Thus, it has been proposed that this animal model could be useful in studying the basis of allergic disease. Two different populations of CD4+ T cells appear to become activated to the inhaled antigen (Renz *et al.*, 1993). CD4+ T cells expressing a $V_{\beta}8.2$ TcR seem important for the induction of IgE synthesis, while CD4+ T cells expressing a $V_{\beta}2$ TcR inhibit the production of IgE *in vivo* (Renz *et al.*, 1993). CD8+ T cells also become activated in this model, and can inhibit IgE synthesis when adoptively transferred to a naive mouse (Renz *et al.*, 1994). At present it is not clear if the CD8+ T cells described by Renz *et al.* (1994), and those identified by McMenamin *et al.* (1991, 1994), are equivalent populations. CD8+ T cells seem to play a role in inhibiting IgE synthesis in other animal models, as well as suggesting they play an integral part in regulating IgE synthesis *in vivo* (reviewed in Kemeny & Diaz-Sanchez, 1993).

The above studies indicate the important role that CD4+ T cells play in the induction of IgE responses to foreign antigens (O'Hehir *et al.*, 1991), although genetic and environmental factors are also important in determining susceptibility to developing allergic disease in humans (reviewed in Holt & McMenamin, 1989; Holt *et al.*, 1990). One of the best studied groups of allergens is that of the house dust mite (HDM), *Dermatophagoides* species. There are seven major HDM allergens that have been characterized to date (Thomas, 1993) and approximately 10% of the population become sensitized to these allergens, displaying symptoms of perennial rhinitis, atopic dermatitis or asthma. Both atopic and non-atopic individuals become sensitized to the aeroallergens of the ubiquitous HDM, but it is the nature of the responses elicited by these two groups which are important in determining the outcome of allergen exposure. HDM-reactive CD4+ T cells isolated from atopic patients predominantly secrete IL-4, IL-5 and IL-10 when activated with HDM antigen *in vitro*, and thus are characterized as being Th2 dominant (Thomas, 1993; Romagnani, 1994). HDM-reactive CD4+ T cells isolated from non-atopic patients, on the other hand, tend to secrete IL-2 and IFN-γ, and thus are Th-1 dominant. Unlike the murine immune system, human CD4+ T cells do not display such strict Th1 and Th2 phenotypes, but a predominance of Th2-like cells during an allergic response could provide the immunological stimulus to drive and maintain a persistent allergen-specific IgE antibody response *in vivo* (Romagnani, 1994). Also, during the effector phase of the allergic response the lymphokines released from Th2 cells could act on other inflammatory cells (e.g. mast cells, basophils, eosinophils) and initiate a self-perpetuating cycle which could sustain the inflammatory response. Two recent studies have been published which support the notion that there is a preferential expansion of Th2-like cells during an allergic response. Robinson *et al.* (1992) demonstrated that there was an increased frequency of T cells in the bronchoalveolar lavage fluid from asthmatic patients that were positive for IL-2, IL-3, IL-4, IL-5 and GM-CSF mRNA. In support of this, Durham *et al.* (1992) have shown that there was a significant increase in the number of mRNA+ cells producing IL-3, IL-4, IL-5 and GM-CSF in nasal biopsies taken from asthmatic vs. control patients following local nasal allergen provocation. The authors noted that allergen provocation usually resulted in tissue eosinophilia, which may have been a consequence of the release of cytokines by infiltrating cells that display a profile similar to that of murine Th2 cells.

Treatment of allergy

Present desensitization therapy is successful for a limited number of HDM allergic patients but more effective methods of modulating the allergic immune response are required. Recently, it has been shown that human HDM-reactive CD4+ T cells can be inactivated *in vitro* by exposing them to supra-optimal concentrations of their cognate peptide (O'Hehir *et al.*, 1991; Higgins *et al.*, 1992). Peptide treatment *in vitro* results in the induction of clonal anergy. During the induction phase of anergy, T cells secrete a range of lymphokines (IL-2, IL-4 and IFN-γ) (O'Hehir *et al.*, 1991). However, when re-stimulated *in vitro*, they selectively down-regulate IL-2 and IL-4 but maintain IFN-γ secretion (O'Hehir *et al.*, 1991). This type of response would therefore be of value in the clinical situation. It has recently been shown that it is possible to inhibit the function of allergen-reactive CD4+ T cells *in vivo* by either intranasal or oral administration of a peptide containing the immunodominant T-cell epitope of Der p 1, p1 111–139, in H-2b mice (Hoyne *et al.*, 1993, 1994a). Following peptide treatment, T cells failed to secrete IL-2 or proliferate when stimulated with antigen *in vitro*. Peptides containing the immunodominant epitope of Der p 1 were more effective in inhibiting T-cell function than those containing only minor epitopes (Hoyne *et al.*, 1994a). In addition, it was found that both intranasal and orally administered peptide could inhibit the response to the whole protein on both naive and sensitized mice (Hoyne *et al.*, 1993, 1994a). Thus, induction of non-responsiveness to one epitope appeared to induce suppression to other potential epitopes on the antigen. However, it remains to be defined how the phenomenon of cross-epitope regulation is mediated *in vivo*. Recently, it has been shown that intranasal peptide treatment induces a strong transient activation in antigen-specific CD4+ T cells, and that within 14 days of treatment, T cells down-regulate the capacity to secrete IL-2, IL-4 and IFN-γ (Hoyne *et al.*, 1994b). Thus, it appears that intranasal peptide may induce clonal anergy in allergen-specific T cells. Further studies are required to determine if CD8+ T cells play a role in regulating the CD4+ T-cell response following intranasal or oral peptide treatment.

Briner *et al.* (1993) have recently demonstrated that subcutaneous administration of peptides derived from the major cat allergen Fel d 1, could inhibit the T-cell responses to the whole allergen in mice. Allergen-specific CD4+ T cells from peptide-treated mice showed down-regulated secretion of IL-2, IL-4 and IFN-γ when stimulated with antigen *in vitro*. However, in these studies, mice were treated with two different peptides, and thus it is difficult to know if one peptide would be as effective as the two, as has previously been found in other studies (Hoyne *et al.*, 1993, 1994a; Metzler & Wraith, 1993).

Conclusions

This chapter has examined the different ways in which the immune system regulates T-cell responses to self and foreign antigens. Transgenic animals have been particularly useful in elucidating the mechanisms that regulate the function of self-reactive T cells *in vivo*. In addition, ways of directly manipulating the immune response in either naive or sensitized animals, to either self or foreign antigens, through the use of antigenic peptides and altered peptide ligands, have been examined. The information obtained from these studies will be important in devising effective strategies for the treatment of allergic diseases in humans. Some of these strategies are already being tested in clinical trials, and the outcomes of these studies are awaited with interest.

References

Acha-Orbea, H., Mitchell, D.J., Timmermann, L. *et al.* (1988) Limited heterogenity of T cell receptors from lymphocytes mediating autoimmune encephalomyelitis allows specific immune intervention. *Cell*, **54**, 263–73.

Adorini, L., Barnaba, V., Bona, C. *et al.* (1990) New perspectives on immunointervention in autoimmune diseases. *Immunol. Today*, **11**, 383–6.

Adorini, L., Appella, E., Doria, G., Cardinaux, F. & Nagy, Z.A. (1989) Competition for antigen presentation in living cells involves exchange of peptides bound by class II MHC molecules. *Nature*, **342**, 800–3.

Adorini, L., Muller, S., Cardinaux, F., Lehmann, P.V., Falcioni, F. & Nagy, Z.A. (1988) *In vivo* competition between self peptides and foreign antigens in T-cell activation. *Nature*, **334**, 623–5.

Aichele, P., Kybruz, D., Ohashi, P. *et al.* (1994) Peptide-induced tolerance to prevent autoimmune diabetes in a transgenic mouse model. *Proc. Nat. Acad. Sci. USA*, **91**, 444–8.

Bitmar, D.M. & Whitacre, C.C. (1988) Suppression of experimental autoimmune encephalomyelitis by the oral administration of myelin basic protein. *Cell. Immunol.*, **112**, 364–70.

von Boehmer, H. (1990) Developmental biology of T cells in T cell-receptor transgenic mice. *Ann. Rev. Immunol.*, **8**, 309–26.

Boussiotis, V.A., Barber, D.L., Nakarai, T. *et al.* (1994) Prevention of T cell anergy by signaling through the gc chain of the IL-2 receptor. *Science*, **266**, 1039–42.

Briner, T.J., Kuo, M.-C., Rogers, B.R. *et al.* (1993) Inhibition of allergen-specific murine T cell responses after subcutaneous injection of T cell epitope-containing peptide. *Proc. Nat. Acad. Sci. USA*, **90**, 7608.

Brodsky, F.M. & Guargliardi, L.E. (1991) The cell biology of processing and presentation. *Ann. Rev. Immunol.*, **9**, 707–44.

Burkly, L.C., Lo, D., Kanagawa, O., Brinster, R.L. & Flavell, R.A. (1989) T-cell tolerance by clonal anergy in transgenic mice with nonlymphoid expression of MHC class II I-E. *Nature*, **342**, 564–6.

Carlow, D.A., Teh, S.J., van Oers, N.S.C., Miller, R.G. & Teh, H.S. (1992) Peripheral tolerance through clonal deletion of mature CD4– CD8+ T cells. *Int. Immunol.*, **4**, 599–604.

Challacombe, S.J. & Tomasi, T.J. (1980) Systemic tolerance and secretory immunity after oral immunization. *J. Exp. Med.*, **152**, 1459–72.

Chen, Y., Kuchroo, V.K., Inobe, J.-I., Hafler, D.A. & Weiner, H.L. (1994) Regulatory T cell clones induced by oral tolerance: suppression of autoimmune encephalomyelitis. *Science*, **265**, 1237–40.

Chen, C. & Nabavi, N. (1994) *In vitro* induction of T cell anergy by blocking B7 and early T cell costimulatory molecule ETC-1/B7-2. *Immunity*, **1**, 147–54.

Cyster, J.G., Hartley, S.B. & Goodnow, C.C. (1994) Competition for follicular niches excludes self-reactive cells from the recirculating B-cell repertoire. *Nature*, **371**, 389–95.

Davis, M. & Bjorkman, P. (1988) T cell antigen receptor genes and T cell recognition. *Nature*, **334**, 395–402.

De Magistris, M.T., Alexander, J., Coggeshall, M. *et al.* (1992) Antigen analog–major histocompatibility complexes act as antagonists of the T cell receptor. *Cell*, **68**, 625–34.

Dick, A.D., Cheng, Y.F., McKinnon, A., Liversidge, J. & Forrester, J.V. (1993) Nasal administration of retinal antigens suppresses the inflammatory response in experimental allergic uveoretinitis. A preliminary report of intranasal induction of tolerance with retinal antigens. *Brit. J. Ophthalmol.*, **77**, 171–81.

Durham, S.R., Ying, S., Varney, V.A. *et al.* (1992) Cytokine messenger RNA expression for IL-3, IL-4, IL-5, and granulocyte/macrophage-colony-stimulating factor in the nasal mucosa after local allergen provocation: realtionship to tissue eosinophilia. *J. Immunol.*, **148**, 2390–4.

Evavold, B.D. & Allen, P.M. (1991) Separation of IL-4 production from Th proliferation by an altered TcR ligand. *Science*, **252**, 1308–10.

Evavold, B.D., Sloan-Lancaster, J., Hsu, B.L. & Allen, P.M. (1993) Separation of T helper 1 clone cytolysis from proliferation and lymphokine production using analog peptides. *J. Immunol.*, **150**, 3131–40.

Ferber, I., Schonrich, G., Schenkel, J., Mellor, A.L., Hammerling, G. & Arnold, B. (1994) Levels of peripheral tolerance induced by different doses of antigen. *Science*, **263**, 674–6.

Fields, L.E. & Loh, D.Y. (1992) Organ injury associated with extrathymic induction of immune tolerance in doubly transgenic mice. *Proc. Nat. Acad. Sci. USA*, **89**, 5730–4.

Gammon, G. & Sercarz, E. (1989) How some T cells escape tolerance induction. *Nature*, **342**, 183–5.

Garside, P., Steel, M., Worthey, E.A. *et al.* (1994) A role for clonal anergy/deletion in oral tolerance. *Immunology*, **83** (Suppl. 1), 46.

Gaur, A., Wiers, B., Liu, A., Rothbard, J. & Fathman, C.G. (1992) Amelioration of autoimmune encephalomyelitis by myelin basic protein synthetic peptide-induced anergy. *Science*, **258**, 1491–4.

Go, C. & Miller, J. (1992) Differential induction of transcription factors that regulate the interleukin 2 gene during anergy induction and restimulation. *J. Exp. Med.*, **175**, 1327–36.

Goodman, T. & Lefrancois, L. (1989) Intraepithelial lymphocytes. Anatomical site, not T cell receptor form, dictates phenotype and function. *J. Exp. Med.*, **170**, 1569–81.

Goodnow, C.C. (1992) Transgenic mice and analysis of B-cell tolerance. *Ann. Rev. Immunol.*, **10**, 489–518.

Guerder, S., Meyerhoff, J. & Flavell, R. (1994) The role of the T cell costimulator B7-1 in autoimmunity and the induction and maintenance of tolerance to peripheral antigen. *Immunity*, **1**, 155–6.

Harding, F.A., McArthur, J.G., Gross, J.A., Raulet, D.H. & Allison, J.P. (1992) CD28-mediated signalling co-stimulates murine T cells and prevents induction of anergy in T cell clones. *Nature*, **356**, 607–9.

Harding, C.V. & Unanue, E.R. (1990) Quantitation of antigen-presenting cell MHC class II/peptide complexes necessary for T-cell stimulation. *Nature*, **346**, 574–6.

Havran, W.L., Grell, S., Duwe, G. *et al.* (1989a) Limited diversity of T-cell receptor gamma-chain expression of murine Thy-1+ dendritic epidermal cells revealed by V gamma 3-specific monoclonal antibody. *Proc. Nat. Acad. Sci. USA*, **86**, 4185–9.

Havran, W.L., Poenie, M., Tigelaar, R.E., Tsien, R.Y. & Allison, J.P. (1989b) Phenotypic and functional analysis of gamma delta T cell receptor-positive murine dendritic epidermal clones. *J. Immunol.*, **142**, 1422–8.

Higgins, J.A., Lamb, J.R., Marsh, S.G.E. *et al.* (1992) Peptide-induced non-responsiveness of HLA-DP restricted human T cells reactive with *Dermatophagoides* spp. (house dust mite). *J. Allergy Clin. Immunol.*, **90**, 749–56.

Holt, P.G., Batty, J.E. & Turner, K.J. (1981) Inhibition of specific IgE responses in mice by pre-exposure to inhaled antigen. *Immunology*, **42**, 409–17.

Holt, P.G. & Leivers, S. (1982) Tolerance induction via antigen inhalation: isotype specificity, stability and involvement of suppressor T-cells. *Int. Arch. Allergy Appl. Immunol.*, **67**, 155–60.

Holt, P.G. & McMenamin, C. (1989) Defence against allergic sensitization in the healthy lung: the role of inhalation tolerance. *Clin. Exp. Allergy*, **19**, 255–62.

Holt, P.G., McMenamin, C. & Nelson, D. (1990) Primary sensitisation to inhalant allergens during infancy. *Ped. Allergy Immunol.*, **1**, 3–13.

Hoyne, G.F., Askonas, B.A., Hetzel, C., Thomas, W.R. & Lamb, J.R. (1994b) Intranasal administration of a peptide derived from house dust mite induces transient activation in CD4+ T cells prior to the development of non-responsiveness *Int. Immunol.*, **8**, 335–42.

Hoyne, G.F., Callow, M.G., Kuhlman, J. & Thomas, W.R. (1993) T cell lymphokine response response to orally administered antigens during priming and unresponsiveness. *Immunology*, **78**, 534–40.

Hoyne, G.F., Callow, M.G., Kuo, M-C. & Thomas, W.R. (1994) Differences in epitopes recognized during oral tolerance and priming. *Immunol. Cell. Biol.*, **72**, 29–33.

Hoyne, G.F., Callow, M.G., Kuo, M-C. & Thomas, W.R. (1994a) Inhibition of T cell responses by feeding peptides containing major and cryptic epitopes. Studies with the *Der p* I allergen. *Immunology*, **83**, 190–5.

Hoyne, G.F., O'Hehir, R.E., Wraith, D.C., Thomas, W.R. & Lamb, J.R. (1993) Inhibition of T cell and antibody responses to the major house dust mite allergen in naive and sensitized mice. *J. Exp. Med.*, **178**, 1783–8.

Husby, S., Mestecky, J., Moldoveneau, Z., Holland, S. & Elson, C.O. (1994) Oral tolerance in humans. T cell but not B cell tolerance after antigen feeding. *J. Immunol.*, **152**, 4663–70.

Ishioka, G.Y., Adorini, L., Guery, J.-C. *et al.* (1994) Failure to demonstrate long-lived MHC saturation both *in vitro* and *in vivo*. Implications for therapeutic potential of MHC-blocking peptides. *J. Immunol.*, **152**, 4310–19.

Jameson, S.C., Carbone, F.R. & Bevan, M.J. (1993) Clone-specific T cell receptor antagonists of major histocompatibility complex class I-restricted cytotoxic T cells. *J. Exp. Med.*, **177**, 1541–50.

Jenkins, M.K. & Schwartz, R.H. (1987) Antigen presentation by chemically modified splenocytes induces antigen-specific T cell unresponsiveness *in vitro* and *in vivo*. *J. Exp. Med.*, **165**, 302–19.

Jenkins, M.K., Ashwell, J.D. & Schwartz, R.H. (1988) Allogeneic non-T spleen cells restore the responsiveness of normal T cell clones stimulated with antigen and chemically modified antigen-presenting cells. *J. Immunol.*, **140**, 3324–30.

Jones-Youngblood. S.L., Wieties, K., Forman, J. & Hammer, R.E. (1990) Effect of the expression of a hepatocyte-specific MHC molecule in transgenic mice on T cell tolerance. *J. Immunol.*, **144**, 1187–95.

Kang, S.-M., Beverly, B., Tran, A.-C., Brorson, B., Schwartz, R.H. & Lenardo, M.J. (1992) Transactivation by AP-1 is a molecular target of T cell clonal anergy. *Science*, **257**, 1134–8.

Kaufman, D.L., Clare-Salzler, M., Tian, J. *et al.* (1993) Spontaneous loss of T-cell tolerance to glutamic acid decarboxylase in murine insulin-dependent diabetes. *Nature*, **366**, 69–72.

Kemeny, D.M. & Diaz-Sanchez, D. (1993). The role of CD8+ T cells in the regulation of IgE. *Clin. Exp. Allergy*, **23**, 466–70.

Kisielow, P., Teh, H.S., Bluthmann, H. & von Boehmer, H. (1988) Positive selection of antigen-specific T cells in thymus by restricting MHC molecules. *Nature*, **335**, 730–3.

Kuchroo, V.K., Greer, J.M., Kaul, D. *et al.* (1994) A single TCR antagonist peptide inhibits experimental allergic encephalomyelitis mediated by a diverse T cell repertoire. *J. Immunol.*, **153**, 3326–33.

Lamb, J.R., Skidmore, B.J., Green, N., Chiller, J.M. & Feldmann, M. (1983) Induction of tolerance in influenza virus-immune T lymphocyte clones with synthetic peptides of influenza hemagglutinin. *J. Exp. Med.*, **157**, 1434–47.

Lefrancois, L. & Goodman, T. (1989) *In vivo* modulation of cytolytic activity and Thy-1 expression in TCR-$\gamma\delta^+$ intraepithelial lymphocytes. *Science*, **243**, 1716–18.

Lefrancois, L., LeCorre, R., Mayo, J., Bluestone, J.A. & Goodman, T. (1990) Extrathymic selection of TCR $\gamma\delta^+$ T cells by class II major histocompatibility complex molecules. *Cell*, **63**, 333–40.

Linsley, P., Wallace, P., Johnson, J. *et al.* (1992) Immunosuppression *in vivo* by a soluble form of the CTLA-4 T cell activation molecule. *Science*, **257**, 792–5.

Linsley, P.S., Brady, W., Grosmaire, L., Aruffo, A., Damle, N.K. & Ledbetter, J.A. (1991a) Binding of the B cell activation antigen B7 to CD28 costimulates T cell proliferation and interleukin 2 mRNA accumulation. *J. Exp. Med.*, **173**, 721–30.

Linsley, P.S., Brady, W., Urnes, M., Grosmaire, L., Damle, N. & Ledbetter, J. (1991b) CTLA-4 is a second receptor for the B cell activation antigen B7. *J. Exp. Med.*, **174**, 561–9.

Lo, D. & Sprent, J. (1986) Identity of cells that imprint H-2-restricted T-cell specificity in the thymus. *Nature*, **319**, 672–5.

Lo, D., Burkly, L.C., Widera, G. *et al.* (1988) Diabetes and tolerance in transgenic mice expressing class II MHC molecules in pancreatic beta cells. *Cell*, **53**, 159–68.

Lo, D., Burkly, L.C., Flavell, R.A., Palmiter, R.D. & Brinster, R.L. (1989) Tolerance in transgenic mice expressing class II major histocompatibility complex on pancreatic acinar cells. *J. Exp. Med.*, **170**, 87–104.

MacLennan, I.C.M., Oldfield, S., Liu, Y.-J. & Lane, P.J.L. (1991) Regulation of B cell populations. *Curr. Top. Pathol.*, **79**, 37–57.

McMenamin, C. & Holt, P.G. (1993) The natural immune response to inhaled soluble protein antigens involves major histocompatibilty complex (MHC) class I-restricted CD8+ T cell-mediated but class II-restricted CD4+ T cell-dependent immune deviation resulting in selective suppression of immunoglobulin E production. *J. Exp. Med.*, **178**, 889–99.

McMenamin, C., Oliver, J., Girn, B. *et al.* (1991) Regulation of T-cell sensitization at epithelial surfaces in the respiratory tract: suppression of IgE responses to inhaled antigens by CD3+ TCR α-/β- lymphocytes (putative γ/δ T cells). *Immunology*, **74**, 234–9.

McMenamin, C., Pimm, C., McKersey, M. & Holt, P.G. (1994) Regulation of IgE responses to inhaled antigen in mice by antigen-specific $\gamma\delta$ T cells. *Science*, **265**, 1869–71.

Markmann, J., Lo, D., Naji, A., Palmiter, R.D., Brinster, R.L. & Heber-Katz, E. (1988) Antigen-presenting function of class I MHC expressing pancreatic β cells. *Nature*, **336**, 476.

Matis, L.A. (1988) Diversity and antigen specificity of the T cell receptor. *Curr. Opin. Immunol.*, **1**, 84–7.

Melamed, D. & Friedman, A. (1993) Direct evidence for anergy in T lymphocytes tolerised by oral administration of ovalbumin. *Eur. J. Immunol.*, **23**, 935–42.

Metzler, B. & Wraith, D.C. (1993) Inhibition of experimental autoimmune encephalomyelitis by inhalation but not oral administration of the encephalitogenic peptide: influence of MHC binding affinity. *Int. Immunol.*, **5**, 1159–68.

Miller, A., Lider, O. & Weiner, H.L. (1991) Antigen-driven bystander suppression after oral administration of antigens. *J. Exp. Med.*, **174**, 791–8.

Miller, A., Lider, O., Abramsky, O. & Weiner, H.L. (1994) Orally administered myelin basic protein in neonates primes for immune responses and enhances experimental autoimmune encephalomyelitis in adult animals. *Eur. J. Immunol.*, **24**, 1026–32.

Miller, J.F.A.P. & Morahan, G. (1992) Peripheral T cell tolerance. *Ann. Rev. Immunol.*, **10**, 51–69.

Morahan, G., Allison, J. & Miller, J.F. (1989) Tolerance of class I histocompatibility antigens expressed extrathymically. *Nature*, **339**, 622–4.

Mosmann, T.R. & Coffman, R.L. (1989) TH1 and TH2 cells: different patterns of lymphokine secretion lead to different functional properties. *Ann. Rev. Immunol.*, **7**, 145–73.

Mowat, A.M. (1985) The role of antigen recognition and suppressor cells in mice with oral tolerance to ovalbumin. *Immunology*, **56**, 253.

Mowat, A.M. (1987) The regulation of immune responses to dietary antigens. *Immunol. Today*, **8**, 93–8.

Mowat, A.M. & Ferguson, A. (1981) Hypersensitivity in the small intestinal mucosa. V. Induction of cell-mediated immunity to a dietary antigen. *Clin. Exp. Immunol.*, **43**, 574–82.

Mowat, A.M. & Ferguson, A. (1982a) Intraepithelial lymphocyte count and crypt hyperplasia measure the mucosal component of the graft-versus-host reaction in mouse small intestine. *Gastroenterology*, **83**, 417–23.

Mowat, A.M. & Ferguson, A. (1982b) Migration inhibition of lymph node lymphocytes as an assay for regional cell-mediated immunity in the intestinal lymphoid tissues of mice immunized orally with ovalbumin. *Immunology*, **47**, 365–70.

Mowat, A.M. & Parrot, D.M. (1983) Immunological responses to fed protein antigens in mice. IV. Effects of stimulating the reticuloendothelial system on oral tolerance and intestinal immunity to ovalbumin. *Immunology*, **50**, 547–54.

Mowat, A.M., Strobel, S., Drummond, H.E. & Ferguson, A. (1982) Immunological responses to fed protein antigens in mice. I. Reversal of oral tolerance to ovalbumin by cyclophosphamide. *Immunology*, **45**, 105–13.

Nossal, G.J.V. (1983) Cellular mechanisms of immunologic tolerance. *Ann. Rev. Immunol.*, **1**, 33–62.

O'Hehir, R.E., Garman, R.D., Greenstein, J.L. & Lamb, J.R. (1991) The specificity and regulation of T-cell responsiveness to allergens. *Ann. Rev. Immunol.*, **9**, 67–95.

O'Hehir, R.E., Yssel, H., Verma, S., de Vries, J.E., Spits, H. & Lamb, J.R. (1991) Clonal analysis of differential lymphokine secretion in peptide and superantigen induced anergy. *Int. Immunol.*, **3**, 819–26.

Ohashi, P.S., Oehen, S., Buerki, K. *et al.* (1991) Ablation of 'tolerance' and induction of diabetes by virus infection in viral antigen transgenic mice. *Cell*, **65**, 305–17.

Oldstone, M.B.A., Nerenberg, M., Southern, P., Price, J. & Lewicki, H. (1991) Virus infection triggers insulin-dependent diabetes mellitus in a transgenic model: role of anti-self (virus) immune response. *Cell*, **65**, 319–31.

Ostrov, D., Kreiger, J., Sidney, J., Sette, A. & Concannon, P. (1993) T cell receptor antagonism mediated by interaction between T cell receptor junctional residues and peptide antigen analogues. *J. Immunol.*, **150**, 4277–87.

Poindexter, N.J., Landon, C., Whiteley, P.J. & Kapp, J.A. (1992) Comparison of the T cell receptors on insulin-specific hybridomas from insulin transgenic and nontransgenic mice. *J. Immunol.*, **149**, 38–44.

Racioppi, L., Ronchese, F., Matis, L.A. & Germain, R.N. (1993) Peptide–major histocompatibility complex class II complexes with mixed agonist/antagonist properties provide evidence for ligand related differences in T cell receptor-dependent intracellular signalling. *J. Exp. Med.*, **177**, 1047–66.

Rammensee, H.G. (1989) Veto function *in vitro* and *in vivo*. *Int. Rev. Immunol.*, **4**, 175.

Ramsdell, F., Lantz, T. & Fowlkes, B.J. (1989) A nondeletional mechanism of thymic self-tolerance, *Science*, **246**, 1039–41.

Renz, H., Lack, G., Saloga, J. *et al.* (1994) Inhibition of IgE production and normalization of airways responsiveness by sensitised CD8 T cells in a mouse model of allergen-induced sensitization. *J. Immunol.*, **152**, 351–60.

Renz, H., Bradley, K., Saloga, J., Loader, J., Larsen, G.L. & Gelfand, E.W. (1993) T cells expressing specific Vβ elements regulate immunoglobulin E production and airways responsiveness *in vivo*. *J. Exp. Med.*, **177**, 1175–80.

Renz, H., Smith, H., Henson, J.E., Ray, B.S., Irvin, C.C. & Gelfand, E.W. (1992) Aerosolized antigen exposure without adjuvant causes increased IgE production and increased airway responsiveness in the mouse. *J. Allergy Clin. Immunol.*, **89**, 1127–30.

Ria, F., Chan, B.M., Scherer, M.T., Smith, J.A. & Gefter, M.L. (1990) Immunological activity of covalently linked T-cell epitopes. *Nature*, **343**, 381–3.

Roberts, J.L., Sharrow, S.O. & Singer, A. (1990) Clonal deletion and clonal anergy in the thymus induced by cellular elements with different radiation sensitivities. *J. Exp. Med.*, **171**, 935–40.

Robinson, D.S., Hamid, Q., Ying, S. *et al.* (1992) Predominant Th2-like bronchoalveolar T-lymphocyte population in atopic asthma. *New Engl. J. Med.*, **326**, 298–304.

Rocha, B. & von Boehmer, H. (1991) Peripheral selection of the T cell repertoire. *Science*, **251**, 1225–8.

Romagnani, S. (1994) Lymphokine production by human T cells in disease states. *Ann. Rev. Immunol.*, **12**, 227–58.

Ruppert, J., Alexander, J., Coggeshall, M. *et al.* (1993) Effect of T cell receptor antagonism on interaction between T cells and antigen presenting cells and on T cell signalling events. *Proc. Nat. Acad. Sci. USA*, **90**, 2671–5.

Schonrich, G., Kalinke, U., Momburg, F. *et al.* (1991a) Down-regulation of T cell receptors on self-reactive T cells as a novel mechanism for extrathymic tolerance induction. *Cell*, **65**, 293–304.

Schonrich, G., Momburg, F., Malissen, M. *et al.* (1991b) Distinct mechanisms for extrathymic T cell tolerance due to differential expression of self antigen. *Int. Immunol.*, **4**, 581–90.

Schwartz, R.H. (1990) A cell culture model for T lymphocyte clonal anergy. *Science*, **248**, 1349–56.

Scott, B., Liblau, R., Degermann, S. *et al.* (1994) A role for non-MHC genetic polymorphism in susceptibility to spontaneous autoimmunity. *Immunity*, **1**, 73–82.

Seder, R.A. & Paul, W.E. (1994) Acquisition of lymphokine producing phenotype by CD4+ T cells. *Ann. Rev. Immunol.*, **12**, 635–74.

Sedgwick, J.D. & Holt, P.G. (1983) Induction of IgE-isotype specific tolerance by passive antigenic stimulation of the respiratory mucosa. *Immunology*, **50**, 625–30.

Sedgwick, J.D. & Holt, P.G. (1984) Suppression of IgE response in inbred rats by repeated respiratory tract exposure to antigen: responder phenotype influences isotype specificity of induced tolerance. *Eur. J. Immunol.*, **14**, 893–7.

Sedgwick, J.D. & Holt, P.G. (1985) Down-regulation of immune responses to inhaled antigen: studies on the mechanism of induced suppression. *Immunology*, **56**, 635–42.

Sloan-Lancaster, J., Evavold, B.D. & Allen, P.M. (1993) Induction of T-cell anergy by altered T cell receptor ligand on live antigen presenting cells. *Nature*, **363**, 156–9.

Sloan-Lancaster, J., Evavold, B.D. & Allen, P.M. (1994a) Th2 clonal anergy as a consequence of partial activation. *J. Exp. Med.*, **180**, 1195–205.

Sloan-Lancaster, J., Shaw, A.S., Rothbard, J. & Allen, P.M. (1994b) Partial T cell signalling: altered phospho-ξ and lack of Zap70 recruitment in APL-induced T cell anergy. *Cell*, **79**, 913–22.

Smilek, D.E., Wraith, D.C., Hodgkinson, S., Dwivedy, S., Steinman, L. & McDevitt, H.O. (1991) A single amino acid change in myelin basic protein peptide confers the capacity to prevent rather than induce experimental autoimmune encephalomyelitis. *Proc. Nat. Acad. Sci. USA*, **88**, 9633–7.

Smith, C.A., Williams, G.T., Kingston, R., Jenkinson, E.J. & Owen, J.J.T. (1989) Antibodies to the CD3/T cell receptor complex induce death by apoptosis in immature T cells in thymic cultures. *Nature*, **337**, 181–4.

Staines, N.A., Harper, N. & Ward, F.J. (1994) Modulation of collagen arthritis by nasal administration of a dominant immunogenic peptide of type II collagen. *Immunology*, **83** (Suppl. 1), 46.

Strobel, S. & Ferguson, A. (1985) Oral tolerance—induction and modulation. *Klin. Padiatr.*, **197**, 297–301.

Surh, C.D. & Sprent, J. (1994) T-cell apoptosis detected *in situ* during positive and negative selection in the thymus. *Nature*, **372**, 100–3.

Tan, P., Anasetti, C., Hansen, J. *et al.* (1993) Induction of alloantigen-specific hyporesponsiveness in human T lymphocytes by blocking interaction of CD28 with its natural ligand B7/BB1. *J. Exp. Med.*, **177**, 165–73.

Teh, H.S., Kisielow, P., Scott, B. *et al.* (1988) Thymic major histocompatibility complex antigens and the alpha beta T-cell receptor determine the CD4/CD8 phenotype of T cells. *Nature*, **335**, 229–33.

Thomas, W.R. (1993) Mite allergens group I–VII. A catalogue of enzymes. *Clin. Exp. Allergy*, **23**, 350–4.

Thomas, W.R., Watkins, M.C. & Asherson, G.L. (1979) Suppression of antibody responses by cells from mice painted with picryl chloride. *Immunology*, **36**, 843–50.

Tisch, R., Yang, X.-D., Singer, S.M., Liblau, R., Fugger, L. & McDevitt, H.O. (1993) Immune response to glutamic acid decarboxylase correlates with insulinitis in non-obese diabetic mice. *Nature*, **366**, 72–5.

Webb, S., Morris, C. & Sprent, J. (1990) Extrathymic tolerance of mature T cells: clonal elimination as a consequence of immunity. *Cell*, **63**, 1249–56.

Weiner, H.L., Friedman, A., Miller, A. *et al.* (1994) Oral tolerance: immunologic mechanisms and treatment of animal and human organ-specific autoimmune diseases by oral administration of autoantigens. *Ann. Rev. Immunol.*, **12**, 809–37.

Wells, H.G. (1911) Studies on the chemistry of anaphylaxis III. Experiments with isolated proteins, especially those of the hens egg. *J. Infec. Dis.*, **8**, 147–53.

Whitacre, C.C., Gienapp, I.E., Orosz, C.G. & Bitmar, D.M. (1991) Oral tolerance in experimental autoimmune encephalomyelitis III. Evidence for clonal anergy. *J. Immunol.*, **147**, 2155–63.

Whiteley, P.J., Poindexter, N.J., Landon, C. & Kapp, J.A. (1990) A peripheral mechanism preserves self-tolerance to a secreted protein in transgenic mice. *J. Immunol.*, **145**, 1376–81.

Wieties, K., Hammer, R.E., Jones-Youngblood, S.L. & Forman, J. (1990) Peripheral tolerance in mice expressing a liver-specific class I molecule: inactivation/deletion of a T cell subpopulation. *Proc. Nat. Acad. Sci. USA*, **87**, 6604–8.

Wraith, D.C., McDevitt, H.O., Steinman, L. & Acha-Orbea, H. (1989b) T cell recognition as the target for autoimmune intervention in autoimmune disease. *Cell*, **57**, 709–15.

Wraith, D.C., Smilek, D.E., Mitchell, D.J., Steinman, L. & McDevitt, H.O. (1989a) Antigen recognition in autoimmune encephalomyelitis and the potential for peptide mediated immunotherapy. *Cell*, **59**, 247–55.

Wyllie, A.H. (1980) Glucocorticoid-induced thymocyte apoptosis is associated with endogenous nuclease activation. *Nature*, **284**, 555–6.

Xu-Amano, J., Kiyono, H., Jackson, R.J. *et al.* (1993) Helper T cell subsets for immunoglobulin A responses: oral immunization with tetanus toxoid and cholera toxoid selectively induces Th2 cells in mucosa associated tissues. *J. Exp. Med.*, **178**, 1309–20.

Yui, K., Katsumata, M., Komori, S., Gill-Morse, L. & Greene, M.I. (1992) Response of Vβ8.1+ T cell clones to self-Mlsla: implications for the origin of autoreactive T cells. *Int. Immunol.*, **4**, 125–33.

Yui, K., Komori, S., Katsumata, M., Siegel, R.M. & Greene, M.I. (1990) Self-reactive T cells can escape clonal deletion in T cell receptor Vβ8.1 transgenic mice. *Proc. Nat. Acad. Sci. USA*, **87**, 7135–9.

Zamvil, S.S. & Steinman, L. (1990) The T lymphocyte in experimental allergic encephalomyelitis. *Ann. Rev. Immunol.*, **8**, 579–622.

Zhang, L., Martin, D.R., Fung-Leung, W.P., Teh, H.S. & Miller, R.G. (1992) Peripheral deletion of mature CD8+ T antigen-specific T cells after *in vivo* exposure to male antigen. *J. Immunol.*, **148**, 3740–5.

PART 2

Inflammatory Cells and Mediators

CHAPTER 9
Human Mast Cells and Basophils

M.K. Church, P. Bradding, A.F. Walls & Y. Okayama

Introduction

The mast cell is a major initiating cell of the early phase of allergic reactions, both in the lung and in many other organs in the body. On cross-linkage of its membrane-bound IgE receptors by specific allergen, this cell releases into the local environment a wide array of preformed granule-associated mediators, together with a number of newly generated mediators. These mediators are responsible for most of the early events which characterize allergic reactions of the lung, nose, eye, intestine and skin (their biological properties will be considered in detail later). It has recently been established that the mast cell is also able to contribute to the chronic inflammatory events of allergic disease by the secretion of cytokines. Thus, this cell has the capacity to make major contributions to both acute and chronic elements of pulmonary disease.

Mast cell development

Although the initial description of the mast cell was made in 1863 by Von Recklinhausen, it was not until 1878 that the cell was named by Paul Ehrlich. While still a medical student at Freiburg University, Ehrlich noticed that the granules of the cell appeared purple in colour when stained with blue aniline dyes. This change in colour, or metachromasia, is now known to represent the interaction of the dyes with the highly acidic heparin proteoglycan which is present in the granules. Ehrlich, however, supposed that the granules contained phagocytosed materials, or nutrients, and hence named the cells 'mastzellen', or 'well-fed cells', from where the English name 'mast cell' has been derived. Ehrlich, in a series of elegant drawings, also described the association of mast cells with blood vessels, inflamed tissues, nerves and neoplastic foci, and provided the first description of mast cell degranulation. In addition, he also described the basophil separately as a metachromatically staining cell which circulated in the blood (Ehrlich, 1879). Although this was originally thought to be a circulating mast cell, it is now known that this is not the case as the mast cell and basophil are only distantly related, being derived from different stem cells.

Mast cells and basophils have many features in common, including the presence of acidic proteoglycan in the granule, their ability to store and release histamine, and their ability to bind immunoglobulin E (IgE) with high affinity to a specific receptor, termed FcεRI, on the cell membrane. However, there are also many differences, including nuclear morphology, location within the body, mediator content and synthesis and responses to non-immunological stimulants and drugs. It is now considered that basophils are terminally differentiated leucocytes which mature in the bone marrow from precursors closely related to those of eosinophils, and are released into the blood stream as fully mature cells (Fig. 9.1) (Galli, 1990). Furthermore, culture of basophils *in vitro* does not give rise to mast cells, even under conditions favourable for mast cell growth (Seder *et al.*, 1991). While basophils are not normally found in extravascular compartments, they may migrate there during late-phase allergic responses, and may be responsible for some of the symptoms at that time (Bochner & Lichtenstein, 1992; Massey & Lichtenstein, 1992; Koshino *et al.*, 1993; Makhdum & Pearce, 1993).

In contrast, mast cells leave the bone marrow and circu-

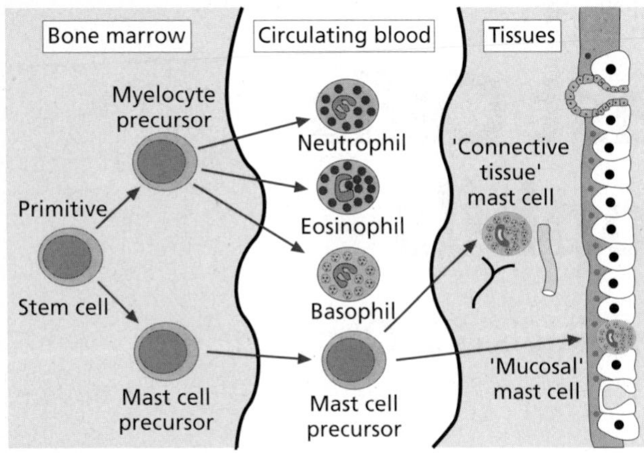

Fig. 9.1 The development of human mast cells from precursors in the bone marrow to mature cells in the tissues.

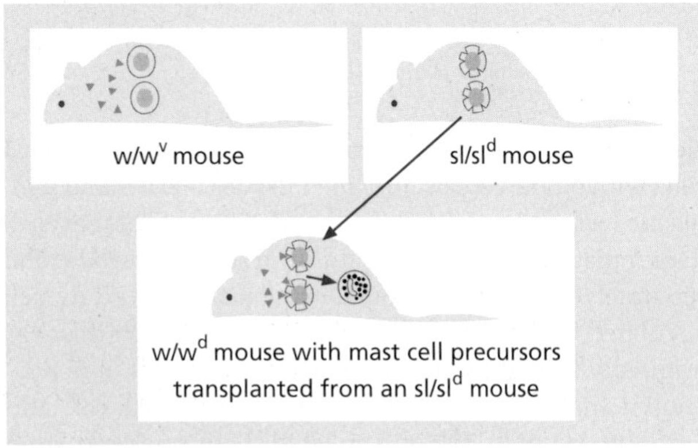

Fig. 9.2 Murine reconstitution experiments to demonstrate that mast cells need stem cell factor (SCF) for maturation. W/W^v mice have SCF, as indicated by the triangles, but no receptors for this ligand on their mast cells. Sl/Sl^d mice have SCF receptors on their mast cells but do not have SCF. Transplantation of immature mast cells from Sl/Sl^d mice to W/W^v mice results in their maturation. (Data from Kitamura *et al.*, 1989.)

late in the blood only as progenitors, and it is not until they enter the tissues that they undergo their terminal differentiation into mature mast cells (Fig. 9.1). When in the blood, mast cell precursors neither possess the FcεRI receptor for IgE nor contain their characteristic neutral proteases or heparin, and thus cannot be readily identified by the usual criteria. However, they can be tentatively identified as mononuclear cells which express mRNA for stem cell factor (SCF), as well as possessing the c-*kit* receptor, a receptor for SCF, a major factor necessary for the maturation of mast cells once in the tissues. In an attempt to detect mast cell progenitor cells in the blood, Ashman *et al.* (1991) performed dual-labelling experiments with YB5.B8, a monoclonal antibody (mAb) against the c-*kit* receptor, and mAb against the cluster determinants, CD33 and CD34. Populations of cells binding YB5.B8, namely YB5.B8+/CD34+/CD33– and YB5.B8+/CD34+/CD33+, were identified based on their pattern of co-expression of the other markers. Both of these cell populations had distinctive two-dimensional light scatter characteristics and the authors suggested that they are likely to correspond to precursor colony-forming cells and maturing mast cells, respectively.

The most elegant studies showing the necessity of SCF in mast cell maturation have been performed by Kitimura and colleagues using mice. They have produced two strains of mouse, W/W^v and Sl/Sl^d, which both show macrocytic anaemia, sterility, lack of hair pigmentation and very few mast cells (Kitamura *et al.*, 1989). When mast cell precursors from Sl/Sl^d are transplanted into W/W^v mice, normal mast cells develop, but when the inverse experiment is performed, no mast cells are found (Fig. 9.2). These results suggest that Sl/Sl^d mice have normal mast cell precursors, but are different in a factor in the microenvironment necessary for their maturation, while W/W^v mice have a normal microenvironment but their mast cell precursors are abnormal. Further genetic studies have shown W/W^v mast cell precursors to be deficient in the c-*kit* receptor, while Sl/Sl^d mice do not produce SCF (Kitamura & Go, 1979; Sonoda *et al.*, 1984; Kanakura *et al.*, 1988; Kitamura *et al.*, 1989). However, the necessity for SCF is not restricted to mice, for human mast cell precursors have repeatedly been shown to require this stromal cell-derived factor for their development (Irani *et al.*, 1992; Dvorak *et al.*, 1993b; Galli *et al.*, 1993; Nilsson *et al.*, 1993).

Mast cell heterogeneity

Mast cells are certainly not a homogeneous population, but differ markedly both between and within species. The earliest suggestion of heterogeneity within the rat mast cell population stems back to the histochemical studies of Maximow in 1906. However, it was not until 1966 that Enerback published a series of papers showing that the mast cells of the intestinal mucosa could be stained metachromatically after fixation in Carnoy's fixative but not after fixation in formaldehyde, while mast cells from a connective tissue source, such as the skin or peritoneal cavity, stained equally well after both types of fixation (Enerback, 1966a,b,c,d). This difference in staining has since been shown to be due to the different proteoglycan content of the two cells in rodents (Razin *et al.*, 1982; Enerback *et al.*, 1985). Furthermore, the studies of Enerback (1966d) showed that the intestinal mast cells did not respond to compound 48/80, a property which was typical of the peritoneal mast cells previously studied with this agent. Thus, the mast cells of the mucosa became known as mucosal mast cells (MMC), or atypical mast cells, whereas those of the peritoneal cavity were termed connective tissue mast cells (CTMC) or typical mast cells. An indication that the development and physiological function of these mast cell sub-types may be different came from the observation that MMC proliferated during parasitic infection (Miller *et al.*, 1986) and are decreased in number with suppression of T-cell function (King *et al.*, 1985). In contrast, the numbers of CTMC are not affected by either of these events. From these observations we can make one general hypothesis, that the 'mucosal' mast cell is associated functionally with the immune system, whereas the 'connective tissue' mast cell is not likely to be so.

By employing Enerback's staining techniques to human mast cells, Stroebel and colleagues (Strobel *et al.*, 1981) suggested a similar subdivision of mast cells in humans. However, two further studies, both of which confirmed the presence of formalin-sensitive and formalin-insensitive subpopulations in humans, failed to find an absolute relationship of histochemical sub-type with anatomical site, both sub-types, for example, being found in the skin (Befus *et al.*, 1985; Marshall *et al.*, 1987). However, the identification of tryptase (Glenner & Cohen, 1960; Schwartz *et al.*, 1981a,b) and chymase (Schechter *et al.*, 1983; Schechter, 1990) as proteases unique to mast cells was to change the criteria by which mast cell heterogeneity was assessed. Tryptase is present in all mast cells whereas chymase is present only in mast cells predominantly associated with connective tissues (Irani *et al.*, 1986). Thus, in 1989, histochemical sub-typing of mast cells was abandoned in favour of immunocytochemical sub-typing into MC_T (those mast cells which contain only tryptase) and MC_{TC} (those mast cells which contain both tryptase and chymase). Further studies (Fig. 9.3) showed that MC_T are preferentially located at mucosal surfaces (Irani *et al.*, 1989a), increase in number in allergic disease (Irani *et al.*, 1987b, 1988, 1989b) and are reduced in number in acquired and chronic immunodeficiency syndromes (Irani *et al.*, 1987a), suggesting that, like rodent MMC, they are acting as an arm of the immune system. In contrast, MC_{TC} are found predominantly in submucosal and connective tissues, are not increased in numbers in areas of heavy lymphocytic infiltration (Irani *et al.*, 1988, 1989a) and are not decreased in number in immunodeficiency syndromes (Irani *et al.*, 1987a). The biological role of this cell is less clear but its associations with fibrotic disease (Walls *et al.*, 1990b) and angiogenesis (Kessler *et al.*, 1976; Rakusan & Campbell, 1991; Duncan *et al.*, 1992; Meininger & Zetter, 1992; Sorbo *et al.*, 1994) indicate that it is likely to play a role in tissue reconstruction.

The discerning reader will now ask whether this means that, in humans, there are only two mast cell subpopulations, in which immunocytochemical identity and functional properties go hand in hand? Sadly this is not the case, for mast cells at different anatomical locations may

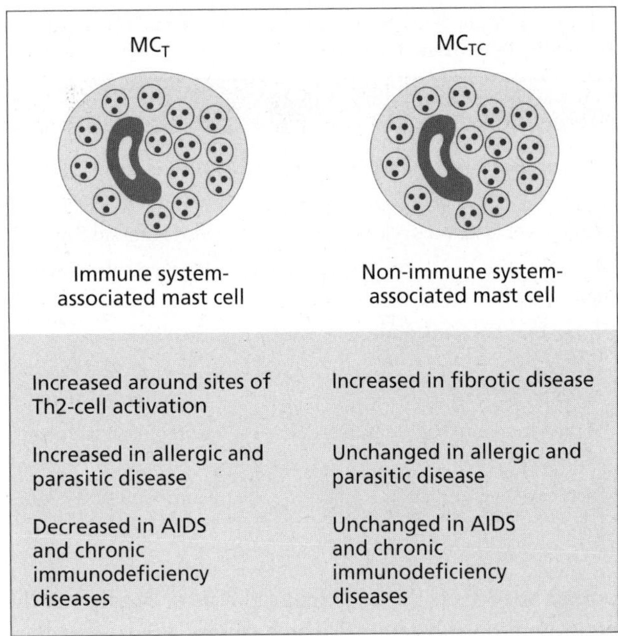

Fig. 9.3 Differential requirements of MC_T and MC_{TC} for development.

respond quite differently to activating agents and modulating drugs even though their immunocytochemical phenotype may be identical. All mast cells bear in their membrane FcεR1, receptors capable of binding with high affinity the Fc portion of IgE. Cross-linkage of two or more IgE molecules to bring their receptors into juxtaposition initiates a sequence of biochemical events which results in degranulation to release histamine, proteases and heparin, and synthesis of prostaglandin D_2 (PGD_2) and leukotriene C_4 (LTC_4) from the membrane-associated phospholipid, arachidonic acid. When this sequence was stimulated in the laboratory by cross-linking the IgE with anti-IgE, it was found that mast cells dispersed from different tissues responded in a quantitatively different manner, both in the extent of histamine release and the time it took to release their histamine (Lowman *et al.*, 1988c; Lau *et al.*, 1994). This bore no relationship to the predominating mast cell type, MC_T or MC_{TC}, within the cell preparation. Thus, it must be hypothesized that factors unique to each tissue microenvironment will affect which genes are expressed in the final mast cell phenotype, i.e. the final physical and functional properties of mast cells within that tissue. Also, diseases such as allergy, parasitic infestation or fibrosis, may affect the maturation of mast cells within a tissue.

In addition to IgE-dependent stimulation, some mast cells may be activated for mediator release by non-immunological secretagogues such as neuropeptides, anaphylatoxins and xenobiotics, including morphine, codeine, muscle relaxants and the histamine releaser, com-

Table 9.1 Comparison between anti-IgE-induced and substance P-stimulated mediator release from human skin mast cells. (After Benyon *et al.*, 1986, 1987, 1989; Church *et al.*, 1989.)

	Anti-IgE	Substance P
Spectrum of mediators released	Preformed mediators, e.g. histamine and proteases, and newly generated mediators, e.g. PGD_2, LTC_4	Preformed mediators, e.g. histamine and proteases
Kinetics of histamine release	Slow, around 5 minutes	Rapid, around 15 seconds
Effect of immunological desensitization or removal of cell-surface IgE	Blockade of cell activation and mediator release	No effect
Effect of the neuropeptide antagonist, SPA	No effect	Reduction of cell activation and mediator release
Calcium requirements	Extracellular and intracellular Ca^{2+}	Intracellular calcium only
Dependency on glucose and oxidative phosphorylation	Complete dependency	Complete dependency
Nature of degranulation	Compound exocytosis	Compound exocytosis

pound 48/80. Of these, perhaps the most studied is the neuropeptide substance P, which causes a weal-and-flare response when injected intradermally into human skin (Hägermark *et al.*, 1978). It has been confirmed, using dispersed skin mast cells, that substance P interacts directly with activation sites on the mast cell membrane to induce mediator release (Lowman *et al.*, 1988a). It has also been shown that the characteristics of substance P skin mast cell activation was quite different from that of IgE-dependent activation (Table 9.1). Anti-IgE-induced mast cell activation is relatively slow, taking minutes to reach completion, requires the presence of extracellular calcium, and results in the release of the full spectrum of preformed and newly generated mast cell mediators. In contrast, activation with substance P and other basic secretagogues is complete within 10–15 seconds, utilizes only intracellular calcium, and results in the release of only preformed mediators (Benyon *et al.*, 1986, 1987, 1989; Church *et al.*, 1989). Exhaustive examination of mast cells dispersed from other organs, including lung, colon, tonsils, adenoids and nasal polyps, many of which show large proportions of MC_{TC}, failed to reveal another mast cell subset which responded to substance P (Lowman *et al.*, 1988c; Rees *et al.*, 1988; Johnston *et al.*, 1993). However, some recent experiments by Ennis have suggested that bronchoalveolar mast cells from asthmatic individuals may respond to substance P, the responsiveness appearing to correlate with asthma severity (M. Ennis, personal communication). The clinical relevance of this observation is not yet understood. However, it must be concluded that the responsiveness to substance P does not follow immunocytochemical sub-typing.

Another example of functional heterogeneity may be explored with the complement anaphylatoxin C5a. When injected into the skin, C5a causes an antihistamine-sensitive weal-and-flare response (Wuepper *et al.*, 1972; Swerlick *et al.*, 1988) suggestive of a mast cell histamine releasing activity. This has recently been confirmed to be dispersed human skin mast cells (El Lati *et al.*, 1994). The characteristics of histamine release are similar to those described for substance P, with the exception that the substance P antagonist, SPA, does not modulate release, suggesting that C5a acts at a different cell-surface activation site (Fig. 9.4). In comparison with the skin, human lung mast cells do not respond to C5a (Schulman *et al.*, 1988). This work has recently been extended (P. Valent *et al.*, personal communication) by the observations that human skin mast cells express the C5a receptor (CD88), whereas mast cells of the lung and uterus do not. As the majority of the uterine mast cells are of the MC_{TC} sub-type, this provides another example of divergence between immunocytochemical and functional heterogeneity.

A particularly pertinent example of functional heterogeneity relates to drug modulation of mediator release (Table 9.2). Mast cells dispersed from human lung, skin

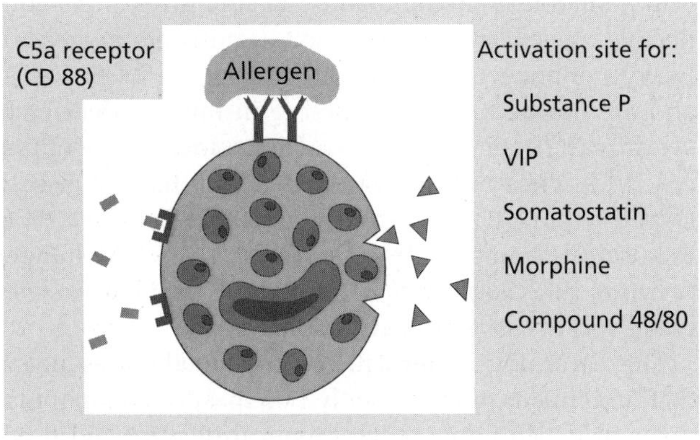

Fig. 9.4 Activation of human skin mast cells by immunological and non-immunological stimuli.

Table 9.2 The effect of anti-allergic drugs on histamine release from human mast cells from lung, colon and skin.

Drug	Lung	Colon	Skin
Salbutamol	Inhibition	Inhibition	Inhibition
Theophylline	Inhibition	Inhibition	Inhibition
Dexamethasone	No effect	No effect	No effect
Sodium cromoglycate	Weak inhibition Tachyphylaxis	Inhibition No tachyphylaxis	No effect

and colon have each been shown to be similarly sensitive to β-stimulants and theophylline-like drugs, concentrations of 10^{-6} mol/l and 5×10^{-4} mol/l, respectively, being effective inhibitors of mediator release (Church & Hiroi, 1987; Okayama & Church, 1992). In contrast, glucocorticoids do not inhibit mast cell degranulation or production of newly generated mediators (Schleimer *et al.*, 1983; Cohan *et al.*, 1989). With anti-allergic drugs, such as sodium cromoglycate and nedocromil sodium, heterogeneity is seen. With lung mast cells, high concentrations of both drugs, up to 100 μmol/l, are required to cause modest inhibition and the cells rapidly become tachyphylactic to the modulatory effects of these drugs (Church & Hiroi, 1987; Okayama *et al.*, 1992; Okayama & Church, 1992). Mediator release from human skin mast cells, in contrast, is not inhibited by either sodium cromoglycate or nedocromil sodium (Clegg *et al.*, 1985; Lowman *et al.*, 1988b; Church *et al.*, 1989; Okayama *et al.*, 1992). A different profile is seen with colonic mast cells (Rees *et al.*, 1988; Okayama *et al.*, 1992), they are both more sensitive to sodium cromoglycate and do not exhibit tachyphylaxis. A similar pattern of activity is seen with mast cells obtained from the airways by bronchoalveolar lavage (Flint *et al.*, 1985b). Thus, again, there is no clear association between immunocytochemical and functional heterogeneity.

Preformed mast cell mediators

The secretory granule of the human mast cell is a complex, with histamine and proteases being ionically bound to a matrix of proteoglycan. Electron microscopy of MC_T shows them to have crystalline intragranular matrices which are seen as scrolls, crystals or whorls (Caulfield *et al.*, 1980). In contrast, MC_{TC}, which contain chymase and carboxypeptidase in addition to tryptase, contain more electron-dense granules in which the crystalline structure, although often just visible, is clouded by the sheer volume of protease (Caulfield *et al.*, 1990). Furthermore, the presence of a different crystalline form, the crystal form, has been reported by Dvorak *et al.* (Dvorak & Kissel, 1991; Dvorak *et al.*, 1991). When mast cell activation occurs, the granules swell, loose their crystalline nature as they become solubilized, and are expelled into the local environment by compound exocytosis (Benveniste *et al.*, 1972; Caulfield *et al.*, 1980, 1990). The granule matrix is then further solubilized by ion exchange, particularly with sodium (Uvnas, 1967), in the extracellular environment.

The mediator most readily associated with the mast cell is the simple diamine, histamine. This is synthesized in the mast cell granule by decarboxylation of histidine, mainly by histidine decarboxylase and, to a lesser extent, by the non-specific decarboxylase, dopa decarboxylase (Schayer, 1963; Beaven, 1978). Histamine is stored in the acid pH of the granules at around 100 mM (equivalent to about 1–4 pg/cell) by ionic linkage with proteoglycans and proteases (Johnson *et al.*, 1980; Lagunoff & Richard, 1983). Once in the extracellular environment, histamine exerts its potent effects, which include contraction of bronchial smooth muscle, increased mucus production, vasodilatation and contraction of post-capillary venular endothelial cells to increase vasopermeability. However, following bronchoprovocation, these effects are of relatively short duration as histamine is rapidly metabolized primarily by histamine-*N*-methyltransferase (around 70%) and, to a lesser extent, by diamine oxidase, sometimes called histaminase (around 30%).

The backbone of the crystalline mast cell granule is proteoglycan which, in human mast cells, is mainly heparin, which constitutes some 75% of the granule proteoglycan, with a mixture of chondroitin sulphates (Stevens *et al.*, 1988b; Thompson *et al.*, 1988). Basophils, in contrast, do not contain heparin, the primary proteoglycan of their granule being chondroitin A (Metcalfe *et al.*, 1984). Proteoglycan comprises a single-chain peptide core which, in humans, is 17.6 kDa containing a glycosaminoglycan attachment region of alternating Ser-Gly residues (Stevens *et al.*, 1988a). The specific glycosaminoglycans attached to these sites determine the nature of the proteoglycan. All glycosaminoglycans contain a variable number of sulphate groups and, hence, are acidic.

Within the granule, the acid nature of the sulphate groups of the glycosaminoglycans provides binding sites for histamine, neutral proteases and acid hydrolases, which it keeps in an inactive state (Fig. 9.5). Thus, the proteoglycan may be viewed as a granular storage matrix. Once released, heparin and, to a lesser effect, chondroitin sulphate may affect the stability or function of other mast cell mediators; for example, its stabilization of the active tetramer of tryptase (Schwartz & Bradford, 1986). Other actions of these proteoglycans include anticoagulant, anticomplement and anti-kallikrein effects, the ability to sequester eosinophil major basic protein, enhancement of

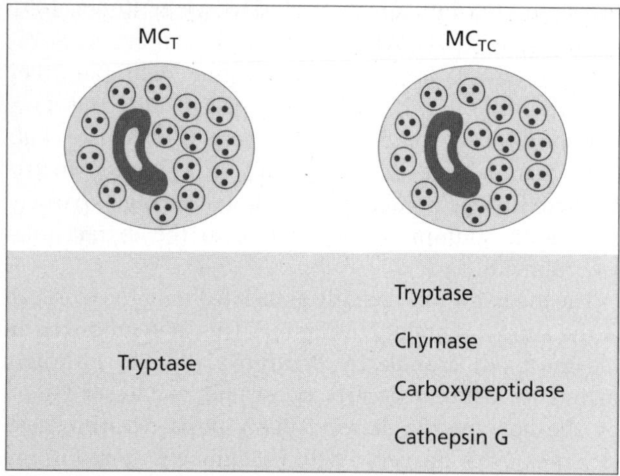

Fig. 9.5 Distribution of neutral proteases in mast cell sub-types.

binding of collagen to fibronectin, and numerous growth factor-enhancing activities.

The major mast cell protease, present in all mast cells, regardless of sub-type, is tryptase. Tryptase is a tetrameric serine protease of around 130 kDa (Schwartz *et al.*, 1981a; Smith *et al.*, 1984; Walls *et al.*, 1990a) which is stored in a fully active form in the granule (Alter *et al.*, 1990). In fact, there are two distinct forms of tryptase, α-tryptase and β-tryptase. The amino-acid sequence of α-tryptase is 90% identical with that of β-tryptase, the first 20 amino acids of the catalytic portions being 100% identical and regions of the substrate binding pocket differing only slightly, α-tryptase having DSCK in residues 217–220 and SWD in residues 242–244, while β-tryptase has DSCQ in residues 218–221 and SWG in residues 243–245 (Miller *et al.*, 1990). Both α- and β-mast cell tryptase are encoded on chromosome 16, showing them to be quite unrelated to lymphocyte tryptases which have been mapped to chromosome 5q11–q12 (Baker *et al.*, 1994). When released into the extracellular environment, the neutral pH allows tryptase to become enzymatically functional. While there appears to be no endogenous inhibitors of tryptase, it is likely to be an enzyme with a very local effect only. This is because, in the absence of heparin, tryptase rapidly dissociates into inactive monomers with altered secondary and tertiary structures (Schwartz & Bradford, 1986; Schwartz *et al.*, 1990). The difficulty of extracting active tryptase from tissues, its relative instability, and the failure, as yet, to clone the enzyme in its fully active tetrameric form has meant that our knowledge of its function is limited. However, some actions pertinent to the airways have been documented (Table 9.3). For example, it is known that tryptase cleaves the bronchodilator peptides, vasoactive intestinal peptide (VIP), peptide histidine methionine (PHM) and the vasodilator calcitonin gene-related peptide (CGRP), but not the bronchoconstrictor neuropeptide, substance P (Tam & Caughey, 1990; Walls *et al.*, 1992b). These observations have led to suggestions that an imbalance of airways neuropeptides may be a factor in bronchial hyperresponsiveness. Furthermore, the report by Sekizawa *et al.* (1989) that tryptase sensitizes bronchial smooth muscle to contractile agents, strengthens the view that tryptase may play a role in asthma. Further actions of tryptase include a kallikrein-like activity (Proud *et al.*, 1988; Walls *et al.*, 1992a), cleavage of matrix components, including 75 kDa gelatinase/type IV collagen, fibronectin (Lohi *et al.*, 1992) and type VI collagen (Kielty *et al.*, 1993), and activation of stromelysin which may, in turn, cleave other matrix components (Gruber *et al.*, 1989). In addition, tryptase is a mitogen for fibroblasts (Ruoss *et al.*, 1991; Hartmann *et al.*, 1992) and in a human epithelial cell line may induce its proliferation, stimulate it to release the granulocyte chemoattractant IL-8 and up-regulate its expression of ICAM-1 (J. Cairns, L. Pearson & A.F. Walls, unpublished observations).

Chymase, which is present only in a subset of pulmonary mast cells, the MC_{TC} subset, is a monomeric protease of 30 kDa (Fraki & Hopsu-Havu, 1972; Wintroub *et al.*, 1986b; Urata *et al.*, 1990) which is stored in the same secretory granules as tryptase (Craig *et al.*, 1988) but is released in a macromolecule complex distinct from tryptase (Goldstein *et al.*, 1992), suggesting that there is no physico-chemical bonding between them. Within the lung, there is a negligible number of MC_{TC} in the epithelial layer, but they are found in large numbers close to submucosal glands and, to a lesser extent, associated with smooth muscle (Matin *et al.*, 1992). Like tryptase, chymase is stored within the granule in its fully active form (Huntley *et al.*, 1985; Goldstein *et al.*, 1992), so that it needs no further processing before release. The enzymatic activities of chymase (Table 9.3) include the degradation of neurotensin (Kinoshita *et al.*, 1991), substance P or VIP (Urata *et al.*, 1990) and the cleavage of angiotensin I to angiotensin II (Reilley *et al.*, 1982; Powers *et al.*, 1985; Urata *et al.*, 1990; Kinoshita *et al.*, 1991). In fact, chymase is more active

Table 9.3 Biological properties of mast cell proteases.

Tryptase	Chymase
Tissue degradation	Tissue degradation
Mast cell degranulation	Mast cell degranulation
Vascular exudation	Vascular exudation
Leucocyte migration and activation	Leucocyte migration
Epithelial cell proliferation	Mucus secretion
ICAM-1 up-regulation	Angiotensin II generation
IL-8 release	Cleavage of cytokines
Bradykinin generation	
Degradation of VIP and CGRP	

See text for definition of abbreviations.

than angiotensin-converting enzyme in this activity, which has led to much interest in chymase from cardiac mast cells. Chymase may also contribute to the purported role of mast cells in tissue remodelling by cleaving type IV collagen (Sage *et al.*, 1979) and splitting the dermal–epidermal junction (Briggman *et al.*, 1984). Actions pertinent to mucosal inflammation include the activation of interleukin-1β (IL-1β) to IL-1 (Mizutani *et al.*, 1991), the degradation of IL-4 (Tunon de Lara *et al.*, 1994a) and the stimulation of secretion from cultured submucosal gland cells (Sommerhoff *et al.*, 1989).

Two other proteinases, carboxypeptidase (Goldstein *et al.*, 1989) and cathepsin G (Schechter *et al.*, 1990), have been associated with human mast cells. Carboxypeptidase is a unique 34.5 kDa metalloproteinase which removes the carboxyl terminal residues from a range of peptides, including angiotensin, Leu^5-enkephalin, kinetensin, neuromedin N and neurotensin (Goldstein *et al.*, 1989; Goldstein *et al.*, 1991; Bunnett *et al.*, 1992), while cathepsin G is a chymotryptic enzyme normally associated with neutrophils. Analysis of cDNA has suggested human skin mast cell cathepsin G to be identical to that reported for neutrophil cathepsin G (Schechter *et al.*, 1994). Interestingly, the genes encoding human mast cell chymase, cathepsin G, T-cell receptor α-/δ-chains and lymphocyte granzymes are closely linked on chromosomal band 14q11.2 (Caughey *et al.*, 1993). Of this group, chymase and cathepsin G are cotranscribed in the human mast cell line HMC-1 and in U-937 cells, while neutrophils and lymphocytes transcribe cathepsin G and granzyme genes, respectively, but not chymase genes, (Caughey *et al.*, 1993). When mast cells are activated, chymase, carboxypeptidase and cathepsin G are released together in a 400–500 kDa complex with proteoglycan and are likely to act in concert with the other enzymes to degrade proteins.

Newly generated mediators

Immunological activation of mast cells induces the liberation of arachidonic acid within the membrane. This phospholipid is then rapidly oxidized down either of two pathways; the cyclo-oxygenase pathway to form PGD_2 or the lipoxygenase pathway to form LTC_4. These are the only two eicosanoids made by the human mast cell (Robinson *et al.*, 1989).

PGD_2 is a potent bronchoconstrictor agent which is rapidly degraded to another bronchoconstrictor agent, 9α,11β-PGF_2 (Hardy *et al.*, 1985; Liston & Roberts, 1985; Beasley *et al.*, 1987). Both of these substances are thought to exert the majority of their bronchoconstrictor actions by the occupation of thromboxane receptors (Beasley *et al.*, 1989a). In addition to its bronchoconstrictor effect, PGD_2 is chemokinetic for human neutrophils (Goetzl & Pickett, 1981), augments LTB_4-induced neutrophilia in the skin (Soter *et al.*, 1983) and is a powerful inhibitor of platelet aggregation.

Leukotriene C_4, or 5(*S*)-hydroxy-6(*R*)-*S*-glutathionyl-7,9-*trans*-11,14-*cis*-eicosatetraenoic acid, is made by a variety of inflammatory cells in the lung, including mast cells and eosinophils. In the extracellular environment, glutamine is removed from the glutathione residue of LTC_4 by γ-glutamine transpeptidase to yield LTD_4, from which glycine is then removed by LTD dipeptidase to yield LTE_4. The physiological effects of the sulphidopeptide leukotrienes include potent contraction of bronchial smooth muscle, contraction of arterial and arteriolar smooth muscle, enhanced permeability of post-capillary venules and enhanced bronchial mucus secretion, most of which, in the airways, are mediated by LTD_4 (Drazen *et al.*, 1980; Lewis *et al.*, 1990). Because of their potent effects on the airways, leukotrienes have long been regarded as important molecules in the pathogenesis of asthma.

Mast cell cytokines

It is now established that mast cells are a source of several multifunctional cytokines. Initial studies demonstrated that many Abelson murine leukaemia virus (A-MuLV)-transformed mouse mast cell lines constitutively express mRNA for granulocyte macrophage colony-stimulating factor (GM-CSF) and IL-4, and release bioactivity indicative of the transcribed proteins (Chung *et al.*, 1986; Brown *et al.*, 1987). A few lines also express mRNA for IL-3. In addition, constitutive expression of mRNA for IL-4 has been demonstrated in non-transformed IL-3-dependent mast cell lines, although no product was found in these studies (Brown *et al.*, 1987). Further studies demonstrated that, in response to FcεRI activation, non-transformed murine mast cell lines or primary cultures of bone marrow-derived mast cells, have the potential to synthesize and secrete many cytokines, including IL-1, IL-2, IL-3, IL-4, IL-5, IL-6, GM-CSF, interferon-γ (IFN-γ), and four members of the intercrine family of cytokines, macrophage inflammatory protein (MIP)-1α, MIP-1β and T-cell activation antigen-3 (TLA-3) (Burd *et al.*, 1989; Plaut *et al.*, 1989). Gordon *et al.* (1990) subsequently demonstrated that mast cells grown *in vitro* or freshly isolated mouse peritoneal mast cells constitutively contained tumour necrosis factor-α (TNF-α) bioactivity and could be induced by IgE-dependent stimulation to generate high levels of TNF-α mRNA. The observations in the above experiments that not all mast cell lines and cultures produced the same pattern of cytokines, and that within primary cultures of bone marrow cultured mast cells (BMCMC) not all cells produce the cytokine mRNA (Gurish *et al.*, 1991), raises the question whether mast cell heterogeneity exists with regard to cytokine production in addition to protease production.

Table 9.4 The cytokine profile of human purified lung mast cells as assessed by the reverse transcriptase polymerase chain reaction.

	IL-2	IL-3	IL-4	IL-5	IL-6	IL-8	IL-10	IL-13	IFN-γ	GM-CSF	TNF-α	APRT	CD4
SCF	−	−	−	+	+	++	+	+	−	+	+	+	−
SCF + anti-IgE	−	+	+	++	+	++	+	++	−	+	+	+	−

Human lung mast cells were purified to greater than 98% by positive affinity selection using the anti-c-*kit* antibody, YB5.B8, coupled to dynabeads. T lymphocytes were similarly removed using anti-CD2. Note the absence of an mRNA signal for CD4, indicating the absence of helper T cells.

Information on human mast cells is more limited. Klein *et al.* showed that degranulation of mast cells in human skin organ cultures induced epxression of ELAM-1 on vascular endothelial cells, an effect which was abrogated by prior administration of either sodium cromoglycate, an inhibitor of mast cell mediator release, or neutralizing antibodies to TNF-α. The same group subsequently demonstrated that human dermal mast cells contain sizeable quantities of TNF-α within granules, which can be released rapidly upon degranulation (Walsh *et al.*, 1991b). Storage of TNF-α, with IgE-dependent release and mRNA induction, has also been demonstrated in human lung mast cells (Ohkawara *et al.*, 1992).

Studies from our own group have provided evidence by the reverse transcriptase polymerase chain reaction (RT-PCR) and *in-situ* hybridization of mRNA for IL-3, IL-4, IL-5, IL-6, IL8, IL-10, IL-13, GM-CSF and TNF-α, by enzyme-linked immunosorbant assay (ELISA) of the secretion of IL-4, IL-5 and TNF-α by purified human lung mast cells and by immunocytochemistry of the presence of IL-4, IL-5, IL-6 and TNF-α in mast cells in bronchial and nasal biopsies (Table 9.4).

Human mast cells isolated from human skin and lung contain immunoreactivity for IL-4 which is lost following IgE-dependent activation, indicative of release (Bradding *et al.*, 1992). IL-4 mRNA is not expressed constitutively but may be demonstrated *in vitro* by RT-PCR 2–4 hours after stimulation of cultured mast cells with anti-IgE (Church *et al.*, 1994; Okayama *et al.*, 1995c). In further, more extensive studies (Okayama *et al.*, 1995b), however, it was found that the mRNA for IL-4 is not expressed constitutively in dispersed human lung mast cells. Furthermore, following cross-linkage of high-affinity Fcε receptors (FcεRI) with anti-IgE, mRNA for IL-4 was detectable in only six out of 13 experiments. No IL-4 protein was detectable by ELISA in these experiments. The reasons for this are not entirely clear but three may be considered: firstly, IL-4 may be produced by mast cells in levels below those detectable by ELISA; secondly, IL-4 is ionically bound to proteoglycan, and is hence not detectable; thirdly, that IL-4 is degraded by the mast cell protease, chymase (Tunon de Lara *et al.*, 1994b). Following provocation of allergic rhinitis, Ying and colleagues found that 20% of cells giving a positive *in situ* hybridization for IL-4 were mast cells (Ying *et al.*, 1994). The presence of IL-4 in mast cells has been demonstrated using immunohistochemistry on nasal and bronchial biopsies from normal subjects, patients with allergic perennial and seasonal rhinitis, and allergic asthma (Bradding *et al.*, 1992, 1993, 1994, 1995). Using two mAb to human IL-4 which identify different epitopes, an interesting pattern has emerged. Mast cells staining with one mAb to IL-4 (3H4) are clearly increased in number, particularly in the epithelium, in those with allergic mucosal diseases compared to normal subjects (Fig. 9.6). Furthermore this mAb gives a characteristic pericellular ring-staining pattern in disease (Bradding *et al.*, 1992, 1993). Although the meaning of this is not entirely understood, one interpretation is that it represents a secreted form of IL-4. Furthermore, there are strong correlations between 3H4+ mast cell numbers and eosinophil numbers in both allergic asthma and allergic rhinitis. Expression of IL-4 immunoreactivity with this antibody in rhinitis is clearly suppressed by a potent topical corticosteroid, fluticasone propionate, following natural seasonal allergen exposure (Bradding *et al.*, 1995). In contrast, a second mAb

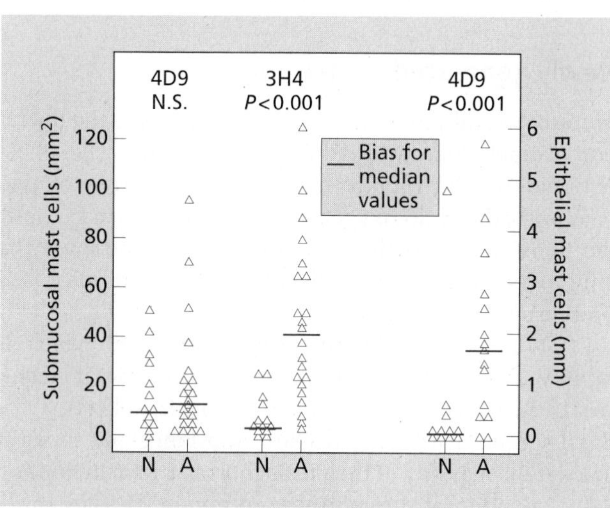

Fig. 9.6 Numbers of mast cells in bronchial biopsies from normal (N) and asthmatic (A) subjects showing immunoreactivity with two antibodies, 4D9 and 3H4, for IL-4.

(4D9) gives a granular cytoplasmic staining pattern in both normals and patients, and stains the same number of mast cells, approximately 75%, in both normals and patients, suggesting that it detects stored IL-4 (Bradding *et al.*, 1992, 1993a).

It has recently been shown (Okayama *et al.*, 1995b) that anti-IgE challenge of purified mast cells from human lung, cultured with SCF and myeloma IgE for 16 hours, results in the strong and consistent expression of mRNA for IL-5 which is evident at 2 hours and which persists for up to 96 hours. In a further study (Okayama *et al.*, 1995a), it was shown by ELISA that IgE-dependent release of IL-5 was variable between tissues ranging from <10 to 3627 pg/10^6 mast cells and that release was enhanced by SCF, which, by itself, stimulated IL-5 mRNA expression but not release of the product. Kinetic studies showed that, whereas IL-5 mRNA was demonstrable within 2 hours, protein secretion occurred only between 8 and 48 hours. Furthermore, cell lysis at the end of an experiment revealed that 44–216 pg IL-5/10^6 mast cells was present, stored within the cell (Fig. 9.7). Whether this represents a stored form of the cytokine in the granule or merely its presence in the cytoplasm following transcription is still to be determined. In biopsies, Ying *et al.* (1994) have described the expression of mRNA for IL-5 in about 10% of nasal mucosal mast cells following allergen challenge. Using

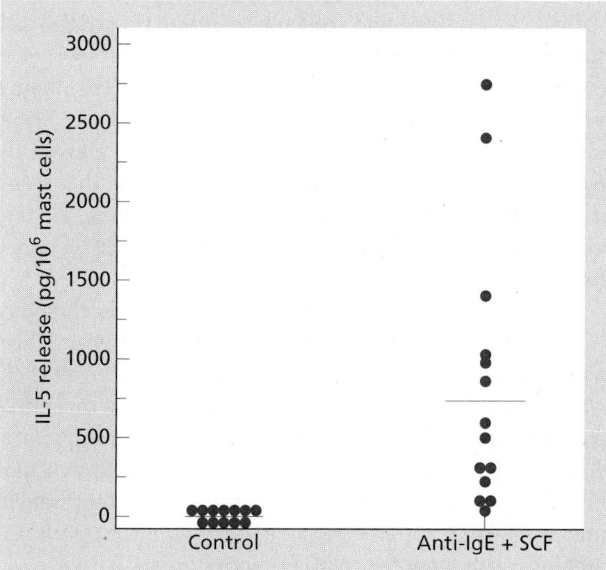

Fig. 9.7 The generation of IL-5 by human lung mast cells by anti-IgE (1 µg/ml) and recombinant human SCF (rhSCF) (50 ng/ml) during a 24-hour incubation period. Mast cells were purified to greater than 98% by positive affinity selection using the anti-c-*kit* antibody, YB5.B8, coupled to dynabeads. T lymphocytes were similarly removed using anti-CD2. Note the absence of an mRNA signal for CD4, indicating the absence of helper T cells.

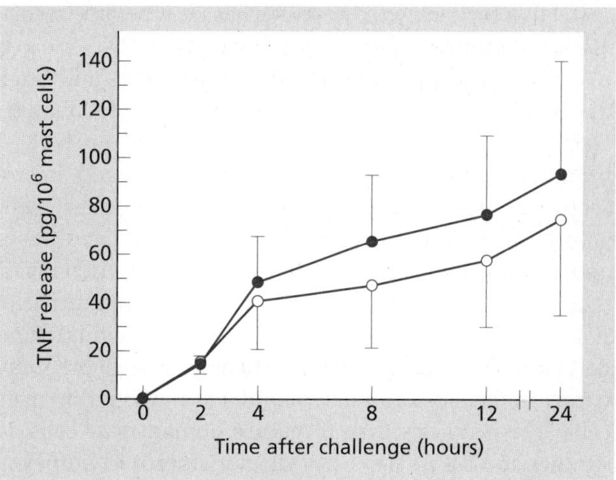

Fig. 9.8 The generation of TNF-α by human lung mast cells by anti-IgE (1 µg/ml) and recombinant human SCF (rhSCF) (50 ng/ml) (closed circles) or SCF alone (open circles) during a 24-hour incubation period. Mast cells were purified to greater than 98% by positive affinity selection using the anti-c-*kit* antibody, YB5.B8, coupled to dynabeads. T lymphocytes were similarly removed using anti-CD2. Note the absence of an mRNA signal for CD4, indicating the absence of helper T cells.

immunocytochemistry, IL-5 has been localized to approximately 10% of mast cells in nasal and bronchial biopsies from normal subjects, patients with allergic perennial and seasonal rhinitis, and allergic asthma (Bradding *et al.*, 1992, 1993, 1994, 1995). There was no obvious difference in the number of mast cells staining for IL-5 in either rhinitis or asthma.

mRNA for IL-6 appears to be constitutively expressed in isolated human lung mast cells cultured with SCF and myeloma IgE (Okayama *et al.*, 1995c). In nasal and bronchial biopsies, IL-6 immunoreactivity is present in approximately 35% of mast cells, numbers which do not change in allergic perennial or seasonal rhinitis or in allergic asthma (Bradding *et al.*, 1992, 1993, 1994, 1995).

Studies *in vitro* have shown that, like IL-5, mRNA for TNF-α is not constitutively expressed but may be activated by either SCF or immunological stimulation. Following immunological activation, expression of TNF-α mRNA was seen within 2 hours and waned slowly by 24 hours. TNF-α protein secretion occurred within 2 hours following anti-IgE stimulation, much more rapidly than that of IL-5. The amounts of TNF-α secreted by human lung mast cells were again variable and dependent on the lung donor, ranging from 7 to 273 pg/10^6 mast cells/24 hours (Fig. 9.8). Examination of nasal and bronchial biopsies by immunocytochemistry has shown TNF-α to be present in approximately 35% of submucosal mast cells, a number which increases significantly in asthma (Bradding *et al.*, 1992, 1993a,b, 1995).

IL-8 is a further cytokine which has now become associated with human mast cells. Möller *et al.* (1993) showed that IL-8 mRNA was expressed in a stimulus- and time-dependent fashion, as detected by Northern blot analysis with an IL-8-specific cDNA probe, in the human HMC-1 immature mast cell line. Also, immunoelectron microscopy of IgE-dependent stimulated-skin mast cells showed IL-8 to be present along cytoplasmic membranes and in intracellular granules. However, in our own investigations of IL-8 immunoreactivity in the nasal mucosa of normal subjects and patients with allergic perennial rhinitis (McNamee *et al.*, 1991), IL-8 was localized predominantly to the nasal epithelium and was not found in mast cells. This suggests that, if mature human mast cells do synthesize IL-8 *in vivo*, they do not store it in sufficient quantities for detection by immunocytochemical techniques.

Colocalization of cytokines within mast cells has shown that some mast cells contain combinations of cytokines while others appear to produce only one cytokine. These observations, plus the predominance of IL-6 positive cells compared with others among the submucosal glands, suggests that heterogeneity exists among human mast cells in cytokine production. However, it is not yet known the nature or reasons for this heterogeneity.

Non-B non-T cell and basophil cytokines

In mice, a population of splenic and bone marrow non-B non-T cells expressing FcεRI are capable of producing IL-4, and in the case of the former IL-3 as well, following IgE-dependent activation (Ben-Sasson *et al.*, 1990; Conrad *et al.*, 1990). The production of IL-4 by these cells is potentiated by either pre-incubation with IL-3 or prior infection of the animal with *Nippostrongylus brasiliensis*. Subsequent characterization of these IL-4-producing cells has demonstrated that they are negative for the expression of c-*kit* and resemble basophils morphologically, suggesting that they are of basophil lineage (Seder *et al.*, 1991). Human bone marrow non-B non-T cells produce IL-4 and IL-5 mRNA, and release IL-4 but not IL-5 protein, following exposure to anti-IgE (Piccinni *et al.*, 1991). The induction of IL-4 mRNA occurs after 48 hours and is potentiated by IL-3.

A recent study by Brunner *et al.* (1993) has confirmed that mature human basophils synthesize and release IL-4. For optimal secretion, priming with IL-3 for 18–48 hours before activation with anti-IgE is required, although low amounts of IL-4 were occasionally detected following incubation with either IL-3 or anti-IgE alone. No spontaneous IL-4 production was detected, and other cytokines known to enhance basophil mediator release, namely IL-5, GM-CSF and nerve growth factor, were inactive. IgE-dependent synthesis and release of IL-4 by IL-3-primed basophils occurred within 2–6 hours, and no IL-4 was stored pre-formed. Stimulation of basophils with a combination of phorbol myristate acetate (PMA) and ionomycin, or ionomycin alone, resulted in IL-4 production of greater or comparable magnitude to that induced by sequential stimulation with IL-3 and anti-IgE. Arock *et al.* (1993) have subsequently confirmed that normal basophils produce IL-4 following activation, and in addition have shown that leukaemic basophils express IL-4 constitutively.

Biological properties of human mast cell cytokines

Each of the cytokines so far identified as human mast cell products are likely to be involved in the pathogenesis of allergic mucosal inflammation. IL-4 activates B cells for Ig secretion through up-regulation of cell-surface MHC class II antigen (Rousset *et al.*, 1988), CD23 (FcεRII) (Vercelli *et al.*, 1988) and CD40 (Clark *et al.*, 1989), and plays a pivotal role in the isotype switching of B cells to IgE synthesis (Del Prete *et al.*, 1988). IL-4 specifically increases expression of vascular cell adhesion molecule-1 (VCAM-1) (Thornhill & Haskard, 1990) involved in the very late antigen (VLA)-4-dependent recruitment of T cells and eosinophils (Thornhill *et al.*, 1991; Schleimer *et al.*, 1992), and induces the expression of the low-affinity IgE receptor (FcεRII, CD23) on monocytes (te Velde *et al.*, 1988). In addition, IL-4 induces fibroblast chemotaxis (Postlethwaite & Seyer, 1991) and collagen secretion (Postlethwaite *et al.*, 1992). Possibly the most important effect of IL-4 is its ability to induce the development of the TH2 phenotype of T cells (Le Gros *et al.*, 1990; Swain *et al.*, 1990), which itself produces IL-4, IL-5 and IL-6 as reviewed by Romagnani (1991). The presence of IL-4 at the onset of an immunological response may therefore dictate whether a cell-mediated (Th1) or humoral (Th2) response develops.

The effects of IL-5 in humans are almost exclusively limited to eosinophils. It is a growth and differentiation factor (Clutterbuck *et al.*, 1989), and activator (Lopez *et al.*, 1988) for eosinophils, and in addition prevents their programmed cell death prolonging survival (Yamaguchi *et al.*, 1991). IL-5 promotes eosinophil adhesion to vascular endothelium through a CD11/CD18-dependent mechanism (Walsh *et al.*, 1991a), and primes eosinophils for chemotaxis in response to other mediators (Warringa *et al.*, 1992a,b) as well as being directly chemotactic itself (Wang *et al.*, 1989). As a consequence, IL-5 is considered to be a pivotal cytokine in allergen- and parasite-mediated eosinophilic responses.

IL-6 has activities on a wide range of cellular processes, including T-cell activation (Tosato & Pike, 1988) and stimulation of Ig production by B cells, and thus it enhances IL-4-dependent IgE synthesis (Jabara *et al.*, 1988). IL-6 is also the most important cytokine responsible for the production of acute-phase proteins by hepatocytes during inflammatory responses. IL-8 belongs to the intercrine family of cytokines and is secreted by a wide variety of cells, including T cells, macrophage/monocytes, endothelium and epithelial cells (Schroder & Christophers, 1989; Smyth *et al.*, 1991; Standiford *et al.*, 1991; Marini *et al.*, 1992). It is a potent chemoattractant for neutrophils (Kunkel *et al.*, 1991) and is also chemotactic for eosinophils after priming with IL-3, IL-5 or GM-CSF (Warringa *et al.*, 1991, 1992).

TNF-α (cachectin) is another cytokine implicated in the pathogenesis of asthma. When administered by inhalation or intravenously to animals, TNF-α increases bronchial responsiveness (Wheeler *et al.*, 1990; Kips *et al.*, 1992). It is a chemoattractant for neutrophils and monocytes (Ming *et al.*, 1987), increases microvascular permeability, enhances both mast cell mediator release (Van Overveld *et al.*, 1992) and eosinophil cytotoxicity (Silberstein & David, 1986; Slungaard *et al.*, 1990). In addition, it has the capacity to up-regulate the leucocyte endothelial cell adhesion molecules (CAM) E-selectin, VCAM-1 and ICAM-1 (Bevilacqua *et al.*, 1989; Osborn *et al.*, 1989; Leung *et al.*, 1991) involved in the recruitment of neutrophils, eosinophils, monocytes and T cells into inflammatory zones. TNF-α also stimulates fibroblast proliferation and secretion of matrix proteins, collagenase and cytokine, including IL-6 (Dayer *et al.*, 1985; Kohase *et al.*, 1986; Mielke *et al.*, 1990; Postlethwaite & Seyer, 1990; Warringa *et al.*, 1992).

Mast cells and basophils in asthma

It is recognized that in addition to contributing to the pathophysiology of allergy, mast cells also play important roles in a number of other physiological, pathological and immunological processes, including tissue remodelling, wound repair, pathological fibrosis, angiogenesis, clotting, and host reactions to certain neoplasms. The ubiquitous distribution of mast cells throughout connective tissues, along epithelial surfaces, and in close proximity to blood vessels, makes their products available to a large number of different cell types, including fibroblasts, glandular epithelial cells, nerves, vascular endothelial cells, smooth muscle cells and other cells of the immune system. This tissue distribution, and the vast array of lipid mediators, proteases, proteoglycans and cytokines identified as potential products of murine and human mast cells, explains how this type of cell could mediate so many diverse effects.

The role of mast cell-derived histamine PGD_2 and LTC_4 in the pathological processes involved in the early-phase airflow obstruction in asthma, namely mucosal oedema due to increased vascular permeability, smooth muscle contraction and excessive mucus secretion, are well established. The recent development of fibreoptic bronchoscopy as a research tool has allowed histological investigation of bronchial biopsies from patients with milder disease (Beasley *et al.*, 1989c). Mast cell numbers are not increased but there is morphological evidence of continuous degranulation (Beasley *et al.*, 1989c; Djukanovic *et al.*, 1990). Basophils are rarely seen (Beasley *et al.*, 1989c).

Fibreoptic bronchoscopy has also allowed the study of bronchoalveolar lavage (BAL) fluid from asthmatic subjects, and again gives us evidence that active inflammation is present (Beasley *et al.*, 1989c). Several groups have shown increased numbers of mast cells, eosinophils and lymphocytes in BAL from unchallenged asthmatic compared with normal controls (Flint *et al.*, 1985a; Casale *et al.*, 1987; Godard *et al.*, 1987; Kirby *et al.*, 1987; Kelly *et al.*, 1989) and increased levels of inflammatory mediators such as histamine (Casale *et al.*, 1987; Kirby *et al.*, 1987), tryptase (Wenzel *et al.*, 1988) and LTE_4 (Lam *et al.*, 1988).

Bronchial provocation in asthma may also provide evidence of the involvement of mast cells. During the early-phase response there is release of a wide range of vasoactive and spasmogenic mediators, which mainly originate from mast cells resident in the airway mucosa. When IgE bound to the high-affinity IgE Fc receptor on mast cells is cross-linked by allergen, a series of membrane and cytoplasmic events utilizing Ca^{2+} and energy-dependent mechanisms culminate in the secretion of pre-formed granule-derived mediators, and the synthesis and release of newly formed lipid products. The measurement of mediators in blood, urine and BAL has provided strong evidence that the early-phase response is predominantly due to the effects of released histamine, PGD_2 and the sulphidopeptide leukotrienes LTC_4, LTD_4 and LTE_4 (slow-reacting substances of anaphylaxis), the latter two being generated from LTC_4 extracellularly (Arm & Lee, 1990). Attenuation of the early-phase response following administration of specific receptor antagonists to these mediators provides further evidence of their role (Rafferty *et al.*, 1987; Beasley *et al.*, 1989b; Taylor *et al.*, 1991).

In addition to these autacoids, other mast cell products are likely to contribute to the asthmatic response. Tryptase and chymase are pre-formed proteases specific for mast cells (Schwartz *et al.*, 1981a; Wintroub *et al.*, 1986a), which are also released following IgE cross-linkage. Tryptase levels are raised at baseline in asthmatic subjects, and rise during the EAR following allergen provocation (Wenzel *et al.*, 1988). Tryptase may generate C3 and bradykinin from their protein precursors, which may act as secondary mediators of smooth muscle contraction and vascular permeability, whilst chymase is a potent secretagogue for

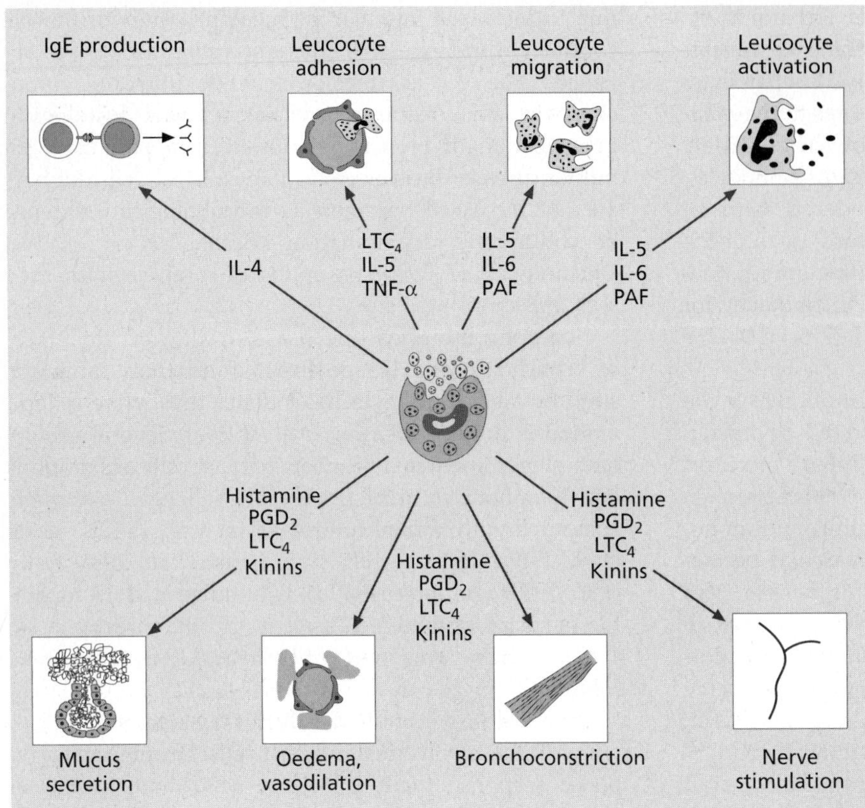

Fig. 9.9 Diagrammatic representation of some of the more prominent actions of mast cells in asthma.

bovine airway submucosal glands (Sommerhoff *et al.*, 1989).

The mast cell contains a virtual pharmacopoeia of biological substances, many of which are capable of inducing the typical pathophysiological changes seen in mucosal inflammation in asthma (Fig. 9.9). The recent identification of mast cells as a source of multifunctional cytokines, which are released in response to IgE-dependent activation, suggests that mast cells may also mediate several aspects of the allergic inflammatory response.

With respect to allergic inflammation, most studies have investigated the role of mast cell cytokines in the rodent model of the IgE-dependent cutaneous late-phase reaction. In mice and rats, this late-phase reaction is similar to that seen in humans, although the infiltrating cells are predominantly neutrophils, which may be a reflection of the general eosinopenia present in normal 'non-atopic' rodents. Studying mice that are normal, genetically mast cell deficient, and genetically mast cell deficient but subsequently replenished with mast cells from normal mice, has demonstrated that the early and late increase in vascular permeability and tissue swelling following IgE-dependent passive cutaneous anaphlylactic reactions is mast cell dependent (Wershil *et al.*, 1987). Furthermore, nearly all the late leucocyte infiltration is also mast cell dependent (Wershil *et al.*, 1991). Higher levels of TNF-α were found in mast cell-reconstituted sites than in mast cell-deficient sites (Gordon & Galli, 1991), and the local administration of neutralizing antibodies to TNF-α reduced leucocyte infiltration by about 50% (Howarth *et al.*, 1991). The recruitment of the remaining leucocytes is likely to be due to other mast cell-derived cytokines. Other studies using this mouse model have also demonstrated that intradermal administration of PMA induces mast cell-dependent neutrophil infiltration (Wershil *et al.*, 1988), while intradermal injection of substance P induces mast-cell dependent eosinophil infiltration (Matsuda *et al.*, 1989). Similarly, in rats, intracutaneous injection of anti-IgE antibodies or compound 48/80, an agent which specifically induces mast cell degranulation, resulted in both early- and late-phase reactions (Tannenbaum *et al.*, 1980). This late-phase cellular infiltration was reproduced by intracutaneous injection of mast cell granules, and was shown to be due to an unidentified granule constituent (Tannenbaum *et al.*, 1980). These studies provide strong evidence that mast cells and their products, including TNF-α, are directly involved in late-phase inflammatory cell recruitment in rodent systems.

The relevance of mast cell cytokines to the inflammatory response during parasite infection, however, is less clear. Nogami *et al.* (1990) demonstrated that in contrast to T-cell deficiency, mast cell deficiency did not prevent marked pulmonary eosinophilia following transnasal infection with *Ascaris suum*.

Although the role of the mast cell in the early response to allergen is well defined and has been described already, studying mast cell dependency in human late-phase reactions, and particularly in chronic allergic inflammation, is more difficult. It has been recognized for many years that human late-phase responses are IgE dependent (Dolovich *et al.*, 1973; Solley *et al.*, 1976), but this does not necessarily implicate mast cells solely in the pathogenesis, as other inflammatory cells, such as macrophages, B cells and possibly eosinophils, can be activated via IgE bound to its low-affinity receptor (FcεRII, CD23). Several studies, however, have demonstrated that intradermal injection of compound 48/80, which produces degranulation of the MC_{TC} subset of mast cells, initiates a late-phase response associated with inflammatory cell infiltration, therefore suggesting that mast cells are directly involved (Atkins *et al.*, 1973; Solley *et al.*, 1976; James *et al.*, 1981).

The study by Klein *et al.* demonstrating that exposure of skin organ cultures to anti-IgE, morphine sulphate, compound 48/80 or A-23187 resulted in expression of endothelial leucocyte adhesion molecule-1 (ELAM-1) on endothelial cells within 2 hours, and that this effect could be inhibited by prior administration of sodium cromoglycate or anti-TNF-α antibodies, provided indirect evidence that mast cell-derived TNF-α is likely to be involved in cutaneous late-phase responses. Leung *et al.* (1991) also reached the conclusion that resident cells within the skin, rather than newly recruited cells, were responsible for TNF-α-induced ELAM-1 expression following intradermal allergen challenge. Subsequently, Walsh *et al.* (1991b) showed that among normal dermal cells, mast cells are the predominant cell type that express both TNF-α protein and TNF-α mRNA, and that induction of ELAM-1 is a direct consequence of release of mast cell TNF-α.

Taken together, these findings indicate that mast cell-derived TNF-α, and probably other mast cell-derived cytokines such as IL-4 and IL-5, are likely to be involved in human late-phase reactions, and therefore, by inference, chronic human allergic inflammation. Many resident and recruited inflammatory cells have the potential to secrete further cytokines in response to mast cell cytokine release. This suggests that the response to release of mast cell cytokines may extend far beyond the changes mediated directly by mast cell cytokines themselves, and has led to the concept of the mast cell–leucocyte cytokine cascade (Galli, 1993).

Mast cell mediators and asthma pathophysiology

The biological activities of a number of mast cell mediators may explain a number of the pathological features present in asthma.

Epithelial damage

The epithelium is fragile and partially denuded even in mild asthmatics. Often the basal cell layer is left intact, suggesting the point of weakness is between this layer and the surface epithelium. Whether this abnormality is primary or secondary is unclear, although evidence suggests the latter may be the case. Although it has been demonstrated that eosinophil products such as major basic protein (MBP), eosinophil cationic protein (ECP) and eosinophil peroxidase (EPO) are cytotoxic to the respiratory epithelium (Ayars *et al.*, 1989; Irani *et al.*, 1989), mast cell products could also be important in this process, although there has been little research in this area. Superoxide produced following mast cell degranulation (Henderson & Kaliner, 1978) may generate highly reactive oxygen species such as hydrogen peroxide, the hydroxyl radical (OH^-) and oxygen free radicals which are able to damage cell membranes, and studies in dogs have shown that proteolytic enzymes such as chymase may also weaken intracellular bonds, resulting in the release of epithelial cells from the basal layer (Briggman *et al.*, 1984).

Epithelial sub-basement membrane thickening

A characteristic histological feature of asthma is thickening of the sub-basement membrane due to type III and V collagen deposition in the lamina reticularis (Roche *et al.*, 1989). The most likely origin for this collagen is proliferating myofibroblasts whose number correlates with the collagen thickness (Brewster *et al.*, 1990). The stimulus for this is not yet clear, but is probably under the control of fibrogenic cytokines which include IL-4 and TNF-α, and possibly mast cell tryptase, heparin and histamine. The effects of mast cells on fibroblasts are described in more detail below.

Mucosal oedema and plasma leakage

Mucosal oedema contributes to the airway narrowing present in asthma. Contraction of endothelial cells in post-capillary venules leads to the formation of gaps, which allow the outflow of plasma. This occurs in response to mediators, such as histamine, prostaglandins, leukotrienes and platelet-activating factor (PAF), released from inflammatory cells, which probably act directly on endothelial cells and bradykinin which may act via neural reflexes. In addition to obstructing the airway lumen, exuded plasma may markedly enhance mucus viscosity. Albumin may increase mucus viscosity through the formation of various protein–glycoprotein complexes (List *et al.*, 1978), which in combination with impaired ciliary motility will promote mucostasis.

Mucus production

Extensive mucus plugging is a characteristic finding in patients dying from asthma, but is also likely to contribute to airways obstruction in stable disease (Cutz *et al.*, 1978). Mucus production in asthmatic airways comes from both hyperplastic goblet cells in the airway epithelium and hypertrophic submucosal glands. The latter are innervated by the parasympathetic nervous system. In addition to cholinergic stimulation, a number of mediators released from inflammatory cells also stimulate mucus secretion. In order of potency these include LTD_4, LTC_4, hydroxyeicosatetraenoic acid, prostanoids and histamine (Shelhamer *et al.*, 1980; Marom *et al.*, 1981, 1982). Canine mast cell chymase is also a potent mucus secretagogue when added to cultures of bovine airway glands (Sommerhoff *et al.*, 1989).

Bronchial hyperresponsiveness

A characteristic pathophysiological feature of asthma is bronchial hyperresponsiveness (BHR) — the exaggerated bronchoconstrictor response of the airways to a wide range of specific and non-specific stimuli (Boushey *et al.*, 1980). Stimuli may act directly, such as the pharmacological compounds histamine and methacholine, or indirectly, such as adenosine, exercise, cold air, bradykinin and sulphur dioxide. BHR is usually expressed as the concentration of histamine or methacholine required to produce a 20% fall in FEV_1 (forced expiratory volume in 1 second; PC_{20}). It is on this background of BHR that natural insults such as exercise, cold air or irritant smoke may induce airway obstruction. The cause of airway narrowing is generally assumed to be bronchoconstriction, although oedema and mucus production may contribute. With respect to asthma, several studies have suggested a cause-and-effect relationship between inflammation and BHR. Following allergen challenge, BHR increases at the time of the late reaction, the time when there is an influx of inflammatory cells, particularly eosinophils, into the airway mucosa. This increase in BHR may last for days or even weeks (Cartier *et al.*, 1982). BAL studies have shown a positive correlation between the number of activated eosinophils and BHR. Furthermore, levels of eosinophil products such as MBP, numbers of epithelial cells, numbers of mast cells and levels of histamine in bronchial lavage also correlate with the degree of BHR (Wardlaw *et al.*, 1988; Beasley *et al.*, 1989d).

Several factors are probably related to the development of BHR in the presence of inflammation. The presence of bronchospastic and mucogenic mediators released by a variety of inflammatory cells, including mast cells, either spontaneously or following exposure to allergen probably contribute. TNF-α induces BHR in mice and sheep, apparently independent of its effects on inflammatory cell recruitment (Wheeler *et al.*, 1990; Kips *et al.*, 1992). Similarly, tryptase has been shown to induce BHR to histamine in dogs (Sekizawa *et al.*, 1989). Tryptase may also contribute to the development of BHR and bronchoconstriction through its degradation of bronchodilator neuropeptides (Caughey *et al.*, 1988; Tam & Caughey, 1990).

IgE production

The recognition that both mast cells and basophils produce IL-4 suggested that they have the potential to influence IgE production by B cells. Gauchat *et al.* (1993) tested this hypothesis recently, using isolated human lung mast cells and peripheral blood basophils. They demonstrated convincingly that both mast cells and basophils express CD40 ligand (CD40L), and are able to provide the cell–cell signal required for IgE production through the interaction of this ligand with CD40 expressed on B cells. Furthermore, in their experimental fluid-phase system basophils induced IgE synthesis without the addition of exogenous IL-4 following stimulation with ionomycin and PMA for 3 hours. In contrast, lung mast cells which were incubated with SCF (c-*kit* ligand) for 72 hours required the addition of exogenous IL-4 in order to induce IgE secretion. These observations therefore open a completely new field in mast cell biology.

Basophil in allergic inflammation

The lack of a specific marker for basophils has hampered their study in allergic diseases, and their relative importance is uncertain. They are only present in very low numbers in peripheral blood, and are not found in normal non-inflamed tissues, indicating they are recruited to sites of inflammation by mediators from other cell types. Several studies have described the presence of basophils at sites of allergic inflammation using metachromatic staining and morphological criteria. In both nasal and cutaneous late-phase responses induced in otherwise asymptomatic patients, basophil recruitment has been reported, although the number of infiltrating basophils compared with neutrophils and eosinophils is tiny (Bascom *et al.*, 1988; Charlesworth *et al.*, 1989b). In patients with symptomatic allergic rhinitis, small numbers of basophils were reported to be present in nasal secretions, while small numbers of mast cells were seen in nasal mucosal scrapings, but neither were present in normal subjects. In patients with symptomatic asthma, however, basophils were almost undetectable in BAL at baseline, but comprised 1% of cells recovered by BAL following allergen challenge, compared with 38% for eosinophils (Heaney *et al.*, 1994). One of the standard morphological criteria for identifying metachromatically staining cells as basophils is the presence of a multilobed nucleus. However, with the introduction of immunohistochemistry to identify mast cells using mAb to mast cell-specific tryptase, it has become apparent that some mast cells, particularly immature mast cells (Irani *et al.*, 1992; Dvorak *et al.*, 1993a), and those cells residing in the epithelium, may also have a lobulated nucleus. This has also been described for up to 15% of mast cells identified by electron microscopy (Kawanami *et al.*, 1985). As the epithelial mast cell population is most likely to account for those cells recovered by lavage procedures, the identification of basophils in the above studies may be an overestimate.

Indirect evidence for the participation of basophils in allergic responses stems from the pattern of mediator release observed during allergen-induced late-phase responses. In both the nose and the skin, a secondary rise occurs in histamine and LTC_4, but not PGD_2, or tryptase (Miller, 1984; Naclerio *et al.*, 1985; Bascom *et al.*, 1988; Shalit *et al.*, 1988; Charlesworth *et al.*, 1989a). It has been suggested that this discriminates between mast cells and basophils as the source of these mediators in the late-phase response, as basophils only produce histamine and LTC_4, while mast cells also produce tryptase and PGD_2. Inhibition of this late histamine rise by corticosteroids also suggests that it may not be due to mast degranulation (Bascom *et al.*, 1988; Charlesworth *et al.*, 1991). It cannot be assumed, however, that mast cells always release their entire armamentarium of mediators on non-immunological stimulation. An example of this is the non-immunological activation of human skin mast cells which causes the preferential release of histamine, with negligible levels of newly generated prostanoids (Benyon *et al.*, 1989). Furthermore, eosinophils which accumulate in the late-phase response in large numbers, also produce LTC_4. Thus, current evidence suggests that the basophil is involved in allergic inflammatory reactions, but proof will have to await the development of a specific immunocytochemical marker for this cell.

Conclusions

As may be seen, the mast cell is a ubiquitous cell which is the source of a wide and unique array of inflammatory mediators, whose actions range from bronchoconstriction to inflammatory cell infiltration and activation. However, its role in asthma must be seen as acting in concert with all the other inflammatory cells which participate in this debilitating disease.

References

Alter, S.C., Kramps, J.A., Janoff, A. & Schwartz, L.B. (1990) Interactions of human mast cell tryptase with biological protease inhibitors. *Arch. Biochem. Biophys.*, **276**, 26–31.

Arm, J.P. & Lee, T.H. (1990) Lipoxygenase mediators. In: *Immunology and Allergy Clinics of North America: Allergic Inflammatory Mediators and Bronchial Hyperresponsiveness* (eds C.W. Bierman & T.H. Lee), pp. 373–81. W.B. Saunders, Philadelphia.

Arock, M., Merle-Béral, H., Dugas, B. *et al.* (1993) IL-4 release by human leukemic and activated normal basophils. *J. Immunol.*, **151**, 1441–7.

Ashman, L.K., Cambareri, A.C., To, L.B., Levinsky, R.J. & Juttner, C.A. (1991) Expression of the YB5.B8 antigen (c-*kit* proto-oncogene product) in normal human bone marrow. *Blood*, **78**, 30–7.

Atkins, P.C., Green, G.R. & Zweiman, B. (1973) Histologic studies of human skin test responses to ragweed, compound 48/80 and histamine. *J. Allergy Clin. Immunol.*, **51**, 263–73.

Ayars, G.H., Altman, L.C., McManus, M.M. *et al.* (1989) Injurious effect of the eosinophil peroxide–hydrogen peroxide–halide system and major basic protein on human nasal epithelium *in vitro*. *Am. Rev. Resp. Dis.*, **140**, 125–31.

Baker, E., Sayers, T.J., Sutherland, G.R. & Smyth, M.J. (1994) The genes encoding NK cell granule serine proteases, human tryptase-2 (TRYP2) and human granzyme A (HFSP), both map to chromosome 5q11-q12 and define a new locus for cytotoxic lymphocyte granule tryptases. *Immunogenetics*, **40**, 235–7.

Bascom, R., Wachs, M., Naclerio, R.M., Pipkorn, U., Galli, S.J. & Lichtenstein, L.M. (1988) Basophil influx occurs after nasal antigen challenge: effects of topical corticosteroid pretreatment. *J. Allergy Clin. Immunol.*, **81**, 580–9.

Beasley, C.R.W., Robinson, C., Featherstone, R.L. *et al.* (1987) 9 alpha, 11 beta-prostaglandin F2, a novel metabolite of prostaglandin D2 is a potent contractile agonist of human and guinea pig airways. *J. Clin. Invest.*, **79**, 978–83.

Beasley, C.R.W., Featherstone, R.L., Church, M.K. *et al.* (1989a) Effect of a thromboxane receptor antagonist on PGD2- and allergen-induced bronchoconstriction. *J. Appl. Physiol.*, **66**, 1685–93.

Beasley, C.R.W., Featherstone, R.L., Church, M.K. *et al.* (1989b) Receptor antagonism of bronchoconstrictor prostanoids *in vitro* and *in vivo* by GR32191: implications for the contribution of these mediators to immediate allergen-induced bronchoconstriction in asthma. *J. Appl. Physiol.*, **66**, 1685–93.

Beasley, C.R.W., Roche, W.R., Roberts, J.A. & Holgate, S.T. (1989c) Cellular events in the bronchi in mild asthma and after bronchial provocation. *Am. Rev. Resp. Dis.*, **139**, 806–17.

Beasley, C.R.W., Roche, W.R., Roberts, J.A. & Holgate, S.T. (1989d) Cellular events in the bronchi in mild asthma and after bronchial provocation. *Am. Rev. Resp. Dis.*, **139**, 806–17.

Beaven, M.A. (1978) Histamine: its role in physiological and pathological processes. *Monogr. Allergy.*, **13**, 1–10.

Befus, A.D., Goodacre, R., Dyck, N. & Bienenstock, J. (1985) Mast cell heterogeneity in man. I. Histologic studies of the intestine. *Int. Arch. Allergy Appl. Immunol.*, **76**, 232–6.

Ben-Sasson, S.Z., Le Gros, G.S., Conrad, D.H., Finkelman, F.D. &

Paul, W.E. (1990) Cross-linking Fc receptors stimulates splenic non-B non-T cells to secrete interleukin-4 and other cytokines. *Proc. Nat. Acad. Sci. USA*, **87**, 1421–5.

Benveniste, J., Henson, P.M. & Cochrane, C.G. (1972) Leucocyte-dependent histamine release from rabbit platelets: the role of IgE, basophils and a platelet activating factor. *J. Exp. Med.*, **136**, 1356–77.

Benyon, R.C., Church, M.K., Clegg, L.S. & Holgate, S.T. (1986) Dispersion and characterization of mast cells from human skin. *Int. Arch. Allergy Appl. Immunol.*, **79**, 332–4.

Benyon, R.C., Lowman, M.A. & Church, M.K. (1987) Human skin mast cells: their dispersion, purification and secretory characteristics. *J. Immunol.*, **138**, 861–7.

Benyon, R.C., Robinson, C. & Church, M.K. (1989) Differential release of histamine and eicosanoids from human skin mast cells activated by IgE-dependent and non-immunological stimuli. *Brit. J. Pharmacol.*, **97**, 898–904.

Bevilacqua, M.P., Stengelin, S., Gimbrone, M.A. Jr & Seed, B. (1989) Endothelial leukocyte adhesion molecule 1: an inducible receptor for neutrophils related to complement regulatory proteins and lectins. *Science*, **243**, 1160–5.

Bochner, B.S. & Lichtenstein, L.M. (1992) Mechanisms of basophil recruitment in allergic diseases. *Clin. Exp. Allergy*, **22**, 973–5.

Boushey, H.A., Holtzman, M.J., Sheller, R. & Nadel, J.A. (1980) State of the art. Bronchial hyperreactivity. *Am. Rev. Resp. Dis.*, **121**, 389–413.

Bradding, P., Feather, I.H., Howarth, P.H. *et al.* (1992) Interleukin 4 is localized to and released by human mast cells. *J. Exp. Med.*, **176**, 1381–6.

Bradding, P., Feather, I.H., Wilson, S. *et al.* (1993a) Immunolocalization of cytokines in the nasal mucosa of normal and perennial rhinitic subjects: the mast cell as a source of IL-4, IL-5 and IL-6 in human allergic mucosal inflammation. *J. Immunol.*, **151**, 3853–65.

Bradding, P., Roberts, J.A., Britten, K.M. *et al.* (1994) Interleukins (IL)-4,-5,-6 and TNFα in normal and asthmatic airways: evidence for the human mast cell as an important source of these cytokines. *Am. J. Respir. Cell. Mol. Med.*, **10**, 471–80.

Bradding, P., Feather, I.H., Wilson, S., Holgate, S.T. & Howarth, P.H. (1995) Cytokine immunoreactivity in seasonal rhinitis: regulation by a topical corticosteroid. *Am. J. Resp. Crit. Care Med.* **151**, 1900–6.

Brewster, C.E., Howarth, P.H., Djukanovic, R., Wilson, J., Holgate, S.T. & Roche, W.R. (1990) Myofibroblasts and subepithelial fibrosis in bronchial asthma. *Am. J. Respir. Cell Mol. Biol.*, **3**, 507–11.

Briggman, R.A., Schechter, N.M., Fraki, J.E. & Lazarus, G.S. (1984) Degradation of the epidermal–dermal junction by a proteolytic enzyme from human skin and human polymorphonuclear leukocytes. *J. Exp. Med.*, **160**, 1027–42.

Brown, M.A., Pierce, J.H., Watson, C.J., Falco, J., Ihle, J.N. & Paul, W.E. (1987) B cell stimulatory factor-1/interleukin-4 mRNA is expressed by normal and transformed mast cells. *Cell*, **50**, 809–18.

Brunner, T., Heusser, C.H. & Dahinden, C.A. (1993) Human peripheral blood basophils primed by interleukin 3 (IL-3) produce IL-4 in response to immunoglobulin E receptor stimulation. *J. Exp. Med.*, **177**, 605–11.

Bunnett, N.W., Goldstein, S.M. & Nakazato, P. (1992) Isolation of a neuropeptide-degrading carboxypeptidase from the human stomach. *Gastroenterology*, **102**, 76–87.

Burd, P.R., Rogers, H.W., Gordon, J.R. *et al.* (1989) Interleukin-3 dependent and independent cell lines stimulated with IgE and antigen express multiple cytokines. *J. Exp. Med.*, **170**, 245–58.

Cartier, A., Thomson, N.C., Frith, P.A., Roberts, R. & Hargreave, F.E. (1982) Allergen-induced increase in bronchial responsiveness to histamine: relationship to the late asthmatic response and change in airway calibre. *J. Allergy Clin. Immunol.*, **70**, 170–7.

Casale, T.B., Wood, D., Richerson, H.B. *et al.* (1987) Bronchoalveolar lavage fluid histamine levels in allergic asthmatics are associated with methacholine bronchial hyperresponsiveness. *J. Clin. Invest.*, **79**, 1197–203.

Caughey, G.H., Schaumberg, T.H., Zerweck, E.H. *et al.* (1993) The human mast cell chymase gene (CMA1): mapping to the cathepsin G/granzyme gene cluster and lineage-restricted expression. *Genomics*, **15**, 614–20.

Caughey, G.H., Leidig, F., Viro, N.F. & Nadel, J.A. (1988) Substance P and vasoactive intestinal peptide degradation by mast cell tryptase and chymase. *J. Pharmacol. Exp. Ther.*, **244**, 133–7.

Caulfield, J.P., El Lati, S.G., Thomas, G. & Church, M.K. (1990) Dissociated human skin mast cells degranulate in response to anti-IgE and substance P. *Lab. Invest.*, **63**, 502–10.

Caulfield, J.P., Lewis, R.A., Hein, A. & Austen, K.F. (1980) Secretion of dissociated human pulmonary mast cells: evidence for solubilization of granule contents before discharge. *J. Cell Biol.*, **85**, 299–311.

Charlesworth, E.N., Hood, A.F., Soter, N.A., Kagey Sobotka, A., Norman, P.S. & Lichtenstein, L.M. (1989a) Cutaneous late-phase response to allergen. Mediator release and inflammatory cell infiltration. *J. Clin. Invest.*, **83**, 1519–26.

Charlesworth, E.N., Kagey-Sobotka, A., Norman, P.S. & Lichtenstein, L.M. (1989b) Effects of cetirizine on mast cell mediator release and cellular traffic during the cutaneous late phase response. *J. Allergy Clin. Immunol.*, **83**, 905–12.

Charlesworth, E.N., Kagey-Sobotka, A., Schleimer, R.P., Norman, P.S. & Lichtenstein, L.M. (1991) Prednisone inhibits the appearance of inflammatory mediators and the influx of eosinophils and basophils associated with the cutaneous late-phase response to allergen. *J. Immunol.*, **146**, 671–6.

Chung, S.W., Wong, P.M.C., Shen-Ong, G., Ruscetti, S., Ishizaka, T. & Eaves, C.J. (1986) Production of granulocyte-macrophage colony-stimulating factor by Abelson virus-induced tumorigenic mast cell lines. *Blood*, **68**, 1074–81.

Church, M.K. & Hiroi, J. (1987) Inhibition of IgE-dependent histamine release from human dispersed lung mast cells by anti-allergic drugs and salbutamol. *Brit. J. Pharmacol.*, **90**, 421–9.

Church, M.K., Okayama, Y. & Bradding, P. (1994) The role of the mast cell in acute and chronic allergic inflammation. In: *Cells and Cytokines in Lung Inflammation* (eds M. Chignard, M. Pretolani, P. Renesto & B.B. Vargaftig), pp. 13–21. Acad Scienc, New York.

Church, M.K., Benyon, R.C., Rees, P.H. *et al.* (1989) Functional heterogeneity of human mast cells. In: *Mast Cell and Basophil Differentiation and Function in Health and Disease* (eds S.J. Galli & K.F. Austen), pp. 161–70. Raven, New York.

Clark, E.A., Shu, G.L., Luscher, B. *et al.* (1989) Activation of human B cells. Comparison of the signal transduced by IL-4 to four different competence signals. *J. Immunol.*, **143**, 3873–80.

Clegg, L.S., Church, M.K. & Holgate, S.T. (1985) Histamine secretion from human skin slices induced by anti-IgE and artificial secretagogues and the effects of sodium cromoglycate and salbutamol. *Clin. Allergy*, **15**, 321–8.

Clutterbuck, E.J., Hirst, E.M. & Sanderson, C.J. (1989) Human interleukin-5 (IL-5) regulates the production of eosinophils in human bone marrow cultures: comparison and interaction with IL-1, IL-3, IL-6, and GMCSF. *Blood*, **73**, 1504–12.

Cohan, V.L., Undem, B.J., Fox, C.C., Adkinson, N.F., Lichtenstein, L.M. & Schleimer, R.P. (1989) Dexamethasone does not inhibit the release of mediators from human mast cells residing in airway, intestine or skin. *Am. Rev. Resp. Dis.*, **140**, 951–4.

Conrad, D.H., Ben-Sasson, S.Z., Le Gros, G.S., Finkelman, F.D. & Paul, W.E. (1990) Infection with *Nippostrongylus brasiliensis* or injection of anti-IgD antibodies markedly enhances Fc-receptor-mediated IL-4 production by splenic non-B non-T cells. *J. Exp. Med.*, **171**, 1497–508.

Craig, S.S., Schechter, N.M. & Schwartz, L.B. (1988) Ultrastructural analysis of human T and TC mast cells identified by immunoelectron microscopy. *Lab. Invest.*, **58**, 682–91.

Cutz, E., Levison, H. & Cooper, D.M. (1978) Ultrastructure of airways in children. *Histopathology*, **2**, 407–21.

Dayer, J.M., Beutler, B. & Cerami, A. (1985) Cachectin/tumor necrosis factor stimulates collagenase and prostaglandin E2 production by human synovial cells and dermal fibroblasts. *J. Exp. Med.*, **162**, 2163–8.

Del Prete, G., Maggi, E., Parronchi, P. *et al.* (1988) IL-4 is an essential cofactor for the IgE synthesis induced *in vitro* by human T-cell clones and their supernatants. *J. Immunol.*, **140**, 4193–8.

Djukanovic, R., Wilson, J.W., Britten, K.M. *et al.* (1990) Quantitation of mast cells and eosinophils in the bronchial mucosa of symptomatic atopic asthmatics and healthy control subjects using immunocytochemistry. *Am. Rev. Resp. Dis.*, **142**, 863–71.

Dolovich, J., Hargreave, F.E., Chalmers, R., Shier, K.J., Gauldie, J. & Bienenstock, J. (1973) Late cutaneous allergic responses in isolated IgE-dependent reactions. *J. Allergy Clin. Immunol.*, **52**, 38–46.

Drazen, J.M., Austen, K.F., Lewis, R.A. *et al.* (1980) Comparative airway and vascular activities of leukotrienes C-1 and D *in vivo* and *in vitro*. *Proc. Nat. Acad. Sci. USA*, **77**, 4354–8.

Duncan, J.I., Brown, F.I., McKinnon, A., Long, W.F., Williamson, F.B. & Thompson, W.D. (1992) Patterns of angiogenic response to mast cell granule constituents. *Int. J. Microcirc. Clin. Exp.*, **11**, 21–33.

Dvorak, A.M., Furitsu, T. & Ishizaka, T. (1993a) Ultrastructural morphology of human mast cell progenitors in sequential cocultures of cord blood cells and fibroblasts. *Int. Arch. Allergy Appl. Immunol.*, **100**, 219–29.

Dvorak, A.M. & Kissel, S. (1991) Granule changes in human skin mast cells characteristic of piecemeal degranulation and associated with recovery during wound healing. *J. Leuk. Biol.*, **49**, 197–210.

Dvorak, A.M., Massey, W., Warner, J.A., Kissel, S., Kagey-Sobotka, A. & Lichtenstein, L.M. (1991) IgE-mediated anaphylactic degranulation of isolated human skin mast cells. *Blood*, **77**, 569–78.

Dvorak, A.M., Mitsui, H. & Ishizaka, T. (1993b) Human and murine recombinant c-*kit* ligands support the development of human mast cells from umbilical cord blood cells: ultrastructural identification. *Int. Arch. Allergy Appl. Immunol.*, **101**, 247–53.

Ehrlich, P. (1878) *Beitrage zur Theorie und Praxis der Histologischen Farburg*. Doctoral Thesis, University of Leipzig.

Ehrlich, P. (1879) Uber die Specifischen Granulationen des Blutes. *Arch. Anat. Physiol. Phys. Abt.*, 571–7.

El Lati, S.G., Dahinden, C.A. & Church, M.K. (1994) Complement peptides C3a- and C5a-induced mediator release from dissociated human skin mast cells. *J. Invest. Dermatol.*, **102**, 803–6.

Enerback, L. (1966a) Mast cells in the gastrointestinal mucosa. IV. Monoamine storing capacity. *Acta Pathol. Microbiol. Scand.*, **67**, 365–79.

Enerback, L. (1966b) Mast cells in the gastrointestinal mucosa. I. Effects of fixation. *Acta Pathol. Microbiol. Scand.*, **66**, 289–302.

Enerback, L. (1966c) Mast cells in the gastrointestinal mucosa. II. Dye binding and metachromatic properties. *Acta Pathol. Microbiol. Scand.*, **66**, 303–12.

Enerback, L. (1966d) Mast cells in the gastrointestinal mucosa. III. Reactivity towards compound 48/80. *Acta Pathol. Microbiol. Scand.*, **66**, 313–22.

Enerback, L., Kolsef, S.O., Kusche, M., Hjerpe, A. & Lindahl, U. (1985) Glycosaminoglycans in rat mucosal mast cells. *Biochem. J.*, **227**, 661–8.

Flint, K.C., Leung, K.B.P., Hudspith, B.N., Brostoff, J., Pearce, F.L. & Johnson, N.M.I. (1985a) Bronchoalveolar mast cells in extrinsic asthma: a mechanism for the initiation of antigen specific bronchoconstriction. *Brit. Med. J.*, **291**, 923–6.

Flint, K.C., Leung, K.B.P., Pearce, F.L., Hudspith, B.N., Brostoff, J. & Johnson, N.M.I. (1985b) Human mast cells recovered from bronchoalveolar lavage: their morphology, histamine release and effects of sodium cromoglycate. *Clin. Sci.*, **68**, 427–32.

Fraki, J.E. & Hopsu-Havu, V.K. (1972) Human skin proteases. Fractionation and characterisation. *Arch. Derm. Forsch.*, **243**, 52–66.

Galli, S.J. (1990) New insight into 'the riddle of the mast cells': microenvironmental regulation of mast cell development and phenotypic heterogeneity. *Lab. Invest.*, **62**, 5–33.

Galli, S.J. (1993) New concepts about the mast cell. *New Engl. J. Med.*, **328**, 257–65.

Galli, S.J., Tsai, M. & Wershil, B.K. (1993) The c-*kit* receptor, stem cell factor, and mast cells. *Am. J. Pathol.*, **142**, 965–74.

Gauchat, J.-F., Henchoz, S., Mazzei, G. *et al.* (1993) Induction of human IgE synthesis in B cells by mast cells and basophils. *Nature*, **365**, 340–3.

Glenner, G.G. & Cohen, L.A. (1960) Histochemical demonstration of a species-specific trypsin-like enzyme in mast cells. *Nature*, **185**, 846–7.

Godard, P., Bousquet, J., Lebel, B. & Michel, F.B. (1987) Bronchoalveolar lavage in the asthmatic. *Bull. Eur. Physiopathol. Resp.*, **23**, 73–83.

Goetzl, E.J. & Pickett, W.C. (1981) Novel structural determinants of the human neutrophil chemotactic activity of leukotriene B. *J. Exp. Med.*, **153**, 482–7.

Goldstein, S.M., Kaempfer, C.E., Kealey, J.T. & Wintroub, B.U. (1989) Human mast cell carboxypeptidase. Purification and characterization. *J. Clin. Invest.*, **83**, 1630–6.

Goldstein, S.M., Leong, J. & Bunnett, N.W. (1991) Human mast cell proteases hydrolyze neurotensin, kinetensin and Leu5-enkephalin. *Peptides*, **12**, 995–1000.

Goldstein, S.M., Leong, J., Schwartz, L.B. & Cooke, D. (1992) Protease composition of exocytosed human skin mast cell protease–proteoglycan complexes: tryptase resides in a complex distinct from chymase and carboxypeptidase. *J. Immunol.*, **148**, 2475–82.

Gordon, J.R. & Galli, S.J. (1991) Release of both preformed and newly synthesized tumor necrosis factor alpha (TNFα)/cachectin by mouse mast cells stimulated via the FcεRI. A mechanism for the sustained action of mast cell-derived TNFα during IgE-dependent biological responses. *J. Exp. Med.*, **174**, 103–7.

Gordon, J.R., Burd, P.R. & Galli, S.J. (1990) Mast cells as a source of multifunctional cytokines. *Immunol. Today*, **11**, 458–64.

Gruber, B.L., Marchese, M.J., Suzuki, K. *et al.* (1989) Synovial procollagenase activation by human mast cell tryptase dependence upon matrix metalloproteinase 3 activation. *J. Clin. Invest.*, **84**, 1657–62.

Gurish, M.F., Ghildyal, N., Arm, J.P. *et al.* (1991) Cytokine mRNA are preferentially increased relative to secretory granule protein mRNA in mouse bone marrow-derived mast cells that have undergone IgE-mediated activation and degranulation. *J. Immunol.*, **146**, 1527–33.

Hägermark, Ö., Hokfelt, T. & Pernow, B. (1978) Flare and itch induced by substance P in human skin. *J. Invest. Dermatol.*, **71**, 233–5.

Hardy, C.C., Robinson, C., Lewis, R.A., Tattersfield, A.E. & Holgate, S.T. (1985) The airway and cardiovascular responses to inhaled prostaglandin I2 in normal and asthmatic man. *Am. Rev. Resp. Dis.*, **131**, 18–21.

Hartmann, T., Ruoss, S.J., Raymond, W.W., Seuwen, K. & Caughey, G.H. (1992) Human tryptase as a potent, cell-specific mitogen: role of signaling pathways in synergistic responses. *Am. J. Physiol. Lung Cell. Mol. Physiol.*, **262**, L528–34.

Heaney, L.G., Cross, L.J.M., Stanford, C.F. & Ennis, M. (1994) Differential reactivity of human bronchoalveolar lavage mast cells to substance P. *Agents Actions*, **41**, C19–21.

Henderson, W.R. & Kaliner, M.A. (1978) Immunologic and non-immunologic generation of superoxide from mast cells and basophils. *J. Clin. Invest.*, **61**, 187–96.

Howarth, P.H., Wilson, S., Lau, L. & Rajakulasingam, K. (1991) The nasal mast cell and rhinitis. *Clin. Exp. Allergy*, **21** (Suppl. 2), 3–8.

Huntley, J.F., Newlands, G.F.J., Gibson, S., Ferguson, A. & Miller, H.R.P. (1985) Histochemical demonstration of chymotrypsin like serine esterases in mucosal mast cells in four species including man. *J. Clin. Pathol.*, **38**, 375–84.

Irani, A.A., Nilsson, G., Miettinen, U. *et al.* (1992) Recombinant human stem cell factor stimulates differentiation of mast cells from dispersed human fetal liver cells. *Blood*, **80**, 3009–21.

Irani, A.M., Bradford, T.R., Kepley, C.L., Schechter, N.M. & Schwartz, L.B. (1989a) Detection of MCT and MCTC types of human mast cells by immunohistochemistry using new monoclonal anti-tryptase and anti-chymase antibodies. *J. Histochem. Cytochem.*, **37**, 1509–15.

Irani, A.A., Butrus, S.I. & Schwartz, L.B. (1988) Distribution of T and TC mast cell subsets in vernal conjunctivitis (VC) and giant papillary conjunctivitis. *NER Allergy Proc.*, **9**, 451. [Abstract.]

Irani, A.A., Craig, S.S., DeBlois, G., Elson, C.O., Schechter, N.M. & Schwartz, L.B. (1987a) Deficiency of the tryptase-positive, chymase-negative mast cell type in gastrointestinal mucosa of patients with defective T lymphocyte function. *J. Immunol.*, **138**, 4381–6.

Irani, A.A., Golzar, N., DeBlois, G., Gruber, B.L. & Schwartz, L.B. (1987b) Distribution of mast cell subtypes in rheumatoid arthritis and osteoarthritis synovia. *Arthritis Rheum.*, **30**, 66.

Irani, A.A., Sampson, H.A. & Schwartz, L.B. (1989b) Mast cells in atopic dermatitis. *Allergy*, **44** (Suppl. 9), 31–4.

Irani, A.A., Schechter, N.M., Craig, S.S., DeBlois, G. & Schwartz, L.B. (1986) Two types of human mast cells that have distinct neutral protease compositions. *Proc. Nat. Acad. Sci. USA*, **83**, 4464–8.

Jabara, H.H., Ackerman, S.J., Vercelli, D. *et al.* (1988) Induction of interleukin-4-dependent IgE synthesis and interleukin-5-dependent eosinophil differentiation by supernatants of a human helper T-cell clone. *J. Clin. Immunol.*, **8**, 437–46.

James, M.P., Kennedy, A.R. & Eady, R.A.J. (1981) A microscopic study of inflammatory reactions in human skin induced by histamine and compound 48/80. *J. Invest. Dermatol.*, **78**, 406–13.

Johnson, R.G., Carty, S.E., Fingerhoff, B.J. & Scarpa, A. (1980) The internal pH of mast cell granules. *FEBS Letts.*, **120**, 75–9.

Johnston, S.L., Price, J.N., Lau, L.C.K. *et al.* (1993) The effect of local hyperthermia on allergen-induced nasal congestion and mediator release. *J. Allergy Clin. Immunol.*, **92**, 850–6.

Kanakura, Y., Thompson, H., Nakano, T. *et al.* (1988) Multiple bidirectional alterations of phenotype and changes in proliferative potential during the *in vitro* and *in vivo* passage of clonal mast cell populations derived from mouse peritoneal mast cells. *Blood*, **72**, 877–85.

Kawanami, O., Ferrans, V.J., Fulmer, J.D. & Crystal, R.G. (1985) Ultrastructure of pulmonary mast cells in patients with fibrotic lung disorders. *Lab. Invest.*, **40**, 717–34.

Kelly, C.A., Stenton, S.C., Ward, C., Bird, G., Hendrick, D.J. & Walters, E.H. (1989) Lymphocyte subsets in bronchoalveolar lavage fluid obtained from stable asthmatics, and their correlations with bronchial responsiveness. *Clin. Exp. Allergy*, **19**, 169–75.

Kessler, D.A., Langer, R.S., Pless, N.A. & Folkman, J. (1976) Mast cells and tumor angiogenesis. *Int. J. Cancer*, **18**, 703–9.

Kielty, C.M., Lees, M., Shuttleworth, C.A. & Woolley, D.E. (1993) Catabolism of intact type VI collagen myofibrils: susceptibility to degradation by serine esterases. *Biochem. Biophys. Res. Commun.*, **191**, 1230–6.

King, S.J., Miller H.R., Newlands, G.F. & Woodbury, R.G. (1985) Depletion of mucosal mast cell protease by glucocorticosteroids: effect on intestinal anaphylaxis in the rat. *Proc. Nat. Acad. Sci. USA*, **82**, 1214–18.

Kinoshita, A., Urata, H., Bumpus, F.M. & Husain, A. (1991) Multiple determinants for the high substrate specificity of an angiotensin-II-forming chymase from the human heart. *J. Biol. Chem.*, **266**, 19192–7.

Kips, J.C., Tavernier, J. & Pauwels, R.A. (1992) Tumor necrosis factor causes bronchial hyperresponsiveness in rats. *Am. Rev. Resp. Dis.*, **145**, 332–6.

Kirby, J.G., Hargreave, F.E., Gleich, G.J. & O'Byrne, P.M. (1987) Bronchoalveolar cell profiles of asthmatic and non-asthmatic subjects. *Am. Rev. Resp. Dis.*, **136**, 379–83.

Kitamura, Y. & Go, S. (1979) Decreased production of mast cells in *Sl/Sld* anemic mice. *Blood*, **53**, 492–7.

Kitamura, Y., Go, S. & Hatanaka, K. (1978) Decrease of mast cells in *W/Wv* mice and their increase by bone marrow transplantation. *Blood*, **52**, 447–52.

Kitamura, Y., Nakayama, H. & Fujita, J. (1989) Mechanism of mast cell deficiency in mutant mice of *W/Wv* and *Sl/Sld* genotype. In: *Mast Cell and Basophil Differentiation and Function in Health and Disease* (eds S.J. Galli & K.F. Austen), pp. 15–25. Raven, New York.

Kohase, M., Henriksen DeStefano, D., May, L.T., Vilcek, J. & Sehgal, P.B. (1986) Induction of beta 2-interferon by tumor necrosis factor: a homeostatic mechanism in the control of cell proliferation. *Cell*, **45**, 659–66.

Koshino, T., Teshima, S., Fukushima, N. *et al.* (1993) Identification of basophils by immunohistochemistry in the airways of post-mortem cases of fatal asthma. *Clin. Exp. Allergy*, **23**, 919–25.

Kunkel, S.L., Standiford, T., Kasahara, K. & Strieter, R.M. (1991) Interleukin-8 (IL-8): the major neutrophil chemotactic factor in the lung. *Exp. Lung Res.*, **17**, 17–23.

Lagunoff, D. & Richard, A. (1983) Evidence for control of mast cell granule protease *in situ* by low pH. *Exp. Cell Res.*, **144**, 353.

Lam, S., Chan, H., LeRiche, J.C., Chan-Yeung, M. & Salari, H. (1988) Release of leukotrienes in patients with bronchial asthma. *J. Allergy Clin. Immunol.*, **81**, 711–17.

Lau, L.C.K., Church, M.K., Walls, A.F. & Howarth, P.H. (1994) Dispersion and characterisation of mast cells from human nasal polyp and the effects of salbutamol and IBMX on histamine secretion induced by anti-IgE (submitted).

Le Gros, G., Ben Sasson, S.Z., Seder, R., Finkelman, F.D. & Paul, W.E. (1990) Generation of interleukin 4 (IL-4)-producing cells *in vivo* and *in vitro*: IL-2 and IL-4 are required for *in vitro* generation of IL-4-producing cells. *J. Exp. Med.*, **172**, 921–9.

Leung, D.Y., Pober, J.S. & Cotran, R.S. (1991) Expression of endothelial-leukocyte adhesion molecule-1 in elicited late phase allergic reactions. *J. Clin. Invest.*, **87**, 1805–9.

Lewis, R.A., Austen, K.F. & Soberman, R.J. (1990) Leukotrienes and other products of the 5-lipoxygenase pathway. Biochemistry and relation to pathobiology in human diseases. *New Engl. J. Med.*, **323**, 645–55.

List, S.J., Findlay, B.P., Forstner, C.G. & Forstner, J.F. (1978) Enhancement of the viscosity of mucus by serum albumin. *Biochem. J.*, **175**, 565–71.

Liston, T.E. & Roberts, L.J. (1985) Transformation of prostaglandin D2 to 9alpha,11beta-(15S)-trihydroxy-prosta-(5Z,13E)-dien-1-oic acid (9alpha,11beta-prostaglandin F2): a unique biologically active prostaglandin produced enzymatically *in vivo* in humans. *Proc. Nat. Acad. Sci. USA*, **82**, 6030–4.

Lohi, J., Harvima, I. & Keski-Oja, J. (1992) Pericellular substrates of human mast cell tryptase: 72 000 Dalton gelatinase and fibronectin. *J. Cell. Biochem.*, **50**, 337–49.

Lopez, A.F., Sanderson, C.J., Gamble, J.R., Campbell, H.D., Young, I.G. & Vadas, M.A. (1988) Recombinant human interleukin-5 is a selective activator of human eosinophil function. *J. Exp. Med.*, **167**, 219–24.

Lowman, M.A., Benyon, R.C. & Church, M.K. (1988a) Characterization of neuropeptide-induced histamine released from human dispersed skin mast cells. *Brit. J. Pharmacol.*, **95**, 121–30.

Lowman, M.A., Benyon, R.C. & Church, M.K. (1988b) Human skin mast cells: effects of salbutamol and sodium cromoglycate on histamine release induced by anti-IgE and substance P. *Skin Pharmacol.*, **1**, 63–4.

Lowman, M.A., Rees, P.H., Benyon, R.C. & Church, M.K. (1988c) Human mast cell heterogeneity: histamine release from mast cells dispersed from skin, lung, adenoids, tonsils and intestinal mucosa in response to IgE-dependent and non-immunological stimuli. *J. Allergy Clin. Immunol.*, **81**, 590–7.

McNamee, L.A., Fattah, L.I., Baker, T.J., Bains, T.J. & Hissey, P.H. (1991) Production, characterization and use of monoclonal antibodies to human interleukin 5 in an enzyme-linked immunosorbant assay. *J. Immunol. Methods*, **141**, 81.

Makhdum, A. & Pearce, F.L. (1993) Histamine release from mast cells and basophils. Hyperosmolar induced histamine release from mast cells: a mechanism for the pathogenesis of exercise-induced asthma. *Agents Actions*, **38** (Suppl. C PT 2), C191–3.

Marini, M., Vittori, E., Hollemborg, J. & Mattoli, S. (1992) Expression of the potent inflammatory cytokines, granulocyte-macrophage-colony-stimulating factor and interleukin-6 and interleukin-8, in bronchial epithelial cells of patients with asthma. *J. Allergy Clin. Immunol.*, **89**, 1001–9.

Marom, Z., Shelhamer, J.H., Bach, M.K., Morton, D.R. & Kaliner, M.A. (1982) Slow reacting substances, leukotrienes C4 and D4, increase the release of mucus from human airways *in vitro*. *Am. Rev. Resp. Dis.*, **126**, 449–51.

Marom, Z., Shelhamer, J.H. & Kaliner, M.A. (1981) Effects of arachidonic acid, monohydroxyeicosantetraenoic acid and prostaglandins on the release of mucus glycoproteins from human airways *in vitro*. *J. Clin. Invest.*, **161**, 657–8.

Marshall, J.S., Ford, G.P. & Bell, E.B. (1987) Formalin sensitivity and differential staining of mast cells in human dermis. *Brit. J. Dermatol.*, **117**, 29–36.

Massey, W.A. & Lichtenstein, L.M. (1992) Role of basophils in human allergic disease. *Blood* **78**, 279–85.

Matin, R., Tam, E.K., Nadel, J.A. & Caughey, G.H. (1992) Distribution of chymase-containing mast cells in human bronchi. *J. Histochem. Cytochem.*, **40**, 781–6.

Matsuda, H., Kawakita, K., Kiso, Y., Nakano, T. & Kitamura, Y. (1989) Substance P induces granulocyte infiltration through degranulation of mast cells. *J. Immunol.*, **142**, 927–31.

Maximow, A. (1906) Uber die zellformen des lockeren bindegewebes. *Arch. F. Mikr. Anat. (Bonn).*, **67**, 680–757.

Meininger, C.J. & Zetter, B.R. (1992) Mast cells and angiogenesis. *Semin. Cancer Biol.*, **3**, 73–9.

Metcalfe, D.D., Bland, C.E. & Wasserman, S.I. (1984) Biochemical and functional characterisation of proteoglycans isolated from basophils of patients with chronic myelogenous leukemia. *J. Immunol.*, **132**, 1943.

Mielke, V., Bauman, J.G., Sticherling, M. *et al.* (1990) Detection of neutrophil-activating peptide NAP/IL-8 and NAP/IL-8 mRNA in human recombinant IL-1 alpha- and human recombinant tumor necrosis factor-alpha-stimulated human dermal fibroblasts. An immunocytochemical and fluorescent *in situ* hybridization study. *J. Immunol.*, **144**, 153–61.

Miller, H.R.P. (1984) The protective mucosal response against gastrointestinal nematodes in ruminants and laboratory animals. *Vet. Immunol. Immunopathol.*, **6**, 167–259.

Miller, H.R.P., King, S.J., Gibson, S., Huntley, J.F., Newlands, G.F.J. & Woodbury, R.G. (1986) Intestinal mucosal mast cells in normal and parasitized rats. In: *Mast Cell Differentiation and Heterogeneity* (eds A.D. Befus, J. Bienenstock & J.A. Denburg), pp. 239–55. Raven, New York.

Miller, J.S., Moxley, G. & Schwartz, L.B. (1990) Cloning and characterization of a second complementary DNA for human tryptase. *J. Clin. Invest.*, **86**, 864–70.

Ming, W.J., Bersani, L. & Mantovani, A. (1987) Tumor necrosis factor is chemotactic for monocytes and polymorphonuclear leukocytes. *J. Immunol.*, **138**, 1469–74.

Mizutani, H., Schechter, N.M., Lazarus, G.S., Black, R.A. & Kupper, T.S. (1991) Rapid and specific conversion of precursor interleukin 1 beta (IL-1 beta) to an active IL-1 species by human mast cell chymase. *J. Exp. Med.*, **174**, 821–5.

Möller, A., Lippert, U., Lessmann, D. *et al.* (1993) Human mast cells produce IL-8. *J. Immunol.*, **151**, 3261–6.

Naclerio, R.M., Proud, D., Togias, A.G. *et al.* (1985) Inflammatory mediators in late antigen-induced rhinitis. *New Engl. J. Med.*, **313**, 65–70.

Nilsson, G., Forsberg, K., Bodger, M.P. *et al.* (1993) Phenotypic characterization of stem cell factor-dependent human foetal liver-derived mast cells. *Immunology*, **79**, 325–30.

Nogami, M., Suko, M., Okudaira, H. *et al.* (1990) Experimental pulmonary eosinophilia in mice by *Ascaris suum* extract. *Am. Rev. Resp. Dis.*, **141**, 1289–95.

Ohkawara, Y., Yamauchi, K., Tanno, Y. *et al.* (1992) Human lung mast cells and pulmonary macrophages produce tumor necrosis factor-α in sensitized lung tissue after IgE receptor triggering. *Am. J. Respir. Cell Mol. Biol.*, **7**, 385–92.

Okayama, Y. & Church, M.K. (1992) Comparison of the modulatory effect of ketotifen, sodium cromoglycate, procaterol and salbutamol in human skin, lung and tonsil mast cells. *Int. Arch. Allergy Appl. Immunol.*, **97**, 216–25.

Okayama, Y., Benyon, R.C., Rees, P.H., Lowman, M.A., Hillier, K. & Church, M.K. (1992) Inhibition profiles of sodium cromoglycate and nedocromil sodium on mediator release from mast cells of human skin, lung, tonsil, adenoid and intestine. *Clin. Exp. Allergy*, **22**, 401–9.

Okayama, Y., Petit-Frère, C., Kassel, O. *et al.* (1995b) The IgE-dependent expression of mRNA for IL-4 and IL-5 in human lung mast cells. *J. Immunol.*, **155**, 1796–808.

Okayama, Y., Lau, L.C.K., Holgate, S.T. & Church, M.K. (1995a) Production of IL-5 by human lung mast cells in response to Fcε receptor cross-linkage and its enhancement by stem cell factor. Submitted for publication.

Okayama, Y., Semper, A., Holgate, S.T. & Church, M.K. (1995c) Multiple cytokine mRNA in human mast cells stimulated via FcεR1. *Int. Arch. Allergy Immunol.*, **107**, 158–9.

Osborn, L., Hession, C., Tizard, R. *et al.* (1989) Direct expression cloning of vascular cell adhesion molecule 1, a cytokine-induced endothelial protein that binds to lymphocytes. *Cell*, **59**, 1203–11.

Piccinni, M.P., Macchia, D., Parronchi, P. *et al.* (1991) Human bone marrow non-B, non-T cells produce interleukin 4 in response to cross-linkage of Fc epsilon and Fc gamma receptors. *Proc. Nat. Acad. Sci. USA*, **88**, 8656–60.

Plaut, M., Pierce, J.H., Watson, C.J., Hanley-Hyde, J., Nordan, R.P. & Paul, W.E. (1989) Mast cell lines produce lymphokines in response to cross linkage of FcεRI or to calcium ionophores. *Nature*, **339**, 64–7.

Postlethwaite, A.E. & Seyer, J.M. (1990) Stimulation of fibroblast chemotaxis by human recombinant tumor necrosis factor alpha (TNF-alpha) and a synthetic TNF-alpha 31–68 peptide. *J. Exp. Med.*, **172**, 1749–56.

Postlethwaite, A.E. & Seyer, J.M. (1991) Fibroblast chemotaxis induction by human recombinant interleukin-4. Identification by synthetic peptide analysis of two chemotactic domains residing in amino acid sequences 70–88 and 89–122. *J. Clin. Invest.*, **87**, 2147–52.

Postlethwaite, A.E., Holness, M.A., Katai, H. & Raghow, R. (1992) Human fibroblasts synthesize elevated levels of extracellular matrix proteins in response to interleukin 4. *J. Clin. Invest.*, **90**, 1479–85.

Powers, J.C., Takumi, T., Harper, J.W. *et al.* (1985) Mammalian chymotrypsin-like enzymes. Comparative reactivities of rat mast cell proteases, human and dog skin proteases and human cathepsin G with peptide-4-nitroanilide substrates and with peptide chloromethyl ketone and sulphonyl fluoride inhibitors. *Biochemistry*, **24**, 2048–58.

Proud, D., Siekierski, E.S. & Bailey, G.S. (1988) Identification of human lung mast cell kininogenase as tryptase and relevance of tryptase kininogenase activity. *Biochem. Pharmacol.*, **37**, 1473–80.

Rafferty, P., Beasley, C.R.W. & Holgate, S.T. (1987) The contribution of histamine to bronchoconstriction produced by inhaled allergen and adenosine 5′-monophosphate in asthma. *Am. Rev. Resp. Dis.*, **136**, 369–73.

Rakusan, K. & Campbell, S.E. (1991) Spatial relationship between cardiac mast cells and coronary capillaries in neonatal rats with cardiomegaly. *Can. J. Physiol. Pharmacol.*, **69**, 1750–3.

Razin, E., Stevens, R.L., Akiyama, F., Schmid, K. & Austen, K.F. (1982) Culture from mouse bone marrow of a subclass of mast cells possessing a distinct chondroitin sulfate proteoglycan with glycosaminoglycans rich in *N*-acetylgalactosamine-4,6-disulphate. *J. Biol. Chem.*, **257**, 7229–36.

Rees, P.H., Hillier, K. & Church, M.K. (1988) The secretory characteristics of mast cells isolated from the human large intestinal mucosa and muscle. *Immunology*, **65**, 437–42.

Reilley, C.F., Tewksbury, D.A., Schechter, N.M. & Travis, J. (1982) Rapid conversion of angiotensin I to angiotensin II by neutrophil and mast cell proteinases. *J. Biol. Chem.*, **257**, 8619–22.

Robinson, C., Benyon, R.C., Holgate, S.T. & Church, M.K. (1989) The IgE- and calcium-dependent release of eicosanoids and histamine from human cutaneous mast cells. *J. Invest. Dermatol.*, **93**, 397–404.

Roche, W.R., Beasley, R., Williams, J.H. & Holgate, S.T. (1989) Subepithelial fibrosis in the bronchi of asthmatics. *Lancet*, **i**, 520–4.

Romagnani, S. (1991) Type 1 T helper and type 2 T helper cells: functions, regulation and role in protection and disease. *Int. J. Clin. Lab. Res.*, **21**, 152–8.

Rousset, F., Malefijt, R.W., Slierendregt, B. *et al.* (1988) Regulation of Fc receptor for IgE (CD23) and class II MHC antigen expression on Burkitt's lymphoma cell lines by human IL-4 and IFN-gamma. *J. Immunol.*, **140**, 2625–32.

Ruoss, S.J., Hartmann, T. & Caughey, G.H. (1991) Mast cell tryptase is a mitogen for cultured fibroblasts. *J. Clin. Invest.*, **88**, 493–9.

Sage, H., Woodbury, R.G. & Bornstein, P. (1979) Structural studies on human type IV collagen. *J. Biol. Chem.*, **254**, 9893–900.

Schayer, R.W. (1963) Histidine decarboxylase in man. *Ann. NY Acad. Sci.*, **103**, 164–78.

Schechter, N.M. (1990) Human chymase. *Monogr. Allergy*, **27**, 114–31.

Schechter, N.M., Fraki, J.E., Geesin, J.C. & Lazarus, G.S. (1983) Human skin chymotryptic proteinase: isolation and relation to cathepsin G and rat mast cell protease. *J. Biol. Chem.*, **258**, 2973–8.

Schechter, N.M., Irani, A.A., Sprows, J.L., Abernethy, J., Wintroub, B.U. & Schwartz, L.B. (1990) Identification of a cathepsin G-like proteinase in the MC_{TC} type of human mast cell. *J. Immunol.*, **145**, 2652–61.

Schechter, N.M., Wang, Z.M., Blacher, R.W., Lessin, S.R., Lazarus, G.S. & Rubin, H. (1994) Determination of the primary structures of human skin chymase and cathepsin G from cutaneous mast cells of urticaria pigmentosa lesions. *J. Immunol.*, **152**, 4062–9.

Schleimer, R.P., Schulman, E.S., MacGlashan, D.W. *et al.* (1983) Effects of dexamethasone on mediator release from human lung fragments and purified human lung mast cells. *J. Clin. Invest.*, **71**, 1830–5.

Schleimer, R.P., Sterbinsky, S.A., Kaiser, J. *et al.* (1992) IL-4 induces adherence of human eosinophils and basophils but not neutrophils to endothelium: association with expression of VCAM-1. *J. Immunol.*, **148**, 1086–92.

Schroder, J.M. & Christophers, E. (1989) Secretion of novel and homologous neutrophil-activating peptides by LPS-stimulated human endothelial cells. *J. Immunol.*, **142**, 244–51.

Schulman, E.S., Post, T.J., Henson, P.M. & Gicias, P.C. (1988) Differential effects of complement peptides, C5a and C5a des arg on human basophil and lung mast cell histamine release. *J. Clin. Invest.*, **81**, 918–23.

Schwartz, L.B. & Bradford, T.R. (1986) Regulation of tryptase from human lung mast cells by heparin. Stabilization of the active tetramer. *J. Biol. Chem.*, **261**, 7372–9.

Schwartz, L.B., Bradford, T.R., Lee, D.C. & Chlebowski, J.F. (1990) Immunologic and physiochemical evidence for conformational changes occurring on conversion of human mast cell tryptase from active tetramer to inactive monomer. Production of monoclonal antibodies recognizing active tryptase. *J. Immunol.*, **144**, 2304–11.

Schwartz, L.B., Lewis, R.A. & Austen, K.F. (1981a) Tryptase from human pulmonary mast cells: purification and characterization. *J. Biol. Chem.*, **256**, 11939–43.

Schwartz, L.B., Riedel, C., Caulfield, J.P., Wasserman, S.I. & Austen, K.F. (1981b) Cell association of complexes of chymase, heparin proteoglycan, and protein after degranulation of rat mast cells. *J. Immunol.*, **126**, 2071–8.

Seder, R.A., Paul, W.E., Dvorak, A.M. *et al.* (1991) Mouse splenic and bone marrow preparation that express high-affinity epsilon receptor and produce interleukin 4 are highly enriched basophils. *Proc. Nat. Acad. Sci. USA*, **88**, 2836–9.

Sekizawa, K., Caughey, G.H., Lazarus, S.C., Gold, W.M. & Nadel, J.A. (1989) Mast cell tryptase causes airway smooth muscle hyperresponsiveness in dogs. *J. Clin. Invest.*, **83**, 175–9.

Shalit, M., Schwartz, L.B., Golzar, N. *et al.* (1988) Release of histamine and tryptase *in vivo* after prolonged cutaneous challenge with allergen in humans. *J. Immunol.*, **141**, 821–6.

Shelhamer, J.H., Marom, Z. & Kaliner, M.A. (1980) Immunologic and neuropharmacologic stimulation of mucous glycoprotein release from human airways *in vitro*. *J. Clin. Invest.*, **66**, 1400–8.

Silberstein, D.S. & David, J.R. (1986) Tumor necrosis factor enhances eosinophil toxicity to *Schistosoma mansoni* larvae. *Proc. Nat. Acad. Sci. USA*, **83**, 1055–9.

Slungaard, A., Vercellotti, G.M., Walker, G., Nelson, R.D. & Jacob, H.S. (1990) Tumor necrosis factor alpha/cachectin stimulates eosinophil oxidant production and toxicity towards human endothelium. *J. Exp. Med.*, **171**, 2025–41.

Smith, T.J., Houghland, M.W. & Johnson, D.A. (1984) Human lung tryptase: purification and characterization. *J. Biol. Chem.*, **259**, 11046–51.

Smyth, M.J., Zachariae, C.O., Norihisa, Y., Ortaldo, J.R., Hishinuma, A. & Matsushima, K. (1991) IL-8 gene expression and production in human peripheral blood lymphocyte subsets. *J. Immunol.*, **146**, 3815–23.

Solley, G.O., Gleich, G.J., Jordan, R.E. & Schroeter, A.L. (1976) The late phase of the immediate wheal and flare skin reaction: its dependence on IgE antibodies. *J. Clin. Invest.*, **58**, 408–20.

Sommerhoff, C.P., Caughey, G.H., Finkbeiner, W.E., Lazarus, S.C., Basbaum, C.B. & Nadel, J.A. (1989) Mast cell chymase. A potent secretagogue for airway gland serous cells. *J. Immunol.*, **142**, 2450–6.

Sonoda, T., Kitamura, Y., Haku, Y., Hara, H. & Mori, K.J. (1984) Proliferation of peritoneal mast cells in the skin of *W/Wv* mice that genetically lack mast cells. *J. Exp. Med.*, **160**, 138–51.

Sorbo, J., Jakobsson, A. & Norrby, K. (1994) Mast-cell histamine is angiogenic through receptors for histamine(1) and histamine(2). *Int. J. Exp. Pathol.*, **75**, 43–50.

Soter, N.A., Lewis, R.A., Corey, E.J. & Austen, K.F. (1983) Local effects of synthetic leukotrienes (LTC4, LTD4, LTE4 and LTB4) in human skin. *J. Invest. Dermatol.*, **80**, 115–19.

Standiford, T.J., Kunkel, S.L., Kasahara, K., Milia, M.J., Rolfe, M.W. & Strieter, R.M. (1991) Interleukin-8 gene expression from human alveolar macrophages: the role of adherence. *Am. J. Respir. Cell Mol. Biol.*, **5**, 579–85.

Stevens, R.L., Avraham, S., Gartner, M.C., Bruns, G.A., Austen, K.F. & Weis, J.H. (1988a) Isolation and characterization of a cDNA which encodes the peptide core of the secretory granule proteoglycan of human promyelocytic leukemia HL-60 cells. *J. Biol. Chem.*, **263**, 7287–91.

Stevens, R.L., Fox, C.C., Lichtenstein, L.M. & Austen, K.F. (1988b) Identification of chondroitin sulfate E proteoglycans and heparin proteoglycans in the secretory granules of human lung mast cells. *Proc. Nat. Acad. Sci. USA*, **85**, 2284–7.

Strobel, S., Miller, H.R.P. & Ferguson, A. (1981) Human intestinal mucosal mast cells: evaluation of fixation and staining techniques. *J. Clin. Pathol.*, **34**, 851–8.

Swain, S.L., Weinberg, A.D., English, M. & Huston, G. (1990) IL-4 directs the development of TH2-like helper effectors. *J. Immunol.*, **145**, 3796–806.

Swerlick, R.A., Yancey, K.B.,Thomas, J. & Lawley, T.J. (1988) A direct *in vivo* comparison of the inflammatory properties of human C5a and C5a des Arg in human skin. *J. Immunol.*, **140**, 2376–81.

Tam, E.K. & Caughey, G.H. (1990) Degradation of airway neuropeptides by human lung tryptase. *Am. J. Respir. Cell Mol. Biol.*, **3**, 27–32.

Tannenbaum, S., Oertel, H., Henderson, W. & Kaliner, M.A. (1980) The biological activity of mast cell granules. I. Elicitation of inflammatory responses in rat skin. *J. Immunol.*, **125**, 325–35.

Taylor, I.K., O'Shaughnessy, K.M., Fuller, R.W. & Dollery, C.T. (1991) Effect of cysteinyl-leukotrience receptor antagonist ICI 204.219 on allergen-induced bronchoconstriction and airway hyperreactivity in atopic subjects. *Lancet*, **337**, 690–4 [see comments].

te Velde, A.A., Klomp, J.P., Yard, B.A., De Vries, J.E. & Figdor, C.G. (1988) Modulation of phenotypic and functional properties of human peripheral blood monocytes by IL-4. *J. Immunol.*, **140**, 1548–554.

Thompson, H.L., Schulman, E.S. & Metcalfe, D.D. (1988) Identification of chondroitin sulfate E in human lung mast cells. *J. Immunol.*, **140**, 2708–13.

Thornhill, M.H. & Haskard, D.O. (1990) IL-4 regulates endothelial cell activation by IL-1, tumor necrosis factor, or IFN-gamma. *J. Immunol.*, **145**, 865–72.

Thornhill, M.H., Wellicome, S.M., Mahiouz, D.L., Lanchbury, J.S., Kyan Aung, U. & Haskard, D.O. (1991) Tumor necrosis factor combines with IL-4 or IFN-gamma to selectively enhance endothelial cell adhesiveness for T cells. The contribution of vascular cell adhesion molecule-1-dependent and -independent binding mechanisms. *J. Immunol.*, **146**, 592–8.

Tosato, G. & Pike, S.E. (1988) Interferon-beta 2/interleukin 6 is a costimulant for human T lymphocytes. *J. Immunol.*, **141**, 1556–62.

Tunon de Lara, J.M., Okayama, Y., McEuen, A.R., Heusser, C.H., Church, M.K. & Walls, A.F. (1994a) Release and inactivation of interleukin-4 by mast cells. In: *Cells and Cytokines in Lung Inflammation* (eds M. Chignard, M. Pretolani, P. Renesto & B.B. Vargaftig), pp. 50–8. Acad Scienc, New York.

Tunon de Lara, J.M., Okayama, Y., McEuen, A.R., Heusser, C.H., Church, M.K. & Walls, A.F. (1994b) Release and inactivation of interleukin-4 by mast cells. *Ann. NY Acad. Sci.*, **725**, 50–8.

Urata, H., Kinoshita, A., Misono, K.S., Bumpus, F.M. & Husain, A. (1990) Identification of a highly specific chymase as the major angiotensin II forming enzyme in the human heart. *J. Biol. Chem.*, **265**, 22348–57.

Uvnas, B. (1967) Mode of binding and release of histamine in mast cell granules of the rat. *Fed. Proc.*, **26**, 219–21.

Van Overveld, F.J., Jorens, P.G., Rampart, M., De Backer, W. & Vermeire, P.A. (1992) Tumor necrosis factor—a novel stimulus for human skin mast cells to secrete histamine and tryptase. *Agents Actions*, **36** (Suppl. C), C256–9.

Vercelli, D., Jabara, H.H., Lee, B.W., Woodland, N., Geha, R.S. & Leung, D.Y. (1988) Human recombinant interleukin 4 induces Fc epsilon R2/CD23 on normal human monocytes. *J. Exp. Med.*, **167**, 1406–16.

Von Recklinhausen, F. (1863) Uber Eiter und Bindewehskorperchen. *Virchows Arch. Pathol. Anat.*, **28**, 157–75.

Walls, A.F., Brain, S.D., Desai, A. *et al.* (1992b) Human mast cell tryptase attenuates the vasodilator activity of calcitonin gene-related peptide. *Biochem. Pharmacol.*, **43**, 1243–8.

Walls, A.F., Bennett, A.R., McBride, H.M., Glennie, M.J., Holgate, S.T. & Church, M.K. (1990a) Production and characterization of monoclonal antibodies specific for human mast cell tryptase. *Clin. Exp. Allergy*, **20**, 581–9.

Walls, A.F., Bennett, A.R., Sueiras-Diaz, J. & Olsson, H. (1992a) The kininogenase activity of human mast cell tryptase. *Biochem. Soc. Trans.*, **20**, 260S.

Walls, A.F., Roberts, J.A., Godfrey, R.C., Church, M.K. & Holgate, S.T. (1990b) Histochemical heterogeneity of human mast cells: disease-related differences in mast cells recovered by bronchoalveolar lavage. *Int. Arch. Allergy Appl. Immunol.*, **92**, 233–41.

Walsh, G.M., Wardlaw, A.J., Hartnell, A., Sanderson, C.J. & Kay, A.B. (1991a) Interleukin-5 enhances the *in vitro* adhesion of human eosinophils, but not neutrophils, in a leucocyte integrin (CD11/18)-dependent manner. *Int. Arch. Allergy Appl. Immunol.*, **94**, 174–8.

Walsh, L.J., Trinchieri, G., Waldorf, H.A., Whitaker, D. & Murphy, G.F. (1991b) Human dermal mast cells contain and release tumor necrosis factor alpha, which induces endothelial leukocyte adhesion molecule 1. *Proc. Nat. Acad. Sci. USA*, **88**, 4220–4.

Wang, J.M., Rambaldi, A., Biondi, A., Chen, Z.G., Sanderson, C.J. & Mantovani, A. (1989) Recombinant human interleukin 5 is a selective eosinophil chemoattractant. *Eur. J. Immunol.*, **19**, 701–5.

Wardlaw, A.J., Dunnette, S., Gleich, G.J., Collins, J.V. & Kay, A.B. (1988) Eosinophils and mast cells in bronchoalveolar lavage in subjects with mild asthma. Relationship to bronchial hyperreactivity. *Am. Rev. Resp. Dis.*, **137**, 62–9.

Warringa, R.A., Koenderman, L., Kok, P.T., Kreukniet, J. & Bruijnzeel, P.L. (1991) Modulation and induction of eosinophil chemotaxis by granulocyte-macrophage colony-stimulating factor and interleukin-3. *Blood*, **77**, 2694–700.

Warringa, R.A., Schweizer, R.C., Maikoe, T., Kuijper, P.H., Bruijnzeel, P.L. & Koendermann, L. (1992a) Modulation of eosinophil chemotaxis by interleukin-5. *Am. J. Respir. Cell Mol. Biol.*, **7**, 631–6.

Warringa, R.A.J., Mengelers, H.J.J., Kuijper, P.H.M., Raaijmakers, J.A.M., Bruijnzeel, P.L.B. & Koenderman, L. (1992b) *In vivo* priming of platelet-activating factor-induced eosinophil chemotaxis in allergic asthmatic individuals. *Blood*, **79**, 1836–41.

Wenzel, S.E., Fowler, A.A. & Schwartz, L.B. (1988) Activation of pulmonary mast cells by bronchoalveolar allergen challenge. *In vivo* release of histamine and tryptase in atopic subjects with and without asthma. *Am. Rev. Resp. Dis.*, **137**, 1002–8.

Wershil, B.K., Mekori, Y.A., Murakami, T. & Galli, S.J. (1987) ^{125}I-fibrin deposition in IgE-dependent immediate hypersensitivity reactions in mouse skin. Demonstration of the role of mast cells using genetically mast cell-deficient mice locally reconstituted with cultured mast cells. *J. Immunol.*, **139**, 2605–14.

Wershil, B.K., Murakami, T. & Galli, S.J. (1988) Mast cell-dependent amplification of an immunologically nonspecific inflammatory response. Mast cells are required for the full expression of cutaneous acute inflammation induced by phorbol 12-myristate 13-acetate. *J. Immunol.*, **140**, 2356–60.

Wershil, B.K., Wang, Z.S., Gordon, J.R. & Galli, S.J. (1991) Recruitment of neutrophils during IgE-dependent cutaneous late phase reactions in the mouse is mast cell-dependent. Partial inhibition of the reaction with antiserum against tumor necrosis factor-alpha. *J. Clin. Invest.*, **87**, 446–53.

Wheeler, A.P., Jesmok, G. & Brigham, K.L. (1990) Tumor necrosis factor's effects on lung mechanics, gas exchange, and airway reactivity in sheep. *J. Appl. Physiol.*, **68**, 2542–9.

Wintroub, B.U., Kaempfer, C.E., Schechter, N.M. & Proud, D. (1986a) Human lung mast cell chymotrypsin-like enzyme: identification and partial characterization. *J. Clin. Invest.*, **77**, 196–201.

Wintroub, B.U., Kaempfer, C.E., Schechter, N.M. & Proud, D. (1986b) Human lung mast cell chymotrypsin-like enzyme: identification and partial characterization. *J. Clin. Invest.*, **77**, 196–201.

Wuepper, K.D., Bokisch, V., Muller-Eberhard, H.J. & Stoughton, R.B. (1972) Cutaneous responses to human C3 anaphylatoxin in man. *Clin. Exp. Immunol.*, **11**, 13–20.

Yamaguchi, Y., Suda, T., Ohta, S., Tominaga, K., Miura, Y. & Kasahara, T. (1991) Analysis of the survival of mature human eosinophils: interleukin-5 prevents apoptosis in mature human eosinophils. *Blood*, **78**, 2542–7.

Ying, S., Durham, S.R., Jacobson, M.R. *et al.* (1994) T lymphocytes and mast cells express messenger RNA for interleukin-4 in the nasal mucosa in allergen-induced rhinitis. *Immunology*, **82**, 200–6.

CHAPTER 10

Eosinophils and the Allergic Inflammatory Response

A.J. Wardlaw, R.M. Moqbel & A.B. Kay

Biology of the eosinophil

Introduction

The term 'eosinophile' was introduced by Ehrlich (1879), who observed that certain cells had numerous intercytoplasmic granules with an affinity for acidic dyes such as eosin. An association between the eosinophil and helminthic disease, allergy and asthma, as well as certain cutaneous and maligant diseases, was then established (Brown, 1898; Ehrlich & Lazarus, 1900). Investigators in the 1960s and 1970s were attracted by the idea that eosinophils could degrade mast cell-derived mediators of anaphylaxis, suggesting that the cell might be important in ameliorating the allergic process (Goetzl *et al.*, 1975). In the mid to late 1970s the observation that eosinophils or their granule-containing proteins were toxic for helminthic parasitic larvae (Butterworth *et al.*, 1974) led to the current, widely held, view that the teleological role of eosinophils is in host defence against worms. Eosinophils are also believed to be major effector cells in producing tissue damage in asthma and related allergic diseases (Gleich & Adolphson, 1986; Wardlaw & Kay, 1987).

This chapter reviews recent findings on the biology of the eosinophil and discusses the possible role of the eosinophil in the pathogenesis of allergic disease.

Morphology and ultrastructure

Morphology of normal mature eosinophils and eosinophil myelocytes

Eosinophils are non-dividing, bone marrow-derived, granule-containing cells, approximately 8 μm in diameter with a bilobed nucleus (Dvorak *et al.*, 1991). One of their most characteristic features is the membrane-bound specific granules, of which there are about 20 per human eosinophil (Fig. 10.1). These are spherical or ovoid and contain a crystalline core surrounded by a less electron dense matrix (Sokol *et al.*, 1991). The core is composed of major basic protein (MBP) and the matrix contains the other three basic granule proteins eosinophil cationic protein (ECP), eosinophil peroxidase (EPO) and eosinophil-derived neurotoxin (EDN or EPX) (Egesten *et al.*, 1986). Eosinophils contain lipid bodies which are the principal store of arachidonic acid esterified into glycerophospholipids (Weller *et al.*, 1991). Lipid bodies are non-membrane bound, roughly spherical and 0.5–2 μm in diameter (Fig. 10.1). There are approximately five lipid bodies per normal eosinophil, but their numbers are increased in activated cells. Lipid bodies contain the enzymes cyclo-oxygenase (prostaglandin endoperoxidase synthase, or PGH synthase) (Dvorak, 1994) and 5-lipoxygenase (Weller & Dvorak, 1994). Eosinophil primary granules lack a core and are of variable size, being often larger than the specific granules. They make up approximately 5% of eosinophil granules. In resting eosinophils primary granules are the sole location of Charcot–Leyden crystal protein (CLC protein) (Dvorak *et al.*, 1988). CLC protein is also found diffusely in the nucleus and cytoplasm in activated eosinophils. Tissue eosinophils contain a number of small granules which stain intensely for acid phosphatase and aryl sulphatase (Parmely & Spicer, 1974; Dvorak *et al.*, 1991), and may also contain catalase (Iozzo *et al.*, 1982).

Eosinophil myelocytes (EM) are larger than the mature

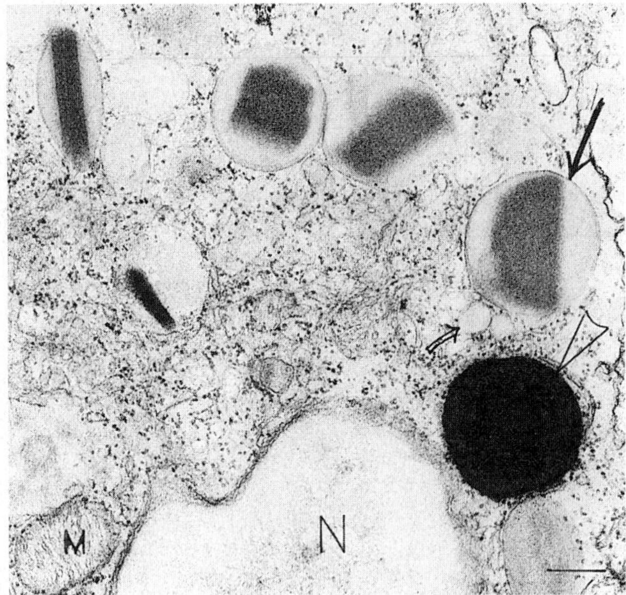

Fig. 10.1 The cytoplasm of a mature peripheral blood eosinophil from a patient with hypereosinophilic syndrome (HES), shows a mixture of bicompartmental secondary granules (closed arrow), several primary granules that do not contain dense central cores, small granules (open arrowhead) and one osmiophilic lipid body. (×14 000). N, nucleus; M, mitochondria; Bar, 0.3 μm. (From Dvorak *et al.*, 1991; courtesy of Dr Ann Dvorak.)

cell and contain a single nucleus with dispersed chromatin (Dvorak *et al.*, 1989) (Fig. 10.2). The cytoplasm contains considerably more biosynthetic structures, such as endoplasmic reticulum. The EM can first be identified when specific core-containing granules appear.

Morphology during activation and degranulation

Morphological markers of activation include increased numbers and size of lipid bodies and increased numbers of primary granules, small granules and vesiculotubular structures. Smooth endoplasmic reticulum and non-membrane-bound cytoplasmic crystals of CLC protein may be observed. Often, particularly in tissue eosinophils, there is a marked reduction in the numbers of specific granules which may also appear translucent as if emptied of their contents.

Many eosinophils at sites of inflammation appear necrotic, with loss of integrity of the granules and plasma membrane and nuclear lysis (Dvorak *et al.*, 1982). In culture, eosinophils undergo apoptosis, a process delayed by growth factor cytokines such as interleukin-5 (IL-5), IL-3 and granulocyte macrophage colony-stimulating factor (GM-CSF) (Yamaguchi *et al.*, 1991; Stern *et al.*, 1992). Apoptotic eosinophils in culture can be indentified by their smaller size, condensed nuclei, characteristic staining with acridine orange, distinct profile of autofluorescence when examined by flow cytometry and DNA degradation.

The most well-characterized form of degranulation is cell secretion, where granules fuse with the plasma membrane around the periphery of the cell with the granule matrix and core contents being extruded. Alternatively granules can fuse intracytoplasmically into large degranulation chambers which open to the outside of the cell through degranulation pores. This is the classic form of regulated secretion, and is well characterized in anaphylactic degranulation of mast cells and basophils (Dvorak, 1991). This process has been shown to occur in eosinophils from patients with inflammatory bowel disease and tissue invasive infections (Dvorak *et al.*, 1993), as well as calcium ionophore-stimulated peripheral blood eosinophils (Henderson & Chi, 1985). It is, however, unusual to see morphological evidence of this type of secretion in eosinophilic inflammation. More commonly observed are appearances consistent with a process known as piecemeal degranulation (PMD), in which granule proteins containing vesicles bud off from the secondary granules, resulting in their gradual emptying. A spectrum of morphologies can be identified, ranging from loss from the core compartment, partial or complete loss from the matrix compartment, to total emptying of the granule contents (Fig. 10.3) (Tai & Spry, 1981).

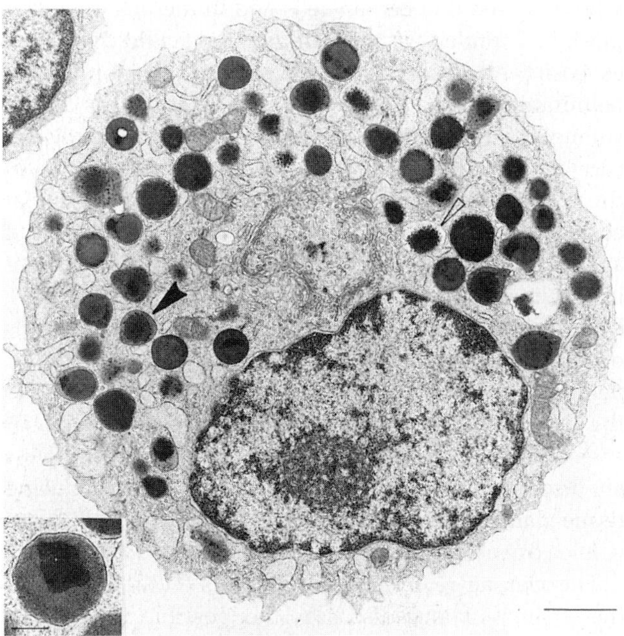

Fig. 10.2 Eosinophilic myelocyte in a 3-week rhIL-3 containing culture of human cord blood mononuclear cells shows an active Golgi area, large mitochondria, dilated cisterns of rough endoplasmic reticulum, and an extensive population of immature and maturing secondary granules with central dense cores (inset, higher magnification of one specific granule with core) and less dense matrix compartments (×10 650, inset ×29 040). (From Dvorak *et al.*, 1991, courtesy of Dr Ann Dvorak.)

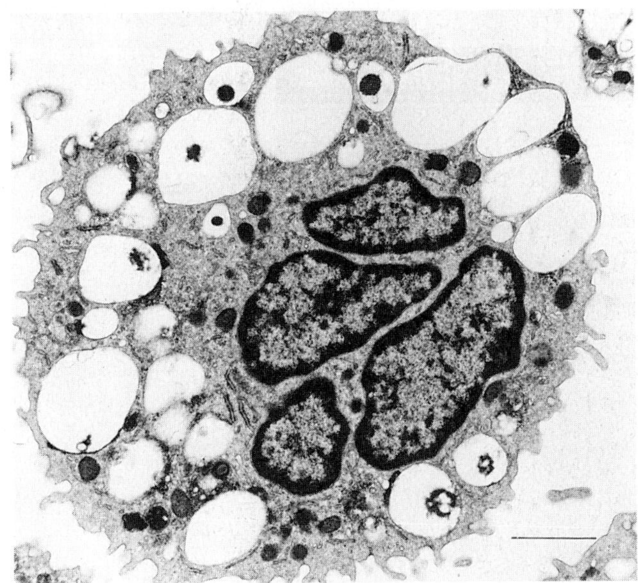

Fig. 10.3 Mature eosinophil grown in rhIL-5 shows polylobed granulocyte nucleus and numerous enlarged, non-fused empty and partially empty secondary granule containers typical of piecemeal degranulation. Partially empty secondary granule containers retain some dense granule material and vesicles (×15 500 before reduction). (From Dvorak *et al.*, 1992, courtesy of Dr Ann Dvorak.)

Eosinophil differentiation and maturation

Eosinophils are derived from haemopoietic stem cells. It is known that all of the young lymphoid and myeloid cells, including eosinophils, are contained within the CD34+ population (Clark & Kamen, 1987; Haylock *et al.*, 1992; Vellenga *et al.*, 1992). Thus, nearly all eosinophil colony-forming cells are CD34+, but this marker is not expressed on the mature cell (Caux *et al.*, 1989). The CD34 molecule is a 115-kDa glycoprotein with three intracellular domains (Greaves *et al.*, 1992). Its precise function is unknown but it has a mucin-like structure and one of its glycoforms is a ligand for L-selectin (Baumheuter *et al.*, 1993).

Exposure of CD34+ cells to IL-3 and GM-CSF, either alone or in combination, leads to progressive commitment to the myeloid lineage, with IL-5 promoting the terminal eosinophil maturation process (Shalit *et al.*, 1995). Interestingly, IL-5 transgenic mice, in which there is overproduction of IL-5, but not apparently GM-CSF and IL-3, have large numbers of blood and tissue eosinophils (Dent *et al.*, 1990; Tominaga *et al.*, 1991). One explanation is that *in vivo* IL-5 may also act at early differentiation steps. These apparent discrepancies between *in vivo* and *in vitro* systems need to be clarified. The description of the human myeloid cell line, AML14, which can be stimulated to produce mRNA for MBP, EPO ECP, EDN and CLC protein, by IL-3, GM-CSF and IL-5, indicates that this may serve as a model for studying cytokine induction of eosinophil growth and differentiation (Paul *et al.*, 1994). However, at the present time, there is little information on the genes that control eosinophil differentiation and maturation and how the level of maturation relates to phenotype, structure and function.

Eosinophil differentiation appears to be closely linked to that of the basophil (Denburg *et al.*, 1985). For example, IL-5 can act as a basophil differentiation factor for HL-60 cells and mature basophils (Denburg *et al.*, 1991). Like eosinophils, basophils contain CLC protein (Ackerman *et al.*, 1982) and MBP (Ackerman *et al.*, 1983). Eosinophil and basophil progenitors (i.e. colony-forming units) have been identified in the blood of patients with allergic rhinitis (Otsuka *et al.*, 1986) and in asthmatics during exacerbations of their disease (Gibson *et al.*, 1990).

Receptors

Receptors involved in eosinophil adhesion and migration

Adhesion receptors

Leucocyte migration from the bone marrow to the blood and then to the tissue is one of the central events of leucocyte biology and essential to the integrity of the immune system. A striking feature of chronic allergic inflammation is the accumulation of activated eosinophils with a relative paucity of neutrophils. As eosinophils generally constitute only a small proportion of the total blood leucocyte count, this suggests a selective process of leucocyte migration.

Preferential eosinophil accumulation at the site of local tissue reactions is believed to be the result of several interrelated events. These include: (i) selective adhesion pathways, (ii) specific chemotactic factors and (iii) enhanced survival by certain cytokines, principally IL-3, IL-5 and GM-CSF.

Stimulated by the possibility that identification of selective migration pathways could lead to selective inhibition of migration without the risk of immunosuppression, the mechanisms involved in the tissue localization of eosinophils have been the subject of intense interest over the past three decades. Neutrophil migration through endothelium has been shown to be a process involving sequential steps, in which the cells are initially lightly tethered to the endothelium and roll along its surface. This is followed by cell activation, mediated by a soluble chemotactic stimulus, which allows a firmer bond to develop between the leucocyte and the endothelial cell and results in successful adhesion and transmigration (Lawrence & Springer 1991; Von Adrian *et al.*, 1991; Springer, 1994). The steps occur in series, so that each is essential for transmigration to occur. In this model, selectivity can be introduced at each of the steps, resulting in considerable

Table 10.1 Eosinophil adhesion receptors and their counter-structures.

Eosinophil receptor	Endothelial receptor	Matrix protein
Integrin		
VLA-4 (α4β1)	VCAM-1	Fibronectin
VLA-6 (α6β1)		Laminin
α4/β7	MAdCAM-1/VCAM-1	Fibronectin
LFA-1	ICAM-1, ICAM-2	
Mac-1	ICAM-1	Fibrinogen
p150, 95	Not known	
Immunoglobulin like		
PECAM	PECAM	
ICAM-3 (binds LFA-1)		
Selectins		
L-selectin	Gly-CAM-1, CD34, MAdCAM-1	
Carbohydrate		
PSGL-1	P-selectin	
ESL-1	E-selectin	
Others		
CD44		Hyaluronate

See text for definition of abbreviations.

diversity in the pattern of signals required for successful emigration. Migration may be modulated at each of the steps, offering a range of targets for pharmacological inhibition. While this staged migration has not been formally shown to occur with eosinophils, it is assumed that the processes are similar. The adhesion receptors involved in eosinophil migration in allergic inflammation are discussed in detail in Chapter 14 and are summarized in Table 10.1.

Eosinophil chemotaxins

Eosinophilia may be the result of selective eosinophil chemoattractants. Numerous candidates have been suggested over the years, but enthusiasm has not been sustained either because of weak activity, lack of selectivity or lack of evidence for their generation during the allergic process. Histamine (Clark *et al.*, 1975) and the eosinophil chemotactic factor anaphylaxis (ECF-A) tetrapeptides (Goetzl *et al.*, 1975) were reported as having *in vitro* chemotactic activity, but were later found to have negligible potency compared with platelet-activating factor (PAF) and C5a (Wardlaw *et al.*, 1986b). Cyclo-oxygenase-derived lipid mediators have no substantive chemotactic activity for eosinophils *in vitro*. Leukotriene B_4 (LTB_4) and various dihydroxyeicosatetraenoic acids (diHETE) (Morita *et al.*, 1990; Sehmi *et al.*, 1991) do have chemotactic activity, but LTB_4 is much more active on guinea pig than human eosinophils and the diHETE were only generated when exogenous arachidonic acid was present. Interestingly, inhaled LTE_4 generated an airway eosinophilia, although it is not clear whether this was a direct or indirect effect (Laitinen *et al.*, 1993). Known eosinophil chemoattractants are summarized in Table 10.2.

In recent years the chemotactic potential of cytokines, particularly growth factors and chemokines, has been explored. GM-CSF, IL-3 and IL-5, as well as being eosinopoietic, enhance the effector function of mature eosinophils in terms of adhesion to human umbilical vein endothelial cells (HUVEC), prolonged survival, mediator release and mobility (Lopez *et al.*, 1988; Wang *et al.*, 1989; Fujisawa *et al.*, 1990; Owen *et al.*, 1990; Walsh *et al.*, 1990).

IL-5 and IL-3 also activate mature basophils but not neutrophils (Bischoff *et al.*, 1990; Bochner *et al.*, 1990; Hirai *et al.* 1990; Shute, 1992; Yamaguchi *et al.*, 1992), and are therefore relatively selective. There is abundant evidence that these cytokines are generated in allergic inflammation (Walker *et al.*, 1991; Robinson *et al.*, 1992). In the Boyden chamber, IL-3, IL-5 and GM-CSF are chemotactic for eosinophils from normal individuals but less active on eosinophils from allergic subjects, possibly as a result of *in vivo* desensitization (Warringa *et al.*, 1991; Sehmi *et al.*, 1992b). Although active at low concentrations, they are only weakly effective when compared with well-documented eosinophil chemoattractants such as PAF. They appear much more active at priming eosinophils *in*

Table 10.2 Eosinophil chemoattractants.

Type	Effectiveness (unprimed)	Commments
Lipids		
PAF	High	Non-selective
LTB_4	Low	Non-selective
LTE_4	NK	Activity reported *in vivo* only
18s, 15s, diHETE	Moderate	Part of guinea pig ECF-A
Small-molecular-weight peptides		
C5a	High	Non-selective
f-MLP	Low	Non-selective
Growth factors		
IL-5	Low	Active only on cells
IL-3	Low	from normals.
GM-CSF	Low	Effective priming agents
IL-2	Low	Possibly mainly
LCF		chemokinetic
Chemokines		
C-C family (not active neutrophils)		
RANTES	High	Active *in vivo* and *in vitro*
MIP-1α	Low/moderate(eos)	Histamine releasers
MCP-3, MCP-4	Moderate	Histamine releasers
Eotaxin	High	Only characterized guinea pigs at present. Active *in vivo* and *in vitro*
C-X-C family		
IL-8	Low	Only active primed cells

vitro for enhanced chemotactic responses to suboptimal concentrations of lipid and low-molecular-weight chemoattractants such as LTB_4 and feu-Met-Leu-Phe (f-MLP) that are otherwise weakly active on unprimed normal eosinophils. Neuropeptides such as substance P (SP), neurokinin A, calcitonin gene-related peptide (CGRP) and cholecystokinin octapeptide had similar modulatory effects on PAF- and LTB_4-induced chemotaxis of human eosinophils (Numao & Agrawal, 1992). IL-5 and GM-CSF also markedly potentiated the transendothelial migration of eosinophils *in vitro* (Ebisawa *et al.*, 1994). This priming effect appears to be relevant *in vivo*, as eosinophils from allergic subjects with a mild to moderate eosinophilia are far more responsive in the Boyden chamber assay to chemotactic stimuli such as PAF than eosinophils from normal subjects (Warringa *et al.*, 1992b). This effect is also seen *in vivo*, as shown by Henocq & Vargaftig (1986), who demonstrated that subcutaneous injections of PAF induced a neutrophil infiltration in normal subjects but an eosinophil-rich infiltration in allergic subjects. It is possible that a selective priming stimulus from growth factors active on mature eosinophils, combining with a non-selective but highly effective chemoattractant, results in selective migration. IL-4 was shown to be chemotactic for eosinophils, but not neutrophils, from patients with atopic dermatitis (Dubois *et al.*, 1994). Eosinophils from normal donors did not respond.

Despite the relative lack of activity of IL-5 in the Boyden chamber, inhalation of IL-5 in animals and humans leads to eosinophil recruitment (Iwama *et al.*, 1992; Terada *et al.*, 1992) and antibodies against IL-5 have been effective at inhibitiing eosinophil migration into the lung of allergen-challenged guinea pigs (Mauser *et al.*, 1993; Van Oosterhout *et al.*, 1993). Antibody-mediated inhibition occurs even when the anti-IL-5 antibody is given at the time of the challenge, so it is not primarily working through an effect on eosinopoiesis. The mechanism for these effects is unclear but there is evidence that IL-5 acts by promoting release of eosinophils from bone marrow.

A new class of relatively cell specific chemotactic peptides are the chemokines or intercrines (reviewed by Baggiolini & Dahinden, 1994). Chemokines are 6–10-kDa basic polypeptides which bind heparin. The family share a common four-cysteine motif and are divided into two subfamilies, based on the position of the first two of the conserved cysteines. In the C-X-C subfamily the cysteines are divided by an amino acid and in the C-C family the cysteines are adjacent (Schall, 1991). The C-X-C family members, such as IL-8, are particularly active on neutrophils and monocytes, although IL-8 has chemotactic activity for primed eosinophils (Sehmi *et al.*, 1993). The C-C family, which include RANTES, as well as being chemotactic for monocytes and CD4+/UCHLI+ 'memory' T cells (Schall *et al.*, 1990), are potent basophil chemotaxins and histamine releasers as well as being chemotactic for eosinophils (Kameyoshi *et al.*, 1992; Rot *et al.*, 1992; Bischoff *et al.*, 1993; Kuna *et al.*, 1993; Dahinden *et al.*, 1994; Jose *et al.*, 1994a,b). As well as being active *in vitro*, RANTES has been shown to result in eosinophil accumulation in the skin of dogs after intradermal injection (Meurer *et al.*, 1993). Other important chemokines active on eosinophils include MCP-3 (Baggiolini & Dahinden 1994; Dahinden *et al.*, 1994) and eostaxin (Jose *et al.*, 1994b). Ying *et al.* (1995) found that exposure to specific allergen induced the transcription of mRNA for MCP-3 and RANTES in the skin of human atopic subjects and that the time-course of appearance of mRNA+ cells for RANTES paralleled the appearance of CD3+, CD4+ and CD8+ cells, whereas the accumulation of eosinophils followed the kinetics of cells mRNA+ for monocyte chemotactic protein-3 (MCP-3). Chemokines are generated by several cell types. For instance, IL-8 is produced by airway epithelial cells (Standiford *et al.*, 1990) and RANTES by eosinophils (Ying *et al.*, 1995). RANTES has also been identified *in vivo* in human nasal polyps (Beck *et al.*, 1994). The eosinophil-active CC chemokines are described in Chapter 22.

Receptors for immunoglobulins

FcγR

Using monoclonal antibodies and functional analysis, three distinct types of Fcγ receptor (FcγR) have been identified on human leucocytes (Fanger *et al.*, 1989; Unkeless, 1989). FcγRI (CD64) is a high-affinity receptor of 72 kDa that is constitutively expressed by monocytes only. FcγRII (CD32) is a low-affinity receptor of 40 kDa and has a wide cellular distribution, including monocytes, neutrophils, eosinophils, platelets and B cells. Only CD32 is constitutively expressed by resting eosinophils to any significant degree (Hartnell *et al.*, 1990). FcγRIII (CD16) is also a low-affinity receptor, of 50–70 kDa, which is constitutively expressed by neutrophils and natural killer (NK) cells. These three receptors are members of the immunoglobulin (Ig) superfamily and have highly homologous extracellular domains (Kinet, 1989). Two isoforms of FcγRIII that are encoded by two distinct genes have been identified (Ravetch & Perussia, 1989; Scallon *et al.*, 1989). FcγRIII-1 (CD16-1) is expressed by neutrophils and has a phosphatidylinositol (PI)-glycan membrane anchor. FcγRIII-1 is shed from neutrophils on stimulation with f-MLP and can be detected in human plasma (Huizinga *et al.*, 1988, 1989, 1990). FcγRIII-2 (CD16-2) is expressed by NK cells and is a transmembrane protein.

Valerius *et al.* (1990) reported that interferon-γ (IFN-γ) enhanced eosinophil FcγRII-dependent antibody-dependent cell-mediated cytotoxicity (ADCC) and that this was accompanied by a modest increase in FcRII expression after 24 hours. Hartnell *et al.* (1992a) demonstated that culture of eosinophils in IFN-γ induced expression *de novo* of FcRI and FcRIII. Eosinophil FcRIII was PI linked and triggered eosinophil membrane depolarization and LTC_4 release.

FcεRI and *FcεRII*

In 1994 Gounni *et al.* described high-affinity IgE receptors on eosinophils from hypereosinophilic patients. However, all subjects had high eosinophil counts in association with the idiopathic hypereosinophilic syndrome (HES), various skin diseases and lymphomas. This observation remains to be confirmed on peripheral blood eosinophils in normal and atopic subjects. Previous studies from these workers had found that eosinophils expressed FcεRII, the low-affinity IgE receptor (Capron *et al.*, 1986a,b; Joualt *et al.*, 1988; Capron *et al.*, 1991), which were identified as CD23. These earlier data are difficult to reconcile with the additional or alternative presence of significant numbers of functional high-affinity IgE receptors on eosinophils. Expression of CD23 by human eosinophils remains to be confirmed by other investigators. Human eosinophils also express the IgE binding molecule Mac-2. In addition, this S-lectin-type moleucle was able to bind radiolabelled IgE and participate in IgE-dependent effector functions of eosinophils (Truong *et al.*, 1993). Mac-2 is also expressed on neutrophils, although neutrophils have no IgE function (Truong *et al.*, 1993). Therefore, while eosinophils are able to participate in IgE-mediated functions, the exact receptor involved remains uncertain.

FcαR

A number of studies have shown that eosinophils possess functional surface IgA receptors (FcαR) (Abu-Ghazaleh *et al.*, 1989; Kita *et al.*, 1991a). IgA, particularly secretory IgA, is effective in stimulating eosinophil degranulation, and IgA-coated Sepharose beads released eosinophil-derived neurotoxin (EDN). This effect was enhanced by pre-incubation of eosinophils with GM-CSF and IL-3.

Monteiro *et al.* (1993) analysed the expression, regulation and biochemical nature of FcαR on eosinophils using the natural IgA ligand and anti-FcαR antibodies. FcαR molecules were detected on eosinophils from normal individuals after *in vitro* activation and unstimulated eosinophils from allergic individuals. The FcαR molecules expressed by eosinophils differed from those on neutrophils and macrophages, and the former had a higher content of N-linked carbohydrate moieities.

Complement receptors

Eosinophils express low levels of CR1 (CD35), a polymorphic single-chain glycoprotein of about 250 kDa that binds the complement fragment C3b (Hartnell *et al.*, 1990). In contrast CR3, which binds to C3bi, is strongly expressed. Complement receptor type 3 (CR3, Mac-1), or CD11b/CD18, is a member of the β2 integrin family of adhesion molecules. This receptor recognizes a number of ligands, such as C3bi, intercellular adhesion molecule-1 (ICAM-1), fibrinogen and polysaccharides (Diamond *et al.*, 1990). This receptor is involved in a number of important eosinophil functions, such as adhesion to endothelial cells (Walsh *et al.*, 1990), and IgE- and IgG-dependent schistosomula killing (Capron & Capron, 1987). Binding of particles via this receptor is a potent stimulus for eosinophils to undergo respiratory burst (Koenderman *et al.*, 1990) and degranulation (Zeiger & Colten, 1977).

In contrast to neutrophils (Berger *et al.*, 1984), short-term stimulation of eosinophils with LTB_4, IL-3, IL-5 and GM-CSF causes only a small increase in CR3 numbers (Fischer *et al.*, 1986; Lopez *et al.*, 1986; Walsh *et al.*, 1990). Hartnell *et al.* (1992b) found that culture of human eosinophils with IL-3 produced a marked dose-dependent up-regulation of CR3 expression. This was dependent on protein and RNA synthesis. IL-5 and GM-CSF had a similar effect on eosinophil CR3 expression but the maximal response to IL-5 was always less than to IL-3 or GM-CSF. Dexamethasone inhibited the IL-3 induced up-regulation of CR3 expression in a dose-dependent manner, with an IC_{50} of 5×10^{-8} M.

Receptors for cytokines and chemokines

In addition to functional surface receptors for immunoglobulins, eosinophils also respond at picomolar concentrations to GM-CSF, IL-3 and IL-5 (Silberstein & David 1986; Owen *et al.*, 1987; Rothenberg *et al.*, 1988, 1989; Her *et al.*, 1991) via high-affinity cytokine receptors which have an average kDa value of 120 pM for the IL-5R, 500 pM for the IL-3R and 50 pM for GM-CSFR. (DiPersio *et al.*, 1988; Lopez *et al.*, 1989; Chihara *et al.*, 1990; Ingley & Young, 1991; Lopez *et al.*, 1991; Migita *et al.*, 1991). Eosinophils and basophils, but not neutrophils, express IL-5R while GM-CSFR is present on both eosinophils and neutrophils with a similar affinity binding value on both (Fig. 10.4). These receptors are composed of heterodimers which share a common β-, but distinct α-chains (Tavernier *et al.*, 1991). The homologous α-chains (60–80 kDa) are specific, and in the case of IL-3 and GM-CSF form a low-affinity association with their receptive cytokines (the human IL-5R α-chain has a high affinity for IL-5). The common β-chain (102–140 kDa) combines with the α-chains to form a higher-affinity binding site (Miyajima *et al.*, 1992).

In addition to the receptors for IL-3, IL-5 and GM-CSF, eosinophils in the HES also expressed functional high-affinity receptors for IL-2 (Rand *et al.*, 1991a). Partially purified supernatants from the U937 cell line, but not GM-CSF, IL-3, IL-5, IFN-γ or the lymphocyte chemotactic factor, were able to enhance CD25 expression on normal density eosinophils after 24–48 hours' incubation (Rand *et al.*, 1991b).

It is increasingly clear that CC or β-chemokines, particularly eotaxin, RANTES, MCP-3 and MCP-4, are of central importance in the promotion of eosinophil recruitment to the site of allergic inflammation (Uguccioni *et al.*, 1996) (see above and Chapter 22). Eotaxin is of particular interest as its activity appears to be exclusively targeted to eosinophils. It is generated by a range of cell types, including epithelial and endothelial cells, as well as eosinophils. mRNA for eotaxin has been detected in eosinophilic lesions in inflammatory bowel disease and nasal polyps (Ponath *et al.*, 1996; Garcia Zepeda, 1996). Mouse eotaxin was generated in the lung after ovalbumin challenge in association with the recruitment of eosinophils and was expressed in a range of tissues after injection of the mice with LPS (Gonzalo *et al.*, 1996). In the guinea pig, the *in vivo* activity of eotaxin was greatly enhanced by pre-

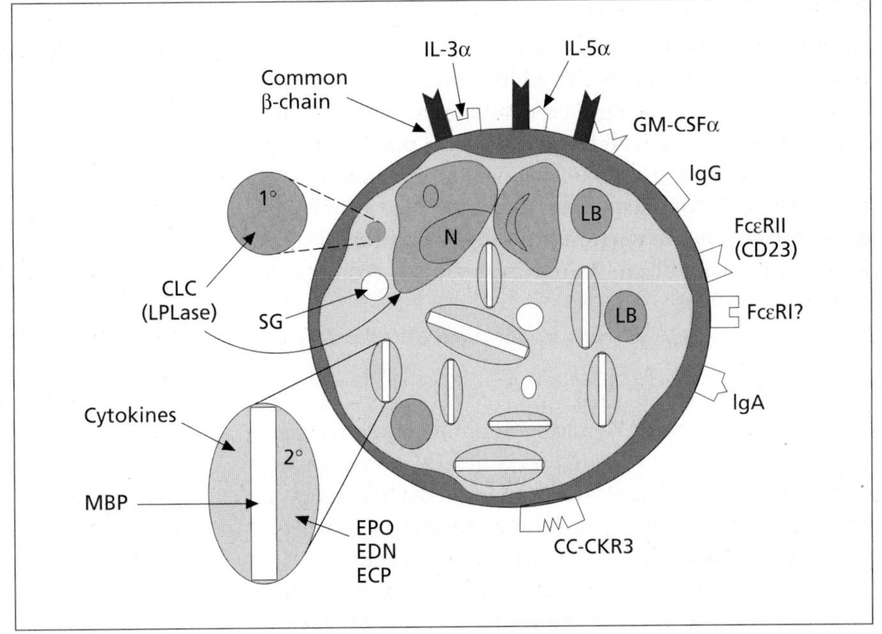

Fig. 10.4 A diagrammatic representation of some of the principal features of the human eosinophil. The characteristic crystalloid secondary (2°) granules contain the four basic proteins, MBP, EPO, EDN and ECP as well as several cytokines. The CLC has LPLase activity and is contained in the primary (1°) granules. Surface receptors for CC-CKR3 and IgFc are also shown. See text for definition of abbreviations.

treatment of the eosinophils with IL-5, again emphasizing the importance of this cytokine as a priming agent for eosinophil migration (Collins *et al.*, 1995). The G-coupled receptor which mediates migration induced by eotaxin, RANTES and MCP-3 has recently been identified and termed CC-chemokine receptor 3 (CC-CKR3) (Daugherty *et al.*, 1996). This receptor appears to be expressed only be eosinophils. It binds eotaxin with a 10-fold greater affinity than RANTES and MCP-3 (kDas of 0.1, 2.7 and 3.1 nm respectively). Binding induced a calcium flux. CC-CKR1, which binds MIP-1α, is also expressed on eosinophils but to a much lower level than CC-CKR3.

Receptors for inflammatory mediators

Eosinophils possess a number of specific receptors for soluble mediators, including LTB_4, PAF, C5a and C3a. Receptors for LTB_4 on guinea pig alveolar and peritoneal eosinophils have been shown to be of both high and low affinity (Sehmi *et al.*, 1992a); however, this has not been confirmed for human eosinophils. Human eosinophils have ben reported to express receptors of two affinities for PAF (Kroegel *et al.*, 1989; Kurihara *et al.*, 1989). Although the presence of a receptor for f-MLP on eosinophils has not been demonstrated directly, there is sufficient evidence to indicate that a low-affinity binding site may be present on eosinophils which is associated with a functional response of eosinophils to high concentrations of this peptide (Yazdanbakhsh *et al.*, 1987). Koenderman *et al.* (1990) have shown that the increase in intracellular Ca^{2+} induced by f-MLP was inhibited by pertussis toxin, suggesting that a guanosine triphosphate (GTP)-binding protein may be involved in f-MLP-mediated cell activation. Receptors for C5a, PAF, f-MLP and LTB_4 have been recognized as belonging to a family of seven transmembrane GTP-binding proteins (Gerard & Gerard 1991; Honda *et al.*, 1991). C5a receptors are involved in stimulation of human eosinophils and inducing their chemotaxis and mediator release, possibly through the activation of phospholipase D (PLD) (Minnicozzi *et al.*, 1990). Eosinophil C3a receptors are also ligands for chemotaxis, mediator release and activation of reactive oxygen radical species production, as well as intracellular Ca^{2+} transport in human eosinophils (Elsner *et al.*, 1994).

Other receptors

Eosinophils express CD4, and eosinophils obtained from HES patients had an elevated level of CD4 immunoreactivity (Lucey *et al.*, 1989a). The expression of CD4 suggests that the eosinophil may provide an additional reservoir for human immunodeficiency virus (HIV) infections.

Human leucocyte antigen (HLA)-DR expression has also been described in eosinophils (Lucey *et al.*, 1989b) following culture in the presence of GM-CSF and 3T3 fibroblasts. Eosinophils can act *in vitro* as relatively weak antigen-presenting cells (Weller *et al.*, 1993).

Nishikawa *et al.* (1992) described the expression *in vivo* of CD69, an early activation marker for lymphocytes (Corte *et al.*, 1981), on lung eosinophils obtained from patients with eosinophilic pneumonia. Hartnell *et al.* (1993) showed that CD69 could be induced on human peripheral blood eosinophils by GM-CSF stimulation as early as 1 hour after incubation, with optimal up-regulation at 24 hours and sustained over 2 days of incubation, *in vitro*. IL-3, IL-5 and IFN-α, but not PAF, also induced eosinophil CD69 expression. This appeared to be protein synthesis dependent and not inhibitable by corticosteroids. *In vivo* expression of this receptor was also seen on eosinophils from bronchoalveolar lavage fluid of mild asthmatic subjects. These two studies suggested that CD69 may be a marker of eosinophil activation by cytokines. However, Walsh *et al.* (1995b) demonstrated that cross-linking of CD69 resulted in apoptosis and cell death of GM-CSF-stimulated eosinophils. Table 10.3 summarizes some of the surface receptors associated with human eosinophils.

Eosinophil mediators

Eosinophils have the capacity to secrete a number of potent mediators (Table 10.4). These include basic proteins stored in eosinophil granules, newly formed membrane-derived lipids, cytokines, various proteases, and products of oxidative metabolism including the superoxide anion and hydrogen peroxide.

Lipid mediators

Eosinophil-derived lipid mediators have recently been reviewed in detail (Weller, 1993). These are principally eicosanoids and PAF.

Table 10.3 Eosinophil receptors other than adhesion molecules.

Immunoglobulin receptors	FcαR, FcεR*, FcγRII (CDw32)
Mediator receptors	IL-5*, IL-3*, GM-CSF, CC-CKR3 (receptor for eotaxin, RANTES and MCP-3), C5a, PAF, f-MLP, LTB_4
Newly expressed receptors	IL-2 (CD25), FcγRIII (CD16), CD4*, ICAM-1, HLA-DR, CD69*
Other receptors	CR1, CR3 (Mac-1), MAC2, CD9*, CD45

* Not expressed on neutrophils.
See text for definition of abbreviations.

Table 10.4 Eosinophil-derived mediators.

Granule-associated mediators	
1 Basic proteins	MBP; ECP; EDN; EPO
2 Enzymes	e.g. lysophospholipase; phospholipase D; arylsulphatase; histaminase; catalase; acid phosphatase; non-specific esterases; glycosaminoglycans; hexosaminidase
3 Cytokines	IL-1α, IL-2; IL-3; IL-4; IL-5; IL-6; IL-8; GM-CSF; TGF-α; TGF-β; TNF-α
4 Chemokines	MIP-1α; RANTES
Membrane-derived mediators	
LTC_4; PAF; 15-HETE; PGE_1; PGE_2; TXB_2	

Eicosanoids

Eicosanoids are oxidation products of arachidonic acid derived from phospholipids by the action of activated phospholipase A2. Eisosanoid formation occurs at the cell membranes and in lipid bodies (Weller & Dvorak, 1985). The principal pathways for the metabolism of arachidonic acid in eosinophils are via the actions of cyclo-oxygenase, which produces the prostaglandins and thromboxanes, and 5- and 15-lipoxygenase, which lead to the generation of leukotrienes and the HETE and diHETE.

Eosinophils can generate picogram quantities of PGE2, PGD_2 and PGF_2 (Hubscher, 1975; Parsons & Roberts, 1988), although the predominant cyclo-oxygenase product was thromboxane B_2 (TXB_2). After stimulation with calcium ionophore, human peripheral blood eosinophils produced over 2 ng of TXB_2 per 10^6 cells (Foegh *et al.*, 1986).

5-Lipoxygenase (Matsumoto *et al.*, 1988) catalyses the oxidation of arachadonic acid at the 5 position to 5S-hydroperoxyeicosatetraenoic acid (5-HPETE) to produce the unstable epoxide LTA_4. The activity of 5-lipoxygenase is dependent on an 18-kDa protein called 5-lipoxygenase activating protein (FLAP) which binds to arachidonic acid (Miller *et al.*, 1990). Neutrophils contain an epoxide hydrolase (LTA hydrolase) which converts LTA_4 to LTB_4, whereas eosinophils have a specific glutathione-*S*-transferase which links glutathione to LTA_4 to produce the stable sulphidopeptide LTC_4 (Samuelsson, 1983). LTC_4 is converted to LTD_4, by the action of γ-glutamyl-transpeptidase, and to LTE_4 by a dipeptidase. LTE_4 is the stable metabolite. Eosinophils generate relatively large amounts (up to 70 ng/106 cells) of the sulphidopeptide LTC_4 after stimulation with the calcium ionophore, but only negligible amounts of LTB_4 (Jorg *et al.*, 1982; Weller *et al.*, 1983). Conversely, neutrophils produce large amounts of LTB_4 but little, if any, LTC_4. Interestingly, guinea pig eosinophils resemble human neutrophils in being able to synthesize LTB_4 but not LTC_4 (Sun *et al.*, 1989). LTC_4, LTD_4 and LTE_4 contain the activity originally known as 'slow-reacting substance of anaphylaxis'. Sulphidopeptide leukotrienes have a number of properties relevant to asthma, including smooth muscle contraction, mucus hypersecretion and increased vascular permeability. In addition to calcium ionophore, human eosinophils can also generate LTC_4 following stimulation by IgG-coated Sepharose beads (Shaw *et al.*, 1985), opsonized zymosan (Brujnzeel *et al.*, 1985) or IgG–*Apergillus fumigatus* immune complexes (Cromwell *et al.*, 1988).

In general, eosinophils from asthmatics generated more LTC_4 than eosinophils from normal donors (Taniguchi *et al.*, 1985; Aizawa *et al.*, 1990; Kohi *et al.*, 1990), although there were exceptions (see below).

Eosinophils, unlike neutrophils, contain large quantities of 15-lipoxygenase, a 70-kDa cytosolic enzyme homologous to 5-lipoxygenase (Sigal *et al.*, 1988b), which catalyses the insertion of an oxygen at position 15 on arachidonic acid to form 15-HPETE and, subsequently, 15-HETE (Sigal *et al.*, 1988a). Eosinophils can generate microgram quantities of 15-HETE (Turk *et al.*, 1982). This may be of importance in asthma, since 15-HETE stimulated mucus production by cultured human airway (Marom *et al.*, 1983).

The dual actions of two lipoxygenase enzymes on a molecule of arachidonic acid gives rise to a further set of compounds termed the lipoxins. Eosinophils can generate lipoxin A_4 (5*S*,6*R*,15*S*-trihydroxy-7,9,13-*trans*-11-*cis*-eicosatetraenoic acid) through the dual actions of 5- and 15-lipoxygenase (Serhan *et al.*, 1987). The activities of lipoxins in relation to eosinophilic inflammation are not entirely clear, but they seem to have a general down-regulatory role; for example, inhibiting neutrophil chemotactic responses to LTB_4 and f-MLP (Lee *et al.*, 1989).

PAF

PAF (1-alkyl-2-acetyl-sn-glycero-3-phosphocholine) is a phospholipid formed by the acetylation of its inactive precursor, lyso-PAF, through the actions of a specific acetyl-transferase. Lyso-PAF is believed to be generated by the cleavage of an acyl group from the C2 position of 1-*O*-alkyl glycerophospholipids by phospholipsae A2. In some situations the acyl group is arachidonic acid so that eicosanoids and PAF may be generated together. Biodegradation occurs as a result of the actions of an acetyl hydrolase which cleaves the acetyl group to generate lyso-PAF (Snyder, 1985). Both of these enzymes are present in eosinophils (Lee *et al.*, 1982, 1984). PAF has a number of pro-inflammatory activities, and in particular acts as a leucocyte chemoattractant and activating agent. Inhalation of PAF causes bronchoconstriction in humans and variable increases in bronchial hyperresponsiveness

(Henson, 1989). Eosinophils can generate substantial quantities of PAF after stimulation with calcium ionophore, zymosan and IgG-coated Sepharose beads (Burke *et al.*, 1990; Cromwell *et al.*, 1990). Much of the PAF remained cell associated.

Eosinophil granule proteins

Eosinophil-specific granules contain four basic proteins. MBP, which makes up 50% of the granule protein, is found in the core of the granule where it accounts for virtually all the protein in the core (Lewis *et al.*, 1978). EPO, ECP and EDN — also known as EPX — are found in the granule matrix (Egesten *et al.*, 1986; Peters *et al.*, 1986). The biology of these proteins has recently been reviewed in detail (Gleich *et al.*, 1994); their functions are summarized in Table 10.5.

MBP

MBP is a single polypetide chain of 117 amino acids, with a molecular weight of 13 801 and a pI of 10.9. It contains 17 arginine residues, which accounts for its basicity, and nine cysteine residues which explains its tendency to form disulphide bonds. The reduced form is as toxic for parasites as the native form but less potent (O'Connell *et al.*, 1983). As well as the mature MBP peptide, the cDNA for MBP encodes for a pre-prosequence which is a putative signal peptide and a 90 amino acid acidic proprotein which may neutralize MBP's toxicity as it is processed through the Golgi and transported to the granule where the prosequence is cleaved (Barker *et al.*, 1988; McGrogan *et al.*, 1988). MBP can also be detected in basophil granules although basophils contain considerably less MBP than eosinophils (Ackerman *et al.*, 1983). Plasma concentrations of MBP are elevated in the sera of pregnant women with a peak 2–3 weeks before parturition. Placental eosinophils are few in number and MBP has been shown by immunofluoresence to be in placental X and giant cells (Maddox *et al.*, 1984). The function of MBP in pregancy is obscure.

ECP

ECP is a single-chain polypetide with a pI in the region of 10.8. On molecular sizing ECP displays marked heterogeneity, probably as a result of differental glycosylation, with molecular-weight bands ranging between 16 000 and 21 400. Two isoforms, ECP-1 and ECP-2, can be identified using heparin Sepharose (Gleich *et al.*, 1986). The ECP cDNA encodes for a leader sequence of 27 amino acids and a mature protein of 133 amino acids with a calculated molecular weight of 15 600 (Barker *et al.*, 1989; Rosenberg *et al.*, 1989a). The amino-acid sequence is 66% homologous to EDN and 31% homologous to human pancreatic ribonuclease. ECP does have ribonuclease activity but it is 100 times less potent than EDN (Slifman *et al.*, 1986). The gene for both EDN and ECP is on chromosome 14q (Hamann *et al.*, 1990). Monoclonal antibodies can distinguish between a form of ECP found in the granules of resting eosinophils (mAb EG1) and a secreted or extracted form of ECP (both mAb EG1 and EG2) (Tai *et al.*, 1984). EG2 also recognizes EDN. The differences between these two forms is not known. There is approximately 25 pg of ECP per eosinophil, which is about an order of magnitude

Table 10.5 Functions of eosinophil granule proteins.

Protein	Function	Reference
MBP	Toxicity towards helminthic parasites such as schistosomulae of *S. mansoni*	Butterworth 1984; Gleich & Adolphson 1986
	Cytotoxicity towards guinea pig and huma airway epithelium at 10 µg/ml	Frigas *et al.*, 1980; Hastie *et al.*, 1987; Hisamatsu *et al.*, 1990
	Bronchoconstriction and increased BHR on inhalation in rats and monkeys	Uchida *et al.*, 1993; Coyle *et al.*, 1993; Gundel *et al.*, 1991
	Non-cytotoxic release of histamine from basophils	Zheutlin *et al.*, 1984
	Strong platelet agonist	Rohrbach *et al.*, 1990
	Activates complement through alternate pathway	Weiler *et al.*, 1992
ECP	Ribonuclease activity (100 times less potent than EDN)	Slifman *et al.*, 1986
	Toxic for helminthic parasites and mammalian epithelial cells	McLaren *et al.*, 1981
	Causes Gordon phenomenon	Fredens *et al.*, 1982
EPO	Toxic for mammalian cells through ability to oxidize halides in presence of H_2O_2 to form reactive hypohalous acids. Thiocyanate, which forms the weak oxidant hypothiocyanous acid, may be preferred halide *in vivo*	Slungaard & Mahoney, 1991
EDN	Only weakly toxic for parasites or mammalian cells	
	Induces Gordon phenomenon	

See text for definition of abbreviations.

less than MBP. ECP exerts its cytotoxic effect through the formation of membrane pores (Young *et al.*, 1986).

EPO

EPO is a haem-containing protein composed of an approximately 14-kDA (light) and a 58-kDa (heavy) subunit, derived from the same strand of mRNA and subsequently cleaved. The cDNA encodes for a 381 leader sequence as well as the light and heavy chains (Ten *et al.*, 1989). EPO shares a 68% amino-acid identity with human neutrophil myeloperoxidase and other peroxidase enzymes and is antigenically similar. The human EPO gene is located on chromosome 17 (Sakamaki *et al.*, 1989). There is approximately 15 pg of EPO per eosinophil.

EDN

EDN, also called EPX (Slifman *et al.*, 1989), is a single-chain peptide with a molecular weight on gel electrophoresis of 18.6 kDa and a calculated molecular weight from the cDNA of 15.5 kDa. Like ECP, it is a member of a ribonuclease multigene family and has marked ribonuclease activity (Slifman *et al.*, 1986; Rosenburg *et al.*, 1989b). EDN expression is not restricted to eosinophils, as it is found in mononuclear cells and possibly neutrophils. It is probably secreted by the liver and the EDN sequence is also identical to human urinary RNase (Beintema *et al.*, 1988).

Cytokines

Eosinophils can synthesize and secrete several important inflammatory and regulatory cytokines. Cytokine mRNA expression has been detected by a combination of *in situ* hybridization, polymerase chain reaction (PCR) and Northern blotting, and protein expression by immunocytochemistry and analysis of supernatants from cell cultures. Many cytokines appear to be stored in specific granules (Moqbel *et al.*, 1994). Several eosinophil cytokines appear to be generated in relatively small amounts and may act in an autocrine fashion, regulating the function of the eosinophil rather than having a wider inflammatory activity. The cytokines generated by eosinophils are summarized in Table 10.6 and are discussed in more detail in a recent comprehensive review (Wardlaw *et al.*, 1995).

Other eosinophil-derived mediators

A major constituent of the human eosinophil is CLC protein. This is a 17.4-kDa hydrophobic protein which

Table 10.6 Cytokine generation by eosinophils.

Cytokine	Comments	Reference
IL-1α	Synthesis triggered by LPS and phorbol esters.	Weller *et al.*, 1993 Del Pozo *et al.*, 1990
TGF-α	mRNA + ve and immunoreactive eosinophils detected in association with healing wounds, HES and squamous carcinoma	Wong *et al.*, 1990, 1993 Todd *et al.*, 1991
TGF-β	Detected in eosinophils in nasal polyps and Hodgkin's lymphoma	Ohno *et al.*, 1992; Kadin *et al.*, 1993
GM-CSF	Secreted in response to IFN-γ and calcium ionophore stimulation	Moqbel *et al.*, 1991; Kita *et al.*, 1991b
IL-2	IL-2 imunoreactivity detected in 10% of peripheral blood eosinophils	Levi-Schaffer *et al.*, 1995
IL-3	IL-3 production inhibited by FK506, rapamycin and cyclosporin	Hom & Estridge 1993
IL-4	75 pg/106 cells detected within eosinophils. mRNA detected by RT-PCR	Moqbel *et al.*, 1995
IL-5	mRNA expression detected in eosinophils by *in situ* hybridization and immunoreactivity in a number of conditions including HES, coeliac disease and BAL cells in asthma. Small amounts released following Fc receptor stimulation	Desreumaux *et al.*, 1992; Broide *et al.*, 1992; Dubucquoi *et al.*, 1994
IL-6	IL-6 stored in unstimulated eosinophil granules	Hamid *et al.*, 1992
IL-8	Stored in eosinophil granules, released by calcium ionophore	Braun *et al.*, 1993
TNF-α	Found in various eosinophilic conditions in association with granules	Costa *et al.*, 1993
MIP-1α/ RANTES	Expression of mRNA in nasal polyp eosinophils, skin eosinophils after allergen challenge and HES eosinophils shown by *in-situ* hybridization	Costa *et al.*, 1993; Ying *et al.*, 1995

was shown to be lysophospholipase (Weller *et al.*, 1980). It has also been shown to be a 16.4-kDa S-type animal lectin (Ackerman *et al.*, 1993).

In addition, the eosinophil contains a number of other granule-stored enzymes whose role in eosinophil function has not been defined (reviewed by Spry, 1988). They include acid phosphatase (large amounts of which have been isolated from eosinophils), collagenase, arylsuphatase B, histaminase, phospholipase D, catalase, non-specific esterases, vitamin B_{12}-binding proteins, and glycosaminoglycans. Eosinophils can undergo a respiratory burst with release of superoxide ion and hydrogen peroxide in response to stimulation (Shult *et al.*, 1985).

Eosinophil activation

Eosinophils from normal individuals circulate in a resting state, in which their effector functions and response to inflammatory mediators are blunted. Exposure to eosinophil-active mediators, either *in vitro* or *in vivo* as they move into sites of inflammation, results in priming which leads to enhancement of some eosinophil effector functions such as chemotaxis. Further stimulation by inflammatory mediators or pertubation of certain membrane receptors results in degranulation of stored proteins and *de novo* synthesis and secretion of mediators, allowing full expression of eosinophil effector functions such as cytotoxicity. The term 'activation' has been used to describe this transition of the eosinophil from a resting through a primed to a secretory state. Activated and degranulating eosinophils have a distinct morphology, which are referred to above.

Eosinophil density

Normal peripheral blood eosinophils are dense cells and can be separated by density gradient centrifugation (Vadas *et al.*, 1979; Gartner 1980). In some eosinophilic diseases a population shift was noted towards a less dense (hypodense) phenotype (Bass *et al.*, 1980). An increased percentage of hypodense eosinophils has been described in asthma, allergic rhinitis and, most spectacularly, HES. The appearance of hypodense cells can, in some circumstances, relate to disease severity. For example Krouwels *et al.* (1995) observed a significant inverse correlation between the number of hypodense eosinophils and the percentage predicted forced expiratory volume in 1 second (FEV_1), FEV_1/FVC ratio and histamine Pc_{20}. They also found an increase in the percentage of hypodense eosinophils after allergen challenge. Eosinophils in tissue have also been found to be predominantly hypodense (Prin *et al.*, 1984). The hypodense peripheral blood eosinophils from patients with HES have evidence of cell swelling, may be vacuolated and have less and smaller specific granules which contain less MBP and ECP (Connell 1968; Peters *et al.*, 1988; Caulfield *et al.*, 1990). These changes may explain the less dense phenotype. Normal-density eosinophils can be made hypodense *in vitro* by stimulation with PAF, C5a and cytokines such as GM-CSF, which suggests a relationship between hypodensity and activation (Kloprogge *et al.*, 1989).

Bass *et al.* (1980) found that normal-density eosinophils from patients with an eosinophilia, compared with normal-density eosinophils from non-eosinophilic subjects, had a reduced surface charge, increased deoxyglucose uptake and increased oxidative metabolism suggestive of activation. Similarly, David *et al.* (1980) found that eosinophils from subjects with an eosinophilia were more cytotoxic for schistosomulae of *Schistosoma mansoni* than eosinophils from normal subjects. However, neither of these studies related their observations to density. In contrast, Pincus *et al.* (1981) found that normal-density eosinophils from patients with an eosinophilia of various causes generated more superoxide after PMA stimulation than eosinophils from normal donors, normal-density eosinophilis from HES donors generated less superoxide. Similarly, normal-density eosinophilis from asthmatics generated less chemiluminescence after zymosan stimulation than eosinophils from normal donors (Shult *et al.*, 1988).

Winquist *et al.* (1982) found that hypodense eosinophils in one patient with HES had increased oxygen consumption and (using the rosette technique) increased expression of IgG and complement receptors, compared with normal-density eosinophils from the same patient. In addition, hypodense eosinophils from two patients with HES had greater oxygen consumption than eosinophils (density not stated) from a number of other eosinophilic patients. However, Hartnell *et al.* (1990) using flow cytometry found no relationship between density and expression of IgG Fc (CD32) receptors or Mac-1, the CR3 receptor. Prin *et al.* (1983) found increased cytotoxicity and increased membrane hexose transport in both normal-density and hypodense cells from patients with a marked eosinophilia and the hypodense cells from the eosinophilic patients were more active than the normal-density cells. However, the hypodense cells were only about 70% pure. In a later study they found reduced respiratory burst activity in hypodense eosinophils which they thought might be due to reduced EPO content (Prin *et al.* 1986). A number of studies have shown that eosinophils from patients with an eosinophilia are more motile and respond differently *in vitro* and *in vivo* to chemotactic stimuli than do eosinophils from normal subjects. They respond better to IL-8, PAF and f-MLP suggesting a priming effect, but less well to IL-5, GM-CSF and IL-3, possibly as a result of *in vivo* desensitization (Sehmi *et al.*, 1993; Wardlaw *et al.*, 1986b; Sehmi *et al.*, 1992b; Warringa *et* al., 1992b; Henocq & Vargaftig, 1986). However, direct comparisons between different density cells from the same donors have not been undertaken. A number of studies have examined PAF and LTC_4 production by eosinophils and related it to density. Findings have been variable, and complicated by the possible metabolism of the lipid mediators or their intracellular retention (Weller *et al.*, 1993). In a detailed study, Hodges *et al.* (1988) compared calcium ionophore-induced LTC_4 generation by hypodense and normal-density eosinophils from asthmatic and normal subjects. They found that hypodense eosinophils released more LTC_4 than normal-density eosinophils from either normal or asthmatic subjects, but that eosinophils of both densities from normal subjects released more LTC_4 than eosinophils from asthmatic subjects. Cromwell *et al.* found that hypodense cells from HES patients generated less PAF after stimulation with IgG-coated beads than normal-density cells from mildly eosinophilic atopic donors but the hypodense cells metabolized PAF to lyso-PAF more rapidly (Cromwell *et al.*, 1990). This highlights the complexity of relating lipid mediator production to activation status.

No conclusive picture therefore emerges from the literature on the relationship between density and the functional capacity of the eosinophil, with apparently different results depending on experimental design. Hypodensity does not therefore appear to be a very reliable marker of eosinophil activation.

Factors which induce eosinophil priming and secretion

A number of inflammatory mediators have been shown to be active on eosinophils, causing enhancement of several eosinophil functions, particularly directional migration, adhesion and cytotoxicity. Many of these are discussed throughout this chapter, particularly in the section dealing with eosinophil chemoattractants (see Table 10.2). A summary of the effects of cytokines on eosinophils is shown in Table 10.7.

Eosinophil mediator release and cytotoxicity

Granule protein release

Substantive secretion of eosinophil granule proteins is observed following interaction of the cell with large opsonized targets, such as a metazoan parasite or Sepharose beads. *In vitro* secretion can be triggered physiologically via IgG and IgA Fc receptors (Winqvist *et al.*, 1982; Shaw *et al.*, 1985; Capron *et al.*, 1988; Abu-Ghazaleh *et al.*, 1989, 1992). Furthermore, eosinophils from patients with an eosinophilia released significantly higher concentrations of their granule proteins (Carlson *et al.*, 1991, 1992; Venge, 1993) than normal cells. Glucocorticosteroids do not suppress immunoglobulin-induced eosinophil degranulation. However, cyclic adenosine monophosphate (cAMP) analogues, phosphodiesterase inhibitors and β-adrenergic agonists inhibit these processes (Kita *et al.* 1991a). Furthermore pretreatment of eosinophils with pertussis toxin abrogates sIgA-induced degranulation and increases in phospholipase C activity. PAF, a potent chemoattractant for eosinophils, induces marginal release of granule proteins (Kroegel *et al.*, 1989a). On the other hand, cytokines, particularly GM-CSF and IL-5 (Kita *et al.*, 1992), can induce substantial eosinophil degranulation, even in the absence of any particulate stimulus.

Priming by cytokines (e.g. IL-5) prior to exposure to a particulate stimulus enhanced the capacity of normal eosinophils to release granule proteins (Fujisawa *et al.*, 1990). Eosinophil degranulation appeared to be dependent on cell–cell contact, with a critical role for β2 integrins. For example, degranulation induced by GM-CSF or PAF was inhibited by antibodies to CD11b/CD18 (Mac-1) (Horie & Kita 1994).

Selective degranulation of the granule proteins has been described. IgE-dependent stimulation was reported to induce the release of MBP and EPO but not ECP, while IgG-coated surfaces induced a selective release of ECP, but not EPO (Capron *et al.*, 1989; Tomassini *et al.*, 1991). IgA, on the other hand, when bound to Sepharose beads, triggered the non-selective release of all granule proteins.

Cromwell *et al.* (1991) studied G protein regulation of eosinophil exocytosis using systems which bypass the initial steps involving surface receptors and their associated G proteins. These involved permeabilization methods, for example bacterial cytolysin, streptolysin-O (SL-O) and patch clamping in the whole-cell configuration. In cells permeabilized with SL-O, secretion was dependent on the presence of both Ca^{2+} and guanine nucleotide (Cromwell *et al.*, 1991). The mechanism closely resembled that of other myeloid cell types, although there were differences, mainly relating to the more extended time over which exocytosis occurs. For example, patch clamp experiments indicated that exocytosis involved fusion of discrete granules with the plasma membrane in two temporally dissociated phases (Nüsse *et al.*, 1990). The first phase involved small granules or vesicles and was at least partly Ca^{2+} dependent. The second phase reflected sequential fusion of all the crystalloid granules as individual units with the plasma membrane and showed an absolute requirement for GTPγS.

Signal transduction

Studies on human, guinea pig and murine eosinophils have indicated that following agonist stimulation, a biochemical cascade is initiated which leads to the regulation

Table 10.7 Effects of cytokines on the effector function of mature human eosinophils.

Effect	Cytokine	Reference
Prolonging survival and viability	IL-3, IL-5, GM-CSF	Owen *et al.*, 1987; Yamaguchi *et al.*, 1991; Rothenberg *et al.*, 1989; Stern *et al.*, 1992
Inducing expression of IL-2 receptors (CD25)	IL-3, GM-CSF	Rand *et al.*, 1991b
Inducing CD69 expression	IL-5, GM-CSF	Hartnell *et al.*, 1993
Inducing expression of CD16	IFN-γ	Hartnell *et al.*, 1992a
Promoting EDN release	GM-CSF	Fujisawa *et al.*, 1990
Promoting and enhancing EDN release by slgA- and IgG-dependent mechanisms	IL-3, IL-5, GM-CSF	Fujisawa *et al.*, 1990
Increasing ADCC cytotoxicity to Daudi lymphoma cells	IL-3, IL-5, IFN-γ	Valerius *et al.*, 1990
Enhancing helminthotoxicity *in vitro*	IL-5, GM-CSF, TNF-α	Silberstein & David, 1986; Owen *et al.*, 1987; Rothenberg *et al.*, 1989
Promoting cytotoxicity towards vascular endothelial cells	TNF-α	Slungaard *et al.*, 1990
Increasing cytotoxicity to opsonized yeast	IL-5	Lopez *et al.*, 1988
Promoting hypodense phenotype	IL-5, GM-CSF	Owen *et al.*, 1987; Rothenberg *et al.*, 1989
Up-regulates hyper-adherence to HUVEC	IL-5	Walsh *et al.*, 1990
Increasing binding of IL-5	GM-CSF	Chihara *et al.*, 1990
Synergizing with IL-5 in inducing ICAM-1 expression	TNF-α	Hansel *et al.*, 1992
Up-regulating LTC_4 production	GM-CSF, TNF-α	Silberstein & David, 1986; Owen *et al.*, 1987; Roubin *et al.*, 1987; Howell *et al.*, 1989
Stimulating oxidative metabolism of eosinophils following adherence	TNF-α, IFN-γ	Slungaard *et al.*, 1990; Dri *et al.*, 1991
Priming for PMA-induced respiratory burst	IL-5	Tagari *et al.*, 1993
Inducing GM-CSF mRNA transcription and translation	IFN-γ	Moqbel *et al.*, 1991
Inducing IL-6 mRNA transcription and translation	IFN-γ	Hamid *et al.*, 1992

See text for definition of abbreviations.

and control of granule- and membrane-derived mediator release. The interaction of agonists with a cell-surface receptor induces the activation of phospholipase C enzyme (PLC) through the action of a Pertussis toxin-sensitive G protein. Among various agonists, PAF and LTB_4 have been shown to activate PLC directly (Kroegel *et al.*, 1989, 1991). For eosinophil exocytosis to occur, uptake of extracellular Ca^{2+} by the cell is supplemented by the intracellular release of Ca^{2+} via inositol triphosphate (IP_3). It is suggested that this pathway may require the activation of an as yet undefined eosinophil Ca^{2+} binding protein, together with a putative, membrane-associated, eosinophil protein (GE) (reviewed by Giembycz & Barnes, 1993). Recent studies have also implicated both PLA_2 and arachidonic acid in eosinophil activation (Aebischer *et al.*, 1993).

The role of tyrosine kinases in IL-5-mediated eosinophil signal transduction has been studied by Pazdrak *et al.* (1995). Many tyrosine kinases have been shown to associate with cytokine receptors. Lyn, a member of the src tyrosine kinase family, has been detected in cells of myeloid origin. Alam *et al.* (1994) detected two species of lyn kinase (56 and 53 kDa) in eosinophils. Both of them were phosphorylated and activated within 1 minute following stimulation of eosinophils with IL-5. Lyn kinase was physically associated with IL-5 β-receptor, as determined by coprecipitation studies. IL-5 also stimulated the binding of GTP to p21 *ras* within 1–3 minutes. The GTP-bound *ras* causes translocation of *raf*-1 to the membrane and its activation. *Raf*-1 then phosphorylates MEK kinase, which subsequently activates MAP kinases. *Raf*-1 and MEK were activated within 3 minutes after IL-5 stimulation, Both 45-

and 41-kDa molecular-weight species of MEK were present and activated in eosinophils. The activity of MAP kinase in eosinophils peaked at 20 minutes. The optimal concentration of IL-5 for stimulation of kinases was 10^{-11} to 10^{-10} M, which is in accordance with other biological activities of this cytokine on eosinophils. Jak2 was found to be physically associated with the eosinophil IL-5 β-receptor and was tyrosine phosphorylated within 3 minutes after IL-5 stimulation. Activated Jak2 underwent autophosphorylation *in situ*, and resulted in expression of *STAT 1* (p91).

Eosinophils and disease

Eosinophilia

The blood eosinophil count represents the balance between the rate of eosinophil migration from the bone marrow and entry into the tissues. Once in the tissue, eosinophils can survive for many days under the influence of locally generated cytokines. Eosinophils can be enumerated in the peripheral blood, either by 'wet counts' in modified Neubauer chambers, differential counts on dried smears or by automated cell counting. Automated counting which uses detection of eosinophil peroxidase is the most accurate method. The normal eosinophil count is (generally taken as) less than 0.4×10^9/l. The eosinophil count varies with age, time of day, exercise and environmental stimuli, particularly allergen exposure. Blood eosinophil counts undergo diurnal variation, being lowest in the morning and highest at night. This effect resulted in a greater than 40% variation in one study (Winkel *et al.*, 1981).

The commonest cause of an eosinophilia worldwide is infection with helminthic parasites The commonest causes of an eosinophilia in developed countries are the atopic allergic diseases, seasonal and perennial rhinitis, atopic dermatitis and asthma. Allergic disease generally results in only a mild increase in eosinophil counts. A moderate or high eosinophil count in asthma raises the possibility of a complication such as Churg–Strauss syndrome or allergic bronchopulmonary aspergillosis (ABPA). Apart from allergic disease and helminthic parasites, a raised eosinophil count, especially a moderate or high count, is unusual and often the result of drug reactions.

The role of eosinophils

Views on the role of eosinophils in health and disease have changed with time. For many years they were thought to ameliorate inflammatory responses, now they are believed to have a tissue-damaging role (Weller & Goetzl, 1979; Gleich, 1990). There is little doubt that eosinophils can cause severe tissue damage under certain circumstances. Persistently high eosinophil counts seen with drug reactions, helminthic parasitic infections, eosinophilic leukaemia and HES are associated with endomyocardial fibrosis. Much of the work undertaken in recent years on eosinophils has been in association with allergic disease and helminthic infection. Recent studies demonstrating that eosinophils are cytokine-producing cells indicate that the cell may have a more complex functional role than previously appreciated. At the same time doubt has been cast on the host defence role of eosinophils in helminthic parasitic disease since, for example, abrogation of the eosinophil response in mice induced by infection with helminthic parasites had no appreciable effect on the course of the disease (Sher *et al.*, 1990). The role of eosinophils in parasistic infections and other diseases has recently been reviewed, and will not be discussed further (Butterworth & Thorne, 1993; Wardlaw *et al.*, 1995).

Eosinophils and allergic inflammation

Pathology of asthma deaths

The association between eosinophils, asthma and allergic disease has been known for many years. It is well established that large numbers of eosinophils together with mononuclear cells are frequently found in and around the bronchi in patients who have died of asthma (Ellis, 1908; Dunnill, 1978; Huber & Koessler 1992). Immunostaining of bronchial tissue from asthma deaths revealed large amounts of MBP deposited in the airway adjacent to areas of desquamated epithelium (Filley *et al.*, 1982). Although an airway eosinophilia is a consistent and often striking finding in asthma deaths it is not universal, with case reports of childhood asthma deaths showing no evidence of airway eosinophilia (Sur *et al.*, 1993).

Peripheral blood eosinophil counts

The presence of increased numbers of peripheral blood eosinophils in both atopic and non-atopic chronic asthma is also well established although this elevation is not as great as that seen in other eosinophil-associated diseases, and the peripheral blood eosinophil count is often normal. Horn and colleagues (1975), in a longitudinal study of 14 oral corticosteroid-dependent asthmatics being treated at a chest clinic, found that eosinophil counts correlated with several measurements of airflow obstruction. Durham & Kay (1985) observed that the degree of bronchial hyperreactivity inversely correlated with the peripheral blood eosinophil count in patients who had a late-phase response after antigen challenge. A similar correlation was observed in a cross-sectional study of asthmatics seen at a routine chest clinic (Taylor & Luksza, 1987). The concentration of ECP in the serum of asthmatics also correlated with the severity of clinical disease, and monitoring of ECP has been suggested as a useful adjunct to clinical assessment (Venge, 1995).

Fibreoptic bronchoscopy studies

A more detailed appreciation of the extent of eosinophil involvement in asthma has come from the use of fibreoptic bronchoscopy to obtain bronchoalveolar lavage (BAL) fluid and endobronchial biopsies from the airways of patients with mild to moderate asthma.

Allergen challenge

Aerosolized challenge of sensitized asthmatics with allergen results in an early phase of bronchoconstriction lasting about 1 hour and returning to baseline. In about 40% of subjects this is followed by a delayed- or late-phase period of airway obstruction, generally increasing up to 6 hours after challenge and lasting up to 12 hours. The late response is associated with the influx of inflammatory cells, thereby more closely mimicking the pathology of clinical asthma (Dolovich *et al.*, 1989; Durham, 1991).

De Monchy *et al.* (1985) observed an increase in the number of eosinophils in BAL fluid and an increase in the ECP/albumin ratio 6 hours after allergen challenge in late responders, but not those subjects who only had a single early response. Diaz and colleagues (1989) studied 14 asthmatics 6 hours after allargen challenge, seven of whom had a late-phase response. They found increased numbers of eosinophils and, to a lesser extent, neutrophils but only in those subjects who had a dual response. Aalbers *et al.* (1993) observed increased numbers of eosinophils in the bronchial wash of dual compared with single responders, the response to allergen challenge having been determined 3–7 weeks before the bronchoscopy. They argued that the increased airway eosinophilia was a predictor of dual response status rather than a consequence of it.

Metzger and coworkers (1987), using a technique of segmental challenge to instill allergen directly into the airways through the bronchoscope, found up to 50% of the lavage cells were eosinophils 24 hours after challenge. Similar findings have been found after allergen challenge to the skin and nose (Frew & Kay 1988; Bentley *et al.*, 1992a). Lam *et al.* (1987) found increased numbers of eosinophils and epithelial cells 24 hours after challenge with plicatic acid in patients with red cedar wood asthma. A BAL neutrophilia was observed after 48 hours. Fabbri and colleagues (1987) observed both an airway eosinophilia and neutrophilia in patients with a late response to challenge with toluene di-isocyanate. A recent detailed kinetic examination of the time-course of the late-phase response in the skin revealed that migration of granulocytes was maximal at 6 hours, with much of the recruitment having occurred by the first hour. Eosinophil infiltration was still present in the skin at 96 hours (Tsicopoulos *et al.*, 1994). Despite the almost invariable finding of an eosinophilia after allergen challenge, the extent to which this is a causal relationship remains uncertain. For example, in the monkey model of asthma (Gundel *et al.*, 1993) the late response appeared to be neutrophil rather than eosinophil related, and not all studies have observed a clear distinction in the BAL cellular profile between single and dual responders (Bentley *et al.*, 1993). Other reasons suggested to explain the development of the late response include the degree of mast cell responsiveness to allergen challenge and the sensitivity of the lung to an inflammatory stimulus (Machado & Stalenheim, 1990).

Clinical disease

An almost invariable increase in the number of eosinophils, often in association with increased numbers of mast cells and epithelial cells, has been observed in BAL fluid and endobronchial biopsies from clinical asthmatics compared with normal controls (Godard *et al.*, 1982; Tomioka *et al.*, 1984; Flint *et al.*, 1985; Kelly *et al.*, 1988; Wardlaw *et al.*, 1988; Beasley *et al.*, 1989; Foresi *et al.*, 1990; and reviewed in Djukanovic *et al.*, 1990). The increase in the number of eosinophils in the asthmatic airway is modest. For example, in BAL fluid this ranged between 1 and 5%, compared with 0–1% in normal controls (Wardlaw *et al.*, 1988). Unlike the allergen challenge studies, increased numbers of airway neutrophils have not generally been observed. One of the most important observations that has emerged from these studies is that even in very mild disease requiring only occasional use of bronchodilators there is clear evidence of airway inflammation with increased numbers of airway eosinophils and BAL epithelial cells. This has led to increased emphasis on the early use of anti-inflammatory drugs, particularly inhaled corticosteroids, in the management of asthma. Airway eosinophils in asthma are activated, as determined by staining with the mAb EG2 and expression of the activation receptor CD69 (Azzawi *et al.*, 1990; Hartnell *et al.*, 1993). The importance of the state of activation of the eosinophils and the extent to which they are releasing their mediators is emphasized by several studies. For example, in the study by Wardlaw *et al.* (1988) the concentration of MBP in the BAL fluid was a better discriminator of disease activity than the BAL eosinophil count. The inhibitory effect of anti-CD18 mAb in the development of allergen-induced bronchial hyperresponsiveness in cyanomolagous monkeys was associated with a decrease in BAL ECP concentrations without any change in the eosinophil count (Wegner *et al.*, 1993). Thus, measurements of eosinophil-associated basic proteins may be a better guide to the degree of eosinophil inflammation than eosinophil numbers. In support of this, Adelroth and coworkers (1990) found that, whereas inhaled corticosteroids had no effect on the number of eosinophils in BAL fluid from asthmatics, they markedly reduced the amounts of ECP in lavage fluid in association with clinical improvement.

Further support for the idea that eosinophil activation and mediator release is required for tissue damage (rather than the presence of eosinophils *per se*) to occur is offered by animal models. For example, IL-5 transgenic mice which have a marked peripheral blood and tissue eosinophilia appear to be healthy (Dent *et al.*, 1990). In addition, when systemically sensitized guinea pigs were challenged by antigen inhalation they developed a BAL eosinophilia without evidence of eosinophil activation and no increase in bronchial hyperresponsiveness. However, after intratracheal challenge with LTB_4, concentrations of MBP and EPO increased in the BAL fluid and the animals developed bronchial hyperresponsiveness (Pretolani *et al.*, 1994).

The specificity of an airway eosinophilia has been addressed by several groups. Allen *et al.* (1990) found that BAL eosinophilia was found in only a restricted range of lung diseases of which asthma is by far the commonest. The difference in airway eosinophils and neutrophils between patients with asthma and smoking-related airway disease was studied by Lacoste *et al.* (1993). They found that both groups of patients had a significant increase in BAL eosinophils compared with normal subjects. There was a significant increase in the concentration of BAL ECP and the number of degranulating eosinophils, but not in the total number of eosinophils, between the asthmatics and patients with smoking-related lung disease. The presence of sputum eosinophilia was noted in seven non-smoking subjects with chronic productive cough, but without evidence of asthma. In this report the presence of a sputum eosinophilia was a marker for corticosteroid responsiveness (Gibson *et al.*, 1989). The specificity of an airway eosinophilia in relation to asthma was also examined by Azzawi *et al.* (1992), who compared the immunohistology of fatal asthma and cystic fibrosis. They found that whereas in 15 patients with asthma there was a mean of 62.7 eosinophils per millimetre length of epithelial basement membrane, in six patients who died of cystic fibrosis there was 1.8 eosinophils, and in normal controls there was 1 eosinophil. A lesser, but often significant, increase in airway eosinophils is seen in atopic non-asthmatics or seasonal asthmatics out of season.

Although most studies have involved atopic asthmatics, airway eosinophila is also a marked feature of intrinsic asthma and isocyanate-induced asthma (Bentley *et al.*, 1992b,c). As well as asthma, eosinophils are also prominent in other forms of allergic inflammation, including allergic rhinitis and atopic dermatitis. Essentially the findings in rhinitis have been similar to those in asthma, with increased numbers of activated eosinophils and eosinophil granule proteins in association with increased numbers of epithelial mast cells (Viegas *et al.*, 1987; Pipkorn *et al.*, 1988; Bentley *et al.*, 1992c). In rhinitis, however, the nasal epithelium generally appears intact. Nasal polyps contain large numbers of activated eosinophils, and the syndrome of aspirin sensitivity, eosinophilia and nasal polyposis is well recognized (Slavin, 1993). In atopic dermatitis a peripheral blood eosinophilia is a common feature and the skin lesions are characterized by marked deposition of eosinophil granule proteins, often in the absence of many intact eosinophils (Leiferman *et al.*, 1985; Bruyjnzeel-Koomen *et al.*, 1988).

An eosinophilia is therefore an almost invariable feature of allergic inflammation. However, if there was a causal relationship between the eosinophil and the pathogenesis of asthma it would be expected that fluctuations in the severity of the disease would be mirrored by fluctuations in the degree of eosinophilia. As discussed above, there was a correlation between the peripheral blood eosinophil count and the FEV_1 in clinical disease and the development of a late-phase response after allergen challenge. In addition, most studies have found a correlation between asthma or rhinitis and the number of hypodense eosinophils in the peripheral blood (Fukuda *et al.*, 1985; Frick *et al.*, 1988, 1989). Bousquet *et al.* (1990) reported a significant correlation, with increasing severity of asthma, between both the airway eosinophil count and BAL ECP concentration. In an electron microscopy study a correlation was observed in 18 asthmatics between the number of epithelial eosinophils and the opening of epithelial tight junctions, which in turn was inversely correlated with the histamine Pc_{20} (Ohashi *et al.*, 1992). Inhibition of an airway eosinophilia by disodium cromoglycate (Diaz *et al.*, 1984), or more effectively corticosteroids (Juniper *et al.*, 1990; Schleimer, 1990), was associated with an improvement in bronchial hyperresponsiveness, symptoms and lung function. Inhibition of migration of eosinophils into the airways of allergen-challenged non-human primates, using a mAb directed against the adhesion molecule ICAM-1, also inhibited the development of airway hyperresponsiveness (Wegner *et al.*, 1990). However, none of these treatments is specific to the eosinophil. Glucocorticoids, for example, probably act to a large extent through inhibition of the release of eosinophil active cytokines from T cells and monocytes (Taylor & Shaw, 1993).

In recent years the T lymphocyte has emerged as important in directing eosinophil function in allergic inflammation. Activated T cells, as defined by the expression of the

IL-2 receptor CD25, are found in increased numbers in the peripheral blood from patients with acute severe asthma and clinical improvment was associated with a decrease in the number of CD25-positive cells in the blood (Corrigan *et al.*, 1988). Similarly, CD25-positive T cells were found in increased numbers in BAL and endobronchial biopsies from asthmatics (Azzawi *et al.*, 1990) and have a Th2-like profile of cytokine mRNA expression (Robinson *et al.*, 1992).

Present evidence suggests that IL-5 plays a critical role in eosinophil-mediated tissue damage. IL-5 mRNA+ cells were detectable in BAL (Robinson *et al.*, 1992) and bronchial biopsies (Hamid *et al.*, 1991) from ongoing steady-state asthmatics, as well as in asthma provoked by inhalational challenge (Bentley *et al.*, 1992b,c). Chronic severe asthmatics had elevated serum concentrations of IL-5 compared with controls, and levels decreased following treatment with corticosteroids (Corrigan *et al.*, 1993). In a placebo-controlled study in moderately severe asthma the numbers of IL-5 mRNA+ cells in BAL also decreased after 2 weeks' treatment with prednisolone (Robinson *et al.*, 1993).

In summary, therefore, eosinophils are almost invariably present in increased numbers at sites of allergic inflammation. They are actively secreting mediators which could cause many of the pathological features of the disease process. The numbers of eosinophils and amounts of eosinophil mediators correlate broadly with disease activity, and effective treatments for asthma, particularly glucocorticoids, reduce the number of tissue and blood eosinophils. There is therefore very good evidence for a pro-inflammatory role for eosinophils in asthma and related diseases. However the evidence still remains circumstantial. In a sense, any further debate becomes sterile until we have conclusive evidence from agents which specifically inhibit eosinophil accumulation or their products in tissue. The emergence of such antagonists from the pharmaceutical locker is keenly awaited.

References

Aalbers, R., Kauffman, H.F., Vrugt, B. *et al.* (1993) Bronchial lavage and bronchoalveolar lavage in allergen-induced single early and dual asthmatic responders. *Am. Rev. Resp. Dis.*, **147**, 76–81.

Abu-Ghazaleh, R.I., Fujisawa, T., Mestecky, J., Kyle, R.A. & Gleich, G.J. (1989) IgA-induced eosinophil degranulation. *J. Immunol.*, **142**, 2393–400.

Abu-Ghazaleh, R.I., Gleich, G.J. & Prendergast, F.G. (1992) Interaction of eosinophil granule major basic protein with synthetic lipid bilayers: a mechanism for toxicity. *J. Membr. Biol.*, **128**, 153–64.

Ackerman, S.J. (1993) Characterization and functions of eosinophil granule proteins. In: *Eosinophils. Biological and Clinical Aspects* (eds S. Makino & T. Fukuda), pp. 33–74. CRC Press, Boca Raton.

Ackerman, S.J., Kephart, G.M., Haberman, T.M., Greipp, P.R. & Gleich, G.J. (1983) Localization of eosinophil granule major basic protein in human basophils. *J. Exp. Med.*, **158**, 946–61.

Ackerman, S.J., Weil, G.J. & Gleich, G.J. (1982) Formation of Charcot–Leyden crystals by human basophils. *J. Exp. Med.*, **155**, 1597–609.

Adelroth, E., Rosenhall, L., Johansson, S., Linden, M. & Venge, P. (1990) Inflammatory cells and eosinophilic activity in asthma investigated by bronchoalveolar lavage. The effects of anti-asthmatic treatment with budesonide or terbutaline. *Am. Rev. Resp. Dis.*, **142**, 91–9.

Aebischer, C.P., Pasche, I. & Jorg, A. (1993) Nanomolar arachidonic acid influences the respiratory burst in eosinophils and neutrophils induced by GTP-binding protein. A comparative study of the respiratory burst in bovine eosinophils and neutrophils. *Eur. J. Biochem.*, **218**, 669–77.

Aizawa, T., Tamura, G., Ohtsu, H. & Takashima, T. (1990) Eosinophil and neutrophil production of leukotriene C4 and B4: comparison of cells from asthmatic subjects and healthy donors. *Ann. Allergy*, **64**, 287–92.

Alam, R., Forsythe, P., Stafford, S. & Fukuda, Y. (1994) Transforming growth factor β abrogates the effects of hematopoietins on eosinophils and induces their apoptosis. *J. Exp. Med.*, **179**, 1041–5.

Allen, J.N., Davis, W.B. & Pacht, E.R. (1990) Diagnostic significance of increased bronchoalveolar lavage fluid eosinophils. *Am. Rev. Resp. Dis.*, **142**, 642–7.

Azzawi, M., Bradley, B., Jeffery, P.K. *et al.* (1990) Identification of activated T lymphocytes and eosinophils in bronchial biopsies in stable atopic asthma. *Am. Rev. Resp. Dis.*, **142**, 1407–13.

Azzawi, M., Johnston, P.W., Majumdar, S., Kay, A.B. & Jeffery, P.K. (1992) T lymphocytes and activated eosinophils in airway mucosa in fatal asthma and cystic fibrosis. *Am. Rev. Resp. Dis.*, **145**, 1477–82.

Baggiolini, M. & Dahinden, C.A. (1994) CC chemokines in allergic inflammation. *Immunol. Today*, **15**, 127–33.

Barker, R.L., Gleich, G.J. & Pease, L.R. (1988) Acidic precursor revealed in human eosinophil granule major basic protein cDNA. *J. Exp. Med.*, **168**, 1493–8.

Barker, R.L., Loegering, D.A., Ten, R.M., Hamann, K.J., Pease, L.R. & Gleich, G.J. (1989) Eosinophil cationic protein cDNA. Comparison with other toxic cationic proteins and ribonucleases. *J. Immunol.*, **143**, 952–5.

Bass, D.A., Grovner, W.H., Lewis, J.G., Szejda, P., DeChatelet, L.R. & McCall, C.E. (1980) Comparison of human eosinophil from normals and patients with eosinophilia. *J. Clin. Invest.*, **66**, 1265–73.

Baumheuter, S., Singer, M.S., Henzel, W. *et al.* (1993) Binding of L-selectin to the vascular sialomucin CD34. *Science*, **262**, 436–8.

Beasley, R., Roche, W.R., Roberts, A.J. & Holgate, S.T. (1989) Cellular events in the bronchi in mild asthma and after bronchial provocation. *Am. Rev. Resp. Dis.*, **139**, 806–17.

Beck, L.A., Schall, T.J. & Beall, L.D. (1994) Detection of the chemokine RANTES and activation of vascular endothelium in nasal polyps. *J. Allergy Clin. Immunol.*, **93**, 234 [abstract].

Beintema, J.J., Hofstenge, J., Wama, M. *et al.* (1988) Amino acid sequence of the non-secretory ribonuclease of human urine. *Biochemistry*, **27**, 4530–8.

Bentley, A.M., Jacobson, M.R., Cumberworth, V. *et al.* (1992a) Immunohistology of the nasal mucosa in seasonal allergic rhinitis: increase in activated eosinophils and epithelial mast cells. *J. Allergy Clin. Immunol.*, **89**, 877–83.

Bentley, A.M., Maestrelli, P., Saetta, M. *et al.* (1992b) Activated T-lymphocytes and eosinophils in the bronchial mucosa in isocyanate-induced asthma. *J. Allergy Clin. Immunol.*, **89**, 821–9.

Bentley, A.M., Menz, G., Storz, C. *et al.* (1992c) Identification of T lymphocytes, macrophages and activated eosinophils in the bronchial mucosa in intrinsic asthma: relationship to symptoms and bronchial hyperresponsiveness. *Am. Rev. Resp. Dis.*, **146**, 500–6.

Bentley, A.M., Meng, Q., Robinson, D.S., Hamid, Q., Kay, A.B. & Durham, S.R. (1993) Increases in activated T lymphocytes, eosinophils and cytokine mRNA expression for the interleukin-5 and granulocyte-macrophage colony-stimulating factor in bronchial biopsies after allergen inhalational challenge in atopic asthmatics. *Am. J. Respir. Cell Mol. Biol.*, **8**, 35–42.

Berger, M., O'Shea, J., Cross, A.S. *et al.* (1984) Human neutrophils increase expression of C3bi as well as C3b receptors upon activation. *J. Clin. Invest.*, **74**, 1566–71.

Bischoff, S.C., Krieger, M., Brunner, T. *et al.* (1993) RANTES and related chemokines activate human basophil granulocytes through different G protein-coupled receptors. *Eur. J. Immunol.*, **23**, 761–7.

Bischoff, S.C., Brunner, T., De Weck, A.L. & Dahinden, C.A. (1990) Interleukin-5 modifies histamine release and leukotriene generation by human basophils in response to diverse agonists. *J. Exp. Med.*, **172**, 1577–82.

Bochner, B.S., McKelvy, A.A., Sterbinsky, S.A. *et al.* (1990) IL-3 augments adhesiveness for endothelium and CD11b expression in human basophils but not neutrophils. *J. Immunol.*, **145**, 1832–7.

Bousquet, J., Chanez, P., Lacoste, J.Y. *et al.* (1990) Eosinophilic inflammation in asthma. *New Engl. J. Med.*, **323**, 1033–9.

Braun, R.K., Franchini, M., Erard, F. *et al.* (1993) Human peripheral blood eosinophils produce and release IL-8 on stimulation with calcium ionophore. *Eur. J. Immunol.*, **23**, 956–60.

Broide, D.H., Paine, M.M. & Firestein, G.S. (1992) Eosinophils express interleukin 5 and granulocyte macrophage-colony stimulating factor mRNA at sites of allergic inflammation in asthmatics. *J. Clin. Invest.*, **90**, 1414–24.

Brown, T.R. (1989) Studies on trichinosis with especial reference to the increase of the eosinophilic cells in the blood and muscle, the origin of these cells and their diagnostic importance. *J. Exp. Med.*, **3**, 315–47.

Bruijnzeel, P.L., Kok, P.T., Hameling, M.L., Kijne, A.M. & Verhagen, J. (1985) Exclusive leukotriene C4 synthesis by purified human eosinophils induced by opsonized zymosan. *FEBS Letts.*, **316**, 350–4.

Bruynzeel-Koomen, C.A.F., Van Wichen, D.F., Spry, C.J.F., Venge, P. & Bruynzeel, P.L.B. (1988) Active participation of eosinophils in patch test reactions to inhalant allergens in patients with atopic dermatitis. *Brit. J. Dermatol*, **118**, 229–38.

Burke, L.A., Crea, R.E.G., Wilkinson, J.R.W., Arm, J.P., Spur, B.W. & Lee, T.H. (1990) Comparison of the generation of platelet activating factor and leukotriene C4 in human eosinophils stimulated by unopsonized zymosan and the calcium inophore A23187: the effects of nedocromil sodium. *J. Allergy Clin. Immunol.*, **85**, 26–35.

Butterworth, A.E. (1984) Cell-mediated damage to helminths. *Adv. Parasitol*, **23**, 143–235.

Butterworth, A.E., Sturrock, R.F., Houba, V. & Rees, P.H. (1974) Antibody-dependent cell-mediated damage to schistosomula *in vitro*. *Nature*, **252**, 503–5.

Butterworth, A.E. & Thorne, K.J.I. (1993) Eosinophils and parasitic disease. In: *Immunopharmacology of Eosinophils* (eds H. Smith & R.M. Cook), pp. 119–50. Academic, London.

Capron, A., Dessaint, J.P., Capron, M., Joseph, M., Ameisen, J.-C. & Tonnel, A.B. (1986a) From parasites to allergy: a second receptor for IgE. *Immunol. Today*, **7**, 15.

Capron, M., Jouault, T., Prin, L. *et al.* (1986b) Functional study of a monoclonal antibody to IgE Fc receptor of eosinophils, platelets, and macrophages. *J. Exp. Med.*, **164**, 72–89.

Capron, M. & Capron, A. (1987) The IgE receptor of human eosinophils. In: *Allergy and Inflammation* (ed. A.B. Kay), pp. 151–9. Academic, London.

Capron, M., Leprevost, Prin, L. *et al.* (1989) In: *Eosinophils and Asthma* (eds J. Morley & I. Colditz), pp. 49–60. Academic, London.

Capron, M., Truong, M.-J., Aldebert, D. *et al.* (1991) Heterogeneous expression of CD23 epitopes by eosinophils from patients. Relationships with IgE-mediated functions. *Eur. J. Immunol.*, **21**, 2423–9.

Carlson, M., Hakansson, L., Peterson, C. & Venge, P. (1991) Secretion of granule proteins from eosinophils and neutrophils is increased in asthma. *J. Allergy Clin. Immunol.*, **87**, 27–33.

Caulfield, J.P., Hein, A., Rothenburg, M.E. *et al.* (1990) A morphometric study of normodense and hypodense human eosinophils that are derived *in vivo* and *in vitro*. *Am. J. Pathol.*, **137**, 27–41.

Caux, C., Favre, C., Saeland, S. *et al.* (1989) Sequential loss of CD34 and class II MHC antigens on purified cord blood hematopoietic progenitors cultured with IL-3: characterization of CD34–, HLA-DR+ cells. *Blood*, **74**, 1287–94.

Chihara, J., Plumas, J., Gruart, V. *et al.* (1990) Characterization of a receptor for interleukin 5 on human eosinophils: variable expression and induction by granulocyte-macrophage colony-stimulating factor. *J. Exp. Med.*, **172**, 1347–51.

Clark, R.A.F., Gallin, J.I. & Kaplan, A.P. (1975) The selective eosinophil chemotactic activity of histamine. *J. Exp. Med.*, **142**, 1462.

Clark, S.C. & Kamen, R. (1987) The human hematopoietic colony stimulating factors. *Science*, **236**, 1229–37.

Collins, P.D., Marleau, S., Griffiths-Johnson, D.A., Jose, P.J. & Williams, T.J. (1996) Cooperation between interleukin-5 and the chemokine eotaxin to induce eosinophil accumulation *in vivo*. *J. Exp. Med.*, **182**, 1169–74.

Connell, J.T. (1968) Morphological changes in eosinophils in allergic disease. *J. Allergy*, **41**, 1–9.

Corrigan, C.J., Haczku, A., Gemou-Engesaeth, V. *et al.* (1993) CD4 T-lymphocyte activation in asthma is accompanied by increased serum concentrations of interleukin-5: effect of glucocorticoid therapy. *Am. Rev. Resp. Dis.*, **147**, 540–7.

Corrigan, C.J., Hartnell, A. & Kay, A.B. (1988) T-lymphocyte activation in acute severe asthma. *Lancet*, **i**, 1129–32.

Corte, G., Moretta, L., Damiani, G., Mingari, M.C. & Bargellesi, A. (1981) Surface antigens specifically expressed by activated T cells in humans. *Eur. J. Immunol.*, **11**, 162–4.

Costa, J.J., Matossian, K., Resnick, M.B. *et al.* (1993) Human eosinophils can express the cytokines tumor necrosis-alpha and macrophage inflammatory protein-1 alpha. *J. Clin. Invest.*, **91**, 2673–84.

Coyle, A.J., Ackerman, S.J. & Irvin, C.G. (1993) Cationic proteins induce airways hyperresponsiveness dependent on charger interactions. *Am. Rev. Resp. Dis.*, **147**, 896–900.

Cromwell, O., Moqbel, R., Fitzharris, P. *et al.* (1988) Leukotriene C4 generation from human eosinophils stimulated with IgG–*Aspergillus fumigatus* antigen immune complexes. *J. Allergy Clin. Immunol.*, **82**, 535–44.

Cromwell, O., Bennett, J.P., Kay, A.B. & Gomperts, B.D. (1991) Mechanisms of granule enzyme secretion from permeabilised guinea pig eosinophils: dependence on Ca^{2+} and guanine nucleotides. *J. Immunol.*, **147**, 1905–11.

Cromwell, O., Wardlaw, A.J., Champion, A., Moqbel, R., Osei, D. & Kay, A.B. (1990) IgG-dependent generation of platelet activating factor by normal and low density human eosinophils. *J. Immunol.*, **145**, 3862–8.

Dahinden, C.A., Geiser, T., Brunner, T. *et al.* (1994) Monocyte chemotactic protein 3 is a most effective basophil and eosinophil activating chemokine. *J. Exp. Med.*, **179**, 751–6.

Daugherty, B.L., Siciliano, S.J., DeMartino, J.A., Malkowitz, L., Sirotina, A. & Springer, M.S. (1996) Cloning, expression and characterization of the human eosinophil eotaxin receptor. *J. Exp. Med.*, **183**, 2349–54.

David, J.R., Vada, M.A., Butterworth, A.E. *et al.* (1980) Enhanced helminthic capacity of eosinophils from patients and eosinophilia. *New Engl. J. Med.*, **303**, 1147–52.

Del Pozo, V., de Andres, B., Martin, E. *et al.* (1990) Murine eosinophils and IL-1: alpha IL-1 mRNA detection by *in situ* hybridization. Production and release of IL-1 from peritoneal eosinophils. *J. Immunol.*, **144**, 3117–22.

De Monchy, J.G.R., Kauffman, H.F., Venge, P. *et al.* (1985) Bronchoalveolar eosinophilia during allergen-induced late asthmatic reactions. *Am. Rev. Resp. Dis.*, **131**, 373–6.

Denburg, J.A., Silver, J.E. & Abrams, J.S. (1991) Interleukin-5 is a human basophilopoietin: induction of histamine content and basophilic differentiation of HL-60 cells and of peripheral blood basophil-eosinophil progenitors. *Blood*, **77**, 1462–8.

Denburg, J.A., Telizyn, S., Messner, H. *et al.* (1985) Heterogeneity of human peripheral blood eosinophil-type colonies: evidence for a common basophil–eosinophil progenitor. *Blood*, **66**, 312–8.

Dent, L.A., Strath, M., Mellor, A.L. & Sanderson, C.J. (1990) Eosinophilia in transgenic mice expressing interleukin 5. *J. Exp. Med.*, **172**, 1425–31.

Desreumaux, P., Janin, A., Dubucquoi, S. *et al.* (1992) Synthesis of interleukin-5 by activated eosinophils in patients with eosinophilic heart diseases. *Blood*, **82**, 1553–60.

Diamond, M.S., Staunton, D.E., De Fougerolles, A.R. *et al.* (1990) ICAM-1 (CD54): a counter-receptor for Mac-1 (CD11b/CD18). *J. Cell Biol.*, **111**, 3219–39.

Diaz, P., Gonzalez, M.C., Galleguillos, F.R. *et al.* (1989) Leukocytes and mediators in bronchoalveolar lavage during late-phase asthmatic reactions. *Am. Rev. Resp. Dis.*, **139**, 1383–9.

Diaz, P., Galleguillos, F.R., Gonzales, M.C., Pantin, C.F. & Kay, A.B. (1984) Bronchoalveolar lavage in asthma: the effect of disodium cromoglycate (cromolyn) on leukocyte counts, immunoglobulins and complement. *J. Allergy Clin. Immunol.*, **74**, 41–8.

DiPersio, J., Billing, P., Kaufman, S., Eghtesady, P., Williams, R.E. & Gasson, J.C. (1988) Characterization of human granulocyte-macrophage colony-stimulating factor receptor. *J. Biol. Chem.*, **263**, 1834–41.

Djukanovic, R., Roche, W.R., Wilson, J.W. *et al.* (1990) Mucosal inflammation in asthma. *Am. Rev. Resp. Dis.*, **142**, 434–57.

Dolovich, J., Hargreave, F.E., Jordana, M. *et al.* (1989) Late-phase airway reaction and inflammation. *J. Allergy Clin. Immunol.*, **83**, 521–4.

Dri, P., Cramer, R., Spessotto, P., Romano, M. & Patriarca, P. (1991) Eosinophil activation on biologic surfaces. *J. Immunol.*, **147**, 613–20.

Dubois, G.R., Bruijnzeel-Koomen, C.A. & Bruijnzeel, P.L. (1994) IL-4 induces chemotaxis of blood eosinophils from atopic dermatitis patients, but not from normal individuals. *J. Invest. Dermatol.*, **102**, 843–6.

Dubucquoi, S., Desreumaux, P., Janin, A. *et al.* (1994) Interleukin 5 synthesis by eosinophils: association with granules and immunoglobulin-dependent secretion. *J. Exp. Med.*, **179**, 703–8.

Dunnill, M.S. (1978) The pathology of asthma. In: *Allergy: Principles and Practice* (eds E. Middleton Jr, C.E. Reed & E.F. Ellis), p. 678. CV Mosby, St Louis.

Durham, S. (1991) The significance of late responses in asthma. *Clin. Exp. Allergy*, **21**, 3–7.

Durham, S.R. & Kay, A.B. (1985) Eosinophils, bronchial hyperreactivity and late-phase asthmatic reactions. *Clin. Allergy*, **15**, 411–8.

Dvorak, A.M. (vol. ed.) (1991) Degranulation of basophils and mast cells. In: *Blood Cell Biochemistry*. Vol. 4. *Basophil and Mast Cell Degranulation and Recovery* (series ed. J.R. Harris), pp. 101–275. Plenum, London.

Dvorak, A.M. (1994) Ultrastructural studies on mechanisms of human eosinophil activation and secretion. In: *Eosinophils in Allergy and Inflammation* (eds G.J. Gleich & A.B. Kay), pp. 159–209. Marcel Dekker, New York.

Dvorak, A.M., Ackerman, S.J. & Weller, P.F. (1991) Subcellular morphology and biochemistry of eosinophils. In: *Blood Cell Biochemistry*. Vol 2. *Megakaryocytes, Platelets, Macrophages and Eosinophils* (ed. J.R. Harris), pp. 237–344. Plenum, London.

Dvorak, A.M., Onderdonk, A.B., McCleod, R.S. *et al.* (1993) Ultrastructural identification of exocytosis of granules from human gut eosinophils *in vivo*. *Int. Arch. Allergy Immunol.*, **102**, 33–45.

Dvorak, A.M., Letourneau, L., Login, G.R., Weller, P.F. & Ackerman, S.J. (1988) Ultrastructural localization of the Charcot–Leyden crystal protein (lysophospholipase) to a distinct crystalloid-free granule population in mature human eosinophils. *Blood*, **72**, 150–8.

Dvorak, A.M., Mihm, M.C. Jr, Osage, J.E., Kwan, T.H., Austen, K.F. & Wintroup, B.U. (1982) Bullous pemphigoid, an ultrastructural study of the inflammatory response: eosinophil, basophil and mast cell granule changes in multiple biopsies from one patient. *J. Invest. Dermatol.*, **78**, 91–101.

Dvorak, A.M., Saito, H., Estrella, P., Kissell, S., Arai, N. & Ishizaka, T. (1989) Ultrastructure of eosinophils and basophils stimulated to develop in human cord blood mononuclear cell cultures containing recombinant human interleukin-5 or interleukin 3. *Lab. Invest.*, **61**, 116–32.

Ebisawa, M., Liu, M.C., Yamada, T. *et al.* (1994) Eosinophil transendothelial migration induced by cytokines. II. Potentiation of eosinophil transendothelial migration by eosinophil-active cytokines. *J. Immunol.*, **152**, 4590–7.

Egesten, A., Alumets, J., von Mecklenburg, C., Plamegren, M. & Olssen, I. (1986) Localization of eosinophil cationic protein, major basic protein and eosinophil peroxidase in human eosinophils by immunoelectron microscopic technique. *J. Histochem. Cytochem.*, **34**, 1399–403.

Ehrlich, P. (1879) Ueber die specifischen granulationen des Blutes. *Arch. Anat. Physiol. Lpz.*, **3**, *Physiol. Abt.*, 571.

Ehrlich, P. & Lazarus, A. (1990) In: *Histology of the Blood: Normal and Pathological* (ed./trans. W. Meyers), p. 148. Cambridge University Press, Cambridge.

Ellis, A.G. (1908) The pathologic anatomy of bronchial asthma. *Am. J. Med. Sci.*, **136**, 407.

Elsner, J., Oppermann, M., Czech, W. *et al.* (1994) C3a activates reactive oxygen radical species production and intracellular calcium transients in human eosinophils. *Eur. J. Immunol.*, **24**, 518–22.

Fabbri, L.M., Boschetto, P. & Zocca, E. (1987) Bronchoalveolar neutrophilia during late asthmatic reactions induced by toluene diisocyanate. *Am. Rev. Resp. Dis.*, **136**, 36–42.

Fanger, M.W., Shen, L., Graziano, R.F. & Guyre, P.M. (1989) Cytotoxicity mediated by human Fc receptors for IgG. *Immunol. Today*, **10**, 92–9.

Filley, W.V., Holley, K.E., Kephart, G.M. & Gleich, G.J. (1982) Identification by immunofluorescence of eosinophil under granule major basic protein in lung tissue of patients with bronchial asthma. *Lancet*, **ii**, 11–16.

Fischer, E., Capron, M., Prin, L., Kusnierz, J.-P. & Kazatchkine, M.D. (1986) Human eosinophils express CR1 and CR3 complement receptors for cleavage fragments of C3. *Cell Immunol.*, **97**, 297–306.

Flint, K.C., Leung, K.B., Hudspith, B.N., Brostoff, J., Pearce, F.L. & Johnson, N.M. (1985) Bronchoalveolar mast cells in extrinsic asthma: a mechanism for the initiation of antigen specific bronchoconstriction. *Brit. Med. J.*, **291**, 923.

Foegh, M.L., Maddox, Y.T. & Ramwell, P.W. (1986) Human peritoneal eosinophils and formation of arachidonate cyclo-oxygenase products. *Scand. J. Immunol.*, **23**, 599–603.

Foresi, A., Berzorelli, G., Pesci, A. *et al.* (1990) Inflammatory markers in bronchoalveolar lavage and in bronchial biopsy in asthma during remission. *Chest*, **98**, 528–35.

Fredens, K., Dahl, R. & Venge, P. (1982) The Gordon phenomenon induced by the eosinophil cationic protein and eosinophil protein X. *J. Allergy Clin. Immunol.*, **70**, 361–6.

Frew, A.J. & Kay, A.B. (1988) The relationship between infiltrating CD4+ lymphocytes, activated eosinophils and the magnitude of the allergen induced late-phase response in man. *J. Immunol.*, **141**, 4158–64.

Frick, W.E., Sedgwick, J.B. & Busse, W.W. (1988) Hypodense eosinophils in allergic rhinitis. *J. Allergy Clin. Immunol.*, **82**, 119–25.

Frick, W.E., Sedgwick, J.B. & Busse, W.W. (1989) The appearance of hypodense eosinophils in antigen-dependent late phase asthma. *Am. Rev. Resp. Dis.*, **139**, 1401–6.

Frigas, E., Loegering, D.A. & Gleich, G.J. (1980) Cytotoxic effects of the guinea pig eosinophil granule major basic protein on tracheal epithelium. *Lab. Invest.*, **42**, 35–43.

Fujisawa, T., Abu-Ghazaleh, R., Kita, H., Sanderson, C.J. & Gleich, G.J. (1990) Regulatory effect of cytokines on eosinophil degranulation. *J. Immunol.*, **144**, 642–6.

Fukuda, T., Dunnette, S.L., Reed, C.E., Ackerman, S.J., Peters, M.S. & Gleich, G.J. (1985) Increased numbers of hypodense eosinophils in the blood of patients with bronchial asthma. *Am. Rev. Resp. Dis.*, **132**, 981–5.

Garcia-Zepeda, E.A., Rothenberg, M.E., Owneby, R.T., Celestin, J., Leder, P. & Luster, A.D. (1996) Human eotaxin is a specific chemoattractant for eosinophil cells and provides a new mechanism to explain tissue eosinophilia. *Nature Mechanism*, **2**, 449–56.

Gartner, I. (1980) Separation of human eosinophils in density gradients of polyvinylpyrrolidone-coated silica gel (Percoll). *Immunology*, **40**, 133–6.

Gerard, N.P. & Gerard, C. (1991) The chemotactic receptor for human C5a and anaphylatoxin. *Nature*, **349**, 614.

Gibson, P.G., Dolovich, J., Girgis-Gabardo, A. *et al.* (1990) The inflammatory response in asthma exacerbation: changes in circulating eosinophils, basophils and their progenitors. *Clin. Exp. Allergy*, **20**, 661–8.

Gibson, P.G., Dolovich, J., Denburg, J., Ramsdale, E.H. & Hargreave, F.E. (1989) Chronic cough: eosinophilic bronchitis without asthma. *Lancet*, **i**, 1346–8.

Giembycz, M.A. & Barnes, P.J. (1993) Stimulus-response coupling in eosinophils: receptors, signal transduction and pharmacological modulation. In: *Immunopharmacology of Eosinophils* (eds H. Smith & R.M. Cook), pp. 91–118. Academic, New York.

Gleich, G.J. (1990) The eosinophil and bronchial asthma: current understanding. *J. Allergy Clin. Immunol.*, **85**, 422–36.

Gleich, G.J., Abu-Ghazaleh, R.I. & Glitz, D.G. (1994) In: *Eosinophils in Allergy and Inflammation* (eds G.J. Gleich & A.B. Kay), pp. 1–20. Marcel Dekker, New York.

Gleich, G.J. & Adolphson, C.R. (1986) The eosinophil leukocyte: structure and function. *Adv. Immunol.*, **39**, 177–253.

Gleich, G.J., Loegering, D.A., Bell, M.P., Checkel, J.L., Ackerman, S.J. & McKean, D.J. (1986) Biochemical and functional similarities between human eosinophil derived neurotoxin and eosinophil cationic protein: homology with ribonuclease. *Proc. Nat. Acad. Sci. USA*, **83**, 3146–50.

Godard, P., Chaintreuil, J., Damon, M. *et al.* (1982) Functional assessment of alveolar macrophages: comparison of cells from asthmatics and normal subjects. *J. Allergy Clin. Immunol.*, **70**, 88–93.

Goetzl, E.J., Wasserman, S.I. & Austen, K.F. (1975) Eosinophil polymorphonuclear leukocyte function in immediate hypersensitivity. *Arch. Pathol.*, **99**, 4.

Gonzalo, J.-A., Jia, G.-Q., Aquirre, V. *et al.* (1996) Mouse eotaxin expression parallels eosinophil accumulation during allergic inflammation but is not restricted to a Th2-type response. *Immunity*, **4**, 1–14.

Gounni, A.S., Lamkhioued, B., Ochiai, K. *et al.* (1994) High-affinity IgE receptor on eosinophils is involved in defence against parasites. *Nature*, **367**, 183–6.

Greaves, M.F., Brown, J., Molgaard, H.V. *et al.* (1992) Molecular features of CD34: a hemopoietic progenitor cell-associated molecule. *Leukemia*, **6** (Suppl. 1), 31–6.

Gundel, R.H., Letts, L.G. & Gleich, G.J. (1991) Human eosinophil major basic protein induces airway constriction and airway hyperresponsiveness in primates. *J. Clin. Invest.*, **87**, 1470–3.

Gundel, R.H., Wegner, C.D. & Letts, L.G. (1993) Eosinophils and neutrophils in a primate model of asthma. In: *Asthma. Physiology, Pharmacology and Treatment* (eds S.T. Holgate, K.F. Austen, L.M. Lichtenstein & A.B. Kay), pp. 173–85. Academic, London.

Hamann, K.J., Gleich, G.J., Checkel, J.L., Loegring, D.A., McCall, J.W. & Barker, R.L. (1990) *In vitro* killing of microfilariae of *Brugia pahangi* and *Brugia malayi* by eosinophil granule proteins. *J. Immunol.*, **144**, 3166–73.

Hamid, Q., Azzawi, M., Ying, S. *et al.* (1991) Expression of mRNA for interleukin-5 in mucosal bronchial biopsies from asthma. *J. Clin. Invest.*, **87**, 1541–6.

Hamid, Q., Barkans, J., Meng, Q. *et al.* (1992) Human eosinophils synthesize and secrete interleukin-6, *in vitro*. *Blood*, **80**, 1496–501.

Hansel, T.T., De Vries, I.J., Carballido, J.M. *et al.* (1992) Induction and function of eosinophil intercellular adhesion molecule-1 and HLA-DR. *J. Immunol.*, **149**, 2130–6.

Hartnell, A., Kay, A.B. & Wardlaw, A.J. (1992a) IFN-gamma induces expression of Fc gammaRIII (CD16) on human eosinophils. *J. Immunol.*, **148**, 1471–8.

Hartnell, A., Kay, A.B. & Wardlaw, A.J. (1992b) Interleukin-3-induced up-regulation of CR3 expression on human eosinophils is inhibited by dexamethasone. *Immunology*, **77**, 488–93.

Hartnell, A., Moqbel, R., Walsh, G.M., Bradley, B. & Kay, A.B. (1990) Fcγ and CD11/CD18 receptor expression on normal density and low density human eosinophils. *Immunology*, **69**, 264–70.

Hartnell, A., Robinson, D.S., Kay, A.B. & Wardlaw, A.J. (1993) CD69 is expressed by human eosinophils activated *in vivo* in asthma and *in vitro* by cytokines. *Immunology*, **80**, 281–6.

Hastie, A.T., Loegering, D.A., Gleich, G.J. & Kueppers, F. (1987) The effect of purified human eosinophil major basic protein on mammalian ciliary activity. *Am. Rev. Resp. Dis.*, **135**, 848–53.

Haylock, D.N., To, L.B., Dowse, T.L., Juttner, C.A. & Simmons, P.J. (1992) *Ex vivo* expansion and maturation of peripheral blood CD34+ cells into the myeloid lineage. *Blood*, **80**, 1405–12.

Henderson, W.R. & Chi, E.Y. (1985) Ultrastructural characterization and morphometric analysis of human eosinophil degranulation. *J. Cell Sci.*, **73**, 33–48.

Henocq, E. & Vargaftig, B.B. (1986) Accumulation of eosinophils in response to intracutaneous PAF-acether and allergens in man. *Lancet*, **i**, 1378–9.

Henson, P.M. (1989) PAF—a perspective. *Am. J. Respir. Cell Mol. Biol.*, **1**, 263–5.

Her, E., Frazer, J., Austen, K.F. & Owen, W.F. (1991) Eosinophil hematopoietins antagonize the programmed cell death of human eosinophils: cytokine and glucocorticoid effects on eosinophils maintained by endothelial cell conditioned medium. *J. Clin. Invest.*, **88**, 1982–7.

Hirai, K., Yamaguchi, M. & Misaki, Y. (1990) Enhancement of human basophil histamine release by interleukin-5. *J. Exp. Med.*, **172**, 1525–8.

Hisamatsu, K., Ganbo, T., Nakazawa, T. *et al.* (1990) Cytotoxicity of human eosinophil granule major basic protein to human nasal sinus mucosa *in vitro*. *J. Allergy Clin. Immunol.*, **86**, 52–63.

Hodges, M.K., Weller, P.F., Gerard, N.P., Ackerman, S.J. & Drazen, J.M. (1988) Heterogenity of leukotriene C4 production by eosinophils from asthmatic and normal subjects. *Am. Rev. Resp. Dis.*, **138**, 799–804.

Hom, J.T. & Estridge, T. (1993) FK506 and rapamycin modulate the functional activities of human peripheral blood eosinophils. *Clin. Immunol. Immunopathol.*, **68**, 293–300.

Honda, Z., Nakamura, M., Miki, I. *et al.* (1991) Cloning by functional expression of platelet activating receptor from guinea pig lung. *Nature*, **349**, 342–6.

Horie, S. & Kita, H. (1994) CD11b/CD18 (Mac-1) is required for degranulation of human eosinophils induced by human recombinant granulocyte-macrophage colony-stimulating factor and platelet-activating factor. *J. Immunol.*, **152**, 5457–67.

Horn, B.R., Robin, E.D., Theodore, J. & Van Kessel, A. (1975) Total eosinophil counts in the management of bronchial asthma. *New Engl. J. Med.*, **292**, 1152.

Howell, C.J., Pujol, J.L., Crea, A.E. *et al.* (1989) Identification of an alveolar macrophage-derived activity in bronchial asthma that enhances leukotriene C4 generation by human eosinophils stimulated by ionophore A23187 as a granulocyte-macrophage colony-stimulating factor. *Am. Rev. Resp. Dis.*, **140**, 1340–7.

Huber, H.L. & Koessler, K.K. (1992) The pathology of bronchial asthma. *Arch. Intern. Med.*, **30**, 689.

Hubscher, T. (1975) Role of the eosinophil in allergic reactions. II. Release of prostaglandins from human eosinophilic leukocytes. *J. Immunol.*, **114**, 1389.

Huizinga, T.W.J., de Hass, M., Kleijer, M., Nuijens, H.H., Roos, D. & Kr.von dem Borne, A.E.G. (1988) The PI-linked receptor FcRIII is released on stimulation of neutrophils. *Nature*, **333**, 667.

Huizinga, T.W.J., de Hass, M., Kleijer, M., Nuijens, J.H., Roos, D. & Kr.von dem Borne, A.E.G. (1990) Soluble Fc gamma receptor III in human plasma originates from release by neutrophils. *J. Clin. Invest.*, **86**, 416–23.

Huizinga, T.W.J., van Kemenade, F., Koenderman, L. *et al.* (1989) The 40 kDa Fc gamma receptor (FcRII) on human neutrophils is essential for the IgG-induced respiratory burst and IgG-induced phagocytosis. *J. Immunol.*, **142**, 2365–9.

Ingley, E. & Young, I.G. (1991) Characterization of a receptor for interleukin-5 on human eosinophils and the myeloid leukemia line HL f60. *Blood*, **78**, 339–44.

Iozzo, R.V., MacDonald, G.H. & Wight, T.N. (1982) Immunoelectron microscopic localization of catalase in human eosinophil leukocytes. *J. Histochem. Cytochem.*, **30**, 697–701.

Iwama, T., Nagai, H., Suda, H., Tsuruoka, N. & Koda, A. (1992) Effect of murine recombinant interleukin 5 on the cell population in guinea pig airways. *Brit. J. Pharmacol.*, **1055**, 19–22.

Jorg, A., Henderson, W.R., Murphy, R.C. & Klebanoff, S.J. (1982) Leukotriene generation by eosinophils. *J. Exp. Med.*, **155**, 390–402.

Jose, P.J., Adcock, I.M., Griffiths-Johnson, D.A. *et al.* (1994a) Eotaxin: cloning of an eosinophil chemoattractant cytokine and increased mRNA expression in allergen-challenged guinea pig lungs. *Biochem. Biophys. Res. Commun.*, **205**, 788–94.

Jose, P.J., Griffiths-Johnson, D.A., Collins, P.D. *et al.* (1994b) Eotaxin: a potent eosinophil chemoattractant cytokine detected in a guinea pig model of allergic airways inflammation. *J. Exp. Med.*, **179**, 881–7.

Joualt, T., Capron, M., Balloul, J.-M., Ameisen, J.-C. & Capron, A. (1988) Quantitative and qualitative analysis of the Fc receptor for IgE (Fc epsilon RII) on human eosinophils. *Eur. J. Immunol.*, **18**, 237–41.

Juniper, E.F., Kline, P.A., Vanzieleghem, A., Ramsdale, H., O'Byrne, P.M. & Hargreave, F.E. (1990) Effect of long term treatment with an inhaled corticosteroid (budesonide) on airway hyperresponsiveness and clinical asthma in non steroid dependent asthmatics. *Am. Rev. Resp. Dis.*, **142**, 832–6.

Kadin, M., Butmarc, J., Elovic, A. & Wong, D.T.W. (1993) Eosinophils are the major source of transforming growth factor-beta 1 in nodular sclerosing Hodgkin's disease. *Am. J. Pathol.*, **142**, 11–16.

Kameyoshi, Y., Dorschner, A., Mallet, A.I., Christophers, E. & Schroder, J.M. (1992) Cytokine RANTES released by thrombin stimulated platelets is a potent attractant for human eosinophils. *J. Exp. Med.*, **176**, 587–92.

Kelly, C., Ward, C., Stenton, C.S., Bird, G. Hendricks, D.J. & Walters, E.H. (1988) Number and activity of inflammatory cells in bronchoalveolar lavage fluid in asthma and their relation to airway hyperresponsiveness. *Thorax*, **43**, 684–92.

Kinet, J.-P. (1989) Antibody–cell interactions: Fc receptors. *Cell*, **57**, 351–4.

Kita, H., Abu-Ghazaleh, R., Gleich, G.J. & Abraham, R.T. (1991a) Regulation of Ig-induced eosinophil degranulation by adenosine 3',5'-cyclic monophosphate. *J. Immunol.*, **146**, 2712–18.

Kita, H., Ohnishi, T., Okubo, Y., Weiler, D., Abrams, J.S. & Gleich, G.J. (1991b) Granulocyte-macrophage colony-stimulating factor and interleukin 3 release from human peripheral blood eosinophils and neutrophils. *J. Exp. Med.*, **174**, 743–8.

Kita, H. *et al.* (1992) Release of granule proteins from eosinophils cultured with IL-5. *J. Immunol.*, **149**, 629–35.

Kloprogge, E., de Leeuw, A.J., de Monchy, J.G.R. & Kauffman, H.F. (1989) Hypodense eosinophilic granulocytes in normal individuals and patients with asthma; generation of hypodense cell populations *in vitro*. *J. Allergy Clin. Immunol.*, **83**, 393–400.

Koenderman, L., Tool, A.T.J., Roos, D. & Verhoeven, A.J. (1990) Priming of the respiratory burst in human eosinophils is accompanied by changes in signal transduction. *J. Immunol.*, **145**, 3883–8.

Kohi, F., Miyagawa, H., Agrawal, D.K., Bewtra, A.K. & Townley, R.G. (1990) Generation of leukotriene B4 and C4 from granulocytes of normal controls, allergic rhinitis and healthy donors. *Ann. Allergy*, **65**, 228–32.

Kroegel, C., Chilvers, E.R., Giembycz, M.A., Challis, R.A.J. & Barnes, P.J. (1991) Platelet activating factor stimulates a rapid accumulation of inositol(1,4,5)trisphosphate in guinea-pig eosinophils: relationship to calcium mobilization and degranulation. *J. Allergy Clin. Immunol.*, **88**, 114–24.

Kroegel, C., Yukawa, T., Dent, G., Venge, P., Chung, K.F. & Barnes, P.J. (1989) Stimulation of degranulation from human eosinophils by platelet activating factor. *J. Immunol.*, **142**, 3518–26.

Krouwels, F.H., Kerstens, L.C.M., van der Maarel, H.M.W., Degenhart, H.J. & Neijens, H.J. (1995) Density of eosinophil reflects activity of disease in allergic asthmatic children. *Clin. Exp. Allergy*, **25**, 1171–81.

Kuna, P., Reddigari, S.R., Schall, I.J., Rucinski, D., Sadick, M. & Kaplan, A.P. (1993) Characterisation of the human basophil response to cytokines, growth factors and histamine releasing factors of the intercrine/chemokine family. *J. Immunol.*, **150**, 1932–43.

Kurihara, K., Wardlaw, A.J., Moqbel, R. & Kay, A.B. (1989) Inhibition of platelet activating factor (PAF) induced chemotaxis and PAF binding to human eosinophils and neutrophils by the specific ginkgolide-derived PAF antagonist BN52021. *J. Allergy Clin. Immunol.*, **83**, 83–90.

Lacoste, J.-Y., Bousquet, J., Chanez, P. *et al.* (1993) Eosinophilic and neutrophilic inflammation in asthma, chronic bronchitis and chronic obstructive pulmonary disease. *J. Allergy Clin. Immunol.*, **92**, 537–48.

Laitinen, L.A., Haahtela, T., Spur, B.W., Laitenen, A., Vilkka, V. & Lee, T.H. (1993) Leukotriene E4 and granulocytic infiltration into asthmatic airways. *Lancet*, **314**, 989–90.

Lam, S., LeRichie, J., Phillips, D. *et al.* (1987) Cellular and protein changes in bronchial lavage fluid after late asthmatic reaction in patients with red cedar wood asthma. *J. Allergy Clin. Immunol.*, **80**, 44.

Lawrence, M.B. & Springer, T.A. (1991) Leukocytes roll on a selectin at physiological flow rates: distinction from and pre-requisite for adhesion through integrins. *Cell*, **65**, 859–73.

Lee, T.-C., Lenihan, D.J., Malone, B., Roddy, L.L. & Wasserman, S.I. (1984) Increased biosynthesis of platelet activating factor in activated human eosinophils. *J. Biol. Chem.*, **259**, 5526–30.

Lee, T.-C., Malone, B., Wasserman S.I., Fitzgerald, V. & Snyder, F. (1982) Activities of enzymes that metabolize platelet-activating factor (1-alkyl-2-acetyl-sn-glycero-3-phosphocholine) in neutrophils and eosinophils from human and the effect of a calcium ionophore. *Biochem. Biophys. Res. Commun.*, **105**, 1303–8.

Lee, T.H., Horton, C.E., Kyan Aung, Haskaard, D., Crea, A.E. & Spur, B.W. (1989) Lipoxin A4 and lipoxin B4 inhibit chemotactic responses of human neutrophils stimulated by leukotriene B4 and *N*-formyl-methionine-leucine-phenylalanine. *Clin. Sci.*, **77**, 195–203.

Leiferman, K.M., Ackerman, S.J., Sampson, H.A., Haugen, H.S., Venenci, P.Y. & Gleich, G.J. (1985) Dermal deposition of eosinophil granule major basic protein in atopic dermatitis. Comparison with onchocerciasis. *New Engl. J. Med.*, **313**, 282–5.

Levi-Schaffer, F., Lacey, P., Severs, N.J. *et al.* (1995) Association of granulocyte-macrophage colony stimulating factor with the crystalloid granulues of human eosinophils. *Blood*, **85**(9), 2579–86.

Lewis, D.M., Lewis, J.C., Loegering, D.A. & Gleich, G.J. (1987) Localization of the guinea pig eosinophil major basic protein to the core of the granule. *J. Cell Biol.*, **77**, 702–13.

Lopez, A.F., Williamson, D.J., Gamble, J.R. *et al.* (1986) Recombinant human granulocyte-macrophage colony-stimulating factor stimulates *in vitro* mature human neutrophil and eosinophil function surface receptor expression and survival. *J. Clin. Invest.*, **78**, 1220.

Lopez, A.F., Vadas, M.A., Woodcock, J. *et al.* (1991) Selective interaction of the human eosinophil interleukin-5 receptor with interleukin-3 and granulocyte-macrophage colony-stimulating factor. *J. Biol. Chem.*, **266**, 24741–7.

Lopez A.F., Eglinton, J.M., Gillis, D., Park, L.S., Clark, S. & Vadas, M.A. (1989) Reciprocal inhibition of binding between interleukin 3 and granulocyte-macrophage colony-stimulating factor to human eosinophils. *Proc. Nat. Acad. Sci. USA*, **86**, 7022–6.

Lopez, A.F., Sanderson, C.J., Gamble, J.R., Campbell, H.D., Young, I.G. & Vadas, M.A. (1988) Recombinant interleukin 5 is a selective activator of human eosinophil function. *J. Exp. Med.*, **167**, 219–24.

Lucey, D.R., Dorsky, D.I., Nicholson-Weller, A. & Weller, P.F. (1989a) Human eosinophils express CD4 protein and bind human immunodeficiency virus 1 gp120. *J. Exp. Med.*, **169**, 327–32.

Lucey, D.R., Nicholson-Weller, A. & Weller, P.F. (1989b) Mature human eosinophils have the capacity to express HLA-DR. *Proc. Nat. Acad. Sci. USA*, **86**, 1348–51.

McGrogan, M., Simonsen, C., Scott, R. *et al.* (1988) Isolation of a complementary DNA clone encoding a precursor to human eosinophil major basic protein. *J. Exp. Med.*, **168**, 2295–308.

Machado, L. & Stalenheim, G. (1990) Factors influencing the occurrence of late bronchial reactions after allergen challenge. *Allergy*, **45**, 268–74.

McLaren, D.J., McKean, J.R., Olsson, I., Venge, P. & Kay, A.B. (1981) Morphological studies on the killing of schistosomula of *Schistosoma mansoni* by human eosinophil and neutrophil cationic proteins *in vitro*. *Parasite Immunol.*, **3**, 359–73.

Maddox, D.E., Kephart, G.M., Coulam, C.B., Butterfield, J.H., Benirschke, K. & Gleich, G.J. (1984) Localization of a molecule immunochemically similar to eosinophil major basic protein in human placenta. *J. Exp. Med.*, **160**, 29–41.

Marom, Z., Shelhamer, J.H., Sun, F. & Kaliner, M. (1983) Human airway monohydroxyeicosatetraenoic acid generation and mucus release. *J. Clin. Invest*, **72**, 122–7.

Matsumoto, T., Funk, C.D., Radmark, O., Hoog, J.O., Jornvall, H. & Samuelsson, B. (1988) Molecular cloning and amino acid sequence of human 5-lipoxygenase. *Proc. Nat. Acad. Sci. USA*, **85**(10), 3406.

Mauser, P.J., Pitman, A., Witt, A. *et al.* (1993) Inhibitory effect of the TRFK-5 anti IL-5 antibody in a guinea pig model of asthma. *Am. Rev. Resp. Dis.*, **148**, 1623–7.

Melani, C., Mattia, G.F., Silvani, A. *et al.* (1993) Interleukin-6 expression in human neutrophil and eosinophil peripheral blood granulocytes. *Blood*, **81**, 2744–9.

Metzger, W.J., Zavala, D., Richerson, H.B. *et al.* (1987) Local allergen challenge and bronchoalveolar lavage of allergic asthmatic lungs: description of the model and local airway inflammation. *Am. Rev. Resp. Dis.*, **135**, 433–40.

Meurer, R., Van Riper, G., Feeney, W. *et al.* (1993) Formation of eosinophilic and monocytic intradermal inflammatory sites in the dog by injection of human RANTES but not human monocyte chemoattractant protein 1, human macrophage inflammatory protein 1 alpha or human interleukin 8. *J. Exp. Med.*, **178**, 1913–21.

Migita, M., Yamaguchi, N., Mita, S. *et al.* (1991) Characterization of the human IL-5 receptors on eosinophils. *Cell. Immunol.*, **133**, 484–97.

Miller, D.K., Gillard, J.W., Vickers, P.J. *et al.* (1990) Identification and isolation of a membrane protein necessary for leukotriene production. *Nature*, **343**, 278–81.

Minnicozzi, M., Anthes, J.C., Siegel, M.I., Billah, M.M. & Egan, R.W. (1990) Activation of phospholipase D in normodense human eosinophils. *Biochem. Biophys. Res. Commun.*, **170**, 540–7.

Miyajima, A., Kitamura, T., Harada, N., Yokota, T. & Arai, K.L. (1992) Cytokine receptors and signal transduction. *Ann. Rev. Immunol.*, **10**, 295–331.

Monteiro, R.C., Hostoffer, R.W., Cooper, M.D., Bonner, J.R., Gartland, G.L. & Kubagawa, H. (1993) Definition of immunoglobulin A receptors on eosinophils and their enhanced expression in allergic individuals. *J. Clin. Invest.*, **92**, 1681–5.

Moqbel, R., Hamid, Q., Ying, S. *et al.* (1991) Expression of mRNA and immunoreactivity for the granulocyte/macrophage-colony stimulating factory in activated human eosinophils. *J. Exp. Med.*, **174**, 749–52.

Moqbel, R., Lacy, P., Levi-Schaffer, F. *et al.* (1994) Interleukin-6 is a granule-associated preformed mediator in eosinophils from asthmatic subjects. *Am. J. Resp. Crit. Care. Med.*, **149**, A836.

Moqbel, R., Ying, S., Barkans, J. *et al.* (1995) Eosinophils transcribe and translate mRNA for IL-4. *J. Allergy Clin. Immunol.*, **95**, 221 [abstract 321.]

Morita, E., Schroder, J.M. & Christophers, E. (1990) Identification of a novel and highly potent eosinophil chemotactic lipid in human eosinophils treated with arachadonic acid. *J. Immunol.*, **144**, 1893–900.

Nishikawa, K., Morii, T., Ako, H., Hamada, K., Saito, S. & Narita, N. (1992) *In vivo* expression of CD69 on lung eosinophils in eosinophilic pneumonia. CD69 as a possible activation marker for eosinophils. *J. Allergy Clin. Immunol.*, **90**, 169.

Numao T. & Agrawal, D.K. (1992) Neuropeptides modulate human eosinophil chemotaxis. *J. Immunol.*, **149**, 3309–15.

Nüsse, O., Lindau, M., Cromwell, O., Kay, A.B. & Gomperts, B.D. (1990) Intracellular application of guanosine-5′-O-(3-thiotriphosphate) induces exocytotic granule fusion in guinea pig eosinophils. *J. Exp. Med.*, **171**, 775–86.

O'Connell, M.C., Ackerman, S.J., Gleich, G.J. & Thomas, L.L. (1983) Activation of basophil and mast cell histamine release by eosinophil granule major basic protein. *J. Exp. Med.*, **157**, 1981.

Ohashi, Y., Motojima, S., Fukuda, T. & Makino, S. (1992) Airway hyperresponsiveness, increased intracellular spaces of bronchial epithelium and increased infiltration of eosinophils and lymphocytes in bronchial mucosa in asthma. *Am. Rev. Resp. Dis.*, **145**, 1469–76.

Ohno, I., Lea, R.G., Flanders, K.C. *et al.* (1992) Eosinophils in chronically inflamed human upper airway tissues express transforming growth factor beta 1 gene. *J. Clin. Invest.*, **89**, 1662.

Otsuka, H., Dolovich, J., Befus, D., Bienenstock, J. & Denburg, J. (1986) Peripheral blood basophils basophil progenitors, and nasal metachromatic cells in allergic rhinitis. *Am. Rev. Resp. Dis.*, **133**, 757–62.

Owen, W.F., Rothenberg, M.E., Silberstein, D.S. *et al* (1987) Regulation of human eosinophil viability, density and function by granulocyte/macrophage colony-stimulating factor in the presence of 3T3 fibroblasts. *J. Exp. Med.*, **166**, 129–41.

Owen, W.F.J., Petersen, J., Sheff, D.M. *et al.* (1990) Hypodense eosinophils and interleukin 5 activity in the blood of patients with the eosinophilia-myalgia syndrome. *Proc. Nat. Acad. Sci. USA*, **87**, 8647–51.

Parmley, R.T. & Spicer, S.S. (1974) Cytochemical ultrastructural identification of a small type granule in human late eosinophils. *Lab. Invest.*, **30**, 557.

Parsons, W.G. & Roberts, L.J. (1988) Transformation of prostaglandin D2 to isomeric prostaglandin F2 compounds by human eosinophils. A potential mast cell–eosinophil interaction. *J. Immunol.*, **141**, 2413.

Paul, C.C., Ackerman, S.J., Mahrer, S., Tolbert, M., Dvorak, A.M. & Baumann, M.A. (1994) Cytokine induction of granule protein synthesis in an eosinophil-inducible human myeloid cell line, AML14. *J. Leuk. Biol.*, **55**, 74–9.

Pazdrak, K., Schreiber, D., Forsythe, P., Justement, L. & Alam, R. (1995) The intercellular signal transduction mechanism of interleukin 5 in eosinophils: the involvement of lyn tyrosine kinase and the Ras-Raf-1-MEK-microtubule associated protein kinase pathway. *J. Exp. Med.*, **181**, 1827–34.

Peters, M.S., Gleich, G.J., Dunnette, S.L. & Fukuda, T. (1988) Ultrastructural study of eosinophils from patients with the hypereosinophilic syndrome: a morphological basis of hypodense eosinophils. *Blood*, **71**, 780–5.

Peters, M.S., Rodriguez, M. & Gleich, G.J. (1986) Localization of human eosinophil granule major basic protein, eosinophil cationic protein and eosinophil-derived neurotoxin by immunoelectron microscopy. *Lab. Invest.*, **54**, 656–62.

Pincus, S.H., Schooley, W.R., DiNapoli, A.M. & Broder, S. (1981) Metabolic heterogeneity of eosinophils from normal and hypereosinophilic patients. *Blood*, **58**, 1175–81.

Pipkorn, U., Karlsson, G. & Enerback, L. (1988) The cellular response of the human allergic mucosa to natural allergen exposure. *J. Allergy Clin. Immunol.*, **82**, 1046–54.

Ponath, P.D., Qin, S., Ringler, D.J. *et al.* (1996) Cloning of the human eosinophil chemoattractant, eotaxin. Expression, receptor binding and functional properties suggest a mechanism for the selective recruitment of eosinophils. *J. Clin. Invest.*, **97**, 604–12.

Pretolani, M., Ruffiç, C., de Silva, L., Joseph, D., Lobb, R. & Vargaftig, B. (1994) Antibody to very late activation antigen 4 prevents antigen-induced bronchial hyperreactivity and cellular infiltration in the guinea-pig airways. *J. Exp. Med.*, **180**, 795–805.

Prin, L., Charon, J., Capron, M. *et al.* (1984) Heterogeneity of human eosinophils. II. Variability of respiratory burst activity related to cell density. *Clin. Exp. Immunol.*, **57**, 735–42.

Prin, L., Capron, M., Gosset, P. *et al.* (1986) Eosinophilic lung disease: immunological studies of blood and alveolar eosinophils. *Clin. Exp. Immunol.*, **63**, 249–57.

Prin, L., Capron, M., Tonnel, A.-B., Bletry, O. & Capron, A. (1983) Heterogeneity of human peripheral blood eosinophils: variability in cell density and cytotoxic ability in relation to the level and the origin or hypereosinophilia. *Int. Arch. Allergy Appl. Immunol.*, **72**, 336–46.

Rand, T.H., Cruickschank, W.W., Center, D.M. & Weller, P.F. (1991a) CD4-mediated stimulation of human eosinophils. Lymphocyte chemoattractant factor and other CD4-binding ligands elicit eosinophil migration. *J. Exp. Med.*, **173**, 1521–28.

Rand, T.H., Silberstein, D.S., Kornfield, H. & Weller, P.F. (1991b) Human eosinophils express functional interleukin-2 receptors. *J. Clin. Invest.*, **88**, 825–32.

Ravetch, J.V. & Perussia, B. (1989) Alternative membrane forms of Fc gamma RIII (CD16) on human natural killer cells and neutrophils. *J. Exp. Med.*, **170**, 481–97.

Robinson, D.S., Hamid, Q., Ying, S. *et al.* (1992) Predominant TH2-type bronchoalveolar lavage T-lymphocyte population in atopic asthma. *New Engl. J. Med.*, **326**, 298–304.

Robinson, D.S., Hamid Q., Ying, S. *et al.* (1993) Prednisolone treatment in asthma is associated with modulation of bronchoalveolar lavage cell interleukin-4, interleukin-5 and interferon-gamma cytokine gene expression. *Am. Rev. Resp. Dis.*, **148**, 401–6.

Rohrbach, M.S., Wheatley, C.L., Slifman, N.R. & Gleich, G.J. (1990) Activation of platelets by eosinophil granule proteins. *J. Exp. Med.*, **172**, 1271–4.

Rosenberg, H.F., Ackerman, S.J. & Tenen, D.G. (1989a) Human eosinophil cationic protein: molecular cloning of a cytotoxin and helminthotoxin with ribonuclease activity. *J. Exp. Med.*, **170(1)**, 163–76.

Rosenburg, H.F., Tenen, D.G. & Ackerman, S.J. (1989b) Molecular cloning of the human eosinophil-derived neurotoxin: a member of the ribonuclease gene family. *Proc. Nat. Acad. Sci. USA*, **86**, 4460–4.

Rot, A., Krieger, M., Brunner, T., Bischoff, S.C., Schall, T.J. & Dahinden, C.A. (1992) RANTES and macrophage inflammatory protein 1 alpha induce the migration and activation of normal human eosinophil granulocytes. *J. Exp. Med.*, **176**, 1489–95.

Rothenburg, M.E., Owen, W.F., Silberstein, D.S. *et al.* (1988) Human eosinophils have prolonged survival, enhanced functional properties and become hypodense when exposed to human interleukin-3. *J. Clin. Invest.*, **81**, 1986–92.

Rothenburg, M.E., Petersen, J., Stevens, R.L. *et al.* (1989) IL-5-dependent conversion of normodense human eosinophils to the hypodense phenotype uses 3T3 fibroblasts for enhanced viability, accelerated hypodensity and sustained antibody-dependent cytotoxicity. *J. Immunol.*, **143**, 2311–16.

Roubin, R., Elsas, P.P., Fiers, W. & Dessein, A.J. (1987) Recombinant human tumour necrosis factor (rTNF) enhances leukotriene biosynthesis in neutrophils and eosinophils stimulated with the calcium ionophore A238127. *Clin. Exp. Immunol.*, **70**, 484–90.

Sakamaki, K., Tomonaga, M., Tsukui, K. & Nagata, S. (1989) Molecular cloning and characterization of a chromosomal gene for human eosinophil peroxidase. *J. Biol. Chem.*, **264**, 16828–36.

Samuelsson, B. (1983) Leukotrienes: mediators of hypersensitivity reactions and inflammation. *Science*, **220**, 568–75.

Scallon, B.J., Scigliano, E., Freedman, V.H. *et al.* (1989) A human immunoglobulin G receptor exists in both polypeptide-anchored and phosphatidylinositol-anchored forms. *Proc. Nat. Acad. Sci. USA*, **86**, 5079–83.

Schall, T.J. (1991) Biology of the RANTES/SIS cytokine family. *Cytokine*, **3**, 165–83.

Schall, T.J., Bacon, K. Toy, K.J. & Goeddel, D.V. (1990) Selective attraction of monocytes and T lymphocytes of memory phenotype by cytokine RANTES. *Nature*, **347**, 669–71.

Schleimer, R.P. (1990) Effects of gluocorticosteroids on inflammatory cells relevant to their therapeutic applications in asthma. *Am. Rev. Resp. Dis.*, **141**, S59–69.

Sehmi, R., Cromwell, O., Taylor, G.W. & Kay, A.B. (1991) The identification of leukotriene B4 and 18 (s) 15 (s)-diHete as the principal eosinophil chemotactic factors released during anaphylaxis of guinea pig lung (ECF-A). *J. Immunol.*, **147**, 2276–83.

Sehmi, R., Cromwell, O., Wardlaw, A.J. Moqbel, R. & Kay, A.B. (1993) Interleukin 8 is a chemoattractant for eosinophils purified from subjects with blood eosinophilia but not from normal healthy subjects. *Clin. Exp. Allergy*, **23**, 1027–36.

Sehmi, R., Rossi, A.G., Kay, A.B. & Cromwell, O. (1992a) Identification of receptors for leukotriene B4 (LTB4) expressed on guinea pig peritoneal eosinophils. *Immunology*, **77**, 129–35.

Sehmi, R., Wardlaw, A.J., Cromwell, O., Waltman, P., Kurihara, K. & Kay, A.B. (1992b) Interleukin 5 (IL-5) selectively enhances the chemotactic response of eosinophils obtained from normal but not eosinophilic donors. *Blood*, **79**, 2952–2959.

Serhan, C.N., Hirsch, U., Palmblad, J. & Samuelsson, B. (1987) Formation of lipoxin A by granulocytes from eosinophilic donors. *FEBS Letts.*, **217**, 242–6.

Shalit, M., Sekhsaria, S. & Malech, H.L. (1995) Modulation of growth and differentiation of eosinophils from human peripheral blood CD34+ cells by IL-5 and other growth factors. *Cell. Immunol.*, **160**, 50–7.

Shaw, R.J., Walsh, G.M., Cromwell, O., Moqbel, R., Spry, C.J.F. & Kay, A.B. (1985) Activated human eosinophils generate SRS-A leukotrienes following physiological (IgG-dependent) stimulation. *Nature*, **316**, 150–2.

Sher, A., Coffman, R.L., Hieny, S. & Cheever, A.W. (1990) Ablation of eosinophil and IgE responses with anti-IL-5 and anti-IL-4 antibodies fails to affect immunity against *Schistosoma mansoni* larvae in the mouse. *J. Immunol.*, **145**, 3911–16.

Shult, P.A., Graziano F.M. & Busse, W.W. (1985) Enhanced eosinophil luminol-dependent chemoluminescence in allergic rhinitis. *J. Allergy Clin. Immunol.*, **77**, 702.

Shult, P.A., Lega, M., Jadid, S. *et al.* (1988) The presence of hypodense eosinophils and diminished chemiluminescence response in asthma. *J. Allergy Clin. Immunol.*, **81**, 430–7.

Shute, J. (1992) Basophil migration and chemotaxis. *Clin. Exp. Allergy*, **22**, 321–3.

Sigal, E., Craik, C.S., Highland, E. *et al.* (1988a) Molecular cloning and primary structure of human 15-lipoxygenase. *Biochem. Biophys. Res. Commun.*, **157**, 457–6.

Sigal, E. Grunberger, D., Cashman, J.R., Craik, C.S., Caughey, G.H. & Nadel, J.A. (1988b) Arachidonate 15-lipoxygenase from human eosinophil enriched leukocytes: partial purification and properties. *Biochem. Biophys. Res. Commun.*, **150**, 376–83.

Silberstein, D.S. & David, J.R. (1986) Tumor necrosis factor enhances eosinophil toxicity to *Schistosoma mansoni* larvae. *Proc. Nat. Acad. Sci. USA*, **83**, 1055–9.

Slavin, R.G. (1993) Upper respiratory tract. In: *Bronchial Asthma. Mechanisms and Therapeutics* (eds E.B. Weiss & M. Stein), pp. 533–44. Little Brown, Boston.

Slifman, N.R., Loegering, D.A., McKean, D.J. & Gleich, G.J. (1986) Ribonuclease activity associated with human eosinophil derived neurotoxin and eosinophil cationic protein. *J. Immunol.*, **137**, 2913–7.

Slifman, N.R., Peterson, C.G.B., Gleich, G.J., Dunette, S.L. & Venge, P. (1989) Human eosinophil-derived neurotoxin and eosinophil protein-X are likely the same protein. *J. Immunol.*, **143**, 2317–2.

Slungaard, A. & Mahoney, J.R. Jr (1991) Thiocyanate is the major substrate for eosinophil peroxidase in physiological fluids: implications for cytotoxicity. *J. Biol. Chem.*, **266**, 4903–10.

Slungaard, A., Vercellotti G.M., Walker, G., Nelson, R.D. & Jacob, H.S. (1990) Tumor necrosis factor alpha/cachectin stimulates eosinophil oxidant production and toxicity towards human endothelium. *J. Exp. Med.*, **171**, 2025–41.

Snyder, F. (1985) Chemical and biochemical aspects of platelet activating factor: a novel class of acetylated ether linked choline-phospholipids. *Med. Res. Rev.*, **5**, 107–40.

Sokol, R.J., Hudson, G., Wales, J. & James, N.T. (1991) Ultrastructural morphometry of human leukocytes in health and disease. *Electron Microsc. Rev.*, **4**, 179–95.

Springer, T.A. (1994) Traffic signals for lymphocyte recirculation and leukocyte emigration: the multistep paradigm. *Cell*, **76**, 301–14.

Spry, C.J.F. (1988) *Eosinophils. A Comprehensive Review and Guide to the Medical Literature.* Oxford University Press, Oxford.

Standiford, T.J., Kunkel, S.L. & Bosha, M.A. (1990) Interleukin-8 gene expression by a pulmonary epithelial cell line: a model for cytokine network in the lung. *J. Clin. Invest.*, **86**, 1945–7.

Stern, M. Meagher, L., Savill, J. & Haslett, C. (1992) Apoptosis in human eosinophils; programmed cell death in the eosinophil leads to phagocytosis by macrophages and is modulated by IL-5. *J. Immunol.*, **148**, 3543–9.

Sun, F.F., Czuk, C.I. & Taylor, B.M. (1989) Arachidonic acid metabolism in guinea pig eosinophils: synthesis of thromboxane B2 and leukotriene B4 in response to soluble or particulate activators. *J. Leuk. Biol.*, **46**, 152.

Sur, S., Crotty, T.B., Kephart, G.M. *et al.* (1993) Sudden onset fatal asthma. A distinct entity with few eosinophils and relatively more neutrophils in the airway submucosa? *Am. Rev. Resp. Dis.*, **148**, 713–19.

Tagari, P., Pecheur, E.I., Scheid, M., Brown, P., Ford-Hutchinson, A.W. & Nicholson, D. (1993) Activation of human eosinophils and differentiated HL-60 cells by interleukin-5. *Int. Arch. Allergy Appl. Immunol.*, **101**, 227–33.

Tai, P.-C. & Spry, C.J.F. (1981) The mechanisms which produce vacuolated and degranulated eosinophils. *Br. J. Haematol.*, **49**, 219–26.

Tai, P.-C., Spry, C.J., Peterson, C., Venge, P. & Olsson, I. (1984) Monoclonal antibodies distinguish between storage and secreted forms of eosinophil cationic protein. *Nature*, **309**, 182–4.

Tan, X., Hsueh, W. & Gonzalez-Crussi, F. (1993) Cellular localization of tumor necrosis factor (TNF)-alpha transcripts in normal bowel and in necrotizing enterocolitis. TNF gene expression by Paneth cells, intestinal eosinophils, and macrophages. *Am. J. Pathol.*, **142**, 1858–65.

Taniguchi, N., Mita, H., Saito, H., Yui, Y., Kajita, T. & Shida, T. (1985) Increased generation of leukotriene C4 from eosinophils in asthmatic patients. *Allergy*, **40**, 571–3.

Tavernier, J., Devos, R., Cornelis, S. *et al.* (1991) A human high affinity interleukin-5 receptor (IL-5R) is composed of an IL-5-specific alpha chain and a beta chain shared with the receptor for GM-CSF. *Cell*, **66**, 1175–84.

Taylor, I.K. & Shaw, R.J. (1993) The mechanism of action of corticosteroids in asthma. *Resp. Med.*, **87**, 261.

Taylor, K.J. & Luksza, A.R. (1987) Peripheral blood eosinophil counts and bronchial hyperresponsiveness. *Thorax*, **42**, 452–6.

Ten, R.M., Pease, L.R., McKean, D.J., Bell, M.P. & Gleich, G.J. (1989) Molecular cloning of the human eosinophil peroxidase. *J. Exp. Med.*, **169**, 1757–69.

Terada, N., Konno, A., Tada, H., Shirotori, K., Ishikawa, K. & Togawa, K. (1992) The effect of recombinant human interleukin-5 on eosinophil accumulation and degranulation in human nasal mucosa. *J. Allergy Clin. Immunol.*, **90**, 160–8.

Todd, R., Donoff, B.R., Chiang, T. *et al.* (1991) The eosinophil as a cellular source of transforming growth factor alpha in healing cutaneous wounds. *Am. J. Pathol.*, **138**, 1307–13.

Tomassini, M., Tsicopoulos, A., Tai, P.C. *et al.* (1991) Release of granule proteins by eosinophils from allergic and non-allergic patients with eosinophils on immunoglobulin-dependent activation. *J. Allergy Clin. Immunol.*, **88**, 365–75.

Tominaga, A., Takaki, S., Koyama, N. *et al.* (1991) Transgenic mice expressing a B cell growth and differentiation factor gene (interleukin 5) develop eosinophilia and autoantibody production. *J. Exp. Med.*, **173**, 429–37.

Tomioka, M., Ida, S., Shindoh, Y., Ishihara, T. & Takashima. T. (1984) Mast cells in bronchoalveolar lumen of patients with bronchial asthma. *Am. Rev. Resp. Dis.*, **129**, 1000–5.

Truong, M.J., Gruart, V., Kusnierz, J.P. *et al.* (1993) Human neutrophils express immunoglobulin E (IgE) binding proteins (Mac-2/epsilon BP) of the S-type lectin family: role in IgE-dependent activation. *J. Exp. Med.*, **177**, 243–8.

Tsicopoulous, A., Hamid Q., Hackzu, A. *et al.* (1994) Kinetics of cell infiltration and cytokine messenger RNA expression after intradermal challenge with allergen and tuberculin in the same atopic individuals. *J. Allergy Clin. Immunol.*, **94**, 764–72.

Turk, J., Maas R.L., Brash, A.R., Roberts, L. & Oates, J.A. (1982) Arachidonic acid and 15-lipoxygenase products from human eosinophils. *J. Biol. Chem.*, **257**, 7068–76.

Uchida, D.A., Ackerman, S.J., Coyle, A.J. *et al.* (1993) The effect of human eosinophil granule major basic protein on rat airways responsiveness *in vivo*: a comparison with polycations. *Am. Rev. Resp. Dis.*, **147**, 982–8.

Uguccioni, M., Loetscher, P., Forssmann, U. *et al.* (1996) Monocyte chemotactic protein 4 (MCP-4), a novel structural and functional analogue of MCP-3 and eotaxin. *J. Exp. Med.*, **183**, 2379–84.

Unkeless, J.C. (1989) Function and heterogeneity of human Fc receptors for immunoglobulin G. *J. Clin. Invest.*, **83**, 355–61.

Vadas, M.A., David, J.P., Butterworth, P., Pisani, N.T. & Siongok, T.A. (1987) A new method for the purification of human eosinophils and neutrophils and a comparison of the ability of these cells to damage schistosomula of *Schistosoma mansoni*. *J. Immunol.* **122**, 1228–36.

Valerius, T., Repp, R., Kalden, J.R. & Platzer, E. (1990) Effects of IFN on human eosinophils in comparison with other cytokines. *J. Immunol.*, **145**, 2950–8.

Van Oosterhout, A.J.M., Ladenius, R.S., Savelkoul, H.F.J., Van Ark, I., Delsman, K.C. & Nijkamp, F.P. (1993) Effect of anti-IL-5 and IL-5 on airway hyperreactivity and eosinophils in guinea pigs. *Am. Rev. Resp. Dis.*, **147**, 548–52.

Vellenga, E., Esselink, M.T., Straaten, J. *et al.* (1992) The supportive effects of IL-7 on eosinophil progenitors from human bone marrow cells can be blocked by anti-IL-5. *J. Immunol.*, **149**, 2992–5.

Venge, P. (1993) Human eosinophil granule proteins: structure, function and release. In: *Immunopharmacology of Eosinophils* (eds H. Smith & R.M. Cook), pp. 43–55. Academic, London.

Venge, P. (1995) Monitoring of asthma inflammation by serum measurements of eosinophil cationic protein (ECP). A new clinical approach to asthma management. *Resp. Med.*, **89**, 1–2.

Viegas, M., Gomez, E., Brooks, J., Gatland, D. & Davies, R.J. (1987) Effect of the pollen season on nasal mast cells. *Brit. Med. J.*, **294**, 414.

Von Adrian, U.H. Chambers, J.D., McEvoy, L.M., Bargatze, R.F., Arfors, K.E. & Butcher, E.C. (1991) Two step model of leukocyte endothelial cell interaction in inflammation: distinct roles for LECAM-1 and the leukocyte 12 integrins *in vivo*. *Proc. Nat. Acad. Sci. USA*, **88**, 7538–42.

Walker, C., Virchow, J.C., Bruijnzeel, P.L.B. & Blaser, K. (1991) T cell subsets and their soluble products regulate eosinophilia in allergic and non allergic asthma. *J. Immunol.*, **146**, 1829–35.

Walsh, G.M., Hartnell, A., Wardlaw, A.J., Kurihara, K., Sanderson, C.J. & Kay, A.B. (1990) IL-5 enhances the *in vitro* adhesion of human eosinophils, but not neutrophils in a leucocyte integrin (CD11/18)-dependent manner. *Immunology*, **71**, 258–65.

Walsh, G.M., Symon, F.A. & Wardlaw, A.J. (1995) Human eosinophils preferentially survive on tissue compared with plasma fibronectin (submitted).

Walsh, G.M., Symon, F.A., Willars, G. & Wardlaw, A.J. (1996) Cross-linking CD69 causes eosinophil apoptosis and cell death *Clin. Exp. Allergy*, **25**, 1128–36.

Wang, J.M., Rambaldi, A., Biondi, A., Chen, Z.G., Sanderson, C.J. & Mantovani, A. (1989) Recombinant human interleukin-5 is a selective eosinophil chemoattractant. *Eur. J. Immunol.*, **19**, 701–5.

Wardlaw, A.J. & Kay, A.B. (1987) The role of the eosinophil in the pathogenesis of asthma. *Allergy*, **42**, 321–35.

Wardlaw, A.J., Cromwell, O., Celestino, D. *et al.* (1986a) Morphological and secretory properties of bronchoalveolar lavage mast cells in respiratory diseases. *Clin. Allergy*, **16**, 163–73.

Wardlaw, A.J., Dunnette, S., Gleich, G.J., Collins, J.V. & Kay, A.B. (1988) Eosinophils and mast cells in bronchoalveolar lavage fluid and mild asthma: relationship to bronchial hyperreactivity *Am. Rev. Resp. Dis.*, **137**, 62.

Wardlaw, A.J., Moqbel, R., Cromwell, O. & Kay A.B. (1986b) Platelet activating factor is a potent chemotactic and chemokineic factor for human eosinophils. *J. Clin. Invest.*, **78**, 1701–6.

Wardlaw, A.J., Moqbel, R. & Kay, A.B. (1995) Eosinophils: biology and function. *Adv. Immunol.* (in press).

Warringa, R.A.J., Koenderman, L., Kok, P.T.M., Krekniet, J. & Bruijnzeel, P.L.B. (1991) Modulation and induction of eosinophil chemotaxis by granulocyte-macrophage colony stimulating factor and interleukin-3. *Blood*, **77**, 2694–700.

Warringa, R.J., Koenderman, L., Kok, P.T.M., Kreukniet, J. & Bruijnzeel, P.L.B. (1992a) Modulation and induction of eosinophil chemotaxis by granulocyte-macrophage colony stimulating factor and interleukin 3. *Blood*, **77**, 2694–700.

Warringa, R.A., Menglers, H.J., Kuijpers, P.H., Raaijmakers, J.A., Bruijnzeel, P.L. & Koenderman, L. (1992b) *In vivo* priming of platelet activating factor induced eosinophil chemotaxis in allergic asthmatic individuals. *Blood*, **79**, 1836–41.

Wegner, C.D., Gundel, R.H., Churchill, L. & Letts, L.G. (1993) Adhesion glycoproteins as regulators of airway inflammation; emphasis on the role of ICAM-1. In: *Asthma; Physiology, Pharmacology and Treatment* (eds S.T. Holgate, K.F. Austen, L.M. Lichtenstein & A.B. Kay), pp. 227–42. Academic, London.

Wegner, C.D., Gundel, R.H., Reilly, P., Haynes, N., Letts, G.L. & Rothlein, R. (1990) ICAM-1 in the pathogenesis of asthma. *Science*, **247**, 416–18.

Weiler, J.M., Edens, R.E. & Gleich, G.J. (1992) Eosinophil granule cationic proteins regulate complement. I: Activity on the alternative pathway. *J. Immunol.*, **149**, 643–8.

Weller, P.F. (1993) Eicosanoids, cytokines and other mediators elaborated by eosinophils. In: *Eosinophils, Biological and Clinical Aspects* (eds S. Makino & T. Fukuda), pp. 125–54. CRC Press, Boca Raton.

Weller, P.F. & Dvorak, A.M. (1985) Arachidonic acid incorporation by cytoplasmic lipid bodies of human eosinophils. *Blood*, **65**, 1269–74.

Weller, P.F. & Dvorak, A.M. (1994) Lipid bodies: intracellular sites for eicosanoid formation. *J. Allergy Clin. Immunol.* (Suppl.), **94**, 1151–6.

Weller, P.F. & Goetzl, E.J. (1979) The regulatory and effector roles of eosinophils. *Adv. Immunol.*, **27**, 339–71.

Weller, P.F., Goetzl, E.J. & Austen, K.F. (1980) Identification of human eosinophils lysophospholipase as the constituent of Charcot–Leyden crystals. *Proc. Nat. Acad. Sci. USA*, **77**, 7440–3.

Weller, P.F., Lee, C.N., Foster, D.W., Corey, E.J., Austen, K.F. & Lewis, R.A. (1983) Generation and metabolism of 5-lipoxygenase pathway leukotrienes by human eosinophils; predominant production of leukotriene C4. *Proc. Nat. Acad. Sci. USA*, **80**, 7625–30.

Weller, P.F., Monahan-Earley, R.A., Dvorak, H.F. & Dvorak, A.M. (1991) Cytoplasmic lipid bodies of human eosinophils: subcellular isolation and analysis of arachidonate incorporation. *Am. J. Pathol.*, **138**, 141–8.

Weller, P.F., Rand, T.H., Barrett, T., Elovic, A., Wong D.T. & Finberg, R.W. (1993) Accessory cell function of human eosinophils. HLA-DR dependent, MHC restricted antigen presentation and IL-1 alpha expression. *J. Immunol.*, **150**, 2554–62.

Winkel, P., Statland, B.E., Saunders, A.M., Osborn, H. & Kupperman, H. (1981) Within day physiologic variation of leukocyte types in healthy subjects as assayed by two automated leukocyte differential analyzers. *Am. J. Clin. Pathol.*, **75**, 693–700.

Winqvist, I., Olofsson, T., Olsson, I., Persson, A.M. & Hallberg, T. (1982) Altered density, metabolism and surface receptors of eosinophils in eosinophilis. *Immunology*, **47**, 531–9.

Wong, D.T.W., Donoff, R.B., Yang, J. *et al.* (1993) Sequential expression of transforming growth factors alpha and beta 1 by eosinophils during cutaneous wound healing in the hamster. *Am. J. Pathol.*, **143**, 130–42.

Wong, D.T.W., Weller, P.F., Gell, S.J. *et al.* (1990) Human eosinophils express transforming growth factor alpha. *J. Exp. Med.*, **172**, 673–9.

Yamaguchi,Y., Suda, T. Ohta, S. *et al.* (1991) Analysis of the survival of mature human eosinophils: interleukin-5. *Blood*, **78**, 2542–7.

Yamaguchi M. Hirai, K., Shoji, S. *et al.* (1992) Haemopoietic growth factors induce human basophil migration *in vitro*. *Clin. Exp. Allergy*, **22**, 379–83.

Yazdanbakhsh, M., Tai, P.-C., Spry, C.J.F., Gleich, G.J. & Roos, D. (1987) Synergism between eosinophil cationic protein and oxygen metabolites in killing of schistosomula of *Schistosoma mansoni*. *J. Immunol.*, **138**, 3443–7.

Ying, S., Taborda-Barata, L., Meng, Q., Humbert, M. & Kay, A.B. (1995) The kinetics of allergen-induced transcription of messenger RNA for monocyte chemotactic protein-3 (MCP-3) and RANTES in the skin of human atopic subjects: relationship to eosinophil, T-cell and macrophage recruitment. *J. Exp. Med.*, **181(6)**, 2153–9.

Young, J.D.E., Peterson, C.G.B., Venge, P. & Cohn, Z.A. (1986) Mechanism of membrane damage mediated by human eosinophil cationic protein. *Nature*, **321**, 613–6.

Zeiger, R.R. & Colten, H.R. (1977) Histamine release from human granulocytes. *J. Immunol.*, **118**, 540.

Zheutlin, L.M., Ackerman, S.J., Gleich, G.J. & Thomas, L.L. (1984) Stimulation of basophil and rat mast cell histamine release by eosinophil derived cationic proteins. *J. Immunol.*, **133**, 2180–5.

CHAPTER 11
The Neutrophil

C. Haslett & E.R. Chilvers

Introduction

Structure and origin

Neutrophilic polymorphonuclear leucocytes are white blood cells originating from the myeloid series in the bone marrow. On electron microscopy, the cells have a mean diameter of about 7 μm and a large number of intracellular granules are seen (Fig. 11.1), the neutrophil being easily distinguished from the eosinophil which has larger, angular granules. When neutrophils are stained for peroxidase, the granules appear heterogeneous with large azurophil (primary) granules which are peroxidase positive, and specific (or secondary) granules which are peroxidase negative. A third type of granule, the tertiary or storage granule, is also now recognized. Azurophil granules generally contain agents that are released into the phagocytic vacuole at the end of the phagocytic process or secreted onto opsonized surfaces. These agents include digestive proteinases and hydrolases and microbicidal proteins, including defensins and bactericidal/permeability inducing protein (BPI). Although specific granules do contain some enzymes such as lysozyme and collagenase together with lactoferrin and vitamin B_{12}-binding protein, they also provide an intracellular reserve of important membrane components, including adhesion molecules, chemotaxin receptors and constituents of the nicotinamide adenine dinuleotide phosphate (NADPH) oxidase. There may be several sub-types of tertiary granule, some are still awaiting definition. While they also contain a small complement of enzymes including gelatinase and hydrolases, they also contain membrane components, for example CR_3, and the cytochrome of NADPH oxidase in a form which can be very rapidly mobilized to the cell surface.

It is likely that most granule contents (Table 11.1) have evolved to aid the neutrophil's rapid migration through tissues and promote effective bacterial killing, but it can readily be appreciated that many of these agents would be highly toxic to normal tissues if released inappropriately or in excessive amounts.

Other subcellular structures, including Golgi apparatus and mitochondria, are not seen in great abundance but human neutrophils do contain significant amounts of endoplasmic reticulum (ER). The plasma membrane is of great importance in this rapidly responsive cell, since it contains the receptors which detect inflammatory events and the molecules involved in transduction of external signals into cellular responses, including locomotion, phagocytosis, secretion and the oxidative burst. Therefore, intimate arrangements must exist between the membrane and primary and tertiary granules which replenish important membrane components and also with the cytoskeletal framework of the cell which resides mainly in the submembrane region and is responsible for complex motility functions.

Neutrophil physiological functions and their role in host defence

The production of neutrophils accounts for more than half of the work of the bone marrow. Constitutive granulocytopoeisis is under the control of general growth factors such as interleukin-3 (IL-3), and granulocyte macrophage colony-stimulating factor (GM-CSF) and granulocyte colony-stimulating factor (G-CSF) which are lineage

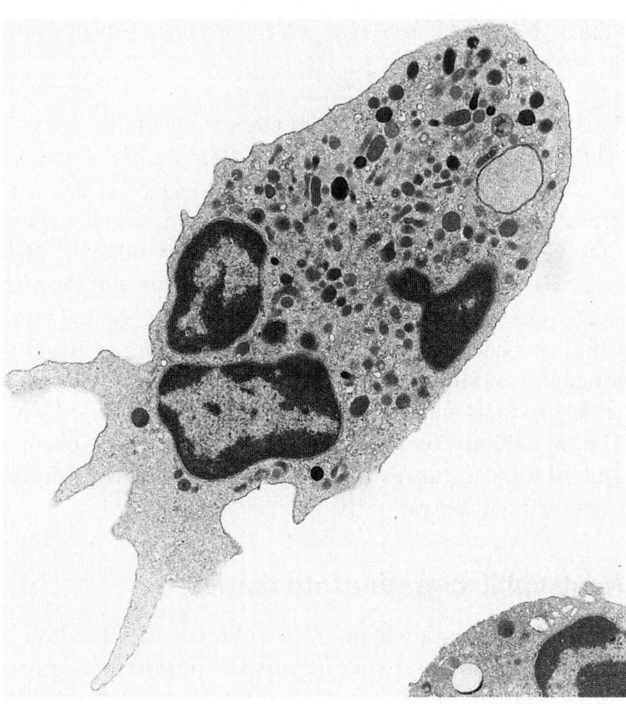

Fig. 11.1 Electron micrograph of an activated human neutrophil granulocyte demonstrating the multilobed nucleus and cytoplasmic granules.

Table 11.1 Some constituents of human neutrophil granules.

Microbicidal enzymes	Lysozyme Myeloperoxidase
Neutral proteinases	Elastase Collagenases Cathepsin G
Acid hydrolases	Cathepsin B, cathepsin D β-Glycerophosphatase Lipases Histonase β-Glucuronidase Neuraminidase
Others	BPI (bactericidal/permeability inducing protein) Defensins Cationic proteins Lactoferrin Vitamin B_{12}-binding protein Chemotaxin receptors C3b receptors Cytochrome B Flavoproteins

specific. Stromal cells in the marrow appear to be a particularly important source of these factors. They are of great relevance to the control of inflammation, as stromal cell release of growth factors is exquisitely sensitive to external agents such as IL-1 and tumour necrosis factor-α (TNF-α) which are released from inflamed sites. Thus, granulocytopoeisis can be increased several-fold during the response to infection and inflammation.

Mature neutrophils exist in the blood compartment under normal circumstances with a half-life of about 6 hours. About half the neutrophils in the vascular compartment at any given time do not circulate, forming the 'marginating pool' of neutrophils that are temporarily sequested in the microvascular beds of the lung, spleen and liver. The function of the marginated pool is uncertain but it may represent a rapidly releasable source of neutrophils mobilized in response to stress or injury, and the presence of large numbers of neutrophils in the pulmonary microvasculature may help support lung defences against the inevitable exposure to inhaled micro-organisms.

There has been little research interest in the physiological fate of the short-lived granulocyte. Until recently, it was thought that the oral cavity or gut served as a sump for effete neutrophils. However, studies with radiolabelled neutrophils have shown that they normally meet their fate in the liver, spleen and bone marrow, and it is likely that they undergo apoptosis or physiological 'programmed cell death' which leads to their recognition and removal by mononuclear phagocytes in these organs (see below).

Why the bone marrow devotes so much work to the production of large numbers of cells with a very short half-life, and which are only occasionally required to protect against bacterial invasion, remains an enigma, but since neutrophil apoptosis and lifespan (see below), and neutrophil production, are both markedly influenced by inflammatory mediators, these processes provide an exquisitely sensitive means for making available or removing enormous numbers of these highly effective bacterial killers at a site of infection. Indeed, neutrophils are ideally suited to their evolutionary role. They are extremely sensitive and respond rapidly to signals generated in infected or injured tissues; they are the first blood cells to migrate to the inflamed site where, using their oxidative responses (see below) and array of granule agents (Table 11.1), are rapidly effective in killing phagocytosed bacteria, particularly streptococci.

Until quite recently the neutrophil was widely perceived as an immutable end-stage cell which digested its way blindly through tissues and killed bacteria, before finally disintegrating. However, it is now clear that the neutrophil is a key player in several aspects of the evolving inflammatory response. Moreover, each stage of its behaviour at the inflamed site, including its final removal, has the potential to be finely controlled in order to limit incidental injury to normal tissues and to facilitate resolution of inflammation and tissue repair, so that tissues can be restored to their normal homeostatic function once the bacterial invasion has been wiped out. For example, the neutrophil can be involved in the initial generation of inflammatory oedema; the migration of monocytes (which subsequently mature into inflammatory macrophages) appears to be dependent upon the initial emigration of neutrophils; and it is now recognized that the neutrophil can generate a variety of important cytokines and chemokines which may amplify inflammation and attract more neutrophils and other cells to the inflamed site. It is also clear that each event of neutrophil behaviour during the inflammatory response—sequestration; adhesion and capillary transmigration; chemotaxis; bacterial phagocytosis; the oxidative burst and granule secretion; and its lifespan and remova—are interlinked and under fine controls which depend on a variety of signalling events linking the cell membrane, cytoskeleton, granules and nucleus. Some of these important pathways are now being dissected at the molecular level (see below).

Neutrophils and inflammatory/allergic disease

Until quite recently the inflammatory response, and the neutrophil specifically, were perceived as serving entirely beneficial roles in host defence, particularly against infection. It is now apparent, however, that they are involved in the pathogenesis of a wide variety of diseases which, now the scourge of bacterial infections is largely overcome in the developed world, are responsible for a considerable burden of mortality and untimely deaths. In the lung these include chronic bronchitis and emphysema, asthma, acute lung injury in the adult and neonate, and a variety of chronic inflammatory/scarring conditions of the lung. While the neutrophil has been specifically implicated in most of these diseases, the size of its contribution in human asthma and other allergies remains uncertain. Most researchers believe that the eosinophilic granulocyte is critically involved in the pathogenesis of asthma (Durham *et al.*, 1989). It is more abundant in the tissues than neutrophils (Laitinen *et al.*, 1992), and its products are thought to be important in the epithelial injury which is an important pathological element in human asthma. However, neutrophils predominate in equine asthma (McGarum *et al.*, 1993) and in some cases of fatal asthma in humans (Sur *et al.*, 1993), and they appear to be necessary for some models of asthma (Murphy *et al.*, 1986). Finally, because neutrophils are much shorter lived than eosinophils, a few neutrophils seen in histological sections may in fact represent, by comparison, a very significant dynamic contribution. Therefore, in an inflammatory response which displays so many examples of redundancy, it would seem prudent, at present, to expect that the neutrophil may play important contributory roles, even in allergic responses in which the eosinophil appears to predominate.

This chapter focuses on the biological events whereby a neutrophil may take part in an inflammatory response as part of an allergic/inflammatory disease process. This will include a brief overview of important events involved in the attraction of neutrophils to inflamed sites (vascular sequestration, adhesion and transmigration in microvessels and subsequent chemotaxis), potential injurious mechanisms, mechanisms controlling neutrophil longevity and the processes whereby they and their histotoxic products may be removed from the inflamed site. The signalling processes that bring about these events, and, in some instances, link with them, will be considered in more detail below.

Neutrophil migration into tissues

Neutrophils migrate to an inflamed focus as a result of a complex interplay between several important events, some occurring simultaneously and others sequentially (Fig. 11.2). These include the 'sensing' by resident macrophages and other tissue cells of phlogistic agents such as bacteria in the tissues, and the subsequent generation of some agents which are directly chemotactic for neutrophils (Table 11.2) and others, for example TNF-α and IL-1, which can stimulate other local cells to release neutrophil chemotaxins and also activate endothelial cells in the local microvessels to express adhesion molecules which are important in neutrophil sequestration and endothelial transmigration events. At the same time, neutrophil chemotaxins activate neutrophil surface molecules that are involved in endothelial adhesion.

Neutrophil chemotactic factors

When injected into tissues many inflammatory agents can cause neutrophil migration, but the number of true chemotaxins, i.e. agents which cause directed migration of neutrophils via ligation of specific neutrophil receptors, is

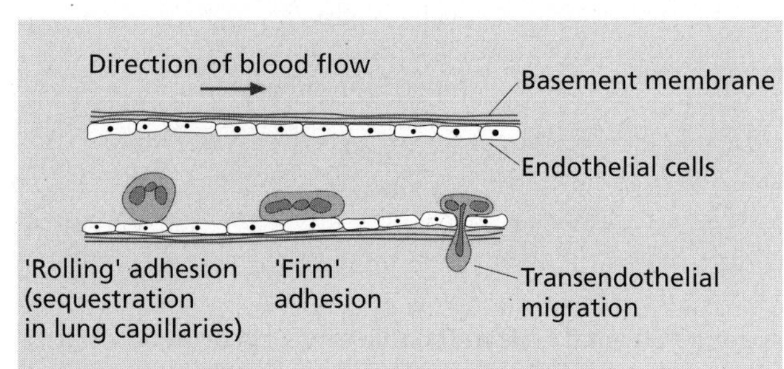

Fig. 11.2 The sequence of events involved in neutrophil sequestration and emigration in microvessels.

Table 11.2 Neutrophil chemotactic factors.

C-X-C chemokines
Interleukin 8 (IL-8)
Neutrophil activating protein-2 (NAP-2)
Granulocyte chemotactic protein-2 (GCP-2)
Epithelial neutrophil activating protein (ENA-78)
Growth-regulated oncogene alpha (GRO-α)
Growth-regulated oncogene beta (GRO-β)
Growth-regulated oncogene gamma (GRO-γ)
Complement cascade
C5a
Leukotriene cascade
Leukotriene B_4 (LTB_4)
Bacterial peptides
Formylated peptides (e.g. f-MLP)

likely to be quite restricted (Table 11.2). These include the complement component C5a, which can be secreted by some cells but is mainly generated by extracellular activation of the complement pathway. Similarly, the leukotriene cascade is activated during most inflammatory processes and leukotriene B_4 (LTB_4) has long been recognized as a specific neutrophil chemotaxin. In the past few years, intense interest has been generated in the role of a new family of chemotaxins—the chemokines (Baggiolini *et al.*, 1989). They are a group of platelet factor 4-like small proteins of molecular weight 8–19 kDa, their structure containing four cystiene residues. The alignment of the residues defines two subgroups—one group ('C-X-C') with the first two cysteines separated by one amino acid, and the other ('C-C') with adjacent cysteines. The C-X-C group (also called the α-chemokines) includes the archetypal neutrophil chemokine IL-8 and two other closely related neutrophil chemotactic peptides, neutrophil-activating peptide-2 (NAP-2) and growth-regulated oncogene-α (GRO-α). The C-C group (β-chemokines) contains agents which are mainly chemotactic for monocytes and eosinophils. The C-X-C chemokines can be generated by a variety of resident cells, including macrophages, fibroblasts and epithelial cells, particularly when they are stimulated with IL-1 or TNF-α. The lung is a potent source of IL-8 (Kunkel *et al.*, 1991). Indeed it is now possible to state with some confidence that IL-8 and other neutrophil chemokines are centrally involved in neutrophil chemotaxis and activation *in vivo*. It can also be appreciated that agents such as IL-1 and TNF-α, which are not themselves specific chemotaxins, may exert major neutrophil recruitment effects *in vivo* through stimulating the release of C-X-C chemokines from other cells. Thus, a phlogistic agent, such as a bacterium, may cause neutrophil chemotaxis by a variety of mechanisms: release from its surface of chemotactic peptides (e.g. formyl-methionyl-leucylphenylalanine, f-MLP); activation of complement to produce C5a; and upon its ingestion by macrophages it may induce the production of LTB_4, C-X-C chemokines and other cytokines like TNF-α and IL-1 which can further amplify neutrophil recruitment by the secondary stimulation of other local cells to produce C-X-C chemokines. Finally, it is important to recognize that neutrophils themselves are a potent source of chemokines including IL-8, thus presenting the opportunity for major positive feedback effects on further neutrophil emigration (Kunkel *et al.*, 1995).

Some of the important receptors with which chemotactic factors interact with the surface of neutrophils have been cloned and sequenced and some of the ligation mechanisms which activate the cell and cause the signalling events responsible for many of its complex functions are beginning to be unravelled (see below).

Neutrophil sequestration in microvessels

The arrest of neutrophils in the microcirculation is a necessary prelude to their transmigration through the endothelium. In most tissues, this occurs in post-capillary venules but in the lung this takes place in the capillary. In systemic vascular beds sequestration results from the expression/activation of neutrophil surface adhesion molecules which ligate counter-receptors on the surface of activated endothelial cells, but in the lung, alterations in neutrophil rheological properties, especially a reduction in their deformability, may play an important contributory role.

Deformability

Reduction in neutrophil deformability is one of the earliest responses of neutrophils to the ligation of chemotactic factors with their surface receptors and results within seconds in a corresponding change of the cytoskeleton of the cell to a more rigid form. The average diameter of a neutrophil is 7.5 μm, whereas that of the pulmonary capillary is 5.5 μm (Schmid-Schonbein *et al.*, 1980). Therefore, in its normal passage through pulmonary capillaries the neutrophil is required to 'squeeze' through, and any reduction in its deformability would greatly enhance sequestration. A variety of chemotactic factors have been shown to cause a mild reduction in neutrophil deformability in a way that correlates directly with vascular sequestration (Worthen *et al.*, 1989; Drost *et al.*, 1992).

Neutrophil–endothelial cell adhesion

This is a complex and multistaged process. In venules a phase of 'rolling' or transient adhesion precedes a second

Table 11.3 Major adhesion molecules involved in neutrophil–endothelial interactions.

	Receptor	Other names	Distribution	Ligand/counter receptor	Promotes adhesion of
Integrin family	LFA-1	CD11a/CD18	All leucocytes	ICAM-1, ICAM-2, ICAM-3	Endothelial cells
	CR3/Mac-1	CD11b/CD18	Granulocytes, monocytes, lymphocytes, NK cells	ICAM-1 iC3b Factor X	Endothelial cells Phagocytic particles
			Granulocytes, monocytes	LPS	
	P150, 95	CD11c/CD18		Endothelial ligand?	Endothelial cells
Immunoglobulin superfamily	ICAM-1	CD54	Endothelial cells, epithelial cells, fibroblasts (inducible by TNF, IL-1)	LFA-1 Mac-1	All leucocytes
Selectin family	E-Selectin	ELAM-1	Endothelium (inducible by TNF, IL-1)	NCA 160 (contains) Lex S Lex (CD15.5 CD15)	Neutrophils Memory T cells
	P-Selectin	CD62 G-MP-140 PADGEM	Endothelium Platelets	S Lex (SCD15)	Neutrophils
	L-Selectin	LECAM-1 Leu-8, Me 14, etc.	Neutrophils Monocytes Lymphocytes	?E Selectin ?P Selectin Lex (CD15)	Endothelium

See text for definition of abbreviations.

stage of 'firm' adhesion, which is essential for transendothelial migration to take place (Lawrence & Springer, 1991). A large array of protein and carbohydrate molecules may be involved in neutrophil–endothelial adhesion (Table 11.3), and it appears that different members of the adhesion molecule repertoire may be involved at different stages of the process. For example, P-selectin and E-selectin can support neutrophil rolling adhesion but do not induce their firm adhesion, which in turn depends on integrin activation.

Selectins

Three members of this family have so far been described, their nomenclature relating to the cell type on which they were first described—P-selectin on activated platelets, E-selectin on activated *e*ndothelium, and L-selectin which was first recognized as having a role in *l*ymphocyte homing. They are structurally related molecules with a C-type lectin domain followed by an epidermal growth factor-like domain and three short consensus repeats. They bind to carbohydrate ligands such as Lewis antigen (Le^x) and their sialylated derivatives (SLe^x and SLe^a) via their lectin domains (Bevilacqua *et al.*, 1991; Rosen, 1993). P-selectin is rapidly translocated to the surface of activated endothelial cells, E-selectin is not expressed on the surface of resting endothelium but is inducible by inflammatory agents such as bacterial lipopolysaccharide, TNF-α and IL-1, whereas L-selectin is constitutively expressed on the neutrophil surface. During neutrophil activation, L-selectin is shed, and it is thought that neutrophil L-selectin interacting with endothelial E-selectin represents a very early event in neutrophil–endothelial adhesion which may also be responsible for subsequent integrin activation (Lo *et al.*, 1991).

In humans, the importance of selectin molecules in neutrophil adhesion is supported by the rare genetic defect, leucocyte adhesion deficiency 2 (LAD2). These individuals lack fucosyl transferase activity, and are unable to express selectin ligands (Etzioni *et al.*, 1992). LAD2 patients suffer recurrent bacterial infections and their infected lesions fail to form pus despite high circulating neutrophil counts.

Integrins

Integrins are heterodimeric glycoproteins comprising an α-subunit, non-covalently linked to a β-subunit. At least eight different β-subunits and 11 α-subunits have now been cloned and sequenced (Hymes, 1992). The leucocyte integrins or $\beta 2$ integrin subfamily, which includes LFA-1 CR3/Mac-1 and P150,95, play a key role in neutrophil adhesion to endothelial cells. Individual leucocyte integrins may serve a number of functions and can bind not only ligands related to endothelial adhesion, but also those related to other important inflammatory events, including a role for CR3 in phagocytosis (Table 11.3). P150,95 has been implicated in endothelial adhesion but the endothelial ligands have not yet been identified. In the two-stage model of neutrophil binding to microvascular endothelial cells, the leucocyte integrins are centrally involved in the 'firm' adhesion stage that precedes, and is necessary for, endothelial transmigration (Lawrence & Springer, 1991). The attachment and detachment processes which must occur during neutrophil movement on the endothelial surface and during transmigration imply on–off switching and/or recycling (Lorant *et al.*, 1991) and other forms of control of integrin function. This is likely to occur by ligand regulation, for example modulation of endothelial surface expression of intercellular adhesion molecule-1 (ICAM-1) by cytokines (see below), and by poorly understood processes controlling integrin receptor function. There is now increasing evidence that interaction of leucocyte integrins with ligand involves exposure of active sites, which then confers functional activity (Figdor *et al.*, 1990).

The central importance of leucocyte integrins in neutrophil emigration is demonstrated by the genetic defect LAD1 in which a deficiency of β2 integrins is associated with a syndrome of recurrent infections from early life (Arnaout, 1990). In this rare condition neutrophils fail to emigrate to infected tissues despite high circulating cell counts, and neutrophils from these patients show a reduced, *ex vivo*, ability to bind to endothelial cells and fail to transmigrate through endothelial monolayers.

The immunoglobulin superfamily

Many receptors involved in cellular recognition processes are members of the immunoglobulin superfamily. The molecular structure of the basic unit of immunoglobulin, termed the Ig-domain, is particularly suited for the recognition of a variety of structures. Their key counter-receptors that mediate neutrophil adhesion and transmigration at the inflamed site are neutrophil 'non-specific cross-reacting antigens' or NCA which display the carbohydrate ligands for selectins (e.g. NCA-160 contains Le^x, Le^a and Sle^x which are recognized by selectins and have been implicated in E-selectin binding) as well as ICAM. ICAM-1 is the major counter-receptor for neutrophil LFA-1 (Staunton *et al.*, 1989), but ICAM-2 and ICAM-3 can also serve as counter-receptors. ICAM-1 is constitutively expressed on the surface of endothelial cells, and is strongly up-regulated in the presence of mediators such as TNF-α, IL-1 and platelet-activating factor (PAF). TNF-α causes a gradually increasing expression of ICAM-1 over 6–24 hours. This observation, together with the fact that ICAM-1 does not support rolling adhesion and is a key ligand for neutrophil integrins, suggests that it is important in the later stages of neutrophil–endothelial interactions, particularly 'firm' adhesion and capillary transmigration (Perry & Granger, 1991).

Neutrophil transmigration of the microvasculature

Since Lord Florey's classical electron microscopical observations, it has been known that neutrophils can 'squeeze' between microvascular endothelial cells by diapedesis. This poorly understood process involves adhesive interactions between ICAM-1 on endothelial cells and the leucocyte integrins.

After endothelial cells, the next 'barrier' to neutrophil emigration is the basement membrane, the broaching of which might be expected to involve significant degradation of connective-tissue matrix proteins. Although neutrophils contain an extensive repertoire of degradative enzymes, there is an intriguing suggestion (Huber & Weiss, 1989) that endothelial cells themselves may play the lead role in local degradation and reformation of the capillary basement membrane during neutrophil transmigration. Similarly, neutrophils can migrate through the tight junctions of intact monolayers of epithelial cells *in vitro* without injuring the monolayer or altering its electrical resistance. Together these observations suggest the remarkable possibility that neutrophils may remain fairly 'silent', at least in terms of a secretory response, during the process of transmigration, but clearly any breakdown in the subtle intracellular control mechanisms that must exist has the potential to result in major neutrophil-induced endothelial, epithelial and connective-tissue damage which represent the key histological features of most inflammatory diseases.

Neutrophil activation and the metabolic burst

Plasma membrane receptors

The neutrophil possesses a broad array of ligand-specific receptors. These can be divided into four main groups:

1 the G-protein-coupled, seven-transmembrane-domain receptors, e.g. for PAF, C5a, substance P and IL-8 (Besemer *et al.*, 1989; Samanta *et al.*, 1989; Baggiolini *et al.*, 1993);

2 the single-transmembrane-domain receptors for many cytokines, e.g. for GM-CSF, hepatocyte growth factor and TNF-α (Liu & Djeu, 1995);

3 the single-transmembrane-domain receptors activated following immobilization by cross-linkage, e.g. the Fc and integrin receptors and the lipopolysaccharide (LPS)–LBP (LPS binding protein) complex receptor, CD14 (Wright *et al.*, 1990, 1991);

4 the intracellular receptors for cell-permeable agents, e.g. glucocorticosteroids.

G proteins

Heterotrimeric G proteins couple many of the plasma membrane receptors to effector (e.g. actin polymerization

(Bengtsson, 1990)) or second-messenger generating systems (e.g. phospholipase C, D and A_2) within the cell (Taylor, 1990). Although a very large number of G proteins have now been identified, only a limited number have been detected in neutrophils and/or HL-60 cells. These include Gi_2 and Gi_3, the dominant G proteins present in the neutrophil, and $G_{16/15}$, G_q/G_{11}, $G_{12/13}$ and Gs. G proteins are activated by guanosine triphosphate (GTP) displacing guanosine diphosphate (GDP) on the α-subunit causing α–βγ subunit dissociation. In most instances the activated GTP-bound α-subunit is thought to be the principal effector molecule; however, especially in haemopoetic cells, the unbound βγ-subunits can also initiate certain responses including PLCβ2 activation (Katz *et al.*, 1992; Lee & Rhee, 1995).

Recent data support the view that the rate of G-protein activation also plays a role in dictating the signalling pathway stimulated by a particular receptor (Jacobs *et al.*, 1995). This system allows different receptors to share a common pool of promiscuous G proteins without losing functional specificity. Other factors that regulate Gα function and Gα–βγ subunit interaction include the ability of the α-subunit to be post-translationally modified by the addition of the fatty acid palmitate (Milligan *et al.*, 1995) or to be ribosylated by mono(adenosine diphosphate (ADP)-ribosyl) transferases. In the neutrophil there is preliminary evidence to indicate that priming by agents such as lipopolysaccaride and TNF-α cause a translocation of $G\alpha i_2$ and $G\alpha i_2$ to the plasma membrane (Yasui *et al.*, 1992; Klein *et al.*, 1995). These observations suggest that regulation of G-protein distribution and for expression may be a significant mechanism underlying neutrophil priming (see below). It is also apparent that the expression of certain G proteins, for example $G\alpha_{16}$, alter quite significantly during neutrophilic differentiation of HL-60 cells (Amatruda *et al.*, 1991).

Lipid-derived second messenger pathways

Phospholipase C

At least 10 mammalian isozymes of phosphoinositide-specific phospholipase C (PLC) have now been identified (PLCβ1–4, PLCγ1–2 and PLCδ1–4) and are responsible for the cleavage of phosphatidylinositol 4,5-bisphosphate (PtdIns(4,5)P_2) to inositol 1,4,5-trisphosphate (Ins-(1,4,5)P_3) and *sn*1,2-diacylglycerol (DAG). To date, no phosphatidylcholine-specific PLC activity has been identified in the neutrophil (Strum *et al.*, 1993). The dominant PLC forms expressed in haematopoietic cells are PLCγ2 and PLCβ2. The former is activated by phosphorylation of Tyr 753 and Tyr 759 by growth-factor receptors and by non-receptor protein tyrosine kinases. In the neutrophil, unlike the situation in most other cell types, receptor-mediated activation of PLCβ2 appears to be mediated principally by βγ dimers rather than GTP-activated Gα subunits (Lee & Rhee, 1995).

PtdIns(4,5)P_2 is also a substrate for phosphatidylinositol 3-kinase (see below), is a membrane attachment site for proteins containing pleckstrin homology (PH) domains, regulates actin polymerization, and acts as a co-factor for PtdCho-specific PLD (Lee & Rhee, 1995).

In vitro studies in neutrophils demonstrate that PLC activity can be induced by GTP analogues (GTP-γ-S >GppNHp >GppCH_2p) and fluoride, and most agonist-stimulated responses are blocked by pre-treatment with pertussis toxin (Cockcroft, 1994). This latter effect is peculiar to haematopoietic cells and implicates a member of the Gi family of G proteins in this pathway, probably Gi_2 or Gi_3. In HL-60 cells, maximal G-protein-stimulated PLC activity is dependent on a cytosolic PtdIns transfer protein that appears to be involved in maintaining PtdIns(4,5)P_2 substrate supply (Thomas *et al.*, 1993).

The Ca^{2+} dependency of PLC activation in neutrophils and HL-60 cells has been much debated (Cockcroft, 1994). While it is clear that receptor-mediated activation of PLC requires the presence of nanomolar levels of Ca^{2+}, and that an elevation in intracellular Ca^{2+} ($[Ca^{2+}]_i$) to micromolar levels potentiates this response, it is now generally agreed that, unlike in many excitable cells, an increase in $[Ca^{2+}]_i$ cannot alone stimulate PLC activity.

The large bulk of the PLC found in these cells is cytosolic and current evidence suggests that one function of the activated G-protein components is to recruit the relevant PLC to the membrane to allow access to its lipid substrate. Certain neutrophil receptors, for example those with intrinsic tyrosine kinase activity or the ability to activate src-related soluble tyrosine kinases, recruit proteins, including PLCγ2, to the cell membrane via activation of an intrinsic SH2 (Src homology) binding domain. This latter pathway is the proposed mechanism whereby cross-linking of the FcγRI and FcγRII molecules results in phosphorylation and activation of PLCγ2.

In neutrophils, f-MLP, C5a, PAF, LTB_4 and IL-8 receptors all activate PLC and result in the hydrolysis of PtdIns(4,5)P_2 to Ins(1,4,5)P_3 and DAG. Stimulation of neutrophils with f-MLP causes a rapid but transient accumulation of Ins(1,4,5)P_3 (maximal at 10 seconds) and a similar rapid increase in DAG mass. Whether the prompt decline in Ins(1,4,5)P_3 levels represents transient production, or receptor-mediated activation of the 3-kinase or 5-phosphatase enzymes responsible for its metabolism, remains to be determined.

Phosphatidylinositol 3-kinase

Phosphatidylinositol 3-kinase (PI3K) is responsible for the conversion of PtdIns(4,5)P_2 to phosphatidylinositol 3,4,5-

trisphosphate (PtdIns(3,4,5)P_3). This lipid has been proposed to mediate a number of intracellular events, including activation of a ribosomal S6 kinase responsible for G1–S phase transition, protein trafficking and various aspects of cytoskeletal function including membrane ruffling (see Malarkey *et al.*, 1995). It also has a particularly important signalling role in the neutrophil (Traynor-Kaplan *et al.*, 1989; Stephens *et al.*, 1993a), where it mediates superoxide generation. While in the majority of cells PI3K activation results from interaction of its regulatory p85 subunit with receptor tyrosine kinases and thereafter binding and stimulation of the p110 catalytic PI3K subunit, the neutrophil contains a novel PI3K activity regulated by βγ-subunits (Stephens *et al.*, 1993b).

Phospholipase D

Ligation of several cell-surface receptors in the neutrophil stimulates phospholipase D (PLD)-mediated cleavage of phosphatidylcholine to generate phosphatidic acid (PA) and its inactive water-soluble headgroup choline. While it is likely that several forms of this enzyme exist (Massenburg *et al.*, 1994), no mammalian form of PLD has yet been cloned. In the presence of ethanol, the phosphatidyl moiety reacts preferentially with this molecule to form phosphatidylethanol, a non-metabolizable product easily separated by thin-layer chromatography. This transphosphatidylation reaction forms the basis of a very sensitive assay of PLD activity in intact cells.

Evidence for agonist-stimulated PLD activity in neutrophils arose from studies demonstrating a rapid and major increase in PA mass following incubation with f-MLP, that could not be attributed to phosphoinositide hydrolysis, with subsequent conversion of DAG to PA. A wide variety of agents are now recognized to stimulate PLD activity in neutrophils, including f-MLP, C5a, ATP, PAF, LTB_4, C3b/bi and IgG-opsonized yeast particles (Thompson *et al.*, 1991). How these receptors trigger PLD activation in neutrophils is not entirely clear, but one or more of the following pathways is thought to be involved: a direct G-protein-mediated linkage, a Ca^{2+}/PKC pathway and a tyrosine kinase-mediated route. PLD activity in granulocytes is also activated in a fairly dramatic way by a cytosolic GTP-bound ADP-ribosylation factor (ARF) (Cockcroft *et al.*, 1994) that requires PtdIns(4,5)P_2 for full activation. Whether these pathways operate in parallel or series is uncertain. The other major regulator of PLD activity in neutrophils is cyclic adenosine monophosphate (cAMP), which may be responsible, at least in part, for limiting the duration of agonist-induced PLD responses (Tyagi *et al.*, 1991).

To date, no second-messenger role has been identified for choline and hence the major active product of PLD activity is believed to be PA. While the conversion of PA to DAG by phosphatidate phosphohydrolase appears to be responsible for the delayed, secondary-phase accumulation of DAG following f-MLP stimulation, PA undoubtedly functions as a signalling molecule in its own right and may well trigger the exocytotic response in these cells. A good correlation also exists between enhanced PLD activity and priming of respiratory burst activity, suggesting that PA is required for competent assembly and activation of the NADPH oxidase.

Phospholipase A_2

Activation of phospholipase A_2 (PLA_2) results in cleavage of arachidonic acid (AA) from the *sn*-2 position of phosphatidylcholine, phosphatidylethanolamine or phosphatidylinositol with release of the corresponding lyso-phospholipid. Among other functions, AA is the major precursor for the biosynthesis of eicosanoids, namely the prostaglandins, leukotrienes and lipoxins. Two isoforms of PLA_2 are recognized, a 110-kDa cytosolic PLA_2 ($cPLA_2$) (Sharp *et al.*, 1991) and a low-molecular-weight (14-kDa) secretory PLA_2 ($sPLA_2$) (Kramer *et al.*, 1989). The former is Ca^{2+} dependent and is responsible for the release of AA from intracellular membrane phospholipids. Full activation of $cPLA_2$ also requires phosphorylation by both MAP kinase-dependent and -independent pathways (Fouda *et al.*, 1995). In intact neutrophils the activation of $cPLA_2$ by f-MLP is rapid (sec) and thought to be G-protein mediated with Ca^{2+} triggering the initial translocation of the enzyme from the cytosol to the membrane to permit this interaction.

The secretory form of PLA_2 is released extracellularly from granules where it targets phospholipids present in the outer leaflet of the cell membrane. The secretory forms of PLA_2 also differ from $cPLA_2$, in that they do not demonstrate selectivity for AA over other fatty acids present at the *sn*-2 position of the phospholipids. Neutrophil priming causes enhanced activity and mobilization of both forms of PLA_2, even in the absence of any change in $[Ca^{2+}]_i$ (Bass *et al.*, 1994; Doerfler *et al.*, 1994; Durstin *et al.*, 1994). Priming also enhances the activity of a further two enzymes involved in the PLA_2–AA–eicosanoid pathway, namely the co-enzyme A-independent transacylase (CoAIT), responsible for maintaining PLA_2 lipid substrate levels (Winkler *et al.*, 1994), and the 5-lipoxygenase-activating protein, FLAP (Pouliot *et al.*, 1994).

Sphingomyelin–ceramide pathway

There has been considerable recent interest in the ability of cell-permeable ceramide analogues to mimic the ability of agents such as TNF-α, nerve growth factor, Fas ligand and IL-1 to induce cell-cycle arrest and/or apoptosis (Kolesnick & Fuks, 1995). From these and other studies, it

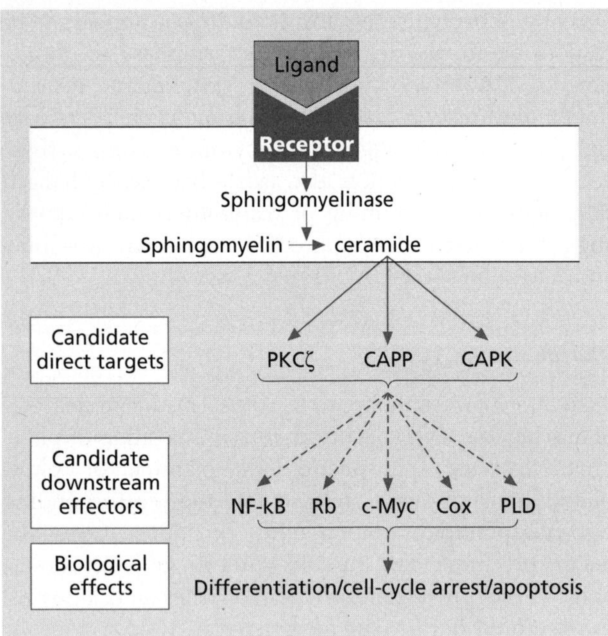

Fig. 11.3 The sphingomyelin–ceramide signalling pathway.

has been proposed that receptor-mediated activation of a neutral membrane-bound and/or a lysosomal acidic form of sphingomyelinase (a sphingomyelin-specific PLC) results in cleavage of the phospholipid sphingomyelin (*N*-acetylsphingosin-1-phosphocholine) to generate ceramide (Fig. 11.3) (Hannun, 1994; Michell & Wakelam, 1994). Of particular relevance to the neutrophil is the recent observation that HL-60 cells possess a variant cytosolic neutral sphingomyelinase that is activated by vitamin D (Okazaki *et al.*, 1994). While the precise mechanisms underlying the signalling effect of ceramide are unclear, at least four target proteins have been identified, including a ceramide-activated protein kinase (CAPK) and protein phosphatase (CAPP), PKC-ζ, and the putative guanine nucleotide exchange factor Vav (Wright & Kolesnick, 1995).

Of relevance to the neutrophil is the recent proposal that the effect of endotoxin in cells may, at least in part, be mediated by its ability to mimic the action of ceramide, since there appears to be a strong structural similarity between these molecules. However, recent studies have shown that ceramide analogues in neutrophils do not mimic the priming or apoptosis-modulating effects of TNF-α or LPS, and hence the importance of this signalling pathway in neutrophils remains uncertain.

Cystolic calcium

Elevation of $[Ca^{2+}]_i$ in the neutrophil stimulates cell polarization, superoxide anion generation, degranulation and aggregation (Pozzan *et al.*, 1983). The immediate Ca^{2+} spike observed following receptor activation results from Ins(1,4,5)P_3-induced Ca^{2+} release from the ER system, with Ca^{2+} influx responsible for the more prolonged phase II elevation in $[Ca^{2+}]_i$. Recent data examining the effects of immune complexes on neutrophil Ca^{2+} responses suggest the presence of more than one Ca^{2+} storage organelle in the neutrophil in addition to multiple influx pathways (Davies & Hallett, 1995; see also O'Flaherty *et al.*, 1988). The precise details of how Ca^{2+} influx is controlled in the neutrophil remain uncertain, but may involve Ins(1,3,4,5)P_4 and/or a discrete 'calcium influx factor' responsible for signalling between the empty Ca^{2+} store and the plasma membrane. Binding of the terminal membrane attack complex (MAC) of complement (C5b–C9) appears to elevate neutrophil $[Ca^{2+}]_i$ via a direct effect on membrane Ca^{2+} permeability (Laffafian *et al.*, 1995). Subsequent and more detailed examination of the effects of $[Ca^{2+}]_i$ in neutrophil activation indicated that Ca^{2+}, although necessary, is not alone sufficient to explain fully the effects of physiological stimuli (Rossi *et al.*, 1988, Gomez-Cambronero *et al.*, 1989). Ca^{2+} also appears to play a role in regulating the rate at which neutrophils undergo apoptosis (Whyte *et al.*, 1992a).

Cyclic ADP ribose (cADPR), synthesized from NAD^+ by ADP-ribosyl cyclase, has also received attention recently regarding its ability to regulate $[Ca^{2+}]_i$ by interacting with certain types of ryanodine receptor (Berridge, 1993; Galione, 1993). This system has been proposed to operate in the same way as Ins(1,4,5)P_3 and Ca^{2+} that co-operate at the Ins(1,4,5)P_3 receptor. Whether this molecule plays a similar role in the neutrophils is, as yet, unclear.

It is important to note that neutrophil activation results also in alterations in the concentration of a variety of other ions aside from Ca^{2+}. For example, a number of peptide and lipid chemoattractants have been shown to induce a rapid (<30 seconds) decline in $[pH]_i$ followed by a PKC-mediated, amiloride-inhibitable (Na^+/H^+ antiport) alkalinization phase (Weisman *et al.*, 1987). The increased intracellular Na^+ concentration resulting from Na^+/H^+ antiport activation is handled largely via enhanced Na^+/K^+ exchange.

Protein phosphorylation

Serine-threonine kinases

The cAMP- and cGMP-dependent protein kinases (PKA and PKG) appear to be mainly involved in inhibiting or terminating neutrophil responses (Moilanen *et al.*, 1993). A number of mechanisms are involved in elevating cAMP in neutrophils, including both receptor (e.g. β_2-adrenoceptor) and Ca^{2+}/calmodulin-dependent activation of adenylyl cyclase (Cooper *et al.*, 1995), Ca^{2+}-mediated inhibition of (type IV) phosphodiesterase activity, and elevation mediated via secondary release of prostanoids (e.g. PGE_2 and PGD_2) and/or adenosine. Elevation in cAMP has been shown to inhibit a wide variety of neutrophil responses, including, for example, chemoattractant-induced Ca^{2+} influx and PLD activation (Takenawa *et al.*, 1986).

While the functional role of cGMP and PKG in neutrophils appears less certain (Zurier *et al.*, 1974; Wenzel-Seifert *et al.*, 1991; Moilanen *et al.*, 1993), nitric oxide (NO) has now been shown to attenuate neutrophil adhesion (Kubes *et al.*, 1991), aggregation, LTB_4 release, degranulation, superoxide anion release and chemotaxis (Moilanen *et al.*, 1993). Neutrophils also have the ability to generate NO (McCall *et al.*, 1989; Wright *et al.*, 1989) and contain both the Ca^{2+}-regulated Ic isoform of NO synthase and, at least in rats, an LPS-inducible and dexamethasone inhibitable, Ca^{2+}-independent NOS (Mariotto *et al.*, 1995).

The neutrophil contains multiple isoforms of protein kinase C, including members of the conventional (cPKC), atypical (aPKC) and novel (nPKC) forms of PKC. It is not suprising therefore that the effects of PKC activation in the neutrophil with agents such as phorbol esters are somewhat complex, causing stimulation of superoxide anion generation, specific granule exocytosis and PLD activity but inhibition of many agonist-initiated events, including chemotaxis, degranulation and Ca^{2+} mobilization (e.g. Naccache *et al.*, 1985). While PKC activation has been shown to result in the phosphorylation of a large number of neutrophil proteins, including myosin light chain, profilin, G-actin, vimentin and lipocortin, the lack of information on the precise functional specificity of the various PKC isoforms present is currently hampering progress in this area.

Phosphotyrosine kinases

Phosphotyrosine kinases and phosphatases are now recognized as playing a crucial role in the regulation of multiple cell functions and have been the focus of intense research over recent years. In the neutrophil, activation of tyrosine kinases occurs as a result of ligand binding to receptors with intrinsic tyrosine kinase activity (e.g. many of the growth factor receptors, including G-CSF and GM-CSF) and through receptor activation of a family of small cytosolic tyrosine kinases (e.g. Lyn, Fyn and Syk), via, as yet, a poorly defined G-protein-mediated mechanism. This latter transduction mechanism is employed, for example, by receptors to f-MLP, IgG, IgE, C5a and substance P. In many systems this results in the tyrosine phosphorylation of a multiple protein substrate including focal adhesion kinase ($p125^{FAK}$), the p85 subunit of phosphatidylinositol 3-kinase ($p85^{PI3K}$) and mitogen-activated

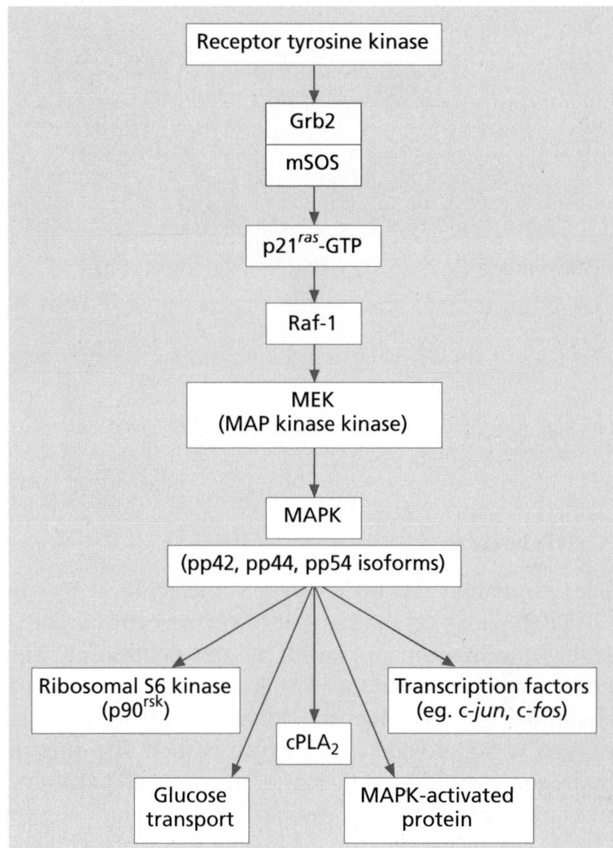

Fig. 11.4 Growth factor-induced activation of the MAP kinase cascade.

protein kinase ($p40^{hera}$, $p42^{erk2}$, $p44^{erk1}$ and $p46^{erk4}$). One of the best characterized signalling cascades triggered by receptor-initiated tyrosine phosphorylation is the ras/raf/MAP kinase (MAPK) pathway depicted in Fig. 11.4. In the neutrophil, PAF has been demonstrated to induce tyrosine phosphorylation of a range of proteins (42–116 kDa), including the $p42^{erk2}$ form of MAP kinase, an effect that is potentiated greatly by pre-treatment with LPS (Fouda *et al.*, 1995).

Tyrosine phosphorylation has also been proposed as playing a role in neutrophil priming (Hallett & Lloyds, 1995). This is based on data showing that tyrosine phosphorylation is triggered by dedicated priming agents and low (priming) concentrations of secretagogue agonists, precedes the priming effect, and if induced with tyrosine phosphatase inhibitors, results in neutrophil priming. In this model it is proposed that tyrosine phosphorylation of a 40–43 kDa (possibly MAPK) or a 72–74 kDa protein allows full activation of the $p47^{phox}$ component of the NADPH oxidase when a Ca^{2+}-mobilizing agonist is subsequently applied.

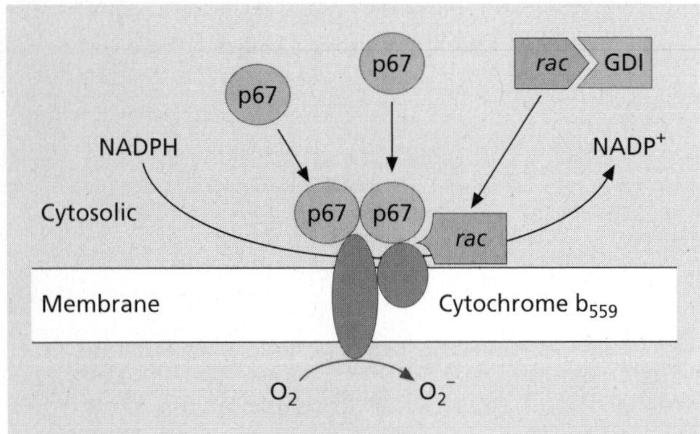

Fig. 11.5 Assembly of the multicomponent NADPH oxidase.

NADPH oxidase

The generation of toxic oxygen metabolites by the NADPH oxidase is the basis of the phagocytic oxidative killing mechanism employed by the neutrophil. This multicomponent enzyme forms an electron-transport chain, using NADPH as the donor to reduce molecular oxygen to superoxide anion which is then dismuted to hydrogen peroxide and thereafter metabolized to hyroxyl free radicals and hypochlorous acid. The enzyme complex (Fig. 11.5) consists of a unique membrane-attached flavocytochrome (cytochrome b_{558}), an associated GTP-binding protein Rap1A, and two cytosolic proteins $p47^{phox}$ and $p67^{phox}$ that bind to cytochrome b_{558} following cell activation (Rotrosen *et al.*, 1993; reviews by Segal & Abo, 1993; Bokoch, 1994). The final component is the GTP-binding protein Rac1/Rac2 ($p21^{rac1}/p21^{rac2}$) that dissociates from its complex with [Rho]GDI and translocates to the plasmalemma and/or membrane-associated cytoskeleton to form an integral part of the NADPH oxidase (Dusi *et al.*, 1995). Rac2 also appears to be regulated by *bcr* that is involved in reciprocal translocation in (Ph)-positive leukaemias, since the neutrophils of *bcr* (–/–) mice show a pronounced increase in reactive oxygen species production and are more sensitive to priming stimuli (Voncken *et al.*, 1995). The importance of these individual components for NADPH oxidase function is indicated by the condition chronic granulomatous disease, where the absence of cytochrome b_{558} (X-linked form), $p47^{phox}$ or $p67^{phox}$ (autosomal forms) results in a disease typified by severe infection.

In the primed state, stimulation of oxidase activity appears directly proportional to the increase in $[Ca^{2+}]_i$ (Hallett *et al.*, 1990). It is clear, however, that a rise in $[Ca^{2+}]_i$ alone is insufficient to stimulate oxidase activity and that PtdIns(3,4,5)P_3 generation and certain protein tyrosine phosphorylation events are also required (Hallett & Lloyds, 1995). The accompanying production of protons is a major factor underlying the transient cytosolic acidification observed under these conditions and triggers activation of a voltage-dependent H^+ current that extrudes protons and maintains intracellular pH (Schumann *et al.*, 1995).

Neutrophil-mediated tissue injury

It can readily be appreciated that the neutrophil possesses considerable capacity for releasing a wide variety of agents with the potential to injure local tissues. However, several other general factors need to be included in the equation determining whether excessive tissue injury occurs (Fig. 11.6).

1 The presence *per se* of neutrophils in tissues does not equate with injury. Models of inflammation *in vivo* exist in which neutrophils emigrate to the lung without any evidence of lung injury, and, as discussed above, neutrophils can migrate through endothelial cells and epithelial monolayers without causing toxic effects. It is now recognized that for maximal injurious potential, the neutrophil requires exposure to the combined effects of 'priming' agents and triggering agents. Priming agents including LPS, TNF-α and PAF, even in large concentrations, do not exert significant neutrophil secretory effects. However, in very low concentrations, they prime or alter the neutrophil's baseline state, such that when the cell is then exposed to a triggering agent such as a chemotaxin (e.g. IL-8, C5a) there is then a maximal secretory and oxidative response (Haslett *et al.*, 1985; Smedly *et al.*, 1986). Thus, we must consider the functional state of the neutrophil at different stages of the inflammatory process. For example, it seems likely that loss of control of neutrophil function

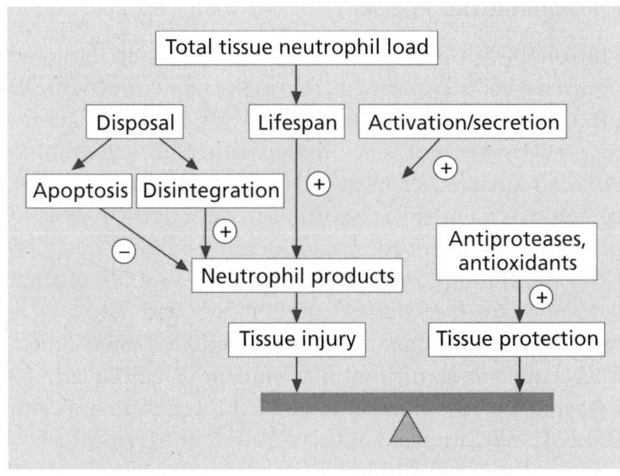

Fig. 11.6 The 'balance' of injurious and protective influences in the determination of excessive inflammatory tissue injury.

during the migratory stage particularly might be expected to cause the type of major endothelial and epithelial injury which characterizes many inflammatory diseases.

2 Even fully primed and triggered neutrophils are unable to degrade matrix (Campbell *et al.*, 1982; Rice & Weiss, 1990) or to injure 'target' cells unless they are in close proximity. The creation of a discrete intercellular microenvironment by neutrophils tightly adherent to endothelial cells, for example, may favour injury by a variety of potential mechanisms:

(a) the local concentrations of histotoxic agents may reach very high levels;

(b) some very labile reactive oxygen intermediates may have a very short distance of tissue activity;

(c) high-molecular-weight proteinase inhibitors, such as α_1-antiproteinase, would tend to be excluded;

(d) some proteinases, such as elastase, are presented in high concentrations on the leading surface of the neutrophil.

Thus, it can be envisaged that tight and prolonged contact of maximally primed and stimulated neutrophils, with endothelium for example, would tend to favour local tissue injury.

The role of apoptosis in the longevity and tissue clearance of neutrophils

Despite the importance of tissue residence time and the rate of removal of neutrophils and their products in the control of neutrophil tissue 'load' (Fig. 11.6), there has been little formal study of the mechanisms controlling these events. It had been widely assumed that neutrophils inevitably undergo necrosis and disintegrate *in situ* (necrosis) before their fragments are removed by local macrophages (Hurley, 1983). However, if this was the rule, healthy tissues would inevitably be exposed to large quantities of injurious neutrophil contents. Although a number of pathological descriptions have favoured neutrophil necrosis as a major mechanism operating in inflammation, most of these examples have been derived from histological observation of diseased tissues rather than 'beneficial' inflammatory responses, such as the response to infection. Furthermore, there has been evidence from the classical observations of Metchnikoff (1986) more than a century ago of an alternative fate for neutrophils, whereby the intact cell is removed by local macrophages. More recently, it has been shown that a major mechanism available for the removal of intact neutrophils and other granulocytes at the inflamed site is the process of apoptosis or programmed cell death, which, by contrast with necrosis, has very different implications for the control of inflammation (Haslett, 1992). There is now clear evidence of a role for apoptosis in the clearance of neutrophils from tissues in a variety of acute inflammatory disorders and their experimental models (Grigg *et al.*, 1991; Cox *et al.*, 1995). Moreover, it appears that apoptosis represents a pivotal control point, controlling the functional longevity of granulocytes, which can be modulated by a variety of inflammatory mediators.

Apoptosis

Unlike necrosis or 'accidental' cell death, Wyllie and his colleagues recognized apoptosis as a process which occurred in situations where death is predictable or physiological, such as thymic involution, or in other situations where cell turnover is physiologically rapid, for example crypt cells in the gut epithelium (Wyllie *et al.*, 1980). During the process of apoptosis, ultrastructural studies show that, in contrast with necrosis, cells shrink yet the plasma membrane remains intact and retains the ability to exclude vital dyes and the cell continues to retain organelles including granules (Fig. 11.7). Apoptotic cells are very rapidly ingested by phagocytes, particularly macrophages, *in vivo*; as an example, in tissue sections of the remodelling embryo, apoptotic cells are rarely seen outside phagocytes. Furthermore, in these examples of programmed cell death there is no evidence of local tissue injury or the induction of an inflammatory response, suggesting that apoptosis may represent a tissue injury-limiting mechanism for the removal of neutrophils.

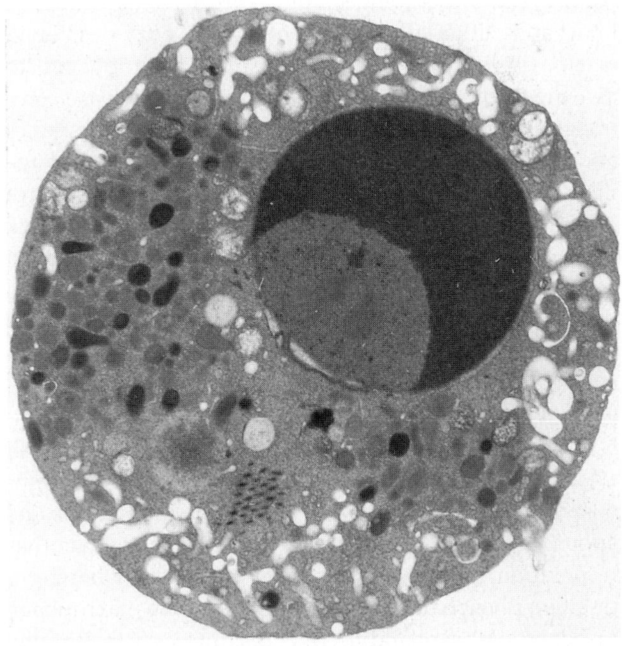

Fig. 11.7 Electron micrograph of an apoptotic human neutrophil. Note the intact cell membrane, the retention of granules as well as the nuclear chomatin condensation and cytoplasmic vacuolation which characterize apoptosis.

Apoptosis and the control of neutrophil functional longevity in tissues

It has been known for several years that a variety of inflammatory mediators, including GM-CSF, are able to prolong the lifespan of cultured neutrophils, as assessed by the necrosis of the cell determined by their inability to exclude vital dyes (Lopez *et al.*, 1986). More recently, it has been discovered that these observations may be explained by inhibition of the process of apoptosis, which precedes necrosis in cultured eosinophils and neutrophils (Brach *et al.*, 1992; Lee *et al.*, 1993). Furthermore, it has been found that GM-CSF, LPS and C5a not only prolong the lifespan of cultured neutrophils by inhibiting apoptosis, but also that this process results in prolongation of neutrophil functional longevity measured by a number of assays including secretion and chemotaxis (Whyte *et al.*, 1993a). The intracellular mechanisms governing the rate of neutrophil apoptosis are poorly understood but involve second messenger signalling, including Ca^{2+} (Whyte *et al.*, 1993b), and in other cells, a range of oncogene products and members of the Bcl-2 family are particularly important in the control of apoptosis (Reed, 1994). However, a specific role for Bcl-2 in the control of apoptosis in mature granulocytes has not been established.

Neutrophil apoptosis and their removal by macrophages

Neutrophils undergoing apoptosis are ingested while still intact and without the leakage of granule enzymes (Savill *et al.*, 1989). The usual response of macrophages to the ingestion of particles *in vitro* is to release pro-inflammatory mediators such as thromboxanes, enzymes and cytokines. However, even maximal macrophage ingestion of apoptotic neutrophils fails to release pro-inflammatory mediators (Meagher *et al.*, 1992). This lack of macrophage responsiveness appears to be determined by the specific recognition employed by macrophages in the uptake of apoptotic neutrophils. Recent work has shown that human monocyte-derived macrophages utilize a novel recognition mechanism involving the integrin $\alpha v \beta 3$ (the vitronectin receptor) and CD36 (thrombospondin receptor) on their surface (Savill *et al.*, 1990, 1992). These molecules appear to link with thrombospondin to bind an as yet unidentified moiety on the apoptotic neutrophil surface. In a murine model, another recognition mechanism has been suggested whereby a putative phosphatidylserine receptor on the macrophage recognizes phosphatidylserine residues which become exposed on the surface of neutrophils during the process of apoptosis (Fadok *et al.*, 1992). The significance of these observations *in vivo* is as yet uncertain; however, there is evidence *in vitro* that the rate of neutrophil ingestion by macrophages can also be modulated by environmental factors and by agents which alter macrophage cAMP (McCutcheon, 1996). Finally, semi-professional phagocytes, such as fibroblasts and mesangial cells, have the capacity to recognize and ingest apoptotic neutrophils *in vitro* but not with the facility or capacity of macrophages (Savill *et al.*, 1992b; Hall *et al.*, 1994). The significance of this observation *in vivo* is uncertain but it could represent a 'back-up' mechanism for the macrophage system.

Thus, apoptosis not only determines the functional longevity of granulocytes at the inflamed site but it can be modulated and controlled by external mediators of relevance to the control of inflammation. In contrast with necrosis, it provides a neutrophil removal mechanism which again is influenced by inflammatory mediators and which, by a variety of mechanisms, would tend to limit rather than promote bystander injury to healthy tissues:

- the cell membrane remains intact and apoptotic neutrophils retain their dangerous contents;
- during the process of apoptosis, the neutrophil loses its ability to mount a secretory response to microenvironmental pro-inflammatory stimuli;
- the macrophage ingests the intact apoptotic neutrophil;
- macrophage phagocytic recognition of apoptotic neutrophils employs novel receptors which fail to trigger a pro-inflammatory macrophage secretory response.

Conclusion

Antineutrophil strategies in the treatment of inflammatory and allergic diseases

It will be appreciated that recent advances in research have identified a number of specific molecular processes and events which could be targetted in the treatment of inflammatory diseases. However, it is important to draw attention to two potential difficulties. Firstly, the efficacy of the inflammatory response in host defence lies, at least in part, in the redundancy of many of its mechanisms. When this redundancy is turned against us in inflammatory disease, the prospects for rational therapeutic treatments directed at a single mediator become daunting. Secondly, effective anti-inflammatory strategies directed against the neutrophil are likely to critically weaken host defences, particularly against bacterial infection. It is probable, therefore, that powerful new treatments directed at the neutrophil will need to be applied during periods of opportunity when inflammatory mechanisms are more critical to the evolution of disease process than they are to the general defence of the host, while at the same time employing approaches to prevent infective complications. Alternatively, it may be possible to develop new strategies directed at boosting tissue protection against inflammatory injury which would not have the same deleterious consequences for host defence.

References

Amatruda, T.T., Steele, D.A., Slepak, V.Z. & Simon, M.I. (1991) Gα16, a G protein α subunit specifically expressed in haematopoietic cells. *Proc. Nat. Acad. Sci. USA*, **88**, 5587–91.

Arnaout, M.A. (1990) Leukocyte adhesion molecules deficiency: its structural basis, pathophysiology and implications for modulating the inflammatory response. *Immunol. Rev.*, **114**, 145–80.

Baggiolini, M., Boulay, F., Badwey, J.A. & Curnutte, J.T. (1993) Activation of neutrophil leukocytes: chemoattractant receptors and respiratory burst. *FASEB J.*, **7**, 1004–10.

Baggiolini, M., Walz, A. & Kunkel, S.L. (1989) Neutrophil-activating peptide/interleukin 8, a novel cytokine that activates neutrophils. *J. Clin. Invest.*, **84**, 1045–9.

Bass, D.A., Seeds, M.C., Jones, D.F., Chilton F.H. & Bauldry, S.A. (1994) Priming of phospholipases A_2 of human neutrophils by tumour necrosis factor. *Chest*, **105**, 99S–100S.

Bengtsson, B. (1990) Correlation between chemotactic peptide-induced changes in chlorotetracycline fluorescence and F-actin content in human neutrophils: a role for membrane-associated calcium in the regulation of actin polymerization. *Exp. Cell Res.*, **191**, 57–63.

Berridge, M.J. (1993) A tale of two messengers. *Nature*, **365**, 388–9.

Besemer, J., Hujber, A. & Kuhn, B. (1989) Specific binding, internalization and degradation of human neutrophil platelet activating factor by human polymorphonuclear leukocytes. *J. Biol. Chem.*, **264**, 17409–15.

Bevilacqua, M., Butcher, E., Furie, B. *et al.* (1991) Selectins: a family of adhesion receptors. *Cell*, **67**, 233.

Bokoch, G.M. (1994) Regulation of the human neutrophil NADPH oxidase by the rac GTP-binding proteins. *Curr. Opin. Cell Biol.*, **6**, 212–18.

Brach, M.A., de Vos, S., Gruss, H.-J. & Herrman, F. (1992) Prolongation of survival of human polymorphonuclear neutrophils by granulocyte-macrophage colony-stimulating factor is caused by inhibition of programmed cell death. *Blood*, **80**, 2920–4.

Campbell, E.J., Senior, R.M., McDonald, J.A. & Cox, D.L. (1982) Proteolysis by neutrophils. Relative importance of cell–substrate contact and oxidative inactivation of proteinase inhibitors *in vivo*. *J. Clin. Invest.*, **70**, 845–52.

Cockcroft, S. (1994) Receptor-mediated signal transduction pathways in neutrophils: regulatory mechanisms that control phospholipases C, D and A_2. In: *Immunopharmacology of Neutrophils* (eds P.G. Helliwell & T.J. Williams). Academic, London.

Cockcroft, S., Thomas, G.M., Fensome, A. *et al.* (1994) Phospholipase D is a downstream effector of ARF in granulocytes. *Science*, **263**, 523–6.

Cooper, D.M.F., Mons, N. & Karpen, J.W. (1995) Adenylyl cyclases and the interaction between calcium and cAMP signalling. *Nature*, **374**, 421–4.

Cox, G., Crossley, J. & Xing, Z. (1995) Macrophage engulfment of apoptotic neutrophils contributes to the resolution of acute pulmonary inflammation *in vivo*. *Am. J. Respir. Cell Mol. Biol.*, **12**, 232–7.

Davies, E.V. & Hallett, M.B. (1995) A novel pathway for Ca^{2+} signalling in neutrophils by immune complexes. *Immunology*, **85**, 538–43.

Doerfler, M.E., Weiss J., Clark, J.D. & Elsbach, P. (1994) Bacterial lipopolysaccharide primes human neutrophils for enhanced release of arachidonic acid and causes phosphorylation of an 85 kD cytosolic phospholipase A_2. *J. Clin. Invest.*, **93**, 1583–91.

Drost, E.M., Selby, C., Lannan, S., Lowe, G.O. & MacNee, W. (1992) Changes in neutrophil deformability following *in vitro* smoke exposure. *Am. J. Respir. Cell Mol. Biol.*, **6**, 287–95.

Durham, S.R., Loegering, D.A., Dunnett, E.S., Gleich, G.J. & Kay, A.B. (1989) Blood eosinophils and eosinophil-derived proteins in allergic asthma. *J. Allergy Clin. Immunol.*, **19**, 3–8.

Durstin, M., Durstin, S., Molski, T.F.P., Becker, E.L. & Sha'afi, R.I. (1994) Cytoplasmic phospholipase A_2 translocates to membrane fraction in human neutrophils activated by stimuli that phosphorylate mitogen-activated protein kinase. *Proc. Nat. Acad. Sci. USA*, **91**, 3142–6.

Dusi, S., Donni, M. & Rossi, F. (1995) Mechanisms of NADPH oxidase activation in human neutrophils: p67phox is required for the translocation of rac 1 but not rac 2 from cytosol to the membrane. *Biochem. J.*, **308**, 991–4.

Etzioni, A., Frydman, M., Pollock, S. *et al.* (1992) Recurrent severe infections caused by a novel leukocyte adhesion deficiency. *New Engl. J. Med.*, **327**, 1789–92.

Fadok, V.A., Savill, J.S., Haslett, C. *et al.* (1992) Different populations of macrophages use either the vitronectin receptor or the phosphatidylserine receptor to recognise and remove apoptotic cells. *J. Immunol.*, **149**, 4029–35.

Figdor, C.E., van Kooyk, Y. & Keizer, G.D. (1990) On the mode of action of LFA-1. *Immunol. Today*, **11**, 277–80.

Fouda, S.I., Molski, T.F.P., Ashour, M.S.-E. & Sha'afi, R.I. (1995) Effect of lipopolysaccharide on mitogen-activated protein kinases and cytosolic phospholipase A_2. *Biochem. J.*, **308**, 815–22.

Galione, A. (1993) Cyclic ADP-ribose: a new way to control calcium. *Science*, **259**, 325–6.

Gomez-Cambronero, J., Durstin, M., Molski, T.F.P., Naccache, P.H. & Sha'afi, R.I. (1989) Calcium is necessary but not sufficient for the platelet-activating factor release in human neutrophils. *J. Biol. Chem.*, **264**, 21699–704.

Grigg, J.M., Savill, J.S., Sarraf, C., Haslett, C. & Silverman, M. (1991) Neutrophil apoptosis and clearance from neonatal lungs. *Lancet*, **338**, 720–2.

Hall, S.E., Savill, J.S., Henson, P.M. & Haslett, C. (1994) Apoptotic neutrophils are phagocytosed by fibroblasts with participation of the fibroblast vitronectin receptor and involvement of a mannose/fucose-specific lectin. *J. Immunol.*, **153**, 3218–27.

Hallett, M.B., Davies, E.V. & Campbell, A.K. (1990) Oxidase activation in individual neutrophils is dependent on the onset and magnitude of the Ca^{2+} signal. *Cell Calcium*, **11**, 655–63.

Hallett, M.B. & Lloyds, D. (1995) Neutrophil priming: the cellular signals that say 'amber' but not 'green'. *Immunol. Today*, **16**, 264–8.

Hannun, Y.A. (1994) The sphingomyelin cycle and the second messenger function of ceramide. *J. Biol. Chem.*, **269**, 3125–8.

Haslett, C. (1992) Resolution of acute inflammation and the role of apoptosis in the tissue fate of granulocytes. *Clin. Sci.*, **83**, 639–48.

Haslett, C., Guthrie, L.A., Kopaniak, M.M., Johnston, R.B. & Henson, P.M. (1985) Modulation of multiple neutrophil functions by preparative methods or trace concentrations of lipopolysaccharide. *Am. J. Pathol.*, **119**, 101–10.

Huber, A.R. & Weiss, S.J. (1989) Disruption of the subendothelial basement membrane during neutrophil diapedesis in an *in vitro* construct of a blood vessel wall. *J. Clin. Invest.*, **83**, 1122–36.

Hurley, J.V. (1983) *Termination of Acute Inflammation. 1. Resolution. Acute inflammation*, 2nd edn., p. 109. Churchill Livingstone, London.

Hymes, R.O. (1992) Integrins: versatility, modulation and signalling in cell adhesion. *Cell*, **69**, 11–25.

Jacobs, A.A., Huber, J.L., Ward, R.A., Klein, J.B. & McLeish, K.R. (1995) Chemoattractant receptor-specific differences in G protein activation rates regulate effector enzyme and functional responses. *J. Leuk. Biol.*, **57**, 679–86.

Katz, A., Wu, D. & Simon, M.I. (1992) Subunits βγ of heterotrimeric G protein activate β2 isoform of phospholipase C. *Nature*, **360**, 686–9.

Klein, J.B., Scherzer, J.A., Harding, G., Jacobs, A.A. & Mcleish, K.R. (1995) TNFα stimulates increased plasma membrane guanine nucleotide binding protein activity in polymorphonuclear leukocytes. *J. Leuk. Biol.*, **57**, 500–6.

Kolesnick, R. & Fuks, Z. (1995) Ceramide: a signal for apoptosis of mitogenesis? *J. Exp. Med.*, **181**, 1949–52.

Kramer, R.M., Hession, C., Johansen, B. *et al.* (1989) Structure and properties of a human non-pancreatic phospholipase A_2. *J. Biol. Chem.*, **264**, 5768–75.

Kubes, P., Suzuki, M. & Grander, D.N. (1991) Nitric oxide: an endogenous modulator of leukocyte adhesion. *Proc. Nat. Acad. Sci. USA*, **88**, 4651–5.

Kunkel, S.L., Lukas, M. & Strieter, R.M. (1995) Expression and biology of neutrophil and endothelial cell-derived cytokines. *Semin. Cell Biol.*, **6** (in press).

Kunkel, S.L., Standiford, T., Kasahara, K. & Strieter, R.M. (1991) Interleukin 8: the major neutrophil chemotactic factor in the lung. *Exp. Lung Res.*, **17**, 17–23.

Laffafian, I., Davies, E.V., Campbell, A.K. & Hallett, M.B. (1995) Complement component C9-dependent cytosolic free Ca^{2+} rise and recovery in neutrophils. *Cell Calcium*, **17**, 279–86.

Laitinen, L.A., Laitinen, A. & Haahtela, T. (1992) A comparative study of the effects of an inhaled corticosteroid, budesonide, and a β_2-agonist, terbutaline, and airway inflammation in newly-diagnosed asthma: a randomised double-blind parallel group controlled trial. *J. Allergy Clin. Immunol.*, **90**, 32–42.

Lawrence, M.B. & Springer, T.A. (1991) Leukocytes roll on a selectin at physiological flow rates: distinction from and prerequisite for adhesion through integrins. *Cell*, **65**, 859–73.

Lee, A., Whyte, M.K.B. & Haslett, C. (1993) Inhibition of apoptosis and prolongation of neutrophil functional longevity by inflammatory mediators. *J. Leuk. Biol.*, **54**, 283–8.

Lee, S.B. & Rhee, S.G. (1995) Significance of PIP_2 hydrolysis and regulation of phospholipase C isoenzymes. *Curr. Opin. Cell Biol.*, **7**, 183–9.

Liu, J.H. & Djeu, J.Y. (1995) Role of cytokines in neutrophil functions. In: *Human Cytokines: Their Role in Disease and Therapy* (eds B.B. Aggarwal & R.K. Puri), pp. 71–86. Blackwell Science, Oxford.

Lo, S.K., Lee, S., Ramos, R.A. *et al.* (1991) Endothelial leukocyte adhesion molecule 1 stimulates the adhesion activity of leukocyte integrin CR3 on human neutrophils. *J. Exp. Med.*, **173**, 1493–500.

Lopez, A.F., Williamson, D.J., Gamble, J.R. *et al.* (1986) Recombinant human granulocyte-macrophage colony-stimulating factor stimulates *in vitro* mature human neutrophil and eosinophil function, surface receptor expression, and survival. *J. Clin. Invest.*, **78**, 1220–8.

Lorant, D.E., Patel, K.D., McIntyre, T.M. *et al.* (1991) Co-expression of GMP-140 and PAF by endothelium stimulated by histamine or thrombin: a juxtacrine system for adhesion and activation of neutrophils. *J. Cell Biol.*, **115**, 223–34.

McCall, T.B., Boughton-Smith, N.K., Palmer, R.M.J., Whittle, B.J.R. & Moncada, S. (1989) Synthesis of nitric oxide from L-arginine by neutrophils. *Biochem. J.*, **261**, 293–6.

McCutcheon, J.C., Fleming, S., Haslett, C. & Dransfield, I. (1996) Macrophage adhesion — a potential regulator of the capacity for recognition of apoptotic cells (submitted).

McGorum, B.C., Dixon, P.M. & Halliwell, R.E.W. (1993) Responses of horses affected with chronic obstructive pulmonary disease to inhalation challenges with mould antigens. *Equine Vet. J.*, **25**, 261–7.

Malarkey, K., Belham, C.M., Paul, A. *et al.* (1995) The regulation of tyrosine kinase signalling pathways by growth factor and G-protein-coupled receptors. *Biochem. J.*, **309**, 361–75.

Mariotto, S., Cuzzolin, L., Adami, A., Del Soldato, P., Suzuki, H. & Benoni, G. (1995) Effect of a new non-steroidal anti-inflammatory drug, nitroflurbiprofen, on the expression of inducible nitric oxide synthase in rat neutrophils. *Br. J. Pharmacol.*, **115**, 225–6.

Massenburg, D., Han, J.S., Liyanage, M. *et al.* (1994) Activation of rat brain phospholipase D by ARFs 1, 5 and 6: separation of ARF-dependent and oleate-dependent enzymes. *Proc. Nat. Acad. Sci. USA*, **91**, 11718–22.

Meagher, L.C., Savill, J.S., Baker, A., Fuller, R.W. & Haslett, C. (1992) Phagocytosis of apoptotic neutrophils does not induce macrophage release of thromboxane B_2. *J. Leuk. Biol.*, **52**, 269–73.

Metchnikoff, E. (1986) *Lectures on the Comparative Pathology of Inflammation. Lecture VII. Delivered at the Pasteur Institute in 1891* (translated F.A. Starling & E.H. Starling). Dover, New York.

Michell, R.H. & Wakelam, M.J.O. (1994) Second messengers: sphingolipid signalling. *Curr. Biol.*, **4**, 370–3.

Milligan, G., Parenti, M. & Magee, A.I. (1995) The dynamic role of palmitoylation in signal transduction. *TIBS*, **20**, 181–6.

Moilanen, E., Vuorinen, P., Kankaanranta, H., Metsa-Ketela, T. & Vapaatalo, H. (1993) Inhibition by nitric oxide-donors of polymorphonuclear leucocyte functions. *Br. J. Pharmacol.*, **109**, 852–8.

Murphy, K.R., Wilson, M.C., Irvin, C.G. *et al.* (1986) The requirement for polymorphonuclear leukocytes in the late asthmatic response and heightened airways reactivity in an animal model. *Am. Rev. Resp. Dis.*, **134**, 62–8.

Naccache, P.H., Molski, T.F.P., Borgeat, P. & Sha'afi, R.I. (1985) Phorbol esters inhibit the fMet-Leu-Phe and leukotriene B_4 stimulated calcium mobilization and enzyme secretion in rabbit neutrophils. *J. Biol. Chem.*, **260**, 2125–32.

O'Flaherty, J.T., Jacobson, D. & Redman, J. (1988) Mechanism involved in the mobilization of neutrophil calcium by 5-hydroxyeicosatetraenoate. *J. Immunol.*, **140**, 4323–8.

Okazaki, T., Bielawska, A., Domae, N., Bell, R.M. & Hannun, Y.A. (1994) Characteristics and partial purification of a novel cytosolic, magnesium-independent, neutral sphingomyelinase activated in early signal transduction of 1α,25-dihydroxy-vitamin D_3-induced HL-60 cell differentiation. *J. Biol. Chem.*, **269**, 4070–7.

Perry, M.A. & Granger, D.N. (1991) Role of CD11/CD18 in shear rate-dependent leukocyte–endothelial cell interactions in cat mesenteric venules. *J. Clin. Invest.*, **87**, 1798–804.

Pouliot, M., McDonald, P.P., Khamzina, L., Borgeat, P. & McColl, S.R. (1994) Granulocyte-macrophage colony-stimulating factor enhances 5-lipoxygenase levels in human polymorphonuclear leukocytes. *J. Immunol.*, **152**, 851–8.

Pozzan, T., Lew, D.P., Wollheim, C.B. & Tsein, R.Y. (1988) Is cytosolic ionized calcium regulating neutrophil activation? *Science*, **221**, 1413–15.

Reed, J.C. (1994) Bcl-2 and the regulation of programmed cell death. *J. Cell Biol.*, **124**, 1–6.

Rice, W.E. & Weiss, S.J. (1990) Regulation of proteolysis at the neutrophil substrate interface by secretory leukoprotease inhibitor. *Science*, **249**, 173–81.

Rosen, S.D. (1993) Cell surface lectins in the immune system. *Semin. Immunol.*, **5**, 237–47.

Rossi, A.G., MacIntyre, D.E. & McMillan, R.M. (1988) Human neutrophil activation: cytosolic free calcium ($[Ca^{2+}]_i$) thresholds for aggregation, degranulation, leukotriene B_4 synthesis and phosphatidate formation. *Biochem. Soc. Trans.*, **16**, 37–8.

Rotrosen, D., Yeung, C.L. & Katkin, J.P. (1993) Production of recombinant cytochrome b_{558} allows reconstitution of the phagocycte NADPH oxidase solely from recombinant proteins. *J. Biol. Chem.*, **268**, 14256–60.

Samanta, A.K., Oppenheim, J.J. & Matsushima, K. (1989) Identification and characterisation of specific receptors for monocyte-derived neturophil chemotactic factor (MDNCF) on human neutrophils. *J. Exp. Med.*, **169**, 1185–9.

Savill, J.S., Dransfield, I., Hogg, N. & Haslett, C. (1990) Macrophage recognition of 'senescent self'; the vitronectin receptor mediates phagocytosis of cells undergoing apoptosis. *Nature*, **342**, 170–3.

Savill, J.S., Hogg, N. & Haslett, C. (1992a) Thrombospondin co-operates with CD36 and the vitronectin receptor in macrophage recognition of aged neutrophils. *J. Clin. Invest.*, **90**, 1513–29.

Savill, J.S., Smith, J., Ren, Y., Sarraf, C., Abbott, F. & Rees, A.J. (1992b) Glomerular mesangial cells and inflammatory macrophages ingest neutrophils undergoing apoptosis. *Kidney Int.*, **42**, 924–36.

Savill, J.S., Wyllie, A.H., Henson, J.E., Henson, P.M. & Haslett, C. (1989) Macrophage phagocytosis of aging neutrophils in inflammation. Programmed cell death in the neutrophil leads to its recognition by macrophages. *J. Clin. Invest.*, **83**, 865–75.

Schmid-Schonbein, G.W., Shih, Y.Y. & Chien, S. (1980) Morphometry of human leukocytes. *Blood*, **56**, 866–75.

Schumann, M.A., Leung, C.C. & Raffin, T.A. (1995) Activation of NADPH-oxidase and its associated whole-cell H^+ current in human neutrophils by recombinant human tumor necrosis factor α and formyl-methionyl-leucyl-phenylalanine. *J. Biol. Chem.*, **270**, 13124–32.

Segal, A.W. & Abo, A. (1993) The biochemical basis of the NADPH oxidase of phagocytes. *TIBS*, **18**, 43–7.

Sharp, J.D., White, D.L., Chiou, X.G. *et al.* (1991) Molecular cloning and expression of human Ca^{2+}-sensitive cytosolic phospholipase A_2. *J. Biol. Chem.*, **266**, 14850–3.

Smedly, L.A., Tonnesen, M.G., Sandhaus, R.A. *et al.* (1986) Neutrophil mediated injury to endothelial cells: enhancement by endotoxin and essential role of neutrophil elastase. *J. Clin. Invest.*, **77**, 1233–43.

Staunton, D.E., Dustin, M.L. & Springer, T.A. (1989) Functional cloning of ICAM-2, a cell adhesion ligand for LFA-1 homologous to ICAM-1. *Nature*, **339**, 61–4.

Stephens, L., Eguinoa, A., Corey, S., Jackson, T. & Hawkins, P.T. (1993a) Receptor stimulated accumulation of phosphatidylinositol(3,4,5)-trisphosphate by G-protein mediated pathways in human myeloid derived cells. *EMBO J.*, **12**, 2265–72.

Stephens, L., Jackson, T.R. & Hawkins, P.T. (1993b) Agonist-stimulated synthesis of phosphatidylinositol-3,4,5-trisphosphate: a new intracellular signalling system? *Biochim. Biophys. Acta*, **1179**, 27–54.

Strum, J.C., Nixon, A.B., Daniel, L.W. & Wykle, R.L. (1993) Evaluation of phospholipase C and D activity in stimulated neutrophils using a phosphono analogue of choline phosphoglyceride. *Biochim. Biophys. Acta*, **1169**, 25–9.

Sur, S., Crotty, T.B. & Kephart, G.M. *et al.* (1993) Sudden-onset fatal asthma. A distant entity with few eosinophils and relatively more neutrophils in the airway submucosa? *Am. Rev. Resp. Dis.*, **148**, 713–9.

Takenawa, T., Ishitoya, J. & Nagai, Y. (1986) Inhibitory effect of prostaglandin E_2, forskolin, and dibutyryl cAMP on arachidonic acid release and inositol phospholipid metabolism in guinea pig neutrophils. *J. Biol. Chem.*, **261**, 1092–8.

Taylor, C.W. (1990) The role of G proteins in transmembrane signalling. *Biochem. J.*, **272**, 1–13.

Thomas, G.M.H., Cunningham, E., Fensome, A. *et al.* (1993) An essential role for phosphatidylinositol transfer protein in phospholipase C-mediated inositol lipid signalling. *Cell*, **74**, 919–28.

Thompson, N.T., Bonser, R.W. & Garland, L.G. (1991) Receptor-coupled phospholipase D and its inhibitors. *TIPS*, **12**, 404–8.

Traynor-Kaplan, A.E., Thompson, B.L., Harris, A.L., Taylor, P., Omann, C.M. & Sklar, L.A. (1989) Transient increases in phosphatidylinositol-3,4-bisphosphate and phosphatidylinositol trisphosphate during activation of human neutrophils. *J. Biol. Chem.*, **264**, 15668–72.

Tyagi, S.R., Olson, S.C., Burnham, D.N. & Lambeth, J.D. (1991) Cyclic AMP-elevating agents block chemoattractant activation of diradylglycerol generation by inhibiting phospholipase D activation. *J. Biol. Chem.*, **266**, 3498–504.

Voncken, J.W., van Schaick, H., Kaartinen, V. *et al.* (1995) Increased neutrophil respiratory burst in *bcr*null mutants. *Cell*, **80**, 719–28.

Weisman, S.J., Punzo, A., Ford, C. & Sha'afi, R.I. (1987) Intracellular pH changes during neutrophil activation: Na^+/H^+ antiport. *J. Leuk. Biol.*, **41**, 25–32.

Wenzel-Seifert, K., Ervens, J. & Seifert, R. (1991) Differential inhibition and potentiation by cell-permenant analogues of cyclic AMP and cyclic GMP and NO-containing compounds of exocytosis in human neutrophils. *Naunyn-Schmiedebergs Arch. Pharmacol.*, **344**, 396–402.

Whyte, M.K.B., Meagher, L.C., Hardwick, S., Savill, J. & Haslett, C. (1993a) Transient elevations of cystolic free calcium retard subsequent apoptosis in neutrophils *in vitro*. *J. Clin. Invest.*, **92**, 446–55.

Whyte, M.K.B., Meagher, L.C., MacDermot, J. & Haslett, C. (1993b) Impairment of function in aging neutrophils is associated with apoptosis. *J. Immunol.*, **150**, 5123–34.

Winkler, J.D., Sung, C.M., Huang, L. & Chilton, F.H. (1994) CoA-independent transacylase activity is increased in human neutrophils after treatment with tumor necrosis factor alpha. *Biochem. Biophys. Acta*, **1215**, 133–40.

Worthen, G.S., Schwab, B., Elson, E.L. & Downey, G.P. (1989) Mechanics of stimulated neutrophils: cell stiffening induces retention in capillaries. *Science*, **245**, 183–6.

Wright, S.D. & Kolesnick, R.N. (1995) Does endotoxin stimulate cells by mimicking ceramide? *Immunol. Today*, **16**, 297–302.

Wright, C.D., Mulsch, A., Busse, R. & Osswald, H. (1989) Generation of nitric oxide by human neutrophils. *Biochem. Biophys. Res. Commun.*, **160**, 813–9.

Wright, S.D., Ramos, R.A., Tobias, P.S., Ulevitch, R.J. & Mathison, J.C. (1990) CD14, a receptor for complexes of lipopolysaccharide (LPS) and LPS binding protein. *Science*, **249**, 1431–3.

Wright, S.D., Ramos, R.A., Hermanowski-Vosatka, A., Rockwell, P. & Detmers, P.A. (1991) Activation of the adhesive capacity of CR3 on neutrophils by endotoxin: dependence on lipopolysaccharide binding protein and CD14. *J. Exp. Med.*, **173**, 1281–6.

Wyllie, A.H., Kerr, J.F.R. & Currie, A.R. (1980) Cell death: the significance of apoptosis. *Int. Rev. Cytol.*, **68**, 251–306.

Yasui, K., Becker, E.L. & Sha'afi, R.I. (1992) Lipopolysaccharide and serum cause the translocation of G-protein to the membrane and prime neutrophils via CD14. *Biochem. Biophys. Res. Commun.*, **183**, 1208–6.

Zurier, R.B., Weissmann, G., Hoffstein, S., Kammerman, S. & Tai, H.H. (1974) Mechanisms of lysosomal enzyme release from human leukocytes. *J. Clin. Invest.*, **53**, 297–309.

CHAPTER 12

Platelets

C.M. Herd & C.P. Page

Introduction

The platelet has been traditionally associated with disorders of the cardiovascular system, and is a well-recognized cell type actively involved in the maintenance of haemostasis and the initiation of repair after tissue injury. However, studies reported by several groups suggest an important role of the platelet in allergic diseases (Capron *et al.*, 1987; Gresele *et al.*, 1987; Page, 1988). This chapter summarizes the experimental and clinical evidence implicating the involvement of this cell in allergic inflammation, in particular in relation to bronchial asthma.

Platelets possess many of the features of classical inflammatory cells such as polymorphonuclear leucocytes (PMN). They are capable of undergoing chemotaxis (Lowenhaupt, 1982), have been shown to phagocytose foreign particles (Mustard & Packham, 1979), contain and release various adhesive proteins, activate complement, interact with parasites, viruses and bacteria, alter vascular tone and enhance vascular permeability (Weksler, 1983). Furthermore, platelets synthesize, store, take up and release a variety of potent inflammatory and/or anaphylactic mediators.

Platelet-derived mediators

Platelets are a rich source of a wide range of biologically active substances that, when released from the cell following activation, are capable of inducing or augmenting inflammatory responses. Platelet-dense granules contain adenosine diphosphate (ADP) and adenosine triphosphate (ATP), 5-hydroxy tryptamine (5-HT) and Ca^{2+}, and the more numerous α-granules store mediators synthesized by the megakaryocyte or taken up from the circulation. α-Granules also contain a variety of proteins, some platelet specific, which include adhesive proteins, the 'anti-heparinoid' platelet factor 4 (PF_4), platelet-derived growth factor (PDGF), β-thromboglobulin (β-TG) and transforming growth factor-β (TGF-β). Figure 12.1 illustrates a variety of platelet-derived mediators which when released following platelet stimulation may play a significant role in asthma and/or inflammation. Table 12.1 summarizes those platelet-derived mediators which are chemotactic for a range of inflammatory cell types.

5-HT, stored in large amounts in human platelets, may contribute to the inflammatory response via its vasoconstrictor properties and ability to increase vascular permeability. Human platelets synthesize, take up and release histamine (Saxena *et al.*, 1989; Mannaioni *et al.*, 1992, 1993), a potent inflammatory mediator capable of inducing bronchoconstriction, vasodilatation, oedema caused by leakage of plasma proteins from post-capillary venules, stimulation of bronchoconstrictor reflexes and mucus secretion. In addition, human platelets activated with thrombin, collagen and platelet-activating factor (PAF) have been shown to liberate a substance that stimulates the release of histamine from mast cells and basophils, platelet-derived histamine releasing factor (PDHRF) (Knauer *et al.*, 1984; Orchard *et al.*, 1986). PDHRF has also been shown to be chemotactic toward eosinophils, and to induce early- and late-onset airway obstruction and airway hyperresponsiveness in experimental animals (Fisher *et al.*, 1990). Adenosine, which can be formed from the nucleotides stored and released by platelets, may play a role in bronchoconstriction (Holgate *et al.*, 1991) and

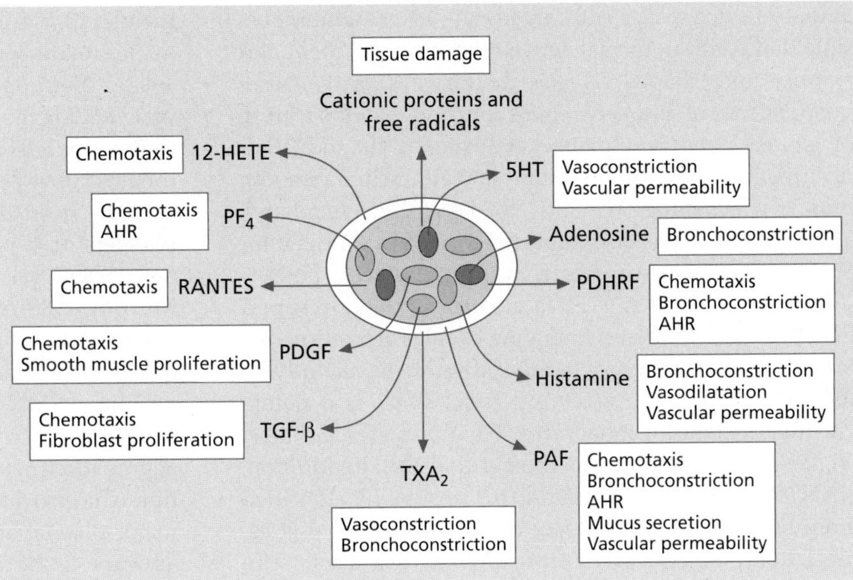

Fig. 12.1 Mediators released from activated platelets that may play a role in asthma and/or allergy.

Table 12.1 Chemotactic factors released from activated platelets. The inflammatory cell(s) type which may be recruited in response to platelet activation and release are listed alongside each mediator.

Mediator	Cell type
PAF	Basophil Eosinophil Fibroblast Monocyte Neutrophil Smooth muscle cell T lymphocyte
PDHRF	Eosinophil
PF_4	Eosinophil Fibroblast Monocyte Neutrophil
PDGF	Fibroblast Monocyte Neutrophil Smooth muscle cell
TGF-β	Fibroblast Neutrophil
RANTES	Basophil Eosinophil Monocyte T lymphocyte
12-HETE	Eosinophil

See text for definition of abbreviations.

receptors for adenosine have been shown to be up-regulated in allergic rabbits compared with normal rabbits (Mustafa *et al.*, 1991).

Platelets contain cationic proteins which can increase vascular permeability (Sasaki *et al.*, 1991), in addition to a cationic protein that cleaves the fifth component of complement to form a factor which is chemotactic for leucocytes (Weksler & Coupal, 1973). The platelet-specific protein PF_4 possesses many properties that suggest a key role in allergy and inflammation. It has been shown to increase the expression of Fc-IgG and Fc-IgE receptors (Chihara *et al.*, 1988) and to stimulate the release of histamine from basophils (Brindley *et al.*, 1983). PF_4 is not only chemotactic for PMN, monocytes and fibroblasts (Deuel *et al.*, 1981), but also for eosinophils (Chihara *et al.*, 1988). The ability of PF_4 to activate eosinophils is of particular interest, as it has been suggested that these cells contribute to the tissue damage observed in asthma which may be associated with airway hyperresponsiveness (Frigas & Gleich, 1986). Furthermore, PF_4 has been shown to increase airway responsiveness in rats (Coyle *et al.*, 1993).

PDGF may act as a mediator of inflammation and repair by affecting vascular tone (Berk *et al.*, 1986), exerting chemotactic effects towards monocytes and neutrophils (Deuel *et al.*, 1982), and by activating monocytes (Tzeng *et al.*, 1985) and neutrophils (Deuel & Huang, 1984). Smooth muscle cells and fibroblasts are strongly attracted to PDGF, suggesting that these cells may migrate to injured sites where subsequent mitogenic stimulation furthers repair processes (Deuel & Huang, 1984). Similarly, TGF-β has been shown to be chemotactic for neutrophils and fibroblasts (Wahl *et al.*, 1987). Bronchial smooth muscle hypertrophy is characteristic of the asthmatic lung at autopsy (Ebina *et al.*, 1990; Carroll *et al.*, 1993) and it is possible that continuous platelet activation, recruitment and extravascular diapedesis into the airways, with consequent release of mitogens, could contribute to this feature of asthma. The role of platelet activation in the induction of myofibroblast proliferation and bronchial smooth muscle thickening remains to be fully elucidated, although PDGF has been reported to act as a mitogen for airway smooth muscle cells in culture (Hirst *et al.*, 1992).

The chemokine RANTES (a member of the IL-8 supergene family), expressed following cellular activation of a broad range of cell types (reviewed in Zhang *et al.*, 1994) including platelets (Kameyoshi *et al.*, 1992), is a potent chemoattractant for monocytes, T lymphocytes (Schall *et al.*, 1990) and basophils (Bischoff *et al.*, 1993). In addition, RANTES is a chemoattractant for eosinophils purified from both normal and atopic donors (Kameyoshi *et al.*, 1992; Rot *et al.*, 1992; Alam *et al.*, 1993), with a similar efficacy to the most potent known eosinophil chemoattractant C5a (Rot *et al.*, 1992). RANTES is able to activate purified eosinophils; it induces the release of eosinophil cationic protein, stimulates the respiratory burst, causes cells to adopt a hypodense phenotype and increases their expression of the cell surface adhesion molecule Mac-1 (CD11b/CD18) (Rot *et al.*, 1992; Alam *et al.*, 1993). An inflammatory infiltrate composed predominantly of eosinophils and monocytes was observed following the intradermal injection of rhRANTES into dogs (Meurer *et al.*, 1993). In addition, RANTES has been shown to release histamine from basophils (Kuna *et al.*, 1992).

Following platelet stimulation and activation, products of the metabolism of membrane arachidonic acid (AA) are synthesized via the enzymes cyclo-oxygenase and lipoxygenase, many of which may contribute to the allergic response. Thromboxane A_2 (TXA_2) and prostaglandin $F_{2\alpha}$ ($PGF_{2\alpha}$) are potent vasoconstrictors and bronchial smooth muscle spasmogens, whereas PGF_2 is a vasodilator and inducer/modulator of pain and fever. It has been suggested that $PGF_{2\alpha}$ may cause heightened reflex bronchoconstriction by sensitizing nerve endings in the airway (O'Byrne *et al.*, 1984). 12-Hydroxyeicosatetraenoic acid (12-HETE) has been shown to exert chemotactic activity towards eosinophils (Goetzl *et al.*, 1977). A recent study in guinea pigs has demonstrated that intravenous administration of the stable metabolite of $PGF_{2\alpha}$, 13,14-dihydro-15-keto-$PGF_{2\alpha}$, induced airway hyperresponsiveness to histamine which was mediated by TXA_2, as shown by inhibition of the response with the TXA_2 antagonists ONO-NT-126 and ONO-8809 (Kurasawa *et al.*, 1994).

Platelets and PMN have been shown to co-operate in processing AA or AA-derived intermediate metabolites into biologically active substances (Marcus, 1990). In the presence of activated platelets, leucocytes can produce increased amounts of leukotrienes due to the ability of platelet 12-hydroperoxyeicosatetraenoic acid (12-HPETE) to stimulate leucocyte 5-lipoxygenase (Maclouf *et al.*, 1982). Neutrophils can utilize AA from stimulated platelets for the synthesis of 5-HETE and leukotriene B_4 (LTB_4) (Marcus *et al.*, 1982), a mediator with a wide pro-inflammatory profile. PAF can also stimulate the synthesis of LTB_4 from these cells (Lin *et al.*, 1982). Conversely, platelets may produce LTC_4 from LTA_4 synthesized by leucocytes via glutathione-*S*-transferase (Maclouf & Murphy, 1988), a powerful bronchial smooth muscle constrictor and proposed mediator of allergic asthma (reviewed in Piacentini & Kaliner, 1991).

Human PMN stimulated *in vitro* by several specific agonists are able to activate co-incubated platelets, inducing aggregation, cytoplasmic Ca^{2+} increase and TXA_2 production (Chignard *et al.*, 1986; Del Maschio *et al.*, 1990). The major platelet activator released by PMN in this system appears to be cathepsin G, a neutral serine protease released from azurophilic granules of activated PMN (Evangelista *et al.*, 1991). TXB_2 production, however, is the result of transcellular metabolism of AA between activated PMN and cathepsin G-stimulated platelets, where platelets use PMN-derived unmetabolized AA to synthesize TXB_2 (Maugeri *et al.*, 1992). Cathepsin G released from activated PMN induces expression of P-selectin on platelet membranes, which modulates cell–cell contact and transcellular metabolism of AA (Maugeri *et al.*, 1994).

Both neutrophils and platelets can liberate PAF from membrane phospholipids in modest amounts in response to activation stimuli (Chignard *et al.*, 1980). The presence, however, of a small number of platelets in a suspension of neutrophils results in the generation of significantly increased amounts of PAF, far in excess of that predicted from the individual cell types (Coeffier *et al.*, 1984). PAF is an extremely potent inflammatory agent and has been implicated as a mediator of inflammation and asthma (reviewed in Page, 1988).

Platelet-membrane proteins

Platelet-surface glycoproteins play a primary role in the adhesion of platelets to exposed subendothelial matrix proteins, interaction with ligands such as collagen and thrombin, and exposure of fibrinogen receptors to facilitate aggregation (reviewed in Tuffin, 1991; Roth, 1992). Several glycoproteins of the integrin superfamily of adhesion receptors are present on the plasma membrane (reviewed in Parmentier *et al.*, 1990). Platelets (and endothelial cells) express an adhesion protein of the selectin family (P-selectin, GMP-140, PADGEM, CD62) following degranulation which permits the interaction of platelets with leucocytes (Parmentier *et al.*, 1990).

The transmembrane 4 superfamily (TM4SF) of membrane proteins, to date, comprises 15 members that are variously expressed on leucocytes and a variety of other mammalian tissues (reviewed in Wright & Tomlinson, 1994). The precise biochemical function of the TM4SF is not yet clear; however, a role in the regulation of cell development, proliferation, activation and motility is suggested from the available data (Wright & Tomlinson, 1994). Expression of CD9 antigen has been described on platelets and functional data suggests a role in signal transduction and cell adhesion. CD63 is expressed on activated platelets and on lysosomal and dense granule membranes in resting platelets. A role of this molecule in cell adhesion of platelets and endothelial cells has been suggested (summarized in Wright & Tomlinson, 1994).

Platelets possess a glycoprotein receptor for the third component of complement (C3b) which resembles that located on mononuclear cells (Yu *et al.*, 1986), and Fc receptors for both IgG and IgE antibodies (Rosenfeld *et al.*, 1985; Joseph *et al.*, 1986). Human platelets can bind IgE *in vitro* and cross-linking of surface-bound IgE with anti-IgE or the specific antigens induces platelet activation and secretion. A specific receptor for the Fc fragment of IgE (FcεRII) has been demonstrated on the platelet membrane which is of low affinity (10^{-7} M) compared with that found on mast cell or basophil surfaces (FcεRI) (10^{-9} M) (Joseph *et al.*, 1986), but of comparable affinity to the IgE receptor located on other inflammatory cell types such as alveolar macrophages and eosinophils (Capron *et al.*, 1986). Only a small number (20–30%) of platelets from normal individuals bind IgE, but more than 50% of the platelets from patients with aspirin-induced asthma, allergic patients and patients with parasitic diseases bind IgE (Maccia *et al.*, 1977; Joseph *et al.*, 1983, 1986).

The physiological relevance of the platelet IgE receptor may be associated with a mechanism for aiding the removal of parasitic infections, as the passive transfer of platelets bearing IgE receptors toward schistosomes to naive rats can protect these animals from parasitic challenge (Bout *et al.*, 1986). The platelet IgE receptor does not appear to be associated in any way with the formation of aggregates, but is linked with the ability of platelets to mount a reaginic antibody-dependent cytotoxic response against helminth parasites, such as *Shistosoma mansoni*, through oxidative killing (Capron *et al.*, 1986).

Platelet activation

A distinction may exist between the mechanism of platelet activation resulting in the generation of free radicals and that resulting in degranulation. Platelets that release free radicals do not aggregate and platelet aggregation itself will inhibit any subsequent free radical release (Page, 1989). This type of activation can be elicited by a range of stimuli thought to be involved in the inflammatory response, including C-reactive protein (Bout *et al.*, 1986), substance P (Damonneville *et al.*, 1990), the complement-derived peptides C3b and C5b-C9, the eosinophil-specific major basic protein (MBP) (Rohrbach *et al.*, 1990), and the cytokines, interferon-γ (IFN-γ) (Pancre *et al.*, 1988) and tumour necrosis factor-α (TNF-α) (Damonneville *et al.*, 1990). Anti-allergic compounds such as disodium cromoglycate (Tsicopoulos *et al.*, 1988) and nedocromil sodium (Thorel *et al.*, 1988) inhibit IgE-dependent release of free radicals from platelets, yet these drugs are ineffective against classical platelet aggregation (Lewis *et al.*, 1984). Furthermore, the therapeutic efficacy of certain antiparasitic drugs such as diethylcarbamazine may, to some extent, be related to their ability to generate free radicals from platelets (Cesbron *et al.*, 1987).

It has been shown that a suppressive lymphokine released by activated mononuclear cells can inhibit the production of cytotoxic free radicals by IgE-coated platelets (Pancre *et al.*, 1986). This lymphokine has been termed 'platelet activity suppressive lymphokine' (PASL), a heat-stable molecule of molecular weight 15 000–20 000 and a product of a T-lymphocyte subpopulation bearing the CD8+ antigen (Pancre *et al.*, 1986). Furthermore, CD4+/CD8– lymphocytes have been observed to release factors, including IFN-γ which can induce cytotoxic activity in normal platelets (Pancre *et al.*, 1987).

Platelets and allergic asthma

Asthma is characterized clinically by hyperresponsiveness of tracheobronchial smooth muscle to various spasmogens, resulting in the widespread narrowing of the airways. In recent years it has been recognized that asthma is a chronic inflammatory disease associated pathologically with eosinophil infiltration and damaged airway epithelium. These underlying inflammatory events are considered important in the development of the enhanced airway responsiveness observed in asthmatic individuals. Airway inflammation is a complex event triggered by inflammatory stimuli interacting with primary effector cells resident in the airway; numerous effector cell types have been implicated. The release of inflammatory mediators from these cells may recruit and activate other effector cells, thus augmenting the inflammatory process. Evidence now exists in support of a role for the platelet in the pathogenesis of asthma—acting as an inflammatory cell, releasing spasmogens and/or interacting with other cell types.

PAF has been suggested as a mediator of asthma, as it can reproduce many of the characteristic features of the disease, including bronchospasm, mucus hypersecretion, increased vascular permeability and increased airway responsiveness, both in experimental animals and humans (reviewed in Page, 1988). PAF may provide the link between platelet activation and allergic asthma (Gresele, 1991), as evidence suggests that the ability of PAF to induce airway hyperresponsiveness and eosinophil infiltration may involve the activation of platelets (Lellouch-Tubiana *et al.*, 1988; Coyle *et al.*, 1990b). The putative interaction between PAF and platelets in the development of airway tissue damage and airway hyperresponsiveness is summarized in Fig. 12.2. The activation of platelets by PAF results in the release of a range of chemotactic factors which attract eosinophils. Once activated, eosinophils are capable of releasing cytotoxic agents such as major basic protein (MBP), eosinophil peroxidase (EPO), eosinophil cationic protein (ECP) and oxygen free radicals (O_2^-), which have been implicated in the pathogenesis of asthma (Frigas & Gleich, 1986).

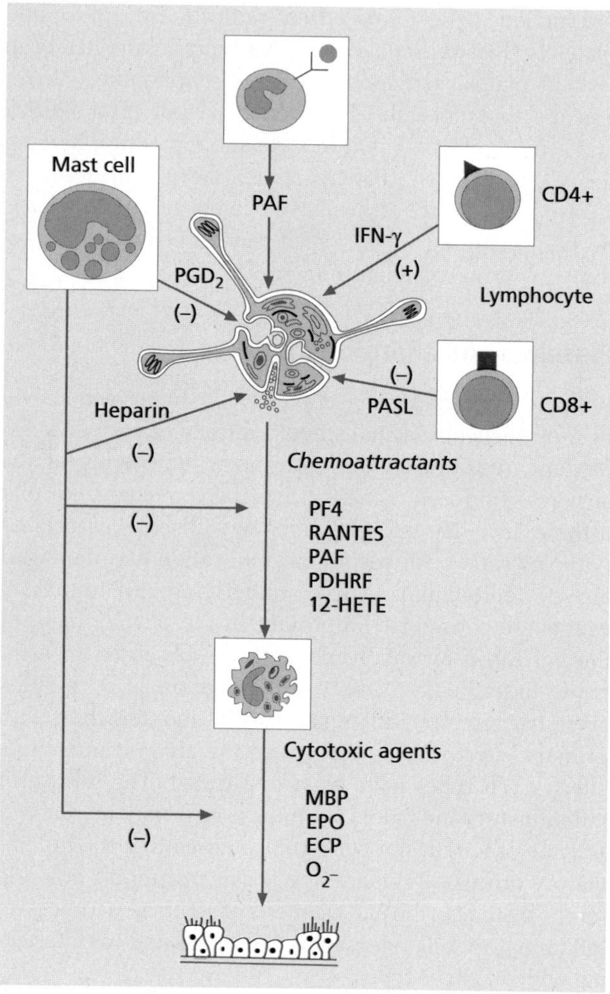

Fig. 12.2 Schematic representation of the possible relationship between PAF release from inflammatory cells, the activation of platelets and recruitment of eosinophils. The resultant release of cytotoxic materials may contribute to the tissue damage underlying airway hyperresponsiveness. By releasing mediators, other inflammatory cells are known to modulate platelet responsiveness.

PAF is released from a number of inflammatory cells in the lung, including alveolar macrophages, eosinophils and neutrophils. Human alveolar macrophages and eosinophils are rich sources of PAF, are present in the airways of asthmatics and are activated following antigen provocation (Metzger *et al.*, 1987; Beasley *et al.*, 1989). Eosinophils obtained from hypereosinophilic patients (including asthmatics) have a greatly enhanced capacity to generate PAF (Lee *et al.*, 1984). In addition, platelets (Chignard *et al.*, 1980; Benveniste *et al.*, 1982a, 1982b) and vascular endothelial cells (Camussi *et al.*, 1983) have been shown to release PAF. All these factors may play a role in the pathophysiology of asthma. Furthermore, isolated lungs from sensitized guinea pigs have been shown to release PAF when challenged with antigen (Fitzgerald *et al.*, 1986).

Animal evidence

Platelets have been observed to undergo diapedesis into the extravascular tissue of the lungs of guinea pigs following challenge with antigen or PAF (Lellouch-Tubiana *et al.*, 1985). The extravasated platelets have been observed in close proximity to bronchial smooth muscle and to infiltrating eosinophils. Treatment of experimental animals with other platelet agonists such as ADP, whilst inducing platelet aggregation in the pulmonary vasculature, does not elicit extravascular diapedesis of platelets and eosinophils (Lellouch-Tubiana *et al.*, 1985), suggesting a possible link between the two cell types. Platelets have also been detected in bronchoalveolar lavage (BAL) fluid obtained from rabbits undergoing late-onset airways obstruction following antigen challenge (Metzger *et al.*, 1987). Further evidence that platelets are involved in experimental allergic responses is the detection of markers of platelet activation, such as PF_4, in plasma following antigen challenge (McManus *et al.*, 1979).

In several animal species, the intravenous injection of selected platelet agonists induces thrombocytopenia associated with bronchospasm (Vargaftig & Lefort, 1979). This also occurs in sensitized animals challenged with specific antigen, which appears to be a platelet-dependent phenomenon since platelet depletion protects against the lethal consequences of the antigen provocation (Pinckard *et al.*, 1977; Halonen *et al.*, 1981). In isolated human bronchus, platelet depletion prevents smooth muscle contraction induced by PAF (Schellenberg *et al.*, 1983). Similarly, the intravenous administration of PAF into guinea pigs induces bronchospasm associated with the accumulation of platelets in the lung (Page *et al.*, 1984); the bronchospasm is platelet dependent since platelet depletion abolishes the response (Vargaftig *et al.*, 1980). Under these circumstances platelet aggregates have been located histologically (Pinckard *et al.*, 1977; Dewar *et al.*, 1984) and by the use of radiolabelled platelets (Page *et al.*, 1984) within the pulmonary vasculature. It has been suggested that this bronchoconstrictor response is reflex in origin; however, peak changes in lung function largely precede detectable accumulation of ^{111}In-labelled platelets in the pulmonary vasculature (Page *et al.*, 1984). Furthermore, several classes of drugs, including the anti-asthma drugs ketotifen and theophylline, inhibit the platelet release reaction *in vitro* and platelet-dependent bronchospasm *in vivo*, but do not affect platelet accumulation within the lung (Page *et al.*, 1985). These observations indicate that platelet-derived mediators contribute to the bronchospasm as well as, or instead of, physical obstruction of pulmonary vessels by platelet aggregates. The dissociation of platelet release and aggregation *in vivo* led to the hypothesis that platelet activation plays a central role in the pathogenesis of asthma (Morley *et al.*, 1984). Furthermore, the pharmacological inhibition of the platelet-release reaction (Chignard *et al.*, 1982; Vargaftig *et al.*, 1982) or TXA_2 production (Chung *et al.*, 1986) can abrogate the bronchospasm, suggesting the response is related to the release of bronchoactive agents from the platelets rather than the retention of platelet aggregates *per se*.

The late-onset response to antigen challenge in rabbits may be abrogated by prior treatment with a selective antiplatelet antiserum (Coyle *et al.*, 1990a). This phenomenon may be attributable to an interaction between platelets and eosinophils, as the antigen-induced pulmonary eosinophil infiltration is inhibited in thrombocytopenic animals (Coyle *et al.*, 1990a). In the guinea pig and rabbit, PAF-induced airway hyperresponsiveness is platelet dependent, since it can be abrogated by rendering animals selectively thrombocytopenic by the intravenous administration of a specific lytic antiplatelet antiserum (Mazzoni *et al.*, 1985; Coyle *et al.*, 1990b). Activation of platelets by PAF differs from activation by other agonists, since ADP, collagen, thrombin or the TXA_2 mimetic U46619, in amounts sufficient to cause comparable pulmonary platelet accumulation *in vivo*, do not induce airway hyperresponsiveness (Sanjar *et al.*, 1989; Smith *et al.*, 1989). Therefore, as with the bronchoconstrictor response, the pulmonary retention of platelets is not the central cause of airway hyperresponsiveness.

A factor released from platelets has been reported to induce airway hyperreactivity (platelet-derived hyperreactivity factor (PDHF)) (Sanjar *et al.*, 1989). PAF injected into thrombocytopenic guinea pigs does not induce an acute bronchoconstrictor response nor enhance airway responsiveness. However, in platelet-depleted guinea pigs, the supernatant obtained from normal guinea pig platelet-rich plasma (PRP) incubated with PAF, induced airway hyperresponsiveness (Sanjar *et al.*, 1989). The generation of PDHF was inhibited by prior incubation of PRP with the stable prostacyclin mimetic iloprost. The secretion or formation of this mediator of hyperresponsiveness appears to be PAF specific, as neither platelet disruption nor activation of platelets with ADP induced its production. The chemical nature of this material remains as yet unidentified. Ketotifen and prednisolone have been shown to inhibit the airway hyperresponsiveness induced by PAF-stimulated platelet supernatants, whereas cromoglycate and aminophylline were without effect (Morley *et al.*, 1989). Similarly, when ketotifen or prednisolone were incubated with PRP prior to the addition of PAF, the injection of supernatants into thrombocytopenic guinea pigs resulted in reduced airway hyperresponsiveness (Morley *et al.*, 1989). In addition, human PDHRF has been shown to induce airway hyperresponsiveness as well as selective pulmonary eosinophil infiltration in allergic rabbits (Fisher *et al.*, 1990; Metzger *et al.*, 1990).

Eosinophils and their products such as MBP have been implicated in the pathogenesis of asthma (Frigas & Gleich, 1986). Platelet depletion has been shown to reduce PAF and antigen-induced eosinophil infiltration into the lungs of experimental animals (Lellouch-Tubiana *et al.*, 1988; Coyle *et al.*, 1990a, 1990b), suggesting a central role for platelets in this response. This finding may have clinical relevance where thromboembolic diseases are often associated with the hypereosinophilic syndrome and patients with eosinophilia have coagulation abnormalities (Elouaer-Blanc *et al.*, 1985). The mechanism by which platelets attract eosinophils into the lung may be via the release of PF_4, which is a powerful eosinophil chemoattractant (Chihara *et al.*, 1988). Both platelet depletion and treatment with the PAF antagonist BN 52021 have been shown to inhibit antigen-induced late-onset airways obstruction, airway hyperresponsiveness and eosinophil infiltration in experimental animals (Coyle *et al.*, 1988; Metzger *et al.*, 1988; Smith *et al.*, 1988; Coyle *et al.*, 1989, 1990a). These findings suggest that antigen-induced release of PAF may play a role in the platelet activation necessary to initiate the eosinophil infiltration into the airways which, in turn, contributes to airway hyperresponsiveness.

Thrombin activation, as evidenced by the presence of fibrinopeptide A, has been described in early- and late-phase allergic responses (Metzger *et al.*, 1983) and may therefore activate platelets during allergen-induced responses. Further evidence in favour of the platelet as an important effector cell in asthma has been provided in *in vitro* studies where platelets potentiate mucous glycoprotein release from tracheal submucosal glands induced by PAF (Sasaki *et al.*, 1989).

Clinical evidence

A number of clinical studies have demonstrated platelet activation in diseases where there is activation of the allergic response, although such diseases are not normally associated with thrombosis. Platelets from asthmatics have been shown to behave abnormally *in vitro*, lacking the second wave of aggregation (Fishel & Zwemer, 1970; Solinger *et al.*, 1973; Maccia *et al.*, 1977; Thompson *et al.*, 1984) or defective release of platelet 5-HT, PF_4 (Maccia *et al.*, 1977) and platelet nucleotides (D'Souza & Glueck, 1977) following stimulation with platelet agonists. These *in vitro* abnormalities are suggestive of overstimulation *in vivo* (Harker *et al.*, 1980).

In asthmatic patients the uptake of 5-HT by platelets has been shown to be reduced, possibly due to exposure of the cells to an increased concentration of this amine (Malmgren *et al.*, 1982). Increased plasma levels of 5-HT have been reported in asthmatics (Bakulin & Joffe, 1979), as well as elevated resting levels of platelet cytoplasmic Ca^{2+} and inositol triphosphate production (Block *et al.*, 1990), findings suggestive of *in vivo* platelet stimulation.

Thrombocytopenia was first reported to accompany asthmatic attacks in 1955 (Storck *et al.*, 1955). Platelet activation *in vivo* during provoked or spontaneous asthmatic attacks has also been shown by the detection of circulating platelet aggregates (Gresele *et al.*, 1982, 1987) and activated platelets in the circulation (Traietti *et al.*, 1984). A number of studies have demonstrated elevated plasma levels of PF_4 and β-TG associated with bronchoconstriction induced by antigen or exercise (Knauer *et al.*, 1981; Gresele *et al.*, 1982, 1985, 1987; Toga *et al.*, 1984; Johnson *et al.*, 1986). Release of these platelet-derived markers was not observed following comparable bronchoconstriction induced by methacholine, suggesting that platelet activation occurs as a consequence of the allergic reaction rather than of the bronchoconstriction.

Evidence of platelet activation has also been reported during exacerbations of nocturnal asthma (Morrison *et al.*, 1991; Gresele *et al.*, 1993) (Fig. 12.3). In another study, increased levels of PF_4 and β-TG have been demonstrated in BAL fluid following antigen challenge in asthmatic subjects (Averill *et al.*, 1992). Platelet markers were significantly elevated during the late inflammatory response to antigen and were significantly correlated with elevations in albumin, eosinophil granule proteins and inflammatory prostanoids (PGE_2 and $PGF_{2\alpha}$). A study investigating the possible involvement of platelets under three different conditions (chronic asthma, bronchial provocation inhaling house dust mite, and status asthmaticus), suggested that platelet activation is sometimes provoked in asthma, but plasma levels of α-derived proteins did not reflect the intensity or severity of asthma (Yamamoto *et al.*, 1993). The authors of this study suggested that PAF is the likely mediator responsible for the platelet activation (Yamamoto *et al.*, 1993).

Both urinary TXB_2 (stable metabolite of TXA_2) (Lupinetti *et al.*, 1989) and plasma 13,14-dihydro-15-keto-

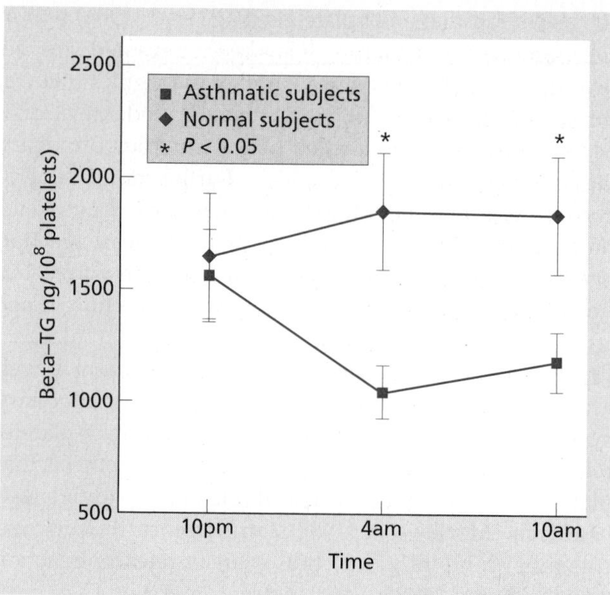

Fig. 12.3 Daily pattern of intraplatelet levels of β- thromboglobulin (β-TG) (mean ± SEM) in asthmatic and normal subjects. A significant difference was observed between asthmatic and control subjects (*$P < 0.05$). (From Gresele *et al.*, 1993.)

$PGF_{2\alpha}$ (stable metabolite of $PGF_{2\alpha}$) (Green *et al.*, 1974) have been shown to increase following bronchial allergen challenge in humans, and in children plasma levels of 13,14-dihydro-15-keto-$PGF_{2\alpha}$ were markedly elevated during asthma attacks (Skona *et al.*, 1988).

Evidence of platelet activation has not been consistently observed (Greer *et al.*, 1984, 1985; Durham *et al.*, 1985; Shephard *et al.*, 1985; Hemmendinger *et al.*, 1989). In other studies pulmonary platelet sequestration was not found to follow antigen challenge in asthmatic volunteers (Ind *et al.*, 1985; Hemmendinger *et al.*, 1989). However, numerous other clinical observations support the proposed role of platelets in asthma. In lung tissue removed at autopsy from patients dying from status asthmaticus, abnormal megakaryocytes have been observed in abundance (Slater *et al.*, 1985; Martin *et al.*, 1987), suggesting a potential abnormality in this system. Platelet survival time in atopic asthmatics is severely shortened, a finding which indicates continuous cell activation (Taytard *et al.*, 1986). Shortened platelet regeneration time, an index of *in vivo* platelet activation associated with accelerated platelet consumption (i.e. increased platelet turnover) (Harker, 1978) has been reported in asthmatics undergoing acute asthma attacks (Gresele *et al.*, 1987), and increased bleeding time has been observed in a group of atopic asthmatics (Szczecklik *et al.*, 1986). In addition, altered responsiveness of platelets from allergic patients has been observed by numerous investigators (reviewed by Gresele *et al.*, 1987), the incidence of which was greatest in patients presenting with high serum IgE titres (Maccia *et al.*, 1977). Furthermore, platelet size (Audera *et al.*, 1988), platelet count and platelet mass (Szczeklik *et al.*, 1986) have been found to be increased in asthmatics.

Accumulated platelets have been observed in the lung microvasculature of patients undergoing bronchial provocation with allergen (Beasley *et al.*, 1989) and have also been detected by electron microscopy in BAL fluid obtained from asthmatics undergoing late-onset airways obstruction following antigen provocation (Metzger *et al.*, 1987). The extravascular platelets in this clinical situation were observed in close association with other inflammatory cells such as the eosinophil (Metzger *et al.*, 1987). In addition, platelets have been observed undergoing diapedesis in sections biopsied from asthmatics (Fig. 12.4) (Page, 1993). Subepithelial extravasation of platelets together with fibrinous material have been observed at sites of denuded epithelium in bronchial biopsies from symptomatic asthmatics (Jeffery *et al.*, 1989). Furthermore, platelets from asthmatic subjects have been shown to migrate *in vitro* in response to antigen, possibly by interaction with platelet-bound antigen-specific IgE (Zhang *et al.*, 1993).

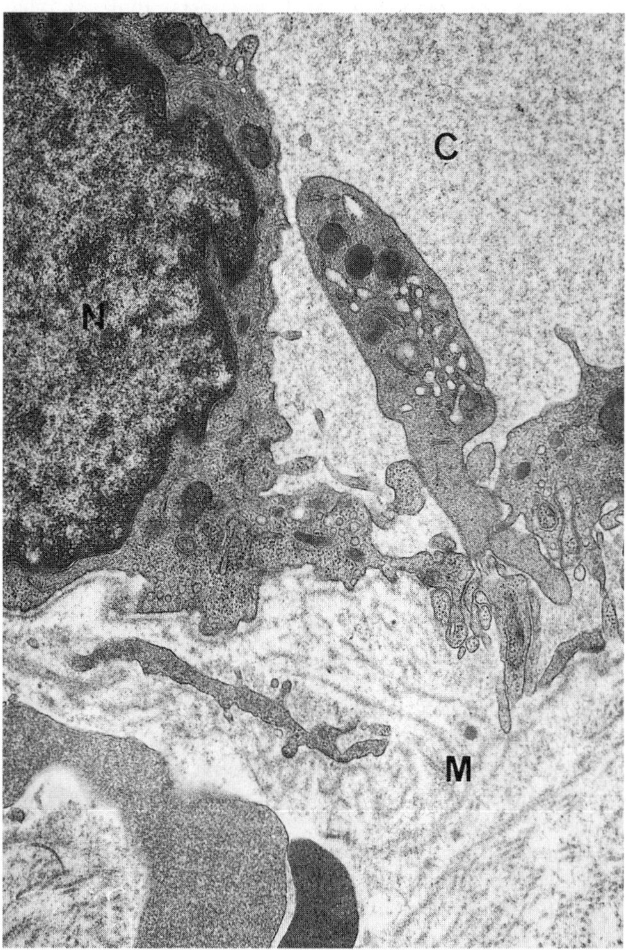

Fig. 12.4 Transmission electron micrograph of a bronchial vessel and an intravascular platelet passing between two adjoining endothelial cells. Endothelial cell nucleus (N), capillary lumen (C) and bronchial mucosa (M) in a biopsy from a subject with mild atopic asthma (glutaraldehyde and osmium tetroxide : uranyl acetate and lead citrate, ×21 600. (Courtesy of Dr P.K. Jeffery, National Heart & Lung Institute, London.)

The fate of platelets in the circulation of asthmatics is unknown, although overt trapping in the pulmonary vasculature is not a feature of either stable asthmatics or those undergoing bronchoconstriction (Gresele *et al.*, 1987).

Therapeutic perspectives

Animal studies have shown that several selective, but structurally unrelated, PAF antagonists inhibit various aspects of asthma pathophysiology, including antigen-induced bronchoconstriction, late-phase response, airway hyperresponsiveness, oedema formation, mucus hypersecretion and pulmonary eosinophil infiltration (reviewed in Heuer, 1992). Pretreatment with BN 52063 has been shown to attenuate the response to PAF in the skin of normal subjects (Chung *et al.*, 1987) and to antigen-induced cutaneous responses in atopic subjects (Roberts *et al.*, 1988b). BN 52063 has also been shown to reduce the bronchoconstrictor response to inhaled PAF in normal volunteers (Roberts *et al.*, 1988a), wherease WEB 2086 (Adamus *et al.*, 1990) and UK-74,505 (O'Connor *et al.*, 1991) completely abolished the response. Furthermore, BN 52063 (Guinot *et al.*, 1987) and BN 52021 (Hsieh, 1991) have been shown to inhibit the immediate bronchoconstrictor response to inhaled allergen, and BN 52063 has been shown to inhibit the platelet activation accompanying exercise-induced bronchoconstriction in asthmatic subjects (Wilkens *et al.*, 1990) (Fig. 12.5). These results suggest that the release of PAF may be central to the platelet activation accompanying exercise-induced bronchoconstriction, as has been suggested in nocturnal attacks of asthma (Gresele *et al.*, 1993). Findings with UK-74,505, the most potent PAF antagonist yet studied in humans (Kuitert *et al.*, 1993), confirm preliminary reports of WEB 2086 (Freitag *et al.*, 1991) and MK-287 (Bel *et al.*, 1991) which have shown no effect on the early or late response to inhaled allergen in mild atopic asthmatics or on the subsequent airway hyperresponsiveness. Treatment with WEB 2086 did not reduce the requirement for inhaled corticosteroid in atopic asthmatics (Spence *et al.*, 1994), although another recent study with WEB 2086 did show a clinical effect in allergic asthmatic patients (Tamura *et al.*, 1994).

The lack of effect of these PAF antagonists in humans, despite achieving plasma levels capable of inhibiting *ex vivo* platelet aggregation induced by PAF, may be due to a

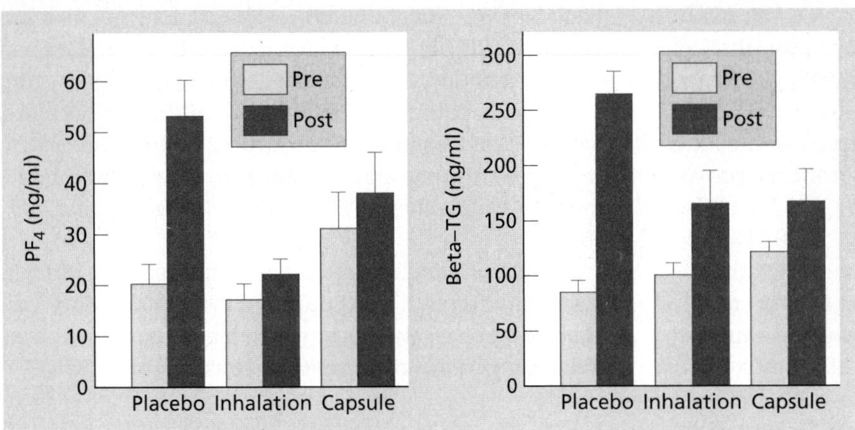

Fig. 12.5 Effects of BN 52063 on the plasma concentrations of platelet factor 4 (PF_4) (left) and β-thromboglobulin (β-TG) (right) (mean ± SEM) before (Pre) and 5 min after (Post) exercise challenge. Note the significant inhibition of increase in protein levels and pretreatment with BN 52063 (*$P < 0.05$). (From Wilkens *et al.*, 1990.)

number of reasons. Firstly PAF may not be as important in asthma as previously thought. Secondly, PAF released *in vivo* is a family of related compounds, whereas PAF antagonists have been developed as antagonists to PAF C_{16}. It is possible, therefore, that other PAF homologues may be of biological significance. Thirdly, current PAF antagonists have not been designed to penetrate cells and thus may not interact with intracellular receptors. As the bulk of PAF appears to be retained intracellularly in a variety of cell types (Bratton & Henson, 1989), PAF antagonists may need to be able to enter cells or PAF synthesis may need to be inhibited, rather than antagonism of its extracellular effects (Stewart & Phillips, 1989).

Treatment of atopic asthmatic individuals with anti-asthma drugs such as glucocorticoids and ketotifen has been shown to correct abnormal platelet survival (Taytard *et al.*, 1987). In asthmatic subjects the anti-allergy drug nedocromil sodium has been shown to inhibit platelet activation induced by PAF *ex vivo* (Roth *et al.*, 1993). In a recent study of mild asthmatics in our laboratory, thrombocytopenia was evident 24 hours following antigen challenge. However, after 6 weeks of treatment with low-dose theophylline, circulating platelet numbers remained unaltered following antigen (C.P. Page *et al.*, unpublished data). Therefore, part of the efficacy of these drugs may reside in their ability to restore normal platelet behaviour.

Conclusion

There is overwhelming evidence that platelets are involved and play an active role in primary defence mechanisms such as antibody-dependent cytotoxicity of parasites. Inappropriate activation of this system in allergic patients may contribute to eosinophil infiltration and subsequent damage to the host tissue, resulting in the heightened airway responsiveness characteristic of bronchial asthma. The recent awareness that platelets are capable of interacting with other inflammatory cells opens up new areas of potential ways to influence the allergic inflammatory response, and suggests that platelets should be considered to play a central role in the allergic process.

References

Adamus, W.S., Heuer, H.O., Meade, C.J. & Schilling, J.C. (1990) Inhibitory effects of the new PAF acether antagonist WEB 2086 on pharmacologic changes induced by PAF inhalation in human beings. *Clin. Pharmacol. Ther.*, **47**, 456–62.

Alam, R., Stafford, S., Forsythe, P. *et al.* (1993) RANTES is a chemotactic and activating factor for human eosinophils. *J. Immunol.*, **150**, 3442–8.

Audera, C., Rocklin, R., Vaillancourt, R., Jakubowski, J.A. & Deykin, D. (1988) Altered arachidonic acid metabolism and platelet size in atopic subjects. *Clin. Immunol. Immunopathol.*, **46**, 352–9.

Averill, F.J., Hubbard, W.C., Proud, D., Gleich, G.J. & Liu, M.C. (1992) Platelet activation in the lung after antigen challenge in a model of allergic asthma. *Am. Rev. Resp. Dis.*, **145**, 571–6.

Bakulin, M.P. & Joffe, E.J. (1979) Content of biologically active substances, histamine and serotonin in patients with bronchial asthma. *Teraput. Arkhiv*, **51**, 45–9.

Beasley, R., Roche, W.R., Roberts, J.A. & Holgate, S.T. (1989) Cellular events in the bronchi in mild asthma and after bronchial provocation. *Am. Rev. Resp. Dis.*, **139**, 806–17.

Bel, E.H., De Smet, M., Rossing, T.H., Timmers, M.C., Dijkman, J.H. & Sterk, P.J. (1991) The effect of a specific oral PAF-antagonist, MK-287, on antigen-induced early and late asthmatic reactions in man. *Am. Rev. Resp. Dis.*, **143**, A811.

Benveniste, J., Chignard, M., le Couedic, J.P. & Vargaftig, B.B. (1982a) Biosynthesis of platelet activating factor (PAF-acether). II. Involvement of phospholipase A_2 in the formation of PAF-acether and lyso-PAF-acether from rabbit platelets. *Thromb. Res.*, **25**, 375–85.

Benveniste, J., Roubin, R., Chignard, M. & Jouvin-Marche, E. (1982b) Release of platelet activating factor (PAF-acether) and 2-lyso-PAF-acether from three cell types. *Agents Actions*, **12**, 711–13.

Berk, B.C., Alexander, R.W., Brock, T.A., Gimbrone, M.A. & Webb, R.C. (1986) Vasoconstriction: a new activity for platelet-derived growth factor. *Science*, **232**, 87–90.

Bischoff, S.C., Krieger, M., Brunner, T. *et al.* (1993) RANTES and related chemokines activate human basophil granulocytes through different G protein-coupled receptors. *Eur. J. Immunol.*, **23**, 761–7.

Block, L.H., Imhof, E., Emmons, L.R., Roth, M. & Perruchoud, A.P. (1990) PAF-dependent phosphatidylinositol turnover in platelets: differences between asthmatics and normal individuals. *Respiration*, **57**, 373–8.

Bout, D., Joseph, M., Pontet, M., Vorng, H., Deslee, D. & Capron, A. (1986) Rat resistance to schistomasiasis: platelet-mediated cytotoxicity induced by C-reactive protein. *Science*, **231**, 153–6.

Bratton, D. & Henson, P.M. (1989) Cellular origins of PAF. In: *Platelet Activating Factor and Human Disease* (eds P.J. Barnes, C.P. Page & P.M. Henson), pp. 23–57. Blackwell Scientific Publications, Oxford.

Brindley, L.L., Sweet, J.M. & Goetzl, E.J. (1983) Stimulation of histamine release from human basophils by human platelet factor 4. *J. Clin. Invest.*, **72**, 1218–23.

Camussi, G., Aglietta, M., Malavasi, F. *et al.* (1983) The release of platelet-activating factor from human endothelial cells in culture. *J. Immunol.*, **131**, 2397–403.

Capron, M., Jouault, T., Prin, L. *et al.* (1986) Functional study of a monoclonal antibody to IgE Fc receptor (FceR2) of eosinophils, platelets and macrophages. *J. Exp. Med.*, **164**, 72–89.

Capron, A., Joseph, M., Ameisen, J.-C., Capron, M., Pancre, V. & Auriault, C. (1987) Platelets as effectors in immune and hypersensitivity reactions. *Int. Arch. Allergy Appl. Immunol.*, **82**, 307–12.

Carroll, N., Elliot, J., Morton, A. & James, J. (1993) The structure of large and small airways in nonfatal and fatal asthma. *Am. Rev. Resp. Dis.*, **147**, 405–10.

Cesbron, J.Y., Capron, A., Vargaftig, B.B. *et al.* (1987) Platelets mediate the action of diethylcarbamazine on Microfillariae. *Nature*, **325**, 533–6.

Chignard, M., le Couedic, J.P., Vargaftig, B.B. & Benveniste, J. (1980) Platelet activating factor (PAF-acether) from platelets: effects of aggregating agents. *Brit. J. Haematol.*, **46**, 455–64.

Chignard, M., Selak, M.A. & Smith, J.B. (1986) Direct evidence for the existence of a neutrophil-derived platelet activator (neutrophilin). *Proc. Nat. Acad. Sci. USA*, **83**, 8609–13.

Chignard, M., Wal, F., Lefort, J. & Vargaftig, B.B. (1982) Inhibition by sulphinpyrazone of the platelet-dependent bronchoconstriction due to platelet activating factor (Paf-acether) in the guinea pig. *Eur. J. Pharmacol.*, **78**, 71–9.

Chihara, J., Fukuda, K., Yasuba, H. *et al.* (1988) Platelet factor 4 enhances eosinophil IgG and IgE Fc receptors and has eosinophil chemotactic activity. *Am. Rev. Resp. Dis.*, **137**, A421.

Chung, K.F., Aizawa, H., Leikauf, G.D., Ueki, I.F., Evans, T.W. & Nadel, J.A. (1986) Airway hyperresponsiveness induced by platelet activating factor: role of thromboxane generation. *J. Pharmacol. Exp. Ther.*, **236**, 580–84.

Chung, K.F., Dent, G., McCusker, M., Guinot, P.H., Page, C.P. & Barnes, P.J. (1987) Effect of a ginkgolide mixture (BN 52063) in antagonising skin and platelet responses in atopic subjects. *Lancet*, **ii**, 248–50.

Coeffier, E., Chignard, M., Delautier, D. & Benveniste, J. (1984) Cooperation between platelets and neutrophils for Paf-acether formation. *Fed. Proc.*, **43**, 781.

Coyle, A.J., Ackerman, S.J. & Irvine, C.G. (1993) Cationic proteins induce airway hyperresponsiveness dependent on charge interactions. *Am. Rev. Resp. Dis.*, **147**, 896–900.

Coyle, A.J., Page, C.P., Atkinson, L., Flanagan, R. & Metzger, W.J. (1990a) The requirement for platelets in allergen-induced late asthmatic airway obstruction. *Am. Rev. Resp. Dis.*, **142**, 587–93.

Coyle, A.J., Page, C.P., Atkinson, L., Sjoerdsma, K., Touvay, C. & Metzger, W.J. (1989) Modification of allergen-induced airway obstruction and airway hyperresponsiveness in an allergic rabbit model by the selective platelet-activating factor antagonist, BN 52021. *J. Allergy Clin. Immunol.*, **84**, 960–7.

Coyle, A.J., Spina, D. & Page, C.P. (1990b) PAF-induced bronchial hyperresponsiveness in the rabbit: contribution of platelets and airway smooth muscle. *Brit. J. Pharmacol.*, **101**, 31–8.

Coyle, A.J., Urwin, S.C., Page, C.P., Touvay, C., Villain, B. & Braquet, P. (1988) The effect of the selective PAF antagonist BN 52021 on PAF and antigen-induced bronchial hyperreactivity and eosinophil accumulation. *Eur. J. Pharmacol.*, **148**, 51–8.

Damonneville, M., Monte, D., Auriault, C. *et al.* (1990) The neuropeptide substance P stimulates the effector functions of platelets. *Clin. Exp. Immunol.*, **81**, 346–51.

Del Maschio, A., Evangelista, V., Rajtar, G., Chen, Z.M., Cerletti, C. & de Gaetano, G. (1990) Platelet activation by polymorphonuclear leukocytes exposed to chemotactic agents. *Am. J. Physiol.*, **258**, H870–9.

Deuel, T.F. & Huang, J.S. (1984) Platelet-derived growth factor: structure, function, and roles in normal and transformed cells. *J. Clin. Invest.*, **74**, 669–76.

Deuel, T.F., Senior, R.M., Chang, D., Griffin, G.L., Heinrickson, R.L. & Kaiser, E.T. (1981) Platelet factor 4 is chemotactic for neutrophils and monocytes. *Proc. Nat. Acad. Sci. USA*, **78**, 4584–7.

Deuel, T.F., Senior, R.M., Huang, J.-S. & Griffin, G.L. (1982) Chemotaxis of monocytes and neutrophils to platelet derived growth factor. *J. Clin. Invest.*, **69**, 1046–9.

Dewar, A., Archer, C.B., Paul, W., Page, C.P., MacDonald, D.M. & Morley, J. (1984) Cutaneous and pulmonary histopahological responses to platelet activating factor (Paf-acether) in the guinea pig. *J. Pathol.*, **144**, 25–34.

D'Souza, L. & Glueck, H.I. (1977) Measurement of nucleotide pools in platelets using high pressure liquid chromatography. *Thromb. Haemost.*, **38**, 990–1001.

Durham, S.R., Dawes, J. & Kay, A.B. (1985) Platelets in asthma. *Lancet*, **i**, 36.

Ebina, M., Yaegashi, H., Chiba, R., Takahashi, T., Motomiya, M. & Tanemura, M. (1990) Hyperreactive site in the airway tree of asthmatic patients revealed by thickening of bronchial muscles. *Am. Rev. Resp. Dis.*, **141**, 1327–32.

Elouaer-Blanc, L., Zafrani, E.S., Farcet, J.P., Saint-Marc Girardin, M.F., Mathiue, D. & Dhumeaux, D. (1985) Hepatic vein obstruction in idiopathic hypereosinophilc syndrome. *Arch. Intern. Med.*, **145**, 751–3.

Evangelista, V., Rajtar, G., de Gaetano, G., White, J.G. & Cerletti, C. (1991) Platelet activation by fMLP-stimulated polymorphonuclear leukocytes: the activity of cathepsin G is not prevented by antiproteinases. *Blood*, **77**, 2379–88.

Fishel, C.W. & Zwemer, R.J. (1970) Aggregation of platelets from *B. pertussis*-injected mice and atopically sensitive human individuals. *Fed. Proc.*, **29**, 640.

Fisher, R.H., Henriksen, R.A., Wirfel-Svet, K.L., Atkinson, L.B. & Metzger, W.J. (1990) Bronchial challenge with platelet-derived histamine releasing factor (PD-HRF) supernatant induces prolonged changes in dynamic compliance (Cdyn) and hyperreactivity in the allergic asthmatic rabbit model. *J. Allergy Clin. Immunol.*, **85**, 261.

Fitzgerald, M.F., Moncada, S. & Parente, L. (1986) The anaphylactic release of platelet activating factor from perfused guinea pig lung. *Brit. J. Pharmacol.*, **88**, 149–53.

Freitag, A., Watson, R.M., Matsos, G., Eastwood, C. & O'Byrne, P.M. (1991) The effect of treatment with an oral platelet activating factor antagonist (WEB 2086) on allergen-induced asthmatic responses in human subjects. *Am. Rev. Resp. Dis.*, **143**, A157.

Frigas, E. & Gleich, G.J. (1986) The eosinophil and the pathophysiology of asthma. *J. Allergy Clin. Immunol.*, **77**, 527–37.

Goetzl, E.J., Woods, J.M. & Gorman, R.R. (1977) Stimulation of human eosinophil and neutrophil polymorphonuclear leukocyte chemotaxis and random migration by 12-L-hydroxy-5,8,10,14-eicosatetraenoic acid. *J. Clin. Invest.*, **59**, 179–83.

Green, K., Hedqvist, P. & Svanborg, N. (1974) Increased plasma levels of 15-keto-13,14-dihydro-prostaglandin F2α after allergen-provoked asthma in man. *Lancet*, 1419–21.

Greer, I.A., Winter, J.H., Gaffney, D. *et al.* (1984) Platelets in asthma [letter]. *Lancet*, **i**, 1479.

Greer, I.A., Winter, J.H., Gaffney, D. *et al.* (1985) Platelet activation in allergic asthma [letter]. *Thromb. Haemost.*, **53**, 438.

Gresele, P. (1991) The platelet in asthma. In: *The Platelet in Health and Disease* (ed. C.P. Page), pp. 132–57. Blackwell Scientific Publications, Oxford.

Gresele, P., Dottorini, M., Selli, M.L. *et al.* (1993) Altered platelet function associated with the bronchial hyperresponsiveness accompanying nocturnal asthma. *J. Allergy Clin. Immunol.*, **91**, 894–902.

Gresele, P., Grasselli, S., Todisco, T. & Nenci, G.G. (1985) Platelets and asthma [letter]. *Lancet*, **i**, 347.

Gresele, P., Ribaldi, E., Grasselli, S., Todisco, T. & Nenci, G.G. (1987) Evidence for platelet activation in asthma. In: *Platelets, Platelet Activating Factor and Asthma. Agents and Actions Supplement*, Vol. 21 (eds M. Schmitz-Schumann, G. Menz & C.P. Page), pp. 119–28. Birkhauser Verlag, Basel.

Gresele, P., Todisco, T., Merante, F. & Nenci, G.G. (1982) Platelet activation and allergic asthma [letter]. *New Engl. J. Med.*, **306**, 549.

Guinot, P., Brambilla, C., Duchier, J., Braquet, P. & Bonvoison B. (1987) Effect of BN 52063, a specific PAF-acether antagonist, on bronchial provocation test to allergen in asthmatic patients. A preliminary study. *Prostaglandins*, **34**, 723–31.

Halonen, M., Palmer, J.D., Lohman, C., McManus, L.M. & Pinckard, R.N. (1981) Differential effects of platelet depletion on the physiologic alterations of IgE anaphylaxis and acetyl glyceryl ether phsophorycholine infusion in the rabbit. *Am. Rev. Resp. Dis.*, **124**, 416–21.

Harker. L.A. (1978) Platelet survival time: its measurement and use. *Prog. Hemost. Thromb.*, **4**, 321–47.

Harker, L.A., Malpass, T.W., Branson, H.E., Hessel, E.A. & Slichter, S.J. (1980) Mechanism of abnormal bleeding in patients undergoing cardiopulmonary bypass: aquired transient platelet dysfunction associated with selective alpha granule release. *Blood*, **56**, 824–34.

Hemmendinger, S., Pauli, G., Tenabene, A. *et al.* (1989) Platelet function: aggregation by PAF or sequestration in lung is not modified during immediate or late allergen-induced bronchospasm in man. *J. Allergy Clin. Immunol.*, **83**, 990–6.

Heuer, H.O. (1992) Current status of PAF antagonists. *Clin. Exp. Allergy*, **22**, 980–3.

Hirst, S.J., Barnes, P.J. & Twort, C.H.C. (1992) Quantifying proliferation of cultured human and rabbit airway smooth muscle cells in response to serum and platelet-derived growth factor. *Am. J. Respir. Cell Mol. Biol.*, **7**, 574–81.

Holgate, S.T., Church, M.K. & Polosa, R. (1991) Adenosine: a positive modulator of airway inflammation in asthma. *Ann. NY Acad. Sci.*, **629**, 227–36.

Hsieh, K.-H. (1991) Effects of a PAF antagonist, BN 52021, on the PAF, methacholine-, and allergen-induced bronchoconstriction in asthmatic children. *Chest*, **99**, 877–82.

Ind, P.W., Peters, A.M., Malik, F., Lavender, J.P. & Dollery, C.T. (1985) Pulmonary platelet kinetics in asthma. *Thorax*, **40**, 412–17.

Jeffery, P.K., Wardlaw, A.J., Nelson, F.C., Collins, J.V. & Kay, A.B. (1989) Bronchial biopsies in asthma: an ultrastructural, quantitative study and correlation with hyperreactivity. *Am. Rev. Resp. Dis.*, **140**, 1745–53.

Johnson, C.E., Belfield, P.W., Davis, S., Cooke, N.J., Spencer, A. & Davies, J.A. (1986) Platelet activation during excercise-induced asthma. Effect of prophylaxis with salbutamol. *Thorax*, **42**, 290–4.

Joseph, M., Capron, A., Ameisen, J.-C. *et al.* (1986) The receptor for IgE on blood platelets. *Eur. J. Immunol.*, **16**, 306–12.

Joseph, M., Auriault, C., Capron, A., Vorng, H. & Viens, P. (1983) A new function for platelets: IgE-dependent killing of schistosomes. *Nature*, **303**, 810–12.

Kameyoshi, Y., Dorschner, A., Mallet, A.I., Christophers, E. & Schroder, J.M. (1992) Cytokine RANTES released by thrombin-stimulated platelets is a potent attractant for human eosinophils. *J. Exp. Med.*, **176**, 587–92.

Knauer, K.A., Kagey-Sobotka, A., Adkinson, N.F. & Lichtenstein, L.M. (1984) Platelet augmentation of IgE-dependent histamine release from human basophils and mast cells. *Int. Arch. Allergy Appl. Immunol.*, **74**, 29–35.

Knauer, K.A., Lichtenstein, L.M., Adkinson, N.F. Jr & Fish, J.E. (1981) Platelet activation during antigen-induced airway reactions in asthmatic subjects. *New Engl. J. Med.*, **304**, 1404–6.

Kuitert, L.M., Hui, K.P., Uthayarkumar, S. *et al.* (1993) Effect of the platelet-activating factor antagonist UK-74,505 on the early and late response to allergen. *Am. Rev. Resp. Dis.*, **147**, 82–6.

Kuna, P., Reddigari, S.R., Schall, T.J., Rucinski, D., Viksman, M.Y. & Kaplan, A.P. (1992) RANTES, a monocyte and T lymphocyte chemotactic cytokine releases histamine from human basophils. *J. Immunol.*, **149**, 636–42.

Kurasawa, M., Yodonawa, S., Inamura, H. & Tsukagoshi, H. (1994) Inhibition by thromboxane antagonists of airway hyperresponsiveness to histamine induced by 13,14-dihydro-15-keto-$PGF_{2\alpha}$ in guinea-pigs. *Clin. Exp. Allergy*, **24**, 669–75.

Lee, T., Lenihan, D.J., Malone, B., Roddy, L.L. & Wasserman, S.I. (1984) Increased biosynthesis of platelet activating factor in activated human eosinophils. *J. Biol. Chem.*, **259**, 5526–30.

Lellouch-Tubiana, A., Lefort, J., Pirotzky, E., Vargaftig, B.B. & Pfister, A. (1985) Ultrastructural evidence for extravascular platelet recruitment in the lung upon intravenous injection of platelet activating factor (PAF-acether) to guinea-pigs. *Brit. J. Exp. Pathol.*, **66**, 345–55.

Lellouch-Tubiana, A., Lefort, J., Simon, M.-T., Pfister, A. & Vargaftig, B.B. (1988) Eosinophil recruitment into guinea pig lungs after PAF-acether and allergen administration. *Am. Rev. Resp. Dis.*, **137**, 948–54.

Lewis, A.J., Dervinis, A. & Chang, J. (1984) The effects of antiallergic and bronchodilator drugs on platelet-activating factor (PAF-acether) induced bronchospasm and platelet aggregation. *Agents Actions*, **15**, 636–42.

Lin, A.H., Morton, D.R. & Gorman, R.R. (1982) Acetyl glyceryl ether phosphorylcholine stimulates leukotriene B_4 synthesis in human polymorphonuclear leukocytes. *J. Clin. Invest.*, **70**, 1058–65.

Lowenhaupt, R.W. (1982) Human platelet chemotaxis can be induced by low molecular substance(s) derived from the interaction of plasma and collagen. In: *Interaction of Platelets and Tumour Cells* (eds G.A. Jamieson & A.R. Scipio), pp. 269–80. Alan R. Liss, New York.

Lupinetti, M.D., Sheller, J.R., Catella, F. & Fitzgerald, G.A. (1989) Thromboxane biosynthesis in allergen-induced bronchospasm: evidence for platelet activation during exercise induced asthma. *Am. Rev. Resp. Dis.*, **140**, 932–5.

Maccia, C.A., Gallagher, J.S., Ataman, G., Gluek, H.I., Brooks, S.M. &

Bernstein, I.L. (1977) Platelet thrombopathy in asthmatic patients with elevated immunoglobulin E. *J. Allergy Clin. Immunol.*, **59**, 101–8.

Maclouf, J.A. & Murphy, R.C. (1988) Transcellular metabolism of neutrophil-derived leukotriene A_4 by human platelets. A potential source of leukotriene C_4. *J. Biol. Chem.*, **263**, 174–81.

Maclouf, J., Fruteau de Laclos, B. & Borgeat, P. (1982) Stimulation of leukotriene biosynthesis in human blood leukocytes by platelet derived 12-hydroperoxy-icosatetraenoic acid. *Proc. Nat. Acad. Sci. USA*, **79**, 6042–6.

McManus, L.M., Morley, C.A., Levine, S.P. & Pinckard, R.N. (1979) Platelet activating factor (PAF) induced release of platelet factor 4 (PF_4) *in vitro* during IgE anaphylaxis in the rabbit. *J. Immunol.*, **123**, 2835–41.

Malmgren, R., Grubbstrom, J., Olsson, P., Theorell, H., Tornling, G. & Unge, G. (1982) Defective serotonin (5-HT) transport mechanism in platelets from patients with endogenous and allergic asthma. *Allergy*, **37**, 29–39.

Mannaioni, P.F., Di Bello, M.G., Gambassi, F., Mugnai, L. & Masini, E. (1992) Platelet histamine: characterization of the proaggregatory effect of histamine in human platelets. *Int. Arch. Allergy Appl. Immunol.*, **99**, 394–6.

Mannaioni, P.F., Di Bello, M.G., Raspanti, S., Pistelli, A. & Masini, E. (1993) Histamine release by human platelets. *Agents Actions*, **38**, C203–5.

Marcus, A.J. (1990) Thrombosis and inflammation as multicellular processes: pathophysiologic significance of transcellular metabolism. *Blood*, **76**, 1903–7.

Marcus, A.J., Broekman, M.J., Safier, L.B. *et al.* (1982) Formation of leukotrienes and other hydroxy acids during platelet-neutrophil interactions *in vitro*. *Biochem. Biophys. Res. Commun.*, **109**, 130–7.

Martin, J.F., Slater, D.N. & Trowbridge, E.A. (1987) Platelet production in the lungs. In: *PAF, Platelets and Asthma. Agents and Actions Supplements*, Vol. 21 (eds M. Schmitz-Schumann, G. Menz & C.P. Page), pp. 37–57. Birkhauser Verlag, Basel.

Maugeri, N., Evangelista, V., Piccardoni, P. *et al.* (1992) Transcellular metabolism of arachidonic acid: increased platelet thromboxane generation in the presence of activated polymorphonuclear leukocytes. *Blood*, **80**, 447–51.

Maugeri, N., Evangelista, V., Celardo, A. *et al.* (1994) Polymorphonuclear leukocyte–platelet interaction: role of P-selectin in thromboxane B_2 and leukotrienes C_4 cooperative synthesis. *Thromb. Haemost.*, **72**, 450–6.

Mazzoni, L., Morley, J., Page, C.P. & Sanjar, S. (1985) Induction of airway hyperreactivity by platelet activating factor in the guinea-pig. *J. Physiol.*, **365**, 107P.

Metzger, W.J., Sjoerdsma, K., Richerson, H.B. *et al.* (1987) Platelets in bronchoalveolar lavage from asthmatic patients and allergic rabbits with allergen-induced late phase responses. *Agents Actions*, **21**, 151–9.

Metzger, W.J., Henriksen, R.A., Atkinson, L.B., Wirfel-Svet, K.L. & Fisher, R.H. (1990) Bronchial challenge with platelet derived histamine releasing factor (PD-HRF) induces a pulmonary eosinophilic infiltrate. *J. Allergy Clin. Immunol.*, **85**, 262A.

Metzger, W.J., Henriksen, R.A., Zaleski, T. & Donnelly, A. (1983) Evidence for platelet release and thrombin generation in early and late asthmatic response. *Clin. Res.*, **31**, 164A.

Metzger, W.J., Sjoerdsma, K., Brown, L., Page, C. & Touvay, C. (1988) The late phase asthmatic response in the allergic rabbit: a role for platelet activating factor (PAF) and modification by a PAF antagonist, gingkolide BN 52021. In: *Gingkolides—Chemistry, Biology, Pharmacology and Clinical Perspectives* (eds P. Braquet), pp. 313–31. J.R. Prous Science, Publisher S.A., Barcelona.

Meurer, R., van Riper, G., Feeney, W. *et al.* (1993) Formation of eosinophilic and monocytic intradermal inflammatory sites in the dog by injection of human RANTES but not human monocyte chemoattractant protein 1, human macrophage inflammatory protein 1α, or human interleukin 8. *J. Exp. Med.*, **178**, 1913–21.

Morley, J., Chapman, I.D., Sanjar, S. & Schaeublin, E. (1989) Actions of ketotifen on PAF-induced airway hyperreactivity in the anesthetised guinea-pig. *Brit. J. Pharmacol.*, **96**, 76P.

Morley, J., Sanjar, S. & Page, C.P. (1984) The platelet in asthma. *Lancet*, **i**, 1142–4.

Morrison, J.F.J., Pearson, S.B., Dean, H.G., Craig, I.R. & Bramley, P.N. (1991) Platelet activation in nocturnal asthma. *Thorax*, **46**, 197–200.

Mustafa, S.J., Ali, S. & Metzger, W.J. (1991) Adenosine induced bronchoconstriction in allergic rabbits: evidence for receptor involvement. *Jpn. J. Pharmacol.*, **52**, 113.

Mustard, J.F. & Packham, M.A. (1979) The reaction of the blood to injury. In: *Inflammation, Immunity and Hypersensitivity* (eds H.Z. Movat), p. 61. Harper & Row, New York.

O'Byrne P.M., Aizawa, H., Bethel, R.A., Chung, K.F., Nadel, J.A. & Holtzman, M.J. (1984) Prostaglandin $F_{2\alpha}$ increases responsiveness of pulmonary airways in dogs. *Prostaglandins*, **28**, 537–43.

O'Connor, B.J., Ridge, S.M., Chen-Wordseil, Y.M., Uden, S., Barnes, P.J. & Chung, K.F. (1991) Complete inhibition of airway and neutrophil responses to inhaled platelet activating factor (PAF) by an oral PAF antagonist UK-74,505. *Am. Rev. Resp. Dis.*, **143**, A156.

Orchard, M.A., Kagey-Sobotka, A., Proud, D. & Lichtenstein, L.M. (1986) Basophil histamine release induced by a substance from stimulated human platelets. *J. Immunol.*, **136**, 2240–4.

Page, C.P. (1988) The involvement of platelets in non-thrombotic processes. *Trends Pharmacol. Sci.*, **9**, 66–71.

Page, C.P. (1989) Platelets as inflammatory cells. *Immunopharmacology*, **17**, 51–9.

Page, C.P. (1993) Platelets. In: *Allergy Illustrated* (eds S.T. Holgate & M.K. Church), pp. 8.1–8.8. Gower Medical, London.

Page, C.P., Paul, W. & Morley, J. (1984) Platelets and bronchospasm. *Int. Arch. Allergy Appl. Immunol.*, **74**, 347–50.

Page, C.P., Tomiak, R.H.H., Sanjar, S. & Morley, J. (1985) Suppression of Paf-acether responses: an anti inflammatory effect of anti-asthma drugs. *Agents Actions*, **16**, 33–5.

Pancre, V., Joseph, M., Capron, A. *et al.* (1988) Recombinant human interferon induced increased IgE receptor expression on human platelets. *Eur. J. Immunol.*, **18**, 829–32.

Pancre, V., Auriault, C., Joseph, M., Cesbon, J.Y., Kusnierz, J.P. & Capron, A. (1986) A suppressive lymphokine of platelet cytotoxic functions. *J. Immunol.*, **137**, 585–91.

Pancre, V., Joseph, M., Mazingue, C., Weitzerbin, J. & Capron, A. (1987) Induction of platelet cytoxic functions by lymphokines: role of interferon gamma. *J. Immunol.*, **138**, 4490–5.

Parmentier, S., Kaplan, C., Catimel, B. & McGregor, J.L. (1990) New families of adhesion molecules play a vital role in platelet functions. *Immunol. Today*, **11**, 225–7.

Piacentini, G.L. & Kaliner, M.A. (1991) The potential roles of leukotrienes in bronchial asthma. *Am. Rev. Resp. Dis.*, **143**, S96–9.

Pinckard, R.N., Halonen, M., Palmer, J.D., Butler, C., Shaw, J.O. & Henson, P.M. (1977) Intravascular aggregation and pulmonary sequestration of platelets during IgE induced systemic anaphylaxis in the rabbit: abrogation of lethal anaphylactic shock by platelet depletion. *J. Immunol.*, **119**, 2185–93.

Roberts, N.M., McCusker, M., Chung, K.F. & Barnes, P.J. (1988a) Effect of a PAF antagonist, BN 52063, on PAF-induced bronchoconstriction in normal subjects. *Brit. J. Clin. Pharmacol.*, **26**, 65–72.

Roberts, N.M., Page, C.P., Chung, K.F. & Barnes, P.J. (1988b) Effect of a PAF antagonist, BN 52063, on antigen-induced, acute, and late-onset cutaneous responses in atopic subjects. *J. Allergy Clin. Immunol.*, **82**, 236–41.

Rohrbach, M.S., Wheatley, C.L., Slifman, N.R. & Gleich, G.J. (1990) Activation of platelets by eosinophil granule proteins. *J. Exp. Med.*, **172**, 1271–4.

Rosenfeld, S.J., Looney, R.J., Leddy, J.P., Phipps, D.C., Abraham, G.N. & Anderson, C.L. (1985) Human platelet Fc receptor for immunoglobin G. *J. Clin. Invest.*, **76**, 2317–22.

Rot, A., Krieger, M., Brunner, T., Bischoff, S.C., Schall, T.J. & Dahinden, C.A. (1992) RANTES and macrophage inflammatory protein 1α induce the migration and activation of normal human eosinophil granulocytes. *J. Exp. Med.*, **176**, 1489–95.

Roth, G.J. (1992) Platelets and blood vessels: the adhesion event. *Immunol. Today*, **13**, 100–5.

Roth M., Soler, M., Lefkowitz, H. *et al.* (1993) Inhibition of receptor-mediated platelet activation by nedocromil sodium. *J. Allergy Clin. Immunol.*, **91**, 1217–25.

Sanjar, S., Smith, D. & Kristersson, A. (1989) Incubation of platelets with PAF produces a factor which causes airway hyperreactivity in guinea-pigs. *Brit. J. Pharmacol.*, **96**, 75P.

Sasaki, M., Paul, W., Douglas, G.J. & Page, C.P. (1991) Cutaneous responses to poly-L-lysine in the rabbit. *Brit. J. Pharmacol.*, **104**, 444P.

Sasaki, T., Shimura, S., Ikeda, K., Sasaki, H. & Takishima, T. (1989) Platelet-activating factor increases platelet-dependent glycoconjugate secretion from tracheal submucosal gland. *Am. J. Physiol.*, **257**, L373–8.

Saxena, S.P., Brandes, L.J., Becker, A.B., Simons, K.J., LaBella, F.S. & Gerrard, J.M. (1989) Histamine is an intracellular messenger mediating platelet aggregation. *Science*, **243**, 1596–9.

Schall, T.J., Bacon, K., Toy, K.J. & Goeddel, D.V. (1990) Selective attraction of monocytes and T lymphocytes of the memory phenotype by cytokine RANTES. *Nature*, **347**, 669–71.

Schellenberg, R.R., Walker, B. & Snyder, F. (1983) Platelet-dependent contraction of human bronchus by platelet activating factor. *J. Allergy Clin. Immunol.*, **71**, 145.

Shephard, E.G., Malan, L., Macfarlane, C.M., Mouton, W. & Joubert, J.R. (1985) Lung function and plasma levels of thromboxane B_2, 6-ketoprostaglandin $F_{1\alpha}$ and β-thromboglobulin in antigen-induced asthma before and after indomethacin pretreatment. *Brit. J. Clin. Pharmacol.*, **19**, 459–70.

Skona, D.P., Page, R., Asman, B., Gillen, L. & Fireman, P. (1988) Plasma elevations of histamine and a prostaglandin metabolite in acute asthma. *Am. Rev. Resp. Dis.*, **137**, 1009–14.

Slater, D., Martin, J. & Trowbridge, A. (1985) The platelet in asthma [letter]. *Lancet*, **i**, 110.

Smith, H.R., Henson, P.M., Clay, K.L. & Larsen, G.L. (1988) Effect of the PAF antagonist L-659,989 on the late asthmatic response and increased airway reactivity in the rabbit. *Am. Rev. Resp. Dis.*, **137**, A283.

Smith, D., Sanjar, S. & Morley, J. (1989) Platelet activation and PAF-induced airway hyperreactivity in the anaesthetised guinea-pig. *Brit. J. Pharmacol.*, **96**, 74P.

Solinger, A., Bernstein, I.L. & Glueck, H.I. (1973) The effect of epinephrine on platelet aggregation in normal and atopic subjects. *J. Allergy Clin. Immunol.*, **51**, 29–34.

Spence, D.P.S., Johnston S.L., Calverley, P.M.A. *et al.* (1994) The effect of the orally active platelet-activating factor antagonist WEB 2086 in the treatment of asthma. *Am. J. Resp. Crit. Care Med.*, **149**, 1142–8.

Stewart, A.G. & Phillips, W.A. (1989) Intracellular platelet-activating factor regulates eicosanoid generation in guinea-pig resident peritoneal macrophages. *Brit. J. Pharmacol.*, **98**, 141–8.

Storck, H., Hoigne, R. & Koller, F. (1955) Thrombocytes in allergic reactions. *Int. Arch. Allergy*, **6**, 372–84.

Szczeklik, A., Milner, P.C., Birch, J., Watkins, J. & Martin, J.F. (1986) Prolonged bleeding time, reduced platelet aggregation, altered PAF-acether sensitivity and increased platelet mass are a trait of asthma and hay fever. *Thromb. Haemost.*, **56**, 283–7.

Tamura, G., Takishima, S., Mue, S. *et al.* (1994) Effectiveness of a potent platelet activating factor (PAF) receptor antagonist, WEB-2086, on asthma: a multicenter, double-blind, placebo-controlled study. *Eur. Resp. J.*, **7**, 152s.

Taytard, A., Guenard, H., Vuillemin, L. *et al.* (1986) Platelet kinetics in stable atopic asthmatic patients. *Am. Rev. Resp. Dis.*, **134**, 983–5.

Taytard, A., Vuillemin, L., Guenarg, H., Rio, P., Vergeret, J. & Ducassou, D. (1987) Platelet kinetics in stable asthma patients: effect of ketotifen. *Am. Rev. Resp. Dis.*, **135**, 388A.

Thompson, J.M., Hanson, H., Bilani, M., Turner-Warwick, M. & Morley, J. (1984) Platelets, platelet activating factor and asthma. *Am. Rev. Resp. Dis.*, **129**, A3.

Thorel, T., Joseph, M., Tsicopoulos, A., Tonnel, A.B. & Capron, A. (1988) Inhibition by nedocromil sodium of IgE mediated activation of human mononuclear phagocytes and platelets in allergy. *Int. Arch. Allergy Appl. Immunol.*, **85**, 232–7.

Toga, H., Ohya, N. & Kitagawa, S. (1984) Clinical studies on plasma platelet factor 4 in patients with bronchial asthma. *Jpn. J. Allergy*, **33**, 474–9.

Traietti, P., Marmaggi, S., Dardes, N., Moscatelli, B., Bologna, E. & Vulterini, S. (1984) Circulating platelet activation in respiratory diseases: differences between arterial and venous blood in cold and asthmatic patients. *Respiration*, **46**, 62–3.

Tsicopoulos, A., Lassalle, P., Joseph, M., Tonnel, T., Dessaint, J.P. & Capron, A. (1988) Effect of disodium cromogycate on inflammatory cells bearing the Fc epsilon receptor Type II (FcRII). *Int. J. Immunopharmacol.*, **10**, 227–36.

Tuffin, D.P. (1991) The platelet surface membrane, ultrastructure, receptor binding and function. In: *The Platelet in Health and Disease* (ed. C.P. Page), pp. 10–60. Blackwell Scientific Publications, Oxford.

Tzeng, D.Y., Deuel, T.F., Huang, J.S. & Boehner, R.L. (1985) Platelet-derived growth factor promotes human peripheral monocyte activation. *Blood*, **66**, 179–83.

Vargaftig, B.B. & Lefort, J. (1979) Differential effects of prostacyclin and prostaglandin E_1 on bronchoconstriction and thrombocytopenia during collagen and arachidonate infusions and anaphylactic shock in the guinea pig. *Prostaglandins*, **18**, 519–28.

Vargaftig, B.B., Lefort, J., Chignard, M. & Benveniste, J. (1980) Platelet activating factor induces a platelet-dependent bronchoconstriction unrelated to the formation of prostaglandin derivatives. *Eur. J. Pharmacol.*, **65**, 185–92.

Vargaftig, B.B., Lefort, J., Wal, F., Chignard, M. & Medeiros, M. (1982) Non-steroidal antiinflammatory drugs if combined with antihistamine and antiserotonin agents interfere with the bronchial and platelet effects of 'platelet activating factor' (PAF-acether). *Eur. J. Pharmacol.*, **82**, 121–30.

Wahl, S.M., Hunt, D.A., Wakefield, L.M. *et al.* (1987) Transforming growth factor type *beta* induces monocyte chemotaxis and growth factor production. *Proc. Nat. Acad. Sci. USA*, **63**, 943–5.

Weksler, B. & Coupal, C.E. (1973) Platelet dependent generation of chemotactic activity in serum. *J. Exp. Med.*, **137**, 1419–30.

Weksler, B.B. (1983) Platelets. In: *Inflammation: Basic Principles and Clinical Correlates* (eds J.I. Gallin, I.M. Golgstein & R. Snyderman). Raven, New York.

Wilkens, J.H., Wilkens, H., Uffman, J., Bovers, J., Fabel, H. & Frolich, J.C. (1990) Effects of a PAF-antagonist (BN 52063) on bronchoconstriction and platelet activation during exercise induced asthma. *Brit. J. Clin. Pharmacol.*, **29**, 85–91.

Wright, M.D. & Tomlinson, M.G. (1994) The ins and outs of the transmembrane 4 superfamily. *Immunol. Today*, **15**, 588–94.

Yamamoto, H., Nagata, M., Tabe, K. *et al.* (1993) The evidence of platelet activation in bronchial asthma. *J. Allergy Clin. Immunol.*, **91**, 79–87.

Yu, G.H., Holers, V.M., Seya, T., Ballard, L. & Atkinson, J.P. (1986) Identification of a thrid component of complement-binding glycoprotein of human platelets. *J. Clin. Invest.*, **78**, 494–501.

Zhang, L., Redington, A.E. & Holgate, S.T. (1994) RANTES: a novel mediator of allergic inflammation? *Clin. Exp. Allergy*, **24**, 899–904.

Zhang, X., Selli, M.L., Baglioni, S. *et al.* (1993) Platelets from asthmatic patients migrate *in vitro* in response to allergen stimulation. *Thromb. Haemost.*, **69**, 916.

CHAPTER 13

Macrophages and Dendritic Cells in Allergic Reactions

P.G. Holt

Introduction

It is now evident that qualitative and quantitative aspects of T-cell dependent allergic responses are regulated by cellular interactions occurring at the 'antigen-presentation' step in the T-cell activation process. In the primary response, the principal antigen presenting cells (APC) are dendritic cells (DC), particularly in the respiratory and gastrointestinal tracts, where they form tightly meshed networks at surfaces in contact with the outside environment. For reactivation of secondary responses, particularly in microenvironments in which tissue is chronically inflamed, the APC requirements of T-memory cells are considerably less stringent, and this function can apparently be served to varying degrees, by any cell expressing surface class II major histocompatibility complex (MHC). The latter category can include monocytes, B cells, mesenchymal cells (including airway and intestinal epithelial cells and keratinocytes), and possibly even eosinophils; however, DC remain the most potent APC.

Recent findings from a number of laboratories have demonstrated that the overall efficiency of the T-cell activation process is subject to regulation by the secreted products of adjacent cells, in particular mature tissue macrophages. This regulation potentially occurs at several different levels, including modulation of the functional phenotype of the APC (in particular DC), and modulation of the capacity of antigen-specific T cells to clonally expand subsequent to T-cell receptor (TcR) ligation.

Responses underlying allergic reactions, which predominantly occur in mucosal/epithelial tissue microenvironments rich in both DC and mature macrophages, are prime candidates for this form of cellular regulation. This chapter focuses on the nature of the interactions between these two cell populations, particularly in relation to regulation of allergic responses to aeroallergens.

Macrophages

Macrophages are widely distributed in virtually all tissues, and are a prominent feature of cellular infiltrates at sites of inflammation. These cells are capable of expressing a large range of effector and immunoregulatory functions, and can respond to changes in their local tissue microenvironment via rapid alterations in their functional phenotype. Data from a number of laboratories have implicated macrophages in allergic responses at several different levels, both as mediators of tissue damage in their own right or indirectly through their capacity to activate adjacent effector cells, and also as host-protective 'dampeners' in allergic inflammation.

The discussion below reviews their known properties in the context of allergic reactions at mucosal surfaces, in particular macrophage populations in the respiratory tract, which have been characterized functionally in more detail than in most other tissues.

Distribution

Four discrete macrophage populations have been identified in the respiratory tract, and they are discussed in detail below.

Pulmonary alveolar macrophages

Pulmonary alveolar macrophages (PAM) comprise the

most widely studied macrophage population in the respiratory tract, and is readily accessible for study in experimental animals and humans, via the bronchoalveolar lavage (BAL) technique. This procedure yields in the order of 0.5–1.0 × 10^6 PAM per normal animal even from species as small as the mouse, and this number can increase on a log scale in response to local inflammatory challenge.

The popular conception of these cells is that of the 'pulmonary frontiersman', patrolling the lumenal surfaces of the peripheral lung within the epithelial lining fluid layer, in search of inhaled particulates. This view is challenged by a small number of careful ultrastructural studies, empolying lung tissue rapidly fixed with glutaraldehyde via perfusion through the vascular bed. This procedure fixes the cells efficiently *in situ* without disturbance to PAM/epithelial cell interactions that follow the more common practise of fixation through the airways, and reveals that about 90% of PAM in resting lung tissue of humans and experimental animals are intimately associated with type 1 alveolar epithelial cells, particularly at alveolar–septal junctions (Brain *et al.*, 1984; Parra *et al.*, 1986; Fig. 13.1).

Airway (lumenal) macrophages

A second macrophage population is found in intimate and stable association with the airway epithelial surface (Brain *et al.*, 1984). This population appears to be derived from PAM, and is likely to predominantly comprise effete 'ageing' cells *en route* to clearance via the mucociliary system (Lehnert *et al.*, 1990).

Airway (mucosal) macrophages

A third macrophage population can be clearly seen in connective tissue surrounding the conducting airways (Holt *et al.*, 1988b), and morphologically appear as typical mature tissue macrophages.

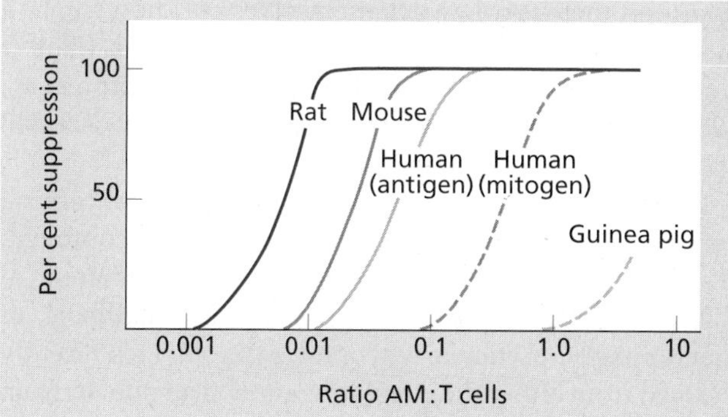

Fig. 13.1 *In vitro* T-cell suppression by alveolar macrophages.

Interstitial macrophages

Lung parenchymal tissues are also rich in macrophages, and these are most prominent at interseptal junctions, below the type 1 alveolar epithelial membrane (Holt & Schon-Hegrad, 1987; Holt *et al.*, 1988b).

Intravascular macrophages

In addition to the populations described above, a further macrophage population has been described in the peripheral lung vascular bed; this does not appear to be part of the marginal monocyte pool, but instead is a resident population of mature macrophages stably associated with the endothelial basement membrane (Warner & Brain, 1986; Winkler, 1989). These cells are not discussed further, as nothing is known with any certainty concerning their functions, but their strategic location suggests a potentially important role in syndromes such as septic shock, as they are clearly capable of phagocytosing particulates (such as bacteria and possibly antigen–antibody complexes) from the circulation. Similarly, they may contribute to the expression of allergic reactivity in the lung via uptake of circulating allergen–antibody complexes, although there is no direct evidence to support this suggestion.

Surface phenotype

Airway mucosal and lung interstitial macrophages in all species examined express a range of surface markers typical of mature mononuclear phagocytes, many of which (such as CD68 and RFD7; Spiteri & Poulter, 1991) are also found on resting PAM. It is noteworthy that PAM do not express certain of the range of surface molecules that are characteristic of mature tissue histiocytes, exemplified by the ED2 marker in the rat (Holt & Schon-Hegrad, 1987; Winkler, 1989), and their overall marker profile appears more closely allied to macrophages from primary lymphoid organs, as opposed to those in peripheral tissues (Bilyk *et al.*, 1988). It is aditionally important to note that resting macrophage populations from lung and airway tissues of humans and experimental animals express few of the surface markers characteristic of monocytes, such as Mac-1 and CD14 (Hance *et al.*, 1985; Bilyk *et al.*, 1988). Surface expression of MHC class II is uncommon on PAM from experimental animals (Holt & Schon-Hegrad, 1987; Bilyk *et al.*, 1988) but not humans (Lipscomb *et al.*, 1986), although (as discussed below) the latter does not necessarily correlate with MHC-dependent antigen presentation activity.

Population dynamics

As PAM are readily accessible via the BAL technique, they have been examined in detail in turnover studies. The overall size of the PAM population remains constant during the steady state. Effete cells are removed to the gastrointestinal tract via the mucociliary elevator (Spritzer *et al.*, 1968), and this is paralleled by traffic of (small numbers of) PAM into the lung interstitium and regional lymph nodes (Corry *et al.*, 1984). The maintenance of this population at a steady level implies the operation of an effective system for rapid replacement of these emigrant PAM.

Until recently, the prevailing view was that this process proceeded in a similar fashion to that described for the majority of peripheral tissues, i.e. recruitment of the majority of 'precursors' from the peripheral blood monocyte pool, supplemented to a small degree by expansion of precursors derived from a local tissue stem cell population (Blussé van Oud Alblas & van Furth, 1979). However, two independent lines of evidence from animal studies have cast doubt on the validity of these assumptions. Firstly, experiments with parabiotic rats (circulations joined via cross-canulation) failed to detect the migration of labelled monocytes from the 'donor' of the pair, into the PAM population of the recipient (Collins & Auclair, 1980; Hance *et al.*, 1985). Secondly, a series of experiments involving the induction of severe monocytopenia with the bone marrow-seeking isotope strontium-89 indicated that interruption of the supply of marrow-derived precursors does not affect the rate of PAM renewal over at least a 30-day period (Sawyer *et al.*, 1982; Oghiso & Kubota, 1986; Sawyer, 1986). Consistent with this finding, monocytopenic human leukaemia patients have been shown to maintain normal numbers of PAM (Golde *et al.*, 1974). These latter data strongly suggest that, in the steady state, PAM renewal proceeds mainly via replication of locally derived precursors. Colony-stimulating factor (CSF)-'sensitive' precursors have been identified within both the PAM and lung interstitial populations (Stanley *et al.*, 1978; Bowden & Adamson, 1980), and constitutive cerebrospinal fluid (CSF) production has been demonstrated in normal lung tissues (Rajavashisth *et al.*, 1987; Troutt & Lee, 1989).

Conversely, when there is local inflammatory stimulation, the contribution of blood monocyte recruitment becomes more significant, and in some circumstances may be the dominant factor in local PAM renewal. These conclusions derive from studies in mice challenged intratracheally with bacillus Calmette-Guérin (BCG) or carbon particles, in which the magnitude and kinetics of the cellular response is markedly attenuated by monocyte depletion (Bowden & Adamson, 1980, 1982; Blussé van Oud Alblas *et al.*, 1983; Evans *et al.*, 1987). In humans, blood monocyte recruitment has been implicated in expansion of PAM populations in a variety of respiratory inflammatory diseases, including asthma (Beasley *et al.*, 1989; Poston *et al.*, 1992) and allergic alveolitis (Hoogsteden *et al.*, 1989); however, increased local proliferation of precursors also appears to play a role in this process, at least in chronic inflammatory lung diseases (Bitterman *et al.*, 1987).

Stimulation of macrophage precursor expansion in the lung is controlled by local production of CSF-1, granulocyte macrophage colony-stimulating factor (GM-CSF) and interleukin-3 (IL-3). The most potent of these factors, CSF-1, is produced mainly by macrophages, particularly in response to stimulation with pro-inflammatory agents such as bacterial lipopolysaccharide (LPS) (Rajavashisth *et al.*, 1987; Kreipe *et al.*, 1990; Wiktor *et al.*, 1990); GM-CSF (which synergizes powerfully with CSF-1) is produced by activated T cells, monocytes and by mesenchymal cells, notably by airway epithelial cells in diseases such as asthma (Sousa *et al.*, 1993); production of IL-3 is restricted to T cells.

Functions of lung macrophage populations

Secretory function(s)

The secretory functions of PAM have been recently reviewed in detail (Sibille & Reynolds, 1990), and a synopsis of their mediator repertoire is given in Table 13.1. This list could be equally applied in a *qualitative* sense to any mononuclear phagocyte population in the lung and/or elsewhere in the body; however, it is becoming clear from the literature that *quantitative* capacity for secretion of individual mediators varies markedly throughout the lifecycle of individual cells as a function of their intrinsic activation/maturation status, and hence extrapolations between macrophage populations in different tissues, or between subpopulations within the same tissue, must be made with caution. In this context, it should be stressed that the only direct functional studies available addressing the secretory functions of lung macrophage populations pertain to PAM, which themselves are known to be a heterogeneous mixture of immature/mature cells (Holt *et al.*, 1982; Shellito & Kaltreider, 1984, 1985; Sandron *et al.*, 1986), and hence must be taken as a very 'broad-brush' approach to a complex problem.

Despite these reservations, recent data concerning certain of these mediators merit individual comment. IL-1 can illustrate some of the complexities inherent in this area. Production of this cytokine is a hallmark of macrophages, particularly 'young' macrophages recently derived from either the circulating monocyte pool or from locally replicated tissue precursors. However, several studies have demonstrated that resident PAM (including

Table 13.1 Alveolar macrophage secretory activity.

Growth factors and cytokines
Fibroblast growth factor
IL-1, IL-6, IL-8, IL-10
IL-1 receptor antagonist
IFN-α, IFN-β, IFN-γ
Macrophage inflammatory proteins (MIP-1 and -2)
PDGF
TGF-α, TGF-β
TNF-α
Enzymes
Acid hydrolases
Angiotensin-converting enzyme
Aryl sulfatase
β-glucronidase
Cathepsin
Collagenase
Elastase
Lysozyme
Plasminogen activator
Other bioactivated proteins
α_1-Protease inhibitor
α_2-Macroglobulin
Coagulation factors
Collagenase inhibitor
Complement factors
Dihydroxyvitamin D_3
Endothelin
Ferretin
Fibronectin
Glutathione
Transferrin
Lipid mediators
Leukotrienes
PAF
Prostaglandins
Thromboxane
Oxidants
Reactive nitrogen intermediates
Reactive oxygen intermediates

See text for definition of abbreviations.

those from humans) have a severely limited capacity for IL-1 production in relation to blood moncoytes tested in parallel (Wewers *et al.*, 1984), indicating that this function is progressively down-regulated during the monocyte-to-macrophage maturation process. Consequently, the results of any individual study on IL-1 production by BAL cells will be largely determined by the relative proportions of resident (mature) PAM and recently recruited (or locally divided) 'monocytes', which will in turn reflect the recent history of exposure of the cell donor to airborne 'irritants' (chemical or antigenic).

There are, in addition, a variety of complex secondary control mechanisms that operate locally at various points in the production/secretion sequence, which regulate the final 'effective' dose of secreted mediator in the lung. A prime example is tumour necrosis factor-α (TNF-α), which (in contrast to IL-1) is produced constitutively at the mRNA level in higher amounts by mature PAM than by monocytes (Martinet *et al.*, 1988). However, on closer examination it became evident that a further level of control for production of this cytokine exists at a point downstream from readoff of the TNF-α gene, preventing secretion of the active product until the PAM receives a *second* inflammatory stimulus such as LPS (Kips *et al.*, 1992).

Transforming growth factor-β (TGF-β) is another cytokine which appears to be produced constitutively by PAM (Yamauchi *et al.*, 1987, 1988), and which (like TNF-α) can rapidly increase in production following local challenge. However, this cytokine is released in an inactive form, and requires enzymatic conversion into its active form after secretion. There is little information on the control of this process in the lung and airways, but some evidence suggests that macrophage-derived enzymes may be involved. Additionally, α_2-macroglobulin, which is produced in substantial quantities by PAM, can reportedly inactivate TGF-β (Hovi *et al.*, 1977; Roberts & Sporn, 1990).

Additionally, it is evident that PAM are capable of secreting a variety of biologically active peptides which were hitherto thought to be restricted to cells of non-bone-marrow origin, such as endothelial cells (notably endothelin; Ehrenreich *et al.*, 1990).

Finally, it is relevant to note that a significant body of opinion favours a direct 'effector' role for the secreted products of PAM in diseases such as allergic asthma. These suggestions arise from experiments in the early 1980s, demonstrating that cross-linking of FcR-bound surface immunoglobulin E (IgE) on PAM with either specific allergen or monoclonal antibody (mAb)–anti-IgE, leads to secretion of inflammatory mediators (Joseph *et al.*, 1980, 1983; Fuller *et al.*, 1986). However, it should be noted that this attractive hypothesis rests almost entirely on *in vitro* observations, which have yet to be followed up in detail by systematic studies on PAM collected after bronchial challenge with allergens.

Immunomodulatory function(s)

Until the relatively recent discovery of the specialized APC role of DC and B lymphocytes, macrophages were believed to be the principal APC population throughout the body, and this view was reinforced by a broad range of experimental data derived from *in vitro* studies with human and animal macrophages, particularly from blood, peritoneal cavity and primary lymphoid organs. The first suspicion that lung macrophages may be in some way different to their 'cousins' in other tissues came from the pioneering studies of Mackaness and colleagues in the early 1970s, which led to the original decription of T-cell-dependent macrophage activation (later to be ascribed to interferon-γ (IFN-γ)) as the primary mechanism of cell-mediated antimicrobial immunity. A key observation in their studies was that the activation of secondary immunity in the pre-immunized host occurred at different rates in different organs; notably, mobilization of secondary T-cell-dependent immunity in the lungs was very slow, and did not occur until influxing blood monocytes, attracted to the site of challenge in the lung, outnumbered the original resident PAM population. This led them to conclude that, unlike macrophages from other organs, those which matured within the peripheral lung compartment had lost their capacity to present antigen to T cells, and hence that the induction of local immunity in this specialized tissue microenvironment depended absolutely on recruitment of fresh monocytes from the peripheral blood compartment (Mackaness, 1971).

Work in the late 1970s extended these observations, and indicated a further level of control in the form of active suppression of T-cell activation by resident PAM (Holt, 1978), and these findings have subsequently been repeated and expanded in a large number of laboratories (reviewed in Holt, 1986, 1993). This form of suppression has been shown to function in all species *except the guinea pig* (which, interestingly, is the easiest species in which to elicit hypersensitivity responses to inhaled antigens), with the proviso that T-cell responses to genuine protein antigens are used as the *in vitro* readout (Upham *et al.*, 1994; Fig. 13.1); reliance on the use of mitogens often produces equivocal results, and indeed PAM preparations (especially from humans) which are suppressive to antigen-driven T-cell proliferation may be permissive/helpful in mitogen responses tested in parallel.

It is now generally accepted that this T-cell-suppressive phenomenon is not the exclusive province of lung macrophages, but instead is a common attribute of 'activated' macrophages, i.e. as macrophages mature from the 'monocyte' through to the 'resident mature tissue mcrophage' stage, they go through a series of functional changes which affect their interactions with T cells. At the extreme end of this spectrum are the classical 'activated/cytotoxic' macrophages which are usually seen only in the context of exposure to adjuvants, microbial pathogens (such as BCG or *Corynebacterium parvum*) or parasites, and which are exquisitely suppressive to T cells; Kupffer cells in the liver and PAM from the lung approach (but do not normally equal) this activation state, presumably due to their constant exposure to 'toxins' arriving via the blood or in inspired air, and are hence normally maintained in a constant T-cell-suppressive state. Recent studies (Bilyk & Holt, 1995) suggest that, in experimental animals, it takes ⩾5 days for incoming (or locally dividing) monocytes to reach a state of activation equivalent to that of the resident PAM population, at least during the steady state.

It is evident that mature resident PAM function poorly as APC for T cells, as well as actively suppressing the overall T-cell activation process. With respect to APC activity, three key functions appear defective. Firstly, uptake/processing of particulate antigens is inefficient in PAM (Weinberg *et al.*, 1981); secondly, they display diminished capacity for clustering (namely active binding) to T cells (Lyons *et al.*, 1986; Gant *et al.*, 1991), possibly due to reduced surface expression of adhesion molecules (Melis *et al.*, 1991); and thirdly, as noted above, PAM produce only low levels of IL-1 (Wewers *et al.*, 1984), which is an obligatory requirement for the induction of IL-2 secretion by T cells.

When considering active suppression of T-cell activation/proliferation, PAM appear to have available a variety of different effector mechanisms, which may be used to varying degrees by PAM from different species, and/or under particular circumstances within an individual species. Those described include the following.

- TGF-β production — this cytokine has been shown to suppress *in vitro* T-cell proliferation (Kehrl *et al.*, 1986), via a mechanism operative late in the activation sequence (Wahl *et al.*, 1988).
- IL-1Ra — produced constitutively by PAM during *in vitro* culture (Moore *et al.*, 1992).
- PGE_2 — selectively suppresses cytokine production by Th2 cells (Betz & Fox, 1991); however, experiments with inhibitors show at best only partial reversal of suppression (Rich *et al.*, 1987).
- Contact-dependent suppression — operative *in vitro* at high PAM/T-cell ratios (Rich *et al.*, 1991), and may be attributable to membrane-bound TGF-β.
- Calcitriol — produced by human PAM (Mason *et al.*, 1984), and in animal systems shown to be a powerful inhibitor of T-cell proliferation (Rigby, 1988).
- Reactive nitrogen intermediates (RNI) — the major product, nitric oxide (NO), has been shown to be a major mediator of PAM suppression of T-cell proliferation in rodents (Kawabe *et al.*, 1992; Bilyk & Holt, 1995), but is of minor importance in humans (Upham *et al.*, 1994).

T-helper cell 'selection' by macrophage-derived cytokines during primary immune responses

Studies from a number of independent laboratories (reviewed in Romagnani, 1992; see also Chapter 6) suggest an important role for cytokines released by macrophages 'activated' by contact with microbial pathogens or parasites, in the regulation of 'bystander' immune responses to environmental antigens encountered concomitant with the infection.

In particular, macrophage-derived IL-12 and IFN-α have been shown to preferentially inhibit the growth of Th2 clones, thus positively 'selecting' for Th1-type immunity.

Selective suppression of T-cell proliferation without disturbance of effector functions

Recent work by the author has involved detailed re-examination of the precise nature of PAM-mediated T-cell suppression, employing rat, mouse and human cells tested in parallel. The impetus for these studies has been a series of observations in the rat model, suggesting that while T cells exposed to mitogen/antigen in the presence of PAM were unable to proliferate, they apparently secreted normal levels of IL-2 (Strickland *et al.*, 1994).

The format of the studies involved sampling of PAM/T-cell cocultures at strategic intervals for assessment of T-cell 'activation' parameters (as listed in Table 13.2), and

Table 13.2 T-cell activation in the presence of PAM.

	Resting T cells	T cells stimulated with mitogen/antigen	
		−PAM	+PAM
Proliferation (^{3}H-DNA synthesis)	−	+++	−
Cell-cycle stage	G0/G1	G0/G1/S/G2M	Predominantly G0/G1
Ca^{2+} flux	−	+	+
Transient TcR modulation			
CD3	−	+	+
TCRαβ	−	+	+
Costimulators			
CD2	+	++	+
CD28	+	+	+
Surface expression of			
'Late' activation antigen	−	+	+
IL2Rα/Rβ	−	+	+
CD4/8	−	+	+
MHC II	−	+	+
Secretion of			
IL-2	−	++	+++
GM-CSF/IL-3	−	++	++
IFN-γ	−	++	+

See text for definition of abbreviations.

finally assessing proliferation via DNA synthesis. The salient results from the study have been successfully replicated in the three species, and are as follows.

- The presence of PAM at levels equivalent to ⩾2.5% total cells per coculture completely inhibited T-cell proliferation as assessed by DNA synthesis, and cell-cycle analysis demonstrated that T cells in the 'blocked' cultures remained in G0/G1.
- The initial Ca^{2+} flux proceeded normally in the presence of PAM.
- Expression of the costimulators CD2 and CD28 remained high in the 'blocked' cultures.
- Transient down-modulation of TcR-associated surface molecules, a normal consequence of T-cell activation, was equivalent in the cultures.
- Surface expression of a variety of molecules associated with activation, notably 'late' activation antigen, IL-2Rα and IL-2Rβ, MHC class II, was comparable in the presence and absence of PAM; equivalent levels of CD4/CD8 co-expression were also seen.
- High levels of cytokine secretion (including IL-2 and IFN-γ) were observed in both sets of cultures.

Furthermore, it was observed that the time of addition of the PAM was critical; if activation was permitted to proceed for >12 hours in the absence of PAM, subsequent proliferation was refractory to the effects of the macrophages. Also, these effects were readily reversible, as removal of the PAM permitted proliferation to proceed normally after an initial latent period; the latter occurred even in the absence of further antigen/mitogen, indicating that optimal 'activating' levels of TcR ligation were achieved during the initial phase of the culture, even in the presence of the 'inhibitory' PAM.

Thus, PAM-mediated T-cell 'suppression' appears to be a potentially much more sophisticated mechanism for maintenance of local immunological homeostasis than has hitherto been appreciated. In principle, it provides the means to permit incoming antigen-specific T-memory cells to carry out their prime host-protective effector functions (namely cytokine release in response to their specific antigens), while at the same time limiting the responses of individual T cells to a 'single hit' by inhibiting local clonal expansion. This can be viewed as an important protective mechanism for prevention of 'overshoot' of cellular immune responses at the delicate blood–air interface in the lung. It can be further speculated that the reversibility of the process provides the means for preservation and expansion of immunological memory against antigens encountered in the lung, as T cells migrating away from this tissue microenvironment are released from suppression and can consequently clonally expand within regional lymph nodes, without the necessity for further antigenic stimulation.

Additionally, there is recent evidence from the rat

Table 13.3 Principal immunoregulatory functions of pulmonary alveolar macrophages.

Inhibition of local T-cell proliferation
Damping mononuclear cell influx during inflammation
Selective suppression of Th2-dependent (local) allergic responses
Damping of local 'antigen-presentation' activity

model that this process operates *in vivo*. Thus, T cells freshly isolated from normal rat lung are extremely heterogeneous with respect to surface expression of CD3 and TcRαβ. In particular, a major subset of these T cells appear analogous to post-activated T cells by these criteria, but DNA analysis indicates that virtually all of the population are in the G0/G1 (i.e. resting) phase of the cell cycle (D. Strickland & P.G. Holt, in preparation). T cells from human parenchymal lung tissue display a variety of different properties consistent with recent activation, and are also predominantly in G0/G1 (Marathias *et al.*, 1991). It is additionally noteworthy that lung T cells from both humans (Holt *et al.*, 1988a) and experimental animals (Strickland *et al.*, 1993) function extremely poorly in T-cell cloning assays.

Regulation of local APC activity

In addition to direct effects on T-cell responses via regulation of T-cell proliferation subsequent to antigenic stimulation, PAM appear capable of controlling the efficiency of the initial antigen presentation step in this process, via modulation of the activity of the principal local APC population, DC. Moreover, this property is shared by airway mucosal macrophages (Holt & Schon-Hegrad, 1987) and interstitial macrophages from peripheral lung tissue (Holt *et al.*, 1985).

This issue is discussed in detail below.

Immunological consequences of in vivo *PAM depletion*

The data reviewed above are based entirely on *in vitro* analysis of PAM isolated by the BAL technique, and the validity of extrapolation of these findings to the situation *in vivo* can be legitimately questioned.

A technique has recently been developed for *in situ* depletion of macrophage populations, which has provided a unique opportunity to address this issue objectively. This 'macrophage suicide technique' involves the use of the drug dichloromethylene diphosphonate (DMDP) encapsulated in liposomes, which are avidly phagocytosed by macrophages; DMDP is converted into a short-range-acting cytotoxin within phagolysozomes, which rapidly kills the phagocytes.

Intratracheal administration of DMDP liposomes reduces the resident PAM population in rats and mice by approximately 90% within a 12-hour period, and they remain severely reduced for weeks thereafter. Examination of 'immune-associated' functions in the respiratory tract of PAM-deficient animals indicates severe disruption of local immunological homeostasis, as follows.

- While primary allergic responses to inhaled antigens remain unaffected, secondary responses against antigens to which the animals were presensitized are grossly amplified, resulting in invasion of the challenged lung with activated T cells, plasma cells and monocytes; both local and systemic antibody responses (measured as serum antibody titres or numbers of specific plasma cells in lung tissue and regional lymph nodes) increase markedly, relative to intact controls (Thepen *et al.*, 1989, 1992).
- The increased secondary response is selective for the Th2 T-cell compartment, as the largest increases observed were for IgE (Thepen *et al.*, 1992).
- T cells from lungs of PAM-deficient animals acquired normal capacity for *in vitro* clonal expansion (Strickland *et al.*, 1993).
- The APC activity of local DC populations increased markedly (Holt *et al.*, 1993; further discussion below).

Collectively, these observations are consistent with a major *in vivo* role for resident PAM, in limiting the magnitude of allergic responses to inhaled antigens which rely upon local activation of T-memory cells.

Modulation of the functional phenotype of PAM populations: the role of local cytokine release during inflammation

PAM down-modulation of T-memory cell reactivation within the lung provides a plausible mechanism for limiting T-cell-mediated damage to host tissue during local immune responses, in particular those to essentially non-pathogenic airborne environmental antigens such as pollen allergens. However, the mechanism proposed above begs the important question of how this form of 'normal immunosuppression' is overcome in the face of challenge with genuinely pathogenic antigens, which require a rapid and effective local T-cell response for host protection.

Several related lines of evidence suggest that the immunomodulatory functions of the PAM population can be modified directly by the effects of certain cytokines, and indirectly via 'dilution' with incoming monocytes attracted via locally generated chemokines.

In indirect 'dilution', as noted above, blood monocytes function effectively as APC or 'accessory cells' for T-cell activation. Consequently, challenge of the lung with inflammatory stimuli that lead to local influx of monocytes into the airways can be expected to dampen the overall suppressive effects of the resident PAM population, and the degree of dampening of this mechanism should reflect the size of the monocyte influx. This has indeed been observed experimentally in animal models involving lung challenge with microbial irritants (Holt, 1978) and inorganic particulates (Bilyk & Holt, 1995). Additionally, data from two independent laboratories indicating diminished T-cell suppressive activity of PAM populations in atopic asthma (Aubas *et al.*, 1984; Gant *et al.*, 1992), a disease characterized by monocytic infiltration of airway tissue (Mattoli *et al.*, 1991; Poston *et al.*, 1992), also appear consistent with this picture. Similar conclusions follow from findings of increased PAM accessory cell functions associated with monocyte influx in sarcoidosis (Lem *et al.*, 1985; Venet *et al.*, 1985; Poulter, 1990) and chronic respiratory infections (Fujiwara *et al.*, 1986; Ina *et al.*, 1991).

However, monocytic infiltration of inflammatory foci are generally part of the delayed component of the host response, often not commencing before ⩾48 hours post-challenge, so the question remaining is how PAM suppression can potentially be bypassed during the early stages of an immunoinflammatory response. It has recently been shown that ⩾12 hours exposure of murine PAM to GM-CSF, particularly in combination with TNF-α, effectively 'deprogrammes' the T-cell-suppressive activity of resident PAM and converts them into 'accessory cells' with T-cell-activating activity equivalent to monocytes (Bilyk *et al.*, 1993). Moreover, TGF-β achieves the same result but without the necessity for a 12-hour pre-exposure period (Bilyk & Holt, 1995).

Thus, it can be hypothesized that local inflammatory responses which involve release of combinations of these cytokines may open up an early 'window' for T-cell activation via modulation of the immunosuppressive activity of PAM (Fig. 13.2). Interestingly, this 'window', at least with respect to the effects of GM-CSF, appears only transient, as PAM become refractory to this cytokine beyond

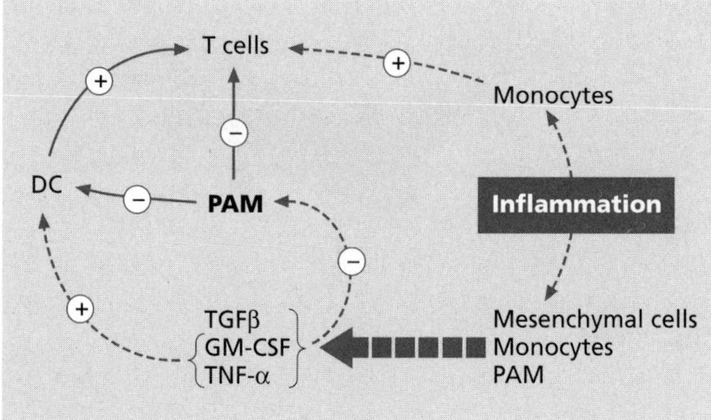

Fig. 13.2 Modulation of T-cell activation by alveolar macrophages in normal vs. inflamed lung. See text for definition of abbreviations.

an initial 48-hour exposure period (reacquiring their suppressive properties), presumably as a result of tachyphylaxis of GM-CSF receptors (Bilyk & Holt, 1995).

Recent reports indicating increased local GM-CSF production in the airway wall of asthmatics (Sousa *et al.*, 1993), and selectively increased GM-CSF and TNF-α production by monocytes and macrophages from asthmatics (Hallsworth *et al.*, 1994), are of further interest.

DC

DC are now generally acknowledged as a highly potent APC population, uniquely specialized for presentation of antigen to naive T cells; the available evidence also suggests that they are more efficient than B cells or monocytes in the delivery of antigen-specific activating signals to T-memory cells (Steinman, 1991).

These cells were originally thought to comprise a very small subpopulation of the bone-marrow-derived mononuclear cell population in a minority of solid tissues, but more recent evidence indicates that they are ubiquitous in the body, and in some tissue microenvironments represent the dominant mononuclear cell type. They are particularly prominent at sites such as the epidermis and the epithelia of the gut and respiratory tracts, which are in direct contact with the outside environment, and it is accordingly axiomatic that they must play a central role in regulation of immunoinflammatory responses to environmental allergens.

The discussion below concentrates mainly on recent findings relevant to the respiratory tract DC populations most likely to be involved in allergy to airborne antigens, and where appropriate draws analogies with their counterparts in the gut and skin.

DC distribution and density in normal lung and airway tissues

The original descriptions of DC in human respiratory tract tissues were in the context of chronic interstitial lung diseases such as histiocytosis X (Cagle *et al.*, 1988; Soler *et al.*, 1989). However, more recent studies have established their presence in both the alveolar and airway wall of normal subjects (reviewed in Holt *et al.*, 1990).

In particular, the development of techniques for sectioning airway epithelium in a plane parallel to the underlying basement membrane (Holt *et al.*, 1990) has only very recently revealed the magnitude of these populations. As shown in Fig. 13.3, immunostaining frozen sections of airway epithelium sectioned in this fashion with mAb anti-class II MHC(Ia) demonstrates the presence of a dense, contiguous network of highly pleiomorphic DC (Fig. 13.3a), which are virtually identical in density and distribution to the familiar Langerhans cell (LC) network

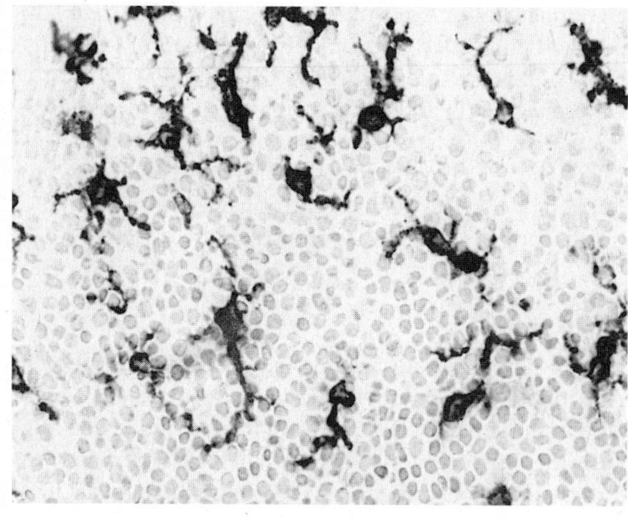

(a)

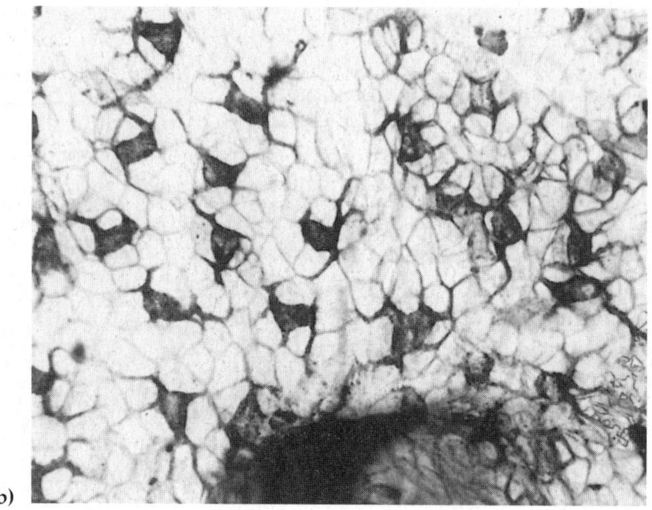

(b)

Fig. 13.3 Dendritic cell networks in the airway epithelium (a) and epidermis (b) revealed by immunostaining for MHC class II antigen.

in the epidermis (Fig. 13.3(b)). In longitudinal sections, these airway DC can be seen in intimate association with the epithelial basement membrane (Holt *et al.*, 1990), which may provide their major anchor point within the epithelium.

In addition to the airway DC population, large numbers of DC are also found within alveolar septal walls (Fig. 13.4).

In normal human subjects and experimental animals, the DC network accounts for close to 100% of Ia immunostaining (Holt *et al.*, 1990), but this fact is only evident when employing this specialized plane of section, which accurately reveals the morphology of individual stained cells. In the large airways of rodents and down to the small bronchioles in humans, the density of these cells is of the order of 500–800 per square millimetre of epithelial surface.

In addition to the conducting airway DC population, large numbers are also found in the alveolar parenchyma (Holt *et al.*, 1990), the epithelium of the nasal mucosa (Fokkens *et al.*, 1989) and turbinates (Nelson *et al.*, 1994a), and they have also been observed in BAL in several species, including humans (van Haarst *et al.*, 1994). Several workers have also reported small numbers of 'immature' DC in BAL fluids of normal animals (Havenith *et al.*, 1992) and humans (Casolaro *et al.*, 1988; van Haarst *et al.*, 1994).

Structure and surface phenotype of lung DC

The identification of DC in respiratory tract tissues relies on the use of a mixture of immunological and morphological characteristics, as no universal surface marker is yet available for any species. Constitutive expression of Ia is generally held to be a hallmark of all DC; however, this is no longer universally tenable in the light of a recent report on the presence of a major subset of Ia-negative DC in the airway epithelium of rats, especially young animals (Nelson *et al.*, 1994a).

A property shared by all mature DC is their characteristic dendriform shape, exhibiting processes which ramify laterally between adjacent epithelial cells (e.g. Fig. 13.3(a)); however, recently blood-derived immature 'precursor' DC within the airway epithelium appear similar in size and shape to monocytes or B cells (McWilliam *et al.*, 1994), and consequently it is necessary to costain with both pan-B-cell and pan-macrophage mAb in order to be sure that these latter cell types are not significant contaminants of any DC population under study.

Lung and airway DC express a variety of cell–cell interaction molecules, including β1 and β2 leucocyte integrins,

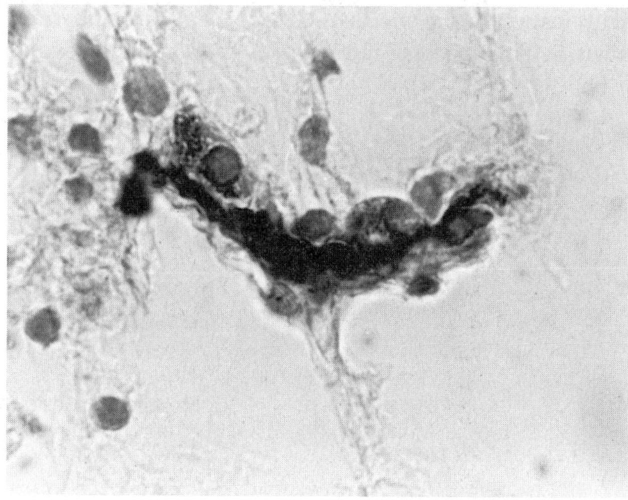

Fig. 13.4 MHC class II-bearing dendritic cell in the alveolar septal wall.

and adhesins such as LFA-1 (leucocyte function associated antigen-1) and ICAM-1 (intercellular adhesion molecule-1) (Schon-Hegrad *et al.*, 1991; Gong *et al.*, 1992; Nicod & El Habre, 1992), the T-200 and S-100 antigens (Sertl *et al.*, 1986) and FcR (Pollard & Lipscomb, 1990; Gong *et al.*, 1992). Considerable variation in intensity of surface expression of these markers is observed within individual respiratory tract DC populations, and also between DC populations at different levels of the respiratory tree (Holt & Schon-Hegrad, 1987; Soler *et al.*, 1989; Winkler, 1989; Schon-Hegrad *et al.*, 1991; Gong *et al.*, 1992), suggesting that the synthesis of these function-associated molecules is under local (tissue microenvironmental) control.

Origin and kinetics of lung DC in the steady state

Limited information is available on the population dynamics of DC in solid tissues, with the exception of the epidermal LC network in the skin. The available evidence (reviewed in Holt *et al.*, 1994) indicates that this population turns over relatively slowly, with a half-life in the order of 15–21 days; by contrast, DC populations from lymphoid organs are more dynamic, and appear to be renewed every 7–10 days.

A detailed study on the origin and turnover of respiratory tract DC populations in rats has recently been carried out by the author's laboratory. A radiation chimera model involving two congenic rats strains differing in a single allele at the CD45 locus was used. The single-allele difference was detectable via surface immunostaining of leucocytes (including DC) with mAb against the two respective CD45.

In employing this system, the supply of precursor DC required to maintain the resident lung populations at steady-state levels was interrupted by bone-marrow depletion with either X-rays or high-dose steroids, and the density of the intra-epithelial and lung parenchymal populations monitored thereafter on a daily basis; some animals were reconstituted with congenic bone marrow.

As shown in Fig. 13.5(a), following interruption of the supply of incoming bone marrow precursors, DC populations in skin, peripheral lung and airway epithelium decline at different rates, the latter reflecting the continuous daily flux of cells emigrating to regional lymph nodes (Steinman, 1991; Holt *et al.*, 1994). It can be seen that this decline is fastest for the airway population, and reconstitution with bone marrow rapidly replenishes these DC (Fig. 13.5(b)). These data provide a close estimate of the steady-state half-life of the airway DC population, at approximately 1.5–2 days; this compares to around 7 days for the deep lung, and >14 days for the epidermis. The only solid tissue containing DC with a comparably rapid turnover time in the steady state is the gut (Holt *et al.*, 1994), emphasizing the importance of DC in antigen surveillance (see further discussion below) at the two major 'front-line' mucosal surfaces of the body.

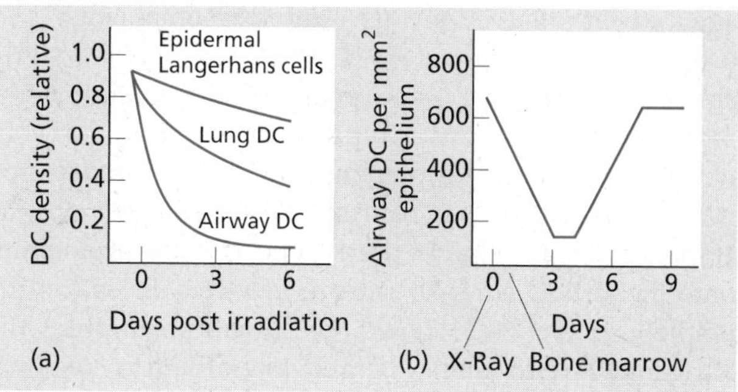

Fig. 13.5 Origin and turnover of DC in the rat. (a) Relative rates of decline in DC density following sublethal X-irradiation. (b) Replenishment of airway DC in X-irradiated animals following bone marrow transplantation. (Based on results in Holt *et al.*, 1994.)

Response of DC to acute and chronic inflammation

There is suggestive evidence from the dermatology literature that LC networks expand at sites of chronic infection, and also in atopic dermatitis lesions (Fokkens *et al.*, 1990); it is also evident that in the latter disease the surface phenotype of the LC changes in response to the inflammatory tissue milieu, notably via expression of the low-affinity receptor for IgE (Fokkens *et al.*, 1990).

There is currently only limited information available on allergic respiratory disease, which suggests upregulation of nasal mucosal DC in rhinitis patients in the pollen season (Fokkens *et al.*, 1989), and increased density of RFD1+ cells in bronchial biopsies from asthmatics (Poulter *et al.*, 1994). However, from animal models, data (discussed below) suggest that such changes in allergic humans are likely, in relation to both chronic and acute challenge.

Firstly, in a study on chronic exposure of animals to pine shavings rich in pleicatic and abietic acids (two of the principal aetiological agents in cedar workers' asthma), the development of airway intra-epithelial eosinophilia associated with focal Ia expression on epithelial cells, with concomitant increases in the density (approximately 50%) of DC, has been reported (Schon-Hegrad *et al.*, 1991). In addition, the DC displayed increased surface expression of a variety of function-associated molecules, including Ia and LFA-1 (Schon-Hegrad *et al.*, 1991).

Secondly, acute challenge of animals with aerosol containing low levels of soluble bacterial LPS resulted in a transient influx of DC, over a time-course resembling that of neutrophils (Schon-Hegrad *et al.*, 1991). In a more detailed follow-up study to characterize this potentially important phenomenon, a more potent inflammatory agent (heat-killed *Moraxella catarrhalis* organisms) was used (McWilliam *et al.*, 1994). The results of this study established that the acute phase of the inflammatory response in the airways contains a hitherto covert, but nevertheless large, DC component, previously undetected because (unlike the neutrophil component of the response) the DC do not proceed beyond the epithelium onto the airway surface; instead, they remain within the epithelium for 24–36 hours, presumably sampling the antigenic environment, before migrating to regional lymph nodes (McWilliam *et al.*, 1994).

Indirect evidence suggests that a similar mechanism exists in the gut, but we have thus far been unable to demonstrate it in the skin (McWilliam *et al.*, 1994), suggesting it may be restricted to the common mucosal immune system.

Sensitivity of DC to steroids

Recent studies in our laboratory have examined the effects of topical and systemic steroids on lung DC populations. The results demonstrate that repeated exposure of normal animals to aerosols containing drugs such as beclomethasone, budesonide or fluticasone are capable of reducing steady-state airway DC population density in the order of 40% within 48 hours, whereas high-dose dexamethasone given systemically can deplete the population by 85–90% over the same time period (Nelson, 1994b). This contrasts with the relatively slower kinetics reported for steroid-mediated down-modulation of LC populations in the skin (reviewed in Holt *et al.*, 1994), and these differences are presumably attributable to the varying turnover times of the different DC populations.

Consistent with this latter view, the locus of action of steroids in this system appears to be at the level of prevention of recruitment of blood-borne DC (Holt *et al.*, 1994). Therefore, it is noteworthy that both systemic and topical steroids are able to virtually ablate the large DC influx into the epithelium during acute inflammation (Nelson, 1994b), reflecting the reliance of this response on incoming precursors.

APC function(s) of DC

Formal proof of the role of DC as the principal APC in respiratory tract tissues has been supplied from three lines of investigation (reviewed in Holt, 1993).

Firstly, cell separation studies on collagenase digests of lung and airway tissue from several species identified local APC as non-adherent, surface Ig negative, non-phagocytic and of ultra-low density on Percoll. Secondly, these cells were potent not only in reactivation of hyperimmune T-memory cells, but also in the induction of primary mixed lymphocyte responses (MLR). Thirdly, these cells were able to efficiently 'acquire' inhaled antigens *in situ*.

It was noteworthy that in the systems tested, the capacity of these respiratory tract DC to activate T cells was negatively related to the density of contaminating macrophages in the preparations. This was observed for both lung parenchymal DC in the presence of PAM or interstitial macrophages (e.g. Holt *et al.*, 1985), and for airway intra-epithelial DC in the presence of airway mucosal macrophages (Holt *et al.*, 1988b).

Regulation of the APC functions of respiratory tract DC *in situ*

It has previously been established that while *in situ* in normal skin, LC are specialized for the uptake and processing of antigen, but do not acquire the ability to efficiently 'present' to T cells until they migrate to regional lymph nodes where they undergo a GM-CSF-dependent process of maturation into potent APC (Steinman, 1991).

It has recently been shown that a similar situation pertains to airway and lung wall DC, which do not express their full potential for T-cell activation until they are cultured with a source of GM-CSF (Fig. 13.6; Holt *et al.*, 1993; see also Tazi *et al.*, 1993 for *in vivo* data). This could represent an important host-protective mechanism, the function of which is to limit the extent of potentially tissue-damaging T-cell activation events within the sensitive airway intra-epithelial microenvironment. This begs the question, however, of the effects of local GM-CSF production, which is known to occur in diseases such as asthma. Are such events part of the 'vicious circle' in atopic disease, in which chronically inflamed tissues become hyperresponsive to an increasingly wide range of erstwhile innocuous antigenic stimuli?

While the latter question remains currently within the realms of speculation, it is evident that nature (not unexpectedly) foresaw the danger, and provided a back-up mechanism to deal with it. This conclusion stems from the results of studies which demonstrate that secreted products from PAM, which include NO and TNF-α, inhibit the capacity of DC to respond to GM-CSF signals *in vitro* (Holt *et al.*, 1993; see also Fig. 13.2); moreover, PAM depletion leads to large-scale up-regulation of the APC activity of lung DC (Holt *et al.*, 1993), suggesting that this mechanism is indeed operative *in vivo*.

Also consistent with this suggestion, immunohistochemical and electron microscopic analyses of the distribution of DC and macrophage populations in respiratory tract tissues demonstrate close juxtaposition of these cell types in the airway mucosa, where they are found on opposite sides of the epithelial basement membrane (Holt & Schon-Hegrad, 1987; Holt *et al.*, 1993). A similar relationship exists in the peripheral lung, where they are closely

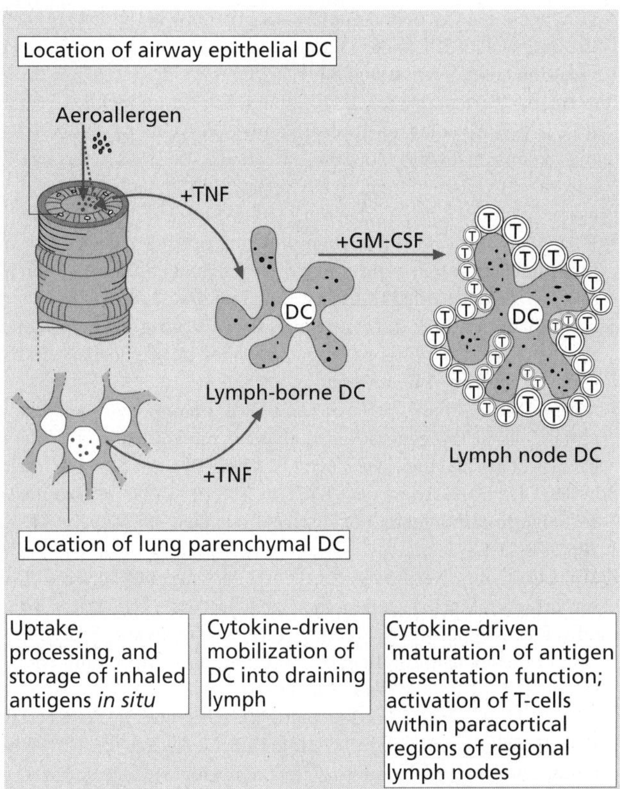

Fig. 13.6 Changes in the functional phenotype of lung DC at different stages of their lifecycle.

apposed at alveolar interseptal junctions (Holt *et al.*, 1993). A comparably intimate relationship is evident between these two cell types in the gastric mucosa, and gut macrophages have been reported to suppress the APC activity of DC in an analogous fashion to that described for their lung counterparts.

T-cell sensitization to aeroallergens during infancy: the significance of DC ontogeny

It is evident from the human seroepidemiological literature that primary sensitization to aeroallergens occurs most commonly during early childhood (Holt, 1994). Given the specialized role of DC as APC for primary sensitization of naive T cells, and the unique distribution of these cells throughout the airway epithelium, it is logical to speculate that airway DC may play a significant role in this process. Accordingly, it is important to determine the functional status of these populations in the neonate.

Currently, no direct information is yet available that is relevant to this issue for humans, although it seems likely from findings of relatively low DC numbers and Ia expression in neonatal human skin and gut, that the respiratory tract DC networks may develop mainly after birth.

A detailed ontogenic study in rats, which provides interesting pointers for future human studies in this area, has recently been completed. This revealed that DC precursors are seeded into airway tissue *in utero*, and by birth the intra-epithelial density of these cells is approximately a third that of adults (Nelson *et al.*, 1994a). However, these cells do not express surface Ia until after birth, and for a prolonged period thereafter (beyond normal weaning) they express much lower levels of Ia than adults (Nelson *et al.*, 1994a).

Sequential sampling studies indicate that Ia expression is first 'switched on' at the base of the nasal turbinates, presumably under the intensive drive from inflammatory stimuli which would be maximal at these sites; Ia expression 'lights up' progressively with time, deeper into the respiratory tree, presumably reflecting variations in net inflammatory stimulation at the different levels (Nelson *et al.*, 1994). The process can be hastened by exogenous IFN-γ, and retarded by steroids, consistent with it being driven by inflammation (Nelson *et al.*, 1994a). Interestingly, Ia expression on epidermal LC in the same animals attains adult-equivalent levels within the first week of life. As airway DC and LC are believed to be derived from identical precursors, it therefore appears likely that tissue-specific mechanism(s) exist within the respiratory tract to suppress Ia expression in the neonatal period.

Functional analyses of neonatal rat airway DC are in progress in the author's laboratory, and results to date suggest they respond poorly to GM-CSF maturation signals; moreover, parallel studies on PAM from neonatal animals indicate at least adult-equivalent levels of DC-suppressive activity, suggesting that the 'balance' between opposing forces in relation to T-cell activation is skewed towards suppression at this early stage of life. Whether a disturbance in this balance predisposes to excessive T-cell sensitization, remains to be established.

Conclusions

The review above argues that the T-cell responses which underlie the induction and expression of allergic diseases in the respiratory tract are regulated by interactions between local populations of DC and macrophages.

At the level of initial T-cell sensitization, the key cell type is the airway intra-epithelial DC, which normally functions as a 'sentinel' in surveillance for foreign antigens/allergens that are sequestered and eventually transported to T cells in regional lymph nodes for 'presentation', after receipt of an obligatory maturation signal based on GM-CSF. Under normal steady-state conditions, it is maintained in the sentinel phenotype via signals from adjacent macrophages, which inhibit its capacity to respond to GM-CSF. Lung-derived macrophages may potentially contribute to this process, particularly at the level of Th1/Th2 selection, provided they receive sufficient stimulation (e.g. from a bystander microbial pathogen) to both initiate secretion of IL-12 (etc.) and migrate to regional lymph nodes.

When considering local reactivation of memory cells in the steady state, resident DC have limited capacity to carry out this function, and any 'successful' stimulatory events will be subject to tight control by local PAM and their mature tissue macrophage counterparts in the lung and airway wall. However, as the strength of local inflammatory stimulation increases, further mechanisms come into play, potentially including:

• recruitment of monocytes (and possibly B cells);
• initiation of GM-CSF production and Ia expression by epithelial cells;
• initiation of production of GM-CSF, TNF-α and TGF-β production by incoming monocytes and resident macrophages;
• temporary 'shut-off' of local macrophage-mediated suppression of T-cell proliferation, permitting local amplification of T-cell responses;
• temporary 'shut-off' of macrophage-mediated mechanisms which prevent *in situ* up-regulation of the APC activity of intra-epithelial DC, in response to locally produced GM-CSF.

With the proviso that these changes are reversible within a relatively short time-frame (e.g. via such mechanisms as GM-CSF receptor tachyphylaxis, as discussed above), they may have no significant pathological sequelae. Conversely, if they persist beyond a critical period, such that this (or a related) cytokine profile becomes more or less 'constitutive' in this tissue microenvironment, chronic inflammatory disease may be the ultimate result. The latter outcome can be viewed as a potentially important contributing factor in the pathogenesis of chronic allergic disease, in the respiratory tract and in other tissues.

References

Aubas, P., Cosso, B., Godard, P., Michel, F.B. & Clot, J. (1984) Decreased suppressor cell activity of alveolar macrophages in bronchial asthma. *Am. Rev. Resp. Dis.*, **130**, 875–8.

Beasley, R., Roche, W.R., Roberts, J.A. & Holgate, S.T. (1989) Cellular events in the bronchi of mild asthmatics after bronchial provocation. *Am. Rev. Resp. Dis.*, **139**, 806–17.

Betz, M. & Fox, B.S. (1991) Prostaglandin E2 inhibits production of Th1 lymphokines but not of Th2 lymphokines. *J. Immunol.*, **146**, 108–13.

Bilyk, N. & Holt, P.G. (1993) Inhibition of the immunosuppressive activity of resident pulmonary alveolar macrophages by granulocyte/macrophage colony-stimulating factor. *J. Exp. Med.*, **177**, 1773–7.

Bilyk, N. & Holt, P.G. (1995) Cytokines modulate the immunosuppressive phenotype of pulmonary alveolar macrophages populations, *Immunology*, **86**, 231–7.

Bilyk, N., MacKenzie, J.S., Papadimitriou, J.M. & Holt, P.G. (1988) Functional studies on macrophage populations in the airways and the lung wall of SPF mice in the steady state and during respiratory virus infection. *Immunology*, **65**, 417–25.

Bitterman, P.B., Saltzman, L.E., Adelberg, S., Ferrans, V.J. & Crystal, R.G. (1987) Alveolar macrophage replication. One mechanism for the expansion of the mononuclear phagocyte population in the chronically inflamed lung. *Am. J. Respir. Cell Mol. Biol.*, **4**, 460–9.

Blussé van Oud Alblas, A., van der Linden-Schrever, B. & van Furth, R. (1983) Origin and kinetics of pulmonary macrophages during an inflammatory reaction induced by intra-alveolar administration of aerosolized heat-killed BCG. *Am. Rev. Resp. Dis.*, **128**, 276–81.

Blussé van Oud Alblas, A. & van Furth, R. (1979) Origin, kinetics, and characteristics of pulmonary macrophages in the normal steady state. *J. Exp. Med.*, **149**, 1504–18.

Bowden, D.H. & Adamson, I.Y.R. (1980) Role of monocytes and interstitial cells in the generation of alveolar macrophages. I. Kinetic studies of normal mice. *Lab. Invest.*, **42**, 511–17.

Bowden, D.H. & Adamson, I.Y.R. (1982) Alveolar macrophage response to carbon in monocyte-depleted mice. *Am. Rev. Resp. Dis.*, **126**, 708–11.

Brain, J.D., Gehr, P. & Kavet, R.I. (1984) Airway macrophages. The importance of the fixation method. *Am. Rev. Resp. Dis.*, **129**, 823–6.

Cagle, P.T., Mattioli, C.A., Truong, L.D. & Greenberg, S.D. (1988) Immunohistochemical diagnosis of pulmonary eosinophilic granuloma on lung biopsy. *Chest*, **94**, 1133–7.

Casolaro, M.A., Bernaudin, J.F., Saltini, C., Ferrans, V.J. & Crystal, R.G. (1988) Accumulation of Langerhans' cells on the epithelial surface of the lower respiratory tract in normal subjects in association with cigarette smoking. *Am. Rev. Resp. Dis.*, **137**, 406–11.

Collins, F.M. & Auclair, L.K. (1980) Mononuclear phagocytes within the lungs of unstimulated parabiotic rats. *J. Reticuloendoth. Soc.*, **27**, 429–41.

Corry, D., Kulkarni, P. & Lipscomb, M.F. (1984) The migration of bronchoalveolar macrophages into hilar lymph nodes. *Am. J. Pathol.*, **115**, 321–8.

Ehrenreich, H., Anderson, R.W., Fox, C.H. *et al.* (1990) Endothelins, peptides with potent vasoactive properties, are produced by human macrophages. *J. Exp. Med.*, **172**, 1741–8.

Evans, M.J., Sherman, M.P., Campbell, L.A. & Shami, S.G. (1987) Proliferation of pulmonary alveolar macrophages during postnatal development of rabbit lungs. *Am. Rev. Resp. Dis.*, **136**, 384–7.

Fokkens, W.J., Bruijnzeel, K.C., Vroom, T.M. *et al.* (1990) The Langerhans cell: an underestimated cell in atopic disease. *Clin. Exp. Allergy*, **20**, 627–38.

Fokkens, W.J., Vroom, T.M., Rijntjes, E. & Mulder, P.G. (1989) CD-1+ (T6), HLA-DR-expressing cells, presumably Langerhans cells, in nasal mucosa. *Allergy*, **44**, 167–72.

Fujiwara, H., Kleinhenz, M.E., Wallis, R.S. & Ellner, J.J. (1986) Increased Interleukin-1 production and monocyte suppressor cell activity associated with human tuberculosis. *Am. Rev. Resp. Dis.*, **133**, 73–7.

Fuller, R.W., Morris, P.K., Richmond, R. *et al.* (1986) Immunoglobulin E-dependent stimulation of human alveolar macrophages: significance in type 1 hypersensitivity. *Clin. Exp. Immunol.*, **65**, 416–26.

Gant, V., Cluzel, M., Shakoor, Z., Rees, P.J., Lee, T.K. & Hamblin, A.S (1992) Alveolar macrophage accessory cell function in bronchial asthma. *Am. Rev. Resp. Dis.*, **146**, 900–4.

Gant, V.A., Shakoor, Z., Barbosa, I.L. & Hamblin, A.S. (1991) Normal and sarcoid alveolar macrophages differ in their ability to present antigen and to cluster with autologous lymphocytes. *Clin. Exp. Immunol.*, **86**, 494–9.

Golde, D.W., Finley, T.N. & Cline, M.J. (1974) The pulmonary macrophage in acute leukemia. *New. Engl. J. Med.*, **290**, 875–8.

Gong, J.L., McCarthy, K.M., Telford, J., Tamatani, T., Miyasaka, M. & Schneeberger, E.E. (1992) Intraepithelial airway dendritic cells: a distinct subset of pulmonary dendritic cells obtained by microdissection. *J. Exp. Med.*, **175**, 797–807.

Hallsworth, M.P., Soh, C.P.C., Lane, S.J., Arm, J.P. & Lee, T.H. (1994) Selective enhancement of GM-CSF, TNF-α, IL-1β and IL-8 production of monocytes and macrophages of astmatic subjects. *Eur. Resp. J.*, **7**, 1096–102.

Hance, A.J., Douches, S., Winchester, R.J., Ferrans, J. & Crystal, R.J. (1985) Characterisation of mononuclear phagocyte subpopulations in the human lung by using monoclonal antibodies: changes in alveolar macrophage phenotype associated with pulmonary sarcoidosis. *J. Immunol.*, **134**, 284–92.

Havenith, C.E., Breedijk, A.J. & Hoefsmit, E.C. (1992) Effect of Bacillus Calmette-Guerin inoculation on numbers of dendritic cells in bronchoalveolar lavages of rats. *Immunobiology*, **184**, 336–47.

Holt, P.G. (1978) Inhibitory activity of unstimulated alveolar macrophages on T-lymphocyte blastogenic response. *Am. Rev. Resp. Dis.*, **118**, 791–3.

Holt, P.G. (1986) Downregulation of immune responses in the lower respiratory tract: the role of alveolar macrophages. *Clin. Exp. Immunol.*, **63**, 261–70.

Holt, P.G. (1993) Regulation of antigen-presenting function(s) in lung and airway tissues. *Eur. Resp. J.*, **6**, 120–9.

Holt, P.G. (1994) Immunoprophylaxis of atopy: light at the end of the tunnel? *Immunol. Today*, **15**, 484–9.

Holt, P.G. & Schon-Hegrad, M.A. (1987) Localization of T cells, macrophages and dendritic cells in rat respiratory tract tissue: implications for immune function studies. *Immunology*, **62**, 349–56.

Holt, P.G., Degebrodt, A., Venaille, T. *et al.* (1985) Preparation of interstitial lung cells by enzymatic digestion of tissue slices: preliminary characterization by morphology and performance in functional assays. *Immunology*, **54**, 139–47.

Holt, P.G., Kees, U.R., Schon-Hegrad, M.A. *et al.* (1988a) Limiting-dilution analysis of T cells extracted from solid human lung tissue: comparison of precursor frequencies for proliferative responses and lymphokine production between lung and blood T cells from individual donors. *Immunology*, **64**, 649–54.

Holt, P.G., Schon-Hegrad, M.A. & Oliver, J. (1988b) MHC class II antigen-bearing dendritic cells in pulmonary tissues of the rat. Regulation of antigen presentation activity by endogenous macrophage populations. *J. Exp. Med.*, **167**, 262–74.

Holt, P.G., Oliver, J., Bilyk, N. *et al.* (1993) Downregulation of the antigen presenting cell function(s) of pulmonary dendritic cells *in vivo* by resident alveolar macrophages. *J. Exp. Med.*, **177**, 397–407.

Holt, P.G., Haining, S., Nelson, D.J. & Sedgwick, J.D. (1994) Origin and steady-state turnover of class II MHC-bearing dendritic cells in the epithelium of the conducting airways. *J. Immunol.*, **153**, 256–61.

Holt, P.G., Schon-Hegrad, M.A. & McMenamin, P.G. (1990) Dendritic cells in the respiratory tract. *Int. Rev. Immunol.*, **6**, 139–49.

Holt, P.G., Warner, L.A. & Papadimitriou, J.M. (1982) Alveolar macrophages. VII. Functional heterogeneity within macrophage populations from rat lung. *Aust. J. Exp. Biol. Med. Sci.*, **60**, 607–18.

Hoogsteden, H.C., van Dongen, J.J., van Hal, P.T., Delahaye, M., Hop, W. & Hilvering, C. (1989) Phenotype of blood monocytes and alveolar macrophages in interstitial lung disease. *Chest*, **95**, 574–7.

Hovi, T., Mosher, D. & Vaheri, A. (1977) Cultured human monocytes synthesize and secrete α_2-macroglobulin. *J. Exp. Med.*, **145**, 1580–9.

Ina, Y., Takada, K., Yamamoto, M., Morishita, M. & Yoshikawa, K. (1991) Antigen-presenting capacity of alveolar macrophages and monocytes in pulmonary tuberculosis. *Eur. Resp. J.*, **4**, 88–93.

Joseph, M., Tonnel, A.B., Capron, A. & Voisin, C. (1980) Enzyme release and superoxide anion production by human alveolar macrophages stimulated with immunoglobulin E. *Clin. Exp. Immunol.*, **40**, 416–22.

Joseph, M., Tonnel, A.B., Torpier, G. & Capron, A. (1983) Involvement of immunoglobulin E in the secretory processes of alveolar macrophages from asthmatic patients. *J. Clin. Invest.*, **71**, 221–30.

Kawabe, T., Isobe, K.I., Hasegawa, Y., Nakashima, I. & Shimokata, K. (1992) Immunosuppressive activity induced by nitric oxide in culture supernatant of activated rat alveolar macrophages. *Immunology*, **76**, 72–8.

Kehrl, J.H., Wakefield, L.M., Roberts, A.B. *et al.* (1986) Production of transforming growth factor beta by human T lymphocytes and its potential role in the regulation of T cell growth. *J. Exp. Med.*, **163**, 1037–50.

Kips, J.C., Tavernier, J. & Pauwels, R.A. (1992) Tumor necrosis factor (TNF) causes bronchial hyperresponsiveness in rats. *Am. Rev. Resp. Dis.*, **145**, 332–6.

Kreipe, H., Radzun, H.J., Heidorn, K. *et al.* (1990) Proliferation, macrophage colony-stimulating factor, and macrophage colony-stimulating factor-receptor expression of alveolar macrophages in active sarcoidosis. *Lab. Invest.*, **62**, 697–703.

Lehnert, B.E., Valdez, Y.E., Sebring, R.J., Lehnert, N.M., Saunders, G.C. & Steinkamp, J.A. (1990) Airway intra-luminal macrophages: evidence of origin and comparisons to alveolar macrophages. *Am. J. Respir. Cell Mol. Biol.*, **3**, 377–91.

Lem, V.M., Lipscomb, M.F., Weissler, J.C. *et al.* (1985) Bronchoalveolar cells from sarcoid patients demonstrate enhanced antigen presentation. *J. Immunol.*, **135**, 1766–71.

Lipscomb, M.F., Lyons, C.R., Nunez, G. *et al.* (1986) Human alveolar macrophages: HLA-DR-positive macrophages that are poor stimulators of a primary mixed leukocyte reaction. *J. Immunol.*, **136**, 497–504.

Lyons, C.R., Ball, E.J., Toews, G.B. *et al.* (1986) Inability of human alveolar macrophages to stimulate resting T cells correlates with decreased antigen-specific T cell-macrophage binding. *J. Immunol.*, **137**, 1173–80.

Mackaness, G.B. (1971) The induction and expression of cell-mediated hypersensitivity in the lung. *Am. Rev. Resp. Dis.*, **104**, 813–28.

McWilliam, A.S., Nelson, D., Thomas, J.A. & Holt, P.G. (1994) Rapid dendritic cell recruitment is a hallmark of the acute inflammatory response at mucosal surfaces. *J. Exp. Med.*, **179**, 1331–6.

Marathias, K.P., Preffer, F.I., Pinto, C. & Kradin, R.L. (1991) Most human pulmonary infiltrating lymphocytes display the surface immune phenotype and functional responses of sensitized T cells. *Am. J. Respir. Cell Mol. Biol.*, **5**, 470–6.

Martinet, Y., Yamaguchi, K. & Crystal, R.G. (1988) Differential expression of the tumor necrosis factor/cachectin gene by blood and lung mononuclear phagocytes. *Am. Rev. Resp. Dis.*, **138**, 659–65.

Mason, R.S., Frankel, T., Chan, Y.L., Lissner, D. & Posen, S. (1984) Vitamin D conversion by sarcoid lymph node homogenate. *Ann. Intern. Med.*, **100**, 59–61.

Mattoli, S., Mattoso, V.L., Soloperto, M., Allegra, L. & Fasoli, A. (1991) Cellular and biochemical characteristics of bronchoalveolar lavage fluid in symptomatic nonallergic asthma. *J. Allergy Clin. Immunol.*, **87**, 794–802.

Melis, M., Gjomarkaj, M., Pace, E., Malizia, G. & Spatafora, M. (1991) Increased expression of leukocyte function associated antigen-1 (LFA-1) and intercellular adhesion molecule-1 (ICAM-1) by alveolar macrophages of patients with pulmonary sarcoidosis. *Chest*, **100**, 910–6.

Moore, S.A., Streiter, R.M., Rolfe, M.W. *et al.* (1992) Expression and regulation of human alveolar macrophage-derived interleukin-1 receptor antagonist. *Am. J. Respir. Cell Mol. Biol.*, **6**, 569–75.

Nelson, D.J., McMenamin, C., McWilliam, A.S., Brenan, M. & Holt, P.G. (1994a) Development of the airway intraepithelial dendritic cell network in the rat from class II MHC (Ia) negative precursors: differential regulation of Ia expression at different levels of the respiratory tract. *J. Exp. Med.*, **179**, 203–12.

Nelson, D., McWilliam, A.S., Haining, S. & Holt, P.G. (1995) Downmodulation of airway intraepithelial dendritic cell populations following local and systemic exposure to steroids. *Am. J. Resp. Crit, Care Med.*, **151**, 475–81.

Nicod, L.P. & El Habre, F. (1992) Adhesion molecules on human lung dendritic cells and their role for T-cell activation. *Am. J. Respir. Cell Mol. Biol.*, **7**, 207–13.

Oghiso, Y. & Kubota, Y. (1986) Heterogeneity in immunologic functions among canine alveolar macrophage subfractions. *Nippon Juigaku Zasshi*, **48**, 1125–34.

Parra, S.C., Burnette, R., Preston Price, H. & Takaro, T. (1986) Zonal distribution of alveolar macrophages, type II pneumocytes, and alveolar septal connective tissue gaps in adult human lungs. *Am. Rev. Resp. Dis.*, **133**, 908–12.

Pollard, A.M. & Lipscomb, M.F. (1990) Characterization of murine lung dendritic cells: similarities to Langerhans cells and thymic dendritic cells. *J. Exp. Med.*, **172**, 159–67.

Poston, R.N., Chanez, P., Lacoste, J.Y., Litchfield, T., Lee, T.H. & Bousquet, J. (1992) Immunohistochemical characterisation of the cellular infiltration in asthmatic bronchi. *Am. Rev. Resp. Dis.*, **145**, 918–21.

Poulter, L.W. (1990) Changes in lung macrophages during disease. *FEMS Microbiol. Immunol.*, **64**, 327–32.

Poulter, L.W., Janossy, G., Power, C., Sreenan, S. & Burke, C. (1994) Immunological/physiological relationships in asthma: potential regulation by lung macrophages. *Immunol. Today*, **15**, 258–61.

Rajavashisth, T.B., Eng, R., Shadduck, R.K. *et al.* (1987) Cloning and tissue specific expression of mouse macrophage colony-stimulating factor mRNA. *Proc. Nat. Acad. Sci. USA*, **84**, 1157–61.

Rich, R.A., Cooper, C., Toossi, Z. *et al.* (1991) Requirement for cell-to-cell contact for the immunosuppressive activity of human alveolar macrophages. *Am. J. Respir. Cell Mol. Biol.*, **4**, 287–94.

Rich, R.A., Tweardy, D.J., Fujiwara, H. & Ellner, J.J. (1987) Spectrum of immunoregulatory functions and properties of human alveolar macrophages. *Am. Rev. Resp. Dis.*, **136**, 258–65.

Rigby, W.F.C. (1988) The immunobiology of vitamin D. *Immunol. Today*, **9**, 54–8.

Roberts, A.B. & Sporn, M.B. (1990) The transforming growth factor-betas. In: *Peptide Growth Factors and their Receptors. Handbook of Experimental Pharmacology* (eds Sporn, M.B.R., Roberts A.B.), pp. 419–72. Springer-Verlag, New York.

Romagnani, S. (1992) Induction of T_H1 and T_H2 responses: a key role for the 'natural' immune response? *Immunol. Today*, **13**, 379–81.

Sandron, D., Reynolds, H.Y., Venet, A., Laval, A.M., Israel-Biet, D. & Chretien, J. (1986) Human alveolar macrophage subpopulations isolated in discontinuous albumin gradients: functional data in normals and sarcoid patients. *Eur. J. Resp. Dis.*, **69**, 226–34.

Sawyer, R.T. (1986) The cytokinetic behaviour of pulmonary alveolar macrophages in monocytopenic mice. *J. Leuk. Biol.*, **39**, 89–99.

Sawyer, R.T., Strausbauch, P.H. & Volkman, A. (1982) Resident macrophage proliferation in mice depleted of blood monocytes by strontium-89. *Lab. Invest.*, **46**, 165–70.

Schon-Hegrad, M.A., Oliver, J., McMenamin, P.G. & Holt, P.G. (1991) Studies on the density, distribution, and surface phenotype of intraepithelial class II major histocompatibility complex antigen (Ia)-bearing dendritic cells (DC) in the conducting airways. *J. Exp. Med.*, **173**, 1345–56.

Sertl, K., Takemura, T., Tschachler, E., Ferrans, V.J., Kaliner, M.A. & Shevach, E.M. (1986) Dendritic cells with antigen-presenting capability reside in airway epithelium, lung parenchyma, and visceral pleura. *J. Exp. Med.*, **163**, 436–51.

Shellito, J. & Kaltreider, H.B. (1984) Heterogeneity of immunological function among subfractions of normal rat alveolar macrophages. *Am. Rev. Resp. Dis.*, **129**, 747–53.

Shellito, J. & Kaltreider, H.B. (1985) Heterogeneity of immunologic function among subfractions of normal rat alveolar macrophages. II. Activation as a determinant of functional activity. *Am. Rev. Resp. Dis.*, **131**, 678–83.

Sibille, Y. & Reynolds, H.Y. (1990) Macrophages and polymorphonuclear neutrophils in lung defense and injury. *Am. Rev. Resp. Dis.*, **141**, 471–501.

Soler, P., Moreau, A., Basset, F. & Hance, A.J. (1989) Cigarette smoking-induced changes in the number and differentiated state of pulmonary dendritic cells/Langerhans cells. *Am. Rev. Resp. Dis.*, **139**, 1112–7.

Sousa, A.R., Lane, S.J., Nakhosteen, J., Yoshimura, T. & Lee, T.H. (1993) GM-CSF expression in bronchial epithelium of asthmatic airways: decrease by inhaled corticosteroids. *Am. Rev. Resp. Dis.*, **147**, 1557–61.

Spiteri, M.A. & Poulter, L.W. (1991) Characterization of immune inducer and suppressor macrophages from the normal human lung. *Clin. Exp. Immunol.*, **83**, 157–62.

Spritzer, A.A., Watson, J.A., Auld, J.A. & Guethoff, M. (1968) Pulmonary macrophage clearance. The hourly rates of transfer of pulmonary macrophages to the oropharynx of the rat. *Arch. Environ. Health*, **17**, 726–30.

Stanley, E.R., Chen, B.D. & Lin, H.-S. (1978) Induction of macrophage production and proliferation by a purified colony-stimulating factor. *Nature*, **274**, 168–70.

Steinman, R.M. (1991) The dendritic cell system and its role in immunogenicity. *Ann. Rev. Immunol.*, **9**, 271–96.

Strickland, D.H., Kees, U.R. & Holt, P.G. (1995) Suppression of T-cell activation by pulomary alveolar macrophages: dissociation of effects on TcR, IL2-R expression, and proliferation. *Eur. Resp. J.* (in press).

Strickland, D.H., Thepen, T., Kees, U.R., Kraal, G. & Holt, P.G. (1993) Regulation of T-cell function in lung tissue by pulmonary alveolar macrophages. *Immunology*, **80**, 266–72.

Tazi, A., Bouchonnet, F., Grandsaigne, M., Boumsell, L., Hance, A.J. & Soler, P. (1993) Evidence that granulocyte macrophage-colony-stimulating factor regulates the distribution and differentiated state of dendritic cells/Langerhans cells in human lung and lung cancers. *J. Clin. Invest.*, **91**, 566–76.

Thepen, T., McMenamin, C., Girn, B., Kraal, G. & Holt, P.G. (1992) Regulation of IgE production in presensitised animals: *in vivo* elimination of alveolar macrophages preferentially increases IgE responses to inhaled allergen. *Clin. Exp. Allergy*, **22**, 1107–14.

Thepen, T., Van Rooijen, N. & Kraal, G. (1989) Alveolar macrophage elimination *in vivo* is associated with an increase in pulmonary immune response in mice. *J. Exp. Med.*, **170**, 499–509.

Troutt, A.B. & Lee, F. (1989) Tissue distribution of murine haemopoietic growth factor mRNA production. *J. Cell Physiol.*, **138**, 38–44.

Upham, J.W., Strickland, D.H., Bilyk, N. & Holt, P.G. (1995) Alveolar macrophages from humans and rodents selectively inhibit T-cell proliferation but permit activation and cytokine secretion. *Immunology*, **84**, 142–7.

van Haarst, J.M.W., Hoogsteden, H.C., de Wit, H.J., Verhoeven, G.T., Havenith, C.E. & Drexhage, H.A. (1994) Dendritic cells and their precursors isolated from human bronchoalveolar lavage: immunocytologic and functional properties. *Am. J. Respir. Cell Mol. Biol.*, **11**, 344–50.

Venet, A., Hance, A.J., Saltini, C., Robinson, B.W.S. & Crystal, R.G. (1985) Enhanced alveolar macrophage-mediated antigen-induced T lymphocyte proliferation in sarcoidosis. *J. Clin. Invest.*, **75**, 293–301.

Wahl, S.M., Hunt, D.A., Wong, H.L. *et al.* (1988) Transforming growth factor-beta is a potent immunosuppressive agent that inhibits IL-1 dependent lymphocyte proliferation. *J. Immunol.*, **140**, 3026–32.

Warner, A.E. & Brain, J.D. (1986) Intravascular pulmonary macrophages: a novel cell removes particles from blood. *Am. J. Physiol.*, **250**, R728–32.

Weinberg, D.S. & Unanve, E.R. (1981) Antigen presenting function of alveolar macrophages: uptake and presentation of Listeria monocytogenes. *J. Immunol.*, **126**, 794–9.

Wewers, M.D., Rennard, S.I., Hance, A.J., Bitterman, P.B. & Crystal, R.G. (1984) Normal human alveolar macrophages obtained by lavage have a limited capacity to release interleukin-1. *J. Clin. Invest.*, **74**, 2208–18.

Wiktor, J.W., Bartocci, A., Ferrante, A.W.J. *et al.* (1990) Total absence of colony-stimulating factor 1 in the macrophage-deficient osteopetrotic (op/op) mouse. *Proc. Nat. Acad. Sci. USA*, **87**, 4828–32.

Winkler, G.C. (1989) Review of the significance of pulmonary intravascular macrophages with respect to animal species and age. *Exp. Cell. Biol.*, **57**, 281–6.

Yamauchi, K., Basset, P., Martinet, Y. & Crystal, R. (1987) Normal human alveolar macrophages express the gene coding for transforming growth factor-beta, a protein with a capacity to suppress fibroblast growth. *Am. Rev. Resp. Dis.*, **135**, A66 [abstract].

Yamauchi, K., Martinet, Y., Basset, P., Fells, G.A. & Crystal, R.G. (1988) High levels of transforming growth factor-beta are present in the epithelial lining fluid of the normal human lower respiratory tract. *Am. Rev. Resp. Dis.*, **137**, 1360–3.

CHAPTER 14

Leucocyte Adhesion in Allergic Inflammation

A. J. Wardlaw

Introduction

Leucocyte migration from the bone marrow into the blood and then into the tissue is one of the central events of leucocyte biology and essential to the integrity of the immune system. This is illustrated by leucocyte adhesion deficiency disease (LAD) type 1, where the inability of neutrophils to enter tissue due to defective expression of the leucocyte integrins leads to severe life-threatening infections and premature death (Anderson & Springer, 1987). A striking feature of allergic inflammation is the accumulation of activated eosinophils and mononuclear cells without increased numbers of neutrophils. As eosinophils make up only a small proportion of the normal leucocyte count, this suggests a selective process of leucocyte migration. Leucocyte migration through endothelium has been shown to be a process involving sequential steps in which the cells are initially lightly tethered to the endothelium and roll along its surface. This is followed by cell activation, mediated by a soluble chemotactic stimulus, which allows a firmer bond to develop between the leucocyte and the endothelial cell resulting in successful adhesion and transmigration (Lawrence & Springer, 1991; Von Adrian *et al.*, 1991). The steps occur in series so that each is essential for transmigration to occur. This means that selectivity can be introduced at each of the steps, resulting in considerable diversity in the pattern of signals at any one inflammatory site. It also implies that migration can be modulated at each of the steps, offering a range of targets for pharmacological inhibition. The receptors and mediators involved in leucocyte migration have, to a large extent, been characterized (Fig. 14.1). Selectins and their counter-receptors, as well as α4 integrins, are thought to mediate the initial attachment and rolling step; a number of chemotactic mediators have been implicated in the activation step, and β2 and α4 integrins expressed on leucocytes, binding to their endothelial adhesion counter-receptors belonging to the immunoglobulin superfamily, are implicated in the firmer adhesion step (Bevilacqua, 1993; Springer, 1994).

Structure and function of leucocyte adhesion receptors

Selectins and their counter-structures

The selectins

The selectins consist of three type 1 glycoprotein membrane receptors, L-selectin, P-selectin (formerly GMP-140) and E-selectin (formerly endothelial leucocyte adhesion molecule 1 (ELAM-1)) (Rosen, 1993). E- and P-selectin are expressed on endothelium, while L-selectin is expressed by all leucocytes. P-selectin is also expressed on platelets. Whereas E-selectin expression is induced on endothelial cells as a result of cytokine-stimulated gene transcription and new protein synthesis (Bevilacqua *et al.*, 1987), P-selectin is stored in cytoplasmic Weibel–Palade bodies and translocated within minutes to the cell surface after stimulation of the endothelium by a variety of mediators, including thrombin, leukotriene C_4 (LTC_4) and histamine (McEver *et al.*, 1989; Geng *et al.*, 1990). L-selectin was first defined by the monoclonal antibody (mAb) MEL 14 in the mouse as a peripheral lymph node T-cell homing receptor which recognized sulphated, fucosylated counter-receptors (addressins) on lymph node high endothelial

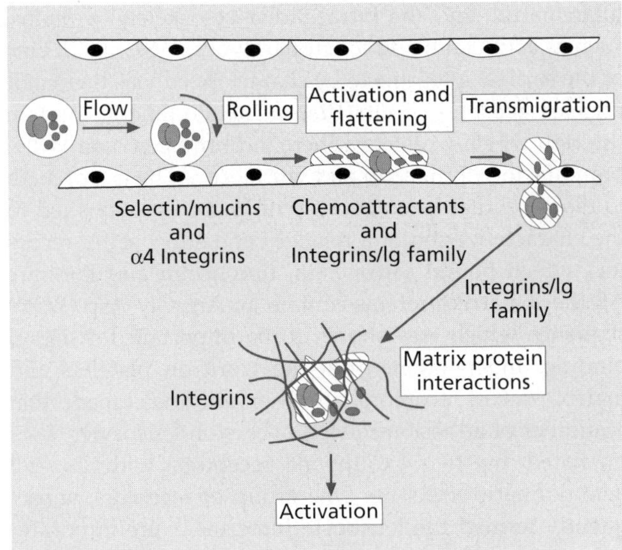

Fig. 14.1 Schematic outline of the stages involved in leucocyte migration and the adhesion receptor families involved.

venules (HEV) (Gallatin *et al.*, 1983). L-selectin is constitutively expressed and shed on cell activation (Kishimoto *et al.*, 1990). The selectins have a common structure characterized by an N-terminal calcium-dependent (C type) lectin domain which binds sugars consisting of a family of sialylated fucosylated glycosaminoglycans typified by the carbohydrate moiety sialyl Lewis x (Springer & Lasky, 1991). Sialylation appears necessary for adhesion, as neuraminidase abolishes selectin-dependent adhesion interactions. Similarly, fucosylation is an important requirement, as shown by patients with a defect in endogeneous fucose metabolism who are immunodeficient as a result of an inabilty of cells to bind through selectins (LAD type 2) (Etzioni *et al.*, 1992). Adjacent to the lectin domain is an epithelial growth factor (EGF)-like domain and a variable number of between two and nine (depending on the selectin) repeated units related to complement binding proteins such as decay accelerating factor (DAF) (Johnston *et al.*, 1989; Tedder *et al.*, 1989). L-selectin has two repeat units, E-selectin 6 and P-selectin 9 (Fig. 14.2).

Selectin counter-structures

Although the adhesion function of the selectins requires binding through sugars, the backbone on which the sugars are presented is important in providing increased specificity and affinity of binding. Three ligands for L-selectin have been identified—glycosylated cell adhesion molecule-1 (GlyCAM-1), CD34 and mucosal addressin cell adhesion molecule (MAdCAM-1). A chimeric molecule comprising the extracellular region of L-selectin attached to the CH2 and CH3 regions of human Fc was used as an immunoaffinity reagent to immunoprecipitate two bands from lysates of HEV organ cultures labelled with $^{S}35$-sulphate or ^{3}H-fucose. The molecular weight of one band was 50 kDa and the other, 90 kDa. The 50-kDa band was identified as a novel mucin-like molecule with two heavily *O*-glycosylated serine threonine-rich domains termed GlyCAM-1 (Lasky *et al.*, 1992). GlyCAM-1 does not have a transmembrane region and appears to be a secreted molecule, although antibodies against it stain the surface of HEV. Sulphation and possibly fucosylation are required for GlyCAM-1 to be functionally active (Imai *et al.*, 1993) The 90-kDa ligand was found to be an HEV-specific glycoform of CD34 (Baumheuter *et al.*, 1993). CD34 is a heavily *O*-glycosylated transmembrane receptor with a mucin-like structure. It is expressed widely on endothelial cells as well as haemopoietic stem cells (Greaves *et al.*, 1992). Only the HEV isoform of CD34 binds L-selectin. Like GlyCAM-1, CD34 has sialylated, sulphated and fucosylated O-linked sugars. A mAb MECA 79 inhibits L-selectin dependent-binding of lymphocytes to HEV and recognizes both CD34 and GlyCAM-1, as well as a number of other proteins (Hemmerich *et al.*, 1994). It may therefore recognize the carbohydrate epitope common to L-selectin ligands.

A third L-selectin ligand is the mouse mucosal lymph node (MLN) addressin MAdCAM-1 (Briskin *et al.*, 1993). MAdCAM-1, as well as containing a region that binds α4β7, has a mucin-like domain. Interestingly, while MAdCAM-1 isolated from mesenteric lymph nodes supports rolling of transfected lymphoid cells, MAdCAM-1

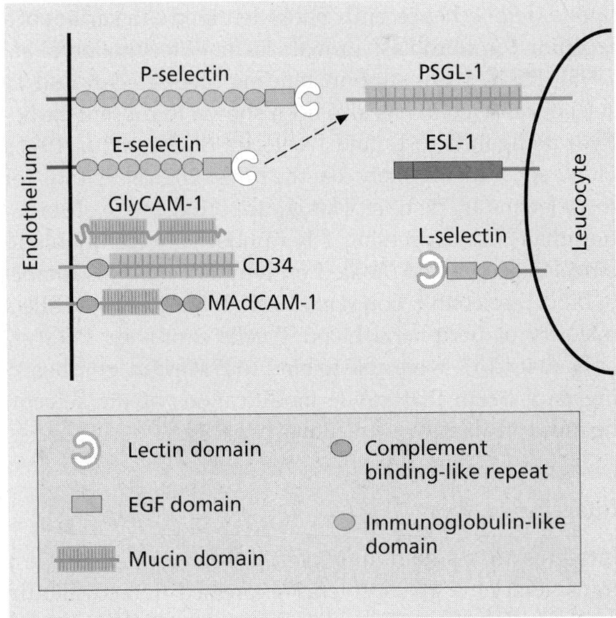

Fig. 14.2 Schematic representation of the structure of the selectins and their ligands. See text for definition of abbreviations.

from cultured endothelioma cells does not. Consistent with this, the MLN MAdCAM-1 was recognized by MECA 79, whereas the endothelioma cells were not recognized by this antibody (Berg *et al.*, 1993). Thus, carbohydrate modifications of MAdCAM-1 by HEV are necessary to support L-selectin binding.

Further insights into the nature of selectin ligands were gained from the cloning of PSGL-1, the receptor for P-selectin (Sako *et al.*, 1993). PSGL-1 was cloned using an expression technique from an HL60 cDNA library which was cotransfected with a cDNA for α(1,3/1,4)fucosyltransferase (3/4FT). PSGL-1 is a mucin-like transmembrane protein which is a homodimer of 220 kDa. Therefore, it has the same structure and molecular weight as the P-selectin ligand described on neutrophils (Moore *et al.*, 1992). As with the L-selectin ligands, sialylation and fucosylation are essential for P-selectin binding (Zhou *et al.*, 1991). As mentioned above, E-selectin, like P-selectin, recognizes an α(2,3) sialylated α 1(1–3) fucosylated lactosaminoglycan moiety which includes sialyl Lewis x. One molecule which carries this epitope is the cutaneous lymphocyte antigen (CLA), recognized by the mAb HECA 452. CLA binds E-selectin and recognizes a distinct subset of peripheral blood T lymphocytes which home to the skin (Picker *et al.*, 1991). In this context, E-selectin is working as a skin vascular addressin for T lymphocytes. Although it might be expected that the ligand for E-selectin would be a mucin, this does not appear to be the case. T-lymphocyte binding to E-selectin was not affected by removal of cell-surface sialomucins by *O*-glycoprotease, whereas binding to P-selectin was abolished (Alon *et al.*, 1994). In addition, the mouse neutrophil E-selectin ligand (ESL-1) has recently been identified as a variant of a receptor for fibroblast growth factor (Steegmaler *et al.*, 1995). PSGL-1 can support binding of E-selectin and L-selectin. L-selectin has also been shown to present carbohydrate ligands to E- and P-selectin (Picker *et al.*, 1991). However, it seems likely that the physiological ligands for the selectins are distinct. This is supported by the observation that CLA-expressing T lymphocytes were unable to bind P-selectin, and PSGL-1 on lymphocytes was unable to bind E-selectin (Alon *et al.*, 1994). Interestingly, while a majority of peripheral blood T cells expressed PSGL-1, only about 15% were able to bind to P-selectin, emphasizing once again that subtle modifications of the selectin ligands can alter their functional capacity.

Integrins

Integrins are a superfamily of α, β, heterodimeric, type 1 transmembrane glycoproteins, expressed non-covalently on the cell surface. They were termed integrins because they were perceived as forming a bridge between an extracellular ligand, particularly proteins of the extracellular matrix, and the intracellular cytoskeletal proteins, such as actin, talin and vinculin (Hynes, 1987, 1992). One of the earliest integrins to be characterized was the major platelet receptor gpIIb/IIIa, a heterodimeric protein through which platelets adhere to fibrinogen, von Willebrand factor, fibronectin and vitronectin. The use of mAb to block cellular interactions with matrix proteins led to the characterization of a related yet distinct set of receptors which bound vitronectin, fibronectin and laminin. All these matrix proteins contain an Arg-Gly-Asp (RGD) sequence which was shown to be important for ligand binding. Independent from the work on platelets and matrix protein receptors, an observation was made that a number of adhesion-related events on leucocytes were mediated by two groups of receptors with an α/β heterodimeric structure. One group of receptors, subsequently termed the leucocyte integrins, were important in leucocyte adhesion to endothelium, T-cell proliferation and cytotoxic T-cell killing. The second group were termed the VLA proteins, because the first two identified, VLA-1 and VLA-2, appear very late after lymphocyte activation. Full characterization of these receptors resulted in a classification based on complementarity at the nucleotide and amino-acid level. Three subfamilies of integrins were defined based on a common β-chain combining with a number of α-chains. Thus, the β1 integrin family consisted of a single β-chain (CD29), combining with six-chains (CD49a–f, α_{1-6}/β1) to form the very late activation (VLA) family, the β2 integrin family (leucocyte integrins; CD18/CD11a–c; LFA-1,Mac-1,p150,95; α_L/β1, α_M/β1, α_X/β1) and the β3 family (cytoadhesions; gpIIb/IIIa, CD41/CD61; vitronectin receptor; $\alpha_V\beta3$, CD51/CD61), of which gpIIb/IIIa is the most abundant platelet receptor playing a crucial role in platelet aggregation. Since that original classification, it has become apparent that the association between α- and β-chains is not as restricted as once thought. In addition, a number of new α- and β-chains have been characterized, giving the integrin family another level of complexity (Fig. 14.3).

Leucocyte integrins

Mac-1 (also known as Mo-1, OKM-1 and complement receptor type 3 (CR3)) was first defined by mAb as a marker for myeloid cells (Springer *et al.*, 1979). LFA-1 was identified by screening the mAb that blocked killing by cytotoxic T lymphocytes of tumour cells (Davignon *et al.*, 1981a,b). It became apparent that these two receptors shared a similar structure, with a high-molecular-weight α-chain and a common β-chain. Characterization of the third member of the family, p150,95, followed shortly (Schwarting *et al.*, 1985; Miller *et al.*, 1986). A fourth member of the subfamily, CD11d/CD18, has been identified which is expressed on tissue macrophages and binds

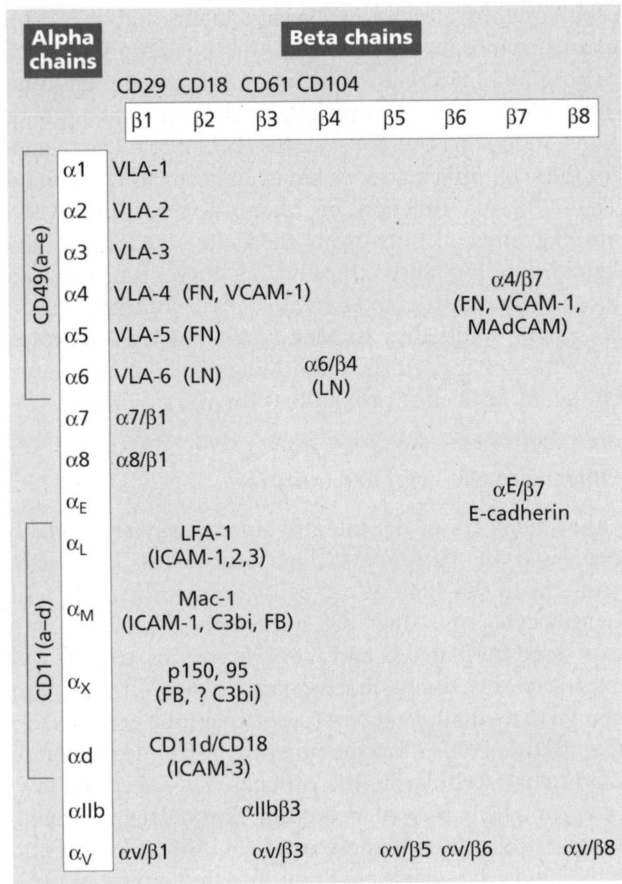

Fig. 14.3 The integrin superfamily. See text for definition of abbreviations.

ICAM-3 (Hogg & Berlin, 1995). Expression of the leucocyte integrins is restricted to cells of the immune system, with LFA-1 expressed by virtually all leucocytes (Krensky *et al.*, 1983) and Mac-1 expressed by myeloid cells, large granular lymphocytes and a subset of B cells (Arnaout & Colten, 1984). p150,95 is expressed on macrophages and is a marker for hairy cell leukaemia. It is only weakly expressed on neutrophils and has been designated CR4 (Myones *et al.*, 1988). The importance of the leucocyte integrins was underlined by the realization that a rare autosomal recessive immunodeficiency disorder, LAD, was due to lack of expression of the three members of the β2 integrins by all leucocytes (Anderson & Springer, 1987). This disease is characterized by life-threatening septicaemia, indolent superficial infections which fail to respond to antibiotics and, commonly, death in early infancy. Neutrophils from LAD patients exhibit a marked *in vitro* defect in adhesion-related functions such as chemotaxis and phagocytosis. Biopsies from infected wounds revealed large numbers of neutrophils in the vasculature but very few in the tissue. The disease is due to mutations in the β2-chain (Wardlaw *et al.*, 1990).

The complete primary structures of the α-subunits of LFA-1 (Larson *et al.*, 1989), Mac-1 (Arnaout *et al.*, 1988; Corbi *et al.*, 1988a) and p150,95 (Corbi *et al.*, 1987) have been determined. The subunits have a molecular weight of 180, 170 and 150 kDa, respectively, which, after deglycosylation, are reduced to 149, 137 and 132 kDa. The common β-subunit has a molecular weight of 95 kDa (78 kDa).

cDNA cloning of the β2-chain revealed a deduced sequence of 769 amino acids with an N-terminal extracellular domain of 677 amino acids with six potential *N*-glycosylation sites, a 23 amino-acid transmembrane domain and a 46 amino-acid cytoplasmic domain (Kishimoto *et al.*, 1987; Law *et al.*, 1987). There was a high cysteine content (7.4%) which was concentrated in a cysteine-rich (20%) region of 186 amino acids, giving the subunit a rigid tertiary structure. There was general homology with the β1 and β3 integrin subunits (37–45% shared identity), with particularly high homology in the cytoplasmic domain, the transmembrane domain and a region of 241 amino acids in the extracellular domain (64%). Cross-linking studies of RGD peptide binding to gpIIb/IIIa suggests that this latter region is important in ligand binding (D'Souza *et al.*, 1988). In addition, in several LAD patients the mutation in the β-chain responsible for the disease is located in this region, suggesting that it is important for α/β association. All 56 cysteine residues are conserved between the three family members. The genes for the α subunits of LFA-1, CR3 and p150,95 have been located to the short arm of chromosome 16 between bands p11 and p13.1 (Corbi *et al.*, 1988b), while the gene for the β2-chain is located to chromosome band 21q/22.3 on chromosome 21 using somatic cell hybrids (Marlin *et al.*, 1986).

The α-subunit cDNA revealed deduced primary structures characterized by long extracellular domains (approximately 1000 amino acids) and short cytoplasmic domains (19–53 amino acids). An important feature of all three α-chains are three homologous repeats that have putative cation-binding sites which are similar to the 'EF-hand loop' found in other calcium-binding proteins such as calmodulin. These sites may account for the magnesium dependency of leucocyte integrin dependent adhesion. Mac-1 and p150,95 α-chains share 63% identity with each other but only 35% identity with the LFA-1 α-subunit. The α-subunits of the integrin superfamily share 25–63% amino-acid identity. There are certain shared features within the superfamily which suggest an evolutionary grouping of the α-chains. Thus, a number of α-chains, such as those of VLA-5, VLA-3, αv/β3 and αIIb/β3, share a sequence in the C-terminal end of the extracellular domain which is post-translationally cleaved, with resulting fragments bridged by a disulphide bond. VLA-4 has a unique cleavage site in the centre of the extracellular domain to give approximately equal sized fragments

(Hemler *et al.*, 1990). The leucocyte integrins do not have a cleavage site but do have a 200 amino-acid region which is present in $\alpha1\beta1$, $\alpha2\beta1$ and $\alpha_E\beta7$ but none of the other α-chains. This region has been termed the I domain, for inserted or interactive domain. A similar domain appears in a number of other proteins, including collagen, various collagen binding proteins such as cartilage matrix proteins and von Willebrand factor and the complement factors B and C2. Recombinant I (or A) domain from Mac-1 contains a novel cation binding site and can bind ICAM-1 and fibrinogen, as well as being the binding site for the hookworm-derived Mac-1 inhibitor NIF (Michishita *et al.*, 1993; Moyle *et al.*, 1994). The crystal structure of the domain has shown that it adopts the dinucleotide binding fold which is a common structural motif in a variety of intracellular enzymes (Lee *et al.*, 1995). A number of ligands or counter-receptors for the leucocyte integrins have been described. LFA-1 was shown to bind to a member of the immunoglobulin gene superfamily called intercellular adhesion molecule-1 (ICAM-1). Since then, two other ICAM-like molecules which bind LFA-1 have been described (ICAM-2, ICAM-3) and ICAM-1 has been shown to bind Mac-1, although with a lower affinity than LFA-1 (Fig. 14.4).

Mac-1 appears to have an extensive range of binding activities. It binds the 'inactivated' opsonic C3b (iC3b) component (Beller *et al.*, 1982). Binding of iC3b does not depend on neutrophil activation but is increased by activation. Although iC3b contains an RGD sequence, binding is not dependent on this region. Neutrophils can also bind fibrinogen through Mac-1 (Altieri *et al.*, 1988; Wright *et al.*, 1988) and *Leishmania* gp63 (Russell & Wright, 1988). These proteins also have RGD sequences, although Mac-1 binding to these proteins does not appear to be RGD dependent. Another binding site on Mac-1 is 'lectin-like' and binds to various ligands such as unopsonized rabbit erythrocytes, bakers' yeast particles and its capsule extract zymosan. In addition, Mac-1 is responsible for neutrophil binding to unstimulated vascular endothelium, plastic and glass surfaces and neutrophil aggregation (Anderson *et al.*, 1986; Wallis *et al.*, 1986). The ligands for these binding activities have not been clearly defined. The adhesive function of Mac-1 appears to involve binding sites distinct from those involved in soluble ligand binding and adhesion, as these functions are blocked by different mAb (Anderson *et al.*, 1986; Dana *et al.*, 1986). Antibodies to Mac-1 also block Fc receptor-mediated phagocytosis, suggesting that the two molecules may be in close proximity (Brown *et al.*, 1988).

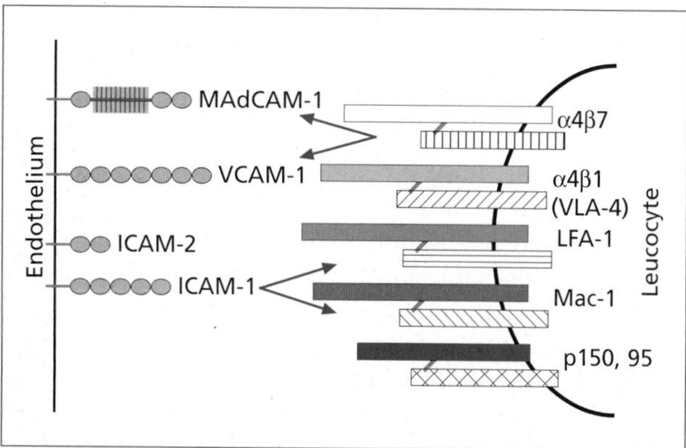

Fig. 14.4 Schematic representation of the structure of leucocyte integrins and their ligands. See text for definition of abbreviations.

Other leucocyte-expressed integrins

Other members of the integrin superfamily are variably expressed by peripheral blood leucocytes. Expression varies with the state of cell activation, particularly with lymphocytes. Of the $\beta3$ integrins, $\alpha^{IIb}/\beta3$ is only expressed by platelets and megakaryocytes, $\alpha^{v}\beta3$ is well expressed by tissue macrophages where it has been shown to mediate phagocytosis of apoptotic granulocytes (Savill *et al.*, 1990). Most members of the $\beta1$ integrin family bind to extracellular matrix proteins. The exception is $\alpha4$ integrin which, as well as binding fibronectin, also binds vascular cell adhesion molecule-1 (VCAM-1). In addition, $\alpha4\beta7$ binds the endothelial lymphocyte homing receptor MAdCAM-1, and $\alpha_E\beta7$, expressed by epithelial T lymphocytes, binds E-cadherin (Cepek *et al.*, 1994). $\alpha4\beta7$ is expressed by lymphocytes, eosinophils and natural killer (NK) cells but not by neutrophils or monocytes (Erle *et al.*, 1994).

$\alpha4\beta1$ was characterized as one of the $\beta1$ (VLA) integrins expressed by T lymphoblastoid cell lines. It has an unusual structure, lacking both an I domain and the disulphide-linked light chain near the C terminus which is seen in several other VLA-α chains. Uniquely, it has a cleavage site in the middle of the protein which yields bands of 80 and 70 kDa in sodium dodecyl sulphate–polyacrylamide gel electrophoresis (SDS–PAGE), as well as a single 150 kDa band (Takada *et al.*, 1989; Hemler *et al.*, 1990). It binds VCAM-1 and the alternatively spliced IIICS region of fibroenctin recognizing an LDV (single letter amino-acid code) motif in both proteins (Elices *et al.*, 1990). $\beta7$ was first identified as a partial cDNA obtained from human lung by the polymerase chain reaction (PCR), using oligonucleotides that recognized highly conserved sequences of integrin β-chains. $\beta7$ is a 798 amino-acid protein (including signal peptide) which is 32–46% homologous to other β-integrin chains. It is most closely related to the $\beta2$ integrin (Erle *et al.*, 1991).

It has recently become clear that, like the selectins, both $\alpha4\beta1$ binding to VCAM-1 and $\alpha4\beta7$ binding to

MAdCAM-1 can participate in rolling interactions and arrest of leucocytes under conditions of flow (Berlin *et al.*, 1995; Kassner *et al.*, 1995).

Regulation of integrin function

A number of leucocyte functions, including migration, as well as needing rapid adherence to endothelium and related structures also requires dis-adherence. An important aspect of integrin function is therefore the regulation of adhesiveness for ligand. On resting cells many integrins are unable to bind ligand. For example, resting T lymphocytes and granulocytes bind to purified ICAM-1 only very weakly. Activation of T lymphocytes, for example by phorbol esters or by cross-linking CD3, caused up-regulation of adhesiveness which in the case of phorbol esters was prolonged, but in the case of a CD3-mediated signal was transient, lasting only about 20 minutes (Dustin & Springer, 1989; Van Kooyk *et al.*, 1989). The mechanisms involved in regulation of integrin function have been intensively studied and the findings reviewed (Diamond & Springer, 1994). A number of models to explain the mechanisms involved in changes in integrin function have been proposed, and there is a consensus that a conformational change in the receptor occurs which alters the structure of the ligand-binding domain, so changing its affinity for ligand. Activation can result in the appearance of neo-epitopes recognized by certain activation-related mAb. For example, NKI-L16, an anti-LFA mAb, binds only poorly to resting lymphocytes, but binds well to phorbol ester-activated cells (Van Kooyk *et al.*, 1991). Other anti-integrin antibodies cause up-regulation of integrin binding. For example, KIM 127 recognizes CD18 and promotes adhesion mediated by LFA-1 and Mac-1 (Robinson *et al.*, 1992). Similarly, changes in the cation can alter affinity of binding with Mn^{2+} stimulating binding (Gailit & Rusholahti, 1988). The regulation of affinity of binding by phorbol esters raised the possibility that phosphorylation of the cytoplasmic domain of the β-subunit was responsible. However, mutagenesis of the major phosphorylation site of the β2-subunit did not alter adhesiveness of LFA-1 for ICAM-1 (Hibbs *et al.*, 1991b). Nonetheless, truncation of the cytoplasmic regions of both the α and β integrin subunits can affect affinity of binding. For example, truncation of the β2-subunit cytoplasmic domain in COS cell transfected with LFA-1 inhibited binding to ICAM-1 (Hibbs *et al.*, 1991). In the case of $\alpha^{IIb}\beta3$, deletion of a highly conserved five-amino-acid membrane proximal region converts the receptor into a constitutively activated form (O'Toole *et al.*, 1991). One possible explanation for these findings is that intracellular protein(s) exist which bind to the cytoplasmic regions of the α- or β-chains. In this model, binding of this putative protein regulated by cell activation would alter the conformation of the extracellular region of the integrin, resulting in either repression or enhancement of adhesion.

In the case of some integrins, cellular activation results in increased expression of the receptor. For Mac-1 this is as a result of recruitment from intracellular stores (Miller *et al.*, 1987). This intracellular pool can be rapidly mobilized in response to stimulus with a number of chemoattractants, including formyl-methionyl-leucyclphenylalanine (f-MLP), C5a, LTB_4 (Fearon & Collins, 1983; Arnout & Colten, 1984; Berger *et al.*, 1984), platelet-activating factor (PAF) (Shalit *et al.*, 1988) and granulocyte macrophage colony-stimulating factor (GM-CSF) (Buckle & Hogg, 1989). There is evidence that the newly expressed receptors are functionally inactive (Buyon *et al.*, 1988; Phillips *et al.*, 1988; Vedder & Harlan, 1988; Nourshargh *et al.*, 1989; Schleiffenbaum *et al.*, 1989), and it appears more likely that functional activation of the receptor is due to a conformational change as discussed above.

Immunoglobulin family members

ICAM-1

It was observed that homotypic aggregation of lymphoid cells was mediated through LFA-1, binding to a counter-structure distinct from itself (Rothlein *et al.*, 1986). mAb were raised against Epstein–Barr virus (EBV) transformed B cells from a patient with LAD; therefore, the cells did not express LFA-1. This panel of mAb was screened for their ability to inhibit LFA-1-dependent homotypic aggregation. One mAb (RR1/1) was characterized which inhibited this function (Rothlein & Springer, 1986). It defined a 76–114-kDa heavily glycosylated single-chain transmembrane receptor with a peptide backbone of 55 kDa, the variable molecular weight being due to different degrees of glycosylation of its eight potential, N-linked, glycosylation sites (Dustin *et al.*, 1986; Rothlein *et al.*, 1986). A number of approaches including binding between purified ICAM-1 and LFA-1, conclusively demonstrated that ICAM-1 was a receptor for LFA-1 (Marlin & Springer, 1987). cDNA cloning of ICAM-1 revealed that it was a member of the immunoglobulin gene superfamily and was thus the first demonstration of an interaction between members of the integrin and immunoglobulin gene families (Dustin *et al.*, 1988b; Simmons *et al.*, 1988; Staunton *et al.*, 1988) ICAM-1 contains five immunoglobulin-like domains, with homology to the neural cell adhesion molecule (NCAM) and myelin-associated protein (MAG), another neural adhesion protein. As well as binding LFA-1 and Mac-1 (Dustin & Springer, 1988; Smith *et al.*, 1989; Diamond *et al.*, 1990), ICAM-1 is also a receptor for *Plasmodium falciparum* (Berendt *et al.*, 1989) and the major group of rhinovirus (Greve *et al.*, 1989; Staunton *et al.*, 1989; Tomassini *et al.*, 1989). A soluble form of ICAM-1 lacking the transmembrane and cytoplasmic domains binds the human rhinovirus inhibiting infection (Marlin *et al.*, 1990). LFA-1, rhinovirus and *P. falciparum* bind to distinct regions of the first two amino-terminal domains of ICAM-1, with the first domain being of particular importance (Staunton *et al.*, 1990), whereas Mac-1 binds to the third amino-terminal domain (Diamond *et al.*, 1991). As a result there is a difference in the pattern of mAb inhibition of ICAM-1/β2 integrin interactions. For example, mAb RR1/1 inhibits LFA-1/ICAM-1 interactions but not Mac-1/ICAM-1 interactions, whereas mAb R6.5 inhibits both. ICAM-1 is a widely expressed molecule and is found on vascular endothelium, leucocytes, dendritic cells, fibroblasts and epithelial cells (Rothlein *et al.*, 1986; Dustin *et al.*, 1988a; Makgoba *et al.*, 1988; Weetman *et al.*, 1989; Vogetseder *et al.*, 1989). In contrast to the integrins, its function appears to be regulated by increased expression rather than a conformational change in constitutively expressed molecules. Expression is increased on most cell types by a number of cytokines, including interleukin-1 (IL-1), tumour necrosis factor (TNF) and interferon-γ (IFN-γ), with some specificity between cytokine and cell type (Dustin *et al.*, 1986; Pober *et al.*, 1986b). For example, keratinocyte ICAM-1 is induced by IFN-γ, and less well by TNF, whereas IFN-γ, TNF and lipopolysaccharide (LPS) are all good inducers of ICAM-1 on fibroblasts. Increased expression *in vitro* is protein synthesis dependent, detectable after about 4 hours and maximal by 24 hours. ICAM-1 has been implicated in a large number of cellular functions, including leucocyte migration, lymphocyte homing, cytotoxic T lymphocytes (CTL) and large granular lymphocyte cytotoxicity, antigen presentation and thymocyte maturation.

Functional studies with lymphocyte cell lines suggested that LFA-1 had ligands other than ICAM-1. Two other ICAMs have been characterized. ICAM-2 is a 60 000-kDa single-chain transmembrane receptor with a peptide backbone of 31 kDa. Like ICAM-1, ICAM-2 is a member of the immunoglobulin superfamily with two immunoglobulin-like domains which are most homologous (35%) to the two amino-terminal domains of ICAM-1. ICAM-2 is constitutively expressed on vascular endothelial cells and expression is not increased by cytokine activation (Staunton *et al.*, 1989). It is also expressed on lymphocytes, monocytes and platelets, but not on neutrophils (de Fougerolles *et al.*, 1991). ICAM-3 is a highly glycosylated protein of 124 kDA which is well expressed on all leucocytes, including neutrophils, but not endothelial cells (de Fougerolles & Springer, 1992). In assays of adhesion of resting lymphocytes to purified LFA-1, ICAM-3 appeared to have the greatest role (compared with ICAM-1 and -2) in modulating lymphocyte function.

VCAM-1

Functional studies with lymphocytic cell lines had demonstrated an adhesion pathway independent of the leucocyte integrins and ICAM-1 (Dustin & Springer, 1988). The endothelial receptor responsible for this pathway was attributed to a 110-kDa protein initially termed INCAM-110 (Rice *et al.*, 1989; Rice & Bevilacqua, 1990). The name vascular cell adhesion molecule-1 was ascribed to a molecule characterized by an elegant functional expression cloning technique (Osborn *et al.*, 1989). VCAM-1 is expressed by endothelial cells as well as fibroblasts and dendritic cells. Its expression is induced on human umbilical vein endothelial cells (HUVEC) by TNF-α and IL-1, with a time-course similar to ICAM-1. IL-4 selectively up-regulates VCAM-1 expression (Thornhill *et al.*, 1991). VCAM-1 is synthesized in two forms, a six-domain and seven-domain form as a result of mRNA splicing (Cybulsky *et al.*, 1991). The seven-domain form is predominant in endothelial cells. Subsequently, VCAM-1 was shown to bind to VLA-4 on the surface of the Jurkat cells (Elices *et al.*, 1990). This pathway has subsequently been shown to be important in monocyte, lymphocyte, eosinophil and basophil adhesion to HUVEC (Campanero *et al.*, 1990; Schwartz *et al.*, 1990; Bochner *et al.*, 1991; Dobrina *et al.*, 1991; Walsh *et al.*, 1991; Weller *et al.*, 1991). Neutrophils do not express VLA-4 (Hemler *et al.*, 1984; Hemler, 1988) and cannot bind to VCAM-1. A possible role for VCAM-1 in mediating selective eosinophil migration in allergic disease has been proposed.

MAdCAM-1

A recent addition to the immunoglobulin-like adhesion receptor family is the MAdCAM-1. To date this has only been identified in mice. It is preferentially expressed on HEV in Peyer's patches and mesenteric lymph nodes. MAdCAM-1 is a type 1 glycoprotein with an interesting structure. It has two N-terminal immunoglobulin domains, most closely related to VCAM-1 and ICAM-1, which bind α4β7, followed by a mucin-like domain which can bind L-selectin, and then closest to the membrane is an immunoglobulin domain related to the third domain of immunoglobulin A1 (IgA1) which is also mucosa related (Berlin *et al.*, 1993; Brisken *et al.*, 1993). It has been identified as a lymphocyte homing receptor, but its role in human leucocyte migration is currently unknown.

Expression of adhesion receptors in allergic inflammation

Selectins

Expression of E-selectin in allergic inflammation has been

studied with variable results. Normal skin endothelium has a low background expression of E-selectin. Expression was increased after allergen challenge, with the kinetics of up-regulation broadly corresponding to the pattern observed *in vitro* with HUVEC (Kyan-Aung *et al.*, 1991). Up-regulation of E-selectin expression was observed after allergen challenge of skin biopsy organ cultures, suggesting that cells resident in the skin (TNF-α from mast cells would be a likely candidate) were able to generate the mediators responsible for increased expression (Leung *et al.*, 1991). In both the upper and lower airway a more complex pattern of expression is observed, with good constitutive staining of E-selectin in the normal airway. This has made it more difficult to demonstrate an increase in expression of these receptors after allergen challenge or in clinical disease. In a study by Bentley *et al.* (1993), E-selectin expression was increased in the airways of intrinsic asthmatics but not extrinsic asthmatics compared with non-asthmatic controls. Similar findings were reported by Montefort *et al.* (1992). In the Bentley study no increases in E-selectin expression were seen after aerosol allergen challenge. But in another study E-selectin expression was increased after segmental allergen challenge through a bronchoscope (Monteforte *et al.*, 1993). P-selectin expression has not been addressed by the above studies; however, a recent study, reported as an abstract, demonstrated expression of P-selectin on the lumenal surface of skin endothelium using immuno-electron microscopy 1 hour after allergen challenge, this had dissipated by 6 hours after challenge (Murphy *et al.*, 1994). Another study reported the translocation of P-selectin to the endothelial cell membrane for up to 1 hour after the injection of the neuropetides substance P (SP), vasoactive intestinal peptide (VIP) and calcitonin gene-related peptide (CGRP) (Smith *et al.*, 1993). In studies carried out by the authors of eosinophil adhesion to nasal polyp endothelium (see below), good expression of E-selectin and P-selectin was found, with on average of about 30% of blood vessels stained. However, it was subsequently discovered that the E-selectin antibody cross-reacted with P-selectin. Using specific anti-E-selectin mAb, rather weaker expression has been found. Unlike the position with HUVEC where P-selectin is only transiently expressed, it was found that P-selectin was consitutively expressed on the cell surface in the chronic inflammation of nasal polyps (Symon *et al.*, 1994).

Expression of integrins and immunoglobulin family adhesion receptors in allergic inflammation

The expression of ICAM-1 and VCAM-1 in allergic inflammation has been investigated by a number of groups. Normal skin endothelium has a low background expression of ICAM-1 and expression is increased after allergen challenge (Kyan-Aung *et al.*, 1991). VCAM-1 expression was weak in both normal and allergen-challenged skin. Good constitutive staining of ICAM-1 was observed in the normal human airway, with increased expression of ICAM-1 in the bronchi of intrinsic, but not extrinsic asthmatics (Bentley *et al.*, 1993). Descriptions of VCAM-1 expression in the upper and lower airways have been variable. Some reports have suggested an increase in asthma and rhinitis, although changes have been small. Increases in expression after allergen challenge have also been reported. Bentley *et al.* (1993) found no significant increases in ICAM-1 and VCAM-1 in endobronchial biopsies after aerosol allergen challenge, but there was a trend towards an increase in VCAM-1 with a good correlation between numbers of airway eosinophils after allergen challenge and expression of VCAM-1. A modest increase (9 vs. 26%) in the number of blood vessels positive for VCAM-1 was also observed after allergen challenge (by applying paper discs to the nasal mucosa) in subjects with allergic rhinitis (Nacleiro *et al.*, 1994). ICAM-1, like E-selectin, was increased after segmental allergen challenge through a bronchoscope (Monteforte *et al.*, 1993). In perennial rhinitis an increase in endothelial expression of ICAM-1 and VCAM-1 was observed compared with normal controls, although VCAM-1 was relatively weak (Monteforte *et al.*, 1992). In the nasal polyp model described above, very weak VCAM-1 has been found, despite strong staining in tonsil tissue as a control. In contrast, Jahnsen *et al.*, using immunofluorescence, found increased expression of VCAM-1 in nasal polyps compared with normal nasal tissue, although only a mean of 5% of blood vessels stained strongly (Jahnsen *et al.*, 1995). Also, Ohkawara *et al.*, in six asthmatics compared with six normal controls, found increased expression of VCAM-1 as well as E-selectin and ICAM-1 in the bronchial submucosa (Ohkawara *et al.*, 1995). Presumably these discrepancies are due to differences in the sensitivity of the staining technique.

ICAM-1 expression on epithelial cells has also been studied. A number of groups have shown increased ICAM-1 on bronchial epithelium in asthma (Bentley *et al.*, 1993; Vignola *et al.*, 1993; Manolitsas *et al.*, 1994). In addition, Ciprandi *et al.* have demonstrated induction of ICAM-1 within 30 minutes of allergen challenge on both nasal and conjunctival epithelium (Ciprandi *et al.*, 1993, 1994). The role of ICAM-1 in epithelial function in allergic disease is unclear, although it could be acting as an accessory molecule for T-cell stimulation. Also, its function as a receptor for the major group of rhinoviruses means that the epithelium in asthmatics may be more vulnerable to viral infection, thus offering an explanation for the vulnerability of asthmatics to viral infections.

Soluble adhesion molecules

Several adhesion molecules can be detected in soluble form circulating in the plasma. In some cases, for example P-selectin and ICAM-1, these appear to be truncated forms of the receptors which have been synthesized from alternatively spliced mRNA and lack a transmembrane domain, leading to secretion rather than membrane expression (Simmons *et al.*, 1988). For other receptors, for example L-selectin and possibly E-selectin, a secreted form is not apparent and the soluble form is the result of proteolytic cleavage. Raised concentrations of circulating adhesion molecules have been detected in a number of diseases (Gearing & Newman, 1993), although concentrations are generally below those required to block leucocyte adhesion to endothelium. Montefort *et al.* (1994) investigated whether concentrations of circulating adhesion molecules may reflect inflammatory activity in asthma. They found that concentrations of E-selectin, ICAM-1 and VCAM-1 were not elevated in stable asthma, but there was a significant increase compared with normal controls in concentrations of sE-selectin and sICAM-1 in patients with acute severe asthma. However, concentrations of these molecules did not correlate with disease severity and were therefore not thought useful in clinical management. Similarly, concentrations of sICAM-1 and sE-selectin were increased in severe atopic dermatitis but did not fall after successful treatment with UVA-1 therapy (Kowalzick *et al.*, 1995). Modest increases in concentrations of sICAM-1 and sE-selectin have also been detected in bronchoalveolar lavage (BAL) fluid after segmental allergen challenge (Georas *et al.*, 1992; Takahashi *et al.*, 1994).

In vivo studies of adhesion receptor antagonists in models of allergic inflammation

In vivo inhibition of selectin interactions

Antibodies against L-selectin partially inhibited rolling of human eosinophils on rabbit mesentery venular endothelium *in vivo*, as shown by intra-vital microscopy (Sriramarao *et al.*, 1994). A number of studies have been performed on wild-caught cyanomologous monkeys with a natural sensitivity to *Ascaris* antigen (Gundel *et al.*, 1993). Inhalation challenge of *Ascaris* antigen in these animals resulted in an airway inflammatory response and increased bronchial hyperresponsiveness (BHR). Different responses were observed depending on whether antigen challenge was single, in which case an early and sometimes dual (early and late) response was observed, or multiple over several days in which case a marked eosinophilia and increased BHR were seen. The pre-challenge state of the animal was also important in determining the response. Some animals had a pre-challenge airway eosinophilia and markedly increased BHR. These animals developed a late response after a single allergen challenge, which was characterized by increased numbers of airway neutrophils. Other animals had a relative paucity of eosinophils in their BAL pre-challenge, but developed a marked airway eosinophilia and increased BHR after multiple allergen challenge. The airway eosinophilia and increased BHR after multiple antigen challenge was inhibited by a mAb against ICAM-1 but not E-selectin (Wegner *et al.*, 1990) In contrast, the airway neutrophilia generated by a single challenge was inhibited by anti-E-selectin but not anti-ICAM-1 (Gundel *et al.*, 1991). This suggests that, in this model at least, BHR was associated with an airway eosinophilia which was mediated in part by ICAM-1, whereas the airway neutrophilia was associated with the development of a late response and mediated by E-selectin.

In vivo inhibition of integrin/immunoglobulin interactions

Animal models of allergic inflammation have provided further information on the relative importance of integrins and their ligands in eosinophil migration. As mentioned above, in the cyanomologous monkey model anti-ICAM-1 was effective at inhibiting eosinophil migration into the airways and the development of BHR. It is of course possible that the antibody was working indirectly on other cell types, rather than blocking eosinophil migration directly. In the same multiple allergen challenge model, anti-Mac-1 mAb inhibited the development of BHR and reduced the levels of eosinophil cationic protein (ECP) in the BAL fluid but did not inhibit the airway eosinophilia. This suggested that Mac-1 was not essential for eosinophil migration, but that Mac-1 may be involved in triggering eosinophil activation and mediator release (Wegner *et al.*, 1993). In a sheep model of allergen challenge, the anti-VLA-4 mAb HP1/2 was able to inhibit the late response to allergen challenge and the development of bronchial hyperresponsiveness when given both intravenously and by inhalation (Abraham *et al.*, 1993). Interestingly, there was little difference between the antibody-treated animals and control animals in the recruitment of eosinophils into BAL, dissociating the airway eosinophilia from the physiological effects of allergen challenge. One explanation suggested by the authors for this apparent discrepancy was that anti-VLA-4 treatment was inhibiting eosinophil activation and mediator release in a similar manner to that observed with the anti-Mac-1 treatment in the monkey model. In support of this hypothesis they observed that eosinophils treated *in vitro* with anti-VLA-4 mAb released less eosinophil peroxidase (EPO) after PAF stimulation than control eosinophils. Consistent with the observation that eosinophil migration was not VLA-4 dependent in this model, no increase in VCAM-1 expression was seen on the airway endothelium. In rats, anti-VLA-4, Mac-1 and LFA-1 were all able to inhibit the early and late response to ovalbumin challenge but had no obvious effect on leucocyte recruitment into the lung, although this was measured 8 hours after challenge before any major cellular recruitment into the lung occurred (Rabb *et al.*, 1994). The mechanism by which the antibodies inhibited the response to antigen challenge in this study is therefore not clear.

A different pattern has been observed in guinea pigs and mice. In guinea pigs, the anti-VLA-4 mAb HP1/2 inhibited the migration of eosinophils into the skin both after injection of chemotactic factors and after passive cutaneous anaphylaxis. Expression of VCAM-1 on skin endothelium was not investigated (Weg *et al.*, 1993). Similarly, HP1/2 was able to inhibit migration of eosinophils into the airway submucosa in sensitized, ovalbumin-challenged guinea pigs. The allergen challenge-induced increase in BHR was also prevented, as was the increase in the concentration of EPO in BAL fluid (Pretolani *et al.*, 1994). In sensitized mice, anti-VLA-4 mAb inhibited eosinophil and T-cell infiltration into the trachea after ovalbumin challenge (Nakajima *et al.*, 1994). Anti-VCAM-1 mAb was also effective and VCAM-1 expression was strongly induced by antigen challenge. Neither the VCAM-1 expression or the eosinophil infiltration was IL-4 dependent. Unlike the monkey model, anti-ICAM-1 and anti-LFA-1 mAb were ineffective at inhibiting eosinophil migration. Lastly, aerosolized anti-VLA-4 mAb inhibited allergen-induced BAL eosinophilia and BHR in rabbits sensitized to house dust mite (Metzger *et al.*, 1994). These studies point to an important role for VLA-4, Mac-1, ICAM-1 and, possibly, VCAM-1 in eosinophil recruitment and activation in allergic inflammation, and offer the possibility that suitably designed adhesion receptor antagonists may be therapeutically effective. They also suggest that there are important species differences in the adhesion receptors used by eosinophils to migrate into antigen-challenged airways.

Role of adhesion receptors in leucocyte migration in allergic disease

Allergic inflammatory reactions are characterized by a distinctive pattern of leucocyte infiltration. In the first few hours after allergen challenge, neutrophils followed by eosinophils appear. By 24 hours, eosinophil accumulation persists together with basophil infiltration but the neutrophil accumulation has subsided. Activated monocytes and Th2-type lymphocytes have appeared. In the chronic disease state neutrophils are relatively scanty and the lesions are characterized by an eosinophil- and mononuclear cell-rich inflammatory process. It has been hypothesized that selective patterns of adhesion receptor expression control this process. The most distinctive feature is the presence of eosinophils and most investigators have concentrated on mechanisms of eosinophil migration.

Eosinophils and basophils

Eosinophil/basophil selectin interactions

The mechanisms involved in eosinophil and basophil recruitment have recently been reviewed (Wardlaw *et al.*, 1994). Eosinophil adhesion to cytokine-stimulated cultured HUVEC can be inhibited by blocking mAb against E- and L-selectin (Weller *et al.*, 1991; Knol *et al.*, 1993). In addition, eosinophils can adhere specifically to COS cells transfected with an E-selectin cDNA (G.M. Walsh & A.J. Wardlaw, unpublished observations), to tissue culture plates coated with either E- or P-selectin and to CHO cells transfected with the P-selectin cDNA (Vadas *et al.*, 1993). Eosinophils express L-selectin in similar amounts to neutrophils and, like neutrophils, L-selectin is shed on eosinophil activation *in vitro* with chemotactic mediators and *in vivo* (Smith *et al.*, 1992). Eosinophil binding to E- and P-selectin does not appear to be affected by the state of activation of the cells. Superficially, at least, eosinophils appear very similar to neutrophils in their selectin interactions, but there is some evidence of subtle but important differences between these two cell types. Whereas neutrophils express large amounts of sialyl Lewis x, eosinophils express relatively little of this sugar moiety. The pattern of inhibition of eosinophil adhesion to HUVEC by a panel of L-selectin antibodies was found to be different between eosinophils and neutrophils (Knol *et al.*, 1994). In addition, neutrophils bound much more avidly than eosinophils to purified E-selectin (Bochner *et al.*, 1994).

A study was reported above, in which the frozen-section, Stamper–Woodruff assay was used to investigate eosinophil adhesion to nasal polyp endothelium (Symon *et al.*, 1994). It was found that eosinophil adhesion was mediated largely by endothelial P-selectin, which was constitutively expressed in this chronic inflammatory model. More recently, neutrophil binding has been compared in the same assay. A striking finding was that eosinophils bound with much greater avidity to the polyp blood vessels than neutrophils. However, the profile of adhesion receptors used by the two cell types was broadly similar, with over 80% inhibition of adhesion by antibodies against P-selectin and PSGL-1. To try and explain this observation, it was hypothesized that there may be differences in the eosinophil and neutrophil P-selectin ligands. The eosinophil P-selectin ligand, characterized using a P-selectin-IgG chimera and a rabbit antiserum against PSGL-1, appeared to be a structural isoform of PSGL-1 which migrates in SDS gels with a calculated molecular weight about 10 kDa higher than neutrophil PSGL-1. In agreement with Wein *et al.* (1995), it was found that under static conditions eosinophils and neutrophils bind to purified soluble P-selectin coated on tissue culture plates with the same avidity. However, selectins function under flow and the Stamper–Woodruff assay is carried out under shear stress conditions. In collaboration with Dr Michael Lawrence of the University of Virginia, a comparison has been made between eosinophil and neutrophil binding to purified P-selectin under flow conditions. In the five subjects studied, it was demonstrated that eosinophils bound to P-selectin with greater avidity than neutrophils at physiological flow rates. This therefore supports the concept that eosinophil PSGL-1 is structurally and functionally distinct from neutrophil PSGL-1, and that the eosinophil receptor supports increased binding to P-selectin in the nasal polyp model (Symon *et al.*, 1996).

Eosinophil/basophil integrin interactions

Eosinophil adhesion to unstimulated HUVEC is enhanced about twofold by stimulation with PAF, IL-5 and other eosinophil active inflammatory mediators, and this enhancement is almost totally inhibited by mAb to the leucocyte integrin Mac-1 binding to an as yet unidentified endothelial ligand (Kimani *et al.*, 1988; Lamas *et al.*, 1988; Walsh *et al.*, 1990). Compared with adhesion to unstimulated HUVEC, eosinophil and basophil adhesion to TNF-α- or IL-1-stimulated HUVEC is markedly increased, and this enhancement can be inhibited by mAb against ICAM-1 and VCAM-1 on the endothelium and LFA-1, Mac-1 and VLA-4 on the leucocyte (Bochner *et al.*, 1991; Dobrina *et al.*, 1991; Walsh *et al.*, 1991). Eosinophil transmigration through endothelial cells using artificial models of the blood vessel wall has also been investigated. These studies have demonstrated that eosinophil transmigration through HUVEC was increased by cytokine stimulation of the endothelium, and that eosinophils from allergic donors showed an increased migration capacity consistent with the idea that eosinophils from subjects with allergic disease are activated (Moser *et al.*, 1992). Similarly, *in vitro* culture of peripheral blood eosinophils from normal donors with GM-CSF, IL-3 and IL-5 increased their migration capacity. The receptors that mediate transmigration of eosinophils through IL-1- or TNF-α-stimulated HUVEC appear to be primarily the leucocyte integrins LFA-1 and Mac-1 on the eosinophil binding to ICAM-1 and possibly other as yet unidentified ligands on the endothelium (Ebisawa *et al.*, 1992). Antibodies against VLA-4 and VCAM-1 did not inhibit IL-1-stimulated transmigration. In contrast, eosinophil migration through IL-4-stimulated HUVEC was partly inhibited by anti-VLA-4 antibodies as well as antibodies against the leucocyte integrins (Schleimer *et al.*, 1992). The hypothesis that VLA-4/VCAM-1 could be a selective pathway of adhesion was strengthened, as discussed above, by the observation that IL-4 selectively induced expression of VCAM-1 on HUVEC (Thornhill *et al.*, 1991).

Eosinophil adhesion to extracellular matrix

After migration through the endothelium the eosinophil and basophil come into contact with the proteins of the extracellular matrix. This is not simply a mesh in which the leucocytes are supported, but a complex network of large fibrillar proteins that have a profound influence on cellular function, mainly through adhesive contacts with integrin receptors expressed both on the surface of resident cells such as fibroblasts and the epithelium as well as leucocytes migrating from the peripheral blood. Tissue eosinophils have an activated phenotype. They express activation receptors such as CD69 (Hartnell *et al.*, 1993), generate mRNA for a number of cytokines that do not appear to be generated by normal peripheral blood eosinophils (Desreumauz *et al.*, 1992) and express the secreted form of ECP as recognized by the mAb EG2 (Azzawi *et al.*, 1990; Bentley *et al.*, 1992). Whether basophils also become activated as they migrate into inflammatory sites is not so clear. The mechanism of eosinophil activation is not well understood. *In vitro* studies suggest that the process of migration through endothelium itself may result in eosinophil activation (Walker *et al.*, 1991). In addition, locally generated chemotactic mediators may be involved. Interaction with the extracellular matrix can result in 'outside in' signalling through integrin receptors, leading to eosinophil and basophil priming and mediator release (Hynes, 1992). There have been relatively few studies of such interactions. Dri *et al.* (1991) studied the production of superoxide by eosinophils resting on different surfaces including endothelial cells and a number of matrix proteins after stimulation with soluble mediators. They found that the nature of the surface influenced the amount of superoxide produced with, for example, endothelial cells inhibiting superoxide production and fibrinogen priming eosinophils for enhanced superoxide generation after stimulation with f-MLP. Anwar *et al.* (1994) demonstrated enhancement of calcium ionophore-stimulated LTC_4 generation by eosinophils adhering to fibronectin when compared with bovine serum albumin (BSA)-coated surfaces, and Neeley *et al.* (1994) have reported that VLA-4-mediated interaction with fibronectin resulted in increased f-MLP-induced eosinophil degranulation. In contrast, Kita *et al.* (1994) found that adherence to fibronectin and laminin inhibited eosinophil-derived neurotoxin (EDN) release stimulated by PAF, C5a and IL-5 but not by phorbol myristate acetate (PMA). The secretogogue used is obviously important in determining the effects of matrix proteins on eosinophil degranulation. When eosinophils were cultured for several days on plasma fibronectin they had increased survival compared with eosinophils cultured on BSA or plastic as a result of autocrine generation of GM-CSF and IL-3. Cytokine release and survival was inhibited by anti-VLA-4 mAb (Anwar *et al.*, 1993). These observations have now been extended to show that tissue fibronectin is considerably more effective than plasma fibronectin at supporting eosinophil survival (Walsh *et al.*, 1995). This is consistent with the idea that survival is a result of triggering through $\alpha4/\beta1$ (VLA-4), as tissue fibronectin contains more of the alternatively spliced 111CS region that contains the binding site for VLA-4 (Mould *et al.*, 1990). In addition to antibodies against VLA-4, survival was also inhibited by antibodies against $\alpha4/\beta7$ and Mac-1, suggesting that survival on fibronectin may be due to triggering through multiple integrin receptors. Eosinophils can adhere to laminin through $\alpha6/\beta1$ (Georas *et al.*, 1993). Laminin also promotes eosinophil survival. As well as being important to eosinophil cytokine generation in disease, the interaction between eosinophils and fibronectin may be a homeostatic mechanism that enables eosinophils to survive for prolonged periods in tissue before undergoing apoptosis and removal.

Monocytes

The specific pathways involved in monocyte adhesion interactions in allergic disease have not been so well studied as those involving eosinophils. Monocytes express VLA-5 as well as VLA-4 and VLA-6, but expression of $\alpha4/\beta7$ is difficult to detect. They express all of the $\beta2$ leucocyte integrin subfamily, as well as $\alpha v/\beta3$. They express L-selectin and can interact with P- and E-selectin (Patarroyo, 1994). They can use both leucocyte integrins and VLA-4 binding to ICAM-1, VCAM-1 and Fn to migrate through HUVEC (Meerschaert & Furie, 1995).

T lymphocytes

A central function of lymphocytes is their ability to re-circulate from the blood into the lymphoid organs and back to blood in search of antigen. Lymphocyte re-circulation is controlled by the interaction between adhesion receptors on lymphocytes (homing receptors) and their counter-receptors (addressins) on vascular endothelium. The lymphoid system can be considered as being divided into three compartments. A primary compartment consisting of the thymus and bone marrow, where lymphocyte differentiation occurs, a secondary compartment consisting of the lymph nodes and specialized aggregates of lymphoid tissue where antigen presentation principally occurs, and a tertiary compartment consisting of the remainder of the body tissues where inflammatory reactions occur and lymphocytes undertake many of their effector functions (Picker & Butcher, 1992). The components of the secondary lymphatic compartment appear to be grouped according to anatomical site and they are linked to specific tertiary lympoid organs. For example, the peripheral lymph nodes (PLN) drain the skin and superficial tissues, Peyers patches (PP) and mesenteric lymph nodes are gut-associated mucosal lymphoid tissues which drain the intestine, and the thoracic hilar lymph nodes form a third group of lymphoid tissues which drain the lung. It has been appreciated for many years that lymphocytes continuously re-circulate between the blood and the secondary lymphoid organs (Gowans, 1957). Naive lymphocytes which have never encountered antigen can circulate widely through different groups of lymph nodes but have a limited ability to migrate into the tissues. In contrast, the migration of lymphoblasts and memory lymphocytes is non-random. These activated lymphocytes preferentially re-circulate back to the lymph nodes in which they first encountered antigen. Thus, lymphoblasts obtained from peripheral lymph nodes in the mouse when radiolabelled and re-injected back into the mouse return to the peripheral lymph nodes. In addition, activated lymphocytes can enter non-specialized lymphoid tissue through post-capillary venules, especially if the tissue is inflamed.

The entry of lymphocytes from the circulation into lymph nodes is controlled by adhesion and transmigration of the lymphocyte through specialized post-capillary venules, found in the T-cell domains of the lymph node cortex, called high endothelial venules (HEV). These endothelial cells have a cuboidal shape, unlike the flat appearance of most venular endothelium (Gowans & Knight, 1964). HEV are found in all secondary lymphoid organs including PLN, PP, tonsils, mesenteric lymph nodes and the small aggregates of lymphoid tissue on mucosal surfaces of the respiratory and gastrointestinal tract termed, respectively, bronchial- and gut-associated lymphoid tissue (BALT and GALT). In addition, HEV-like vessels are seen in chronically inflamed tissue, such as the synovium associated with rheumatoid arthritis.

The basis for many of the studies that have characterized the pattern of lymphocyte re-circulation is the Stamper–Woodruff frozen section assay (Stamper & Woodruff, 1976). This is an *ex vivo* assay in which lymphocytes, obtained either from lymph nodes or the peripheral blood, are layered on frozen sections of lymph nodes. Under appropriate conditions the lymphocytes adhere to

HEV and this can be inhibited by anti-adhesion mAb. *In vivo* studies in rats and mice investigating the inhibitory effects of these blocking mAb on lymphocyte re-circulation have generally confirmed the findings obtained with the frozen section assay. Thus, the PLN, T-lymphocyte homing receptor was defined as L-selectin and the gut mucosal homing receptor was characterized as α4/β7 (Holzmann *et al.*, 1989). CD44 and LFA-1 appear to act as accessory adhesion receptors that strengthen the adhesive process without controlling selectivity of attachment (Jalkanen *et al.*, 1987).

A number of studies have suggested that there is selective lymphocyte homing to the lung (Spencer & Hall, 1984; der Brugge-Gamelkoorn *et al.*, 1986). For example, McDermott & Bienenstock (1979) found that lymphoblasts from the lung of rats localized poorly to the intestine, but entered lung-associated lymph nodes 10 times better than lymphoblasts from PLN and three times better than lymphoblasts from mesenteric nodes.

The role of lymphocyte homing receptors in sensitization to allergens and the localization of T cells in the airways in asthma or other types of allergic inflammation has not been well defined, although as mentioned above the CLA antigen appears to act as a homing receptor for a subset of T cells that preferentially localize to the skin (Picker *et al.*, 1991a). BAL T cells in normal subjects as well as asthmatics are mostly memory cells and express CD69. Increased numbers of CD25-positive T cells are seen in BAL fluid in asthma (Corrigan & Kay, 1992). T cells in BAL fluid from allergen-challenged mice were L-selectin negative and expressed increased amounts of VLA-4, although a variable pattern of adhesion receptor expression was observed on these cells (Kennedy *et al.*, 1995).

Summary and conclusions

Considerable progress has been made in our understanding of the molecular mechansisms involved in leucocyte adhesion interactions. Migration through endothelium is a staged process, with each stage offering a level of control over the cell specificity and degree of migration. This also offers a wide range of targets for pharmacological intervention. Although the structure and function of the receptors involved in leucocyte migration have been well characterized, the contribution each makes to the pattern of leucocyte accumulation in disease, and in particular allergic disease, has been less well studied. Most work has been undertaken on selective patterns of eosinophil receptor usage and a number of differences from neutrophils have been identified. These include VLA-4/VCAM-1 interactions, which are also likely to be involved in monocyte, T-lymphocyte and basophil recruitment, as well as potentially important differences in the pattern of selectin interactions. Relatively little work has been undertaken on T-lymphocyte and monocyte adhesion interactions in allergic disease and this is an interesting area for further study, although selective antagonists are likely to be needed for conclusive results. Results using mAb in a number of animal models already offer the hope that this approach may be successful. The development of drugs that can be tested in the clinic are awaited with considerable interest.

References

Abraham, W.M., Sielczak, M.W., Ahmed, A. *et al.* (1993) α4 integrins mediate antigen-induced late bronchial responses and prolonged airway hyperresponsiveness in sheep. *J. Clin. Invest.*, 776–87.

Alon, R., Rossiter, H., Wang, X., Springer, T.A. & Kupper, T.S. (1994) Distinct cell surface ligands mediate T lymphocyte attachment and rolling on P and E-selectin under physiological flow. *J. Cell Biol.*, **127**, 1485–95.

Altieri, D.C., Bader, R., Mannucci, P.M. & Edgington, T.S. (1988) Oligospecificity of the cellular adhesion receptor Mac-1 encompasses an inducible recognition specificity for fibrinogen. *J. Cell Biol.*, **107**, 1893–900.

Anderson, D.C., Miller, L.J., Schmalsteig, F.C., Rothlein, R. & Springer, T.A. (1986) Contributions of the Mac-1 glycoprotein family to adherence-dependent granulocytic functions: structure–function assessments employing sub-unit specific monoclonal antibodies. *J. Immunol.*, **137**, 15–27.

Anderson, D.C. & Springer, T.A. (1987) Leukocyte adhesion deficiency: an inherited defect in the Mac-1, LFA-1 and p150,95 glycoproteins. *Ann. Rev. Med.*, **38**, 175–94.

Anwar, A.R.E., Cromwell, O., Walsh, G.M., Kay, A.B. & Wardlaw A.J. (1993) Adhesion to fibronectin prolongs eosinophil survival. *J. Exp. Med.*, **177**, 839–43.

Anwar, A.R.E., Cromwell, O., Walsh, G.W., Kay, A.B. & Wardlaw, A.J. (1994) Adhesion to fibronectin primes eosinophils via α4/β1. *Immunology*, **82**, 222–8.

Arnaout, M.A. & Colten, H.R. (1984) Complement C3 receptors: structure and function. *Mol. Immunol.*, **21**, 1191–9.

Arnaout, M.A., Gupta, S.K., Pierce, M.W. & Tenen, D.G. (1988) Amino acid sequence of the alpha subunit of human leukocyte adhesion receptor Mo1 (complement receptor type 3) *J. Cell. Biol.*, **106**, 2153–8.

Azzawi, M., Bradley, B., Jeffery, P.K. *et al.* (1990) Identification of activated T lymphocytes and eosinophils in bronchial biopsies in stable atopic asthma. *Am. Rev. Resp. Dis.*, **142**, 1407–13.

Baumheuter, S., Singer, M.S., Henzel, W. *et al.* (1993) Binding of L-selectin to the vascular sialomucin CD34. *Science*, **262**, 436–8.

Beller, D.I., Springer, T.A. & Schreiber, R.D. (1982) Anti-Mac-1 selectivity inhibits the mouse and human type three complement receptor. *J. Exp. Med.*, **156**, 1000–9.

Bentley, A.M., Menz, G., Storz, C. *et al.* (1992) Identification of T lymphocytes, macrophages and activated eosinophils in the bronchial mucosa in intrinsic asthma: relationship to symptoms and bronchial hyperresponsiveness. *Am. Rev. Resp. Dis.*, **146**, 500–6.

Bentley, A.M., Durham, S.R., Robinson, D.S. *et al.* (1993) Expression of endothelial and leukocyte adhesion molecules, intercellular adhesion molecule-1, E-selectin and vascular cell adhesion molecule-1 in the bronchial mucosa in steady state and allergen induced asthma. *J. Allergy Clin. Immunol.*, **92**, 857–68.

Berendt, A.R., Simmons, D.L., Tansy, J., Newbold, C.I. & Marsh, K.

(1989) Intercellular adhesion molecule-1 is an endothelial cell adhesion receptor for *Plasmodium falciparum*. *Nature*, **341**, 57–9.

Berg, E.L., McEvoy, L.M., Berlin, C., Bargatze, R.F. & Butcher, E.C. (1993) L-selectin mediated lymphocyte rolling on MAdCAM-1. *Nature*, **366**, 695–8.

Berger, M., O'Shea, J., Cross, A.S. *et al.* (1984) Human neutrophils increase expression of C3bi as well as C3b receptors upon activation. *J. Clin. Invest.*, **74**, 1566–71.

Berlin, C., Berg, E.L., Briskin, M.J. *et al.* (1993) α4β7 integrin mediates lymphocyte binding to the mucosal vascular addressin MAdCAM-1. *Cell*, **74**, 185–95.

Berlin, C., Bargatze, R.F., Campbell, J.J. *et al.* (1995) α4 integrin mediates lymphocyte attachment and rolling under physiologic flow. *Cell*, **80**, 413–22.

Bevilacqua, M.P. (1993) Endothelial leukocyte adhesion molecules. *Ann. Rev. Immunol.*, **11**, 767–804.

Bevilacqua, M.P., Pober, J.S., Mendrick, D.L., Cotran, R.S. & Gimbrone, M.A. (1987) Identification of an inducible endothelial leukocyte adhesion molecule ELAM-1. *Proc. Nat. Acad. Sci. USA*, **84**, 9238–42.

Bochner, B.S., Lusckinskas, F.W., Gimbrone, M.A. *et al.* (1991) Adhesion of human basophils and eosinophils to IL-1 activated human vascular endothelial cells: contribution of endothelial cell adhesion molecules. *J. Exp. Med.*, **173**, 1552.

Bochner, B.S., Sterbinsky, S.A., Bickel, C.A., Werfel, S., Wein, M. & Newman, W. (1994) Differences between human eosinophils and neutrophils in the function and expression of sialic acid containing counterligands for E-selectin. *J. Immunol.*, **152**, 774–82.

Briskin, M.J., McEvoy, L.M. & Butcher, E.C. (1993) MAdCAM-1 has homology to immunoglobulin and mucin-like adhesion receptors and IgA-1. *Nature*, **363**, 461–4.

Brown, E.J., Bohnsack, J.F. & Gresham, H.D. (1988) Mechanism of inhibition of immunoglobulin G-mediated phagocytosis by monoclonal antibodies that recognize the Mac-1 antigen. *J. Clin. Invest.*, **81**, 365–75.

Buckle, A.M. & Hogg, N. (1989) The effect of IFN-gamma and colony stimulating factors on the expression of neutrophil cell membrane receptors. *J. Immunol.*, **143**, 2295–301.

Buyon, J.P., Abramson, S.B., Phillips, M.R. *et al.* (1988) Dissociation between increased surface expression of gp165/95 and homotypic neutrophil aggregation. *J. Immunol.*, **140**, 3156–60.

Campanero, M.R., Puliod, R., Ursa, M.A. *et al.* (1990) An alternative leukocyte adhesion mechanism, LFA-1/ICAM-1 independent, triggered through the human VLA-4 integrin *J. Cell Biol.*, **110**, 2157–65.

Cepek, K.L., Shaw, S.K., Parker, C.M. *et al.* (1994) Adhesion between epithelial cells and T lymphocytes mediated by E-cadherin and the αEβ7 integrin. *Nature*, **372**, 190–3.

Ciprandi, G., Buscaglia, S., Pesce, G.P., Villaggio, B., Bagnesco, M. & Canonica, G.W. (1993) Allergic subjects express intracellular adhesion molecule 1 (ICAM-1 or CD54) on epithelial cells of conjunctiva after allergen challenge. *J. Allergy Clin. Immunol.*, **91**, 783–92.

Ciprandi, G., Pronzato, C., Ricca, V., Passalacqua, G., Bagnasco, M. & Canonica, G.W. (1994) Allergen specific challenge induces intercellular adhesion molecule-1 (ICAM-1/CD54) expression on nasal epithelial cells in allergic subjects. Relationship with early and late inflammatory phenomena. *Am. J. Resp. Crit. Care Med.*, **150**, 1653–9.

Corbi, A.L., Kishimoto, T.K., Miller, L.J. & Spriner, T.A. (1988a) The human leukocyte adhesion glycoprotein Mac-1 (complement receptor type 3, CD11b) alpha subunit. Cloning, primary structure, and relation to the integrins, von Willebrand factor and factor B. *J. Biol. Chem.*, **263**, 12403–11.

Corbi, A.L., Larson, R.S., Kishimoto, T.K., Springer, T.A. & Morton, C.C. (1988b) Chromosomal location of the genes encoding the leukocyte adhesion receptors LFA-1, Mac-1 and p150,95; identification of a gene cluster involved in cell adhesion. *J. Exp. Med.*, **176**, 1597–607.

Corbi, A.L., Miller, L.J., O'Connor, K., Larson, R.S. & Springer, T.A. (1987) cDNA cloning and complete primary stucture of the alpha subunit of a leukocyte adhesion glycoprotein, p150,95. *EMBO J.*, **6**, 4023–8.

Corrigan, C.J. & Kay, A.B. (1992) T lymphocytes in asthma. In: *Basic Mechanisms and Clinical Management* (eds P.J. Barnes, I.W. Rodger & N.C. Thomson), pp. 125–42. Academic, London.

Cybulsky, M.I., Fries, J.W.U., Williams, A.J. *et al.* (1991) Gene structure, chromosomal location and basis for alternative RNA splicing of the human VCAM-1 gene. *Proc. Nat. Acad. Sci. USA*, **88**, 7859.

Dana, N., Styrt, B., Griffin, J., Todd, R.F. III, Klempner, M. & Amaout, M.A. (1986) Two functional domains in the phagocyte membrane glycoprotein Mo1 identified with monoclonal antibodies. *J. Immunol.*, **137**, 3259–63.

Davignon, D., Martz, E., Reynolds, T., Kurzinger, K. & Springer, T.A. (1981a) Monoclonal antibody to a novel lymphocyte function associated antigen (LFA-1): mechanisms of blocking of T lymphocyte-mediated killing and effects on other T and B lymphocyte functions. *J. Immunol.*, **127**, 590–5.

Davignon, D., Martz, E., Reynolds, T., Kurzinger, K. & Springer, T.A. (1981b) Lymphocyte function associated antigen 1 (LFA-1); a surface antigen distinct from Lyt-2,3 that participates in T lymphocyte-mediated killing. *Proc. Nat. Acad. Sci. USA*, **78**, 4535–9.

de Fougerolles, A.R. & Springer, T.A. (1992) Intercellular adhesion molecule 3, a third adhesion counter receptor for lymphocyte function-associated molecule-1 on resting lymphocytes. *J. Exp. Med.*, **175**, 185–90.

de Fougerolles, A.R., Stacker, S.A., Schwarting, R. & Springer, T.A. (1991) Characterisation of ICAM-2 and evidence for a third counter-receptor for LFA-1. *J. Exp. Med.*, **174**, 253–67.

Desreumauz, P., Janin, A. & Colomble, J.F. (1992) Interleukin 5 messenger RNA expression by eosinophils in the intestinal mucosa of patients with coeliac disease. *J. Exp. Med.*, **175**, 293–6.

Diamond, M.S. & Springer, T.A. (1994) The dynamic regulation of integrin adhesiveness. *Curr. Biol.*, **4**, 506–17.

Diamond, M.S., Staunton, D.E., de Fougerolles, A.R. *et al.* (1990) ICAM-1 (CD54): a counter-receptor for Mac-1 (CD11b/CD18). *J. Cell Biol.*, **111**, 3129–39.

Diamond, M.S., Staunton, D.E., Marlin, S.D. & Springer, T.A. (1991) Binding of the integrin Mac-1 (CD11b/CD18) to the third immunoglobulin-like domains of ICAM-1 (CD54) and its regulation by glycosylation. *Cell*, **65**, 961–71.

Dobrina, A., Menegazzi, R., Carlos, T.M. *et al.* (1991) Mechanisms of eosinophil adherence to cultured vascular endothelial cells: eosinophils bind to the cytokine induced endothelial ligand vascular cell adhesion molecule-1 via the very late antigen-4 receptor. *J. Clin. Invest.*, **88**, 20.

Dri, P., Cramer, R., Spessotto, P., Romano, M. & Patriarca, P. (1991) Eosinophil activation on biologic surfaces. *J. Immunol.*, **147**, 613–20.

D'Souza, S.E., Ginsberg, M.H., Burke, T.A., Lam, S.C.T. & Plow, E.F. (1988) Localisation of a ARG-GLY-ASP recognition site within an integrin adhesion receptor. *Science*, **242**, 91–3.

Dustin, M.L., Rothlein, R., Bhan, A.K., Dinarello, C.A. & Springer, T.A. (1986) Induction by IL-1 and interferon-gamma: tissue distribution, biochemistry and function of natural adherence molecule (ICAM-1). *J. Immunol.*, **137**, 245–54.

Dustin, M.L., Singer, K.H., Tuck, D.T. & Springer, T.A. (1988a) Adhesion of T lymphoblasts to epidermal keratinocytes is regulated by interferon gamma and is mediated by intercellular adhesion molecule-1 (ICAM-1). *J. Exp. Med.*, **167**, 1323–40.

Dustin, M.L. & Springer, T.A. (1988) Lymphocyte function associated antigen-1 (LFA-1) interaction with intercellular adhesion molecule-1 (ICAM-1) is one of at least three mechanisms for lymphocyte adhesion to cultured endothelial cells. *J. Cell Biol.*, **107**, 321–31.

Dustin, M.L. & Springer, T.A. (1989) T cell receptor cross-linking transiently stimulates adhesiveness through LFA-1. *Nature*, **341**, 619–24.

Dustin, M.L., Staunton, D.E. & Springer, T.A. (1988b) Supergene families meet in the immune system. *Immunol. Today*, **9**, 213–15.

Ebisawa, M., Bochner, B.S., Georas, S.N. & Schleimer, R.P. (1992) Eosinophil transendothelial migration induced by cytokines. Role of the endothelial and eosinophil adhesion molecules in IL-1b induced transendothelial migration. *J. Immunol.*, **149(12)**, 4021–8.

Elices, M.J., Osbourn, L., Takada, Y. *et al.* (1990) VCAM-1 on activated endothelium interacts with the leukocyte integrin VLA-4 at a site distinct from the VLA-4/fibronectin binding site. *Cell*, **60**, 577–84.

Erle, D.J., Briskin, M.J., Butcher, E.D., Garcia-Pardo, A., Lazarovits, A.I. & Tidswell, M. (1994) Expression and function of the MAdCAM-1 receptor integrin α4/β7 on human leukocytes. *J. Immunol.*, **153**, 517–28.

Erle, D.J., Ruegg, C., Sheppard, D. & Pytela, R. (1991) Complete amino acid sequence of an integrin β subunit (β7) identified in leukocytes. *J. Biol. Chem.*, **266**, 11009–16.

Etzioni, A., Frydman, M., Pollack, S. *et al.* (1992) Severe recurrent chest infections due to a novel adhesion molecule defect. *New Engl. J. Med.*, **327**, 1789–92.

Fearon, D.T. & Collins, L.A. (1983) Increased expression of C3b receptors on polymorphonuclear leukocytes induced by chemotactic factors and by purification procedures. *J. Immunol.*, **130**, 370–5.

Gailit, J. & Rusholahti, E. (1988) Regulation of the fibronectin receptor affinity by divalent cations. *J. Biol. Chem.*, **263**, 12927–32.

Gallatin, W.M., Weissman, I.L., Butcher, E.C. (1983) A cell surface molecule involved in organ-specific homing of lymphocytes. *Nature*, **303**, 30–4.

Gearing, A.J. & Newman, W. (1993) Circulating adhesion molecules in disease. *Immunol. Today*, **14**, 506–12.

Geng, J.G., Bevilacqua, M.P., Moore, K.L. *et al.* (1990) Rapid neutrophil adhesion to activated endothelium mediated by GMP-140. *Nature*, **343**, 757–60.

Georas, S.N., Liu, M.C., Newman, W., Beall, L.D., Stealey, B.A. & Bochner, B.S. (1992) Altered adhesion molecule expression and endothelial cell activation accompany the recruitment of human granulocytes to the lung after segmental antigen challenge. *Am. J. Respir. Cell Mol. Biol.*, **7**, 261–9.

Georas, S.N., McIntyre, W.B., Ebisawa, M. *et al.* (1993) Expression of a functional laminin receptor a6b1 (very late activation antigen-6) on human eosinophils. *Blood*, **82**, 2872–9.

Gowans, J.L. (1957) The effect of the continous re-infusion of lymph and lymphocytes on the output of lymphocytes from the thoracic duct of unanaesthetized rats. *Brit. J. Exp. Pathol.*, **38**, 67–78.

Gowans, J.L. & Knight, E.J. (1964) The route of re-circulation of lymphocytes in the rat. *Proc. Roy. Soc. Service. Bull.*, **159**, 257–90.

Greaves, M.F., Brown, J., Molgaard, H.V. *et al.* (1992) Molecular features of CD34; a hemopoietic progenitor cell-associated molecule. *Leukemia*, **6**, 31.

Greve, J.M., Davies, G., Meyer, A.M. *et al.* (1989) A major human rhinovirus receptor is ICAM-1. *Cell*, **56**, 839–47.

Gundel, R.H., Wegner, C.D. & Letts, L.G. (1993) Eosinophils and neutrophils in a primate model of asthma. In: *Asthma: Physiology, Pharmacology and Treatment* (eds J.T. Holgate, K.F. Austen, L.M. Lichtenstein & A.B. Kay), pp. 173–85. Academic, London.

Gundel, R.H., Wegner, C.D., Torcellini, C.A. *et al.* (1991) ELAM-1 mediates antigen-induced acute airway inflammation and late phase obstruction in monkeys. *J. Clin. Invest.*, **88**, 1407–11.

Hartnell, A., Robinson, D.S., Kay, A.B. & Wardlaw, A.J. (1993) CD69 is expressed by human eosinophils activated *in vivo* in asthma and *in vitro* by cytokines. *Immunology*, **80**, 281–6.

Hemler, M.E. (1988) Adhesive protein receptors on haemopoietic cells. *Immunol. Today*, **9**, 109–13.

Hemler, M.E., Sanchez-Madrid, F., Flotte, T.J. *et al.* (1984) Glycoproteins of 210 000 and 130 000 molecular weight on activated T cells: cell distribution and antigenic relation to components on resting cells and T cell lines. *J. Immunol.*, **132**, 3011–18.

Hemler, M.E., Elices, M.J., Parker, C. & Takada, Y. (1990) Structure of the integrin VLA-4 and its cell–cell and cell–matrix adhesion functions. *Immunol. Rev.*, **114**, 45–65.

Hemmrich, S., Butcher, E.C. & Rosen, S.D. (1994) Sulphation-dependent recognition of high endothelial venules (HEV)-ligands by L-selectin and MECA 79, an adhesion blocking monoclonal antibody. *J. Exp. Med.*, **180**, 2219–26.

Hibbs, M.L., Jakes, S., Stacker, S.A., Wallace, R.W. & Springer, T.A. (1991a) The cytoplasmic domain of the integrin lymphocyte function-associated antigen 1β subunit: sites required for binding to intercellular adhesion molecule 1 and the phorbol ester-stimulated phosphorylation site. *J. Exp. Med.*, **174**, 1227–38.

Hibbs, M.L., Xu, H., Stacker, S.A. & Springer, T.A. (1991b) Regulation of adhesion to ICAM-1 by the cytoplasmic domain of LFA-1 integrin beta subunit. *Science*, **251**, 1611–13.

Hogg, H. & Berlin, C. (1995) Structure and function of adhesion receptors in leukocyte trafficking. *Immunol. Today*, **16**, 327–30.

Holzmann, B., McIntyre, B.W. & Weissman, I.L. (1989) Identification of a murine Peyer's patch specific lymphocyte homing receptor as an integrin molecule with an α chain homologous to VLA-4α. *Cell*, **56**, 37–46.

Hynes, R.O. (1987) Integrins: a family of cell surface receptors. *Cell*, **48**, 549–54.

Hynes, R.O. (1992) Integrins: versatility, modulation and signalling in cell adhesion. *Cell*, **69**, 11–25.

Imai, Y., Lasky, L.A. & Rosen, S.D. (1993) Sulphation requirement for GlyCAM-1, an endothelial ligand for L-selectin. *Nature*, **361**, 555–7.

Jahnsen, F.L., Haraldsen, G., Aanesen, J.P., Haye, R. & Brandtzeg, P. (1995) Eosinophil infiltration is related to increased expression of vascular cell adhesion molecule-1 in nasal polyps. *Am. J. Respir. Cell Mol. Biol.*, **12**, 624–32.

Jalkanen, S., Bargatze, R.F., de los Toyos, J.M. & Butcher, E.C. (1987) Lymphocyte recognition of high endothelium: antibodies to distinct epitopes of an 85–95 kd glycoprotein antigen differentially inhibit binding to lymph node, mucosal or synovial endothelial cells. *J. Cell Biol.*, **105**, 983–90.

Johnston, G.I., Cook, G.R. & McEver, R.P. (1989) Cloning of GMP-140, a granule membrane protein of platelets and endothelium; a sequence similarity to proteins involved in cell adhesion and inflammation. *Cell*, **56**, 1033–44.

Kassner, A.R., Carr, M.W., Finger, E.B., Hemler, M.E. & Springer, T.A. (1995) The integrin VLA-4 supports tethering and rolling in flow on VCAM-1. *J. Cell Biol.*, **128**, 1243–53.

Kennedy, J.D., Hatfield, C.A., Fidler, S.F. *et al.* (1995) Phenotypic characterisation of T lymphocytes emigrating into lung tissue and the airway lumen after antigen inhalation in sensitised mice. *Am. J. Respir. Cell Mol. Biol.*, **12**, 613–23.

Kimani, G., Tonnensen, M.G. & Henson, P.M. (1988) Stimulation of eosinophil adherence to human vascular endothelial cell *in vitro* by platelet activating factor. *J. Immunol.*, **140**, 3161.

Kishimoto, T.K., Jutila, M.A. & Butcher, E.C. (1990) Identification of a human peripheral lymph node homing receptor; a rapidly down regulated adhesion molecule. *Proc. Nat. Acad. Sci. USA*, **87**, 2244–8.

Kishimoto, T.K., O'Connor, K., Lee, A., Roberts, T.M. & Springer, T.A. (1987) Cloning of the beta subunit of the leukocyte adhesion proteins; homology to an extracellular matrix receptor defines a novel supergene family. *Cell*, **48**, 681–90.

Kita, H., Horie, S. & Gleich, G.J. (1994) Laminin and fibronectin inhibit adhesion and degranulation of eosinophils. *J. Allergy Clin. Immunol.*, **93**, 212 [abstract].

Knol, E.F., Tackey, F., Tedder, T.F. *et al.* (1994) Comparison of human eosinophil and neutrophil adhesion to endothelial cells under non-static conditions; the role of L-selectin. *J. Immunol.*, **153**, 2161–67.

Knol, E.F., Kansas, G.S., Tedder, T.F., Schleimer, R.P. & Bochner, B.S. (1993) Human eosinophils use L-selectin to bind to endothelial cells under non static conditions. *J. Allergy Clin. Immunol.*, **91**, 334.

Kowalzick, L., Kleinheinz, A., Neuber, K., Weichenthal, M., Kohler, I. & Ring, J. (1995) Elevated serum levels of soluble adhesion molecules ICAM-1 and ELAM-1 in patients with severe atopic eczema and influence of UVA-1 treatment. *Dermatology*, **190**, 14–18.

Krensky, A.M., Sanchez-Madrid, F., Robbins, E., Nagy, J., Springer, T.A. & Burakoff, S.J. (1983) The functional significance, distribution and structure of LFA-1, LFA-2, and LFA-3: cell surface antigens associated with CTL-target interactions. *J. Immunol.*, **131**, 611–16.

Kyan-Aung, U., Haskard, D.O., Poston, R.N., Thornhill, M.H. & Lee, T.H. (1991) Endothelial leukocyte adhesion molecule-1 and intercellular adhesion molecule-1 mediated the adhesion of eosinophils to endothelial cells *in vitro* and are expressed by endothelium in allergic cutaneous inflammation *in vivo*. *J. Immunol.*, **146**, 521–8.

Lamas, A.M.C., Mulroney, C.M. & Schleimer, R.P. (1988) Studies of the adhesive interaction between purified human eosinophils and cultured vascular endothelial cells. *J. Immunol.*, **140**, 1500.

Larson, R.S., Corbi, A.L., Berman, L. & Springer, T.A. (1989) Primary structure of the LFA-1 alpha subunit. An integrin with an embedded domain defining a protein superfamily. *J. Cell Biol.*, **108**, 703–12.

Lasky, L.A., Singer, M.S. & Dowbenko, D. (1992) An endothelial ligand for L-selectin is a novel mucin like molecule. *Cell*, **69**, 927–38.

Law, S.K.A., Gagnon, J., Hildreth, J.E.K., Wells, C.E., Willis, A.C. & Wong, A.J. (1987) The primary structure of the beta subunit of the cell surface adhesion glycoproteins LFA-1, CR3 and p150,95 and its relationship to the fibronectin receptor. *EMBO J.*, **6**, 915–19.

Lawrence, M.B. & Springer, T.A. (1991) Leukocytes roll on a selectin at physiological flow rates: distinction from and pre-requisite for adhesion through integrins. *Cell*, **65**, 859–73.

Lee, J.O., Rieu, P., Arnaout, M.A. & Liddington, R. (1995) Crystal structure of the A domain from the α subunit of integrin CR3 (CD11b/CD18). *Cell*, **80**, 631–8.

Leung, Y.M., Pober, J.S. & Cotran, R.S. (1991) Expression of endothelial-leukocyte adhesion molecule-1 in elicited late phase allergic reactions. *J. Clin. Invest.*, **87**, 1805–9.

McDermott, M.R. & Bienenstock, J. (1979) Evidence for a common mucosal immunologic system. I. Migration of B immunoblasts into intestinal, respiratory and genital tissues. *J. Immunol.*, **122**, 1892–8.

McEver, R.P., Beckstead, J.H., Moore, K.L., Marshall-Carlson, L. & Bainton, D.F. (1989) GMP-140, a platelet α-granule membrane protein, is also synthesised by vascular endothelial cells and is localised in Weibel–Palade bodies. *J. Clin. Invest.*, **84**, 92.

Makgoba, M.W., Sanders, M.E., Ginther, G.E. *et al.* (1988) ICAM-1, a ligand for LFA-1 dependent adhesion of B, T and myeloid cells. *Nature*, **331**, 86–8.

Manolitsas, N.D., Trigg, C.J., McAulay, A.E. *et al.* (1994) The expression of intercellular adhesion molecule-1 and the bi-integrins in asthma. *Eur. Resp. J.*, **7**, 1439–44.

Marlin, S.D., Morton, C.C., Anderson, D.C. & Springer, T.A. (1986) Definition of the genetic defect and chromosomal mapping of α and β subunits of the lymphocyte function-associated antigen-1 (LFA-1) by complementation in hybrid cells. *J. Exp. Med.*, **164**, 855–67.

Marlin, S.D. & Springer, T.A. (1987) Purified intercellular adhesion molecule 1 (ICAM-1) is a ligand for lymphocyte function-associated antigen 1 (LFA-1). *Cell*, **51**, 813–19.

Marlin, S.D., Staunton, D.E., Springer, T.A., Stratowa, C., Sommergruber, W. & Merluzzi, V. (1990) A soluble form of intercellular adhesion molecule-1 inhibits rhinovirus infection. *Nature*, **344**, 70–2.

Meerschaert, J. & Furie, M.B. (1995) The adhesion molecules used by monocytes for migration across endothelium include CD11a/CD18, CD11b/CD18 and VLA-4 on monocytes and ICAM-1, VCAM-1 and other ligands on endothelium. *J. Immunol.*, **154**, 4099–112.

Metzger, W.J., Ridgr, V., Tollefson, V., Arrheius, T., Gaeta, F.C.A. & Elices, M. (1994) Anti-VLA-1 antibody and CS1 peptide inhibitor modify airway inflammation and bronchial airway hyperresponsiveness (BHR) in the allergic rabbit. *J. Allergy Clin. Immunol.*, **93**, 183 [abstract].

Michishita, M., Videm, V. & Arnaout, M.A. (1993) A novel divalent cation-binding site in the A domain of the β2 integrin CR3 (CD11b/CD18) is essential for ligand binding. *Cell*, **72**, 857–67.

Miller, L.J., Bainton, D.F., Borregaard, N. & Springer, T.A. (1987) Stimulated mobilisation of monocyte Mac-1 and p150,95 adhesion proteins from an intracellular vascular compartment to the cell surface. *J. Clin. Invest.*, **80**, 535–44.

Miller, L.J., Schwarting, R. & Springer, T.A. (1986) Regulated expression of the Mac-1, LFA-1p150,95 glycoprotein family during leukocyte differentation. *J. Immunol.*, **137**, 2891–900.

Montefort, S., Feather, I.H. & Wilson, S.J. (1992) The expression of leukocyte endothelial adhesion molecules is increased in perennial allergic rhinitis. *Am. J. Respir. Cell Mol. Biol.*, **7**, 393–8.

Montefort, S., Roche, W.R., Howarth, P.H. *et al.* (1992) Intercellular adhesion molecule-1 (ICAM-1) and endothelial leucocyte adhesion molecule-1 (ELAM-1) expression in the bronchial mucosa of normals and asthmatic subjects. *Eur. Resp. J.*, **5**, 815–23.

Montefort, S., Gratziou, C., Goulding, D. *et al.* (1993) Upregulation of leukocyte–endothelial cell adhesion molecules 6 hours after local allergen challenge of sensitised asthmatic airways. *J. Clin. Invest.*, **93**, 1411–21.

Montefort, S., Lai, C.K.W., Kapahi, P. *et al.* (1994) Circulating adhesion molecules in asthma. *Am. J. Resp. Crit. Care Med.*, **149**, 1149–52.

Moore, K.L., Stults, N.L., Disaz, S. *et al.* (1992) Identification of a specific glycoprotein ligand for P-selectin (CD62) on myeloid cells. *J. Cell Biol.*, **118**, 445–6.

Moser, R., Fehr, J., Olgati, L. & Bruijnzeel, P.L.B. (1992) Migration of primed human eosinophils across cytokine activated endothelial cell monolayers. *Blood*, **79**, 2937–45.

Mould, A.P., Wheldon, A., Komoriya, E.A., Wayner, E.A., Yamada, K.M. & Humphries, M.J. (1990) Affinity chromatic isolation of the melanoma adhesion receptor for the IIICS region of fibronectin and its identification as the integrin α4β1. *J. Biol. Chem.*, **265**, 4020.

Moyle, M., Foster, D.L., McGrath, D.E. *et al.* (1994) A hookworm glycoprotein that inhibits neutrophil functions is a ligand for the integrin CD11b/CD18. *J. Biol. Chem.*, **269**, 10008–15.

Murphy, G., Leventhal, L. & Zweiman, B. (1994) Endothelial CD62 and E-selectin expression in developing late-phase IgE mediated skin reactions. *J. Allergy Clin. Immunol.*, **93**, 183 [abstract].

Myones, B.L., Daizell, J.G., Hogg, N. & Ross, G.D. (1988) Neutrophil and monocyte cell surface p150,95 has iC3b-receptor (CR4) activity resembling CR3. *J. Clin. Invest.*, **82**, 640–51.

Nacleiro, R.M., Bochner, B.S. & Baroody, F.M. (1994) Upregulation of vascular cell adhesion molecule-1 (VCAM-1) after nasal allergen challenge. *J. Allergy Clin. Immunol.*, **93**, 183 [abstract].

Nakajima, H., Sano, H., Nishimura, T., Yoshida, S. & Iwanoto, I. (1994) Role of vascular cell adhesion molecule 1/very late antigen 4 and intercellular adhesion molecule 1 interactions in antigen-induced eosinophil and T cell recruitment into the tissue. *J. Exp. Med.*, **179**, 1145–54.

Neeley, S.P., Hamann, K.J., Dowling, T., McAllister, K.T., White, S.R. & Leff, A.R. (1994) Augmentation of stimulated eosinophil degranulation by VLA-4 (CD49d)-mediated adhesion to fibronectin. *Am J. Respir. Cell Mol. Biol.*, **11**, 206–13.

Nourshargh, S., Rampart, M., Hellewell, P.G. *et al.* (1989) Accumulation of ^{111}In-neutrophils in rabbit skin in allergic and non allergic inflammatory reactions *in vivo*. *J. Immunol.*, **142**, 3193–8.

O'Toole, T.E., Mandelman, D., Forsyth, J., Shattil, S.J., Plow, E.F. & Ginsberg, M.H. (1991) Modulation of the affinity of integrin a $^{IIb}\beta3$ (gpIIb–IIIa) by the cytoplasmic domain of a Iib. *Science*, **254**, 845–7.

Ohkawara, Y., Yamauchi, K., Maruyama, N. *et al.* (1995) *In situ* expression of the cell adhesion molecules in bronchial tissues from asthmatics with air flow limitation: *in vivo* evidence of VCAM-1/VLA-4 interaction in selective eosinophil infiltration. *Am. J. Respir. Cell Mol. Biol.*, **12**, 4–12.

Osbourn, L., Hession, C., Tizard, R. *et al.* (1989) Direct expression cloning of vascular adhesion molecule 1, a cytokine induced endothelial protein that binds to lymphocytes. *Cell*, **59**, 1203–11.

Patarroyo, M. (1994) Adhesion molecules mediating recruitment of monocytes to inflamed tissue. *Immunobiology*, **191**, 474–7.

Phillips, M.R., Buyon, J.P., Winchester, R., Weissman, G. & Abramson, S.B. (1988) Upregulation of the iC3b receptor (CR3) is neither necessary nor sufficient to promote neutrophil aggregation. *J. Clin. Invest.*, **82**, 495–501.

Picker, L.J. & Butcher, E.C. (1992) Physiological and molecular mechanisms of lymphocyte homing. *Ann. Rev. Immunol.*, **10**, 561–91.

Picker, L.J., Kishimoto, T.K., Smith, C.W., Warnock, R.A. & Butcher, E.C. (1991a) ELAM-1 is an adhesion molecule for skin-homing T cells. *Nature*, **349**, 796.

Picker, L.J., Warnock, R.A., Burns, A.R., Doerschuk, C.M., Berg, E.L. & Butcher, E.C. (1991b) The neutrophil selectin LECAM-1 presents carbohydrate ligands to the vascular selectins ELAM-1 and GMP-140. *Cell*, **66**, 921–33.

Pober, J.S., Gimbrone, M.A. Jr, Lapierre, L.A. *et al.* (1986b) Overlapping patterns of activation by human endothelial cells by interleukin-1, tumor necrosis factor and immune interferon. *J. Immunol.*, **137**, 1893–6.

Pretolani, M.C., Ruffie, C., de Silva, L., Joseph, D., Lobb, R. & Vargaftig, B. (1994) Antibody to very late activation antigen 4 presents antigen-induced bronchial hyperreactivity and cellular infiltration in the guinea pig airways. *J. Exp. Med.*, **180**, 795–805.

Rabb, H.A., Olivenstein, R., Issekutz, T.B., Renzl, P.M. & Martin, J.G. (1994) The role of the leucocyte adhesion molecules VLA-4, LFA-1 and Mac-1 in allergic airway responses in rat. *Am. J. Resp. Crit. Care Med.*, **149**, 1186–91.

Rice, G.E. & Bevilacqua, M.P. (1989) An inducible endothelial cell surface glycoprotein mediates melanoma adhesion. *Science*, **246**, 1303–74.

Rice, G.E., Munro, J.M. & Bevilacqua, M.P. (1990) Inducible cell adhesion molecule-110 (INCAM-110) is an endothelial receptor for lymphocytes. II. A CD11/Cd18-independent adhesion mechanism. *J. Exp. Med.*, **171**, 1369–74.

Robinson, M.K., Andrew, D., Rosen, H. *et al.* (1992) Antibody against the Leu-cam b chain CD18 promotes both LFA-1 and CR3 dependent adhesion events. *J. Immunol.*, **148(4)**, 1080–5.

Rosen, S.D. (1993) Cell surface lectins in the immune system. *Semin. Immunol.*, **5**, 237–47.

Rothlein, R., Dustin, M.L., Martin, S.D. & Springer, T.A. (1986) A human inter-cellular adhesion molecule (ICAM-1) distinct from LFA-1. *J. Immunol.*, **137**, 1270–4.

Rothlein, R. & Springer, T.A. (1986) The requirement for lymphocyte function associated antigen 1 in homotypic leukocyte adhesion stimulated by phorbol ester. *J. Exp. Med.*, **163**, 1132–49.

Russell, D.G. & Wright, S.D. (1988) Complement receptor type 3 (CR3) binds to an arg-gly-asp containing region of the major surface glycoprotein, gp63, of *Leishmania* promastigotes. *J. Exp. Med.*, **168**, 279–92.

Sako, D., Chang, X.J. & Barone, K.M. (1993) Expression cloning of a functional glycoprotein ligand for P-selectin. *Cell*, **75**, 1179.

Savill, J., Dransfield, I., Hogg, N. & Haslett, C. (1990) Vitronectin receptor-mediated phagocytosis of cells undergoing apoptosis. *Nature*, **343**, 170–3.

Scheiffenbaum, B., Moser, R., Patarroyo, M. & Fehr, J. (1989) The cell surface glycoprotein Mac-1 (CD11b/CD18) mediates neutrophil adhesion and modulates degranulation independently of its quantitative cell surface expression. *J. Immunol.*, **142**, 3537–45.

Schleimer, R.P., Sterbinsky, S.A., Kaiser, J. *et al.* (1992) Il-4 induces adherence of human eosinophil and basophils but not neutrophils to endothelium. *J. Immunol.*, **148**, 1086–92.

Schwarting, R., Stein, H. & Wang, C.Y. (1985) The monoclonal antibodies αS-HCL-1 (αLeu 14) and αS-HCL-3 (α Leu-M%) allow the diagnosis of hairy cell leukaemia. *Blood*, **65**, 974–83.

Schwartz, B.R., Wayner, E.A., Carlos, T.M., Ochs, H.D. & Harlan, J.M. (1990) Idenification of surface proteins mediating adherence of CD11/18-deficient lymphoblastoid cells to cultured endothelium. *J. Clin. Invest.*, **85**, 2019–22.

Shalit, M., Von Allmen, C., Atkins, P.C. & Zweiman, B. (1988) Platelet activating factor increases expression of complement receptors on human neutrophils. *J. Leuk. Biol.*, **44**, 212–17.

Simmons, D., Makgoba, M.W. & Seed, B. (1988) ICAM-1 an adhesion ligand of LFA-1 is homologous to the neural cell adhesion molecule NCAM. *Nature*, **331**, 624–7.

Smith, C.H., Barker, J.N.W.N., Morris, R.W., MacDonald, D.M. & Lee, T.H. (1993) Neuropeptides induce rapid expression of endothelial cell adhesion molecules and elicit granulocytic infiltration in human skin. *J. Immunol.*, **151**, 3274–82.

Smith, C.W., Marlin, S.D., Rothlein, R., Toman, C. & Anderson, D.C. (1989) Cooperative interactions of LFA-1 and Mac-1 with intercellular adhesion molecule-1 in facilitating adherence and transendothelial migration of human neutrophils *in vitro*. *J. Clin. Invest.*, **83**, 2008–17.

Smith, J.B., Kunjummen, R.D., Kishimoto, T.K. & Anderson, D.C. (1992) Expression and regulation of L-selectin on eosinophils from human adults and neonates. *Ped. Res.*, **32**, 465–71.

Spencer, J. & Hall, J.G. (1984) Studies on the lymphocytes of sheep. IV. Migration patterns of lung-associated lymphocytes efferent from the caudal medistinal lymph node. *Immunology*, **52**, 1–5.

Springer, T.A. (1994) Traffic signals for lymphocytic recirculation and leukocyte emigration: the multistep paradigm. *Cell*, **76**, 301–14.

Springer, T.A. & Lasky, L.A. (1991) Sticky sugars for selectins. *Nature*, **349**, 425–34.

Springer, T.A., Galfre, G., Secher, D.S. & Milstein, C. (1979) Mac-1: a macrophage differentiation antigen identified by monoclonal antibody. *Eur. J. Immunol.*, **9**, 301–16.

Sriramarao, P., von Adrian, U.H., Butcher, E.C., Bourdon, M.A. & Broide, D.H. (1994) L-selectin and very late antigen-4 integrin promote eosinophil rolling at physiological sheer street rate *in vivo*. *J. Immunol.*, **153**, 4238–46.

Stamper, H.B. Jr & Woodruff, J.J. (1976) Lymphocyte homing into the lymph nodes: *in vitro* demonstration of the selective affinity of recirculating lymphocytes for high-endothelial venules. *J. Exp. Med.*, **144**, 828.

Staunton, D.E., Dustin, M.L., Erickson, H.P. & Springer, T.A. (1990) The arrangement of the immunoglobulin like domains of ICAM-1 and the binding sites for LFA-1 and rhinovirus. *Cell*, **61**, 243–54.

Staunton, D.E., Dustin, M.L. & Springer, T.A. (1989) Functional cloning of ICAM-2, a cell adhesion ligand for LFA-1 homologous to ICAM-1. *Nature*, **339**, 61–4.

Staunton, D.E., Marlin, S.D., Stratowa, C., Dustin, M.L. & Springer, T.A. (1988) Primary structure of intercellular adhesion molecule 1 (ICAM-1) demonstrates interaction between members of the immunoglobulin and integrin supergene families. *Cell*, **52**, 925–33.

Steegmaler, M., Levinovitz, A., Isenmann, S. *et al.* (1995) The E-selectin ligand ESL-1 is a variant of a receptor for fibroblast growth factor. *Nature*, **373**, 615–20.

Symon, F.A., Lawrence, M.B., Williamson, M.L., Walsh, G.M., Watson, S.R. & Wardlaw, A.J. (1996) Functional and structural characterization of the eosinophil P-selectin ligand. *J. Immunol.*, **157**, (in press).

Symon, F.A., Walsh, G.M., Watson, S. & Wardlaw, A.J. (1994) Eosinophil adhesion to nasal polyp endothelium is P-selectin dependent. *J. Exp. Med.*, **180**, 371–6.

Takada, Y., Elices, M.J., Crouse, C. & Hemler, M.E. (1989) The primary structure of the α4 subunit of VLA-4; homology to other integrins and a possible cell–cell adhesion function. *EMBO J.*, **8**, 1361.

Takahashi, N., Liu, M.C., Proud, D., Yu, X.-Y., Hasegawa, S. & Spannhake, E.W. (1994) Soluble intercellular adhesion molecule-1 in bronchoalveolar lavage fluid of allergic subjects following segmental antigen challenge. *Am. J. Resp. Crit. Care Med.*, **150**, 704–9.

Tedder, T.F., Issacs, T., Ernst, G., Demetri, G., Alder, G. & Disteche, C. (1989) Isolation and chromosomal localisation of cDNAs encoding a novel human lymphocyte cell surface molecule, LAM-1; homology with the mouse lymphocyte homing receptor and other human adhesion molecules. *J. Exp. Med.*, **170**, 123–33.

Thornhill, M.H., Wellicome, S.M., Mahiouz, D.L., Lanchbury, J.S., Kyan-Aung, U. & Haskard, D.O. (1991) Tumor necrosis factor combines with IL-4 or IFN-α to selectively enhance endothelial cell adhesiveness for T cells. *J. Immunol.*, **146**, 592.

Tomassini, J.E., Graham, D., DeWitt, C.M., Lineberger, D.W., Rodkey, J.A. & Colonno, R.J. (1989) cDNA cloning reveals that the major group rhinovirus receptor on HeLa cells is intercellular adhesion molecule 1. *Proc. Nat. Acad. Sci. USA*, **86**, 4907–11.

Vadas, M.A., Lucas, C.M., Gamble, J.R., Lopez, A.F., Skinner, M.P. & Berndt, M.C. (1993) Regulation of eosinophil function by P-selectin. In: *Eosinophils in Allergy and Inflammation* (eds G.J. Gleich & A.B. Kay), pp. 69–80. Marcel Dekker, New York.

Van der Brugge-Gamelkoorn, G.J. & Glaassen, E., Sminia, T. (1986) Anti-TNP forming cells in bronchus associated lymphoid tissue (BALT) and paratracheal lymph note (PTLN) of the rat after intratracheal priming and boosting with TNP-KLH. *Immunology*, **57**, 405–9.

Van Kooyk, Y., Weder, P., Hogervorst, F. *et al.* (1991) Activation of LFA-1 through a Ca^{2+} dependent epitope stimulates lymphocyte adhesion. *J. Cell Biol.*, **112**, 345–54.

Van Kooyk, Y., van de Wiel-van Kemenade, P., Weder, P., Kuijpers, T.W. & Figdor, C.G. (1989) Enhancement of LFA-1 mediated cell adhesion by triggering through CD2 or CD3 on T lymphocytes. *Nature*, **342**, 811–13.

Vedder, N.B. & Harlan, J.M. (1988) Increased surface expression of CD11b/CD18 (Mac-1) is not required for stimulated neutrophil adherence to cultured endothelium. *J. Clin. Invest.*, **81**, 676–82.

Vignola, A.M., Campbell, A.M., Chanez, P. *et al.* (1993) HLA-DR and ICAM-1 expression on bronchial epithelial cells in asthma and chronic bronchitis. *Am. Rev. Resp. Dis.*, **147**, 529–34.

Vogetseder, W., Feichtinger, H., Schultz, T.F. *et al.* (1989) Expression of 7F7-antigen, a human adhesion molecule identical to intercellular adhesion molecule-1 human carcinoma and their stromal fibroblasts. *Int. J. Cancer*, **43**, 768–73.

Von Adrian, U.H., Chambers, J.D. & McEvoy, L.M. (1991) Two step model of leukocye endothelial cell intraction with inflammation; distinct roles for LECAM-1 and the leukocyte 12 integrins *in vivo*. *Proc. Nat. Acad. Sci. USA*, **88**, 7538–42.

Walker, C., Virchow, J.C., Bruijnzeel, P.L.B. & Blasser, K. (1991) T cell subsets and their soluble products regulate eosinophilia in allergic and non allergic asthma. *J. Immunol.*, **146**, 1829–35.

Wallis, W.J., Hickstein, D.D., Schwartz, B.R. *et al.* (1986) Monoclonal antibody-defined functional epitopes on the adhesion promoting glycoprotein complex (Cdw 18) of human neutrophils. *Blood*, **67**, 1007–13.

Walsh, G.M., Hartnell, A., Mermod, J.J., Kay, A.B. & Wardlaw, A.J. (1991) Human eosinophil, but not neutrophil adherence to IL-1 stimulated HUVEC is a4b1 (VLA-4) dependent. *J. Immunol.*, **146**, 3419–23.

Walsh, G.M., Hartnell, A., Wardlaw, A.J., Kurihara, K., Sanderson, C.J. & Kay, A.B. (1990) Il-5 enhances the *in vitro* adhesion of human eosinophils, but not neutrophils in a leucocyte integrin (CD11/18) dependent manner. *Immunology*, **71**, 258–65.

Walsh, G.M., Symon, F.A. & Wardlaw, A.J. (1995) Human eosinophils preferentially survive on tissue compared with plasma fibronectin *Clin. Exp. Allergy*, **25**, 1128–36..

Wardlaw, A.J., Hibbs, M.L., Stacker, S.A. & Springer, T.A. (1990) Distinct mutations in two patients with leukocyte adhesion deficiency and their functional correlates. *J. Exp. Med.*, **172**, 335–45.

Wardlaw, A.J., Walsh, G.M. & Symon, F.A. (1994) Mechanisms of eosinophil and basophil migration. *Allergy*, **49**, 797–807.

Weetman, A.P., Cohen, S., Mategoba, M.W. & Borysiewicz, L.K. (1989) Expression of an intercellular adhesion molecule-1, ICAM-1, by human thyroid cells. *J. Endocrinol.*, **122**, 185–91.

Weg, V.B., Williams, T.J., Lobb, P.R. & Nourshargh, S. (1993) A monoclonal antibody recognizing the very late activation antigen-4 inhibits eosinophil accumulation *in vivo*. *J. Exp. Med.*, **177**, 561–6.

Wegner, C.D., Grundel, R.H., Reilly, P., Haynes, N., Letts, G.L. & Rothlein, R. (1990) ICAM-1 in the pathogenesis of asthma. *Science*, **247**, 416–18.

Wegner, C.D., Gundel, R.H., Churchill, L. & Letts, L.G. (1993) Adhesion glycoproteins as regulators of airway inflammation; emphasis on the role of ICAM-1. In: *Asthma: Physiology, Pharmacology and Treatment* (eds S.T. Holgate, K.F. Austen, L.F. Lichtenstern & A.B. Kay), pp. 227–42. Academic, London.

Wein, M., Sterbinsky, S.A., Bickel, C.A., Schleimer, R.P. & Bochner, B.S. (1995) Comparison of human eosinophil and neutrophil ligands for P-selectin: ligands for P-selectin differ from those for E-selectin. *Am. J. Respir. Cell Mol. Biol.*, **12**, 315–19.

Weller, P.F., Rand, T.H., Golez, S.E., Chi-Rosso, G. & Lobb, R.R. (1991) Human eosinophil adherence to vascular endothelium mediated by binding to vascular cell adhesion molecule-1 and endothelial leukocyte adhesion molecule 1. *Proc. Nat. Acad. Sci. USA*, **88**, 7430.

Wright, S.D., Weitz, J.I., Huang, A.J., Levin, S.M., Silverstein, S.C. & Loike, J.D. (1988) Complement receptor type three (CD11b/CD18) of human polymorphonuclear leukocytes recognises fibrinogen. *Proc. Nat. Acad. Sci. USA*, **85**, 7734–8.

Zhou, Q., Moore, K.L., Smith, D.F., Varki, A., McEver, R.P. & Cummings, R.D. (1991) The selectin GMP-140 bind to sialylated fucoslyated, lactose amionoglycans on both myeloid and non myeloid cells. *J. Cell Biol.*, **115**, 557–64.

CHAPTER 15

Airway Epithelium in Asthma

L.A. Cohn, B.M. Fischer, T.M. Krunkosky, D.T. Wright & K.B. Adler

Introduction

Asthma is characterized by hyperresponsivness of the respiratory airways to multiple stimuli. It may be regarded as a complex of conditions which cause limitation to airflow that is temporally variable and reversible (Moser, 1994). Although asthma is a common disease affecting approximately 5% of the population, the pathophysiology is far from clear. It may be broadly divided into atopic or non-atopic forms. Each form results in narrowing of airway diameter as a result of contraction of smooth muscle, vascular congestion and oedema of bronchial walls, and hypersecretion of tenacious mucus. Historically, attention has centred on contraction of bronchial smooth muscle, but it is now recognized that inflammation of the airways is crucial to development of the disease, and even very mild asthma in asymptomatic individuals is characterized by chronic inflammation of the airways (Beasley *et al.*, 1993).

In the airways of asthmatic patients there are a variety of inflammatory mediators, which may play an important role in disease development. Inflammatory cells are the major source of these mediators, but they also may be produced by the airway epithelial cells themselves. Thus, the epithelium of the airways is both a target and an effector in asthma. As a target, mediators released from inflammatory cells alter the function and viability of epithelial cells. As an effector, the epithelium itself releases mediators which then act in either a paracrine or autocrine fashion to propagate pathophysiological changes occurring during the asthmatic attack.

Airway anatomy

The airways are composed of conducting, transitional and respiratory zones (West, 1985; Wang, 1994). The airways become smaller in diameter but more numerous as they branch from one zone to the next. The conducting zone extends from the trachea through the main bronchi, lobar and segmental bronchi, and includes the small bronchioles. The transitional zone is composed of terminal and respiratory bronchioles, while the respiratory zone is made up of alveoli. The framework of the trachea is composed of incomplete cartilaginous rings connected posteriorly by the trachealis muscle. The trachea and bronchi provide the rigid conducting system of the respiratory tree. The conducting airways are lined by a pseudostratified columnar epithelium that is situated on top of a basement membrane. Seromucous glands lie within the submucosal layer. Circular bundles of smooth muscle surround the bronchi down to the level of the terminal bronchiole. The conducting airways and associated smooth muscle are surrounded by connective tissue containing nerves, blood vessels and lymphatics. Clinical symptoms of asthma (bronchospasm and bronchoconstriction) are associated with medium-sized bronchi, where only minimal amounts of cartilage are found.

The pseudostratified columnar epithelium lining the conducting airways is composed of three main cell types: 'ciliated', 'goblet' and 'basal' (Reznik, 1990; Rose, 1992; Wang, 1994). Ciliated cells are columnar in shape. Their apical cilia beat in a co-ordinated metachronal manner within an overlying mucous layer to propel particulates crainiad where they can be expectorated or swallowed. Cilia plus mucus make up the mucociliary escalator clearance system of the airways. Mucus is composed of water, lipid and high-molecular-weight mucin glycoproteins. The amount, physicochemical properties and proteins expressed in mucus may change with disease. Basal cells may be progenitors for the ciliated and goblet cells of the conducting airway epithelium. These cells develop a strong attachment with the underlying basal lamina via formation of hemidesmosomes, while ciliated and goblet cells do not form hemidesmosomes with the basal lamina (Kawanami *et al.*, 1979; Evans & Plopper, 1988; Evans *et al.*, 1989). Adjacent cells are attached to each other by desmosomes. This phenomenon is important to epithelial shedding: basal cells tend to remain attached and begin epithelial regeneration after injury.

Pathophysiology

As mentioned above, asthma may be regarded as a complex of conditions which result in a common symptomatology and pathology. A useful way to divide asthma is into either atopic or non-atopic types. In the allergic type, exposure of a previously sensitized individual to an allergen (antigen) causes an immediate hypersensitivity reaction in the airways. In comparison with non-atopic asthma, patients with allergic asthma tend to develop disease at a younger age and often have a personal or family history of allergy or atopy. They may have increased serum immunoglobulin E (IgE) concentrations, and often have positive reactions to either an interdermal injection of a specific antigen (weal and flare) or to provocative inhalation of an antigen (decreased forced expiratory volumes). Non-atopic asthma lacks these features and may follow exercise, exposure to cold air, or exposure to various chemicals and drugs (Moser, 1994). It may be difficult to assign an individual to either type as there is overlap of these broad classifications.

Asthma is allergic in nature in approximately 25–35% of patients, and an allergic component may be contributory in approximately another 33% (Moser, 1994). When the allergic asthmatic is exposed to an inhaled allergen, cross-linking of IgE on the surface of mast cells leads to their degranulation and *de novo* synthesis and release of inflammatory mediators (e.g. eicosanoids). Clinical signs may develop within minutes (early reaction). In 30–50% of patients, a second wave of bronchoconstriction (the late reaction) develops in 6–10 hours. Theoretically, interaction between epithelial cells and infiltrating or resident inflammatory cells produce mediators causing an intense local reaction, which may then be amplified by both cellular mediators and neural reflexes (McFadden, 1994). These mediators lead to an increase in airway resistance, a decrease in expiratory volume and flow rates, hyperinflation of the lungs, altered elastic recoil and respiratory muscle function, mismatching of ventilation and perfusion, and hypoxia.

The pathology of asthma has been extensively described (reviewed by Beasley *et al.*, 1993; Hogg, 1993). The airways of patients who have died of asthma are characterized by a marked inflammatory process with massive submucosal cell infiltrate primarily composed of eosinophils. There is deposition of collagen beneath the true basement membrane, increased smooth muscle thickness due to hyperplasia, tissue oedema and vascular congestion. The airways may be occluded with thick, tenacious mucous plugs containing eosinophils, macrophages, plasma cells and epithelial cells. The bronchial epithelial cells show marked detachment, leaving denuded areas. Biopsies of mildly to moderately affected asthma patients have similar pathological changes, including mucosal infiltration of activated eosinophils, mast cells (often degranulated) in the lamina propria, goblet cell hyperplasia, epithelial damage and denudation. Sputum from asthmatics may contain Curschmann's spirals (mucoid casts), creola bodies (sloughed epithelial clumps) and Charcot–Leyden crystals (eosinophil remnants). Bronchoalveolar lavage (BAL) fluid yields increased epithelial cells, mast cells, eosinophils and T lymphocytes.

The presence of inflammatory cells and mediators does not fully explain the pathogenesis of asthma. Disease severity and the degree of inflammatory infiltrate do not always correlate (McFadden, 1994). Patients with mast cell disease, atopy or other inflammatory airway diseases may have the same types of cellular infiltrates and/or mediators present both systemically and in the airways, yet they do not develop the bronchial hyperresponsiveness that characterizes asthmatic airways (Bousquet *et al.*, 1990, 1994; Bentley *et al.*, 1992; Djukanovic *et al.*, 1992; McFadden, 1994). On the other hand, some clinically normal non-asthmatics without inflammation do have bronchial hyperresponsiveness when challenged with appropriate stimuli (Power *et al.*, 1993). What is clear is that further investigation of inflammatory cells, epithelial cells and mediators released from both is needed to develop a more adequate explanation of asthma. Only with a better understanding of disease pathogenesis will better therapeutic options become likely.

Cells and mediators in asthma

As previously described, there are a variety of resident cells in the airways, including tracheal–bronchial epithelium, submucosal glands, bronchial smooth muscle, endothelium, fibroblasts, nervous tissues and alveolar macrophages. These cells release a variety of inflammatory mediators including cytokines and lipid mediators. It is the network of interactions between mediators and cells

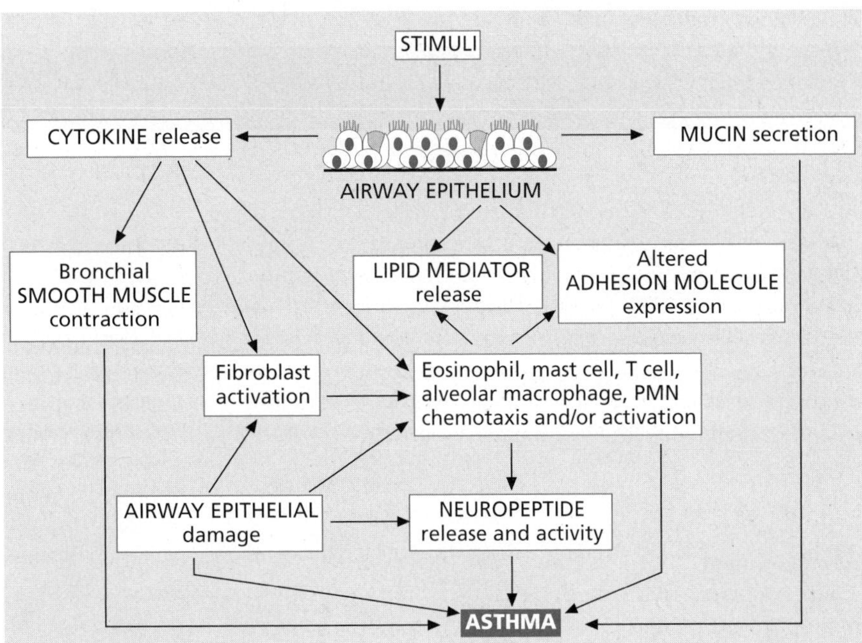

Fig. 15.1 Airway epithelium in asthma network. Upon exposure to a stimulant (e.g. allergen), the airway epithelium will participate in a complicated network of cellular and mediator interactions, culminating in the clinical symptoms which constitute the asthmatic response.

that perpetuates the asthmatic reaction (Fig. 15.1). Some of these cellular mediators are chemotactic for leucocytes and other inflammatory cells. This results in influx of eosinophils, monocytes, lymphocytes, mast cells and others. The infiltrating cells also release a variety of mediators, including oxidants, preformed granular mediators, lipid mediators and cytokines. This results in perpetual stimulation of resident and infiltrating cells. The interrelationships among and between these cells and the epithelium are complicated and difficult to dissect.

Airway epithelium plays a pivotal role in the inflammatory network seen in airways during asthma. The airway epithelium is the first tissue layer to encounter environmental stimuli such as inhaled allergens or microbes. In response to these stimuli the epithelium will hypersecrete mucus, increase mucociliary escalator activity, release a variety of inflammatory mediators which act in a paracrine, autocrine or endocrine fashion, or even die. The different mediators associated with asthma and their relationships with infiltrating and resident cell populations, especially the airway epithelium, will be discussed. Often, there is overlap in the types of mediators released by infiltrating cells and by the epithelium itself. To avoid redundancy, specific effects of relevant mediators produced by more than one cell in the asthmatic airway have been outlined in Tables 15.1, 15.2, 15.4, 15.6 and 15.7.

Lipid mediators

Lipid mediators (prostaglandins (PG), leukotrienes (LT), hydroxyeicosatetraenoic (HETE) acids and platelet-activating factor (PAF)) are major mediators in the asthmatic response. Both infiltrating inflammatory cells and the airway epithelial cells themselves produce these mediators when appropriately stimulated. Bronchoconstriction, alteration of vascular and epithelial permeability, leucocyte chemotaxis and mucin hypersecretion may be caused by lipid mediators relevant to the asthmatic response. The different lipid mediators produced by the airway epithelium and their effects are summarized in Table 15.1. Some cytokines from inflammatory cells upregulate epithelial production of lipid mediators (Hoeck *et al.*, 1993; Wu *et al.*, 1993a and b). Some eicosanoids may attenuate the asthmatic response, in addition to their pro-inflammatory effects. It is important to remember that these lipid mediators interact intimately with cytokines and other cellular mediators such as histamine and growth factors to create the complex network of interactions seen in asthma (Fig. 15.2).

Epithelial-derived factors

The airway epithelium itself is purported to release factors which modulate bronchial smooth muscle tone and alter bronchial contractility. Both relaxing and constrictive factors have been described (Bertrand & Tschirhart, 1993), but these factors have not been clearly identified, even by type — eicosanoid, cytokine, etc. It has long been known that removal of the airway epithelium augments bronchial smooth muscle contraction in response to bronchoconstrictive agents such as methacholine (Raeburn, 1990; Coyle *et al.*, 1993). This has been speculated to be

Table 15.1 Lipid mediators in asthma.

Lipid mediator	Source in airways	Effects associated with the epithelium	Other relevant effects in asthma	References
Prostaglandins (PG) and thromboxanes (TX)				
PGD_2	Epithelium Mast cells	Stimulates chloride secretion	Bronchoconstrictor Vasodilator Increases vascular permeability	O'Byrne, 1990; Djukanovic *et al.*, 1990
PGE_2	Epithelium AM Mast cells Smooth muscle	Believed to be a major component of EpDRF Produced in response to many secretagogues oxidants, bradykinin, LTC_4 Stimulates chloride secretion Decreases mucus secretion	Counteracts bronchoconstrictor responses and relaxes bonchial smooth muscle Decreases release of acetylcholine from airway nerves Produced by airway smooth muscle cells *in vitro*	Marom *et al.*, 1981; Eling *et al.*, 1986; O'Byrne, 1990; Prie *et al.*, 1990; Delamere *et al.*, 1993; McKinnon *et al.*, 1993
$PGF_{2\alpha}$	Epithelium AM	Mediates oxidant-induced mucin secretion Stimulates chloride secretion	Bronchoconstrictor	Adler *et al.*, 1990
PGI_2	Epithelium	Believed to be a major component of EpDRF	Counteracts bronchoconstrictor responses and relaxes bronchial smooth muscle	O'Byrne, 1990; Prie *et al.*, 1990
TXA_2/B_2	Epithelium AM Mast cells	Important mediator of PAF and cytokine-induced effects in the respiratory system Production induced by oxidants	Bronchoconstrictor Increased urinary concentration in allergen bronchoprovocation in atopic asthmatics Vasoconstrictor	Kumlin *et al.*, 1992; McKinnon *et al.*, 1993; Kruse-Elliott & Olson, 1993
Leukotrienes (LT) (sulphidopeptide leukotrienes or cysteinyl leukotrienes)				
LTB_4	Epithelium AM Eosinophils	Oxidants induce its production	Potent PMN chemoattractant Primes eosinophils AM are a major source of LTB_4 in the airways	O'Byrne, 1990; Piacentini & Kaliner, 1991; McKinnon *et al.*, 1993
LTC_4	Epithelium Mast cells AM Eosinophils	Production induced by PAF and oxidants Stimulates mucus secretion Stimulates chloride secretion	Eosinophils are a major source in asthmatics Very potent bronchoconstrictor Alters vascular permeability	Leikauf *et al.*, 1986; Adler *et al.*, 1987; Piacentini & Kaliner, 1991; McKinnon *et al.*, 1993
LTD_4	Epithelium Mast cells	Production induced by PAF and oxidants Stimulates mucus secretion Stimulates chloride secretion Stimulates mucociliary escalator at low doses and inhibits at high doses	Augments proliferative effects of IGF on airway smooth muscle Very potent bronchoconstrictor Increases vascular permeability Produces prolonged airway hyperreactivity Enhances AM production of PAF	Leikauf *et al.*, 1986; Adler *et al.*, 1987; Piacentini & Kaliner, 1991; Smith, 1992; Lin *et al.*, 1993; McKinnon *et al.*, 1993; Noveral *et al.*, 1994
LTE_4	Epithelium Mast cells	Production induced by PAF and oxidants Stimulates mucus secretion Stimulates chloride secretion	Bronchoconstrictor Increased urinary concentration in allergen bronchoprovacation in atopic asthmatics Arterial levels may reflect severity of asthmatic attack and this response can be altered by corticosteroids Alters vascular permeability	Leikauf *et al.*, 1986; Adler *et al.*, 1987; Piacentini & Kaliner, 1991; Kumlin *et al.*, 1992; McKinnon *et al.*, 1993; Shindo *et al.*, 1994

Continued

Table 15.1 *Continued.*

Lipid mediator	Source in airways	Effects associated with the epithelium	Other relevant effects in asthma	References
HETE (hydroxy eicosatetraenoic acids)				
5-HETE	Eosinophils Epithelium	Production stimulated by PAF and ROS	Increases PAF-induced PMN degranulation	Adler *et al.*, 1992
12-HETE	Epithelium	Production stimulated by PAF and ROS Stimulates mucus secretion	Bronchoconstrictor	Adler *et al.*, 1992
15-HETE	Epithelium Eosinophils	Major AA metabolite released by asthmatic bronchi as compared with lung parenchyma Mediates PAF-induced mucin secretion Stimulates mucin secretion Production induced by IL-5, IFN-γ and ROS	Bronchoconstrictor	Kumlin *et al.*, 1990; Adler *et al.*, 1992; Goswami *et al.*, 1993; Wu *et al.*, 1993a,b
Platelet-activating factor (PAF)	Epithelium Eosinophils AM Neutrophils Platelets Endothelium Mast cells	Stimulates mucin production Produced in response to oxidants Stimualtes ROS production by epithelium 'Primary' mediator of asthma and other respiratory diseases Stimulates eicosanoid production by epithelium Alters epithelial permeability Impairs mucociliary clearance	Important networking between PAF and TNF-α in respiratory diseases Production stimulated by TNF-α in many cell types in the airways Chemoattractant for eosinophils to the airways Primes eosinophils Increases vascular permeability Bronchoconstrictor Mediates cytokine-induced cardiopulmonary changes Stimulates LTC_4 release by eosinophils Produces prolonged airway hyperreactivity	Camussi *et al.*, 1987; Djukanovic *et al.*, 1990a; Piacentini & Kaliner, 1991; Adler *et al.*, 1992; Kinnula *et al.*, 1992; Smith, 1992; Kruse-Elliott *et al.*, 1993; Wright *et al.*, 1994

See text for definition of abbreviations.

due to the loss of an epithelial-derived relaxing factor (EpDRF). There is some thought that EpDRF is a group of compounds working together, some of which may be PGE_2 and PGI_2 (Prie *et al.*, 1990). β_2-agonists are used therapeutically to treat asthma; β_2-adrenoceptors have been identified on both airway epithelial cells and bronchial smooth muscle cells. When the airway epithelium is removed there is diminished relaxation of the bronchi in response to β-agonists. It is possible that β-agonists stimulate EpDRF release, in addition to direct effects on bronchial smooth muscle (Morrison *et al.*, 1993).

There also has been circumstantial evidence of an epithelial-derived contracting factor (EpDCF). The contractile activity of EpDCF is believed to be related in part to epithelial-derived LT and neuropeptides, such as calcitonin gene-related peptide (CGRP) (Barnes, 1991; Bertrand & Tschirhart, 1993). Endothelin-1 is a potent bronchoconstrictive agent; bronchial epithelial cells isolated from asthmatic patients express mRNA for the endothelin-1 precursor and release high levels of endothelin. Hydrocortisone, a glucocorticosteroid used effectively in the treatment of asthma, inhibits the release of biologically active endothelin from bronchial cells (Vittori *et al.*, 1992). It is quite possible that the airway epithelium is central to the maintenance of smooth muscle tone through both the relaxation effects of EpDRF and the contractile effects of EpDCF. In asthma, the epithelium is damaged and often large sections are shed. This damage may cause

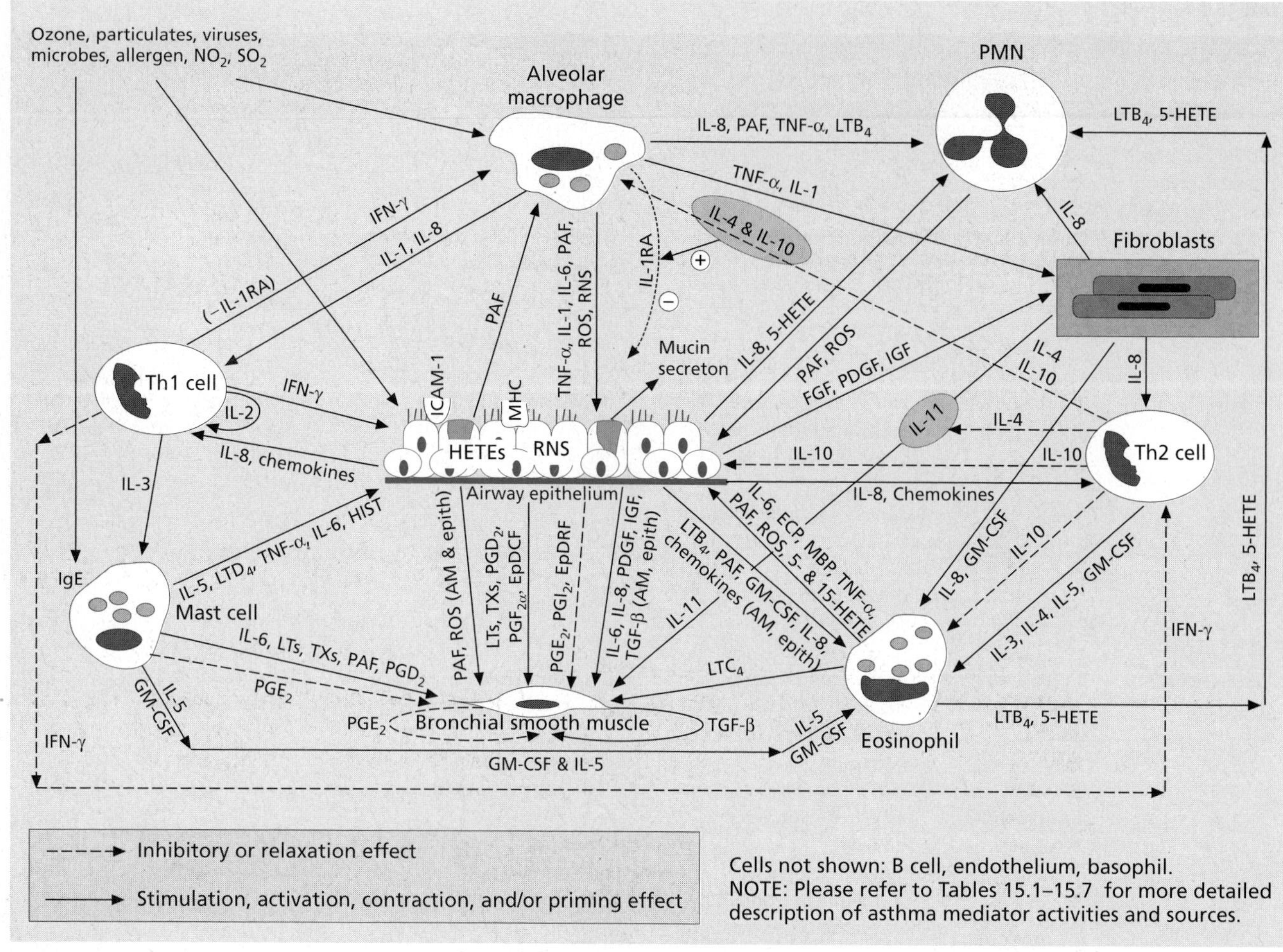

Fig. 15.2 Cytokines in asthma. See text for definition of abbreviaitons.

perturbations in this system of counter-balances, furthering the bronchial hyperresponsiveness which characterizes asthma.

Reactive nitrogen/oxygen species

Reactive nitrogen (RNS) and oxygen (ROS) species may target the airway epithelium and/or be produced by the airway epithelium. Recent work has demonstrated the importance of nitric oxide (NO) in asthma, both as a therapeutic agent and as a mediator (Hamid *et al.*, 1993). Preliminary studies from our laboratory implicate airway epithelial-derived NO as an important intracellular mediator involved in mucin hypersecretion (Fischer *et al.*, 1995; Wright *et al.*, 1996). NO can modulate ciliary beating in response to inflammatory mediators (Jain *et al.*, 1993). Although NO has been identified as the endothelial-derived relaxing factor (EDRF), it does not appear to be the EpDRF (Bertrand & Tschirhart, 1993). Bronchial muscle tone is minimally affected by inhalation of NO in asthmatic patients (Pfeffer *et al.*, 1994). NO derived either from the epithelium itself or from activated macrophages may contribute to epithelial damage in asthma. There is evidence of macrophage activation in asthma (Chanez *et al.*, 1991), and the inducible form of NO synthase is a source of large quantities of NO from activated macrophages. NO can combine with superoxide to form peroxynitrite, a potent oxidant. Peroxynitrite also may decompose to hydroxyl radical, the most reactive and potentially damaging of all the reactive oxygen species (Beckman *et al.*, 1990).

ROS (i.e. superoxide anion, hydrogen peroxide, hypochlorous acid) are produced by the respiratory burst of activated phagocytic cells (eosinophils, neutrophils, macrophages) (Babior, 1984; Lehrer *et al.*, 1988) and by the airway epithelial cells themselves (Kinnula *et al.*, 1992). It has been speculated that these molecules play an important role in the pathogenesis of asthma (Barnes, 1990). They are certainly capable of producing many of the changes associated with asthma, including mucus hyper-

Table 15.2 Cytokines in asthma.

Cytokine	Relevant sources	Effects associated with airway epithelium	Other relevant effects	References
Tumour necrosis factor-α (TNF-α)	Epithelium Endothelium Mast cells Eosinophils AM BAL leucocytes	Alteration of epithelial permeability Stimulates mucin secretion Stimulates endothelin synthesis Up-regulates ICAM-1 surface expression Stimulates epithelial migration, but negatively influences epithelial proliferation and defect repair Stimulates production of IL-6, IL-8 and GM-CSF by epithelium May abrogate cilia bioelectrical properties	Chemotactic for MON and PMN Stimulates PMN release of LTB_4 and PAF Stimulates PAF release in the lung/alveoli Up-regulates VCAM-1 expression on endothelium with IL-4 Increases pulmonary vascular permeability TNF-α production by AM enhanced by PAF Elevated levels in BALF from asthmatics.	Ming *et al.*, 1987; Camussi *et al.*, 1989; Mullin & Snock, 1990; Wegner *et al.*, 1990; Thornhill *et al.*, 1991; Cromwell *et al.*, 1992; Endo *et al.*, 1992; Gosset *et al.*, 1992; Cembrzynska-Nowak *et al.*, 1993; Ito *et al.*, 1993; Levine *et al.*, 1993; Bradding *et al.*, 1994
Interleukins (IL)				
IL-1, IL-1β, IL-1α	Endothelium MON MAC AM	Stimulates epithelial production of IL-6, IL-8 and GM-CSF Stimulates mucin secretion Stimulates endothelin synthesis Up-regulates ICAM-1 surface expression Stimulates EpDRF release	Activates T lymphocytes to express IL-2 Induces PMN transepithelial and transendothelial migration Primes eosinophils Its effects are mitigated by endogenous IL-1RA secreted by AM Stimulates airway smooth muscle hyperplasia and hypertrophy *in vitro*	Gosset *et al.*, 1988; Wegner, 1990; Cromwell *et al.*, 1992; Endo *et al.*, 1992; Levine *et al.*, 1993; Bittleman *et al.*, 1994; De *et al.*, 1994; Kline *et al.*, 1994; Tamaoki *et al.*, 1994
IL-2	Th1 lymphocytes	Stimulates airway hyperresponsiveness	Autocrine growth factor Stimulates formation of NK cells	Munakata *et al.*, 1993
IL-3	T lymphocytes Mast cells	Increases EOS and mast cells in airways and lung	Important for mast cell and basophil activation Enhances EOS tissue survival Important for B-cell differentiation and inducing immunoglobulin secretion	Barnes, 1994
IL-4	Mast cells Th2 lymphocytes	IL-4 and VCAM-1 important for EOS accumulation in BALF or airways	Up-regulates VCAM-1 expression on endothelium with TNF-α Stimulates B cells to produce IgE Suppresses IL-1, IL-6, and IL-8 production by AM Inhibits AM proliferation and TNF-α production Primes EOS for IL-8-induced chemotaxis Effects on B cells and AM counteracted by IFN-γ Inhibits cytokine-induced IL-11 production in fibroblasts Up-regulates IL-1RA production	Thornhill *et al.*, 1991; Trow *et al.*, 1993; Bradding *et al.*, 1994; Fukuda *et al.*, 1994; Kline *et al.*, 1994; Lehnert *et al.*, 1994; Ohta *et al.*, 1994
IL-5	Mast cells Th2 lymphocytes	Associated with eosinophilic inflammation in the airways	Important in eosinophil differentiation, survival, priming and activation	Sanderson, 1992; Wu *et al.*, 1993a; Bradding *et al.*, 1994; Schweizer *et al.*, 1994

Continued p. 270

Table 15.2 *Continued.*

Cytokine	Relevant sources	Effects associated with airway epithelium	Other relevant effects	References
		Stimulates AA release and 15-HETE production Potent inducer of lung inflammation, and increased inflammatory cells in BALF, and desquamation of bronchial epithelial cells	Primes EOS for chemokine-induced chemotaxis, calcium mobilization, and increases in F-actin content	
IL-6	Epithelium AM Mast cells Fibroblasts Endothelium Th2 lymphocytes Eosinophils	Up-regulation of both mRNA and protein in bronchial epithelium of asthmatics that is inhibited by Corticosteroids Stimulates endothelin synthesis Stimulates mucin secretion and *MUC-2* gene expression Histamine stimulates IL-6 release *in vitro*	Promotes B-cell maturation and immunoglobulin synthesis Acute-phase response protein Production stimulated by IL-1, TNF-α and IFN-γ IL-4 suppresses IL-6 production by AM Stimulates airway smooth muscle hyperplasia and hypertrophy *in vitro*	Endo *et al.*, 1992; Bradding, 1994; De *et al.*, 1994; Levine *et al.*, 1994; Marini *et al.*, 1992; Ohta *et al.*, 1994
IL-8 and chemokines RANTES, MIP-1α, GRO, GRO, MIP-2, MIP-1β	Epithelium AM Fibroblasts	TNF-α and IL-1 stimulate epithelial IL-8 production Stimulates endothelin synthesis	IL-8 potent chemoattractant for PMN IL-8 IL-8 chemoattractant for EOS primed with IL-4 or IL-5 RANTES potent chemoattractant for EOS T-lymphocyte chemoattractants Smooth muscle spasmogen Stimulates histamine release from IL-3-activated basophils MIP-1α chemotactic for eosinophils	Cromwell *et al.*, 1992; Endo *et al.*, 1992; Marini *et al.*, 1992; Bellini *et al.*, 1993; Alam *et al.*, 1994; Kunkel *et al.*, 1994; Schweizer *et al.*, 1994
IL-10	Th2 lymphocytes	Inhibits TNF-α-induced mucin secretion	'Anti-inflammatory' effects in asthma Suppresses IL-1, IL-6 and IL-8 production by AM Inhibits EOS survival and cytokine production in response to endotoxin Reduces numbers of EOS and lymphocytes in BAL in response to allergen Abrogates endotoxin-induced TNF-α production by AM Up-regulates IL-1RA production	Armstrong & Miller, 1994; Kline *et al.*, 1994; Levine *et al.*, 1994b; Ohta *et al.*, 1994; Woolley *et al.*, 1994
IL-11	Epithelium Fibroblasts	Production stimulated by RSV	Increases airway smooth muscle responsiveness to histamine IL-1α and TGF-β stimulate IL-11 production by fibroblasts, that is inhibitable by IL-4	Trow *et al.*, 1993; Einarsson *et al.*, 1994
Granulocyte macrophage colony-stimulating factor (GM-CSF)	Epithelium AM Eosinophils T lymphocytes Fibroblasts Mast cells	Increased expression in bronchial epithelium of asthmatics. Epithelial production of GM-CSF inhibited by corticosteroids	Important for eosinophil activation and survival in asthma	Vancheri *et al.*, 1989; Solopereto *et al.*, 1991; Cromwell *et al.*, 1992; Marini *et al.*, 1992; Sousa *et al.*, 1993

Continued

Table 15.2 *Continued.*

Cytokine	Relevant sources	Effects associated with airway epithelium	Other relevant effects	References
Interferon-γ (IFN-γ)	Th1 lymphocytes	Stimulates cytokine release and ICAM-1 expression Increases MHC1 and II expression on epithelial cells IFN-γ-treated cells are able to present antigen to T cells, but at a lower efficiency than MON Stimulates AA release and 15-HETE production Decreases airway hyperresponsiveness *in vitro* by an epithelial-dependent mechanism	Inhibitory effect on Th2 lymphocytes Enhances AM release of TNF-α Increases MHC I and II expression on AM Up-regulates IL-1RA production Elevated levels in BALF from asthmatics	Rossi *et al.*, 1990; Wegner *et al.*, 1990; Mezzetti *et al.*, 1991; Cerembryznska-Nowak *et al.*, 1993; Munakata *et al.*, 1993; Wu *et al.*, 1993b; Kline *et al.*, 1994
Growth factors Platelet-derived growth factor (PDGF) Transforming growth factor-β (TGF-β) Insulin-like growth factors (IGF) Fibroblast growth factors (FGF)	AM Epithelium Eosinophils Smooth muscle	TGF-β important for squamous differentiation of bronchial epithelium Ozone exposure stimulates gene expression for TGF-β2 and PDGF *in vitro* IGF important in airway epithelial repair after injury TGF-β1 stimulates integrin expression	*PDGF* Stimulates fibroblast proliferation and collagen secretion Stimulates ASM proliferation *FGF* Regulates fibrinogenesis *TGF-β* Secreted by ASM cells and stimulates their proliferation Stimulates collagen secretion by fibroblasts that is enhanced by insulin *IGF* Stimulates ASM proliferation and hypertrophy Stimulates fibroblast proliferation	Masui *et al.*, 1986; Hirst *et al.*, 1992; Sheppard *et al.*, 1992; Cambrey *et al.*, 1993; Ashe *et al.*, 1994; Black *et al.*, 1994; Krupsky *et al.*, 1994; Michelson *et al.*, 1994; Noveral *et al.*, 1994; Ohno *et al.*, 1994

See text for definition of abbreviations.

secretion, cytotoxicity, impaired mucociliary clearance and bronchial smooth muscle contraction (Burman & Martin, 1986; Phipps *et al.*, 1986; Adler *et al.*, 1990; Kobayashi *et al.*, 1991; Simon *et al.*, 1991; Lansing *et al.*, 1993). The respiratory epithelium may have a role in protection from ROS as well. The airway epithelium has potent antioxidant capacity (Cohn *et al.*, 1994). Because of its anatomical position, the antioxidative properties of the epithelium may be important in protecting underlying tissues such as smooth muscle from the luminal oxidant burden associated with inflammation and activation of phagocytic cells. If epithelial shedding diminishes the antioxidant capacity of the airways, there may be increased oxidative stress, promoting asthma.

Cytokines

Cytokines are regulatory proteins released by a wide variety of cell types. There is a complex network of interactions between the airway epithelium, other resident and infiltrating cells, and cytokines. As summarized in Table 15.2, there are many pluripotent cytokines involved in asthma. As listed in Table 15.3, the airway epithelium is a source of several cytokines, including: tumour necrosis factor-α (TNF-α), interleukin-6 (IL-6), IL-8, granulocyte macrophage colony-stimulating factor (GM-CSF) and insulin-like growth factor-1 (IGF-1). Each of these cytokines may play an important part in the epithelium's central role in asthma. For example, IL-6 generated by the

Table 15.3 Airway cells and the cytokines they produce.

Cell or tissue type	Cytokines
Epithelium	TNF-α, IL-6, IL-8, IL-11, GM-CSF, growth factors
Endothelium	TNF-α, IL-1, IL-6
Mast cells	TNF-α, IL-3, IL-4, IL-5, IL-6, GM-CSF
Alveolar macrophage/ monocyte	TNF-α, IL-1, IL-1RA, IL-6, IL-8, GM-CSF, growth factors
Fibroblasts	IL-6, IL-8, IL-11, GM-CSF
Eosinophils	TNF-α, IL-6, GM-CSF, growth factors
Th1 lymphocytes	IL-2, IFN-γ
Th2 lymphocytes	IL-4, IL-5, IL-6, IL-10
T lymphocytes	IL-3, GM-CSF

See text for definition of abbreviations.

epithelium can be important in immunoglobulin production in the airway, and also can stimulate smooth muscle proliferation and hypertrophy. Likewise, IL-8 is a potent chemoattractant for neutrophils, lymphocytes and eosinophils. Epithelial-derived GM-CSF is important for eosinophil activation and survival in the asthmatic airways. Epithelial-derived growth factors function in both repair of the epithelium, and at the same time alter airway smooth muscle growth. Similarly, cytokines elaborated by other cell types act on the epithelium to stimulate several important components of the asthmatic response, including: mucin hypersecretion, cytokine production, adhesion molecule expression, altered epithelial permeability and autacoid production. Certain cytokines allow the airway epithelial cells themselves to express major histocompatibility antigens, thereby causing the epithelial cells to present antigen (Rossi *et al.*, 1990; Kalb *et al.*, 1991). Antigen presentation to lymphocytes potentiates the cell-mediated hypersensitivity responses observed in asthma (Poulter *et al.*, 1994). IL-12, IL-13, IL-14, and IL-15 have recently been identified; however, their importance in the asthmatic response is still under investigation. Consequently, as summarized in Fig. 15.2, the epithelium plays a central and pivotal role in the control of airway inflammation and hyperresponsiveness in asthma.

Adhesion molecules

Inflammatory cell infiltration is regulated to some degree by adhesion molecules. In the inflamed lung, haematogenous inflammatory cells (eosinophils and neutrophils) must undergo vascular margination, diapedesis (trans-endothelial migration) and interstitial migration to reach sites of inflammation such as the epithelial surface. The first crucial step in this process involves the interaction of the leucocyte and the endothelium, and has been termed the 'leucocyte–endothelial cell adhesion cascade' (Albelda *et al.*, 1994). This 'cascade' is essential to airway inflammation and the adhesion molecules involved in this process have been studied extensively (Table 15.4). The local environment and cytokines regulate adhesion molecules, which in turn regulate the cascade (Dayer *et al.*, 1993; Resnick & Weller, 1993; Strieter *et al.*, 1993; Walker & Virchow, 1993).

The airway hyperresponsiveness of asthma has been associated with an increase in intercellular adhesion molecule-1 (ICAM-1) expression (Wegner *et al.*, 1990; Gundel *et al.*, 1993). ICAM-1 is part of the immunoglobulin supergene family which functions in leucocyte–endothelium and leucocyte–epithelium interactions (Calderon & Lockey, 1992). ICAM-1 is expressed on neutrophils, eosinophils, pulmonary endothelial and epithelial cells, and several other tissues throughout the body (Wegner *et al.*, 1990; Kishimoto & Rothlein, 1994). ICAM-1 is the receptor/ligand for leucocyte cell adhesion molecules on lymphocytes and macrophages (Calderon & Lockey, 1992). ICAM-1 can be up-regulated by a number of inflammatory mediators associated with asthma (Rothlein *et al.*, 1988; Wawryk *et al.*, 1991; Lassalle *et al.*, 1993). BAL fluids, sputum and sera from asthmatics display increased surface or soluble expression of ICAM-1 and endothelial leucocyte adhesion molecule/E-selectin (ELAM-1) (Hansel *et al.*, 1991; Hansel & Walker, 1992; Kroegel *et al.*, 1992; Lassalle, *et al.*, 1993; Kobayashi *et al.*, 1994; Mengelers *et al.*, 1994; Montefort *et al.*, 1994; Pretolani *et al.*, 1994). Bronchial biopsies from asthmatic patients display elevated surface expression of ICAM-1, class II human leucocyte antigen (HLA-DR) on epithelial cells and a significant increase in ELAM-1, vascular adhesion molecule-1 (VCAM-1) and ICAM-1 on endothelial cells (Bentley *et al.*, 1993; Vignola *et al.*, 1993, 1994; Gosset *et al.*, 1994). Up-regulation of these cellular adhesion molecules on the epithelial cells promotes epithelial interaction with inflammatory cells. Allergen-induced bronchial hyperresponsiveness in rats can be inhibited when the animals are pretreated with ICAM-1 antibodies (Sun *et al.*, 1994), suggesting that the epithelial component of the interaction controls inflammatory cell association and subsequent effects. Rabb *et al.* illustrated that airway changes in allergen-challenged rats depend upon adhesion molecules in early- as well as late-phase cellular responses (Rabb *et al.*, 1994). Thus, adhesion molecules can alter airway responses not only via changes in cellular migration but also by altering the function of inflammatory cells already present in the airway.

The majority of epithelial cells recovered in the BAL of asthmatics are columnar cells (Laitinen *et al.*, 1985). Columnar bronchial epithelial cells have less contact with the basement membrane than basal cells. Basal cells interact with the basement membrane through integrin molecules in the hemidesmosomes. Integrins are trans-

Table 15.4 Leucocyte–endothelial interactions.

Adhesion molecule	Ligand	Distribution	Function	References
Immunoglobulin supergene family				
ICAM-1	LFA-1 (CD11a/CD18) Mac-1 (CD11b/CD18)	Endothelium Lymphocytes Respiratory epithelium Other tissues	Adherence and emigration	Rothlein *et al.*, 1986; Calderon & Lockey, 1992; Kishimoto & Rothlein, 1994
ICAM-2	LFA-1 (CD11a/CD18)	Endothelium Mononuclear leucocytes	Adherence and emigration	Yong & Khwaja, 1990; Korthuis *et al.*, 1994
ICAM-3	LFA-1 (CD11a/CD18)	Lymphocytes Monocytes Neutrophils	?	Dussis-Anagnostopoulou *et al.*, 1993; Kishimoto & Rothlein, 1994
PECAM-1	PECAM-1	Leucocytes Platelets	Leucocyte adhesion Leucocyte chemotaxis	Newman, 1994
VCAM-1	VLA-4 (CD49d/CD29)	Endothelium	Adherence	Sanchez-Madrid & Corbi, 1992; Dean *et al.*, 1993
Integrin family				
LFA-1, CD11a/CD18	ICAM-1 ICAM-2	All leucocytes	Adherence and emigration	Leff *et al.*, 1991
Mac-1, CD11b/CD18	ICAM-1 iC3b fibronectin	Granulocytes Monocytes	Adherence and emigration	Korthuis *et al.*, 1994
p150,95, CD11c/CD18	iC3b	Macrophages Monocytes Granulocytes	Postulated that it down-regulates activated leucocytes	Korthuis *et al.*, 1994
VLA-4 (CD49d/CD29)	VCAM-1	Fibronectin Fibroblasts	Adherence	Elices *et al.*, 1990
Selectin family				
P-selectin PADGEM	Sialyl Lewis-x	Stimulated endothelium Activated platelets	Rolling/margination	Korthuis *et al.*, 1994
L-selectin LECAM-1	P-selectin E-selectin Mannose-6-phosphate Fructose-6-phosphate	Lymphocytes Neutrophils Monocytes	Rolling/margination	Gundel *et al.*, 1993; Korthuis *et al.*, 1994
E-selectin ELAM-1	Sialyl Lewis-x	Endothelium	Rolling/margination	Korthuis *et al.*, 1994

See text for definition of abbreviations.

membrane glycoproteins, which link the intracellular cytoskeleton with the extracellular matrix. In the lung they bind to basement membrane proteins (laminin, collagen, fibronectin) or inflammatory matrix proteins (fibrinogen, fibronectin, vitronectin, thrombospondin) (Albelda, 1991) (Table 15.5). Columnar cells adhere to the basal cells through the integral proteins in desmosomes and gap junctions (Roche *et al.*, 1993). The importance of these adhesive proteins in epithelial desquamation in the asthmatic lung is still unclear, but it is possible that integrin attachments and alterations in these integrins are the keys to desquamation of viable epithelial cells in asthma. After shedding of epithelial cells the denuded basement membrane must undergo wound healing. It has been suggested that adhesion molecules aid the epithelial cells to migrate and re-populate these injured areas (Albelda, 1991; Calderon & Lockey, 1992).

Preformed mediators

Eosinophils, mast cells, neutrophils and macrophages possess preformed mediators within cytoplasmic granules. When these cells are appropriately stimulated, their granular contents may be released. All of these cell types

Table 15.5 Bronchial epithelial integrins.

Integrin subunits	Ligand	Reference
α1/β1	Laminin/collagen	Tournier *et al.*, 1992
α2/β1	Collagen/laminin	Albelda, 1991; Mette *et al.*, 1993; Roche *et al.*, 1993
α3/β1	Laminin/collagen/ fibronectin	Albelda, 1991; Mette *et al.*, 1993
α5/β1	Fibronectin RGD site	Albelda, 1991; Mette *et al.*, 1993
αv/β1	Fibronectin	Albelda, 1991; Sheppard *et al.*, 1992; Mette *et al.*, 1993
α6/β1	Laminin	Tournier *et al.*, 1992; Mette *et al.*, 1993; Roche *et al.*, 1993
β3	Dependent on α-subunit	Sheppard *et al.*, 1992
α6/β4	Laminin	Tournier et al., 1992; Mette *et al.*, 1993; Roche *et al.*, 1993
β5	Dependent on α-subunit	Sheppard *et al.*, 1992
β6	Dependent on α-subunit	Sheppard *et al.*, 1992

RGD, adhesive tripeptide arginine, glycine, aspartic acid.

are involved in the inflammatory response associated with asthma, and many of the granular mediators exert marked effects on the respiratory epithelium. Eosinophils and mast cells have long been linked to allergic asthma. On bronchial biopsy the submucosa of asthmatics is infiltrated with eosinophils and the epithelial lining has elevated numbers of eosinophils and mast cells (Laitinen *et al.*, 1993; Pesci *et al.*, 1993; Bradding *et al.*, 1994). Eosinophilia and mild mastocytosis may be found in BAL fluid from asthmatic patients (Djukanovic *et al.*, 1990a,b; Bradley *et al.*, 1991; Bousquet *et al.*, 1994; Bradding *et al.*, 1994). Both the eosinophils and mast cells found in asthmatic airways are in an activated state with evidence of degranulation (Bousquet *et al.*, 1990; Djukanovic *et al.*, 1990b; Soloperto *et al.*, 1991). The airway epithelial cells themselves produce and release factors which are chemotactic for eosinophils and which enhance their survival in the airways (Masuda *et al.*, 1992; Koyama *et al.*, 1993). Although neutrophil accumulation is not a typical characteristic of asthma, the inflammatory reaction of the late asthmatic response may include neutrophils (Metzger *et al.*, 1986; Murray *et al.*, 1986). Macrophages are numerically the largest cellular component of the BAL in both normal and asthmatic subjects; newly recruited monocytes join a resident population of pulmonary tissue macrophages (Djukanovic *et al.*, 1990). Stimulated airway epithelial cells release factors which are chemotactic for both neutrophils and monocytes (Koyama *et al.* 1989; Nakamura *et al.*, 1991).

The granular products of these cells may damage the epithelium and mucociliary escalator, act as mucus secretagogues, affect bronchial tone and alter ion secretion (Table 15.6). Eosinophil granule contents, particularly major basic protein (MBP), are likely to play a key role in the epithelial damage that is a characteristic feature of asthmatic airways (Motojima *et al.*, 1989). An intact epithelium affords some protection from preformed granular mediators. The barrier function of intact airway epithelium prevents luminal elastase released by activated neutrophils from causing tissue damage. Exposure of the basolateral surface, as occurs in areas of epithelial denudation, allows elastase to detach epithelial cells from their subjacent matrix (Rickard *et al.*, 1992). The epithelium is a not only a physical barrier in the protection of smooth muscle from constrictive mediators, but also a metabolic barrier which can degrade many of the mediators. Airway epithelial cells contain histaminases which may inactivate histamine and therefore attenuate its bronchoconstrictive properties (Lindstrom *et al.*, 1991).

Neuropeptides

The respiratory tract is extensively innervated. In addition to the classical adrenergic and cholinergic systems, neuropeptides (synthesized in nerve cell bodies and transported through the dendrites) released upon stimulation of peptidergic motor or sensory nerves modulate a number of lung functions. Epithelial interactions with neuropeptides may be relevant to the asthmatic response. Some studies have found that depletion of neuropeptides blunts airway hyperresponsiveness to repeated antigen exposure (Matsuse *et al.*, 1991), while other studies did not (Ingenito *et al.*, 1991; Lai, 1991). Epithelial denudation which accompanies asthma not only alters barrier and secretory functions, but also exposes nerve endings and may initiate neurogenic inflammatory pathways. An axonal reflex involving the stimulation of neuropeptide release has been suggested to contribute to the pathogenesis of asthma (Barnes, 1987, 1991). Inflammatory cells and mediators which would not normally contact nerve endings under the epithelial cells could contact and stimulate such nerves in areas of epithelial denudation. Some of the most relevant neuropeptides in the respiratory system can be grouped as contractile neuropeptides (substance P (SP) and neurokinin A (NKA)) or inhibitory neuropeptides (vasoactive intestinal peptide (VIP) and peptide histidine isoleucine (PHI)). As a general rule, the contractile peptides are bronchoconstrictive, act as mucus secreta-

Table 15.6 Pre-formed granular mediators in asthma.

Mediator	Source	Mucous effects	Bronchial effect	Vascular effects	Other effects
Elastase	PMN	Secretagogue (Varsano *et al.*, 1987; Breuer *et al.*, 1989; Kim *et al.*, 1989; Sommerhoff *et al.*, 1990)			Causes epithelial detachment from extracellular matrix Increases epithelial permeability (Rickard & Rennard, 1989; Amitani *et al.*, 1991)
Cathepsin G	PMN Mast cells	Secretagogue (Varsano *et al.*, 1987; Breuer *et al.*, 1989; Kim *et al.*, 1989; Sommerhoff *et al.*, 1990)			
Histamine	Mast cell Basophil	Secretagogue (Parke 1978; Shelhamer *et al.*, 1980)	Bronchoconstrictor (Rosa & McDowall, 1951; Thomson, 1987) Primary mediator of allergic asthma	Increases vascular permeability (White *et al.*, 1987)	Stimulates chloride ion secretion by epithelium (Marin *et al.*, 1977)
Tryptase	Mast cell		Enhances histamine-induced bronchoconstriction (Sekizawa *et al.*, 1989)		Inactivates VIP, PHM, and CGRP (Tam & Caughey, 1992)
Chymase	Mast cell	Secretagogue (Sommerhoff *et al.*, 1989)			Causes epithelial detachment from extracellular matrix (Schwartz, 1992)
ECP	Eosinophil	Secretagogue (Lundgren *et al.*, 1991)			
MBP	Eosinophil		Enhances responsiveness to constrictors (Uchida *et al.*, 1993; Coyle *et al.*, 1994).		Stimulates chloride ion secretion by epithelium (Lundgren *et al.*, 1991) Cytotoxic to airway epithelium (Motojima *et al.*, 1989). Impairs mucociliary clearance (Hastie *et al.*, 1987)

CGRP, calcitonin gene-related peptide; ECP, eosinophilic cationic protein; MBP, major basic protein; PHM, peptide histidine methionine; PMN, polymorphonuclear neutrophilic leucocyte; VIP, vasoactive intestinal peptide.

gogues and act to increase vascular permeability. The inhibitory peptides are bronchodilators, have variable effects on mucus and are vasodilators (Table 15.7) (Webber, 1988; Amin *et al.*, 1989). The CGRP causes migration of bronchial epithelial cells. In areas of epithelial denudation, CGRP peptide may be crucial for the epithelium to repair itself (Sanghavi *et al.*, 1994). Neuropeptides in the lung have been reviewed (Barnes, 1991).

The ability of airway epithelial cells to degrade neuropeptides may be important in asthma. Many neuropeptides are cleaved by neural endopeptidase (NEP); specific neuropeptides may be cleaved by other substances as well (i.e. VIP is degraded by tryptase, SP is degraded by angiotensin-converting enzyme (ACE) — see Table 15.7). NEP is a membrane-bound enzyme found on a number of cell types, including airway epithelial cells (Choi *et al.*, 1990; Lilly *et al.*, 1993). In the microenvironment of the inflamed airway, loss of epithelia will lead to loss of NEP. While this will affect the degradation of both contractile and inhibitory peptides, there is preferential degradation of inhibitory peptides. The inhibitory peptide VIP is subject to degradation by mast cell products chymase and tryptase (Caughey *et al.*, 1988; Tam & Caughey, 1992; Lilly *et al.*, 1993b), which may both be elevated in asthmatic airways (Wenzel *et al.*, 1988; Liu *et al.*, 1990). On the other hand, the contractile peptides are not significantly degraded by mast cell products. Even enzymes such as ACE do not function effectively when SP is presented

Table 15.7 Neuropeptides in asthma.

Neuropeptide	Location	Degradation	Bronchial effects	Mucin effects	Vascular effectrs	Other effects
SP	C fibre afferent nerves in airway epithelium Near blood vessels Within bronchial smooth muscle (Springall *et al.*, 1988)	NEP ACE from serosal surface chymase (Lilly *et al.*, 1993)	Bronchoconstriction (Sekizawa *et al.*, 1987)	Stimulates mucin secretion (Barnes *et al.*, 1986; Basbaum *et al.*, 1988; Lundgren *et al.*, 1989; Mizoguchi & Hicks, 1989)	Vasodilatation (Pernow, 1985) Increases microvascular permeability (Lundberg *et al.*, 1983)	Stimulates chloride ion secretion by epithelium (Mizoguchi & Hicks, 1989) Increases ciliary beat frequency (Wong *et al.*, 1991)
NKA	Co-localizes with SP	NEP (Frossard *et al.*, 1989)	Bronchoconstriction (Martling *et al.*, 1987)	Stimulates mucin secretion (<SP) (Barnes, 1991)	Vasodilatation (<SP) (Barnes, 1991)	
CGRP	Sensory nerves primarily along bronchial vessels (Lundberg *et al.*, 1985)	Moderate degradation by NEP (Nadel, 1992)	Bronchoconstriction (Palmer *et al.*, 1987; Bannenberg *et al.*, 1994)		Vasodilatation (Marling *et al.*, 1988; McCormack *et al.*, 1989) No affect on microvascular permeability (Rogers *et al.*, 1988)	Initiates migration of epithelial cells in wound repair (Sanghavi *et al.*, 1994)
VIP	In airway walls Within smooth muscle Around vasculature Around mucous glands Beneath epithelium. (Springall *et al.*, 1988)	NEP Tryptase Chymase (Lilly, Drazen *et al.*, 1993a)	Bronchodilatation (Palmer *et al.*, 1986)	Decreases secretion from epithelial cells (Amin *et al.*, 1989) Increases secretion from glands (Peatifield *et al.*, 1983)	Vasodilatation (Laitinen *et al.*, 1987)	Stimulates fluid and chloride transport in epithelium (Nathanson *et al.*, 1983)
PHI	Co-localizes with VIP (Barnes 1991)		Bronchodilatation (Palmer *et al.*, 1986)	Decreases secretion from epithelial cells (Webber 1988)	Vasodilatation (<VIP) (Barnes 1991)	

See text for definition of abbreviations.

along the luminal surface of the airway epithelium (Stimler-Gerard, 1987; Honda *et al.*, 1991; Lilly *et al.*, 1993a). Therefore, in the inflamed asthmatic airway, there may be more functional contractile neuropeptide than inhibitory peptide, contributing to bronchoconstriction as well as mucus hypersecretion and vascular oedema.

Conclusions

The airway epithelium is intimately involved in the pathogenesis of asthma. As a target of lipid and granular mediators, cytokines, ROS, RNS and neuropeptides, it may increase mucus secretion, alter ion and water transport, increase or decrease mucociliary escalator function, or be directly damaged. As an effector, the epithelium produces lipid mediators, cytokines and ROS, which target the epithelium in an autocrine fashion, but which also act in a paracrine manner to affect the function of nearby nervous, vascular and muscle tissues as well as inflammatory cells. Epithelial cells can themselves present antigen to T-lymphocytes, potentiating asthmatic responses. Epithelial expression of adhesion molecules can potentiate disease by permitting infiltration of inflammatory cells. Changes in adhesion molecules may influence epithelial shedding but may also facilitate epithelial repair through migration of epithelial cells. The epithelium serves as a physical barrier between mediators and underlying target tissues (i.e. smooth muscle, vasculature). As a physical barrier it diminishes the opportunity for allergen exposure to underlying antigen-presenting cells and diminishes exposure of other cell types to luminally released mediators. As a metabolic barrier, the epithelium actually degrades compounds such as neuropeptides, histamines and others. The epithelial lining of the airways can potentiate damage and/or protect from damage associated with asthma. There is much to be learned before the role of airway epithelial cells in asthma pathogenesis is fully understood.

Acknowledgements

Supported by: National Institutes of Health Grants HL36982, HL08647 and HL09063; a grant from Hoffman La Roche Incorporated, Nutley, NJ; a grant from Glaxo Wellcome Incorporated, RTP, NC; and a grant from the State of North Carolina.

References

Adler, K.B., Akley, N.J. & Glasgow, W.C. (1992) Platelet-activating factor provokes release of mucin-like glycoproteins from guinea pig respiratory epithelial cells via a lipoxygenase-dependent mechanism. *Am. J. Respir. Cell Mol. Biol.*, **6**, 550–6.

Adler, K.B., Holden-Stauffer, W.J. & Repine, J.E. (1990) Oxygen metabolites stimulate release of high-molecular-weight glycoconjugates by cell and organ cultures of rodent respiratory epithelium via an arachidonic acid-dependent mechanism. *J. Clin. Invest.*, **85**, 75–85.

Adler, K.B., Schwarz, J.E., Anderson, W.H. & Welton, A.F. (1987) Platelet activating factor stimulates secretion of mucin by explants of rodent airways in organ culture. *Exp. Lung Res.*, **13**, 25–43.

Alam, R., York, J., Boyars, M. *et al.* (1994) The involvement of chemokines in bronchial asthma. The detection of mRNA for MCP-1, MCP-3, RANTES, MIP-1alpha and IL-8 in bronchoalveolar lavage cells, and the measurement of RANTES and MIP-1 in the lavage fluid. *Am. J. Resp. Crit. Care Med.*, **149**, A951.

Albelda, S.M. (1991) Endothelial and epithelial cell adhesion molecules. *Am. J. Respir. Cell Mol. Biol.*, **4**, 195–203.

Albelda, S.M., Smith, C.W. & Ward, P.A. (1994) Adhesion molecules and inflammatory injury. *FASEB J.*, **8**, 504–12.

Amin, D.N., Goswami, S., Maayani, S. & Marom, Z. (1989) Functional antagonism between neurotransmitters in the control of mucous glycoprotein secretion in a model of epithelial cells. *Am. Rev. Resp. Dis.*, **139**, A410.

Amitani, R., Rutman, R.W.A., Read, R. *et al.* (1991) Effects of human neutrophil elastase and *Peudomonas aeruginosa* proteinases on human respiratory epithelium. *Am. J. Respir. Cell Mol. Biol.*, **4**, 26–32.

Armstrong, L. & Millar, A.B. (1994) Reduction of LPS-induced tumor necrosis factor-alpha (TNF-alpha) release by macrophages/monocytes in response to interleukin-10 (IL-10). *Am. J. Resp. Crit. Care Med.*, **149**, A1066.

Ashe, W.S., Retsch-Bogart, G.Z., Moats-Staats, B.M., Stiles, A.D. & Leigh, M.W. (1994) The role of insulin-like growth factors in the repair of airway epithelium following acute injury. *Am. J. Resp. Crit. Care Med.*, **149**, A710.

Babior, B.M. (1984) The respiratory burst of phagocytes. *J. Clin. Invest.*, **73**, 599–601.

Bannenberg, G., Kimland, M., Ryrfeldt, A., Lundberg, J.M. & Moldeus, P. (1994) Sensory neuropeptide-mediated bronchoconstriction of the guinea pig lung by diamide; a comparison to hydrogen peroxide. *Eur. J. Pharmacol.*, **270**, 175–82.

Barnes, P.J. (1987) Neuropeptides in human airways: function and clinical implications. *Am. Rev. Resp. Dis.*, **136**, S77–83.

Barnes, P.J. (1990) Reactive oxygen species and airway inflammation. *Free Radic. Biol. Med.*, **9**, 235–43.

Barnes, P.J. (1991) Neuropeptides and asthma. *Am. Rev. Resp. Dis.*, **143**, S28–32.

Barnes, P.J. (1994) Cytokines as mediators of chronic asthma. *Am. J. Resp. Crit. Care Med.*, **150**, S42–9.

Barnes, P.J., Dewar, A. & Rogers, D.F. (1986) Effect of substance P, muscarinic and adrenergic stimulation *in vitro*. *Brit. J. Pharmacol.*, **89**, 767P.

Basbaum, C., Carlson, D., Davidson, E., Verdugo, P. & Gail, D.B. (1988) Cellular mechanisms of airway secretion. *Am. Rev. Resp. Dis.*, **137**, 479–85.

Beasley, R., Burgess, C., Crane, J., Pearce, N. & Roche, W. (1993) Pathology of asthma and its clinical implications. *J. Allergy Clin. Immunol.*, **92**, 148–54.

Beckman, J.S., Beckman, T.W., Chen, J., Marshall, P.A. & Freeman, B.A. (1990) Apparent hydroxyl radical production by peroxynitrite: implications for endothelial injury from nitric oxide and superoxide. *Proc. Nat. Acad. Sci. USA*, **87**, 1620–4.

Bellini, A., Yoshimura, H., Vittori, E., Marini, M. & Mattoli, S. (1993) Bronchial epithelial cells of patients with asthma release chemoattractant factors for T lymphocytes. *J. Allergy Clin. Immunol.*, **92**, 412–24.

Bentley, A.M., Menz, G., Storz, C. *et al.* (1992) Identification of T lymphocytes, macrophages and activated eosinophils in the bronchial mucosa of intrinsic asthma: relationship to symptoms and bronchial responsivness. *Am. Rev. Resp. Dis.*, **146**, 500–6.

Bentley, A.M., Durham, S.R., Robinson, D.S. *et al.* (1993) Expression of endothelial and leukocyte adhesion molecules, intercellular adhesion molecule-1, E-selectin, and vascular cell adhesion molecule-1 in the bronchial mucosa in steady-state and allergen-induced asthma. *J. Allergy Clin. Immunol.*, **92**, 857–68.

Bertrand, C. & Tschirhart, E. (1993) Epithelial factors: modulation of the airway smooth muscle tone. *Fundam. Clin. Pharmacol.*, **7**, 261–73.

Bittleman, D.B., Thomas, M.D. & Casale, M.D. (1994) Interleukin-1a induces potent and distinct signals for neutrophil transendothelial and transepithelial migration. *Am. J. Resp. Crit. Care Med.*, **149**, A231.

Black, P.N., Young, P.G., Scott, L., Merrilees, M.J. & Skinner, S.J.M. (1994) Is transforming growth factor-beta an autocrine growth factor for airway smooth muscle? *Am. J. Resp. Crit. Care Med.*, **149**, A302.

Bousquet, J., Chanez, P., Lacoste, J.Y. *et al.* (1990) Eosinophilic inflammation in asthma. *New Engl. J. Med.*, **323**, 1033–9.

Bousquet, J., Chanez, P., Vignola, A.M., Lacoste, J.Y. & Michel, F.B. (1994) Eosinophil inflammation in asthma. *Am. J. Resp. Crit. Care Med.*, **150**, S33–8.

Bradding, P., Roberts, J.A., Britten, K.M. *et al.* (1994) Interleukin-4, -5, and -6 and tumor necrosis factor-α in normal and asthmatic airways: evidence for the human mast cell as a source of these cytokines. *Am. J. Respir. Cell Mol. Biol.*, **10**, 471–80.

Bradley, B.L., Azzawi, M., Jacobson, M. *et al.* (1991) Eosinophils, T-lymphocytes, mast cells, neutrophils and macrophages in bronchial biopsy specimens from atopic subjects with asthma: comparison with biopsy specimens from atopic subjects without asthma and normal control subjects and relationship to bronchial hyperresponsiveness. *J. Allergy Clin. Immunol.*, **88**, 661–74.

Breuer, R., Christensen, T.G., Niles, R.M., Stone, P.J. & Snider, G.L. (1989) Human neutrophil elastase causes glycoconjugate release from the epithelial cell surface of hamster trachea in organ culture. *Am. Rev. Resp. Dis.*, **139**, 779–82.

Burman, W.J. & Martin, W.J. (1986) Oxidant-mediated ciliary dysfunction. Possible role in airway disease. *Chest*, **89**, 410–13.

Calderon, E. & Lockey, R.F. (1992) A possible role for adhesion molecules in asthma. *J. Allergy Clin. Immunol.*, **90**, 852–65.

Cambrey, A.D., Kwon, O.J., McAnulty, R.J. *et al.* (1993) Release of fibroblast proliferative activity from cultured human airway epithelial cells: a role for insulin-like growth factor 1 (IGF-1). *Am. Rev. Resp. Dis.*, **147**, A277.

Camussi, G., Bussolino, F., Salvidio, G. & Baglioni, C. (1987) Tumor necrosis factor/cachectin stimulates peritoneal macrophages, polymorphonuclear neutrophils, and vascular endothelial cells to synthesize and release platelet activating factor. *J. Exp. Med.*, **166**, 1390–404.

Camussi, G., Tetta, C., Bussolino, F. & Baglioni, C. (1989) Tumor necrosis factor stimulates human neutrophils to release leukotriene B4 and platelet activating factor. *J. Biochem.*, **182**, 661–6.

Caughey, G.H., Leidig, F., Viro, N.F. & Nadel, J.A. (1988) Substance P and vasoactive intestinal peptide degradation by mast cell tryptase and chymase. *J. Pharmacol. Exp. Ther.*, **244**, 133–7.

Cembrzynska-Nowak, M., Szklarz, E., Inglot, A.D. & Teodorczyk-Injeyan, J.A. (1993) Elevated release of tumor necrosis factor-alpha and interferon-gamma by bronchoalveolar leukocytes from patients with bronchial asthma. *Am. Rev. Resp. Dis.*, **147**, 291–5.

Chanez, P., Bousquet, J., Couret, I. *et al.* (1991) Increased numbers of hypodense alveolar macrophages in patients with bronchial asthma. *Am. Rev. Resp. Dis.*, **144**, 923–30.

Choi, H.S., Lesser, M., Cardozo, C. & Orlowski, M. (1990) Immunohistochemical localization of endopeptidase 24.15 in rat trachea, lung tissue, and alveolar macrophages. *Am. J. Respir. Cell Mol. Biol.*, **3**, 619–24.

Cohn, L.A., Kinnula, V.L. & Adler, K. (1994) Antioxidant properties of guinea pig tracheal epithelial cells *in vitro*. *Am. J. Physiol.*, **266**, L397–404.

Coyle, A.J., Mitzner, W. & Irvin, C.G. (1993) Cationic proteins alter smooth muscle function by an epithelium-dependent mechanism. *J. Appl. Physiol.*, **74**, 1761–8.

Coyle, A.J., Uchida, D., Ackerman, S.J., Mitzner, W. & Irvin, C.G. (1994) Role of cationic proteins in the airway: hyperresponsiveness due to airway inflammation. *Am. J. Resp. Crit. Care Med.*, **150**, S63–71.

Cromwell, O., Hamid, Q., Corrigan, C.J. *et al.* (1992) Expression and generation of interleukin-8, IL-6 and granulocyte-macrophage colony-stimulating factor by bronchial epithelial cells and enhancement by IL-1 beta and tumour necrosis factor-alpha. *Immunology*, **77**, 330–7.

Dayer, J.M., Isler, P. & Nicod, L.P. (1993) Adhesion molecules and cytokine production. *Am. Rev. Resp. Dis.*, **148**, S70–4.

De, S., Zelazny, E., Souhrada, J.F. & Souhrada, M. (1994) Interleukin-1beta (IL-1beta) and interleukin-6 (IL-6) induce both hyperplasia and hypertrophy of cultured guinea pig airway smooth muscle (ASM) cells. *Am. J. Resp. Crit. Care Med.*, **149**, A707.

Dean, D.C., Iademarco, M.F., Rosen, G.D. & Sheppard, A.M. (1993) The Integrin α4β1 and its counter receptor VCAM-1 in development and immune function. *Am. Rev. Resp. Dis.*, **148**, S43–6.

Delamere, F., Holland, E., Patel, S., Pavord, I. & Know, A. (1993) Production of PGE_2 by cultured airway smooth muscle cells and its inhibition by prostaglandin synthetase inhibitors. *Am. Rev. Resp. Dis.*, **147**, A845.

Djukanovic, R., Roche, W.R., Wilson, J.W. *et al.* (1990a) Mucosal inflammation in asthma. *Am. Rev. Resp. Dis.*, **142**, 434–57.

Djukanovic, R., Wilson, J.W., Britten, K.M. *et al.* (1990b) Quantification of mast cells and eosinophils in the bronchial mucosa of symptomatic atopic asthmatics and healthy control subjects using immunohistochemistry. *Am. Rev. Resp. Dis.*, **142**, 863–71.

Djukanovic, R., Lai, C.K., Wilson, J.W. *et al.* (1992) Bronchial mucosal manifestations of atopy: a comparison of markers of inflammation between atopic asthmatics, atopic nonasthmatics and healthy controls. *Eur. Resp. J.*, **5**, 538–44.

Dussis-Anagnostopoulou, I., Kaklamanis, L., Cordell, J. *et al.* (1993) ICAM-3 expression on endothelium in lymphoid malignancy. *Am. J. Pathol.*, **143**, 1040–3.

Einarsson, O., Panuska, J., Zhu, Z., Landry, M. & Elias, J. (1994) Respiratory syncytial virus stimulation of interleukin-11 production by airway epithelial cells and lung fibroblasts. *Am. J. Resp. Crit. Care Med.*, **149**, A47.

Elices, M.J., Osborn, L., Takada, Y. *et al.* (1990) VCAM-1 on activated endothelium interacts with the leukocyte integrin VLA-4 at the site distinct from the VLA-4/fibronectin binding site. *Cell*, **60**, 577–84.

Eling, T.E., Danilowicz, R.M., Henke, D.C., Sivarajah, K., Yankaskas, J.R. & Boucher, R.C. (1986) Arachidonic acid metabolism by canine tracheal epithelial cells: product formation and relationship to chloride secretion. *J. Biol. Chem.*, **261**, 12841–9.

Endo, T., Uchida, Y., Matsumoto, H. *et al.* (1992) Regulation of endothelin-1 synthesis in cultured guinea pig airway epithelial cells by various cytokines. *Biochem. Biophys. Res. Commun.*, **186**, 1594–9.

Evans, M.J., Cox, R.A., Shami, S.G., Wilson, B. & Plopper, C.G. (1989) The role of basal cells in attachment of columnar cells to the basal lamina of the trachea. *Am. J. Resp. Cell Mol. Biol.*, **1**, 463–9.

Evans, M.J. & Plopper, C.G. (1988) The role of basal cells in adhesion of columnar epithelium to airway basement membrane. *Am. Rev. Resp. Dis.*, **138**, 481–3.

Fischer, B.M., Krunkosky, T.M., Wright, D.T., Dolan-O'Keefe, M. & Adler, K.B. (1995) Tumor necrosis factor alpha (TNFα) stimulates mucin secretion and gene expression in airway epithelium *in vitro*. *Chest*, **107(3)**, 1335–55.

Frossard, N., Rhoden, K.J. & Barnes, P.J. (1989) Influence of epithelium on guinea pig airway responses to tachykinins: role of endopeptidase and cyclooxygenase. *J. Pharmacol. Exp. Ther.*, **248**, 292–8.

Fukuda, T., Fukushima, Y., Asakawa, J. *et al.* (1994) IL-4, VCAM-1 expression and eosinophil accumulation in airways of asthmatics. *Am. J. Resp. Crit. Care Med.*, **149**, A956.

Gosset, P., Lassalle, P., Tonnel, A.B. *et al.* (1988) Production of an interleukin-1 inhibitory factor by human alveolar macrophages from mammals and allergic asthmatic patients. *Am. Rev. Resp. Dis.*, **138**, 40–6.

Gosset, P., Tillie-Leblond, I., Janin, A. *et al.* (1994) Increased expression of ELAM-1, ICAM-1, and VCAM-1 on bronchial biopsies from allergic asthmatic patients. *Ann. NY Acad. Sci.*, **725**, 163–72.

Gosset, P., Isicopoulos, A., Wallaert, B., Joseph, M., Capron, A. & Tonnel, A.B. (1992) Tumor necrosis factor alpha and interleukin-6 production by human mononuclear phagocytes from allergic asthmatics after IgE-dependent stimulation. *Am. Rev. Resp. Dis.*, **146**, 768–74.

Goswami, S.K., Gollub, E., Vanderhoek, J.Y. & Marom, Z. (1993) 15-HETE (hydroxy eicosatetraenoic acid) enhances mucus like glycoprotein (MLGP) secretion from an epithelial cell line via protein kinase C (PKC). *Am. Rev. Resp. Dis.*, **147**, A439.

Gundel, R.H., Wegner, C.D. & Letts, L.G. (1993) Adhesion molecules in a primate model of allergic asthma: clinical implications for respiratory care. *Springer Semin. Immunopathol.*, **15**, 75–88.

Hamid, Q., Springall, D.R., Riveros-Moreno, V. *et al.* (1993) Induction of nitric oxide synthase in asthma. *Lancet*, **342**, 1510–13.

Hansel, T.T. & Walker, C. (1992) The migration of eosinophils into the sputum of asthmatics: the role of adhesion molecules. *Clin. Exp. Allergy*, **22**, 345–56.

Hansel, T.T., Braunstein, J.B., Walker, C. *et al.* (1991) Sputum eosinophils from asthmatics express ICAM-1 and HLA-DR. *Clin. Exp. Immunol.*, **86**, 271–7.

Hastie, A.T., Loegering, D.A., Gleich, G.J. & Kueppers, F. (1987) The effect of purified human eosinophil major basic protein on mammalian ciliary activity. *Am. Rev. Resp. Dis.*, **135**, 848–53.

Hirst, S.J., Barnes, P.J. & Twort, C.H. (1992) Quantifying proliferation of cultured human and rabbit airway smooth muscle cells in response to serum and platelet-derived growth factor. *Am. J. Respir. Cell Mol. Biol.*, **7**, 574–81.

Hirst, S.J., Barnes, P.J. & Twort, C.H. (1994) Proliferation of human and rabbit airway smooth muscle in culture by platelet-derived growth factor isoforms. *Am. J. Resp. Crit. Care Med.*, **149**, A302.

Hoeck, W.G., Ramesha, C.S., Chang, D.J., Fan, N. & Heller, R.A. (1993) Cytoplasmic phospholipase A2 activity and gene expression are stimulated by tumor necrosis factor: dexamethasone blocks the induced synthesis. *Biochemistry*, **90**, 4475–9.

Hogg, J.C. (1993) Pathology of asthma. *J. Allergy Clin. Immunol.*, **92**, 1–5.

Honda, I., Kohrogi, H., Yamaguchi, T., Ando, M. & Araki, S. (1991) Enkephalinase inhibitor potentiates substance P-induced and capsaicin-induced bronchial smooth muscle contractions in humans. *Am. Rev. Resp. Dis.*, **143**, 1416–18.

Ingenito, E.J., Pliss, L.B., Martins, M.A. & Ingram, R.H. (1991) Effects of capsaicin on mechanical, cellular, and mediator responses to antigen in sensitized guinea pigs. *Am. Rev. Resp. Dis.*, **143**, 527–77.

Ito, H., Romberger, D.J., Rennard, S.I. & Spurzem, J.R. (1993) TNF-α bronchial epithelial cell migration and attachment to fibronectin. *Am. Rev. Resp. Dis.*, **147**, A46.

Jain, B., Rubinstein, I., Robbins, R.A., Leise, K.L. & Sisson, J.H. (1993) Modulation of airway epithelial cell ciliary beat frequency by nitric oxide. *Biochem. Biophys. Res. Commun.*, **191**, 83–8.

Kalb, T.H., Chuang, M.T., Marom, Z. & Mayer, L. (1991) Evidence for accessory cell function by class II MHC antigen-expressing airway epithelial cells. *Am. J. Respir. Cell Mol. Biol.*, **4**, 320–9.

Kawanami, O., Ferrans, V.J. & Crystal, R.G. (1979) Anchoring fibrils in the normal canine respiratory system. *Am. Rev. Resp. Dis.*, **120**, 595–611.

Kim, K.C., Nassiri, J. & Brody, J.S. (1989) Mechanisms of airway goblet cell mucin release: studies with cultured tracheal surface epithelial cells. *Am. J. Respir. Cell Mol. Biol.*, **1**, 137–43.

Kinnula, V.L., Adler, K.B., Akley, N.J. & Crapo, J.D. (1992) Release of reactive oxygen species by guinea pig tracheal epithelial cells *in vitro*. *Am. J. Physiol.*, **262**, L708–12.

Kishimoto, T.K. & Rothlein, R. (1994) Integrins, ICAMs, and selectins: role and regulation of adhesion molecules in neutrophil recruitment to inflammatory sites. *Adv. Pharmacol.*, **25**, 117–69.

Kline, J.N., Monick, M.M. & Hunninghake, G.W. (1994) Regulation of interleukin-1 receptor antagonist by TH1 and TH2 cytokines. *Am. J. Resp. Crit. Care Med.*, **149**, A263.

Kobayashi, T., Hashimoto, S., Imai, K. *et al.* (1994) Elevation of serum soluble intercellular adhesion molecule-1 (sICAM-1) and sE-selectin levels in bronchial asthma. *Clin. Exp. Immunol.*, **96**, 110–15.

Kobayashi, K., Cartana, N., Soloni, F. & Wanner, A. (1991) Reversible H_2O_2 induced inhibition of airway ciliary function: role of protein kinase C. *Am. Rev. Resp. Dis.*, **143**, A137.

Korthuis, R.J., Anderson, D.C. & Granger, D.N. (1994) Role of neutrophil-endothelial cell adhesion in inflammatory disorders. *J. Crit. Care*, **9**, 47–71.

Koyama, S., Rennard, S.I., Shoji, S. *et al.* (1989) Bronchial epithelial cells release chemoattractant activity for monocytes. *Am. J. Physiol.*, **257**, L130–6.

Koyama, S., Fujimoto, K., Sato, E. *et al.* (1993) Bradykinin stimulates bronchial epithelial cells to release eosinophil chemotactic activity. *Am. Rev. Resp. Dis.*, **147**, A241.

Kroegel, C., Virchow, J.C. Jr, Kortsik, C. & Matthys, H. (1992) Cytokines, platelet activating factor and eosinophils in asthma. *Resp. Med.*, **86**, 375–89.

Krupsky, M., Fine, A., Poliks, C. & Goldstein, R. (1994) Transforming growth factor-beta and insulin interact to induce large increases in collagen production by human fibroblasts. *Am. J. Resp. Crit. Care Med.*, **149**, A626.

Kruse-Elliott, K.T. & Olson, N.C. (1993) CGS 8515 and indomethacin attenuate cytokine-induced cardioplumonary dysfunction in pigs. *Am. J. Physiol.*, **264**, H1076–86.

Kruse-Elliott, K.T., Pino, M.V. & Olson, N.C. (1993) Effect of PAF receptor antagonism on cardiopulmonary alterations during coinfusion of TNF-alpha and IL-1 alpha in pigs. *Am. J. Physiol.*, **264**, L175–82.

Kumlin, M., Ohlson, E., Bjorck, T. *et al.* (1990) 15-(S)-hydroxyeicosatetraenoic acid (15-HETE) is the major arachidonic acid metabolite in human bronchi. *Adv. Prost. Thromb. Leuk. Res.*, **21**, 441–4.

Kumlin, M., Dahlen, B., Bjorck, T., Zetterstrom, O., Granstrom, E. & Dahlen, S.-E. (1992) Urinary excretion of leukotriene E4 and 11-dehydro-thromboxane B2 in response to bronchial provocations with allergen, aspirin, leukotriene D4, and histamine in asthmatics. *Am. Rev. Resp. Dis.*, **146**, 96–103.

Kunkel, S.L., Burdick, M.D. & Strieter, N.W. (1994) The role of MIP-1a in eosinophil recruitment into the airway of asthmatic mice. *Am. J. Resp. Crit. Care Med.*, **149**, A529.

Lai, Y.L. (1991) Endogenous tachykinins in antigen-induced acute bronchial responses of guinea pigs. *Exp. Lung Res.*, **17**, 1047–60.

Laitinen, L.A., Heino, M., Laitinen, A., Kava, T. & Haahtela, T. (1985) Damage of the airway epithelium and bronchial reactivity in patients with asthma. *Am. Rev. Resp. Dis.*, **131**, 599–606.

Laitinen, L.A., Laitinen, A. & Haahtela, T. (1993) Airway mucosal inflammation even in patients with newly diagnosed asthma. *Am. Rev. Resp. Dis.*, **147**, 697–704.

Laitinen, L.A., Laitinen, A., Salonen, R.O. & Widdicombe, J.G. (1987) Vascular actions of airway neuropeptides. *Am. Rev. Resp. Dis.*, **136**, S59–64.

Lansing, M.W., Ahmed, A., Cortes, A., Sielczak, M.W., Wanner, A. & Abraham, W.M. (1993) Oxygen radicals contribute to antigen-induced airway hyperresponsiveness in conscious sheep. *Am. Rev. Resp. Dis.*, **147**, 321–6.

Lassalle, P., Gosset, P., Delneste, Y. *et al.* (1993) Modulation of adhesion molecule expression on endothelial cells during the late asthmatic reaction: role of macrophage-derived tumor necrosis factor-alpha. *Clin. Exp. Immunol.*, **94**, 105–10.

Leff, A.R., Hamann, K.J. & Wegner, C.D. (1991) Inflammation and cell–cell interactions in airway hyperresponsiveness. *Am. J. Physiol.*, **260**, L189–206.

Lehnert, B.E., Valdez, Y.E., Lehnert, N.M. & Englen, M.D. (1994) Inhibition of alveolar macrophage proliferation and tumor necrosis factor-α production by interleukin-4. *Am. J. Resp. Crit. Care Med.*, **149**, A1101.

Lehrer, R.I., Ganz, T., Selsted, M.E., Babior, B.M. & Curnutte, J.T. (1988) Neutrophils and host defense. *Ann. Intern. Med.*, **109**, 127–42.

Leikauf, G.D., Ueki, I.F., Widicombe, J.H. & Nadel, J.A. (1986) Alteration of chloride secretion across canine tracheal epithelium by lipoxygenase products of arachidonic acid. *Am. J. Physiol.*, **250**, F47–53.

Levine, S.J., Larivée, P., Logun, C. & Shelhamer, J.H. (1994a) IL-6 induces respiratory mucous glycoprotein secretion and MUC-2 gene expression by human airway epithelial cells. *Am. J. Resp. Crit. Care Med.*, **149**, A27.

Levine, S.J., Logun, C. & Shelhamer, J.H. (1994b) IL-10 inhibits TNF-alpha mediated respiratory mucous glycoprotein secretion by human airway epithelial cells. *Am. J. Resp. Crit. Care Med.*, **149**, A986.

Levine, S.J., Logun, C., Larivée, P. & Shelhamer, J.H. (1993a) TNF-α induces secretion of respiratory mucous glycoprotein from human airways *in vitro*. *Am. Rev. Resp. Dis.*, **147**, A1011.

Levine, S.J., Logun, C., Larivée, P. & Shelhamer, J.H. (1993b) IL-1β induces secretion of respiratory mucous glycoprotein from human airways *in vitro*. *Am. Rev. Resp. Dis.*, **147**, A437.

Lilly, C.M., Drazen, J.M. & Shore, S.A. (1993a) Peptidase modulation of airway effects of neuropeptides. *Proc. Soc. Exp. Biol. Med.*, **203**, 388–404.

Lilly, C.M., Martins, M.A. & Drazen, J.M. (1993b) Peptidase modulation of the effects of vasoactive intestinal peptide. Pulmonary relaxation in tracheal perfused guinea pig lungs. *J. Clin. Invest.*, **91**, 235–43.

Lin, Y.G., Wong, L.B., Mussatto, D.J., Daza, A.V. & Yeates, D.B. (1993) Responses of tracheal ciliary beat frequency, tracheal mucus velocity, bronchial mucociliary clearance and lung resistance to low dose leukotriene D4. *Am. Rev. Resp. Dis.*, **147**, A296.

Lindstrom, E.G., Andersson, R.G., Granerus, G. & Grundstrom, N. (1991) Is the airway epithelium responsible for histamine metabolism in the trachea of guinea pigs? *Agents Actions*, **33**, 170–2.

Liu, M.C., Bleecker, E.R., Lichenstein, L.M. *et al.* (1990) Evidence for elevated levels of histamine, prostaglandin D_2 and other bronchoconstricting prostaglandins in the airways of subjects with mild asthma. *Am. Rev. Resp. Dis.*, **142**, 126–32.

Lundberg, J.M., Anders, F., Hua, X., Hokfelt, T. & Fischer, J.A. (1985) Coexistence of substance P and calcitonin gene-related peptide-like immunoreactivities in sensory nerves in relation to cardiovascular and bronchoconstrictor effects of capsaicin. *Eur. J. Pharmacol.*, **108**, 315–19.

Lundberg, J.M., Saria, A., Brodin, E., Rusells, S. & Folkers, R. (1983) A substance P antagonist inhibits vagally induced increase in vascular permeability and bronchial smooth muscle contraction in the guinea pig. *Proc. Nat. Acad. Sci. USA*, **80**, 1120–4.

Lundgren, J.D., Davey, R.T., Lundgren, B. *et al.* (1991) Eosinophil cationic protein stimulates and major basic protein inhibits airway mucus secretion. *J. Allergy Clin. Immunol.*, **87**, 689–98.

Lundgren, J.D., Wiedermann, C.J., Logun, C., Plutchok, J., Kaliner, M. & Shelhamer, J.H. (1989) Substance P receptor-mediated secretion of glycoconjugates from feline airways *in vitro*. *Exp. Lung Res.*, **15**, 17–29.

McCormack, D.G., Salonen, R.O. & Barnes, P.J. (1989) Effects of sensory neuropeptides on canine bronchial and pulmonary vessels *in vitro*. *Life Sci.*, **45**, 2405–12.

McFadden, E.R. (1994) Asthma: morphologic–physiologic interactions. *Am. J. Resp. Crit. Care Med.*, **150**, S23–6.

McKinnon, K.P., Madden, M.C., Noah, T.L. & Devlin, R.B. (1993) *In vitro* ozone exposure increases release of arachidonic acid products from a human bronchial epithelial cell line. *Toxicol. Appl. Pharmacol.*, **118**, 215–23.

Marin, M.G., Davis, B. & Nadel, J.A. (1977) Effect of histamine on electrical and ion transport properties of tracheal epithelium. *J. Appl. Physiol.*, **42**, 735–8.

Marini, M., Vittori, E., Hollemborg, J. & Mattoli, S. (1992) Expression of the potent inflammatory cytokines, granulocyte-macrophage-colony-stimulating factor and interleukin-6 and interleukin-8, in bronchial epithelial cells of patients with asthma. *J. Allergy Clin. Immunol.*, **89**, 1001–9.

Marling, C., Saria, A., Fischer, J.A., Hokfelt, T. & Lundberg, J.M. (1988) Calcitonin gene-related peptide and lung: neuronal coexistence with substance P, release by capsaicin and vasodilatory effect. *Regul. Pept.*, **20**, 125.

Martling, C.-R., Theordorsson-Norheim, E. & Lundberg, J.M. (1987) Occurrence and effects of multiple tachykinins: substance P, neurokinin A, neuropeptide K in human lower airways. *Life Sci.*, **40**, 1633–43.

Marom, Z., Shellmamer, J.H. & Kaliner, M. (1981) Effects of arachidonic acid, monohydroxyeicosatetraenic acids and prostaglandins on the release of mucous glycoproteins from human airways *in vitro*. *J. Clin. Invest.*, **67**, 1695–702.

Masuda, T., Suda, Y., Shimura, S. *et al.* (1992) Airway epithelial cells enhance eosinophil survival. *Respiration*, **59**, 238–42.

Masui, T., Wakefield, L.M., Lechner, J.F., LaVeck, M.A., Sporn, M.B. & Harris, C.C. (1986) Type β transforming growth factor is the primary differentiation-inducing serum factor for normal human bronchial epithelial cells. *Proc. Nat. Acad. Sci. USA*, **83**, 2438–42.

Matsuse, T., Thomson, R.J., Chen, X.R., Salari, H. & Schellenberg, R.R. (1991) Capsaicin inhibits airway hyperresponsiveness but not lipoxygenase activity or eosinphilia after repeated aerosolized antigen in guinea pigs. *Am. Rev. Resp. Dis.*, **144**, 368–72.

Mengelers, H.J., Miakoe, T., Brinkman, L., Hooibrink, B., Lammers, J.W. & Koenderman, L. (1994) Immunophenotyping of eosinophils recovered from blood and BAL of allergic asthmatics. *Am. J. Resp. Crit. Care Med.*, **149**, 345–51.

Mette, S.A., Pilewski, J., Buck, C.A. & Albelda, S.M. (1993) Distribution of integrin cell adhesion receptors on normal bronchial epithelial cells and lung cancer cells *in vitro* and *in vivo*. *Am. J. Resp. Crit. Care Med.*, **8**, 562–72.

Metzger, W.J., Richerson, H.B., Warden, K., Monick, M. & Hunninghake, G.W. (1986) Bronchoalveolar lavage of allergic asthmatic patients following allergen provocation. *Chest*, **89**, 477–83.

Mezzetti, M., Soloperto, M.B., Fasoli, A. & Mattoli, S. (1991) Human bronchial epithelial cells modulate CD3 and mitogen-induced DNA synthesis in T cells but function poorly as antigen-presenting cells compared to pulmonary macrophages. *J. Allergy Clin. Immunol.*, **87**, 930–8.

Michelson, P.H., McKinnon, K.P., Reed, W., Carter, J.D. & Devlin, R.B. (1994) Growth factor production in human airway epithelial cells exposed to ozone *in vitro*. *Am. J. Resp. Crit. Care Med.*, **149**, A316.

Ming, W.J., Bersani, L. & Mantovani, A. (1987) Tumor necrosis factor is chemotactic for monocytes and polymorphonuclear leukocytes. *J. Immunol.*, **138**, 1469–74.

Mizoguchi, H. & Hicks, C.R. (1989) Effects of subtance P (SP) on ion transport and glycoconjugate release in the isolated ferret trachea. *Am. Rev. Resp. Dis.*, **139**, A475.

Montefort, S., Lai, C.K.W., Kapahi, P. *et al.* (1994) Circulating adhesion molecules in asthma. *Am. J. Respir. Crit. Care Med.*, **149**, 1149–52.

Morrison, K.J., Gao, Y. & Vanhoutte, P.M. (1993) β-Adrenoceptors and the epithelial layer in airways. *Life Sci.*, **52**, 2123–30.

Moser, K.M. (1994) Asthma. In: *Harrison's Principles of Internal Medicine* (eds K.J. Isselbacher, E. Braunwald, J.D. Wilson, J.B. Martin, A.S. Fauci & D.L. Kasper), pp. 1167–72. McGraw-Hill, New York.

Motojima, S., Frigas, E., Loegering, D.A. & Gleich, G.J. (1989) Toxicity of eosinophil cationic proteins for guinea pig tracheal epihelium *in vitro*. *Am. Rev. Resp. Dis.*, **139**, 801–5.

Mullin, J.M. & Snock, K.V. (1990) Effect of tumor necrosis factor on epithelial tight junctions and transepithelial permeability. *Cancer Res.*, **50**, 2172–6.

Munakata, M., Chen, H., Ukita, H., Masaki, Y., Homma, Y. & Kawakami, Y. (1993) Effect of interleukin-2 (IL-2) and interferon gamma (IFN-γ) on guinea-pig airway strips. *Am. Rev. Resp. Dis.*, **147**, A1013.

Murray, J.J., Tonel, A.B., Brash, A.R. *et al.* (1986) Release of prostaglandin D_2 into human airways during acute allergen challenge. *New Engl. J. Med.*, **315**, 800–4.

Nadel, J.A. (1992) Regulation of neurogenic inflammation by neutral endopeptidase. *Am. Rev. Resp. Dis.*, **145**, S48–52.

Nakamura, H., Yoshimura, K., Jaffe, H.A. & Crystal, R.G. (1991) Interleukin-8 gene expression in human bronchial epithelial cells. *J. Biol. Chem.*, **266**, 19611–17.

Nathanson, I., Widdicombe, J.H. & Barnes, P.J. (1983) Effect of vasoactive intestinal peptide on ion transport across dog tracheal epithelium. *J. Appl. Physiol.*, **55**, 1844–8.

Newman, P.J. (1994) The role of PECAM-1 in vascular cell biology. *Ann. NY Acad. Sci.*, **714**, 165–74.

Noveral, J.P., Cohen, P., Bhala, A., Hintz, R.L. & Grunstein, M.M. (1994) Regulation of airway smooth muscle cell proliferation by insulin-like growth factors (IGFs) and IGF-binding proteins: modulatory role of leukotriene D4. *Am. J. Resp. Crit. Care Med.*, **149**, A301.

O'Byrne, P. (1990) Eicosanoids and inflammatory cells in asthma. *Agents Actions Suppl.*, **31**, 85–101.

Ohno, I., Yamauchi, K., Tamura, G. *et al.* (1994) Expression of TNF, TGFβ1 and PDGF-B by eosinophils in asthmatic bronchial tissues. *Am. J. Resp. Crit. Care Med.*, **149**, A957.

Ohta, T., Yamashita, N., Maruyama, M., Matsui, S., Sugiyama, E. & Kobayashi, M. (1994) Suppressive effect of interluekin-4 (IL-4) and IL-10 on IL-1, IL-6, and IL-8 production by human alveolar macrophages. *Am. J. Resp. Crit. Care Med.*, **149**, A677.

Palmer, J.B., Cuss, F.M. & Barnes, P.J. (1986) VIP and PHM and their role in non-adrenergic inhibitory responses in isolated human airways. *J. Appl. Physiol.*, **61**, 1322–8.

Palmer, J.B.D., Cuss, F.M.C., Mulderry, P.K. *et al.* (1987) Calcitonin gene-related peptide is localised to human airway nerves and potently constricts human airway smooth muscle. *Br. J. Pharmacol.*, **91**, 95–101.

Parke, D.V. (1978) Pharmacology of mucus. *Br. Med. J.*, **34**, 89–94.

Peatfield, A.C., Barnes, P.J., Bratcher, C., Nadel, J.A. & Davis, B. (1983) Vasoactive intestinal peptide stimulates tracheal submucosal gland secretion in ferret. *Am. Rev. Resp. Dis.*, **128**, 89–93.

Pernow, B. (1985) Role of tachykinins in neurogenic inflammation. *J. Immunol.*, **135**, 812S–15S.

Pesci, A., Foresi, A., Bertorelli, G., Chetta, A. & Oliveri, D. (1993) Histochemical characteristics and degranulation of mast cells in epithelium and lamina propria of bronchial biopsies from asthmatic and normal subjects. *Am. Rev. Resp. Dis.*, **147**, 684–9.

Pfeffer, K.D., Ellison, G. & Day, R.W. (1994) The effect of inhaled nitric oxide in pediatric asthma. *Am. J. Resp. Crit. Care Med.*, **149**, A199.

Phipps, R.J., Denas, S.M., Sielczak, M.W. & Wanner, A. (1986) Effects of 0.5 ppm ozone on glycoprotein secretion, ion and water fluxes in sheep trachea. *J. Appl. Physiol.*, **60**, 918–27.

Piacentini, G.L. & Kaliner, M.A. (1991) The potential role of leukotrienes in bronchial asthma. *Am. Rev. Resp. Dis.*, **143**, S96–9.

Poulter, K.W., Janossy, G., Power, C., Sreenan, S. & Burke, C. (1994) Immunological/physiological relationships in asthma: potential regulation by lung macrophages. *Immunol. Today*, **15**, 258–61.

Power, C., Sreenan, S., Hurson, B., Burke, C. & Poulter, L.W. (1993) Distribution of immunocompetent cells in bronchial wall of clinically healthy subjects showing bronchial hyperresponsiveness. *Thorax*, **48**, 1125–9.

Pretolani, M.G., Ruffie, C., Joseph, D. *et al.* (1994) Role of eosinophil activation in the bronchial reactivity of allergic guinea pigs. *Am. J. Resp. Crit. Care Med.*, **149**, 1167–74.

Prie, S., Cadieux, A. & Sirois, P. (1990) Removal of guinea pig bronchial and tracheal epithelium potentiates the contractions to leukotrienes and histamine. *Eicosanoids*, **3**, 29–37.

Rabb, H.A., Olivenstein, R., Issekutz, T.B., Renzi, P.M. & Martin, J.G. (1994) The role of the leukocyte adhesion molecules VLA-4, LFA-1, and Mac-1 in allergic airway responses in the rat. *Am. J. Resp. Crit. Care Med.*, **149**, 1186–91.

Raeburn, D. (1990) Putative role of epithelial derived factors in airway smooth muscle reactivity. *Agents Actions Suppl.*, **31**, 259–74.

Resnick, M.B. & Weller, P.F. (1993) Mechanisms of eosinophil recruitment. *Am. J. Respir. Cell. Mol. Biol.*, **8**, 349–55.

Reznik, G.K. (1990) Comparative anatomy, physiology, and function of the upper respiratory tract. *Environ. Health Perspect.*, **85**, 171–6.

Rickard, K. & Rennard, S. (1989) Neutrophil elastase causes detachment of bronchial epithelial cells from extracellular matrix. *Am. Rev. Resp. Dis.*, **139**, A406.

Rickard, K.A., Taylor, J. & Rennard, S.I. (1992) Observations of development of resistance to detachment of cultured bovine epithelial cells in response to protease treatment. *Am. J. Respir. Cell Mol. Biol.*, **6**, 414–20.

Roche, W.R., Montefort, S., Baker, J. & Holgate, S.T. (1993) Cell adhesion molecules and the bronchial epithelium. *Am. Rev. Resp. Dis.*, **148**, s79–82.

Rogers, D.F., Carstairs, J.R., Alton, E.W., Dewar, A. & Barnes, P.J. (1988) Tachykinins and mucus secretion in human bronchi *in vitro*. *Am. Rev. Resp. Dis.*, **137**, 12.

Rosa, L.M. & McDowall, R.J.S. (1951) The action of local hormones on the isolated human bronchus. *Acta Allergol.*, **4**, 293–304.

Rose, M. (1992) Mucins: structure, function, and role in pulmonary diseases. *Am. J. Physiol.*, **263**, L413–29.

Rossi, G.A., Sacco, O., Balbi, B. *et al.* (1990) Human ciliated bronchial epithelial cells: expression of the HLA-DR antigens and of the HLA-DR alpha gene, modulation of the HLA-DR antigens by gamma-interferon and antigen-presenting function in the mixed leukocyte reaction. *Am. J. Respir. Cell Mol. Biol.*, **3**, 431–9.

Rothlein, R., Czajkowski, M., O'Neill, M.M., Marlin, S.D., Mainolfi, E. & Merluzzi, V.J. (1988) Induction of intercellular adhesion molecule 1 on primary and continuous cell lines by pro-inflammatory cytokines. Regulation by pharmacologic agents and neutralizing antibodies. *J. Immunol.*, **141**, 1665–9.

Rothlein, R., Dustin, M.L., Marlin, S.D. & Springer, T.A. (1986) A human intercellular adhesion molecule (ICAM-1) distinct from LFA-1. *J. Immunol.*, **137**, 1270–4.

Sanchez-Madrid, F. & Corbi, A.L. (1992) Leukocyte integrins: structure, function and regulation of their activity. *Semin. Cell Biol.*, **3**, 199–210.

Sanderson, C.J. (1992) Interleukin-5, eosinophils and disease. *Blood*, **79**, 3101–9.

Sanghavi, J.N., Rabe, K.F., Kim, J.S., Magnussen, H., Leff A.R. & White, S.R. (1994) Migration of human and guinea pig airway epithelial cells in response to calcitonin gene related peptide. *Am. J. Respir. Cell Mol. Biol.*, **11**, 181–7.

Schwartz, L.B. (1992) Cellular inflammation in asthma: neutral proteases of mast cells. *Am. Rev. Resp. Dis.*, **145**, S18–21.

Schweizer, R.C., Welmers, B.A.C., Zanen, P. *et al.* (1994) Chemokine induced responses in normal human eosinophils: effect of priming with IL-5 on chemotaxis, Ca^{2+} mobilization, and actin polymerization. *Am. J. Resp. Crit. Care Med.*, **149**, A515.

Sekizawa, K., Caughey, G.H., Lazarus, S.C., Gold, W.M. & Nadel, J.A. (1989) Mast cell tryptase causes airway smooth muscle hyperresponsiveness in dogs. *J. Clin. Invest.*, **83**, 175–9.

Sekizawa, K., Tamaoki, J., Graf, P.D., Basbaum, C.B., Borson, D.B. & Nadel, J.A. (1987) Enkephalinase inhibitor potentiates mammalian tachykinin-induced contraction in ferret trachea. *J. Pharmacol. Exp. Ther.*, **243**, 1211–17.

Shelhamer, J.H., Marom, Z. & Kaliner, M. (1980) Immunologic and neuropharmacologic stimulation of mucous glycoprotein release from human airways *in vitro*. *J. Clin. Invest.*, **66**, 1400–8.

Sheppard, D., Cohen, D.S., Wang, A. & Busk, M. (1992) Transforming growth factor β differentially regulates expression of integrin subunits in guinea pig airway epithelial cells. *J. Biol. Chem.*, **267**, 17409–14.

Shindo, K., Fukumura, M., Miyakawa, K., Sumitomo, M. & Ito, A. (1994) Plasma levels of leukotriene E4 during clinical course of bronchial asthma and the effect of oral predisolone. *Am. J. Resp. Crit. Care Med.*, **149**, A945.

Simon, R., Edwards, J., Reza, M. & Kunkel, R. (1991) Injury of rat pulmonary alveolar epithelial cells by H_2O_2: dependence on phenotype and catalase. *Am. J. Physiol.*, **260**, L318–25.

Smith, L.J. (1992) Bioactive mediators of asthma. *Chest*, **101**, 381S–4S.

Soloperto, M., Mattoso, V.L., Fasoli, A. & Mattoli, S. (1991) A bronchial epithelial cell-derived factor in asthma that promotes eosinophil activation and survival as GM-CSF. *Am. J. Physiol.*, **260**, L530–8.

Sommerhoff, C.P., Caughey, G.H., Finkbeiner, W.E., Lazarus, S.C., Basbaum, C.B. & Nadel, J.A. (1989) Mast cell chymase. A potent secretagogue for airway gland serous cells. *J. Immunol.*, **142**, 2450–6.

Sommerhoff, C.P., Nadel, J.A., Basbaum, C.B. & Caughey, G.H. (1990) Neutrophil elastase and cathepsin G stimulate secretion from cultured bovine airway gland serous cells. *J. Clin. Invest.*, **85**, 682–9.

Sousa, A.R., Poston, R.N., Lane, S.J., Nakhosteen, J.A. & Lee, T.H. (1993) Detection of GM-CSF in asthmatic bronchial epithelium and decrease by inhaled corticosteroids. *Am. Rev. Resp. Dis.*, **147**, 1557–61.

Springall, D.R., Bloom, S.R. & Polak, J.M. (1988) Distribution, nature, and origin of peptide containing nerves in mammalian airways. In: *The Airways: Neural Control in Health and Disease* (eds M.A. Kaliner & P.J. Barnes), pp. 299–341. Marcel Dekker, New York.

Stimler-Gerard, N.P. (1987) Neutral endopeptidase-like enzyme controls the contractile activity of substance P in guinea pig lung. *J. Clin. Invest.*, **79**, 1819–25.

Strieter, R.M., Lukacs, N.W., Standiford, T.J. & Kunkel S.L. (1993) Cytokines and lung inflammation: mechanisms of neutrophil recruitment to the lung. *Thorax*, **48**, 765–9.

Sun, J., Elwood, W., Haczku, A., Barnes, J.P., Hellewell, P.G. & Chung, K.F. (1994) Contribution of intercellular adhesion molecule-1 in allergen-induced airway hyperresponsiveness and inflammation in sensitized brown-norway rats. *Int. Arch. Allergy Immunol.*, **104**, 291–5.

Tam, E.K. & Caughey, G.H. (1992) Degradation of neuropeptides by human lung triptase. *Am. J. Respir. Cell Mol. Biol.*, **3**, 27–32.

Tamaoki, J., Yamawaki, I., Takeyama, K., Chiyotani, A., Yamauchi, F. & Konno, K. (1994) Interleukin-1β inhibits airway smooth muscle contraction via epithelium-dependent mechanism. *Am. J. Resp. Crit. Care Med.*, **149**, 134–7.

Thomson, N.C. (1987) Mediators and inflammation in the airways. *Brit. J. Clin. Pract.*, **S53**, 44–52.

Thornhill, M.H., Wellicome, S.M., Mahiouz, D.L., Lanchbury, J.S.S., Kyan-Aung, V. & Haskard, D.O. (1991) Tumor necrosis factor combines with IL-4 or IFN-γ to selectively enhance endothelial cell adhesiveness for T cells: the contribution of vascular adhesion molecule-1-dependent and -independent binding mechanisms. *J. Immunol.*, **146**, 592–8.

Tournier, J.M., Goldstein, G.A., Hall, D.E., Damsky, C.H. & Basbaum, C.B. (1992) Extracellular matrix proteins regulate morphologic and biochemical properties of tracheal gland serous cells through integrins. *Am. J. Respir. Cell Mol. Biol.*, **6**, 461–71.

Trow, T.K., Zheng, T., Whiting, N. *et al.* (1993) Cytokine regulation of human lung fibroblast interleukin-11 production. *Am. Rev. Resp. Dis.*, **147**, A230.

Uchida, D.A., Ackerman, S.J., Coyl, A.J. *et al.* (1993) The effect of human eosinophil granule major basic protein on airway responsiveness in the rat *in vivo*. A comparison with polycations. *Am. Rev. Resp. Dis.*, **147**, 982–8.

Vancheri, C., Gauldie, J., Bienenstock, J. *et al.* (1989) Human lung fibroblast-derived granulocyte-macrophage colony stimulating factor (GM-CSF) mediates eosinophil survival *in vitro. Am. J. Respir. Cell Mol. Biol.*, **1**, 289–95.

Varsano, S., Basbaum, C.B., Forsberg, L.S., Borson, D.B., Caughey, G.H. & Nadel, J.A. (1987) Dog tracheal epithelial cells in culture synthesize sulfated macromolecular glyconconjugates and release them from the cell surface upon exposure to extracellular proteinases. *Exp. Lung Res.*, **13**, 157–84.

Vignola, F.B., Campbell, A.M., Chanez, P. *et al.* (1993) HLA-DR and ICAM-1 expression on bronchial epithelial cells in asthma and chronic bronchitis. *Am. Rev. Resp. Dis.*, **148**, 689–94.

Vignola, F.B., Chanez, P., Campbell, A.M. *et al.* (1994) Quantification and localization of HLA-DR and intercellular adhesion molecule-1 (ICAM-1) molecules on bronchial epithelial cells of asthmatics using confocal microscopy. *Clin. Exp. Immunol.*, **96**, 104–9.

Vittori, E., Marini, M., Fasoli, A., De Franchis, R. & Mattoli, S. (1992) Increased expression of endothelin in bronchial epithelial cells of asthmatic patients and effect of corticosteroids. *Am. Rev. Resp. Dis.*, **146**, 1320–5.

Walker, C. & Virchow, J.C. Jr (1993) T-cells and endothelial cells in asthma. *Allergy*, **48**, 24–31.

Wang, N.-S. (1994) Anatomy. In: *Pulmonary Pathology* (eds D.H. Dail & S.P. Hammar), pp. 21–44. Springer-Verlag, New York.

Wawryk, S.O., Cockerill, P.N., Wicks, I.P. & Boyd, A.W. (1991) Isolation and characterization of the promoter region of the human intercellular adhesion molecule-1 gene. *Int. Immunol.*, **3**, 83–93.

Webber, S.E. (1988) The effects of peptide histidine isoleucine and neuropeptide Y on mucus volume output by the ferret trachea. *Br. J. Pharmacol.*, **95**, 49–54.

Wegner, C.D., Gundel, R.H., Reilly, P., Haynes, N., Letts, L.G. & Rothlein, R. (1990) Intercellular adhesion molecule-1 (ICAM-1) in the pathogenesis of asthma. *Science*, **247**, 456–9.

Wenzel, S.E., Fowler, A.A. & Schwartz, L.B. (1988) Activation of pulmonary mast cells by bronchoalveolar allergen challenge: *in vivo* release of histamine and tryptase in atopic subjects with and without asthma. *Am. Rev. Resp. Dis.*, **137**, 1002–8.

West, J.B. (1985) Structure and function—how the architecture of the lung subserves its function. In: *Respiratory Physiology—The Essentials*, (ed. J.B. West) pp. 1–10. Williams & Wilkins, Baltimore.

White, M.V., Slater, J.E. & Kaliner, M.A. (1987) Histamine and asthma. *Am. Rev. Resp. Dis.*, **135**, 1165–76.

Wong, L.B., Miller, I.F. & Yeates, D.B. (1991) Pathways of substance P stimulation of canine tracheal ciliary beat frequency. *J. Appl. Physiol.*, **70**, 267–73.

Woolley, M.J., Woolley, K.L., Otis, J., Conlon, P.D., O'Byrne, P.M. & Jordana, M. (1994) Inhibitory effects of IL-10 on allergen-induced airway inflammation and airway responses in brown norway rats. *Am. J. Resp. Crit. Care Med.*, **149**, A760.

Wright, D.T., Adler, K.B., Akley, N.J., Dailey, L.A. & Friedman, M. (1994) Ozone stimulates release of platelet activating factor and activates phospholipases in guinea pig tracheal epithelial cells in primary culture. *Toxicol. Appl. Pharmacol.*, **127**, 27–36.

Wright, D.T., Li, C., Fischer, B.M. *et al.* (1996) Reactive oxygen species provoke secretion of respiratory mucin and activate phospholipase C in airway epithelial cells *in vitro* via a mechanism dependent on nitric oxide. *Am. J. Physiol. (Lung Cell. Molec. Physiol.)* (in press).

Wu, T., Larivée, P., Logun, C. & Shelhamer, J.H. (1993a) The effect of interleukin-5 on arachidonate metabolism in human tracheal epithelial cells. *Am. Rev. Resp. Dis.*, **147**, A1011.

Wu, T., Lawrence, M., Logun, C. & Shelhamer, J. (1993b) Interferon-gamma increases 15-HETE production in human tracheal epithelial cells: involvement of cytosolic phospholipase A2 activation. *Am. Rev. Resp. Dis.*, **147**, A437.

Yong, K. & Khwaja, A. (1990) Leukocyte cellular adhesion molecules. *Blood Rev.*, **4**, 211–25.

CHAPTER 16

Endothelial Cells in Allergy

A.-B. Tonnel, P. Jeannin, S. Molet, P. Gosset, Y. Delneste, B. Wallaert & M. Joseph

Introduction

Until recently, endothelial cells have received limited attention in monographs on allergy and, more particularly, asthma. An excellent and very comprehensive work on 'pulmonary endothelium in health and disease' published in 1987 did not refer to asthma in its subject index (Ryan, 1987). However, in the past few years more attention has been paid to this area. Progress in the understanding of the dynamic process which leads to the establishment of inflammatory conditions, and which is largely dependent on the filter function of vascular endothelium between the bloodstream and surrounding tissues, has focused investigations on the pathogenesis of bronchial asthma towards endothelial cells. Besides their various physiological functions in vasomotricity, in gaseous and liquid exchanges and in haemostasis, these cells also restrict or allow the influx of blood leucocytes into tissues through modulation of the expression of adhesion molecules and through the secretion of cytokines with activating or inhibitory properties for the migrating cells.

The mechanisms by which leucocytes adhere to, and then migrate through, the vascular endothelium have long been a matter of debate. However, it has been generally admitted that sticking of leucocytes to the endothelium preceded the migration of inflammatory cells through capillary walls (Clark & Clark, 1935). From the concept put forward by E. Metchnikoff a century ago, that leucocyte emigration was the result of chemotactic attraction from outside the vessel wall, the controversy has remained until recently concerning the precise primary modification inducing increased adhesion of leucocytes to endothelium: either an enhancement of adhesive properties of migrating cells, or an alteration in the surface of endothelial cells, or both of these events.

When considering the physiopathology of bronchial asthma, initially the endothelium was mainly associated with plasma exudation, with protein leakage and leucocyte sticking and migration, at the level of post-capillary venules (Persson, 1986, 1991). The process, which appeared largely passive for endothelial cells, was through the intercellular junctions of which leucocytes were moving by diapedesis. The resulting oedema was considered to increase plasma proteins in airways, and had a dual role: protective by chelating ferric ions, unavailable for the production of damaging free radicals (Lamm *et al.*, 1988), and negative by increasing mucus viscosity (Forstner *et al.*, 1977).

For a few years, a better understanding of the inflammatory processes involved in bronchial asthma had resulted from pathological studies obtained from bronchial biopsies (Jeffery *et al.*, 1989), as well as bronchoalveolar findings in asthmatics (Bousquet *et al.*, 1990) or post-mortem histological analysis (Saetta *et al.*, 1991). All these studies showed that the bronchial inflammation is mainly characterized by a cell infiltration in which mast cells, T lymphocytes and activated eosinophils predominate (Corrigan & Kay, 1992; Robinson *et al.*, 1992). In fact, to explain the constitution of the cell infiltration inside the bronchial mucosa in asthmatic patients and its relative specificity, several successive and concomitant events, linked to the behaviour of the endothelial cell, are worth taking into consideration.

• The endothelial cell can be seen to be an active participant in the development of the allergic inflammatory reaction, by the production of pro-inflammatory mediators or through the expression of adhesion molecules at its surface.

• The vascular endothelium represents a target for the different cell types involved in allergy.

• Both aspects of the role of endothelial cells in asthma explain, at least in part, the observations obtained *in vitro* in animal models and in allergic patients.

The endothelial cell as an active partner in allergic inflammation

The endothelial cell directly participates in the development of inflammation. By producing vasoactive products, it is capable of intrinsic modulation of the vascular tone. Pro-relaxant factors like prostacyclin and endothelial-derived relaxing factor, that are at least in part composed of nitric oxide, are released upon various stimuli (hypoxia, acetylcholine, bradykinin, thrombin and also mediators present in allergic inflammation, such as histamine and serotonin). The effects of these relaxant factors, which determine local vasodilatation with an accumulation of fluid and plasma proteins, are counter-balanced by pro-contractile factors such as endothelin-1, which elicit potent and prolonged vasoconstrictive properties. Moreover, besides vasoactive components, the endothelial cell has the capacity to generate mediators directly implied in the allergic reaction, including phospholipid mediators such as platelet-activating factor (PAF), cytokines and chemokines. Lastly, endothelium has been proved to control inflammation by its ability to express endothelial cell surface molecules that support the adhesion of blood leucocytes and their further emigration towards the sites of the allergen conflict (Albelda, 1991). These various factors give the endothelial cell a crucial role in the development of the allergic inflammatory reaction.

Production of pro-inflammatory mediators by the endothelial cell

Some acute endothelial responses occur within the first 15 minutes following an environmental injury. Among pro-inflammatory mediators, local generation of PAF has been evidenced (Lewis *et al.*, 1988) as a consequence of hydrogen peroxide production. Endothelial cells can also generate the peptide leukotrienes LTC_4 and LTD_4, from LTA_4 provided by neutrophils (Feinmark & Cannon, 1986). These components interfere in the allergic reaction: for example, PAF which is produced by the vascular endothelium was shown to exert a potent chemotactic activity to eosinophils and their further emigration through human umbilical vein endothelial cell (HUVEC) preparations. This eosinophil transendothelial migration was blocked in the presence of the PAF-receptor antagonist WEB 2086, which did not affect neutrophil migration (Casale *et al.*, 1993).

Endothelial cells are both a source and a target for cytokines and chemokines. In response to injury or inflammatory stimuli, endothelial cells demonstrate long-term complex responses that require *de novo* mRNA expression and protein synthesis (Gerritsen & Bloor, 1993). Following exposure to interleukin-1 (IL-1) α/β and tumour necrosis factor-α (TNF-α), endothelial cells participate in inflammatory reactions through the release of colony-stimulating factors (CSF), not only granulocyte macrophage colony-stimulating factor (GM-CSF) but also CSF and macrophage colony-stimulating factor (M-CSF). If endothelial cells do not constitutively secrete IL-1, it seems that TNF-α may activate endothelial cells to release IL-1 by a mechanism that is dependent on protein synthesis. TNF-α and other cytokines also induce structural changes in the endothelial cells by a rearrangement of actin and the loss of tight junctions that are responsible for plasma protein leakage. IL-6, which is secreted mainly by cells of monocyte and macrophage lineage, is also produced by endothelial cells. IL-6 production by endothelial cells is triggered by several mediators, including histamine (Delneste *et al.*, 1994).

Several chemokines have been identified as secreted by endothelial cells like IL-8 and RANTES. IL-8, first characterized as a product of lipopolysaccharide (LPS)-activated monocytes, is effectively secreted by a number of cell types including endothelial cells. It was initially considered as a chemoattractant for neutrophils, but it also exerts chemotactic activities towards T lymphocytes (Larsen *et al.*, 1989) and eosinophils (Collins *et al.*, 1993; Erger & Casale, 1995) and therefore is directly implicated in allergic inflammation. Similarly, RANTES is recognized to be a chemoattractant *in vitro* and an activating factor for human eosinophils (Alam *et al.*, 1993) with a more efficient migratory response after eosinophil priming with IL-5 (Schweizer *et al.*, 1994). Moreover, intradermal injection of human RANTES in dogs demonstrated a local eosinophil infiltration, pointing to a potential role in allergic diseases (Meurer *et al.*, 1993). A number of potential sources of RANTES have been identified, including endothelial cells. Indeed it was known that little or no RANTES was generated after stimulation of HUVEC with interferon-γ (IFN-γ), IL-1 or TNF-α. However, in a recent study, Marfaing-Koka *et al.* (1995) observed the direct role of endothelial cells in the production of RANTES: its production by endothelial cells was potentiated by a combination of TNF-α and IFN-γ, and the synergistic effect was detected at relatively low concentrations of each cytokine. In addition, IL-4 and IL-13 inhibited the effects of TNF-α and IFN-γ on RANTES secretion. Therefore, the vascular endothelium appears to be a direct participant in the secretion of a large series of chemokines.

Expression of adhesion molecules on endothelial cells

The evidence of increased adhesion of leucocytes, and particularly of neutrophils (reviewed in Worthen *et al.*, 1987), under the effect of chemotactic factors or cell activators, was one of the first acquisitions of tissue-culture technology. Therefore, it is possible that endothelial cells could also be activated to become more adhesive for leucocytes (Bevilacqua *et al.*, 1985; Gamble *et al.*, 1985) through a dramatic increase in cell surface expression of adhesion molecules upon the effect of various stimuli (Albelda & Buck, 1990; Osborn, 1990; Wardlaw, 1990). This characteristic is the hallmark of endothelial cells in the inflammatory process. Some adhesion molecules, such as P-selectin, are immediatly but transiently expressed; others are delayed and prolonged over a period of hours to days. Leucocyte integrins, selectins, members of the immunoglobulin supergene family and specific carbohydrates are the main actors in the adhesion processes between endothelial cells and leucocytes, mainly eosinophils, T lymphocytes and basophils, which represent the major cell types implicated in allergic inflammation (Table 16.1).

The selectins are considered to play a crucial role in the initial binding of leucocytes to endothelium. The identification of E-selectin (previously named ELAM-1) on endothelial cells was originally performed by using monoclonal antibodies generated against cytokine-activated endothelial cells. E-selectin is an induced adhesion structure; after exposure to endotoxin, IL-1 or TNF-α, cultured endothelial cells synthesize and express E-selectin, with the main expression between 4 and 6 hours. E-selectin, which was initially reported to support neutrophil adhesion, was later shown to participate in the adhesion of most circulating leucocytes (monocytes, eosinophils, basophils and some subsets of T lymphocytes). Another selectin, P-selectin (GMP140), is also found on endothelial cells and platelets (McEver *et al.*, 1989). Upon activation by thrombin or histamine, P-selectin primarily found in α-granules, is rapidly redistributed to the surface of platelets. In endothelial cells, P-selectin is also found under a storage form in Weibel–Palade bodies and is rapidly expressed within 15 minutes after activation. Both E- and P-selectins are considered to play an essential role in the first step of leucocyte rolling at the surface of the vascular endothelium. Interestingly, mediators that stimulate P-selectin are also responsible for endothelial retraction, with a subsequent increase in vascular permeability.

Among the adhesion molecules belonging to the immunoglobulin supergene family, intercellular adhesion molecule-1 and -2 (ICAM-1 and ICAM-2), vascular cell adhesion molecule-1 (VCAM-1) and platelet endothelial cell adhesion molecule-1 (PECAM-1 or CD3) are present at the surface of the vascular endothelium. ICAM-1 (CD54) is constitutively expressed at a low level on unstimulated endothelial cells; its expression is largely enhanced after stimulation by IL-1 and TNF-α, with a different pattern compared with that for E-selectin. Overexpression of ICAM-1 increases progressively and peaks at a maximum value at the 24th hour. ICAM-1 and ICAM-2, also present on endothelial cells, interact with most leucocytes through binding with β2 integrins represented by the complex CD11a/CD18 (LFA-1), CD11b/CD18 (Mac-1 or CR3) and CD11c/CD18 (also registered as gp 150–95). The second step in the adhesion process, named ‘firm adhesion’, mainly results from the interaction ICAM-1/β2 integrins.

The third cytokine-inducible endothelial adhesion molecule is VCAM-1, initially denoted INCAM-110. Like ICAM-1, the expression of VCAM-1 is up-regulated in the

Table 16.1 Adhesion molecules present on endothelial cells and their counter-ligands.

	Expressed on:			
	Endothelial cells	Other cells	Induced by	Counter-ligand
Selectins				
E-selectin (ELAM-1)	+		IL-1, TNF-α	Sialyl-Lewis x/a
P-selectin (GMP140)	+	Platelets	Thrombin, histamine	Sialyl-Lewis x/L-selectin
Immunoglobulin supergene family				
ICAM-1	+	Epithelial cells (eosinophils, macrophages)	TNF, IL-1, IFN-γ	LFA-1/Mac 1
ICAM-2	+	–	Constitutive	LFA-1
VCAM-1	+	(Lymphocytes)	TNF, IL-1, IL-4	VLA-4
PECAM-1	+	Platelets (neutrophils, subsets of T cells)	Constitutive	PECAM-1

See text for definition of abbreviations.

presence of IL-1 and TNF-α (Osborn *et al.*, 1989; Briscoe *et al.*, 1992; Ebisawa *et al.*, 1992; Petzelbauer *et al.*, 1993), with maximal activity reached by 6–12 hours. Of particular interest is the capacity of IL-4 and IL-13, two cytokines directly implicated in allergy, to enhance VCAM-1 expression on endothelial cells. This effect of IL-4 on VCAM-1 expression differentiates this adhesion molecule from ICAM-1 and E-selectin which are insensitive to IL-4. The counter-ligand for VCAM-1 is the α4 β1 integrin, also called very late antigen-4 (VLA-4 or CD29/CD49d), which is present on lymphocytes, monocytes, but not neutrophils. VCAM-1 is also involved in eosinophil and basophil adhesion to activated endothelium.

Lastly, platelet endothelial cell adhesion molecule-1 (PECAM-1), a member of the same immunoglobulin supergene family, is also found on endothelial cells, platelets and some leucocytes. Its role is less well defined; it binds to glycosaminoglycans or to PECAM-1 itself by a homotypic adhesion process. It appears to contribute to endothelial cell-to-cell adhesion, and perhaps participates in the control of vascular permeability (Newman & Albelda, 1992).

In allergic inflammation, continuous exchanges do exist between soluble mediators generated by peripheral blood leucocytes or cells present, into bronchial mucosa and the endothelial surface. All these factors constantly mediate, modulate and alter the expression of adhesion molecules. Leucocytes must first adhere to the vascular lumen, then migrate between endothelial cells in order to constitute the cell infiltration characteristic of the allergic process. Therefore, during the development of the allergic reaction, mediators of allergy, cytokines, chemokines and cell adhesion molecules expressed on endothelial cells and on leucocytes (like integrins and L-selectin) interfere bidirectionally to induce, regulate and eventually reverse the cellular influx. Moreover, processes that regulate cell trafficking differ according to the cell type implicated: eosinophils, T lymphocytes and basophils respond to different leucocyte–endothelial cell adhesion pathways, which may explain the apparent selectivity of migration.

Specificity and selectivity of adhesion processes with each of the cells involved in allergic inflammation

Adhesion molecules controlling lymphocyte migration

Although activated T lymphocytes represent a major component of cell infiltrates seen in allergic asthma, little is known about the control of lymphocyte migration in the airway mucosa. The selectin and CD18 integrin pathways, as well as other pathways not used by neutrophils, including the α4 β1 integrin (VLA-4) and α4 β7 integrins—which preferentially bind to the endothelial cells' counter-ligands VCAM-1 and mucosal addressin cell adhesion molecule 1 (MAdCAM-1)—have been implicated in lymphocyte migration through the endothelial barrier.

However, evidence exists for a selectivity of lymphocyte traffic that is supported by the fact that naive and memory T lymphocytes have different recirculation pathways: memory lymphocytes are programmed so as to be predisposed to return to the tissue where they were first exposed to the allergen (e.g. skin or respiratory mucosa) (Mackay *et al.*, 1992). In the skin, T lymphocytes localized at the site of the allergen conflict were shown to express a carbohydrate termed 'cutaneous lymphocyte-associated antigen' (CLA). CLA represents a homing structure that primarily interacts during the rolling step with E-selectin (Berg *et al.*, 1991). In the second phase of transmigration, CLA engagement is required for using the VLA-4/VCAM-1 pathway (Santamaria-Babi *et al.*, 1995). Therefore, CLA-dependent transendothelial T-cell migration appears to be a complex system, in which mutual interactions between CLA and E-selectin as well as VLA-4/CAM-1 are successively involved in T-lymphocyte homing.

Lymphocyte chemoattractants are also implicated in lymphoaccumulation at inflammatory sites. A number of chemokines, some of which are produced by endothelial cells, are found to be chemoattractive for lymphocyte subpopulations. Macrophage chemotactic peptide-1 (MCP-1) is a major lymphocyte chemoattractant; macrophage inflammatory protein-1β (MIP-1β) enhances the binding of CD8+ cells to VCAM-1 (Tanaka *et al.*, 1993); RANTES selectively attracts the memory T lymphocytes (Schall *et al.*, 1990).

In allergic asthma the exact traffic signals for lymphocyte emigration are presently unknown. Specific bronchial homing molecules, which might explain the influx of activated T lymphocytes in target tissues, remain to be discovered. Conditions of lymphocyte recirculation in asthmatics are also incompletely understood. However, some indirect data indicate that T lymphocytes in bronchial asthma have the capacity to circulate and migrate towards other parts of the mucosal-associated lymphoid tissue (MALT). In a propective study, the histological abnormalities of the minor salivary glands (MSG) in a series of 58 asthmatics (29 with allergic asthma, 29 with non-allergic asthma) were compared with 15 healthy subjects and 15 patients with chronic obstructive pulmonary disease (COPD) (Wallaert *et al.*, 1994). The results are summarized in Table 16.2: 43 of 58 asthmatics patients (74%) presented MSG abnormalities with a large T-lymphocyte infiltration, with partly degranulated mast cells and basement membrane thickening. Abnormalities were more often observed in non-allergic (97%) than in allergic asthmatics (52%, $n<0.01$). They were practically absent in the two control groups (6%, $n<0.001$ vs. asthmatics). Thus,

Table 16.2 Minor salivary gland abnormalities in patients with bronchial asthma, chronic obstructive pulmonary disease (COPD) or in healthy subjects.

	Patients with allergic asthma ($n = 29$)	Patients with non-allergic asthma ($n = 29$)	Patients with COPD ($n = 15$)	Healthy subjects ($n = 15$)
Lymphocyte infiltration	9/29	24/29	1/15	1/15
Mean Chisholm's score*	0.45 ± 0.14	1.5 ± 0.18	0.07 ± 0.07	0.07 ± 0.07
Eosinophils	1/29	1/29	0/15	0/15
Mast cells	13/29	27/29	3/15	4/15
Basement membrane thickening	11/29	26/29	1/15	0/15
Vascular wall oedema	1/29	14/29	0/15	0/15
ICAM-1 expression (on vascular sections)	0/6	10/16	0/4	0/4

* The Chisholm score is the number of focal inflammatory cell agregates containing 50 or more lymphocytes or plasma cells in each 4-mm^2 area of salivary gland.

these intriguing observations showed that, except for eosinophil infiltration which was absent in MSG, the glandular tissue of MSG in bronchial asthma expressed an airway-like inflammation which might be due to the homing of T lymphocytes in another part of the MALT system. Interestingly, endothelial changes with turgescent endothelial cells, vascular wall oedema and narrowing of capillary and venule lumens were detectable in 15 patients (26%). Morphological alterations of vessels—the vascular expression of ICAM-1 observed mainly in non-allergic asthmatics—supports the hypothesis that endothelial cells were activated and suggests that at least an ICAM-1-dependent pathway may be involved in the T-lymphocyte sequestration into the MSG tissue of asthmatics.

Adhesion molecules controlling basophil recruitment

The mechanisms by which circulating human basophils migrate in allergic tissues are progressively identified. Several studies specified that basophils were involved in the late-phase reaction. After nasal allergen challenge, the analysis of mediators locally released showed two peaks of histamine in lavage fluids. The first is related to a local mast cell degranulation, and the second, which is not accompanied by a rise in PGD_2 and tryptase, is considered to be basophil dependent (Naclerio *et al.*, 1994). Similar results were reported for the late asthmatic response in allergic asthmatics (Guo *et al.*, 1994). These data suggest, therefore, that circulating basophils were actively recruited during the late phase, implying the existence of specific adherence and migration process across the vascular barrier. Effectively, Bochner (Bochner *et al.*, 1988; Bochner & Schleimer, 1994) showed that human basophils were able to adhere to cultured HUVEC, this process resulting from both the activation of the basophil and the previous activation of HUVEC.

Adhesion molecules controlling eosinophil recruitment

All recent studies emphasize the prominent role of eosinophils in allergy and their marked accumulation at the sites of allergic inflammation (Resnick & Weller ,1993). Many structures expressed on the surface of eosinophils, particularly after eosinophil activation, are susceptible to interact with counter-ligands on endothelial cells and on extracellular matrix components (Table 16.3) (Moser *et al.*, 1992a,b).

Like other leucocytes, eosinophils express the β2 integrins (LFA-1, Mac-1, gp 150-95) which are able to bind, among others, ICAM-1. When eosinophils are exposed to a range of chemotactic or activating stimuli, expression of CD11b rapidly increased (Hartnell *et al.*, 1990; Walker *et al.*, 1993); an up-regulation of CD11b levels is also induced by IL-5, GM-CSF and PAF addition (Warringa *et al.*, 1991), with additive or synergistic effects when various combinations are used. In parallel, Hansel *et al.* (1991) reported

Table 16.3 Eosinophil adherence to human endothelial cells.

Adhesion molecules expressed on:	
Eosinophils	**Endothelial cells**
β2 integrins	
CD11a/CD18 (LFA-1)	ICAM-1 and ICAM-2
CD11b/CD18 (Mac-1)	ICAM-1
α4 integrins	
VLA-4	VCAM-1
α4 β7	MAdCAM
L-selectin	Sialoglycoproteins

See text for definition of abbreviations.

that eosinophils from sputum, nasal polyps and bronchoalveolar lavage (BAL) from asthmatics demonstrated a marked increase in CD11b (Mac-1) compared with blood eosinophils.

However, other adhesion receptors present on eosinophils appear to be more specific: they are represented by the group of α4 integrins. Part of the specificity may be explained by the presence of a counter-receptor for VCAM-1; the VLA-4 present on eosinophils but not on neutrophils (Bochner *et al.*, 1991; Dobrina *et al.*, 1991; Walsh *et al.*, 1991a). Integrin α4 β7 also binds VCAM-1 and fibronectin and acts as a homing receptor for MAdCAM. It was first thought that α4 β7 was restricted to a subset of lymphocytes with a particular tropism for gut mucosa. More recent studies have shown that α4 β7 is detected on eosinophils. Moreover, experimental studies with monoclonal antibodies to α4 integrins blocked eosinophil infiltration in allergy lung models (Lobb & Hember, 1994). More interestingly, α4 integrin antagonists have been synthesized and inhibited binding to components of the extracellular matrix, more precisely at the level of the α4 recognition motif.

L-selectin acts differently; it is likely to be involved in leucocyte rolling on the vessel wall, a process that precedes firm adhesion and extravasation. L-selectin, unlike the two other selectins (P- and E-selectins) is constitutively expressed at the surface of most leucocytes, and eosinophils from peripheral blood currently express L-selectin. However, after cellular activation, L-selectin is shed. Effectively after allergen challenge, eosinophils that migrate into the alveolar spaces have a lower expression of L-selectin. This down-regulation of L-selectin allows eosinophils to detach themselves from the endothelial surface; this de-adhesion after shedding of L-selectin favours the subsequent migration (Mengelers *et al.*, 1993).

The issue of eosinophil migration is now still more comlicated. Indeed, cytokines active on eosinophil trafficking were originally considered to be derived predominantly from lymphocytes and mast cells: they are now known to be elaborated by many other cell types, including the eosinophil itself. Eosinophils synthesize and store in their granules several important inflammatory and regulating cytokines, including IL-1, IL-3, IL-5, IL-6, IL-8, GM-CSF, TGF-α, TNF-α and MIP-1α (Wong *et al.*, 1990; Moqbel *et al.*, 1991; Desreumaux *et al.*, 1992; Hamid *et al.*, 1992; Braun *et al.*, 1993). Human eosinophils also synthesize IL-4 and RANTES in airway tissue and/or in late-phase reaction lesions (Moqbel *et al.*, 1995; Ying *et al.*, 1995). Thus, eosinophils are certainly contributing in the modification of their own environment and facilitate, by autocrine cytokine release, emigration through the vascular endothelium.

The vascular endothelium as a target organ of allergic inflammation

The endothelial cell has not only a modulatory role on emigrating leucocytes but also appears to be as sensitive to leucocyte cytokines. Various models of endothelial cell monolayers *in vitro* have provided information on the behaviour of the endothelium behaviour in the presence of leucocyte products, showing that this cell type is not only a source but also a target of activating mediators (Fig. 16.1). These observations have been important in the understanding of the physiopathology of vascular endothelium in inflammatory reactions.

Interaction between macrophages and endothelial cells

In asthmatics, alveolar macrophages (AM) stimulated *in vitro* with an anti-human immunoglobulin E (IgE) immune serum or with IgE-related allergens produced large amounts of TNF-α and IL-6, with amplification in the case of costimulation with IFN-γ. Increased release of TNF-α and IL-6 by AM was observed in patients who developed a late asthmatic response (Gosset *et al.*, 1991). After bronchial allergen challenge, a BAL performed 18 hours after allergen exposure allowed the recovery of AM that produced large amounts of TNF-α and IL-6 (a 10–12-fold increase when compared with patients studied at baseline or exhibiting only an immediate bronchospastic response). The direct addition of AM supernatants on endothelial cell cultures mediated an enhanced expression of ICAM-1 and E-selectin, which was completely abolished in the presence of anti-TNF-α antibodies. Results suggest, therefore, that macrophages might partic-

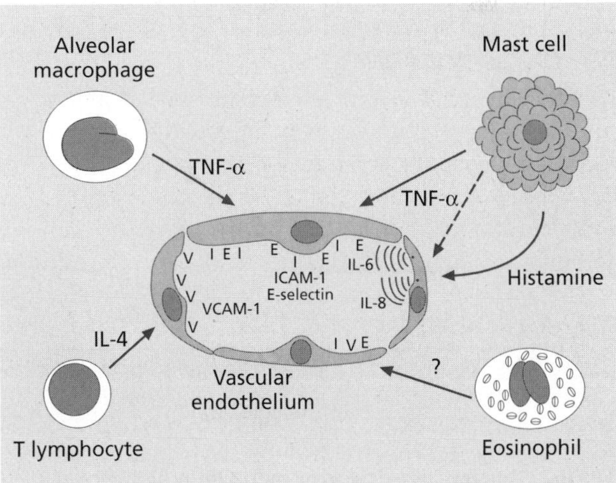

Fig. 16.1 Schematic representation of interactions between the endothelial cell and the main cell types involved in allergic inflammation. See text for definition of abbreviations.

ipate in the induction of the local inflammation reaction observed in bronchial asthma, namely by their capacity to induce expression of cell adhesion molecules in their near environment (Lassalle *et al.*, 1993).

Interaction between mast cells and endothelial cells

Among mast cell mediators, histamine interacts directly with endothelial cells. Histamine is known to induce early changes on endothelium, such as an increased permeability, a transient expression of P-selectin and the secretion and/or the surface expression of early mediators (e.g. prostaglandin I_2 (PGI_2), PAF and LTB_4) (Falus & Meretey, 1992).

However, later effects of histamine on endothelial cells, in particular on cytokine production, had not been evaluated. A study performed by Jeannin *et al.* (1994) aimed to assess the action of histamine on IL-8 and IL-6 production by human endothelial cells. HUVEC were incubated in the presence of increasing amounts of histamine (from 10^{-7} to 10^{-3} M) and both interleukins measured in the supernatants after culture for 6 and 24 hours (Jeannin *et al.*, 1994). IL-8 secretion by histamine-stimulated HUVEC was concentration dependent, with the highest amount of IL-8 obtained with a histamine concentration of 10^{-3} M. However, after a 24-hour incubation, lower concentrations of histamine (10^{-6} M) also induced a significant increase in IL-8 production (Fig. 16.2). IL-8 neosynthesis was assessed by Northern blot analysis: when endothelial cells were cultured for 4 hours in the presence of histamine, there was an increase of 1.8 kb mRNA expression compared with basal expression in resting cells. Moreover, histamine and TNF-α (a mediator present in mast cell granules and released concomitantly with histamine) had synergistic effects on IL-8 production. TNF-α used alone at 50 U/ml induced a modest but significant IL-8 production by endothelial cells, largely enhanced in the case of co-incubation with histamine.

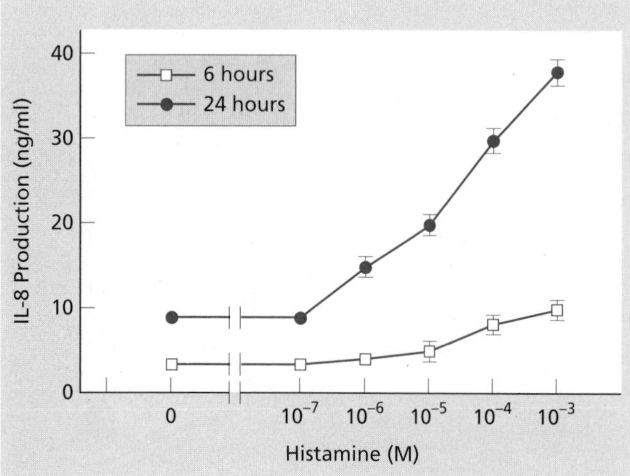

Fig. 16.2 Concentration-dependent induction by histamine of IL-8 production from human umbilical vein endothelial cell (HUVEC) monolayers. IL-8 was measured by an immunoassay in supernatants at the end of a 6- or 24-hour incubation with the indicated concentrations of histamine.

IL-8 production by endothelial cells in the presence of histamine probably reflects its *in vivo* activity at inflammatory sites. Although it was difficult to exactly define histamine concentrations in the target organs, concentrations of histamine (from 10^{-6} to 10^{-4} M) are compatible with those measured in tissues after mast cell degranulation. Furthermore, as histamine-induced IL-8 production by endothelial cells was detected from 4 to 24 hours after stimulation, it might participate in the late-phase reaction: IL-8 exerts a chemotactic activity for neutrophils, eosinophils and basophils *in vitro*. IL-8 has also been demonstrated to modulate basophil histamine release. This point is important in allergic rhinitis, where different observations suggest that basophils are implicated as effector cells in the late-phase reaction (Naclerio, 1990).

The same results were obtained for IL-6. After incubation with increasing concentrations of histamine, IL-6 was also secreted by endothelial cells, with the same timespan and at similar concentrations as for IL-8 (Delneste *et al.*, 1994).

Interaction between eosinophils and endothelial cells

It has been known for a long time that proteins from eosinophil granules possess the ability to activate other cells associated with allergic inflammation. Micromolar concentrations of major basic protein (MBP) and eosinophil peroxidase (EPO) affect the functional activities of basophils and neutrophils. MBP stimulates histamine release from human basophils and rat mast cells (O'Donnell *et al.*, 1983); it also activates neutrophils by enhancing the expression of CR3 and gp 150-95 (Moy *et al.*, 1993). All these experiments indicated that MBP and various eosinophil products were capable of activating other participants of the inflammatory reaction.

To test whether eosinophils and their degranulation products were likely to interfere with vascular endothelium, the effects of eosinophil supernatants on the cell adhesion molecule expression of HUVEC preparations were evaluated. Eosinophils from patients with circulating hypereosinophilia (hypereosinophilic syndrome, chronic eosinophilic pneumonia, allergic asthma, various atopic diseases, including atopic dermatitis), purified by adsorption of CD16 (FcγRIII)-positive cells on magnetic beads, were stimulated via IgE or IgG activation. Supernatants were transferred to HUVEC monolayers and the subsequent expression of ICAM-1, E-selectin and VCAM-1 measured by enzyme-linked immunosorbent assay (ELISA) after 6 and 24 hours. With 1-hour supernatants,

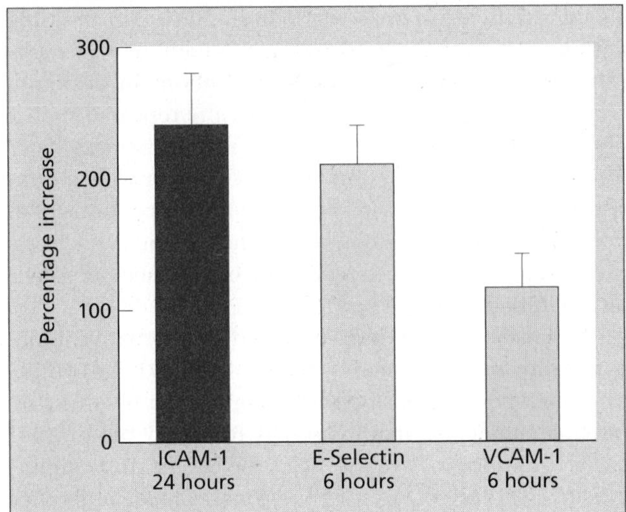

Fig. 16.3 Adhesion molecule expression induced on HUVEC monolayers by supernatants of purified eosinophils from patients with hypereosinophilic diseases of various aetiologies. Enhancement of adhesion molecule expression was evaluated after 6 hours for E-selectin and VCAM-1, after 24 hours for ICAM-1.

a clear-cut enhancement of ICAM-1 and E-selectin was obtained with IgE-dependent stimulation. VCAM-1 expression compared with unstimulated eosinophils did not significantly vary. In contrast, with eosinophil supernatants collected after 18 hours, the expression of the three cell adhesion molecules was largely enhanced (200%), with similar levels in all conditions (Fig. 16.3).

The addition of eosinophil supernatants on endothelial cells appears, therefore, to largely enhance adhesion molecule expression, the role of contaminant cells being ruled out by the high degree of purity of the eosinophil preparation. The present problem is to identify the factor(s) present in eosinophil supernatants that is (are) responsible for the overexpression of adhesion molecule. Several potential candidates have been discussed: arachidonic acid metabolites and PAF-acether are not involved; the role of basic proteins or of cytokines produced after eosinophil activation, or the association of both, is presently under investigation. Whatever their exact nature, it appears that eosinophils, recovered from patients with hypereosinophilia, have the capacity to directly activate the vascular endothelium and to create a kind of autoamplification loop in the inflammatory process.

Interaction between T lymphocytes and endothelial cells

Lymphokines also up-regulate, but to a lesser extent, adhesion molecule expression on endothelial cells. IFN-γ modulates ICAM-1 and human leucocyte antigen (HLA) class II expression, favouring mainly the adherence of neutrophils and T lymphocytes. IL-4, a lymphokine with a broad range of immune functions, specifically up-regulates VCAM-1 expression, allowing preferential eosinophil, basophil, and T-lymphocyte adhesion on endothelium (Masinovski *et al.*, 1990; Thornhill *et al.*, 1990; Schleimer *et al.*, 1992).

The inflammatory response in allergic diseases is characterized by infiltrates of activated T lymphocytes (Corrigan & Kay, 1992). In bronchial asthma, activated T cells secrete IL-3, IL-4, IL-5 or GM-CSF (Robinson *et al.*, 1992). Therefore, T lymphocytes appear to be among the most important cells able to promote and regulate cellular events of the inflammatory reaction. In this context, the activation of endothelial cells by T-cell-derived lymphokines, produced by peripheral blood T cells from mite-sensitive asthmatics, has been explored in the presence of the related allergen presented by paraformaldehyde-fixed antigen-presenting cells (Delneste *et al.*, 1995). T-lymphocyte supernatants from these patients induced an increase in VCAM-1 (Fig. 16.4) and ICAM-1 expression, but not in E-selectin. IL-6 synthesis by endothelial cells was also significantly enhanced. The induction of VCAM-1 expression was inhibited by adding neutralizing antibodies against IL-4, whereas IL-6 and ICAM-1 expression were inhibited by anti-IFN-γ. An enhanced production of both lymphokines was in fact detected in the supernatants

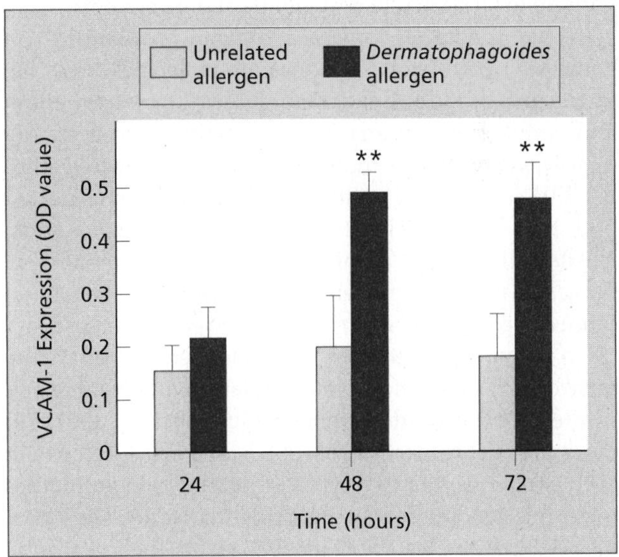

Fig. 16.4 VCAM-1 expression induced on HUVEC monolayers after addition of supernatants of T lymphocytes incubated in the presence of *Dermatophagoides pteronyssinus* allergen (dark bars) or in the presence of an unrelated allergen (light bars) (**$P > 0.001$ compared with unrelated allergen). Supernatants of activated T lymphocytes were collected after 24, 48 and 72 hours.

of allergen-stimulated T cells from allergic subjects, compared with unstimulated cells from asthmatics or allergen-stimulated cells from healthy controls.

Endothelial cells in asthma: experimental and clinical approaches

Histopathological studies performed on patient biopsies, and therapeutic effects of antibodies directed against some of the adhesion structures present on endothelial cells, have led to a better, although incomplete and sometimes controversial, understanding of the role of endothelial cells in allergic diseases.

Experimental models of asthma

Several animal models have been used (guinea pigs, sheep and primates) for evaluating endothelial and/or epithelial adhesion molecules in the experimental situations compared with acute or chronic asthma.

In primate models of asthma, it is possible to reproduce acute or chronic airway responses consecutive to an allergen inhalation (Wegner *et al.*, 1991). A single inhalation of *Ascaris suum* antigens in Cyanomolgus monkeys induced a rapid and short neutrophil infiltration, followed by long-term eosinophil infiltration (6 hours to 6–7 days), and only a weak increase in bronchial hyperresponsiveness (BHR). In contrast, repeated antigen exposure produced a massive and pure eosinophil infiltration alongside a severe increase in airways responsiveness thought to be related to eosinophil cationic proteins.

In the model of repeated antigen inhalations, an enhanced expression of adhesion molecules was detected on bronchial biopsies (ICAM-1 on epithelium and endothelium of airways, E-selectin only on airway microvessels). When monkeys were administered anti-ICAM-1 monoclonal antibodies, this treatment corrected both the eosinophil infiltration and BHR (Wegner *et al.*, 1990). In the case of a unique *Ascaris* antigen inhalation, bronchial challenge in sensitized animals resulted in an immediate bronchoconstriction followed, in some cases, by a late-phase response characterized by an acute neutrophilic infiltration, well correlated with the intensity of the bronchospastic response (Gundel *et al.*, 1991). To determine the respective role of ICAM-1 and E-selectin in both situations, the two types of neutralizing antibodies were injected intravenously prior to *Ascaris* challenge: ICAM-1 antibodies were ineffective on the neutrophil infiltration in airways, while anti-E-selectin antibodies clearly inhibited the late-phase bronchoconstriction as well as the number of neutrophils and myeloperoxidase activity present in BAL fluids. In this model of experimental acute asthma, E-selectin appears, therefore, to be playing a crucial role in the allergen-induced late bronchoconstriction response, while in the model of multiple antigen inhalations, ICAM-1 was predominatly implicated in BHR and eosinophil infiltration. In addition, when allergen exposure was chronically repeated with a persistent inflammation and airway responsiveness, daily intravenous administration of anti-ICAM-1 and E-selectin antibodies given *a posteriori*, failed to reverse both phenomena, suggesting that an anti-adhesion molecule treatment would be unable to reverse an established persistent airway inflammation (Gundel *et al.*, 1992).

More recent studies have explored an alternative adhesion pathway represented by the VCAM-1/VLA-4 couple. In guinea pigs the eosinophil accumulation obtained by passive cutaneous anaphylaxis is inhibited by an anti-VLA-4 antibody (Weg *et al.*, 1993). In ovalbumin-sensitized guinea pigs, anti-VLA-4 monoclonal antibodies also blocked the eosinophil influx into alveolar spaces, as well as the bronchial hyperreactivity obtained in response to carbachol (Pretolani *et al.*, 1994). Similar results were obtained in rats and sheep challenged with allergen: treatment with an anti-VLA-4 monoclonal antibody restricted the accumulation of lymphocytes and eosinophils in BAL, 24 hours after aerosol ovalbumin challenge (Richards *et al.*, 1995); in sheep, monoclonal antibodies to VLA-4 also prevented the late-phase bronchospastic response and BHR but without any effect on eosinophil attraction (Abraham *et al.*, 1994). In fact, multiple experimental models that are presently tested are directed against endothelial cell adhesion molecules and also against integrins (from the group of $\alpha4$ integrins such as VLA-4 or $\alpha4$ $\beta7$, or belonging to the complex CD11/CD18). Several methods for administration must presently be evaluated: the question of the best route of administration—systemic or inhaled—is still debated and changes according to the choosen target, circulating blood leucocytes, endothelial cells or airway epithelial cells.

Adhesion molecule expression on the microvasculature in allergic diseases

After the initial demonstration in 1990 (Wegner *et al.*, 1990) that the intravenous administration of antibodies against ICAM-1 and E-selectin could prevent the development of bronchial hyperresponsiveness and cell infiltration in sensitized monkeys, many studies were initiated in patients with allergic rhinitis or allergic asthma. Some of the studies evaluated adhesion molecule expression at baseline, others after allergen challenge.

The analysis of mechanisms for the accumulation of inflammatory cells at the site of a cutaneous late-phase allergic reaction allowed a demonstration, for the first time in humans, of the important role of adhesion molecules (Leung *et al.*, 1991). In this study, expression of ELAM-1 (named E-selectin here) was quantified in sequential skin biopsies from patients with respiratory allergy, between 20 minutes and 24 hours after intradermal allergen challenge. In all seven atopics tested, allergen injection determined the appearance of E-selectin on endothelial cells, and simultaneously the influx of inflammatory cells: E-selectin expression was detected 3 and 4 hours after allergen administration, increased in intensity at 6 hours and declined after 24 hours, reproducing the well-known kinetics of E-selectin expression. Cytokines involved in the process were identified as IL-1 and TNF-α, as proved by the inhibition of allergen-induced E-selectin expression when skin biopsies were incubated with a combination of anti-TNF-α and anti-IL-1 antibodies. Many cells types are potentially presumed to secrete IL-1 and TNF-α. Klein *et al.* (1989) and Walsh *et al.* (1991b) have reported the presence of preformed TNF-α in mast cells of human skin fragments and its release upon allergen challenge. Both suggested that up-regulation of E-selectin on endothelial cells by antigen addition could be related to TNF-α release from IgE-triggered mast cells.

In perennial allergic rhinitis, immunostaining of nasal biopsies showed that the number of endothelial cells expressing ICAM-1 and VCAM-1 were significantly elevated (Montefort *et al.*, 1992a). Another study carried out by Lee *et al.* (1994) compared data obtained at baseline and after nasal challenge: in this study ICAM-1 appeared as the adhesion molecule predominantly expressed in endothelial cells of the nasal mucosa but was considered as constitutive, while similar expression levels were observed both in allergic and non-allergic patients. More interestingly, when patients were allergen challenged, a second set of biopsies performed at 24 hours showed no significant changes in ICAM-1 and E-selectin but an enhanced percentage of vessels expressing VCAM-1. The low expression of E-selectin may be explained by the timing of the study: biopsies were performed at 24 hours after challenge, i.e. at a period when E-selectin, which is known to be induced early (between 4 and 6 hours), already declined.

Results obtained in asthma confirm this modulation of cell adhesion molecules on the microvasculature. In allergic asthmatic patients, Gosset *et al.* (1995) found that ICAM-1 and to a lesser degree E-selectin and VCAM-1 were overexpressed at the surface of the vascular endothelium when studied at baseline (Fig. 16.5). An increased expression of ICAM-1 on the bronchial epithelium was also detectable.

The authors' results differ from those reported by Bentley *et al.* (1993) and Montefort *et al.* (1992b), who saw no difference between normal donors and asthmatics. Many points may explain these apparent discrepancies. Most of the patients were symptomatic at the time of bronchoscopy and the Aas (symptom) score was higher. In contrast, in the non-allergic asthma group, adhesion molecule expression in bronchial biopsies was not significantly different from the control population: as patients in this subgroup demonstrated a higher degree of severity, a probable role for corticosteroids, used more largely in intrinsic asthma, is therefore suggested.

There is also evidence that endothelial activation occurs within the human airways after local allergen challenge. By using an endobronchial allergen instillation (Montefort *et al.*, 1994a), it is possible to compare, in the same patient, morphological and histochemical modifications consecutive to allergen challenge. Biopsies were performed 6 hours after challenge and compared with specimens recovered at the same time-point from saline-instilled bronchial segments. In parallel with a submucosal infiltration with neutrophils, eosinophils, mast cells and CD3+ lymphocytes, a marked increase in ICAM-1 and E-selectin

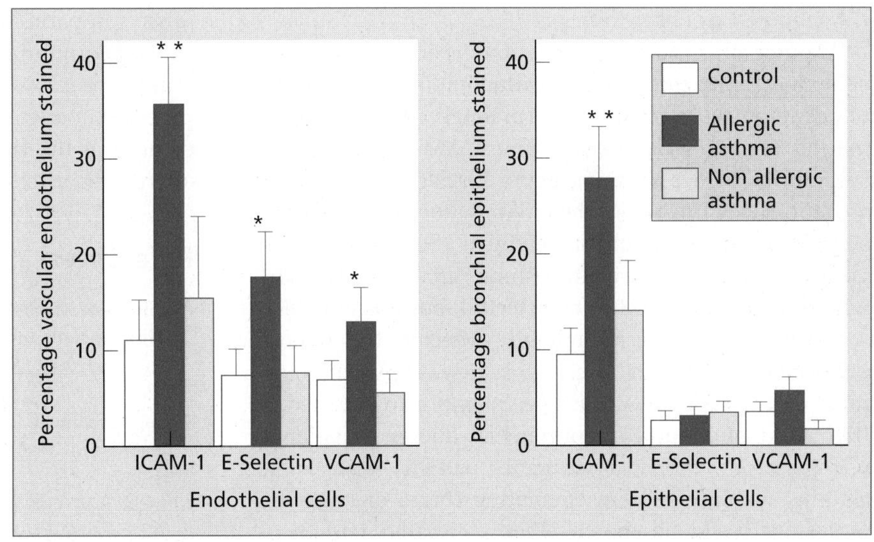

Fig. 16.5 Adhesion molecule expression quantified on sections of bronchial biopsies from allergic and non-allergic asthmatics. Comparison of endothelial and epithelial staining ($*P < 0.05$, $**P < 0.01$ compared with controls).

but not VCAM-1 was detectable on the microvasculature. The mechanisms sustaining the dissociation of VCAM-1 and ICAM-1 expressions are not completely understood, since ICAM-1 and VCAM-1 have theoretically similar patterns of up-regulation. Nevertheless, it seems possible to postulate that, following allergen exposure, cell emigration through the vascular endothelium proceeds in two successive steps: an early up-regulation of E-selectin and ICAM-1 which is responsible for the eosinophil and T-cell response at 6 hours, followed by a second step with the enhancement of VCAM-1 persistent for 24 hours that may account for a more selective eosinophil and basophil attraction by interaction with VLA-4. Another important issue was represented by the relationships between an enhanced expression of adhesion molecules and the level of air-flow limitation. In asthmatic patients, monitored with a peak-flow meter, Ohkawara *et al.* (1995) performed BAL procedures and bronchial biopsies as soon as peak expiratory flow values were below 80% of the control values. In these conditions, they clearly demonstrated a marked up-regulation of ICAM-1, VCAM-1 and E-selectin in vascular endothelial cells, concomitant with local eosinophil accumulation. Interestingly, immunoelectron microscopy allowed the detection of specific immunoreactivity for the three molecules, especially for VCAM-1, in the perinuclear space and on the luminal surface of endothelial cells, suggesting active *in vivo* synthesis by the bronchial microvasculature. Nevertheless, this up-regulation of adhesion molecules in submucosal tissues of bronchi are not specific for allergic or non-allergic asthma. In patients with chronic obstructive bronchitis (Di Stefano *et al.*, 1994), a quantitative analysis by immunohistochemical techniques demonstrated an enhanced expression of E-selectin on bronchial vessels and of ICAM-1 on basal epithelial cells. The increased number of vessels positive for E-selectin was correlated with the level of airway obstruction and with the number of neutrophils present in the submucosa of bronchitics.

Another approach to the role of adhesion molecules in asthma is represented by the evaluation of soluble forms of adhesion molecules. Not surprisingly, during inflammation, serum levels of circulating ICAM-1, VCAM-1, E-selectin, as well as the leucocyte L-selectin, have been measured as witnesses of the inflammatory process, of its severity or reversal under treatment (Seth *et al.*, 1991; Gearing *et al.*, 1992). In acute asthma, circulating ICAM-1 (cICAM-1) and E-selectin (cE-selectin), but not VCAM-1, were enhanced, which probably reflected the intense inflammatory reaction occurring in airways. An enhancement of a soluble form of E-selectin was also detected in BAL fluid after local endobronchial allergen challenge (Georas *et al.*, 1992). However, in patients with stable asthma, no difference in circulating forms of adhesion molecules could be shown when compared with non-atopic asthmatics and healthy subjects (Montefort *et al.*, 1994b).

There was also no correlation between the concentrations of the three circulating adhesion molecules or between serum levels and the degree of severity of the disease. A significant rise in serum levels of the soluble form of ICAM-1 was observed in dual asthmatic responders; it was associated with the up-regulation of ICAM-1 on peripheral blood T lymphocytes and the secondary decrease in ICAM-1 expression on CD8+ and CD4+ T cells at the time when the late bronchospastic reaction developed (De Rose *et al.*, 1994).

Nevertheless, even if measurements of circulating adhesion molecules are devoid of any diagnostic use, it would be worth elucidating their precise role in allergic inflammation; a potential blocking effect on counter-receptors present on leucocytes and a consecutive down-regulating function in cell recruitments might be postulated.

Conclusion

Vascular endothelium appears to be both a target and an effector of allergic inflammation, particularly at the level of bronchial mucosa in asthma. The balance between secreted mediators and adhesion molecule expression has to be very precisely regulated in endothelial cells as well as in migrating leucocytes. Therefore, among the many functions carried out by the microvasculature, it does assist complex and persistent interactions between the vascular endothelium and the neighbouring structures: endothelial cells secrete components that modify the reactivity of circulating and/or migrating cells. In contrast, endothelial cell behaviour, namely in the field of adhesion molecule expression, is constantly modified or adapted in reaction to the large panel of mediators, cytokines and chemokines, released during the allergic conflict. As always in pathological situations, dysregulation of such a refined equilibrium leads to the overexpression of inflammatory processes with detrimental effects for patients. A precise knowledge of these complex interactions will be of help in the therapy, and possibly the prophylaxis of allergic disorders.

References

Abraham, W.M., Sielczak, M.W., Ahmed, A. *et al.* (1994) Alpha-4 integrins mediate antigen-induced late bronchial responses and prolonged airway hyperresponsiveness in sheep. *J. Clin. Invest.*, **93**, 776–87.

Alam, R., Stafford, P., Forsythe, P. *et al.* (1993) RANTES is a chemotactic and activating factor for human eosinophils. *J. Immunol.*, **150**, 3442–7.

Albelda, S.M. (1991) Endothelial and epithelial cell adhesion molecules. *Am. J. Respir. Cell Mol. Biol.*, **4**, 195–203.

Albelda, S.M. & Buck, C.A. (1990) Integrins and other cell adhesion molecules. *FASEB J.*, **4**, 2868–80.

Bentley, A.M., Durham, S.R., Robinson, D.S. *et al.* (1993) Expression of endothelial and leukocyte adhesion molecules (ICAM-1, E-selectin and VCAM-1) in the bronchial mucosa in steady state and allergen induced asthma. *J. Allergy Clin. Immunol.*, **92**, 857–68.

Berg, E.L., Yoshino, T., Rott, L.S. *et al.* (1991) The cutaneous lymphocyte antigen is a skin lymphocyte homing receptor for the vascular lectin endothelial cell leukocyte adhesion molecules. *J. Exp. Med.*, **174**, 1461–6.

Bevilacqua, M.P., Pober, J.S., Wheeler, M.E., Cotran, R.S. & Gimbrone, M.J. (1985) Interleukin-1 acts on cultured human vascular endothelium to increase the adhesion of polymorphonuclear leukocytes, monocytes and related leukocyte cell lines. *J. Clin. Invest.*, **76**, 2003–11.

Bochner, B.S. & Schleimer, R.P. (1994) The role of adhesion molecules in human eosinophil and basophil recruitment. *J. Allergy Clin. Immunol.*, **94**, 427–38.

Bochner, B.S., Luscinskas, F.W., Gimbrone, M.A. *et al.* (1991) Adhesion of human basophils, eosinophils, and neutrophils to interleukin 1-activated human vascular endothelial cells: contributions of endothelial cell adhesion molecules. *J. Exp. Med.*, **173**, 1553–7.

Bochner, B.S., Peachell, P.T., Brown, K.E. & Schleimer, R.P. (1988) Adherence of human basophils to cultured umbilical vein endothelial cells. *J. Clin. Invest.*, **81**, 1355–64.

Bousquet, J., Chanez, P., Lacoste, J.Y. *et al.* (1990) Eosinophilic inflammation in asthma. *New Engl. J. Med.*, **323**, 1033–9.

Braun, R.K., Franchini, M., Erard F., Rihs, S. *et al.* (1993) Human peripheral blood eosinophils produce and release interleukin 8 on stimulation with calcium ionophore. *Eur. J. Immunol.*, **23**, 956–60.

Briscoe, D.M., Cotran, R.S. & Pober, J.S. (1992) Effects of tumor necrosis factor, lipopolysaccharide, and IL-4 on the expression of vascular cell adhesion molecule-1 *in vivo*. *J. Immunol.*, **149**, 2954–60.

Casale, T.B., Erger, R.A. & Little, M.M. (1993) Platelet-activating factor-induced human eosinophil transendothelial migration: evidence for a dynamic role of the endothelium. *Am. J. Respir. Cell Mol. Biol.*, **8**, 77–82.

Clark, E.R. & Clark, E.L. (1935) Observations on changes in blood vascular endothelium in the living animal. *Am. J. Anat.*, **57**, 385–438.

Collins, P.D., Weg, W.B., Gaccioli, L.H., Watson, M.L., Moqbel, R. & Williams, T.J. (1993) Eosinophil accumulation induced by human interleukin 8 in guinea pig *in vivo*. *Immunology*, **79**, 312–18.

Corrigan, C.J. & Kay, A.B. (1992) T cells and eosinophils in the pathogenesis of asthma. *Immunol. Today*, **13**, 501–6.

De Rose, V., Rolla, G., Bucca, C. *et al.* (1994) Intercellular adhesion molecule-1 is upregulated on peripheral blood T lymphocyte subsets in dual asthmatic responders. *J. Clin. Invest.*, **94**, 1840–5.

Delneste, Y., Jeannin, P., Gosset, P. *et al.* (1995) Allergen-stimulated T lymphocytes from allergic patients induce vascular cell adhesion molecule-1 (VCAM-1) expression and IL-6 production by endothelial cells. *Clin. Exp. Immunol.*, **101**, 167–71.

Delneste, Y., Lassalle, P., Jeannin, P., Joseph, M., Tonnel, A.B. & Gosset, P. (1994) Histamine induces IL-6 production by human endothelial cells. *Clin. Exp. Immunol.*, **98**, 344–9.

Desreumaux, P., Janin, A., Colombel, J.F. *et al.* (1992) Interleukin-5 messenger RNA expression by eosinophils in the intestinal mucosa of patients with coeliac disease. *J. Exp. Med.*, **175**, 293–6.

Di Stefano, A., Maestrelli, P., Poggeri, A. *et al.* (1994) Upregulation of adhesion molecules in the bronchial mucosa of subjects with chronic obstructive bronchitis. *Am. J. Resp. Crit. Care Med.*, **149**, 803–10.

Dobrina, A., Menegazzi, R., Carlos, T.M. *et al.* (1991) Mechanisms of eosinophil adherence to cultured vascular endothelial cells. Eosinophils bind to the cytokine-induced endothelial ligand VCAM-1 via the very late activation antigen-4 integrin receptor. *J. Clin. Invest.*, **88**, 20–6.

Ebisawa, M., Bochner, B.S., Georas, S.N. & Schleimer, R.P. (1992) Eosinophil transendothelial migration induced by cytokines. I. Role of endothelial and eosinophil adhesion molecules in IL-1β-induced transendothelial migration. *J. Immunol.*, **149**, 4021–5.

Erger, R.A. & Casale, T.B. (1995) Interleukin-8 is a potent mediator of eosinophil chemotaxis through endothelium and epithelium. *Am. J. Physiol.*, **268**, L117–22.

Falus, A. & Meretey, K. (1992) Histamine: an early messenger in inflammatory and immune reaction. *Immunol. Today*, **13**, 154–8.

Feinmark, S.J. & Cannon, P.J. (1986) Endothelial cell leukotriene C4 synthesis results from intercellular transfer of LTA4 synthesized by polymorphonuclear leukocytes. *J. Biol. Chem.*, **261**, 16466–72.

Forstner, J.F., Jabbal, I., Findlay, B.P. & Forstner, G.G. (1977) Interaction of mucins with calcium, H^+ ion and albumin. *Mod. Probl. Paed.*, **19**, 54–65.

Gamble, J.R., Harlan, J.M., Klebanoff, S.J. & Vadas, M.A. (1985) Stimulation of the adherence of neutrophils to umbilical vein endothelium by human recombinant tumor necrosis factor. *Proc. Nat. Acad. Sci.*, **82**, 8667–71.

Gearing, A.J.H., Hemingway, I., Pigott, R., Hughes, J., Rees, A.J. & Cashman, S.J. (1992) Soluble forms of vascular adhesion molecules, E selectin, ICAM-1 and VCAM-1: pathological significance. *Ann. NY Acad. Sci.*, **667**, 324–31.

Georas, S.N., Liu, M.C., Newman, W. *et al.* (1992) Altered adhesion molecule expression and endothelial cell activation accompanies the recruitment of human granulocytes to the lung after segmental antigen challenge. *Am. J. Respir. Cell Mol. Biol.*, **7**, 261–9.

Gerritsen, M.E. & Bloor, C.M. (1993) Endothelial cell gene expression in response to injury. *FASEB J.*, **7**, 523–32.

Gosset, P., Tillie Leblond, I., Janin, A. *et al.* (1995) Expression of E-selectin, ICAM-1 and VCAM-1 on bronchial biopsies from allergic and non-allergic asthmatic patients. *Int. Arch. Allergy Immunol.*, **106**, 69–77.

Gosset, P., Tsicopoulos, A., Wallaert, B., Joseph, M., Tonnel, A.B. & Capron, A. (1991) Increased secretion of tumor necrosis factor and interleukin 6 by alveolar macrophages during late asthmatic reaction after bronchial allergen challenge. *J. Allergy Clin. Immunol.*, **88**, 561–71.

Gundel, R.H., Wegner, C.D., Torcellini, C.A. *et al.* (1991) Endothelial leukocyte adhesion molecule-1 mediates antigen-induced acute airway inflammation and late-phase airway obstruction in monkeys. *J. Clin. Invest.*, **88**, 1407–11.

Gundel, R.H., Wegner, C.D., Torcellini, C.A. & Letts, L.G. (1992) The role of intercellular adhesion molecule-1 in chronic airway inflammation. *Clin. Exp. Allergy*, **22**, 569–75.

Guo, C.B., Liu, M.C., Galli, S.J., Bochner, B.S., Kagey, S.A. & Lichtenstein, L.M. (1994) Identification of IgE-bearing cells in the late-phase response to antigen in the lung as basophils. *Am. J. Respir. Cell Mol. Biol.*, **10**, 384–90.

Hamid, Q., Barkans, J., Meng, Q. *et al.* (1992) Human eosinophils synthesize and secrete interleukin-6 *in vitro*. *Blood*, **80**, 1496–501.

Hansel, T.T., Braunstein, J.B., Walker, C. *et al.* (1991) Sputum eosinophils from asthmatics express ICAM-1 and HLA-DR. *Clin. Exp. Immunol.*, **86**, 271–7.

Hartnell, A., Moqbel, R., Walsh, G.M., Bradley, B. & Kay, A.B. (1990) Fc gamma and CD11/CD18 receptor expression on normal density and low density eosinophils. *Immunology*, **69**, 264–70.

Jeannin, P., Delneste, Y., Gosset, P. *et al.* (1994) Histamine induces Interleukin-8 secretion by endothelial cells. *Blood*, **84**, 2229–33.

Jeffery, P.K., Wardlaw, A., Nelson, F.C., Collins, J.V. & Kay, A.B. (1989) Bronchial biopsies in asthma: an ultrastructural quantification study and correlation with hyperreactivity. *Am. Rev. Resp. Dis.*, **140**, 1745–53.

Klein, L.M., Lavker, R.M., Mates, W.L. & Murphy, G.F. (1989) Degranulation of human mast cells induces an endothelial antigen central to leukocyte adhesion. *Proc. Nat. Acad. Sci. USA*, **86**, 8972–6.

Laitinen, L.A. & Laitinen, A. (1987) Is asthma also a vascular disease? *Am. Rev. Resp. Dis.*, **135**, A474.

Lamm, W.J.E., Selfe, S. & Albert, R.K. (1988) Pharmacologic and pulmonary physiologic effects of leukotrienes binding to albumin. *Am. Rev. Resp. Dis.*, **137**, 398 [abstract].

Larsen, C.G., Anderson, A.O., Appella, E., Oppenheim, J.J. & Matsushima, K. (1989) The neutrophil-activating peptide (NAP-1) is also chemotactic for T-lymphocytes. *Science*, **243**, 1464–6.

Lassalle, P., Gosset, P., Delneste, Y. *et al.* (1993) Modulation of adhesion molecule expression on endothelial cells during the late asthmatic reaction: role of macrophage-derived tumour necrosis factor-alpha. *Clin. Exp. Immunol.*, **94**, 105–10.

Lee, B.J., Naclerio, R.M., Bochner, B.S., Taylor, R.M., Lim, M.C. & Baroody, F. (1994) Nasal challenge with allergen up-regulates the local expression of vascular endothelial adhesion molecules. *J. Allergy Clin. Immunol.*, **94**, 1006–16.

Leung, D.Y.M., Pober, J.S. & Cotran, R.S. (1991) Expression of endothelial–leukocyte adhesion molecule-1 in elicited late phase allergic reactions. *J. Clin. Invest.*, **87**, 1805–9.

Lewis, M.S., Whatley, R.E., Cain, P., Mclntyre, T.M., Prescott, S.M. & Zimmerman, G.A. (1988) Hydrogen peroxide stimulates the synthesis of platelet activating factor by endothelium and induces endothelial cell dependent adhesion. *J. Clin. Invest.*, **82**, 2045–55.

Lobb, R.R. & Hember, M.E. (1994) The pathophysiologic role of α4 integrins *in vivo*. *J. Clin. Invest.*, **94**, 1722–8.

McEver, R.P., Beckstead, J.H., Moore, K.L., Marshall-Carlson, L. & Bainton, D.F. (1989) GMP-140, a platelet-α granule membrane protein, is also synthesized by vascular endothelial cells and is localized in Weibel–Palade bodies. *J. Clin. Invest.*, **84**, 92–9.

Mackay, C.R., Marston, W.L., Dudler, L., Spertini, O., Tedder, T.F. & Hein, W.R. (1992) Tissue specific migration pathways by phenotypically distinct subpopulations of memory T-cells. *Eur. J. Immunol.*, **22**, 887–95.

Marfaing-Koka, A., Devergne, O., Gorgone, G. *et al.* (1995) Regulation of the production of the RANTES chemokine by endothelial cells—synergistic induction by IFN-gamma plus TNF-alpha and inhibition by IL-4 and IL-13. *J. Immunol.*, **154**, 1870–8.

Masinovski, B., Urdal, D. & Gallatin, W.M. (1990) IL-4 acts synergistically with IL-1β to promote lymphocyte adhesion to microvascular endothelium by induction of vascular cell adhesion molecule-1. *J. Immunol.*, **145**, 2886–93.

Mengelers, H.J.J., Maikoe, T., Hooibrink, B. *et al.* (1993) Down modulation of L-selectin expression on eosinophils recovered from bronchoalveolar lavage fluid after allergen provocation. *Clin. Exp. Allergy*, **23**, 196–204.

Meurer, R., Van Riper, G., Feeney, W. *et al.* (1993) Formation of eosinophilic and monocytic intradermal inflammatory sites in the dog by injection of human RANTES but not human MCP-1, human MIP-1α or human IL-8. *J. Exp. Med.*, **178**, 1913–21.

Montefort, S., Feather, I.H., Wilson, S.J. *et al.* (1992a) The expression of leukocyte–endothelial adhesion molecules is increased in perennial allergic rhinitis. *Am. J. Respir. Cell Mol. Biol.*, **7**, 393–8.

Montefort, S., Roche, W.R., Howarth, P.H. *et al.* (1992b) Intercellular adhesion molecule-1 (ICAM-1) and endothelial leucocyte adhesion molecule-1 (ELAM-1) expression in the bronchial mucosa of normal and asthmatic subjects. *Eur. Resp. J.*, **5**, 815–23.

Montefort, S., Gratziou, C., Goulding, D. *et al.* (1994a) Bronchial biopsy evidence for leukocyte infiltration and upregulation of leukocyte–endothelial cell adhesion molecules 6 hours after local allergen challenge of sensitized asthmatic airways. *J. Clin. Invest.*, **93**, 1411–21.

Montefort, S., Lai, C.K., Kapahi, P. *et al.* (1994b) Circulating adhesion molecules in asthma. *Am. J. Resp. Crit. Care Med.*, **149**, 1149–52.

Moqbel, R., Hamid, Q. & Ying, S. (1991) Expression of mRNA and immunoreactivity for the granulocyte macrophage-colony stimulating factor (GM-CSF) in activated human eosinophils. *J. Exp. Med.*, **174**, 749–52.

Moqbel, R., Ying, S., Barkans, J. *et al.* (1995) Identification of mRNA for interleukin-4 in human eosinophils with granule localization and release of the translated product. *J. Immunol.*, **155**, 4939–47.

Moser, R. Fehr, J. & Bruijnzeel, P.L.B. (1992a) IL-4 controls the selective endothelium-driven transmigration of eosinophils from allergic individuals. *J. Immunol.*, **149**, 1432–8.

Moser, R., Fehr, J., Olgiati, L. & Bruijnzeel, P.L. (1992b) Migration of primed human eosinophils across cytokine-activated endothelial cell monolayers. *Blood*, **79**, 2937–45.

Moy, J.N., Thomas, L.L. & Wisler, L.C. (1993) Eosinophil major basic protein enhances the expression of neutrophil CR3 and p 150-95. *J. Allergy Clin. Immunol.*, **92**, 598–604.

Naclerio, R.M. (1990) The role of histamine in allergic rhinitis. *J. Allergy Clin. Immunol.*, **86**, 628–35.

Naclerio, R.M., Baroody, F.M., Kagey-Sobotka, A. & Lichtenstein, L.M. (1994) Basophils and eosinophils in allergic rhinitis. *J. Allergy Clin. Immunol.*, **94**, 1303–9.

Newman, P.J. & Albelda, S.M. (1992) Cellular and molecular aspects of PCAM-1. *Nouv. Rev. Fr. Hematol.*, **34**, S7–11.

O'Donnell, M.A., Ackerman, S.J., Gleich, G.J. & Thomas, L.L. (1983) Activation of basophil and mast cell histamine release by eosinophil granule proteins. *J. Exp. Med.*, **157**, 1981–8.

Ohkawara, Y., Yamauchi, K., Maruyama, N. *et al.* (1995) *In situ* expression of the cell adhesion molecules in bronchial tissues from asthmatics with air flow limitation: *in vivo* evidence of VCAM-1/VLA-4 interaction in selective eosinophil infiltration. *Am. J. Respir. Cell Mol. Biol.*, **12**, 4–12.

Osborn, L. (1990) Leukocyte adhesion to endothelium in inflammation. *Cell*, **62**, 3–6.

Osborn, L., Hession, C., Tizard, R. *et al.* (1989) Direct expression cloning of vascular cell adhesion molecule-1 (VCAM-1), a cytokine-induced endothelial protein that binds to lymphocytes. *Cell*, **59**, 1203–1211.

Persson, C.G.A. (1986) Role of plasma exudation in asthmatic airways. *Lancet*, **i**, 1126–9.

Persson, C.G.A. (1991) Tracheobronchial microcirculation in asthma. In: *Asthma. Its Pathology and Treatment Lung Biology in Health and Disease* (eds M.A. Kalmer, P.J. Barnes & C.G.A. Persson), pp. 209–29. Marcel Dekker, New York.

Petzelbauer, P., Bender, J.R., Wilson, J. & Pober, J.S. (1993) Heterogeneity of dermal microvascular endothelial cell antigen expression and cytokine responsiveness *in situ* and in cell culture. *J. Immunol.*, **151**, 5062–72.

Pretolani, M., Ruffié, C., Lapa e Silva, J.R., Joseph, D., Lobb, R.R. & Vargaftig, B.B. (1994) Antibody to very late activation antigen 4 prevents antigen induced bronchial hyperreactivity and cellular infiltration in the guinea pig airways. *J. Exp. Med.*, **180**, 795–805.

Resnick, M.B. & Weller, P.F. (1993) Mechanisms of eosinophil recruitment. *Am. J. Respir. Cell Mol. Biol.*, **8**, 345–55.

Richards, I.M., Kolbasa, K.P., Hatfield, C.A. *et al.* (1996) VLA-4 dependent eosinophil and lymphocyte accumulation in the lungs and airway lumen of ovalbumin-sensitized Brown Norway rats. In: *Cytokines and Adhesion Molecules in Lung*, (eds M. Chignard, M. Pretolani & B.B. Vargaftig). New York Academy of Sciences, New York (in press).

Robinson, D.S., Hamid, Q., Ying, S. *et al.* (1992) Predominant Th2-like bronchoalveolar T-lymphocyte population in atopic asthma. *New Engl. J. Med.*, **326**, 298–304.

Ryan, U.S. (1987) *Lung Biology in Health and Disease*, Vol. 32 *Pulmonary Endothelium in Health and Disease* (Series ed. C. Lenfant). Marcel Dekker, New York.

Saetta, M., Distefano, A., Rosina, C., Thiene, G. & Fabbri, L.M. (1991) Quantitative structural analysis of peripheral airways and arteries in sudden fatal asthma. *Am. Rev. Resp. Dis.*, **143**, 138–43.

Santamaria-Babi, L.F., Moser, R., Perez-Soler, M.T., Picker, L.J., Blaser, K. & Hauser, C. (1995) Migration of skin-homing T cells across cytokine-activated human endothelial cell layers involves interaction of the cutaneous lymphocyte-associated antigen (CLA), the very late antigen-4 (VLA-4), and the lymphocyte function-associated antigen-1 (LFA-1). *J. Immunol.*, **154**, 1543–50.

Schall, T.J., Bacon, K., Toy, K.J. & Goeddel, D.V. (1990) Selective attraction of monocytes and T-lymphocytes of the memory phenotype by cytokine RANTES. *Nature*, **347**, 669–71.

Schleimer, R.P., Sterbinsky, S.A., Kaiser, J. *et al.* (1992) IL-4 induces adherence of human eosinophils and basophils but not neutrophils to endothelium. Association with expression of VCAM-1. *J. Immunol.*, **148**, 1086–92.

Schweizer, R.C., Walmers, B.A.C., Raaijmakers, J.A., Zanen, P., Lammers, J.W.J. & Koenderman, L. (1994) RANTES and Interleukin 8 induced responses in normal human eosinophils: effects of priming with interleukin 5. *Blood*, **83**, 3697–704.

Seth, R., Raymond, F.D. & Makgoba, M.W. (1991) Circulating ICAM-1 isoforms: diagnostic propects for inflammatory and immune disorders. *Lancet*, **338**, 83–4.

Tanaka, Y., Adams, D.H., Hubscher, S., Hirano, H., Siebenlist, U. & Shaw, S. (1993) T cell adhesion induced by proteoglycan immobilized MIP-1β. *Nature*, **361**, 79–82.

Thornhill, M.H., Kyan-Aung, U. & Haskard, D.O. (1990) IL-4 increases human endothelial cell adhesiveness for T cells but not for neutrophils. *J. Immunol.*, **144**, 3060–5.

Walker, C., Rihs, S., Braun, R.K., Betz, S. & Bruijnzeel, P.L. (1993) Increased expression of CD11b and functional changes in eosinophils after migration across endothelial cell monolayers. *J. Immunol.*, **150**, 4061–71.

Wallaert, B., Janin, A., Lassalle, P. *et al.* (1994) Airway like inflammation of the salivary gland in bronchial asthma. *Am. J. Resp. Crit. Care Med.*, **150**, 802–9.

Walsh, G.M., Mermod, J.J., Hartnell, A., Kay, A.B. & Wardlaw, A.J. (1991a) Human eosinophil, but not neutrophil, adherence to IL-1-stimulated human umbilical vascular endothelial cells is alpha 4 beta 1 (very late antigen-4) dependent. *J. Immunol.*, **146**, 3419–23.

Walsh, L.J., Trinchieri, G., Waldorf, H.A., Whitaker, D. & Murphy, G.F. (1991b) Human dermal mast cells contain and release tumor necrosis factor α, which induces endothelial leukocyte adhesion molecule-1. *Proc. Nat. Acad. Sci. USA*, **88**, 4220–4.

Wardlaw, A. (1990) Leukocyte adhesion to endothelium. Review. *Clin. Exp. Immunol.*, **20**, 619–26.

Warringa, R.A.J., Koenderman, L., Kok, P.T.M., Kreukniet, J. & Bruijnzeel, P.L.B. (1991) Modulation and induction of eosinophil chemotaxis by granulocyte macrophage colony stimulating factor and IL-3. *Blood*, **77**, 2694–700.

Weg, W.B., Williams, T.J., Lobb, R.R. & Nourshargh, S. (1993) A monoclonal antibody recognizing very late activation antigen-4 inhibits eosinophil activation *in vivo*. *J. Exp. Med.*, **177**, 561–6.

Wegner, C.D., Gundel, R.H., Reilly, P., Haynes, N., Letts, L.G. & Rothlein, R. (1990) Intercellular adhesion molecule-1 (ICAM-1) in the pathogenesis of asthma. *Science*, **247**, 456–9.

Wegner, C.D., Torcellini, C.A., Clarke, C.C., Letto, L.G. & Gundel, R.H. (1991) Effects of single and multiple inhalations of antigen on airway responsiveness in monkeys. *J. Allergy Clin. Immunol.*, **87**, 835–41.

Wong, D.T., Weller, P.F., Galli, S.J. *et al.* (1990) Human eosinophils express transforming growth factor-α. *J. Exp. Med.*, **172**, 673–81.

Worthen, G.S., Lien, D.C., Tonnesen, M.G. & Hensen, P.M. (1987) Interaction of leukocytes with the pulmonary endothelium. In: *Pulmonary Endothelium in Health and Disease* (ed. U.S.R. Ryan), pp. 123–60. Marcel Dekker, New York.

Ying, S., Taborda-Barata, L., Meng, Q., Humbert, M. & Kay, A.B. (1995) The kinetics of allergen-induced transcription of messenger RNA for monocyte chemotactic protein-3 (MCP-3) and RANTES in the skin of human atopic subjects: relationship to eosinophil, T-cell and macrophage recruitment. *J. Exp. Med.*, **181**, 2153–9.

CHAPTER 17

Fibroblasts and Bronchial Asthma

W.R. Roche

Introduction

Bronchial asthma has recently been redefined as a chronic inflammatory disorder of the airways which is manifested clinically as episodic wheezing and altered bronchial reactivity (Barnes, 1989). This has highlighted the importance of cellular changes in the bronchial wall in the pathogenesis of the clinical disease state. The characteristic eosinophil-rich inflammatory cell infiltration of the airway wall which is associated with bronchial asthma has attracted much attention as the underlying mechanism for the reduction in airway calibre (Djukanovic *et al.*, 1990). However, the documentation of allergic-type inflammation in association with atopy alone (Bradley *et al.*, 1991; Djukanovic *et al.*, 1992) or with mild asthma in the absence of current symptoms (Beasley *et al.*, 1989) shows the need for careful evaluation of the direct role of inflammatory cell infiltration in the production of clinical disease.

Structural remodelling of the airway wall is currently regarded as a potential pathway through which inflammation may indirectly produce the physiological abnormalities that characterize asthma. These abnormalities in airway function in asthma may be divided into two arbitrary categories: the episodic reductions in airway calibre and the underlying abnormalities in baseline airway function and reactivity. The contribution of the structural cells of the airway wall to the pathogenesis of bronchial asthma must be considered under these headings, although this distinction is artificial and acute events and chronic alterations interact to produce the spectrum of clinical presentations that we know as asthma.

The persistent features of bronchial asthma include increased airway reactivity with loss of the normal plateau in the provocative dose–response curve. There is an increase in bronchial smooth muscle mass in asthma, due to the concomitant processes of hyperplasia and hypertrophy (Ebina *et al.*, 1993), but there is no consistent evidence of abnormalities in the response of the individual muscle cells. An alternative approch to understanding the role of airway remodelling uses a mathematical model of the human tracheobronchial tree (Wiggs *et al.*, 1992). This method allowed Wiggs *et al.* to reproduce the characteristic spirometric response to bronchial provocation in asthma by introducing a small reduction in lung recoil and thickening of the airway walls into the equation. Thickening of the walls of the more peripheral airways was of particular importance in enhancing the effect of smooth muscle contraction. The increase in airway wall thickness is likely to be at least partly responsible for the altered airway responses to a given dose of histamine or methacholine in asthma. Airway thickening internal to the smooth muscle can greatly exaggerate the effect of smooth muscle contraction on the airway calibre, while airway thickening external to the smooth muscle may make the airway refractory to the forces generated by pulmonary elastic recoil which help maintain patency of the airways.

Remodelling of the airway is also likely to be the mechanism of the exaggerated decline in pulmonary function associated with asthma (Peat *et al.*, 1987), and probably contributes to the development of fixed airway obstruction in patients with severe unremitting disease. Thus, any process which contributes to thickening of the walls of the conducting airways may be of considerable clinical importance in determining not only the degree of bronchial hyperreactivity but also its potentially fatal nature.

The structural components of the airway which undergo specific changes in asthma are the bronchial epithelium, the epithelial basement membrane and its associated mesenchymal cell population, the subepithelial vasculature, bronchial gland mass, smooth muscle and the extracellular matrix (Dunnill, 1960). All these structures may be involved in changes in the smaller bronchioles, except for the bronchial glands which are confined to the cartilaginous airways. The understanding of the composition and clinical importance of the extracellular matrix and fixed cell populations of the bronchi is less developed than the knowledge of the inflammatory cells in asthma. Nevertheless, the studies performed to date have already resulted in new findings and a revision of the paradigm of the pathogenesis of the tissue changes associated with bronchial asthma (Roche *et al.*, 1989). The components of the extracellular matrix are briefly reviewed below and their role in the disease state is then discussed.

Collagens

The collagens form the structural protein framework of the tissues, by forming large homopolymers and by interacting with other components of the extracellular matrix. Collagens contribute to the mechanical properties of the resultant matrix and provide it with many of the structural advantages of composite materials. The collagens derive their properties from two basic molecular motifs: the closely wound triple helix and globular 'non-collagenous' domains at one or both ends of the subunit chain (Chu *et al.*, 1990).

The collagens may be divided into two subfamilies: the fibrillar collagens, such as types I, II, III, V and XI, and the non-fibrillar collagens, including types IV, VI and VII. These distinctions are based on the ultrastructural appearances of fibrils formed by the staggered assembly of collagen triple helices. The fibrils are formed, after enzymatic cleavage of the C--and N-terminal peptides, by aggregation in the extracellular matrix in intimate contact with the parent cell. This classification has value in distinguishing between the major structural and functional roles of the collagens but cannot be regarded as absolute, as collagen fibrils may be heterogeneous in their composition and non-fibrillar collagens may be closely associated with the formation of collagen fibrils (Linsenmayer *et al.*, 1990).

The non-fibrillar collagens have helical domains of various lengths but retain their terminal peptides which are available for non-covalent and disulphide-bonded homopolymerization, and the binding of other collagen species, matrix components and cells. These collagen types are particularly associated with basement membranes (Fig. 17.1), where their greater molecular complexity and physical flexibility contribute to both structural and functional characteristics. Although a quantitatively small component of the interstitial compartment, they also contribute to molecular and cellular adhesive mechanisms in this site.

Basement membranes

The basement membranes beneath epithelia have a number of functions, including the provision of mechanical support for the overlying cells, permeability to nutrients and molecular sieving, anchorage of the epithelial cells and the underlying matrix, and signalling for cellular differentiation, migration and division (Martinez-Hernandez & Amenta, 1983). The structure of epithelial basement membranes is similar to that of vascular endothelium and of the basal lamina of smooth muscle and Schwann cells. Transmission electron microscopy demonstrates three layers in the basement membrane: two apparently homogeneous thin sheets, the lamina lucida immediately beneath the epithelium and the outer lamina densa and, external to these, fibrillar lamina reticularis, which is composed of condensed interstitial components (Fig. 17.2).

Type IV collagen forms the basic framework of the basement membrane by the formation of an open polygonal meshwork composed of collagen fibres polymerized at amino- and carboxy-terminals and by lateral associations (Abrahamson, 1987; Yurchenco, 1990). Tetramers can be formed by flexible linear collagen IV molecules joined at the N-terminals, initially by non-covalent bonds and subsequently by covalent and disulphide bond formation. The carboxy-terminal non-collagenous domains self-associate into dimers, which are also stabilized by disulphide bonds. These domains probably also determine the side-by-side bonding of collagen IV molecules involved in the production of laterally associated polymers (Yurchenco & Ruben, 1987).

Laminin is a large-molecular-weight species with multiple binding sites, which is important in the assembly of the basement membrane. This large glycoprotein (molecular mass *c.* 800 kDa) is an asymmetrical cruciate shape with one long arm. It is formed from three subunits, one A chain and two smaller B chains, which are joined by disulphide bonds (Sasaki *et al.*, 1988). Laminin aggregates into small polymers, which in turn form larger complexes in the presence of divalent cations. The bonds between ends of the arms of the molecule allow it to form an open lattice structure. This capacity to form homopolymers may be important in the formation of some basement membranes which are synthesized before collagen IV deposition. Separate sites on the laminin molecule bind heparin sulphate proteoglycans, entactin and collagen IV. Laminin is also

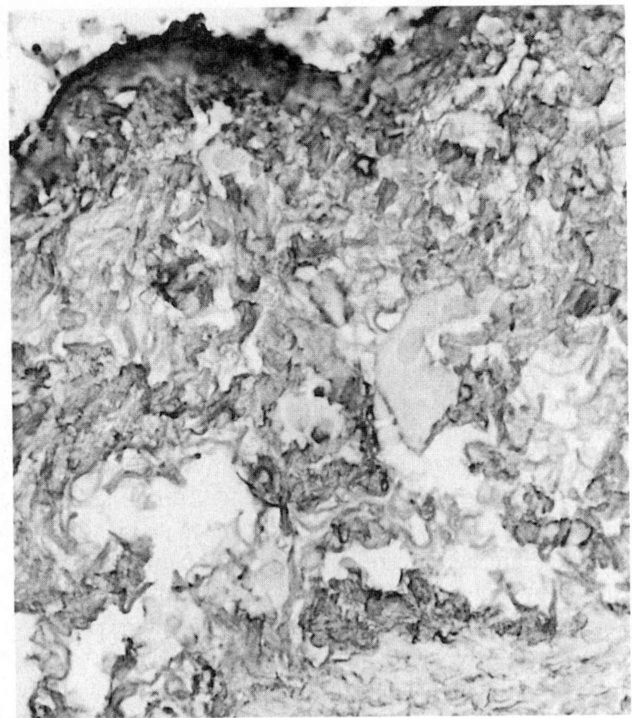
(a)

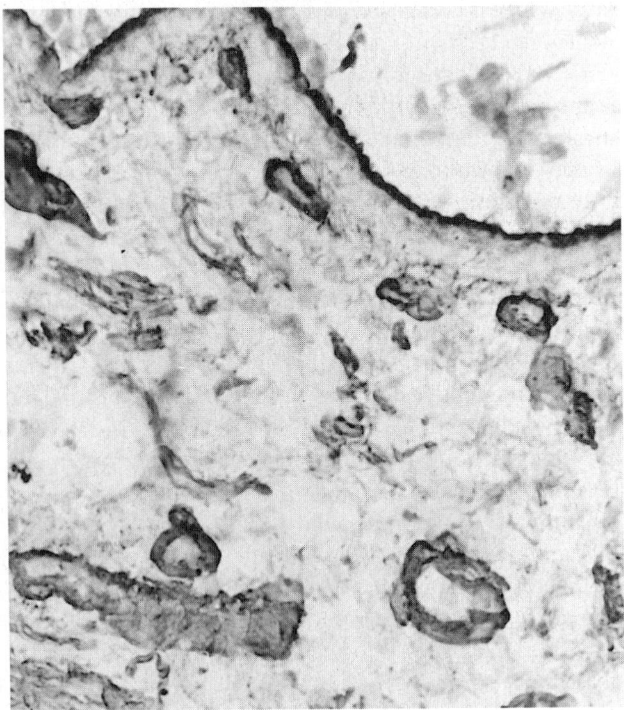
(b)

Fig. 17.1 Immunohistochemistry showing collagen III in the subepithelial zone and interstitium (a) and collagen IV confined to epithelial and vascular basement membranes (b) in bronchial tissue from an asthmatic subject. (Immunoperoxidase, H_2O_2/diaminobenzidine, ×720.)

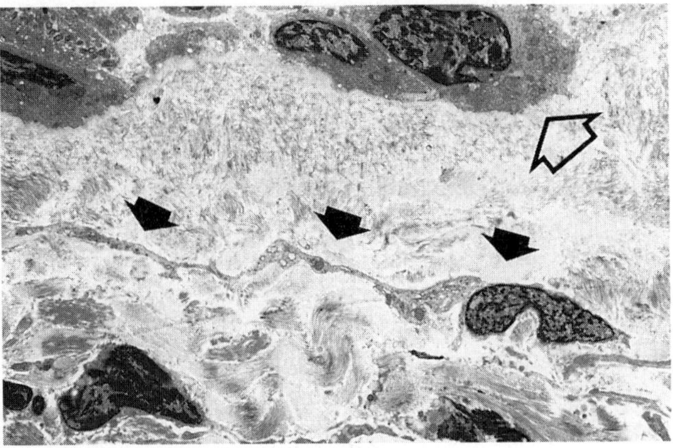

Fig. 17.2 Bronchial biopsy specimen from an asthmatic subject showing the lamina reticularis beneath the bronchial epithelium (open arrow) and a bronchial myofibroblast with a cytoplasm extending from the nucleus forming a thin layer (solid arrows) beneath the lamina reticularis. (Electron microscopy, uranyl acetate and lead citrate, ×5000.)

bound by integrin and non-integrin receptors on cell membranes, which are important for both cell structure and function (Beck *et al.*, 1990).

The basement membrane contains a heterogeneous group of other glycoproteins with adhesive and other properties. These include fibronectin, a large multispliced molecule which has domains for binding to cell membrane receptors, collagen and heparan sulphate proteoglycans (Hynes, 1985), and entactin or nidogen, a sulphated glycoprotein which binds to the central portion of the laminin molecule. Entactin also binds collagen IV and has an RDG (Arg-Gly-Asp) sequence which may allow it to be bound by cell-surface integrin molecules (Mann *et al.*, 1989). The proteoglycans of the basement membrane differ from the glycoproteins, in that the sugar molecules form linear chains of repeated disaccharide sequences bound to specific core proteins (Fransson *et al.*, 1986). These molecules have at least four roles in the basement membrane: the cross-linkage of basement membrane molecules including collagen, fibronectin, laminin and proteoglycans themselves; the determination of the electrical charge of the basement membrane by virtue of their highly anionic glycosaminoglycan chains; transmembrane receptors for cell adhesion and signal transduction; and as a repository for growth factors such as fibroblast growth factor and transforming growth factor-β (TGF-β) (Yamaguchi *et al.*, 1990). The glycosaminoglycan side chains of heparin and heparan sulphate are composed of repeated α1–4 linked L-iduronic acid *N*-acetylglucosamine disaccharides which are sulphated to varying degrees, by *N*-deacetylation yielding *N*-sulpho-D-glucosamine, *O*-sulphation of the uronic acid residues at C2 and of the glucosamine residues at C6 (Conrad,

1989). These chains are linked to the core protein by a galactosyl-galactosyl-xylosyl-serine linkage (Lindahl & Roden, 1966). Although the basic disaccharide repeats distinguish between the major glycosaminoglycan families, the variable lengths of side chains, sites and extent of sulphation and degree of epimerization to L-iduronic acid cause difficulty in subclassification of the molecular species.

In keeping with the stratified nature of the overlying bronchial epithelium (Evans *et al.*, 1989), the bronchial basement membrane is anchored to the underlying connective tissue by collagen VII fibres, similar to the arrangement found in skin (Wetzels *et al.*, 1991). Collagen VII is confined to the basement membranes of multilayered epithelia, probably reflecting the greater mechanical forces which these structures experience (Montefort *et al.*, 1992). In contrast, the basement membrane of the single-layered alveolar epithelium is devoid of collagen VII.

Extracellular matrix alterations in bronchial asthma

Early pathological studies of asthma fatalities showed a characteristic histological change of apparent thickening of the bronchial basement membrane (Dunnill, 1960). Studies based on tinctorial methods had indicated that the apparent basement membrane thickening did not involve the intrinsic basement membrane components but the significance of this was not appreciated (Crepea & Harman, 1955). More recently, examination by electron microscopy of biopsy material obtained from two children with asthma undergoing thoracotomy and from asthma fatalities, showed increased fibrillar collagen deposition in the lamina reticularis (Cutz *et al.*, 1978).

The application of electron microscopy and immunohistochemistry to endoscopic bronchial biopsy specimens, from subjects with mild atopic asthma and normal controls, confirmed the thickening of the lamina reticularis beneath the basement membrane (Roche *et al.*, 1989) (Figs 17.1 & 17.2). In normal subjects this layer measured 4 μm deep, while in subjects with mild asthma it extended to approximately twice that depth beneath the epithelium. This is an early event in asthma, occurring in patients with a short clinical history, in mild disease and in children (Cutz *et al.*, 1978). These appearances are not due to an increase in the basement membrane-specific proteins but are due to the deposition of interstitial collagens III and V, fibronectin and, to a lesser extent, collagen I, beneath the bronchial epithelial basement membrane (Roche *et al.*, 1989). Collagens type I, III and V, and fibronectin, were also detected in the lamina reticularis of normal subjects, suggesting that the alteration in asthma is a quantitative rather than a qualitative change. However, more recent studies have demonstrated the presence of abundant immunoreactivity for the glycoprotein tenascin in association with the lamina reticularis in asthma (Laitinen & Laitinen, 1994). This glycoprotein is expressed in embryonic organogenesis and in wound healing and is thought to play an important role in the regulation of epithelial–mesenchymal interactions and in modulation of cellular adhesion to the extracellular matrix. The presence of tenascin in asthma may be indicative of an important interaction between the bronchial epithelium and its underlying matrix.

The early appearance of sub-epithelial fibrosis in asthma was confirmed by study of subjects who had developed asthma after occupational exposure to toluene diisocyanate (Saetta *et al.*, 1992). Subjects with as little as 3 years' exposure and with symptoms for less than 1 year exhibited sub-epithelial collagen deposition. Allergen avoidance for 6 months induced a regression towards normal in the collagen thickness, although there was persistence of the bronchial inflammatory cell infiltrate. In contrast, inhaled corticosteroids reduce bronchial inflammation but appear not to affect the extent of sub-epithelial fibrosis (Jeffrey *et al.*, 1992).

The influence of excessive sub-epithelial collagen deposition on airway diameter and function is uncertain. Although decreased distensibility of the airway wall has been decribed *in vivo* (Wilson *et al.*, 1993), the relative contribution of components of the wall to this effect is uncertain. Studies of the smaller airways in autopsy lungs have shown that all compartments of the airway, including the adventitial tissue, are increased in asthma (Kuwano *et al.*, 1993). While the characteristic band of collagen beneath the epithelium of large bronchi may have little effect on airway resistance in the patent airway, the mechanical properties of this layer might lead to airway wall infolding and exaggerate the effects of smooth muscle contraction. Furthermore, this process extends to small bronchioles where it may contribute to airway thickening, which underlies the asthmatic response to inhaled provocants.

Bronchial myofibroblasts

The recognition of the apparent basement membrane thickening in asthma as the accumulation of interstitial collagens in the lamina reticularis led to the search for the origin of this material. Interstitial fibrillar collagens are usually deposited by fibroblasts and excessive production may occur in response to cytokines (Kovacs, 1991). The peculiar restriction of the fibrotic process to this layer suggested that either there was a specific directional stimulus for collagen deposition by the fibroblasts of the lamina propria, or that there was a unique cell population in association with the lamina reticularis.

The histological appearances of bronchial asthma share

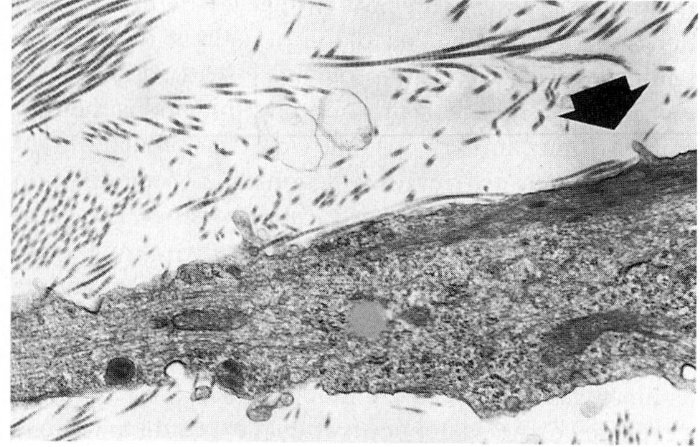

Fig. 17.3 Bronchial myofibroblast cytoplasm showing contractile filaments beneath the cell membrane and surrounding collagen fibrils. (Electron microscopy, uranyl acetate & lead citrate, ×20 000.)

some similarities with an uncommon bowel condition called collagenous colitis (Rams *et al.*, 1987). This condition is characterized by a dense band of fibrosis beneath the bronchial epithelium and a scattered infiltrate of eosinophil leucocytes. The collagens deposited are types I and III, and this is associated with ultrastructural evidence of activation of a unique fibroblast population (Hwang *et al.*, 1986). These cells are termed *pericryptal myofibroblasts* and are present in the intestine of normal subjects and at least some animals.

The term myofibroblast was coined to describe a cell found in the granulation tissue of healing wounds (Gabbiani *et al.*, 1971). These cells have features akin to both fibroblasts and smooth muscle. The synthetic capacity of the myofibroblast is reflected in the presence of numerous polyribosomes in its cytoplasm. The contractile forces which these cells exert are generated by arrays of thin filaments with focal densities in the cytoplasm, similar to those seen in smooth muscle (Fig. 17.3). These cells express, to a variable extent, cytoskeletal components normally associated with smooth muscle (Skalli *et al.*, 1989). Thus, immunohistochemistry may demonstrate the muscle-specific intermediate filament, desmin, and the smooth muscle-associated isotype of the contractile protein, actin (α-smooth muscle actin), as positive, singly or together, or negative in the cytoplasm of individual myofibroblasts.

The myofibroblasts of wound healing are thought to be derived from resident cells at the site of injury, although the mode of induction of this phenotype is uncertain (Sappino *et al.*, 1990). Constitutive myofibroblasts are also recognized. These cells apparently maintain their phenotype in the absence of inflammation or wound healing. In the rabbit intestine, the pericryptal cells form a self-renewing population, distinct from the colonic epithelium and other cells of the lamina propria (Pascal *et al.*, 1968). A monoclonal antibody, PR 2D3, raised to rectal tissue scrapings, was found to decorate these cells in the human colonic mucosa. This antibody appeared to react with a 140-kDa membrane protein, which was shared with smooth muscle cells (Richman *et al.*, 1987).

Ultrastructural analysis of bronchial biopsy specimens from normal and asthmatic subjects revealed thin cytoplasmic strands running parallel to and beneath the bronchial epithelium (Brewster *et al.*, 1990) (Figs 17.2, 17.3). Examination of multiple grids revealed that these cytoplasmic strands were extensions from cells with elongated, partially crenated nuclei, which lay in a horizontal plane beneath the epithelium. The collagen of the lamina reticularis was denser above these cells. The cytoplasm contained ribosomes and thin filaments with focal densities (Fig. 17.3), indicating that these cells were myofibroblasts. The cytoplasmic processes of these cells extend for up to 50 μm on either side of the nucleus and overlap without forming intercellular junctions, thus constituting a discontinuous cytoplasmic network through which inflammatory cells must pass in order to reach the bronchial epithelium. Others have subsequently described similar cells in the rat trachea (Evans *et al.*, 1993), and this network of cells may be analogous to the network of contractile interstitial cells in the alveolar septae (Adler *et al.*, 1989).

Myofibroblasts were present in the bronchial mucosa of both normal and asthmatic subjects. Immunohistochemical analysis showed that there was a median of five myofibroblasts per millimetre of epithelial basement membrane in normal subjects and eight per millimetre in asthmatics (Fig. 17.4). These numbers are consistent with the ultrastructural appearances of elongated sheets of cytoplasm in the region of 100 μm in diameter forming an overlapping myofibroblast layer beneath the bronchial epithe-

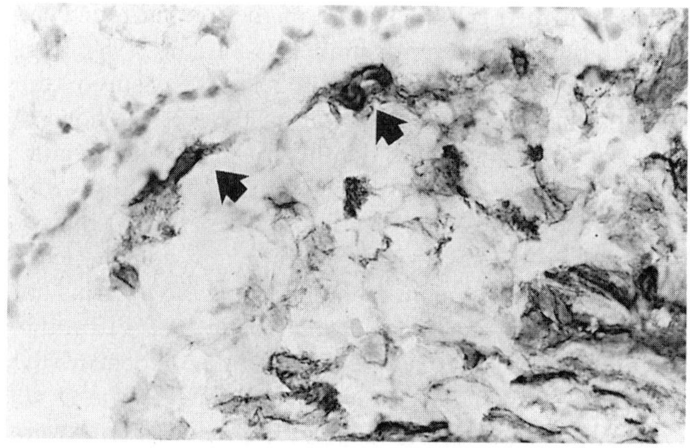

Fig. 17.4 Bronchial myofibroblasts beneath the lamina reticularis of the bronchial basement membrane in an asthmatic subject. (Monoclonal antibody PR 2D3, immunoperoxidase, H_2O_2/diaminobenzidine, ×1150.)

lium. The number of myofibroblasts in individual subjects correlated strongly with the depth of collagen beneath the bronchial epithelium, suggesting that the sub-epithelial myofibroblast is responsible for the synthesis of the interstitial collagens of the lamina reticularis (Brewster *et al.*, 1990).

Proliferative and fibrogenic cytokines in the airway

The increase in sub-epitheial myofibroblast numbers may be a reflection of the range of peptide and other mediators which are released in the bronchial mucosa in asthma. Fibroblast replication may be stimulated by a variety of factors which are potentially active in the bronchial mucosa, including: histamine (Norrby, 1980), mast cell heparin (Roche, 1985), mast cell tryptase (Ruoss *et al.*, 1991), interleukin-1 (IL-1) (Rupp *et al.*, 1986), IL-4 (Monroe *et al.*, 1988), platelet-derived growth factor (Shimokado *et al.*, 1985), fibroblast growth factor (Burgess & Maciag, 1989) and endothelin (Simonson *et al.*, 1989). These may be derived from the inflammatory cell infiltrate or from resident cell populations such as the bronchial epithelium or myofibroblasts themselves, in response to agents released during the inflammatory response.

The increase in sub-epithelial collagen in asthmatic subjects may be due to increased synthesis, decreased degradation of pro-collagens in the cytoplasm, or reduced proteolysis of extracellular collagen. A number of potentially fibrogenic cytokines which act to increase collagen synthesis may act in the bronchial mucosa. TGF-β is a potent stimulator of both collagen and fibronectin synthesis by fibroblasts (Ignotz & Massagné, 1986), and high levels of TGF-β have been reported in the airways (Yamauchi *et al.*, 1988). IL-4, which may be derived from T lymphoctes or mast cells, appears to be central to the immunological abnormalities and may also contribute to deposition of excessive amounts of collagen and fibronectin in the extracellular matrix (Gillery *et al.*, 1992). Similarly, mast cells have been shown to contain fibroblast growth factor (Qu *et al.*, 1995). This aspect of the cell biology of asthma is still largely unexplored and the relative contribution of individual cytokines is unknown.

Cellular signals from the extracellular matrix

Apart from the provision of mechanical support to the tissues, the extracellular matrix is increasingly recognized as functioning as a source of signals for cellular localization, migration, differentiation and activation. These signals may result from the interaction of specific cell-surface receptors with components of the matrix or from the exposure of bioactive molecules which have accumulated as complexes with matrix components. Extracellular matrix molecules can reorganize the actin cytoskeleton in fibroblasts which constitutively express β1 integrins, with the formation of focal contacts which link matrix glycoproteins, integrins, actin-binding proteins and the cytoskeleton (Turner & Burridge, 1991). β1 integrins are expressed as very late antigen (VLA) cell membrane proteins by T lymphocytes in response to activation signals. This allows the T lymphocyte to bind to cell-matrix components and this interaction may stimulate the secretion of cytokines and enhance lymphocyte responsiveness (Yamada *et al.*, 1991).

Similarly, the survival and function of eosinophil leucocytes is modulated by the presence of extracellular matrix components, such as fibronectin. Their secretion of superoxide radicals (O^{-}_2) in response to tumour necrosis factor, platelet-activating factor (PAF), lipopolysaccharide and substance P, has been shown to be inhibited by matrix components (Dri *et al.*, 1991). The expression of α4 β1 integrin by eosinophil leucocytes is one mechanism whereby the matrix may affect the responses of these important effector cells in asthma (Bochner *et al.*, 1991). Unlike many cell-surface receptors, the integrins do not possess protein kinase activity, as the intracellular signal transduction of many of the responses which are mediated or modulated by extracellular matrix involve phosphorylation steps, and the integrins must be capable of regulation of kinases. The localization of regulatory protein kinases at the intracellular sites of adhesion plaques may be one mechanism of this response (Schaller *et al.*, 1992). Conversely, intracellular events, such as the cell cycle, may modulate the adhesive functions of the cell membrane integrins by phosphorylation of either the α- or β-chain (Shaw *et al.*, 1990). Phosphorylation of integrins can also be induced by exposure to inflammatory cytokines and can enhance the adhesiveness of cells to the extracellular matrix, although phosphorylation is not universally required for activation of integrin-mediated adhesion.

The extracellular matrix may also play a role in the biology of the mast cell, which is one of the cells central to the pathogenesis of asthma. Mast cells exhibit different phenotypes in the tissues, as determined by their neutral protease expression. The mast cell found in skin and connective tissue contains both chymase and tryptase in its granules (MC_{TC}). These cells express α6 integrins and adhere to laminin, at least partially via a Ca^{2+}-dependent mechanism (Walsh *et al.*, 1991). Degranulated mast cells appear to lose their laminin receptors. Laminin has also been shown to be chemotactic for murine mast cells (Thompson *et al.*, 1989) and synthesis of laminin by mast cells has been reported (Thompson *et al.*, 1991). The interaction of mast cells with laminin may facilitate the recruitment of mast cells in some allergic disorders, such as atopic conjunctivitis. However, the modulation of adhesion to matrix may be more important in bronchial asthma and rhinitis, where there is no overall increase in mast cell number but mast cells both degranulate and migrate through the laminin-rich basement membrane into the bronchial epithelium.

The extracellular matrix also acts as a repository for growth factors, which are mainly bound to proteoglycans. The principal growth factors which are found in the matrix are basic fibroblast growth factor (FGF-2) (Folkman *et al.*, 1988) in basement membranes and TGF-β in the interstitium (Heine *et al.*, 1987). FGF-2 is an angiogenic and highly mitogenic growth factor with activity for a range of epithelial, mesenchymal and neural cells. It belongs to the heparin-binding family of fibroblast growth factors and its biological activity is potentiated by heparan sulphate proteoglycans which may protect FGF-2 from proteolytic degradation in the extracellular matrix (Salsela *et al.*, 1988). The stored FGF-2 in the matrix may be released by enzyme action and the free molecule may be bound by cell-surface proteoglycans. The latter alter the conformation of FGF-2, thus enhancing its interaction with high-affinity receptors (Prestrelski *et al.*, 1992). Similarly, the TGF-β receptors include a transmembrane proteoglycan, β-glycan (Andres *et al.*, 1991). TGF-β binds to the core protein of β-glycan and also to the core proteins of the small extracellular proteoglycans biglycan and decorin. These interstitial proteoglycans inhibit the biological activity of TGF-β and may have a therapeutic role in the control of abnormal matrix deposition (Border *et al.*, 1992).

The specialized fibroblast population beneath the bronchial epithelium may also be an important source of cytokines. Membrane appositions of eosinophil leucocytes and myofibroblasts are frequently observed in the bronchial mucosa (Fig. 17.1). This close contact may allow for the stimulation of the eosinophils by both high local concentrations of cytokines and direct cell–cell contact. T lymphocytes and mast cells also come into close contact with myofibroblasts before infiltrating the overlying epithelium. The cytokine repertoire of fibroblasts is large: chemotactic cytokines (Strieter *et al.*, 1989; Yoshimura *et al.*, 1989) include IL-8 and monocyte chemotactic factor; colony-stimulating factors (Vancheri *et al.*, 1989) such as granulocyte-macrophage colony-stimulating factor (GM-CSF) which is a potent priming and survival agent for eosinophils; lymphocyte activators such as IL-1 and IL-6 (Elias *et al.*, 1989; Elias & Reynolds, 1990); stem cell factor for mast cell proliferation, differentiation and migration (Nocka *et al.*, 1990); and scatter factor/hepatocyte growth factor for epithelial cell migration, growth and morphogenesis (Montesano *et al.*, 1991).

The expression of cytokines by fibroblasts is stimulated by cytokines, such as IL-1 and tumour necrosis factor-α (Elias & Reynolds, 1990), which are secreted by a range of inflammatory cells. This process may amplify a network of cytokine signals in the bronchial mucosa and contribute significantly to the characteristic inflammatory infiltrate in asthma. Fibroblasts grown from nasal polyp material have been shown to secrete higher levels of cytokines than those derived from normal nasal mucosa (Vancheri *et al.*, 1991), suggesting that their response to inflammatory messages is prolonged and that they may thereby sustain persistent inflammatory reactions long after allergen exposure. Furthermore, cell–cell interactions between fibroblasts and inflammatory effector cells, such as eosinophils, may enhance the effects of soluble cytokines alone. Murine 3T3 fibroblasts have been reported to produce a prolongation of the survival of human eosinophils in the presence of GM-CSF in excess of that obtained with GM-CSF alone (Owen *et al.*, 1987).

Conclusions

Fibroblasts act to produce clinically relevant abnormalities in the airways by alterations in the extracellular matrix, which is an important source of signals for cellular activation, and via structural changes involving the amount and relative distribution of components of the matrix. The specialized fibroblasts which exist beneath the bronchial epithelium appear to be involved in the characteristic alterations in the lamina reticularis beneath the bronchial epithelium in asthma. Although bronchial myofibroblasts cannot respond to specific allergens, the allergen-induced release of cytokines from cells bearing antigen receptors may stimulate the myofibroblast to secrete a wide range of pro-inflammatory cytokines. The position of these cells in the bronchial mucosa allows for local cytokine production, combined with matrix alterations, which may lead to the perpetuation of the process of allergic inflammation.

References

Abrahamson, D.R. (1987) Structure and development of the glomerular capillary wall and basement membrane. *Am. J. Physiol.*, **22**, F783–94.

Adler, K.B., Low, R.B., Leslie, K.O., Mitchell, I.J. & Evans, J.N. (1989) Contractile cells in normal and fibrotic lung. *Lab. Invest.*, **60**, 473–485.

Andres, J.L., Ronnstrand, L., Chiefetz, S. & Massagne, J. (1991) Purification of the transforming growth factor-β (TGF-β) binding proteoglycan β-glycan. *J. Biol. Chem.*, **266**, 23282–7.

Barnes, P.J. (1989) A new approach to the treatment of asthma. *New Engl. J. Med.*, **321**, 1517–27.

Beasley, R., Roche, W.R., Roberts, J.A. & Holgate, S.T. (1989) Cellular events in the bronchi in mild asthma and after bronchial provocation. *Am. Rev. Resp. Dis.*, **139**, 806–13.

Beck, K., Hunter, I. & Engel, J. (1990) Structure and function of laminin: anatomy of a multidomain glycoprotein. *FASEB J.*, **4**, 148–60.

Bochner, B.S., Luscinskas, F.W., Gimbrone, M.A. Jr *et al.* (1991) Adhesion of human basophils, eosinophils, and neutrophils to interleukin 1-activated human vascular endothelial cells: contributions of endothelial cell adhesion molecules. *J. Exp. Med.*, **173**, 1553–7.

Border, W.A., Noble, N.A., Yamamoto, T. *et al.* (1992) Natural inhibitor of transforming growth factor-β protects against scarring in experimental renal disease. *Nature*, **360**, 361–4.

Bradley, B.L., Azzawi, M., Jacobson, M. *et al.* (1991) Eosinophils, T-lymphocytes, mast cells, neutrophils and macrophages in bronchial biopsy specimens from atopic subjects with asthma: comparison with biopsy specimens from atopic subjects without asthma and normal control subjects and relationship to bronchial hyperresponsiveness. *J. Allergy Clin. Immunol.*, **88**, 661–74.

Brewster, C.E.P., Howarth, P.H., Djukanovic, R., Wilson, J.W., Holgate, S.T. & Roche, W.R. (1990) Myofibroblasts and subepithelial fibrosis in bronchial asthma. *Am. J. Respir. Cell Mol. Biol.*, **3**, 507–11.

Burgess, W.H. & Maciag, T. (1989) The heparin-binding (fibroblast) growth factor family of proteins. *Ann. Rev. Biochem.*, **58**, 575–606.

Chu, M.-L., Pau, T.-C., Conway, D. *et al.* (1990) Structure of type VI collagen. *Ann. NY Acad. Sci.*, **580**, 55–63.

Conrad, H.E. (1989) Structure of heparan sulphate and dermatan sulphate. *Ann. NY Acad. Sci.*, **556**, 18–28.

Crepea, S.B. & Harman, J.W. (1955) Pathology of bronchial asthma; significance of membrane changes in asthma and non-allergic pulmonary disease. *J. Allergy*, **26**, 453–60.

Cutz, E., Levison, H. & Coopr, D.M. (1978) Ultrastructure of airways in children with asthma. *Histopathology*, **2**, 407–21.

Djukanovic, R., Roche W.R., Wilson, J.W. *et al.* (1990) State of the art. Mucosal inflammation in asthma. *Am. Rev. Resp. Dis.*, **142**, 434–57.

Djukanovic, R., Lai, C.W.K., Wilson, J.W. *et al.* (1992) Bronchial mucosal manifestations of atopy: a comparison of markers of inflammation between atopic asthmatics, atopic non-asthmatics and healthy controls. *Eur. Resp.*, **5**, 538–44.

Dri, P., Cramer, R., Spessotto, P., Romano, M. & Patriarca, P. (1991) Eosinophil activation on biologic surfaces. Production of O^-_2 in response to physiologic soluble stimuli is differentially modulated by extracellular matrix components and endothelial cells. *J. Immunol.*, **147**, 613–20.

Dunnill, M.S. (1960) The pathology of asthma, with special references to changes in the bronchial mucosa. *J. Clin. Pathol.*, **13**, 27–33.

Ebina, M., Takakashi, T., Chiba, T. & Motomiya, M. (1993) Cellular hypertrophy and hyperplasia of airway smooth muscles underlying bronchial asthma. *Am. Rev. Resp. Dis.*, **148**, 720–6.

Elias, J.A. & Reynolds, M.M. (1990) Interleukin-1 and tumour necrosis factor synergistically stimulate lung fibroblast Interleukin-1α production. *Am. J. Respir. Cell Mol. Biol.*, **3**, 13–20.

Elias, J.A., Trinchieri, G., Beck, J.M. *et al.* (1989) A synergistic interaction of IL-6 and IL-1 mediates the thymocyte-stimulating activity produced by recombinant IL-1-stimulated fibroblasts. *J. Immunol.*, **142**, 509–14.

Evans, M.J., Cox, R.A., Shami, S.G., Wilson, B. & Plopper, C.G. (1989) The role of basal cells in attachment of columnar cells to the basal lamina of the trachea. *Am. J. Respir. Cell Mol. Biol.*, **1**, 463–9.

Evans, M.J., Guha, S.C., Cox, R.A. & Moller, P.C. (1993) Attenuated fibroblast sheath around the basement membrane zone in the trachea. *Am. J. Respir. Cell Mol. Biol.*, **8**, 188–92.

Folkman, J., Klagsbrun, M., Sasse, J., Wadziniski, M., Ingber, D. & Vodavsky, I. (1988) A heparin-binding angiogenic protein—basic fibroblastic growth factor—is stored within basement membrane. *Am. J. Pathol.*, **130**, 393–400.

Fransson, L.-A., Carlstedt, I., Coster, L. & Malmstrom, A. (1986) The functions of the heparan sulphate proteoglycans. *Ciba Found. Symp.*, **124**, 125–42.

Gabbiani, G., Ryan, G.B. & Majuo, G. (1971) Presence of modified fibroblasts in granulation tissue and their possible role in wound contraction. *Experientia*, **27**, 549–50.

Gillery, P., Fertin, C., Nicolas, J.F. *et al.* (1992) Interleukin-4 stimulates collagen gene expression in human fibroblast monolayer cultures. Potential role in fibrosis. *FEBS Letts.*, **302**, 231–4.

Heine, U.L., Flanders, K., Roberts, A.B., Munoz, E.F. & Sporn, M.B. (1987) Role of transforming growth factor-β in the development of the mouse embryo. *J. Cell Biol.*, **105**, 2861–76.

Hwang, W.S., Kelly, J.K., Shaffer, E.A. & Hershfield, N.B. (1986) Collagenous colitis, a disease of the pericryptal fibroblast sheath. *J. Pathol.*, **149**, 33–40.

Hynes, R.O. (1985) Molecular biology of fibronectin. *Ann. Rev. Cell Biol.*, **1**, 67–90.

Ignotz, R.A. & Massagné, J. (1986) Tranforming growth factor-β stimulates the expression of fibronectin and collagen and their incorporation into the extracellular matrix. *J. Biol. Chem.*, **261**, 4337–45.

Jeffrey, P.K., Godfrey, R.W., Adelroth, E., Nelson, F., Rogers, A. & Johansson, S.-A. (1992) Effects of treatment on airway inflammation and thickening of basement membrane reticular collagen in asthma. A quantitative light and electron microscopic study. *Am. Rev. Resp. Dis.*, **145**, 890–9.

Kovacs, E.J. (1991) Fibrogenic cytokines: the role of immune mediators in the development of scar tissue. *Immunol. Today*, **12**, 17–23.

Kuwano, K., Bosken, C.H., Pare, P.D., Bai, T.R., Wiggs, B.R. & Hogg, J.C. (1993) Small airways dimensions in asthma and chronic obstructive pulmonary disease. *Am. Rev. Resp. Dis.*, **148**, 1220–5.

Laitinen, L.A. & Laitinen, A. (1994) Structural and cellular changes in asthma. *Eur. Resp. Rev.*, **4**, 348–51.

Lindahl, U. & Roden, L. (1966) The chondroitin 4-sulphate-protein linkage. *J. Biol. Chem.*, **241**, 2113–19.

Linsenmayer, T.F., Fitch, J.M. & Birk, D.E. (1990) Heterotypic collagen fibrils and stabilizing collagens. Controlling elements in corneal morphogenesis. *Ann. NY Acad. Sci.*, **580**, 143–60.

Mann, K., Deutzmann, R., Aumailley, M. *et al.* (1989) Amino acid sequence of mouse nidogen, a multidomain basement membrane protein with binding activity for laminin, collagen IV and cells. *EMBO J.*, **8**, 65–72.

Martinez-Hernandez, A. & Amenta, P.S. (1983) The basement membrane in pathology. *Lab. Invest.*, **48**, 656–77.

Monroe, J.G., Haldar, S., Prystowsky, M.B. & Lammie, P. (1988) Lymphokine regulation of inflammatory processes: interleukin-4 stimulated fibroblast proliferation. *Clin. Immunol. Immunopathol.*, **49**, 292–8.

Montefort, S., Roberts, J.A., Beasley, R., Holgate, S.T. & Roche, W.R. (1992) The site of disruption of the bronchial epithelium in asthmatic and non-asthmatic subjects. *Thorax*, **47**, 499–503.

Montesano, R., Matsumoto, K., Nakamura, T. & Orci, L. (1991) Identification of fibroblast-derived epithelial morphogen as hepatocyte growth factor. *Cell*, **67**, 901–8.

Nocka, K., Buck, J., Levi, E., Tan, J. & Besmer, P. (1990) Candidate ligand for the *c-kit* transmembrane kinase receptor: KL, a fibroblast-derived growth factor stimulates mast cells and erythroid progenitors. *EMBO J.*, **9**, 3287–94.

Norrby, K. (1980) Mast cell histamine, a local mitogen acting via H_2 receptors in nearby tissue cells. *Virchows Arch. [B]*, **34**, 13–20.

Owen, W.F. Jr, Rothenberg, M.E., Silberstein, D.S. *et al.* (1987) Regulation of human eosinophil viability, density and function by granulocyte/macrophage colony-stimulating factor in the presence of 3T3 fibroblasts. *J. Exp. Med.*, **166**, 129–41.

Pascal, R.P., Kaye, G.I. & Lane, N. (1968) Colonic pericryptal fibroblast sheath replication, migration and cytodifferentiation of a mesenchymal cell system in adult tissue. I Autoradiographic studies of normal rabbit colon. *Gastroenterology*, **54**, 836–51.

Peat, J.K., Woolcock, A.J. & Culen, K. (1987) Rate of decline of lung function in subjects with asthma. *Eur. J. Resp. Dis.*, **70**, 171–9.

Prestrelski, S.J., Fox, F.M. & Arakawa, T. (1992) Binding of heparin to basic fibroblast growth factor induces a conformational change. *Arch. Biochem. Biophys.*, **293**, 314–19.

Qu, Z., Lieber, J.M., Powers, M.R. *et al.* (1995) Mast cells are a major source of fibroblast growth factor in chronic inflammation and cutaneous hemangioma. *Am. J. Pathol.*, **147**, 564–73.

Rams, H., Rogers, A.I. & Ghandur-Mnaymeh, L. (1987) Collagenous colitis. *Ann. Intern. Med.*, **106**, 108–13.

Richman, P.I., Tilly, R., Jass, J.R. & Bodmer, W.F. (1987) Colonic pericryptal sheath cells: characterisation of cell type with new monoclonal antibody. *J. Clin. Pathol.*, **40**, 593–600.

Roche, W.R. (1985) Mast cells and tumors. The specific enhancement of tumor proliferation *in vitro*. *Am. J. Pathol.*, **119**, 57–64.

Roche, W.R., Beasley, R., Williams, J.H. & Holgate, S.T. (1989) Subepithelial fibrosis in the bronchi of asthmatics. *Lancet*, **i**, 520–4.

Ruoss, S.J., Hartmann, T. & Caughey, G.H. (1991) Mast cell tryptase is a mitogen for cultured fibroblasts. *J. Clin. Invest.*, **88**, 493–9.

Rupp, E.A., Cameron, P.M., Ranawat, C.S., Schmidt, J.A. & Bayne, E.K. (1986) Specific bioactivities of monocyte derived interleukin-1α and interleukin-1β are similar to each other on cultured murine thymocytes and on cultured human connective tissue cells. *J. Clin. Invest.*, **78**, 836–9.

Saetta, M., Maestrelli, P., Di Stefano, A. *et al.* (1992) Effect of cessation of exposure to toluene diisocyanate (TDI) on bronchial mucosa of subjects with TDI-induced asthma. *Am. Rev. Resp. Dis.*, **145**, 169–74.

Salsela, O., Moscatelli, D., Sommer, A. & Rifkin, D.B. (1988) Endothelial cell-derived heparan sulfate binds basic fibroblast growth factor and protects it from proteolytic degradation. *J. Cell Biol.*, **107**, 743–751.

Sappino, A.P., Schürch, W. & Gabbiani, G. (1990) Differentiation repertoire of fibroblastic cells. Expression of cytoskeletal proteins as a marker of phenotypic modulations. *Lab. Invest.*, **63**, 144–61.

Sasaki, M., Kleinman, H.K., Huber, H., Deutzmann, R. & Yamada, Y. (1988) Laminin, a multidomain protein: the A chain has a unique globular domain and homology with the basement membrane proteoglycan and the laminin B chains. *J. Biol. Chem.*, **263**, 16536–44.

Schaller, M.D., Borgman, C.A., Cobb, B.S., Vines, R.R., Reynolds, A.B. & Parsons, J.T. (1992) PP125^{FAK}, a structurally distinctive protein tyrosine kinase associated with focal adhesions. *Proc. Nat. Acad. Sci. USA*, **89**, 5192–6.

Shaw, L.M., Messier, J.M. & Mercurio, A.M. (1990) The activation dependent adhesion of macrophages to laminin involves cytoskeletal anchoring and phosphorylation of the α6β1 integrin. *J. Cell Biol.*, **110**, 2167–74.

Shimokado, K., Raines, E.W., Madtes, D.K., Barrett, T.B., Benditt, E.P. & Ross, R. (1985) A significant part of macrophage-derived growth factor consists of at least two forms of PDGF. *Cell*, **43**, 277–86.

Simonson, M.S., Wann, S., Mene, P. *et al.* (1989) Endothelin stimulates phospholipase C, Na^+/H^+ exchange, *c-fos* expression, and mitogenesis in rat mesangial cells. *J. Clin. Invest.*, **83**, 708–12.

Skalli, O., Schürch, W., Seemayer, T. *et al.* (1989) Myofibroblasts from diverse pathological settings are heterogenous in their content of actin isoforms and intermediate filament proteins. *Lab. Invest.*, **60**, 275–85.

Strieter, R.M., Phan, S.H., Showell, H.J. *et al.* (1989) Monokine-induced neutrophil chemotactic factor gene expression in human fibroblasts. *J. Biol. Chem.*, **264**, 10621–6.

Thompson, H.L., Burbelo, P.D., Gabriel, G., Yamada, Y. & Metcalfe, D.D. (1991) Murine mast cells synthesize basement membrane components. A potential role in early fibrosis. *J. Clin. Invest.*, **87**, 619–23.

Thompson, H.L., Burbelo, P.D., Yamada, Y., Kleinman, H.K. & Metcalfe, D.D. (1989) Mast cells chemotax to laminin with enhancement after IgE-mediated activation. *J. Immunol.*, **143**, 4188–92.

Turner, C.E. & Burridge, K. (1991) Transmembrane molecular assemblies in cell–extracellular matrix interactions. *Curr. Opin. Cell Biol.*, **3**, 849–53.

Vancheri, C., Gauldie, J., Bienenstock, J. *et al.* (1989) Human lung fibroblast-derived granulocyte-macrophage colony stimulating factor (GM-CSF) mediates eosinophil survival *in vitro*. *Am. J. Respir. Cell Mol. Biol.*, **1**, 289–95.

Vancheri, C., Ohtoshi, T., Cox, G. *et al.* (1991) Neutrophilic differentiation induced by human upper airway fibroblast-derived granulocyte/macrophage colony-stimulating factor (GM-CSF). *Am. J. Respir. Cell Mol. Biol.*, **4**, 11–17.

Walsh, L.J., Kaminer, M.S., Lazarus, G.S., Lavker, R.M. & Murphy, G.F. (1991) Role of laminin in localization of human dermal mast cells. *Lab. Invest.*, **65**, 433–40.

Wetzels, R.H.W., Robben, H.C.M., Leigh, I.M., Schaafsura, H.E., Vooijs, G.P. & Ramaekers, F.C.S. (1991) Distribution pattern of type VII collagen in normal and malignant human tissues. *Am. J. Pathol.*, **139**, 451–9.

Wiggs, B.R., Bosken, C., Pare, P.D., James, A. & Hogg, J.C. (1992) A model of airway narrowing in asthma and in chronic obstructive pulmonary disease. *Am. Rev. Resp. Dis.*, **145**, 1251–8.

Wilson, J.W., Li, X. & Pain, MCF. (1993) The lack of distensibility of asthmatic airways. *Am. Rev. Resp. Dis.*, **148**, 806–9.

Yamada, A., Nojima, Y., Sugita, K., Dang, N.H., Schlossman, S.F. & Morimoto, C. (1991) Cross-linking of VLA/CD29 molecule has a co-mitogenic effect with anti-CD3 on CD4 cell activation in serum-free culture system. *Eur. J. Immunol.*, **21**, 319–25.

Yamaguchi, Y., Mann, D.M. & Ruoslathi, E. (1990) Negative regulation of transforming growth factor-β by the proteoglycan decorin. *Nature*, **346**, 281–4.

Yamauchi, K., Martinet, Y., Busset, P., Fells, G.A. & Crystal, R.G. (1988) High levels of tranforming growth factor-β are present in the epithelial lining of the normal lower respiratory tract. *Am. Rev. Resp. Dis.*, **137**, 1360–3.

Yoshimura, T., Yuhki, N., Moore, S.K., Appella, E., Lerman, M.I. & Leonard, E.J. (1989) Human monocyte chemoattractant protein-1 (MCP-1). Full length c-DNA cloning, expression in mitogen-stimulated blood mononuclear leukocytes, and sequence similarity to murine competence gene JE. *FEBS Letts.*, **244**, 487–93.

Yurchenco, P.D. (1990) Assembly of basement membrane. *Ann. NY3 Acad. Sci.*, **580**, 195–213.

Yurchenco, P.D. & Ruben, G.C. (1987) Basement membrane structure *in situ*: evidence for lateral associations in the type IV collagen network. *J. Cell Biol.*, **105**, 2559–68.

CHAPTER 18

Complement and Antigen–Antibody Complexes

W.J. Schwaeble & K. Whaley

Introduction

The complement system comprises a group of 22 plasma proteins with an associated group of cell-membrane proteins which act as receptors for activation peptides of the plasma system and/or are regulators of complement activation. The system is activated by contact with bacteria and other micro-organisms, tissue breakdown products and antigen–antibody (Ag/Ab) complexes. Activation leads to the assembly of multimolecular enzymes that activate the third (C3) and the fifth (C5) complement components. The plasma system may be activated by either of two pathways, the classical and the alternative, as a result of which multimolecular enzymes that activated C3 and C5 are generated. Activated C3 (C3b) binds to the surface of micro-organisms and other activators and promotes their phagocytosis and killing by neutrophils and macrophages. Following activation of C5 the cytolytic membrane attack complex (MAC), consisting of activated C5 (C5b), C6, C7, C8 and C9, is generated (reviewed in Law & Reid, 1988; Weiler, 1993). During complement activation a number of biological activities are generated. These include the pro-inflammatory peptides (anaphylatoxins) C4a, C3a and C5a, which are released from the N termini of the α-chains of C4, C3 and C5, C3b and iC3b (factor I cleaved, inactivated C3b) which are involved in neutrophil activation and the MAC which at sublethal concentrations will activate inflammatory cells to release inflammatory mediators. Covalent binding of C4b and C3b (opsonization) is important for the phagocytosis of micro-organisms, retaining Ag/Ab complexes in solution or for solubilizing insoluble Ag/Ab complexes. In addition to the cytolytic pro-inflammatory and opsonic activities, there is evidence that complement peptides C3a, C5a, C3dg/C3d and C3e have immunoregulatory activities (Law & Reid, 1988).

Nomenclature

Classical and terminal complement components are designated by a number prefixed by a letter. The first four components are numbered C1, C4, C2, C3. They are numbered in the order of their discovery, not their position in the reaction sequence. Components of the alternative pathway are designated by letters (factors B, P, D). Cleavage fragments are indicated by a suffixed lower case letter (e.g. C3a and C3d are fragments of C3). Enzymatically inactivated C3b is iC3b, whereas fluid-phase C3b, which has lost its ability to bind to surfaces due to hydrolysis of its internal thiolester group, is called C3bi. Peptide chains of complement components are suffixed by a Greek letter as C4α, C4β and C4γ, the α-chain being the largest and the γ-chain the smallest. C3 receptors are CR1, CR2, CR3 and CR4 and have been assigned CD numbers, as have other membrane complement regulatory proteins (e.g. CD46, CD59). Table 18.1(a) lists the components of the classical and alternative pathway and the membrane attack complex, as well as the regulatory protein, membrane proteins and complement receptors (Table 18.1(b)) known as of 1995.

Table 18.1(a) Serum proteins.

Component	Serum concentration (μg/ml)	M_r	Chain structure	Cleavage fragments	Biological activities
Classical pathway					
Clq	70–300	460 000	18 (6 × 3)	—	Binds to antibody and other activators
Clr	34–100	83 000	1	—	Activates Cls
Cls	30–80	85 000	1	—	Activates C4 and C2
C4	350–600	204 000	3	C4a	Anaphylatoxin
				C4b	Binds covalently to membrane Binds to C2
				C4c	
				C4d	
C2	15–30	102 000	1	C2a	Enzymatic site of C4b2a Binds to C4b
				C2b	Binds to C4b
Alternative pathway					
B	140–240	1000 000	1	Ba	Chemotactic
				Bb	Enzymatic site of C3bBb
P	20–30	56 500	4	—	Stabilizes C3bBb
D	1–2	24 000	1	—	Cleaves B to Ba and Bb
Third component					
C3	1299–1500	190 000	2	C3a	Anaphylatoxin
				C3b	Part of alternative pathway Part of C5 convertase Interacts with CR1 (CD35) Solubilization of Ag/Ab complexes Opsonic fragment
				C3d, C3d, g	Interacts with CR2 (CD21)
				'C3e', C3d-K	Leucocytosis
				C3f	
Terminal pathway or membrane attack complex (MAC)					
C5	70–85	196 000	2	C5a	Anaphylatoxin, chemotaxis
				C5b	Formation of MAC
C6	60–70	125 000	1	—	Part of MAC
C7	55–70	120 000	1	—	Part of MAC
C8	55–80	150 000	3	—	Part of MAC
C9	50–160	66 000	1	—	Part of MAC
Control					
C1 inhibitor (C1-INH)	180–275	105 000	1	—	Stoichiometric inhibitor of C1
C4 binding protein (C4bp)	250	550 000	7	—	Cofactor for factor I in C4b degrading, decay of C4b2a
Factor H	300–560	150 000	1	—	Cofactor for factor I in C3b degradation, decay of C3bBb
Factor I	34–50	100 000	2	—	Degrades C3b and C4b
Anaphylatoxin inactivator	35	310 000	—	—	Inactivates C3a and C5a to $C3a_{desarg}$ and $C5a_{desarg}$
S protein (vitronectin)	150–500	83 000	—	—	Controls membrane insertion of MAC

Table 18.1(b) Receptor proteins.

Membrane receptor	M_r	Chain structure	Primary ligand(s)	Biological activities	Primary cellular location
CR1 (CD35)	160 000–250 000	1	C3b, C4b	Ag/Ab complex transport	Monocytes, RBC, B cells
CR2 (CD21)	140 000	1	C3d, C3dg, iC3b	B-cell regulation	B cells
			Adherence		Monocytes, PMN
CR3 (CD11b/CD18)	265 000	2	iC3b		Macrophages
CR4	260 000	1	C3dg		Platelets
cC1qR	56 000	1	Collagenous region of aggregated C1q	Unknown	Monocytes
gC1qR	33 000	1	'Globular heads' of C1q	Unknown	Monocytes, B cells, T cells, PMN
Decay accelerating factor (DAF, CD55)	70 000	1	C4b2a, C3bBb	Decay of convertase	RBC, platelets
Membrane cofactor protein cMCP,CD46	45 000–70 000	1	C3b, C4b	1	PMN, monocytes
C3a receptor	?	?	C3a, C4a?	Mast cell degranulation	PMN, mast cells?
C5a receptor	45 000	1	C5a, $C5a_{desarg}$?	Mast cell degranulation	PMN, mast cells? monocytes, platelets
Homologous restriction factor (HRF)	65 000	1	C8, C9	Homologous lysis	RBC
CD59	19 000	1	C8, C9	Homologous lysis	Monocytes, RBC, T cells

RBC, red blood cells; PMN, polymorphonucleocytes.

The classical pathway of complement activation

Components

The first component of complement (C1) is composed of three subunits, the subcomponent C1q (460 kDa) and the pro-enzymes C1r and C1s (found as a Ca^{2+}-dependent 360-kDa $C1r_2C1s_2$ complex). The C1q subcomponent is a hexameric macromolecule with six globular heads linked via six collagen-like stalks to a fibril-like central region (Law & Reid, 1988) formed out of 18 polypeptide chains (six A-, six B- and six C-chains). Each of the three different chains of C1q is approximately 225 amino-acid residues long with an N-terminal collagen-like region and a C-terminal globular region. The pro-enzymes C1r and C1s are single chains of approximately 83 kDa which are activated by the splitting of a single peptide bond, in both cases, to yield non-catalytic α-chains of approximately 56 kDa, disulphide bonded to catalytic β-chains of approximately 27 kDa.

C2 and C4 are the constituents of the classical pathway convertase. C4 is a heterotrimeric glycoprotein (C4a, C4β, C4γ) of approximately 200 kDa, formed from a single precusor molecule (pro-C4) by post-translational modification. Pro-C4 is encoded by an mRNA species of 5.5 kb and the order of the chains in the precursor (NH_2-β-α-γ-COOH) was later confirmed by nucleotide sequence analysis of the cDNA for C4 and amino-acid sequencing of biosynthetically labelled C4 (Goldberger & Colton, 1980).

The α-chain of C4 contains an internal thiolester bond which is essential for the covalent binding of activated C4 (C4b) to targets of complement activation. C4 in plasma comprises the products of two C4 gene loci, C4A and C4B. The amino-acid differences between C4A and C4B lie in the thiolester-containing region of the α-chain and regulate the covalent binding reaction. Thus, C4A is more effective at forming amide bonds than C4B, while C4B may be slightly more effective at forming ester bonds than C4A (Dodds *et al.*, 1985; Carroll *et al.*, 1990).

C2 is a single-chain zymogen of 102 kDa. The serine protease domain is located at the C-terminal portion of the molecule and contributes the enzymatically active site in the C4b2a complex, the C3 convertase of the classical pathway.

C3 is a dimeric glycoprotein of 190 kDa composed of a disulphide-linked α-chain (120 kDa) and β-chain (70 kDa), both formed from a single-chain precursor which is encoded by an mRNA of 5.2 kb. Like C4, the α-chain of C3 contains an internal thiolester bond which is important for the covalent binding of activated C3 (C3b) to targets of complement activation.

Activation of the classical pathway

The classical pathway is activated when Ag–Ab complexes containing immunoglobulin G (IgG) (subclasses IgG1, IgG2 and IgG3) or IgM antibody interact with the first component (C1). Each of the globular heads of C1q can bind to the Fc region of immunoglobulin, the CH2 domain of IgG, or the CH3 domain of IgM, but multivalent attachment of C1q is required for C1 activation. In solution, IgM exists as a pentameric, planar molecule to which C1q binds weakly. Once a molecule of IgM antibody binds to a multivalent antigen it assumes a 'staple' conformation which allows at least two C1q heads to bind to separate Fc pieces. Thus, a single pentameric IgM molecule is sufficient to activate C1. Natural antibodies are of the IgM class and are therefore extremely efficient complement activators. As IgG is monomeric, at least two molecules are required to cross-link the globular heads of C1q and activate C1. On particulate antigens several thousand IgG molecules may have to bind to ensure that two are within 40 nm of each other to form a stable binding site for C1q. Therefore, on particulate antigens, IgG antibody is a far less efficient complement activator than IgM. When IgG binds to soluble antigens, complexes formed at equivalence or in the zone of slight antibody excess are better activators of C1 than those formed in antigen excess or marked antibody excess, again because at this ratio the IgG molecules are closest together.

Following binding to antibody, C1q undergoes a conformational change, which results in activation of C1r. It is thought that one molecule of C1r in the tetramer activates the other C1r by proteolysis. Activated C1r has one natural substrate, C1s, which is converted to its proteolytically active form as a result of a single proteolytic cleavage. Activated C1s, the active 'extrovert' enzyme of C1, has two natural substrates, C4 and C2. Activated C1s cleaves a 6-kDa fragment, C4a, from the amino-terminus of the α-chain of C4, and an internal thiolester bond in the a'-chain of the major product C4b is exposed (Fig. 18.1). This thiolester links the sulphydryl group of the cysteine in position 991 to the carbonyl group of a glutamine residue in position 994. Nucleophilic attack of the thiolester bond by exposed hydroxyl groups or amino groups on nearby surfaces results in the formation of ester or amide bonds, respectively. Thus, for a few microseconds, nascent C4b with an exposed thiolester is able to bind covalently to targets. C4b which does not form ester or amide bonds within this period loses its binding site, as the thiolester reacts with water to become inactive fluid-phase C4b in which the thiolester becomes hydrolysed and the residue corresponding to 994 becomes glutamate.

C2 binds to C4b in a Mg^{2+}-dependent reaction to form a pro-convertase, before being cleaved by activated C1s into C2b, which bears the original C4b binding site, and C2a which develops a binding site for C4b and also expresses serine protease activity. The C4b2a complex is the classical pathway C3 convertase which cleaves the α-chain of C3 to release a 9-kDa fragment, C3a, from the amino-terminus and exposes an internal thiolester bond in the α-chain of C3b. As with C4b, the thiolester becomes the subject of nucleophilic attack and forms covalent ester and amide

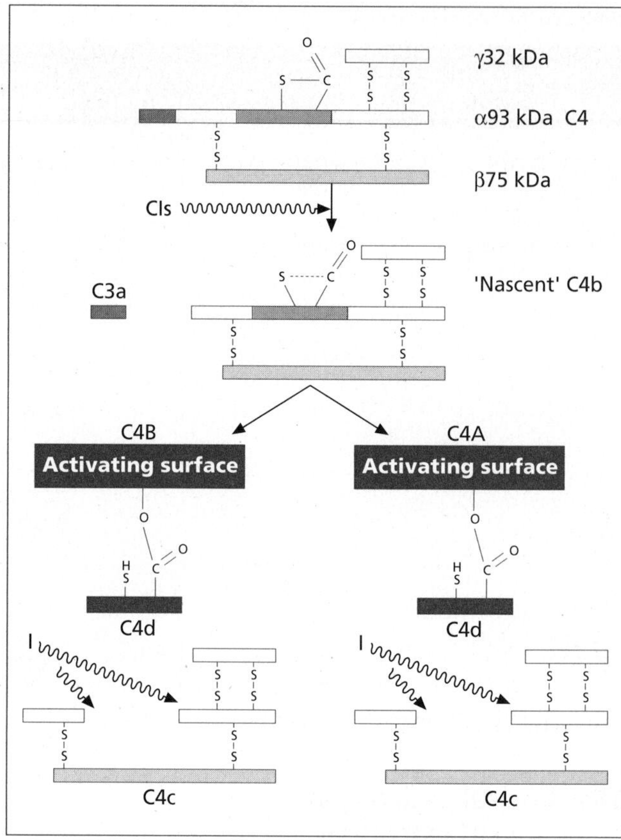

Fig. 18.1 Activation of C4 by C1s involves cleavage of the N terminus of the α-chain to release C4a (6 kDa). A thiolester bond in the α-chain of C4b reacts with hydroxyl groups to form ester bonds or amino groups to form amide bonds. Although both C4A and C4B can form either type of bond, C4A has a greater propensity to form amide bonds than C4B. Thus, C4a is shown as forming amide bonds and C4B as forming ester bonds. Inactivation of C4b occurs by enzymatic attack of factor I and a cofactor (C4bp or membrane cofactor protein) to release C4c and leave C4d bound to the target. Disulphide bridges are shown schematically.

bonds with surface hydroxyl or amino groups; respectively usually ester bonds are formed. Only a small proportion (up to 10%) of C3 binds covalently to a complement-activating surface. The thiolester of the majority of the activated C3 reacts with water, so that inactive fluid-phase C3b is formed. Some C3 binds to C4b in C4b2a and acts as a receptor for C5. This complex, C4b2a3b, is the classical pathway C5 convertase. C5 binds to C3b in the C5 convertase and C2a cleaves the C5 α-chain to release a 12-kDa peptide, C5a, from the amino-terminus of C5 and the major cleavage product, C5b is available for the assembly of the cytolytic membrane attack complex. The activation sequence of the classical pathway is summarized in Fig. 18.2.

The classical pathway can also be activated in the absence of antibody or Ag/Ab complexes. C-reactive

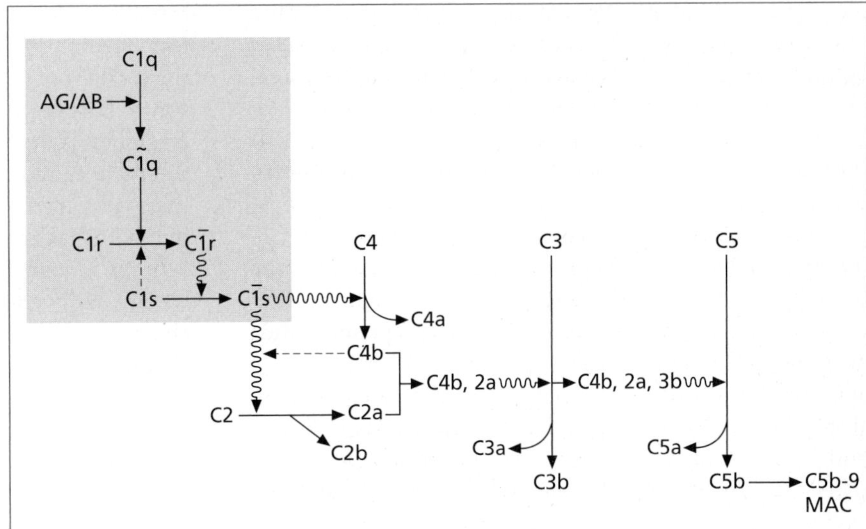

Fig. 18.2 Classical pathway activation by antigen–antibody complexes. The shaded area represents the processes involved in the activation of C1. The dashed arrow indicates the facilitation of C1s-mediated activation of C2 by C4b. (From Whaley, 1987.)

protein (CRP), an acute-phase reactant, binds to bacterial capsular polysaccharides to form a C1-activating particle (Claus *et al.*, 1977). Serum CRP levels increase dramatically during the early phase of infection due to cytokine-stimulated hepatic synthesis. This mechanism plays an important role in host defence during the early stages of the humoral immune response. Certain viruses (Cooper *et al.*, 1976) and Gram-negative bacteria (Cias & Loos, 1987) can bind and activate C1 directly, while Gram-positive bacteria will only activate the classical pathway when antibacterial antibody is present (Cias & Loos, 1987). Mitochondria will bind C1 and activate the classical pathway (Giclas *et al.*, 1979). It has been suggested that such complement activation is important in the pathogenesis of tissue injury following myocardial infarction (Yashuda *et al.*, 1990). It has recently become clear that another route of complement activation exists, distinct from the accepted knowledge of activation of the classical or alternative pathways. The serum collectin, mannose-binding lectin (MBL) binds to mannose- or glucosamine-rich surfaces, and activates complement (Lu *et al.*, 1990). MBL is similar in overall shape to C1q, and consists of six globular heads, linked together by collagenous helices. In MBL, each globular head contains three C-type lectin domains, which bind to carbohydrate structures on yeasts, bacteria and viruses. Further studies showed that MBL appeared to act very similarly to C1q, in that purified MBL, bound via its lectin domains to a suitable target, can bind and activate C1r and C1s. More recent work, however, has indicated that in physiological conditions, MBL is likely to activate complement not via C1r and C1s, but via one or more distinct proteases, which are homologous to C1r and C1s. These proteases are known as MASPs (MBL-associated serine proteases). Human MASP-1 has been sequenced at the cDNA level, and is highly homologous to C1r or C1s (including an identical mosaic domain structure). Activated MASP-1, like C1s, cleaves C2 and C4, and it has also been reported to cleave C3 directly at a low rate (Matsushita & Fujita, 1995). MASP-1 forms complexes with C1-inh, and is also reported to interact with the protease α2-macroglobulin, but the latter is unlikely to be physiologically relevant (M. Matsushita, personal communication). The mechanism of complement activation by MBL thus appears to be similar in mechanism to C1q-C1r-C1s interaction. The C1r-C1s complex has, however, a defined stoichiometry of 2C1r + 2C1s, and the mechanism by which C1r and C1s appear to be activated requires the interaction of several protease molecules with 1 C1q molecule. If MASP-1 is the only protease associated with MBL, it is difficult to envisage how a fixed MBL : protease stoichiometry of 1 : 4 could be achieved. MASP-1 alone could not form a tetramer to resemble the C1r2-C1s2 complex. It is likely, therefore, that another protease exists, which may be an equivalent of C1r.

A second related protease, MASP-2 has been identified (Thiel *et al.*, 1995). A partial peptide sequence of MASP-2 has been established and cDNA clones for MASP-2 were isolated using randomized oligonucleotides derived from these peptide sequences. We have cloned the entire coding sequence for MASP-2 from 3 different human liver cDNA libraries. The derived peptide sequence of 622 amino acids is very similar to C1r, MASP-1 and C1s, with C1r showing the highest degree (>75%) of homology (W.J. Schwaeble, unpublished observations).

Regulation of the classical pathway

Classical pathway activation is localized by the binding of

antibody to target antigen and the extreme lability of the thiolester bonds of C4b and C3b, which focuses subsequent activation of the cascade onto the site of initial interaction with C1. The short half-lives (approximately 90 seconds at 37°C) of the C3 and the C5 convertases also limit complement activation. In addition, there are a series of plasma and membrane proteins which regulate complement activation. C1 activation is regulated by C1-inhibitor, which is a classical serine protease inhibitor (SERPIN) and binds covalently to the active sites of the C1r and C1s subcomponents of C1 and so prevents further activation of C4 and C2 (Harpel & Cooper, 1975).

C1 inhibitor, a 105-kDa glycoprotein, regulates the classical pathway by binding stoichiometrically (1:1) to C1r and C1s, leading to permanent inactivation of these proteins. During enzyme–inhibitor interaction, C1 inhibitor is cleaved at the C-terminal end and a covalent bond is formed between enzyme and inhibitor (He *et al.*, 1996).

C1 inhibitor acts as a 'false' substrate, becomes cleaved by the enzyme and forms an acyl intermediate. The covalently linked C1r–C1s–C1 inhibitor complex (molar ratio 1:1:2) dissociates from the C1 complex, leaving C1q bound to the Ag–Ab complex. C1 inhibitor also acts as an inhibitor of a number of proteases generated during activation of the Hageman factor-dependent pathways.

Classical pathway activation is also controlled by C4 binding protein (C4bp), a macromolecule of 550 kDa formed out of six α-chains (70 kDa) and one β-chain (45 kDa). It regulates the classical pathway by disassembling the C4b2a complex and prevents binding of C2 to C4b and acts as a cofactor for factor I in the inactivation of C4b. The α′-chain of C4b is cleaved twice to release C4c into the fluid phase, leaving C4d covalently attached to the surface. Thus, assembly of C4bC2a is restricted. C4bp also binds to C4b which is part of C4b2a, and increases the rate of decay in this already very unstable enzyme.

The serine protease factor I is a dimeric glycoprotein of 100 kDa which regulates complement activation by cleaving C3b and C4b, thus converting them to haemolytically inactive forms. The factor I precursor peptide is a single-chain molecule encoded by a 2.4-kb mRNA (Catterall *et al.*, 1987).

Three membrane proteins, decay accelerating factor (DAF), membrane cofactor protein (MCP) and complement receptor type 1 (CR1), are the principle regulators of the expression of C3 and C5 convertases on host cells. CR1 possesses both cofactor and decay accelerating activities.

C3 degradation

Membrane-bound C3b can be inactivated slowly by factor I, but a rapid and effective inactivation requires the binding of cofactors like factor H or the membrane cofactors CR1 or MCP. In the presence of any one of these cofactors, factor I produces two closely adjacent cleavages in the α-chain of C3b, releasing a fragment of 3 kDa (Harrison & Lachmann, 1980; see Fig. 18.3). The residual iC3b fragment is functionally different from C3b. The iC3b fragment cannot interact with factor B to form the alternative pathway C3 convertase, nor can it recognize C5, so that both classical and alternative pathway C5 convertase activity is lost. Binding to CR1 is also greatly reduced when C3b is converted to iC3b. iC3b consists of two α-chain fragments (68 kDa and 43 kDa) and the intact β-chain. A further cleavage of the α-chain is produced, possibly by factor I using CR1 as its cofactor (Medof

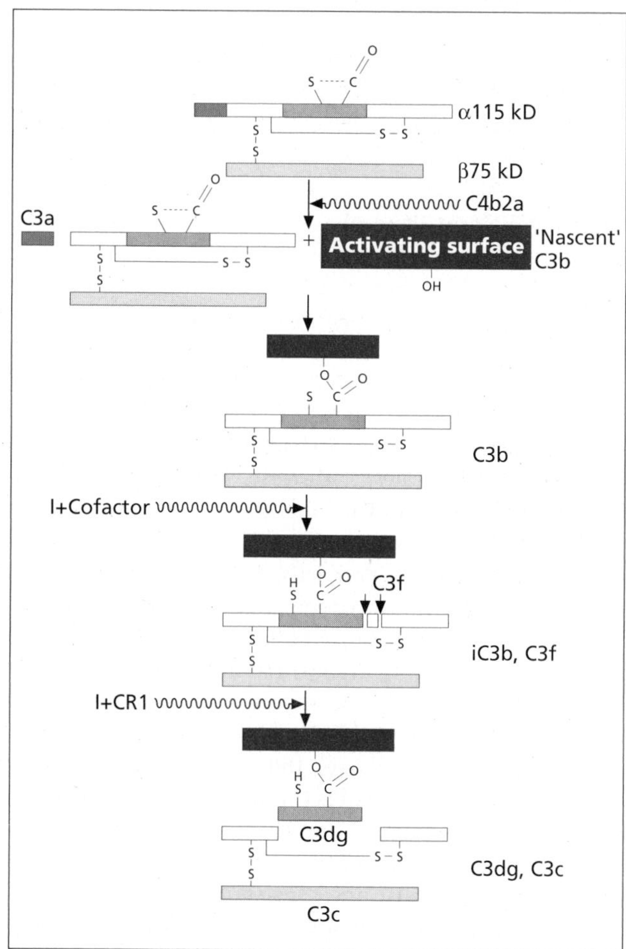

Fig. 18.3 Activation of C3 by C3 convertases (C4b2a or C3bBbP) results in the release of C3a (9 kDa) from the N terminus of the α-chain. The thiolester bond of the α-chain of C3b forms covalent (ester or amide) bonds with the complement activating surface. Inactivation of C3b occurs in two stages, both of which are catalysed by factor I. In the first step, involving factor H or membrane cofactor protein as cofactor, two closely adjacent cleavages occur in the α-chain to release a small fragment (C3f, 3 kDa) and iC3b is formed which cannot bind C5 or factor B. A further cleavage, possibly involving CR1 as a cofactor, releases C3c and leaves C3dg bound to the target. The cross-hatched region is C3dg.

et al., 1982). This cleavage results in the release of C3c (135 kDa) and leaves the C3 -fragments called C3dg, C3d, and C3dk (28–38 kDa), which contain the thiolester, covalently bound to the complement-activating surface (Fig. 18.3).

The alternative pathway of complement activation

Components

In addition to C3 (see above) the alternative pathway comprises the following components:

- factor B is a single-chain zymogen of 90 kDa encoded by an mRNA of 2.4 kb;
- factor D is a single-chain serine protease of 24 kDa which circulates in enzymatically active form;
- properdin is a single-chain glycoprotein of approximately 53 kDa which is encoded by a 1.6 kb mRNA. It is present in plasma as a polydispersed mixture of cyclic polymers, mainly dimers, trimers, and tetramers, in the ratio 20 : 54 : 26 (Nolan *et al.*, 1991).

Activation of the alternative pathway

Alternative pathway activation can occur in the absence of immunoglobulin. The activation involves three processes: initiation, amplification and recognition. Initiation of alternative pathway activation starts from a continuous low-grade fluid phase turnover as the thiolester of C3 undergoes spontaneous hydrolysis to form C3(H_2O) which, for less than 1 second, can bind factor B to form the C3(H_2O)B complex in which factor B is susceptible to cleavage and activation by factor D to form C3(H_2O)Bb, the C3 convertase of the alternative pathway. Amplification is achieved by a positive-feedback loop in which factor B complexes with C3b, generated after the cleavage of C3 by the C3(H_2O)Bb complex. Again, the C3bB complex becomes a substrate for the serine protease factor D and develops C3 convertase activity after conversion to C3bBb. This convertase cleaves C3 in exactly the same site as the classical pathway C3 convertase, C4b2a, so that more C3b is generated (Law & Reid, 1988). Thus, a positive-feedback or amplification loop is formed (Fig. 18.4). C3bBb is a fairly unstable complex with a half-life of approximately 90 seconds at 37°C. The convertase is stabilized by the non-covalent binding of properdin to form the complex C3bBbP.

Although C3b is an integral part of the alternative pathway C3 convertase, C5 cleavage can only occur when a second C3b molecule has bound to the original C3b molecule to act as a receptor for C5 prior to C5 cleavage by Bb (Fig. 18.4). Thus, the alternative pathway C5 convertase is ($(C3b)_n$BbP), and cleaves in exactly the same position as the classical pathway C5 convertase.

Regulation of the alternative pathway

The fluid-phase regulators of the alternative pathway are the serum protease factor I (see above) and the two variants of factor H (M_r 155 kDa and M_r 43 kDa), which are the alternative pathway analogues of C4bp (Schwaeble *et al.*, 1991). Low-grade fluid-phase turnover is held in check by factor I, which inactivates C3b in the presence of its plasma cofactor, factor H (Whaley & Ruddy, 1976a; Misasi *et al.*, 1989). Factor H binds to C3b and thereby catalyses the factor I-mediated cleavage of the α-chain of C3, which is cleaved twice (Fig. 18.3) to form haemolytically inactive iC3b. When C3b is formed, it can bind to any surface including pathogens and host cells, and discrimination of self and non-self surfaces occurs through the affinity with which factor H binds to native C3b. On host cell membranes factor H will bind to C3b with approximately 100 times the affinity of factor B (Kazatchkine *et al.*, 1979), thus the balance favours C3b degradation. However, on the surface of alternative pathway activators the affinity of

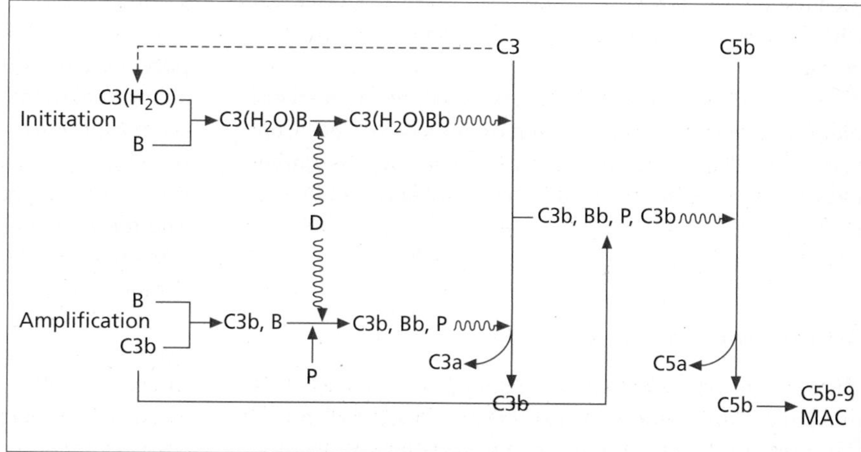

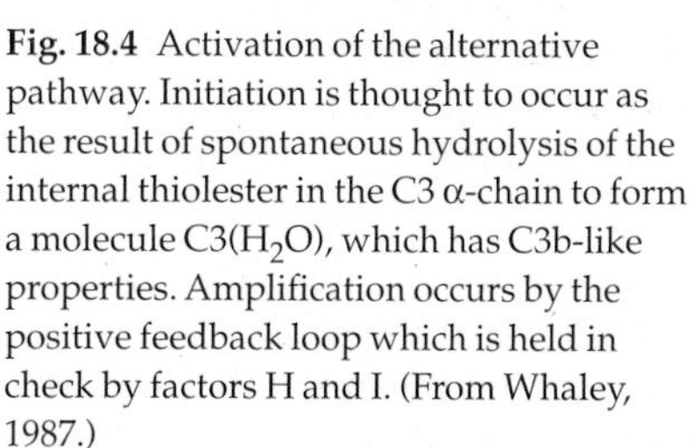

Fig. 18.4 Activation of the alternative pathway. Initiation is thought to occur as the result of spontaneous hydrolysis of the internal thiolester in the C3 α-chain to form a molecule C3(H_2O), which has C3b-like properties. Amplification occurs by the positive feedback loop which is held in check by factors H and I. (From Whaley, 1987.)

factor H for C3b is decreased to a level which is similar to that of factor B for C3b, so that the balance is shifted away from regulation to amplification. In this way amplification is confined to the surface of the activating agent. The surface structures which determine whether it is an alternative pathway activator or a non-activator must be diverse, but absence of sialic acid has been shown to be such a factor.

Factor H performs a further important regulatory step, as it can accelerate the decay of the C3 convertase by displacing Bb from the complexes (Whaley & Buddy, 1976a). Absence of either factor I or factor H results in uncontrolled turnover of the alternative pathway. Because C3b is an integral component of the C5 convertases of both classical and alternative pathways, the binding of factor H to C3b also regulates C5 convertase activity (Whaley & Ruddy, 1976b). Thus, factor H plays a key role in regulating the expression of the alternative pathway C3 convertase activity and also the activities of the C5 convertases of both classical and alternative pathways.

In addition to the fluid-phase regulatory components of complement, the cells of the host are protected from complement attack by the presence of cell-membrane regulatory proteins. These include CR1, DAF, MCP and CD59. DAF accelerates the decay of both classical and alternative pathway C3 and C5 convertases but has no cofactor activity. MCP is a cofactor for factor I in the degradation of C4b and C3b but has no decay acceleration activity. In contrast, CR1 possesses the activities of DAF and MCP. CD59 limits the insertion of C9 into the membrane attack complex and thereby protects cells from lysis (reviewed in Law & Reid, 1988).

Teminal activation sequence

Components

C5 is a disulphide-linked heterodimer formed of a single chain by co- and postsynthetic cleavage of 196-kDa precursor encoded by a 5.5-kb-long mRNA. Unlike C4 and C3, the α-chain of C5 does not contain a thiolester bond.

C6 (M_r 120 kDa) and C7 (M_r 110 kDa) are single-chain molecules, while C8 is a three-chain molecule (C8α, C8β, C8γ) of 150 kDa which requires a complex assembly mechanism, as—like C1q—the chains are encoded by different genes.

C9 is a single chain molecule of M_r 71 kDa.

Activation of the terminal cascade

Once C5 has been cleaved by C5 convertases, the MAC is assembled from C5, C6, C7, C8 and C9. C6, C7, C8 and C9 are structurally homologous amphipathic molecules. They are relatively hydrophobic, with amino- and carboxyl-termini which contain repetitive hydrophilic sequences. Cleavage of C5 by either the classical or the alternative pathway C5 convertase results in the formation of C5a and the larger fragment C5b. Although C5 is structurally similar to C4 and C3, it lacks an internal thiolester bond (Lundwall *et al.*, 1985). C5b remains bound to the C3b subunit of the C5 convertase and acts as a receptor for C6. The C5b binding site for C6 decays rapidly, having a half-life of approximately 2 minutes at 37°C. The C5b6 complex may remain bound to C3b and serve as an acceptor for C7, or if C7 does not bind it is released into the fluid phase where it can complex with C7 and be inserted into other cell membranes for subsequent binding of C8 and C9. This process is called reactive lysis (Lachmann & Thompsen, 1970). The binding of C7 to C5b6 produces an irreversible transition from hydrophilic precursor to the amphiphilic C5b67 complex. This transition is achieved by conformational changes, which expose internal hydrophobic domains in C6 and C7. As a result of this change the C5b67 complex becomes inserted into the cell membrane and its ability to bind C8 and C9 remains for long periods. If the complement-activating agent does not possess a lipid bilayer (e.g. immune complexes or zymosan particles), the C5b67 complex is incapable of binding and is released into the fluid phase where it can bind to host cells and target them for destruction. 'Innocent bystander lysis' is prevented by a number of proteins (summarized below). C8 binds the C5b67 complex by its β-chain while the C8α–γ subunit becomes inserted into the cell membrane. Formation of the C5b–8 complex in the membrane creates small pores of approximately 100 nm diameter which probably result from the aggregation of two or more C5b–8 complexes (Podack, 1986). The formation of C5b–8 pores in certain *in vitro* systems (e.g. complement activation on the surface of sheep erythrocytes) results in 'low-grade lysis'. For rapid lysis C9 must be incorporated into the C5b–8 complex. C9 binds to C8α–γ and undergoes a conformational change, which exposes a second C9 binding site to which a second molecule of C9 binds and undergoes the same changes. Thus, a tubular polymer consisting of 10–16 C9 molecules forms, having an internal diameter of 9–12 nm, and an everted lip on the outer aspect of the cell membrane, with an external diameter of 22 nm (Tschopp, 1984). As show in Fig. 18.5, C9 polymer penetrates the cell membrane and produces lysis. The mechanism of lysis is still unclear. The formation of transmembrane channels in anucleated cells may result in osmotic lysis. When large numbers of MAC are inserted into a cell membrane, a dramatic increase in surface area occurs in the absence of osmotic swelling. This swelling may disrupt the integrity of the cell membrane and cause cell death independently of ion fluxes through transmembrane channels (Esser *et al.*, 1979). Membrane C5b–9 pores

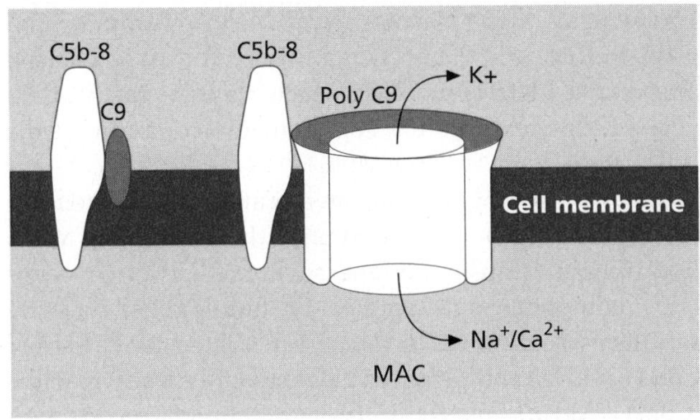

Fig. 18.5 A model of the membrane attack complex (MAC), in which C5b–8 directs polymerization of poly C9 channels which transverse the cell membrane.

allow entry of Na^+ and Ca^{2+} and efflux of K^+ ions. Increased intracellular Ca^{2+} is associated with random triggering of a number of intracellular pathways and rapid depletion of adenosine triphosphate (ATP) and high-energy phosphates. All these factors may contribute to cell death. Damage to the cell membrane by the MAC does not always result in cell death: there is good evidence that cells may recover. Recovery is associated with 'capping' and vesiculation of the MAC and associated cell membrane. Non-lethal complement attack of neutrophils and macrophages results in secretion of inflammatory mediators, such as arachidonic acid metabolites and toxic oxygen radicals.

Regulation of the terminal cascade

The potent effects of the MAC require that its activity is regulated to prevent the damage to host cells. Autologous or homologous complement-mediated cell lysis is prevented by membrane-associated 'homologous restriction factors' present on various blood cells and the vascular endothelium. The major proteins involved are homologous restriction factor (HRF), also denoted as C8/C9 binding protein of 60 kDa (Hänsch *et al.*, 1987), and CD59 (protectin) which has an M_r of 18–20 kDa. Both HRF and CD59 are associated with cell membranes via a glycosylphosphatidylinositol moiety (Rosse, 1990a). Also, both HRF and CD59 have a widespread cell-surface and tissue distribution and bind to the C5b–8 complex, thus preventing the polymerization of C9 which is essential for the formation of effective transmembrane channels. S-protein (vitronectin) is a serum protein of 84 kDa involved in the protection of autologous cells from complement-mediated cell lysis. Vitronectin binds to the fluid-phase C5b–9 complex and prevents the transition of this complex within the cell membrane and the subsequent formation of the lytic complement pore by polymerization of C9. Another plasma protein of 80 kDa, denoted Sp40 : 40 (clusterin), has been found associated with the C5b–9 complex (Murphy *et al.*, 1988). Structural analysis of Sp40 : 40 revealed putative hydrophobic binding domains (Jenne & Tschopp, 1989), which may associate with high-density lipoprotein particles and may thereby constitute the active inhibitor of the cytolytic complex.

Complement receptors and membrane regulatory molecules

Receptors for C3b and C4b and their cleavage fragments

Four different receptor molecules (termed CR1–4) have been described for the subfragments of C3 generated during complement activation. Two of these cellular receptors, CR1 (CD35) and CD2 (CD21), are single-chain molecules which belong to the gene family of complement control proteins (CCP). CR1 has complement regulatory activity by binding to C3b, iC3 and C4b and serving as a cofactor in the factor I-mediated conversion of C3b and C4b to haemolytically inactive iC3b and C4d (after release of C4c), respectively. CR1 is present on erythrocytes, phagocytes, B-lymphocytes and glomerular epithelial cells. Beside its complement regulatory activity, CR1 plays an important role in mediating the adherence of opsonized bacteria, viruses and Ag/Ab complexes to cells. This facilitates phagocytosis and the clearance of micro-organisms and immune complexes.

CR2 binds to C3d, C3dg and iC3b. Moreover, the Epstein–Barr virus (EBV) binds to CR2 and requires CR2 as a receptor to enter the cell. CR2 is expressed on B lymphocytes, phagocytes, glial cells and epithelial cells in the nasopharynx. CR2 plays an important role in the control of B-cell proliferation. Cross-linking of CR2 by aggregated C3d is required for activated B lymphocytes to progress from G0 to G1 in the cell cycle (Melchers *et al.*, 1985). Thus, C3d and C3dg may regulate antibody production.

The complement receptors CR3 and CR4 are closely related heterodimers which belong to the intergrin family. As β2 integrins, they share an identical β-chain of 95 kDa (CD18), but differ in their α-chains (CD11b in CR3 and CD11c in CR4). It has been clearly shown that both receptors bind to iC3b, but it appears more than likely that other non-complement proteins may also act as ligands for these adhesion-mediating receptors. A well-characterized non-complement ligand of CR3 is intercellular adhesion molecule-1 (ICAM-1, CD54). The binding of the ligands occurs in a divalent-cation-dependent manner and mediates at least two activities: (i) the binding of iC3b-coated targets; and (ii) in cooperation with CR1, ligand binding leading to an enhanced ingestion in phagocytes (Weitzman & Law, 1993).

Receptors for anaphylatoxins

The receptors of the anaphylatoxins C3a, C4a and C5a have been characterized by binding and cross-linking studies and all appear to have an M_r of approximately 90 kDa. The C5a receptor was recently cloned and identified as a member of the rhodopsin supergene family, alongside the formyl peptide receptor and the β-adrenergic receptor (Gerard & Gerard, 1991). Studies on receptor antagonists and receptor blockade by domain-specific antibodies will influence strategies to cope with the undesirable side-effects of anaphylatoxins (Köhl & Bitter-Suermann, 1993).

Receptors for C1q

Two different surface receptors have recently been described for C1q. One binds to the collagenous region of the C1q macromolecule (cC1qR), while the other binds to the globular heads of C1q (gC1qR). cC1qR has a molecular weight of 56 kDa, and also binds to the collagenous region of C1q-related peptides like conglutinin, lung surfactant protein A and mannan binding protein (Holmskov *et al.*, 1994). Amino-acid sequence data (Malhotra *et al.*, 1990) obtained for the cC1qR indicated that C1qR was closely related to a published cDNA-derived sequence claimed (McCauliffe *et al.*, 1990) to be a component of Ro/SS-A, a ribonucleoprotein autoantigen, but now known to be calreticulin (Michalck *et al.*, 1992). gC1qR with a molecular weight of 33 kDa has recently been cloned and the peptide sequence derived, but it does not share homology with any known protein (Ghebrehiwet *et al.*, 1994). However, the mechanisms by which these two different C1q receptors are bound to the cell surface, and the possible pathways of signal transduction, remain to be clarified.

It has been reported that binding of aggregated C1q to C1q receptors triggers a variety of biological activities, depending on the cell type; for example, the enhanced ingestion of pathogens in phagocytes and the enhanced generation of toxic oxygen radicals in neutrophils, eosinophils, endothelial cells and vascular smooth muscle cells (Tenner, 1989).

Membrane-anchored regulatory molecules

In addition to receptor molecules for complement activation products, membrane-anchored down-regulators of complement activation are expressed on the surface of most cells to prevent autologous lysis during activation.

DAF, a glycoprotein of 70 kDa, shortens the half-lives of C3 and C5 convertases of both activation pathways by binding to C3b and C4b with the disruption of the enzyme complexes. DAF is composed of four CCP repeat units and attached to the plasma membrane via glycophosphotidyl inositol (GPI) anchoring. This type of anchoring allows a fast lateral mobility which makes it easily available for down-regulating complement activation on the cell surface.

MCP is a single-chain membrane glycoprotein of 58/63 kDa which is inserted into the membrane via a hydrophobic transmembrane anchor. MCP down-regulates complement activation of autologous cells by serving as a cofactor in the factor I-mediated conversion of C3b (178 kDa) and C4b (185 kDa) to cytolytically inactive iC3b (175 kDa) and the C4b degradation products C4d (45 kDa) and C4c (140 kDa), respectively.

Biological activities

Lysis

Lysis of cells is due to the formation of MAC on cell membranes. Lysis of microbes is important in host defence, but spontaneous lysis of host erythrocytes occurs in patients with paroxysmal noctural haemoglobulinuria, a rare disorder in which the phosphatidyl inositol-anchored membrane proteins, including DAF, HRF and CD59, are deficient. Lysis may also be seen in individuals suffering from cobra bites due to intense fluid-phase complement activation and the occurrence of reactive lysis. Insertion of a large number of MAC into membranes of nucleated cells may result in cell death, but at lower concentrations cell activation may occur. In neutrophils and mononuclear phagocytes this leads to the production of inflammatory mediators, including prostaglandins, toxic oxygen metabolites and cytokines.

Opsonization

Fragments of C3 are deposited on activating surfaces such as effete red cells, bacteria and Ag/Ab complexes. Phagocytic cells then ingest these opsonized substances and phagocytosed bacteria may be killed intracellularly.

Clearance of immune complexes

Complement plays an important role in the clearance of immune complexes. The alternative pathway increases the solubility of immune complexes and the classical pathway prevents large insoluble Ag/Ab complexes from being formed. Ag/Ab complexes opsonized by C3b may then be cleared from the blood by binding to erythrocytes by CR1 and being transported to the liver for removal. Phagocytes will ingest aggregated C3b opsonized complexes.

Anaphylatoxin activity

C4a, C3a and C5a are anaphylatoxins; C4a is the weakest and C5a is the most potent. Anaphylatoxins cause: (i) mast cell degranulation with the release of histamine and other mast cell granule mediators; (ii) increased vascular permeability; and (iii) smooth muscle contraction. Anaphylatoxins are regulated by an inactivator (carboxypeptidase N), which circulates in its active form to remove the carboxyl-terminal arginine within seconds of anaphylatoxins formed. Thus, C3a becomes $C3_{desarg}$, which has no anaphylatoxic activity (Köhl & Bitter-Suermann, 1993).

Chemotactic activity

C5a and $C5a_{desarg}$ may attract certain cells into the area of inflammation. C5a has both anaphylatoxic and chemotactic activity; C3a and C4a have no chemotactic activity. C5a requires a cofactor, vitamin D binding protein, for this activity.

Neutrophil and monocytic activity

C5a and $C5a_{desarg}$ regulate monocyte and neutrophil activity. C5a may cause augmented cell adherence, production of toxic oxygen species, degranulation and release of intracellular enzymes from granulocytes, and initiation of other metabolic events. In this respect, these anaphylatoxins have similar activities to sublytic amounts of the C5b–9 complex.

Leucocytosis

A fragment of iC3, C3e, was thought to induce leucocytosis. However, this peptide has never been characterized or mapped onto the C3 molecule. Another fragment called C3d-K, which is produced by treating iC3b with kallikrein, also causes leucocytosis and inhibits T-cell reponses. C3d-K is identical to C3dg, with the exception that it contains an additional nine amino acids on its amino-terminal end. This nonapeptide is thought to be responsible for bone-marrow release of leucocytes.

Immune response

Interaction with CR2/CD21 regulates antibody production, by a direct effect on the cell-cycle progression in activated B cells by C3d (Melchers *et al.*, 1985), and the requirement of iC3b or C3dg for the B-cell response to a soluble T-cell-dependent antigen (Weisman *et al.*, 1990). Additional complement components and fragments such as C4a, C3a and C5a may also play a role in the regulation of antibody production.

Miscellaneous biological activities

Hereditary angioedema, which results from C1-inhibitor deficiency, may be mediated by a kinin-like substance released from C2. A fragment of factor B may cause increased spreading and adherence of macrophages. Complement may also neutralize viruses or—in the case of human immunodeficiency virus (HIV) — may contribute alternative infection pathways for opsonized viral particles via complement receptors.

Complement deficiencies

Most of the constituents of the complement system, including plasma components and membrane regulators and receptors, have been cloned and their gene loci localized (Table 18.2).

Inherited complete or partial deficiencies of single complement components have been reported for most constituents (Rosen, 1993), as summarized in Table 18.3. The deficiencies can be conveniently grouped according to the most prominent symptoms. A deficiency of a protein of the classical pathway (C1, C4, C2) usually results in Ag/Ab complex disease, presenting frequently as discoid or systemic lupus erythematosus, which is often antinuclear antibody negative. Deficiencies of alternative pathway components (properdin and factor D) are rare and no deficiency of factor B has yet been described. The symptoms experienced by either properdin- or factor D-deficient individuals emphasizes the importance of the alternative activation pathway of complement in the immune defence. Approximately 50% of the patients suffer pyogenic infections, particularly with meningococci. Susceptibility to infection with *Neisseria* is also found in patients with deficencies of the terminal components (C5, C6, C7 and C8). Patients with deficiencies of C3, factor H and factor I are predisposed to a broader range of bacterial infections, particularly from pyogenic bacteria. Finally, most individuals with C9 deficiency are asymptomatic, although some reports from Japan suggest that C9 deficiency causes an increased susceptibility to *Neisseria* infections.

C1 deficiency

Deficiencies have been described for all the three subcomponents of the first component of complement. For C1q, the major subcomponent of C1, two different types of deficiencies have been described. In one type of C1q deficiency, C1q is present at normal serum levels, but this C1q is deficient in terms of inducing classical pathway activation. The second type of C1q deficiency is characterized by a total lack of C1q in the serum. In both cases, the defect is

Table 18.2 Chromosomal localization of proteins and receptors associated with the activation and control of the human serum complement system.

Plasma components	Chromosomal localization
Classical pathway	
C1q (A, B and C chains)	1p34–1p36.5
C1r	12p13
C1s	12p13
C4	6p21.3
C2	6p21.3
Alternative pathway	
Factor B	6p21.3
Factor D	Unknown
C3	19
Terminal pathway	
C5	9q32–9q34
C6	5q
C7	5q
C8 (α- and β-chains)	1q
C8γ	9
C9	5
Control (fluid phase)	
Factor H	1q32
Factor I	4
C4 binding protein	1q32
C1 inhibitor	11
S protein (vitroneotin)	Unknown
Sp40, 40	Unknown
Anaphylatoxin inactivator	Unknown
Control (membrane bound)	
DAF (CD55)	1q132
MCP (CD46)	1q32
HRF (65-kDa homologous restriction factor)	Unknown
CD59 (protectin, HRF20, MACIF)	11p
Complement receptors	
CR1 (CD35)	1q32
CR2 (CD21)	1q32
CR3 (CD11b/CD18)	16p11–16p13.1 (CD11a, b and c)
CR4 (CD11c/CD18)	21q22.1 (CD18)
CR5	Unknown
C5a receptor	Unknown
C3a receptor	Unknown
C1q receptor	Unknown

See text for definition of abbreviations.

inherited phenotypically as an autosomal recessive. In only one case could the molecular basis of a deficiency be ascertained, to a premature stop codon in the β-chain resulting in a failure of C1q synthesis and assembly. This mutation leads to a loss of a Taq 1 cleavage site, so that the defect can be detected by restriction fragment length polymorphism (RFLP) (Reid & Thompson, 1983).

Several cases of deficiencies of the C1r subcomponent have been described. These deficiencies are consistently associated with a deficiency in C1s. At present, the molecular basis for C1r/C1s deficiencies is unknown.

In general, deficiencies in the first component of complement may lead to severe Ag/Ab complex disease with symptoms of systemic lupus erythematosis (SLE) with severe glomerulonephritis.

C1-inhibitor deficiency

Hereditary C1-inhibitor deficiency or hereditary angioedema (HAE) is an autosomal dominant disease that is characterized by recurrent episodes of subcutaneous and submucosal oedema. Biochemically, HAE can be subdivided into type I HAE in which there are low serum levels of functionally normal C1- inhibitor, and type II HAE with normal or elevated serum levels mainly of dysfunctional C1-inhibitor protein. A limited number of reports of gene mutations accounting for HAE have recently been described. In type I HAE, deletions of exon 4 or exon 7, or exon duplications, have been reported (Siddique *et al.*, 1991, 1993). Intragenic Alu repeats in the human C1 inhibitor locus seem to predispose for deleterious rearrangements (Stoppa-Lyonnet *et al.*, 1990). Exon deletions give rise to truncated mRNA transcripts with very low abundance. This is probably due to instability of the truncated mRNA. Other mutations producing type I HAE include those affecting donor splice sites (Siddique *et al.*, 1991) and point mutations, particularly in exon 8 (Tosi, 1993). Point mutations occurring in the active site (Arg 444) cause type II HAE. Type II HAE is also caused by exon 8 mutations affecting the hinge region (Tosi, 1993). These include point mutations and triplet insertions.

Aquired C1 inhibitor deficiency is usually associated with monoclonal gammopathy. These monoclonal antibodies have specificity for native C1 inhibitor. C1 inhibitor in the sera of these patients is usually in the cleaved form (96 kDa) and is unreactive with these antibodies. It is thought that the antibodies permit cleavage of C1 inhibitor by C1s, but inhibit the formation of the enzyme/inhibitor complex. Thus, C1 inhibitor is converted to a substrate. The majority of these antibodies appear to recognize an epitope in the distal region (He *et al.*, 1996).

Treatment of C1 inhibitor deficiency includes the use of fresh frozen plasma or C1 inhibitor concentrate for acute attacks, and the use of tranexamic acid and/or androgens (danazol, stanazol) for prophylaxis. Home therapy with C1 inhibitor concentrate is under consideration.

Table 18.3 Complement deficiency syndromes.

Missing complement	Cases reported	Mode of inheritance	Functional defect	Associated disease
Classical pathway				
C1 (C1q, Clr/Cls)	31	Autosomal recessive	Impaired immune complex handling and loss of classical pathway	ICD/ICTD (48%). Infection with encapsulated bacteria (22%). Both 18%. Healthy 12%
C4	21	Autosomal recessive		
C2	109	Autosomal recessive		
Alternative pathway				
D	3	X-linked	Impaired complement activation in the absence of specific antibody	Infection (usually meningococcal) 74%. Healthy 26%
P	70	Autosomal recessive		
C3	19	Autosomal recessive	Absent classical and alternative pathway activity. Impaired immune complex handling. Absent serum bactericidal activity. Impaired opsonization/ phagocytosis. Impaired chemotaxis	ICD/ICTD 79%. Infections with encapsulated bacteria 71%
Terminal sequence				
C5	27	Autosomal recessive	Impaired chemotaxis. Absent serum bactericidal activity	Infection (*Neisseria* spp. especially meningococcal 59%)
C6	77	Autosomal recessive	Absent serum bactericidal activity	ICD/ICTD 4%. Both 1%. Healthy 25%
C7	73	Autosomal recessive		
C8	73	Autosomal recessive		
C9	18	Autosomal recessive	Reduced serum bactericidal activity	Healthy 92%. Infection 8%
Plasma proteins				
C1 inhibitor	Many	Autosomal, dominant or acquired	Lack of regulation of C1 activation and of enzymes in Hageman factor-dependent results in generation of inflammatory mediator	Hereditary angioedema. ICD/ ICTD 2–5%
C4bp	3	Autosomal recessive	Impaired regulation of C4b2a	Angioedema + Behçet's-like syndrome in one patient
Factor H	13	Autosomal recessive	Uncontrolled alternative pathway turnover → secondary deficiencies of C3 and factor B	ICD/ICTD 40%. ICD/ICTD + infections with encapsulated or ganisms 40%. Healthy 20%
Factor I	14	Autosomal recessive	Uncontrolled alternative pathway turnover → secondary deficiencies of C3 and factor B	Infections with encapsulated organisms 100%
Membrane proteins				
DAF/CD59/HRF	Many	Acquired	Impaired regulation of C3 and C5 convertases of both pathways and impaired regulation of MAC assembly → lysis of blood cells	Paroxysmal nocturnal haemoglobinuria
CR3	>20	Autosomal recessive	Impaired neutrophil adhesive functions, e.g. margination, chemotaxis, iC3b-mediated opsonization, and phagocytosis	Infections (*Staphylococcos aureus*, *Pseudomonas* sp.) 100%

ICD, immune complex disease; ICTD, immune complex-type disease. See text for other definitions of abbreviations.

C4 deficiency

C4 is encoded by two (presumably duplicated) genes, C4A and C4B, in the class III region of the major histocompatibility complex (MHC) on the short arm of chromosome 6. The presence of two functional C4 genes is peculiar to humans. The C4B gene is centromeric (towards HLA-DR) and the C4A gene is telomeric (towards HLA-B). The translation products of both genes differ in only four amino acids in the α-chain between residues 1101 and

1106. However, both isoforms of C4 differ considerably in their biological properties. C4A is reactive with amino groups and C4B with hydroxyl side chains (Hauptmann *et al.*, 1988).

Both C4A and C4B are highly polymorphic and to date not less than 35 different alleles have been described (Rosen, 1993b).

Approximately 1.5 kb 3′ to each C4 gene lies a gene for P-450 21-hydroxylase. The 21-hydroxylase gene 3′ to C4A is a pseudogene, and only deletions in the 21-hydroxylase gene 3′ to C4B results in congenital adrenal hyperplasia.

There is extraordinarily high frequency of C4 null alleles in the population, with the consequence that only 65% of individuals express both genes. However, complete C4 deficiencies are very rare. Almost all patients with complete C4 deficiency have systemic or discoid lupus with or without associated glomerulonephritis. C4A null alleles are found in almost all patients with idiopathic SLE.

C2 deficiency

Unlike C4, C2 exhibits very little polymorphism and complete C2 deficiency is relatively common in the Caucasian population. The gene encoding C2 is located in the MHC class III region, telomeric to the genes encoding C4 and factor B (Dunham *et al.*, 1987). C2 mRNA codes for three different polypeptides of M_r 84 kDa, 79 kDa and 70 kDa, from which only the 84-kDa form is secreted, while the other forms remain cell associated (Perlmutter *et al.*, 1984).

C2 deficiency (C2QO) is almost invariably linked with slow factor B (BfS), C4A4 and C4B2 (Awdeh *et al.*, 1981). In cell cultures from C2-deficient individuals, no biosynthesis of C2 can be detected, although the C2 mRNA content is normal. There is consistently a 28-bp deletion at the 3′ end of exon 6, so that faulty splicing leads to a loss of exon 6, thereby generating a frameshift and stop codon 14 bp distal to the end of exon 5 (Johnson & Colten, unpublished observation). One in 100 Caucasians bears the C2QO gene, so that 1 in 10 000 is completely C2 deficient. Probably close to half these individuals are perfectly healthy; the others present with lupus-like disease and/or severe bacterial infections, polymyositis, Hench–Schönlein purpura and other forms of vasculitis. Heterozygous C2 deficiency is present with increased frequency in patients with SLE and juvenile rheumatoid arthritis.

C3 deficiency

C3 has a well-defined polymorphism and two common alleles, designated S and F for fast and slow mobility. Several rare variants are also known. C3-deficient patients have very little or no detectable C3. Almost all C3-deficient individuals suffer from recurrent pyogenic infections and to a certain extent from immune complex disease, particulary membranoproliferative glomerulonephritis. Botto *et al.* (1990) described a 61-bp deletion in one patient. This deletion in exon 18 resulted from a faulty donor splice site in intron 18 that caused a premature stop codon 17 bp 3′ to the deletion. The same investigators detected in two other C3-deficient individuals another deletion, comprising 700 bp which encompasses exons 22 and 23 and causes a stop codon 5′ of the deletion (Botto *et al.*, 1990). In surveying an Afrikaaner population, two further proposti were found with the same genetic defect, as was found in the original Afrikaaner girl. This strongly suggests a founder effect in the Afrikaaner population where the gene defect has a high incidence.

Factor H deficiency

At least eight factor H-deficient families have been documented and the deficiency is inherited in an autosomal recessive fashion (Sim *et al.*, 1993). In all of these patients low serum levels of factor H antigen are present. It is not known whether all the affected individuals have a complete or an incomplete deficiency of the 155-kDa variant of factor H with normal levels of the 43-kDa factor H variant. It is likely that the deficiencies are due to mutations in the factor H gene which affect expression. In addition to human factor H deficiencies, an inherited factor H deficiency has been described in pigs which consistently leads to lethal glomerulonephritis (Hogasen *et al.*, 1994). Absence of factor H in humans is strongly associated with recurrent bacterial infections, particularly meningitis, and with glomerulonephritis. Kidney damage is likely to arise from Ag/Ab complex deposition.

Factor I deficiency

Complete factor I deficiencies result in uncontrolled turnover of the alternative pathway, with secondary deficiencies of C3 and factor B due to depletion. These patients have a high incidence of Ag/Ab complex disease and severe systemic bacterial infections (meningitis, septicaemia, septic arthritis).

Deficiencies in factor B, factor P and factor D

Deficiencies of the alternative pathway components factor D and factor P have been documented, but there are no reported cases of primary factor B deficiency. Factor D deficiency is associated with recurrent meningitis, septicaemia and respiratory infections, while a large proportion of patients with factor P deficiency develop meningococcal disease (75% mortality; Schwaeble *et al.*,

1993)). Some patients with factor P deficiency are asymptomatic and others may develop less severe bacterial infections of the lower respiratory tract.

Deficiencies in C5, C6, C7, C8 and C9

Deficiencies of C5, C6, C7, C8β, C8α and C9 have been reported and are all associated with increased risk of systemic *Neisseria* infection, usually meningococcal meningitis. In contrast to the high mortality seen in patients with factor P deficiency, meningitis in these patients has a lower mortality and tends to be recurrent.

Deficiency in C4bp

Deficiency of C4bp has been reported in one kindred in association with Behçet's syndrome and angioedema (Trapp *et al.*, 1987).

Deficiencies in DAF, HRF and CD59

A deficiency in DAF, HRF and CD59 occurs in patients with paroxysmal noctural haemoglobinuria (Hänsch *et al.*, 1987). In this aquired clonal disorder of bone marrow cells, GPI-anchored proteins cannot be inserted in the cell membrane, so that they are unduly susceptible to complement lysis (Rosse, 1990b). Thus, any complement activation will generate C5b–9 complexes which may be formed on erythrocytes or other blood cells and result in their lysis as GPI-anchored membrane complement control proteins are not expressed.

Leucocyte adhesion deficiencies

The complement receptors type 3 (CR3) and type 4 (CR4 or p150–95) and LFA-1 are members of the integrin family of cell-membrane proteins (Anderson & Springer, 1987). Deficiency occurs as part of the leucocyte adhesion deficiency syndrome, in which patients are unable to synthesize normal amounts of the functional active β-chain (CD18) of the heterodimer which all three molecules have in common. This results in a leucocyte adhesion defect in which leucocytes cannot adhere to endothelial cells. Leucocyte migration is impaired, as well as bacterial adhesion and killing. Delayed umbilical cord separation, recurrent bacterial infections of soft tissues, mucosal surfaces and intestinal tract occur, often progressing to necrosis.

References

Anderson, D.C. & Springer, T.A. (1987) Leucocyte adhesion deficiency: an inherited defect in the Mac-1, LFA-1, and p150,95 glycoproteins. *Ann. Rev. Med.*, **38**, 1975–94.

Awdeh, Z.L., Raum, D.D., Glass, D. *et al.* (1981) Complement: human histocompatibility antigen haplotypes in C2 deficiency. *J. Clin. Invest.*, **67**, 581–3.

Botto, M., So, A.K., Fong, K.Y. *et al.* (1991) Homozygous hereditary C3 deficiency due to partial gene deletion. In: *XIV International Complement Workshop*, 15–20 September, Cambridge, England.

Botto, M., Fong, K.Y., So, A.K., Rudge, A. & Walport, M. (1990) Molecular basis of heriditary C3 deficiency. *J. Clin. Invest.*, **86**, 1158–63.

Carroll, M., Fathallah, D., Bergamaschini, L., Alicot, E. & Isenman, D. (1990) Substitution of a single aminoacid (aspartic acid for histidine) converts the functional activity of human complement C4B to C4A. *Proc. Nat. Acad. Sci. USA*, **87**, 6868–72.

Catterall, C.F., Lyons, A., Sim, R.B., Day, A.J. & Harris, T.J.R. (1987) Characterization of the primary amino acid sequene of human complement control protein factor I from analysis of cDNA clones. *Biochem. J.*, **242**, 849–56.

Cias, F. & Loos, M. (1987) Complement and bacteria. In: *Complement in Health and Disease* (ed. K. Whaley), pp. 201–31. MTP, Lancaster.

Claus, D.R., Siege, L.J., Petras, K., Skor, D., Osmond, P. & Gewurz, H. (1977) Complement activation by interaction of multiple poly anions and poly cations in the presence of C-reactive protein. *J. Immunol.*, **118**, 83–7.

Cooper, N.R., Jensen, F.C., Welsh, R.M. & Oldstone, M.B.A. (1976) Lysis of RNA tumour viruses by human serum: direct antibody-independent triggering of the classical pathway. *J. Exp. Med.*, **144**, 970–84.

Dodds, A.W., Law, S.K.A. & Porter, R.R. (1985) The origin of the very variable haemolytic activities of the common human complement component C4 allotypes including C4-A6. *EMBO J.*, **4**, 2239–44.

Dunham, I., Sargent, C.A., Trowsdale, J. & Campbell, R.D. (1987) Molecular mapping of the human major histocompatibility complex by pulsed-field gel electrophoresis. *Proc. Nat. Acad. Sci. USA*, **84**, 7237–41.

Esser, A.F., Kolb, W.P., Podack, E.R. & Müller-Eberhard, H.J. (1979) Molecular reorganisation of lipid bilayers by complement: a possible mechanism by membranolysis. *Proc. Nat. Acad. Sci. USA*, **76**, 1410–14.

Gerard, N.P. & Gerard, C. (1991) The chemotactic receptor for human C5a and anaphylatoxin. *Nature*, **349**, 614–17.

Ghebrehiwet, B., Lim, B.-L., Peerschke, E.I.B., Willis, A.C. & Reid, K.B.M. (1994) Isolation, cDNA cloning, and overexpression of a 33 kDa cell surface glycoprotein that binds to the globular 'heads' of C1q. *J. Exp. Med.*, **179**, 1809–21.

Giclas, P.C., Pinkard, R.N. & Olson, M.S. (1979) *In vivo* activation of complement by isolated heart subcellular membranes. *J. Immunol.*, **122**, 146–51.

Goldberger, G. & Colton, H.R. (1980) Precursor complement protein (pro-C4) is converted *in vitro* to native C4 by plasmin. *Nature*, **286**, 515–16.

Hänsch, G.M., Schönermark, S. & Roelcke, D. (1987) Paroxysmal noctural haemoglobinuria type III. Lack of erythrocyte membrane protein restricting the lysis by C5b–9. *J. Clin. Invest.*, **80**, 7–12.

Harpel, P.C. & Cooper, N.R. (1975) Synthesis of human plasma C1 inactivator–enzyme interaction. I. Mechanisms of interaction with C1s, plasmin, and trypsin. *J. Clin. Invest.*, **55**, 593–604.

Harrison, R.A. & Lachmann, P.J. (1980) The physiological breakdown of the third component of complement. *Mol. Immunol.*, **17**, 9–20.

Hauptmann, G., Tappeiner, G. & Schifferli, J.A. (1988) Inherited deficiency of the fourth component of human complement. *Immunodef. Rev.*, **1**, 32–42.

He, S., Tsang, S., North, J., Chohan, N., Sim, R.B. & Whaley, K. (1996)

Epitope mapping of C1 inhibitor autoantibodies from patients with acquired C1 inhibitor deficiency. *J. Immunol.*, **156**, 2009–13.

Hogasen, K., Jansen, J.H., Möllnes, T.E. & Harboe, M. (1994) Heriditary porcine membranoproliferative glomerulonephritis (MPGN) type II is caused by factor H deficiency. *Clin. Exp. Immunol.*, **97** (5th European Meeting on Complement in Human Disease, Abstract 53).

Holmskov, U., Malhotra, R., Sim, R.B. & Jesenius, J.C. (1994) Collectins, collageous C-type lectins of the immune defense system. *Immunol. Today*, **15**, 67–70.

Jenne, D.E. & Tschopp, J. (1989) Molecular structure and functional characterization of a human complement cytolysis inhibitor found in blood and seminal plasma: identity to sulfated glycoprotein-2, a constituent of rat testis fluid. *Proc. Nat. Acad. Sci. USA*, **86**, 7123–7.

Ji, Y.-H., Fujita, T., Hatsuse, H., Takahashi, A., Matsushita, M. & Kawakami, M. (1993) Activation of the C4 and C2 components of complement by a proteinase in serum, bactericidal factor, Ra Reactive Factor. *J. Immunol.*, **150**, 517–78.

Kazatchkine, M.D., Fearon, D.T. & Austen, K.F. (1979) Human alternative complement pathway: membrane associated sialic acid regulates the competition between B and β1H for cell bound C3b. *J. Immunol.*, **122**, 75–81.

Köhl, J. & Bitter-Suermann, D. (1993) Anaphylatoxins. In: *Complement in Health and Disease* (eds K. Whaley, M. Loos & J.M. Weiler), 2nd edn, pp. 299–324. Kluwer Academic, Lancester.

Lachmann, P.J. & Thompsen, R.A. (1970) Reactive lysis: the complement mediated lysis of unsensitized cells. II. The characterization of activated reactor as C5b and the participation of C8 and C9. *J. Exp. Med.*, **131**, 643–57.

Law, A. & Reid, K.B.M. (1988) *Complement.* IRL Press, Oxford.

Lu, J., Thiel, S., Wiedemann, H., Timpl, R. & Reid, K.B.M. (1990) Binding of the pentamer/hexamer forms of mannan-binding protein to zymosan activates the proenzyme $C1r_2C1s_2$ complex, of the classical pathway of complement, without development of C1q. *J. Immunol.*, **144**, 2287–94.

Lundwall, A.B., Wetsel, R.A., Kristensen, T. *et al.* (1985) Isolation and sequence analysis of a cDNA clone encoding the fifth complement component. *J. Biol. Chem.*, **260**, 2108–12.

McCauliffe, D.P., Lux, F.A., Lieu, T.S. *et al.* (1990) Molecular cloning, expression, and chromosome 19 localisation of a human Ro/SS-A autoantigen. *J. Clin. Invest.*, **85**, 1379–82.

Malhotra, R., Thiel, S., Reid, K.B.M. & Sim, R.B. (1990) Human leucocyte C1q receptor binds to other soluble proteins with collagen domains. *J. Exp. Med.*, **173**, 955–9.

Matsushita, M. & Fujita, T. (1995) Cleavage of the third component of complement (C3) by Mannose-binding protein-associated serine protease (MASP) with subsequent complement activation. *Immunobiology.*, **194**, 443–7.

Medof, M.E., Iida, K., Mold, C. & Nussenzweig, V. (1982) Unique role for the complement receptor CR1 in the degradation of C3b associated with immune complexes. *J. Exp. Med.*, **156**, 1739–54.

Melchers, F., Erdei, A., Schulz, T. & Dierich. M.P. (1985) Growth control of activated, synchronized murine B cells by the C3d fragment of human complement. *Nature*, **317**, 264–7.

Michalck, M., Milner, R.E., Burns, K. & Opas, M. (1992) Calreticulin. *Biochem. J.*, **285**, 681–93.

Misasi, R., Huemer, H.P., Schwaeble, W., Sölder, E., Larcher, C. & Dierich, M.P. (1989) Human complement factor H: an additional gene product of 43 kDa isolated from human plasma shows cofactor activity for the cleavage of the third component of complement. *Eur. J. Immunol.*, **19**, 1765–8.

Murphy, B.F., Kirszbaum, L., Walker, I.D. & d'Apice, A.J. (1988) SP40–40, a newly identified normal human serum protein found in the SC5b–9 complex of complement and in the immune deposits in glomerulonephritis. *J. Clin. Invest.*, **81**, 1858–64.

Nolan, K.F., Schwaeble, W., Kaluz, S., Dierich, M.P. & Reid, K.B.M. (1991) Molecular cloning of the cDNA coding for properdin, a positive regulator of the alternative pathway of human complement. *Eur. J. Immunol.*, **21**, 771–6.

Perlmutter, D.H., Cole, F.S., Goldberger, G. & Colten, H.R. (1984) Distinct primary translation products of human liver mRNA give rise to secreted and cell associated form of complement C2. *J. Biol. Chem.*, **259**, 10380–5.

Podack, E.R. (1986) Assembly and functions of the terminal components. In: *Immunology of the Complement System* (ed. G.D. Ross), pp. 115–137. Academic, Orlando.

Reid, K.B.M. & Thompson, R.A. (1983) Characterisation of a nonfunctional form of C1q found in patients with a genetically linked deficiency of C1q activity. *Mol. Immunol.*, **20**, 1117–25.

Rosen, F.S. (1993) Genetic deficiencies of the complement system: an overview. In: *Complement in Health and Disease* (eds K. Whaley, M. Loos & J.M. Weiler), 2nd edn, pp. 159–97. Kluwer Academic, Lancaster.

Rosse, W.F. (1990a) Phosphatidylinositol-linked proteins and paroxysmal noctural haemoglobinuria. *Blood*, **75**, 1595–601.

Rosse, W.F. (1990b) Phosphatidylinositol-linked proteins and paroxysmal noctural haemoglobinuria. *Blood*, **75**, 1595–601.

Schwaeble, W., Dippold, W., Schäfer, M.K.-H. *et al.* (1993) Properdin, a positive regulator of complement activation, is expressed in human T-cell lines and peripheral blood T-cells. *J. Immunol.*, **151**, 2521–8.

Schwaeble, W., Zwirner, J., Schulz, T.F., Linke, R.P., Dierich, M.P. & Weiss, E.H. (1987) Human complement factor H: expression of an additional truncated gene product of 43-kDa in human liver. *Eur. J. Immunol.*, **17**, 1485–9.

Siddique, Z., McPhaden, A.R. & Whaley, K. (1993) C1-inhibitor gene nucleotide insertion causes type II heriditary angio-oedema. *Hum. Genet.*, **92**, 189–90.

Siddique, Z., McPhaden, A.R., Lappin, D.F. & Whaley, K. (1991) An RNA splice site mutation in the C1-inhibitor gene causes type I heriditary angio-oedema. *Hum. Genet.*, **88**, 231–2.

Sim, R.B., Kölble, K., McAleer, M.A., Dominguez, O. & Dee, V.M. (1993) Genetics and deficiencies of the soluble regulatory proteins of the complement system. *Int. Rev. Immunol.*, **10**, 65.

Stoppa-Lyonnet, D., Carter, P.E., Meo, T. & Tosi, M. (1990) Clusters of intragenic Alu repeats predispopse the human C1 inhibitor locus to deleterious rearrangements. *Proc. Nat. Acad. Sci. USA*, **87**, 1551–5.

Tenner, A. (1989) C1q interaction with cell surface receptors. *Behring Inst. Mitt.*, **84**, 220.

Thiel, S., Jensen, T.V., Laursen S.B., Willis, A. & Jensenius, J.C. (1995) Identification of a new Mannan-binding protein associated serine protease. *J. Immunol.*, **86**, 101 [abstract].

Tosi, M. (1993) Molecular genetics of C1-inhibitor and hereditary angio-oedema. In: *Complement in Health and Disease* (eds K. Whaley, M. Loos & J.M. Weiler), 2nd edn, pp. 245–67. Kluwer Academic, Lancaster.

Trapp, R.G., Fletcher, M., Forrisal, J. & West, C.D. (1987) C4 binding protein deficiency in a patient with Behçet's disease. *J. Rheumatol.*, **14**, 135–8.

Tschopp, J. (1984) Ultrastructure of the membrane attack complex of complement. Heterogeniety of the complex caused by different degrees of C9 polymerisation. *J. Biol. Chem.*, **259**, 7857–63.

Weiler, J.M. (1993) Introduction to complement. In: *Complement in Health and Disease* (eds K. Whaley, M. Loos & J.M. Weiler), 2nd edn, pp. 1–35. Kluwer Academic, Lancaster.

Weisman, H.F., Bartow, T., Leppo, M.K. *et al.* (1990) Soluble human complement receptor type 1: *in vivo* inhibitor of complement surpressing post-ischemic myocardial inflammation and necrosis. *Science*, **249**, 146–53.

Weitzman, J.B. & Law, S.K.A. (1993) CR3 and its relationship with other phagocytic receptors. In: *Complement in Health and Disease* (eds K. Whaley, M. Loos & J.M. Weiler), 2nd. edn, pp. 269–97. Kluwer Academic, Lancaster.

Whaley, K. (1987) Biochemistry and reaction mechanisms of complement. In: *Complement in Health and Disease.* (ed K. Whaley). MTP, Lancaster.

Whaley, K. & Ruddy, S. (1976a) Modulation of the alternative complement pathway by beta 1H globin. *J. Exp. Med.*, **144**, 1147–63.

Whaley, K. & Ruddy, S. (1976b) Modulation of C3b hemolytic activity by a plasma protein distinct from C3b inactivator. *Science*, **193**, 1011–13.

Yashuda, M., Takeuchi, K., Hiruma, M. *et al.* (1990) The complement system in ischaemic heart disease. *Circulation*, **81**, 156–63.

CHAPTER 19

Intrinsic Coagulation/ Bradykinin-Forming Cascade

A.P. Kaplan, M. Silverberg & S. Reddigari

Introduction

The plasma kinin-forming system consists of three essential plasma proteins, which interact in a complex fashion once they are bound to certain negatively charged surfaces or macromolecular complexes. These are coagulation factor XII (Hageman factor or HF), prekallikrein and high-molecular-weight kininogen (HK). Once factor XII is activated to factor XIIa, it converts plasma prekallikrein to kallikrein and kallikrein digests HK to liberate bradykinin. Factor XIIa also converts coagulation factor XI to factor XIa to continue the intrinsic coagulation cascade. The interactions of all four of these proteins to initiate blood clotting is known as 'contact activation', thus the formation of bradykinin is a cleavage product of the initiating step of this cascade (Fig. 19.1).

Protein constituents and mechanisms of activation

Factor XII

Factor XII circulates as a single-chain zymogen which possesses no detectable enzymatic activity (Silverberg & Kaplan, 1982). It has a molecular weight of 80 000 on sodium dodecyl sulphate (SDS) gel electrophoresis (Revak *et al.*, 1974), it is synthesized in the liver, and circulates in plasma at a concentration of 30–35 μg/ml. Its primary sequence is known from analysis of complementary DNA (cDNA) isolated from human liver cDNA libraries (Cool *et al.*, 1985; Que & Davie, 1986) and from direct protein-sequence data (Fujikawa & McMullen, 1983; McMullen & Fujikawa, 1985). The 596 amino acids present account for a molecular weight of 66 915; the remainder (16.8%) is carbohydrate. The protein has distinct domains homologous to fibronectin, plasminogen and plasminogen activators (Cool *et al.*, 1985; Castellino & Beals, 1987) at its N-terminal end, while the C terminus has the catalytic domain. This latter portion is homologous to serine proteases such as pancreatic trypsin, and even more so to the catalytic domain of plasminogen activators.

Factor XII is unusual because it is capable of autoactivating, once bound to initiating 'surfaces' (Silverberg *et al.*, 1980a; Tankersley & Finlayson, 1984). Thus, factor XII that is bound undergoes a conformational change which renders it a substrate for factor XIIa (Griffin, 1978). Gradually, all of the bound factor XII can be converted to factor XIIa. Whether plasma normally has a trace of factor XIIa present is unknown, but if so, its concentration is less than 0.01% of factor XII. The alternative is that the first molecule of factor XIIa is formed by interaction of two factor XII zymogen molecules on the surface, but this presumes some minimal activity present in the zymogen. If so, it is below our limits of detection, and the former scenario is favoured (Silverberg & Kaplan, 1982).

Activation of factor XII is due to cleavage of the molecule at a critical Arg-Val bond (Fujikawa & McMullen, 1983) contained within a disulphide bridge; the resulting factor XIIa is a two-chain, disulphide-linked 80-kDa enzyme, consisting of a heavy chain of 50 kDa and a light chain of 28 kDa (Revak *et al.*, 1977). The light chain contains the enzymatic active site (Meier *et al.*, 1977) and is at the carboxyl-terminal end, while the heavy chain contains the binding site for the surface and is at the amino-terminal end (Pixley *et al.*, 1987). Further cleavage can

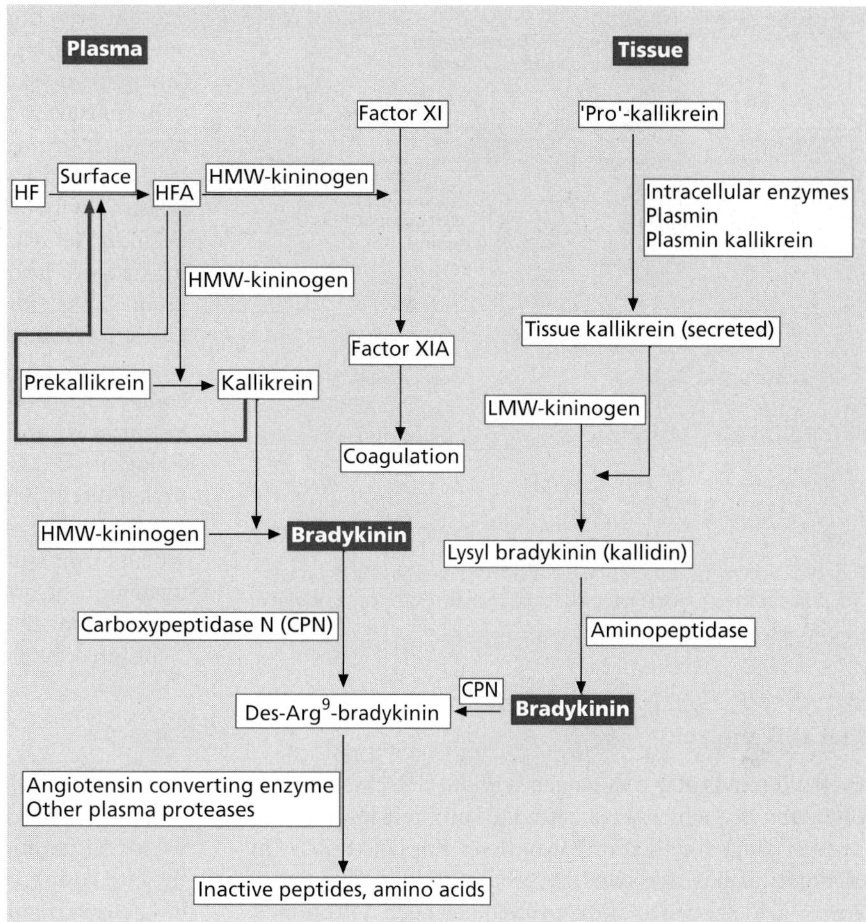

Fig. 19.1 Outline of the plasma tissue pathways of kinin formation and degradation. LMW, low molecular weight; HMW, high molecular weight.

occur at the C-terminal end of the heavy chain, to produce a series of fragments of activated factor XII which retain enzymatic activity (Kaplan & Austen, 1970, 1971). The most prominent of these is a 30-kDa species termed factor XIIf. Careful examination of factor XIIf on SDS gels in the absence of reduction reveals a doublet, in which the higher band at 30 kDa is gradually converted to the lower band which has a molecular weight of 28.5 kDa (Dunn & Kaplan, 1982). Reduced gels demonstrate that these species are composed of the light chain of factor XIIa and a very small piece of the original heavy chain. These fragments lack the binding site to the surface and lose much of the ability of factor XIIa to convert factor XI to factor XIa and do not participate in factor XII autoactivation. However, these fragments remain potent activators of prekallikrein (Kaplan & Austen, 1970). Thus, formation of factor XIIf allows bradykinin production to continue until the enzyme is inactivated and the reactions can proceed at sites distant from the initiating surface. A diagrammatic representation of the cleavages in factor XII to generate factor XIIa and factor XIIf is shown in Fig. 19.2.

Once factor XIIa interacts with prekallikrein, rapid conversion to kallikrein ensues, followed by an important positive feedback in which kallikrein digests surface-bound factor XII to form factor XIIa and then factor XIIf (Cochrane *et al.*, 1973; Meier *et al.*, 1977; Dunn *et al.*, 1982). This reaction is 50–100 times more rapid than the autoactivation reaction (Dunn *et al.*, 1982; Tankersley & Finlayson, 1984). Thus, quantitatively, most of the factor XIIa or factor XIIf activity generated when plasma is activated is a result of kallikrein activation of factor XII. However, the autoactivation phenomenon can be demonstrated in plasma that is congenitally deficient in prekallikrein (Fletcher trait) and cannot therefore generate any bradykinin (Wuepper, 1973; Saito *et al.*, 1974; Weiss *et al.*, 1974). Nevertheless, clotting (i.e. conversion of factor XI to factor XIa by factor XIIa) does proceed, albeit at a much slower rate, and the partial thromboplastin time (PTT) can be shown to progressively shorten as the time of incubation of the plasma with the surface is increased prior to recalcification. This is likely to be due to factor XII autoactivation on the surface. As more factor XIIa forms, the rate of factor XI activation increases and the PTT approaches normal.

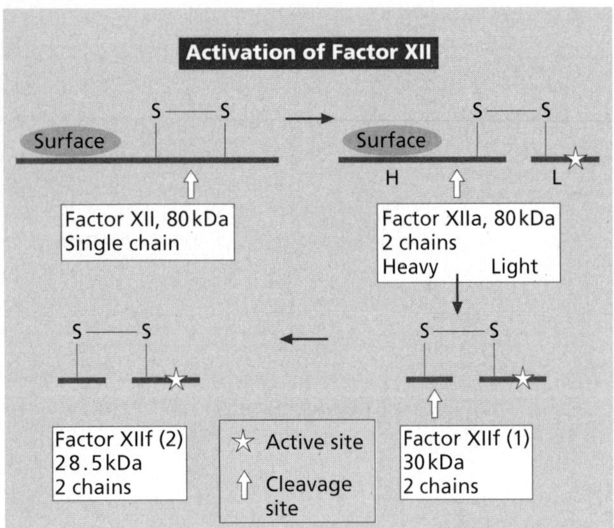

Fig. 19.2 Schematic representation of cleavages occurring in factor XII, which activates it to factor XIIa, and then further cleaves it to the two forms of factor XIIf.

Prekallikrein

Prekallikrein is also a zymogen without detectable proteolytic activity, which is converted to kallikrein by cleavage during contact activation (Mandle & Kaplan, 1977). On SDS gels, it has two bands at 88 and 85 kDa. The entire amino-acid sequence of the protein has been determined by a combination of direct protein sequencing and amino-acid sequence prediction from cDNA isolated from a λgt-11 expression library (Chung *et al.*, 1986). A signal peptide of 19 residues (which is cleaved off prior to secretion) is followed by the sequence of the mature plasma prekallikrein which has 619 amino acids with a calculated molecular weight of 69 710. In addition, there is 15% carbohydrate. The heterogeneity on SDS gel electrophoresis is not reflected in the amino-acid sequence, thus it may be due to variation in glycosylation. Activation of prekallikrein by factor XIIa or factor XIIf is due to cleavage of a single Arg-Ile band within a disulphide bridge, such that a heavy chain of 56 kDa is disulphide linked to a light chain of either 33 or 36 kDa, each of which has a diisopropyl fluorophosphate (DFP)-inhibitable active site (Mandle & Kaplan, 1977; Bouma *et al.*, 1980). This light-chain heterogeneity reflects the two forms of the zymogen.

The amino-acid sequence of the kallikrein heavy chain is unusual and is homolgous only to the corresponding portion of factor XI. It has four tandem repeats, each containing approximately 90–91 amino acids. The presence of six cysteines per repeat suggests a repeating structure with three disulphide loops. It is postulated that a gene coding for the ancestor of this repeat sequence duplicated, and then the entire segment duplicated again to give the present structure. The light chain, containing the active site, is homologous to many of the catalytic domains of other enzymes of the coagulation cascade.

In contrast to factor XII, prekallikrein does not circulate as a separate protein. It is bound to HK in a 1 : 1 bimolecular complex through a site on its heavy chain. The binding is firm, with a dissociation constant of 12–15 nmol/l (Mandle *et al.*, 1976; Bock *et al.*, 1985), and this is unchanged upon conversion of prekallikrein to kallikrein. Thus, at plasma concentration of prekallikrein (35–50 μg/ml) and HK, about 80–90% of the prekallikrein is normally complexed (Scott & Colman, 1980). During contact activation, the prekallikrein–HK complex binds to surfaces, and the binding is primarily through HK (Wiggins *et al.*, 1977), although some interaction of prekallikrein with the surface can be inferred (Rosing *et al.*, 1985). The dissociation of 10–20% of the kallikrein which forms from the surface may serve to propagate the formation of bradykinin in the fluid phase and at sites distant from the initiating reaction (Cochrane & Revak, 1980; Silverberg *et al.*, 1980b).

Factor XI

Coagulation factor XI is the second substrate of factor XIIa (Fig. 19.1), but it has no role in bradykinin formation. Factor XI is unique among the clotting factors, because the circulating zymogen consists of two identical chains linked by disulphide bonds (Bouma & Griffin, 1977; Kurachi & Davie, 1977). The dimer has an apparent molecular weight of 160 kDa on SDS gel electrophoresis, but reveals a single 80-kDa protein upon reduction. Factor XI activation follows the familiar pattern of cleavage of a single peptide band (Arg–Ile) wthin a disulphide bridge, to yield an animo-terminal heavy chain of 50 kDa and a disulphide-linked light chain of 33 kDa. Since both subunits can be cleaved by factor XIIa and each resultant light-chain bears a functional active site, factor XIa is a four-chain protein with two active sites. The concentration in plasma is only 4–8 μg/ml, the lowest of these proteins, and the heavy chain(s), like that of kallikrein, binds to the light chain of HK. Thus, factor XI and HK also circulate as a complex (Thompson *et al.*, 1977). The dissociation constant is 70 nmol/l (Tait & Fujikawa, 1987), which is high enough to ensure that virtually all the factor XI is complexed. The molar ratio of the complex can consist of one or two molecules of HK per factor XI because of the dimeric nature of factor XI (Warn-Cramer & Bajaj, 1985). The binding site for HK on factor XI has been localized to the first (N-terminal) tandem repeat (Baglia *et al.*, 1989). The factor XI–HK complex binds to the surface and conversion to factor XIa must occur on the surface; fluid-phase conversion by factor XIIf is only 2–4% of that of surface-bound factor XIIa (Kaplan & Austen, 1971). The primary function of factor XIa is to activate factor IX to IXa, which is the first Ca^{2+}-dependent reaction in the intrinsic coagulation cascade.

The amino-acid sequence of human factor XI has been determined by translation of a cDNA insert obtained from a λgt-11 cDNA library prepared from human liver poly (A) RNA (Fujikawa *et al.*, 1986). It has a 19-amino-acid leader peptide, followed by a 60% amino-acid sequence for each of the two chains of the mature protein. The amino-acid sequence of the heavy chain of factor XIa, like that of kallikrein, has four tandem repeats of about 90 amino acids with six cysteines per repeat, implying three disulphide bands. Unpaired cysteines in the first and fourth repeats are postulated to form the interchain disulphide bridges between monomers to produce the homodimer. The striking similarity in structure between prekallikrein and factor XI is shown in Fig. 19.3.

HK

HK circulates as a 115-kDa glycoprotein when examined under reducing conditions by SDS gel electrophoresis (Colman & Muller-Esterl, 1988). Its apparent molecular weight by gel filtration is aberrant, at about 200 000, indicative of a large partial specific volume due to its conformation in solution (Mandle *et al.*, 1976). It circulates in plasma at a concentration of 70–90 μg/ml (Proud *et al.*, 1980; Adam *et al.*, 1985; Berrettini *et al.*, 1986; Reddigari & Kaplan, 1989b) and forms non-covalent complexes with both prekallikrein and factor XI with dissociation constants of 15 nmol/l (Bock & Shore, 1983; Bock *et al.*, 1985) and 70 nmol/l (Thompson *et al.*, 1979; Tait & Fujikawa, 1987), respectively. There is sufficient HK in plasma to theoretically bind both factor XII substrates, and the excess HK (about 10–20%) circulates uncomplexed. The complexes of HK with prekallikrein or factor XI are formed with the light-chain region of HK; the isolated light chain (after reduction and alkylation) possesses the same binding characteristics as the whole molecule (Thompson *et al.*, 1978, 1979). HK functions as a coagulation cofactor and this activity resides in the light chain (Thompson *et al.*, 1978), which consists of a basic (histidine-rich) amino-terminal domain that binds to initiating surfaces (Ikari *et al.*, 1981), and a carboxyl-terminal domain that binds prekallikrein or factor XI (Tait & Fujikawa, 1986). The one cysteine in the light chain links it to the heavy chain. The prekallikrein binding site maps to residues 194–224 (Tait & Fujikawa, 1986, 1987) and factor XI binds to the same region, but with a broader span encompassing residues 185–242 (Tait & Fujikawa, 1987). Since they overlap, one molecule of HK binds either prekallikrein or factor XI, but not both.

During contact activation, kallikrein cleaves HK in two positions within a disulphide bridge; first at the C-terminal Arg-Ser (Mori & Nagasawa, 1981; Mori *et al.*, 1981) and then at the N-terminal Lys-Arg to release the nonapeptide bradykinin (Arg-Pro-Pro-Gly-Phe-Ser-Pro-Phe-Arg). A two-chain disulphide-linked kinin-free HK results, consisting of a heavy chain of 65 000 and a light chain variously reported at molecular weights of 56 000–62 000. A subsequent further cleavage of the light chain yields a final product of 46 000–49 000 (Schiffman *et al.*, 1980; Mori *et al.*, 1981; Mori & Nagasawa, 1981; Bock & Shore, 1983; Reddigari & Kaplan, 1988), which retains all light-chain functions. Tissue kallikrein can also digest HK to liberate kallidin or Lys-bradykinin, leaving the heavy-chain disulphide linked to the 56–62-kDa light chain; the additional cleavage of the light chain is not made by this

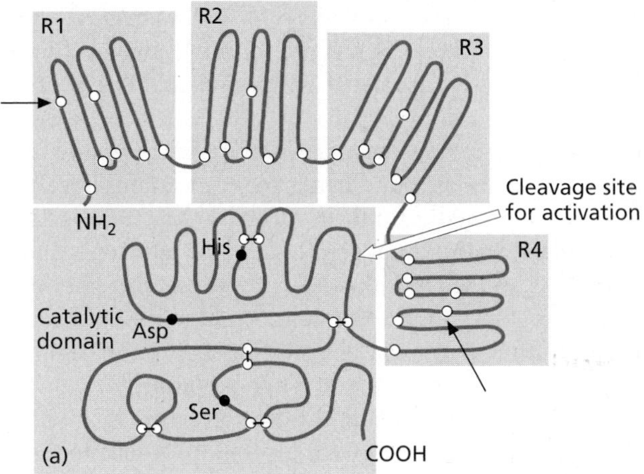

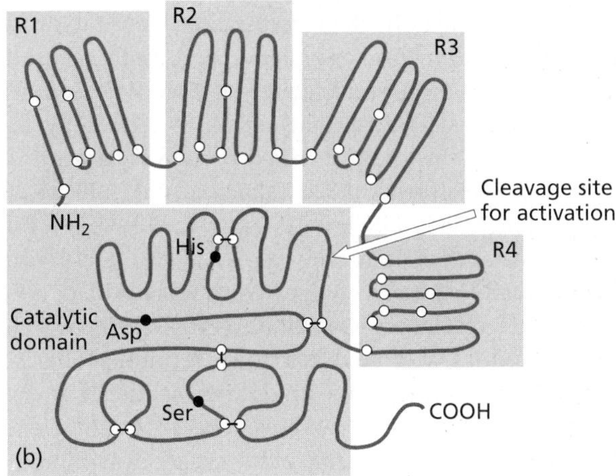

Fig. 19.3 Schematic diagram of the protein chains of factor XI (a) and prekallikrein (b), showing the structural domains inferred from sequence homologies. The catalytic triad residues are shown by solid circles, half-cysteines are indicated by open circles, and the cleavage sites leading to activation by activated factor XII are marked with open arrows. The solid arrows indicate the unmatched half-cysteines that might be involved in interchain disulphide bonds. (After Fujikawa *et al.*, 1986.)

enzyme (Reddigari & Kaplan, 1988). It is important to note that tissue kallikrein is a kinin-forming enzyme that is immunologically unrelated to plasma kallikrein. It is secreted by various organs or cells, such as salivary glands, kidney, pancreas, prostate, pituitary gland and neutrophils, and is found in high concentrations in saliva, urine and prostatic fluid. Its primary substrate is low-molecular-weight kininogen (LK), but it releases kallidin from HK or LK. Kallidin has properties that are very similar to bradykinin, but it is slightly less potent. A plasma amino peptidase (Guimaraes *et al.*, 1973) removes the N-terminal Lys to convert it to bradykinin.

HK has a very unusual domain structure (Fig. 19.4). Domain 5, the histidine-rich region at the N-terminal end of the light chain, binds to initiating surfaces, while the binding of prekallikrein or factor XI at the C-terminal domain 6 of the light chain account for the cofactor function of HK in intrinsic coagulation and kinin generation. The complete amino-acid sequence of HK has been determined as translated from the cDNA, as well as by direct sequence analysis of the purified protein (Kitamura *et al.*, 1985; Lottspeich *et al.*, 1985; Takagaki *et al.*, 1985; Kellermann *et al.*, 1986). HK has 626 amino acids with a calculated molecular weight of 69 896. It has 40% carbohydrate, an unusually high percentage, which when added, gives a molecular weight close to that observed. The heavy chain of 362 residues is derived from the N terminus. This is followed by the nine-residue bradykinin sequence and then the light chain of 265 residues. The N-terminal end is blocked with pyroglutamic acid (cyclic glutamine). The carbohydrate is distributed via three N-linked glycosidic linkages on the heavy chain and nine O-linked glycosidic

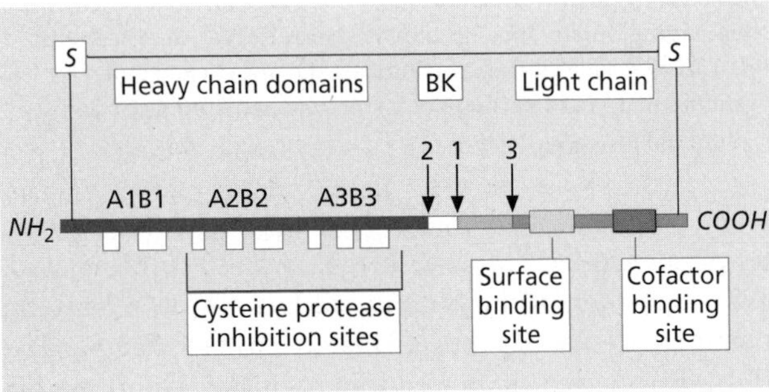

Fig. 19.4 The structure of high-molecular-weight kininogen (HK). The heavy-chain region consists of three homologous domains—A1B1, A2B2 and A3B3—of which the latter two are sulphydryl protease inhibition sites. The small rectangles under the heavy-chain region represent the eight intra-heavy-chain disulphide bonds. The light-chain region of HK, which contains the binding sites for surface and prekallikrein or factor XI, is located towards the C-terminal end of the protein. The heavy and light chains are held together by the ninth disulphide bond. The arrowheads labelled 1, 2 and 3 indicate the sites and the order in which plasma kallikrein cleaves HK. BK, bradykinin.

linkages on the light chain. The heavy chain has three contiguous and homologous 'apple'-type domains consisting of residues 1–116, 117–238 and 239–360 (Fig. 19.4). There are 17 cysteines, one of which is disulphide linked to the light chain and the other from light disulphide loops within these domains (Kellermann *et al.*, 1986). These three domains are homologous to a family of small (12–13 kDa) cysteine protease inhibitors called cystatins, which inactivate certain intracellular cathepsins. Domains 2 and 3 (but not 1) retain this function; for example, native HK can bind and inactivate two molecules of the sulphydryl-containing protease papain (Gounaris *et al.*, 1984; Muller-Esterl *et al.*, 1985a; Higashiyama *et al.*, 1986; Ishiguro *et al.*, 1987). Limited proteolysis of the heavy chain can occur at susceptible bonds that separate the domains, so that individual domains can be isolated. Cleavage at these sites may occur under certain pathological conditions.

LK and kininogen genes

LK, a second kininogen of molecular weight 68 kDa, is digested by tissue kallikrein to yield Lys-bradykinin, and a kinin-free kininogen consisting of a 65-kDa heavy-chain disulphide linked to a light chain of only 4 kDa (Jacobsen & Kritz, 1967; Lottspeich *et al.*, 1984; Muller-Esterl *et al.*, 1985b; Kellermann *et al.*, 1986; Johnson *et al.*, 1987). LK is *not* cleaved by plasma kallikrein. The amino-acid sequence of HK and LK are identical from the amino terminus through the bradykinin sequence plus the next 12 residues (Muller-Esterl *et al.*, 1985b). Then the sequence diverges, because the light chains of the two kininogens have no homology whatsoever. Thus, LK does not bind to surfaces or to prekallikrein or factor XI. The kininogens are produced from a single gene thought to have originated by two successive duplications of a primordial cystatin-like gene (Kitamura *et al.*, 1985). As represented in Fig. 19.5, there are 11 exons. The first nine code for the heavy chain and each of the three domains in this portion of the protein is represented by three exons. The 10th exon codes for bradykinin and the light chain of HK, while the light chain of LK is encoded by exon 11. The mRNA for HK and LK are produced by alternative splicing at a point 12 amino acids beyond the bradykinin sequence, which provides alternative light-chain moieties (Fig. 19.5).

Mechanisms of contact activation

Initiating surfaces

Contact activation was initially observed by the interaction of blood with glass surfaces (Margolis, 1958); subsequently, finely divided kaolin was used extensively as an experimental surface and for coagulation assays such

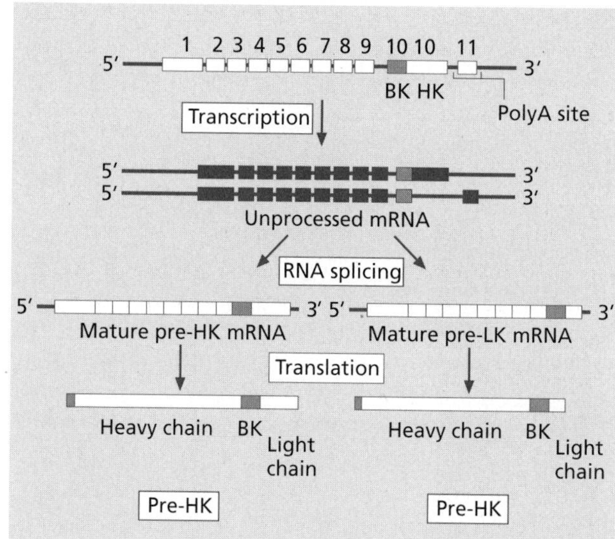

Fig. 19.5 The gene for high-molecular-weight kininogen (HK). The boxes labelled 1–9 represent the exon coding for the heavy chain of both HK and low-molecular-weight kininogen (LK). Exon 10 codes for the bradykinin (BK) sequence and the light chain of HK, whereas exon 11 codes for the light chain of LK. The mature mRNAs are assembled by alternative splicing events in which the light-chain sequences are attached to the 3′ end of the 12-amino-acid common sequence C terminus to BK.

as the PTT (Proctor & Rapaport, 1961). Ellagic acid (Ratnoff & Crum, 1964), a tannin-like substance used as a component of many commercial assay systems, was purported to be a soluble initiator, but was later shown to form large sedimentable aggregates catalysed by trace heavy metal ions; therefore, it is also a particulate (Bock *et al.*, 1981). More recently, dextran sulphate (Kluft, 1978; Fujikawa *et al.*, 1980) and sulphatide (Fujikawa *et al.*, 1980) have been used to study contact activation. Sulphatide, a naturally occurring sphingolipid bearing a galactose sulphate group, is found in small quantities in nerve tissue where it is too diluted by other lipids to be an effective activator. However, when purified, it can form highly charged micelles which are very efficient initiators (Tans & Griffin, 1982; Griep *et al.*, 1985). Dextran sulphate is a truly soluble activator and a close homologue of naturally occurring sulphated mucopolysaccharides. High-molecular-weight preparations of 500 kDa are typically used (Fujikawa *et al.*, 1980; Silverberg & Kaplan, 1982; Tankersley & Finlayson, 1984), but in a study of factor XII autoactivation (Silverberg & Diehl, 1987b), much smaller fractions were effective down to as low as 5 kDa. The rate of factor XII activation increased markedly with dextran sulphate at 10 kDa (or more), where the theoretical number of factor XII molecules capable of binding per particle increased from one to two, and similar results were seen with heparin. This presumably provides a critical intermolecular interaction required for optimal autoactivation.

Naturally occurring polysaccharides are effective if they are highly sulphated, and include heparin and chondroitin sulphate E (described in rodent mucosal mast cells) (Hojima *et al.*, 1984). Other mucopolysaccharides known to catalyse factor XII autoactivation are dermatan sulphate, keratin polysulphate or chondroitin sulphate C (Brunnée *et al.*, 1995). The basement membrane of endothelial cell matrix may support contact activation, but this has not been demonstrated *in vivo*. Collagen, long thought to be an initiator, was proven to be ineffective and the activity reported was likely to be due to contaminating matrix proteins. One pathophysiological substance very likely to initiate contact activation *in vivo* is endotoxin (Pettinger & Young, 1970; Morrison & Cochrane, 1974; Roeise *et al.*, 1988), and there is good reason to believe that the contact cascade is activated in septic shock and the observed symptoms are due, in part, to the generation of bradykinin (Mason *et al.*, 1970; Kaufman *et al.*, 1991). Crystals of uric acid and pyrophosphate can also initiate kinin formation via this pathway (Kellermeyer & Breckenridge, 1965; Ginsberg *et al.*, 1980).

Activation mechanisms and regulation

The various interactions of these constituents are shown in Fig. 19.6, which also includes those steps that can be inhibited by the C1 inhibitor (C1 INH). The slow autoactivation of factor XII is shown, as well as the kallikrein feedback loop to generate factor XIIa. This reciprocal reaction is so fast that if plasma concentration of factor XII and prekallikrein are mixed, assuming one activated molecule of XII per millilitre, there is 50% activation in 13 seconds (Tankersley & Finlayson, 1984). This represents a starting concentration of active enzyme of 5×10^{-13}%. The source of this infinitesimal amount of active enzyme is unknown, but may be formed by other plasma proteases, e.g. plasmin. In fact, very slow turnover of the cascade may always be occurring which is controlled by plasma inhibitors (Weiss *et al.*, 1986). Introduction of a surface or other polyanionic substance could accelerate many thousand-fold the baseline turnover of factor XII and prekallikrein to ignite the cascade. The addition of the cofactor HK (which was not included in the aforementioned kinetic analysis) accelerates these reactions even further, but requires the surface to be present. The surface appears to create a local milieu in the contiguous fluid (Griffin & Cochrane, 1976; Griep *et al.*, 1985; Silverberg & Diehl, 1987a) phase where the local concentrations of reactants are greatly increased, which increases the rates of the reciprocal interaction. In addition, factor XII, when bound, undergoes a conformational change that renders it more susceptible to cleavage (Griffin, 1978). The alterna-

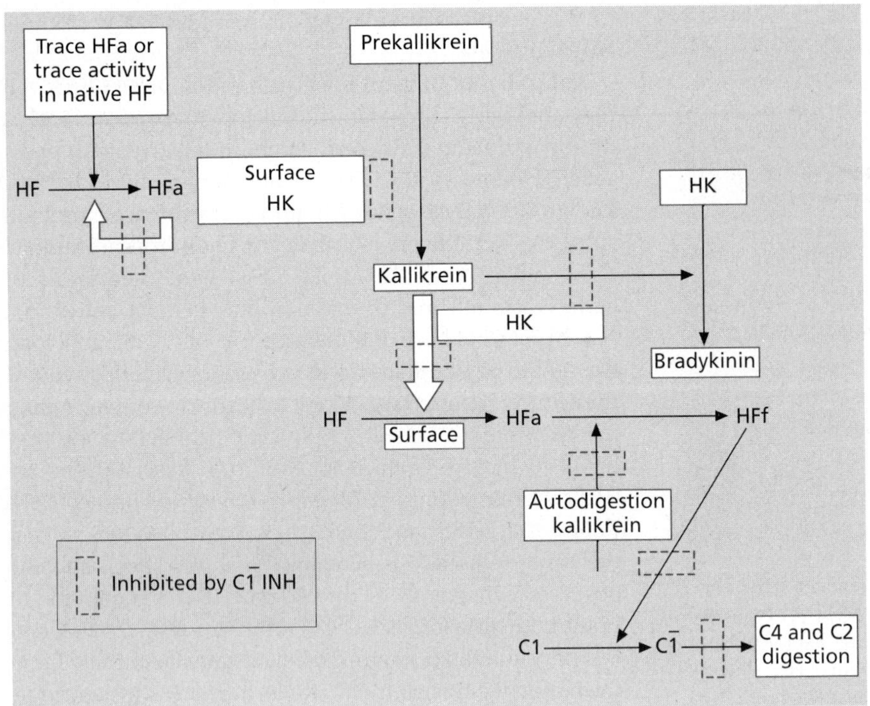

Fig. 19.6 The plasma kinin-forming cascade depicting the initiating autoactivation step, the positive feedback involving kallikrein and a linkage to the complement cascade. All steps inhibitable by C1 INH are shown. HF, Hageman factor.

tive idea (McMillin *et al.*, 1974; Ratnoff & Saito, 1979; Kurachi *et al.*, 1980) that binding of factor XII induces a conformational change that exposes an active site has essentially been disproven. Inhibitors such as C1 INH are not bound to the surface, thus the balance between activation and inactivation is upset. The effect of dilution on plasma also diminishes the effect of inhibitors far more than any slowing of enzymatic reaction rates. The net effect is, therefore, a marked augmentation of reaction rate. Using dextran sulphate, the effect of the surface upon factor XIIa conversion of prekallikrein to kallikrein was 70-fold (Tankersley & Finlayson, 1984), while the effect upon digestion of factor XII by kallikrein was as much as 3000–12 000-fold (Tankersley & Finlayson, 1984; Rosing *et al.*, 1985). This latter reaction is about 2000-fold more rapid than the rate of factor XII autoactivation, and this kinetic dominance means that prekallikrein must be considered to be a coagulation factor. As indicated earlier, the PTT of prekallikrein-deficient plasma is much prolonged, but does autocorrect as factor XII autoactivates on the surface. On the other hand, factor XII-deficient plasma has a markedly abnormal PTT and does not autocorrect and is essentially devoid of intrinsic clotting or kinin formation. Alternatively, purified factor XII preparations activate when tested with a surface or polyanion under physiological conditions (Silverberg *et al.*, 1987a,b; Tans *et al.*, 1983; Tankersley & Finlayson, 1984), whereas prekallikrein does not. Hence, factor XII is considered to be an absolute requisite for intrinsic coagulation, while prekallikrein acts as an accelerator.

In plasma, the involvement of an additional protein was indicated by the discovery of individuals whose plasma had a very prolonged PTT and who generated no bradykinin upon incubation with kaolin, but were not deficient in factor XII or prekallikrein (Colman *et al.*, 1975; Wuepper *et al.*, 1975; Donaldson *et al.*, 1976). This phenomenon was explained by the identification of HK as a non-enzymatic cofactor in contact activation. It appeared to accelerate activation of both factor XII and prekallikrein as well as factor XI (Griffin & Cochrane, 1976; Meier *et al.*, 1977; Revak *et al.*, 1977; Wiggins *et al.*, 1977). The discovery that prekallikrein and factor XII circulate bound to HK provided the mechanistic key to the explanation (Mandle *et al.*, 1976; Thompson *et al.*, 1977). One function of HK is to present the substrates of factor XIIa in a conformation that facilitates their activation. Thus, prekallikrein that is bound to a surface in the absence of HK is not subsequently activated by factor XIIa (Silverberg *et al.*, 1980b). A synthetic peptide encompassing the HK binding site for prekallikrein can interfere with contact activation by competitively interfering with the binding of prekallikrein to the HK light chain (Tait & Fujikawa, 1987) and, similarly, a monoclonal antibody to this binding site inhibits coagulation and kinin formation in plasma (Reddigari & Kaplan, 1989a). Factor XI activation is almost totally dependent upon the formation of a surface-binding complex with

HK. HK also augments the rate of factor XII activation in plasma (Revak *et al.*, 1977; Wiggins *et al.*, 1977), although it does not augment the activity of kallikrein against synthetic substrates. The effect seems to be largely indirect. Firstly, it is required for efficient formation of kallikrein in surface-activated plasma. Secondly, since kallikrein can dissociate from surface-bound HK, it can interact with surface-bound factor XII on an adjacent particle, thereby disseminating the reaction (Wiggins *et al.*, 1977; Cochrane & Revak, 1980; Silverberg *et al.*, 1980b). As a result, the effective kallikrein/factor XII ratio is increased in the presence of HK. Finally, in plasma, HK can displace other adhesive glycoproteins such as fibrinogen from binding to the surface (Schmaier *et al.*, 1984). These data indicate that HK must also be considered to be a coagulation cofactor, because it is required for the generation of kallikrein (a factor XII activator), as well as the activation of factor XI. HK-deficient plasma has a profoundly prolonged activated PTT that is almost as abnormal as that of factor XII deficiency (Colman *et al.*, 1975; Wuepper *et al.*, 1975; Donaldson *et al.*, 1976).

Regulation of contact activation occurs via plasma protease inhibitors. A summary of the major control proteins of this pathway is given in Table 19.1. The C1 INH is a major inhibitor of factor XIIa or XIIf (Forbes *et al.*, 1970; Schreiber *et al.*, 1973; de Agostini *et al.*, 1984; Pixley *et al.*, 1985) and it is not active against other coagulation enzymes, except for a weak inhibition of factor XIa. The inhibitor is cleaved by the protease and then binds at the active site of the protease in a 1 : 1 molar covalent complex that completely inactivates the enzyme (Travis & Salvesen, 1983). Antithrombin III (AT III), which is a critical control protein for much of the coagulation cascade, makes a minor contribution to factor XIIa (f) inactivation (Stead *et al.*, 1976; de Agostini *et al.*, 1984; Pixley *et al.*, 1985; Cameron *et al.*, 1989). Heparin can augment the inhibition by AT III, although the magnitude of augmentation has been reported to vary. Heparin can also function as an activating polyanion for contact activation (Hojima *et al.*, 1984; Silverberg & Diehl, 1987b). Curiously, α_2-macroglobulin, which is an inhibitor of broad reactivity with enzymes, does not significantly inhibit any of the forms of activated factor XII.

Kallikrein is inhibited by both C1 INH and α_2-macroglobulin (Gigli *et al.*, 1970; McConnell, 1972; Harpel, 1974), which together account for over 90% of the inhibitory activity of plasma (Schapira *et al.*, 1982; van der Graaf *et al.*, 1983). α_2-Macroglobulin does *not* bind to the active site, but traps the protease within its structure so as to sterically interfere with its ability to cleave large protein substrates (Barrett & Starkey, 1973). About one-third of the enzyme's activity on small synthetic substrates is retained since the active site is available, although the activity on its natural substrates is <1%. Although these two inhibitors contribute roughly equally when kallikrein is added to plasma (Schapira *et al.*, 1982; van der Graaf *et al.*, 1983; Harpel *et al.*, 1985), when a surface such as kaolin is added, 70–80% of the kallikrein formed is bound to C1 INH (Harpel *et al.*, 1985). The reason for this difference is unknown. Conversely, at low temperatures, C1 INH is less effective, and much of the kallikrein inhibition is mediated by α_2-macroglobulin (Harpel *et al.*, 1985). A major inhibitor of factor XIa is α_1-antitrypsin (Heck & Kaplan, 1974; Scott *et al.*, 1982b). This is unusual and represents the only major role for this inhibitor in the coagulation cascade. Other factor XIa inhibitors are C1 INH (Meijers *et al.*, 1988) and AT III (Scott *et al.*, 1982b), and here too the magnitude of heparin enhancement of AT III function is disputed (Scott *et al.*, 1982a; Beeler *et al.*, 1985).

Activation on a surface occurs very quickly, while inhibition has a slower reaction rate. In plasma of patients with hereditary angioedema in which C1 inhibitor is absent or dysfunctional, the amount of surface needed to produce maximal activation is 10–20-fold less than that needed to activate normal plasma (Cameron *et al.*, 1989).

Table 19.1 Plasma inhibitors of enzymes of contact activation: percentage inhibition in normal human plasma.

	Enzyme			
	Factors			Factor
Inhibitor	XIIa	XIIf	Kallikrein	XIa
C1 inhibitor	91.3	93	52 (84)*	8
Antithrombin III†	1.5	4	ND	16
α_2-macroglobulin	4.3	—	35 (16)*	—
α_1-protease inhibitor	—	—	ND	68
α_2-antiplasmin	3.0	3	ND	8

ND, not determined separately.
* Data obtained from generation of kallikrein *in situ*.
† Data are for results obtained in the absence of added heparin.

Bradykinin: functions and control mechanisms

The functions of bradykinin include venular dilatation, increased vascular permeability (Regoli & Barabe, 1980), constriction of uterine and gastrointestinal smooth muscle, constriction of coronary and pulmonary vasculature, bronchoconstriction, and activation of phospholipase A_2 to augment arachidonic acid metabolism. It acts in most tissues via B_2 receptors, and selective B_2-receptor antagonists have been recently synthesized. In plasma, bradykinin is first digested by carboxypeptidase N (also known as angiotension-converting enzyme (ACE)) (Erdos & Sloane, 1962), which removes the C-terminal Arg leaving des-Arg9 bradykinin (Sheikh & Kaplan, 1986b).

This peptide lacks the inflammatory function of bradykinin (vasodilatation, increased permeability) that is evident in skin or smooth muscle, but can interact with B_1 receptors in the vasculature to cause hypotension. B_1 receptors are induced during inflammatory conditions (Regoli & Barabe, 1980), while B_2 receptors are synthesized constitutively. When serum is examined, the rate of removal of the C-terminal Arg is more rapid than can be attributed to carboxypeptidase N (Sheikh & Kaplan, 1989). This may be due to secretion (from cells) or activation of carboxypeptidase U, a newly described exopeptidase (Wang *et al.*, 1994). The next cleavage is by ACE, which digests des-Arg9 bradykinin (Arg-Pro-Pro-Gly-Phe-Ser-Pho-Phe) via its tripeptidase activity (Sheikh & Kaplan, 1986a) (dipeptidase activity converts angiotensin I to angiotensin II) to yield Arg-Pro-Pro-Gly-Phe + Ser-Pro-Phe. These products are inactive on both B_1 and B_2 receptors. Further slow digestion leads to the final products of Arg-Pro-Pro, plus one mole each of the amino acids Gly, Ser, Pro and Arg, and two moles of Phe (Sheikh & Kaplan, 1989).

In vivo, kinin degradation occurs rapidly along endothelial cells of the pulmonary vasculature. However, here, the predominant enzyme is ACE, which acts as a dipeptidase if the C-terminal Arg is present to remove Phe-Arg. The resultant heptapeptide is cleaved once again at the C-terminal end to liberate Ser-Pro, leaving the pentapeptide Arg-Pro-Pro-Gly-Phe (Sheikh & Kaplan, 1986a). These peptides are further metabolized to Arg-Pro-Pro and free amino acids as indicated above. The cough and angioedema associated with the use of ACE inhibitors for treatment of heart failure, hypertension, diabetes or scleroderma may be due to inhibition of kinin inactivation and accumulation of bradykinin, as conversion to angiotensin II is prevented.

Assembly along endothelial cell surfaces

All the components of the contact activation cascade can be found along the surface of endothelial cells, as shown diagrammatically in Fig. 19.7. Schmaier *et al.* (1988) and Van Iwaarden *et al.* (1988) first described binding of HK to human umbilical vein endothelial cells in a zinc-dependent reaction. This binding was demonstrated subsequently by immunochemical staining of umbilical veins after incubation with HK (Nishikawa *et al.*, 1992) and binding was shown to be saturable, reversible, dependent on 15–50 μmol/l zinc (normal plasma concentration) and fulfilling the characteristics of a receptor. There are 1×10^6 to 1×10^7 binding sites (an unusually large number) with a high-affinity kDa of approximately 40–50 nmol/l. Binding is seen with each chain of HK (i.e. heavy and light chains), thus a complex interaction with subsites within the receptor seems likely (Reddigari *et al.*, 1993a). A similar complex interaction has been observed with platelets, although the binding site number is far less. Since prekallikrein and factor XI circulate bound to HK, these are brought to the endothelial cell surface via HK (Berrettini *et al.*, 1992). There are no separate receptor sites for either prekallikrein or factor XI. When binding of factor XII was examined, binding characteristics of a receptor, which was strikingly similar to that seen with HK, including a requirement for zinc, was found (Reddigari *et al.*, 1993b). It was then demonstrated that HK and factor XII can compete for binding at a comparable molar basis, suggesting that they bind to the same receptor (Reddigari *et al.*, 1993b).

It has also been demonstrated that factor XII can slowly autoactivate when bound to endothelial cells (Reddigari *et al.*, 1993b), and that addition of kallikrein can digest bound HK to liberate bradykinin at a rate proportional to the kallikrein concentration and with a final bradykinin level dependent on the amount of bound HK. Thus, activation of the cascade along the endothelial cell surface is likely; bradykinin is liberated and then interacts with the B_2 receptors to increase permeability. Bradykinin can also stimulate cultured endothelial cells to secrete tissue plasminogen activator (Smith *et al.*, 1985), prostaglandin I_2 (prostacyclin) and thromboxane A_2 (Hong, 1980; Crutchly *et al.*, 1983), and can thereby modulate platelet function and stimulate local fibrinolysis.

Clinical considerations

Kinin formation in hereditary angioedema

The pathogenesis of hereditary angioedema (HAE) suggests liberation of a kinin that has variously been considered to be a product of the second component of complement or produced by contact activation. As shown in Fig. 19.7, if C1 INH is either absent (type I) or dysfunctional (type II), there is insufficient inhibition of all the activated forms of factor XII, kallikrein or activated C1 (specifically C1r and C1s, each of which is inhibited by C1 INH). The production of bradykinin is markedly augmented under these conditions and it has been shown that addition of dextran sulphate at concentrations insufficient to activate normal plasma leads to complete digestion of HK in HAE plasma within a few minutes. Thus, seemingly insignificant trauma or infections may be sufficient to initiate an attack in such patients.

Soon after C1 INH deficiency was shown to be the cause of HAE, evidence was presented to suggest that cleavage of C2 (Donaldson, 1968) or C2b (Donaldson *et al.*, 1977) would generate a kinin that was responsible for the symptoms. Attempts to produce this kinin by cleavage of C2 or C2b have, in general, been negative (Fields *et al.*, 1983), nor has such a kinin been shown to circulate in patients during

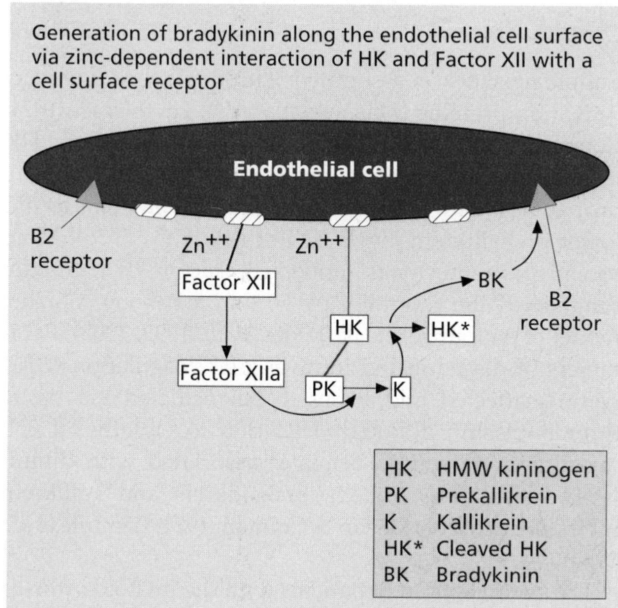

Fig. 19.7 Assembly of the proteins involved in bradykinin formation along the endothelial cell surface. A common receptor binds factor XII and HK requiring zinc ion. Bradykinin, once liberated, acts on the B_2 receptor to activate endothelial cells and increase vascular permeability.

an attack. However, synthesis of overlapping peptides within the C2b portion of the molecule revealed a sequence which possessed kinin-like peptides (Strang *et al.*, 1988), although enzymatic cleavage of the protein to release this peptide has not yet been achieved.

Activated kallikrein has been shown to be present in markedly augmented amounts in blister fluids derived from patients, and bradykinin has been reported to be the major kinin found when HAE plasma is activated (Curd *et al.*, 1980). The bulk of evidence favours a major role for bradykinin in causing the symptoms of HAE (Fields *et al.*, 1983). However, the presence of an additional kinin-like fragment, derived from C2 by a mechanism that is not yet understood, is possible. If so, synergy between the two kinins might occur. Use of B_2-receptor antagonists in such patients, once they are available for human use, should help settle the question.

Complement is nevertheless clearly activated in HAE, and this may be due to the autoactivation of C1r when C1 INH is absent. C4 levels are diminished, presumably due to consumption by C1s in HAE patients even when they are asymptomatic; with attacks of swelling, C4 levels approach zero and C2 levels diminish. As seen in Fig. 19.7, this process may be augmented by factor XIIf (HFf), which has been shown to enzymatically cleave and activate C1r, and to a lesser degree, C1s (Ghebrehiwet *et al.*, 1983). Use of androgenic therapeutic agents (danazol, stanozolol) may increase synthesis of C1 INH sufficiently to prevent swelling. Levels of C4 and C1 INH increase; however, the magnitude may not parallel the clinical effect. Use of agents which inhibit plasminogen activation (e-amino caproic acid, tranexamic acid) are also effective therapeutic agents which prevent formation of plasmin; they may also have direct inhibitory effects on C1 activation (Soter *et al.*, 1975). Plasmin is also an enzymatic activator of factor XII (Kaplan & Austen, 1971) and might thereby contribute to HFf production and bradykinin formation, or it might digest C2b to yield a kinin-like fragment (Strang *et al.*, 1988).

Contact activation in allergic diseases

By analogy with observations using dextran sulphate, naturally occurring glycosaminoglycans or proteoglycans may be able to induce contact activation. Heparin proteoglycan from the Furth murine mastocytoma has been tested for its ability to activate a mixture of factor XII and prekallikrein. There is progressive conversion of prekallikrein to kallikrein as the concentration of mast cell heparin is increased. The potency of heparin proteoglycan equals that of dextran sulphate and its activity is inhibited by heparinase I or II, but not by heparitinase or chondroitinase ABC. Of the glycosaminoglycans that have been tested, heparin, dermatan sulphate, keratin polysulphate and chondroitin sulphate C are positive in the assay (in that order), while heparan sulphate and chondroitin sulphate A are negative. Collagen types I, III, IV and V, laminin, fibronectin and vitronectin are also negative. Activation can then occur by release of heparin and/or other mucopolysaccharides secreted by mast cells and basophils upon exposure to plasma proteins and via interaction of these proteins with exposed connective tissue proteoglycans during tissue injury. The proteins of the kinin-forming system have been shown to be present in interstitial fluid of rabbit skin, thus the source may not solely be dependent upon exudation and activation of plasma.

Any aspect of inflammation which leads to dilution of plasma constituents or exclusion of inhibitors will augment contact activation, since inhibitory functions are very dependent upon concentration. Thus, the degree of activation of plasma can be shown to be related directly to dilution. Once levels of C1 INH are less than 25% of normal (i.e. a 1:4 dilution), patients with HAE are prone to attacks of swelling.

Activation of the plasma and tissue kinin-forming systems have been observed in allergic reactions in the nose, lungs and skin, and include the immediate reaction as well as the late-phase reaction, although the contributions of the plasma and tissue kallikrein pathways to each aspect of allergic inflammation are likely to be quite different. Antigen challenge of the nose, followed by nasal lavage, revealed an increase in Tosyl Arginine Methyl Ester (TAME) esterase activity which is largely attributable to kallikrein(s) (Proud *et al.*, 1983). The activation was seen during the immediate response as well as the late-phase reaction (Creticos *et al.*, 1984). Both LK and HK were shown to be present in nasal lavage fluid (Baumgarten *et al.*, 1985), and fractionation of nasal washings demonstrated evidence of both tissue kallikrein (Baumgarten *et al.*, 1986a) and plasma kallikrein (Baumgarten *et al.*, 1986b). Tissue kallikrein can be secreted by glandular tissue as well as by infiltrating cells such as neutrophils, and will cleave LK to yield kallidin. Plasma kallikrein will digest HK to yield bradykinin directly. High-performance liquid chromatographic (HPLC) analysis of kinins in nasal washings revealed both kallidin and bradykinin; the latter can be formed from kallidin by aminopeptidase action; however, a portion of the bradykinin is also likely to be the direct result of plasma kallikrein activity. Tissue kallikrein has also been found in bronchoalveolar lavage fluids of asthmatics (Christiansen *et al.*, 1987).

Studies of the allergen-induced late-phase reactions in the skin (Atkins *et al.*, 1987) have demonstrated the presence of kallikrein–C1 INH and activated factor XII–C1 INH complexes in induced blisters observed for an 8-hour period (Fig. 19.4). Elevated levels of these complexes were seen between 3 and 6 hours, coincident with the late-phase response, and were specific for the antigen to which the patient was sensitive (Fig. 19.8).

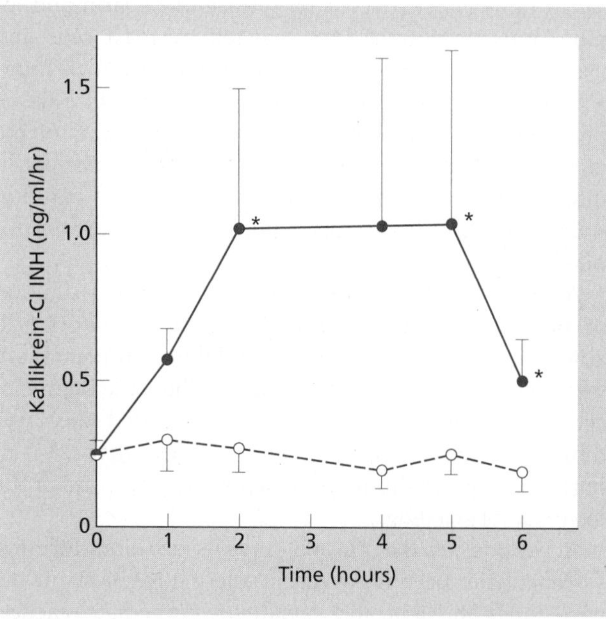

Fig. 19.8 Formation of kallikrein–C1 INH complexes during the course of an induced cutaneous late-phase reaction to ragweed pollen.

Other disorders

Endotoxic shock is associated with depletion of contact activation proteins (Mason *et al.*, 1970; Hirsh *et al.*, 1974; Robinson *et al.*, 1975; O'Donnell *et al.*, 1976) and serial HK levels have prognostic value (Hirsh *et al.*, 1974), since a drop to near zero usually indicates a fatal outcome as did lower prekallikrein levels (O'Donnell *et al.*, 1976). More recently, a monoclonal antibody to factor XII markedly diminished the mortality by 50% in a baboon monkey model of endotoxic shock (Pixley *et al.*, 1992, 1993). Parameters of disseminated intravascular coagulation (DIC) were unaffected and likely to be mediated via tissue thromboplastin, although DIC due to endothelial cell injury and/or endotoxaemia is associated with diminished levels of factor XII, prekallikrein and kallikrein inhibiting activity (Mason & Colman, 1971; Lämmle *et al.*, 1984).

The synovial fluid of patients with rheumatoid arthritis has been shown to contain plasma kallikrein which can activate stromelysin and convert procollagenase to collagenase (Nagase *et al.*, 1982). Uric acid and pyrophosphate cystals can act as surfaces for contact activation (Kellermeyer & Breckenridge, 1965; Ginsberg *et al.*, 1980) and many contribute to the inflammation seen in gout or pseudogout, but it should be noted that at least one case of gout (Londino & Luparello, 1984) and one of rheumatoid arthritis (Donaldson *et al.*, 1972) have been reported in factor XII-deficient subjects.

Pancreatitis, particularly acute haemorrhagic pancreatitis, is associated with the release of large quantities of tissue kallikrein; thus, kallidin and/or bradykinin may contribute to the pooling of fluid within the abdominal cavity and the hypotension that can result. Finally, rodent models of hypertension have revealed that the effects of ACE inhibitors are reversed by B_2-receptor antagonists, suggesting that prevention of bradykinin degradation by ACE may be important in lowering blood pressure apart from inhibition of angiotensin II formation (Hecker *et al.*, 1994).

References

Adam, A., Albert, A., Calay, G., Closset, J., Damas, J. & Franchimont, P. (1985) Human kininogens of low and high molecular mass: quantification by radioimmunoassay and determination of reference values. *Clin. Chem.*, **31**, 423–6.

Atkins, P.C., Miragliotta, G., Talbot, S.F., Zweiman, B. & Kaplan, A.P. (1987) Activation of plasma Hageman factor and kallikrein in ongoing allergic reactions in the skin. *J. Immunol.*, **139**, 2744–8.

Baglia, F.A., Sinha, D. & Walsh, P.N. (1989) Functional domains in the heavy-chain region of factor XI: a high molecular weight kininogen-binding site and a substrate binding site for factor IX. *Blood*, **74**, 244–51.

Barrett, A.J. & Starkey, P.M. (1973) The interaction of α_2-macroglobulin with proteinases. *Biochem. J.*, **133**, 709–24.

Baumgarten, C.R., Nichols, R.C., Naclerio, R.M., Lichtenstein, L.M., Norman, P.S. & Proud, D. (1986a) Plasma kallikrein during experimentally-induced allergic rhinitis: role in kinin formation and contribution to TAME-esterase activity in nasal secretions. *J. Immunol.*, **137**, 977–82.

Baumgarten, C.R., Nichols, R.C., Naclerio, R.M. & Proud, D. (1986b) Concentrations of glandular kallikrein in human nasal secretions increase during experimentally-induced allergic rhinitis. *J. Immunol.*, **137**, 1323–8.

Baumgarten, C.R., Togias, A.G., Naclerio, R.M., Lichtenstein, L.M., Norman, P.S. & Proud, D. (1985) Influx of kininogens into nasal secretions after antigen challenge of allergic individuals. *J. Clin. Invest.*, **76**, 191–7.

Beeler, D.L., Marcum, J.A., Schiffman, S. & Rosenberg, R.D. (1985) Interaction of factor XIa and antithrombin in the presence and absence of heparin. *Blood*, **67**, 1488–92.

Berrettini, M., Lammle, B., White, T. *et al.* (1986) Detection of *in vitro* and *in vivo* cleavage of high molecular weight kininogen in human plasma immunoblotting with monoclonal antibodies. *Blood*, **68**, 455–62.

Berrettini, M., Schleef, R.R., Heeb, M.J., Hopmeier, P. & Griffin, J.H. (1992) Assembly and expression of intrinsic factor IX activator complex on the surface of cultured human endothelial cells. *J. Biol. Chem.*, **267**, 19833–9.

Bock, P.E. & Shore, J.D. (1983) Protein–protein interaction of blood coagulation. Characterization of a fluorescein-labeled human high molecular weight kininogen light chain as a probe. *J. Biol. Chem.*, **258**, 15079–86.

Bock, P.E., Shore, J.D., Tans, G. & Griffin, J.H. (1985) Protein–protein interactions in contact activation of blood coagulation. Binding of high molecular weight kininogen and the 5-(iodoacetamido) fluorescein-labeled kininogen light chain to prekallikrein, kallikrein, and the separated kallikrein heavy and light chains. *J. Biol. Chem.*, **260**, 12434–43.

Bock, P.E., Srinivasan, K.R. & Shore, J.D. (1981) Activation of intrinsic blood coagulation by ellagic acid: insoluble ellagic acid metal ion complexes are the activating species. *Biochemistry*, **20**, 7258–71.

Bouma, B.N. & Griffin, J.H. (1977) Human blood coagulation factor XI: purification, properties, and mechanism of activation by factor XII. *J. Biol. Chem.*, **252**, 6432–7.

Bouma, B.N., Miles, L.A., Barretta, G. & Griffin, J.H. (1980) Human plasma prekallikrein. Studies of its activation by activated factor XII and of its inactivation by diisopropyl phosphofluoridate. *Biochemistry*, **19**, 1151–60.

Brunnée, T., Reddigari, S.R., Shibayama, Y., Salerno, V., Kaplan, A.P. & Silverberg, M. (1995) Activation of the contact system by glycosaminoglycan derived from mast cell proteoglycan. (Submitted).

Cameron, C.L., Fisslthaler, B., Sherman, A., Reddigari, S. & Silverberg, M. (1989) Studies on contact activation: effects of surfaces and inhibitors. *Med. Prog. Tech.*, **15**, 53–62.

Castellino, F.J. & Beals, J.M. (1987) The genetic relationships between the kringle domains of human plasminogen, prothrombin, tissue plasminogen activator, urokinase, and coagulation factor XII. *J. Mol. Evol.*, **26**, 358–69.

Christiansen, S.C., Proud, D. & Cochrane, C.G. (1987) Detection of tissue kallikrein in the bronchoalveolar lavage fluids of asthmatic subjects. *J. Clin. Invest.*, **79**, 188–97.

Chung, D.W., Fujikawa, K., McMullen, B.A. & Davie, E.W. (1986) Human plasma prekallikrein, a zymogen to a serine protease that contains four tandem repeats. *Biochemistry*, **25**, 2410–17.

Cochrane, C.G. & Revak, S.D. (1980) Dissemination of contact activation in plasma by plasma kallikrein. *J. Exp. Med.*, **152**, 608–19.

Cochrane, C.G., Revak, S.D. & Wuepper, K.D. (1973) Activation of Hageman factor in solid and fluid phases. *J. Exp. Med.*, **138**, 1564–83.

Colman, R.W. & Muller-Esterl, W. (1988) Nomenclature of kininogens. *Thromb. Haemost.*, **60**, 340–1.

Colman, R.W., Bagdasarian, A., Talamo, R.C. *et al.* (1975) Williams trait: human kininogen deficiency with diminished levels of plasminogen proactivator and prekallikrein associated with abnormalities of the Hageman factor dependent pathways. *J. Clin. Invest.*, **56**, 1650–62.

Cool, D.E., Edgell, C.S., Louie, G.V., Zoller, M.J., Brayer, G.D. & MacGillivray, R.T.A. (1985) Characterization of Human Blood Coagulation Factor XII cDNA. *J. Biol. Chem.*, **25**, 13666–76.

Creticos, P.S., Peters, S.P., Adkinson, N.F. Jr *et al.* (1984) Peptide leucotriene release after antigen challenge in patients sensitive to ragweed. *New Engl. J. Med.*, **310**, 1626–30.

Crutchly, D.J., Ryan, J.W., Ryan, U.S. & Fisher, G.H. (1983) Bradykinin induced release of prostacyclin and thromboxanes from bovine pulmonary artery endothelial cells. *Biochim. Biophys. Acta*, **751**, 99–107.

Curd, J.G., Prograis, L.F. Jr, & Cochrane, C.G. (1980) Detection of active kallikrein in induced blister fluids of hereditary angioedema patients. *J. Exp. Med.*, **152**, 742–7.

de Agostini, A., Lijnen, H.R., Pixley, R.A., Colman, R.W. & Schapira, M. (1984) Inactivation of factor XII active fragment in normal plasma. Predominent role of Cl-inhibitor. *J. Clin. Invest.*, **73**, 1542–9.

Donaldson, V.H. (1968) Mechanisms of activation of C1 esterase in hereditary angioneurotic edema plasma *in vitro*: the role of Hageman factor, a clot-promoting agent. *J. Exp. Med.*, **127**, 411–29.

Donaldson, V.H., Glueck, H.I. & Fleming, T. (1972) Rheumatoid arthritis in a patient with Hageman trait. *New Engl. J. Med.*, **386**, 528–30.

Donaldson, V.H., Glueck, H.I. & Miller, M.A. (1976) Kininogen deficiency in Fitzgerald trait: role of high molecular weight kininogen in clotting and fibrinolysis. *J. Lab. Clin. Med.*, **89**, 327–37.

Donaldson, V.H., Rosen, F.S. & Bing, D.H. (1977) Role of the second component of complement (C2) and plasmin in kinin release in hereditary angioneurotic edema (H.A.N.E.) plasma. *Trans. Assoc. Am. Phys.*, **40**, 174–83.

Dunn, J.T. & Kaplan, A.P. (1982) Formation and structure of human Hageman factor fragments. *J. Clin. Invest.*, **70**, 627–31.

Dunn, J.T., Silverberg, M. & Kaplan, A.P. (1982) The cleavage and formation of activated Hageman factor by autodigestion and by kallikrein. *J. Biol. Chem.*, **275**, 1779–84.

Erdos, E.G. & Sloane, G.M. (1962) An enzyme in human plasma that inactivates bradykinin and kallidins. *Biochem. Pharmacol.*, **11**, 585–92.

Fields, T., Ghebrehiwet, B. & Kaplan, A.P. (1983) Kinin formation in hereditary angioedema plasma: evidence against kinin derivation from C2 and in support of 'spontaneous' formation of bradykinin. *J. Allergy Clin. Immunol.*, **72**, 54–60.

Forbes, C.O., Pensky, J. & Ratnoff, O.D. (1970) Inhibition of activated Hageman factor and activated plasma thromboplastin antecedent by purified C1 inactivator. *J. Lab. Clin. Med.*, **76**, 809–15.

Fujikawa, K., Chung, D.W., Hendrickson, L.E. & Davie, E.W. (1986) Amino acid sequence of human factor XI, a blood coagulation factor with four tandem repeats that are highly homologous with plasma prekallikrein. *Biochemistry*, **25**, 2417–24.

Fujikawa, K., Heimark, R.L., Kurachi, K. & Davie, E.W. (1980) Activation of bovine factor XII (Hageman factor) by plasma kallikrein. *Biochemistry*, **19**, 1322–30.

Fujikawa, K. & McMullen, B.A. (1983) Amino acid sequence of Human b-Factor XIIa. *J. Biol. Chem.*, **258**, 10924–33.

Ghebrehiwet, B., Randazzo, B.P., Dunn, J.T., Silverberg, M. & Kaplan, A.P. (1983) Mechanism of activation of the classical pathway of complement by Hageman factor fragment. *J. Clin. Invest.*, **71**, 1450–6.

Gigli, I., Mason, J.W., Coleman, R.W. & Austen, K.F. (1970) Interaction of plasma kallikrein with the C1 inhibitor. *J. Immunol.*, **104**, 574–81.

Ginsberg, M., Jaques, B., Cochrane, C.G. & Griffin, J.H. (1980) Urate crystal dependent cleavage of Hageman factor in human plasma and synovial fluid. *J. Lab. Clin. Med.*, **95**, 497–506.

Gounaris, A.D., Brown, M.A. & Barrett, A.J. (1984) Human plasma α_1-cystein proteinase inhibitor. Purification by affinity chromatography, characterization, and isolation of an active fragment. *Biochem. J.*, **221**, 445–52.

Griep, M.A., Fujikawa, K. & Nelsestuen, G.L. (1985) Binding and activation properties of human factor XII, prekallikrein and derived peptides with acidic lipid vesicles. *Biochemistry*, **24**, 4124–30.

Griffin, J.H. (1978) Role of surface in surface-dependent activation of Hageman factor (blood coagulation Factor XII). *Proc. Nat. Acad. Sci. USA*, **75**, 1998–2002.

Griffin, J.H. & Cochrane, C.G. (1976) Mechanisms for the involvement of high molecular weight kininogen in surface-dependent reactions of Hageman factor. *Proc. Nat. Acad. Sci. USA*, **73**, 2554–8.

Guimaraes, J.A., Borges, D.R., Prado, E.S. & Prado, J.L. (1973) Kinin converting aminopeptidase from human serum. *Biochem. Pharmacol.*, **22**, 403–14.

Harpel, P.C. (1974) Circulatory inhibitors of human plasma kallikrein. In: *Chemistry and Biology of the Kallikrein–Kinin System in Health and Disease* (eds J.J. Pisano & K.F. Austen), p. 169. US Government Printing Office, Washington, DC.

Harpel, P.C., Lewin, M.F. & Kaplan, A.P. (1985) Distribution of plasma kallikrein between C1 inactivator and α_2-macroglobulin–kallikrein complexes. *J. Biol. Chem.*, **260**, 4257–63.

Heck, L.W. & Kaplan, A.P. (1974) Substrates of Hageman factor: I. Isolation and characterization of human factor XI (PTA) and inhibition of the activated enzyme by α_1-antitrypsin. *J. Exp. Med.*, **140**, 1615–30.

Hecker, M., Porsti, I. & Busse, R. (1994) Mechanisms involved in the angiotensin II-dependent hypotensive action of ACE inhibitors. In: *Brazilian Journal of Medical and Biological Research — Proceedings of 'Kinin 93 Brazil'* (eds C.A.M. Sampaio, A.C.M. Daiva & L.J. Greene), pp. 1917–21. Associacao Brasileira de Divulgacao Cientifica, Sao Paulo, Brazil.

Higashiyama, S., Ohkubo, I., Ishiguro, H., Kunimatsu, M., Sawaki, K. & Sasaki, M. (1986) Human high molecular weight kininogen as a thiol protease inhibitor: presence of the entire inhibition capacity in the native from of heavy chain. *Biochemistry*, **25**, 1669–75.

Hirsh, E.F., Nakajima, T., Oshima, G., Erdos, E.G. & Herman, M. (1974) Kinin-system responses in sepsis after trauma in man. *J. Surg. Res.*, **17**, 147–53.

Hojima, Y., Cochrane, C.G., Wiggins, R.C., Austen, K.F. & Stevens, R.L. (1984) *In vitro* activation of the contact (Hageman factor) system of plasma by heparin and chondroitin sulfate E. *Blood* , **63**, 1453–9.

Hong, S.L. (1980) Effect of bradykinin and thrombin on prostacyclin synthesis in endothelial cells from calf and pig aorta and human umbilical cord vein. *Thromb. Res.*, **18**, 787–95.

Ikari, N., Sugo, T., Fujii, S., Kato, H. & Iwanaga, S. (1981) The role of bovine high molecular weight kininogen in contact-mediated activation of bovine factor XII: interaction of HMW kininogen with kaolin and plasma prekallikrein. *J. Biochem.*, **89**, 1699–709.

Ishiguro, H., Higashiyama, S., Ohkubo, I. & Sasaki, M. (1987) Mapping of functional domains of human high molecular weight and low molecular weight kininogens using murine monoclonal antibodies. *Biochemistry*, **26**, 7021–9.

Jacobsen, S. & Kritz, M. (1967) Some data on two purified kininogens from human plasma. *Brit. J. Pharmacol.*, **29**, 25–36.

Johnson, D.A., Salveson, G., Brown, M. & Barrett, A.J. (1987) Rapid isolation of human kininogens. *Thromb. Res.*, **48**, 187–93.

Kaplan, A.P. & Austen, K.F. (1970) A prealbumin activator of prekallikrein. *J. Immunol.*, **105**, 802–11.

Kaplan, A.P. & Austen, K.F. (1971) A prealbumin activator of prekallikrein II: derivation of activators of prekallikrein from active Hageman factor by digestion with plasmin. *J. Exp. Med.*, **133**, 696–712.

Kaufman, N., Page, J.D., Pixley, R.A., Schein, R., Schmaier, A.H. & Colman, R.W. (1991) α_2 macroglobulin–kallikrein complexes detect contact system activation in hereditary angioedema and human sepsis. *Blood*, **77**, 2660–7.

Kellermann, J., Lottspeich, F., Henschen, A. & Muller-Esterl, W. (1986) Completion of the primary structure of human high molecular weight kininogen. The amino acid sequence of the entire heavy chain and evidence for its evolution by gene triplication. *Eur. J. Biochem.*, **154**, 471–8.

Kellermeyer, R.W. & Breckenridge, R.T. (1965) The inflammatory process in acute gouty arthritis, I. Activation of Hageman factor by sodium urate crystals. *J. Lab. Clin. Med.*, **63**, 307–15.

Kitamura, N., Kitagawa, H., Fukushima, D., Takagaki, Y., Miyata, T. & Nakanishi, S (1985) Structural organization of the human kininogen gene and a model for its evolution. *J. Biol. Chem.*, **260**, 8610–17.

Kluft, C. (1978) Determination of prekallikrein in human plasma: optimal conditions for activating prekallikrein. *J. Lab. Clin. Med.*, **91**, 83–93.

Kurachi, K. & Davie, E.W. (1977) Activation of human factor XI (plasma thromboplastin antecedent) by factor XII (activated Hageman factor). *Biochemistry*, **16**, 5831–9.

Kurachi, K., Fujikawa, K. & Davie, E.W. (1980) Mechanism of activation of bovine factor XI by factor XII and factor XII_a. *Biochemistry*, **19**, 1330–8.

Lämmle, B., Tran, T.H., Ritz, R. & Duckert, F. (1984) Plasma prekallikrein, factor XII, antithrombin III, C_1-inhibitor and α_2-macroglobulin in critically ill patients with suspected disseminated intravascular coagulation (DIC). *Am. J. Clin. Pathol.*, **82**, 396–404.

Londino, A. & Luparello, F.J. (1984) Factor XII deficiency in a man with gout and angioimmunoblastic lymphadenopathy. *Arch. Intern. Med.*, **144**, 1497–8.

Lottspeich, F., Kellermann, J., Henschen, A., Foertsch, B. & Muller-Esterl, W. (1985) The amino acid sequence of the light chain of human high molecular mass kininogen. *Eur. J. Biochem.*, **152**, 307–14.

Lottspeich, F., Kellermann, J., Henschen, A., Rauth, G. & Muller-Esterl, W. (1984) Human low-molecular-mass kininogen. Amino-acid sequence of the light chain; homology with other protein sequences. *Eur. J. Biochem.*, **142**, 227–32.

McConnell, D.J. (1972) Inhibitors of kallikrein in human plasma. *J. Clin. Invest.*, **51**, 1611–23.

McMillin, C.R., Saito, H., Ratnoff, O.D. & Walton, A.G. (1974) The secondary structure of human Hageman factor (factor XII) and its alteration by activating agents. *J. Clin. Invest.*, **54**, 1312–22.

McMullen, B.A. & Fujikawa, K. (1985) Amino acid sequence of the heavy chain of human a-factor XIIa (activated Hageman factor). *J. Biol. Chem.*, **260**, 5328–41.

Mandle, R.J. Jr, Colman, R.W. & Kaplan, A.P. (1976) Identification of prekallikrein and HMW-kininogen as a complex in human plasma. *Proc. Nat. Acad. Sci. USA*, **73**, 4179–83.

Mandle, R.J.J. & Kaplan, A.P. (1977) Hageman factor substrates. II. Human plasma prekallikrein. Mechanism of activation by Hageman factor and participation in Hageman factor-dependent fibrinolysis. *J. Biol. Chem.*, **252**, 6097–104.

Margolis, J. (1958) Activation of plasma by contact with glass: evidence for a common reaction which releases plasma kinin and initiates coagulation. *J. Physiol*, **144**, 1–22.

Mason, J.N. & Colman, R.W. (1971) The role of Hageman factor in disseminated intravascular coagulation induced by sepsis, neoplasia, or liver disease. *Thromb. Diath. Haemorrh.*, **26**, 325–31.

Mason, J.W., Kleeberg, U.R., Dolan, P. & Colman, R.W. (1970) Plasma kallikrein and Hageman factor in gram-negative bacteremia. *Ann. Intern. Med.*, **73**, 545–51.

Meier, H.L., Pierce, J.V., Colman, R.W. & Kaplan, A.P. (1977) Activation and function of human Hageman factor. The role of high molecular kininogen and prekallikrein. *J. Clin. Invest.*, **60**, 18–31.

Meijers, J.C., Vlooswijk, R.A.A. & Bouma, B.N. (1988) Inhibition of human blood coagulation factor XIa by C1 Inhibitor. *Biochemistry*, **27**, 959–63.

Mori, K. & Nagasawa, S. (1981) Studies on human high molecular weight (HMW) kininogen. II. Structural change in HMW kininogen by the action of human plasma kallikrein. *J. Biochem.*, **89**, 1465–73.

Mori, K., Sakamoto, W. & Nagasawa, S. (1981) Studies on human high molecular weight (HMW) kininogen III. Cleavage of HMW kininogen by the action human salivary kallikrein. *J. Biochem.*, **90**, 503–9.

Morrison, D.C. & Cochrane, C.G. (1974) Direct evidence for Hageman factor (factor XII) activation by bacterial lipopolysaccharides (endotoxins). *J. Exp. Med.*, **140**, 797–811.

Muller-Esterl, W., Fritz, H., Machleidt, I.W. *et al.* (1985a) Human plasma kininogens are identical with α_2-cysteine protease inhibitors. Evidence from immunological, enzymological, and sequence data. *FEBS Letts.*, **182**, 310–14.

Muller-Esterl, W., Rauth, G., Lottspeich, F., Kellermann, J. & Henschen, A. (1985b) Limited proteolysis of human low-molecular mass kininogen by tissue kallikrein. Isolation and characterization of the heavy and light chains. *Eur. J. Biochem.*, **149**, 15–22.

Nagase, H., Cawston, J.E., DeSilva, M. & Barrett, A.J. (1982) Identification of plasma kallikrein as an activator of latent collagenase in rheumatoid synovial fluid. *Biochim. Biophys. Acta*, **707**, 133–42.

Nishikawa, K., Kuna, P., Calcaterra, E., Kaplan, A.P. & Reddigari, S.R. (1992) Generation of the vasoactive peptide bradykinin from human high molecular weight kininogen bound to human umbilical vein endothelial cells. *Blood*, **80**, 1980–8.

O'Donnell, T.F., Clowes, G.H.J., Talamo, R.C. & Colman, R.W. (1976) Kinin activation in the blood of patients with sepsis. *Surg. Gynecol. Obstet.*, **143**, 539–45.

Pettinger, M.A. & Young, R. (1970) Endotoxin-induced kinin (bradykinin) formation: activation of Hageman factor and plasma kallikrein in human plasma. *Life Sci.*, **9**, 313–22.

Pixley, R.A., De La Cadena, R.A., Page, J.D. *et al.* (1992) Activation of the contact system in lethal hypotensive bacteremia in a baboon model. *Am. J. Pathol.*, **140**, 897–906.

Pixley, R.A., De La Cadena, R.A., Page, J.D. *et al.* (1993) The contact system contributes to hypotension but not disseminated intravascular coagulation in lethal bacterimia. *In vivo* use of a monoclonal anti Factor XII antibody to block contact activation in baboons. *J. Clin. Invest.*, **92**, 61–8.

Pixley, R.A., Schapira, M. & Colman, R.W. (1985) The regulation of human factor XII by plasma proteinase inhibitors. *J. Biol. Chem.*, **260**, 1723–9.

Pixley, R.A., Stumpo, L.G., Birkmeyer, K., Silver, L. & Colman, R.W. (1987) A monoclonal antibody recognizing an icosapeptide sequence in the heavy chain of human factor XII inhibits surface-catalyzed activation. *J. Biol. Chem.*, **262**, 10140–5.

Proctor, R.R. & Rapaport, S.J. (1961) The partial thromboplastin time with kaolin: a simple screening test for first stage clotting deficiencies. *Am. J. Clin. Pathol.*, **35**, 212–19.

Proud, D., Pierce, J.V. & Pisano, J.J. (1980) Radioimmunoassay of human high molecular weight kininogen in normal and deficient plasma. *J. Lab. Clin. Med.*, **95**, 563–74.

Proud, D., Togias, A.G., Naclerio, R.M., Crush, S.A., Norman, P.S. & Lichtenstein, L.M. (1983) Kinins are generated *in vivo* following nasal airway challenge of allergic individuals with allergen. *J. Clin. Invest.*, **72**, 1678–85.

Que, B.G. & Davie, E.W. (1986) Characterization of a cDNA coding for human factor XII (Hageman factor). *Biochemistry*, **8**, 1525–8.

Ratnoff, O.D. & Crum, J.D. (1964) Activation of Hageman factor by solutions of ellagic acid. *J. Lab. Clin. Med.*, **63**, 359–77.

Ratnoff, O.D. & Saito, H. (1979) Amidolytic properties of single chain activated Hageman factor. *Proc. Nat. Acad. Sci. USA*, **76**, 1461–3.

Reddigari, S.R. & Kaplan, A.P. (1988) Cleavage of high molecular weight kininogen by purified kallikreins and upon contact activation of plasma. *Blood*, **71**, 1334–40.

Reddigari, S.R. & Kaplan, A.P. (1989a) Monoclonal antibody to human high molecular weight kininogen recognizes its prekallikrein binding site and inhibits its coagulant activity. *Blood*, **74**, 695–702.

Reddigari, S.R. & Kaplan, A.P. (1989b) Quantification of human high molecular weight kininogen by immunoblotting with a monoclonal anti-light chain antibody. *J. Immunol. Meth.*, **119**, 19–25.

Reddigari, S.R., Miragliotta, G., Kuna, P., Nishikawa, K. & Kaplan, A.P. (1993a) Human high molecular weight kininogen binds to human umbilical vein endothelial cells via its heavy and light chains. *Blood*, **81**, 1306–11.

Reddigari, S.R., Shibayama, Y., Brunnee, T. & Kaplan, A.P. (1993b) Human Hageman factor (FXII) and high molecular weight kininogen compete for the same binding site on human umbilical vein endothelial cells. *J. Biol. Chem.*, **268**, 11982–7.

Regoli, D. & Barabe, J. (1980) Pharmacology of bradykinin and related kinins. *Pharmacol. Rev.*, **32**, 1–46.

Revak, S.D., Cochrane, C.G. & Griffin, J.H. (1977) The binding and cleavage characteristics of human Hageman factor during contact activation: a comparison of normal plasma with plasma deficient in factor XI, prekallikrein or high molecular weight kininogen. *J. Clin. Invest.*, **58**, 1167–75.

Revak, S.D., Cochrane, C.G., Johnston, A.R. & Hugli, T.E. (1974) Structural changes accompanying enzymatic activation of human Hageman factor. *J. Clin. Invest.*, **54**, 619–27.

Robinson, J.A., Klodynicky, M.L., Loeb, H.S., Recic, M.R. & Gunnar,

R.M. (1975) Endotoxin, prekallikrein, complement, and systemic vascular resistances. Sequential measurement in man. *Am. J. Med.*, **59**, 61–7.

Roeise, O., Bouma, B.N., Stadaas, J.O. & Aasen, A.O. (1988) Dose dependence of endotoxin-induced activation of the plasma contact system: an *in vitro* study. *Circ. Shock*, **26**, 419–30.

Rosing, J., Tans, G. & Griffin, J.H. (1985) Surface-dependent activation of human factor XII by kallikrein, and its light chain. *Eur. J. Biochem.*, **151**, 531–8.

Saito, H., Ratnoff, O.D. & Donaldson, V.H. (1974) Defective activation of clotting, fibrinolytic and permeability-enhancing systems in human Fletcher trait. *Circ. Res.*, **34**, 641–51.

Schapira, M., Scott, C.F. & Colman, R.W. (1982) Contribution of plasma protease inhibitors to the inactivation of kallikrein in plasma. *J. Clin. Invest.*, **69**, 462–8.

Schiffman, S., Mannhalter, C. & Tynerk, D. (1980) Human high molecular weight kininogen. Effects of cleavage by kallikrein on protein structure and procoagulant activity. *J. Biol. Chem.*, **255**, 6433–8.

Schmaier, A.H., Kuo, A., Lundberg, D., Murray, S. & Cines, D.B. (1988) The expression of high molecular weight kininogen on human umbilical vein endothelial cells. *J. Biol. Chem.*, **263**, 16327–33.

Schmaier, A.H., Silver, L., Adams, A.L. *et al.* (1984) The effects of high molecular weight kininogen on surface-adsorbed fibrinogen. *Thromb. Res.*, **33**, 51–7.

Schreiber, R.D., Kaplan, A.P. & Austen, K.F. (1973) Inhibition by C1 INH of Hageman factor fragment activation of coagulation, fibrinolysis, and kinin generation. *J. Clin. Invest.*, **52**, 1402–9.

Scott, C.F. & Colman, R.W. (1980) Function and immunochemistry of prekallikrein–high molecular weight kininogen complex in plasma. *J. Clin. Invest.*, **65**, 413–21.

Scott, C.F., Schapira, M. & Colman, R.W. (1982a) Effect of heparin on the inactivation of human factor XIa by antithrombin III. *Blood*, **60**, 940–7.

Scott, C.F., Schapira, M., James, H.L., Cohen, A.B. & Colman, R.W. (1982b) Inactivation of factor XIa by plasma protease inhibitors. Predominant role of α_1-protease inhibitor and protective effect of high molecular weight kininogen. *J. Clin. Invest.*, **69**, 844–52.

Sheikh, I.A. & Kaplan, A.P. (1986a) Studies of the digestion of bradykinin, lysylbradykinin and des-arg^9 bradykinin by angiotensin converting enzyme. *Biochem. Pharmacol.*, **35**, 1951–6.

Sheikh, I.A. & Kaplan, A.P. (1986b) Studies of the digestion of bradykinin, lysylbradykinin and kinin degradation products by carboxypeptidases A, B and N. *Biochem. Pharmacol.*, **35**, 1957–63.

Sheikh, I.A. & Kaplan, A.P. (1989) The mechanism of digestion of bradykinin and lysylbradykinin (kallidin) in human serum: the role of carboxy-peptidase, angiotensin converting enzyme, and determination of final degradation products. *Biochem. Pharmacol.*, **38**, 993–1000.

Silverberg, M. & Diehl, S.V. (1987a) The activation of the contact system of human plasma by polysaccharide sulfates. *Ann. NY Acad. Sci.*, **516**, 268–79.

Silverberg, M. & Diehl, S.V. (1987b) The autoactivation of factor XII (Hageman factor) induced by low Mr heparin and dextran sulphate. *Biochem. J.*, **248**, 715–20.

Silverberg, M., Dunn, J.T., Garen, L. & Kaplan, A.P. (1980a) Autoactivation of human Hageman factor. *J. Biol. Chem.*, **255**, 7281–6.

Silverberg, M. & Kaplan, A.P. (1982) Enzymatic activities of activated and zymogen forms of human Hageman factor (factor XII). *Blood*, **60**, 64–70.

Silverberg, M., Nicoll, J.E. & Kaplan, A.P. (1980b) The mechanism by which the light chain of cleaved HMW-kininogen augments the activation of prekallikrein, factor XI, and Hageman factor. *Thromb. Res.*, **20**, 173–89.

Smith, D., Gilbert, M. & Owen, W.G. (1985) Tissue plasminogen activator release *in vivo* in response to vasoactive agents. *Blood*, **66**, 835–9.

Soter, N.A., Austen, K.F. & Gigli, I. (1975) Inhibition by E-aminocaproic acid of the activation of the first component of the complement system. *J. Immunol.*, **114**, 928–32.

Stead, N., Kaplan, A.P. & Rosenberg, R.D. (1976) Inhibition of activated factor XII by antithrombin-heparin cofactor. *J. Biol. Chem.*, **251**, 6481–8.

Strang, C.J., Cholin, S., Spragg, J. *et al.* (1988) Angioedema induced by a peptide derived from complement component C2. *J. Exp. Med.*, **168**, 1685–98.

Tait, J. & Fujikawa, K. (1986) Identification of the binding site plasma prekallikrein in human high molecular weight kininogen. *J. Biol. Chem.*, **261**, 15396–401.

Tait, J.F. & Fujikawa, K. (1987) Primary structure requirements for the binding of human high molecular weight kininogen to plasma prekallikrein and factor XI. *J. Biol. Chem.*, **262**, 11651–6.

Takagaki, Y., Kitamura, N. & Nakanishi, S. (1985) Cloning and sequence analysis of cDNAs for high molecular weight and low molecular weight prekininogens. *J. Biol. Chem.*, **260**, 8601–9.

Tankersley, D.L. & Finlayson, J.S. (1984) Kinetics of activation and autoactivation of human factor XII. *Biochemistry*, **23**, 273–9.

Tans, G. & Griffin, J.H. (1982) Properties of sulfatides in factor XII dependent contact activation. *Blood*, **59**, 69–75.

Tans, G., Rosing, J. & Griffin, J.D. (1983) Sulfatide dependent autoactivation of human blood coagulation factor XII (Hageman factor). *J. Biol. Chem.*, **258**, 8215–22.

Thompson, R.E., Mandle, R.J. Jr & Kaplan, A.P. (1977) Association of factor XI and high molecular weight kininogen in human plasma. *J. Clin. Invest.*, **60**, 1376–80.

Thompson, R.E., Mandle, R.J. & Kaplan, A.P. (1978) Characterization of human high molecular weight kininogen. Procoagulant activity associated with the light chain of kinin-free high molecular weight kininogen. *J. Exp. Med.*, **147**, 488–99.

Thompson, R.E., Mandle, R.J. & Kaplan, A.P. (1979) Studies of the binding of prekallikrein and factor XI to high molecular weight kininogen and its light chain. *Proc. Nat. Acad. Sci. USA*, **76**, 4862–6.

Travis, J. & Salvesen, G.S. (1983) Human plasma proteinase inhibitors. *Ann. Rev. Biochem.*, **52**, 655–709.

van der Graaf, F., Koedam, J.A. & Bouma, B.N. (1983) Inactivation of kallikrein in human plasma. *J. Clin. Invest.*, **71**, 149–58.

Van Iwaarden, F., deGroot, P.G. & Bouma, B.N. (1988) The binding of high molecular weight kininogen to cultured human endothelial cells. *J. Biol. Chem.*, **263**, 4698–703.

Wang, W., Hendriks, D.K. & Scharpé, S.S. (1994) Carboxypeptidase U, a plasma carboxypeptidase with high affinity for plasminogen. *J. Biol. Chem.*, **269**, 15937–44.

Warn-Cramer, B.J. & Bajaj, S.P. (1985) Stoichiometry of binding of high molecular weight kininogen to factor XI/XIa. *Biochem. Biophys. Res. Commun.*, **133**, 417–22.

Weiss, A.S., Gallin, J.I. & Kaplan, A.P. (1974) Fletcher factor deficiency. A diminished rate of Hageman factor activation caused by absence of prekallikrein with abnormalities of coagulation, fibrinolysis, chemotactic activity, and kinin generation. *J. Clin. Invest.*, **53**, 622–33.

Weiss, R., Silverberg, M. & Kaplan, A.P. (1986) The effect of C1 inhibitor upon Hageman factor autoactivation. *Blood*, **68**, 239–43.

Wiggins, R.C., Bouma, B.N., Cochrane, C.G. & Griffin, J.H. (1977) Role of high molecular weight kininogen in surface-binding and activation of coagulation factor XIa and prekallikrein. *Proc. Nat. Acad. Sci. USA*, **77**, 4636–40.

Wuepper, K.D. (1973) Prekallikrein deficiency in man. *J. Exp. Med.*, **138**, 1345–55.

Wuepper, K.D., Miller, D.R. & LaCombe, M.J. (1975) Flaujeac trait. Deficiency of human plasma kininogen. *J. Clin. Invest.*, **56**, 1663–72.

CHAPTER 20

Cytokines (Interleukins)

C.J. Corrigan

Introduction

Cytokines are soluble proteins or glycoproteins produced by leucocytes, and in many cases other cell types, which act as chemical communicators between cells, but generally not as effector molecules in their own right. Most are secreted, but some can be expressed on the cell membrane, and others are held in reservoirs in the extracellular matrix. Cytokines bind to specific receptors on the surface of target cells which are coupled to intracellular signal transduction and second messenger pathways. Most cytokines are growth and/or differentiation factors and they generally act on cells within the haematopoietic system, although some have systemic effects. Over the last 15 years, cytokines have been given various names. 'Lymphokines' were originally defined as cell-free soluble factors generated by sensitized T lymphocytes in response to specific antigen (Dumonde *et al.*, 1969). The terms 'cytokine' and 'interleukin' served to broaden this definition to include factors originating from many different cell types (Aarden *et al.*, 1979). Cytokines were defined initially on the basis of their activities, but the cloning of the genes for these products has greatly facilitated their classification, and cytokine expression both *in vitro* and *in vivo* can now be studied at the gene, mRNA or protein level. Identification of cytokine genes has also allowed examination of the factors regulating the production of different cytokines. Two particularly striking functional features of cytokines are their extensive pleiotropy and their redundancy; most cytokines have multiple functions, and any one function can generally be mediated by more than one cytokine (Paul, 1989).

In contrast to hormones, which are carried by the bloodstream throughout the entire body, cytokines, with certain exceptions, tend to mediate localized effects. Studies involving administration of recombinant cytokines *in vivo* have shown that their half-life in the circulation is brief, typically less than 30 minutes, substantiating the notion that re-circulation is not usually a fundamental aspect of cytokine physiology. Cytokines are highly potent mediators and exert their actions by binding to high-affinity receptors (K_d typically 10^{-11} mol/l) expressed at low numbers (typically 100–1000 receptors per cell) on different cell types. These receptors generally consist of two or more chains, each containing single membrane-spanning domains. Frequently one, and sometimes both of these receptor chains belong to a family of cytokine receptors characterized by a degree of structural homology in their extracellular domains, including conservation of key cysteine residues and the expression of a common pentameric amino acid motif adjacent to the cell membrane. Although most cytokines are glycoproteins, glycosylation is generally not required for biological function, since non-glycosylated forms generally retain all biological activites. T-lymphocyte-derived cytokine genes exist as single copies in the haploid genome and generally show a related genomic organization consisting of four exons and introns. Several T-cell-derived cytokine genes (including the genes encoding interleukin-3 (IL-3), IL-4, IL-5, IL-13, granulocyte macrophage colony-stimulating factor (GM-CSF), macrophage colony-stimulating factor (M-CSF) and its receptor) are clustered on the long arm of human chromosome 5 (Arai *et al.*, 1990).

The current system of cytokine nomenclature pays little attention to any systematic relationships between individual molecules. This is a reflection of the different historical approaches to naming new cytokines, which were based either on their cell of origin or the bioassay by which they were initially defined. The interleukin nomenclature, which merely assigns a sequential number to new factors, is a potentially rational system, but it has not been universally applied to all new factors. Thus, although IL-8 was the first member of the chemokine cytokine family to be described, none of the other chemokines has been given an interleukin number. Other attempts to impose order on cytokine nomenclature by grouping cytokines as lymphokines (lymphocyte-derived) or monokines (monocyte-derived) have usually proved misleading when sensitive detection systems are used.

With the availability of large quantitites of recombinant cytokines, X-ray and nuclear magnetic resonance (NMR) studies have generated accurate structures for many molecules, and these have been used to model the structures of related cytokines. Further homologies derived from studying gene organization, chromosomal location and receptor usages have allowed most cytokines to be placed into one of at least six different families. These families are listed in Table 20.1.

Although it is possible to list the specific properties of any given cytokine, delineation of their role *in vivo* is complicated by the tendency of cytokines to affect the expression of other cytokines and/or their receptors. In addition, it is clear that there are no circumstances *in vivo* in which cytokines are produced individually. Rather they are produced together with other cytokines in patterns characteristic of the particular stimulus or disease. From experiments using cytokine proteins as agonists, or by blocking cytokine production or action with drugs or monoclonal antibodies, the contributions which many individual cytokines can make to particular aspects of immunity, inflammation and haematopoiesis are now beginning to be delineated. Evidence from such experiments can allow hypotheses to be constructed, which can be tested in animal models or in human disease. One good example of this type of analysis has been the description of the Th1- and Th2-like cytokine patterns (Mosmann & Coffman, 1989b). It is a major triumph of cytokine biology that diseases including asthma and allergic inflammation are now regarded as 'Th2-like diseases'.

Table 20.1 Structural families of cytokines.

Family	Members	Receptor superfamily*
Haematopoietins (4α-helical bundles)	IL-2, IL-3, IL-4, IL-5, IL-6, IL-7, IL-9, IL-13, G-CSF, GM-CSF, CNTF, OSM, LIF, erythropoietin	Cytokine receptor
	IFN-α/β/γ, IL-10	Interferon receptor
	M-CSF	Protein tyrosine kinase receptor
EGF (β-pleated sheet)	EGF, TGF-α	Protein tyrosine kinase receptor
β-trefoil	FGF-α/β, IL-1α/1β, IL-1RA	Immunoglobulin
TNF (jelly roll motif)	TNF-α/β	Nerve growth factor receptor
Cysteine knot	TGF-β1/β2/β3	Protein tyrosine kinase receptor
	PDGF	
	NGF	Nerve growth factor receptor

*See Table 20.2.
See text for definition of abbreviations.

Regulation of cytokine production and activity

Gene expression

There is good evidence for the constitutive expression of cytokines such as M-CSF, G-CSF, stem cell factor (SCF), IL-6 and erythropoeitin which are necessary to maintain a steady state of haematopoiesis. In addition to constitutive expression, there is increasing evidence that several cytokines are stored pre-synthesized, either in cytoplasmic granules (e.g. GM-CSF, transforming growth factor-β (TGF-β), platelet-derived growth factor (PDGF)), as membrane proteins (e.g. tumour necrosis factor-α (TNF-α), IL-β, TGF-α) or as a complex with cell-surface binding proteins or extracellular matrix (e.g. TGF-β, IL-8) (Jyung & Mustoe, 1993; Massague & Pandiella, 1993; Tanaka *et al*., 1993). These pools of cytokine protein are available for rapid release in response to stimulation. Most cytokines, however, are not constitutively expressed but are rapidly synthesized in response to stimulation. The stimuli for gene expression may include infectious agents such as bacteria, viruses, fungi and parasites, as well as mechanical injury and toxic stimuli. In addition to classical antigen, infectious agents also contain many non-specific cytokine-inducing molecules, such as endotoxins. In many cells, cytokines potently induce the expression of other cytokines. Some of these (IL-1, TNF and interferon-γ (IFN-γ)) are particularly potent inducers of cytokine gene expression, and have been referred to as 'pro-inflammatory' cytokines.

For most cytokines, the nature and extent of the transcription factors which regulate expression of their genes are not fully characterized. The specific consensus nucleotide recognition sequences for known transcription factors can be identified in genomic DNA, and simple experiments using reporter genes linked to the 5′ sequences of these genes can support a role for particular transcription factors. The precise biochemistry of the regulatory processes imposed even by the known transcription factors is, however, extremely complex. For example, induction of IL-2 gene transcription requires both constitutive (NFAT-1 and NFIL-2A) and inducible factors (AP-1 and NFκB). The importance of other regulatory sequences outside the 5′ regions is largely unknown.

In addition to these positive stimuli, several mediators act to limit or prevent cytokine gene expression, or to limit cytokine action. The classical inhibitors of cytokine gene expression are the glucocorticoids which are widely used as anti-inflammatory drugs. The glucocorticoid receptor complex binds to glucocorticoid response elements present in the promotor regions of many cytokine genes, including IL-1, IL-2, IL-3, IL-6, IL-8 and IFN-γ. Newer immunusuppressive drugs, including cyclosporin A, FK-506 and rapamycin, also act via modulating cytokine gene transcription.

Processing

Control of cytokine function can also be achieved by regulating the processing of precursor forms. Many cytokines, including TGF-α, IL-1β, IL-1α and TNF-α, are produced initially as integral membrane proteins which require proteolytic cleavage in order to release the active molecule. Alternatively, cytokines such as TGF-β are synthesized initially as biologically inactive precursors which must be enzymatically processed to the active form. The identity of many of the processing enzymes is unknown, although the cysteine protease which mediates the processing of IL-1β, known as ICE, has been cloned recently (Thornberry *et al.*, 1992).

Sequestration

Some cytokine growth factors, such as TGF-β and IL-1, are sequestered on extracellular matrix in connective tissues, skin and bone (Tanaka *et al.*, 1993). This produces a sink of active cytokine which can be released rapidly when the matrix is disrupted during tissue injury or repair. Other cytokines, such as GM-CSF, IL-3 and SCF, are localized in stromal cell layers in bone marrow where they stimulate haematopoeisis (Gordon *et al.*, 1987).

Soluble binding proteins

Several binding proteins for cytokines are found in blood and tissue fluids. Some of these are secreted forms of cytokine cell membrane receptors (see below), whereas others such as α_2-macroglobulin bind a range of cytokines (James, 1990). These binding proteins may serve as passive carriers of these cytokines, either extending their half-life or promoting their excretion, or they may function as circulating inhibitors limiting the systemic effects of the cytokines. It is important to consider the possible effects of these binding proteins in modulating the potential effects of both locally and systemically released cytokines.

Cytokine receptor antagonists

At the present time, the only naturally occurring cytokine receptor antagonist that has been identified is the IL-1 receptor antagonist. It is structurally related to IL-1α and IL-1β and binds to IL-1 receptors, but does not cause signal transduction, thereby acting as a classical competitive antagonist (Eisenberg *et al.*, 1990).

Cytokine receptor modulation

Control of cytokine function can also be achieved by modulation of the numbers of cytokine receptors on the cell surface, which may be affected through gene expression, internalization or receptor shedding. Modulation of the affinity of a receptor or its function can also be brought about by receptor phosphorylation, or through competition for shared receptor chains or signal transduction molecules (Ullrich & Schlessinger, 1990).

Cytokine receptors

The receptors for many cytokines have now been cloned. Certain analogies of their primary structure have allowed grouping into 'superfamilies' based on common homology regions (Table 20.2). These regions may form discrete structural units or 'domains'. The most common domains established by their tertiary structure include immunoglobulin constant region-like domains (C1 and C2), complement control protein domains, fibronectin type III (FNIII) domains and cytokine receptor domains (CK).

The cytokine receptor superfamily

The extracellular regions of proteins of the cytokine receptor superfamily all contain combinations of CK, FNIII and, in some cases, C2 immunoglobulin domains. The CK domain has a length of approximately 100 amino acids with a characteristic Cys-X-Trp motif and three other conserved Cys residues. The FNIII domain was first identified in the extracellular matrix protein fibronectin. It includes the Trp-Ser-X-Trp-Ser (WSXWS) motif required for ligand binding and signal transduction.

Some members of the cytokine receptor superfamily (e.g. G-CSF receptor) comprise a single polypeptide chain

Table 20.2 Cytokine receptor superfamilies.

Superfamily	Receptors for	Common structure
Cytokine receptor (haematopoietic receptor)	IL-2 (β-, γ-chains), IL-4, IL-3 (α-, β-chains), IL-5 (α-, β-chains), IL-6, gp130, IL-9, IL-12, G-CSF, GM-CSF, CNTF, LIF, erythropoietin (?IL-7)	Single spanning membrane glycoproteins with CK, FNIII and C2 Ig domains. Receptors often heterodimers or trimers of single protein subunits
Interferon receptor (cytokine receptor type II)	IFN-α/β/γ, IL-10	Single spanning membrane glycoproteins with FNIII domains
Immunoglobulin	IL-1, IL-6, FGF, PDGF, M-CSF, SCF (c-*kit*)	Domains containing the 'immunoglobulin fold'
Protein tyrosine kinase receptor	EGF (class I), insulin (class II), PDGF, M-CSF, SCF (c-*kit*) (class III), FGF (class IV)	Intracellular protein tyrosine kinase domains. Class III and III and IV also have 'immunoglobulin folds'
Nerve growth factor receptor	NGF, TNF-I/II	Three or four cysteine-rich repeats in extracellular part of molecule
G-protein-coupled seven transmembrane spanning receptor	C5a, PAF, f-MLP, IL-8 and other chemokines	Short extracellular N-terminus, seven transmembrane domains with three extra- and four intracellular loops
Complement control protein	IL-2 (α-chain), proteins controlling the complement cascade	Multiple repeats of characteristic short domains

C2Ig, C2-like immunoglobulin fold.
See text for other definitions of abbreviations.

which binds to its ligand with high affinity in isolation. For other receptors, binding studies have revealed the existence of more than one binding affinity for ligand. Typically, these are high (K_d 10–100 pmol/l) and low- (K_d 1–10 pmol/l) affinity binding sites. For these receptors, additional subunits have been identified which are required for high-affinity receptor expression. Furthermore, some of these subunits are shared by more than one cytokine receptor, giving rise to heterodimeric and in some cases heterotrimeric structures. The arrangement of these multi-subunit receptors may explain some of the functional cross-reactivity and redundancy characteristic of cytokines. Examples of this phenomenon (explained in fuller detail in succeeding sections) include the following.

- *Receptors which share the GM-CSF receptor β-chain*. IL-3, IL-5 and GM-CSF each have a unique and specific low-affinity receptor with short intracytoplasmic regions which are unable to transduce an activation signal. Association of these chains with a second β-chain common to all three receptors converts this low-affinity binding to high-affinity binding, although the β-chain does not bind ligand (Hayashida *et al*., 1990). The β-chain has a much larger intracytoplasmic portion and is able to transduce an activation signal.
- *Receptors which share the IL-6 receptor β-chain (gp130)*. The receptors for IL-6, ciliary neurotrophic factor (CNTF), leukaemia inhibitory factor (LIF) and oncostatin M (OSM) share a common signalling subunit known as gp130. The IL-6 receptor binds to IL-6 with low affinity but is unable to transduce an activation signal. This IL-6/IL-6 receptor complex binds two gp130 molecules, which then dimerize, resulting in tyrosine phosphorylation of the gp130 proteins and subsequent signal transduction.
- *Receptors which share the IL-2 receptor γ-chain*. The IL-2 receptor is a complex of three polypeptide chains (Minami *et al*., 1993). The α-chain (Tac, CD25 or p55, not a member of the cytokine receptor superfamily) binds IL-2 with low affinity (K_d 1.4×10^{-8} mol/l), but does not transduce a signal. The other two components of the receptor are the β-chain (p75) and the γ-chain (p64). The β-chain binds IL-2 with intermediate affinity (K_d 1.2×10^{-7} mol/l) but the γ-chain does not bind IL-2. Receptor complexes comprising α/γ or β/γ heterodimers bind IL-2 with an affinity of approximately 10^{-9} mol/l. The high-affinity receptor complex is an α/β/γ heterotrimer (K_d 1.3×10^{-11} mol/l). Both β/γ and α/β/γ complexes are able to mediate signal transduction. The β-chain is also a component of the IL-15 receptor, whereas the γ-chain is also a functional component of the receptors for IL-4, IL-7 and IL-15.

There are no consensus sequence motifs in the intracytoplasmic portions of cytokine receptor superfamily molecules associated with known enzymatic activity, so that other membrane enzymes, such as tyrosine kinases or phosphatases, must associate with the ligand/receptor complexes for signal transduction. Downstream events following ligand binding are not well defined, although tyrosine phosphorylation of several cellular proteins has been described in association with the response to IL-2, IL-3, IL-4, IL-5, IL-6, IL-7, G-CSF, GM-CSF, LIF, CNTF and erythropoietin. The substrates include phosphatidyl inositol 3 kinase (PI_3K), $p120^{GAP}$, Raf-1 kinase and the JAK kinases. In addition, cytokine receptor chains may themselves be phosphorylated on binding ligand, probably by association with, or indirect activation of, protein tyrosine kinases such as $p56^{lck}$ (IL-2 receptor β-chain).

Many proteins of the cytokine receptor superfamily are secreted as soluble forms, produced by alternative splicing of their mRNA transcripts to produce proteins lacking the transmembrane region and the cytoplasmic proximal charged residues which anchor the protein in the membrane. Soluble receptors for several cytokines, including those for IL-4, IL-5, IL-7, IL-9, GM-CSF, G-CSF and LIF, have been described. The precise function of these soluble receptors *in vivo* is not yet established. They may act as antagonists by competitive ligand binding, although the affinity of cytokines for soluble receptors is generally low. Alternatively, soluble receptors could act as transport proteins to carry cytokines to remote sites, where they might be required for biological activity or alternatively might be removed from the body. Finally, soluble receptors complexed with cytokines may act as agonists. For example, the IL-6/IL-6 receptor complex binds to surface gp130 molecules and transduces a signal (Taga *et al.*, 1989).

The interferon receptor superfamily

The members of this family are single spanning transmembrane glycoproteins, characterized by either one (IFN-γ and IL-10 receptors) or two (IFN α/β receptors) homologous extracellular regions of approximately 200 amino acids, each of which has two FNIII domains. Signal transduction by the interferon receptor superfamily involves phosphorylation and activation of JAK and TYK2 protein tyrosine kinases.

The immunoglobulin superfamily

The immunoglobulin superfamily is the largest known superfamily. At least 40% of known leucocyte membrane polypeptides contain one or more immunoglobulin superfamily domains. Cytokine receptors with similar domains in their extracellular sequences include the receptors for IL-1, IL-6, FGF, PDGF, M-CSF and SCF (c-*kit*). The immunoglobulin domains are characterized by a structural unit of approximately 100 amino acids, with a distinct folding pattern known as the immunoglobulin fold.

Other cytokine receptor superfamilies

Proteins comprising the protein tyrosine kinase receptor superfamily all have a large glycosylated extracellular binding domain, a single transmembrane domain and an intracellular tyrosine kinase catalytic domain. They have been divided into four subgroups (Table 20.2), according to the degree of oligomerization induced by ligand binding. A significant feature of signal transduction by these receptors is autophosphorylation.

Proteins of the nerve growth factor (NGF) receptor superfamily are characterized by three or four cysteine-rich repeats of about 40 amino acids in the extracellular part of the molecule. The family includes the receptor for NGF and the type I and II receptors for TNF-α/β (TNF receptors I/II). One unusual feature of this superfamily is that some of the receptors bind more than one ligand. For example, both TNF-α and TNF-β bind to TNF receptors I and II with high affinity, even though these two cytokines show only 31% amino-acid sequence homology. The mode of signal transduction by this superfamily of molecules has not been elucidated. The leucocyte surface glycoproteins CD27, CD30, CD40 and Fas antigen belong to this superfamily.

The seven-transmembrane-spanning receptor superfamily is part of a very large family of receptors related to rhodopsin. It includes receptors for the C5a component of complement, IL-8 and many of the chemokines, as well as platelet-activating factor and formyl-methionyl-leucylphenylalanine (f-MLP). The receptors have a characteristic structure of a relatively short acidic extracellular N-terminal sequence, followed by seven transmembrane-spanning domains with three extracellular and three intracellular loops. These receptors are coupled to heterotrimeric guanosine triphosphate (GTP) binding proteins, which induce phosphatidylinositol 4,5-biphosphate (PIP_2) hydrolysis and activate kinases, phosphatases and ion channels.

The α-chain (p55) of the IL-2 receptor has two domains belonging to the complement control protein superfamily which are involved in ligand binding. The complement control binding superfamily domain is also known as the short consensus repeat, and is found in many proteins which control the complement cascade, including factor H, which is solely composed of 20 adjacent domains, and factors B and C2 with three domains. The CD35 and L-selectin cell-surface molecules also belong to this superfamily.

Properties of individual cytokines

An account of those cytokines which may play a role in asthmatic and allergic inflammation is given below. This is followed by a synopsis of how these cytokines may inter-

Table 20.3 Physicochemical properties and gene chromosomal location of selected cytokines.

Cytokine	Amino acids	MW (kDa)*	Chromosomal location
IL-1α	159	17.5	2q12–q21
IL-1β	153	17.3	2q13–21
IL-2	133	15–20	4q26–q27
IL-3	133	14–30	5q23–31
IL-4	129	15–19	5q31
IL-5	115	45**	5q23–q31
IL-6	183†	26	7p21–p14
IL-7	152	20–28	8q12–q13
IL-9	126	32–39	5q31.1
IL-10	160	39–40‡	1 (syntenic)
IL-11	179	23	19q13.3–13.4
IL-12 p35§	196	30–33	?
IL-12 p40§	306	35–44	?
IL-13	112	9–17	5q31
IL-14	483	60	?
IL-15 (simian)	114	14–15	?
TNF-α	157 (mature) ǁ	52¶	6p21.3
IFN-γ	143 (mature)	40–70	12q24.1
GM-CSF	127 (mature)	22	5q21–q32
SCF	248/220††	36	12q22–q24

See text for definition of abbreviations.
*Variability in molecular weight reflects variable glycosylations.
† Following cleavage of a 29-amino-acid signal peptide.
‡ Homodimeric form active.
§ Heterodimer of disulphide-linked chains, neither of which has biological activity alone.
ǁ Secreted as a pro-peptide with a membrane anchor domain and processed by proteolytic cleavage of 76 terminal amino acids.
¶ Normally secreted as a homodimer; monomeric TNF-α is not biologically active.
** Antiparallel homodimer.
†† Long and short membrane-bound forms following removal of signal peptide.

act in regulating the presence or absence and clinical severity of these diseases. Some basic physicochemical properties of selected cytokines and the chromosomal locations of their genes are listed in Table 20.3.

The 'pro-inflammatory' cytokines: IL-1, TNF-α and IL-6

These three cytokines are grouped together because they exert a broad range of pro-inflammatory properties both locally and systemically, and are probably responsible for many of the systemic features of the immune responses against invading organisms and tumours, such as cachexia, fever, neutrophilia and the acute-phase response.

IL-1 is a product of many cell types, and exerts a broad spectrum of biological activity (mainly stimulatory) on immune cells as well as cells outside the immune system (reviewed by Durum *et al.*, 1986; Dinarello, 1994). A remarkable feature of IL-1 regulation is the existence of a powerful natural inhibitor, the IL-1 receptor antagonist (IL-1RA), that has a structure which is similar to that of IL-1β. The two molecular forms of IL-1 (termed IL-1α and IL-1β), and the receptor antagonist IL-1RA, are encoded by three separate genes. IL-1α and IL-1β show only 20% homology in their amino-acid sequences. Despite this, they exert similar, if not identical, biological properties. Many cells express both types of IL-1 but the relative proportions of IL-1α and IL-1β vary. Expression of IL-1RA can be induced principally in monocytes by many stimuli, and this natural antagonist is also constitutively expressed in neutrophils, keratinocytes and epithelial cells. IL-1α and IL-1β are initially translated as pro-peptides which are cleaved by neutral proteases. This process occurs primarily extracellularly, when the proteases are released from the producing cell along with the pro-peptides. IL-1α and IL-1β lack signal peptides, so that the precise mechanism of this secretion is uncertain.

IL-1α/β are secreted by many cell types, including monocyte/macrophages, keratinocytes, kidney mesangial cells, corneal epithelium, T lymphocytes, large granular lymphocytes, B lymphocytes, astrocytes, endothelial cells, Langerhans cells, dendritic cells, thymic epithelial cells, fibroblasts, neutrophils, eosinophils and smooth muscle cells. Monocyte/macrophages and keratinocytes are probably the major biological sources of IL-1 *in vivo*. Secretion is induced by many agents including microbial products (toxins, haemagglutinins), and endogenous agents including C5a, TNF-α, TGF-β, IL-1 itself and probably other T-lymphocyte-derived cytokines. T lymphocytes also induce the production of IL-1 by monocytes during antigen-specific cell contact. IL-1 is also found in normal amniotic fluid, sweat, and dermal and brain tissue.

IL-1 receptors comprise two high-affinity receptors, termed IL-1RI and II (CDw121a/b) (McMahan *et al.*, 1991). Both receptors are members of the immunoglobulin gene superfamily, and both bind to IL-1α and IL-1β as well as IL-1RA. The IL-1RI transmits cellular signals directly via its cytoplasmic portion, whereas the IL-1RII has only a very short intracytoplasmic domain which probably does not transmit an intracellular signal. Its function is therefore unclear, although it may exist in a soluble form and thereby regulate IL-1 antagonism or act as an IL-1 carrier protein. Neither receptor has intrinsic protein kinase activity, although receptor-mediated cellular activation causes rapid phosphorylation of various protein substrates on serine/threonine residues, followed by expression of the transcription factors AP-1, NFκB and NF-IL-6.

Type I IL-1 receptors are widely distributed on many cells, including T cells, B cells, monocyte/macrophages, basophils, neutrophils, eosinophils, dendritic cells, fibroblasts, endothelial cells and neural cells. The type II receptor is expressed on T cells, B cells, monocytes and keratinocytes.

IL-1 stimulates all aspects of haemopoiesis, and has been used therapeutically following bone marrow transplantation. It exerts cytostatic effects on tumour cell lines *in vitro*, and enhances cell-mediated immune rejection of many tumours.

Monocytes/macrophages respond to IL-1 with increased synthesis of other cytokines, including IL-1 itself, IL-6, IL-8 and TNF-α, as well as prostaglandins, plasminogen activator and proteases. IL-1 exerts effects on cartilage and bone metabolism and fibroblast growth and proliferation. These properties, added to its ability to induce fever, acute-phase protein synthesis and corticotrophin-releasing factor from the hypothalamus, implicate IL-1 in the genesis of many of the local and systemic features of acute and chronic inflammation.

IL-1 is a growth factor for immature and mature thymocytes, and a cofactor for the induction of proliferation and IL-2 secretion by peripheral blood CD4 and CD8 T cells following engagement of their antigen receptors, although IL-6 can substitute for this function in some systems. Th2-like T-lymphocyte clones are more dependent on IL-1 for proliferation in response to antigen-primed antigen-presenting cells when compared with Th1-like clones. For example, IL-1RA blocked proliferation of Th2-like, but not Th1-like, clones *in vitro* (Abbas *et al.*, 1991). IL-1 is also a growth factor for pre-B cells and 'virgin' mature B cells, in synergy with other cytokines. It can also exert indirect stimulatory effects on B-cell function through the release of other cytokines such as IL-6.

TNF-α originates principally from macrophages and was originally defined as an activity which induced haemorrhagic necrosis of certain tumours *in vivo*. The actions of TNF-α are reviewed by Old (1985). TNF-α shares many activities with TNF-β (lymphotoxin), since both molecules bind to the same receptor. The principal source of TNF-β is, however, the T lymphocyte.

The genes encoding TNF-α and TNF-β are closely linked and situated within the major histocompatability (MHC) encoding complex. Like IL-1, TNF-α is secreted as a pro-peptide but in this case with a membrane anchor domain, which is processed by proteolytic cleavage of the terminal 76 amino acids. The mature TNF-α protein trimerizes *in vivo*. This allows aggregation of its receptors, which is essential for signal transduction (Jones *et al.*, 1989), and is a unique feature of the activity of this cytokine.

The potential sources of TNF-α *in vivo* are wide, although monocytes/macrophages are the principal source, and can be induced to secrete TNF-α in the presence of both endogenous and exogenous agents similar to those which induce IL-1. Secretion of TNF-α by monocytes/macrophages is greatly enhanced by other cytokines, including IL-1, GM-CSF and IFN-γ. Activated T lymphocytes and mast cells also secrete TNF-α. In addition, hepatocytes, thymic and splenic stromal cells and kidney tubule epithelial cells also naturally express TNF-α, even in the absence of disease.

Two receptor proteins (type I, CD120a and type II, CD120b) for TNF have been described. Both bind to TNF-α and TNF-β with high affinity. The receptor proteins, which are of molecular size 55 and 75 kDa, are members of the NGF receptor superfamily (Table 20.2). TNF receptors are present on nearly all cell types with few exceptions, such as erythrocytes and resting T cells. Although most cells expressing TNF receptors express both receptor forms, these appear to exert distinct functions in different target cells (Tartaglia & Goeddel, 1992). For example. The 55-kDa protein mediates TNF-induced cytotoxicity, antiviral effects and fibroblast proliferation, whereas the 75-kDa protein mediates enhancement of T-lymphocyte proliferation.

TNF-α causes regression of some tumours both *in vivo* and *in vitro*. This is not a reproducible effect on particular histological types, and appears to occur somewhat at random. TNF-α has no similar action on normal cells. The mechanism of induced necrosis is poorly understood, although it is greatly enhanced by inhibitors of protein synthesis, which has lead to the suggestion that protection against the inhibitory properties of TNF-α are conferred by one or more unidentified proteins which tumour cells lack.

TNF-α has many systemic effects that are similar to those of IL-1, including the induction of cachexia, fever, and acute-phase protein production in the liver. It also inhibits bone resorption and synthesis and induces proliferation of fibroblasts. TNF-α acts on vascular endothelial cells, inducing or up-regulating the expression of many adhesion molecules, including intercellular adhesion molecule-1 (ICAM-1), vascular adhesion molecule-1 (VCAM-1) and E-selectin. This in turn enhances the adhesion of many granulocytes, including neutrophils and eosinophils. TNF-α enhances the expression of class I and II MHC molecules. In particular, it increases the expression of class II MHC molecules on antigen-presenting cells. In addition, it enhances IL-1 release by these cells. It also acts as a costimulatory factor for activated T lymphocytes, enhancing proliferation and expression of receptors for IL-2.

The cytokine IL-6 has a broad spectrum of effects overlapping those of IL-1 and TNF-α. IL-6 was originally and independently described for its antiviral activity (originally called IFN-β_2), its effects on hepatocytes and its growth-promoting effects on B lymphocytes and plasmacytomas. It is made by monocytes/macrophages, T lymphocytes, B lymphocytes, and many other cells including bone marrow stromal cells, fibroblasts, keratinocytes, mesangial cells, astrocytes and endothelial cells. It is secreted as an autocrine growth factor by plasmacytoma cells and other tumours such as Kaposi's sarcoma.

High-affinity (K_d 10^{-11} mol/l) IL-6 receptors are formed by the non-covalent association of two subunits. The α-chain (CD126) binds to IL-6 with low affinity (K_d 10^{-9} mol/l), but does not signal. The β-chain (CD130, gp130) does not itself bind IL-6, but associates with the α-chain/IL-6 complex and is responsible for signal transduction. IL-6 receptors are expressed on activated but not resting B lymphocytes and plasma cells, T lymphocytes, monocytes and many other target cells of the 'acute-phase response'. IL-6 enhances proliferation and immunoglobulin M (IgM) synthesis by late-activated B lymphocytes. It also acts as a costimulator for antigen-presenting cell activated T lymphocytes and can increase the activity of cytotoxic T lymphocytes.

IL-2 and IL-15

IL-2 was first isolated in 1983 and was classically described as a T-lymphocyte growth factor. It is now clear that IL-2 stimulates the growth and differentiation of T cells, B cells, natural killer (NK) cells, lymphokine-activated killer (LAK) cells, monocytes/macrophages and oligodendrocytes (reviewed by Smith, 1988). Activated T lymphocytes are a major source of IL-2, but B lymphocytes can also be induced to secrete IL-2 under some conditions *in vitro*. IL-2 activates various immune cells, including helper and cytotoxic T lymphocytes, B lymphoctyes, macrophages and NK cells. It functions as an autocrine growth factor for T cells in isolation and also exerts paracrine effects on other T cells. IL-2 is secreted by antigen-activated T lymphocytes 4–12 hours following activation. This is later accompanied by up-regulation of high-affinity IL-2 receptors on the same cells. Binding of IL-2 to this receptor induces proliferation of T lymphocytes, secretion of cytokines and enhanced expression of receptors for other growth factors such as insulin. The IL-2 receptor complex is subsequently removed from the T-lymphocyte surface by internalization. Activated B lymphocytes also express high-affinity IL-2 receptors, which mediate differentiation and immunoglobulin secretion of mature cells. IL-2 also acts on monocytes, enhancing IL-1 secretion, cytotoxicity and phagocytosis. The response of NK cells to IL-2 is characterized by the secretion of IFN-γ, proliferation and enhanced cytolytic activity. IL-2 administered therapeutically to patients with tumours results in lymphocytosis, which is often accompanied by a peripheral blood eosinophilia, which may be secondary to the release of IL-5 from activated T lymphocytes.

Table 20.4 Structural subunits of the interleukin (IL)-2 receptor.

	Subunit		
	α	β	γ
IL-2 binding affinity (nmol/l)	10	1000	None
Size (kDa)	55	75	64
Signal transduction	No	Yes	Yes

The receptor complex for IL-2 is composed of three polypeptide chains termed α (CD25, Tac, p55), β (CD122, p75) and γ. Both the α- and β-chains bind IL-2 in isolation, but with low affinity. The γ-chain does not bind IL-2 alone. Intermediate affinity (K_d 10^{-9} mol/l) IL-2 receptor complexes are formed from α/γ and β/γ heterodimers. The high-affinity (K_d 1.3×10^{-11} mol/l) receptor complex is a α/β/γ heterotrimer (Table 20.4). The β- and γ-chains are members of the haematopoietic growth receptor superfamily. The α-chain is not a member of this superfamily, but has two extracellular domains with homology to the complement control protein (Table 20.2).

In terms of signal transduction, the α-chain of the receptor alone is unable to transduce any signal, despite its ability to bind IL-2. There are some cell lines that exhibit only intermediate-affinity IL-2 binding and lack the α-chain of the receptor. These cell lines retain their ability to respond to IL-2, indicating that the α-chain is dispensable for signal transduction. The β-chain, on the other hand, is an essential component for signal transduction, and the intracellular domain has critical sequences necessary for inducing growth-promoting signals (Hatakeyama *et al.*, 1989). The γ-chain also appears to be important for signal transduction, since a mutant IL-2 protein with an Asp substitution at residue Gln141 is specifically defective in interaction with the γ-chain (Zurawski & Zurawski, 1992). This mutant protein is defective in receptor activation and is an antagonist of native IL-2. The expression of the α-chain is highly inducible in T lymphocytes following activation via their antigen receptors. Its expression is not restricted to T lymphocytes, since B lymphocytes and some haematopoetic cells can also express the α-chain. The β-chain is expressed constitutively in T lymphocytes, while the γ-chain is expressed in T lymphocytes, B lymphocytes and NK cells.

IL-15 was first isolated from the simian kidney epithelial cell line CB1/EBNA (Carson *et al.*, 1994). It shares many of the properties of IL-2, including all its effects on T-lymphocyte proliferation and the generation of LAK cells. Messenger RNA encoding IL-15 has been found in a wide variety of human cells, including peripheral blood mononuclear cells, placental cells, skeletal muscle cells, hepatocytes, lung cells, kidney epithelial cells and bone marrow stromal cells. It is synthesized in particular abundance by epithelial cells and monocytes. The β- and γ-chains of the IL-2 receptor are both components of the IL-15 receptor, although the α-chain is not. It seems likely, therefore, that IL-15 can substitute for many of the functions of IL-2 in cells which express IL-2 receptors. This may explain why mice rendered IL-2 deficient by gene targetting are normal in respect of thymic and peripheral T-lymphocyte subset composition (Schorle *et al.*, 1991).

IL-4 and IL-13

IL-4 was first identified in 1982 in mice as a B-lymphocyte stimulatory factor. It is synthesized by Th2-like CD4 T lymphocytes and certain subpopulations of thymocytes (CD4–CD8–α/β receptor-positive cells and CD3+, CD4+, CD8– cells), as well as some CD8 T-lymphocyte clones, eosinophils and cells of the mast cell and basophil lineages. Synthesis is induced by stimulation of the antigen receptor in T lymphocytes and by IgE Fc receptor cross-linking in mast cells and basophils.

IL-4 plays an important role in many phases of B-lymphocyte activation. It increases expression of class II MHC molecules on resting B lymphocytes, as well as enhancing expression of CD23, the low-affinity (FCεRII) receptor, CD40 and the α-chain of the IL-2 receptor. It is an effective costimulator of B lymphocytes activated by exposure to specific antigen or anti-CD40 antibodies. It promotes immunoglobulin synthesis by B lymphocytes and plays a central role in immunoglobulin class switching, promoting switching of activated B lymphocytes to the synthesis of IgG4 and IgE (reviewed by Paul, 1992). This switching to IgE synthesis is accompanied by germline ε-chain synthesis. In contrast, IL-4 inhibits many of the functions of IL-2-activated B lymphocytes. IL-4 also regulates many phases of T-lymphocyte development, stimulating growth of helper and cytotoxic T cells and augmenting the proliferation of thymocytes. It promotes the development of Th2-like CD4 T lymphocytes and inhibits the development of Th1-like cells (LeGros *et al.*, 1990; Swain *et al.*, 1990). It potently enhances the cytolytic activity of CD8 cytotoxic T cells.

IL-4 exerts complex regulatory effects on monocytes/macrophages (reviewed by Figdor & de Velde, 1992). It enhances the surface expression of class II MHC molecules and the antigen-presenting capability of macrophages, but inhibits macrophage colony formation and release of cytokines such as TNF-α, IL-1, IL-12, IFN-γ and IL-8 by these cells. IL-4 also acts on other haematopoietic cells, acting in synergy with colony-stimulating factors to promote the growth of various cell types, especially mast cells and myeloid and erythroid progenitors, in concert with cytokines such as G-CSF, IL-6 and erythropoietin (reviewed by Rennick *et al.*, 1992).

IL-13 shares many of the properties of IL-4 *in vitro* (reviewed by Punnonen *et al.*, 1994). It is synthesized by activated CD4 and CD8 T lymphocytes and is a product of Th1-, Th2- and Th0-like CD4 T-lymphocyte clones (Mosmann & Coffman, 1989b). Like IL-4, it induces the synthesis of IgE, IgG4 and IgM by B lymphocytes cultured in the presence of activated CD4 T-lymphocyte clones or anti-CD40 antibody. This is accompanied by germline ε-chain synthesis. This effect is not mediated through enhanced IL-4 production, since anti-IL-4 monoclonal antibodies fail to inhibit IL-13-mediated IgE sythesis (Punnonen *et al.*, 1993). Thus, IL-13 may play as important a role as IL-4 in the induction and maintenance of inappropriate IgE synthesis in atopic patients. IL-13 exerts a similar range of activities to IL-4 on monocytes/macrophages. Like IL-4, IL-13 inhibits the secretion of IFN-γ and IL-12 by monocytes. Thus, both IL-4 and IL-13 promote the development of Th2-like CD4 T lymphocytes, both by a direct effect and by inhibition of synthesis of IFN-γ and IL-12, which inhibit Th2-like, but promote Th1-like, T-cell development.

Despite these similar effects on B lymphocytes, the functions of IL-4 and IL-13 are not identical. In particular, IL-13 exerts no growth-promoting effects on T lymphocytes, while the murine analogue of IL-13 exerts no effects on murine B lymphocytes, which is consistent with the fact that IgE synthesis cannot be induced in IL-4-deficient mice, a critical difference when studying IgE regulation in murine systems.

IL-10

The discovery of IL-10 emerged in part from an analysis of activities expressed by Th2-like murine CD4 T-lymphocyte clones which supressed cytokine production by Th1-like cells (reviewed by Moore *et al.*, 1993). IL-10 forms non-covalent homodimers which are required for activity. It shows strong sequence homology at the DNA and protein sequence levels to an open reading frame termed BCRF1 in the Epstein–Barr virus genome, a product of which displays some of the properties of human IL-10 (Moore *et al.*, 1990). It is expressed by a diversity of cell types, including CD4+ and CD8+ T lymphocytes, monocytes/macrophages, kerationocytes, activated B lymphocytes and B-cell lymphomas (reviewed by Moore *et al.*, 1993). In this respect IL-10 is not strictly a Th2-like cytokine in humans.

The properties of IL-10 are diverse. This cytokine suppresses some immune responses and augments others. IL-10 inhibits cytokine synthesis by Th1-like T lymphocytes and NK cells. This effect on T cells is partly an indirect effect through impairment of the antigen-presenting function of macrophages and dendritic cells, but not B cells. IL-10 also inhibits the production of many inflammatory cytokines, including TNF-α, IL-1, IL-6, IL-8 and GM-CSF by monocytes/macrophages (Fiorentino *et al.*, 1991a,b).

In contrast to these suppressive effects on cell-mediated immunity, IL-10 exerts a wide range of immunostimulatory effects on B lymphocytes (reviewed by Moore *et al.*, 1993). IL-10 augments the expression of MHC class II molecules by B lymphocytes, the proliferation and differentiation of B cells into plasma cells and the synthesis of IgM, IgG and IgA. It augments the proliferation of thymocytes in concert with IL-2, and may therefore play a role in T-cell development. It also stimulates murine mast cells, and synergizes with IL-3 and IL-4 to induce the proliferation of several murine mast cell lines.

IL-3, IL-5 and GM-CSF

These cytokines are considered together in view of their numerous shared properties. These shared properties result from the fact that the cytokines utilize a common signal-transducing β-chain in their heterodimeric receptors (Lopez *et al.*, 1991). In addition, the genes encoding IL-3, IL-5 and GM-CSF are clustered together on human chromosome 5. Also clustered at this location are the genes for IL-4, M-CSF and the M-CSF receptor (reviewed by Arai *et al.*, 1990; also see above). A unique feature of IL-5 is its homodimeric structure, with each chain of the homodimer arranged in opposing directions. Both chains are required for biological activity.

Activated T lymphocytes are the major physiological source of IL-3, IL-5 and GM-CSF. In addition, mucosal and connective tissue mast cells secrete small amounts of these cytokines following cross-linking of their surface IgE receptors. GM-CSF is also secreted by monocytes, fibroblasts and endothelial cells.

IL-3, IL-5 and GM-CSF exert most of their effects on granulocytic haematopoietic cell lines. All three cytokines act as eosinophil differentiation factors, although IL-5 acts specifically on late committed eosinophil precursors. In addition, IL-5 is the only cytokine which acts specifically on mature eosinophil granulocytes. IL-5 is the predominant regulator of eosinophilia, as shown in mice overexpressing IL-5 transgenes (Dent *et al.*, 1990). In contrast, mice overexpressing IL-3 or GM-CSF show only modest eosinophilia but succumb early owing to massive tissue infiltration and destruction by myeloid cells, especially neutrophils and macrophages. While IL-5 has clear effects in inducing the differentiation of murine B lymphocytes into immunoglobulin-producing plasma cells, the role of IL-5 in human B-cell growth and differentiation remains somewhat controversial. While apparently devoid of any apparent direct effect on B cells, IL-5 does induce differentiation of human B cells activated with mitogens or T-lymphocyte clones (Yokota *et al.*, 1986).

In contrast to IL-5, IL-3 and GM-CSF exert a broad range of effects on many cell types (reviewed by Clark & Kamen, 1987). IL-3 promotes survival, proliferation and differentiation of pluripotential stem cells and committed precursors of the granulocyte/macrophage, erythroid, eosinophil, megakaryocyte, mast cell and basophil lineages. It also enhances myeloid end cell functions, such as phagocytosis by eosinophils and monocyte cytotoxicity. GM-CSF prolongs the survival and enhances the function of mature leucocytes and their progenitors, including granulocytes, monocytes and eosinophils. Unlike IL-3, GM-CSF shows no activity on mast cells or pluripotential stem cells, but can serve as a growth factor for endothelial cells, erythroid cells and T cells.

IL-9

The cytokine IL-9 was first identified as a novel haematopoietic growth factor stimulating the proliferation of a megakaryoblastic leukaemia cell line (Yang *et al.*, 1989). It supports the growth of certain CD4 T-lymphocyte clones but not cytolytic CD8 T-lymphocyte clones. In mice, it enhances the growth of bone marrow-derived mast cell lines in response to IL-3 (Hültner *et al.*, 1990). Human IL-9 also supports erythroid colony formation in the presence of erythropoietin. In the murine system, at least, IL-9 appears to be secreted predominantly by Th2-like CD4 T-lymphocyte clones. Recent reports suggest that IL-9 may be involved in the regulation of IgE synthesis, since it augments IL-4-mediated IgE synthesis by human B cells (Dugas *et al.*, 1993). This, along with its effects on mast cell differentiation, provides a potential role for IL-9 in the pathogenesis of atopy and allergic inflammation.

IL-12

IL-12 is a heterodimer composed of two disulphide-linked polypeptide chains of molecular weights 35 and 40 kDa. IL-12 was initially recognized as a cytokine capable of synergizing with IL-2 to augment cytotoxic T-lymphocyte responses, and also as an inducer of IFN-γ synthesis by resting human peripheral blood mononuclear cells *in vitro*. It also enhances the lytic activity of NK and LAK cells independently of IL-2 (Kobayashi *et al.*, 1989; Stern *et al.*, 1990). These activities suggest that IL-12 plays an important role in defence against intracellular pathogens and other infections such as malaria (Sedegah *et al.*, 1994). It is secreted by antigen-presenting cells, including B lymphocytes and monocytes/macrophages. Its receptor is expressed on T cells and NK cells. One component of this receptor is related to gp130 (see above).

Perhaps the most important potential role of IL-12 is its effect in modulating the nature of T-cell responses to external antigens. In particular, IL-12 induces the development of Th1-like CD4 T-cell reponses while inhibiting the differentiation of Th2-like cells (Manetti *et al*., 1993). One mechanism of this activity may be the early priming of undifferentiated T-helper cells for IFN-γ secretion (Manetti *et al*., 1994). Furthermore, it directly inhibits the synthesis of IgE by IL-4-stimulated human B lymphocytes (Kiniwa *et al*., 1992). This effect might be expected to be further enhanced by its induction of release of IFN-γ, which also inhibits IgE synthesis, by mononuclear cells.

These properties of IL-12 indicate that it may play a critical role in directing the development of Th1-like T-cell responses against intracellular pathogens, while inhibiting the development of Th2-like responses and IgE synthesis. IL-12 may play an important role in inhibiting inappropriate IgE synthesis and allergic inflammation as a result of allergen exposure (see also Chapter 6).

IFN-γ

This cytokine was originally identified as a product of mitogen-stimulated T lymphocytes which inhibited viral replication in fibroblasts. To date, CD4+ (particularly 'Th1-like') and CD8+ T lymphocytes and NK cells are the only known sources. IFN-γ is a pleiotropic cytokine involved in the regulation of many phases of immune and inflammatory responses. IFN-γ is a heavily glycosylated homodimer formed by the antiparallel association of its two monomers. These are secreted as precursors of 166 amino acids which undergo signal peptide removal (20 amino acids) and further post-translational N-terminal cleavage (three amino acids) forming the mature 143-amino-acid protein.

The IFN-γ receptor is a single transmembrane protein, a member of the cytokine receptor type II superfamily (Table 20.2). Although the receptor binds IFN-γ with high affinity, signal transduction requires a species-specific accessory protein which associates with the extracellular domain of the receptor. This subunit is encoded by a gene on chromosome 21 and has been termed the IFN-γ receptor β-chain. The receptor is expressed on a wide variety of cells, including T cells, B cells, monocytes/macrophages, dendritic cells, granulocytes and platelets, but not erythrocytes. Many somatic cells, such as epithelial and endothelial cells, as well as many tumour cells, also express receptors.

The properties of IFN-γ have been reviewed by Trinchieri & Perussia (1985). IFN-γ potently activates macrophages, stimulating tumoricidal and microbicidal activities often secondary to the release of other cytokines such as IL-1, TNF-α, IL-6 and IL-8. It modulates class I and II MHC molecule expression, including up-regulation of class II molecules on monocytes/macrophages and dendritic cells, and induces *de novo* expression on epithelial, endothelial and other cells, rendering them capable of antigen presentation.

IFN-γ is a prototype Th1-like cytokine which promotes the development of Th1-like CD4+ T cells but inhibits that of Th2-like T cells (Swain *et al*., 1991). It is also a powerful and relatively specific inhibitor of IL-4-induced IgE and IgG4 synthesis by B lymphocytes, although at higher concentrations it non-specifically inhibits the production of all antibody isotypes. IFN-γ augments cytotoxic immune responses against intracellular organisms and tumours mediated by NK cells and cytotoxic T lymphocytes. Like IL-12, IFN-γ has the propensity to promote cell-mediated cytotoxic responses while inhibiting allergic inflammation and IgE synthesis.

Summary

At the start of this chapter it was emphasized that it is unwise, when assessing the roles of cytokines in immune responses and other inflammatory processes, to consider the properties of individual cytokines in isolation. Nevertheless, it is possible to construct hypotheses based on a consideration of these properties regarding the possible role of individual cytokines in asthmatic and allergic inflammation (Table 20.5). These should not be regarded as didactic, but simply as a basis for future laboratory and clinical experiments.

With regard to the pathogenesis of atopy, IL-4 and IL-13 are heavily implicated since only these cytokines can bring about IgE synthesis in B lymphocytes through switching (see also Chapter 6). Other cytokines, such as

Table 20.5 Cytokines which may be implicated in atopy, asthma and allergic inflammation.

Function	Cytokines implicated
General 'pro-inflammatory' cytokines	IL-1α/β, TNF-α/β, IL-6, IFN-γ
'Atopy' cytokines	
Promoters	IL-4, IL-13, IL-9
Inhibitors	IFN-γ, IL-12
Eosinophil-active cytokines	IL-3, IL-5, GM-CSF, IL-4, RANTES,* MCP-3*
'Th2-like' cytokines	IL-4, IL-5, IL-13, IL-9 (?)
Mast cell developmental cytokines	IL-3, IL-9, SCF (c-*kit*)

See text for definition of abbreviations.
*Chemokines: see Chapter 22.

IL-9, may amplify this process without directly regulating switching. Cytokines such as IL-12 and IFN-γ inhibit IgE production, and might be implicated in inhibiting inappropriate IgE responses in non-atopic individuals.

The concept of the division of CD4 T lymphocytes into two broad functional groups, based on their patterns of cytokine secretion, represents a significant milestone in our understanding of the operation of cytokine networks. CD4+ T lymphocytes can be classified as 'Th1-like' (prototype cytokine IFN-γ) or 'Th2-like' (prototype cytokines IL-4 and IL-5), based on the predominant cytokines which they secrete (for further details see Chapter 3). It is remarkable that these broad divisions of T-lymphocyte function correspond to the time-honoured division of immune responses into 'cell-mediated' (involving cytotoxic T cells and NK cells) and 'humoral' (involving antibodies) although, as would be expected from the pleiotropic nature of cytokines, these divisions are not absolute. Immune responses against viruses and other intracellular pathogens are associated with elevated synthesis of Th1-like cytokines, particularly IFN-γ which, along with IL-12 released from infected macrophages, would be expected to promote cell-mediated cytotoxicity. Th2-like cytokines are more facilitatory to antibody synthesis by B lymphocytes (and are absolutely required in the case of IgE) and would be expected to promote humoral responses as well as IgE synthesis. Asthmatic and allergic inflammation are also associated with Th2-like patterns of cytokine secretion, although there is little evidence, with the notable exception of IgE, that humoral responses play a significant role in the pathogenesis of these diseases. Elevated secretion of IL-5 and IL-4 by Th2-like T lymphocytes probably initiates the selective accumulation of tissue eosinophils and inappropriate IgE responses associated with allergy and asthma (see Chapter 90).

The mechanisms by which particular antigens induce Th1-like or Th2-like responses is only partly understood, and may depend on factors such as the local cytokine microenvironment under which antigen exposure first occurs, the nature of the antigen-presenting cells and the amount and extent of exposure (see Chapter 7). Once established, Th1- and Th2-like responses are mutually inhibitory. For example, IFN-γ, a Th1-like cytokine, suppresses Th2-like T-cell development and inhibits IgE synthesis, whereas IL-4 promotes Th2-like development but inhibits secretion of IFN-γ by Th1-like T cells and macrophages. Local IL-12 secretion may also have an important role to play in the inhibition of Th2-like responses.

One longstanding challenge in the pathogenesis of asthmatic and allergic inflammation has been to explain the specific accumulation of tissue eosinophils in these diseases. As mentioned above, IL-5 may play a critical role in this process, whereas other cytokines acting on eosinophils (although, unlike IL-5, not specifically on these cells) such as IL-3 and GM-CSF may also be required. A recent exciting observation has been that some β-chemokines specifically attract eosinophils (see Chapters 10 & 22) and an appraisal of the role of these factors in asthma pathogenesis is now urgently required.

It is to be hoped that these hypothetical 'frameworks' will form the basis for further investigation of asthma pathogenesis and guide future therapy. Switching of T-cell responses from Th1-like to Th1-like, and the blocking of cytokine production or action with drugs or monoclonal antibodies, seem exciting prospects in this regard.

References

Aarden, L.A., Brummer, T.K., Cerottini, J.-C. *et al.* (1979) Revised nomenclature for antigen-non-specific T-cell proliferation and helper factors. *J. Immunol.*, **123**, 2928–9.

Abbas, A.K., Williams, M.E., Burstien, H.J., Chang, T.-L., Bossu, P. & Lichtman, A.H. (1991) Activation and functions of CD4+ T cell subsets. *Immunol. Rev.*, **136**, 5–22.

Arai, K., Lee, F., Miyajima, A., Miyatake, S., Arai, N. & Yokota, T. (1990) Cytokines: co-ordinators of immune and inflammatory responses. *Ann. Rev. Biochem.*, **59**, 783–802.

Carson, W.E., Giri, J.G., Lindemann, M.J. *et al.* (1994) Interleukin (IL) 15 is a novel cytokine that activates human natural killer cells via components of the IL-2 receptor. *J. Exp. Med.*, **180**, 1395–403.

Clark, S.C. & Kamen, R. (1987) The human hematopoietic colony-stimulating factors. *Science*, **236**, 1229–37.

Dent, L.A., Strath, M., Mellor, A.L. & Sanderson, C.J. (1990) Eosinophilia in transgenic mice expressing interleukin 5. *J. Exp. Med.*, **172**, 1425–31.

Dinarello, C. (1994) The biological properties of interleukin-1. *Eur. Cytokine Netw.*, **5**, 517–31.

Dugas, B., Renauld, J.P., Bonnefoy, J.Y. *et al.* (1993) Interleukin-9 potentiates the interleukin-4-induced immunoglobulin (IgG, IgM and IgE) production by normal human B lymphocytes. *Eur. J. Immunol.*, **23**, 1687–92.

Dumonde, D.C., Wolstencraft, R.A., Panayi, G.S., Matthew, M., Morley, J. & Howson, W.T. (1969) 'Lymphokines': non-antibody mediators of cellular immunity generated by lymphocyte activation. *Nature*, **224**, 38–42.

Durum, S.K., Schmidt, J.A. & Oppenheim, J.J. (1986) Interleukin 1: an immunological perspective. *Ann. Rev. Immunol.*, **3**, 263–87.

Eisenberg, S.P., Evans, R.J., Arend, W.P. *et al.* (1990) Primary structure and functional expression from complementary DNA of a human interleukin-1 receptor antagonist. *Nature*, **343**, 341–6.

Figdor, C. & de Velde, A. (1992) Regulation of human monocyte phenotype and function by IL-4. In: *IL-4: Structure and Function* (ed. H. Spits), p. 187. CRC Press, Boca Raton.

Fiorentino, D.F., Zlotnik, A., Mosmann, T.R., Howard, M. & O'Garra, A. (1991a) IL-10 inhibits cytokine production by activated macrophages. *J. Immunol.*, **147**, 3815–22.

Fiorentino, D.F., Zlotnik, A., Vieira, P. *et al.* (1991b) IL-10 acts on the antigen-presenting cell to inhibit cytokine production by Th1 cells. *J. Immunol.*, **146**, 3444–51.

Gordon, M.Y., Riley, G.P., Watt, S. & Greaves, M.F. (1987) Compartmentalization of a haematopoietic' growth factor (GM-CSF) by glycosaminoglycans in the bone marrow microenvironment. *Nature*, **326**, 403–5.

Hatakeyama, M., Mori, H., Doi, T. & Taniguchi, T. (1989) A restricted cytoplasmic region of IL-2 receptor β chain is essential for growth signal transduction but not for ligand binding and internalization. *Cell*, **59**, 837–45.

Hayashida, K., Kitamura, T., Gorman, D.M., Arai, K.I., Yokota, T. & Miyajima, A. (1990) Molecular cloning of a second subunit of the receptor for human granulocyte-macrophage colony-stimulating factor (GM-CSF): reconstitution of a high-affinity GM-CSF receptor. *Proc. Nat. Acad. Sci. USA*, **87**, 9655–9.

Hültner, L., Druez, C., Moeller, J. *et al.* (1990) Mast cell growth-enhancing activity (MEA) is stucturally related and functionally identical to the novel mouse T cell growth factor P40/TCGF III (interleukin 9). *Eur. J. Immunol.*, **20**, 1413–16.

James, K. (1990) Interactions between cytokines and alpha$_2$-macroglobulin. *Immunol. Today*, **11**, 163–6.

Jones, E.Y., Stuart, D.I. & Walker, N.P.C. (1989) Structure of tumour necrosis factor. *Nature*, **338**, 225–8.

Jyung, R.W. & Mustoe, T.A. (1993) In: *Clinical Applications of Cytokines* (ed J.J. Oppenheim). Oxford University Press, Oxford.

Kiniwa, M., Gately, M., Gubler, U., Chizzonite, R., Fargeas, C. & Delespesse, G. (1992) Recombinant interleukin-12 suppressed the synthesis of immunoglubulin E by interleukin-4 stimulated human lymphocytes. *J. Clin. Invest.*, **90**, 262–6.

Kobayashi, M., Fitz, L., Ryan, M. *et al.* (1989) Identification and purification of natural killer cell stimulatory factor (NKSF), a cytokine with multiple biologic effects on human lymphocytes. *J. Exp. Med.*, **170**, 827–45.

Le Gros, G., Ben Sasson, S.Z., Seder, R., Finkelman, F.D. & Paul, W.E. (1990) Generation of interleukin 4 (IL-4) producing cells *in vivo* and *in vitro*: IL-2 and IL-4 are required for *in vitro* generation of IL-4 producing cells. *J. Exp. Med.*, **172**, 921–9.

Lopez, A.F., Vadas, M.A., Woodcock, J.M. *et al.* (1991) Interleukin-5, interleukin-3, and granulocyte macrophage colony stimulating factor cross-compete for binding to cell surface receptors on human eosinophils. *J. Biol. Chem.*, **266**, 24741–7.

McMahan, C.J., Slack, J.L., Moslwy, B. *et al.* (1991) A novel IL-1 receptor, cloned from B cells by mammalian expression, is expressed in many cell types. *EMBO J.*, **10**, 2821–32.

Manetti, R., Parronchi, P., Giudizi, M.G. *et al.* (1993) Natural killer cell stimulatory factor (interleukin 12 (IL-12)) induces T helper type 1 (Th1)-specific immune responses and inhibits the development of IL-4 producing Th cells. *J. Exp. Med.*, **177**, 1199–204.

Manetti, R., Gerosa, F., Giudizi, M.G. *et al.* (1994) Interleukin 12 induces stable priming for interferon gamma (IFN-gamma) production during differentiation of human T helper (Th) cells and transient IFN-gamma production in established Th2 cell clones. *J. Exp. Med.*, **179**, 1273–83.

Massague, J. & Pandiella, A. (1993) Membrane-anchored growth factors. *Ann. Rev. Biochem.*, **62**, 515–41.

Minami, Y., Kono, T., Miyazaki, T. & Taniguchi, T. (1993) The IL-2 receptor complex: its structure, function, and target genes. *Ann. Rev. Immunol.*, **11**, 213–44.

Moore, K.W., O'Garra, A., de Waal Malefyt, R., Vieira, P. & Mosmann, T.R. (1993) Interleukin-10. *Ann. Rev. Immunol.*, **11**, 165–90.

Moore, K.W., Vieira, P., Fiorentino, D.F., Trounstine, M.L., Khan, T.A. & Mosmann, T.R. (1990) Homology of cytokine synthesis inhibitory factor (IL-10) to the Epstein–Barr virus gene BCRFI. *Science*, **248**, 1230–4.

Mosmann, T. & Coffman, R.L. (1989a) Heterogeneity of cytokine secretion patterns and functions of helper T cells. *Adv. Immunol.*, **46**, 111–47.

Mosmann, T.R. & Coffman, R.L. (1989b) Th1 and Th2 cells: different patterns of cytokine secretion lead to different functional properties. *Ann. Rev. Immunol.*, **7**, 145–73.

Old, L.J. (1985) Tumor necrosis factor (TNF). *Science*, **230**, 630–2.

Paul, W.E. (1989) Pleiotropy and redundancy: T-cell-derived lymphokines in the immune response. *Cell*, **57**, 521.

Paul, W.E. (1992) The role of IL-4 in the regulation of B cell development, growth, and differentiation. In: *IL-4: Structure and Function* (ed H. Spits), p. 57. CRC Press, Boca Raton.

Punnonen, J., Aversa, G., Cocks, B.G. *et al.* (1993) Interleukin 13 induces interleukin-4-independent IgG4 and IgE synthesis and CD23 expression by human B cells. *Proc. Nat. Acad. Sci. USA*, **90**, 3730–4.

Punnonen, J., Aversa, G., Cocks, B.G. & de Vries, J.E. (1994) Role of interleukin-4 and interleukin-13 in synthesis of IgE and expression of CD23 by human B cells. *Allergy*, **49**, 576–86.

Rennick, D., Moore, J.G. & Thompson-Snipes, L. (1992) IL-4 and hematopoiesis. In: *IL-4: Structure and Function* (ed. H. Spits), p. 151. CRC Press, Boca Raton.

Schorle, H., Holtschke, T., Hunig, T., Schimpl, A. & Horak, I. (1991) Development and function of T-cells in mice rendered interleukin-2 deficient by gene targeting. *Nature*, **352**, 621–4.

Sedegah, M., Finkelman, F. & Hoffman, S.L. (1994) Interleukin 12 induction of interferon gamma-dependent protection against malaria. *Proc. Nat. Acad. Sci. USA*, **91**, 10700–2.

Smith, K.A. (1988) Interleukin-2: inception, impact, and implications. *Science*, **240**, 1169–76.

Stern, A.S., Podlanski, F.J., Hulmes, J.D. *et al.* (1990) Purification to homogeneity and partial characterization of cytotoxic lymphocyte maturation factor from human B-lymphoblastoid cells. *Proc. Nat. Acad. Sci. USA*, **87**, 6808–12.

Swain, S.L., Bradley, L.M., Croft, M. *et al.* (1991) Helper T-cell subsets: phenotype, function and the role of lymphokines in regulating their development. *Immunol. Rev.*, **123**, 115–44.

Swain, S.L., Weinberg, A.D., English, M. & Huston, G. (1990) IL-4 directs the development of Th2-like helper effectors. *J. Immunol.*, **145**, 3796–806.

Taga, T., Hibi, M., Hirata, Y. *et al.* (1989) Interleukin-6 triggers the association of its receptor with a possible signal transducer. *Cell*, **58**, 573–81.

Tanaka, Y., Adams, D.H. & Shaw, S. (1993) Proteoglycans on endothelial cells present adhesion-inducing cytokines to leukocytes. *Immunol. Today*, **14**, 111–15.

Tartaglia, L.A. & Goeddel, D.V. (1992) Two TNF receptors. *Immunol. Today*, **13**, 151–3.

Thornberry, N.A., Bull, H.G., Calacay, J.R. *et al.* (1992) A novel heterodimeric cysteine protease is required for interleukin-1 beta processing in monocytes. *Nature*, **356**, 768–74.

Trinchieri, G. & Perussia, B. (1985) Immune interferon: a pleiotropic lymphokine with multiple effects. *Immunol. Today*, **6**, 131.

Ullrich, A. & Schlessinger, J. (1990) Signal transduction by receptors with tyrosine kinase activity. *Cell*, **61**, 203–12.

Yang, Y.C., Ricciardi, S., Ciarletta, A., Calvetti, I., Kelleher, K. & Clark, S.C. (1989) Expression cloning of a cDNA encoding a novel human hematopoietic growth factor: human homologue of murine T-cell growth factor P40. *Blood*, **74**, 1880–4.

Yokota, T., Otsuka, T., Mosmann, T. *et al.* (1986) Isolation and characterization of a human interleukin cDNA clone, homologous to mouse B-cell stimulatory factor 1, that expresses B-cell and T-cell-stimulating activities. *Proc. Nat. Acad. Sci. USA*, **83**, 5894–8.

Zurawski, S.M. & Zurawski, G. (1992) Receptor antagonist and selective agonist derivatives of mouse interleukin-2. *EMBO J.*, **11**, 3905–10.

CHAPTER 21

Role of IL-5, IL-3 and GM-CSF in the Pathophysiology of Asthma and Allergy

A.B. Kay

Introduction

Over the past decade there has been increasing interest in interleukin-5 (IL-5), IL-3 and granulocyte macrophage colony-stimulating factor (GM-CSF) — related cytokines with multiple overlapping biological activities relevant to inflammation, allergy and asthma. The genes encoding IL-3, IL-5 and GM-CSF are clustered together on human chromosome 5, together with IL-4, macrophage colony-stimulating factor (M-CSF) and the M-CSF receptor (see Chapter 76). IL-5, IL-3 and GM-CSF were initially described as haemopoietic growth factors but are now known to have a wide range of potent effects which include cell activation, mobilization and survival. IL-5 is more restricted in its properties, acting predominantly on cells of the eosinophil/basophil lineage. Each receptor for these cytokines is composed of a ligand-specific α-chain which binds the cognate ligand with low affinity, and a common β-chain, which, although failing to bind to the ligand itself, confers high-affinity binding on the α-chain (Lopez *et al.*, 1992). The sharing of the β-chain may explain the cross-competition between IL-5, IL-3 and GM-CSF. The common β-chain is required for high-affinity binding and it is also essential for signal transduction (Lopez *et al.*, 1991). A diagrammatic representation of this subfamily of receptors is shown in Fig. 21.1.

The biological responses of neutrophils, monocytes and eosinophils to these cytokines is reflected by their receptor expression. Neutrophils only express the GM-CSF receptor (R) α-chain and the common β-chain, whereas monocytes express the GM-CSFR and the IL-3R α-chains in excess over the β-chain (Fig. 21.2). Eosinophils express the GM-CSF, IL-3 and IL-5 receptor α-chains in similar numbers to the β-chain. Thus, IL-5 production results in the stimulation of eosinophils but not neutrophils, whereas production of GM-CSF or IL-3 will lead to the stimulation of neutrophils or monocytes (Lopez *et al.*, 1992).

IL-5 has a novel dimer configuration and exists in an antiparallel (head to tail) fashion (Milburn *et al.*, 1993). The homodimers are disulphide linked and the molecule is highly homologous between species. Both chains are required for biological activity. The crystal structure of IL-5 shows a striking similarity to the cytokine fold found in GM-CSF and human growth hormone (Fig. 21.3).

Biological activities IL-5

IL-3, IL-5 and GM-CSF exert most of their effects on granulocytic cells and there is abundant evidence that these cytokines are generated in allergic inflammation (Fig. 21.4). All three cytokines can serve as eosinophil differentiation factors, although IL-5 acts specifically on late committed eosinophil precursors (reviewed in Wardlaw *et al.*, 1995). IL-3 is a multilineage haemopoietic factor, whereas granulocyte colony-stimulating factor (G-CSF) and IL-5 are lineage-specific haemopoietic factors for neutrophils and eosinophils, respectively. Present evidence suggests that GM-CSF and IL-3 commit CD34+, CD33– progenitor cells to an eosinophil lineage and that IL-5 brings about terminal differentiation of CD34–, CD33+ cells derived from CD34+, CD33– precursors (Ema *et al.*, 1990). Therefore, IL-5 is the only cytokine which acts selectively on mature eosinophil granulocytes and is the predominant regulator of eosinophilia as demonstrated in mice over-expressing IL-5 transgenes (Dent *et al.*, 1990). In contrast,

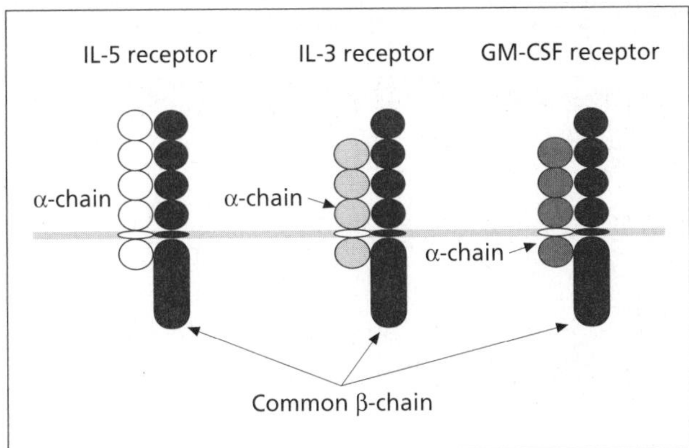

Fig. 21.1 Schematic illustration of molecular components for the IL-5, GM-CSF and IL-3 receptors, complex. (Modified from Takatsu, 1995.) See text for definition of abbreviations.

mice overexpressing IL-3 or GM-CSF show only modest eosinophilia but succumb early owing to massive tissue infiltration and destruction by myeloid cells, especially neutrophils and macrophages.

IL-5 also enhances the effector function of mature eosinophils in terms of adhesion, survival, mediator release and mobility (Lopez *et al.*, 1988; Wang *et al.*, 1989; Fujisawa *et al.*, 1990; Owen *et al.*, 1990; Walsh *et al.*, 1990a,b). For example, IL-5 potentiated integrin-dependent adhesion of eosinophils to plasma-coated glass and human microvascular endothelial cells (Walsh *et al.*, 1990b). These effects were not observed with neutrophils. IL-5 also enhanced the generation of superoxide radical and of leukotriene C_4 (LTC_4). *In vitro* cytotoxicity against helminthic targets, and IgA- and IgG-dependent degranulation of eosinophils, were also enhanced by IL-5.

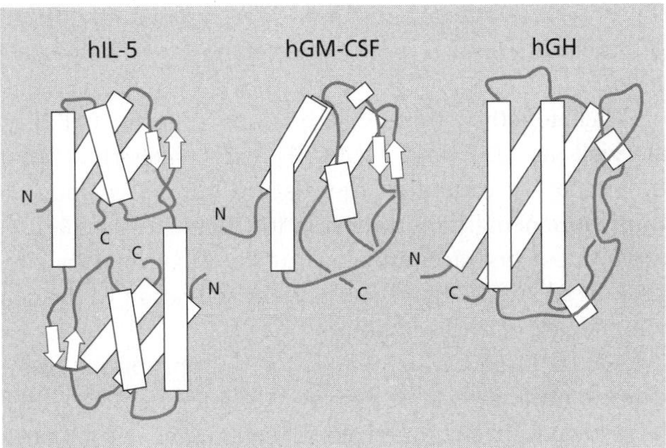

Fig. 21.3 Schematic illustration of tertiary structure of hIL-5 molecule in comparison to hGM-CSF and human growth hormone (hGH). Boxes and arrows indicate α-helices and β-strands, respectively. The drawing was prepared based on the analysis of the crystal structure of hIL-5. (From Takatsu, 1995.) See text for definition of abbreviations.

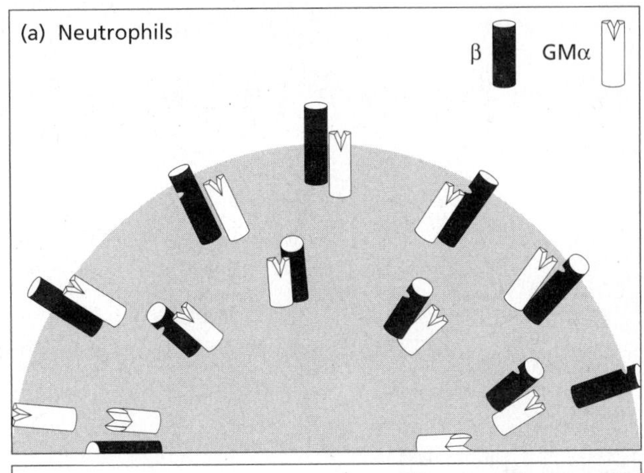

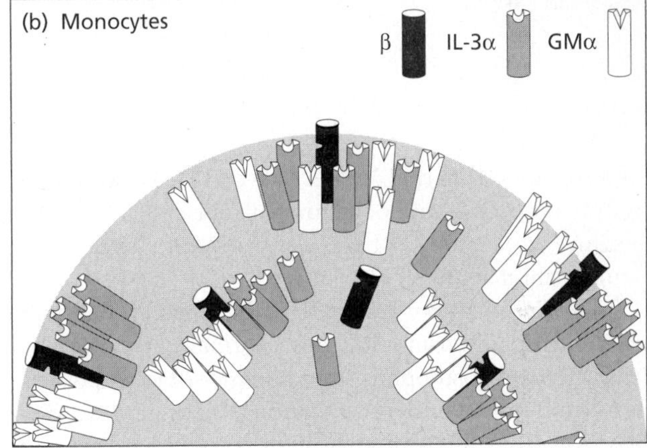

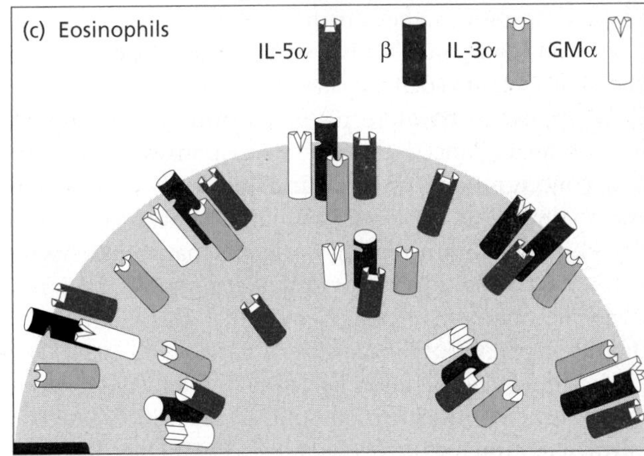

Fig. 21.2 Proposed expression of the different receptor α-chains and common β-chain on human neutrophils (a), monocytes (b) and eosinpohils (c). (From Lopez *et al.*, 1992).

Eosinophil-active IL-5 production from human T cells was enhanced by leukotriene B_4 (LTB_4), but not by the stereoisomer 5s,12s-dihydroxy-6,8,10,14-ETE (Yamaoka & Kolb, 1993), suggesting a further link between Th2-type cytokines and allergic inflammation. Culture of eosinophils for several days with IL-5 resulted in at least 50% release of total granule proteins into the culture

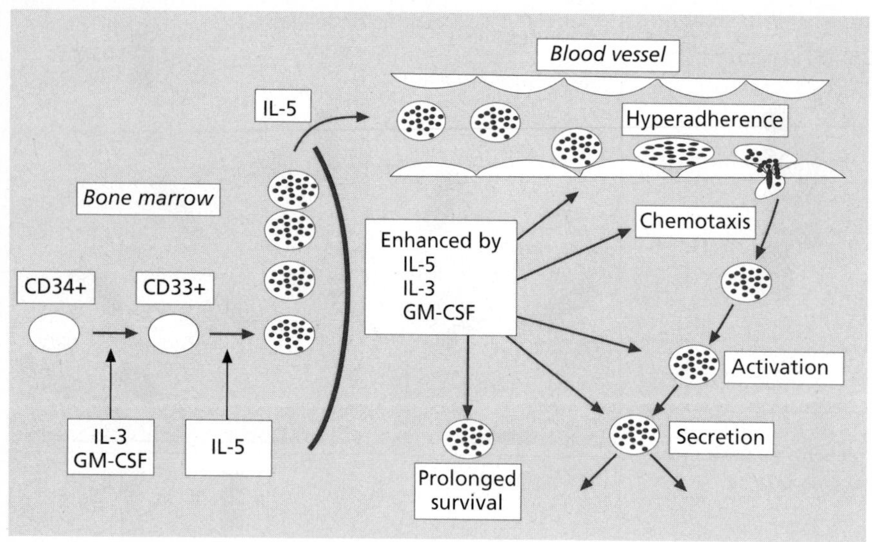

Fig. 21.4 Diagrammatic representation of the effects of IL-5, IL-3 and GM-CSF on eosinophil function.

supernatants (Kita *et al.*, 1992). IL-5 and IL-3 also activate mature basophils but not neutrophils (Bischoff *et al.*, 1990; Bochner *et al.*, 1990; Hirai *et al.*, 1990; Shute, 1992; Yamaguchi *et al.*, 1992).

In Boyden chamber assays, IL-3, IL-5 and GM-CSF were chemotactic for eosinophils from normal individuals but less active on eosinophils from allergic subjects, possibly as a result of *in vivo* desensitization (Warringa *et al.*, 1991; Sehmi *et al.*, 1992). Although these cytokines are active at low concentrations, they are in general only weakly effective when compared with well-documented eosinophil chemoattractants such as platelet-activating factor (PAF). They appear to be more potent in priming eosinophils *in vitro* for enhanced chemotactic responses to suboptimal concentrations of lipid and low-molecular-weight chemoattractants such as LTB_4 and formyl-methionyl-leucyl-phenylalunine (f-MLP)—agents that are otherwise weakly active in unprimed normal eosinophils. IL-5 and GM-CSF markedly potentiated the transendothelial migration of eosinophilia *in vitro* (Ebisawa *et al.*, 1994). The evidence for co-operation between IL-5 and the chemokine *eotaxin* in inducing eosinophil accumulation *in vivo* is particularly interesting (Collins *et al.*, 1995) Thus, IL-5 acts predominently by mobilizing eosinophils from the bone marrow with eotaxin facilitating egress of eosinophils into the site of allergic tissue reactions.

Despite the relative lack of chemotactic activity of IL-5, inhalation of IL-5 in animals and humans leads to eosinophil recruitment (Iwama *et al.*, 1992; Terada *et al.*, 1992), and antibodies against IL-5 have been found to be effective at inhibiting eosinophil migration into the lung of allergen-challenged guinea pigs (Mauser *et al.*, 1993; Van Ooseterhout *et al.*, 1993). Antibody-mediated inhibition occurs even when the anti-IL-5 antibody was given at the time of the challenge, so it appears to be working primarily through an effect on eosinopoiesis. A possible explanation of the apparent discrepancy between the *in vivo* and *in vitro* findings is that IL-5 may be a more effective chemoattractant *in vivo* than *in vitro*. Alternatively, IL-5 priming of adhesion to vascular endothelium may be important in eosinophil transmigration after allergen challenge. In a monkey model of asthma an antibody to IL-5 produced prolonged production of eosinophils and inhibited bronchial hyperresponsiveness, suggesting that anti-IL-5 may be inhibiting eosinophil release from the bone marrow (Mauser *et al.*, 1995).

IL-5, IL-3 and GM-CSF not only activate mature eosinophils but they also delay programmed cell death (apoptosis), thus prolonging survival of the cell *in vitro* (Owen *et al.*, 1987; Rothenberg *et al.*, 1988, 1989; Her *et al.*, 1991; Stern *et al.*, 1992). Apoptosis of eosinophils and their ingestion by macrophages has also been observed in allergic inflammation in atopic subjects *in vivo* (Kay *et al.*, 1996).

Taken together, these observations suggest that IL-5, as well as IL-3 and GM-CSF, exert important pro-inflammatory effects on the mature human eosinophil, thus influencing their adhesion to the microvasculature, recruitment and accumulation in the inflammatory site, prolonged survival and subsequent activation of the cell with release of their mediators.

IL-5, IL-3 and GM-CSF bind to the appropriate leucocyte membrane via high-affinity cytokine receptors which have been fully characterized (DiPersio *et al.*, 1988; Lopez *et al.*, 1989; Chihara *et al.*, 1990; Ingley & Young, 1991; Lopez *et al.*, 1991, Migita *et al.*, 1991). All of these receptors are of single high affinity for each cytokine, with an average k_d value of 120 pmol/l for the IL-5R, 500 pmol/l for the IL-3R and 50 pmol/l for GM-CSFR. Eosinophils and basophils, but not neutrophils, express IL-5R, while

GM-CSFR is present on both eosinophils and neutrophils with a similar affinity binding value on both.

Most of the IL-5R mRNA encodes a soluble isoform which has inhibitory activity in an IL-5-dependent eosinophil differentiation assay (Tavernier *et al.*, 1992). The α-chain of IL-5 is encoded on chromosome 3 and occurs as two soluble isoforms (S1 and S2), produced by 'normal' or no splicing, respectively. The membrane-anchored form of the IL-5R is produced by alternative splicing (Tavernier *et al.*, 1992). IL-5R α-chain mRNA was down-regulated by transforming growth factor-β1 (TGF-β1) (Zanders, 1994). Since TGF-β induced eosinophil apoptosis (Alam *et al.*, 1994), this raises the possibility that soluble IL-5R acts at several levels of control, including eosinophil survival, expression of the membrane-anchored IL-5R and terminal eosinophil differentiation steps.

Cell source of IL-5

T cells are a major source of IL-5, as are mast cells and eosinophils (Fig. 21.5). Corrigan *et al.* (1995) demonstrated that purified CD4+ cells from patients with exacerbations of asthma were mRNA+ for IL-5 and spontaneously released this cytokine, together with GM-CSF, into the culture supernatant. Eosinophil-active cytokines, including IL-5, were produced by CD4+, and to a lesser extent from CD8+ T-cell lines obtained from bronchoalveolar lavage (BAL) from atopic asthmatics. IL-5 concentrations were significantly higher in atopic asthmatics compared with atopic and non-atopic controls (Till *et al.*, 1995). This

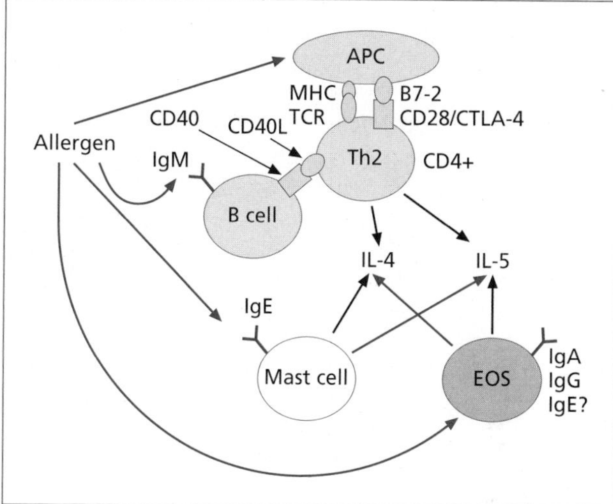

Fig. 21.5 Diagrammatic representation of the allergen-induced release of IL-5 and IL-4 from CD4+ and CD8+ Th2-type T cells, mast cells and eosinophils. Allergen presentation via MHC/TCR and the costimulatory molecules B7-2/CD28/CTLA-4 are also shown. See text for definition of abbreviations.

suggests that overproduction of IL-5 by asthmatic CD4+ T cells may be a fundamental abnormality in this disease. Ying *et al.* (1995) investigated the phenotype of cells expressing mRNA encoding IL-5 in BAL and bronchial biopsies from mild atopic asthmatic patients and compared the results with non-asthmatic controls. CD3+ T cells were the most abundant cell expressing IL-4 and IL-5 mRNA in BAL and bronchial biopsies from allergic asthma. Fewer, but detectable numbers of tryptase-positive mast cells and EG2+ eosinophils also expressed these transcripts. It is well known that viral infections exacerbate asthma and that cytotoxic cells provide basic immunity against viral infections through MHC class I-restricted mechanisms. Therefore, it was of particular interest that in a murine model of airway hyperresponsiveness viral-specific CD8+ cells elaborated IL-5 and induced airway eosinophilia (Coyle *et al.*, 1995). However, in bronchial biopsies from asthma, including virus-associated intrinsic asthma (see below), the majority of mRNA for IL-5 was colocalized to CD4+ cells, with a relatively small contribution from CD8+ cells (S. Ying *et al.*, unpublished). T cells were also the principal source of IL-5 mRNA in allergen-induced rhinitis (Ying *et al.*, 1993).

Eosinophils infiltrating mucosa of patients with active coeliac disease were also shown to express mRNA for IL-5 (Desreumaux *et al.*, 1992) and IL-5 mRNA+ cells were found in diseased, but not normal, tissue and were absent after treatment with a gluten-free diet. By *in situ* hybridization, mRNA was identified in peripheral blood eosinophils from the hypereosinophilic syndrome. IL-5 (together with GM-CSF) mRNA expression in eosinophils was also demonstrated, *in vivo*, in BAL cells obtained from asthmatic subjects (Broide *et al.*, 1992), suggesting that eosinophil IL-5 and GM-CSF expression at sites of allergic inflammation in asthma may provide a combined autocrine pathway, thus maintaining the viability and effector function of the recruited eosinophils. IL-5 released following stimulation of immunoglobulin A (IgA)-, IgE- or IgG-antigen complexes was colocalized to eosinophilic granules by immunogold staining (Dubucquoi *et al.*, 1994).

IL-5 mRNA expression in allergic disease *in vivo*

It is now well established that cells mRNA+ for IL-4 and IL-5 predominate in blood and tissues in atopic allergy and helminthic parasitic infections. Allergen-specific T-cell clones derived from the peripheral blood of atopic donors secreted a type 2 pattern of cytokines, whereas bacterial antigen-specific clones secreted a type 1 pattern (Parronchi *et al.*, 1991). Skin-biopsy (Kay *et al.*, 1991) and nasal-biopsy (Durham *et al.*, 1992) specimens and BAL cells obtained from atopic asthmatics (Robinson *et al.*, 1992) contained an inflammatory infiltrate rich in cells expressing mRNA encoding predominantly IL-3, IL-4, IL-5 and GM-CSF, but not IL-2 or IFN-γ. Conversely, the cells infiltrating tuberculin reactions expressed IFN-γ and IL-2, but with little IL-4 and IL-5 (Tsicopoulos *et al.*, 1992).

Evidence for believing that IL-5 plays a critical role in asthma comes from the following clinical studies. Using the technique of *in situ* hybridization, the numbers of IL-5 mRNA cells were elevated in BAL and bronchial biopsies from baseline asthma as compared with controls (Hamid *et al.*, 1991). After allergen challenge there was an increase in mRNA+ cells for IL-5 (and GM-CSF) in bronchial biopsies from atopic asthmatics (Bentley *et al.*, 1993). Also, following segmental lavage, IL-5 protein product was observed, together with eosinophils, after antigen challenge (Ohnishi *et al.*, 1993). Of particular interest is the relationship between symptomatology and IL-5 mRNA expression. By the use of *in situ* hybridization, Robinson *et al.* (1993c) found that there were elevated numbers of mRNA cells for IL-3, IL-4, IL-5 and GM-CSF when symptomatic asthmatics were compared with asymptomatic subjects (Fig. 21.7). Furthermore, there was a significant correlation between IL-5 mRNA+ cells and both the degree of airflow obstruction and bronchial hyperresponsiveness (Fig. 21.6). There was also a strong correlation between IL-4 and IL-5 mRNA+ cells suggesting, but not proving, that these cytokines were co-expressed by the same Th2-type T cells. Using a semiquantitative reverse transcriptase-polymerase chain reaction (RT-PCR) method, Corrigan *et al.* (1996) confirmed that IL-5 mRNA correlated with disease severity, whereas IL-4 mRNA

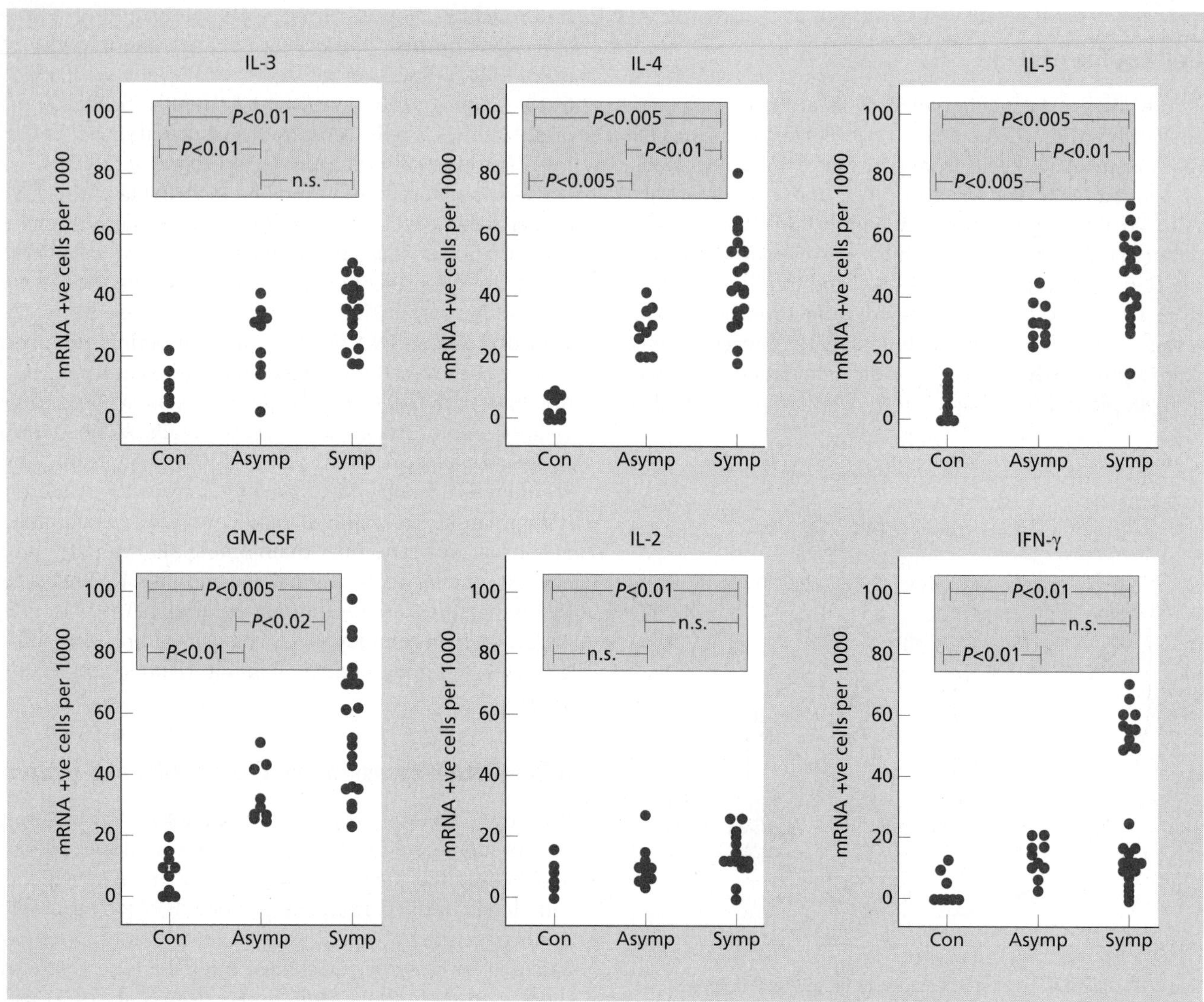

Fig. 21.6 Numbers of BAL cells per 1000 giving positive *in situ* hybridization signals for mRNA for Th1- and Th2-type cytokines from normal controls (c), asthmatics without symptoms (AS, $n = 10$) and from subjects with symptomatic asthma (S, $n = 19$). Median bars are indicated. n.s., Not significant. (Adapted from Robinson *et al.*, 1993b,c.)

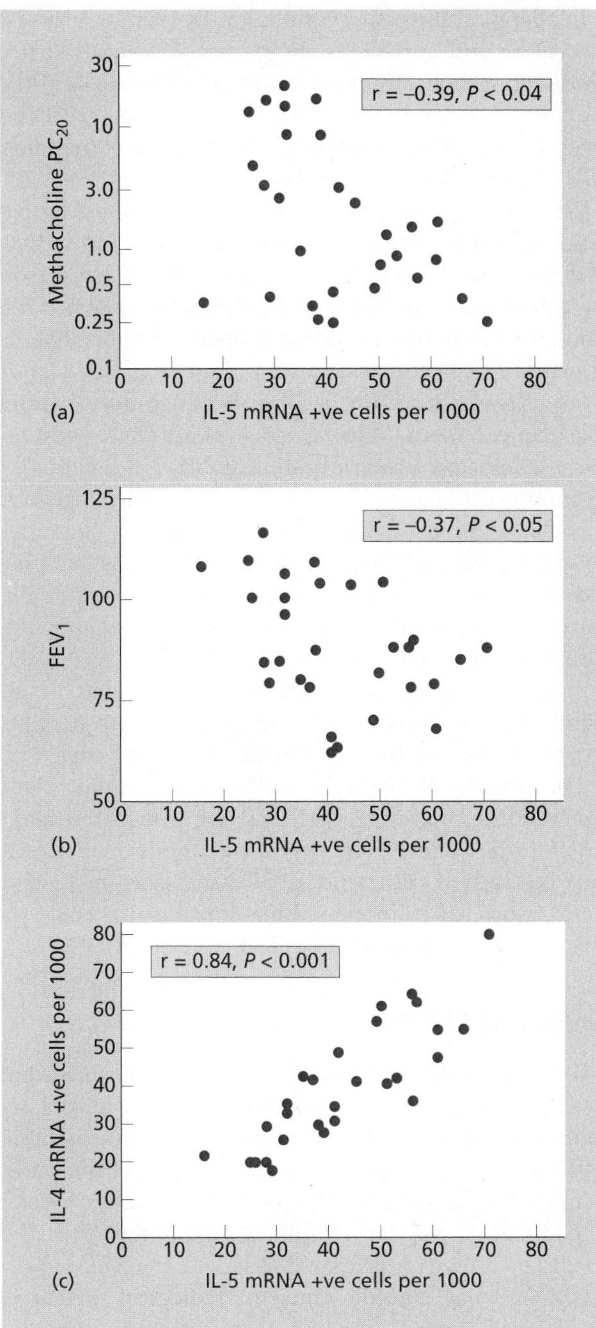

Fig. 21.7 Associations between numbers of BAL cells expressing cytokine mRNA and clinical measures of asthma. (a) Relationship between cells positive for IL-5 mRNA and airway methacholine responsiveness (log PC_{20}). (b) Relationship between cells positive for IL-5 mRNA and FEV_1. (c) Relationship between numbers of cells expressing mRNA for IL-5 and numbers expressing mRNA for IL-4. (From Robinson *et al.*, 1993b,c.)

expression correlated with serum IgE concentrations. This indicates that IL-4 is necessary, but not sufficient, for the effector limb of the asthma process, and that IL-5 and eosinophil mobilizing events are required for full expression of the disease. As discussed elsewhere, these workers also observed that IL-5 and IL-4 were equally elevated at the mRNA and protein product levels in both atopic and non-atopic (intrinsic) asthmatics (Alexander *et al.*, 1994; Humbert *et al.*, 1996a).

Support for IL-5-dependent mechanisms in asthma also comes from studies using anti-asthma drugs. The effect of prednisolone on IL-5 gene expression in symptomatic chronic asthmatics was evaluated in BAL and endobronchial biopsy specimens, taken before and after 2 weeks of therapy in a double-blind placebo-controlled parallel group study (Robinson *et al.*, 1993b; Bentley *et al.*, 1996). Patients receiving prednisolone improved, as shown by decreases in airflow obstruction and bronchial responsiveness to inhaled methacholine. This was not observed in patients receiving placebo (Fig. 21.8). Between-group comparison showed a significant fall in the numbers of BAL cells per 1000, with positive *in situ* hybridization signals for mRNA for IL-5 with prednisolone treatment. There was also a reduction in BAL eosinophils in prednisolone-treated patients when compared with those receiving placebo. Concentrations of IL-5 protein product in serum have been analysed by an enzyme-linked immuno-sorbent assay (ELISA) method and have also been shown to decrease after treatment with prednisolone (Corrigan *et al.*, 1993). Similar observations have been made in childhood asthma (Gemou-Engesaeth *et al.*, 1996).

In vitro IL-5 production by CD4+ cells is also inhibited by the immunosuppressants cyclosporin A and FK-506 (Mori *et al.*, 1995). Meng *et al.* (1996) observed that cyclosporin A, together with dexamethasone and rapamycin, inhibited IL-5-induced eosinophil survival and degranulation. Such observations have led to the development of treatment strategies for chronic corticosteroid-dependent asthmatics using immunosuppressants such as cyclosporin A. Thus, cyclosporin A was shown to improve lung function and decrease exacerbations in chronic asthmatics (Alexander *et al.*, 1992) and to reduce oral prednisolone requirements by >60% over a 9-month period (Lock *et al.*, 1996).

The mechanism of corticosteroid-resistant asthma is unknown but it is of considerable interest that, unlike steroid-sensitive asthmatics, resistant patients did not have a decrease in IL-5 mRNA+ cells in BAL after 7 days of oral prednisolone (Leung *et al.*, 1995). This suggests that steroid resistance in these subjects may be associated with dysregulation of cytokine expression.

It was recently suggested that the whole mucosal immune system is involved in asthma and atopy, since IL-3, IL-5 and GM-CFS immunoreactive mast cells and eosinophils were detected in duodenal biopsies of volunteers who did not have gastrointestinal symptoms (Wallaert *et al.*, 1995).

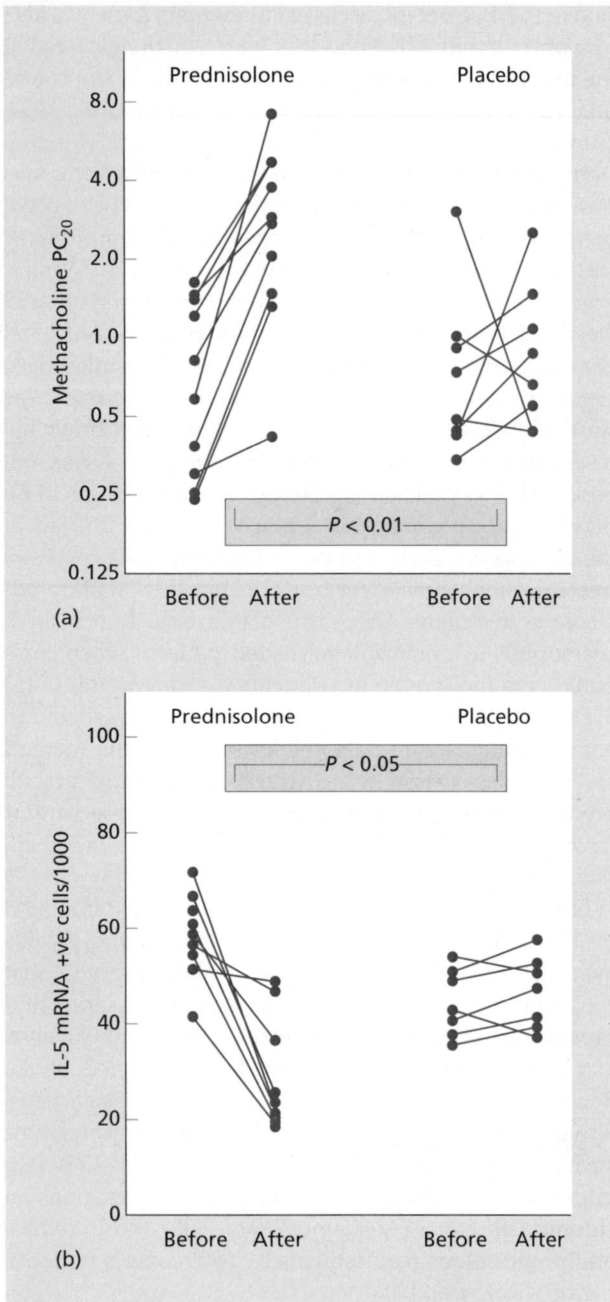

Fig. 21.8 Effect of prednisolone treatment on bronchial hyperreactivity and IL-5 gene expression in asthma. (a) Methacholine airway reactivity before and after 2 weeks of treatment of symptomatic asthmatic subjects with either prednisolone (0.6 mg/kg per day) or placebo in a double-blind study (PC_{20}, concentration of methacholine producing a 20% fall in FEV_1 from baseline value). (b) Numbers of BAL cells per 1000 total on cytocentrifuge preparations giving positive signals for IL-5 mRNA by *in-situ* hybridization after either prednisolone or placebo treatment. Comparison of treatments is by Mann–Whitney U test on the differences before and after prednisolone or placebo treatment. (From Robinson *et al.*, 1993b.)

In allergic rhinitis successful immunotherapy was also associated with a decrease in grass pollen-induced IL-5 production by peripheral blood mononuclear cells (Till *et al.*, 1996). Similar results have been obtained with IL-4 (Secrist *et al.*, 1993), suggesting that this form of treatment down-regulates Th2-type cells.

When recombinant human IL-5 (rhIL-5) was administered repeatedly onto the nasal mucosa of individuals with Japanese cedar pollinosis outside the pollen season, the numbers of eosinophils and epithelial cells and the amount of eosinophil cationic protein, secretory IgA (S-IgA) and IgA in the nasal lavage fluid increased significantly (Terada *et al.*, 1992). Responsiveness to histamine was also enhanced. When S-IgA was administered onto the nasal mucosa after application of rhIL-5, the amount of eosinophil cationic protein (ECP) in the nasal lavage fluid was also significantly increased. The authors suggested that IL-5 enhanced the release of ECP from eosinophils activated by S-IgA and/or IgA, and that epithelial damage to the nasal mucosa preceded the development of nasal hyperreactivity to histamine.

Increased expression of mRNA IL-5R (soluble (s) and membrane (m) anchored) has recently been observed in bronchial biopsies from asthmatics (Ploysongsang *et al.*, 1995). Virtually all the IL-5R mRNA was associated with eosinophils, suggesting that this cell type is the major target for IL-5 effects. Of interest was an inverse relationship between IL-5Rm and IL-5Rs. Increases in IL-5Rm were associated with poor lung function, whereas the reverse was observed with IL-5Rs (Yasruel *et al.*, 1967).

Biology of GM-CSF

GM-CSF is produced by a wide variety of cells, including T cells, monocytes, macrophages, eosinophils, fibroblasts, epithelial and endothelial cells (reviewed by Cousins *et al.*, 1994), and is a glycoprotein with an apparent molecular weight of 23–28 kDa. In transgenic mice, overexpression of GM-CSF is associated with accumulation of macrophages in the eyes and striated muscle (Lang *et al.*, 1987).

GM-CSF has a wide range of biological effects on several cell types, including monocytes/macrophages, neutrophils and eosinophils. (Moqbel *et al.*, 1991; Levi-Shaffer, 1995). The properties include maturation and differentiation of precursor myoloid cells, as well as hyperadherence, and increased responses to chemotaxis, oxidative metabolism and lipid and granule mediator release. IL-3 has very similar properties but its principal source is mainly T cells, mast cells and eosinophils, and it acts predominantly on the monocyte/macrophage and eosinophil (reviewed by Robinson *et al.*, 1993a).

Role of GM-CSF and IL-3 in allergy and asthma

In asthma the production of GM-CSF by macrophages and epithelial cells is generally up-regulated; effects that can be inhibited by corticosteroids (Robinson *et al.*, 1992b; Lane *et al.*, 1993; Nakamura *et al.*, 1993; Sousa *et al.*, 1993; Hallsworth *et al.*, 1994; Woolley *et al.*, 1994). The eosinophil is also an important source of GM-CSF in the inflammatory response characteristic of asthma (Broide *et al.*, 1992). Wang *et al.* (1994) observed enhanced epithelial immunostaining in mild asthmatics for GM-CSF and IL-8. This was suppressed by treatment with inhaled corticosteroids. Interestingly, GM-CSF expression correlated with airway hyperresponsiveness as measured by the histamine PC_{20}. The recent description of GM-CSF mutants with poor receptor binding may have therapeutic promise (Hercus *et al.*, 1994).

Cells mRNA+ for IL-3 are also generally unregulated in asthma and models of atopic inflammation (Kay *et al.*, 1991; Robinson *et al.*, 1992). In 'baseline' asthma, expression of IL-3, unlike IL-5 and GM-CSF, does not correlate with clinical features (Robinson *et al.*, 1993c). Also, after inhalational allergen challenge the numbers of mRNA+ cells for IL-5, but not IL-3, increase in bronchoalveolar fluid (Bentley *et al.*, 1993).

IL-5 and GM-CSF in 'intrinsic asthma'

Intrinsic asthma is sometimes considered as a distinct clinicopathological entity, since these patients are skin test negative to common aeroallergens and their disease does not appear to be exacerbated by exposure to agents such as pollens, mites and animal danders (unlike the majority of asthmatics who tend to be atopic). Furthermore, their serum IgE concentrations are within the normal range. Humbert *et al.* (1996a,b) have recently shown that the expression of mRNA and protein product for IL-4 and IL-5, as well as the numbers of FcεRI-bearing mast cells, macrophages and eosinophils, were similar in bronchial biopsies taken from atopic (extrinsic) and non-atopic (intrinsic) asthmatics. Since a marked eosinophilia was a feature of both variants of the disease, these data suggest that a Th2 response with local IgE production, possibly directed against viral or even autoantigens, may be operative in both intrinsic and atopic (extrinsic) asthmatics.

One unexpected, and as yet unexplained, feature of intrinsic asthma is an increase (compared with atopic asthma) in the number of bronchial mucosal cells expressing mRNA for the α-GM-CSF receptor (Kotsimbos *et al.*, 1996). Furthermore, the cells expressing α-GM-CSF were largely CD68+ (i.e. macrophages). The possibility exists that, in intrinsic asthma, the putative distinct antigen(s) operative leads to the release of interferon-γ (IFN-γ) with subsequent activation of macrophages (Walker *et al.*, 1991, 1992).

Summary

There is compelling evidence that the IL-5, IL-3 and GM-CSF eosinophil-associated group of cytokines plays a critical role in the pathogenesis of allergic inflammation and asthma. Their major effects relate to eosinophil differentiation, recruitment, activation and prolonged survival. IL-5 is of particular interest, since expression of this cytokine correlates with many features of the asthma process and inhibition of IL-5 production in a primate model of asthma reduces allergen-provoked airway hyperresponsiveness and eosinophilia. Studies with anti-IL-5 and IL-5 antagonists hold promise for the development of future therapies.

References

Alam, R., Forsythe, P., Stafford, S. & Fukuda, Y. (1994) Transforming growth factor β abrogates the effects of haematopoietins on eosinophils and induces their apoptosis. *J. Exp. Med.*, **179**, 1041–5.

Alexander, A.G., Barkans, J., Moqbel, R., Barnes, N.C., Kay, A.B. & Corrigan, C.J. (1994) Serum interleukin-5 concentrations in atopic and non-atopic patients with glucocorticoid-dependent chronic severe asthma. *Thorax*, **49**, 1231–4.

Alexander, A.G., Barnes, N.C. & Kay, A.B. (1992) Trial of cyclosporin A in corticosteroid-dependent chronic severe asthma. *Lancet*, **339**, 324–8.

Bentley, A.M., Hamid, Q., Robinson, D.S. *et al.* (1996) Prednisolone treatment in asthma: reduction in the numbers of eosinophils, T cells, tryptase-only positive mast cells (MC_T) and modulation of interleukin-4, interleukin-5 and interferon-gamma cytokine gene expression within the bronchial mucosa. *Am. J. Resp. Crit. Care Med.*, **153**, 551–6.

Bentley, A.M., Qiu Meng, Robinson, D.S., Hamid, Q., Kay, A.B. & Durham, S.R. (1993) Increases in activated T lymphocytes, eosinophils and cytokine messenger RNA for IL-5 and GM-CSF in bronchial biopsies after allergen inhalation challenge in atopic asthmatics. *Am. J. Respir. Cell Mol. Biol.*, **8**, 35–42.

Bischoff, S.C., Brunner, T., De Weck, A.L. & Dahinden, C.A. (1990) Interleukin-5 modifies histamine release and leukotriene generation by human basophils in response to diverse agonists. *J. Exp. Med.*, **172**, 1577–82.

Bochner, B.S., McKelvy, A.A., Sterbinsky, S.A. *et al.* (1990) IL-3 augments adhesiveness for endothelium and CD11b expression in human basophils but not neutrophils. *J. Immunol.*, **145**, 1832–7.

Broide, D.H., Paine, M.M. & Firestein, G.S. (1992) Eosinophils express interleukin 5 and granulocyte macrophage-colony stimulating factor mRNA at sites of allergic inflammation in asthmatics. *J. Clin. Invest.*, **90**, 1414–24.

Chihara, J., Plumas, J., Gruart, V. *et al.* (1990) Characterization of a receptor for interleukin 5 on human eosinophils: variable expression and induction by granulocyte-macrophage colony-stimulating factor. *J. Exp. Med.*, **172**, 1347–51.

Collins, P.D., Marleau, S., Griffith-Johnson, D.A., Jose, P.J. & Williams, T.J. (1995) Cooperation between interleukin-5 and the chemokine eotaxin to induce eosinophil accumulation *in vivo*. *J. Exp. Med.*, **182**, 1169–74.

Corrigan, C.J., Haczku, A., Gemou-Engesaeth, V. *et al.* (1993) CD4 T-lymphocyte activation in asthma is accompanied by increased serum concentrations of interleukin-5: effect of glucocorticoid therapy. *Am. Rev. Resp. Dis.*, **147**, 540–7.

Corrigan, C.J., Hamid, Q., North, J. *et al.* (1995) Peripheral blood CD4, but not CD8 T lymphocytes in patients with exacerbation of asthma transcribe and translate messenger RNA encoding cytokines which prolong eosinophil survival in the context of a Th2-type pattern: effect of glucocorticoid therapy. *Am. J. Respir. Cell Mol. Biol.*, **12**, 567–78.

Corrigan, C.J., Humbert, M., Durham, S.R. *et al.* (1996) Relationship of bronchial mucosal IL-5 mRNA expression with disease severity and IL-4 mRNA expression with serum IgE concentrations in atopic and non-atopic asthmatics. *J. Allergy Clin. Immunol.*, **97** [abstract].

Cousins, D.J., Staynov, D.Z. & Lee, T.H. (1994) Regulation of interleukin-5 and granulocyte-macrophage colony-stimulating factor expression. *Am. J. Resp. Crit. Care Med.*, **150**, S50–3.

Coyle, A.J., Erard, F., Bertrand, C., Walti, S., Pircher, H. & Le Gros, G. (1995) Virus-specific CD8+ cells can switch to interleukin 5 production and induce airway eosinophilia. *J. Exp. Med.*, **181**, 1229–33.

Dent, L.A., Strath, M., Mellor, A.L. & Sanderson, C.J. (1990) Eosinophilia in transgenic mice expressing interleukin 5. *J. Exp. Med.*, **172**, 1425–31.

Desreumaux, P., Janin, A. & Colomble, J.F. (1992) Interleukin 5 messenger RNA expression by eosinophils in the intestinal mucosa of patients with coeliac disease. *J. Exp. Med.*, **175**, 293–6.

DiPersio, J., Billing, P., Kaufman, S., Eghtesady, P., Williams, R.E. & Gasson, J.C. (1988) Characterization of human granulocyte-macrophage colony-stimulating factor receptor. *J. Biol. Chem.*, **263**, 1834–41.

Dubucquoi, S., Desreumaux, P., Janin, A. *et al.* (1994) Interleukin 5 synthesis by eosinophils: association with granules and immunoglobulin-dependent secretion. *J. Exp. Med.*, **179**, 703–8.

Durham, S.R., Ying, S., Varney, V.A. *et al.* (1992) Cytokine messenger RNA expression for IL-3, IL-4, IL-5 and GM-CSF in the nasal mucosa after local allergen provocation: relationship to tissue eosinophilia. *J. Immunol.*, **148**, 2390–4.

Ebisawa, M., Liu, M.C., Yamada, T. *et al.* (1994) Eosinophil transendothelial migration induced by cytokines. II. Potentiation of eosinophil transendothelial migration by eosinophil-active cytokines. *J. Immunol.*, **152**, 4590–7.

Ema, H., Suda, T., Nagayoshi, K., Miura, Y., Civin, C.I. & Nakauchi, H. (1990) Target cells for granulocyte colony-stimulating factor, interleukin-3, and interleukin-5 in differentiation pathways of neutrophils and eosinophils. *Blood*, **76**, 1956–61.

Fujisawa, T., Abu-Ghazaleh, R., Kita, H., Sanderson, C.J. & Gleich, C.J. (1990) Regulatory effect of cytokines on eosinophil degranulation. *J. Immunol.*, **144**, 642–6.

Gemou-Engesaeth, V., Bush, A., Kay, A.B., Hamid, Q. & Corrigan, C.J. (1996) Inhaled glucocorticoid therapy of childhood asthma is associated with reduced peripheral blood T cell activation and 'Th2-type' cytokine mRNA expression. (Submitted.)

Hallsworth, M.P., Soh, C.P., Lane, S.J., Arm, J.P. & Lee, T.H. (1994) Selective enhancement of GM-CSF, TNF-alpha, IL-1 beta and IL-8 production by monocytes and macrophages of asthmatic subjects. *Eur. Resp. J.*, **7**, 1096–102.

Hamid, Q., Azzawi, M., Ying, S. *et al.* (1991) Expression of mRNA for interleukin-5 in mucosal bronchial biopsies from asthma. *J. Clin. Invest.*, **87**, 1541–6.

Her, E., Frazer, J., Austen, K.F. & Owen, W.F. (1991) Eosinophil hematopoietins antagonize the programmed cell death of human eosinophils: cytokine and glucocorticoid effects on eosinophils maintained by endothelial cell conditioned medium. *J. Clin. Invest.*, **88**, 1982–7.

Hercus, T.R., Bagley, C.J., Cambareri, B. *et al.* (1994) Specific human granulocyte-macrophage colony-stimulating factor antagonists. *Proc. Nat. Acad. Sci. USA*, **91**, 5838–42.

Hirai, K., Yamaguchi, M. & Misaki, Y. (1990) Enhancement of human basophil histamine release by interleukin-5. *J. Exp. Med.*, **172**, 1525–8.

Humbert, M., Durham, S.R., Ying, S. *et al.* (1996a) IL-4 and IL-5 mRNA and protein in bronchial biopsies from atopic and non-atopic asthmatics: evidence against 'intrinsic' asthma being a distinct immunopathological entity. *Am. J. Resp. Crit. Care Med.* (in press).

Humbert, M., Grant, J.A., Taborda-Barata, L. *et al.* (1996b) High affinity IgE receptor (FcεRI) bearing cells in bronchial biopsies from atopic and non-atopic asthma. *Am. J. Resp. Crit. Care Med.*, **153**, 1931–7.

Ingley, E. & Young, I.G. (1991) Characterization of a receptor for interleukin-5 on human eosinophils and the myeloid leukemia line HL-60. *Blood*, **78**, 339–44.

Iwama, T., Nagai, H., Suda, H., Tsuruoka, N. & Koda, A. (1992) Effect of murine recombinant interleukin 5 on the cell population in guinea pig airways. *Brit. J. Pharmacol.*, **1055**, 19.

Kay, A.B., Ying, S., Varney, V. *et al.* (1991) Messenger RNA expression of the cytokine gene cluster, IL-3, IL-4, IL-5 and GM-CSF in allergen-induced late-phase cutaneous reactions in atopic subjects. *J. Exp. Med.*, **173**, 775–8.

Kay, A.B., Meng, Q., Taborda-Barata, L. & Ying, S. (1996) Apoptosis of neutrophils (Neu) and eosinophils (Eos) and their ingestion by macrophages is associated with the resolution of allergen-induced cutaneous late phase response (LPR). *J. Allergy Clin. Immunol.*, **97** [abstract].

Kita, H. Weiler, D.A., Abu-Ghazaleh, R., Sanderson, C.J. & Gleich, G.J. (1992) Release of granule proteins from eosinophils cultured with IL-5. *J. Immunol.*, **149**, 629–35.

Kotsimbos, A.T.C., Humbert, M., Minshall, E. *et al.* (1997) Upregulation of αGM-CSF-receptor in non-atopic but not in atopic asthma. (Submitted).

Lane, S.J., Wilkinson, J.R., Cochrane, G.M., Lee, T.H. & Arm, J.P. (1993) Differential *in vitro* regulation by glucocorticoids of monocyte-derived cytokine generation in glucocorticoid-resistant bronchial asthma. *Am. Rev. Resp. Dis.*, **147**, 690–6.

Lang, R.A., Metcalf, D., Cuthbertson, R.A. *et al.* (1987) Transgenic mice expressing a haemopoietic growth factor gene (GM-CSF) develop accumulations of macrophages, blindness, and a fatal syndrome of tissue damage. *Cell*, **51**, 675–86.

Leung, D.Y.M., Martin, R.J., Szeflre, S.J. *et al.* (1995) Dysregulation of interleukin-4, interleukin-5 and interferon-gamma gene expression in steroid-resistant asthma. *J. Exp. Med.*, **181**, 33–40.

Levi-Schaffer, F., Lacey, P., Severs, N.J. *et al.* (1995) Association of granulocyte-macrophage colony-stimulating factor with the crystalloid granules of human eosinophils. *Blood*, **85**, 2579–86.

Lock, S.H., Kay, A.B. & Barnes, N.C. (1996) Double-blind, placebo-controlled study of cyclosporin A as a corticosteroid-sparing agent in corticosteroid-dependent asthma. *Am. J. Resp. Crit. Care Med.*, **153**, 509–14.

Lopez, A.F., Vadas, M.A., Woodcock, J. *et al.* (1991) Selective interaction of the human eosinophil interleukin-5 receptor with interleukin-3 and granulocyte-macrophage colony-stimulating factor. *J. Biol. Chem.*, **266**, 24741–7.

Lopez, A.F., Eglinton, J.M., Gillis, D., Park, L.S., Clark, S. & Vadas, M.A. (1989) Reciprocal inhibition of binding between interleukin 3 and granulocyte-macrophage colony-stimulating factor to human eosinophils. *Proc. Nat. Acad. Sci. USA*, **86**, 7022–6.

Lopez, A.F., Elliott, M.J., Woodcock, J. & Vadas, M.A. (1992) GM-CSF, IL-3 and IL-5: cross-competition on human haemopoietic cells. *Immunol. Today*, **13**, 495–500.

Lopez, A.F., Sanderson, C.J., Gamble, J.R., Campbell, H.D., Young, I.G. & Vadas, M.A. (1988) Recombinant interleukin 5 is a selective activator of human eosinophil function. *J. Exp. Med.*, **167**, 219–24.

Mauser, P.J., Pitman, A.M., Fernandez, X. *et al.* (1995) Effects of an antibody to interleukin-5 in a monkey model of asthma. *Am. J. Resp. Crit. Care Med.*, **152**, 467–72.

Mauser, P.J., Pitman, A., Witt, A. *et al.* (1993) Inhibitory effect of the TRFK-5 anti IL-5 antibody in a guinea pig model of asthma. *Am. Rev. Resp. Dis.*, **148**, 1623–27.

Meng, Q., Ying, S., Assoufi, B., Moqbel, R. & Kay, A.B. (1996) Effects of dexamethasone, cyclosporine A and rapamycin on eosinophil degranulation and survival. *J. Allergy Clin. Immunol.*, **97**, 277, [abstract].

Migita, M., Yamaguchi, N., Mita, S. *et al.* (1991) Characterization of the human IL-5 receptors on eosinophils. *Cell Immunol.*, **133**, 484–97.

Milburn, M.V., Hassell, A.M., Lambert, M.H. *et al.* (1993) A novel dimer configuration revealed by the crystal structure of 2.4 A resolution of human interleukin-5. *Nature*, **363**, 172–6.

Moqbel, R., Hamid, Q., Ying, S. *et al.* (1991) Expression of mRNA and immunoreactivity for the granulocyte-macrophage colony-stimulating factor in activated human eosinophils. *J. Exp. Med.*, **174**, 749–52.

Mori, A., Suko, M., Nishizaki, Y. *et al.* (1995) IL-5 production by CD4+ T cells of asthmatic patients is suppressed by glucocorticoids and the immunosuppressants FK506 and cyclosporin A. *Int. Immunol.*, **7**, 449–57.

Nakamura, Y., Ozaki, T., Kamei, T. *et al.* (1993) Increased granulocyte-macrophage colony-stimulating factor production by mononuclear cells from peripheral blood of patients with bronchial asthma. *Am. Rev. Resp. Dis.*, **147**, 87–91.

Ohnishi, T., Kita, H., Weiler, D. *et al.* (1993) IL-5 is the predominant eosinophil-active cytokine in the antigen-induced pulmonary late-phase reaction. *Am. Rev. Resp. Dis.*, **147**, 901–7.

Owen, W.F., Rothenberg, M.E., Silberstein, D.S. *et al.* (1987) Regulation of human eosinophil viability, density and function by granulocyte/macrophage colony-stimulating factor in the presence of 3T3 fibroblasts. *J. Exp. Med.*, **166**, 129–41.

Owen, W.F.J., Petersen, J., Sheff, D.M. *et al.* (1990) Hypodense eosinophils and interleukin 5 activity in the blood of patients with the eosinophilia-myalgia syndrome. *Proc. Nat. Acad. Sci. USA*, **87**, 8647–51.

Parronchi, P., Macchia, D., Piccinni, M.P. *et al.* (1991) Allergen- and bacterial antigen-specific T lymphocyte clones established from atopic donors show a different profile of cytokine production. *Proc. Nat. Acad. Sci. USA*, **88**, 4538–42.

Ploysongsang, Y., Humberet, M., Ying, S. *et al.* (1995) Increased expression of interleukin-5 receptor gene in asthma. *J. Allergy Clin. Immunol.*, **95**, 279 [abstract 555].

Robinson, D.S., Durham, S.R. & Kay, A.B. (1993a) Cytokines in asthma. *Thorax*, **48**, 845–53.

Robinson, D.S., Hamid, Q., Ying, S. *et al.* (1993b) Prednisolone treatment in asthma is associated with modulation of bronchoalveolar lavage cell interleukin-4, interleukin-5 and interferon-gamma cytokine gene expression. *Am. Rev. Resp. Dis.*, **148**, 401–6.

Robinson, D.S., Ying, S., Bentley, A.M. *et al.* (1993c) Relationship among numbers of bronchoalveolar lavage cells expressing messenger ribonucleic acid for cytokines, asthma symptoms, and airway methacholine responsiveness in atopic asthma. *J. Allergy Clin. Immunol.*, **92**, 397–403.

Robinson, D.S., Hamid, Q., Ying, S. *et al.* (1992) Predominant T_{H2}-type bronchoalveolar lavage T-lymphocyte population in atopic asthma. *New Engl. J. Med.*, **326**, 298–304.

Rothenburg, M.E., Owen, W.F., Silberstein, D.S. *et al.* (1988) Human eosinophils have prolonged survival, enhanced functional properties and become hypodense when exposed to human interleukin-3. *J. Clin. Invest.*, **81**, 1986–92.

Rothenburg, M.E., Petersen, J., Stevens, R.L. *et al.* (1989) IL-5-dependent conversion of normodense human eosinophils to the hypodense phenotype uses 3T3 fibroblasts for enhanced viability, accelerated hypodensity and sustained antibody-dependent cytotoxicity. *J. Immunol.*, **143**, 2311–16.

Secrist, H., Chelen, C.J., Wen, Y., Marshall, J.D. & Umetsu, D.T. (1993) Allergen immunotherapy decreases interleukin-4 production in CD4+ T-cells from allergic individuals. *J. Exp. Med.*, **178**, 2123–30.

Sehmi, R., Wardlaw, A.J., Cromwell, O., Kurihara, K., Waltmann, P. & Kay, A.B. (1992) Interleukin-5 (IL-5) selectively enhances the chemotactic response of eosinophils obtained from normal but not eosinophilic subjects. *Blood*, **79**, 2952–9.

Shute, J. (1992) Basophil migration and chemotaxis. *Clin. Exp. Allergy*, **22**, 321–3.

Sousa, A.R., Poston, R.N., Lane, S.J., Nakhosteen, J.A. & Lee, T.H. (1993) Detection of GM-CSF in asthmatic bronchial epithelium and decrease by inhaled corticosteroids. *Am. Rev. Resp. Dis.*, **147**, 1557–61.

Stern, M., Meagher, L., Savill, J. & Haslett, C. (1992) Apoptosis in human eosinophils: programmed cell death in the eosinophil leads to phagocytosis by macrophages and is modulated by IL-5. *J. Immunol.*, **148**, 3543.

Takatsu, K. (1995) *Interleukin-5 and its Receptor System: From Genes to Disease*. R.G. Landes, Austin, Texas.

Tavernier, J., Tuypens, T., Plaetinck, G., Verhee, A., Fiers, W. & Devos, R. (1992) Molecular basis of the membrane-anchored and two soluble isoforms of the human interleukin 5 receptor alpha subunit. *Proc. Nat. Acad. Sci. USA*, **89**, 7041–5.

Terada, N., Konno, A., Tada, H., Shirotori, K., Ishikawa, K. & Togawa, K. (1992) The effect of recombinant human interleukin-5 on eosinophil accumulation and degranulation in human nasal mucosa. *J. Allergy Clin. Immunol.*, **90**, 160–8.

Till, S.J., Li, B., Durham, S. *et al.* (1995) Secretion of the eosinophil-active cytokines interleukin-5, granulocyte/macrophage colony-stimulating factor and interleukin-3 by bronchoalveolar lavage CD4+ and CD8+ T cell lines in atopic asthmatics, and atopic and non-atopic controls. *Eur. J. Immunol.*, **25**, 2727–31.

Till, S.J., Corrigan, C., Huston, D. *et al.* (1996) Grass pollen induced IL-5 production by peripheral blood mononuclear cells (PBMC) is increased in allergic rhinitis and inhibited by immunotherapy (IT). *J. Allergy Clin. Immunol.*, **97** [abstract] (in press).

Tsicopoulos, A., Hamid, O., Varney, V. *et al.* (1992) Preferential mRNA expression of Th1-type cells (IFNγ+, IL-2+), in classical delayed-type (tuberculin) hypersensitivity reactions in human skin. *J. Immunol.*, **148**, 2058–61.

Van Oosterhout, A.J., Ladenius, R.S., Savelkoul, H.F., Van Ark, I.,

Delsman, K.C. & Nijkamp, F.P. (1993) Effect of anti-IL-5 and IL-5 on airway hyperreactivity and eosinophils in guinea pigs. *Am. Rev. Resp. Dis.*, **147**, 548.

Walker, C., Bode, E., Boer, L., Hansel, T.T., Blaser, K. & Virchow, J.-C. (1992) Allergic and non-allergic asthmatics have distinct patterns of T-cell activation and cytokine production in peripheral blood and bronchoalveolar lavage. *Am. Rev. Resp. Dis.*, **146**, 109–15.

Walker, C., Virchow, J.C., Bruijnzeel, P.L.B. & Blaser, K. (1991) T cell subsets and their soluble products regulate eosinophilia in allergic and non allergic asthma. *J. Immunol.*, **146**, 1829–35.

Wallaert, B., Desreumaux, P., Copin, M.C. *et al.* (1995) Immunoreactivity for interleukin-3 and 5 and granulocyte/macrophage colony-stimulating factor of intestinal mucosa in bronchial asthma. *J. Exp. Med.*, **182**, 1897–904.

Walsh, G.M., Hartnell, A., Moqbel, R. *et al.* (1990a) Receptor expression and functional status of cultured human eosinophils derived from umbilical cord blood mononuclear cells. *Blood*, **76**, 105–11.

Walsh, G.M., Hartnell, A., Wardlaw, A.J., Kurihara, K., Sanderson, C.J. & Kay, A.B. (1990b) IL-5 enhances the *in vitro* adhesion of human eosinophils, but not neutrophils in a leucocyte integrin (CD11/18)-dependent manner. *Immunology*, **71**, 258–65.

Wang, J.H., Trigg, C.J., Devalia, J.L., Jordan, S. & Davies, R.J. (1994) Effect of inhaled beclomethasone dipropionate on expression of proinflammatory cytokines and activated eosinophils in the bronchial epithelium of patients with mild asthma. *J. Allergy Clin. Immunol.*, **94**, 1025–34.

Wang, J.M., Rambaldi, A., Biondi, A., Chen, Z.G., Sanderson, C.J. & Mantovani, A. (1989) Recombinant human interleukin-5 is a selective eosinophil chemoattractant. *Eur. J. Immunol.*, **19**, 701–5.

Wardlaw, A.J., Moqbel, R., Kay, A.B. (1995) Eosinophils: biology and role in disease. *Adv. Immunol.*, **60**, 151–266.

Warringa, R.A.J., Koenderman, L., Kok, P.T.M., Krekniet, J. & Bruijnzeel, P.L.B. (1991) Modulation and induction of eosinophil chemotaxis by granulocyte-macrophage colony stimulating factor and interleukin-3. *Blood*, **77**, 2694–700.

Woolley, K.L., Adelroth, E., Woolley, M.J., Ellis, R., Jordana, M. & O'Byrne, P.M. (1994) Granulocyte-macrophage colony-stimulating factor, eosinophils and eosinophil cationic protein in subjects with and without mild, stable, atopic asthma. *Eur. Resp. J.*, **7**, 1576–84.

Yamaguchi, M., Hirai, K., Shoji, S. *et al.* (1992) Haemopoietic growth factors induce human basophil migration *in vitro*. *Clin. Exp. Allergy*, **22**, 379–83.

Yamaoka, K.A. & Kolb, J.P. (1993) Leukotriene B_4 induces interleukin-5 generation from human T lymphocytes. *Eur. J. Immunol.*, **23**, 2392–8.

Yasruel, Z., Humbert, M., Kotsimbos, A.T.C. *et al.* (1997) Expression of membrane-bound and soluble interleukin-5 α receptor mRNA in the bronchial mucosa of atopic and non-atopic asthmatics. *Am J. Resp. Crit. Care Med.* (in press).

Ying, S., Durham, S.R., Barkans, J. *et al.* (1993) T cells are the principal source of interleukin-5 mRNA in allergen-induced rhinitis. *Am. J. Respir. Cell Mol. Biol.*, **9**, 356–60.

Ying, S., Durham, S.R., Corrigan, C.J., Hamid, Q. & Kay, A.B. (1995) Phenotype of cells expressing mNA for TH2-type (interleukin-4 and interleukin-5) and TH1-type (interleukin-2 and interferon-gamma) cytokines in bronchoalveolar lavage and bronchial biopsies from atopic asthmatics and normal control subjects. *Am. J. Respir. Cell Mol. Biol.*, **12**, 477–87.

Zanders, E.D. (1994) Interleukin-5 receptor alpha chain mRNA is down-regulated by transforming growth factor beta 1. *Eur. Cytokine Netw.*, **5**, 35–42.

CHAPTER 22
Chemokines

C.A. Dahinden

Introduction

Effectors of allergic inflammation

Allergic diseases are inflammatory pathologies. This notion is now well accepted by researchers and physicians alike, and has led to the recommendation that anti-inflammatory therapy should constitute the first line of treatment in allergic disease. Under experimental-challenge conditions, the allergic reaction can be divided into an early phase induced by IgE-mediated mast cell activation leading to vasodilatation and oedema, and into a late phase characterized by a cellular infiltration composed of eosinophils, basophils and mononuclear cells, in particular T-helper cells secreting a 'Th2-type' of cytokine profile (Frigas & Gleich, 1986; Frew & Kay, 1988; Kay *et al.*, 1991; Kay, 1992; Gao *et al.*, 1994). The late phase is thought to be responsible for the clinically more relevant chronic inflammatory process and thus the major symptoms in allergic patients, since these effector leucocytes release inflammatory mediators such as leukotriene C_4 (LTC_4) and cytotoxic products, leading to tissue damage. Obviously, these leucocytes must be attracted and activated by host-derived factors, since the cellular infiltrate occurs late after antigen exposure. Furthermore, several eosinophilic inflammatory pathologies can occur even in the absence of specific IgE and allergen; for example, in 'intrinsic' asthma and certain types of intestinal inflammation. The major problem in our understanding of the pathogenesis of allergic diseases, and the future design of more specific anti-allergic drugs, is in defining the mechanisms leading to the relative selective attraction of eosinophils, basophils and lymphocyte subsets, and their subsequent activation at an inflammatory site.

Inflammation is the response of the macro-organism to injury by a variety of exogenous (microbial, chemical, physical) or endogenous (immunological, neurological) disturbances, and is characterized by infiltration of effector leucocytes into the affected tissue. The inflammatory response involves a complex interaction between different leucocyte types and endothelial as well as mesenchymal cells by means of cell adhesion molecules and a host of soluble humoral and cell-derived mediators, cytokines and growth factors. Most of these mechanisms are presumably in common to all types of inflammatory responses, and thus operate also in allergic diseases. Yet, depending on the stimulus, the histology of the inflamed tissue differs strongly. For example, acute tissue injury, common bacterial infections or antigen-antibody (Ag/ab)-complex deposition leads to a neutrophilic infiltrate, while mononuclear cells predominate in infections with intracellular pathogens or delayed-type hypersensitivity, in marked contrast to the eosinophilic inflammation characteristic of helminth infections or immediate-type hypersensitivity disease. Until recently, however, the mechanism for the selective recruitment of the distinct effector leucocytes into an inflammatory site has remained obscure, since most pro-inflammatory cytokines, mediators and chemoattractants are rather pleiotropic. The biological activities of chemokines, which constitute an increasingly large family of homologous cytokines with partially distinct, partially overlapping target cell selectivities, now offer a plausible explanation for the induction of these different pathologies, including allergic inflammation.

Modulation of effector cell functions

The biological activities of the chemokines cannot be discussed in isolation from other cytokine networks regulating inflammation and host defence, as summarized in Fig. 22.1. In order to emigrate from the bloodstream, leucocytes have first to engage with endothelial cells through the interaction of selectins with cell-surface glycoproteins, leading to rolling of cells on the blood vessel wall (Springer, 1994). Firm adhesion and transendothelial migration requires expression and activation of integrins and adhesion molecules (intercellular adhesion molecule (ICAM) and vascular cell adhesion molecule (VCAM)) on leucocytes and endothelial cells, respectively. Some selectivity may due to the expression of VCAM, whose ligand very late antigen-4 (VLA-4, CD29/49d) is expressed by eosinophils, basophils, monocytes and activated lymphocytes, but not neutrophils. Importantly, VCAM is induced selectively by interleukin-4 (IL-4) or IL-13 (Schleimer *et al.*, 1992), key cytokines in allergic disease, which are produced, for example, by activated Th2 cells and basophils (Dahinden *et al.*, 1992; Brunner *et al.*, 1993; Brunner & Dahinden, 1993; Gauchat *et al.*, 1993). Furthermore, in order to interact with high affinity with adhesion molecules, the leucocyte integrins have to be activated by cell agonists, in particular chemotactic factors including chemokines.

Certain chemokines may be expressed differentially by endothelial cells themselves upon activation, and are possibly presented in an anchoraged manner (see below) to responding leucocyte subsets (Rot, 1992; Gilat *et al.*, 1994; Marfaing-Koka *et al.*, 1995).

Another group of cytokines, belonging mainly to the haematopoietic growth factor (HGF) family, also strongly affects the response of effector leucocytes to different cell agonists, including chemokines. Most growth factors not only act on progenitors increasing the pool of the corresponding leucocyte types, but also enhance all functions (adherence, diapedesis, chemotaxis, exocytosis, mediator formation, cytotoxicity) of the mature effector cells. They also change their function in a qualitative manner, since leucocytes release lipid mediators (e.g. leukotrienes) in response to chemokines and all other endogenous agonists, such as C5a, only in the presence of an appropriate priming cytokine (Dahinden *et al.*, 1993; Dahinden, 1994). However, the target cell profiles of priming cytokines are partially distinct. Of particular relevance to allergic inflammation are IL-3 and IL-5, which act on eosinophils and basophils, but not neutrophils (Bischoff *et al.*, 1990a,b). Granulocyte macrophage colony-stimulating factor (GM-CSF), which is expressed in response to many pro-inflammatory stimuli, acts on all myeloid cell types (Dahinden *et al.*, 1988). By contrast, the neurotrophic cytokine nerve growth factor (NGF) acts on basophils only, indicating an interaction between the nervous system and inflammatory responses involving basophils (Bischoff & Dahinden, 1992b). Thus, the profile of priming cytokines, for example the presence of GM-CSF, IL-3 and IL-5 in allergic inflammation, may be another important mechanism regulating the distinct inflammatory pathologies of different aetiologies.

Structure and function of chemokines

Chemokine subfamilies

The chemokine family of cytokines represents a new class of structurally related, cell-derived, relatively cationic,

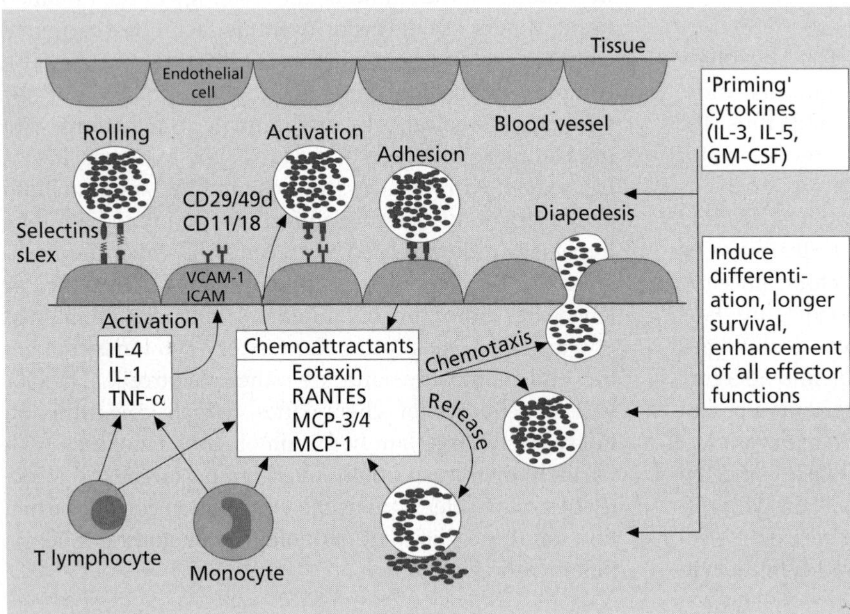

Fig. 22.1 Mechanism of attraction and activation of basophil and eosinophil leucocytes at allergic inflammatory sites.

peptides of approximately 8–10 kDa molecular weight which play key roles in the orchestration of inflammatory reactions and immune responses. Their primary and best studied function is the attraction and activation of different leucocyte types. Most chemokines act on one or more cell types in a fashion similar to that of the classical chemotactic factors, such as C5a, but with a more restricted target cell profile. The best-studied chemokine family member, IL-8, has all the properties of a neutrophil chemoattractant: inducing changes in cell shape; integrin up-regulation and activation; chemotaxis; a transient rise in intracellular free Ca^{2+} ($[Ca^{2+}]_i$); granule exocytosis and a respiratory burst. For details, the reader is referred to several recent reviews (Oppenheim *et al.*, 1991; Schall, 1991; Schall *et al.*, 1993; Schall & Bacon, 1994; Baggiolini *et al.*, 1994).

The first chemokines have been identified from the supernatant of activated mononuclear cells, implicating their function in the amplification and modulation of inflammatory reactions. More recent studies, however, have clearly shown that most chemokines are produced by a variety of resident tissue cells and thus can also act as primary mediators of inflammation. At least 19 human chemokines have been identified to date by cloning or by biochemical purification and amino-acid sequencing (Fig. 22.2). They all share variable degrees of sequence identity of at least 20%, and have similar secondary and tertiary structures, indicating that they have arisen from a common ancestral gene. All (except lymphotactin) have four conserved cysteines forming the characteristic disulphide bonds, a short amino-terminal and a longer carboxyl-terminal sequence. Nuclear magnetic resonance spectroscopy and X-ray crystallography of several chemokines have shown that chemokines have a conformationally disordered amino-terminal domain, followed by a core structure consisting of a triple-stranded antiparallel β-sheet arranged in a Greek key, on top of which lies a long C-terminal α-helix (Lodi *et al.*, 1994; Shaw *et al.*, 1994; Clore & Gronenborn, 1995).

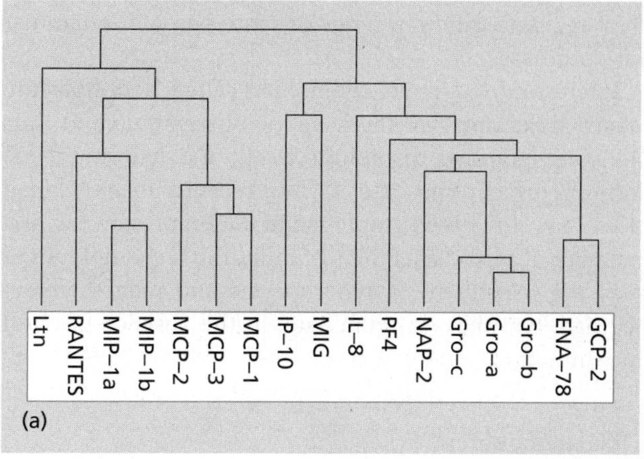

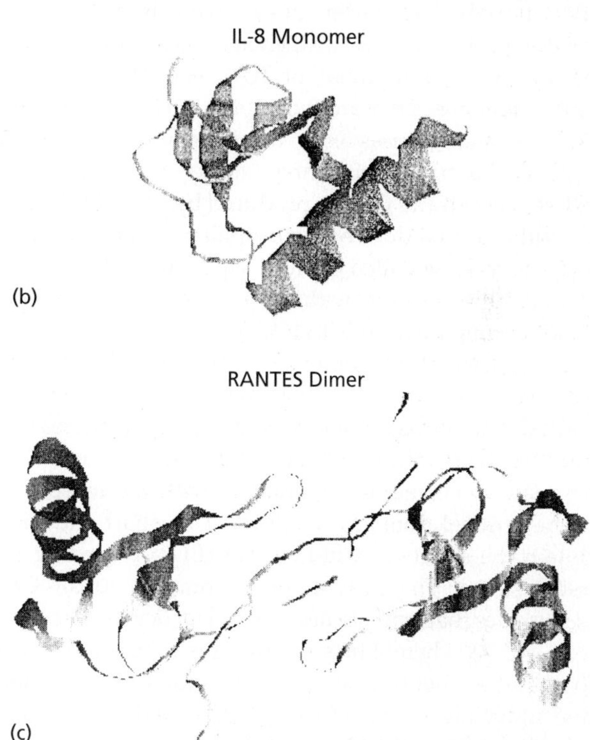

Fig. 22.2 The chemokine family of chemokines. (a) Homology tree of the cloned human chemokines. (b) Tertiary structure of the IL-8 monomer as a prototype of the members of the chemokine family. (c) Quaternary structure of the RANTES dimer representative for the configuration of CC chemokines.

The chemokines can be divided into two subfamilies based on the arrangement of the first two cysteines, which are either separated by one amino acid (CXC chemokines) or are adjacent (CC chemokines). The utility and the solid foundation of this separation of chemokines into these two subfamilies is supported by differences in the chromosomal location of their genes, quaternary structure and bioactivity profiles. All CXC chemokines are 24–84% identical to each other and are encoded by genes clustered on chromosome 4q12–q21, while CC chemokines sharing 25–71% sequence identities are encoded on chromosome 17. Despite similar tertiary structures of all chemokines, and the fact that all CXC chemokines are 20–40% identical to all CC chemokines, the quaternary structures of the dimers is entirely different and is globular in the case of CXC chemokines, but elongated and cylindrical in CC chemokines, although at physiological concentrations chemokines are likely to act as monomers (Paolini *et al.*, 1994). Finally CXC chemokines activate predominantly neutrophils, while CC chemokines act on monocytes, lymphocyte subsets, and, as discussed in more detail here, on basophil and eosinophil granulocytes, but not on neutrophils (Baggiolini & Dahinden, 1994). Thus, CXC chemokines can be regarded as primary mediators of acute inflammatory reactions in response to tissue injury and common bacterial infections, while CC chemokines may regulate different types of more chronic inflammatory processes.

Interestingly, a novel chemokine called lymphotactin, which lacks one cysteine near the N terminus and thus the corresponding disulphide bond, and whose gene is located on chromosome 1, has recently been cloned (Kelner *et al.*, 1994). Lymphotactin may represent the first member of a third chemokine family, the C chemokines. It may act selectively on lymphocytes and may therefore regulate lymphocyte trafficking, in the absence of overt inflammation.

CXC chemokines

After the initial characterization of the first chemotactic cytokine, IL-8, several CXC chemokines with biological activities similar to those of IL-8 were discovered in rapid succession. They are neutrophil-activating protein-2 (NAP-2), which arises from the N-terminal processing of platelet basic protein, three closely related proteins, GRO-α, GRO-β and GRO-γ, produced by a variety of cells, an epithelial cell-derived neutrophil-activating protein, ENA-78, and a so-called granulocyte chemotactic protein-2 (GCP-2). IL-8 shares with these chemokines sequence identities ranging from 24 to 46%. Two G-protein-coupled, seven-transmembrane-domain receptors for IL-8 have been characterized. Binding and functional studies showed that one receptor is selective for IL-8, whereas the other has high affinity for several CXC chemokines. The main site of chemokine interaction with the receptor is the N-terminal domain, which must be short and must contain the sequence Glu-Leu-Arg (ELR) preceding the first cysteine. The ELR motif is common to all CXC chemokines that activate neutrophil leucocytes. The functions of CXC chemokines lacking this motif, and which do not attract neutrophils, platelet factor-4 (PF-4), monokine inducible by interferon-γ (MIG) and interferon-γ-inducible protein (IP-10), are still unclear. PF-4 and IP-10 might play a role by binding to proteoglycans rather than by interacting with a specific receptor (Luster *et al.*, 1995), although weak lymphocyte and monocyte chemotactic activity has been proposed for IP-10 and IL-8 (Larsen *et al.*, 1989; Taub *et al.*, 1993a).

CC chemokines

The first CC chemokine was identified by differential hybridization cloning, and was termed LD78. Several cDNA isoforms of a closely related chemokine, Act-2, were later described, and two similar proteins, macrophage inflammatory protein-1α (MIP-1α) and MIP-1β, were purified from the culture medium of lipopolysaccharide (LPS)-stimulated mouse macrophages. On the basis of amino-acid identities of more than 70%, the murine and human proteins are considered as homologues, and the terms human MIP-1α and MIP-1β are commonly used instead of LD78 and Act-2. The best characterized CC chemokine is monocyte chemotactic protein-1 (MCP-1), which was purified and cloned from different sources. Other CC chemokines, I-309, RANTES and HC14, were purified or cloned as products of activated T cells. HC14, also termed MCP-2, was isolated along with a novel CC chemokine, MCP-3, from osteosarcoma cell cultures, which was subsequently cloned and expressed. The sequence identities of CC chemokines with MCP-1 are between 29 and 71%. MCP-2 (HC14) and MCP-3 are 62 and 71% identical with MCP-1.

MCP-1, the best-studied member of the CC chemokine subfamily, is chemotactic for monocytes, but not for neutrophils, and was initially considered as a counterpart of IL-8. As judged from stimulus-dependent $[Ca^{2+}]_i$ changes and chemotaxis experiments, monocytes respond to all CC chemokines, with the possible exception of I-309. While the view that CXC chemokines act on neutrophils and CC chemokines on monocytes is still valid, recent studies revealed that CC chemokines have a much wider range of biological activities as they also activate some lymphocytes types, and in particular basophil and eosinophil leucocytes.

It is important to realize that the known chemokines available from the public data banks do not reflect the true picture of the redundancy within this already remarkably large family of cytokines, particularly in the CC chemokine subfamily and probably also the novel C chemokine group. There is unpublished information indicating that by high-output sequencing of cDNA, no less than 11 novel CC chemokines have been discovered, raising the number of CC chemokines to 18 subfamily members.

Activation of basophils and eosinophils

Eosinophils and basophils are developmentally, phenotypically and functionally closely related cell types, despite their distinct staining characteristics. With very few exceptions, they respond to the same profile of cytokines and cell agonists in a similar fashion, and express similar adhesive molecules and receptors (Dahinden, 1994). Thus, human basophils have much more in common with human eosinophils than with human tissue mast cells, and are likely to be attracted at inflammatory sites together with eosinophils, although this issue is still controversial due to the lack of a specific immunological marker for basophils. Basophils are prominent sources of inflammatory mediators found in allergic late-phase reactions (histamine and LTC_4), and eosinophils contain several cytotoxic cationic proteins, indicating that the basophil could be primarily involved in generating secondary mediators, while the eosinophil is the primary cytotoxic effector cell leading to the epithelial damage associated with, for example, bronchial hyperreactivity in asthma.

Unfortunately, the fact that basophils, like mast cells, constitutively express the high-affinity receptor for IgE and contain histamine in their granules, often resulted in the erroneous conclusion found in most immunology textbooks, that basophils and mast cells function in a similar fashion. It is important to note that the only cytokine yet identified to influence human mast cell function is the c-*kit* ligand (or stem cell growth factor) (Bischoff & Dahinden, 1992a), and that chemokines, as far as they have been examined, do not activate mast cells in the human system, and therefore do not appear to regulate the allergic immediate reaction. However, mast cells may generate certain chemokines as demonstrated in murine mast cell lines and primary mast cells, thereby contributing to the late-phase reaction, although in humans it is still uncertain whether mast cells can express chemokines.

Several humoral and cell-derived chemotactic agonists not belonging to the chemokine family, including the complement products C5a, $C5a_{desarg}$ and C3a, *N*-formyl-methionyl-peptides (bacterial product analogues) and platelet-activating factor (PAF), can also activate basophils and eosinophils (Kurimoto *et al.*, 1989, 1991; Brunner *et al.*, 1991; Takafuji *et al.*, 1991, 1992, 1994; Bürgi *et al.*, 1994). Most of these chemoattractants act on all myeloid cell types, in particular C5a and formylpeptides, but there are also certain selectivities outside the chemokine family. For example, C3a is a most potent degranulating agent for eosinophils which can also activate basophils, but not neutrophils. PAF is a particularly potent chemotactic factor for eosinophils, while LTB_4 is a strong chemoattractant for neutrophils with negligable effects on eosinophils and basophils.

CXC chemokines

Although the first chemokines identified to affect basophil and eosinophil functions belong to the CXC family, they are rather ineffective stimuli. Basophils and eosinophils express functional IL-8 receptors, as shown by changes in $[Ca^{2+}]_i$ and by binding studies. However, exocytosis and leukotriene formation in basophils, and chemotaxis of basophils and eosinophils, only occurs in a significant manner if the cells have been exposed to appropriate priming cytokines, such as IL-3, IL-5 or GM-CSF, or if the cells have been isolated from allergic individuals (Dahinden *et al.*, 1989, 1991b; Kernen et al., 1991; Krieger *et al.*, 1992a; Bruijnzeel *et al.*, 1993).

Other neutrophil chemoattractants of the CXC family exhibit barely measurable effects even in primed cells, and binding studies on leukaemic basophils are consistent with a predominant expression of the IL-8 receptor type which is relatively specific for IL-8 (IL-8RA). The bioactivities of CXC chemokines which do not activate neutrophils, such as the identification of connective tissue activating peptide III (CTAP-III) as a histamine releasing factor, or PF-4 as an eosinophil chemoattractant, reported in earlier studies may be due to non-specific charge effects of high concentrations of these proteins, since they do not induce Ca^{2+} fluxes in basophils or eosinophils characteristic of that induced by chemotactic agonists, and since they do not compete with IL-8 binding to its receptor. Alternatively, these platelet products may have been contaminated with other chemokines, such as RANTES known to be present in platelets.

Depending on the experimental conditions, IL-8 can also inhibit histamine release in response to the same or other chemokines at concentrations which were 10–100 times lower than those needed to induce exocytosis (Bischoff *et al.*, 1991; Alam *et al.*, 1992b). The mechanism(s) and the significance of these findings are unclear and may be due to homologous and heterologous desensitization of chemokine receptors. In conclusion, it is still unclear whether CXC chemokines play any role in allergic inflammation, and whether the effects would be pro- or anti-inflammatory, despite the fact that IL-8 can be found in allergic inflammatory lesions.

CC chemokines

The potential role of CC chemokines in allergic inflammation became apparent only recently, when three independent groups found that MCP-1 is nearly as effective as C5a and much more potent than IL-8 as a stimulus of exocytosis for human basophils (Alam *et al.*, 1992c; Bischoff *et al.*, 1992; Kuna *et al.*, 1992a). MCP-1 induces high levels of histamine release from normal, i.e. non-primed, cells. After priming with IL-3, IL-5 or GM-CSF, the release of histamine is enhanced, and production of LTC_4 is observed in addition. This need for priming basophils to allow the production of lipid mediators is a general phenomenon observed with all endogenous humoral and cell-derived agonists, including chemokines. Further studies showed that histamine release is also obtained after stimulation with two other CC chemokines, RANTES and MIP-1α, but not with MIP-1β (Alam *et al.*, 1992a; Kuna *et al.*, 1992b; Bischoff *et al.*, 1993). A direct comparison brought up a remarkable difference in the response pattern of basophils to CC chemokines: MCP-1 is highly effective as an inducer of mediator release but only has moderate chemotactic activity, while RANTES is the most effective basophil chemoattractant and a weak stimulus of release. MIP-1α has relatively weak chemotactic and activating properties, but acts at lower concentrations, indicating that this chemokine may activate a yet unexplored effector func-

Table 22.1 The bioactivity and efficacy of chemokines.

Chemokine	Basophils Chemotaxis	Basophils Mediator release	Eosinophils Chemotaxis	Eosinophils Mediator release	Neutrophils Chemotaxis	Neutrophils Mediator release
I-309	−	−	−	−	−	−
MIP-1β	−	−	−	−	−	−
MIP-1α	+	+	+	+	−	−
RANTES	+++	+	+++	+	−	−
MCP-1	+	+++	−	−	−	−
MCP-2	++	++	++	−	−	−
MCP-3	+++	+++	+++	+	−	−
MCP-4	+++	++	+++	+	−	−
Eotaxin	+++	+	+++	+	−	−
IL-8	+	+	(+)	−	+++	+++
ELR-CXC	(+)	−	−	−	+++	+

ELR-CXC, CXC chemokines other than IL-8 containing an ELR motif before the first cysteine; −, no activity; +, activity, number of + symbols represents efficacy. See text for definition of abbreviations.

tion. RANTES and MIP-1α by themselves induce weak histamine release in basophils from selected donors only, and consistent mediator release is only observed with primed cells, as found for the CXC chemokine IL-8.

Unlike basophils, eosinophils do not respond at all to MCP-1, at least at concentrations up to 50 nmol/l (Rot *et al.*, 1992). Thus, basophils and their mediators, such as histamine, may also play a role in pathological processes in which eosinophils are not involved, since MCP-1 is expressed in many inflammatory conditions characterized by monocytic infiltrates such as arteriosclerotic plaques (Nelken *et al.*, 1991). However, eosinophils are strongly activated by several other CC chemokines, much more efficiently than by CXC chemokines, in a manner similar to basophils. As in basophils, the most potent eosinophil chemoattractant is regulated upon activation, normal T cell expressed and secreted (RANTES (Kameyoshi *et al.*, 1992; Rot *et al.*, 1992; Alam *et al.*, 1993; Ebisawa *et al.*, 1994; Schweizer *et al.*, 1994). RANTES has a similar efficacy to attract eosinophils as the most effective pleiotropic leucocyte agonists C5a and PAF, and has all the properties of an eosinophil chemotactic and activating factor, inducing changes in cell shape, actin polymerization, integrin up-regulation, exocytosis of eosinophil cationic proteins and a respiratory burst. However, compared with C5a or C3a, RANTES is a relatively weak stimulus of exocytosis and of leukotriene formation, even when the eosinophils are primed (Rot *et al.*, 1992). In synergy with IL-5, RANTES strongly promotes endothelial transmigration of eosinophils *in vitro* (Ebisawa *et al.*, 1994). Importantly, RANTES induces an eosinophilic infiltrate in dog skin *in vivo*, in contrast to several other human chemokines tested (Meurer *et al.*, 1993). Thus, RANTES has all the properties to attract the predominant leucocyte types found in exudates of allergic inflammatory sites. MIP-1α also attracts eosinophils and induces some degranulation at low concentrations, although with considerably lower efficacy than RANTES (Rot *et al.*, 1992). Furthermore, as in basophils, MIP-1β does not activate eosinophils. Moreover, an excess of MIP-1β does not alter the dose dependency of MIP-1α-induced eosinophil activation, indicating that MIP-1β does not act as an MIP-1α antagonist and does not strongly interact with MIP-1α receptors on eosinophils (unpublished observations).

The bioactivity and target cell profile of the two CC chemokines that are closely related to MCP-1, MCP-2 and MCP-3 (Van Damme *et al.*, 1992; Minty *et al.*, 1993), have been studied more recently. It has been interesting to find that MCP-3 is a very effective agonist of basophil mediator release and a powerful chemoattractant for basophils as well as eosinophils, and thus combines the bioactivities of the only distantly related CC chemokines MCP-1 and RANTES (Dahinden *et al.*, 1994; see Table 22.1). Therefore, MCP-3 may be of particular importance in allergic inflammation, since this chemokine strongly attracts and activates all effector cell types (eosinophils, basophils, lymphocytes and monocytes) thought to be primarily involved in allergic late-phase reactions. It is also important to note that MCP-3 is much more restricted in its expression than MCP-1, which is induced by a variety of pro-inflammatory stimuli. In the murine system, a novel MCP termed MARK, possibly representing the murine homologue of MCP-3, has been recently cloned (Kulmburg *et al.*, 1992; Thirion *et al.*, 1994), and appears to be relatively selectively expressed by murine mast cells, further supporting the suggested importance of MCP-3 in allergic inflammation. In the bronchoalveolar lavage (BAL) fluids of a guinea pig model of eosinophilic inflammation, an MCP-homologue, called eotaxin, with reportedly potent and specific eosinophil chemotactic activity *in vitro* and *in vivo*, has recently been characterized (Jose *et al.*, 1994; Rothenberg *et al.*, 1995). Eotaxin may represent the guinea pig homologue of MCP-3. Alternatively, a yet to be identified human eotaxin may also exist (see above), particularly since eotaxin is the only MCP not sharing an Ala-Gln signal peptide cleavage site as all the other human and animal MCP, and eotaxin has therefore only seven instead of 10 amino acids N-terminal to the first cysteine. In any case, all available data point to a key role of certain MCP homologues in mediating allergic and other eosinophilic inflammatory processes.

MCP-2, which has similar degrees of sequence identities to both MCP-1 and MCP-3 of approximately 60%, shares the target profile of MCP-3 rather than that of MCP-1, and activates basophils and eosinophils, albeit much less efficiently (Weber *et al.*, 1995). In the group of monocyte chemotactic proteins, MCP-2 is the weakest stimulus of basophil mediator release and priming is needed for an efficient response. Under certain experimental conditions, MCP-2 can also inhibit the action of the more effective MCP analogues, and it is possible that MCP-2, which is a interferon-γ-inducible chemokine, may have an inhibitory effect in allergic disease *in vivo*.

The effects of the various CC chemokines on basophil and eosinophil leucocytes are summarized in Table 22.1. The authors found that, using cells from the same unselected donors under identical experimental conditions, the order of efficacy of mediator release in basophils was found to be as follows: MCP-1 = MCP-3 > MCP-2 > IL-8 = RANTES > MIP-1α; MIP-1β and I-309 inactive. The efficacies of chemotaxis for basophils and eosinophils was: RANTES = MCP-3 > MCP-2 > MIP-1α > MCP-1 (in basophils, no activity in eosinophils). Similar findings have been reported by independent studies. Some minor differences in the order of potency reported by others (Alam *et al.*, 1994) are probably due to differences in experimental conditions and the chemokine preparations used. Thus, the different chemokines not only have distinct target cell selectivities, but each agonist has its characteristic profile for promoting the various effector functions. The chemokines are therefore particularly adapted to fine tune inflammatory reactions of diverse aetiologies.

Although it could be anticipated that MCP-3 is a strong stimulus of release given its sequence identity of over 70% with MCP-1, it was surprising to find that MCP-3 has the same chemoattractant properties as RANTES, with which it shares only 25% sequence identity. Interestingly, diverging effects were also observed for the highly homologous pair MIP-1α and MIP-1β, of which only MIP-1α activates basophils and eosinophils. It thus appears that sequence similarity is not necessarily predictive for the capacity of different CC chemokines to elicit one or the other effector functions in basophils and eosinophils. The bioactivity profile of a certain chemokine and its capacity to interact with different chemokine receptors may rather depend on discrete amino-acid motifs. The fact that the effects of a certain CC chemokine depend on short amino-acid motifs rather than on overall sequence similarities, also makes it problematic to assign to an animal chemokine its corresponding human homologue, particularly in a family of similar proteins as large as that of the CC chemokines. This may also limit interpretations of *in vivo* studies and of pharmacological interventions in animal models of allergic disease.

Activation of monocytes and lymphocytes

As eosinophils and basophils, monocytes and lymphocytes are activated by CC chemokines rather than CXC chemokines. The different CC chemokines activate monocytes in the fashion typical for chemotactic agonists interacting with seven-transmembrane, G-protein-coupled receptors, inducing the same set of cellular responses as IL-8 on neutrophils, albeit with distinct efficacies depending on the chemokine (Oppenheim *et al.*, 1991; Schall *et al.*, 1993; Baggiolini *et al.*, 1994; Schall & Bacon, 1994; Vaddi & Newton, 1994; Uguccioni *et al.*, 1995). The best studied and most potent monocyte attracting and activating chemokine is MCP-1, which also induces monocytic infiltrates in animal models *in vivo*. In contrast to eosinophils and basophils, MIP-1β is active on monocytes. Most, if not all, CC chemokines also attract different lymphocyte subpopulations with distinct target cell selectivities. RANTES is a most effective lymphocyte chemotaxin with some selectivity for T-helper memory cells (Schall *et al.*, 1990; Taub *et al.*, 1993c), and also acts *in vivo* in a humanized mouse model (Murphy *et al.*, 1994). MIP-1α and MIP-1β attract lymphocyte subsets of the CD-8 and the CD-4 subset, respectively, particularly if the cells have been activated (Schall *et al.*, 1993; Tanaka *et al.*, 1993; Taub *et al.*, 1993a,c). Recent studies indicate that MCP-1, -2 and -3 also potently activate lymphocyte clones and attract blood lymphocytes, in conflict with earlier studies in which MCP-1 was inactive (Carr *et al.*, 1994; Loetscher *et al.*, 1994). Finally, CC chemokines may also affect the function and trafficking of B cells and natural killer (NK) cells (Maghazachi *et al.*, 1994). Although it is clear that CC chemokines are key regulators of lymphocyte migration, the selectivity of the individual family members for different lymphocyte subpopulations is a controversial issue, and most information depends on chemotaxis experiments only. It is likely that, depending on the activation state and the phenotype of the lymphocyte, the expression of different chemokine receptors, and therefore their responsiveness to chemokines, can change (Xu *et al.*, 1995). Lymphocytes are by themselves important sources of different CC chemokines and these may play a yet undetermined autocrine role in lymphocyte functions. It is also unknown to what extent chemokines regulate lymphocyte functions other than chemotaxis and adherence.

Adhesive interactions

Many chemokines have been isolated by using their interaction with heparin, and chemokines are known to bind to negatively charged proteoglycans in the extracellular matrix and on the cellular glycocalyx (Huber *et al.*, 1991; Rot, 1992; Gilat *et al.*, 1994; Witt & Lander, 1994). Thus, chemokines may also act in an anchoraged manner, for example on endothelial cells, or be presented in a more stable gradient in the tissue. A promiscuous 'receptor' for chemokines, the Duffy antigen, present on erythrocytes and endothelial cells, may represent a similar anchor or also a sink for chemokines in the bloodstream (Horuk *et al.*, 1993; Neote *et al.*, 1994; Peiper *et al.*, 1995). Finally, some chemokines, such as PF-4 or IP-10, have been found to be antiangiogenic (Maione *et al.*, 1990; Hoogewerf *et al.*, 1995; Luster *et al.*, 1995) by interacting with proteoglycans, thereby displacing other cytokines needing interactions with proteoglycans (e.g. other chemokines and even basic fibroblast growth factor). Thus, some chemokines may act primarily as anti-inflammatory peptides by binding to proteoglycans.

Chemokine receptors

Functional characterization

The responses of basophils, eosinophils and monocytes to CC chemokines are prevented by pretreatment of the cells with *Bordatella pertussis* toxin (Bischoff *et al.*, 1993), suggesting that they are mediated by G-protein-coupled, seven-transmembrane domain receptors. The same type of receptors are involved in the activation of neutrophils and basophils by CXC chemokines (Krieger *et al.*, 1992a).

A rapid and transient rise in $[Ca^{2+}]_i$ is one of the early events observed after stimulation of leucocytes with chemotactic agonists. In contrast to functional responses such as chemotaxis or exocytosis, the $[Ca^{2+}]_i$ changes induced by different CC chemokines in basophils, eosinophils and monocytes are similar in extent and kinetics, and real-time recordings of the transients are often used to monitor receptor activation. When the same receptor is stimulated twice within a short time with receptor saturating concentrations of the same agonist, the second $[Ca^{2+}]_i$ transient is prevented as a consequence of desensitization.

Desensitization after repeated stimulation is a sensitive test for receptor usage by different or related chemotactic agonists. Stimulation with different CC chemokines does not affect the response to other agonists, including C5a, C3a, formyl-peptides and PAF and vice versa, indicating that basophils, eosinophils and monocytes express distinct CC chemokine receptors. In cells in which both CXC and CC chemokines induce Ca^{2+} transients, for example in basophils, there is no cross-desensitization between IL-8 and all the active CC chemokines, indicating that CXC and CC chemokines act on different chemokine receptors. The results obtained with CC chemokines in basophils and eosinophils presented synoptically in Fig. 22.3, however, suggest the existence of several CC chemokine receptors with partially distinct, partially overlapping ligand specificities. A complete desensitization of the second response is always obtained when the same chemokine is applied twice. In basophils, sequential stimulation with different chemokines yields the following patterns of desensitization: MCP-1 and MIP-1α prevent their own response only, RANTES prevents in addition the response to MIP-1α, while MCP-3 desensitizes the cells to all CC chemokines tested. In eosinophils (which do not respond to MCP-1) there is full cross-desensitization between MCP-3 and RANTES, while MIP-1α again only prevents its own response. As in basophils, full and partial desensitization toward MIP-1α is observed with RANTES and MCP-3, respectively.

The data matrix in Table. 22.1 suggests the existence of at least three CC chemokine receptors: an *MCP-1 receptor* activated by MCP-1 and MCP-3 is expressed on basophils but not on eosinophils; a *RANTES receptor* which responds to RANTES and MCP-3 and is expressed in both cell types; and an *MIP-1α receptor*, also present in both cell types, that is activated by MIP-1α, RANTES and, less efficiently, by MCP-3 (Fig. 22.4). MCP-2 has a similar target cell profile, but acts less strongly. The functions elicited by CC chemokines in basophils indicate that the three receptors may have different signalling properties. Release responses appear to be mediated largely through the MCP-1 receptor, and chemotaxis through the RANTES receptor. The role of the MIP-1α receptor is still unclear. It may serve other, unknown functions, since MIP-1α is a considerably weaker chemoattractant than RANTES and MCP-3. Desensitization experiments with combinations of two stimuli (Fig. 22.3) could also be taken to suggest the existence of an additional receptor on basophils that is selective for MCP-3, because no CC chemokine, except for MCP-3 itself, prevents the $[Ca^{2+}]_i$ change induced by MCP-3. This possibility is unlikely, however, since the response to MCP-3 is abrogated after prestimulation with both MCP-1 and RANTES.

Interestingly, the desensitization patterns in monocytes differs markedly (Bischoff *et al.*, 1993; Uguccioni *et al.*, 1995). For example, MIP-1α, and even MIP-1β, potently inhibits the RANTES response, in marked contrast to the situation observed in basophils and eosinophils. There is

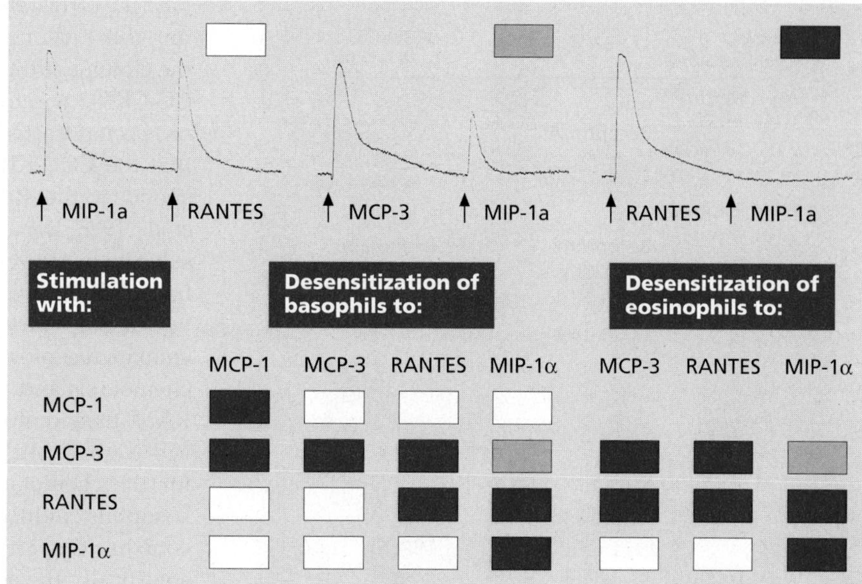

Fig. 22.3 Desensitization of the intracellular calcium transients between different CC-chemokines in basophils and eosinophils. The upper part shows representative tracings for no desensitization (symbolized by a white box); partial desensitization (light green box); and complete desensitization (dark green).

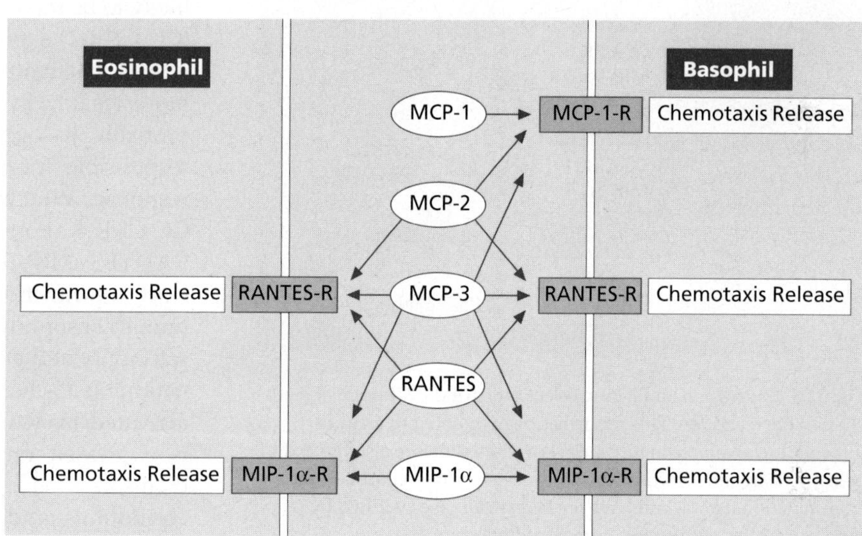

Fig. 22.4 Minimal receptor model for CC-chemokines on basophils and eosinophils: The MCP-1 receptor activated by MCP-1, MCP-3 and more weakly by MCP-2 (and MCP-4) is expressed only on basophils and mediates predominantly release; the RANTES receptor activated by RANTES, MCP-3 and more weakly by MCP-2 is expressed on both cell types and mediates predominantly chemotaxis; The MIP-1α receptor, also expressed on both cell types, is activated by MIP-1α and RANTES, more weakly by MCP-3 and promotes comparably weak chemotactic and release responses.

also cross-desensitization between MIP-1α and MIP-1β. Monocytes may therefore express different sets of chemokine receptors than eosinophils and basophils. Binding studies, mostly performed with monocytes, also indicate the presence of different receptors with partially overlapping ligand selectivities. On monocytic THP cells three receptors have been suggested: a specific MCP-1 receptor; a receptor binding MCP-1, MIP-1α and RANTES; and a common MIP-1α/MIP-1β receptor (Kelvin *et al.*, 1993).

Cloned chemokine receptors

Consistent with functional and binding studies, six different chemokine receptors have been cloned up to now—two for CXC and four for CC chemokines. The current knowledge about the ligand selectivities and the pattern of expression is summarized in Fig. 22.5, but this must be regarded as preliminary because the CC chemokine receptors have been characterized only very recently (Gao *et al.*, 1993; Neote *et al.*, 1993; Schall *et al.*, 1993; Charo *et al.*, 1994; reviewed in Horuk, 1994; Murphy, 1994; Yamagami *et al.*, 1994; Combardiere *et al.*, 1995). Most of the receptors have been isolated from cDNA of mononuclear cells and are strongly expressed in monocytes. It is likely that more receptors for CC chemokines will be identified. In particular, the postulated RANTES/MCP-3 receptor on eosinophils, which may be the major receptor mediating chemotaxis and which is not desensitized by MIP-1α, remains to be defined. As anticipated, novel members of the CC-chemokine family have been cloned and expressed. Of particular importance for allergic inflam-

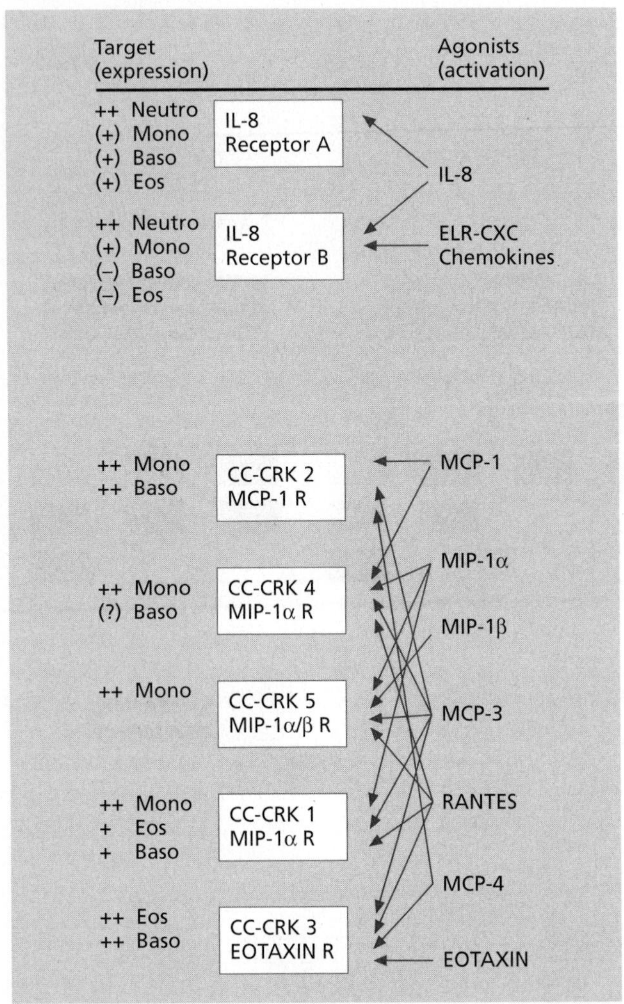

Fig. 22.5 Expression and ligand selectivities of the different cloned chemokine receptors. This figure has been updated to include information available in July 1996. For discussion see also the text below. The ligand selectivities of the receptors are in part derived from functional data, and have not been in all cases verified by binding studies with receptor transfectants.

mation is the identification of human eotaxin, which is a potent chemoattractant for eosinophils (Ponath *et al.*, 1996a) and basophils (C. Dahinden, unpublished observations). Human eotaxin is highly homologous to other MCP-chemokines, but has only eight amino acids before the first cysteine and lacks a N-terminal glutamine. This may be one of the reasons why eotaxin, in contrast to other MCPs, does not activate mononuclear cells (Ponath *et al.*, 1996; Uguccioni *et al.*, 1996), since deletion of the glutamine from MCP-1 reduces its histamine releasing and monocyte activity by approximately 100-fold (Weber *et al.*, 1996). Another MCP-homologue, MCP-4 has been cloned, which has a similar bioactivity profile to MCP-3. MCP-4 is even more potent than MCP-3 in attracting eosinophils (Uguccioni *et al.*, 1996) and basophils, but is a weaker inducer of histamine release than MCP-3 (C. Dahinden, unpublished observations). The original paper reporting the cloning of the CC-chemokine receptor 3 claiming that CC-CKR-3 is activated by RANTES, MIP-1α and MIP-1β, has been retracted (Combadiere *et al.*, 1995). It is now clear that the CC-CKR-3 is the eotaxin receptor which corresponds to the 'RANTES receptor' in Fig. 22.4 (Daugherty *et al.*, 1996; Ponath *et al.*, 1996b). The eotaxin receptor is selectively expressed at high levels in eosinophils and basophils (C. Dahinden, unpublished observations), but not or only very weakly on other leucocyte types. The eotaxin receptor (CC-CKR-3) mediates predominantely chemotaxis and is activated by eotaxin, MCP-3, MCP-4, RANTES and more weakly by MCP-2, but not by MCP-1, MIP-1α and MIP-1β, and is responsible to a large degree for the chemotactic responses of both eosinophils and basophils induced by all CC-chemokines. Thus, the eotaxin receptor is a potential drug target to inhibit specifically the accumulation of these leucocyte types in allergic diseases. The release responses of basophils are likely to be mediated by activation of the MCP-1 receptor (CC-CKR-2) expressed on basophils, but not eosinophils, which is activated most strongly by MCP-1 and -3, and more weakly by MCP-2 and -4. Eosinophils, and most probably basophils, also express CC-CKR-1, which is responsible for the MIP-1α and part of the RANTES response. Whether basophils also express the receptor CC-CKR-4 (Power *et al.*, 1995), which is activated by RANTES, MIP-1α and MCP-1 is uncertain at this time since the functional profile of the MCP-homologues on human basophils more closely correspond to the ligand selectivity of the MCP-1 receptor (see CC-CKR-2). Finally, another CC-chemokine receptor, CC-CKR-5, which is activated by RANTES, MIP-1α and MIP-1β, and which is expressed on monocytes has recently been cloned (Samson *et al.*, 1996). CC-CKR-5 is not expressed on eosinophils and basophils explaining why these cell types, in contrast to monocytes, do not respond to MIP-1β (Rot *et al.*, 1992).

In any case, the emergence of a large CC chemokine family and a corresponding (may be less abundant) set of partially selective, partially promiscuous receptors, which can be differentially expressed in the tissue and on leucocytes, suggests an unique cytokine network capable of regulating and fine tuning all kinds of inflammatory pathologies.

Structure and function of chemokines

There is increasing evidence that the N terminus of CC chemokine is important for bioactivity, despite the lack of a conserved motif in this region, as is the case for CXC chemokines (Zhang *et al.*, 1994; Gong & Clark-Lewis, 1995). It is important to realize that binding to and activation of the receptors is likely to depend on distinct structures of the chemokine, as has been demonstrated for the interaction of C5a with the C5a receptor (Gerard & Gerard, 1994). Changing the length of the N terminus can inhibit bioactivity and even result in antagonists. It has recently been found that deletion of a single amino acid at the N terminus of MCP-1 not only strongly inhibits its histamine-releasing activity, but at the same time confers to the peptide a novel activity on eosinophils, indicating that N-terminal processing may be another way of regulating the bioactivity and target cell profile of CC chemokines (Weber *et al.*, 1996).

Expression of chemokines in allergy

Histamine-releasing factors

The fact that cell-derived factors can induce histamine release in basophils has been known for many years, and several laboratories have attempted to characterize these factors, operationally termed 'histamine releasing factors' (HRF) (Thueson *et al.*, 1979; Schulman *et al.*, 1988; Alam *et al.*, 1984, 1987, 1989; Baeza *et al.*, 1989; Kuna *et al.*, 1989; Sampson *et al.*, 1989; Kaplan *et al.*, 1994; Ezeanuzie & Assem, 1995). Functionally, histamine-releasing factors can be divided into IgE-independent factors and an IgE-dependent factor which has been characterized very recently (Liu *et al.*, 1986; Lichtenstein, 1988; MacDonald *et al.*, 1995). It is highly likely that most, if not all, the IgE-independent histamine-releasing activity is due to CC chemokines, with some possible synergism between priming cytokines and chemokine agonists in crude supernatants. Several studies indicate that HRF is related to disease severity and response of the patient to therapeutic interventions (Alam *et al.*, 1984, 1987; Brunet *et al.*, 1992). Thus, the measurement of distinct CC chemokines specifically expressed in allergic diseases may provide finally the long-searched-for and heavily needed laboratory parameter for monitoring the severity of allergic disease, and for a more objective measure of the patient's response to immunotherapy and pharmacotherapy. Finally, other undefined bioactivities, such as eosinophilotactic factors of anaphylaxis, can most likely also be attributed to CC chemokines.

Chemokine expression and function *in vivo*

Although there is an increasing number of studies demonstrating the expression of CC chemokines in inflammatory pathologies of diverse aetiologies (Antoniades *et al.*, 1992), including allergic diseases, there is still little information on their importance *in vivo*. It is important to realize that chemokines need generally higher concentrations to induce a response than other cytokines, and thus the mere demonstration of CC chemokines *in vivo* using sensitive methods does not prove their involvement in the pathological process under study. Several chemokines, in particular IL-8 and MCP-1, are induced by many pro-inflammatory stimuli. Nevertheless, there is also increasing evidence that the different chemokines, in particular CC chemokines, can be separately expressed (Rathanaswami *et al.*, 1993; Brown *et al.*, 1994; Conlon *et al.*, 1995).

MCP-1 is expressed in bronchial tissue from asthmatic subjects (Sousa *et al.*, 1994), and in a model of allergic late-phase reactions in the skin MCP-3 and RANTES were found to be expressed with a kinetics that would explain the infiltration of eosinophils and lymphocytes, respectively (Ying *et al.*, 1995). MIP-1α and RANTES have been identified in the exudate after nasal and ocular challenge of allergic individuals (Bitticks *et al.*, 1994; Chihata *et al.*, 1995). It should be noted, however, that the main eosinophil chemoattractant chemokine may not have been identified yet. It is also intriguing that RANTES is induced by interferon-γ and found in granulomatous diseases with no eosinophil infiltration (Devergne *et al.*, 1994). It is possible that the presence of priming cytokines is needed for eosinophil accumulation *in vivo*, or that interferon-γ induces an antagonistic cytokine for eosinophils.

Conclusions

Although the study of the biochemistry and the biology of chemokines is still in its inception, there is increasing evidence that the members of the CC chemokine family are key regulators in allergic inflammation and other chronic inflammatory processes. The fact that different chemokines attract and activate distinct cell types, and also activate different effector functions, indicates that chemokine receptor antagonists could be designed that intervene in different inflammatory disorders in a much more specific manner than that of presently available drugs. Furthermore, the selective expression of certain chemokines could provide more disease-specific laboratory parameters for the diagnosis and monitoring of allergic diseases.

Acknowledgements

Dr M. Weber is thanked for his help with this chapter. The work is supported by a grant from the National Swiss Science Foundation.

References

Ahuja, S.K., Gao, J.K. & Murphy, P.M. (1994) Chemokine receptors and molecular mimicry. *Immunol. Today*, **15**, 281–7.

Alam, R., Forsythe, P.A., Lett-Brown, M.A. & Grant, J.A. (1989) Cellular origin of histamine releasing factor produced by peripheral blood mononuclear cells. *J. Immunol.*, **142**, 3951–6.

Alam, R., Forsythe, P., Lett-Brown, M.A. & Grant, J.A. (1992a) Macrophage inflammatory protein-1 is an activator of basophils and mast cells. *J. Exp. Med.*, **176**, 781–6.

Alam, R., Forsythe, P.A., Lett-Brown, M.A. & Grant, J.A. (1992b) Interleukin-8 and RANTES inhibit basophil histamine release induced with monocyte chemotactic and activating factor/monocyte chemoattractant peptide-1 and histamine releasing factor. *Am. J. Respir. Cell. Mol. Biol.*, **7**, 427–33.

Alam, R., Lett-Brown, M.A., Forsythe, P.A. *et al.* (1992c) Monocyte chemotactic and activating factor is a potent histamine releasing factor basophils. *J. Clin. Invest.*, **89**, 723–8.

Alam, R., Forsythe, P., Stafford, S. *et al.* (1994) Monocyte chemotactic protein-2, monocyte chemotactic protein-3, and fibroblast-induced cytokine. Three new chemokines induce chemotaxis and activation of basophils. *J. Immunol.*, **153**, 3155–9.

Alam, R., Kuna, P., Rozniecki, J. & Kuzminska, B. (1987) The magnitude of the spontaneous production of histamine releasing factor (HRF) by lymphocytes *in vitro* correlates with the state of bronchial hyperreactivity in asthmatic patients. *J. Allergy Clin. Immunol.*, **79**, 103–8.

Alam, R., Rozniecki, J. & Selmaj, K. (1984) A mononuclear cell-derived histamine releasing factor (HRF) in asthmatic patients. Histamine release from basophils *in vitro*. *Ann. Allergy*, **53**, 66–9.

Alam, R., Stafford, S., Forsythe, P. *et al.* (1993) RANTES is a chemotactic and activating factor for human eosinophils. *J. Immunol.*, **150**, 3442–8.

Alam, R., Welter, J.B., Forsythe, P.A., Lett-Brown, M.A. & Grant, J.A. (1989b) Comparative effect of recombinant IL-1, -2, -3, -4, and -6, IFN-γ, granulocyte-macrophage colony-stimulating factor, tumor necrosis factor-α, and histamine-releasing factors on the secretion of histamine from basophils. *J. Immunol.*, **142**, 3431.

Antoniades, H.N., Neville-Golden, J., Galanopoulos, T., Kradin, R.L., Valente, A.J. & Graves, D.T. (1992) Expression of monocyte chemoattractant protein 1 mRNA in human idiopathic pulmonary fibrosis. *Proc. Nat. Acad. Sci. USA*, **89**, 5371–5.

Baeza, M.L., Reddigari, S., Haak-Frendscho, M. & Kaplan, A.P. (1989) Purification and further characterization of human mononuclear cell histamine-releasing factor. *J. Clin. Invest.*, **83**, 1204–10.

Baggiolini, M. & Dahinden, C.A. (1994) CC chemokines in allergic inflammation. *Immunol. Today*, **15**, 127–33.

Baggiolini, M., Dewald, B. & Moser, B. (1994) Interleukin-8 and related chemotactic cytokines — CXC and CC chemokines. *Adv. Immunol.*, **55**, 97–179.

Bischoff, S.C., Baggiolini, M., de Weck, A.L. & Dahinden, C.A. (1991) Interleukin-8: inhibitor and inducer of histamine and leukotriene release in human basophils. *Biochem. Biophys. Res. Commun.*, **179**, 628–33.

Bischoff, St C., Brunner, Th., de Weck, A.L. & Dahinden, C.A. (1990b) Interleukin 5 modifies histamine release and leukotriene generation by human basophils in response to diverse agonists. *J. Exp. Med.*, **172**, 1577–82.

Bischoff, S.C. & Dahinden, C.A. (1992a) C-kit ligand: a unique potentiator of mediator release by human lung mast cells. *J. Exp. Med.*, **175**, 237–244.

Bischoff, S.C. & Dahinden, C.A. (1992b) Effect of nerve growth factor on the release of inflammatory mediators by mature human basophils. *Blood*, **79**, 2662–9.

Bischoff, S.C., Krieger, M., Brunner, Th. & Dahinden, C.A. (1992) Monocyte chemotactic protein-1 is a potent activator of human basophils. *J. Exp. Med.*, **175**, 1271–5.

Bischoff, S.C., Krieger, M., Brunner, Th. *et al.* (1993) RANTES and related chemokines activate human basophil granulocytes through different G protein-coupled receptors. *Eur. J. Immunol.*, **23**, 761–7.

Bischoff, S.C., de Weck, A.L. & Dahinden, C.A. (1990a) Interleukin-3 and granulocyte/macrophage-colony-stimulating factor render human basophils responsive to low concentrations of complement component C3a. *Proc. Nat. Acad. Sci. USA*, **87**, 6813–17.

Bitticks, L., Hilsmeier, K., Schreiber, D. & Sim, T. (1994) Secretion profile of IL-1β, GM-CSF, and chemokines (IL-8, MIP-1, and RANTES) in allergen-induced nasal responses: inhibition by topical steroids. *J. Allergy Clin. Immunol.*, **93**, 270.

Brown, Z., Gerritsen, M.E., Carley, W.W., Strieter, R.M., Kunke, S.L. & Westwick, J. (1994) Chemokine gene expression and secretion by cytokine-activated human microvascular endothelial cells. Differential regulation of monocyte chemoattractant protein-1 and interleukin-8 in response to interferon-gamma. *Am. J. Pathol.*, **145**, 913–21.

Bruijnzeel, P.L.B., Kuijper, P.H.M., Rihs, S., Betz, S., Warringa, R.A.J. & Keonderman, L. (1993) Eosinophil migration in atopic dermatitis 1: increased migratory responses to *N*-formyl-methionyl-leucyl-phenylalanine, neutrophil-activating factor, platelet activating factor, and platelet factor 4. *J. Invest. Dermatol.*, **100**, 137–42.

Brunet, C., Bedard, P.M., Lavoie, A., Jobin, M. & Hebert, J. (1992) Allergic rhinitis to ragweed pollen. II. Modulation of histamine-releasing factor production by specific immunotherapy. *J. Allergy Clin. Immunol.*, **89**, 87–94.

Brunner, T. & Dahinden, C.A. (1993) Regulation of basophil effector functions by cytokines. *ACI News*, **56**, 175–80.

Brunner, Th., Heusser, T.H. & Dahinden, C.A. (1993) Human peripheral blood basophils primed by interleukin 3 (IL-3) produce IL-4 in response to immunoglobulin E receptor stimulation. *J. Exp. Med.*, **177**, 605–11.

Brunner, Th., de Weck, A.L. & Dahinden, C.A. (1991) Platelet-activating factor induces mediator release by human basophils primed with IL-3, granulocyte-macrophage colony-stimulating factor, or IL-5. *J. Immunol.*, **147**, 237–42.

Bürgi, B., Brunner, T. & Dahinden, C.A. (1994) The degradation product of the C5a anaphylatoxin $C5a_{desarg}$ retains basophil-activating properties. *Eur. J. Immunol.*, **24**, 1583–9.

Carr, M.W., Roth, S.J., Luther, E., Rose, S.S. & Springer, T.A. (1994) Monocyte chemoattractant protein 1 acts as a T-lymphocyte chemoattractant. *Proc. Nat. Acad. Sci. USA*, **91**, 3652–6.

Charo, I.F., Myers, S.J., Herman, A., Franci, C., Connolly, A.J. & Coughlin, S.R. (1994) Molecular cloning and functional expression of two monocyte chemoattractant protein 1 receptors reveals alternative splicing of the carboxyl-terminal tails. *Proc. Nat. Acad. Sci. USA*, **91**, 2752–6.

Chihara, J., Yamada, H., Takamura, E., Yoshino, K. & Nakajima, S. (1995) Possible presence of RANTES in tears of patients with allergic conjunctivitis (letter). *Int. Arch. Allergy Immunol.*, **106**, 428.

Clore, G.M. & Gronenborn, A.M. (1995) Three-dimensional structures of alpha and beta chemokines. *FASEB J.*, **9**, 57–62.

Combadiere, C., Ahuja, S.K. & Murphy, P.M. (1995) Cloning and functional expression of a human eosinophil CC chemokine receptor. *J. Biol. Chem.*, **270**, 16491–4.

Conlon, K., Lloyd, A., Chattopadhyay, U. *et al.* (1995) CD8+ and CD45RA+ human peripheral blood lymphocytes are potent sources of marcophage inflammatory protein 1 alpha, interleukin-8 and RANTES. *Eur. J. Immunol.*, **25**, 751–6.

Dahinden, C.A. (1994) Regulation of leukotriene production by cytokines. In: *Advances in Prostaglandin, Thromboxane, and*

Leukotriene Research, Vol. 22 (ed. S.E. Dahlen *et al.*), pp. 327–39. Raven Press, New York.

Dahinden, C.A., Geiser, T., Brunner, T. *et al.* (1994) Monocyte chemotactic protein 3 is a most effective basophil- and eosinophil-activating chemokine. *J. Exp. Med.*, **179**, 751–6.

Dahinden, C.A., Bischoff, S.C., Brunner, Th., Krieger, M., Takafuji, S. & de Weck, A.L. (1991a) Regulation of mediator release by human basophils: importance of the sequence and time of addition in the combined action of different agonists. *Int. Arch. Allergy Appl. Immunol.*, **94**, 161–4.

Dahinden, C.A., Brunner, T., Krieger, M., Bischoff, S.C. & de Weck, A.L. (1992) Cytokines in allergic inflammation. In: *Progress in Immunology VIII. Proceedings of the 8th International Congress of Immunology Budapest, 1992*, pp. 411–18.

Dahinden, C.A., Krieger, M., Brunner, Th. & Bischoff, S.C. (1993) Basophil activation by members of the chemokine superfamily. *Adv. Exp. Med. Biol.*, **351**, 99–110.

Dahinden, C.A., Krieger, M., Brunner, T., Takafuji, S. & Bischoff, S.C. (1991b) Factors promoting histamine and leukotriene release. In: *New Trends in Allergy III, Munich 1990*, pp. 138–42. Springer Verlag, Berlin.

Dahinden, C.A., Kurimoto, Y., de Weck, A.L., Lindley, I., Dewald, B. & Baggiolini, M. (1989) The neutrophil-activating peptide NAF/NAP-1 induces histamine and leukotriene release by interleukin-3 primed basophils. *J. Exp. Med.*, **170**, 1787–92.

Dahinden, C.A., Zingg, J., Maly, F.E. & de Weck, A.L. (1988) Leukotriene production in human neutrophils primed by recombinant human granulocyte/macrophage colony-stimulating factor and stimulated with the complement component C5a and fMLP as second signals. *J. Exp. Med.*, **167**, 1281–95.

Daugherty, B.L., Siciliano, S.J., DeMartino, J.A., Malkowitz, L., Sirotina, A. & Springer, M.S. (1996) Cloning, expression and characterization of the eosinophil eotaxin receptor. *J. Exp. Med.*, **183**, 2349–54.

Devergne, O., Marfaing-Koka, A., Schall, T.J. *et al.* (1994) Production of the RANTES chemokine in delayed-type hypersensitivity reactions: involvement of macrophages and endothelial cells. *J. Exp. Med.*, **179**, 1689–94.

Ebisawa, M., Yamada, T., Bickel, C., Klunk, D. & Schleimer, R.P. (1994) Eosinophil transendothelial migration induced by cytokines. III. Effect of the chemokine RANTES. *J. Immunol.*, **153**, 2153–60.

Ezeamuzie, I.C. & Assem, E.S. (1985) A study of histamine release from basophils by products of lymphocyte stimulation. *Agents Actions*, **13**, 222–30.

Frew, A.J. & Kay, A.B. (1988) The relationship between CD4+ lymphocytes, activated eosinophils and the magnitude of the allergen-induced late phase skin reaction in man. *J. Immunol.*, **141**, 4158–64.

Frigas, E. & Gleich, G.J. (1986) The eosinophil and the pathophysiology of asthma. *J. Allergy Clin. Invest.*, **77**, 527–37.

Gao, J.L., Kuhns, D.B., Tiffany, H.L. *et al.* (1993) Structure and functional expression of the human macrophage inflammatory protein 1 alpha/RANTES receptor. *J. Exp. Med.*, **177**, 1421–7.

Gao, C.B., Liu, M.C., Galli, S.J., Bochner, B.S., Kagey-Sobotka, A. & Lichtenstein, L.M. (1994) Identification of IgE-bearing cells in the late-phase response to antigen in the lung as basophils. *Am. J. Respir. Cell. Mol. Biol.*, **10**, 384–90.

Gauchat, J.-F., Henchoz, S., Mazzel, G. *et al.* (1993) Induction of human IgE synthesis in B cells by mast cells and basophils. *Nature*, **365**, 340–3.

Gerard, C. & Gerard, N.P. (1994) C5A anaphylatoxin and its seven transmembrane-segment receptor. *Ann. Rev. Immunol.*, **12**, 775–808.

Gilat, D., Hershkoviz, R., Mekori, Y.A., Vlodavsky, I. & Lider, O. (1994) Regulation of adhesion of CD4+ T lymphocytes to intact or heparinase-treated subendothelial extracellular matrix by diffusable or anchored RANTES and MIP-1β. *J. Immunol.*, **153**, 4899–906.

Gong, J.H. & Clark-Lewis, I. (1995) Antagonists of monocyte chemoattractant protein 1 identified by modification of functionally critical NH2-terminal residues. *J. Exp. Med.*, **181**, 631–40.

Griffiths-Johnson, D.A., Collins, P.D., Rossi, A.G., Jose, P.J. & Williams, T.J. (1993) The chemokine, eotaxin, activates guinea-pig eosinophils *in vitro* and causes their accumulation into the lung *in vivo*. *Biochem. Biophys. Res. Commun.*, **197**, 1167–72.

Hoogewerf, A.J., Leone, J.W., Reardon, I.M. *et al.* (1995) CXC chemokines connective tissue activating peptide-III and neutrophil activating peptide-2 are heparin/heparan sulfate-degrading enzymes. *J. Biol. Chem.*, **270**, 3268–77.

Horuk, R. (1994) The interleukin-8-receptor family: from chemokines to malaria. *Immunol. Today*, **15**, 169–74.

Horuk, R., Chitnis, C.E., Darbonne, W.C. *et al.* (1993) A receptor for the malarial parasite *Plasmodium vivax*: the erythrocyte chemokine receptor. *Science*, **261**, 1182–4.

Huber, A.R., Kunkel, S.L., Todd III, R.F. & Weiss, S.J. (1991) Regulation of transendothelial neutrophil migration by endogenous interleukin-8. *Science*, **254**, 99–102.

Jose, P.J., Griffiths-Johnson, D.A., Collins, P.D. *et al.* (1994) Eotaxin: a potent eosinophil chemoattractant cytokine detected in a guinea pig model of allergic airways inflammation. *J. Exp. Med.*, **179**, 881–7.

Kameyoshi, Y., Dorschner, A., Mallet, A.I., Christophers, E. & Schroder, J.M. (1992) Cytokine RANTES released by thrombin-stimulated platelets is a potent attractant for human eosinophils. *J. Exp. Med.*, **176**, 587–92.

Kaplan, A.P., Kuna, P. & Reddigari, S.R. (1994) Chemokines as allergic mediators—relationship to histamine-releasing factors. *Allergy*, **49**, 495–501.

Kay, A.B. (1992) 'Helper' (CD4+) T cells and eosinophils in allergy and asthma. *Am. Rev. Resp. Dis.*, **145**, S22–6.

Kay, A.B., Ying, S., Varney, V. *et al.* (1991) Messenger RNA expression of the cytokine gene cluster, IL-3, IL-4, IL-5 and GM-CSF, in allergen-induced late-phase reactions in atopic subjects. *J. Exp. Med.*, **173**, 775–8.

Kelner, G.S., Kennedy, J., Bacon, K.B. *et al.* (1994) Lymphotactin: a cytokine that represents a new class of chemokine. *Science*, **266**, 1395–9.

Kelvin, D.J., Wang, J.M., McVicar, D. & Oppenheim, J.J. (1993) Promiscuity of ligand binding in the human chemokine beta receptor family. *Adv. Exp. Med. Biol.*, **351**, 147–53.

Kernen, P., Wymann, M.P., von Tscharner, V. *et al.* (1991) Shape changes, exocytosis and cytosolic free calcium changes in stimulated human eosinophils. *J. Clin. Invest.*, **87**, 2012–17.

Krieger, M., Brunner, Th., Bischoff, S.C. *et al.* (1992a) Activation of human basophils through the interleukin 8 receptor. *J. Immunol.*, **8**, 2662–7.

Krieger, M., von Tscharner, V. & Dahinden, C.A. (1992b) Signal transduction for interleukin-3 dependent leukotriene synthesis in normal human basophils: opposing role of tyrosine kinase and protein kinase C. *Eur. J. Immunol.*, **22**, 2907–13.

Kulmburg, P.A., Huber, N.E., Scheer, B.J., Wrann, M. & Baumruker, T. (1992) Immunoglobulin E plus antigen challenge induces a novel intercrine/chemokine in mouse mast cells. *J. Exp. Med.*, **176**, 1773–8.

Kuna, P., Alam, R., Kuzminska, B. & Rozniecki, J. (1989) The effect of preseasonal immunotherapy on the production of histamine-releasing factor (HRF) by mononuclear cells from patients with seasonal asthma: results of a double-blind, placebo-controlled, randomized study. *J. Allergy Clin. Immunol.*, **83**, 816–24.

Kuna, P., Reddigari, S.R., Rucinski, D., Oppenheim, J.J. & Kaplan, A.P. (1992a) Monocyte chemotactic and activating factor is a potent histamine-releasing factor for human basophils. *J. Exp. Med.*, **175**, 489–93.

Kuna, P., Reddigari, S.R., Schall, T.J., Rucinski, D., Viksman, M.Y. & Kaplan, A.P. (1992b) RANTES, a monocyte and T lymphocyte chemotactic cytokine releases histamine from human basophils. *J. Immunol.*, **149**, 636–42.

Kurimoto, Y., de Weck, A.L. & Dahinden, C.A. (1989) Interleukin 3-dependent mediator release in basophils triggered by C5a. *J. Exp. Med.*, **170**, 467–79.

Kurimoto, Y., de Weck, A.L. & Dahinden, C.A. (1991) The effect of interleukin 3 upon IgE-dependent and IgE-independent basophil degranulation and leukotriene generation. *Eur. J. Immunol.*, **21**, 361–8.

Larsen, C.G., Anderson, A.O., Appella, E., Oppenheim, J.J. & Matsushima, K. (1989) The neutrophil-activating protein, (NAP-1) is also chemotactic for T lymphocytes. *Science*, **243**, 1464–6.

Lichtenstein, L.M. (1988) Histamine releasing factor and IgE heterogeneity. *J. Allergy Clin. Immunol.*, **81**, 814–20.

Liu, M.C., Proud, D., Lichtenstein, L.M. *et al.* (1986) Human lung macrophage-derived, histamine-releasing activity is due to IgE-dependent factors. *J. Immunol.*, **136**, 2588–95.

Lodi, P.J., Garrett, D.S., Kuszewski, J. *et al.* (1994) High-resolution solution structure of the beta chemokine hMIP-1 beta by multidimensional NMR. *Science*, **263**, 1762–7.

Loetscher, P., Seitz, M., Clark-Lewis, I., Baggiolini, M. & Moser, B. (1994) Monocyte chemotactic proteins MCP-1, MCP-2, and MCP-3 are major attractants for human CD4+ and CD8+ T lymphocytes. *FASEB J.*, **8**, 1055–60.

Lukacs, N.W., Strieter, R.M., Shaklee, C.L., Chensue, S.W. & Kunkel, S.L. (1995) Macrophage inflammatory protein-1α influences eosinophil recruitment in antigen-specific airway inflammation. *Eur. J. Immunol.*, **25**, 245–51.

Luster, A.D., Greenberg, S.M. & Leder, P. (1995) The IP-10 chemokine binds to a specific cell surface heparan sulfate site shared with platelet factor 4 and inhibits endothelial cell proliferation. *J. Exp. Med.*, **182**, 219–31.

MacDonald, S., Rafnar, R., Langdon, J. & Lichtenstein, L.M. (1995) Molecular identification of an IgE-dependent histamine releasing factor. *Science*, **269**, 688–90.

Maghazachi, A.A., al Aoukaty, A. & Schall, T.J. (1994) C-C chemokines induce the chemotaxis of NK and IL-2-activated NK cells. Role for G proteins. *J. Immunol.*, **153**, 4969–77.

Maione, T.E., Gray, G.S., Petro, J. *et al.* (1990) Inhibition of angiogenesis by recombinant human platelet factor-4 and related peptides. *Science*, **247**, 77–9.

Marfaing-Koka, A., Devergne, O., Gorgone, G., *et al.* (1995) Regulation of the production of the RANTES chemokine by endothelial cells. Synergistic induction by IFN-gamma plus TNF-alpha and inhibition by IL-4 and IL-13. *J. Immunol.*, **154**, 1870–8.

Meurer, R., Van-Riper, G., Feeney, W. *et al.* (1993) Formation of eosinophilic and monocytic intradermal inflammatory sites in the dog by injection of human RANTES but not human monocyte chemoattractant protein 1, human macrophage inflammatory protein 1 alpha, or human interleukin 8. *J. Exp. Med.*, **178**, 1913–21.

Minty, A., Chalon, P., Guillemot, J.C. *et al.* (1993) Molecular cloning of the MCP-3 chemokine gene and regulation of its expression. *Eur. Cytokine Netw.*, **4**, 99–110.

Murphy, P.M. (1994) The molecular biology of leukocyte chemoattractant receptors. *Ann. Rev. Immunol.*, **12**, 593–633.

Murphy, W.J., Taub, D.D., Anver, M. *et al.* (1994) Human RANTES induces the migration of human T lymphocytes into the peripheral tissues of mice with severe combined immune deficiency. *Eur. J. Immunol.*, **24**, 1823–7.

Myers, S.J., Wong, L.M. & Charo, I.F. (1995) Signal transduction and ligand specificity of the human monocyte chemoattractant protein-1 receptor in transfected embryonic kidney cells. *J. Biol. Chem.*, **270**, 5786–92.

Nelken, N.A., Coughlin, S.R., Gordon, D. & Wilcox, J.N. (1991) Monocyte chemoattractant protein-1 in human atheromatous plaques. *J. Clin. Invest.*, **88**, 1121–7.

Neote, K., DiGregorio, D., Mak, J.Y., Horuk, R. & Schall, T.J. (1993) Molecular cloning, functional expression, and signaling characteristics of a C-C chemokine receptor. *Cell*, **72**, 415–25.

Neote, K., Mak, J.Y., Kolakowski, L.F. Jr & Schall, T.J. (1994) Functional and biochemical analysis of the cloned Duffy antigen: identity with the red blood cell chemokine receptor. *Blood*, **84**, 44–52.

Oppenheim, J.J., Zachariae, C.O., Mukaida, N. & Matsushima, K. (1991) Properties of the novel proinflammatory supergene 'intercrine' cytokine family. *Ann. Rev. Immunol.*, **9**, 617–48.

Paolini, J.F., Willard, D., Consler, T., Luther, M. & Krangel, M.S. (1994) The chemokines IL-8, monocyte chemoattractant protein-1, and I-309 are monomers at physiologically relevant concentrations. *J. Immunol.*, **153**, 2704–17.

Peiper, S.C., Wang, Z.X., Neote, K. *et al.* (1995) The Duffy antigen/receptor for chemokines (DARC) is expressed in endothelial cells of Duffy negative individuals who lack the erythrocyte receptor. *J. Exp. Med.*, **181**, 1311–17.

Ponath, P.D., Qin, S., Ringler, D.J. *et al.* (1996a) Cloning of the human eosinophil chemoattractant, eotaxin. Expression, receptor binding, and functional properties suggest a mechanism for the selective recruitment of eosinophils. *J. Clin. Invest.*, **97**, 604–12.

Ponath, P.D., Qin, S., Post, T.W. *et al.* (1996b) Molecular cloning and characterization of a human eotaxin receptor expressed selectively on eosinophils. *J. Exp. Med.*, **183**, 2437–48.

Power, C.A., Meyer, A., Nemeth, K. *et al.* (1995) Molecular cloning and functional expression of a novel CC chemokine receptor cDNA from a human basophilic cell line. *J. Biol. Chem.*, **270**, 19495–500.

Rathanaswami, P., Hachicha, M., Sadick, M., Schall, T.J. & McColl, S.R. (1993) Expression of the cytokine RANTES in human rheumatoid synovial fibroblasts. Differential regulation of RANTES and interleukin-8 genes by inflammatory cytokines. *J. Biol. Chem.*, **268**, 5834–9.

Rot, A. (1992) Endothelial cell binding of NAP-1/IL-8: role in neutrophil emigration. *Immunol. Today*, **13**, 291–4.

Rot, A., Krieger, M., Brunner, Th., Bischoff, S.C., Shall, T. & Dahinden, C.A. (1992) Rantes and MIP-1α induce the migration and activation of normal human eosinophil granulocytes. *J. Exp. Med.*, **176**, 1489–95.

Rothenberg, M.E., Luster, A.D., Lilly, C.M., Drazen, J.M. & Leder, P. (1995) Constitutive and allergen-induced expression of eotaxin mRNA in the guinea pig lung. *J. Exp. Med.*, **181**, 1211–16.

Sampson, H.A., Broabent, K.R. & Bernhisel-Broadbent, J. (1989) Spontaneous basophil histamine release and histamine releasing factor in patients with atopic dermatitis and food hypersensitivity. *New Engl. J. Med.*, **321**, 228–32.

Samson, M., Labbe, O., Mollereau, C., Vassart, G. & Parmentier, M. (1996) Molecular cloning and functional expression of a new human CC-chemokine receptor gene. *Biochemistry*, **35**, 3362–7.

Schall, T.J. (1991) Biology of the RANTES/SIS cytokine gene family. *Cytokine*, **3**, 165–83.

Schall, T.J. & Bacon, K.B. (1994) Chemokines, leukocyte trafficking, and inflammation. *Curr. Opin. Immunol.*, **6**, 865–73.

Schall, T.J., Bacon, K., Camp, R.D., Kaspari, J.W. & Goeddel, D.V. (1993) Human macrophage inflammatory protein alpha (MIP-1 alpha) and MIP-1 beta chemokines attract distinct populations of lymphocytes. *J. Exp. Med.*, **177**, 1821–6.

Schall, T.J., Bacon, K., Toy, K.J. & Goeddel, D.V. (1990) Selective attraction of monocytes and T lymphocytes of the memory phenotype by cytokine RANTES. *Nature*, **347**, 669–71.

Schall, T.J., Mak, J.Y., DiGregorio, D. & Neote, K. (1993) Receptor/ligand interactions in the C-C chemokine family. *Adv. Exp. Med. Biol.*, **351**, 29–37.

Schleimer, R.P., Sterbinsky, S.A., Kaiser, J. *et al.* (1992) IL-4 induces adherence of human eosinophils and basophils but not neutrophils to endothelium: association with expression of VCAM-1. *J. Immunol.*, **148**, 1086–92.

Schulman, E.S., McGettigan, M.C., Post, T.J., Vigderman, R.J. & Shapiro, S.S. (1988) Human monocytes generate basophil histamine releasing activities. *J. Immunol.*, **7**, 2369–75.

Schweizer, R.C., Welmers, B.A., Raaijmakers, J.A., Zanen, P., Lammers, J.W. & Koenderman, L. (1994) RANTES- and interleukin-8-induced responses in normal human eosinophils: effects of priming with interleukin-5. *Blood*, **83**, 3697–704.

Shaw, J.P., Kryger, G., Cleasby, A. *et al.* (1994) Crystallization and preliminary X-ray diffraction studies of human RANTES. *J. Mol. Biol.*, **242**, 589–90.

Sousa, A.R., Lane, S.J., Nakhosteen, J.A., Yoshimura, T., Lee, T.H. & Poston, R.N. (1994) Increased expression of the monocyte chemoattractant protein-1 in bronchial tissue from asthmatic subjects. *Am. J. Respir. Cell. Mol. Biol.*, **10**, 142–7.

Springer, T.A. (1994) Traffic signals for lymphocyte recirculation and leukocyte emigration: the multistep paradigm. *Cell*, **76**, 301–14.

Takafuji, S., Bischoff, S.C., de Weck, A.L. & Dahinden, C.A. (1991) Interleukin 3 and interleukin 5 prime normal human eosinophils to produce leukotriene C4 in response to soluble agonists. *J. Immunol.*, **147**, 3855–61.

Takafuji, S., Bischoff, S.C., de Weck, A.L. & Dahinden, C.A. (1992) Opposing effects of tumor necrosis factor-α and nerve growth factor upon leukotriene C4 production by human eosinophils triggered with *N*-formyl-methionyl-leucyl-phenylalanine. *Eur. J. Immunol.*, **22**, 969–74.

Takafuji, S., Tadokoro, K., Ito, K. & Dahinden, C.A. (1994) Degranulation from human eosinophils stimulated with C3a and C5a. *Int. Arch. Allergy Immunol.*, **104**, s27–9.

Tanaka, Y., Adams, D.H., Hubscher, S., Hirano, H., Siebenlist, U. & Shaw, S. (1993) T cell adhesion induced by proteoglycan-immobilized cytokine MIP-1β. *Nature*, **361**, 79–82.

Taub, D.D., Conlon, K., Lloyd, A.R., Oppenheim, J.J. & Kelvin, D.J. (1993a) Preferential migration of activated CD4+ and CD8+ T cells in response to MIP-1 alpha and MIP-1 beta. *Science*, **260**, 355–8.

Taub, D.D., Lloyd, A.R., Conlon, K. *et al.* (1993b) Recombinant human interferon-inducible protein 10 is a chemoattractant for human monocytes and T lymphocytes and promotes T cell adhesion to endothelial cells. *J. Exp. Med.*, **177**, 1809–14.

Taub, D.D., Lloyd, A.R., Wang, J.M., Oppenheim, J.J. & Kelvin, D.J. (1993c) The effects of human recombinant MIP-1 alpha, MIP-1 beta, and RANTES on the chemotaxis and adhesion of T cell subsets. *Adv. Exp. Med. Biol.*, **351**, 139–46.

Thirion, S., Nys, G., Fiten, P., Masure, S., Van Damme, J. & Opdenakker, G. (1994) Mouse macrophage derived monocyte chemotactic protein-3: cDNA cloning and identification as MARC/FIC. *Biochem. Biophys. Res. Commun.*, **201**, 493–9.

Thueson, D.O., Speck, L.S., Lett-Brown, M.A. & Grant, J.A. (1979) Histamine-releasing activity (HRA). I. Production by mitogen- or antigen-stimulated human mononuclear cells. *J. Immunol.*, **123**, 626–32.

Uguccioni, M., D'Apuzzo, M., Loetscher, M., Dewald, B. & Baggiolini, M. (1995) Actions of the chemotactic cytokines MCP-1, MCP-2, MCP-3, RANTES, MIP-1 alpha and MIP-1 beta on human monocytes. *Eur. J. Immunol.*, **25**, 64–8.

Uguccioni, M., Loetscher, P., Forssmann, U. *et al.* (1996) Monocyte chemoattractant protein 4 (MCP-4), a novel structural and functional analog of MCP-3 and eotaxin. *J. Exp. Med.*, **183**, 2379–84.

Vaddi, K. & Newton, R.C. (1994) Regulation of monocyte integrin expression by β-family chemokines. *J. Immunol.*, **153**, 4721–32.

Van Damme, J., Proost, P., Lenaerts, J.P. & Opdenakker, G. (1992) Structural and functional identification of two human, tumor-derived monocyte chemotactic proteins (MCP-2 and MCP-3) belonging to the chemokine family. *J. Exp. Med.*, **176**, 59–65.

Weber, M., Uguccioni, M., Baggiolini, M., Clark-Lewis, I. & Dahinden, C.A. (1996) Deletion of the NH_2-terminal residue converts monocyte chemotactic protein 1 from an activator of basophil mediator release to an eosinohpil chemoattractant. *J. Exp. Med.*, **183**, 681–5.

Weber, M., Uguccioni, M., Ochensberger, B., Baggiolini, M., Clark-Lewis, I. & Dahinden, C.A. (1995) The monocyte chemotactic protein MCP-2 activates human basophil and eosinophil leukocytes similar to MCP-3. *J. Immunol.*, **154**, 4166–72.

Witt, D.P. & Lander, A.D. (1994) Differential binding of chemokines to glycosaminoglycan subpopulations. *Curr. Biol.*, **4**, 394–400.

Xu, L., Kelvin, D.J., Ye, G.Q., Taub, D.D., Ben-Baruch, A., Oppenheim, J.J. & Wang, J.M. (1995) Modulation of IL-8 receptor expression on purified human T lymphocytes is associated with changed chemotactic responses to IL-8. *J. Leukocyte Biol.*, **57**, 335–42.

Yamagami, S., Tokuda, Y., Ishii, K., Tanaka, H. & Endo, N. (1994) cDNA cloning and functional expression of a human monocyte chemoattractant protein 1 receptor. *Biochem. Biophys. Res. Commun.*, **202**, 1156–62.

Ying, S., Taborda-Barata, L., Meng, Q., Humbert, M. & Kay, A.B. (1995) The kinetics of allergen-induced transcription of messenger RNA for monocyte chemotactic protein-3 and RANTES in the skin of human atopic subjects: relationship to eosinophil, T cell, and macrophage recruitment. *J. Exp. Med.*, **181**, 2153–9.

Zhang, Y.J., Rutledge, B.J. & Rollins, B.J. (1994) Structure/activity analysis of human monocyte chemoattractant protein-1 (MCP-1) by mutagenesis. Identification of a mutated protein that inhibits MCP-1-mediated monocyte chemotaxis. *J. Biol. Chem.*, **269**, 15918–24.

CHAPTER 23

Lipid Mediators—Leukotrienes, Prostanoids and Platelet-Activating Factor

S.M.S. Nasser & T.H. Lee

Introduction

The leukotrienes and prostanoids (prostaglandins and thromboxane) form part of a family of oxygenated fatty acids found in virtually every mammalian cell. Physiologically these products of arachidonic acid metabolism participate in many normal processes, which include body temperature regulation, the coagulation cascade, control of parturition, blood pressure maintenance and mediation of the immune system. Pathologically, these lipid mediators have been incriminated in a wide range of diseases, including asthma, psoriasis, rheumatoid arthritis, inflammatory bowel disease and malignancy.

Much of the early work on prostaglandins was carried out by three groups led by Sune Bergstrom, Bengt Samuelsson and John Vane. Bergstrom determined the structure and the biological role of the prostaglandins and discovered that they are synthesized *in vivo* from dietary polyunsaturated fatty acids; Samuelsson determined the metabolic fate and disposition of the prostaglandins; and Vane demonstrated the ability of anti-inflammatory substances, such as aspirin, to inhibit prostaglandin synthesis. However, the original investigation of these compounds began in 1930, with the work of Raphael Kurzok and Charles Lieb, who studied the ability of human semen either to relax or to contract isolated strips of uterine tissue. Three years later, Goldblatt and von Euler independently observed a similar phenomenon using human seminal plasma and extracts from sheep seminal vesical glands. Von Euler therefore coined the term prostaglandin, believing that he had isolated a product of the prostate gland.

Leukotrienes were discovered during the elucidation of a mixture of compounds referred to as the slow-reacting substance of anaphylaxis or SRS-A. In 1938, Feldberg and Kellaway coined the term SRS to define the smooth-muscle contracting activity found in the effluent of the perfused lungs of guinea pigs and cats following treatment with cobra venom. In 1940, Kellawey and Trethewie found that smooth-muscle contractions in anaphylaxis were caused not only by histamine but also in part by a slow-reacting substance. Brocklehurst (1956) unmasked the SRS by demonstrating that the contraction it produced on the isolated guinea pig ileum was not inhibited by an antihistamine added to the organ bath. He also showed that the pattern of contraction was different from bradykinin, substance P and 5-hydroxytryptamine and added the suffix 'A' to indicate that this was a particular slow-reacting substance associated with anaphylaxis. The 1960s and the 1970s saw the purification and description of many biological and physicochemical properties of SRS-A by Orange, Austen, Murphy (Orange & Austen, 1969; Orange *et al.*, 1973), Morris *et al.* (1980), Lewis (1980a) and others. The covalent structure and total synthesis of SRS-A and its identification as a mixture of the sulphidopeptide leukotrienes, leukotriene C_4 (LTC_4), and its biologically active metabolites LTD_4 and LTE_4, was achieved by Samuelsson *et al.* (1980) and Corey *et al.* (1980).

The leukotrienes and the prostanoids are not preformed, but upon cell activation are synthesized *de novo*. The primary substrate fatty acid which acts as a precursor for leukotrienes and prostanoids is 5,8,11,14-eicosatetraenoic acid (arachidonic acid). Arachidonic acid is released from nuclear membrane phospholipids. Subsequent oxidative metabolism of this polyunsaturated fatty acid by the lipoxygenase pathway yields the leukotrienes, and by the cyclo-oxygenase pathway leads to prostanoid synthesis.

Leukotrienes

Biosynthesis

Samuelsson conceived the term leukotriene to describe a family of compounds each containing three conjugated double bonds and derived from the conversion of arachidonic acid by 5-lipoxygenase (5-LO) in leucocytes. He subjected arachidonic acid to the actions of various lipoxygenases and found that rabbit polymorphonuclear leucocytes (PMN) metabolized arachidonate to a family of dihydroxy acids that showed triple spectrophotometric absorption peaks at 259, 269 and 279 nm. These triple peaks suggested the existence of triple conjugated double bonds in these compounds. Arachidonic acid is a 20-carbon polyunsaturated fatty acid released from membrane phospholipids by the action of phospholipase A_2. The enzyme 5-LO catalyses the first step in arachidonic acid metabolism (Fig. 23.1) by inserting oxygen at C-5 to produce the unstable intermediate 5S-hydroperoxyeicosatetraenoic acid (5-HPETE). This is either reduced to the alcohol 5S-hydroxyeicosatetraenoic acid (5-HETE) or converted by 5-LO via a dehydrase step to a C-5,6-transepoxide with three conjugated (7,9-*trans*,11-*cis*) olefinic bonds, and a fourth, unconjugated double bond at C-14. This compound was the first leukotriene described and designated LTA_4. Subsequent metabolism of LTA_4 takes place via two alternative enzymatic pathways, either by an epoxide hydrolase to 5S,12R-dihydroxyeicosatetraenoic acid (LTB_4) or by opening the epoxide by a glutathione S-transferase termed LTC_4 synthase to LTC_4. In the absence of either activated enzyme system, LTA_4 degrades spontaneously to 6-*trans*-LTB_4, which has significantly less bioactivity. LTC_4 is subsequently cleaved to form the 6R-S-cysteinylglycine analogue, LTD_4 by removal of glutamic acid from the peptide by γ-glutamyltranspeptidase. LTD_4 is further cleaved by a dipeptidase to remove glycine to form its 6R-S-cysteinyl analogue (LTE_4). These latter three compounds are known collectively as the sulphidopeptide or cysteinyl leukotrienes, because of the presence of a peptide linked to the eicosanoid backbone through a thiolether link at C-6. The structure of the leukotrienes is shown in Fig. 23.2. The sulphidopeptide leukotrienes comprise the activity previously recognized as the SRS-A.

Although the enzyme 5-LO is the rate-limiting step for leukotriene formation, it requires the association of an additional factor. Mammalian osteosarcoma cells transfected with 5-LO express active enzyme in broken cell preparations but no leukotriene metabolites on stimulation with the calcium ionophore A23187 (Rouzer *et al.*, 1988). In addition, a new class of indole leukotriene biosynthesis inhibitor MK-886 was found to act only on intact PMN but had no direct inhibitory effect on soluble 5-LO activity (Gillard *et al.*, 1989). A membrane protein of M_r 18 kDa was identified with high affinity for MK-886 from rat and human leucocytes, and it was demonstrated that expression of both 5-LO and this MK-886 binding protein was necessary for leukotriene synthesis. This was confirmed by its specific labelling with a ^{125}I-radiolabelled photoaffinity probe and by its retention on agarose gels to which analogues of MK-886 had been bound. This protein was termed 5-lipoxygenase-activating protein (FLAP) (Miller *et al.*, 1990). Using hydrophobic moment analysis, three hydrophobic regions of 20–30 residues were proposed which predicted three transmembrane domains connected by two hydrophilic loops. In osteosarcoma cells transfected with 5-LO or FLAP alone and stimulated with the calcium ionophore A23187, no arachidonic acid metabolites were detected. By contrast, A23187 treatment of cell lines expressing both 5-LO and FLAP resulted in significant production of 5-LO products (Dixon *et al.*,

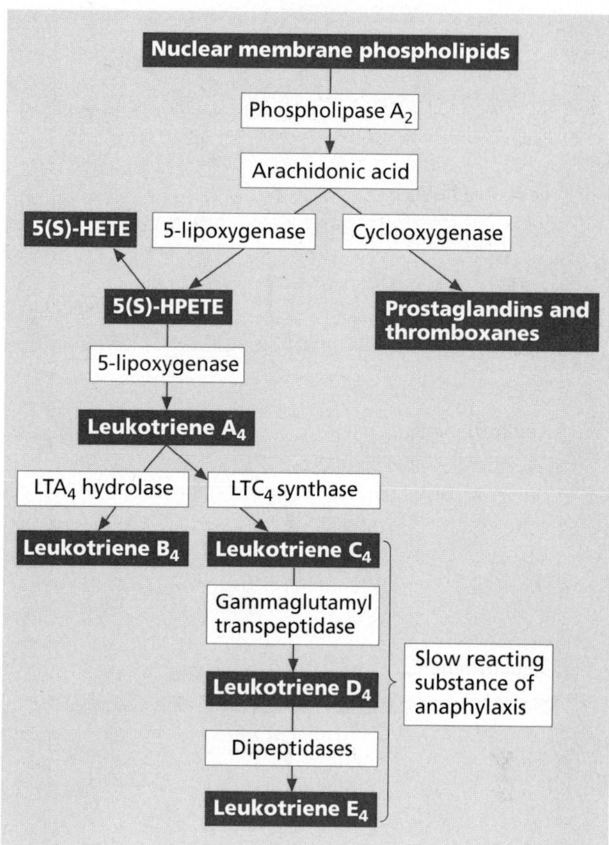

Fig. 23.1 Leukotriene biosynthesis from nuclear membrane phospholipids and arachidonic acid via the 5-lipoxygenase pathway. 5(*S*)-HPETE, 5(*S*)-hydroperoxyeicosatetraenoic acid; 5(*S*)-HETE, 5(*S*)-hydroxyeicosatetraenoic acid.

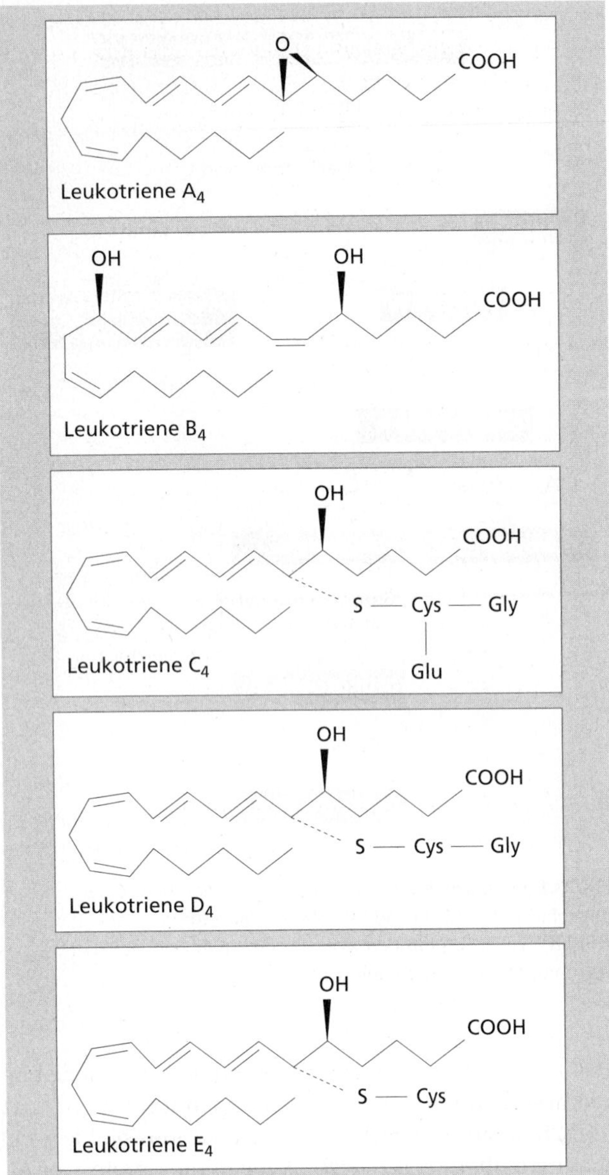

Fig. 23.2 Chemical structure of the leukotrienes.

1990). The human pro-myelocytic cell lines U937 express FLAP but not 5-LO, and are unable to synthesize leukotrienes after A23187 stimulation but do so after transfection by a retroviral vector encoding 5-LO mRNA (Kargman *et al.*, 1993). Human B-lymphocyte lines and normal human tonsillar B lymphocytes have 5-LO activity and can produce LTB_4 upon cell activation (Jakobsson *et al.*, 1991), but five T-cell lines were found to express only FLAP and not 5-LO and therefore were unable to generate leukotrienes upon cell activation (Jakobsson *et al.*, 1992).

The mechanism of cellular activation and subsequent leukotriene generation is believed to arise as a result of translocation of 5-LO from cytosolic to membrane compartments, to bring the enzyme into close proximity with FLAP which acts as an anchor for 5-LO and provides access to substrate and other components of leukotriene synthesis. In osteosarcoma cells expressing 5-LO but not FLAP, 5-LO is able to associate with cell membranes following A23187 stimulation and this is not inhibited by MK-886. This has led the authors to conclude that 5-LO membrane association and activation can be divided into a two-stage process: (i) Ca^{2+}-dependent movement of 5-LO to membrane without product formation which can occur in the absence of FLAP, and (ii) activation of 5-LO with product formation which is FLAP dependent and inhibited by MK-886 (Kargman *et al.*, 1992). High levels of FLAP were expressed in SF9 insect cells transfected with recombinant baclovirus and this system was used to demonstrate that FLAP specifically binds [^{125}I] L-739,059, a photoaffinity analogue of arachidonic acid. This binding is inhibited by both arachidonic acid and MK-886 and suggests that FLAP may activate 5-LO by bringing enzyme and substrate together (Mancini *et al.*, 1993). Ultracentrifugation (Peters-Golden & McNish, 1993) and immunoelectron microscopy studies have demonstrated that on cellular activation 5-LO translocates to the nuclear envelope which is also the location of FLAP (Woods *et al.*, 1993). The situation in resting cells is still uncertain, and 5-LO may be located in the cytosol (Rouzer & Kargman, 1988) or nuclear euchromatin (Woods *et al.*, 1994).

Cellular sources

Because of the requirement to express both 5-LO and FLAP, the range of cells known to synthesize leukotrienes is limited. Cells of myeloid lineage provide the major source of leukotriene production, although recently B lymphocytes have also been shown to be capable of generating small quantities of leukotrienes (Jakobsson *et al.*, 1991). Cells can be divided by their ability to preferentially synthesize LTB_4 or the cysteinyl leukotrienes, LTC_4, LTD_4 and LTE_4, depending on the intracellular predominance of either LTA_4 epoxide hydrolase or LTC_4 synthase. Monocytes, alveolar macrophages and peripheral blood netrophils preferentially generate LTB_4, whereas eosinophils, mast cells and basophils preferentially generate cysteinyl leukotriene products. Monocytes and macrophages have the capacity to generate both LTB_4 and LTC_4. Peripheral blood monocytes in adherent monolayers produce 68 ng LTB_4 and 30 ng LTC_4 per 10^6 cells on stimulation with the ionophore A23187 (Williams *et al.*, 1984). LTB_4 is the major lipoxygenase product of alveolar macrophages which generate 17–30 ng/10^6 cells in response to calcium ionophore A23187 stimulation (Fels *et al.*, 1982). Peripheral blood neutrophils from normal donors produce about 48 ng $LTB_4/10^6$ cells, with only one-

Table 23.1 Cellular source of human leukotriene generation.

Cell	Predominant leukotriene product	Activating stimulus	Approximate amount generated/ 10^6 cells
Neutrophils	LTB_4	A23187	50 ng
	LTC_4	A23187	10 ng
Eosinophils	LTB_4	A23187	10 ng
	LTC_4	A23187	40 ng
Peripheral blood	LTB_4	A23187	70 ng
monocytes	LTC_4		30 ng
Alveolar macrophages	LTB_4	A23187	30 ng
Mast cells	LTC_4	A23187 or anti-IgE	20 ng
Basophils	LTC_4	A23187	10 ng

A23187, divalent calcium ionophore.

seventh as much $LTC_4/10^6$ cells after A23187 stimulation. Eosinophils from the same subjects preferentially synthesize LTC_4 and produce 38 ng $LTC_4/10^6$ cells and about 6 ng $LTB_4/10^6$ in response to A23187 stimulation (Weller *et al.*, 1983). Activation of leucocytes is accompanied by respiratory burst activity with reduction of oxygen to form superoxide anion (O_2^-) and hydrogen peroxide (H_2O_2) and the release of cytoplasmic contents, including eosinophil peroxidase (EPO) from eosinophils and myeloperoxidase (MPO) from neutrophils or monocytes. This leads to oxidative degradation of the cysteinyl leukotrienes and acts as a control over their biological effects. EPO or MPO catalyse the oxidation of halides by H_2O_2 to form hypohalous acids such a HOCl, HOBr or HOI, which readily degrade cysteinyl leukotrienes to their inactive sulphoxide derivatives and to 6-*trans*-stereoisomers of LTB_4 (Henderson *et al.*, 1982; Henderson & Klebanoff, 1983). Human lung mast cells release 22 ng $LTC_4/10^6$ cells, with similar amounts released in response to either IgE- or calcium ionophore A23187-mediated degranulation (Peters *et al.*, 1984). Basophils obtained from the peripheral blood of patients with chronic myelogenous leukaemia were found to release LTB_4 (Rothenberg *et al.*, 1987). Basophils also release LTC_4, but unlike mast cells do not produce prostaglandin D_2 (PGD_2). Local instillation of specific allergen into the nasal mucosa of sensitive subjects leads to recovery of histamine, PGD_2 and LTC_4 from nasal secretions during the early-phase, but only histamine and LTC_4 during the late-phase reaction. These findings suggest that mast cell degranulation is important in the early-phase response to allergen and that basophils mediate the late reaction (Naclerio *et al.*, 1983; Creticos *et al.*, 1984). B lymphocytes produce only small amounts of LTB_4 and 5-HETE upon stimulation with A23187, in comparison to the amounts produced by the sonicates of these cells. However, pre-incubation with a glutathione-depleting agent prior to stimulation leads to similar amounts of LTB_4 generated by the intact cells as are formed by the sonicated cells. T lymphocytes express the FLAP gene but not the 5-LO gene and therefore do not generate leukotrienes (Jakobsson *et al.*, 1992). Guinea pig lung parenchyma has been shown to convert LTA_4 to LTB_4, LTC_4, LTD_4 and LTE_4 (Sirois *et al.*, 1985) and human lung parenchyma converts LTC_4 to LTD_4 and LTE_4 (Aharony *et al.*, 1985; Conroy *et al.*, 1989).

Unlike 5-LO, LTC_4 synthase and LTA_4 hydrolase, which convert LTA_4 to LTC_4 and LTB_4, respectively, are widely distributed. Thus, LTA_4 released by a cell capable of generating 5-LO products, may be utilized for further metabolism by other cells without the enzyme 5-LO. Such transcellular metabolism can lead to the generation of LTC_4 by platelets, (Edenius *et al.*, 1988; Maclouf & Murphy, 1988), mast cells (Dahinden *et al.*, 1985), airway epithelium and vascular endothelial cells (Feinmark & Cannon, 1986), or to the generation of LTB_4 by erythrocytes from LTA_4 supplied by neutrophils (McGee & Fitzpatrick, 1986) (Fig. 23.3).

Leukotriene metabolism and elimination

Removal of the leukotrienes from sites of inflammation requires rapid inactivation by specific and appropriately located enzymes. LTB_4–20-hydroxylase (P-450_{LTB}) is located exclusively in neutrophil microsomes and converts LTB_4 by ω-oxygenation to 20-OH–LTB_4, which has substantially less PMN leucocyte chemotactic and activating activity than LTB_4. Further metabolism takes place by oxidation to 5S,12R-dihydroxy-20-aldehyde-6,14-*cis*-8,10-*trans*-eicosatetraenoic acid (20-CHO–LTB_4), which has no biological activity. This is followed by irreversible conversion to 20-carboxy-6,14-*cis*-8,10-*trans*-eicosatetraenoic acid (20-COOH–LTB_4). 20-CHO–LTB_4 can be converted via an alternative pathway by an aldehyde reductase in the microsomes back to 20-OH–LTB_4, thereby allowing tightly regulated LTB_4 degradation.

LTC_4 can be bioconverted by three major metabolic pathways. The first comprises conversion of LTC_4 by peptide cleavage to LTD_4 and then to LTE_4 by the action of γ-glutamyl transpeptidase and one of a variety of dipeptidases, respectively. This does not require activation of the cells involved and may only result in some loss of biological activity. The second pathway involves the oxidative metabolism of the cysteinyl leukotrienes and depends on the production of hydrogen peroxide by the respiratory burst and secretion of cell-specific peroxidase, which occurs only in the extracellular microenvironment of activated neutrophils, eosinophils and monocytes. A peroxidase–hypochlorous acid reaction then transforms

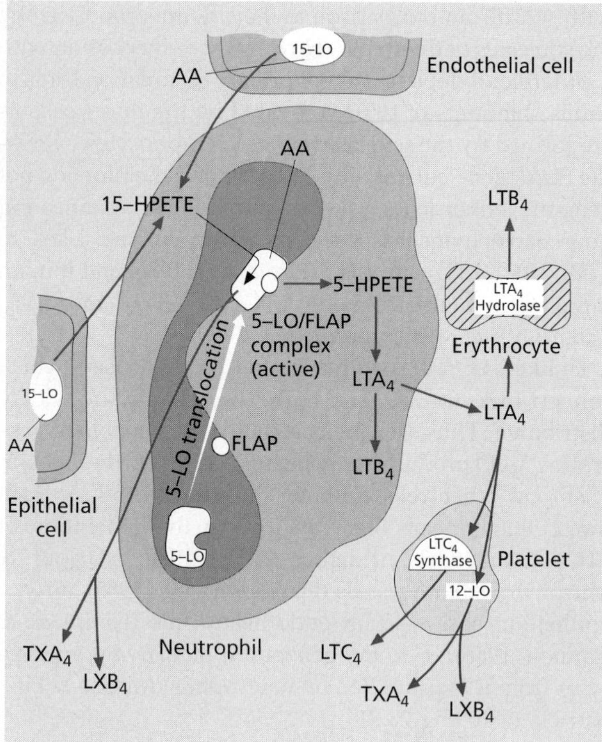

Fig. 23.3 Transcellular biosynthesis of leukotrienes and lipoxins by cell–cell interaction between polymorphonuclear (PMN) leucocytes and platelets for cysteinyl leukotriene production or PMN leucocytes and either platelets, epithelial or endothelial cells for lipoxin generation. Human 5-hypoxygenase (5-LO) is located in the cytosol or nuclear euchromatin of the resting cell, and upon activation is translocated to form a complex with 5-LO activating protein (FLAP) to express enzymatic activity. Endothelial and epithelial cells contain 15-LO and platelets contain both 12-LO and leukotriene C_4 (LTC_4) synthetase activity.

LTC_4, LTD_4 and LTE_4 to their respective S-diastereoisomeric sulphoxides and to the 6-*trans*-(C1–12)-diastereoisomers of LTB_4. Each of the S-diastereomeric sulphoxides is then converted to its respective sulphone, which results in considerable loss of bioactivity. The 6-*trans*-LTB_4-diastereoisomers are not immunoreactive in a sulphidopeptide leukotriene assay and are non-spasmogenic. The sulphoxides are fully immunoreactive but possess less than 5% spasmogenic activity. The third pathway involves β-oxidation and elimination leading to carboxylation, hydroxylation and the gradual shortening of the ω-segment of the molecule. A fraction of infused LTE_4 is excreted unchanged in urine and because this fraction remains constant urinary concentrations of LTE_4 have been used to reflect systemic synthesis of LTC_4. It is likely that cellular activation leads not only to enhanced leukotriene release but also to the increased capacity to degrade them.

Biological activity

LTB_4

LTB_4 acts at the level of the microvasculature by increasing leucocyte adherence to endothelium (Hoover *et al.*, 1984) and enhancing cutaneous microvascular permeability by the secondary action of an unidentified neutrophil-derived factor (Bray *et al.*, 1981; Issekutz, 1981). Other activities include potent chemotaxis for neutrophils, mediated by a subset of high-affinity receptors and chemokinetic and weak chemotactic activity for eosinophils (Palmer *et al.*, 1980; Nagy *et al.*, 1982). LTB_4 is chemokinetic for monocytes (Palmer *et al.*, 1980); enhances expression of CR1 and CR3 receptors on neutrophils and eosinophils (Nagy *et al.*, 1982; Lee *et al.*, 1988); aggregates neutrophils (Ford-Hutchinson *et al.*, 1980); and releases lysosomal enzymes and generates superoxide via a subset of low-affinity receptors (Goldman & Goetzl, 1984). LTB_4 is bronchoconstricting, especially when administered intravenously, and this action is mediated indirectly through the action of thromboxane A_2 (TXA_2) synthesized locally in lung tissue (Sirois *et al.*, 1982). LTB_4 also has immunoregulatory functions. At concentrations of 10^{-12} to 10^{-8} mol/l, LTB_4 significantly enhances natural killer cytotoxicity for virus-infected cells and the tumour

Table 23.2 Biological activity of leukotriene B_4.

Activity	Reference
Increase leucocyte adherence to endothelium	Hoover *et al.*, 1984
Increase microvascular permeability (secondary action)	Bray *et al.*, 1981; Issekutz, 1981
Neutrophil chemotaxis and weak eosinophil chemotaxis	Palmer *et al.*, 1980; Nayy *et al.*, 1982
Monocyte chemokinesis	Palmer *et al.*, 1980
Enhanced expression of CR1 and CR3 receptors on neutrophils and eosinophils	Nagy *et al.*, 1982; Lee *et al.*, 1988
Neutrophil aggregation	Ford-Hutchinson *et al.*, 1980
Lysosomal release and superoxide generation	Goldman & Goetzl, 1984
Bronchoconstriction via secondary release of TXA_2	Sirois *et al.*, 1982
Enhanced NK cell cytotoxicity for virus-infected and tumour cells	Rola-Pleszczynski, 1985
Induction of suppressor T lymphocytes	Atluru & Goodwin, 1986
Enhances IgG production by human B lymphocytes and augments IL-2 and IFN-γ production by T lymphocytes	Rola-Pleszczynski *et al.*, 1986

See text for definition of abbreviations.

cell line K-562 (Rola-Pleszczynski, 1985). It induces increased numbers of suppressor T lymphocytes from precursors (Atluru & Goodwin, 1986). It directly increases immunoglobulin G (IgG) production by highly purified human tonsillar B lymphocytes and augments IL-2 and interferon-γ (IFN-γ) production in human T lymphocytes (Rola-Pleszczynski *et al.*, 1986).

Cysteinyl leukotrienes

LTD_4 and with lesser potency LTC_4 and LTE_4 augment post-capillary dermal venular permeability when administered locally to guinea pigs, as shown by the leakage of intravenously administered dye (Drazen *et al.*, 1980a; Lewis *et al.*, 1980b). The cysteinyl leukotrienes increase microvascular permeability influenced by the contraction of adjacent endothelial cells (Drazen *et al.*, 1980a; Joris *et al.*, 1987) and augment leucocyte adhesion to endothelial cells (McIntyre *et al.*, 1986). The local application of the cysteinyl leukotrienes to the buccal mucosa produces submucosal oedema in hamsters (Dahlén *et al.*, 1981) and subcutaneous injection in humans produces dermal oedema sustained for 2–4 hours (Soter *et al.*, 1983). As little as 10^{-9} mol/l LTC_4 and LTD_4 have been postulated to stimulate mucus secretion from studies of bronchial mucosal explants, and this may contribute to the excess mucus secretion found in bronchial asthma (Marom *et al.*, 1982b). This is a non-stereospecific effect and is therefore unlikely to be receptor mediated (Coles *et al.*, 1983). The cysteinyl leukotrienes are potent contractile agonists for bronchial smooth muscle in isolated human lobar and segmental bronchi, with LTC_4 and LTD_4 reported to be approximately 1000 times more potent than histamine in contracting human bronchi *in vitro* (Dahlén *et al.*, 1980).

Table 23.3 Biological activity of cysteinyl leukotrienes.

Activity	Reference
Augment post-capillary dermal vascular permeability in guinea pigs	Drazen *et al.*, 1980a; Lewis *et al.*, 1980a
Increased microvascular permeability	Drazen *et al.*, 1980a; Joris *et al.*, 1987
Increase leucocyte adhesion to endothelial cells	McIntyre *et al.*, 1986
Increase mucus secretion	Marom *et al.*, 1982a
Potent contractile agonists for bronchial smooth muscle	Dahlen *et al.*, 1980
Vasoconstriction	Camp *et al.*, 1983; Soter *et al.*, 1983
Coronary vasoconstriction in sheep	Michelassi *et al.*, 1982
Systemic vasoconstriction in rats	Pfeffer *et al.*, 1983
Renal vasoconstriction in rats	Badr *et al.*, 1984
Recruit granulocytes into the lamina propria of asthmatic airways (LTE_4)	Laitenen *et al.*, 1993

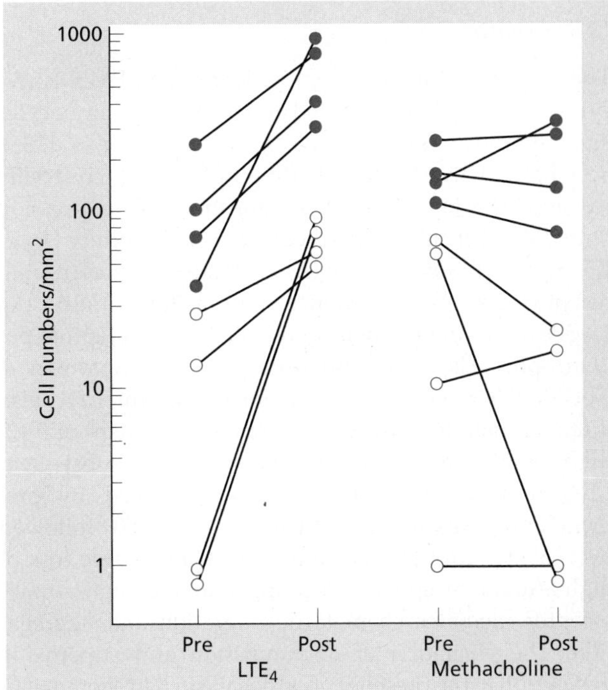

Fig. 23.4 Change in the number of eosinophils (closed circles) and neutrophils (neutrophils) in the lamina propria of airways mucosa before and after provocation with inhaled LTE_4 or methacholine (Laitinen *et al.*, 1993).

Studies using inhaled cysteinyl leukotrienes have demonstrated the potency of these mediators, both in normal and asthmatic subjects, in causing bronchoconstriction, with LTC_4 being the most potent and LTE_4 being the least active (Adelroth *et al.*, 1986; Drazen, 1988; Arm *et al.*, 1990). LTC_4 and, to a lesser extent, LTD_4 have demonstrated vasoconstrictor properties in guinea pig skin after intradermal injection (Drazen *et al.*, 1980a; Lewis *et al.*, 1980b), and in normal human skin by blanching of an elicited weal at the injection site (Camp *et al.*, 1983; Soter *et al.*, 1983). Coronary vasoconstriction has been demonstrated in sheep after direct infusion into a coronary vessel *in vivo* (Michelassi *et al.*, 1982). In the rat, intravenous infusion of LTC_4 led to systemic vasoconstriction (Pfeffer *et al.*, 1983) and renal vasoconstriction (Badr *et al.*, 1984). Recently, LTE_4 has been demonstrated to recruit granulocytes and particularly eosinophils into the lamina propria of asthmatic airways (Laitinen *et al.*, 1993) (Fig. 23.4).

Receptors

The leukotriene receptors have not been cloned but data from novel pharmacological antagonists indicate that leukotrienes mediate their actions through specific receptor interactions.

LTB_4 receptors

The LTB_4 receptor was initially identified in PMN leucocytes and later demonstrated in eosinophils, monocytes and lymphocytes (Rola-Pleszczynski *et al.*, 1986). Scatchard analysis of the binding of $[^3H]LTB_4$ to freshly isolated PMN leucocytes has demonstrated the expression of two distinct subsets of receptors. A high-affinity (K_d of 0.5–5 nmol/l), low-density (20×10^3 sites per neutrophil) receptor has been identified and a low-affinity (K_d 15–500 nmol/l), high-density ($40–400 \times 10^3$ receptors per neutrophil) class has also been detected (Goldman & Goetzl, 1982). These two receptor classes for LTB_4 also differ in their stereospecificity for stereoisomers of 5,12-diHETE. A decreased chemotactic response to subsequent LTB_4 termed deactivation, can be achieved by pre-incubating PMN leucocytes with 1×10^{-8} LTB_4 followed by washing, and this is paralleled by a selective loss of high-affinity receptors indicating that the high-affinity receptor mediates chemotactic migration and aggregation. The elicitation of degranulation and superoxide generation in the presence of cytochalasin B in chemotactically deactivated PMN leucocytes which do not express high-affinity receptors and the requirement of significantly higher concentrations of LTB_4 than for chemotaxis implies that degranulation is mediated by the low-affinity receptor for LTB_4 (Goldman & Goetzl, 1984). Using differentiated HL-60 cells which respond by chemotaxis to LTB_4, it was found that LTB_4 stimulated a dose-dependent increase in guanosine triphosphate (GTP) hydrolysis and guanosine 5′[γ-thio]triphosphate binding. This indicates that LTB_4 receptors on HL-60 cells are coupled to a G protein. Both pertussis and cholera toxin were able to inhibit this effect, indicating that the G protein contains an α-subunit (McLeish *et al.*, 1989).

Cysteinyl leukotriene receptors

The evidence for separate cysteinyl leukotriene receptors is supported by differences in biological activity of the individual leukotrienes, the effects of leukotriene receptor antagonists and by radioligand binding studies. Much of this evidence comes from work carried out in the guinea pig lung which supports the existence of distinct receptors for LTC_4, LTD_4 and LTE_4. The evidence for human tissue is more limited and remains a matter of debate. Certainly, in human lung a ligand-specific and stereospecific LTD_4 receptor is recognized and this is known to be regulated by GTP implying association with a GTP binding protein.

In guinea pig lung the existence of separate receptors for LTC_4, LTD_4 and LTE_4 has been demonstrated by physiological and radioligand binding studies. The rank order of potency of the sulphidopeptide leukotrienes for contracting tracheal spirals ($LTE_4 > LTD_4 = LTC_4$), is different from that for contracting parenchymal strips ($LTD_4 > LTE_4 > LTC_4$), thereby suggesting three separate receptors (Drazen *et al.*, 1983; Lee *et al.*, 1984). Furthermore, whereas LTC_4 and LTE_4 elicit monophasic contraction in peripheral airway strips, LTD_4 evokes a biphasic response (Drazen *et al.*, 1980). Evidence for a separate LTE_4 receptor in guinea pig lung is provided by the reported enhanced histamine responsiveness by LTE_4 in a time- and dose-dependent manner, an effect that could not be reproduced by LTC_4 and LTD_4 despite eliciting the same magnitude of contraction of trachea smooth muscle as LTE_4 (Lee *et al.*, 1984). Studies in guinea pig lung tissue in the presence of L-serine borate, which blocks the conversion of LTC_4 to LTD_4, showed that the LTD_4/LTE_4 antagonist FPL 55712 was unable to antagonize the contractile activity of LTC_4 (Snyder & Krell, 1984). Other selective LTD_4 antagonists have been shown to antagonize LTD_4-induced contraction of guinea pig tracheal strips but had little or no effect on the contractile effects mediated by LTC_4 (Fleisch *et al.*, 1985; Snyder *et al.*, 1987). In guinea pig uterus, specific binding of $[^3H]LTD_4$ could not be detected but specific and saturable binding of $[^3H]LTC_4$ was observed and reversed with unlabelled LTC_4 (Levinson, 1984). The binding of $[^3H]LTD_4$ and $[^3H]LTE_4$, but not $[^3H]LTC_4$, in guinea pig lung was enhanced by divalent ions and the rate of dissociation was accelerated by either NaCl or GTP providing further evidence for a multireceptor theory (Pong & DeHaven, 1983).

Despite the evidence for distinct receptor sub-types, it is likely that cross-reactivity exists between the different cysteinyl leukotrienes and their receptor types. Several studies have now provided evidence for the heterogeneity of LTD_4 receptors, both in the guinea pig lung as well as across other tissues and species (Fleisch *et al.*, 1982; Krell *et al.*, 1983; Hua *et al.*, 1985). Radioligand receptor binding assays with guinea pig trachea (Krell *et al.*, 1983) and lung membranes (Aharony *et al.*, 1989), using specific LTD_4 receptor antagonists, support the existence of at least two distinct receptors for LTD_4, with LTE_4 preferentially interacting with only a subset of LTD_4 receptors. This contrasts with the evidence in studies of human airways. Responses elicited by LTC_4 and LTD_4 are both inhibited to a similar degree by agents that are selective LTD_4 receptor antagonists, with the inference that all the biological effects attributed to LTC_4 can be explained by the bioconversion of LTC_4 to LTD_4 (Drazen & Austen, 1987). Using radiolabelled LTD_4 binding displacement assays, it was demonstrated that LTE_4 binds to the identical receptor as LTD_4 (Cheng & Townley, 1984). However, these studies may be flawed because the prevention of metabolic conversion of LTC_4 to LTD_4 was not demonstrated experimentally, and this could explain the discrepancy in the literature.

Actions in bronchial asthma

It was the lasting contractile property of SRS-A at very low concentrations which originally generated interest in these lipid compounds as putative mediators in bronchial asthma.

Isolated tracheal, bronchial or parenchymal tissues from guinea pigs (Piper & Samhoun, 1981), dogs (Johnson *et al.*, 1983) and rats (Szarek & Evans, 1988) have been found to contract in response to LTC_4 at nanomolar concentrations. In guinea pig tissue, LTC_4 and LTD_4 are approximately equipotent as contractile agonists, with EC_{50} values of 0.1–1 nmol/l. LTE_4 is less potent in the same model, with EC_{50} values of 30–100 nmol/l (Dahlen, 1983; Drazen & Austen, 1987).

Similar effects of the cysteinyl leukotrienes have been demonstrated in studies *in vitro* of human bronchus (Dahlen *et al.*, 1980) and tracheal smooth muscle (Jones *et al.*, 1982). The contractile action of LTC_4 is at least 1000 times more potent than histamine in causing muscle contraction, and LTD_4 has a similar potency to LTC_4. Hanna and coworkers (1981) found a lower contractile activity of LTC_4 and LTD_4 than that of histamine. This contrasts with the findings of Chagnon and coworkers (1985), who showed that LTA_4, LTC_4, and LTD_4 are at least 200 times more potent than histamine in human lung parenchyma *in vitro*. The release of LTC_4, LTD_4 and LTE_4 was demonstrated *in vitro* in isolated bronchi from two birch pollen-sensitive asthmatic subjects after antigen challenge, and the amount of leukotriene released was found to correlate with the contraction evoked by allergen (Dahlen *et al.*, 1983). In the guinea pig, pretreatment with a cyclo-oxygenase inhibitor led to a diminished LTC_4- and LTD_4-induced contractile response in isolated perfused lung, suggesting that bronchoconstrictor prostanoids are released by leukotriene action and contribute significantly to their contractile activity (Piper & Samhoun, 1981). By contrast, in isolated human lung tissue indomethacin pretreatment had no effect on the contractile response to antigen induced by leukotriene release, which could be abolished by a leukotriene biosynthesis inhibitor (Dahlen *et al.*, 1983).

In humans, *in vivo* studies of inhaled leukotrienes have demonstrated potent stimulation of contractile activity in the airways in both normal and asthmatic subjects. Inhalation of nebulized solutions of leukotrienes leads to airway obstruction measured by falls in specific airway conductance or flow as measured from full or partial expiratory flow–volume curves. In five normal subjects the potency of LTC_4 was from 600 to 9500 times greater than that of histamine, with 20 μg/ml LTC_4 and 2–10 mg/ml histamine concentrations required to produce a 30% fall in expiratory flow rate at 30% of baseline vital capacity above residual volume ($\dot{V}_{30}$) (Weiss *et al.*, 1982a). In the same study, LTD_4 was 6000-fold more potent than histamine (Weiss *et al.*, 1983). If data on normal subjects from different sources are combined (Holroyde *et al.*, 1981; Weiss *et al.*, 1982a; Weiss *et al.*, 1983; Barnes *et al.*, 1984a; Smith *et al.*, 1985; Adelroth *et al.*, 1986; Kern *et al.*, 1986; Bel *et al.*, 1987), inhaled LTC_4 and LTD_4 in normal subjects are 2000 times more potent than histamine or methacholine in producing airway obstruction. LTE_4, on the other hand, is only 40- to 60-fold more potent than histamine but produces longer lasting bronchoconstriction (Davidson *et al.*, 1987; O'Hickey *et al.*, 1988). Despite the similar potencies for LTC_4 and LTD_4, the time-course of their action is different. LTC_4 has a slower onset of action (10–15 minutes) than LTD_4 and LTE_4 (4–6 minutes), but the response for LTC_4 is more prolonged (20–40 minutes) (Weiss *et al.*, 1983; Drazen, 1988). The reason for this difference in time-course response is unclear, but may be related either to the action of the cysteinyl leukotrienes at different receptors, or because LTC_4 requires metabolism to LTD_4 prior to action at a specific receptor site. The discrepancy in the literature on the potency of the cysteinyl leukotrienes using a variety of measures of bronchoconstriction is likely to be due to differences in these parameters as measures of constriction at different sites within the lung. Changes in $\dot{V}_{30}$ are mediated by bronchoconstricting agonists considered to act at a peripheral site of action, whereas forced expiratory volume in 1 second (FEV_1) and SGaw are measures of a central site of action. Inhalation of LTC_4 and LTD_4 in normal subjects produced a fall in V_{30} with little effect on FEV_1 (Holroyde *et al.*, 1981). Similarly, Weiss *et al.* (1982b) demonstrated that a 50-fold greater concentration of LTC_4 was required to achieve a 20% fall in FEV_1 compared to the concentration required to cause a 30% fall in $\dot{V}_{30}$. These studies on normal subjects suggested a predominantly peripheral site of action for LTC_4 and LTD_4. In asthmatic subjects, inhalation of LTC_4 and LTD_4 showed similar effects on SGaw and $\dot{V}_{30}$ (Barnes *et al.*, 1984c; Smith *et al.*, 1985; Kern *et al.*, 1986), indicating that the site of LTC_4 and LTD_4 bronchoconstrictor activity in asthma is likely to be in both central and peripheral airways (Barnes *et al.*, 1984a; Pichurko *et al.*, 1989; Molfino *et al.*, 1992).

Asthmatic airways also respond by bronchoconstriction to inhaled leukotrienes, but in contrast to normal airways they exhibit smaller responses when a comparison to a reference agonist is made. LTC_4 and LTD_4 have been reported to be of the order of 40-fold (Adelroth *et al.*, 1986) to 140-fold (Griffin *et al.*, 1983) more potent than histamine or methacholine in their bronchoconstrictor effects on asthmatic airways, which compares with 600- to 9500-fold for LTC_4 (Weiss *et al.*, 1982a) and 6000-fold for LTD_4 (Weiss *et al.*, 1983) in normal airways compared to histamine. A correlation between the airway responsiveness to methacholine (Adelroth *et al.*, 1986) and histamine (Barnes *et al.*, 1984b) with the airway responsiveness to LTC_4 and LTD_4

has been established, but these studies also confirmed the relative lack of airway responsiveness to LTC_4 and LTD_4 in asthmatic subjects when compared to normal subjects (Barnes *et al.*, 1984b). The data for LTE_4 is more limited. Using $\dot{V}_{30}$ as a measure of airways obstruction, LTE_4 was 39-fold more potent than histamine in normal subjects and 14-fold more potent than histamine in asthmatic subjects (Davidson *et al.*, 1987). Using a 35% fall in specific airways conductance as a measure of bronchoconstriction, however, the relative potency of LTE_4 was found to be two to three times greater in asthmatic than in normal individuals (O'Hickey *et al.*, 1988). In view of the discordance in the literature, a more extensive study was performed to compare the relative potencies of LTC_4, LTD_4 and LTE_4 and the reference agonists histamine and methacholine in the same normal and asthmatic individuals (Arm *et al.*, 1990). The airways of the subjects with asthma were approximately 14-fold, 15-fold, sixfold, ninefold and 219-fold more responsive to histamine, methacholine, LTC_4, LTD_4 and LTE_4, respectively, than for normal subjects. Furthermore, as the airway hyperresponsiveness to histamine and methacholine increased, so too did the potency of LTE_4 in contrast to LTD_4 and LTE_4 which decreased. Therefore, the results of these studies taken together suggest that, compared to normals, asthmatic airways are relatively less responsive to LTC_4 and LTD_4 but have a disproportionate hyperresponsiveness to the bronchoconstricting effects of LTE_4. This indicates an important role for LTE_4 in bronchial asthma, which may be due to its relative stability amongst the cysteinyl leukotrienes and because it persists for the longest time at the site of release (Lam *et al.*, 1988).

A subset of asthmatics develops bronchospasm on ingestion of aspirin and other cyclo-oxygenase inhibitors. These subjects are unusually sensitive to the bronchoconstrictor effects of inhaled LTE_4, which is 1870 times more potent than histamine in aspirin-sensitive subjects and only 145 times more potent than histamine in asthmatics who are aspirin tolerant (Arm *et al.*, 1989). Following aspirin desensitization, there was a mean 20-fold decrease in airway responsiveness to LTE_4 but no change in histamine responsiveness. In aspirin-sensitive subjects, this selective hyperresponsiveness is exclusive to LTE_4 and not found with LTC_4 (Christie *et al.*, 1993), suggesting an important role in this form of asthma.

Airway responsiveness

Bronchial hyperresponsiveness to contractile agonists such as histamine and methacholine and to non-specific irritants is a key pathophysiological feature of asthma. Studies *in vitro* on guinea pig ileum have demonstrated that SRS-A enhanced the contractile response to histamine (Brocklehurst, 1962). Pretreatment of guinea pig spirals with a contracting dose of LTE_4 accentuated the subsequent contractile response to histamine in a time- and dose-dependent fashion (Lee *et al.*, 1984). LTC_4 and LTD_4 did not enhance histamine responsiveness in parenchymal strips. Indomethacin pretreatment abolished the hyperresponsiveness to histamine, despite a lack of effect on the contractile activity of LTE_4. A further study in guinea pig tracheal spirals demonstrated enhanced contractile activity to histamine following LTC_4 only in the presence of 0.1 mmol/l Ca^{2+} ions and this effect was blocked by the leukotriene antagonist FPL 55712 (Creese & Bach, 1983). This airways hyperresponsiveness found in guinea pig tracheal spirals is specific for histamine and is not found with carbachol or substance P. Furthermore, the effect is blocked not only by indomethacin but also by a TXA_2/PGH_2 (TP) receptor antagonist (GR32191). Pretreatment with LTE_4 induces a similar effect on isolated human bronchus, with a fourfold leftward displacement of the histamine dose–response curve. This effect is blocked by GR32191, suggesting that the observed LTC_4/LTE_4-induced hyperresponsiveness to histamine found in human and guinea pig trachea is mediated by the secondary generation of cyclo-oxygenase products (Jacques *et al.*, 1991).

In normal subjects, inhalation of either a subthreshold dose of LTD_4 (Barnes *et al.*, 1984b) or bronchoconstricting doses of LTC_4, LTD_4 or LTE_4 (Arm *et al.*, 1988; O'Hickey *et al.*, 1991) did not significantly enhance airways responsiveness to subsequent histamine inhalation. Inhalation of a bronchoconstricting dose of LTD_4 produced an approximately twofold increase in airways responsiveness to methacholine (Kern *et al.*, 1986). In an earlier study, inhalation of a bronchoconstricting dose of LTD_4 led to significantly increased airway methacholine responsiveness, which was maximal at 7 days in six out of eight subjects and persisted for 2–3 weeks in five subjects (Kaye & Smith, 1990). Interestingly, in the same study the degree and duration of changes in methacholine airway responses were similar to those found after platelet-activating factor (PAF) inhalation.

In asthmatic subjects, pre-inhalation of LTE_4 which caused a 41% fall in specific airways conductance produced a dose- and time-dependent increase in histamine responsiveness, which reached a peak of 3.5-fold at 7 hours after LTE_4 inhalation (Arm *et al.*, 1988). A subsequent study by the same authors found that each of the cysteinyl leukotrienes, LTC_4, LTD_4 and LTE_4, produced an approximately three- to fourfold increase in histamine responsiveness at 4 hours after inhalation in seven asthmatic individuals (O'Hickey *et al.*, 1991) (Fig. 23.5). The magnitude of this enhanced histamine responsiveness is similar to that observed after inhaled allergen challenge (Cockcroft *et al.*, 1977; Cartier *et al.*, 1982). Prior inhalation of LTC_4 was found to have no effect on the

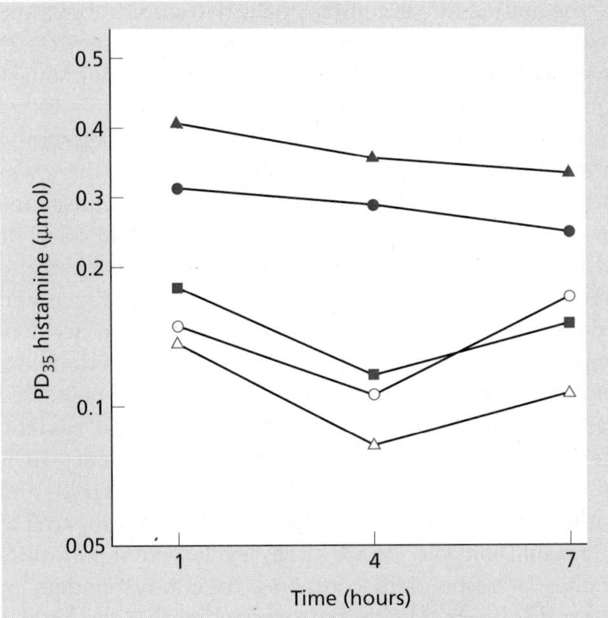

Fig. 23.5 Time-course of changes in airway histamine responsiveness after inhalation of phosphate-buffered saline (closed triangles), methacholine (closed circles), LTC_4 (open triangles), LTD_4 (closed squares) and LTE_4 (open circles). Each point represents the geometric mean for seven subjects with asthma. (From O'Hickey *et al.*, 1991.)

airways response to inhalation of distilled water in nine asthmatic subjects (Bianco *et al.*, 1985). Pre-dosing with indomethacin significantly inhibited the LTE_4-induced hyperresponsiveness to histamine in eight asthmatic subjects (Christie *et al.*, 1992a). Indomethacin was also found to inhibit the increase in airway responsiveness following inhaled allergen provocation in seven atopic subjects, without an effect on either the early or late asthmatic reaction (Kirby *et al.*, 1989). This suggests that the cysteinyl leukotrienes are important mediators in the enhanced airways responsiveness which is so characteristic of asthma and they may exert part of this effect through the secondary generation of cyclo-oxygenase pathway-derived products.

Asthmatic airways are more sensitive to bronchoconstricting agonists such as histamine and methacholine than normal airways, with a leftward shift in the dose–response curve and a greater absolute response. Normal airways are found to reach a plateau of maximum bronchoconstriction at mild degrees of airway narrowing. In a study of eight normal subjects, LTD_4 was found to produce a maximal response plateau at a higher level than methacholine. The addition of methacholine at the top of the LTD_4 plateau caused a further fall of 6.6% and 4.8% in FEV_1 and expiratory flow at 40% vital capacity ($\dot{V}_{40}$-*P*), respectively (Bel *et al.*, 1987). This effect could be demonstrated for at least 3 days following LTD_4 inhalation. A later study by the same group reported that prior administration of budesonide for 6 days could diminish the maximal response to LTD_4 in eight non-asthmatic subjects by 7.9% and 8.4% for FEV_1 and $\dot{V}_{40}$-*P*, respectively (Bel *et al.*, 1989).

Airway secretions

In bronchial asthma, abnormalities of airway mucociliary function are suggested by the clinical observation of excessive tracheobronchial secretions which are difficult to clear and may contribute to bronchial obstruction. The cysteinyl leukotrienes can influence both the mucus secretion and composition as well as mucociliary transport within the airways. Cultured human airway explants when exposed to LTC_4 and LTD_4 increased the rate of secretion of radiolabelled glucosamine as part of a high-molecular-weight glycoprotein by 15 and 26%, respectively (Marom *et al.*, 1982a; Coles *et al.*, 1983). Repeated stimulation of the explants led to diminished radiolabelled product secretion with the ratio of bound radiolabel to protein remaining unchanged, suggesting that LTC_4 and LTD_4 stimulate secretion rather than *de novo* mucus synthesis (Marom *et al.*, 1982a). LTC_4 was found to have 1000-fold more potent secretagogue effects on mucus secretion than LTD_4 when injected into the artery supplying the cervical canine trachea (Johnson & McNee, 1983). *In vitro* studies on cultured airway goblet cells demonstrated enhanced mucin release by the action of physiological concentrations of LTC_4 and LTD_4 (Kim *et al.*, 1989). LTC_4 and LTD_4 also mediate an increase in chloride flux of isolated canine tracheal epithelium, which induces an increase in the short-circuit ionic current (Leikauf *et al.*, 1986) and is accompanied by enhanced fluid secretion (Johnson *et al.*, 1983). In sheep allergic to *Ascaris suum*, concentrations of LTD_4 as low as 25 µg/ml produced significant decreases in tracheal mucus velocity, with the maximum effect observed at 3 hours after leukotriene challenge (Russi *et al.*, 1985). The overall effect of the leukotrienes therefore leads to a thickening of the mucous gel layer and a decrease in tracheal mucus velocity. Cysteinyl leukotrienes were detected in the sputum of 16 out of 25 patients with cystic fibrosis and one out of five patients with chronic bronchitis (Cromwell *et al.*, 1982). In a more recent study of 30 children with cystic fibrosis, urinary LTE_4 levels were found to correlate with sputum LTE_4 values, and one-third of the children with cystic fibrosis had urinary LTE_4 greater than 200 pmol/mol creatinine compared to only 3% of normal children (Sampson *et al.*, 1990). The same group reported that in a study of 13 children with cystic fibrosis the logarithm of sputum LTE_4 levels and total cysteinyl leukotriene levels correlated with the overall severity of pulmonary disease, as assessed by Chrispin–Norman chest radiograph scores (Spencer *et al.*, 1992). These findings suggest that cysteinyl leukotrienes may have a role in the sputum abnormalities characteristic of cystic fibrosis and chronic bronchitis.

Leukotriene release in disease

Leukotrienes have been detected in a variety of biological fluids by employing sensitive assay systems to detect picogram quantities, such as high-performance liquid chromatography (HPLC), radioimmunoassay and fast-atom -bombardment mass spectrometry. Bronchoalveolar lavage (BAL) has been used as a tool to obtain fluid in pulmonary disease states. Because the ratio of the volume of lavage fluid instilled to that recovered is not always constant, BAL suffers from the drawback that it is not easy to interpret the absolute values given and the results are usually expressed in terms of amounts per volume recovered. Urine is a more reliable biological fluid and amounts of mediator are easily standardized by expressing quantities per milligram of creatinine, which is excreted in a relatively constant fashion throughout a 24-hour period (Smith *et al.*, 1992). Maltby found that by infusing three subjects with three doses of radiolabelled LTC_4, it was possible to recover a constant 4.1–6.3%, regardless of the amount infused, in the form of LTE_4, the most stable of the cysteinyl leukotrienes (Maltby *et al.*, 1990). Radiolabelled LTC_4 instilled into the airways of asthmatics, non-asthmatics and asthmatics challenged with allergen was found to be excreted in a constant fashion in all three groups, with LTE_4 as the major metabolite (Westcott *et al.*, 1993). Christie and colleagues found a significant correlation between the dose of inhaled LTC_4 and the amounts excreted as urinary LTE_4 (Christie *et al.*, 1994). These studies provide strong evidence for the utility of urinary LTE_4 as a marker of pulmonary cysteinyl leukotriene release.

Clinical asthma

On BAL, 15 out of 17 asthmatic subjects with mild to severe disease were found to have detectable LTE_4 in BAL fluid, but there was no correlation between LTE_4 levels and pulmonary function. None of the group of nine control subjects had detectable LTE_4 (Lam *et al.*, 1988b). In a study by Wardlaw *et al.* (1989), eight symptomatic asthmatic subjects had significantly higher levels of LTB_4 and LTC_4 in BAL fluid than a control group of 14 without asthma. A comparison of 11 healthy with 11 atopic subjects with mild asthma found no difference in cysteinyl leukotriene, histamine or PAF levels between the two groups, but there was a higher level of PGD_2 and a lower level of LTB_4 in the asthmatic group (Crea *et al.*, 1992). These findings are in contrast to the two studies above and may be due to selection of very mild asthmatic subjects. In a study using urinary LTE_4 as a marker for pulmonary cysteinyl leukotriene release, Smith and colleagues found no difference in baseline urinary levels of LTE_4 between 17 normal and 31 asthmatic subjects. In addition, there was no correlation between urinary LTE_4 levels as measured in picograms per milligram of creatinine and baseline airways responsiveness to histamine or FEV_1 as a percentage of predicted values (Crea *et al.*, 1992). Drazen and coworkers examined 72 subjects presenting to accident and emergency and classified 22 patients with a doubling of peak expiratory flow rate (PEFR) following nebulized salbutamol as responders, and 19 patients with a less than 25% increase in PEFR as non-responders. Urinary LTE_4 levels were assayed by pre-column extraction, HPLC and radioimmunoassay in these two groups and compared to 13 normal controls. Urinary LTE_4 levels were significantly higher in responders compared to non-responders or normal subjects. The authors concluded that the highest levels of LTE_4 found in those with acute reversible airflow obstruction were consistent with a bronchospastic role for cysteinyl leukotrienes in spontaneous acute asthma (Drazen *et al.*, 1992).

Allergen-induced asthma

Leukotriene release has been measured in studies employing various bronchial-challenge procedures. Wenzel and colleagues reported that using HPLC the predominant leukotriene in BAL fluid in atopic asthmatic subjects after endobronchial bronchial allergen challenge is LTC_4, and there was an approximate ninefold rise in levels compared to baseline. Measurable levels of LTC_4 at baseline were found in nine of 11 atopic asthmatic subjects but in only one of seven atopic non-asthmatic subjects and one of six non-atopic subjects. There was only a slight rise in BAL LTC_4 levels after allergen in the atopic non-asthmatic group and no change in the non-atopic samples (Wenzel *et al.*, 1990). In a further study by Wenzel and colleagues, the levels of prostaglandin D_2 (PGD_2), TXB_2, LTC_4 and histamine were measured in BAL fluid before and 5 minutes after endobronchial allergen challenge in three groups of atopic subjects: seven non-asthmatic; six asthmatic subjects without a late asthmatic response; and six asthmatic subjects with a late asthmatic response. LTC_4 was detected in nine out of the 12 asthmatic subjects but in only one out of seven subjects without asthma. Significant increases in all mediator levels were observed in both groups with asthma post-allergen challenge compared to the non-asthmatic group. Interestingly, the asthmatic group without a late asthmatic response recorded significantly higher levels of all four mediators post-challenge than the groups with a late response and the non-asth-

Table 23.4 Release of leukotrienes into biological fluids.

Disease	Biological fluid	Leukotriene release
Asthma		
Clinical disease	BAL	LTE_4 detected in mild asthma/severe
Symptomatic	BAL	LTB_4/LTC_4
Acute	Urine	LTE_4—highest levels in patients responding to β_2-agonist treatment
Allergen challenge		
Early-allergen response	BAL	LTC_4 increases ninefold
	Urine	LTE_4 increases 2–4 hours after allergen challenge
Aspirin sensitive	Urine	LTE_4 sixfold higher at baseline and increases a further fourfold after aspirin challenge
Exercise induced	Nasal lavage	LTC_4 levels increase after lysine-aspirin challenge
	BAL	LTB_4 rises 12-fold and LTC_4 rises fivefold after isocapnic hyperventilation
	Urine	LTE_4 found to increase 1.7-fold in only one study of children with severe asthma
Cryptogenic fibrosing alveolitis	BAL	LTB_4 detected
Persistent pulmonary hypertension	BAL	LTC_4 and LTD_4 detected in newborn infants
Adult respiratory distress syndrome	Pulmonary oedema fluid	LTD_4 increased fourfold
Rheumatoid arthiritis	Synovial fluid	LTB_4 detected in active disease
Gouty arthiritis	Joint fluid	LTB_4 levels significantly increased
Psoriasis	Skin chamber fluid	LTB_4, LTC_4 and LTD_4 levels detected in increased quantities
Inflammatory bowel disease	Infestinal mucosal fluid	LTB_4 detected in both ulcerative colitis and Crohn's disease
Acute myocardial infarction	Urine	LTE_4 levels raised and return to normal day 3
Hepatorenal syndrome	Urine	LTE_4 levels elevated threefold

matic controls (Wenzel *et al.*, 1991). In a study of 17 allergic asthmatic subjects undergoing allergen provocation, there was a fall in FEV_1 within the first 2 hours of between 25 and 59%, and this was accompanied by a rise in urinary LTE_4 levels from 46 to 92 ng over a 12-hour collection period. Methacholine challenge alone, which led to similar falls in FEV_1, did not significantly change urinary LTE_4 excretion. There was a significant correlation between the decrease in FEV_1 during the early asthmatic response, the excretion of urinary LTE_4 and the airways reactivity. No correlation was found between urinary LTE_4 excretion and the severity of late response to allergen, but there was a significant prolonged elevated urinary LTE_4 excretion in those patients with the most severe late asthmatic responses (Westcott *et al.*, 1991). Manning and colleagues studied 18 asthmatic subjects who were divided into three groups: those with an isolated early asthmatic response (EAR); those with an isolated late asthmatic response (LAR); and a third group with a dual asthmatic response (DAR). Urinary LTE_4 rose significantly from baseline values only in the two groups with an EAR, with a rise from 150 to 1816 pg/mg creatinine in the group with an isolated EAR and a rise from 66 to 174 pg/mg creatinine in the group with an EAR preceding a LAR. No increase in urinary LTE_4 was found in the group with an isolated LAR. Furthermore, the degree of maximum bronchoconstriction during the EAR correlated with urinary LTE_4 release, suggesting that the cysteinyl leukotrienes are only released during the EAR and that they contribute significantly to the bronchoconstriction found during this phase of the asthmatic response (Manning *et al.*, 1990a). Several subsequent studies have also documented urinary LTE_4 release 2–4 hours following specific bronchial allergen challenge (Taylor *et al.*, 1989; Hui *et al.*, 1991a; Kumlin *et al.*, 1992a; Nasser *et al.*, 1994b).

Exercise-induced asthma

Pliss and colleagues found increases in BAL fluid levels of LTB_4 from 10 to 121 pg/ml and immunoreactive cysteinyl leukotrienes from 46 to 251 pg/ml following isocapnic hyperventilation as a model for exercise-induced asthma. There were also increases in eosinophil and epithelial cell numbers, but no changes in prostaglandin or histamine levels were detected (Pliss *et al.*, 1990). A further study was unable to find evidence for mast cell-derived mediator release with no increase in BAL fluid histamine, tryptase,

PGD_2 or LTC_4 following treadmill exercise in seven atopic asthmatic subjects. However, the sensitivity of the LTC_4 assay in this study may not have been sufficient to detect any LTC_4 released (Broide *et al.*, 1990). Urinary levels of LTE_4 were not found to increase in a study of six asthmatic subjects after treadmill exercise, leading to a mean 22% fall in FEV_1 (Smith *et al.*, 1991). However, small increases in urinary LTE_4 (14.3 before and 24.3 ng/mg creatinine after exercise) were found in eight out of 10 children with severe asthma following exercise, which produced a 60% fall in FEV_1 but no increases in urinary LTE_4 in seven children with moderate asthma who experienced only a 24% fall in FEV_1 (Kikawa *et al.*, 1991). Despite the conflicting evidence, pharmacological studies have indicated an important role for cysteinyl leukotrienes in exercise-induced bronchospasm. It is likely that our inability to detect these mediators consistently in biological fluids may be because whole-body cysteinyl leukotriene release does not change significantly after exercise, which may be further modified by changes in bronchial or pulmonary blood flow in response to airway cooling and local changes in pH and osmolarity. Furthermore, the modest local increases in cysteinyl leukotriene release in exercise-induced asthma are likely to be difficult to detect with currently employed assays.

Aspirin-sensitive asthma

The cysteinyl leukotrienes have considerable importance in the pathogenesis of aspirin-sensitive asthma (ASA). Mean resting urinary LTE_4 levels in ASA subjects are significantly higher than in normals or non-ASA. Christie and colleagues found sixfold higher urinary LTE_4 levels in ASA subjects compared to non-ASA controls. Furthermore, oral aspirin challenge which led to a mean 21% fall in FEV_1 in six ASA subjects resulted in a fourfold increase in urinary LTE_4 values over baseline values. There was no such increase in urinary LTE_4 levels in the control subjects and no fall in FEV_1 on aspirin ingestion (Christie *et al.*, 1991b). Smith and colleagues reported that baseline urinary LTE_4 levels in 10 ASA subjects were 101 pg/mg creatinine compared to 43 pg/mg creatinine in 31 non-ASA subjects and 34 pg/mg creatinine in 17 normals. There was substantial overlap between the groups and no correlation was found between urinary LTE_4 and histamine PD_{20} or baseline FEV_1, and so measurement of LTE_4 in a single sample of urine does not predict the degree of resting airflow obstruction, the degree of bronchial hyperresponsiveness or diagnose aspirin sensitivity (Smith *et al.*, 1992). Subsequent studies have affirmed these findings (Knapp *et al.*, 1992; Kumlin *et al.*, 1992a; Sladek & Szczeklik, 1993). Recent studies have also confirmed increased urinary LTE_4 levels in ASA subjects following lysine-aspirin bronchial challenge (Christie *et al.*, 1992c; Sladek *et al.*, 1994). Nasal lavage mediator levels have been studied in aspirin-sensitive rhinosinusitis. Following lysine-aspirin challenge increased levels of both histamine and LTC_4 were detected in nasal lavage samples in three out of four ASA subjects with both naso-ocular symptoms and a bronchospastic reaction. No increases in these mediators were found in normals or non-aspirin-sensitive subjects or aspirin-sensitive subjects in whom lysine-aspirin did not provoke naso-ocular symptoms (Ferreri *et al.*, 1988; Picado *et al.*, 1992).

Other diseases

Leukotrienes have also been recovered in a number of other non-allergic disease states. Increased quantities of LTB_4 were detected in lavage fluid of patients with cryptogenic fibrosing alveolitis and correlated with the recovery of polymorphonuclear leucocytes in BAL fluid, suggesting that leukotriene release may be responsible for granulocyte recruitment in this disease (Wardlaw *et al.*, 1989).

LTC_4 and LTD_4 have been found in increased concentrations in the lung lavage fluids of newborn infants with persistent pulmonary hypertension requiring assisted ventilation (Stenmark *et al.*, 1983). In the adult respiratory distress syndrome (ARDS), LTD_4 was detected in fourfold higher concentrations in pulmonary oedema fluid compared to patients with cardiogenic pulmonary oedema. Furthermore, the LTD_4 levels correlated with the ratio of oedema fluid to plasma concentrations of albumin, suggesting that cysteinyl leukotrienes contribute to the permeability defect which allows accumulation of protein-rich fluid in ARDS (Matthay *et al.*, 1984).

Small quantities of LTB_4 have been detected in the synovial fluid of joints from patients with active rheumatoid arthritis (Davidson *et al.*, 1983). In gouty joint effusions, significantly higher quantities of LTB_4 are detected than those found in either normal or rheumatoid joints. This may be due, in part, to monosodium urate crystals which have been shown to inhibit metabolism and biological deactivation of LTB_4 by polymorphonuclear granulocytes (Rae *et al.*, 1982).

Skin chamber fluid from abraded psoriatic skin lesions contains significantly higher quantities of LTB_4 (Brain *et al.*, 1984) and immunoreactive LTC_4 and LTD_4 (Brain *et al.*, 1985) than that from normal skin, and this may partly explain the characteristic intra-epidermal neutrophil infiltration and local vasodilatation found in psoriasis. By measuring the incorporation of radiolabelled thymidine, picomolar to nanomolar concentrations of LTB_4 were found to increase DNA synthesis in cultured epidermal keratinocytes *in vitro*. The peptide leukotrienes LTC_4 and LTD_4 were less potent than LTB_4, but also stimulated keratinocyte DNA synthesis. This finding may relate to the excessive epidermal hyperplasia seen in psoriasis (Kragballe *et al.*, 1985).

Both LTB_4 and the cysteinyl leukotrienes are generated and released *in vitro* in greater quantities from intestinal mucosa obtained from patients with ulcerative colitis and Crohn's disease (Sharon & Stenson, 1984; Peskar *et al.*, 1986; Lauritsen *et al.*, 1987). Intestinal mucosa from patients with inflammatory bowel disease was found to contain 50-fold higher quantities of LTB_4 per gram of tissue than that from normal mucosa (Sharon & Stenson, 1984). The use of rectal pouches has allowed the measurement of mediator levels *in vivo* in inflammatory bowel disease and has demonstrated significantly higher LTB_4 levels in active ulcerative colitis (Lauritsen *et al.*, 1987). Treatment with either prednisolone or aminosalicylic acid decreased the generation of LTB_4 *in vivo* which was associated with clinical improvement. Pretreatment levels of both PGE_2 and LTB_4 were significantly higher in patients not responding to 5-aminosalicylic acid or prednisolone treatment, and the authors of the study suggested that intraluminal levels of these mediators are more useful predictors of relapsing ulcerative colitis than clinical indices of disease severity (Lauritsen *et al.*, 1986).

Levels of urinary LTE_4 were found to be raised in a study of 16 patients presenting with acute myocardial infarction with a fall to normal levels by day 3. Similar elevated levels of urinary LTE_4 were found in unstable angina, with a reduction to normal levels once the chest pain had resolved. Treatment with thrombolytic agents leading to early coronary reperfusion resulted in a faster decline in LTE_4 levels compared to patients who did not receive such treatment, suggesting that cardiac ischaemia and necrosis was responsible for the cysteinyl leukotriene release (Carry *et al.*, 1992).

In hepatorenal syndrome and decompensated liver disease, the rate of urinary LTE_4 excretion per hour is threefold higher than that found in compensated liver disease. The additional finding of reduced renal clearance of a radiolabelled LTC_4 infusion in one such patient suggested that the increased excretion of urinary LTE_4 is due to excessive production or reduced metabolism of LTE_4 and not due to reduced renal clearance of LTE_4 (Moore *et al.*, 1990).

The fact that LTC_4 and LTD_4 are potent renal vasoconstrictors suggests that these mediators may modulate glomerular function and be involved in the pathogenesis of this disease.

Pharmacological modulation of leukotriene action

Over recent years, a further and very important source of evidence has been reported in support of the role of leukotrienes in both allergic and non-allergic disease using pharmacological modulation of both experimentally induced and naturally occuring symptoms. Most of the work with leukotriene antagonists and 5-LO inhibitors focuses on asthma, employing allergen provocation, aspirin challenge in aspirin-sensitive subjects, exercise challenge, isocapnic hyperventilation and the inhalation of cold dry air. However, because these models may only mirror the acute inflammatory effects of asthma and bear little relationship to the chronic structural changes characteristic of the disease, the developmental process of these drugs has placed greater emphasis on the investigation of day-to-day asthma, the steroid sparing and bronchodilator effects of these agents. Increasingly, other diseases are being studied using these therapeutic agents as their wider import is recognized.

Leukotriene action can be pharmacologically modulated by antagonism at the receptor site or by inhibition of their biosynthesis. LTD_4 receptor antagonists have been developed for use in human trials, but thus far LTB_4 receptor antagonists have not been evaluated in humans. 5-LO inhibition can be achieved either by direct interference with its enzymatic properties or via secondary inhibition by blocking its binding to FLAP and thereby inhibiting 5-LO activation.

Leukotriene antagonists

The potency of LTD_4 receptor antagonists is measured by the rightward shift of the dose–response curve to inhaled LTD_4 achieved by pre-dosing with the antagonist. Based on studies with antihistamines (Brik *et al.*, 1987) and β-antagonists (Cubeddu *et al.*, 1985), a rightward shift of at least 20-fold is required for adequate inhibition of cysteinyl leukotriene effects in humans. The first antagonist to be evaluated was the hydroxyacetophenone FPL 55712, which had selective activity as an inhibitor of SRS-A even before the chemical structure of SRS-A was elucidated (Augstein *et al.*, 1973). However, clinically it proved disappointing in asthma because of low potency, a short half-life and bioavailability only by inhalation (Lee *et al.*, 1981). Other first-generation LTD_4 antagonists to be evaluated in humans include L-648,051 (Jones *et al.*, 1986), L-649,923 (Barnes *et al.*, 1987). LY-171,883 (Phillips *et al.*, 1988), LY-170,680 (Wood-Baker *et al.*, 1991) and SK&F 104,353 (Joos *et al.*, 1991). These compounds were of modest potency with a rightward shift in the LTD_4 dose–response curve of three- to 10-fold with poor to moderate clinical efficacy in early trials. Recently a second generation of highly selective antagonists with up to 100-fold greater potency than FPL 55712 have been developed. The most potent of these compounds includes: ICI 204,219, which is up to 1000-fold more potent that FPL 55712 in inhibiting contraction of guinea pig tracheal and parenchymal strips (Krell *et al.*, 1990); ONO 1078, which inhibited both LTC_4 and LTD_4 in guinea pigs and demonstrated 100-fold greater potency than FPL 55712 in isolated human bronchus (Yamaguchi *et al.*, 1992); MK-571, MK-679 and MK-476, which are members of a whole family of quinolone-derived LTD_4 antagonists which demonstrate a 44- to 84-fold rightward shift in the LTD_4 dose–response curve in asthmatic subjects (Kips *et al.*, 1991). MK-571 is a racaemic mixture which is potent, selective and orally active, although early trials used intravenous delivery to correlate drug levels with clinical efficacy. MK-679 is the R-enantiomer of MK-571, which was withdrawn following trials suggesting liver dysfunction in a subgroup of patients. Promising results in clinical trials reported using MK-476, which is a structural modification of MK-679 and a highly potent and selective LTD_4 antagonist, have shown promise (Ford-Hutchinson, 1990; Manning *et al.*, 1990c).

Allergen-induced asthma

Several studies have evaluated anti-leukotriene therapy in the allergen-induced asthma model. In early studies LY-171,883, which has a similar structure to FPL 55712 and L-649,923, had no effect on baseline lung function or the LAR but demonstrated a slight reduction in the EAR (Britton *et al.*, 1987; Fuller *et al.*, 1989). In a study of 10 asthmatics, a single oral dose of 40 mg ICI 204,219, a highly selective and potent LTD_4 antagonist, attenuated the EAR by 80% and the LAR by 50% and suppressed the allergen-induced rise in non-specific bronchial reactivity at 6 hours post-challenge (Taylor *et al.*, 1991a). An inhaled formulation of ICI 204,219 was not so effective but still significantly inhibited the EAR but not the LAR (O'Shaughnessy *et al.*, 1993). A further study using a single inhaled dose of 40 mg ICI 204,219 displaced the allergen dose–response curve to inhaled cat allergen 10-fold compared to placebo (Findlay *et al.*, 1992), the same inhaled formulation has been shown to shorten the recovery time of the EAR from 60 to 40 minutes (Dahlen *et al.*, 1994). The quinolone derivative MK 571 substantially inhibited the EAR by 88% and the LAR by 63% when the AUC (area under curve) of the FEV_1 time curve was analysed (Rasmussen *et al.*, 1992).

Exercise challenge and isocapnic hyperventilation

Exercise is a potent stimulus for bronchoconstriction in asthma, especially in younger patients. The degree of bronchospasm achieved by exercise can be mimicked by isocapnic hyperventilation in a controlled situation, provided respiratory heat exchange is matched in a time-dependent manner. These two stimuli are considered to stimulate similar if not identical pathological mechanisms for the initiation of bronchoconstriction. In a study of 20 asthmatic subjects treated for 2 weeks with LY-171,883, bronchoconstriction induced by isocapnic hyperventilation of cold air was reduced marginally, with an increase in the geometric mean respiratory heat loss required to reduce FEV_1 by 20%. In this study the most reactive subjects demonstrated greatest protection (Israel *et al.*, 1989). Inhaled SK&F 104,353, a weak LTD_4 antagonist, was found to reduce the exercise-induced bronchoconstrictor response from 29 to 20%, with an efficacy comparable to disodium cromoglycate (Robuschi *et al.*, 1992). An oral 20-mg dose of ICI 204,219 was found to have no effect on resting airway calibre 2 hours after dosing but reduced the fall in FEV_1 from 36 to 21.6% produced by treadmill exercise challenge in eight asthmatic subjects respiring cold dry air (Finnerty *et al.*, 1992). Inhaled ICI 204,219 halved the fall in FEV_1 induced by exercise in a study of nine subjects undergoing exercise challenge (Makker *et al.*, 1993). MK-571 produced similar results, with a 70% attenuation of the exercise-induced decrease in FEV_1 in 12 asthmatic subjects and a marked reduction in recovery time from 33 to 8 minutes (Manning *et al.*, 1990b). Despite the potency of these LTD_4 antagonists, they were unable to completely inhibit the bronchoconstrictor response to exercise, suggesting that other mediators such as mast cell-derived histamine or prostaglandins are involved in the pathogenesis of this form of asthma.

ASA

ASA is probably the most leukotriene-dependent model currently available for the evaluation of anti-leukotriene therapy in asthma. The weakly potent LTD_4 antagonist SK&F 104,353, administered by the inhaled route, was shown to inhibit the bronchoconstrictor response to ingested aspirin by a mean 47% in five out of six subjects (Christie *et al.*, 1991a). In a study of eight subjects with ASA, MK-0679 was found to improve baseline pulmonary function and block the airways obstruction produced by inhaled lysine-aspirin with a median 4.4-fold rightward shift in the dose–response curve, with most complete protection in the three subjects who failed to drop their FEV_1 by 20% to a predetermined maximum dose of lysine-aspirin (Kumlin *et al.*, 1992b).

Bronchodilator effect

Isolated human bronchi of 3–12 mm in diameter were found to have a high degree of intrinsic bronchomotor tone, averaging more than 50% of the available maximal constrictor response to 30 mmol/l $BaCl_2$. Pre-incubation in the presence of ICI 204,219 or SKF 104,353 relaxed the bronchi, and this effect was found to be additive with a histamine H_1 antagonist, leading to the conclusion that intrinsic bronchomotor tone is due to the continual production of cysteinyl leukotrienes and histamine (Ellis & Undem, 1994). A number of studies have now been reported that support a role for cysteinyl leukotrienes in the maintenance of intrinsic bronchial muscle tone. An intravenous infusion of the LTD_4 antagonist MK-0679 was carried out in a study of nine asthmatic patients with FEV_1 ranging from 40 to 80% of predicted values. Fifteen minutes after the end of the infusion, mean FEV_1 rose 15.8% and 7.8% with 500-mg and 125-mg doses of MK-0679, and fell 2.6% after placebo infusion (Impens *et al.*, 1993). In a separate study an oral dose of 40 mg ICI 204,219, produced a significant resting increase in FEV_1 compared to placebo, with the effect persisting after inhaled salbutamol (Hui & Barnes, 1991b). The additive effect of inhaled β_2-agonist administration was confirmed in a study of 12 male asthmatic patients. The maximum bronchodilatation achieved from the start of a 6-hour intravenous infusion of MK-571 was 22%, compared to 1.3% after placebo. Salbutamol administered at 5–6 hours from the start of the infusion produced additive bronchodilatation. Overall the degree of bronchodilatation was inversely correlated with baseline FEV_1, suggesting a major contribution from cysteinyl leukotrienes in resting airway tone (Gaddy *et al.*, 1992). A recent study reported that a single oral dose of MK-0476 produced a mean 12% increase in FEV_1 in moderate asthmatics, with the effect persisting up to 6 hours (Sorkness *et al.*, 1994). The magnitude of cysteinyl leukotriene effect on the intrinsic airway tone in ASA has been reported in one study using a single dose of 825 mg MK-0679 in eight subjects with ASA. This led to a mean peak improvement in FEV_1 of 18% with a range of 5–34%, and correlated strongly with the severity of asthma (Dahlen *et al.*, 1993a).

Trials in chronic asthma

Experimental models provide an indication of the efficacy of novel treatments for asthma. Prior to obtaining registration for a product it is essential, however, to demonstrate efficacy in large numbers of patients with asthma in their normal environment. There are still relatively few leukotriene antagonists which have reached this stage in the development process and few studies have been reported. In a multicentre placebo-controlled study, 138 patients with asthma received 600 mg LY-171,883 twice a day for 6 weeks. After active treatment, mean FEV_1 rose significantly compared to placebo from 73.8 to 83.3% of predicted values. Significant improvements were also recorded in the severity of daytime and nocturnal wheeze and breathlessness, with a reduction in β_2-agonist use, but there was no change in cough or chest tightness (Cloud *et al.*, 1989). Treatment with MK-571 for 2 weeks at 75 mg three times a day followed by 4 weeks of treatment with 150 mg three times a day produced a mean 8–14% improvement in FEV_1 and a 30% reduction in morning and evening symptom scores and an approximately 30% reduction in salbutamol usage (Gaddy *et al.*, 1991). In a cross-over study of 11 asthmatic subjects, 1 week's treatment with ONO-1078 led to significant improvement in methacholine PC_{20}- FEV_1 compared to placebo, but there was no change in resting FEV_1 or forced vital capacity (FVC) during that period (Fujimura *et al.*, 1993). A 6-week treatment period with ICI 204,219 produced a significant amelioration in daytime asthma scores, nocturnal awakenings and morning peak flow recordings in mild to moderate asthmatic subjects (Spector *et al.*, 1992). A more recent placebo-controlled dose-ranging study with twice-daily ICI 204,219 in 266 subjects with moderate asthma, found treatment with 40 mg was linearly more effective than 20 mg or 10 mg without any increase in adverse effects. Compared to placebo there was a significant reduction in nocturnal awakenings (by 46%), first morning asthma symptoms, daytime asthma scores (by 26%) and salbutamol use (by 30%), and an increase in FEV_1 (by 11%) and evening peak expiratory flow rates (Spector *et al.*, 1994). The only study so far reported which has added an LTD_4 antagonist to existing therapy with inhaled steroids used 10 days' treatment with RG 12525, which produced significant improvement in FEV_1 in stable asthmatic subjects (Wahedna *et al.*, 1992).

The paucity of trial data in chronic asthma makes it difficult to accurately predict the role of leukotriene antagonists in the treatment of chronic asthma, whether as bronchodilator or anti-inflammatory therapy and whether they have a role in replacing existing treatments such as inhaled corticosteroids or theophyllines. Further and large scale studies, some of which are currently underway, are required to answer these vital questions.

Leukotriene biosynthesis inhibitors

Leukotriene biosynthesis inhibitors may be theoretically more effective than LTD_4 receptor antagonists in preventing the pathophysiological consequences of leukotriene release within the airways, because of the dual prevention of both cysteinyl leukotriene and LTB_4 generation. It is postulated that 5-LO contains a non-haem iron which is normally in the dormant ferrous state (Fe^{2+}) and upon activation by hydroperoxides, adenosine triphosphate (ATP) and Ca^{2+} is converted to the active ferric form (Fe^{3+}). The activated 5-LO translocates, possibly due to a change from a hydrophilic to a hydrophobic conformation to the nuclear membrane, where it comes into contact with the transmembrane FLAP. At this point the enzyme is ready to act on the substrate arachidonic acid, which is then oxidized stereoselectively by a free radical process involving removal of the 7H(S) hydrogen of arachidonic acid followed by peroxidation of the complex and then oxidation of the iron in 5-LO with simultaneous reduction of the hydroperoxide radical to give 5-HPETE. There are, therefore, a number of possible mechanisms to inhibit the action of 5-LO. Direct inhibition of the enzyme can be accomplished by 'redox inhibitors', which can act either by chelation or reduction of the non-haem iron (e.g. acetohydroxamic acids such as BW A4C and hydroxyurea derivatives such as zileuton and BW70C) or by a 'non-redox' mechanism through anti-oxidant/free radical scavenger activity on radical intermediates of 5-LO (e.g. flavonoids, nafazatrom (BAY-G576), naphthalene derivatives such as RS-43,179 and Wy-47,288 and the enantioselective, competitive and reversible inhibitor, ZD2138, a methoxytetrahydropyran). Another mechanism by which 5-LO inhibition can be achieved is through the use of substrate analogues such as eicosatetraynoic acid (ETYA) and prostacyclin analogues. Indirect 5-LO inhibition is accomplished using compounds that bind with high affinity to 5-LO-activating protein; for example, indole derivatives such as MK-886 and quinolone/indole hybrids such as MK-0591. Some 5-LO inhibitors have more than one mode of action. At low concentrations of racaemic Wy-50,295, inhibition of 5-LO translocation predominates, but at higher concentrations its activity as an arachidonic acid analogue becomes significant (Evans *et al.*, 1991). Although it is well recognized that hydroxamic acids and hydroxyureas chelate the essential iron at the active site of the enzyme, there is now evidence to suggest that they also have antioxidant activity (Garland & Salmon, 1991). Clinical trials involving 5-LO inhibitors have followed the pattern set by the cysteinyl leukotriene antagonists, with early studies using compounds with weak activity such as piriprost demonstrating negligible clinical usefulness (Mann *et al.*, 1986), and later more potent compounds reported to have useful clinical activity.

Allergen-induced asthma

Several studies have reported the effect of 5-LO inhibition on the allergen-induced model of asthma. The iron-chelator zileuton (A-64077) was given to nine asthmatic subjects in a single-dose placebo-controlled cross-over study. Although there was almost complete loss of *ex vivo* LTB_4 generation in whole blood and an approximate 50% reduction in the rise of urinary LTE_4, there was no significant reduction in the early or late asthmatic response and no decrease in the airway responsiveness to methacholine (Hui *et al.*, 1991a). The potent and selective non-redox 5-LO inhibitor ZD2138 was evaluated in a study of eight asthmatic subjects and, despite an 82% reduction in *ex vivo* whole-blood LTB_4 generation and an overall 72% inhibition of the rise in urinary LTE_4 excretion, there was no inhibition of the allergen-induced early- or late-asthmatic response (Nasser *et al.*, 1994b). In a separate study of eight atopic men, 500 mg of the FLAP inhibitor MK-886 was given 1 hour before and 250 mg 2 hours after allergen inhalation. Compared to placebo premedication, MK-886 inhibited the EAR by 58% and the LAR by 44%, this was accompanied by a 54.2% inhibition of A23187-stimulated whole blood LTB_4 generation and a 51.5% inhibition of the rise in urinary LTE_4 during the EAR and 80% during the LAR. However, there was no significant difference in the PC_{20} histamine at 30 hours after allergen challenge compared to placebo (Friedman *et al.*, 1993). The FLAP inhibitor MK-0591 (250 mg) was given as three doses at 24, 12 and 1.5 hours before allergen inhalation. For 24 hours after allergen inhalation LTB_4 synthesis was inhibited by 96% and urinary LTE_4 excretion by 84%. The EAR to allergen was inhibited by 79% and the LAR delayed by 3 hours, but there was no effect on airway responsiveness to histamine 24 hours post-allergen challenge (Diamant *et al.*, 1993). Another FLAP inhibitor BAY ×1005 has similar potency to MK-0591, and when administered to atopic asthmatic subjects as a single dose of 750 mg orally 4 hours before allergen challenge was found to inhibit the EAR by 68%. This was associated with an 87% reduction in urinary LTE_4 excretion during the first 2 hours after allergen challenge but this study did not report on the LAR or the effect on allergen-induced airway responsiveness (Dahlén *et al.*, 1993b).

Exercise challenge and isocapnic hyperventilation

Premedication with a single dose of 800 mg zileuton in 13 subjects with asthma inhibited *ex vivo* whole-blood LTB_4 generation by 74% without affecting TXB_2 levels. This led to an increase of 47% in the amount of cold dry air required to reduce FEV_1 by 10%, with an increase in minute ventilation from 27.5 to 39.8 l/min (Israel *et al.*, 1990). A further study of 24 subjects with mild asthma, premedicated for 2 days with zileuton 2.4 g/day, demonstrated a 40% inhibition of the exercise-induced bronchospasm. In addition, there was significant protection against the fall in FVC compared to placebo (Meltzer *et al.*, 1994).

ASA

The effect of aspirin ingestion was examined in eight subjects with the syndrome of aspirin sensitivity and hyperexcretion of urinary LTE_4 after premedication with zileuton or placebo. Zileuton reduced baseline urinary LTE_4 excretion by 70% and prevented the fall in FEV_1 in response to aspirin challenge. There was additional protection against the development of nasal, gastrointestinal and dermal symptoms in response to aspirin ingestion (Israel *et al.*, 1993a). Similar results were reported for ZD2138 (Fig. 23.6), which was shown to protect against aspirin-induced asthma in a study involving seven subjects with ASA and hyperexcretion of urinary LTE_4. In response to aspirin challenge, the fall in FEV_1 was 20.3%

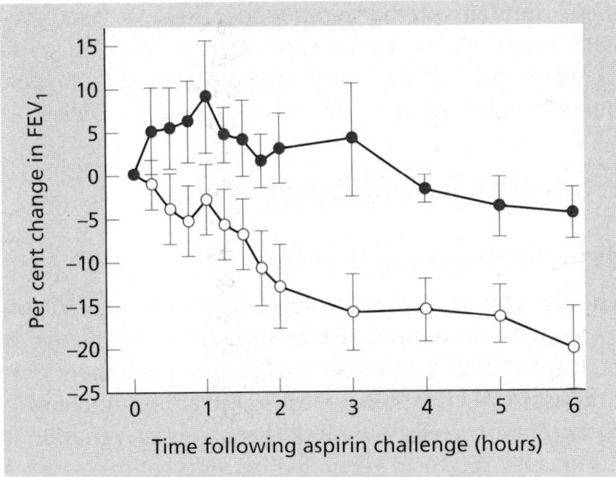

Fig. 23.6 Bronchoprotection by 5-lipoxygenase inhibition against the decrease in forced expiratory volume in 1 second (FEV_1) induced by oral aspirin challenge in seven subjects with aspirin-sensitive asthma. The subjects were premedicated with either ZD2138 (closed circles) or placebo (open circles). (From Nasser *et al.*, 1994a.)

after placebo and 4.9% 4 hours following ZD2138 premedication. This was associated with a reduction in the systemic symptoms after active treatment which also inhibited *ex vivo* LTB_4 generation in whole blood by 72% at 12 hours and urinary LTE_4 by 74% at 6 hours (Nasser *et al.*, 1994a).

Bronchodilator effect

Bronchodilatation in response to 5-LO inhibition would be expected to occur in situations where baseline leukotriene synthesis was high and responsible for significant intrinsic bronchoconstrictor tone. In a study of chronic asthma in patients treated with salbutamol only, baseline FEV_1 increased by 15% within 1 hour of zileuton administration (Israel *et al.*, 1993b). In ASA subjects administration of ZD2138 lead to an approximate 10% increase in FEV_1 compared to baseline within 4 hours. However, in this study, baseline FEV_1 was significantly lower than on the placebo day and bronchodilatation may have represented a regression to normal FEV_1 values (Nasser *et al.*, 1994a).

Trials in chronic asthma

In a multicentre study, 139 asthmatic patients with a baseline predicted FEV_1 of 40–75%, who were not taking oral or inhaled corticosteroids, were placed on placebo or zileuton 2.4 g or 1.6 g/day for 4 weeks. Patients treated with zileuton had a 0.32 l or 13.6% improvement in FEV_1 after 4 weeks, which was significantly better than with placebo. There was also a significant improvement in asthmatic symptom scores and reduction in β_2-agonist use in subjects on the higher dose of zileuton. In addition, there was a reduction in urinary LTE_4 levels with a greater decrease in the higher dose group (Israel *et al.*, 1993b). In an extension of this study, 398 asthmatic patients previously stabilized on salbutamol with moderately severe asthma (baseline FEV_1 61%) were treated for 13 weeks with 2.4 or 1.6 g/day or placebo. In the subjects taking 2.4 g/day there was a sustained increase in FEV_1 of 0.25 l, compared to a 0.08 l increase in the patients who completed the placebo arm of the study. A recently reported study of 109 asthmatic subjects taking 400–1600 μg of either beclomethasone or budesonide with baseline FEV_1 50–75% were placed on placebo or 125 mg MK-0591 twice daily. After 4 weeks' treatment, FEV_1 rose 6.8% in the MK-0591-treated group compared to 0.6% for the placebo group. In addition, there was a rise in morning PEFR of 19% and evening PEFR of 13% in the MK-0591-treated group, compared to a fall in morning and evening PEFR of 5% and 6%, respectively, in the placebo-treated group. There was also a reduction in β_2-agonist use in subjects on active treatment (Chapman *et al.*, 1994).

Other diseases

In a double-blind placebo-controlled study of eight patients suffering from allergic rhinitis, oral administration of a single dose of 800 mg zileuton led to significant attenuation of allergen-induced nasal congestion, and this was associated with inhibition of leukotriene release into nasal lavage fluid (Knapp, 1990).

The acetohydroxamic acid 5-LO inhibitor BWA4C has been shown to reduce LTB_4 synthesis in inflamed colonic resection tissue in patients with inflammatory bowel disease in a dose-dependent fashion (Hawthorne *et al.*, 1992). In an open study of 11 subjects with active ulcerative colitis treated with zileuton 800 mg for 28 days, there was a reduction in symptom scores in all patients and improvement in gross mucosal appearance, although no change on histological examination was found (Collawn *et al.*, 1992).

Lonapalene (6-chloro-2,3-dimethoxynapthalene-dio-diacetate), a selective inhibitor of 5-LO, was applied as a topical 2% ointment onto psoriatic plaques for 28 days. Compared to vehicle-treated sites, there was significant reduction in skin chamber fluid LTB_4 levels by 4 days with a reduction in clinical scores in seven out of nine subjects at 14 and 28 days (Jones *et al.*, 1986). A 2% ointment of R 68,151, a selective 5-LO inhibitor, was applied twice daily for 4 weeks on psoriatic plaques in 44 patients and compared to placebo ointment in a further 44 patients. The active group experienced an improvement in mean symptom scores for scaling, of 46% against 6% for the placebo group and 34% for erythema compared to a deterioration of 3% for the placebo-treated group. In 27% of subjects in the active group the lesions either disappeared or showed marked improvement compared to 8% of vehicle-treated plaques (Degreef *et al.*, 1990).

Twenty-four patients with active rheumatoid arthritis were randomized to receive zileuton 800 mg twice daily or placebo for 4 weeks. There was an improvement in clinical variables in both groups, with a non-statistically significant trend towards greater improvement in joint-swelling index and patient assessment of the number of painful joints in the zileuton group (Weinblatt *et al.*, 1992).

In conclusion, there appear to be many theoretical reasons to suggest that leukotriene biosynthesis inhibitors would be more effective than cysteinyl leukotriene receptor antagonists. Biosynthesis inhibitors block generation of the full spectrum of 5-LO products, which include not only cysteinyl leukotrienes but also other inflammatory mediators such as LTB_4 and 5-HETE (Jones *et al.*, 1988), as well as some of the effects of PAF (Anderson & Fennessy, 1988; Lundgren *et al.*, 1990). Conversely, leukotriene antagonists can only effectively prevent the action of leukotrienes at one receptor. In addition, cysteinyl leukotriene receptor antagonists appear to prolong the half-lives of leukotrienes by interfering with their elimination (Denzlinger *et al.*, 1991). In practice, this has not been found to be the case in clinical studies, with receptor antagonists showing very effective inhibition of cysteinyl leukotriene-mediated disease processes. Several mechanisms may account for this. Firstly, although there is good inhibition of *ex vivo* whole-blood LTB_4 and urinary LTE_4 release, current 5-LO inhibitors may not yet be potent enough to provide effective inhibition of intra-airway leukotriene biosynthesis. Secondly, the presence of even small quantities of generated leukotriene may prove sufficient to exert pathological effects. Thirdly, inhibition of 5-LO may interfere with the synthesis of dual lipoxygenase products such as lipoxin A_4, which may have a moderating influence on cysteinyl leukotriene action (Christie *et al.*, 1992b). Fourthly, there is a theoretical possibility that 5-LO inhibition may lead to shunting of arachidonic acid towards the generation of pro-inflammatory cyclo-oxygenease products. It has been speculated that the ideal compound to modulate the effects of leukotrienes in asthma would possess both leukotriene receptor antagonism and 5-LO synthesis inhibitory activity (Snyder & Fleisch, 1989), because these activities may be functionally additive (Redkar-Brown & Aharony, 1989). Over the next few years the place of these compounds in the treatment of asthma is likely to be established, but first more clinical studies are required to define whether they have corticosteroid-sparing activity and whether they lead to long-term symptomatic improvement. In addition, biopsy studies should be undertaken to determine whether they have anti-inflammatory effects. The promise shown by these anti-leukotriene compounds must be tempered with a note of caution, because leukotrienes are just one of many pro-inflammatory mediators in asthma, and monotherapy with these agents may prove insufficient.

Prostaglandins and thromboxanes

Biosynthesis and cellular source

The products of the cyclo-oxygenase pathway should now be known as compounds arising from the action of prostaglandin H synthases (PGHS) on arachidonic acid. In contrast to 5-LO, this enzyme is found almost universally in mammalian cells, although there is great variation in the specific products generated by different cell sources. Mast cells preferentially generate PGD_2, platelets predominantly generate TXA_2 vascular endothelial cells and both vascular and non-vascular smooth muscle synthesize prostacyclin (PGI_2), macrophages generate $PGF_{2\alpha}$ PGE_2 and TXA_2, and epithelial cells generate PGE_2. Mast cells are the source of PGD_2 released from human lung fragments (Lewis *et al.*, 1982; Holgate *et al.*, 1984b) in response to IgE-dependent and calcium ionophore A23187 stimulation, and this is then metabolized by an nicotinamide adenine dinucleotide phosphate (NADPH)-dependent 11-keto-reductase to the active metabolite 9_{α},11_{β}-PGF_2 which has bronchoconstrictor activity (Beasley *et al.*, 1987a,b). However, neutrophils, eosinophils and basophils do not generate significant quantities of prostanoid products.

Role of PGHS

The prostanoids are formed by the metabolic pathway outlined in Fig. 23.7. Prostanoid synthesis is initiated by hormone-activated mobilization of esterified arachidonate from one or more of a number of precursor phospholipids by phospholipase activity. Arachidonate is converted by the cyclo-oxygenase action of PGHS to the prostaglandin endoperoxides PGG_2 and then onto PGH_2 by a peroxidase reaction. PGH_2 is then rapidly isomerized or reduced by cell-specific synthases (isomerases) or reductases to the major biologically active prostanoids PGD_2, $PGF_{2\alpha}$ and TXA_2 which have bronchoconstrictor properties, and PGE_2 and prostacyclin (PGI_2) which have inhibitory or 'bronchoprotective' properties (Samuelsson *et al.*, 1978; Uotila & Vapaatalo, 1984). It has recently been discovered that mammalian cells contain two isoforms of PGHS, referred to as PGHS-1 and PGHS-2, with 61% homology between their amino-acid sequences (Hla & Neilson, 1992). The two isoforms have conservation of the amino-acid sequences required for both cyclooxygenase and peroxidase activities and similar affinity for and capacity to convert arachidonic acid to PGH_2 (Meade *et al.*, 1993). The differences between these

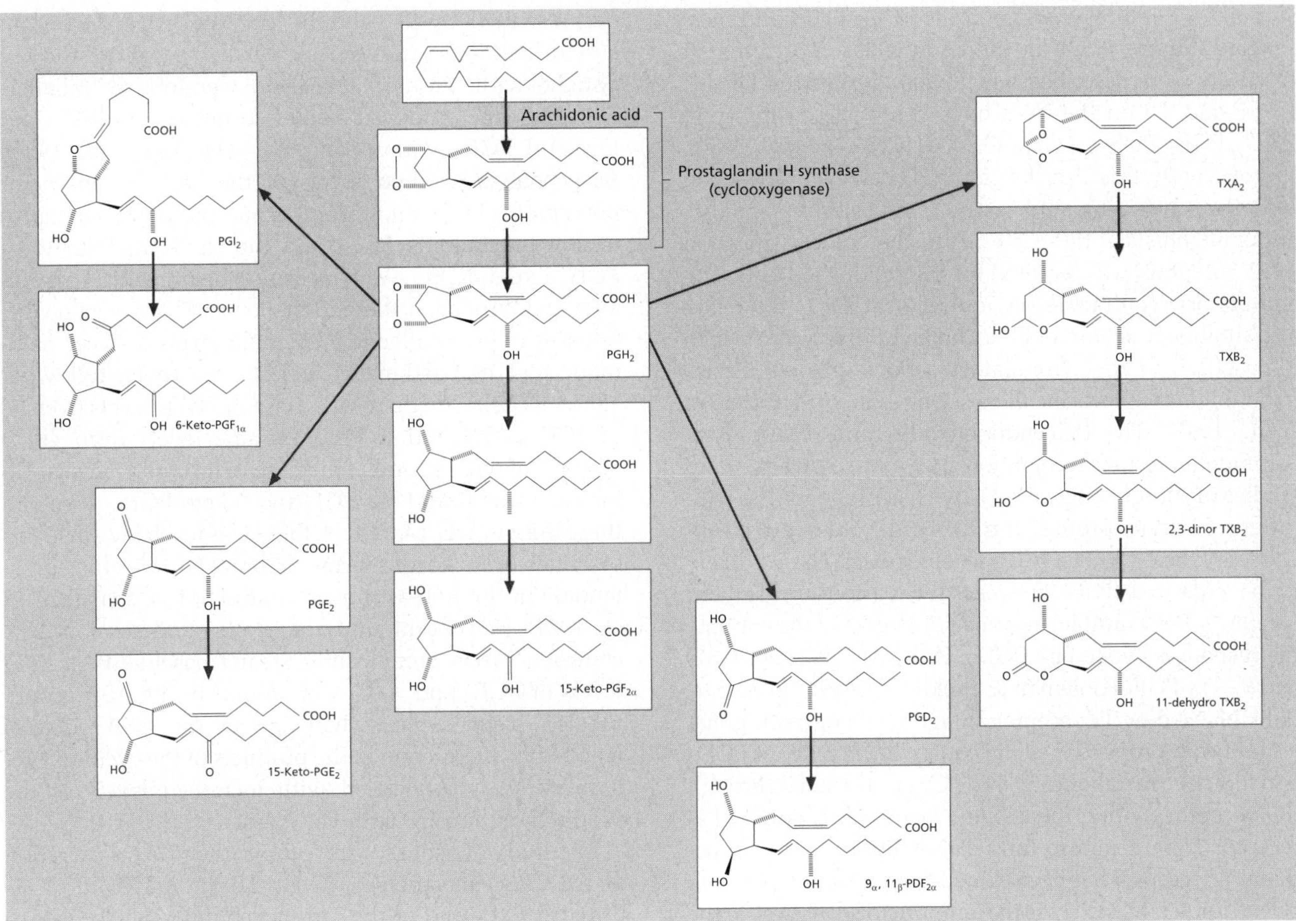

Fig. 23.7 Prostanoid biosynthetic pathway. Cyclo-oxygenase catalyses the first two steps and converts arachidonic acid to the endoperoxides prostaglandin G_2 (PGG_2) and PGH_2, which are then enzymatically transformed to the prostaglandins, prostacyclin and thromboxanes by the action of the respective synthesis.

two isoforms of PGHS appear to involve their regulation and cell expression. PGHS-1 is expressed constitutively at varying levels in virtually all mammalian tissues. For example, vascular endothelial cells (DeWitt *et al.*, 1983) and platelets (Funk *et al.*, 1991) express high baseline levels of enzyme, with only minor increases induced by hormonal or growth factor stimulation of two- to fourfold (DeWitt, 1991; Oshima *et al.*, 1991). PGHS-2, on the other hand is relatively undetectable in the majority of tissues, but its expression increases substantially in situations associated with cell replication and differentiation and in response to inflammation and mitogenic stimuli, with typical increases of 10- to 80-fold (Kujubu *et al.*, 1991; 1993). For example, growth factors such as phorbol esters and interleukin-1 induce PGHS-2 in fibroblasts (Kujubu *et al.*, 1991; O'Banion *et al.*, 1992) and endotoxin can stimulate PGHS-2 expression in monocytes and macrophages (Lee *et al.*, 1992; O'Sullivan *et al.*, 1992). Thus far only a limited number of tissues have been examined for PGHS-2 activity, but it is likely to be found under appropriate stimulatory conditions in as many cell types as PGHS-1. A further regulatory property of PGHS-2 is that its induced expression can be completely inhibited by anti-inflammatory glucocorticoids such as dexamethasone (Masferrer *et al.*, 1992). It has therefore been hypothesized that the constitutively expressed PGHS-1 is a housekeeping gene involved in the production of prostanoids to regulate normal cellular function, and that inducible PGHS-2 is involved in the production of prostanoids that mediate inflammatory and mitogenic responses.

Receptors

Following intracellular synthesis, prostanoids leave the cell probably by facilitated diffusion (Smith, 1986). Outside the cell prostanoids act either on the parent and or neighbouring cells in an autocrine or paracrine fashion through specific G-protein-linked prostanoid receptors, to stimulate or inhibit changes in the levels of second messengers (Smith, 1989). In the early 1980s, five different receptors were described which were designated DP, EP, FP, IP and TP on the basis of preferential sensitivity to PGD_2, PGE_2, $PGF_{2\alpha}$, PGI_2 and TXA_2 (Coleman *et al.*, 1984). More recently, this classification has been extended using radioligand-binding studies and more selective agonists and antagonists at these sites. A further subclassification of EP receptors was required for the actions of PGE_2. The stimulatory/contractile actions occur at EP-1, the relaxant/inhibitory actions at EP-2 and an EP-3 receptor which is proposed to have stimulatory actions in some tissues and inhibitory effects in others (Dong *et al.*, 1986; Coleman *et al.*, 1987). The PG endoperoxides and TXA_2 share common molecular recognition sites in the airways. From studies of a large range of selective receptor agonists with differing activity profiles, it is likely that at least two subclasses of the TXA/PGH (TP) receptor exist. There is likely to be cross-reactivity between the various prostanoid receptors. For example, in guinea pig treachea the contractile responses evoked by PGD_2, $PGF_{2\alpha}$ (Jones *et al.*, 1982) and 9_α,11_β-PGF_2 (Coleman & Sheldrick, 1989) can be partially blocked by TP receptor antagonists, suggesting that a significant proportion of the contractile activity of PGD_2 and its active metabolite 9_α, 11_β-PGF_2 is mediated through this receptor. Within the last few years a functional EP-3 receptor from a mouse lung cDNA library and a functional TP receptor has been cloned from a human placenta cDNA library. In each case the amino acid sequences of the receptors have encoded proteins predicted to be members of the G-protein-linked receptor superfamily with seven transmembrane domains. With further cloning of prostanoid receptors using cDNA probes, it should be possible to study the regulation of prostanoid receptor gene expression, prepare specific antagonists for possible clinical use and prepare antipeptide antibodies for immunolocalization in different tissue types.

Release of prostanoids into biological fluids

There is substantial evidence for prostanoid release in asthma both in disease and in response to allergen challenge. Bronchoalveolar levels of the bronchoconstrictor prostanoids PGD_2, 9_α,11_β-PGF_2 and $PGF_{2\alpha}$ were simultaneously profiled using gas chromatography–mass spectrometry. Compared to normal individuals, levels of these prostanoids were found to be from 12 to 22 times higher in asthmatic airways. Levels of PGD_2 and 9_α,11_β-PGF_2 were 10-fold higher in asthmatic subjects compared to patients with allergic rhinitis, distinguishing subjects with lower airways disease from other atopic conditions. When all 12 normal, 11 allergic rhinitis and 15 mild asthmatic individuals were considered together, an inverse correlation was found between the dose of methacholine required to decrease FEV_1 by 20% and the levels of BAL bronchoconstrictor mediators (Liu *et al.*, 1990). In a separate study of patients with chronic stable asthma, endobronchial allergen challenge produced a 150-fold increase in BAL fluid levels of PGD_2 within 9 minutes (Murray *et al.*, 1986). Bronchoalveolar fluid levels of the bronchoconstrictor prostanoids PGD_2 and thromboxane and the bronchoprotective prostanoids PGE_2 and the stable metabolite of PGI_2, 6-keto-$PGF_{1\alpha}$, were measured before and 5 minutes after endobronchial allergen challenge. There were no differences in pre-challenge prostanoid levels between asthmatic and non-asthmatic subjects. However, following allergen challenge there was a rise in PGD_2 levels from 97 to 1053 pg/ml and in thromboxane levels from 46 to 150 pg/ml with a parallel increase in histamine levels. No increase was found for PGI_2 and 6-keto-$PGF_{1\alpha}$ levels in these individuals. Moreover, there was no change in levels of either bronchoconstrictor or bronchoprotective prostanoids in the non-asthmatic control subjects (Wenzel *et al.*, 1989). In a recent study of 10 ASA and six non-ASA control subjects, significantly greater baseline BAL fluid levels of PGE_2 and TXB_2 were found in the ASA group. Inhaled lysine-aspirin challenge in the ASA subjects resulted in a reduction in the products of the cyclo-oxygenase pathway associated with increased levels of the products of the 5-LO pathway (Sladek *et al.*, 1994).

In a study of acute severe asthma, the urinary excretion of the TXA_2 metabolites, TXB_2, 2,3-dinor-TXB_2 and 11-dihydro TXB_2 and of the prostacyclin metabolites 6-oxo-$PGF_{1\alpha}$ and 2,5-dinor-6-oxo-$PGF_{1\alpha}$ were measured using gas chromatography–mass spectrometry. Both the levels of TXB_2 and prostacyclin metabolites were found to be significantly higher in patients with acute severe asthma compared to a non-smoking control population (Taylor *et al.*, 1991b). Seven atopic asthmatic subjects were predosed with either placebo or low-dose aspirin followed by allergen challenge and urinary metabolites of the major cyclo-oxygenase product of platelets, TXA_2 were measured using the technique of gas chromatography–negative ion, chemical ionization–mass spectrometry. After placebo pre-dosing followed by allergen challenge, there was a rise in urinary excretion of 2,3-dinor-TXB_2 from 76 to 216 pg/mg creatinine and 11-dehydro-TXB_2 from 396 to 627 pg/mg creatinine. Pre-dosing with low-dose aspirin suppressed excretion of thromboxane metabolites and prevented the rise in the urinary excretion of TXA_2 metabolites without altering the level of bronchoconstriction after allergen inhalation, suggesting that although platelets are activated by allergen challenge, the platelet-derived product TXA_2 is not important in the early bronchoconstrictor response (Lupinetti *et al.*, 1989). A similar study of 10 atopic asthmatics found increases in urinary levels of 11-dehydro-TXB_2 from 585 to 1500 pg/mg creatinine at 2 hours after allergen inhalation, but no increase during the late-phase response (Sladek *et al.*, 1990).

Using radioimmunoassay, plasma concentrations of the stable metabolite of $PGF_{2\alpha}$ were measured in 15 infants during acute asthma. The mean level of 13,14-dihydro-15-keto $PGF_{2\alpha}$ was 1470 ng/l, compared to 25.5 ng/l after resolution of airways obstruction, with the highest levels obtained from those infants positive for respiratory syncytial virus (Skoner *et al.*, 1989a). A further study by the same authors reported similar results using 13,14-dihydro-15-keto $PGF_{2\alpha}$, but in addition found that baseline levels of this metabolite of $PGF_{2\alpha}$ were similar between normal and asthmatic children (Skoner *et al.*, 1989b).

Pharmacological properties of prostanoids in asthma

PGD₂

The endoperoxide PGH_2 undergoes non-oxidative isomerization to PGD_2 by the action of unidentified glutathione-dependent and glutathione-independent PGD synthases (Smith *et al.*, 1991). Initial studies indicating the possible role of PGD_2 as a bronchoactive mediator demonstrated bronchoconstrictor actions in the dog (Fitzgerald *et al.*, 1983). In addition, PGD_2 was found to be released from activated rat peritoneal mast cells (Roberts *et al.*, 1979) and during pulmonary anaphylaxis in the guinea pig (Robinson *et al.*, 1984). PGD_2 is the most abundant eicosanoid generated from anti-IgE- (Lewis *et al.*, 1982) and ionophore-stimulated (Holgate *et al.*, 1984a) human pulmonary mast cells. When administered by aerosol to both normal and asthmatic subjects, PGD_2 is a potent contractile agent and elicits a rapidly developing bronchoconstriction (Hardy *et al.*, 1984; Beaseley *et al.*, 1987a,b). In asthmatic subjects it has a potency of approximately 3.5 and 10 times greater than $PGF_{2\alpha}$ and histamine, respectively, with the maximal effect evident 3 minutes following inhalation. The same study reported a significant correlation between airways responsiveness to PGD_2 and methacholine (Hardy *et al.*, 1984). Inhaled PGD_2 was administered in a dose that caused no measurable bronchoconstriction to six mild asthmatic subjects, immediately before each dose of histamine or methacholine. The results demonstrated an approximate two-fold enhancement of bronchial responsiveness to subsequent histamine and methacholine inhalation (Fuller *et al.*, 1986). A further study conducted in asthmatic subjects suggested that sequential doses of PGD_2 followed by histamine are additive and therefore enhanced airway responsiveness was a physiological effect rather than a pharmacological one (Hardy *et al.*, 1986). There is also some evidence to suggest that PGD_2 may enhance the bronchoconstrictor activity of LTC_4 in asthmatic airways (Phillips & Holgate, 1989). Metabolism of PGD_2 yields $9_{\alpha},11_{\beta}$-PGF_2, which has similar bronchoconstrictor potency to PGD_2 and may play a significant role in the biological activity of PGD_2 (Beasley *et al.*, 1987a,b).

PGF₂α

Human lung parenchymal, and to a lesser extent bronchial tissue fragments, spontaneously release $PGF_{2\alpha}$ under resting conditions, leading to the suggestion that this prostanoid, together with PGE_2, may be important in maintaining bronchial tone (Schulman *et al.*, 1982; Cuthbert & Gardiner, 1983). $PGF_{2\alpha}$ has contractile activity on isolated human airway tissue (Sweatman & Collier, 1968; Orehek *et al.*, 1973) and causes bronchoconstriction *in vivo*, with asthmatic subjects demonstrating greater sensitivity to the effects of inhaled $PGF_{2\alpha}$ than normal control subjects. In a study of 10 asthmatic and 10 healthy controls, it was reported that asthmatic subjects were 10 times more sensitive to histamine but 8000 times more sensitive to the bronchoconstrictor action of inhaled $PGF_{2\alpha}$ (Mathe *et al.*, 1973). Furthermore, whereas the healthy controls had reproducible decreases in SGaw in response to repeated $PGF_{2\alpha}$ challenge, the asthmatic subjects demonstrated tachyphylaxis (Mathe & Hedqvist, 1975). Other studies have also reported similar responses to $PGF_{2\alpha}$ inhalation in asthmatic subjects but with wide interstudy variation in the degree of hyperreactivity ranging from 150- (Smith *et al.*, 1975) to 8000-fold (Mathe *et al.*, 1973) greater sensitivity compared to non-asthmatic subjects. In studies of asthmatic individuals examining the effect of $PGF_{2\alpha}$ on airways responsiveness, inhalation of a non-bronchoconstricting dose of $PGF_{2\alpha}$ led to a fourfold enhancement of bronchial responsiveness to histamine (Walters *et al.*, 1981; Heaton *et al.*, 1984), but had no effect on subsequent methacholine provocation (Heaton *et al.*, 1984).

TXA₂

The enzymes responsible for catalysing the conversion of PGH_2 to TXA_2, TXA synthases, have now been cloned from human platelets (Yokoyama *et al.*, 1991) and lung (Ohashi *et al.*, 1992), and it has been confirmed that this enzyme is a member of the cytochrome P-450 family. The half-life of TXA_2 is only about 30 seconds *in vivo* and therefore much of the information about its biological activity comes from studies employing synthetic compounds that are stable analogues of the TXA_2 structure, such as the long-acting thromboxane mimetic U-46619. TXA_2 is readily degraded to its more stable and relatively inactive metabolite TXB_2, which can be measured in biological fluids such as BAL and urine. In a study of isolated human, bronchus, the rank order of contractile potency for prostanoids was U-46619 >> 9_{α}, 11_{β}-PGF_2 = $PGF_{2\alpha}$ >

$PGD_2 > PGE_2 > PGI_2$ (Coleman & Sheldrick, 1989). Interestingly, this is almost exactly the reverse of the rank order for the magnitude of spontaneous prostanoid release from lung parenchymal fragments, which is 6-keto-$PGF_{1\alpha}$ (stable metabolite of prostacyclin) $> PGE_2 = PGF_{2\alpha} > PGD_2 > TXB_2$ (Schulman *et al.*, 1982). A single oral dose of the specific and potent TP receptor antagonist GR 32191 in a study of nine asthmatic subjects had no effect on basal airway calibre and produced no effect on the position or slope of the dose–response curve to methacholine (Beasley *et al.*, 1989). This suggests that the most potent bronchoconstricting prostanoids are released in the smallest quantities under resting conditions and are therefore unlikely to play a role in resting airway tone. The TP receptor antagonist AH 23848 was shown to antagonize the contractile activity of the prostanoids but demonstrated no activity against carbachol-induced contractions (Coleman & Sheldrick, 1989), suggesting that the major bronchoconstrictor action of the prostanoids is mediated through the TP receptor. In a study of 13 asthmatic and six normal subjects, the bronchoconstricting effect of U46619 was found to be 178-fold greater than methacholine. Furthermore, inhalation of a subthreshold dose of U46619 was found to double the subsequent bronchoconstrictor response to methacholine. This effect was transient and only apparent if methacholine challenge took place within 1 hour before U46619 inhalation (Jones *et al.*, 1992).

PGE_2

PGE_2 is spontaneously released from both human bronchial smooth muscle and lung parenchymal tissue (Schulman *et al.*, 1982). Further sources include macrophages (Macdermot *et al.*, 1984), epithelial (Churchill *et al.*, 1989) and endothelial cells. Prostanoids of the E series are usually described as having relaxant properties on airway smooth muscle. Inhalation of 55 μg PGE_1 and PGE_2 in normal subjects increased SGaw by 10 and 18%, respectively, and in asthmatic subjects by 41 and 39%, respectively (Smith *et al.*, 1975). However, the effect of PGE_2 on human smooth muscle is much more complex. Inhalation in normal subjects produces an initial bronchoconstriction within 5 minutes, followed by bronchodilatation peaking at 15 minutes and returning to baseline after 30 minutes (Walters & Davies, 1982). In asthmatic subjects the response to inhaled PGE_2 is more often biphasic, with the degree of initial bronchoconstriction inversely related to resting airway tone and enhanced following bronchodilatation with the anticholinergic agent ipratropium bromide (Walters & Davies, 1982). Additionally, PGE_2 has paradoxical effects against the bronchoconstrictor activity of histamine and methacholine, protecting against bronchoconstriction during the bronchodilator phase and enhancing bronchial responsiveness to these reference agents if administered after the end of this phase (Walters *et al.*, 1982). Further evidence of the possible modulatory role played by PGE_2 in bronchial asthma and other inflammatory diseases comes from its *in vitro* effect in reducing mucus secretion (Marom *et al.*, 1981).

A number of studies have examined the usefulness of PGE_2 in various models of asthma. Inhaled PGE_2 decreased the maximal fall in exercise-induced FEV_1 by 63% and reduced the duration of exercise-induced bronchoconstriction (Melillo *et al.*, 1994). This effect is comparable to that found with leukotriene receptor antagonists (Manning *et al.*, 1990b), sodium cromoglycate (Robuschi *et al.*, 1992) and β_2-agonists (Anderson *et al.*, 1979). There was no effect on methacholine-induced airways responsiveness. Inhaled PGE_2 has also been shown to protect against the early- and late-phase bronchoconstriction induced by allergen (Pavord *et al.*, 1993), inhalation of ultrasonically nebulized distilled water (Pasargiklian *et al.*, 1976) and sodium metabisulphite (Pavord *et al.*, 1991), and protect against the allergen-induced rise in bronchial responsiveness (Pasargiklian *et al.*, 1976).

Although PGE_2 appears to play a bronchoprotective role in asthma, its therapeutic use is unfortunately limited by its short half-life, the initial cough and bronchoconstrictor effect and by the retrosternal soreness that results from inhalation.

PGI_2 (prostacyclin)

Prostacyclin is generated by macrophages and constitutes a major product of endothelial cells with potent cyclic adenosine monophosphate (cAMP)-dependent smooth-muscle relaxant activity for the maintenance of vascular patency. The hydrolysis product of PGI_2, 6-keto-$PGF_{1\alpha}$, is released into biological fluids such as BAL and provides a reliable index of PGI_2 generation and release. This metabolite has been detected as the major cyclo-oxygenase product released from both resting and allergen-stimulated fragments of human bronchi, although the cells responsible for this remain unidentified (Schulman *et al.*, 1982). In studies of airway smooth muscle, PGI_2 was found to cause relaxation of guinea pig tracheal strips and of isolated precontracted human bronchus, although smooth-muscle contraction was also sometimes seen (Gardiner & Collier, 1980). In a study of eight asthmatic and 10 normal controls, the effects of inhaled PGI_2 and its hydrolysis product 6-oxo-$PGF_{1\alpha}$ on airway calibre were examined. Inhalation of both cyclo-oxygenase products caused cough and retrosternal discomfort and no consistent effect was found in either group, except for reproducible bronchodilatation in two asthmatic subjects (Hardy *et al.*, 1985). The same group went on to examine the effect of doubling doses of both prostanoids using different parameters of airway calibre in mild asthmatic subjects. In doses of up to 500 μg/ml PGI_2 there was no effect on SGaw, but a concentration-dependent fall in FEV_1 and a reduction in the maximum flow rate at 30% of vital capacity ($V_{max}30$) was observed in all subjects. In two out of the four subjects there was an increase in residual volume and reduction in vital capacity without a change in total lung capacity. Furthermore, PGI_2 but not 6-oxo-$PGF_{1\alpha}$ protected against PGD_2- and methacholine-induced bronchoconstriction, as measured using any parameter of airway calibre (Hardy *et al.*, 1988). An explanation of these seemingly paradoxical results may be that the principal action of PGI_2 in the airways is to cause vasodilatory mucosal engorgement and hence a reduction in small-airway calibre as measured by FEV_1 and $V_{max}30$, but protect against the spasmogenic effects of other mediators by increasing their clearance from receptor sites by increasing blood flow.

Pharmacological modulation of prostanoid action

Non-steroidal anti-inflammatory drugs (NSAID) have been in clinical use for a considerable time, and until very recently they have been our only means of affecting either the biosynthesis or the action of specific prostanoids. Given the diverse and often opposite actions of the prostanoid compounds, this deficiency of pharmacological products has been a considerable drawback and prevented a more complete understanding of prostanoid action in allergic disease. More recently, thromboxane synthesis inhibitors and receptor antagonists have been developed to block the action of bronchoconstricting prostanoids, whilst sparing the bronchoprotective compounds such as PGE_2 and PGI_2. The elucidation of the differential amino-acid sequences of PGHS-1 and PGHS-2 will allow the development of more selective inhibitors of each isoform and provide us with the opportunity to test new hypotheses.

Resting airway calibre

Indomethacin was found to augment the dose-dependent decrement in dynamic compliance and pulmonary conductance in response to LTC_4 administered to mechanically ventilated guinea pigs (Leitch *et al.* 1983). A similar effect has not been found on studies on human bronchial tissue (Brink *et al.*, 1980; Cuthbert & Gardiner, 1983). In addition, there was no effect on the resting airway calibre of asthmatic subjects treated with cyclo-oxygenase inhibitors (Curzen *et al.*, 1987), thromboxane synthetase inhibitors (Fujimura *et al.*, 1986; Fujimura *et al.*, 1990a) or thromboxane receptor antagonists (Fujimura *et al.*, 1991).

Allergen challenge

In asthmatic subjects pretreatment with 50 mg indomethacin for 4 days significantly increased the airway response to allergen when measures of PD_{20} FEV_1 and PD_{35} SGaw were taken into account (Fish *et al.*, 1981). In a separate study of seven asthmatic subjects exhibiting DAR, 2 days pretreatment with indomethacin 50 mg twice daily had no effect on the allergen-induced EAR or LAR (Kirby *et al.*, 1989). In contrast to these results, Curzen and colleagues reported the effects of pretreatment with the more potent cyclo-oxygenase inhibitor flurbiprofen on the allergen-induced bronchoconstricor response. At a dose of 150 mg daily for 3 days, flurbiprofen and terfenedine reduced the mean maximal fall in FEV_1 by 21 and 43%, respectively. However, the combination of the two drugs did not have an additive effect on the allergen-induced bronchoconstrictor response (Curzen *et al.*, 1987). The thromboxane receptor antagonist GR 32191 administered at a dose of 80 mg to asthmatic subjects produced a variable degree of inhibition of the EAR to inhaled allergen (Beasley *et al.*, 1989). In a study of 12 asthmatic subjects, the specific thromboxane synthetase inhibitor CGS 13080 was administered at a dose of 200 mg four times daily, for 2 days before and 1 day after allergen challenge. Despite significant attenuation of the rise in serum TXB_2 levels, there was only a small, though significant, attenuation of the EAR but there was no effect on the late response to allergen (Manning *et al.*, 1991).

Bronchial hyperresponsiveness

There is considerable evidence for the involvement of prostanoids in bronchial hyperresponsiveness. Indomethacin 50 mg, administered four times daily for 3 days to asthmatic subjects, led to a significant reduction in the airway sensitivity to inhaled histamine (Walters, 1983). This was supported by a further study in which flurbiprofen was administered to asthmatic subjects at a dose of 150 mg daily for 3 days and led to a mean 3.3-fold reduction in airway response to histamine (Curzen *et al.*, 1987). However, the specific thromboxane synthetase inhibitor CGS 13080 demonstrated no effect on baseline or post-allergen airway responsiveness to histamine (Manning *et al.*, 1991).

In open studies, the thromboxane synthetase inhibitor OKY-046 in both oral (Fujimura *et al.*, 1986) and inhaled (Fujimura *et al.*, 1990a) forms reduced the bronchial hyperresponsiveness to acetylcholine in asthmatic subjects. Early studies using cyclo-oxygenase inhibitors failed to demonstrate any effect on the airway hyperresponsiveness to methacholine (Curzen *et al.*, 1987). Similarly, 3 weeks' treatment with the TP receptor antagonist GR32191 160 mg daily (Stenton *et al.*, 1992), and 1 week's therapy with the thromboxane synthetase inhibitor UK-38,485 (Gardiner *et al.*, 1993), demonstrated no reduction in the airway sensitivity to inhaled methacholine. In contrast to these findings, the TP receptor antagonist AA-2414 was found to reduce methacholine-induced airway responsiveness in asthmatic subjects (Fujimura *et al.*, 1991), but this effect was not found in patients with chronic bronchitis or bronchiectasis (Fujimura *et al.*, 1990b).

Exercise-induced asthma

A single dose of the potent cyclo-oxygenase inhibitor flurbiprofen, 150 mg 2 hours before exercise, led to a 31% inhibition of the mean maximal fall in FEV_1 (Finnerty & Holgate, 1990). In contrast, the less potent cyclo-oxygenase inhibitior indomethacin, administered at a dose of 50 mg for 3 days, provided no protection against the exercise-induced fall in FEV_1 (O'Byrne & Jones, 1986). The TP receptor antagonist GR32191 administered as a single dose of 120 mg 1 hour prior to treadmill exercise in 12 asthmatic subjects demonstrated no protection compared to placebo (Finnerty *et al.*, 1991). Similar results were obtained with BAY U3405 also a TP receptor antagonist, which despite demonstrating effective inhibition of PGD_2-induced bronchoconstriction, produced no effect on the exercise-induced decrease in airway calibre (Magnussen *et al.*, 1992). Part of the mechanism of exercise-induced asthma is therefore likely to involve vascular dilatation which may involve prostacyclin; this is supported by the available data indicating the possible benefit from cyclo-oxygenase inhibitors and the ineffectiveness of TP receptor blockade.

Refractory period

Following repeated challenges to a variety of stimuli such as exercise, inhaled hypertonic saline and distilled water, there is a reduced bronchoconstrictor response during a subsequent refractory period. There is evidence that release of prostanoids may be involved in the mechanism of this effect. Pretreatment with indomethacin in asthmatic subjects abolishes the refractoriness to exercise (O'Byrne & Jones, 1986), hypertonic saline callenge (Hawksworth *et al.*, 1992) and distilled water challenge (Mattoli *et al.*, 1987).

PAF

In 1972, Benveniste, Henson and Cochrane coined the term 'platelet-activating factor' for the soluble factor released from IgE-stimulated basophils and which was found to aggregate rabbit platelets. In 1979, Demopoulos, Pinckard and Hanahan described a semisynthetic phosphoacylglycerol, 1-*O*-alkyl-2-acetyl-*sn*-glycero-3-phosphocholine, or AGEPC, which was able to aggregate platelets, release serotonin and had the same physicochemical properties as PAF. In 1980, Hanahan and colleagues purified and characterized PAF from activated basophils and concluded that AGEPC and PAF comprised the same compound.

Biosynthesis

PAF is not a single molecule and should be considered as a family of structurally related autacoid phopholipids synthesized by inflammatory cells, which have platelet-stimulating and neutrophil-priming activity and whose main members include 1-*O*-hexadecyl-2-acetyl-*sn*-glycero-3-phosphorylcholine and 1-*O*-octadecyl-2-acetyl-*sn*-glycero-3-phosphorylcholine. Currently, there is no generally accepted nomenclature to classify the extensive molecular heterogeneity of PAF. The most commonly recognized chemical structure of PAF is shown in Fig. 23.8.

Cell stimulation leads to the release of alkylacylglycerophosphocholine from cell membranes, which can be converted to PAF via one of two metabolic pathways (Fig. 23.9). The 'remodelling pathway' involves a structural modification of a pre-existing ether-linked phospholipid that forms part of the structure of membranes. The initial step is catalysed by the action of phopholipase A_2 on 1-alkyl-2-acyl-glycerophosphocholine, a membrane phospholipid (Hanahan, 1986; Sturk *et al.*, 1989). This deacylation results in lyso-PAF formation and the release of arachidonic acid which has phospholipase A_2 inhibitory activity, thereby reducing further PAF synthesis, or arachidonic acid may act as the substrate for subsequent eicosanoid synthesis. Lyso-PAF is then acetylated by a specific lyso-PAF acetyltransferase to form 1-*O*-alkyl-2-acetyl-*sn*-glycero-3-phosphocholine-PAF. PAF can subse-

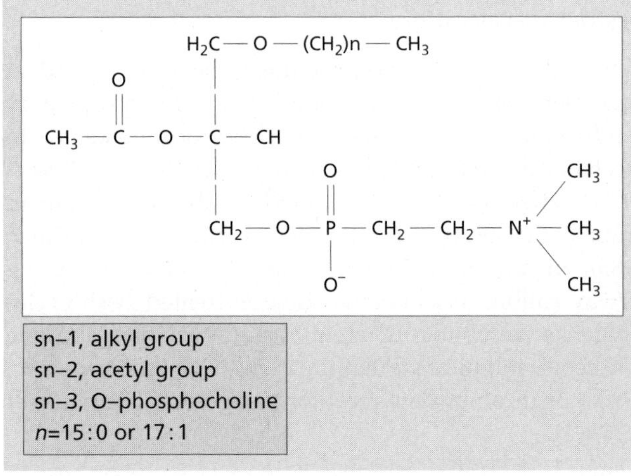

Fig. 23.8 Chemical structure of platelet-activating factor.

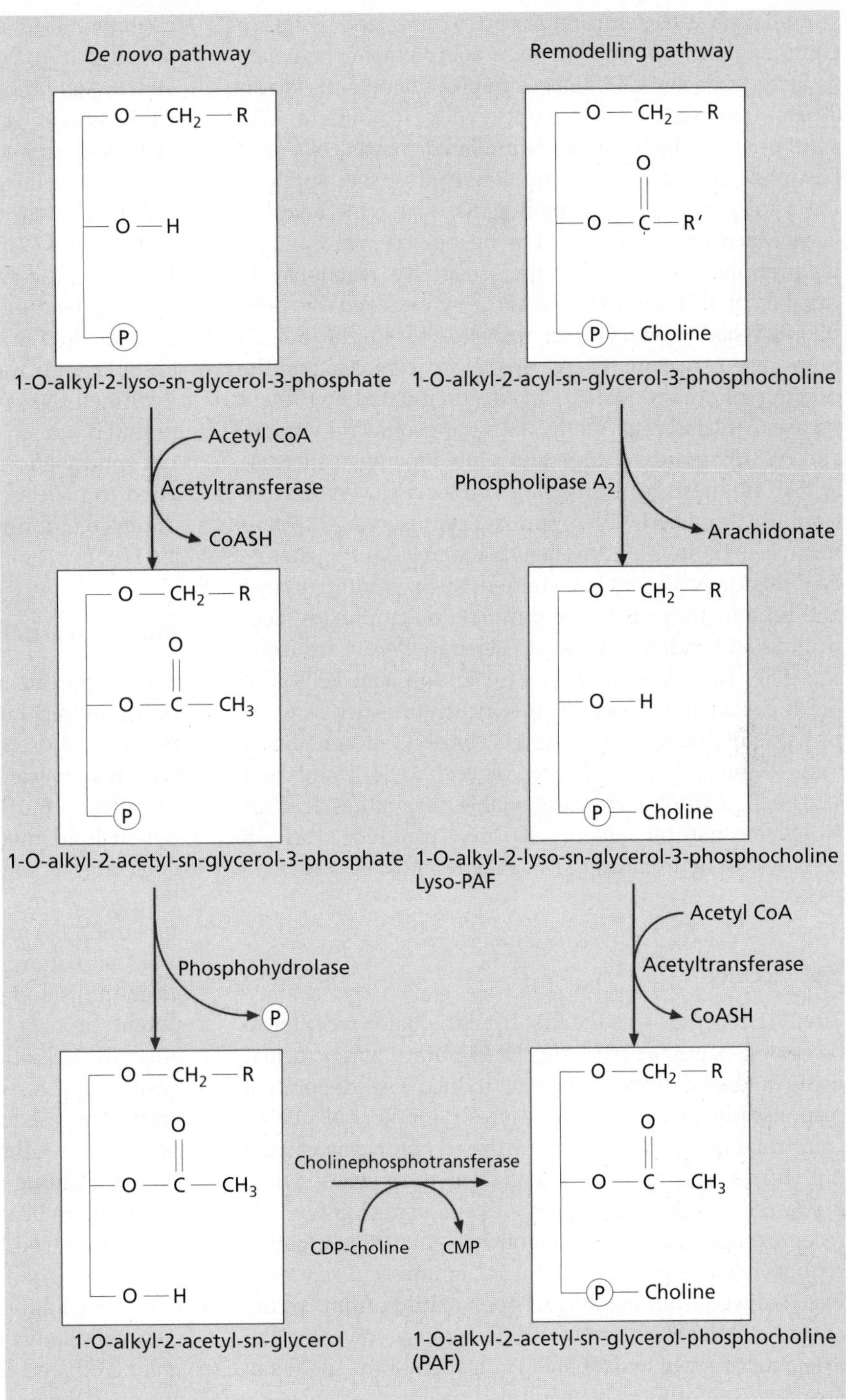

Fig. 23.9 Biosynthetic pathways of platelet-activating factor (PAF) denoting the '*de novo*' and 'remodelling' routes.

quently be remetabolized back to its precursor lyso-PAF by the action of a specific PAF-acetylhydrolase. The other route for PAF biosynthesis is known as the '*de novo*' pathway and begins with an intermediate in the synthesis of ether-linked membrane phospholipids. This is acetylated by a specific acetyltransferase and the phosphate is removed by a phosphohydrolase from the *sn*-3 carbon to form alkylacetylglycerol, which is subsequently converted by cholinephosphotransferase to PAF.

Cellular release

Numerous cell types are capable of PAF synthesis by specific agonist–receptor interactions. Many phagocytic stimuli such as bacteria and parasites opsonized by IgG or complement, immune complexes, complement chemotactic factors C5a and C3a, and eosinophil chemotactic factor-A can stimulate inflammatory cells to initiate PAF synthesis. Antigen or IgE-stimulated mast cells and basophils generate PAF (Schulman *et al.*, 1983), supporting a role for PAF in the pathogenesis of acute anaphylaxis. Macrophages activated by opsonized zymosan and by immune complex in hypersensitivity reactions are capable of PAF synthesis. PAF is synthesized by peripheral blood monocytes in response to 4β-phorbol-12-myrestate-13-acetate (PMA), opsonized zymosan and the calcium ionophore A23187, an effect regulated by protein kinase C (Elstad *et al.*, 1991). Both unopsonized zymosan and A23187 induce a dose- and time-dependent increase in PAF synthesis by eosinophils (Burke *et al.*, 1990). Neutrophils stimulated with opsonized zymosan, A23187 and formyl-methionyl-leucyl-phenylalanine (f-MLP) generate PAF (Sisson *et al.*, 1987). Cytokines such as interleukin-1 and tumour necrosis factor stimulate macrophages, neutrophils and endothelial cells to generate PAF (Camussi *et al.*, 1987; Bussolino *et al.*, 1988). Endothelial cells also produce PAF in response to specific stimuli such as vasopressin, angiotensin II, thrombin, bradykinin and histamine (Camussi *et al.*, 1983; Prescott *et al.*, 1984; McIntyre *et al.*, 1985). Lymphocytes are unable to synthesize PAF. However, natural killer cells may produce PAF in response to IgG binding to Fc receptors (Malavasi *et al.*, 1986).

PAF receptor

The PAF receptor was the first lipid mediator receptor to be cloned. A guinea pig lung cDNA library was screened using a phage clone shown to induce PAF-dependent responses in *Xenopus laevis* oocytes (Honda *et al.*, 1991). Confirmation of the identity of the receptor was carried out based on its pharmacological properties when expressed in COS-7 cells or oocytes and using known PAF receptor agonists and antagonists. A 3020-nucleotide sequence was reported and the 342-amino-acid sequence was deduced from the longest open reading frame of the cloned cDNA. Hydropathy profile analysis revealed the existence of seven hydrophobic transmembrane segments characteristic of G-protein-coupled receptors suggesting that like previously described receptors such as adrenergic 1,2 and muscarinic acetylcholine receptors, the PAF receptor belongs to the G-protein-linked receptor superfamily.

The human PAF receptor cDNA was isolated from a human leucocyte cDNA library using a 0.8-kb fragment of the guinea pig PAF receptor cDNA as a probe. Both the guinea pig and human PAF receptor were shown to possess seven putative transmembrane domains, both contained 342 amino-acid residues and demonstrated 83% homology in amino-acid sequence (Nakamura *et al.*, 1991). Activation of the receptor yielded inositol 1,4,5-triphosphate (IP_3) in the transfected oocytes and COS-7 cells and guanosine 5′-*O*-(2-thio)biphosphate injection into these cells inhibited a PAF-induced Cl^- current, providing evidence that PAF stimulates phosphoinositide turnover via G proteins. When expressed in CHO cells the PAF receptor couples with various second messenger systems, leading to phospholipase C activation, inhibition of adenylate cyclase and activation of the MAP kinase cascade and arachidonate release. A subsequent study identified the PAF receptor cytoplasmic tail as not being required for forward signal transduction. The several phosphorylation sites on the cytoplasmic tail were postulated to play a critical role in the rapid agonist-induced desensitization so characteristic of PAF activity (Takano *et al.*, 1994).

Biological activity

Soon after the identification of this pro-inflammatory phospholipid mediator, PAF was found to have activity beyond the originally described platelet aggregation and was demonstrated to possess a unique profile of biological effects. Furthermore, it was found to be the most potent lipid mediator known with biological responses detectable at concentrations as low as 10^{-14} mol/l and an ED_{50} value for guinea pig platelet activation of about 3×10^{-10} mol/l. The actions of PAF include the recruitment and activation of inflammatory cells, in particular eosinophils and neutrophils (Barnes *et al.*, 1988). PAF has potent bronchoconstrictor activity *in vivo* but *in vitro* effects on smooth-muscle preparations are negligible, suggesting that airway narrowing may be the result of secondary release of spasmogens or the induction of airway oedema secondary to microvascular leakage (Denjean *et al.*, 1983; Chung *et al.*, 1986; Cuss *et al.*, 1986). PAF inhalation induces bronchoconstriction within 2–3 minutes and this is followed by the rapid development of tachyphylaxis (Cuss *et al.*, 1986). Increases in airway responsiveness to reference agonists such as histamine and methacholine were originally described in both the guinea pig (Mazzoni *et al.*, 1985) and the dog (Chung *et al.*, 1986). Later studies observed that inhaled PAF induced a long-lasting increase in airway responsiveness in normal subjects and other investigators subsequently reported similar findings (Chung *et al.*, 1989; Kaye & Smith, 1990). However, the majority of clinical studies on normal subjects have found that the increase in bronchial responsiveness was either absent or only transient (Jenkins *et al.*, 1989; Spencer *et al.*, 1990). Furthermore, in asthmatic subjects inhalation of PAF does not increase airway responsiveness (Chung *et al.*, 1989) and does not lead to late-asthmatic responses

(Lai *et al.*, 1990). PAF produces a receptor-mediated increase in airway microvascular leakage with a 1000-fold greater potency than histamine (Evans *et al.*, 1987). PAF has been detected in the BAL fluid from asthmatic airways (Stenton *et al.*, 1990a). Inhalation of PAF aerosol leads to a twofold increase in neutrophil recovery from BAL fluid but no change in eosinophil recruitment in normal volunteers (Wardlaw *et al.*, 1990). Intracutaneous injection of PAF induces a dual skin response in human subjects, similar to that observed after allergen (Basran *et al.*, 1984), and an eosinophil-rich infiltrate into the skin of allergic subjects, but not of normal subjects (Henocq & Vargaftig, 1988). This raises the possibility of selective recruitment of eosinophils in allergic subjects. Furthermore, eosinophils from atopic subjects release more PAF than those from normal subjects, thus providing a possible positive-feedback loop for continuing inflammation (Lee *et al.*, 1984a). The activation of inflammatory cells leads to the release of other inflammatory mediators, such as the products of both the cyclo-oxygenase (Chung *et al.*, 1986) and the lipoxygenase (Voelkel *et al.*, 1982) pathways and the release of oxygen free radicals (Rouis *et al.*, 1988).

A number of studies have identified the link between PAF and leukotriene synthesis. PAF inhalation stimulates increased biosynthesis of the bronchoconstrictor eicosanoid TXA_2 and the cysteinyl leukotrienes (Taylor *et al.*, 1991c). LTD_4 receptor antagonists reduce the bronchoconstrictor response to inhaled PAF in normal volunteers (Kidney *et al.*, 1993; Spencer *et al.*, 1991), whereas GR 32191B, a thromboxane receptor antagonist, had little effect (Stenton *et al.*, 1990b). This suggests that the cysteinyl leukotrienes may be important in mediating the bronchoconstricor effects to PAF.

PAF receptor antagonists

PAF is an inflammatory mediator which mimics many of the characteristic features of asthma; however, its role remains uncertain and unproven. PAF and its metabolite lyso-PAF have been demonstrated in BAL fluid from stable atopic asthmatic subjects (Stenton *et al.*, 1990a) and in plasma from asthmatic subjects during both early (Chan-Yeung *et al.*, 1991) and late responses to inhaled allergen (Nakamura *et al.*, 1987). Using potent and specific PAF receptor antagonists it should be possible to further elucidate the role of PAF in the pathophysiology of asthma. A number of PAF receptor antagonists have now been evaluated. BN 52063 is a ginkgolide mixture and inhibits PAF-induced weal and flare and platelet aggregatory responses *ex vivo* (Chung *et al.*, 1987). In a subsequent study, this compound demonstrated inhibitory activity against the late-phase cutaneous response to allergen in atopic subjects, with only a 50% reduction in the early weal response. This effect may have resulted from the inhibition of cutaneous eosinophil infiltration (Roberts *et al.*, 1988b). However, in a study of eight normal subjects, inhaled PAF-induced broncoconstriction as measured by V_{30}-P was reduced from 47% after placebo ingestion to 36% at 2 hours after BN 52063. The characteristic neutropenia that occurs within a few minutes of PAF inhalation and the rebound neutrophilia were not affected by the PAF receptor antagonist (Roberts *et al.*, 1988a). WEB 2086 is a hetrazepine compound which inhibits the allergen-induced late response in allergic sheep (Abraham *et al.*, 1989). In human subjects WEB 2086 prevents PAF-induced bronchoconstriction (Adamus *et al.*, 1990) and prevents the histamine hyperresponsiveness induced by PAF *in vitro* (Johnson *et al.*, 1990). In a study of eight mild atopic asthmatic subjects, 1 week's treatment with WEB 2086, 300 mg daily, did not attenuate the allergen-induced early or late responses or the subsequent histamine bronchial hyperresponsiveness (Freitag *et al.*, 1993). In a subsequently reported study of 65 asthmatic subjects, 6 weeks' treatment with WEB 2086, 120 mg daily, did not significantly reduce the requirement for inhaled corticosteroids compared to placebo treatment (Spence *et al.*, 1994). The dihydropyridine compound UK74,505 is a specific and potent PAF receptor antagonist which has 10-fold greater inhibition of PAF-induced aggregation of washed rabbit platelets than WEB 2086 (Alabaster *et al.*, 1991). In a study of 12 normal subjects, inhalation of PAF induced broncoconstriction for 60 minutes, neutropenia at 5 minutes, rebound neutrophilia at 2 hours and stimulated the production of urinary eicosanoids. Premedication with the PAF antagonist UK74,505 completely abolished the bronchoconstrictor response, neutropenia and the rebound neutrophilia, and significantly reduced urinary levels of LTE_4 and 2,3-dinor-TXB_2 (O'Connor *et al.*, 1994). However, in a separate study of eight atopic asthmatic subjects there was no inhibition of the early or late-response to allergen and no difference in histamine airways responsiveness following the late response (Kuitert *et al.*, 1993).

References

Abraham, W.M., Stevenson, J.S. & Garrido, R. (1989) A possible role for PAF in allergen-induced late responses: modification by a selective antagonist. *J. Appl. Physiol.*, **66**, 2351–7.

Adamus, W.S., Heuer, H.O., Meade, C.J. & Schilling, J.C. (1990) Inhibitory effects of the new PAF acether antagonist WEB-2086 on pharmacologic changes induced by PAF inhalation in human beings. *Clin. Pharmacol. Ther.*, **47**, 456–62.

Adelroth, E., Morris, M.M., Hargreave, F.E. & O'Byrne, P.M. (1986) Airway responsiveness to leukotrienes C_4 and D_4 and to methacholine in patients with asthma and normal controls. *New Engl. J. Med.*, **315**, 480–4.

Aharony, D., Catanese, C.A. & Falcone, R.C. (1989) Kinetic and pharmacologic analysis of [^{3}H]leukotriene E_4 binding to receptors on guinea pig lung membranes: evidence for selective binding to a subset of leukotriene D_4 receptors. *J. Pharmacol. Exp. Ther.*, **248**, 581–8.

Aharony, D., Dobson, P.T. & Krell, R.D. (1985) *In vitro* metabolism of [^{3}H]-peptide leukotrienes in human and ferret lung: a comparison with the guinea pig. *Biochem. Biophys. Res. Commun.*, **131**, 892–8.

Alabaster, V.A., Keir, R.F., Parry, M.J. & de Souza, R.N. (1991) UK-74,505, a novel and selective PAF antagonist, exhibits potent and long lasting activity *in vivo*. *Agents Actions Suppl.*, **34**, 221–7.

Anderson, G.P. & Fennessy, M.R. (1988) Lipoxygenase metabolites as mediators of platelet activating factor-induced increased airways responsiveness to histamine in the guinea-pig. *Agents Actions Suppl.*, **23**, 195–200.

Anderson, S., Seale, J.P., Ferris, L., Schoeffel, R. & Lindsay, D.A. (1979) An evaluation of pharmacotherapy for exercise-induced asthma. *J. Allergy Clin. Immunol.*, **64**, 612–24.

Arm, J.P., O'Hickey, S.P., Hawksworth, R.J. *et al.* (1990) Asthmatic airways have a disproportionate hyperresponsiveness to LTE_4, as compared with normal airways, but not to LTC_4, LTD_4, methacholine, and histamine. *Am. Rev. Resp. Dis.*, **142**, 1112–18.

Arm, J.P., O'Hickey, S.P., Spur, B.W. & Lee, T.H. (1989) Airway responsiveness to histamine and leukotriene E_4 in subjects with aspirin-induced asthma. *Am. Rev. Resp. Dis.*, **140**, 148–53.

Arm, J.P., Spur, B.W. & Lee, T.H. (1988) The effects of inhaled leukotriene E_4 on the airway responsiveness to histamine in subjects with asthma and normal subjects. *J. Allergy Clin. Immunol.*, **82**, 654–60.

Atluru, D. & Goodwin, J.S. (1986) Leukotriene B_4 causes proliferation of interleukin 2-dependent T cells in the presence of suboptimal levels of interleukin 2. *Cell. Immunol.*, **99**, 444–52.

Augstein, J., Farmer, J.B., Lee, T.B., Sheard, P. & Tattersall, M.L. (1973) Selective inhibitor of slow reacting substance of anaphylaxis. *Nature New Biol.*, **245**, 215–17.

Badr, K.F., Baylis, C., Pfeffer, J.M. *et al.* (1984) Renal and systemic hemodynamic responses to intravenous infusion of leukotriene C_4 in the rat. *Circ. Res.*, **54**, 492–9.

Barnes, N., Piper, P.J. & Costello, J. (1987) The effect of an oral leukotriene antagonist L-649,923 on histamine and leukotriene D_4-induced bronchoconstriction in normal man. *J. Allergy Clin. Immunol.*, **79**, 816–21.

Barnes, N.C., Piper, P.J. & Costello, J.F. (1984a) Comparative effects of inhaled leukotriene C_4, leukotriene D_4, and histamine in normal human subjects. *Thorax*, **39**, 500–4.

Barnes, N.C., Piper, P.J. & Costello, J.F. (1984b) Actions of inhaled leukotrienes and their interactions with other allergic mediators. *Prostaglandins*, **28**, 629–30.

Barnes, N.C., Watson, A., Piper, P.J. & Costello, J.F. (1984c) Action of inhaled leukotriene C and D on large and small airways. Effect of pre-inhalation of leukotriene D on histamine dose-response curve. *Am. Rev. Resp. Dis.*, **129**, A1.

Barnes, P.J., Chung, K.F. & Page, C.P. (1988) Platelet-activating factor as a mediator of allergic disease. *J. Allergy Clin. Immunol.*, **81**, 919–34.

Basran, G.S., Page, C.P., Paul, W. & Morley, J. (1984) Platelet-activating factor: a possible mediator of the dual response to allergen? *Clin. Allergy*, **14**, 75–9.

Beasley, C.R., Robinson, C., Featherstone, R.L. *et al.* (1987a) 9 alpha, 11 beta-prostaglandin F_2, a novel metabolite of prostaglandin D_2 is a potent contractile agonist of human and guinea pig airways. *J. Clin. Invest.*, **79**, 978–83.

Beasley, C.R., Varley, J., Robinson, C. & Holgate, S.T. (1987b) Cholinergic-mediated bronchoconstriction induced by prostaglandin D_2 and its initial metabolite 9_n,11_β-PGF_2 and PGF_{2n} in asthma. *Am. Rev. Resp. Dis.*, **136**, 1140–44.

Beasley, R.C., Featherstone, R.L., Church, M.K. *et al.* (1989) Effect of a thromboxane receptor antagonist on PGD_2- and allergen-induced bronchoconstriction. *J. Appl. Physiol.*, **66**, 1685–93.

Bel, E.H., van der Veen, H., Dijkman, J.H. & Sterk, P.J. (1989) The effect of inhaled budesonide on the maximal degree of airway narrowing to leukotriene D_4 and methacholine in normal subjects *in vivo*. *Am. Rev. Resp. Dis.*, **139**, 427–31.

Bel, E.H., van der Veen, H., Kramps, J.A., Dijkman, J.H. & Sterk, P.J. (1987) Maximal airway narrowing to inhaled leukotriene D_4 in normal subjects. Comparison and interaction with methacholine. *Am. Rev. Resp. Dis.*, **136**, 979–84.

Benveniste, J., Henson, P.M. & Cochrane, C.G. (1972) Leukocyte-dependent histamine release from rabbit platelets. The role of IgE, basophils, and a platelet-activating factor. *J. Exp. Med.*, **136**, 1356–77.

Bianco, S., Robuschi, M., Vagh, A. *et al.* (1985) In: *Progress in Respiratory Research*, Vol. 19, *Asthma and Bronchial Hyperreactivity* (eds. H. Herzog & A.P. Perruchoud), pp. 82–6. Karger, Basel.

Brain, S.D., Camp, R.D., Black, A.K., Dowd, P.M., Greaves, M.W. & Ford-Hutchinson, A.W. (1985) Leukotrienes C_4 and D_4 in psoriatic skin lesions. *Prostaglandins*, **29**, 611–19.

Brain, S., Camp, R., Dowd, P., Black, A.K. & Greaves, M. (1984) The release of leukotriene B_4-like material in biologically active amounts from the lesional skin of patients with psoriasis. *J. Invest. Dermatol.*, **83**, 70–3.

Bray, M.A., Cunningham, F.M., Ford-Hutchinson, A.W. & Smith, M.J. (1981) Leukotriene B_4: a mediator of vascular permeability. *Brit. J. Pharmacol.*, **72**, 483–6.

Brik, A., Tashkin, D.P., Gong H. Jr, Dauphinee, B. & Lee, E. (1987) Effect of cetirizine, a new histamine H_1 antagonist, on airway dynamics and responsiveness to inhaled histamine in mild asthma. *J. Allergy Clin. Immunol.*, **80**, 51–6.

Brink, C., Grimaud, C., Guillot, C. & Orehek, J. (1980) The interaction between indomethacin and contractile agents on human isolated airway muscle. *Brit. J. Pharmacol.*, **69**, 383–8.

Britton, J.R., Hanley, S.P. & Tattersfield, A.E. (1987) The effect of an oral leukotriene D_4 antagonist L-649,923 on the response to inhaled antigen in asthma. *J. Allergy Clin. Immunol.*, **79**, 811–16.

Brocklehurst, W.E. (1956) *A Slow Reacting Substance in Anaphylaxis—SRS-A. Ciba Symposium on Histamine*. J & A Churchill, London.

Brocklehurst, W.E. (1962) Slow reacting substance and related compounds. *Prog. Allergy*, **6**, 539–58.

Broide, D.H., Eisman, S., Ramsdell, J.W., Ferguson, P., Schwartz, L.B. & Wasserman, S.I. (1990) Airway levels of mast cell-derived mediators in exercise-induced asthma. *Am. Rev. Resp. Dis.*, **141**, 563–8.

Burke, L.A., Crea, A.E., Wilkinson, J.R., Arm, J.P., Spur, B.W. & Lee, T.H. (1990) Comparison of the generation of platelet-activating factor and leukotriene C_4 in human eosinophils stimulated by unopsonized zymosan and by the calcium ionophore A23187: the effects of nedocromil sodium. *J. Allergy Clin. Immunol.*, **85**, 26–35.

Bussolino, F., Camussi, G. & Baglioni, C. (1988) Synthesis and release of platelet-activating factor by human vascular endothelial cells treated with tumor necrosis factor or interleukin 1 alpha. *J. Biol. Chem.*, **263**, 11856–61.

Camp, R.D.R., Coutts, A.A., Greaves, M.W., Kay, A.B. & Walport, M.J. (1983) Response of human skin to intradermal injection of leukotrienes C_4, D_4 and B_4. *Brit. J. Pharmacol.*, **80**, 497–502.

Camussi, G., Aglietta, M., Malavasi, F., Tetta, C., Piacibello, W. &

Sanavio, F. (1983) The release of platelet-activating factor from human endothelial cells in culture. *J. Immunol.*, **131**, 2397–403.

Camussi, G., Bussolino, F., Salvidio, G. & Baglioni, C. (1987) Tumor necrosis factor/cachectin stimulates peritoneal macrophages, polymorphonuclear neutrophils, and vascular endothelial cells to synthesize and release platelet-activating factor. *J. Exp. Med.*, **166**, 1390–404.

Carry, M., Korley, V., Willerson, J.T., Weigelt, L. & Ford-Hutchinson, A.W. (1992) Increased urinary leukotriene excretion in patients with cardiac ischemia. *In vivo* evidence for 5-lipoxygenase activation. *Circulation*, **85**, 230–6.

Cartier, A., Thomson, N.C., Frith, P.A., Roberts, R. & Hargreave, F.E. (1982) Allergen-induced increase in bronchial responsiveness to histamine: relationship to the late asthmatic response and change in airway caliber. *J. Allergy Clin. Immunol.*, **70**, 170–7.

Chagnon, M., Gentile, J., Gladu, M. & Sirois, P. (1985) The mechanism of action of leukotrienes A_4, C_4 and D_4 on human lung parenchyma *in vitro*. *Lung*, **163**, 55–62.

Chan-Yeung, M., Lam, S., Chan, H., Tse, K.S. & Salari, H. (1991) The release of platelet-activating factor into plasma during allergen-induced bronchoconstriction. *J. Allergy Clin. Immunol.*, **87**, 667–73.

Chapman, K.R., Friedman, B.S., Shingo, S., Heyse, J., Reiss, T. & Spector, R. (1994) The efficacy of an oral inhibitor of leukotriene synthesis (MK-0591) in asthmatics treated with inhaled steroids. *Am. J. Resp. Crit. Care Med.*, **149**, A215.

Cheng, J.B. & Townley, R.G. (1984) Evidence for a similar receptor site for binding of [^{3}H] leukotriene E_4 and [^{3}H] leukotriene D_4 to the guinea-pig crude lung membrane. *Biochem. Biophys. Res. Commun.*, **122**, 949–54.

Christie, P.E., Hawksworth, R., Spur, B.W. & Lee, T.H. (1992a) Effect of indomethacin on leukotriene E_4-induced histamine hyperresponsiveness in asthmatic subjects. *Am. Rev. Resp. Dis.*, **146**, 1506–10.

Christie, P.E., Schmitz-Schumann, M., Spur, B.W. & Lee, T.H. (1993) Airway responsiveness to leukotriene C_4 (LTC_4), leukotriene E_4 (LTE_4) and histamine in aspirin-sensitive asthmatic subjects. *Eur. Resp. J.*, **6**, 1468–73.

Christie, P.E., Smith, C.M. & Lee, T.H. (1991a) The potent and selective sulfidopeptide leukotriene antagonist, SK&F 104353, inhibits aspirin-induced asthma. *Am. Rev. Resp. Dis.*, **144**, 957–8.

Christie, P.E., Spur, B.W. & Lee, T.H. (1992b) The effects of lipoxin A_4 on airway responses in asthmatic subjects. *Am. Rev. Resp. Dis.*, **145**, 1281–4.

Christie, P.E., Tagari, P., Ford-Hutchinson, A.W. *et al.* (1991b) Urinary leukotriene E_4 concentrations increase after aspirin challenge in aspirin-sensitive asthmatic subjects. *Am. Rev. Resp. Dis.*, **143**, 1025–9.

Christie, P.E., Tagari, P., Ford-Hutchinson, A.W., Black, C., Markendorf, A. & Lee, T.H. (1992c) Urinary leukotriene E_4 after lysine-aspirin inhalation in asthmatic subjects. *Am. Rev. Resp. Dis.*, **146**, 1531–4.

Christie, P.E., Tagari, P., Ford-Hutchinson, A.W., Black, C., Markendorf, A. & Lee, T.H. (1994) Increased urinary LTE_4 excretion following inhalation of LTC_4 and LTE_4 in asthmatic subjects. *Eur. Resp. J.*, **7**, 907–13.

Chung, K.F., Aizawa, H., Leikauf, G.D., Ueki, I.F., Evans, T.W. & Nadel, J.A. (1986) Airway hyperresponsiveness induced by platelet-activating factor: role of thromboxane generation. *J. Pharmacol. Exp. Ther.*, **236**, 580–4.

Chung, K.F. & Barnes, P.J. (1989) Effects of platelet activating factor on airway calibre, airway responsiveness, and circulating cells in asthmatic subjects. *Thorax*, **44**, 108–15.

Chung, K.F., Cuss, F.M. & Barnes, P.J. (1989) Platelet activating factor: effects on bronchomotor tone and bronchial responsiveness in human beings. *Allergy Proc.*, **10**, 333–7.

Chung, K.F., Dent, G., McCusker, M., Guinot, P., Page, C.P. & Barnes, P.J. (1987) Effect of a ginkgolide mixture (BN 52063) in antagonising skin and platelet responses to platelet activating factor in man. *Lancet*, **i**, 248–51.

Churchill, L., Chilton, F.H., Resau, J.H., Bascom, R., Hubbard, W.C. & Proud, D. (1989) Cyclooxygenase metabolism of endogenous arachidonic acid by cultured human tracheal epithelial cells. *Am. Rev. Resp. Dis.*, **140**, 449–59.

Cloud, M.L., Enas, G.G., Kemp, J. *et al.* (1989) A specific LTD_4/LTE_4-receptor antagonist improves pulmonary function in patients with mild, chronic asthma. *Am. Rev. Resp. Dis.*, **140**, 1336–9.

Cockcroft, D.W., Ruffin, R.E., Dolovich, J. & Hargreave, F.E. (1977) Allergen-induced increase in non-allergic bronchial reactivity. *Clin. Allergy*, **7**, 503–13.

Coleman, R.A., Humphrey, P.P.A., Kennedy, I. & Lumley, P. (1984) Prostanoid receptors — the development of a working classification. *Trends Pharmacol. Sci.*, **5**, 303–6.

Coleman, R.A., Kennedy, I. & Sheldrick, R.L.G. (1987) Prostanoids and related compounds. In: *Advances in Prostaglandin, Thromboxane and Leukotriene Research*, Vol. 17 (eds B. Samuelsson, R. Paoletti & P.W. Ramwell), pp. 467–70. Raven, New York.

Coleman, R.A. & Sheldrick, R.L.G. (1989) Prostanoid-induced contraction of human bronchial smooth muscle is mediated by TP-receptors. *Brit. J. Pharmacol.*, **96**, 688–92.

Coles, S.J., Neill, K.H., Reid, L.M. *et al.* (1983) Effects of leukotrienes C_4 and D on glycoprotein and lysozyme secretion by human bronchial mucosa. *Prostaglandins*, **25**, 155–70.

Collawn, C., Rubin, P., Perez, N. *et al.* (1992) Phase II study of the safety and efficacy of a 5-lipoxygenase inhibitor in patients with ulcerative colitis. *Am. J. Gastroenterol.*, **87**, 342–6.

Conroy, D.M., Piper, P.J., Samhoun, M.N. & Yacoub, M. (1989) Metabolism and generation of cysteinyl containing leukotrienes by human airways *in vitro*. *Brit. J. Pharmacol.*, **96**, 72P.

Corey, E.J., Niwa, H., Falck, JR., Mioskowski, C., Arai, Y. & Marfat, A. (1980) Recent studies on the chemical synthesis of eicosanoids. *Adv. Prostaglandin Thromboxane Res.*, **6**, 19–25.

Crea, A.E., Nakhosteen, JA. & Lee, T.H. (1992) Mediator concentrations in bronchoalveolar lavage fluid of patients with mild asymptomatic bronchial asthma. *Eur. Resp. J.*, **5**, 190–5.

Creese, B.R. & Bach, M.K. (1983) Hyperreactivity of airway smooth muscle produced *in vitro* by leukotrienes. *Prostagland. Leukotrienes Med.*, **11**, 161–9.

Creticos, P.S., Peters, S.P., Adkinson N.F. Jr *et al.* (1984) Peptide leukotriene release after antigen challenge in patients sensitive to ragweed. *New Engl. J. Med.*, **310**, 1626–30.

Cromwell, O., Walport, M.J., Taylor, G.W., Morris, H.R., O'Driscoll, B.R. & Kay, A.B. (1982) Identification of leukotrienes in the sputum of patients with cystic fibrosis. *Adv. Prostaglandin Thromboxane Leukotriene Res.*, **9**, 251–7.

Cubeddu, L.X., Carr M.E. Jr & Fuenmayor, N.J. (1985) Beta blockade by oral propranolol and labetalol. *Clin Pharmacol. Ther.*, **37**, 277–83.

Curzen, N., Rafferty, P. & Holgate, S.T. (1987) Effects of a cyclo-oxygenase inhibitor, flurbiprofen, and an H_1 histamine receptor antagonist, terfenadine, alone and in combination on allergen induced immediate bronchoconstriction in man. *Thorax*, **42**, 946–52.

Cuss, F.M., Dixon, C.M. & Barnes, P.J. (1986) Effects of inhaled platelet activating factor on pulmonary function and bronchial responsiveness in man. *Lancet*, **ii**, 189–92.

Cuthbert, N.J. & Gardiner, P.J. (1983) Endogenous generation of cyclooxygenase products by human isolated lung tissue. *Brit. J. Pharmacol.*, **80**, 496P.

Dahinden, C.A., Clancy, R.M., Gross, M., Chiller, J.M. & Hugli, T.E. (1985) Leukotriene C_4 production by murine mast cells: evidence for a role for extracellular leukotriene A_4. *Proc. Nat. Acad. Sci. USA*, **82**, 6632–6.

Dahlén, B., Margolskee, D.J., Zetterstrom, O. & Dahlen, S.E. (1993a) Effect of the leukotriene receptor antagonist MK-0679 on baseline pulmonary function in aspirin sensitive asthmatic subjects. *Thorax*, **48**, 1205–10.

Dahlén, B., Zetterstrom, O., Björck, T. & Dahlen, S.E. (1994) The leukotriene-antagonist ICI-204,219 inhibits the early airway reaction to cumulative bronchial challenge with allergen in atopic asthmatics. *Eur. Resp. J.*, **7**, 324–31.

Dahlén, S.E. (1983) Pulmonary effects of leukotrienes. *Acta Physiol. Scand. Suppl.*, **512**, 1–51.

Dahlén, S.E., Björk, J., Hedqvist, P. *et al.* (1981) Leukotrienes promote plasma leakage and leukocyte adhesion in postcapillary venules: *in vivo* effects with relevance to the acute inflammatory response. *Proc. Nat. Acad. Sci. USA*, **78**, 3887–91.

Dahlén, S.E., Dahlén, B., Ihre, E. *et al.* (1993b) The leukotriene biosynthesis inhibitor BAY ×1005 is a potent inhibitor of allergen-induced airway obstruction and leukotriene formation in man. *Pulmon. Pharmacol.*, **6**, 87–96.

Dahlén, S.E., Hansson, G., Hedqvist, P., Björck, T., Granstrom, E. & Dahlen, B. (1983) Allergen challenge of lung tissue from asthmatics elicits bronchial contraction that correlates with the release of leukotrienes C_4, D_4, and E_4. *Proc. Nat. Acad. Sci. USA*, **80**, 1712–16.

Dahlén, S.E., Hedqvist, P., Hammarstrom, S. & Samuelsson, B. (1980) Leukotrienes are potent constrictors of human bronchi. *Nature*, **288**, 484–6.

Davidson, A.B., Lee, T.H., Scanlon, P.D. *et al.* (1987) Bronchoconstrictor effects of leukotriene E_4 in normal and asthmatic subjects. *Am. Rev. Resp. Dis.*, **135**, 333–7.

Davidson, E.M., Rae, S.A. & Smith, M.J. (1983) Leukotriene B_4, a mediator of inflammation present in synovial fluid in rheumatoid arthritis. *Ann. Rheum. Dis.*, **42**, 677–9.

Degreef, H., Dockx, P., De Doncker, P., De Beule, K. & Cauwenbergh, G. (1990) A double-blind vehicle-controlled study of R 68 151 in psoriasis: a topical 5-lipoxygenase inhibitor. *J. Am. Acad. Dermatol.*, **22**, 751–5.

Demopoulos, C.A., Pinckard, R.N. & Hanahan, D.J. (1979) Platelet-activating factor. Evidence for 1-O-alkyl-2-acetyl-sn-glyceryl-3-phosphorylcholine as the active component (a new class of lipid chemical mediators). *J. Biol. Chem.*, **254**, 9355–8.

Denjean, A., Arnoux, B., Masse, R., Lockhart, A. & Benveniste, J. (1983) Acute effects of intratracheal administration of platelet-activating factor in baboons. *J. Appl. Physiol. Resp. Environ. Exercise Physiol.*, **55**, 799–804.

Denzlinger, C., Grimberg, M., Kapp, A., Haberl, C. & Wilmanns, W. (1991) Effect of the leukotriene receptor antagonists FPL 55712, LY 163443, and MK-571 on the elimination of cysteinyl leukotrienes in the rat. *Brit. J. Pharmacol.*, **102**, 865–70.

DeWitt, D.L. (1991) Prostaglandin endoperoxide synthase: regulation of enzyme expression. *Biochim. Biophys. Acta*, **1083**, 121–34.

DeWitt, D.L., Day, J.S., Sonnenburg, W.K. & Smith, W.L. (1983) Concentrations of prostaglandin endoperoxide synthase and prostaglandin I_2 synthase in the endothelium and smooth muscle of bovine aorta. *J. Clin. Invest.*, **72**, 1882–8.

Diamant, Z., Timmers, M.C., van der Veen, H. *et al.* (1993) The effect of MK-0591, a potent oral leukotriene biosynthesis inhibitor, on allergen-induced airway responses in asthmatic subjects. *Am. Rev. Resp. Dis.*, **147**, A446.

Dixon, R.A.F., Diehl, R.E., Opas, E. *et al.* (1990) Requirement of a 5-lipoxygenase-activating protein for leukotriene synthesis. *Nature*, **343**, 282–4.

Dong, Y.J., Jones, R.L. & Wilson, N.H. (1986) Prostaglandin E receptor subtypes in smooth muscle: agonist activities of stable prostacyclin analogues. *Brit. J. Pharmacol.*, **87**, 97–107.

Drazen, J.M. (1988) Comparative contractile responses to sulfidopeptide leukotrienes in normal and asthmatic human subjects. *Ann. NY Acad. Sci.*, **524**, 289–97.

Drazen, J.M. & Austen, K.F. (1987) Leukotrienes and airway responses. *Am. Rev. Resp. Dis.*, **136**, 985–98.

Drazen, J.M., Austen, K.F., Lewis, R.A. *et al.* (1980) Comparative airway and vascular activities of leukotrienes C-1 and D *in vivo* and *in vitro*. *Proc. Nat. Acad. Sci. USA*, **77**, 4354–8.

Drazen, J.M., Lewis, R.A., Austen, K.F. & Corey, E.J. (1983) In: *Leukotrienes and Prostacyclin* (eds F. Berti, G. Folco & G.P. Velo), pp. 125–34. Plenum, New York.

Drazen, J.M., O'Brien, J., Sparrow, D., Weiss, S.T., Martins, M.A. & Israel, E. (1992) Recovery of leukotriene E_4 from the urine of patients with airway obstruction. *Am. Rev. Resp. Dis.*, **146**, 104–8.

Edenius, C., Heidvall, K. & Lindgren, J.A. (1988) Novel transcellular interaction: conversion of granulocyte-derived leukotriene A_4 to cysteinyl-containing leukotrienes by human platelets. *Eur. J. Biochem.*, **178**, 81–6.

Ellis, J.L. & Undem, B.J. (1994) Role of cysteinyl-leukotrienes and histamine in mediating intrinsic tone in isolated human bronchi. *Am. J. Resp. Crit. Care Med.*, **149**, 118–22.

Elstad, M.R., Mclntyre, T.M., Prescott, S.M. & Zimmerman, G.A. (1991) Protein kinase C regulates the synthesis of platelet-activating factor by human monocytes. *Am. J. Respir. Cell Mol. Biol.*, **4**, 148–55.

Evans, J.F., Leville, C., Mancini, J.A. *et al.* (1991) 5-Lipoxygenase-activating protein is the target of a quinolone class of leukotriene biosynthesis inhibitors. *Mol. Pharmacol.*, **40**, 22–7.

Evans, T.W., Chung, K.F., Rogers, D.F. & Barnes, P.J. (1987) Effect of platelet-activating factor on airway vascular permeability: possible mechanisms. *J. Appl. Physiol.*, **63**, 479–84.

Feinmark, S.J. & Cannon, P.J. (1986) Endothelial cell leukotriene C_4 synthesis results from intercellular transfer of leukotriene A_4 synthesized by polymorphonuclear leukocytes. *J. Biol. Chem.*, **261**, 16466–72.

Feldberg, W. & Kellaway, C.H. (1938) Liberation of histamine and formation of lysocithin-like substances by cobra venom. *J. Physiol.*, **94**, 187–226.

Fels, A.O., Pawlowski, N.A., Cramer, E.B., King, T.K., Cohn, Z.A. & Scott, W.A. (1982) Human alveolar macrophages produce leukotriene B_4. *Proc. Nat. Acad. Sci. USA*, **79**, 7866–70.

Ferreri, N.R., Howland, W.C., Stevenson, D.D. & Spiegelberg, H.L. (1988) Release of leukotrienes, prostaglandins, and histamine into nasal secretions of aspirin-sensitive asthmatics during reaction to aspirin. *Am. Rev. Resp. Dis.*, **137**, 847–54.

Findlay, S.R., Barden, J.M., Easley, C.B. & Glass, M. (1992) Effect of the oral leukotriene antagonist, ICI 204,219, on antigen-induced bronchoconstriction in subjects with asthma. *J. Allergy Clin. Immunol.*, **89**, 1040–5.

Finnerty, J.P. & Holgate, S.T. (1990) Evidence for the roles of histamine and prostaglandins as mediators in exercise-induced asthma: the inhibitory effect of terfenadine and flurbiprofen alone and in combination. *Eur. Resp. J.*, **3**, 540–7.

Finnerty, J.P., Twentyman, O.P., Harris, A., Palmer, J.B. & Holgate, S.T.

(1991) Effect of GR32191, a potent thromboxane receptor antagonist, on exercise induced bronchoconstriction in asthma. *Thorax*, **46**, 190–2.

Finnerty, J.P., Wood-Baker, R., Thomson, H. & Holgate, S.T. (1992) Role of leukotrienes in exercise-induced asthma. Inhibitory effect of ICI 204,219, a potent leukotriene D_4 receptor antagonist. *Am. Rev. Resp. Dis.*, **145**, 746–9.

Fish, J.E., Ankin, M.G., Adkinson F. Jr & Peterman, V.I. (1981) Indomethacin modification of immediate-type immunologic airway responses in allergic asthmatic and non-asthmatic subjects. *Am. Rev. Resp. Dis.*, **123**, 609–14.

Fitzgerald, G.A., Maas, R.L., Lawson, J.A., Oates, J.A., Roberts, L.J. & Brash, A.R. (1983) Aspirin inhibits endogenous prostacyclin and thromboxane biosynthesis in man. *Adv. Prostaglandin Thromboxane Leukotriene Res.*, **11**, 265–6.

Fleisch, J.H., Rinkema, L.E. & Baker, S.R. (1982) Evidence for multiple leukotriene D_4 receptors in smooth muscle. *Life Sci.*, **31**, 577–81.

Fleisch, J.H., Rinkema, L.E., Haisch, K.D. *et al.* (1985) LY171883, 1-2-hydroxy-3-propyl-4,4-(tetrazol-5-yl) butoxy-phenyl-ethanone, an orally active leukotriene D_4 antagonist. *J. Pharmacol. Exp. Ther.*, **233**, 148–57.

Ford-Hutchinson, A.W. (1990) In: *Advances in Prostaglandin, Thromboxane, and Leukotriene Research*, Vol. 21 (eds B. Samuelsson, P.W. Ramwell, R. Paoletti, G. Folco & E. Granström), pp. 9–16. Raven Press, New York.

Ford-Hutchinson, A.W., Bray, M.A., Doig, M.V., Shipley, M.E. & Smith, M.J.H. (1980) Leukotriene B, a potent chemokinetic and aggregating substance released from polymorphonuclear leukocytes. *Nature*, **286**, 264–5.

Freitag, A., Watson, R.M., Matsos, G., Eastwood, C. & O'Byrne, P.M. (1993) Effect of a platelet activating factor antagonist, WEB 2086, on allergen induced asthmatic responses. *Thorax*, **48**, 594–8.

Friedman, B.S., Bel, E.H., Buntinx, A. *et al.* (1993) Oral leukotriene inhibitor (MK-886) blocks allergen-induced airway responses. *Am. Rev. Resp. Dis.*, **147**, 839–44.

Fujimura, M., Nishioka, S., Kumabashiri, I., Matsuda, T. & Mifune, J. (1990a) Effects of aerosol administration of a thromboxane synthetase inhibitor (OKY-046) on bronchial responsiveness to acetylcholine in asthmatic subjects. *Chest*, **98**, 276–9.

Fujimura, M., Sakamoto, S., Kamio, Y. & Matsuda, T. (1993) Effect of a leukotriene antagonist, ONO-1078, on bronchial hyperresponsiveness in patients with asthma. *Resp. Med.*, **87**, 133–8.

Fujimura, M., Sakamoto, S. & Matsuda, T. (1990b) Attenuating effect of a thromboxane synthetase inhibitor (OKY-046) on bronchial responsiveness to methacholine is specific to bronchial asthma. *Chest*, **98**, 656–60.

Fujimura, M., Sakamoto, S., Saito, M., Miyake, Y. & Matsuda, T. (1991) Effect of a thromboxane A_2 receptor antagonist (AA-2414) on bronchial hyperresponsiveness to methacholine in subjects with asthma. *J. Allergy Clin. Immunol.*, **87**, 23–7.

Fujimura, M., Sasaki, F., Nakatsumi, Y. *et al.* (1986) Effects of a thromboxane synthetase inhibitor (OKY-046) and a lipoxygenase inhibitor (AA-861) on bronchial responsiveness to acetylcholine in asthmatic subjects. *Thorax*, **41**, 955–9.

Fuller, R.W., Black, P.N. & Dollery, C.T. (1989) Effect of the oral leukotriene D_4 antagonist LY171883 on inhaled and intradermal challenge with antigen and leukotriene D_4 in atopic subjects. *J. Allergy Clin. Immunol.*, **83**, 939–44.

Fuller, R.W., Dixon, C.M., Dollery, C.T. & Barnes, P.J. (1986) Prostaglandin D_2 potentiates airway responsiveness to histamine and methacholine. *Am. Rev. Resp. Dis.*, **133**, 252–4.

Funk, C.D., Funk, L.B., Kennedy, M.E., Pong, A.S. & Fitzgerald, G.A. (1991) Human platelet/erythroleukemia cell prostaglandin G/H synthase: cDNA cloning, expression, and gene chromosomal assignment. *FASEB J.*, **5**, 2304–12.

Gaddy, J., McCreedy, W., Margolskee, D., Williams, V. & Busse, W. (1991) A potent leukotriene D_4 antagonist (MK-571) significantly reduces airway obstruction in mild to moderate asthma. *J. Allergy Clin. Immunol.*, **87**, A306.

Gaddy, J.N., Margolskee, D.J., Bush, R.K., Williams, V.C. & Busse, W.W. (1992) Bronchodilation with a potent and selective leukotriene D_4 (LTD_4) receptor antagonist (MK-571) in patients with asthma. *Am. Rev. Resp. Dis.*, **146**, 358–63.

Gardiner, P.J. & Collier, H.O.J. (1980) Specific receptors for prostaglandins in airways. *Prostaglandins*, **19**, 819–41.

Gardiner, P.V., Young, C.L., Holmes, K., Hendrick, D.J. & Walters, E.H. (1993) Lack of short-term effect of the thromboxane synthetase inhibitor UK-38,485 on airway reactivity to metacholine in asthmatic subjects. *Eur. Resp. J.*, **6**, 1027–30.

Garland, L.G. & Salmon, J.A. (1991) Hydroxamic acids and hydroxureas as inhibitors of arachidonate 5-lipoxygenase. *Drugs Future*, **16**, 547–58.

Gillard, J., Ford-Hutchinson, A.W., Chan, C. *et al.* (1989) L-663,536 (MK-886) (3-[1-(4-chlorobenzyl)-3-t-butyl-thio-5-isopropylindol-2-yl]-2,2-dimethyl-propanoic acid), a novel, orally active leukotriene biosynthesis inhibitor. *Can. J. Physiol. Pharmacol.*, **67**, 456–64.

Goldblatt, M.W. (1933) A depressor substance in seminal fluid. *J. Soc. Chem. Ind.*, **52**, 1056–61.

Goldman, D.W. & Goetzl, E.J. (1982) Specific binding of leukotriene B_4 to receptors on human polymorphonuclear leukocytes. *J. Immunol.*, **129**, 1600–4.

Goldman, D.W. & Goetzl, E.J. (1984) Selective transduction of human polymorphonuclear leukocyte functions by subsets of receptors for leukotriene B_4. *J. Allergy Clin. Immunol.*, **74**, 373–7.

Griffin, M., Weiss, J.W., Leitch, A.G. *et al.* (1983) Effects of leukotriene D on the airways in asthma. *New Engl. J. Med.*, **308**, 436–9.

Hanahan, D.J. (1986) Platelet activating factor: a biologically active phosphoglyceride. *Ann. Rev. Biochem.*, **55**, 483–509.

Hanahan, D.J., Demopoulos, C.A., Liehr, J. & Pinckard, R.N. (1980) Identification of platelet activating factor isolated from rabbit basophils as acetyl glyceryl ether phosphorylcholine. *J. Biol. Chem.*, **255**, 5514–16.

Hanna, C.J., Bach, M.K., Pare, P.D. & Schellenberg, R.R. (1981) Slow-reacting substances (leukotrienes) contract human airway and pulmonary vascular smooth muscle *in vitro*. *Nature*, **290**, 343–4.

Hardy, C.C., Bradding, P., Robinson, C. & Holgate, S.T. (1986) The combined effects of two pairs of mediators, adenosine with methacholine and prostaglandin D_2 with histamine, on airway calibre in asthma. *Clin. Sci.*, **71**, 385–92.

Hardy, C.C., Bradding, P., Robinson, C. & Holgate, S.T. (1988) Bronchoconstrictor and antibronchoconstrictor properties of inhaled prostacyclin in asthma. *J. Appl. Physiol.*, **64**, 1567–74.

Hardy, C., Robinson, C., Lewis, R.A., Tattersfield, A.E. & Holgate, S.T. (1985) Airway and cardiovascular responses to inhaled prostacyclin in normal and asthmatic subjects. *Am. Rev. Resp. Dis.*, **131**, 18–21.

Hardy, C.C., Robinson, C., Tattersfield, A.E. & Holgate, S.T. (1984) The bronchoconstrictor effect of inhaled prostaglandin D_2 in normal and asthmatic men. *New Engl. J. Med.*, **311**, 209–13.

Hawksworth, R.J., O'Hickey, S.P. & Lee, T.H. (1992) The effects of indomethacin on the refractory period to hypertonic saline-induced bronchoconstriction. *Eur. Resp. J.*, **5**, 963–6.

Hawthorne, A.B., Broughton-Smith, N.K., Whittle, B.J.R. & Hawkey, C.J. (1992) Colorectal leukotriene B_4 synthesis *in vitro* in inflammatory bowel disease: inhibition by the selective 5-lipoxygenase inhibitor BWA4C. *Gut*, **33**, 513–17.

Heaton, R.W., Henderson, A.F., Dunlop, L.S. & Costello, J.F. (1984) The influence of pretreatment with prostaglandin F_2 alpha on bronchial sensitivity to inhaled histamine and methacholine in normal subjects. *Brit. J. Dis. Chest.*, **78**, 168–73.

Henderson, W.R., Jorg, A. & Klebanoff, S.J. (1982) Eosinophil peroxidase-mediated inactivation of leukotrienes B_4, C_4, and D_4. *J. Immunol.*, **128**, 2609–13.

Henderson, W.R. & Klebanoff, S.J. (1983) Leukotriene production and inactivation by normal, chronic granulomatous disease and myeloperoxidase-deficient neutrophils. *J. Biol. Chem.*, **258**, 13522–7.

Henocq, E. & Vargaftig, B.B. (1988) Skin eosinophilia in atopic patients. *J. Allergy Clin. Immunol.*, **81**, 691–5.

Hla, T. & Neilson, K. (1992) Human cyclooxygenase-2 cDNA. *Proc. Nat. Acad. Sci. USA*, **89**, 7384–8.

Holgate, S.T., Burns, G.B., Robinson, C. & Church, M.K. (1984a) Anaphylactic- and calcium-dependent generation of prostaglandin D_2 (PGD_2), thromboxane B_2 and other cyclooxygenase products of arachidonic acid by dispersed human lung mast cells and relationship to histamine release. *J. Immunol.*, **133**, 2138–44.

Holgate, S.T., Burns, G.B., Robinson, C. & Church, M.K. (1984b) Anaphylactic- and calcium-dependent generation of prostaglandin D_2 (PGD_2), thromboxane B_2, and other cyclooxygenase products of arachidonic acid by dispersed human lung cells and relationship to histamine release. *J. Immunol.*, **133**, 2138–44.

Holroyde, M.C., Altounyan, R.E.C., Cole, M., Dixon, M. & Elliott, E.V. (1981) Bronchoconstriction produced in man by leukotrienes C and D. *Lancet*, **ii**, 17–18.

Honda, Z., Nakamura, M., Miki, I. *et al.* (1991) Cloning by functional expression of platelet-activating factor receptor from guinea-pig lung. *Nature*, **349**, 342–6.

Hoover, R.L., Karnovsky, M.J., Austen, K.F., Corey, E.J. & Lewis, R.A. (1984) Leukotriene B_4 action of endothelium mediates augmented neutrophil/endothelial adhesion. *Proc. Nat. Acad. Sci. USA*, **81**, 2191–3.

Hua, X.Y., Dahlen, S.E., Lundberg, J.M., Hammarstrom, S. & Hedqvist, P. (1985) Leukotrienes C_4, D_4 and E_4 cause widespread and extensive plasma extravasation in the guinea pig. *Naunyn-Schmiedebergs Arch. Pharmacol.*, **330**, 136–41.

Hui, K.P. & Barnes, N.C. (1991a) Lung function improvement in asthma with a cysteinyl-leukotriene receptor antagonist. *Lancet*, **337**, 1062–3.

Hui, K.P., Taylor, I.K., Taylor, G.W., Rubin, P., Kesterson, J. & Barnes, N.C. (1991b) Effect of a 5-lipoxygenase inhibitor on leukotriene generation and airway responses after allergen challenge in asthmatic patients. *Thorax*, **46**, 184–9.

Impens, N., Reiss, T.F., Teahan, J.A. *et al.* (1993) Acute bronchodilation with an intravenously administered leukotriene D_4 antagonist, MK-679. *Am. Rev. Resp. Dis.*, **147**, 1442–6.

Israel, E., Dermarkarian, R., Rosenberg, M., Sperling, R., Taylor, G. & Rubin, P. (1990) The effects of a 5-lipoxygenase inhibitor on asthma induced by cold, dry air. *New Engl. J. Med.*, **323**, 1740–4.

Israel, E., Juniper, E.F., Callaghan, J.T. *et al.* (1989) Effect of a leukotriene antagonist, LY171883, on cold air-induced bronchoconstriction in asthmatics. *Am. Rev. Resp. Dis.*, **140**, 1348–53.

Israel, E., Fischer, A.R., Rosenberg, M.A. *et al.* (1993a) The pivotal role of 5-lipoxygenase products in the reaction of aspirin-sensitive asthmatics to aspirin. *Am. Rev. Resp. Dis.*, **148**, 1447–51.

Israel, E., Rubin, P., Kemp, J.P. *et al.* (1993b) The effect of inhibition of 5-lipoxygenase by zileuton in mild-to-moderate asthma. *Ann. Intern. Med.*, **119**, 1059–66.

Issekutz, A.C. (1981) Vascular responses during acute neutrophilic inflammation. Their relationship to *in vivo* neutrophil emigration. *Lab. Invest.*, **45**, 435–41.

Jacques, C.A., Spur, B.W., Johnson, M. & Lee, T.H. (1991) Mechanism of LTE_4-induced histamine hyperresponsiveness in guinea-pig tracheal and human bronchial smooth muscle, *in vitro*. *Brit. J. Pharmacol.*, **104**, 859–66.

Jakobsson, P.J., Odlander, B., Steinhilber, D., Rosen, A. & Claesson, H.E. (1991) Human B lymphocytes possess 5-lipoxygenase activity and convert arachidonic acid to leukotriene B_4. *Biochem. Biophys Res. Commun.*, **178**, 302–8.

Jakobsson, P.J., Steinhilber, D., Odlander, B., Radmark, O. & Claesson, H.E. (1992) On the expression and regulation of 5-lipoxygenase in human lymphocytes. *Proc. Nat. Acad. Sci. USA*, **89**, 3521–5.

Jenkins, J.R., Lai, C.K.W. & Holgate, S.T. (1989) Effect of increasing doses of platelet-activating factor (PAF) on normal human airways. *J. Allergy Clin. Immunol.*, **83**, 282.

Johnson, H.G. & McNee, M.L. (1983) Secretogogue responses of leukotriene C_4, D_4: comparison of potency in canine trachea *in vivo*. *Prostaglandins*, **25**, 237–43.

Johnson, P.R., Armour, C.L. & Black, J.L. (1990) The action of platelet activating factor and its antagonism by WEB 2086 on human isolated airways. *Eur. Resp. J.*, **3**, 55–60.

Johnson, H.G., McNee, M.L., Johnson, M.A. & Miller, M.D. (1983) Leukotriene C_4 and dimethylphenylpiperazinium-induced responses in canine airway tracheal muscle contraction and fluid secretion. *Int. Arch. Allergy Appl. Immunol.*, **71**, 214–18.

Jones, G.H., Venuti, M.C., Young, J.M. *et al.* (1986) Topical non-steroidal antipsoriatic agents. 1. 1,2,3,4-Tetraoxygenated naphthalene derivatives. *J. Med. Chem.*, **29**, 1504–11.

Jones, T.R., Guindon, Y., Young, R. *et al.* (1986) L-648,051, Sodium-4-[3-(4-acetyl-3-hydroxy-2-propylphenoxy)-propylsulfonyl]-gamma-oxo-benzene butanoate: a leukotriene O_4 receptor antagonist. *Am. J. Physiol. Pharmacol.*, **64**, 1535–42.

Jones, G.L., Saroea, H.G., Watson, R.M. & O'Byrne, P.M. (1992) Effect of an inhaled thromboxane mimetic (U46619) on airway function in human subjects. *Am. Rev. Resp. Dis.*, **145**, 1270–4.

Jones, R.L., Peesapati, V. & Wilson, N.H. (1982) Antagonism of the thromboxane-sensitive contractile systems of the rabbit aorta, dog saphenous vein and guinea-pig trachea. *Brit. J. Pharmacol.*, **76**, 423–38.

Jones, T.R., Charette, L. & Denis, D. (1988) Antigen-induced contraction of guinea-pig isolated trachea: studies with novel inhibitors and antagonists of arachidonic acid metabolites. *Brit. J. Pharmacol.*, **95**, 309–21.

Jones, T.R., Davis, C. & Daniel, E.E. (1982) Pharmacological study of the contractile activity of leukotriene C_4 and D_4 on isolated human airway smooth muscle. *Can. J. Physiol. Pharmacol.*, **60**, 638–43.

Joos, G.F., Kips, J.C., Pauwels, R.A. & Van Der Straeten, M.E. (1991) The effect of aerosolized SK&F 104353-Z2 on the bronchoconstrictor effect of leukotriene D_4 in asthmatics. *Pulmon. Pharmacol.*, **4**, 37–42.

Joris, I., Majno, G., Corey, E.J. & Lewis, R.A. (1987) The mechanism of vascular leakage induced by leukotriene E_4. Endothelial contraction. *Am. J. Pathol.*, **126**, 19–24.

Kargman, S., Rousseau, P., Reid, G.K. *et al.* (1993) Leukotriene synthesis in U937 cells expressing recombinant 5-lipoxygenase. *J. Lipid Mediators*, **7**, 31–45.

Kargman, S., Vickers, P.J. & Evans, J.F. (1992) A23187-induced translocation of 5-lipoxygenase in osteosarcoma cells. *J. Cell Biol.*, **119**, 1701–9.

Kaye, M.G. & Smith, L.J. (1990) Effects of inhaled leukotriene D_4 and platelet-activating factor on airway reactivity in normal subjects. *Am. Rev. Resp. Dis.*, **141**, 993–7.

Kellawey, C.H. & Trethewie, W.R. (1940) The liberation of a slow reacting smooth muscle stimulating substance of anaphylaxis. *Q. J. Exp. Physiol.*, **30**, 124–45.

Kern, R., Smith, L.J., Patterson, R., Krell, R.D. & Bernstein, P.R. (1986) Characterization of the airway response to inhaled leukotriene D_4 in normal subjects. *Am. Rev. Resp. Dis.*, **133**, 1127–32.

Kidney, J.C., Ridge, S.M., Chung, K.F. & Barnes, P.J. (1993) Inhibition of platelet-activating factor-induced bronchoconstriction by the leukotriene D_4 receptor antagonist ICI 204,219. *Am. Rev. Resp. Dis.*, **147**, 215–17.

Kikawa, Y., Hosoi, S., Inoue, Y. *et al.* (1991) Exercise-induced urinary excretion of leukotriene E_4 in children with atopic asthma. *Ped. Res.*, **29**, 455–9.

Kim, K.C., Nassiri, J. & Brody, J.S. (1989) Mechanisms of airway goblet cell mucin release: studies with cultured tracheal surface epithelial cells. *Am. J. Respir. Cell Mol. Biol.*, **1**, 137–43.

Kips, J.C., Joos, G.F., De Lepeleire, I. *et al.* (1991) MK-571, a potent antagonist of leukotriene D_4-induced bronchoconstriction in the human. *Am. Rev. Resp. Dis.*, **144**, 617–21.

Kirby, J.G., Hargreave, F.E., Cockcroft, D.W. & O'Byrne, P.M. (1989) Effect of indomethacin on allergen-induced asthmatic responses. *J. Appl. Physiol.* **66**, 578–83.

Knapp, H.R. (1990) Reduced allergen-induced nasal congestion and leukotriene synthesis with an orally active 5-lipoxygenase inhibitor. *New Engl. J. Med.*, **323**, 1745–48.

Knapp, H.R., Sladek, K. & Fitzgerald, G.A. (1992) Increased excretion of leukotriene E_4 during aspirin-induced asthma. *J. Lab. Clin. Med.*, **119**, 48–51.

Kragballe, K., Desjarlais, L. & Voorhees, J.J. (1985) Leukotrienes B_4, C_4 and D_4 stimulate DNA synthesis in cultured human epidermal keratinocytes. *Brit. J. Dermatol.*, **113**, 43–52.

Krell, R.D., Aharony, D., Buckner, C.K. *et al.* (1990) The preclinical pharmacology of ICI 204,219. A peptide leukotriene antagonist. *Am. Rev. Resp. Dis.*, **141**, 978–87.

Krell, R.D., Tsai, B.S., Berdoulay, A., Barone, M. & Giles, R.E. (1983) Heterogeneity of leukotriene receptors in guinea-pig trachea. *Prostaglandins*, **25**, 171–8.

Kuitert, L.M., Hui, K.P., Uthayarkumar, S., Burke, W., Newland, A.C. & Unden, S. (1993) Effect of the platelet-activating factor antagonist UK-74,505 on the early and late response to allergen. *Am. Rev. Resp. Dis.*, **147**, 82–6.

Kujubu, D.A., Fletcher, B.S., Varnum, B.C., Lim, R.W. & Herschman, H.R. (1991) TIS10, a phorbol ester tumor promoter-inducible mRNA from Swiss 3T3 cells, encodes a novel prostaglandin synthase/cyclooxygenase homologue. *J. Biol. Chem.*, **266**, 12866–72.

Kujubu, D.A., Reddy, S.T., Fletcher, B.S. & Herschman, H.R. (1993) Expression of the protein product of the prostaglandin synthase-2/TIS10 gene in mitogen-stimulated Swiss 3T3 cells. *J. Biol. Chem.*, **268**, 5425–30.

Kumlin, M., Dahlen, B., Bjorck, T., Zetterstrom, O., Granstrom, E. & Dahlen, S.E. (1992a) Urinary excretion of leukotriene E_4 and 11-dehydro-thromboxane B_2 in response to bronchial provocations with allergen, aspirin, leukotriene D_4, and histamine in asthmatics. *Am. Rev. Resp. Dis.*, **146**, 96–103.

Kumlin, M., Johansson, H., Larsson, C. *et al.* (1992b) The leukotriene antagonist MK-0679 improves baseline pulmonary function and blocks aspirin-induced airways obstruction in aspirin-sensitive asthmatics. *Am. Rev. Resp. Dis.*, **145**, A15.

Kurzrok, R. & Lieb, C.C. (1930) Biochemical studies of human semen: II. The action of semen on the human uterus. *Proc. Soc. Exp. Biol. Med.*, **28**, 268–72.

Lai, C.K., Jenkins, J.R., Polosa, R. & Holgate, S.T. (1990) Inhaled PAF fails to induce airway hyperresponsiveness to methacholine in normal human subjects. *J. Appl. Physiol.*, **68**, 919–26.

Laitinen, L.A., Laitinen, A., Haahtela, T., Vilkka, V., Spur, B.W. & Lee, T.H. (1993) Leukotriene E_4 and granulocytic infiltration into asthmatic airways. *Lancet*, **341**, 989–90.

Lam, S., Chan, H., LeRiche, J.C., Chan-Yeung, M. & Salari, H. (1988) Release of leukotrienes in patients with bronchial asthma. *J. Allergy Clin. Immunol.*, **81**, 711–17.

Lauritsen, K., Laursen, L.S., Bukhave, K. & Rask-Madsen, J. (1986) Effects of topical 5-aminosalicylic acid and prednisolone on prostaglandin E_2 and leukotriene B_4 levels determined by equilibrium *in vivo* dialysis of rectum in relapsing ulcerative colitis. *Gastroenterology*, **91**, 834–44.

Lauritsen, K., Laursen, L.S., Bukhave K. & Rask-Madsen, J. (1987) *In vivo* effects of orally administered prednisolone on prostaglandin and leucotriene production in ulcerative colitis. *Gut*, **28**, 1095–9.

Lee, T.H., Sethi, T., Crea, A.E. *et al.* (1988) Characterization of leukotriene B_3: comparison of its biological activities with leukotriene B_4 and leukotriene B_5 in complement receptor enhancement, lysozyme release and chemotaxis of human neutrophils. *Clin. Sci.*, **74**, 467–75.

Lee, S.H., Soyoola, E., Chanmugam, P. *et al.* (1992) Selective expression of mitogen-inducible cyclooxygenase in macrophages stimulated with lipopolysaccharide. *J. Biol. Chem.*, **267**, 25934–8.

Lee, T.C., Lenihan D.J., Malone, B., Roddy, L.L. & Wasserman, S.I. (1984a) Increased biosynthesis of platelet activating factor in activated human eosinophils. *J. Biol. Chem.*, **259**, 5526–30.

Lee, T.H., Austen, K.F., Corey, E.J. & Drazen, J.M. (1984b) Leukotriene E_4-induced airway hyperresponsiveness of guinea pig tracheal smooth muscle to histamine and evidence for three separate sulfidopeptide leukotriene receptors. *Proc. Nat. Acad. Sci. USA*, **81**, 4922–5.

Lee, T.H., Walport, M.J., Wilkinson, A.H., Turner-Warwick, M. & Kay, A.B. (1981) Slow reacting substance of anaphylaxis antagonist FPL 55712 in chronic asthma. *Lancet*, **ii**, 304–5.

Leikauf, G.D., Ueki, I.F., Widdicombe, J.H. & Nadel, J.A. (1986) Alteration of chloride secretion across canine tracheal epithelium by lipoxygenase products of arachidonic acid. *Am. J. Physiol.*, **250**, F47–53.

Leitch, A.G., Corey, E.J., Austein, K.F. & Drazen, J.M. (1983) Indomethacin potentiates the pulmonary response to aerosol leukotriene C_4 in the guinea pig. *Am. Rev. Resp. Dis.*, **128**, 639–43.

Levinson, S.L. (1984) Peptidoleukotriene binding in guinea pig uterine membrane preparations. *Prostaglandins*, **28**, 229–40.

Lewis, R.A., Austen, K.F., Drazen, J.M., Clark, D.A., Marfat, A. & Corey, E.J. (1980a) Slow reacting substance of anaphylaxis: identification of leukotriene C-1 and D from human and rat sources. *Proc. Nat. Acad. Sci. USA*, **77**, 3710–14.

Lewis, R.A., Drazen, J.M., Austen, K.F., Clark, D.A. & Corey, E.J. (1980b) Identification of the C(6)-S-conjugate of leukotriene A with cysteine as a naturally occuring slow reacting substance of anaphylaxis (SRS-A). Importance of the 11-*cis*-geometry for biological activity. *Biochem. Biophys. Res. Commun.*, **96**, 271–7.

Lewis, R.A., Soter, N.A., Diamond, P.T., Austen, K.F., Oates, J.A. & Roberts, L.J. (1982) Prostaglandin D_2 generation after activation of rat and human mast cells with anti-IgE. *J. Immunol.*, **129**, 1627–31.

Liu, M.C., Bleecker, E.R., Lichtenstein, L.M. *et al.* (1990) Evidence for elevated levels of histamine, prostaglandin D_2, and other bronchoconstricting prostaglandins in the airways of subjects with mild asthma. *Am. Rev. Resp. Dis.*, **142**, 126–32.

Lundgren, J.D., Kaliner, M., Logun, C. & Shelhamer, J.H. (1990) Platelet activating factor and tracheobronchial respiratory glycoconjugate release in feline and human explants: involvement of the lipoxygenase pathway. *Agents Actions*, **30**, 329–37.

Lupinetti, M.D., Sheller, J.R., Catella, F. & Fitzgerald, G.A. (1989) Thromboxane biosynthesis in allergen-induced bronchospasm. Evidence for platelet activation. *Am. Rev. Resp. Dis.*, **140**, 932–5.

Macdermott, J., Kelsey, C.R., Waddell, K.A. *et al.* (1984) Synthesis of leukotriene B_4, and prostanoids by human alveolar macrophages: analysis by gas chromatography/mass spectrometry. *Prostaglandins*, **27**, 163–79.

McGee, J.E. & Fitzpatrick, F.A. (1986) Erythrocyte–neutrophil interactions: formation of leukotriene B_4 by transcellular biosynthesis. *Proc. Nat. Acad. Sci. USA*, **83**, 1349–53.

McIntyre, T.M., Zimmerman, G.A., Satoh, K. & Prescott, S.M. (1985) Cultured endothelial cells synthesize both platelet-activating factor and prostacyclin in response to histamine, bradykinin, and adenosine triphosphate. *J. Clin. Invest.*, **76**, 271–80.

McIntyre, T.M., Zimmerman, G.A. & Prescott, S.M. (1986) Leukotrienes C_4 and D_4 stimulate human endothelial cells to synthesize platelet-activating factor and bind neutrophils. *Proc. Nat. Acad. Sci. USA*, **83**, 2204–8.

McLeish, K.R., Gierschik, P., Schepers, T., Sidiropoulos, D. & Jakobs, K.H. (1989) Evidence that activation of a common G-protein by receptors for leukotriene B_4 and *N*-formylmethionyl-leucyl-phenylalanine in HL-60 cells occurs by different mechanisms. *Biochem. J.*, **260**, 427–34.

Maclouf, J.A. & Murphy, R.C. (1988) Transcellular metabolism of neutrophil-derived leukotriene A_4 by human platelets. *J. Biol. Chem.*, **263**, 174–81.

Magnussen, H., Boerger, S., Templin, K. & Baunack, A.R. (1992) Effects of a thromboxane-receptor antagonist, BAY u 3405, on prostaglandin D_2- and exercise-induced bronchoconstriction. *J. Allergy Clin. Immunol.*, **89**, 1119–26.

Makker, H.K., Lau, L.C., Thomson, H.W., Binks, S.M. & Holgate, S.T. (1993) The protective effect of inhaled leukotriene D_4 receptor antagonist ICI 204,219 against exercise-induced asthma. *Am. Rev. Resp. Dis.*, **147**, 1413–18.

Malavasi, F., Tetta, C., Funaro, A. *et al.* (1986) Fc receptor triggering induced expression of surface activation antigens and release of platelet-activating factor in large granular lymphocytes. *Proc. Nat. Acad. Sci. USA*, **83**, 2443–7.

Maltby, N.H., Taylor, G.W., Ritter, J.M., Moore, K., Fuller, R.W. & Dollergy, C.T. (1990) Leukotriene C_4 elimination and metabolism in man. *J. Allergy Clin. Immunol.*, **85**, 3–9.

Mancini, J.A., Abramovitz, M., Cox, M.E. *et al.* (1993) 5-Lipoxygenase-activating protein is an arachidonate binding protein. *FEBS Letts.*, **318**, 277–81.

Mann, J.S., Robinson, C., Sheridan A.Q., Clement, P., Bach, M.K. & Holgate, S.T. (1986) Effect of inhaled piriprost (U-60,257) a novel leukotriene inhibitor, on allergen and exercise-induced bronchoconstriction in asthma. *Thorax*, **41**, 746–52.

Manning, P.J., Stevens, W.H., Cockcroft, D.W. & O'Byrne, P.M. (1991) The role of thromboxane in allergen-induced asthmatic responses. *Eur. Resp. J.*, **4**, 667–72.

Manning, P.J., Rokach, J., Malo, J.L. *et al.* (1990a) Urinary leukotriene E_4 levels during early and late asthmatic responses. *J. Allergy Clin. Immunol.*, **86**, 211–20.

Manning, P.J., Watson, R.M., Margolskee, D.J., Williams, V.C. & Schwartz, J.I. (1990b) Inhibition of exercise-induced bronchoconstriction by MK-571, a potent leukotriene D_4-receptor antagonist [see comments]. *New Engl. J. Med.*, **323**, 1736–9.

Manning, P.J., Watson, R.M., Margolskee, D.J., Williams, V.C., Schwartz, J.I. & O'Byrne, P.M. (1990c) Inhibition of exercise-induced bronchoconstriction by MK-571, a potent leukotriene D_4 antagonist. *New Engl. J. Med.*, **323**, 1736–39.

Marom, Z., Shelhamer, J.H. & Kaliner, M. (1981) Effects of arachidonic acid, monohydroxyeicosatetraenoic acid and prostaglandins on the release of mucous glycoproteins from human airways *in vitro*. *J. Clin. Invest.*, **67**, 1695–702.

Marom, Z., Shelhamer, J.H., Bach, M.K., Morton, D.R. & Kaliner, M. (1982a) Slow-reacting substances, leukotrienes C_4 and D_4, increase the release of mucus from human airways *in vitro*. *Am. Rev. Resp. Dis.*, **126**, 449–51.

Marom, Z., Shelhamer, J.H., Bach, M.K. Morton, D.R. & Kaliner, M. (1982b) Slow-reacting substances, leukotrienes C_4 and D_4, increase the release of mucus from human airways *in vitro*. *Am. Rev. Resp. Dis.*, **126**, 449–51.

Masferrer, J.L., Seibert, K., Zweifel, B. & Needleman, P. (1992) Endogenous glucocorticoids regulate an inducible cyclooxygenase enzyme. *Proc. Nat. Acad. Sci. USA*, **89**, 3917–21.

Mathe, A.A. & Hedqvist, P. (1975) Effect of prostaglandins F_2 alpha and E_2 on airway conductance in healthy subjects and asthmatic patients. *Am. Rev. Resp. Dis.*, **111**, 313–20.

Mathe, A.A., Hedqvist, P., Holmgren, A. & Svanborg, N. (1973) Bronchial hyperreactivity to prostaglandin F_2 and histamine in patients with asthma. *Brit. Med. J.*, **1**, 193–6.

Matthay, M.A., Eschenbacher, W.L. & Goetzl, E.J. (1984) Elevated concentrations of leukotriene D_4 in pulmonary edema fluid of patients with the adult respiratory distress syndrome. *J. Clin. Immunol.*, **4**, 479–83.

Mattoli, S., Foresi, A., Corbo, G.M., Valente, S. & Ciappi, G. (1987) The effect of indomethacin on the refractory period occurring after the inhalation of ultrasonically nebulized distilled water. *J. Allergy Clin. Immunol.*, **79**, 678–83.

Mazzoni, L., Morley, J., Page, C.P. & Sanjar, S. (1985) Induction of airway hyperreactivity by platelet activating factor in the guinea pig. *J. Physiol.*, **365**, 107P.

Meade, E.A., Smith, W.L. & DeWitt, D.L. (1993) Expression of the murine prostaglandin (PGH) synthase-1 and PGH synthase-2 isozymes in cos-1 cells. *J. Lipid Mediators*, **6**, 119–29.

Melillo, E., Woolley, K.L., Manning, P.J., Watson, R.M. & O'Byrne, P.M. (1994) Effect of inhaled PGE_2 on exercise-induced bronchoconstriction in asthmatic subjects. *Am. J. Resp. Crit. Care Med.*, **149**, 1138–41.

Meltzer, S.S., Rechsteiner, E.A., Johns, M.A., Cohn, J. & Bleecker, E.R. (1994) Inhibition of exercise-induced asthma by zileuton, a 5-lipoxygenase inhibitor. *Am. J. Resp. Crit. Care Med.*, **149**, A215.

Michelassi, F., Landa, L., Hill, R.D., Lowenstein, E., Watkins, W.D. & Petkau, A.J. (1982) Leukotriene D_4: a potent coronary artery vasoconstrictor associated with impaired ventricular contraction. *Science*, **217**, 841–3.

Miller, D.K., Gillard, J.W., Vickers, P.J. *et al.* (1990) Identification and isolation of a membrane protein necessary for leukotriene production. *Nature*, **343**, 278–81.

Molfino, N.A., Slutsky, A.S., Hoffstein, V. *et al.* (1992) Changes in cross-sectional airway areas induced by methacholine, histamine and LTC_4 in asthmatic subjects. *Am. Rev. Resp. Dis.*, **146**, 577–80.

Moore, K.P., Taylor, G.W., Maltby, N.H., Siegers, D., Fuller, R.W. & Dollery, C.T. (1990) Increased production of cysteinyl leukotrienes in hepatorenal syndrome. *J. Hepatol.*, **11**, 263–71.

Morris, H.R., Taylor, G.W., Piper, P.J. & Tippins, J.R. (1980) Structure of slow reacting substance of anaphylaxis from guinea-pig lung. *Nature*, **385**, 104–6.

Murray, J.J., Tonnel, A.B., Brash, A.R. *et al.* (1986) Release of prostaglandin D_2 into human airways during acute antigen challenge. *New Engl. J. Med.*, **315**, 800–4.

Naclerio, R.M., Meier, H.L., Kagey-Sobotka, A., Adkinson N.F., Jr Meyers, D.A. & Lichtenstein, L.M. (1983) Mediator release after nasal airway challenge with allergen. *Am. Rev. Resp. Dis.*, **128**, 597–602.

Nagy, L., Lee, T.H., Goetzl, E.J., Pickett, W.C. & Kay, A.B. (1982) Complement receptor enhancement and chemotaxis of human neutrophils and eosinophils by leukotrienes and other lipoxygenase products. *Clin. Exp. Immunol.*, **47**, 541–7.

Nakamura, M., Honda, Z., Izumi, T. (1991) Molecular cloning and expression of platelet-activating factor receptor from human leukocytes. *J. Biol. Chem.*, **266**, 20400–5.

Nakamura, T., Morita, Y., Kuriyama, M., Ishihara, K., Ito, K. & Miyamoto, T. (1987) Platelet-activating factor in late asthmatic response. *Int. Arch. Allergy Appl. Immunol.*, **82**, 57–61.

Nasser, S.M., Bell, G.S., Foster, S. *et al.* (1994a) Effect of the 5-lipoxygenase inhibitor ZD2138 on aspirin-induced asthma. *Thorax*, **49**, 749–56.

Nasser, S.M., Bell, G.S., Hawaksworth, R.J. *et al.* (1994b) Effect of the 5-lipoxygenase inhibitor ZD2138 on allergen-induced early and late asthmatic responses. *Thorax*, **49**, 743–8.

O'Banion, M.K., Winn, V.D. & Young, D.A. (1992) cDNA cloning and functional activity of a glucocorticoid-regulated inflammatory cyclooxygenase. *Proc. Nat. Acad. Sci. USA*, **89**, 4888–92.

O'Byrne, P.M. & Jones, G.L. (1986) The effect of indomethacin on exercise-induced bronchoconstriction and refractoriness after exercise. *Am. Rev. Resp. Dis.*, **134**, 69–72.

O'Connor, B.J., Uden, S., Carty, T.J., Eskra, J.D., Barnes, P.J. & Chung, K.F. (1994) Inhibitory effect of UK74,505, a potent and specific oral platelet activating factor (PAF) receptor antagonist, on airway and systemic responses to inhaled PAF in humans. *Am. J. Resp. Crit. Care Med.* **150**, 35–40.

O'Hickey, S.P., Arm, J.P., Rees, P.J., Spur, B.W. & Lee, T.H. (1988) The relative responsiveness to inhaled leukotriene E_4, methacholine and histamine in normal and asthmatic subjects. *Eur. Resp. J.*, **1**, 913–17.

O'Hickey, S.P., Hawksworth, R.J., Fong, C.Y., Arm, J.P., Spur, B.W. & Lee, T.H. (1991) Leukotrienes C_4, D_4, and E_4 enhance histamine responsiveness in asthmatic airways. *Am. Rev. Resp. Dis.*, **144**, 1053–7.

O'Shaughnessy, K.M., Taylor, I.K., O'Connor, B., O'Connell, F. & Thomson, H. (1993) Potent leukotriene D_4 receptor antagonist ICI 204,219 given by the inhaled route inhibits the early but not the late phase of allergen-induced bronchoconstriction. *Am. Rev. Resp. Dis.*, **147**, 1431–5.

O'Sullivan, M.G., Chilton, F.H., Huggins E.M., Jr & McCall, C.E. (1992) Lipopolysaccharide priming of alveolar macrophages for enhanced synthesis of prostanoids involves induction of a novel prostaglandin H synthase. *J. Biol. Chem.*, **267**, 14547–50.

Ohashi, K., Ruan, K.H., Kulmacz, R.J., Wu, K.K. & Wang, L.H. (1992) Primary structure of human thromboxane synthase determined from the cDNA sequence. *J. Biol. Chem.*, **267**, 789–93.

Orange, R.P. & Austen, K.F. (1969) Slow reacting substance of anaphylaxis. *Adv. Immunol.* **10**, 105–44.

Orange, R.P., Murphy, R.C., Karnovsky, M.J. & Austen, K.F. (1973) The physiochemical characteristics and purification of slow-reacting substance of anaphylaxis. *J. Immunol.*, **110**, 760–70.

Orehek, J., Douglas, J.S., Lewis, A.J. & Bouhuys, A. (1973) Prostaglandin regulation of airway smooth muscle tone. *Nature New Biol.*, **245**, 84–5.

Oshima, T., Yoshimoto, T., Yamamoto, S., Kumegawa, M., Yokoyama, C. & Tanabe, T. (1991) cAMP-dependent induction of fatty acid cyclooxygenase mRNA in mouse osteoblastic cells (MC3T3-E1). *J. Biol. Chem.*, **266**, 13621–6.

Palmer, R.M.J., Stepney, R.J., Higgs, G.A. & Eakins, K.E. (1980) Chemokinetic activity of arachidonic acid lipoxygenase products on leukocytes of different species. *Prostaglandins*, **20**, 411–18.

Pasargiklian, M., Bianco, S. & Allegra, L. (1976) Clinical, functional and pathogenetic aspects of bronchial reactivity to prostaglandins F_2alpha, E_1, and E_2. *Adv. Prostaglandin Thromboxane Res.*, **1**, 461–75.

Pavord, I.D., Wisniewski, A., Mathur, R., Wahedna, I., Knox, A.J. & Tattersfield, A.E. (1991) Effect of inhaled prostaglandin E_2 on bronchial reactivity to sodium metabisulphite and methacholine in patients with asthma. *Thorax*, **46**, 633–7.

Pavord, I.D., Wong, C.S., Williams, J. & Tattersfield, A.E. (1993) Effect of inhaled prostaglandin E_2 on allergen-induced asthma. *Am. Rev. Resp. Dis.*, **148**, 87–90.

Peskar, B.M., Dreyling, K.W., Peskar, B.A., May, B. & Goebell, H. (1986) Enhanced formation of sulfidopeptide-leukotrienes in ulcerative colitis and Crohn's disease: inhibition by sulfasalazine and 5-aminosalicylic acid. *Agents Actions*, **18**, 381–3.

Peters, S.P., MacGlashan D.W. Jr, Schulman, E.S. *et al.* (1984) Arachidonic acid metabolism in purified human lung mast cells. *J. Immunol.* **132**, 1972–9.

Peters-Golden, M. & McNish, R.W. (1993) Redistribution of 5-lipoxygenase and cytosolic phospholipase A_2 to the nuclear fraction upon macrophage activation. *Biochem. Biophys. Res. Commun.*, **196**, 147–53.

Pfeffer, M.A., Pfeffer, J.M., Lewis, R.A., Braunwald, E., Corey, E.J. & Austen, K.F. (1983) Systemic hemodynamic effects of leukotrienes C_4 and D_4 in the rat. *Am. J. Physiol.*, **244**, H628–33.

Phillips, G.D. & Holgate, S.T. (1989) Interaction of inhaled LTC_4 with histamine and PGD_2 on airway caliber in asthma. *J. Appl. Physiol.*, **66**, 304–12.

Phillips, G.D., Rafferty, P., Robinson, C. & Holgate, S.T. (1988) Dose-related antagonism of leukotriene D_4-induced bronchoconstriction by p.o. administration of LY-171883 in nonasthmatic subjects. *J. Pharmacol. Exp. Ther.*, **246**, 732–8.

Picado, C., Ramis, I., Rosellò, J. *et al.* (1992) Release of peptide leukotriene into nasal secretions after local instillation of aspirin in aspirin-sensitive asthmatic patients. *Am. Rev. Resp. Dis.*, **145**, 65–9.

Pichurko, B.M., Ingram R.H. Jr, Sperling, R. *et al.* (1989) Localization of the site of the bronchoconstrictor effects of leukotriene C_4 compared with that of histamine in asthmatic subjects. *Am. Rev. Resp. Dis.*, **140**, 334–9.

Piper, P.J. & Samhoun, M.N. (1981) The mechanism of action of leukotrienes C_4 and D_4 in guinea-pig isolated perfused lung and parenchymal strips of guinea pig, rabbit and rat. *Prostaglandins*, **21**, 793–803.

Pliss, L.B., Ingenito, E.P., Ingram R.H., Jr & Pichurko, B. (1990) Assessment of bronchoalveolar cell and mediator response to isocapnic hyperpnea in asthma. *Am. Rev. Resp. Dis.*, **142**, 73–8.

Pong, S.S. & DeHaven, R.N. (1983) Characterization of a leukotriene D_4 receptor in guinea pig lung. *Proc. Nat. Acad. Sci. USA*, **80**, 7415–19.

Prescott, S.M., Zimmerman, G.A. & McIntyre, T.M. (1984) Human endothelial cells in culture produce platelet-activating factor (1-alkyl-2-acetyl-sn-glycero-3-phosphocholine) when stimulated with thrombin. *Proc. Nat. Acad. Sci. USA*, **81**, 3534–8.

Rae, S.A., Davidson, E.M. & Smith, M.J. (1982) Leukotriene B_4, an inflammatory mediator in gout. *Lancet*, **ii**, 1122-4.

Rasmussen, J.B., Eriksson, L.O., Margolskee, D.J., Tagari, P. & Williams, V.C. (1992) Leukotriene D_4 receptor blockade inhibits the immediate and late bronchoconstrictor responses to inhaled antigen in patients with asthma. *J. Allergy Clin. Immunol.*, **90**, 193–201.

Redkar-Brown, D.G. & Aharony, D. (1989) Inhibition of antigen-induced contraction of guinea pig trachea by ICI 198,615. *Eur. J. Pharmacol.*, **165**, 113–21.

Roberts, L.J., Lewis, R.A., Oates, J.A. & Austen, K.F. (1979) Prostaglandin thromboxane, and 12-hydroxy-5,8,10,14-eicosatetraenoic acid production by ionophore-stimulated rat serosal mast cells. *Biochim. Biophys. Acta*, **575**, 185–92.

Roberts, N.M., McCusker, M., Chung, K.F. & Barnes, P.J. (1988a) Effect of a PAF antagonist, BN52063, on PAF-induced bronchoconstriction in normal subjects. *Brit. J. Clin. Pharmacol.*, **26**, 65–72.

Roberts, N.M., Page, C.P., Chung, K.F. & Barnes, P.J. (1988b) Effect of a PAF antagonist, BN52063, on antigen-induced, acute, and late-onset cutaneous responses in atopic subjects. *J. Allergy Clin. Immunol.*, **82**, 236–41.

Robinson, C., Hoult, J.R., Waddell, K.A., Blair, I.A. & Dollery, C.T. (1984) Total profiling by GC/NICIMS of the major cyclo-oxygenase products from antigen and leukotriene-challenged guinea-pig lung. *Biochem. Pharmacol.*, **33**, 395–400.

Robuschi, M., Riva, E., Fuccella, L.M. *et al.* (1992) Prevention of exercise-induced bronchoconstriction by a new leukotriene antagonist (SK&F 104353). A double-blind study versus disodium cromoglycate and placebo. *Am. Rev. Resp. Dis.*, **145**, 1285–8.

Rola-Pleszczynski, M. (1985) Differential effect of leukotriene B_4 on T4+ and T8+ lymphocyte phenotype and immunoregulatory functions. *J. Immunol.*, **135**, 1357–60.

Rola-Pleszczynski, M., Chavaillaz, P.A. & Lemaire, I. (1986) Stimulation of interleukin 2 and interferon gamma production by leukotriene B_4 in human lymphocyte cultures. *Prostaglandins Leukotrienes Med.*, **23**, 207–10.

Rothenberg, M.E., Caulfield, J.P., Austen, K.F. *et al.* (1987) Biochemical and morphological characterization of basophilic leukoyctes from two patients with myelogenous leukemia. *J. Immunol.*, **138**, 2616–25.

Rouis, M., Nigon, F. & Chapman, M.J. (1988) Platelet activating factor is a potent stimulant of the production of active oxygen species by human monocyte-derived macrophages. *Biochem. Biophys. Res. Commun.*, **156**, 1293–301.

Rouzer, C.A. & Kargman, S. (1988) Translocation of 5-lipoxygenase to the membrane in human leukocytes challenged with ionophore A23187. *J. Biol. Chem.*, **263**, 10980–8.

Rouzer, C.A., Rands, E., Kargman, S., Jones, R.E., Register, R.B. & Dixon, R.A. (1988) Characterization of cloned human leukocyte 5-lipoxygenase expressed in mammalian cells. *J. Biol. Chem.*, **263**, 10135–40.

Russi, E.W., Abraham, W.M., Chapman, G.A., Stevenson, J.S., Codias, E. & Wanner, A. (1985) Effects of leukotriene D_4 on mucociliary and respiratory function in allergic and nonallergic sheep. *J. Appl. Physiol.*, **59**, 1416–22.

Sampson, A.P., Spencer, D.A., Green, C.P., Piper, P.J. & Price, J.F. (1990) Leukotrienes in the sputum and urine of cystic fibrosis children. *Brit. J. Clin. Pharmacol.*, **30**, 861–9.

Samuelsson, B., Goldyne, M., Granström, E., Hamberg, M. Hammarström, S. & Malmsten, C. (1978) Prostaglandins and thromboxanes. *Ann. Rev. Biochem.*, **47**, 997–1029.

Samuelsson, B., Hammarstrom, S., Murphy, R.C. & Borgeat, P. (1980) Leukotrienes and slow reacting substance of anaphyaxis (SRS-A). *Allergy*, **35**, 375–81.

Schulman, E.S., Adkinson N.F., Jr & Newball, H.H. (1982) Cyclooxygenase metabolites in human lung anaphylaxis: airway vs. parenchyma. *J. Appl. Physiol. Resp. Environ. Exercise Physiol.*, **53**, 589–95.

Schulman, E.S., MacGlashanD.W., Jr Schleimer, R.P. *et al.* (1983) Purified human basophils and mast cells: current concepts of mediator release. *Eur. J. Res. Dis. Suppl.*, **128**, 53–61.

Sharon, P. & Stenson, W.F. (1984) Enhanced synthesis of leukotriene B_4 by colonic mucosa in inflammatory bowel disease. *Gastroenterology*, **86**, 453–60.

Sirois, P., Brousseau, Y., Salari, H. & Borgeat, P. (1985) Correlation between the myotropic activity of leukotriene A_4 on guinea-pig lung, trachea and ileum and its biotransformation *in situ*. *Prostaglandins*, **30**, 21–36.

Sirois, P., Roy, S., Borgeat, P., Picard, S. & Vallerand, P. (1982) Evidence for a mediator role of thromboxane A_2 in the myotropic action of leukotriene B_4 (LTB_4) on the guinea-pig lung. *Prostaglandins Leukotrienes Med.*, **8**, 157–70.

Sisson, J.H., Prescott, S.M., McIntyre, T.M. & Zimmerman, G.A. (1987) Production of platelet-activating factor by stimulated human polymorphonuclear leukocytes. Correlation of synthesis with release, functional events, and leukotriene B_4 metabolism. *J. Immunol.*, **138**, 3918–26.

Skoner, D.P., Fireman, P., Davis, H.W., Wall, R. & Caliguri, L.A. (1989a) Increases in plasma concentrations of a prostaglandin metabolite in acute airway obstruction. *Arch. Dis. Childhood*, **64**, 1112–17.

Skoner, D.P., Page, R., Asman, B. *et al.* (1989b) Plasma elevations of histamine and a prostaglandin metabolite in acute asthma. *Am. Rev. Respir. Dis.*, **137**, 1009–14.

Sladek, K. & Szczeklik, A. (1993) Cysteinyl leukotrienes overproduction and mast cell activation in aspirin-provoked bronchospasm in asthma. *Eur. Resp. J.*, **6**, 391–9.

Sladek, K., Dworski, R., Fitzgerald, G.A. *et al.* (1990) Allergen-stimulated release of thromboxane A_2 and leukotrine E_4 in humans. Effect of indomethacin. *Am. Rev. Resp. Dis.*, **141**, 1441–5.

Sladek, K., Dworski, R., Soja, J., Sheller, J.R., Nizankowska, E. & Oates, J.A. (1994) Eicosanoids in bronchoalveolar lavage fluid of aspirin-intolerant patients with asthma after aspirin challenge. *Am. J. Resp. Crit. Care Med.*, **149**, 940–6.

Smith, A.P., Cuthbert, M.F. & Dunlop, L.S. (1975) Effects of inhaled prostaglandins E_1, E_2, and F_2 alpha on the airway resistance of healthy and asthmatic man. *Clin. Sci. Mol. Med.*, **48**, 421–30.

Smith, C.M., Christie, P.E., Hawksworth, R.J., Thien, F. & Lee, T.H. (1991) Urinary leukotriene E_4 levels after allergen and exercise challenge in bronchial asthma. *Am. Rev. Resp. Dis.*, **144**, 1411–13.

Smith, C.M., Hawksworth, R.J., Thien, F.C., Christie, P.E. & Lee, T.H. (1992) Urinary leukotriene E_4 in bronchial asthma. *Eur. Resp. J.*, **5**, 693–9.

Smith, L.J., Greenberger, P.A., Patterson, R., Krell, R.D. & Bernstein, P.R. (1985) The effect of inhaled leukotriene D_4 in humans. *Am. Rev. Resp. Dis.*, **131**, 368–72.

Smith, W.L. (1986) Prostaglandin biosynthesis and its compartmentation in vascular smooth muscle and endothelial cells. *Ann. Rev. Physiol.*, **48**, 251–62.

Smith, W.L. (1989) The eicosanoids and their biochemical mechanisms of action. *Biochem. J.*, **259**, 315–24.

Smith, W.L., Marnett, L.J. & DeWitt, D.L. (1991) Prostaglandin and thromboxane biosynthesis. *Pharmacol. Ther.*, **49**, 153–79.

Snyder, D.W. & Fleisch, J.H. (1989) Leukotriene receptor antagonists as potential therapeutic agents. *Ann. Rev. Pharmacol. Toxicol.*, **29**, 123–43.

Snyder, D.W., Giles, R.E., Keith, R.A., Yee, Y.K. & Krell, R.D. (1987) *In vitro* pharmacology of ICI 198,615: a novel, potent selective peptide leukotriene antagonist. *J. Pharmacol. Exp. Ther.*, **243**, 548–56.

Snyder, D.W. & Krell, R.D. (1984) Pharmacological evidence for a distinct leukotriene C_4 receptor in guinea-pig trachea. *J. Pharmacol. Exp. Ther.*, **231**, 616–22.

Sorkness, C.A., Reeiss, T.F., Zhang, J. *et al.* (1994) Bronchodilation with a selective and potent leukotriene D_4 (LTD_4) antagonist (MK-0476) in patients with asthma. *Am. J. Resp. Crit. Care Med.*, **149**, A216.

Soter, N.A., Lewis, R.A., Corey, E.J. & Austen, K.F. (1983) Local effects of synthetic leukotrienes (LTC_4, LTD_4, LTE_4, and LTB_4) in human skin. *J. Invest. Dermatol.*, **80**, 115–19.

Spector, S.L., Glass, M., Minkwitz, M.C., & ICI Asthma Trial Group (1992) The effect of six weeks of therapy with oral doses of ICI 204,219 in asthmatics. *Am. Rev. Resp. Dis.*, **145**, A16.

Spector, S.L., Smith, L.J., Glass, M. & Accolate Asthma Trialists Group (1994) Effects of 6 weeks therapy with oral doses of ICI 204,219, a leukotriene D_4 receptor antagonist in subjects with bronchial asthma. *Am. J. Resp. Crit. Care Med.*, **150**, 618–23.

Spence, D.P., Johnston, S.L., Claverley, P.M. *et al.* (1994) The effect of the orally active platelet-activating factor antagonist WEB 2086 in the treatment of asthma. *Am. J. Resp. Crit. Care Med.*, **149**, 1142–8.

Spencer, D.A., Evans, J.M., Green, S.E., Piper, P.J. & Costello, J.F. (1991) Participation of the cysteinyl leukotrienes in the acute bronchoconstrictor response to inhaled platelet activating factor in man. *Thorax*, **46**, 441–5.

Spencer, D.A., Green, S.E., Evans, J.M., Piper, P.J. & Costello, J.F. (1990) Platelet activating factor does not cause a reproducible increase in bronchial responsiveness in normal man. *Clin. Exp. Allergy*, **20**, 525–32.

Spencer, D.A., Sampson, A.P., Green, C.P., Costello, J.F., Piper, P.J. & Price, J.F. (1992) Sputum cysteinyl-leukotriene levels correlate with the severity of pulmonary disease in children with cystic fibrosis. *Ped. Pulmonol.*, **12**, 90–4.

Stenmark, K.R., James, S.L., Voelkel, N.F., Toews, W.H., Reeves, J.T. & Murphy, R.C. (1983) Leukotriene C_4 and D_4 in neonates with hypoxemia and pulmonary hypertension. *New Engl. J. Med.*, **309**, 77–80.

Stenton, S.C., Court, E.N., Kingston, W.P. *et al.* (1990a) Platelet-activating factor in bronchoalveolar lavage fluid from asthmatic subjects. *Eur. Resp. J.*, **3**, 408–13.

Stenton, S.C., Ward, C., Duddridge, M., Harris, A., Palmer, J.B. & Hendrick, D.J. (1990b) The actions of GR32191B, a thromboxane receptor antagonist, on the effects of inhaled PAF on human airways. *Clin. Exp. Allergy*, **20**, 311–17.

Stenton, S.C., Young, C.A., Harris, A., Palmer, J.B., Hendrick, D.J. & Walters, E.H. (1992) The effect of GR32191 (a thromboxane receptor antagonist) on airway responsiveness in asthma. *Pulmon. Pharmacol.*, **5**, 199–202.

Sturk, A., ten Cate, J.W., Hosford, D., Mencia-Huerta, J.M. & Braquet, P. (1989) The synthesis, catabolism, and pathophysiological role of platelet-activating factor. *Adv. Lipid Res.*, **23**, 219–76.

Sweatman, W.J. & Collier, H.O. (1968) Effects of prostaglandins on human bronchial muscle. *Nature*, **217**, 69.

Szarek, J.L. & Evans, J.N. (1988) Pharmacologic responsiveness of rat parenchymal strips, bronchi, and bronchioles. *Exp. Lung Res.*, **14**, 575–85.

Takano, T., Honda, Z., Sakanaka, C. *et al.* (1994) Role of cytoplasmic tail phosphorylation sites of platelet-activating factor receptor in agonist-induced desensitization. *J. Biol. Chem.*, **269**, 22453–8.

Taylor, I.K., O'Shaughnessy, K.M., Fuller, R.W. & Dollery, C.T. (1991a) Effect of cysteinyl-leukotriene receptor antagonist ICI 204,219 on allergen-induced bronchoconstriction and airway hyperreactivity in atopic subjects. *Lancet*, **337**, 690–4.

Taylor, I.K., Ward, P.S., O'Shaughnessy, K.M. *et al.* (1991b) Thromboxane A_2 biosynthesis in acute asthma and after antigen challenge. *Am. Rev. Resp. Dis.*, **143**, 119–25.

Taylor, G.W., Taylor, I., Black, P., Maltby, N.H., Turner, N. & Fuller, R.W. (1989) Urinary leukotriene E_4 after antigen challenge and in acute asthma and allergic rhinitis. *Lancet*, **i**, 584–8.

Taylor, I.K., Ward, P.S., Taylor, G.W., Dollery, C.T. & Fuller, R.W. (1991c) Inhaled PAF stimulates leukotriene and thromboxane A_2 production in humans. *J. Appl. Physiol.*, **71**, 1396–402.

Uotila, P. & Vapaatalo, H. (1984) Synthesis, pathways and biological implications of eicosanoids. *Ann. Clin. Res.*, **16**, 226–33.

Voelkel, N.F., Worthen, S., Reeves, J.T., Henson, P.M. & Murphy, R.C. (1982) Nonimmunological production of leukotrienes induced by platelet-activating factor. *Science*, **218**, 286–9.

von Euler, U.S. (1983) History and development of prostaglandins. *Gen. Pharmacol.*, **14**, 3–6.

Wahedna, I., Wisniewski, A.F.Z., Wong, C.S. & Tattersfield, A.E. (1992) Effect of multiple doses of RG 12525, an oral leukotriene D_4 antagonist, in chronic asthma. *Am. Rev. Resp. Dis.*, **145**, A16.

Walters, E.H. (1983) Prostaglandins and the control of airways responses to histamine in normal and asthmatic subjects. *Thorax*, **38**, 188–94.

Walters, E.H., Bevan, C., Parrish, R.W., Davies, B.H. & Smith, A.P. (1982) Time-dependent effect of prostaglandin E_2 inhalation on airway responses to bronchoconstrictor agents in normal subjects. *Thorax*, **37**, 438–42.

Walters, E.H. & Davies, B.H. (1982) Dual effect of prostaglandin E_2 on normal airways smooth muscle *in vivo*. *Thorax*, **37**, 918–22.

Walters, E.H., Parrish, R.W., Bevan, C. & Smith, A.P. (1981) Induction of bronchial hypersensitivity: evidence for a role of prostaglandins. *Thorax*, **36**, 571–4.

Wardlaw, A.J., Chung, K.F., Moqbel, R. *et al.* (1990) Effects of inhaled PAF in humans on circulating and bronchoalveolar lavage fluid neutrophils. Relationship to bronchoconstriction and changes in airway responsiveness. *Am. Rev. Resp. Dis.*, **141**, 386–92.

Wardlaw, A.J., Hay, H., Cromwell, O., Collins, J.V. & Kay, A.B. (1989) Leukotrienes, LTC_4 and LTB_4, in bronchoalveolar lavage in bronchial asthma and other respiratory diseases. *J. Allergy Clin. Immunol.*, **84**, 19–26.

Weinblatt, M.E., Kremer, J.M., Coblyn, J.S. *et al.* (1992) Zileuton, a 5-lipoxygenase inhibitor in rheumatoid arthritis. *J. Rheumatol.*, **19**, 1537–41.

Weiss, J.W., Drazen, J.M., Coles, N. *et al.* (1982a) Bronchoconstrictor effects of leukotriene C in humans. *Science* **216**, 196–8.

Weiss, J.W., Drazen, J.M., McFadden E.R., Jr, *et al.* (1983) Airway constriction in normal humans produced by inhalation of leukotriene D. Potency, time course, and effect of aspirin therapy. *JAMA*, **249**, 2814–17.

Weiss, J.W., Drazen, J.M., McFadden E.R. Jr, Weller, P.F., Corey, E.J. & Lewis, R.A. (1982b) Comparative bronchoconstrictor effects of histamine, leukotriene C, and leukotriene D in normal human volunteers. *Trans. Assoc. Am. Physicians*, **95**, 30–5.

Weller, P.F., Lee, C.W., Foster, D.W., Corey, E.J., Austen, K.F. & Lewis, R.A. (1983) Generation and metabolism of 5-lipoxygenase pathway leukotrienes by human eosinophils: predominant production of leukotriene C_4. *Proc. Nat. Acad. Sci. USA*, **80**, 7626–30.

Wenzel, S.E., Larsen, G.L., Johnston, K., Voelkel, N.F. & Westcott, J.Y. (1990) Elevated levels of leukotriene C_4 in bronchoalveolar lavage fluid from atopic asthmatics after endobronchial allergen challenge. *Am. Rev. Resp. Dis.*, **142**, 112–19.

Wenzel, S.E., Westcott, J.Y. & Larsen, G.L. (1991) Bronchoalveolar lavage fluid mediator levels 5 minutes after allergen challenge in atopic subjects with asthma: relationship to the development of late asthmatic responses. *J. Allergy Clin. Immunol.*, **87**, 540–8.

Wenzel, S.E., Westcott, J.Y., Smith, H.R. & Larsen, G.L. (1989) Spectrum of prostanoid release after bronchoalveolar allergen challenge in atopic asthmatics and in control groups. An alteration in the ratio of bronchoconstrictive to bronchoprotective mediators. *Am. Rev. Resp. Dis.*, **139**, 450–7.

Westcott, J.Y., Smith, H.R., Wenzel, S.E., Larsen, G.L., Thomas, R.B. & Felsien, D. (1991) Urinary leukotriene E_4 in patients with asthma. Effect of airways reactivity and sodium cromoglycate. *Am. Rev. Resp. Dis.*, **143**, 1322–8.

Westcott, J.Y., Voelkel, N.F., Jones, K. & Wenzel, S.E. (1993) Inactivation of leukotriene C_4 in the airways and subsequent urinary leukotriene E_4 excretion in normal and asthmatic subjects. *Am. Rev. Resp. Dis.*, **148**, 1244–51.

Williams, J.D., Czop, J.K. & Austen, K.F. (1984) Release of leukotrienes by human monocytes on stimulation of their phagocytic receptor for particulate activators. *J. Immunol.*, **132**, 3034–40.

Wood-Baker, R., Phillips, G.D., Iucas, R.A., Turner, G.A. & Holgate, S.T. (1991) The effect of inhaled LY-170,680 on leukotriene D_4-induced bronchoconstriction in healthy volunteers. *Drug Invest.*, **3**, 239–47.

Woods, J.W., Coffey, M.J., Singer, I.I. & Peters-Golden, M. (1994) 5-Lipoxygenase is located in the euchromatin of the nucleus in resting human alveolar macrophages and translocates to the nuclear envelope with cell activation. *Am. J. Resp. Crit. Care Med.*, **149**, A233.

Woods, J.W., Evans, J.F., Ethier, D. *et al.* (1993) 5-Lipoxygenase and 5-lipoxygenase-activating protein are localized in the nuclear envelope of activated human leukocytes. *J. Exp. Med.*, **178**, 1935–46.

Yamaguchi, T., Kohrogi, H., Honda, I. *et al.* (1992) A novel leukotriene antagonist. ONO-1078, inhibits and reverses human bronchial contraction induced by leukotrienes C_4 and D_4 and antigen *in vitro*. *Am. Rev. Resp. Dis.*, **146**, 923–9.

Yokoyama, C., Miyata, A., Ihara, H., Ullrich, V. & Tanabe, T. (1991) Molecular cloning of human platelet thromboxane A synthase. *Biochem. Biophys. Res. Commun.*, **178**, 1479–84.

PART 3

Pharmacology

CHAPTER 24
Histamine and Antihistamines

F.E.R. Simons

Introduction

H_1-receptor antagonists are among the most widely used medications in the world. This chapter reviews the molecular basis for their action, and their clinical pharmacology, efficacy in allergic disorders and adverse effects. The first-generation, relatively sedating H_1-receptor antagonists will be discussed briefly, and the role of the second-generation, relatively non-sedating H_1 antagonists (Fig. 24.1) will be discussed in greater detail and future directions for H_1 antagonist research will be identified.

Molecular basis for action of H_1 antagonists

H_1 receptors have been defined pharmacologically by the actions of their respective agonists and antagonists. There is little evidence that peripheral and central H_1 receptors differ (Ter Laak *et al.*, 1993). There is a possibility that isoforms of H_1 receptors, or perhaps different subtypes of H_1 receptors, may exist (Ruat *et al.*, 1990).

The gene encoding the human histamine H_1 receptor has been cloned, and has been expressed in heterologous cell lines (De Backer *et al.*, 1993; Chowdhury *et al.*, 1994; Fukui *et al.*, 1994). It is located on the short arm of chromosome 3. The human histamine H_1 receptor shows 70–80% homology with the H_1 receptors from other species, approximately 45% homology with the muscarinic receptor, and no homology with the H_2 receptor. Histamine receptors belong to a family of G-protein-coupled receptors. The histamine H_1 receptor has been linked to multiple signalling events, including phosphoinositol hydrolysis, cyclic adenosine monophosphate (cAMP) accumulation, arachidonic acid release and calcium flux.

Histamine mediates a variety of physiological and pathological responses in different tissues and cells and is an important chemical mediator of inflammation in allergic disease (Hill, 1990; Levi *et al.*, 1991; Pearce, 1991; Simons & Simons, 1994). Acting via H_1 receptors and inositol phospholipid hydrolysis, it plays an important role in causing smooth-muscle contraction in the respiratory and gastrointestinal tracts and in causing pruritus and sneezing via sensory nerve stimulation (Table 24.1). It induces vascular endothelium to release nitric oxide that stimulates guanalyl cyclase and increases cyclic guanosine monophosphate (cGMP) levels in vascular smooth muscle, causing vasodilatation. Acting via H_1 and H_2 receptors, it causes hypotension, tachycardia, flushing and headache. Activation of H_2 receptors alone causes an increase in gastric acid secretion and numerous other pharmacological responses. H_3-receptor stimulation may have negative modulatory effects.

In the central nervous system (CNS), histamine is a neurotransmitter and can be readily demonstrated by immunohistochemical techniques. It is synthesized *in situ* from L-histidine by specific L-histidine decarboxylase and metabolized exclusively by specific histamine *N*-methyltransferase. Studies of human cerebrospinal fluid (CSF) suggest that brain histaminergic activity increases with age (Prell & Green, 1994).

Mechanisms of action of H_1 antagonists

Three important features of the chemical structure of H_1 antagonists are: the presence of multiple aromatic or heterocyclic rings and alkyl substituents; the basicity of the nitrogen group; and the nature of the linkage atom X,

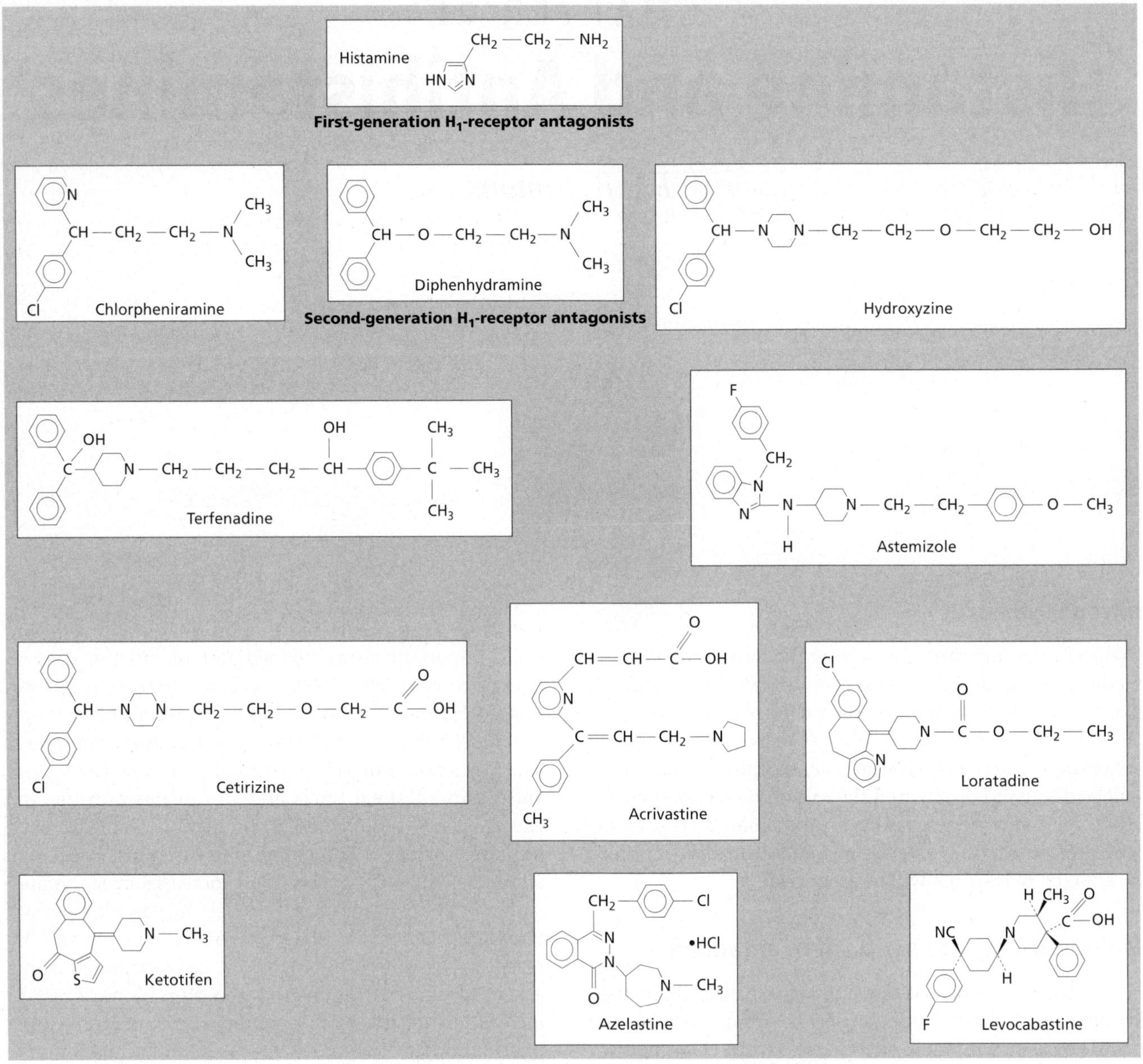

Histamine

First-generation H_1-receptor antagonists

Chlorpheniramine

Diphenhydramine

Hydroxyzine

Second-generation H_1-receptor antagonists

Terfenadine

Astemizole

Cetirizine

Acrivastine

Loratadine

Ketotifen

Azelastine

Levocabastine

Fig. 24.1 Chemical structure of histamine, the general structure for H_1-receptor antagonists, and the structures of selected first- and second-generation H_1-receptor antagonists.

which historically was used to categorize H_1-receptor antagonists into six groups — ethanolamines, ethylene diamines, alkylamines, piperazines, piperidines and phenothiazines. Medications within each class may vary in their efficacy and adverse effect profile. Some of the newer second-generation H_1-receptor antagonists do not fit readily into the traditional classification system; for example, terfenadine, astemizole loratidine, ketofifer and levocabastine contain a piperidine ring, but are not typical piperidines. Loratadine is related to azatadine, cetirizine is an active human metabolite of hydroxyzine and acrivastine is structurally similar to triprolidine.

Histamine H_1 antagonists are highly selective for H_1 receptors, having little effect on H_2 or H_3 receptors. First-generation H_1 antagonists may also activate muscarinic cholinergic, 5-hydroxytryptamine (serotonin) or α-adrenergic receptors, whereas few of the second-generation H_1 antagonists have any of these properties. First-generation H_1-receptor antagonists also cross the blood–brain barrier readily (Yanai *et al.*, 1992). While H_1 selectivity may contribute to the low CNS toxicity of the second-generation H_1 antagonists, H_1 antagonism alone may cause sedation, and lack of CNS toxicity is likely to be due primarily to their inability to cross the tightly fused outer membranes of the endothelial cells lining the brain capillaries (Nicholson *et al.*, 1991; Timmerman, 1992).

The precise structural requirements for H_1 selectivity and affinity are being elucidated; for example, the α-α-biphenyl-4-piperidino-methanol moiety is the pharmacophore for H_1 activity of terfenadine and the phenylbutanol moiety prevents terfenadine from crossing the blood–brain barrier (Casy, 1991; Zhang *et al.*, 1993).

H_1-receptor blockade

At low concentrations, H_1 antagonists are competitive antagonists of histamine (Fig. 24.2). They bind to H_1 receptors but do not activate them, thus preventing histamine binding and action. At higher concentrations, some second-generation H_1 antagonists, such as terfenadine, astemizole and loratadine, also exhibit non-competitive inhibition. The binding of most H_1 antagonists is readily reversible, but some, such as terfenadine and astemizole, do not readily dissociate from H_1 receptors (Simons & Simons, 1994).

During the immediate hypersensitivity reaction, after histamine is released from mast cells, tissue histamine concentrations theoretically reach 10^{-5} to 10^{-3} mol/l. The concentration of an H_1 antagonist achieved in tissue varies with its physicochemical properties, pharmacokinetics and dose; however, peak concentrations seldom exceed 10^{-6} mol/l (Andersson *et al.*, 1994; Simons *et al.*,

Table 24.1 Histamine receptors in humans.

	H_1	H_2	H_3
Location	Bronchial and gastrointestinal smooth muscle, brain	Gastric mucosa, uterus, brain	Brain, bronchial smooth muscle
Function	Constrict smooth muscle (vascular and bronchial) ↑ Vascular permeability ↑ Pruritus ↑ Pain ↑ Cyclic guanosine monophosphate ↑ Prostaglandin generation ↓ Atrioventricular node conduction time Activation of airway vagal afferent nerves ↑ Glycoprotein secretion (bronchial goblet cells) Stimulation of cough receptors ↑ Histidine uptake ↑ Hypotension ↑ Flushing ↑ Headache ↑ Tachycardia ↑ Release of mediators of inflammation* ↑ Recruitment of inflammatory cells*	↑ Gastric acid secretion ↑ Vascular permeability Activates adenylate cyclase Chonotropic action in atrial muscle Inotropic action in ventricular muscle Bronchial smooth-muscle relaxation ↑ Cyclic adenosine monophosphate ↑ Mucus secretion Lipolytic effect in fat cells Stimulation of T-suppressor cells ↓ Basophil histamine release ↓ Neutrophil and basophil chemotaxis and enzyme release Inhibit cytotoxicity and proliferation of lymphocytes Inhibit natural killer cells ↑ Hypotension ↑ Flushing ↑ Headache ↑ Tachycardia	Vasodilatation of cerebral vessels Prevents excessive bronchoconstriction Negative feedback ↓ Neurogenic microvascular leakage ↓ Sympathetic transmission in perivascular nerves
Agonists	2-Methylhistamine Betahistine 2-Pyridylethylamine 2-Thiazolylethylamine	4(5)-Methylhistamine Betazole Dimaprit Impromidine	α-Methylhistamine
Antagonists†	Chlorpheniramine Diphenhydramine Hydroxyzine Terfenadine Astemizole Loratadine Cetirizine	Cimetidine Ranitidine Famotidine Nizatidine Etintidine	Thioperamide Impromidine Betahistine

*Not antagonized by all H_1-receptor antagonists.

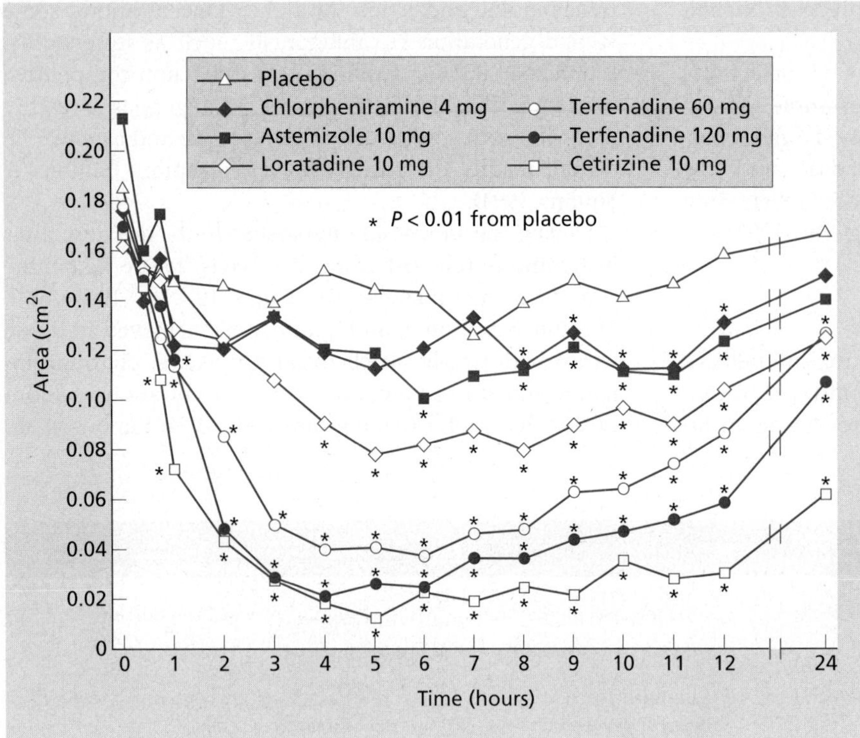

Fig. 24.2 In a single-dose, double-blind, seven-way, cross-over study in 20 healthy male subjects, mean weal areas were measured after epicutaneous histamine phosphate 1 mg/ml before and up to 24 hours after a single oral dose of placebo or H_1-receptor antagonist. The rank order of suppression was, from most effective to least effective: cetirizine 10 mg > terfenadine 120 mg > terfenadine 60 mg > loratadine 10 mg > astemizole 10 mg > chlorpheniramine 4 mg > placebo. (Redrawn with permission from Simons *et al.*, 1990.)

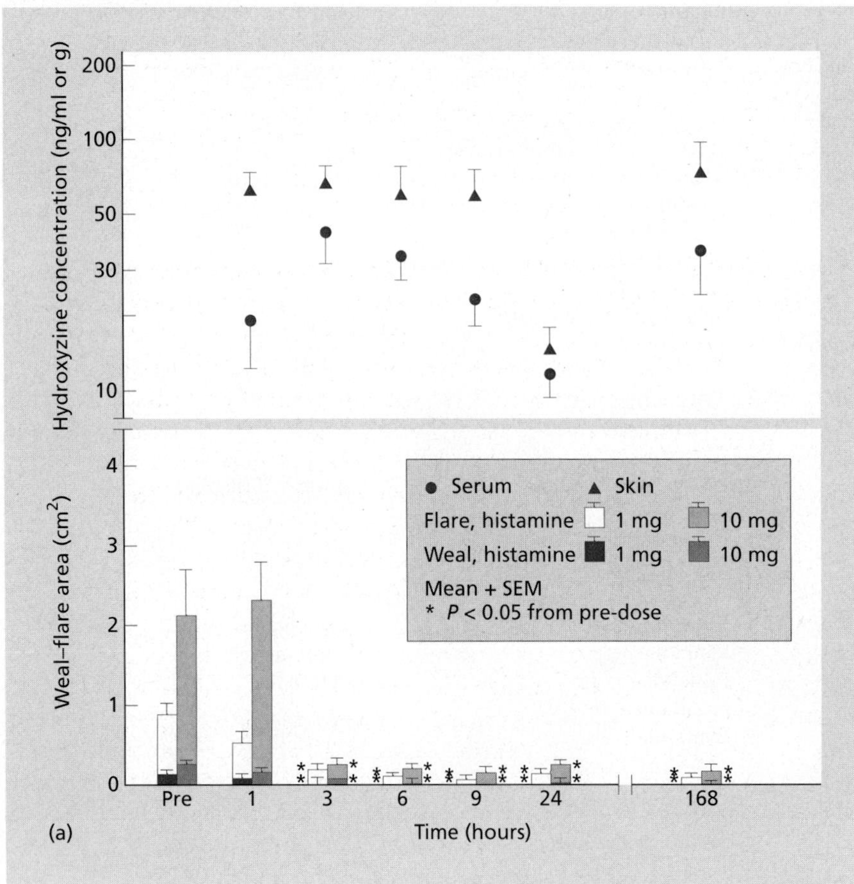

Fig. 24.3 (a) Skin and serum hydroxyzine concentrations vs. time plots and weal-and-flare areas after epicutaneous tests with histamine 1 mg/ml and 10 mg/ml. Tests were performed at baseline and 1, 3, 6, 9 and 24 hours after the initial dose of hydroxyzine 50 mg. Subjects then took hydroxyzine 50 mg at 21.00 hours for 6 consecutive days, and the tests were repeated at 168 hours (steady-state), exactly 12 hours after the seventh and last dose.

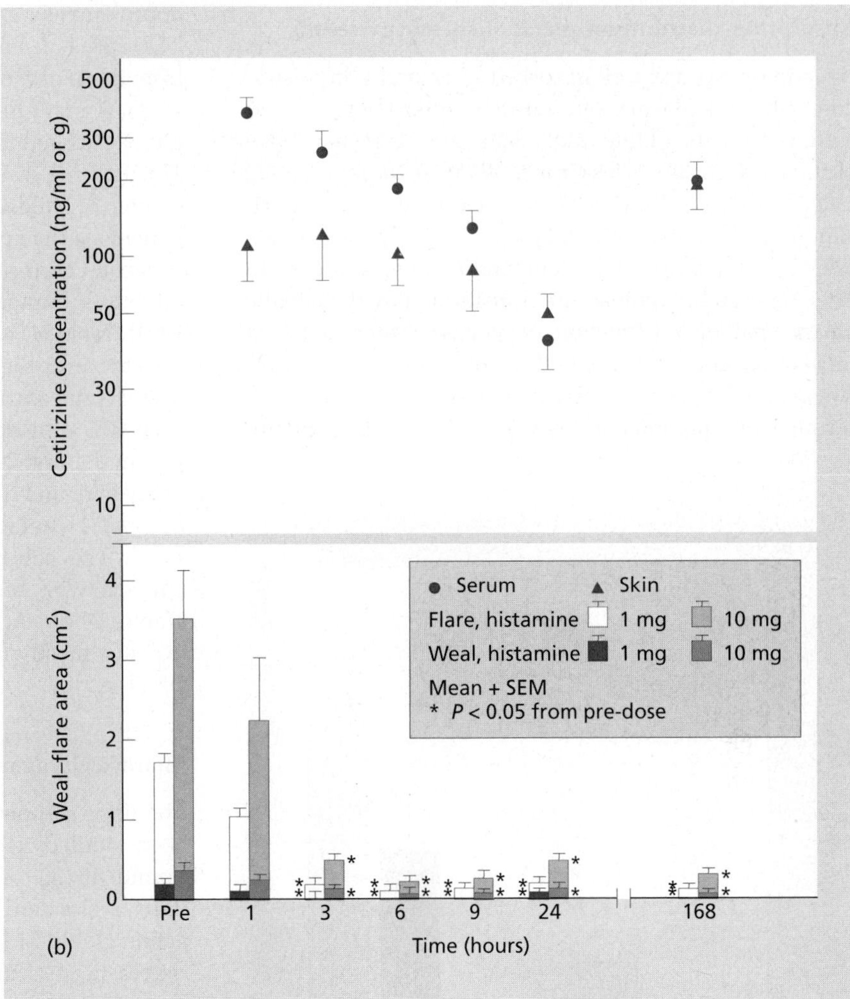

Fig. 24.3 (b) Skin and serum cetirizine concentrations vs. time plots and weal-and-flare areas after epicutaneous tests with histamine 1 mg/ml and 10 mg/ml. Tests were performed at baseline and 1, 3, 6, 9 and 24 hours after the initial dose of cetirizine 10 mg. Subjects then took cetirizine 10 mg at 21.00 hours for 6 consecutive days, and the tests were repeated at 168 hours (steady state), exactly 12 hours after the seventh and last dose. (Redrawn with permission from Simons *et al.*, 1995.)

1995) (Fig. 24.3). For H_1 antagonists such as terfenadine, astemizole and loratadine, tissue concentrations of active H_1 antagonist metabolite(s) may be more relevant than those of the parent compound.

Anti-allergic effects

In vitro, many H_1 antagonists prevent release of mediators of inflammation from human basophils and mast cells. These effects vary with the stimulus for mediator release, the mediator being measured and the H_1-antagonist concentration; for some H_1 antagonists, the concentrations required are up to 1000 times higher than can be achieved *in vivo* after usual doses. The biochemical mechanisms by which H_1 antagonists inhibit mediator release do not involve H_1-receptor antagonism, rather, the H_1 antagonists form ionic associations with cell membranes, prevent calcium binding and inhibit membrane-related activities (Rimmer & Church, 1990; Bousquet *et al.*, 1992).

In vivo, pretreatment with some second-generation H_1 antagonists decreases mediator release after antigen challenge on the nasal mucosa or skin of patients naturally sensitized to the antigen. For example, in patients with allergic rhinitis, pretreatment with terfenadine or loratadine reduces histamine and prostaglandin D_2 (PGD_2) release into nasal secretions (Bousquet *et al.*, 1988; Naclerio *et al.*, 1990; Wagenmann *et al.*, 1994) (Fig. 24.4). An H_1 antagonist may inhibit mediator release more effectively in one organ than in another. In the skin, pretreatment with cetirizine decreases histamine, platelet-activating factor (PAF) and PGD_2 release after antigen challenge, and inhibits eosinophil, neutrophil and basophil migration induced by antigen or by PAF (Michel *et al.*, 1988; Charlesworth *et al.*, 1989), but in patients with allergic rhinitis, cetirizine is less effective in inhibiting mediator release (Naclerio *et al.*, 1989) and does not inhibit eosinophil migration into nasal fluid (Klementsson *et al.*, 1990). The relative importance of the anti-allergic effects of H_1 antagonists in contributing to their overall clinical efficacy is unknown (Janssens & Howarth, 1993).

Absorption, distribution, metabolism and excretion

H_1 antagonists are well absorbed after oral administration, with peak plasma concentrations often being reached within 2 hours (Table 24.2) (Paton & Webster, 1985; McTavish & Sorkin, 1989; Grant *et al.*, 1990; McTavish *et al.*, 1990; Brogden & McTavish, 1991; Dechant & Goa, 1991; Simons & Simons, 1991; Janssens, 1993; Spencer *et al.*, 1993; Haria *et al.*, 1994). Protein binding ranges from 87 to 99%. Most H_1 antagonists are transformed by the hepatic microsomal mixed-function oxygenase system. Plasma concentrations are relatively low after single oral doses, which indicates considerable first-pass hepatic extraction. Terminal elimination half-life values are variable, and are approximately 24 hours for some H_1 antagonists (Table 24.2). The half-life values of active metabolites may differ from those of the parent compound; for example, astemizole has a half-life of 1.1 days, whereas its active metabolite, *N*-desmethylastemizole, has a half-life of 9.5 days. The half-life values for some H_1 antagonists may be shorter in children, and prolonged in the elderly and in patients with hepatic dysfunction or those receiving ketoconazole, erythromycin or other microsomal oxygenase inhibitors (Simons & Simons, 1991; Honig *et al.*, 1993, 1994) (Table 24.3).

Cetirizine, the active carboxylic acid metabolite of hydroxyzine, is not metabolized to any great extent *in vivo*; 60% of a dose is excreted unchanged in the urine within the first 24 hours. Plasma concentrations are relatively high and the volume of distribution is smaller than for other H_1 antagonists (Watson *et al.*, 1989; Spencer *et al.*, 1993). The half-life of cetirizine may be prolonged in patients with renal insufficiency (Spencer *et al.*, 1993) (Table 24.4). Acrivastine and levocabastine are also excreted mostly unchanged in the urine (Dechant & Goa, 1991).

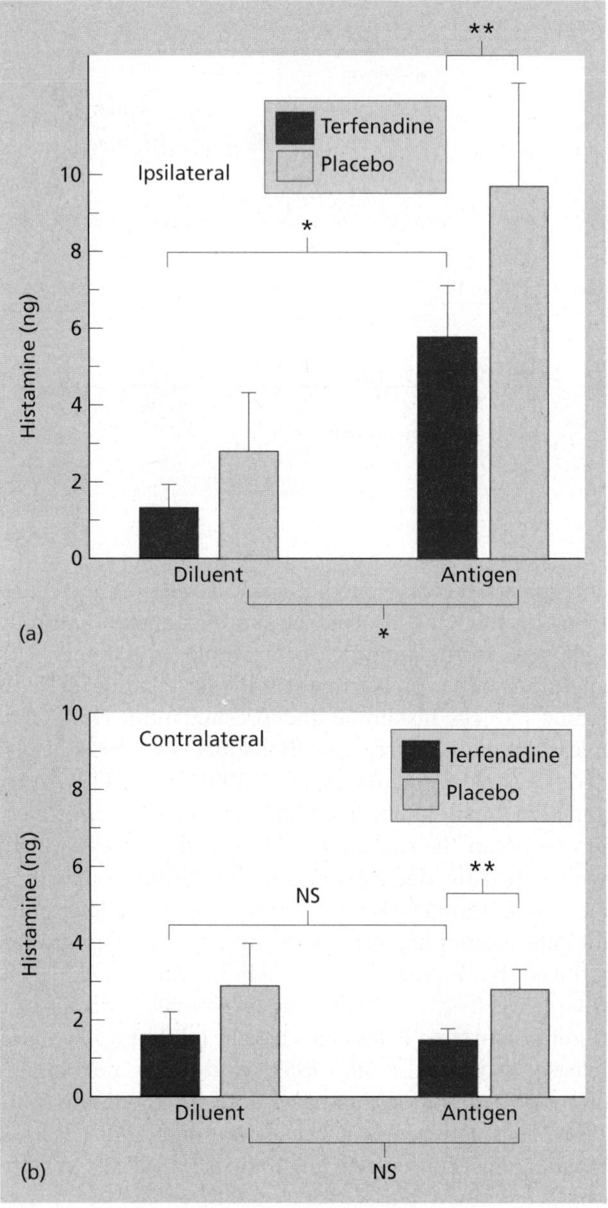

Fig. 24.4 In a double-blind, placebo-controlled study in subjects with allergic rhinitis, antigen was administered on a filter-paper disc unilaterally to the middle portion of the anterior nasal septum, 2 hours after the subject ingested terfenadine 60 mg or placebo. (a) Ipsilateral: histamine values were significantly increased compared with those after diluent challenge after both placebo and terfenadine treatments. Terfenadine premedication caused a significant reduction in antigen-induced histamine release compared with placebo. Levels of histamine were not significantly different after diluent challenges ($P = 0.12$). (b) Contralateral: antigen challenge did not induce a significant increase in histamine after placebo or terfenadine treatments. The amount of histamine after diluent challenges was not significantly different between treatments ($P = 0.35$). After antigen challenge, histamine levels were significantly lower in the terfenadine-treated group ($n = 12$). * $P < 0.05$, antigen vs. diluent; ** $P < 0.05$, terfenadine vs. placebo; NS, not statistically significant. Terfenadine also markedly reduced the number of sneezes and partially decreased the lateral and contralateral secretion rates without affecting the increase in nasal airway resistance (not shown). (Redrawn with permission from Wagenmann *et al.*, 1994.)

Pharmacodynamics

The dose–response relationships of H_1 antagonists have been studied using inhibition of the histamine-, compound 48/80-, codeine- or antigen-induced weal and flare, a standardized biological assay of peripheral H_1 action (Table 24.2). H_1 antagonists decrease weal size by decreasing vascular permeability and leakage of plasma proteins, and decrease flare size by decreasing the vasodilatation caused by the histamine-induced axon reflex. All H_1 antagonists inhibit the histamine-induced weal and

Table 24.2 Relative benefits of second-generation H_1-receptor antagonists in current use.

	Absorption not affected by food	Serum elimination $t_{1/2}$ (active metabolite $t_{1/2}$) (h) single-dose studies	Some potential for drug interactions	Prompt onset of action	24-hour duration of action	Once/day dosing recommended by manufacturer	Effect disappears in ≤ 1 week after short course	No loss of efficacy over time	Anti-allergic effects *in vivo*	Efficacy well documented in most allergic disorders
Terfenadine	✓	19.5 (17)	✓	✓	✓*	✓*	✓	✓	✓	✓
Astemizole	?	1.1 d (9.5 d)	✓	?	✓	✓	✗	✓	✓	✓
Loratadine	✓	10.0 (21)	✓	✓	✓	✓	✓	✓	✓	✓
Cetirizine	✓	9	✗	✓	✓	✓	✓	✓	✓	✓
Acrivastine	✓	2.3 (2.3)	✗	✓	✗	✗	✓	min	min	min
Ketotifen	✓	15.7	✓	✓	min	✗	min	min	✓	min
Ebastine	✓	— (14)	✓	✓	✓	✓	min	min	min	min
Azelastine	✓	22 (54)	✓	✓	min	✗	✗	min	✓	min
Levocabastine†	n/a	33	✗	✓	✗	✗	min	min	✓	min

✓, yes; ✗, no; ?, conflicting information; min, more information needed; n/a, not applicable.
* 120-mg once-daily dose used in some countries.
† Topical, for allergic rhinoconjunctivitis only.

Table 24.3 Interaction of terfenadine* 60 mg q. 12 hours for 7 days with other pharmacological agents in healthy subjects.

Drug co-administered for 7 days	Dose (mg)	Number of subjects with ↑ terfenadine parent compound	Significant ECG changes
Macrolide antibiotics			
Erythromycin	500 q. 8 h	3/9	Yes
Clarithromycin	500 q. 12 h	4/6	Yes
Azithromycin	500 load 250 o.d.	0/6	No
Imidazole antifungals			
Ketoconazole	200 q. 12 h	6/6	Yes
Itraconazole	200 o.d.	6/6	Yes
Fluconazole	200 o.d.	0/6	No
H_2-receptor antagonists			
Cimetidine	600 q. 12 h	1/6	No
Ranitidine	150 q. 12 h	1/6	No
Other			
Naringenin (Grapefruit juice)	240 ml† q. 12 h	6/6	Yes

* Drug interactions have been more thoroughly studied for terfenadine than for any other H_1-receptor antagonist.
† Large amount required.
q., every; o.d., once a day.

Table 24.4 Elimination half-life of cetirizine in healthy young adults, elderly adults and children, and in subjects with renal dysfunction or hepatic dysfunction.

Study participants	$t_{1/2}\beta$ (h)
Healthy adults	6.5–11
Healthy elderly	11.8
Healthy children*	5*–7.1†
Hepatic dysfunction	13.8–14.3
Renal dysfunction	20–20.9

* Age 2–4 years.
† Mean age 8 years.
$t_{1/2}\beta$, elimination half-life.

flare to some extent, but the magnitude of the effect, the time to peak effect, and the duration of effect are dose related. Weal-and-flare inhibition correlates with relief of symptoms of allergic rhinitis (Howarth *et al.*, 1984; Watson *et al.*, 1989). It usually begins within 1 hour and is maximal 5–7 hours after the dose, several hours after the peak plasma concentrations (Simons *et al.*, 1990). The delay in response is probably not due to delay in the medication reaching the skin, as skin concentrations are as high as or higher than plasma concentrations throughout the dosing interval (Simons *et al.*, 1995). There is therefore a pharmacodynamic, as well as a pharmacological, rationale for giving an H_1 antagonist *before* an anticipated allergic reaction, whenever possible, in order to provide maximum efficacy.

H_1-antagonist effects persist even when plasma concentrations become undetectable, probably due to high tissue/plasma concentration ratios and, for some medications, the presence of active metabolites. The duration of action of a single dose, whether assessed subjectively using amelioration of symptoms such as itching of the skin or nose, sneezing and rhinorrhea, or objectively using inhibition of the weal-and-flare response, is more prolonged than might be expected from consideration of the terminal elimination half-life value, and for many H_1 antagonists, including older ones such as chlorpheniramine and hydroxyzine, it is approximately 24 hours (Simons & Simons, 1991). Despite differences in pharmacokinetics and pharmacodynamics, once-daily dosing is possible with many H_1 antagonists (Table 24.5). The main rationale for using timed-release formulations of older medications such as chlorpheniramine is to reduce the CNS dysfunction associated with peak serum and tissue concentrations, rather than to achieve prolonged duration of action.

A 7-day course of an H_1 antagonist such as terfenadine or loratadine causes histamine blockade for a further 7 days after the H_1 antagonist is stopped; therefore, these medications should be discontinued at least 1 week before skin tests or inhalation challenge tests with histamine or antigen (Labrecque *et al.*, 1993). A short course of astemizole causes more prolonged histamine blockade, and these tests should be interpreted with caution even 4–6 weeks after astemizole has been discontinued (Lantin *et al.*, 1990; Malo *et al.*, 1990) (Fig. 24.5).

Chronic administration of H_1 antagonists does not lead to autoinduction of hepatic metabolism or increase the rate of elimination of these medications (Bantz *et al.*, 1987; Simons *et al.*, 1988; Watson *et al.*, 1989). In studies of 4–12 weeks' duration during which compliance was closely monitored, peripheral H_1 blockade in the skin

Table 24.5 Formulations and dosages of representative H_1-receptor antagonists.

H_1-receptor antagonist	Formulation	Recommended dose
First generation		
Chlorpheniramine maleate (Chlor-Trimeton)	Tablets 4 mg, 8 mg†, 12 mg† Syrup 2.5 mg/5 ml Parenteral solution 10 mg/ml	Adult: 8–12 mg b.i.d.† Paediatric*: 0.35 mg/kg/24 h
Hydroxyzine hydrochloride (Atarax)	Capsules 10, 25, 50 mg Syrup 10 mg/5 ml	Adult: 25–50 mg q.d. (h) b.i.d. Paediatric: 2 mg/kg/24 h
Diphenhydramine hydrochloride (Benadryl)	Capsules 25 or 50 mg Elixir 12.5 mg/5 ml Syrup 6.25 mg/5 ml Parenteral solution 50 mg/ml	Adult: 25–50 mg t.i.d. Paediatric: 5 mg/kg/24 h
Second generation		
Terfenadine (Seldane)	Tablets 60 mg, 120 mg Suspension 30 mg/5 ml	Adult: 60 mg b.i.d. *or* 120 mg q.d. Paediatric: (3–6 yr): 15 mg b.i.d. (7–12 yr): 30 mg b.i.d.
Astemizole (Hismanal)	Tablets 10 mg Suspension 10 mg/5 ml	Adult: 10 mg q.d. Paediatric: 0.2 mg/kg/24 h
Loratadine (Claritin)	Tablets 10 mg Syrup 1 mg/ml	Adult: 10 mg q.d. Paediatric: (2–12 yr): 5 mg/d (>12 yr and >30 kg): 10 mg/d
Cetirizine (Reactine)	Tablets 10 mg	Adult: 5–10 mg q.d.
Acrivastine (Semprex)	Tablets 8 mg**	Adult: 8 mg t.i.d.
Ketotifen (Zaditen)	Tablets 1 mg; 2 mg† Suspension?	Patients > 3 yr: 1 mg b.i.d. or 2 mg q.d.† 4 mg q.i.d.† is used in urticaria
Ebastine (Ebastel)	Tablet 10 mg	Adult: 10 mg q.d.
Azelastine (Astelin)	Nasal solution 0.1% (0.137 mg/spray)	Topical: 2 sprays in each nostril q.d. or b.i.d.
Levocabastine (Livostin)	Microsuspension 50 µg/spray	Topical: 2 sprays in each nostril b.i.d.–q.i.d.

* For patients ≤ 40 kg.
** In combination with pseudo-ephedrine 60 mg.
† Timed release.
q.d., once daily; b.i.d., twice daily; t.i.d., three times daily; q.i.d., four times daily.

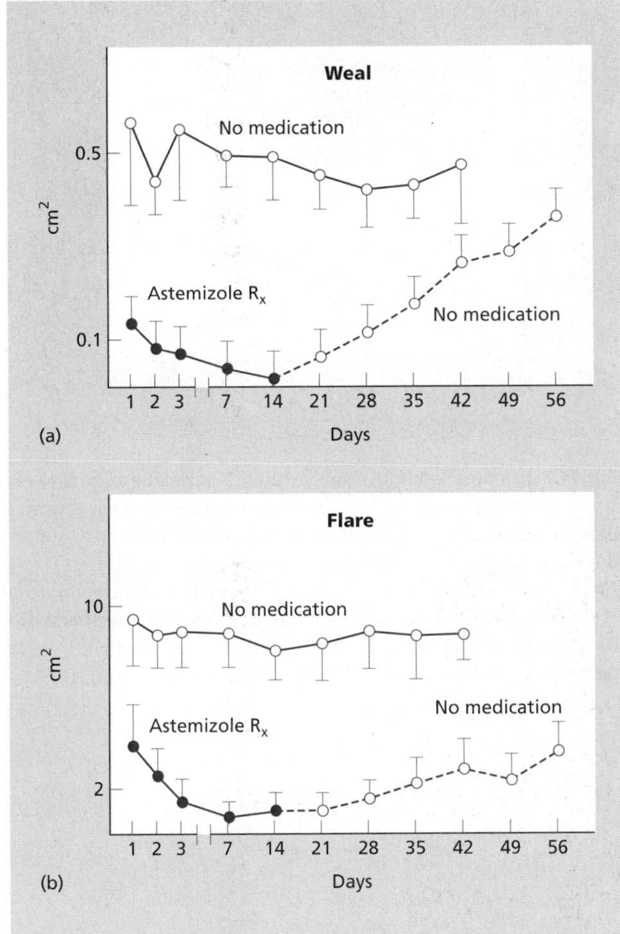

Fig. 24.5 The histamine-induced weal and flare were monitored over 8 weeks in control subjects (top line in each graph) and in patients treated with astemizole 30 mg on day 1, followed by 10 mg on days 2–14, inclusive (bottom line on each graph). The astemizole treatment was discontinued on day 14. Astemizole produced inhibition of skin tests starting 24 hours after the loading dose on day 1, peaking at the end of treatment on day 14, and disappearing very slowly during the following 6 weeks when no treatment was given. Flares were inhibited for a longer period of time than weals. Values are expressed as mean ± 2 SEM. (Redrawn with permission from Lantin *et al.*, 1990.)

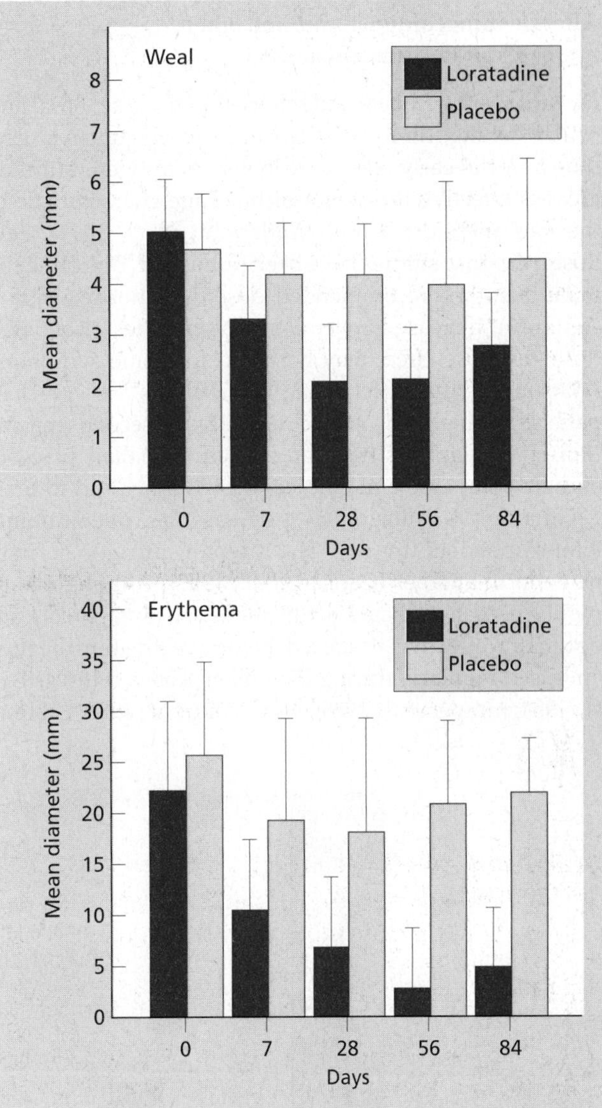

Fig. 24.6 Weal and flare induced by histamine in 20 patients who received either placebo or loratadine 10 mg daily for 12 weeks. The patients treated with loratadine had significantly smaller weal-and-flare reactions after 7 days. This effect was maximal at 28 days and lasted throughout the study. Subsensitivity to loratadine did not develop during the 12-week period. (Redrawn with permission from Bousquet *et al.*, 1990.)

(Simons *et al.*, 1988; Watson *et al.*, 1989; Bousquet *et al.*, 1990) (Fig. 24.6) and efficacy in allergic rhinitis (Juniper *et al.*, 1988) did not decrease significantly. Development of tolerance to adverse CNS effects may (Levander *et al.*, 1991) or may not occur (Goetz *et al.*, 1989).

Efficacy of H_1 antagonists in allergic disorders

The rationale for H_1-antagonist use in allergic rhinitis, asthma, urticaria or atopic dermatitis is that in these disorders local challenge with histamine reproduces some of the symptoms; challenge with antigen or other relevant stimulus may result in local or systemic increase in histamine concentrations; and histamine concentrations may increase spontaneously during active disease. Also, pretreatment with an H_1 antagonist prevents or decreases symptoms after challenge with histamine, antigen or other relevant stimulus, and an H_1 antagonist may relieve naturally occurring symptoms.

Allergic rhinoconjunctivitis and other upper respiratory tract disorders

H_1 antagonists prevent and relieve the sneezing, nasal and ocular itching, rhinorrhea, tearing and conjunctival erythema of the early allergic response to antigen, but they are less effective for the nasal blockage characteristic of the late allergic reaction (Andersson *et al.*, 1994). Few dose–response studies have been published. Doubling the manufacturers' recommended dose does not result in a significant increase in overall symptom relief, although a dose–response effect may be noted for some symptoms (Watson *et al.*, 1989; Stern *et al.*, 1990; Falliers *et al.*, 1991). In patients with allergic rhinoconjunctivitis, second-generation H_1 antagonists have greater efficacy than placebo, and are comparable in efficacy to each other and to first-generation H_1 antagonists such as chlorpheniramine. Non-responders to one H_1 receptor antagonist may respond to another (Carlsen *et al.*, 1993). Although commonly used as 'rescue' medications, H_1 antagonists are optimally effective if started before pollination begins, and used regularly during the pollen season (Howarth *et al.*, 1984; Juniper *et al.*, 1988; Del Carpio *et al.*, 1989; Gibbs *et*

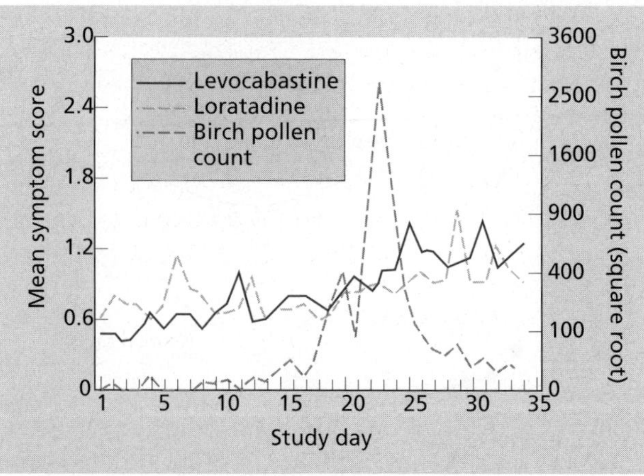

Fig. 24.7 In a double-blind, double-dummy, parallel-group, 5-week study, 47 subjects received levocabastine eye drops and nasal spray plus an oral placebo and 48 subjects received loratadine 10 mg once daily plus placebo eye drops and nasal spray. No statistically significant differences were observed between the efficacy of the oral H_1 antagonist and the topical H_1 antagonist. The adverse effects did not differ between the two groups of subjects. (Redrawn with permission from Odebäck *et al.* (Swedish GP Allergy Team), 1994.)

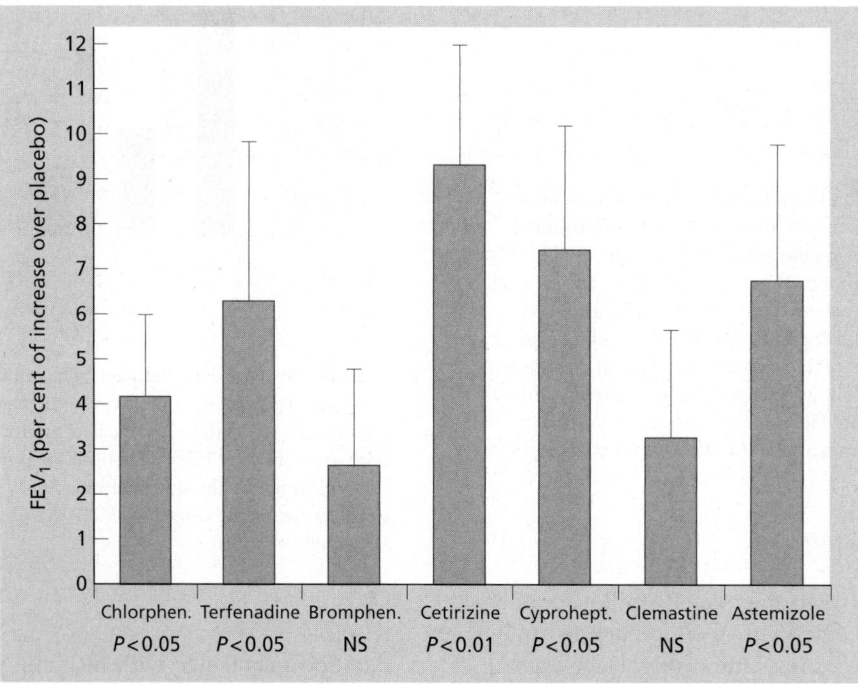

Fig. 24.8 In a single-blind, placebo-controlled study, 20 volunteers with stable asthma received chlorpheniramine (4 mg), terfenadine (60 mg), brompheniramine (4 mg), cetirizine (10 mg), cyproheptadine (4 mg), clemastine (1 mg) or astemizole (10 mg). Subjects had forced expiratory volume in 1 second (FEV_1) measurements, bronchial challenge with histamine phosphate in doubling concentrations of 0.03–32 mg/ml, and epicutaneous tests with doubling concentrations of histamine phosphate from 2 to 32 mg/ml. All H_1 antagonists had some bronchodilator effect (shown). The mean increase in FEV_1 ranged from 2.58% after brompheniramine to 9.28% after cetirizine. All H_1-receptor antagonists displaced the histamine concentration–response curve to the right, but only cetirizine and terfenadine had a significant effect. There was good correlation between the protective effect of the H_1 antagonists in the skin and in the airways ($r = 0.85$, $P < 0.01$). (Reprinted with permission from Wood-Baker & Holgate, 1993.)

al., 1989; Brooks *et al.*, 1990; Falliers *et al.*, 1991; Levander *et al.*, 1991). Some H_1 antagonists, including the newer medications levocabastine and azelastine, have been developed for topical application to the nasal mucosa and/or conjunctivae (McTavish & Sorkin, 1989; Berdy *et al.*, 1991; Dechant & Goa, 1991; Weiler *et al.*, 1991; Frostad & Olsen, 1993), and are as effective or more effective than oral H_1-receptor antagonists (Sohoel *et al.*, 1993; Odebäck *et al.*, 1994) (Fig. 24.7).

In order to provide increased relief of nasal blockage, H_1 antagonists are marketed in fixed-dose combinations with decongestants such as pseudoephedrine (Storms *et al.*, 1989). In patients with seasonal allergic rhinoconjunctivitis, H_1 antagonists and intranasal cromolyn provide comparable relief (Orgel *et al.*, 1991; Frostad & Olsen, 1993). H_1 antagonists are less effective than intranasal glucocorticoids, especially for nasal blockage, but when given concomitantly with intranasal glucocorticoids they may enhance relief of allergic conjunctivitis symptoms (Juniper *et al.*, 1989). In contrast to their role in the treatment of allergic rhinitis, H_1 antagonists have little benefit in the treatment of upper respiratory tract infections (Gaffey *et al.*, 1988; Smith & Feldman, 1993). They are also of unproven benefit in otitis media (Cantekin *et al.*, 1983).

Asthma

Pretreatment with an H_1 antagonist may provide some protection against bronchospasm induced by histamine, exercise, hyperventilation of cold, dry air, hypertonic or hypotonic saline, distilled water, adenosine-5′-monophosphate or allergen. The amount of protection varies with the H_1 antagonist, the dose and the stimulus used (Brik *et al.*, 1987; Rafferty & Holgate, 1987; Town & Holgate, 1990; Wood-Baker & Holgate, 1993) (Fig. 24.8).

The bronchodilator effect of H_1-receptor antagonists varies from one medication to another (Wood-Baker & Holgate, 1993). They relieve mild chronic asthma symptoms, but the clinical importance of the effect is small, and generally obtained only with doses higher than those used in allergic rhinitis (Dijkman *et al.*, 1990; Rafferty *et al.*, 1990). Previous concerns about potential drying of secretions, bronchoconstriction or other adverse effects of H_1 antagonists in asthma have not been substantiated.

Chronic urticaria

In patients with chronic urticaria, H_1 antagonists relieve pruritus and reduce the number, size and duration of urticarial lesions (Cainelli *et al.*, 1986; Grant *et al.*, 1988; Juhlin & Arendt, 1988; Advenier & Queille-Roussel, 1989; Belaich *et al.*, 1990; Brunet *et al.*, 1990; Yang *et al.*, 1991; Sharpe & Shuster, 1993) (Fig. 24.9). The second-generation antagonists such as terfenadine, astemizole, loratadine,

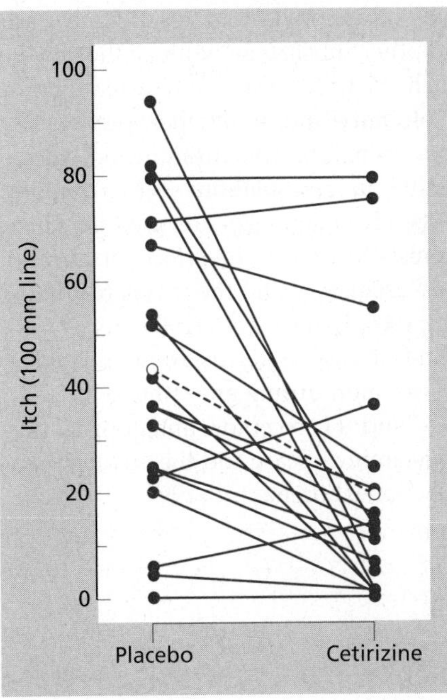

Fig. 24.9 In a double-blind, placebo-controlled, cross-over study, the effect of cetirizine 10 mg at night was studied in 19 patients with dermographic urticaria. Each treatment was given for 7 days, with a 3-day washout in between. Compared to the washout period and to placebo treatment, cetirizine significantly reduced subjectively assessed wealing, itching (shown) and number of nights disturbed; it also significantly decreased the objective response to wealing produced by a spring-loaded stylus and increased the weal threshold calculated from the force–response curve. (Redrawn with permission from Sharpe & Shuster, 1993.)

cetirizine and ketotifen, are probably as effective as their predecessors, although in one study, terfenadine, 120 mg daily, was less effective than hydroxyzine, 100 mg daily (Brunet *et al.*, 1990).

In some patients with urticaria refractory to treatment with an H_1 antagonist alone, concurrent treatment with an H_2 antagonist such as cimetidine or ranitidine enhances relief of pruritus and weal formation (Paul & Bödeker, 1986; Bleehen *et al.*, 1987). In addition to a direct effect on H_2 receptors, which comprise 10–15% of all histamine receptors on the vasculature, this effect may be due in part to the ability of H_2 antagonists to inhibit the metabolism of H_1 antagonists in the hepatic cytochrome P-450 system, leading to elevated plasma and tissue H_1-antagonist concentrations (Simons *et al.*, 1995b).

Anaphylaxis

In patients with anaphylactic or anaphylactoid reactions, the initial treatment of choice is epinephrine, but H_1 antagonists are useful in the ancillary treatment of pruritus, urticaria and angioedema. They are also used for prophylaxis of anaphylactoid reactions to radiocontrast media and other substances. Some of the newer H_1 antagonists, such as terfenadine and astemizole, have low aqueous solubility, and unlike their predecessors such as diphenhydramine, chlorpheniramine or hydroxyzine, are not available in formulations for parenteral use. In anaphylaxis, H_2 antagonists are used concurrently with H_1 antagonists to reduce the effects of histamine on the peripheral vasculature and the myocardium (Marshall & Lieberman, 1989; Lorenz *et al.*, 1990).

Histamine release and histamine-related symptoms are not uncommon during anaesthesia and surgery (Fig. 24.10). H_1- and H_2-receptor antagonists decrease the extent of histamine release and the incidence and severity of these reactions (Lorenz *et al.*, 1994).

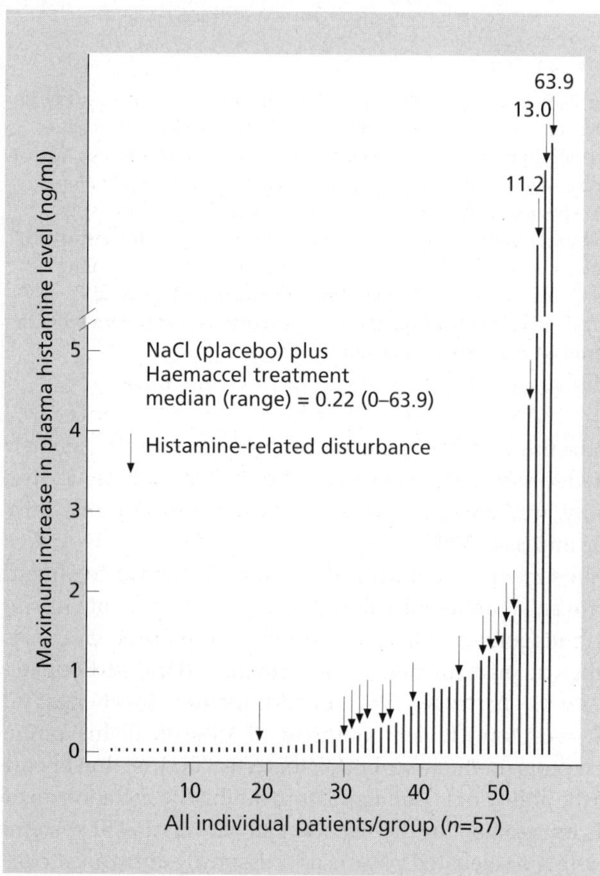

Fig. 24.10 Histamine release is a common event during anaesthesia and surgery. Clinically relevant or life-threatening histamine-related cardiorespiratory disturbances occurred in 26% of subjects who received haemaccel without antihistamines (shown), 8% of those who received Ringer's lactate without antihistamines, and 2% or less of those who received antihistamines ($P < 0.0001$). (Redrawn with permission from Lorenz *et al.*, 1994.)

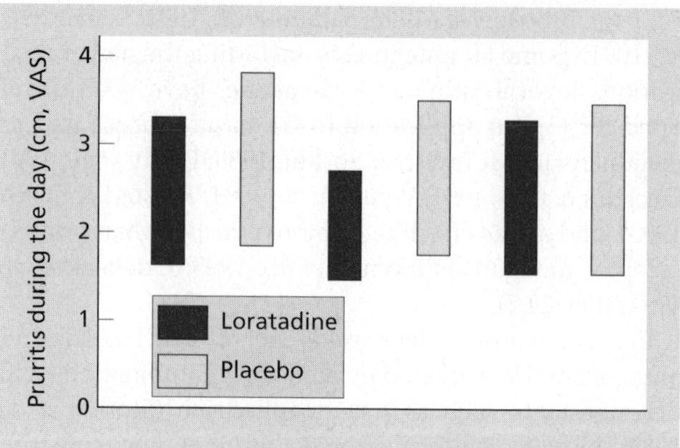

Fig. 24.11 In a double-blind, placebo-controlled, six-period, multi-cross-over design study in 16 subjects, loratadine 10 mg or placebo were given every day, alternating between loratadine and placebo every 2 weeks. Pruritus was recorded by the patients every morning and every evening on a 10-cm visual analogue scale. Loratadine, in comparison to placebo, significantly improved pruritus and the severity of the inflammatory lesions. Nine of the 16 subjects were classified as loratadine responders; one of the 16 was a non-responder. Loratadine has some therapeutic effect on pruritus in subjects with atopic dermatitis. (Redrawn with permission from Langeland *et al.*, 1994.)

Atopic dermatitis

In atopic dermatitis, second-generation H_1 antagonists have not been optimally investigated. During some short-term studies in small numbers of patients, they have generally been less effective for relief of pruritus than first-generation H_1 antagonists such as diphenhydramine or hydroxyzine (Advenier & Queille-Roussel, 1989; Berth-Jones & Graham-Brown, 1989). During other placebo-controlled studies, the efficacy of second-generation H_1 antagonists has been convincingly demonstrated (Hannuksela *et al.*, 1993; Langeland *et al.*, 1994) (Fig. 24.11) and is dose related (Hannuksela *et al.*, 1993).

Adverse effects

First-generation H_1 antagonists

Even in recommended doses, first-generation H_1 antagonists such as triprolidine, diphenhydramine, hydroxyzine or chlorpheniramine often produce adverse CNS effects such as somnolence, diminished alertness, slow reaction time or impairment of cognitive function (Fig. 24.12). The effect is similar to that produced by alcohol or by a major tranquillizer (Roehrs *et al.*, 1993). Gastrointestinal upset, appetite stimulation or anticholinergic effects such as dry mouth, blurred vision, urinary retention or impotence may also be noted; the incidence of these adverse effects

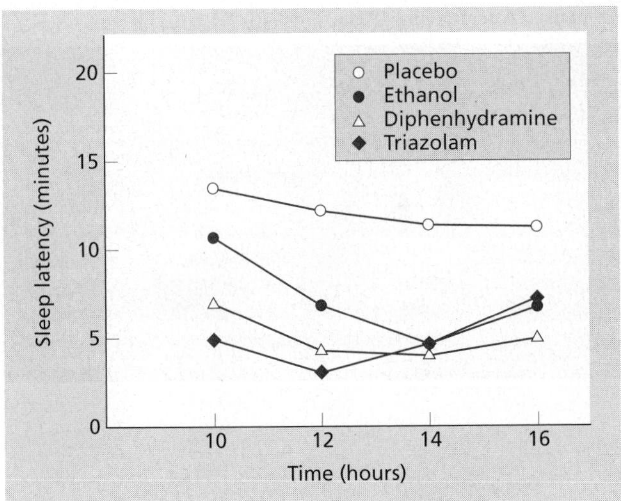

Fig. 24.12 Sleep latency was measured 1, 3, 5 and 7 hours after placebo, triazolam 0.2 mg, diphenhydramine 50 mg or ethanol 0.6 g/kg at 09.00 hours in a double-blind, cross-over study in 12 healthy subjects. The sedative effects of diphenhydramine were similar to those of triazolam and ethanol, and were significantly greater than those produced by placebo. (Redrawn with permission from Roehrs *et al.*, 1993.)

varies with the medications. Rarely, jaundice, cytopenias and apnoea have been reported. After overdose, in addition to sedation or coma, paradoxical stimulatory CNS effects or neuropsychiatric effects such as seizures, dyskinesia, dystonia, hallucinations or psychosis may occur (Meltzer, 1991; Simons, 1994b). Tachycardia is common, and prolongation of the QTc interval, heart block and arrhythmias are occasionally reported.

First-generation H_1 antagonists are still used because they are effective and inexpensive. Some physicians recommend giving these medications at bedtime only, because H_1 blockade may be maintained the next morning and somnolence is of no concern during the night (Paton & Webster, 1985; Goetz *et al.*, 1991; Alford *et al.*, 1992); indeed, some of the older H_1 antagonists are the most widely used non-prescription sleeping aids in the world. Others advise regular daytime use, anticipating that tolerance will develop to the adverse CNS effects, but not to the peripheral H_1 blockade (Levander *et al.*, 1991). These creative dosing schedules require further study, as some individuals may not be free from CNS adverse effects the morning after taking an H_1-antagonist dose at bedtime (Goetz *et al.*, 1991; Alford *et al.*, 1992), and tolerance to the CNS effects of these medications does not necessarily occur (Goetz *et al.*, 1989). Impairment of CNS function has been documented in the absence of CNS symptoms (Goetz *et al.*, 1989; Seidel *et al.*, 1990), and in epidemiological studies some older H_1 antagonists have been implicated as a cause of traffic fatalities (Cimbura *et al.*, 1982).

Second-generation H_1 antagonists

Second-generation H_1-antagonists such as terfenadine, astemizole, loratadine and cetirizine have similar adverse CNS effects to placebo and significantly fewer CNS adverse effects than their predecessors, as documented by electroencephalographic monitoring, sleep latency studies and standardized performance tests, ranging from simple-reaction-time tests to complex sensorimotor tasks such as computer-monitored driving (Bradley & Nicholson, 1987; Bhatti & Hindmarch, 1989; Meador *et al.*, 1989; Seidel *et al.*, 1990; Goetz *et al.*, 1991; Meltzer, 1991; Rombaut *et al.*, 1991; Alford *et al.*, 1992; Rombaut & Hindmarch, 1994; Simons, 1994a,b) (Table 24.6). These objective findings, mostly obtained in healthy volunteers, may be of even greater significance in patients with allergic rhinoconjunctivitis or urticaria, disorders which themselves may affect the duration and quality of nocturnal sleep and subsequent daytime CNS function.

There are relatively few published studies of the potential adverse CNS effects of acrivastine, ketotifen, azelastine or levocabastine; the latter two medications do not seem to cause CNS dysfunction when administered topically (Rombaut *et al.*, 1991; Simons, 1994a).

When the recommended doses of second-generation H_1-antagonists are exceeded, some impairment of CNS function may occur (Bradley & Nicholson, 1987; Bhatti & Hindmarch, 1989). Most of the newer H_1 antagonists do not enhance the CNS effects of alcohol, diazepam or other CNS-active substances when co-administered with these substances (Bhatti & Hindmarch, 1989; Meltzer, 1991; Simons, 1994a). The decongestant component of second-generation H_1-antagonist-decongestant formulations may cause insomnia and other CNS-stimulatory symptoms (Storms *et al.*, 1989).

Astemizole and ketotifen, like the first-generation H_1 antagonist cyproheptadine, may cause appetite stimulation and inappropriate weight gain (Grant *et al.*, 1990; Janssens, 1993). Intranasal azelastine or levocabastine occasionally cause mucosal irritation. Sensitization has not been observed during short-term use (McTavish & Sorkin, 1989; Dechant & Goa, 1991), in contrast to the sensitization reported after topical application of older H_1 antagonists to the skin. Azelastine may cause a transient bitter or metallic taste perception even when administered intranasally (McTavish & Sorkin, 1989).

Rarely, the second-generation H_1-antagonists terfenadine and astemizole have been reported to cause potentially fatal adverse cardiovascular effects (Table 24.6) (Simons, 1994a). After overdose, or when administered

Table 24.6 Relative risks of second-generation H_1-receptor antagonists in current use. (After Simons, 1994a.)

	Adequate number of objective, double-blind, placebo-controlled CNS studies	Absence of CNS effects after manufacturer's recommended doses in majority of studies	Absence of CNS effects when recommended doses are exceeded	At recommended doses, absence of interaction with alcohol or other CNS-active drugs	Absence of potential cardiac problems under usual circumstances	Absence, to date, of cardiac problems after overdose or when concomitantly administered with cyto-chrome P-450 inhibitors*	Absence of other adverse effects, e.g. weight gain
Terfenadine	✓	✓	✗	✓	✓	✗	✓
Astemizole	✓	✓	✓	✓	✓	✗	✗
Loratadine	✓	✓	✗	✓	✓	✓	✓
Cetirizine	✓	✓	✗	✓	✓	✓	✓
Acrivastine	✗	min	✗	✗	✓	✓	min
Ketotifen	✗	✗	✗	min	✓	min	✗
Ebastine	✗	✓	✗	✓	✓	min	min
Azelastine	✗	min	min	min	✓	min	✗
Levocabastine	✗	min	min	min	✓	✓	min

✓, yes; ✗, no; ?, conflicting information; min, more information needed.

*The database in terms of patient days of use varies considerably from one medication to another, being largest for terfenadine, cetirizine, loratadine and astemizole. Little information has been published on the central nervous system (CNS) effects of azelastine and levocabastine.

concomitantly with macrolide antibiotics such as erythromycin or clarithromycin, imidazole antifungal medications such as ketoconazole or itraconazole, or other medications that inhibit the hepatic mixed-function oxygenase cytochrome P-450 system, they may cause a prolonged QTc interval (Honig *et al.*, 1993, 1994), polymorphic ventricular tachycardia (*torsade de pointes*) and other cardiac arrhythmias. QTc prolongation after terfenadine overdose or concomitant administration of a cytochrome P-450 inhibitor is due to accumulation of the parent compound terfenadine, which is not readily detectable in plasma after recommended doses. Terfenadine, but not its active metabolite terfenadine carboxylate, has been shown to block the outward (delayed) rectifier potassium (I_K) current of the ventricular myocyte (Rampe *et al.*, 1993; Woosley *et al.*, 1993) (Fig. 24.13). Patients with hepatic dysfunction, or cardiac disorders associated with prolonged QTc interval, or metabolic disorders such as hypokalaemia or hypomagnesaemia, may be especially prone to adverse cardiovascular effects from H_1 antagonists. In pharmacoepidemiology studies, the incidence of arrhythmias found during terfenadine treatment did not exceed the incidence noted during treatment with older H_1 antagonists (Hanrahan *et al.*, 1992; Pratt *et al.*, 1994). In dose–response studies of loratadine, cetirizine or acrivastine on the QTc interval, no adverse effects were found (Sanders *et al.*, 1992; Affrime *et al.*, 1993; Sale *et al.*, 1994).

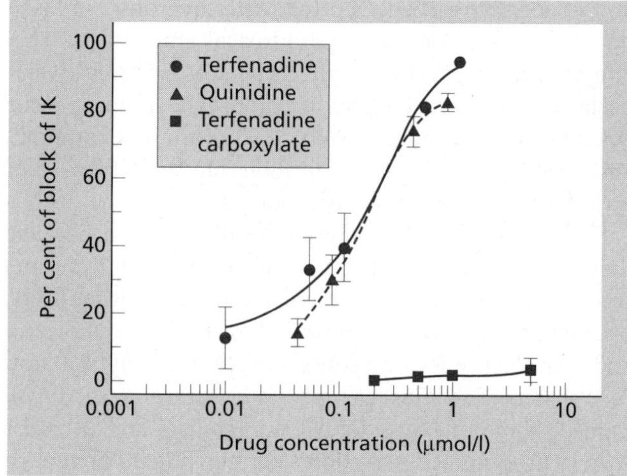

Fig. 24.13 The comparative effects of terfenadine, terfenadine carboxylate and quinidine on the delayed rectifier potassium current (I_K) are shown. The data were obtained using isolated feline ventricular myocytes grown in culture and studied using whole-cell single-suction pipette patch-clamp techniques. Percentage block of maximum I_K was as a function of the concentration of each medication. Terfenadine parent compound at a concentration of 1 μmol/l had a similar effect to 0.83 μmol/l quinidine, but up to 5 μmol/l terfenadine carboxylate (acid metabolite) did not have this effect. Between three and six cells were studied at each concentration. (Redrawn with permission from Woosley *et al.*, 1993.)

After overdose of a second-generation H_1 antagonist such as terfenadine or astemizole, prompt administration of activated charcoal may reduce absorption from the gastrointestinal tract (Laine *et al.*, 1994). Most second-generation H_1 antagonists are not dialysable (Simons, 1994a,b). Continuous electrocardiographic monitoring should be performed for 24 hours or until normalization of the QTc interval, with institution of cardioversion and pacing, if necessary. Most anti-arrhythmic medications are contraindicated; some, such as quinidine or amiodarone, may prolong the QTc interval further.

Use of H_1-antagonists during pregnancy

Available information does not permit identification of the safest H_1 antagonists for use during pregnancy. Tripelennamine, a relatively ineffective older H_1 antagonist, is often recommended, as there are no animal or human data implicating it as a teratogen (Schatz *et al.*, 1993). H_1-receptor antagonists are excreted in breast milk and other H_1-antagonists ingested by a nursing mother can cause sedation or irritability in the infant (Ito *et al.*, 1993).

Conclusions

The second-generation H_1 antagonists are supplanting their predecessors in the treatment of allergic rhinoconjunctivitis and chronic urticaria. Their use can be justified mainly on the basis of a more favourable benefit/risk ratio, predominantly due to reduced CNS toxicity. They are more expensive than the least expensive first-generation H_1-receptor antagonists. Directions for future H_1-antagonist research should include: additional dose–response studies in patients with allergic disorders, especially in children and in the elderly; further objective studies of adverse effects; studies of topical mucosal application of H_1 antagonists; and studies of H_1-antagonist enantiomers and active metabolites. With the cloning of the gene encoding the H_1 receptor, and increased understanding of the precise structural requirements for H_1-receptor activity, H_1 antagonists with an even more favourable therapeutic index may be developed.

Acknowledgement

The assistance of Ms L.L. McNiven is gratefully acknowledged.

References

Advenier, C. & Queille-Roussel, C. (1989) Rational use of antihistamines in allergic dermatological conditions. *Drugs*, **38**, 634–44.

Affrime, M.B., Lorber, R., Danzig, M., Cuss, F. & Brannan, M.D. (1993) Three month evaluation of electrocardiographic effects of loratadine in humans. *J. Allergy Clin. Immunol.*, **91**, 259.

Alford, C., Rombaut, N., Jones, J., Foley, S., Idzikowski, C. & Hindmarch, I. (1992) Acute effects of hydroxyzine on nocturnal sleep and sleep tendency the following day: a C-EEG study. *Hum. Psychopharmacol. Clin. Exp.*, **7**, 25–35.

Andersson, M., Greiff, L. & Svensson, C. (1994) Allergic rhinoconjunctivitis: the role of histamine. *Mediat. Inflamm.*, **3**, 171–5.

Bantz, E.W., Dolen, W.K., Chadwick, E.W. & Nelson, H.S. (1987) Chronic chlorpheniramine therapy: subsensitivity, drug metabolism, and compliance. *Ann. Allergy*, **59**, 341–6.

Belaich, S., Bruttmann, G., DeGreef, H. *et al.* (1990) Comparative effects of loratadine and terfenadine in the treatment of chronic idiopathic urticaria. *Ann. Allergy*, **64**, 191–4.

Berdy, G.J., Abelson, M.B., George, M.A., Smith, L.M. & Giovanoni, R.L. (1991) Allergic conjunctivitis: a survey of new antihistamines. *J. Ocular Pharmacol.*, **7**, 313–24.

Berth-Jones, J. & Graham-Brown, R.A.C. (1989) Failure of terfenadine in relieving the pruritus of atopic dermatitis. *Brit. J. Dermatol.*, **121**, 635–7.

Bhatti, J.Z. & Hindmarch, I. (1989) The effects of terfenadine with and without alcohol on an aspect of car driving performance. *Clin. Exp. Allergy*, **19**, 609–11.

Bleehen, S.S., Thomas, S.E., Greaves, M.W. *et al.* (1987) Cimetidine and chlorpheniramine in the treatment of chronic idiopathic urticaria: a multi-centre randomized double-blind study. *Brit. J. Dermatol.*, **117**, 81–8.

Bousquet, J., Campbell, A. & Michel, F.-B. (1992) Antiallergic activities of antihistamines. In: *Therapeutic Index of Antihistamines* (eds M.K. Church & J.-P. Rihoux), pp. 57–96. Hogrefe & Huber Publishers, Lewiston, NY.

Bousquet, J., Chanal, I., Skassa-Brociek, W., Lemonier, C. & Michel, F.B. (1990) Lack of subsensitivity to loratadine during long-term dosing during 12 weeks. *J. Allergy Clin. Immunol.*, **86**, 248–53.

Bousquet, J., Lebel, B., Chanal, I., Morel, A. & Michel, F.-B. (1988) Antiallergic activity of H_1-receptor antagonists assessed by nasal challenge. *J. Allergy Clin. Immunol.*, **82**, 881–7.

Bradley, C.M. & Nicholson, A.N. (1987) Studies on the central effects of the H_1-antagonist, loratadine. *Eur. J. Clin. Pharmacol.*, **32**, 419–21.

Brik, A., Tashkin, D.P., Gong H. Jr, Dauphinee, B. & Lee, E. (1987) Effect of cetirizine, a new histamine H_1 antagonist, on airway dynamics and responsiveness to inhaled histamine in mild asthma. *J. Allergy Clin. Immunol.*, **80**, 51–6.

Brogden, R.N. & McTavish, D. (1991) Acrivastine. A review of its pharmacological properties and therapeutic efficacy in allergic rhinitis, urticaria and related disorders. *Drugs*, **41**, 927–40.

Brooks, C.D., Karl, K.J. & Francom, S.F. (1990) Profile of ragweed hay fever symptom control with terfenadine started before or after symptoms are established. *Clin. Exp. Allergy*, **20**, 21–6.

Brunet, C., Bédard, P.-M. & Hébert, J. (1990) Effects of H_1-antihistamine drug regimen on histamine release by nonlesional skin mast cells of patients with chronic urticaria. *J. Allergy Clin. Immunol.*, **86**, 787–93.

Cainelli, T., Seidenari, S., Valsecchi, R. & Mosca, M. (1986) Double-blind comparison of astemizole and terfenadine in the treatment of chronic urticaria. *Pharmatherapeutica*, **4**, 679–86.

Cantekin, E.I., Mandel, E.M., Bluestone, C.D. *et al.* (1983) Lack of efficacy of a decongestant–antihistamine combination for otitis media with effusion ('secretory' otitis media) in children. *New Engl. J. Med.*, **308**, 297–301.

Carlsen, K.H., Kramer, J., Fagertun, H.E. & Larsen, S. (1993) Loratadine and terfenadine in perennial allergic rhinitis. Treatment of nonresponders to the one drug with the other drug. *Allergy*, **48**, 431–6.

Casy, A.F. (1991) Antagonists of H_1 receptors of histamine: recent developments. In: *Histamine and Histamine Antagonists* (ed. B. Uvnäs), pp. 549–72. Springer-Verlag, Berlin.

Charlesworth, E.N., Kagey-Sobotka, A., Norman, P.S. & Lichtenstein, L.M. (1989) Effect of cetirizine on mast cell-mediator release and cellular traffic during the cutaneous late-phase reaction. *J. Allergy Clin. Immunol.*, **83**, 905–12.

Chowdhury, B.A., Kaliner, M.A. & Fraser, C.M. (1994) Cloning of a gene encoding the human H_1 histamine receptor. *J. Allergy Clin. Immunol.*, **93**, 215.

Cimbura, G., Lucas, D.M., Bennett, R.C., Warren, R.A. & Simpson, H.M. (1982) Incidence and toxicological aspects of drugs detected in 484 fatally injured drivers and pedestrians in Ontario. *J. Forensic Sci.*, **27**, 855–67.

De Backer, M.D., Gommeren, W., Moereels, H. *et al.* (1993) Genomic cloning, heterologous expression and pharmacological characterization of a human histamine H_1 receptor. *Biochem. Biophys. Res. Commun.*, **197**, 1601–8.

Dechant, K.L. & Goa, K.L. (1991) Levocabastine. A review of its pharmacological properties and therapeutic potential as a topical antihistamine in allergic rhinitis and conjunctivitis. *Drugs*, **41**, 202–24.

Del Carpio, J., Kabbash, L., Turenne, Y. *et al.* (1989) Efficacy and safety of loratadine (10 mg once daily), terfenadine (60 mg twice daily), and placebo in the treatment of seasonal allergic rhinitis. *J. Allergy Clin. Immunol.*, **84**, 741–6.

Dijkman, J.H., Hekking, P.R.M., Molkenboer, J.F. *et al.* (1990) Prophylactic treatment of grass pollen-induced asthma with cetirizine. *Clin. Exp. Allergy*, **20**, 483–90.

Falliers, C.J., Brandon, M.L., Buchman, E. *et al.* (1991) Double-blind comparison of cetirizine and placebo in the treatment of seasonal rhinitis. *Ann. Allergy*, **66**, 257–62.

Frostad, A.B. & Olsen, A.K. (1993) A comparison of topical levocabastine and sodium cromoglycate in the treatment of pollen-provoked allergic conjunctivitis. *Clin. Exp. Allergy*, **23**, 406–9.

Fukui, H., Fujimoto, K., Mizuguchi, H. *et al.* (1994) Molecular cloning of the human histamine H_1 receptor gene. *Biochem. Biophys. Res. Commun.*, **201**, 894–901.

Gaffey, M.J., Kaiser, D.L. & Hayden, F.G. (1988) Ineffectiveness of oral terfenadine in natural colds: evidence against histamine as a mediator of common cold symptoms. *Ped. Infect. Dis. J.*, **7**, 223–8.

Gibbs, T.G., McDonnell, K.A., Stokes, T. & Graham, A.A. (1989) Acrivastine in two doses compared with placebo in a multicentre, parallel group study for the treatment of seasonal allergic rhinitis. *Brit. J. Clin. Pract.*, **43**, 11–14.

Goetz, D.W., Jacobson, J.M., Murnane, J.E. *et al.* (1989) Prolongation of simple and choice reaction times in a double-blind comparison of twice-daily hydroxyzine versus terfenadine. *J. Allergy Clin. Immunol.*, **84**, 316–22.

Goetz, D.W., Jacobson, J.M., Apaliski, S.J., Repperger, D.W. & Martin, M.E. (1991) Objective antihistamine side effects are mitigated by evening dosing of hydroxyzine. *Ann. Allergy*, **67**, 448–54.

Grant, J.A., Bernstein, D.I., Buckley, C.E. *et al.* (1988) Double-blind comparison of terfenadine, chlorpheniramine, and placebo in the treatment of chronic idiopathic urticaria. *J. Allergy Clin. Immunol.*, **81**, 574–9.

Grant, S.M., Goa, K.L., Fitton, A. & Sorkin, E.M. (1990) Ketotifen. A review of its pharmacodynamic and pharmacokinetic properties, and therapeutic use in asthma and allergic disorders. *Drugs*, **40**, 412–48.

Hannuksela, M., Kalimo, K., Lammintausta, K. *et al.* (1993) Dose ranging study: cetirizine in the treatment of atopic dermatitis in adults. *Ann. Allergy*, **70**, 127–33.

Hanrahan, J.P., Choo, P.W., Carlson, W., Greineder, D., Faich, G.A. & Platt, R. (1992) Antihistamine-associated sudden death, ventricular arrhythmias, syncope and QT-interval prolongation: a comparison of terfenadine and other antihistamines. *Post-Marketing Surveillance*, **6**, 23–4.

Haria, M., Fitton, A. & Peters, D.H. (1994) Loratadine. A reappraisal of its pharmacological properties and therapeutic use in allergic disorders. *Drugs*, **48**, 617–37.

Hill, S.J. (1990) Distribution, properties, and functional characteristics of three classes of histamine receptor. *Pharmacol. Rev.*, **42**, 45–83.

Honig, P.K., Wortham, D.C., Zamani, K. & Cantilena, L.R. (1994) Comparison of the effect of the macrolide antibiotics erythromycin, clarithromycin and azithromycin on terfenadine steady-state pharmacokinetics and electrocardiographic parameters. *Drug Invest.*, **7**, 148–56.

Honig, P.K., Wortham, D.C., Zamani, K., Conner, D.P., Mullin, J.C. & Cantilena, L.R. (1993) Terfenadine–ketoconazole interaction. Pharmacokinetic and electrocardiographic consequences. *JAMA*, **269**, 1513–18.

Howarth, P.H., Emanuel, M.B. & Holgate, S.T. (1984) Astemizole, a potent histamine H_1-receptor antagonist: effect in allergic rhinoconjunctivitis, on antigen and histamine-induced skin weal responses and relationship to serum levels. *Brit. J. Clin. Pharmacol.*, **18**, 1–8.

Ito, S., Blajchman, A., Stephenson, M., Eliopoulos, C. & Koren, G. (1993) Prospective follow-up of adverse reactions in breast-fed infants exposed to maternal medication. *Am. J. Obstet. Gynecol.*, **168**, 1393–9.

Janssens, M.M.-L. (1993) Astemizole. A nonsedating antihistamine with fast and sustained activity. *Clin. Rev. Allergy*, **11**, 35–63.

Janssens, M.M.-L. & Howarth, P.H. (1993) The antihistamines of the nineties. *Clin. Rev. Allergy*, **11**, 111–53.

Juhlin, L. & Arendt, C. (1988) Treatment of chronic urticaria with cetirizine dihydrochloride a non-sedating antihistamine. *Brit. J. Dermatol.*, **119**, 67–71.

Juniper, E.F., Kline, P.A., Hargreave, F.E. & Dolovich, J. (1989) Comparison of beclomethasone dipropionate aqueous nasal spray, astemizole, and the combination in the prophylactic treatment of ragweed pollen-induced rhinoconjunctivitis. *J. Allergy Clin. Immunol.*, **83**, 627–33.

Juniper, E.F., White, J. & Dolovich, J. (1988) Efficacy of continuous treatment with astemizole (Hismanal) and terfenadine (Seldane) in ragweed pollen-induced rhinoconjunctivitis. *J. Allergy Clin. Immunol.*, **82**, 670–5.

Klementsson, H., Andersson, M. & Pipkorn, U. (1990) Allergen-induced increase in nonspecific nasal reactivity is blocked by antihistamines without a clear-cut relationship to eosinophil influx. *J. Allergy Clin. Immunol.*, **86**, 466–72.

Labrecque, M., Ghezzo, H., L'Archevêque, J., Trudeau, C., Cartier, A. & Malo, J.-L. (1993) Duration of effect of loratadine and terfenadine administered once a day for one week on cutaneous and inhaled reactivity to histamine. *Chest*, **103**, 777–81.

Laine, K., Kivistö, K.T. & Neuvonen, P.J. (1994) The effect of activated charcoal on the absorption and elimination of astemizole. *Human Exp. Toxicol.*, **13**, 502–5.

Langeland, T., Fagertun, H.E. & Larsen, S. (1994) Therapeutic effect of loratadine on pruritus in patients with atopic dermatitis. A multi-crossover-designed study. *Allergy*, **49**, 22–6.

Lantin, J.P., Huguenot, C.H. & Pécoud, A. (1990) Effect of the H_1-antagonist astemizole on the skin reactions induced by histamine, codeine, and allergens. *Curr. Ther. Res.*, **47**, 683–92.

Levander, S., Stahle-Bäckdahl, M. & Hägermark, O. (1991) Peripheral antihistamine and central sedative effects of single and continuous oral doses of cetirizine and hydroxyzine. *Eur. J. Clin. Pharmacol.*, **41**, 435–9.

Levi, R., Rubin, L.E. & Gross, S.S. (1991) Histamine in cardiovascular function and dysfunction: recent developments. In: *Histamine and Histamine Antagonists* (ed. B. Uvnäs), pp. 347–83. Springer-Verlag, Berlin.

Lorenz, W., Duda, D., Dick, W. *et al.* (1994) Incidence and clinical importance of perioperative histamine release: randomised study of volume loading and antihistamines after induction of anaesthesia. *Lancet*, **343**, 933–40.

Lorenz, W., Ennis, M., Doenicke, A. & Dick, W. (1990) Perioperative uses of histamine antagonists. *J. Clin. Anesthesia*, **2**, 345–60.

McTavish, D., Goa, K.L. & Ferrill, M. (1990) Terfenadine: an updated review of its pharmacological properties and therapeutic efficacy. *Drugs*, **39**, 552–74.

McTavish, D. & Sorkin, E.M. (1989) Azelastine: a review of its pharmacodynamic and pharmacokinetic properties, and therapeutic potential. *Drugs*, **38**, 778–800.

Malo, J.-L., Fu, C.L., L'Archevêque, J., Ghezzo, H. & Cartier, A. (1990) Duration of the effect of astemizole on histamine-inhalation tests. *J. Allergy Clin. Immunol.*, **85**, 729–36.

Marshall, C. & Lieberman, P. (1989) Analysis of 3 pretreatment procedures to prevent anaphylactoid reactions to radiocontrast in previous reactors. *J. Allergy Clin. Immunol.*, **83**, 254.

Meador, K.J., Loring, D.W., Thompson, E.E. & Thompson, W.O. (1989) Differential cognitive effects of terfenadine and chlorpheniramine. *J. Allergy Clin. Immunol.*, **84**, 322–5.

Meltzer, E.O. (1991) Comparative safety of H_1 antihistamines. *Ann. Allergy*, **67**, 625–33.

Michel, L., De Vos, C., Rihoux, J.-P., Burtin, C., Benveniste, J. & Dubertret, L. (1988) Inhibitory effect of oral cetirizine on *in vivo* antigen-induced histamine and PAF-acether release and eosinophil recruitment in human skin. *J. Allergy Clin. Immunol.*, **82**, 101–9.

Naclerio, R.M., Kagey-Sobotka, A., Lichtenstein, L.M., Freidhoff, L. & Proud, D. (1990) Terfenadine, an H_1 antihistamine, inhibits histamine release *in vivo* in the human. *Am. Rev. Resp. Dis.*, **142**, 167–71.

Naclerio, R.M., Proud, D., Kagey-Sobotka, A., Freidhoff, L., Norman, P.S. & Lichtenstein, L.M. (1989) The effect of cetirizine on early allergic response. *Laryngoscope*, **99**, 596–9.

Nicholson, A.N., Pascoe, P.A., Turner, C. *et al.* (1991) Sedation and histamine H_1-receptor antagonism: studies in man with the enantiomers of chlorpheniramine and dimethindene. *Brit. J. Pharmacol.*, **104**, 270–76.

Odebäck, P. & the Swedish GP Allergy Team (1994) Topical levocabastine compared with oral loratadine for the treatment of seasonal allergic rhinoconjunctivitis. *Allergy*, **49**, 611–15.

Orgel, H.A., Meltzer, E.O., Kemp, J.P., Ostrom, N.K. & Welch, M.J. (1991) Comparison of intranasal cromolyn sodium, 4%, and oral terfenadine for allergic rhinitis: symptoms, nasal cytology, nasal ciliary clearance, and rhinomanometry. *Ann. Allergy*, **66**, 237–44.

Paton, D.M. & Webster, D.R. (1985) Clinical pharmacokinetics of H_1-receptor antagonists (the antihistamines). *Clin. Pharmacokinet.*, **10**, 477–97.

Paul, E. & Bödeker, R.H. (1986) Treatment of chronic urticaria with terfenadine and ranitidine. A randomized double-blind study in 45 patients. *Eur. J. Clin. Pharmacol.*, **31**, 277–80.

Pearce, F.L. (1991) Biological effects of histamine: An overview. *Agents Actions*, **33**, 4–7.

Pratt, C.M., Hertz, R.P., Ellis, B.E., Crowell, S.P., Louv, W. & Moyé, L. (1994) Risk of developing life-threatening ventricular arrhythmia associated with terfenadine in comparison with over-the-counter antihistamines, ibuprofen and clemastine. *Am. J. Cardiol.*, **73**, 346–52.

Prell, G.D. & Green, J.P. (1994) Measurement of histamine metabolites in brain and cerebrospinal fluid provides insights into histaminergic activity. *Agents Actions*, **41**, C5–8.

Rafferty, P. & Holgate, S.T. (1987) Terfenadine (Seldane) is a potent and selective histamine H_1 receptor antagonist in asthmatic airways. *Am. Rev. Resp. Dis.*, **135**, 181–4.

Rafferty, P., Jackson, L., Smith, R. & Holgate, S.T. (1990) Terfenadine, a potent histamine H_1-receptor antagonist in the treatment of grass pollen sensitive asthma. *Brit. J. Clin. Pharmacol.*, **30**, 229–35.

Rampe, D., Wible, B., Brown, A.M. & Dage, R.C. (1993) Effects of terfenadine and its metabolites on a delayed rectifier K^+ channel cloned from human heart. *Mol. Pharmacol.*, **44**, 1240–5.

Rimmer, S.J. & Church M.K. (1990) The pharmacology and mechanisms of action of histamine H_1-antagonists. *Clin. Exp. Allergy*, 20, 3–17.

Roehrs, T., Zwyghuizen-Doorenbos, A. & Roth, T. (1993) Sedative effects and plasma concentrations following single doses of triazolam, diphenhydramine, ethanol and placebo. *Sleep*, **16**, 301–5.

Rombaut, N., Bhatti, J.Z., Curran, S. & Hindmarch, I. (1991) Effects of topical administration of levocabastine on psychomotor and cognitive function. *Ann. Allergy*, **67**, 75–9.

Rombaut, N.E.I. & Hindmarch, I. (1994) Psychometric aspects of antihistamines: a review. *Hum. Psychopharmacol. Clin. Exp.*, **9**, 157–69.

Ruat, M., Bouthenet, M.L., Schwartz, J.-C. & Ganellin, C.R. (1990) Histamine H_1-receptor in heart: unique electrophoretic mobility and autoradiographic localization. *J. Neurochem.*, **55**, 379–85.

Sale, M.E., Barbey, J.T., Woosley, R.L. *et al.* (1994) The electrocardiographic effects of cetirizine in normal subjects. *Clin. Pharmacol. Ther.*, **56**, 295–301.

Sanders, R.L., Dockhorn, R.J., Alderman, J.L., McSorley, P.A., Wenger, T.L. & Frosolono, M.F. (1992) Cardiac effects of acrivastine compared to terfenadine. *J. Allergy Clin. Immunol.*, **89**, 183.

Schatz, M., Hoffman, C.P., Zeiger, R.S., Falkoff, R., Macy, E. & Mellon, M. (1993) The course and management of asthma and allergic diseases during pregnancy. In: *Allergy Principles and Practice* (eds E. Middleton C.E. Jr, Reed, E.F. Ellis, N.F. Adkinson J.W. Jr, Yunginger & W.W. Busse), pp. 1301–42. Mosby-Year Book, St Louis.

Seidel, W.F., Cohen, S., Bliwise, N.G. & Dement, W.C. (1990) Direct measurement of daytime sleepiness after administration of cetirizine and hydroxyzine with a standardized electroencephalographic assessment. *J. Allergy Clin. Immunol.*, **86**, 1029–33.

Sharpe, G.R. & Shuster, S. (1993) The effect of cetirizine on symptoms and wealing in dermographic urticaria. *Brit. J. Dermatol.*, **129**, 580–3.

Simons, F.E.R. (1994a) H_1-receptor antagonists. Comparative tolerability and safety. *Drug Safety*, **10**, 350–80.

Simons, F.E.R. (1994b) The therapeutic index of newer H_1-receptor antagonists. *Clin. Exp. Allergy*, **24**, 707–23.

Simons, F.E.R., McMillan, J.L. & Simons, K.J. (1990) A double-blind, single-dose, crossover comparison of cetirizine, terfenadine, loratadine, astemizole, and chlorpheniramine versus placebo: suppressive effects on histamine-induced wheals and flares during 24 hours in normal subjects. *J. Allergy Clin. Immunol.*, **86**, 540–47.

Simons, F.E.R., Murray, H.E. & Simons, K.J. (1995a) Quantitation of H_1-receptor antagonists in skin and serum. *J. Allergy Clin. Immunol.*, **95**, 759–64.

Simons, F.E.R., Sussman, G.L. & Simons, K.J. (1995b) Effect of the H_2-antagonist cimetidine on the pharmacokinetics and pharmacodynamics of the H_1-antagonists hydroxyzine and cetirizine in patients with chronic urticaria. *J. Allergy Clin. Immunol.*, **95**, 685–93.

Simons, F.E.R. & Simons, K.J. (1991) Pharmacokinetic optimisation of histamine H_1-receptor antagonist therapy. *Clin. Pharmacokinet.*, **21**, 372–93.

Simons, F.E.R. & Simons, K.J. (1994) The pharmacology and use of H_1-receptor antagonist drugs. *New Engl. J. Med.*, **330**, 1663–70.

Simons, F.E.R., Watson, W.T.A. & Simons, K.J. (1988) Lack of subsensitivity to terfenadine during long-term terfenadine treatment. *J. Allergy Clin. Immunol.*, **82**, 1068–75.

Smith, M.B.H. & Feldman, W. (1993) Over-the-counter cold medications. A critical review of clinical trials between 1950 and 1991. *JAMA*, **269**, 2258–63.

Sohoel, P., Freng, B.A., Kramer, J. *et al.* (1993) Topical levocabastine compared with orally administered terfenadine for the prophylaxis and treatment of seasonal rhinoconjunctivitis. *J. Allergy Clin. Immunol.*, **92**, 73–81.

Spencer, C.M., Faulds, D. & Peters, D.H. (1993) Cetirizine. A reappraisal of its pharmacological properties and therapeutic use in selected allergic disorders. *Drugs*, **46**, 1055–80.

Stern, M.A., Rosenberg, R.M., Smith, R. & Fidler, C. (1990) A comparative study of terfenadine at two dose levels in the management of hayfever. *Brit. J. Clin. Pract.*, **44**, 359–63.

Storms, W.W., Bodman, S.F., Nathan, R.A. *et al.* (1989) SCH 434: a new antihistamine/decongestant for seasonal allergic rhinitis. *J. Allergy Clin. Immunol.*, **83**, 1083–90.

Ter Laak, A.M., Donné-Op den Kelder, G.M., Bast, A. & Timmerman, H. (1993) Is there a difference in the affinity of histamine H_1 receptor antagonists for CNS and peripheral receptors? An *in vitro* study. *Eur. J. Pharmacol.*, **232**, 199–205.

Timmerman, H. (1992) Factors involved in the incidence of central nervous system effects of H_1-blockers. In: *Therapeutic Index of Antihistamines* (eds M.K. Church & J.-P. Rihoux), pp. 19–31. Hogrefe & Huber Publishers, Lewiston, NY.

Town, G.I. & Holgate, S.T. (1990) Comparison of the effect of loratadine on the airway and skin responses to histamine, methacholine, and allergen in subjects with asthma. *J. Allergy Clin. Immunol.*, **86**, 886–93.

Wagenmann, M., Baroody, F.M., Kagey-Sobotka, A., Lichtenstein, L.M. & Naclerio, R.M. (1994) The effect of terfenadine on unilateral nasal challenge with allergen. *J. Allergy Clin. Immunol.*, **93**, 594–605.

Watson, W.T.A., Simons, K.J., Chen, X.Y. & Simons, F.E.R. (1989) Cetirizine: a pharmacokinetic and pharmacodynamic evaluation in children with seasonal allergic rhinitis. *J. Allergy Clin. Immunol.*, **84**, 457–64.

Weiler, J.M., Meltzer, E.O., Dockhorn, R., Widlitz, M.D., D'Eletto, T.A. & Freitag, J.J. (1991) A safety and efficacy evaluation of azelastine nasal spray in seasonal allergic rhinitis. *J. Allergy Clin. Immunol.*, **87**, 219.

Wood-Baker, R. & Holgate, S.T. (1993) The comparative actions and adverse effect profile of single doses of H_1-receptor antihistamines in the airways and skin of subjects with asthma. *J. Allergy Clin. Immunol.*, **91**, 1005–14.

Woosley, R.L., Chen, Y., Freiman, J.P. & Gillis, R.A. (1993) Mechanism of the cardiotoxic actions of terfenadine. *JAMA*, **269**, 1532–6.

Yanai, K., Watanabe, T., Yokoyama, H. *et al.* (1992) Mapping of histamine H_1 receptors in the human brain using [^{11}C]Pyrilamine and positron emission tomography. *J. Neurochem.*, **59**, 128–36.

Yang, W.H., Drouin, M.A., Copeland, D. *et al.* (1991) Double-blind multicentre study of ketotifen (Zaditen) in chronic idiopathic urticaria. *J. Allergy Clin. Immunol.*, **87**, 224.

Zhang, M.Q., ter Laak, A.M. & Timmerman, H. (1993) Structure–activity relationships within a series of analogues of the histamine H_1-antagonist terfenadine. *Eur. J. Med. Chem.*, **28**, 165–73.

CHAPTER 25

Vascular Permeability and Plasma Exudation

C.G.A. Persson

Introduction

The mucosal output in inflammatory airway diseases consists of cells and secretions. In addition, there is a significant output emanating directly from the subepithelial microcirculation. Thus, microvascular-epithelial exudation of 'bulk' plasma has now been well demonstrated in asthma and rhinitis. Luminal entry of plasma emerges as a specific physiological response that may show the distribution, the intensity and the time-course of different inflammatory processes in the airways. The plasma exudate is also a significant inflammatory factor in its own right, because it contains peptide mediators, adhesive proteins, proteases, cytokines, immunoglobulins, etc. These plasma-derived effector solutes may, in fact, decide much of the molecular disease milieu *in vivo*. This chapter discusses mechanisms of microvascular–epithelial exudation of plasma in upper and lower airways. The emphasis is on the role of the exudate in mucosal defence, epithelial repair and airways inflammation.

Focus on gross functions in complex *in vivo* biosystems

The bulk of novel information on airway epithelium and vascular endothelium now emanates from studies employing reductive biological science approaches and cell-culture techniques. However exciting and important, the novel molecular and cellular approaches may not always be applied with complete success unless the gross physiology and pathophysiology of the airway mucosa have first been well assessed. Somewhat conservatively, therefore, the present discussion will adhere to the experimental strategy of having the proper *in vivo* function established first. The point may be illustrated by an example: one current paradigm is that the airway barrier is abnormally pervious to inhaled molecules in asthma and rhinitis. Accordingly, reductive science approaches now provide data explaining how and by what mechanisms the perviousness is produced. At the same time, however, new functional *in vivo* studies employing increasingly improved physiological methods demonstrate that the absorption rate across the mucosa, if it is at all altered, may actually be decreased in rhinitis and asthma (Persson *et al.*, 1995a). The present focus does not reduce the need for critical comparisons between animal and human findings. Recent concept testing has thus demonstrated that neurogenic inflammation (exudation), which is a major mechanism in guinea pig and rat airways, is not present in human airways (Greiff *et al.*, 1995). In airways subjected to inflammatory provocation and in airways affected by an inflammatory process, the plasma exudation process dramatically alters the composition of proteins, cytokines and peptide mediators in the lamina propria, in the epithelial basement membrane, in the epithelium and on the mucosal surface. This microcirculation plasma-derived molecular milieu (Table 25.1) may affect cellular inflammatory activities in ways which may be difficult to reproduce *in vitro*. The exuded plasma lays down important adhesive proteins such as fibronectin and fibrin(ogen). It provides proteases, antiproteases, binding proteins and immunoglobulins. The extravasated bulk plasma contains many cytokines including growth factors. Some of the plasma proteins, notably α_2-macroglobulin, are known to bind, carry and target numerous cytokines. The plasma-derived peptide

Table 25.1 Contents of extravasated plasma.

Proteins
Adhesive molecules (fibrinogen, fibronectin, etc.)
Proteases, antiproteases
Cytokine modulating proteins
Immunoglobulins
Other
Cytokines
Growth factors (PDGF, IGF, TGF-β, etc.)
Interleukins
Several cytokines bound, carried and targetted by α_2-macroglobulin and other plasma proteins
Peptides
Complement fragments
Bradykinins
Fibrinolysis peptides
Other

IGF, insulin-like growth factor; PDGF, platelet-derived growth factor; TGF-β, transforming growth factor-β.

mediators are not confined to the bradykinins. Fibrinolysis peptides, complement fragments and many more biologically active molecules are dynamically produced by the extravasated protein systems in contact with airway tissue and surface components. The essential but complex, and as yet only partly understood, contributions from the microcirculation should probably affect our strategy in exploring the pathophysiology and pharmacology of inflammatory processes. The *in vivo* approach involving tissues with intact microcirculation may still have a prime role in this exploratory research.

Exudation of plasma as an airway end-organ response

The classical signs of inflammation, 'rubor', 'dolor', 'calor', 'tumor' and 'functio laesa', seem of limited help in identifying the active inflammtory process in the airways. Rubor may characterize an airway embarrassed by irritants that increase blood flow but do not produce inflammation. Besides, the airway mucosal blood flow is already so rich under baseline conditions that moderate changes in flow may not be critical to airway functions in inflammation. This notion is supported by the observation that topical vasoconstrictors, such as oximetazoline, may not affect the inflammatory stimulus-induced plasma exudation in human nasal airways (Persson *et al.*, 1992).

Dolor and calor, pain and heat, cannot be regarded as characteristic features of the inflammatory condition in asthma and rhinitis. In contrast, 'tumor' is clearly important. However, what is behind the visible swelling? The airway mucosa may be swollen due to intravascular pooling of blood, as in the venous sinuses of the nose. This particular kind of thickening is abrogated by sympathomimetic α-receptor agonists. Long-term treatment with topical steroids also inhibits the congestion but this result may reflect the anti-inflammatory efficacy of these drugs rather than any direct vasoconstrictor action. The 'swelling' that is observed through the bronchoscope may be composed of several factors. Congestion may contribute. Airway remodelling with increased numbers of vessels and cells and an abnormal extracellular matrix may well contribute. Also, simple bronchoconstriction that moves a normal, or thickened mucosa regularly, or irregularly, inwards to reduce the patency of the airway lumen may be quite difficult to distinguish from the other causes of tumefaction.

The most common interpretation of the cause of airway swelling is oedema, which simply means that the extravascular tissue holds abnormally large amounts of extravascular fluid. Considerable or sustained extravasation of plasma is normally expected to produce tissue oedema. However, the notion that airway oedema is a major component of asthma and allergic rhinitis is now based more on hypothetical reasoning coupled with selected histological pictures than on irrefutable quantitative research. The most active microcirculation in airway disease would be the capillary–venular plexus residing in the lamina propria, sometimes reaching superficially to penetrate part of the epithelial basement membrane. The acute mucosal challenge-induced increase in vascular permeability, causing extravasation of plasma from the superficial microcirculation, may not produce mucosal oedema but may rather result in luminal entry of 'bulk' plasma. Hence, extravasation of plasma in airway tissues may not always be equated with airway oedema.

Plasma extravasation and, in the airways, mucosal exudation of plasma deserves attention as a breaking point demonstrating that cellular and other mechanisms of inflammation have reached the activity level where tissue end organs become significantly affected. Plasma exudation thus differs from many other airway end organ responses by being rather specific to inflammation (Persson *et al.*, 1992). Bronchial tone, dilatation of venous sinuses, airway secretion and blood flow are all increased both by inflammation and by simple irritant type of provocations, which also evoke neural reflex activity. The most powerful airway reflexes are coughs and sneezes but, again, these reflexes are not exclusive to inflammation, nor are they always induced by inflammation.

The final classical sign, 'functio laesa', is true in the general sense that asthmatic airway inflammation may be a major cause of breathing difficulties. However, in more specific terms this sign seems difficult to reconcile with most cases of asthma and rhinitis where hyper- rather than hypofunction of airway end organs may be prevalent. The increased ability to respond to inhaled stimuli is reflected both by the well known phenomenon of non-specific hyperresponsiveness and by specific hyperresponsiveness of individual mucosal end organs such as the secretory apparatus, the sensory innervation and the microcirculation (Persson *et al.*, 1992).

Exudation pathways and mechanisms

The acute plasma exudation response to airway mucosal challenges involves a series of events which all occur within minutes after challenge. By indirect, cellular release mechanisms, the inflammatory challenge results in increased mucosal tissue levels of vasoactive agents—such an agent itself may constitute a directly acting challenge. The vascular permeability-increasing agents act on the venular wall endothelium that is equipped with a great variety of cell-surface receptors. Through receptor stimulation the cell-to-cell contact is lost at distinct points in the walls of the post-capillary venules. The mechanism of interendothelial gap formation has been widely accepted as a contractile event but the gaps might also be produced by reduced adhesion along tiny stretches of the endothelial cell-to-cell junctions. Through these gaps or holes in the venular wall, non-sieved plasma is moved by the hydrostatic pressure gradient that exists between the venules (about 20 cmH_2O) and the extravascular tissue. The extravasation is a dramatic event that locally abolishes the colloid osmotic pressure gradient between the microvessels and the tissue. During the first 10–20 seconds after challenge the airway lamina propria is flooded with the plasma exudate. Apparently unhindered, the exudate then passes through the epithelial basement membrane and further up between epithelial cells that normally are separated at the base. At the apical pole circumference the epithelial cells are tightly connected. However, not even the tight junctions of an intact epithelial lining are significant obstacles to the further flux of exudate into the airway lumen. The luminal entry of plasma appears to be a self-sustained process, occurring as long as sufficient amounts of plasma press upon the basolateral aspects of columnar epithelial cells (Fig. 25.1).

The bulk plasma that is moved to the mucosal surface is not identical to circulating plasma. Promptly after extravasation several protein systems of the blood plasma will be activated, generating a great variety of peptides and oligoproteins. The extravasated plasma will also have excellent opportunities to interact with interesting cell-derived molecules that are present or released in the lamina propria. For example, several plasma proteins, from the 70-kDa albumin to the 700-kDa α_2-macroglobulin, are avid binders of different molecules such as mediators, cytokines and drugs. The tissue flooding with plasma is not merely a passive lavage. In addition, the extra-

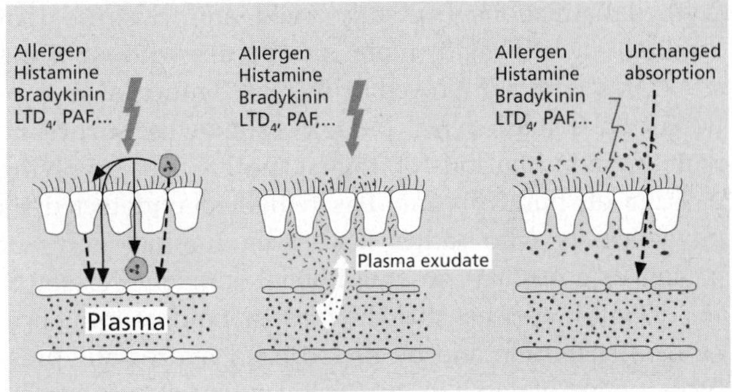

Fig. 25.1 Challenge with allergen and leukotriene-type mediators and several other pro-inflammatory factors produces dose-dependent luminal entry of 'bulk' plasma, without disrupting the epithelial lining and without increasing the absorption ability of the airway mucosa. Thus, all plasma protein systems, irrespective of molecular size, may appear on the surface of the intact airway mucosa.

vasated plasma may offer specific piggy-back riding to the airway surface ('lamina propria lavage') (Persson, 1994). In airway disease conditions, simple histamine challenges, which produce graded exudations of bulk plasma, may through this action also increase, dose dependently, airway lavage fluid levels of select cytokines such as interleukin-6 (Persson *et al.*, 1995b), that are known to be bound by plasma proteins such as α_2-macroglobulin. A potentially very effective lamina propria lavage, induced by the plasma exudation process, may need to be considered in studies of disease mechanisms and drug effects involving techniques such as bronchial and nasal lavages and biopsies.

Erjefält *et al.* (1995), employing colloidal gold (5 nm in diameter) as plasma tracer, have recently observed that the plasma exudate is moved between all epithelial cells in the area and all around each cell. Hence, the burden on each unit length of cell junctions would also be minute at pronounced rates of exudation of bulk plasma. This possibility tallies with previous observations, demonstrating the non-injurious nature of the mucosal exudation process (Persson *et al.*, 1992; Persson, 1994). A mechanism has also been discovered by which the extravasated plasma may pass through epithelial tight junctions (Persson *et al.*, 1995a). Using intact airway tube preparations mounted in organ baths to allow separate regulation of mucosal and serosal bathing fluids, it has thus been demonstrated that a slightly increased hydrostatic pressure load (<5 cmH_2O) on the basolateral aspects of the airway epithelial lining cells is sufficient for moving macromolecular solutes to the mucosal surface. Indeed, this hydraulic process is reversible and repeatable, much in the same way as the *in vivo* exudation evoked by challenge with histamine-type mediators. Furthermore, both *in vitro* and *in vivo* the epithelial junctions evidently yield and close so that luminal entry of macromolecules occurs without being associated with or followed by increased mucosal absorption of polar solutes (Fig. 25.1). It is somewhat surprising that this non-injurious epithelial mechanism, involving passage of 'bulk' plasma, has remained undetected by physiologists who rather have seen luminal entry of plasma as a mechanism of epithelial damage (Persson *et al.*, 1995a). It appears that the plasma exudate influence, by its distribution and by its localized hydrostatic pressure, opens valve-like paracellular pathways for its luminal entry (Fig. 25.1). The ease with which extravasated plasma enters the airway lumen is underscored by the observation that the regional lymph protein transport may be unchanged at inflammatory stimulus-induced exudation of plasma in the guinea pig tracheal mucosa (Erjefält *et al.*, 1993a). As demonstrated in both nasal and tracheobronchial airways, acute exudation of bulk plasma is associated with an unchanged rate of mucosal absorption of hydrophilic solutes (Persson *et al.*, 1992; Persson, 1994) (Fig. 25.1). These observations provide functional *in vivo* evidence that epithelial tight junctions have a valve-like mechanism that is readily opened by plasma that approaches from beneath. Luminal entry of bulk plasma is now forwarded as a major mucosal defence mechanism that neutralizes offending agents on the airway surface even before they penetrate into the tissue (Persson *et al.*, 1991).

Taken together, the experimental data indicate that the active physiological and pharmacological regulation of mucosal exudation of plasma takes place at the level of the endothelial cells of the microvascular wall. This is the site where inflammatory agents produce small, round interendothelial holes initiating the whole airways exudation process. It seems functionally relevant that mediators and drugs shall not act on the epithelial lining cells to selectively regulate the epithelial passage of plasma into the lumen. A tightening effect on the epithelium in this respect would not be a desirable drug action, because it would increase the likelihood of oedema formation in the airway mucosa.

Challenge- and disease-induced plasma exudation responses

A non-specific contractile and secretory mediator, such as acetylcholine or its analogues (methacholine, carbachol, etc.), is without exudative effects in the airways (Persson *et al.*, 1991, 1992; Persson, 1994). Furthermore, irritants such as nicotine and capsaicin that evoke strong neurogenic responses, are without exudative effects in human nasal airways (Greiff *et al.*, 1995). This latter observation is in sharp contrast to findings in guinea pig airways, where capsaicin and nicotine produce pronounced exudation responses. Hence, plasma exudation in human airways is more specific to inflammation than in rodent airways, because simple neural reflex mechanisms may not produce this response.

The human nasal mucosa lends itself to airway-specific, well-controlled challenge and lavage studies. To take advantage of these possibilities a nasal pool technique has been developed (Greiff *et al.*, 1990). Using a compressible nasal pool device, it is possible fill the entire ipsilateral nasal cavity with fluid and solutes. A large airway mucosal surface area can thus be exposed to defined concentrations of agents and tracers. After a selected mucosal exposure time the pool fluid may, almost quantitatively, be recovered into the device. Thus, the exposed mucosal surface is also gently lavaged by the nasal pool fluid, providing the opportunity to sample mucosal indices selectively from the area of interest. This gentle lavage procedure can be carried out numerous times in sequence without causing undue changes in mucosal function. The technique also allows exposure of the same airway mucosal surface area at repeated provocations. It has not been possible to attain similarly controlled experimental conditions in human tracheobronchial airways. However, many mechanisms of the airway mucosa in health and disease can be examined in the nose, and the findings can be extrapolated to apply also to the lower airways (Persson *et al.*, 1992).

Using the nasal pool device, Greiff *et al.* (1990) and Svensson *et al.* (1995) have demonstrated graded exudative effects of different mucosal surface concentrations of histamine. Between 20 μg/ml and 2000 μg/ml this amine produces fivefold to more than 100-fold increases in lavage fluid levels of plasma proteins (albumin to α_2-macroglobulin). Mediators such as histamine, bradykinin and leukotriene D_4 produce graded exudative responses over a wide range of concentrations in both guinea pig and human airways. Histamine, bradykinin and paf acether are about equally potent when applied on the airway mucosa, whereas leukotriene D_4 is about 100-fold more potent than either of these agents. In addition, select cytokines and proteases may induce plasma exudation in the airways. Presumably, most exudative agents somehow act through activation of appropriate receptors on vascular permeability-regulating endothelial cells.

Allergen challenge in subjects with allergic airway disease may produce both immediate- and late-phase plasma exudation responses. Similarly, in sensitized guinea pigs allergen challenge produces dual plasma exudation responses (Erjefält *et al.*, 1993b). (Neurogenic exudation is not involved in the allergic response, even of guinea pig airways.) If the allergen challenge is given to the whole guinea pig lung, involving also the peripheral parenchymal tissue, the late-phase exudation appears to be sustained for about 20 hours. If only the large tracheobronchial airway is challenged the immediate, airway-specific exudation phase is over in about an hour. Then follows a late airway exudation phase that peaks about 5 hours after challenge and then fades off (Erjefält *et al.*, 1993b).

The occupational small-molecular-weight chemical, toluenediisocyanate (TDI), which differs from allergens, produces a strong and sustained plasma exudation response also in airways that have not previously been exposed to TDI, and thus have not been sensitized to this reactive agent. Within a wide dose range, 3 nl to 30 μl, TDI produces dose-dependent plasma exudation into guinea pig tracheobronchial airways of previously unexposed guinea pigs. These doses, applied restrictedly on the large tracheobronchial airways of guinea pigs, may be compared to the accepted exposure level which corresponds to a daily human body burden of about 15 μl TDI. The acute TDI-induced sustained plasma exudation response in non-sensitized guinea pigs peaks 5 hours after challenge and continues for about 15 additional hours.

Guinea pigs that receive repeated challenges with 3 nl of TDI on the large tracheobronchial airways develop an increased inflammatory responsiveness to TDI (Erjefält & Persson, 1992). Thus, challenge with exceedingly low doses of TDI (0.3 nl) in the sensitized animals is associated with pronounced eosinophilia and a marked and sustained exudative response. This TDI-induced plasma exudation response, in contrast to that observed in non-sensitized animals, is inhibited by glucocorticoid pretreatment (Erjefält *et al.*, 1992). In patients with occupational asthma it has also been demonstrated that exposure to the occupational agent produces a late-phase response that encompasses a plasma exudation process. TDI challenge-induced plasma exudation in patients with occupational asthma due to this chemical is also inhibited by pretreatment with inhaled glucocorticoids (Fabbri & Mapp, 1991).

Plasma exudation in inflammatory airway diseases was first demonstrated through determination of plasma proteins in sputum samples obtained in asthma and chronic bronchitis (Persson, 1988). Almost equally early it was observed that steroid treatment significantly reduces the sputum level of different plasma indices (Persson, 1988). Interestingly, the inhibition of exudation seems to occur without concomitant reduction of sputum levels of secretory indices. Indeed, the latter may increase along with reduced sputum volume (Persson, 1988). The relatively poor antisecretory effect of glucocorticosteroids adds to a long list of significant qualitative differences between airway secretory and exudative processes, and supports' the notion that the plasma exudation response may reflect airway inflammation better than other physiological end organ responses in the airways.

Albumin is usually the only plasma protein that has been analysed in the numerous bronchoalveolar lavage fluids (BALF) obtained from asthmatic lungs. However, BALF levels of albumin alone may not always be a useful indicator of the plasma exudation process. Indeed, it has now been demonstrated in studies of the acute response to allergen challenge that BALF albumin may be unchanged, whereas large plasma proteins, such as fibrinogen and α_2-macroglobulin, are significantly increased (Salomonsson *et al.*, 1992; Svensson *et al.*, 1995). Such a result could even be expected because the inflammatory stimulus-induced luminal entry of plasma is almost a bulk flux of proteins with little size restriction and, differing from albumin, low concentrations of the much larger plasma proteins are normally present. Furthermore, BALF contains material that has accumulated on the surface for variable and unknown periods of time. An additional confounding factor concerns the fact that BALF variably samples both airway and alveolar lining surface material. This latter aspect may pose a general problem, in as much as asthma is an airway and not a pulmonary disease. In the nose where airway-specific challenge and lavage are readily feasible, and where the problem of varying baselines can be eliminated, albumin may well reflect the plasma exudation response (Persson *et al.*, 1992). Indeed, albumin and α_2-macroglobulin were highly correlated in nasal lavage liquids after allergen challenge in the nose, whereas in corresponding bronchial experiments, involving the same patients, allergen challenge only increased BALF α_2-macroglobulin (Svensson *et al.*, 1995).

Roles of exuded plasma

The recent observations on mucosal exudation mechanisms in animal and human airways (Persson *et al.*, 1991, 1992, 1995a; Persson, 1994) call for a revision of many of the previously proposed roles of plasma exudation in airway diseases. Increased microvascular permeability in the airways may no longer be equated with airway oedema without reservation. The presence of plasma proteins in the airway lumen may no longer be interpreted as a sign of epithelial damage. More specifically, just because plasma is exuded into the airway lumen, this may no longer tell us anything about the perviousness of the airway mucosa to inhaled molecules. It may also be difficult to make conclusions about the occurrence of tracheobronchial plasma exudation merely from measurements of BALF levels of albumin, and it may be a complete mistake to conclude that a protein that did increase in BALF must come from a cellular source just because the level of albumin did not exhibit a simultaneous increase. Further, knowledge on whether plasma exudation has occurred or not may be needed to properly interpret the appearance of many cellularly derived indices, including cytokines, on the mucosal surface; in particular, we may need to distinguish when the indices merely have been carried from the lamina propria to the surface by the exudate.

Even if plasma extravasation in the airways does not always produce mucosal oedema, there are several other sequelae to consider. Extravasated plasma may deposit its targeting and carrier proteins as well as its fibrinous macromolecules in the lamina propria, the basement membrane, and both in and on the epithelium. Plasma may thus be an important source, providing adhesive protein components to the mucosal extracellular matrix. By continuously supplying these proteins, together with plasma-derived growth factors, and together with important complement fragments, kinins, fibrinolysis peptides, etc., the extravasation process in the airways may be crucial to airway cellular inflammatory processes and to airway remodelling processes. The luminal entry of extravasated plasma is not only a mechanism that reduces the tendency to oedema formation in the airways. Plasma-derived fibrin, fibronectin and other proteins in the epithelium and on the mucosal surface may govern an important part of the traffic and the activity of leucocytes in airway inflammation. Plasma-derived mediators and cytokines, a great variety of active oligoproteins and peptides, may, together with the cellular products, be important factors in almost all facets of mucosal surface inflammation (Persson, 1986, 1994).

By their physical properties and interactions, plasma exudates may further impede the patency of the airway passages in several ways (Persson, 1986). Against a background of stagnated exudate–mucus material in the lumen, a pronounced exudation response in an attack of asthma may cause extremely severe obstruction of the bronchi, and also in instances when bronchial smooth-muscle contraction is increased only slightly (Persson, 1986).

Absorption, exudation and epithelial restitution

Severe airway infections caused by human influenza virus may be associated with extensive airway epithelial damage and shedding, but the extent of increased mucosal absorption under these conditions has been little studied. It has recently been demonstrated that common cold virus inoculation may produce significant disease symptoms, hyperresponsiveness and exudation of plasma macromolecules without causing appreciable increases in the human nasal airway absorption permeability. Corona-virus-induced nasal infection is thus associated with plasma exudation responses, both at baseline and at challenge with histamine, which are significantly greater than the corresponding normal values (Greiff *et al.*, 1994). The hyperresponsiveness to histamine probably reflects true changes in the responsive endorgan (microcirculation), since increased penetration and absorption of topical challenge agents may not apply in the common cold (Greiff *et al.*, 1994).

Using the controlled conditions that are offered by the nasal pool technique (Greiff *et al.*, 1990), Greiff *et al.* (1993) have further observed that the nasal absorption rate of a small hydrophilic tracer (^{52}Cr-EDTA) is abnormally slow in subjects with allergic rhinitis. Thus, late in the Swedish birch pollen season, when eosinophilic exudative inflammation would have been present for several weeks, the allergic airway mucosa exhibited an increased functional tightness. In a separate study quite similar findings have now been obtained concerning peptide absorption across the allergic nasal mucosa (Greiff *et al.*, 1995). During the Swedish pollen season, rhinitic individuals also develop a significantly increased responsiveness to histamine challenge, expressed as abnormally increased plasma exudation (Svensson *et al.*, 1995). Since absorption of histamine would be decreased in these patients, the recorded hyperresponsiveness may be an underestimation of the change that had occurred in the airway microcirculation. It may not be feasible to have perfectly controlled conditions for studies of absorption across a defined bronchial mucosal surface *in vivo* in humans. However, in a recent study Halpin *et al.* (1993) made serious attempts to correct for mucociliary transport of the inhaled absorption tracer and could demonstrate that the absorption permeability in asthma may be reduced. It appears that a new paradigm on airway tightness in allergic inflammation is under development.

These clinical observations on reduced absorption permeability in asthma and rhinitis prompt questions about 'mediators' of tightness rather than permeability. It has been clearly demonstrated that luminal entry of plasma does not cause epithelial disruption, nor is it associated with an increased absorption ability of the airway mucosa (Persson *et al.*, 1992). Is it then possible that the plasma exudation process under some circumstances may impede airway absorption? Another thought-provoking finding concerns the association between increased epithelial damage and shedding and normal or reduced absorption rates in chronic inflammatory airway disease. A decreased absorption ability would certainly not be compatible with extensively denuded basement membranes in the airways. Perhaps then the new absorption data should be taken as support for the possibility that extensive denudation in specimens of asthmatic bronchi may be an artefact of the biopsy procedure rather than a true reflection of the *in situ* condition. A further potentially linked question, and one that may not have received sufficient attention, concerns the epithelial repair or restitution process that would be set in motion as soon as shedding occurs. Can increased knowledge about repair after shedding provide explanations to the well-maintained barrier functions in diseased airways?

Jonas Erjefält *et al.* (1994, 1995a,b) have recently examined effects induced by and following from gentle epithelial cell removal *in vivo* in guinea pig trachea. The employed *in vivo* model mimics epithelial shedding by not causing bleeding or damage to the basement membrane. Two important findings are the promptness and the high speed by which epithelial restitution starts and proceeds, respectively. The immediate physiological and cellular *in vivo* responses to denudation are severalfold. The microcirculation responds by exuding bulk plasma (Erjefält *et al.*, 1994) and, with little delay, large numbers of neutrophils (Erjefält *et al.*, 1995a,b) are extravasated (no bleeding occurs). Secretion is induced (Erjefält *et al.*, 1995). Eosinophil traffic and activation are also induced (Erjefält *et al.*, 1995a,b). Thus, a plasma-derived fibrin–fibronectin gel increasingly rich in neutrophils and eosinophils soon covers the denuded basement membrane (Fig. 25.2). This provisional cover is maintained and continuously supplied with plasma until a new tight epithelium has been established. The intact epithelial cells bordering the denuded area also respond immediately after loosing their neighbour cells. Secretory and ciliated cells (*sic*, ciliated cells do partake as progenitors for the new epithelium (Svensson *et al.*, 1995)), and probably also basal cells, dedifferentiate, flatten and migrate over the membrane. The migration rate is particularly fast during the first minutes after denudation. The speed of migration, most likely aided by *in vivo*-specific factors, is so high (~3 μm/min) that shedding, even of clusters of epithelial cells, would result in de-epithelialized basement membranes only for quite brief periods of time. Hence, epithelial shedding even to the extent of denudation of limited areas may occur *in vivo*, with little consequence to the mucosal barrier functions. Defence and protection during the restitution process would be well catered for by the leucocyte-rich plasma-derived gel. This gel, with its content of plasma-derived migration promoters such as fibronectin, fibrin and growth factors, is also a highly suitable supramembranal milieu for high-speed epithelial restitution. (*In vitro* studies dealing with epithelial repair demonstrate only relatively slow events.) Another conclusion concerns all those physiological and cellular effects that may be evoked by the shedding of airway epithelial cells. Experimental *in vivo* data (Erjefält *et al.*, 1994, 1995a,b) suggest that plasma exudation, secretory effects, traffic, activation and necrosis of eosinophils, neutrophil recruitment and activation can be caused simply by the shedding of epithelial cells. Hence, these well-known characteristics of asthmatic airways may now be regarded as potential sequelae to desquamation.

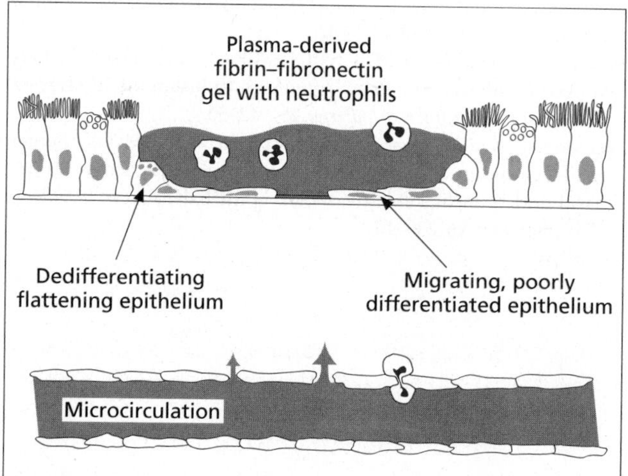

Fig. 25.2 Epithelial restitution in the airways. After denudation epithelial restitution occurs speedily under the provisional cover of a plasma-derived and leucocyte-rich gel. (From an original drawing by Jonas Erjefält.)

Complete denudation with loss of both columnar and basal cells may not be the most common kind of shedding. Columnar cells may be rather more easily shed (Evans & Plopper, 1989; Montefort *et al.*, 1992) and thus leave a cobblestone surface of basal cells behind. What happens to the basel cells when they loose their columnar neighbours? This question is currently being addressed in experiments involving both animal and human airways (Erjefält, 1995c). It appears that the basal cells promptly undergo flattening and that, within minutes, they establish extensive contact with each other. Airway basal cells may thus be well suited to keep up the barrier function and cover the basement membrane fully at shedding of ciliated and secretory cells. Indeed, this newly proposed role of the basal cell (Erjefält, 1995c) may be a major function of these cells, in addition to its role in anchoring of columnar epithelium (Evans *et al.*, 1989). The new flat epithelium that is established after shedding or denudation frequently consists of cells that have a larger apical surface than the normal columnar epithelium. As a consequence, a reduced junctional length of the epithelium per unit mucosal surface area would be available for solute absorption. Speculatively, this change might explain in part the observations of reduced absorption in desquamative airway disease. (The limited barrier defect of epithelial cell removal may also have to change our view on the role of epithelial shedding in respiratory defence (Persson *et al.*, 1995a)!)

The new findings on basal cell responses and on re-epithelialization in a plasma-derived gel *in vivo* after denudation may in part explain why increased absorption permeability has not been widely demonstrated in allergic and other inflammatory airway diseases where epithelial cells are frequently being shed. Perhaps also the clues to explain an increased absorption tightness, some of the pathophysiological effects, and some of the cellular pathology in asthma and rhinitis can be found among mucosal exudation and epithelial restitution mechanisms as they evolve under proper *in vivo* conditions.

Acknowledgements

This work was supported by the Swedish Medical Research Council project 8308, the Medical Faculty, University of Lund; Astra Draco, Lund; and the Swedish Association Against Asthma and Allergy. Mai Broman is thanked for the secretarial work.

References

Erjefält, I. & Persson, C.G.A. (1992) Increased sensitivity to toluene diisocyanate (TDI) in airways previously exposed to low doses of TDI. *Clin. Exp. Allergy*, **22**, 854–62.

Erjefält, I., Luts, A. & Persson, C.G.A. (1993a) Appearance of airway absorption and exudation tracers in guinea-pig tracheobronchial lymph nodes. *J. Appl. Physiol.*, **74**, 817–24.

Erjefält, I., Greiff, L., Alkner, U. & Persson, C.G.A. (1993b) Allergen-induced biphasic plasma exudation responses in guinea pig large airways. *Am. Rev. Resp. Dis.*, **148**, 695–701.

Erjefält, J.S., Erjefält, I., Sundler, F. & Persson, C.G.A. (1994) Microcirculation-derived factors in airway epithelial repair *in vivo*. *Microvasc. Res.*, **48**, 161–78.

Erjefält, J.S., Erjefält, I., Sundler, F. & Persson, C.G.A. (1995a) Epithelial pathways for luminal entry of bulk plasma. *Clin. Exp. Allergy*, **25**, 187–95.

Erjefält, J.S., Erjefält, I., Sundler, F. & Persson, C.G.A. (1995b) *In vivo* restitution of airway epithelium. *Cell Tissue Res.*, **281**, 305–16.

Erjefält, J.S., Greiff, L., Sundler, F. & Persson, C.G.A. (1995c) Basal cells promptly flatten out at detachment of columnar epithelium in human and guinea-pig airways. *Eur. Resp. J.*, **8**, 207s.

Erjefält, J.S., Sundler, F. & Persson, C.G.A. (1996) Eosinophils, neutrophils and venular gaps in the airway mucosa at epithelial removal–restitution. *Am. J. Resp. Crit. Care Med.*, **153**, 1666–74.

Evans, M.J. & Plopper, C.G. (1989) The role of basal cells in adhesion of columnar epithelium to airway basement membrane. *Am. Rev. Resp. Dis.*, **138**, 481–83.

Fabbri, L.M. & Mapp, C. (1991) Bronchial hyperresponsiveness, airway inflammation and occupational asthma induced by toluene diisocyanate. *Clin. Exp. Allergy*, **21**, 42–7.

Greiff, L., Alkner, U., Pipkorn, U. & Persson, C.G.A. (1990) The 'nasal pool' device applies controlled concentrations of solutes on human nasal airway mucosa and samples its surface exudations/secretions. *Clin. Exp. Allergy*, **20**, 253–9.

Greiff, L., Andersson, M., Åkerlund, A. *et al.* (1994) Microvascular exudative hyperresponsiveness in human coronavirus-induced common cold. *Thorax*, **49**, 121–7.

Greiff, L., Svensson, C., Andersson, M. & Persson, C.G.A. (1995a) Effects of topical capsaicin in seasonal allergic rhinitis. *Thorax*, **50**, 225–9.

Greiff, L., Lundin, S., Svensson, C. *et al.* (1995b) Peptide absorption in human allergic airways. *Eur. Resp. J.*, (abstract), (in press).

Greiff, L., Wollmer, P., Svensson, C., Andersson, M. & Persson, C.G.A. (1993) Effect of seasonal allergic rhinitis on airway mucosal absorption of chromium-51-labelled EDTA. *Thorax*, **48**, 648–50.

Halpin, D.M.G., Currie, D., Jones, B., Leigh, T.R. & Evans, T.W. (1993) Permeability of bronchial mucosa to ^{113m}In-DTPA in asthma and the effects of salmeterol. *Eur. Resp. J.*, **6**(17), 512s.

Montefort, S., Roberts, J.A., Beasley, R., Holgate, S.T. & Roche, W.R. (1992) The site of disruption of the bronchial epithelium in asthmatic and non-asthmatic subjects. *Thorax*, **47**, 499–503.

Persson, C.G.A. (1986) The role of plasma exudation in asthmatic airways. *Lancet*, **11**, 1126–9.

Persson, C.G.A. (1988) Plasma exudation and asthma. *Lung*, **166**, 1–23.

Persson, C.G.A. (1994) Airway epithelium and microcirculation. *Eur. Resp. Rev.*, **4**, **23**, 352–62.

Persson, C.G.A., Erjefält, I., Alkner, U. *et al.* (1991) Plasma exudation as a first line respiratory mucosal defence. *Clin. Exp. Allergy*, **21**, 17–24.

Persson, C.G.A., Svensson, C., Greiff, L. *et al.* (1992) The use of the nose to study the inflammatory response of the respiratory tract. Editorial. *Thorax*, **47**, 993–1000.

Persson, C.G.A., Andersson, M., Greiff, L. *et al.* (1995a) Airway permeability. *Clin. Exp. Allergy*, **23**, 807–14.

Persson, C.G.A., Alkner, U., Andersson, M., Greiff, L., Linden, M. & Svensson, C. (1995b) Histamine-challenge-induced 'lamina propria lavage' and mucosal out-put of IL-6 in human airways. *Eur. Resp. J.* [abstract], **8**, 1255.

Salomonsson, P., Grönneberg, R., Gilljam, H. *et al.* (1992) Bronchial exudation of bulk plasma at allergen challenge in allergic asthma. *Am. Rev. Resp. Dis.*, **146**, 1535–42.

Svensson, C., Andersson, M., Greiff, L., Alkner, U. & Persson, C.G.A. (1995a) Exudative hyperresponsiveness to histamine in seasonal allergic rhinitis. *Clin. Exp. Allergy*, **25**, 942–50.

Svensson, C., Grönneberg, R., Andersson, M. *et al.* (1995b) Allergen challenge-induced exudation of α_2-macroglobulin across human nasal and bronchial microvascular–epithelial barriers. *J. Allergy Clin. Immunol.*, **96**, 239–46.

CHAPTER 26
Neuropeptides

M.G. Belvisi & A.J. Fox

Introduction

In addition to the classical autonomic nervous system that encompasses the sympathetic and parasympathetic innervation, another neural pathway exists in a subpopulation of primary sensory neurones that can be stimulated electrically or by capsaicin to release neuropeptides. These peptides include the tachykinins substance P (SP) and neurokinin A (NKA), NKB as well as calcitonin gene-related peptide (CGRP). The local release of these neuropeptides from sensory nerves results in a series of responses, termed 'neurogenic inflammation', in various effector tissues. These responses can occur in various organs, including the airways, eye, heart, skin and the gastrointestinal and genitourinary tracts (Barnes *et al.*, 1990). Furthermore, it is now recognized that there are a multitude of peptides released from parasympathetic and sympathetic, in addition to sensory, neurones and that in many cases the neuropeptides are localized with classical neurotransmitters. This chapter discusses the location, release, activation of cell-surface receptors, the signal transduction mechanisms and the effector responses of neuropeptides with special reference to the respiratory tract.

Tachykinins

The tachykinins are a family of peptides characterized by the common C-terminal sequence Phe-X-Gly-Leu-Met-NH_2. To date three principal tachykinins have been described in mammals — SP, NKA and NKB — which are encoded by two different genes, preprotachykinin I (PPT-I) and preprotachykinin II (PPT-II). PPT-II is transcribed to give one mRNA encoding NKB. In contrast, the primary transcript of PPT-I is alternatively spliced to produce three mRNA encoding different precursor proteins — α-PPT which is cleaved to produce SP alone, β-PPT which gives rise to both SP and NKA, and γ-PPT which is processed to give SP and NKA. In addition, two N-terminal extended forms of NKA have recently been isolated, termed neuropeptide K (NPK) and neuropeptide-γ (NP-γ), which are derived from β-PPT and γ-PPT respectively. Whilst both NPK and NP-γ have biological activity, whether they are precursors of NKA or have transmitter function in their own right remains to be established. The significance of the alternate splicing of the PPT-I gene is also uncertain, although the relative expression of the different mRNA shows marked species dependency (Maggi *et al.*, 1993).

Localization

Tachykinins are found almost exclusively in neurones, both in the central nervous system and in the periphery. Whilst the PPT-II gene and hence NKB is expressed solely in the brain and spinal cord, PPT-I is found both centrally and peripherally, and so SP and NKA have a more widespread distribution. In the periphery SP and NKA are localized almost exclusively to intrinsic nerves of the gut and to sensory nerves. For both visceral and somatic sensory nerves they are found in a subpopulation of small-diameter afferent fibres, conducting in the C- and possibly Aδ-fibre range, which are sensitive to the excitatory and toxic effects of capsaicin (Holzer, 1991). Immunohistochemical studies have shown SP and NKA, and in some cases also NPK or NP-γ, to be present in a number of peripheral tissues including skin, joints, urogenital tract, heart, eye and respiratory tract. In all cases the sensitivity of this staining to pretreatment with capsaicin confirms the sensory origin of the peptides (Holzer, 1988). The cell bodies of these neurones are located in the dorsal root and cranial ganglia which express the PPT-I gene but not the PPT-II gene, as would be expected given the patterns of peptide expression.

SP, NKA and also NPK have been shown to be present in airways from a number of species, including guinea pig, rat and humans (Lundberg *et al.*, 1984a; Martling *et al.*, 1987). However, it has been demonstrated that levels in human airways are influenced by factors such as age, cigarette smoking and pathology. Sensory fibres containing SP and NKA are distributed within the epithelium and smooth muscle, around submucosal glands and blood vessels, and within airway ganglia (Lundberg *et al.*, 1984a; Kummer *et al.*, 1992). Ligation and retrograde tracer experiments have shown that the majority of these fibres are of vagal origin, with their cell bodies in the nodose and jugular ganglia. There is, however, a small proportion of fibres innervating the lungs which originate from spinal dorsal root ganglia, in keeping with the persistence of lower airway reflexes seen after vagotomy in some animal experiments (Widdicombe, 1954).

Demonstration of a Ca^{2+}-dependent release is a prerequisite for considering a substance as a neurotransmitter. For both SP and NKA, a number of studies have shown such a release from the peripheral terminals of sensory nerves. Thus, the release of both peptides has been demonstrated in tissues such as lung, heart, skin, bladder and ureter in response to either antidromic nerve stimulation or capsaicin (Helme *et al.*, 1986; Hua *et al.*, 1986; Franco-Cereceda, 1988; Saira *et al.*, 1988). Moreover, release has also been demonstrated following a noxious heat stimulus in the skin, and, in the lung, following application of substances such as bradykinin and histamine, which have been shown to stimulate sensory nerves (Saria *et al.*, 1988). Little evidence exists for a physiological release of NPK and NP-γ, the N-terminal extended forms of NKA. Thus, although depolarization-evoked release of NPK has been demonstrated in rat substantia nigra, Hua *et al.* (1986) failed to detect any release from guinea pig spinal cord or ureter despite the presence of significant tissue levels of the peptide.

Metabolism

Tachykinins may be degraded by at least two enzymes: angiotensin-converting enzyme (ACE), also known as kininase I or EC 3.4.15.1, and neutral endopeptidase (NEP, enkephalinase or EC 3.4.24.11), although the latter appears to be most important. The activity of these peptidases and their effect on endogenous tachykinin activity has been most studied in the airways. Similar effects, however, would undoubtedly be seen in other tissues (e.g. skin, eye, bladder) receiving tachykininergic innervation. In the airways large amounts of NEP are found in the epithelium whilst ACE is located predominantly in the vascular endothelium (Johnson *et al.*, 1985). In keeping with this, ACE inhibitors such as captopril enhance bronchoconstriction evoked by intravenous but not inhaled SP (Lotvall *et al.*, 1990). Numerous studies have shown that inhibitors of NEP such as thiorphan or phosphoramidon increase bronchoconstrictor responses to tachykinins in guinea pigs both *in vitro* and *in vivo* (Lotvall *et al.*, 1990; Maggi *et al.*, 1990). A similar enhancement is seen *in vitro* after removal of the epithelium (Devillier *et al.*, 1988). These inhibitors also enhance both excitatory-non-adrenergic non-cholinergic (e-NANC) bronchoconstriction and the bronchoconstrictor response to capsaicin in guinea pig airways (Dusser *et al.*, 1988; Maggi *et al.*, 1990). Taken together these data indicate that epithelial NEP regulates the activity of endogenous tachykinins in the airways. This could have implications for airway diseases like asthma, in which the epithelium is often denuded in patients even with relatively mild disease. This would therefore remove the major site of tachykinin metabolism, thereby potentiating the effects of endogenously released peptides (Barnes, 1986).

Receptors

Tachykinin effects are mediated in the majority of cases through their common C-terminal sequence via an interaction with three different receptor types, NK_1, NK_2 and NK_3, which show preferential affinity for the natural ligands, SP, NKA and NKB, respectively. This classification has been confirmed by the development of highly selective synthetic agonists and antagonists (Table 26.1), and ultimately with the isolation and cloning of all three receptor proteins (Maggi *et al.*, 1993). Each belongs to the G-protein-coupled family of receptors, and activation leads to phosphoinositide hydrolysis and increased levels of intracellular Ca^{2+}. With the widespread use of the newly available selective ligands, notably the non-peptide antagonists CP-96,345, RP67580, SR 48968 and SR 140333, it has become apparent that the classification of these receptors may be more complicated. Thus, species variants of the NK_1 receptor appear to exist, with CP96,345 showing higher affinity at the human and guinea pig receptor compared to the rat, the reverse holding for RP67,580. Molecular studies have shown that these differences in affinity are accounted for by variations of a single amino acid in the structure of the receptor between species (Fong *et al.*, 1992). Intraspecies heterogeneity may also exist with the proposal of a 'septide-sensitive' receptor being present in a number of tissues, including guinea pig

Table 26.1 Pharmacology of tachykinin receptors.

	NK_1	NK_2	NK_3
Agonist order of potency	SP > NKA = NKB	NKA > NKB >> SP	NKB > NKA >> SP
Selective agonists	SP methyl ester [Sar^9]SP-sulphone Septide GR73632	[β-Ala^8]NKA(4-10) [Nle^{10}]NKA(4-10) GR64349	Senktide [$MePhe^7$]NKB
Selective antagonists	CP96,345 CP99,994 RP67580 GR82334 FK888 SR140,333 CGP47899	SR48,968 MEN10,376 MEN10,207 R396 L659,877	CAM-4547 SR 142801

ileum and bronchi (Maggi *et al.*, 1993). Similarly, heterogeneity has been proposed within the NK_2 sub-type with NK_{2A} receptors being present in tissues, including the trachea, from human, guinea pig and rabbit and NK_{2B} in those from rat and hamster (Maggi *et al.*, 1993). It remains to be established whether these pharamcological differences are also reflected at the molecular level.

With a few exceptions (e.g. myenteric neurones) NK_3 receptor expression is confined to the brain and spinal cord, whilst NK_1 and NK_2 receptors have a wide distribution centrally and peripherally. Autoradiographic and binding studies have demonstrated the existence of neurokinin receptors in a variety of peripheral tissues, consistent with the distribution of tachykinins in sensory nerves. In particular, NK_1 binding sites have been localized in a number of species to the vascular endothelium of major arteries, blood vessels in the skin, joints and cranium, and smooth muscle of the iris. In the gut, NK_1 and NK_2 receptors have been localized to the longitudinal and circular smooth-muscle layers as well as to the duodenal mucosa (for a review see Hall, 1994), whilst in the urogenital tract both receptor types are present on the smooth muscle from the bladder and ureter, and also in the submucosal layer (Sann *et al.*, 1992).

In the respiratory tract autoradiographic studies using [^{125}I]Bolton-Hunter-SP and, more recently, [^{3}H]FK888 have shown NK_1 receptors to be widespread throughout guinea pig and human lungs, with a high density in smooth muscle from trachea to small bronchioles, submucosal glands and vascular endothelium (Carstairs & Barnes, 1986; Miyayasu *et al.*, 1993). Other studies have confirmed the presence of NK_1 receptors on human vascular endothelium but there is some debate concerning the presence of any binding site on human bronchial smooth muscle (Goldie, 1990; Walsh *et al.*, 1994). A different approach using an anti-substance P anti-idiotypic antibody directed against the ligand binding site of the receptor has, however, shown extensive labelling in human airway smooth muscle, submucosal glands and epithelium that could represent binding to NK_1 or NK_2 receptors (Fischer *et al.*, 1992). In spite of considerable evidence for the existence of functional NK_2 receptors on airway smooth muscle, binding studies have until recently failed to confirm this, primarily due to the lack of a selective radioligand. However, using a novel ligand, ^{125}I-[Lys^5,Tyr(I_2)^7,$MeLeu^9$,Nle^{10}]-NKA(4–10), NK_2 binding sites have now been demonstrated on guinea pig bronchial smooth muscle (Burcher *et al.*, 1994), although there are no reports as yet of their presence in human airways.

Functional effects of tachykinins

Non-adrenergic non-cholinergic mechanisms and capsaicin-sensitive sensory nerves

In a number of peripheral tissues nerve stimulation results in effects that are not blocked by cholinergic or adrenergic blocking drugs. There is now considerable evidence that these non-adrenergic non-cholinergic (NANC) mechanisms result from the release of other transmitters from autonomic nerves, and in many cases are due to the release of neuropeptides from capsaicin-sensitive sensory nerves. The use of capsaicin has been invaluable in delineating these mechanisms, due to its varying effects on this subpopulation of sensory neurones. Thus, at low concentrations it causes excitation with the release of sensory neuropepetides both centrally and peripherally, and at higher concentrations it causes a functional desensitization. Both of these actions appear to result from the receptor-mediated activation of a cation channel (Bevan & Szolcsanyi, 1990). When given systemically it can cause a depletion of the peptide content and neuronal degeneration, depending on age and species (Holzer, 1991). Capsaicin is widely held to act principally on unmyelinated C fibres, althouth in the skin it also excites polymodal nociceptors conducting in the Aδ range (Szolcsyani *et al.*, 1988). In the airways, single-fibre recording experiments have shown that in the guinea pig it selectively excites C fibres with no effect on Aδ-fibres (Fox *et al.*, 1993).

Excitatory NANC mechanisms have been described most fully in the airways. Electrical stimulation of guinea pig bronchi *in vitro* or vagus nerve *in vivo* produces a bronchoconstrictor response with a component that is not blocked by atropine (Lundberg *et al.*, 1983). Similarly, vagal stimulation or capsaicin may evoke plasma extravasation, mucus secretion and bronchial vasodilatation in different species that are unaffected by atropine (Lundberg *et al.*, 1983; Widdicombe, 1991; Ramnarine & Rogers, 1994). These effects are, however, abolished by pretreatment with capsaicin (Lundberg *et al.*, 1983; Kuo *et al.*, 1990) and inhibited by neurokinin receptor antagonists (e.g. Bertrand *et al.*, 1993a; Lou *et al.*, 1993; Ramnarine *et al.*, 1994), indicating that they result from the release of tachykinins from sensory nerves. Moreover, as described below, they may be mimicked by exogenous administration of SP or NKA. The release of tachykinins may occur as a result of direct stimulation of the sensory nerve endings or as a result of a local 'axon reflex'. Similar NANC mechanisms have been described in other tissues, such as the eye, urogenital tract and, most notably, the skin (Fig. 26.1), and their discovery has led to the acceptance of a dual function of sensory nerves combining the classical afferent role and an efferent role resulting from the antidromic release of neuropeptides (for review see Holzer, 1988; Barnes *et al.*, 1990; Maggi, 1991a). Collectively these effects are referred to as 'neurogenic inflammation' and the role of this phenomenon in pathological processes will be discussed more fully later.

Tachykinins as neuromodulators

The first report that suggested tachykinins may have a neuromodulatory role in the peripheral nervous system was in the guinea pig myenteric plexus, where SP was found to evoke the release of acetylcholine (ACh) (Yau & Youther, 1982). A similar phenomenon exists in the respiratory tract. Exogenous tachykinins have been demonstrated to facilitate cholinergic neurotransmission in rabbit and guinea pig airways via a pre-junctional, post-ganglionic mechanism (Tanaka & Grondstan, 1986; Armour *et al.*, 1991; Belvisi, 1994; Belvisi *et al.*, 1994). In a recent study, experiments using selective tachykinin agonists and antagonists suggested the presence of both NK_1 and NK_2 (NK_{2A} subtype) receptors on cholinergic nerve terminals in rabbit bronchi (Belvisi *et al.*, 1994). Exogenous tachykinins also potentiate cholinergic neurotransmission at pre- and post-ganglionic nerve terminals in guinea pig trachea and bronchi via activation of an NK_1 receptor (Hall *et al.*, 1989; Watson *et al.*, 1993; Belvisi *et al.*, 1994).

Facilitatory effects of tachykinins on cholinergic neurotransmission may have physiological relevance, as there has been some suggestion that endogenous tachykinins facilitate cholinergic contractile responses in airway smooth muscle. NEP is a major enzyme involved in the breakdown of tachykinins (Erdös & Skidgel, 1989). Inhibition of this enzyme by phosphoramidon would be expected to augment the actions of endogenously released tachykinins. In guinea pig trachea, phosphoramidon facilitates contractile responses evoked by preganglionic vagal nerve stimulation (PGS) and not transmural stimulation of the trachea, an effect which is blocked by capsaicin pretreatment or an NK_1 antagonist (Watson *et al.*, 1993). These results suggest that there is release of endogenous tachykinins during pre- but not postganglionic nerve stimulation in guinea pig trachea, suggesting that there are facilitatory tachykinin receptors at the level of the parasympathetic ganglia (Watson *et al.*, 1993).

In contrast, in human bronchial rings *in vitro* none of the selective tachykinin receptor agonists had any effect on cholinergic neurotransmission (Belvisi *et al.*, 1994). However, it has previously been shown that NKA produces potentiation of the contractile response to electrical field stimulation (EFS) in human bronchi, but only in the presence of K^+ channel blockade (Black *et al.*, 1990). This points to a neuromodulatory role for NKA in human airways, only in situations where the K^+ channel activity is decreased.

However, tachykinin receptor activation in the airways leads to phosphoinositide hydrolysis and the formation of inositol (1,4,5) triphophate and diglyceride, with the subsequent release of Ca^{2+} from intracellular stores which activates protein kinase C (PKC) (Grandordy *et al.*, 1988). The cell-signalling mechanisms involved in tachykinin-induced neuromodulation are unknown. Such a sequence of events occurring on cholinergic neurones could ultimately lead to the phosphorylation of, as yet unidentified, proteins present in the nerve terminal which could enhance cholinergic neurotransmission.

Therefore, it seems that tachykinins may play an important role in modulating cholinergic neurotransmission in animal airways with no demonstrable effect on human airways. Whilst this seems to rule out a role for endogenous tachykinins in the modulation of neurotransmission in normal human airways, it does not exclude a role for tachykinins as neuromodulators under pathophysiological conditions.

Effects on smooth muscle

The ability to evoke a rapid contraction of gastrointestinal smooth muscle originally gave tachykinins their name, and it has since become apparent that they are potent spasmogens in a variety of different tissues. This effect may be of considerable importance in the respiratory tract, and SP and NKA have been shown to contract airway smooth muscle from a number of species including humans. In isolated human bronchi tachykinin-evoked contraction is mediated via an NK_2 receptor. Thus, NKA is consistently more potent than SP or NKB (Advenier *et al.*, 1987; Frossard & Barnes, 1991), and the NK_2-selective agonist [Nle^{10}]-NKA(4–10) is a potent spasmogen whilst the NK_1-selective [Pro^9]-SP sulphone and NK_3-selective [$MePhe^7$]-NKB are essentially inactive (Naline *et al.*, 1989; Dion *et al.*, 1990). Moreover, the high affinity of the non-peptide NK_2 antagonist SR 48,968 suggests that the receptor present belongs to the NK_{2A} subtype (Advenier *et al.*, 1992; Ellis *et al.*, 1993). The effect of tachykinins after inhalation in humans is less clear cut. Initial studies showed that SP and NKA had no effect on airway calibre in normal subjects, whilst bronchoconstriction was seen with inhalation of NKA but not SP in asthmatics (Joos *et al.*, 1987). Others, however, have shown a bronchoconstrictor effect of SP in more severe asthmatics, and also of NKA in normal and asthmatic subjects (for review see Joos *et al.*, 1994). In the guinea pig, bronchoconstriction evoked by exogenous tachykinins *in vitro* and *in vivo* involves both NK_1 and NK_{2A} receptors (Ireland *et al.*, 1991; Maggi *et al.*, 1991; Bertrand et al, 1993a). However, capsaicin or vagal stimulation-evoked bronchoconstriction is inhibited principally by NK_2 antagonists such as MEN 10,376 and SR 48,968, and to a lesser extent by the NK_1 antagonists CP-96,345 or CP-99,94, but abolished by a combination of the two (Maggi *et al.*, 1991; Bertrand *et al.*, 1993a; Foulon *et al.*, 1993; Lou *et al.*, 1993), implying a predominant involvement of NK_2 receptors in NANC bronchoconstriction. In contrast to the bronchoconstrictor activity in the guinea pig and human, tachykinins and capsaicin cause a relaxation of rat and mouse trachea, an effect which is mediated via NK_1-receptor-mediated prostaglandin release from the epithelium (Devillier *et al.*, 1992; Manzini, 1992).

NANC contractions of smooth muscle resulting from tachykinin release from sensory nerves have been described in a number of other tissues. For example, capsaicin-evoked contractions of the rabbit iris are inhibited by NK_1-receptor antagonists, and exogenous tachykinins cause contractions via NK_1 and NK_3 receptors (Hall, 1994). In the rat bladder capsaicin evokes a biphasic contraction, the first phase of which is blocked by NK_1 antagonists and the later phase by NK_2 antagonists, supporting a role for endogenous tachykinins in the micturition reflex (Maggi, 1991b).

Vascular effects of tachykinins

Substance P is one of the most hypotensive agents known and this effect is considered to be due largely to its vasodilator action on large blood vessels mediated by the release of nitric oxide (NO) from the endothelium. However, tachykinins also have potent effects on the microvasculature, namely vasodilatation and increases in vascular permeability, which underlie the phenomenon of neurogenic inflammation.

Skin

Intradermal injection of capsaicin or antidromic stimulation of peripheral sensory nerves produces a characteristic 'triple response' consisting of a local reddening, a weal and a flare spreading far from the initial stimulus. These responses result from arteriolar vasodilatation and increased vascular permeability of post-capillary venules leading to leakage of plasma proteins. It is now established that this neurogenic inflammation involves sensory nerves. Thus, there is a huge literature to show that it is abolished by systemic or local pretreatment with capsaicin or by sensory denervation (see Holzer, 1988). Furthermore, the vasodilatation and plasma extravasation are mimicked by intradermal injection of SP and blocked by tachykinin receptor antagonists (Lembeck *et al.*, 1982; Foreman *et al.*, 1983; Yonehara *et al.*, 1992), indicating that they result from SP release. Information obtained from the use of selective agonists and antagonists indicates that the microvascular leak at least is mediated by NK_1 receptors (Lembeck *et al.*, 1992). These receptors are located on the endothelial cells of both arterioles and venules, and vasodilatation mediated by SP is secondary to the release of NO. The flare, but not the reddening or weal, evoked by capsaicin is inhibited by local anaesthetics indicating the involvement of nerve conduction (Jancso *et al.*, 1968). A similar inhibitory effect of tetrodotoxin on sensory nerve-mediated effects is seen in other tissues and these actions are therefore considered to be due to an 'axon reflex'. Here, stimulation of the sensory fibre ending leads to orthodromic impulse generation centrally, and also antidromic impulses to axon collaterals innervating the blood vessel or other cell type, thereby enabling the spread of the flare to areas not directly affected by the original noxious stimulus (Fig. 26.1). It is possible that other mediators are also involved in these vascular effects. Thus, the flare but not the weal evoked by injection of SP into human skin is inhibited by capsaicin and local anaesthetics (Foreman *et al.*, 1983). SP does not itself excite

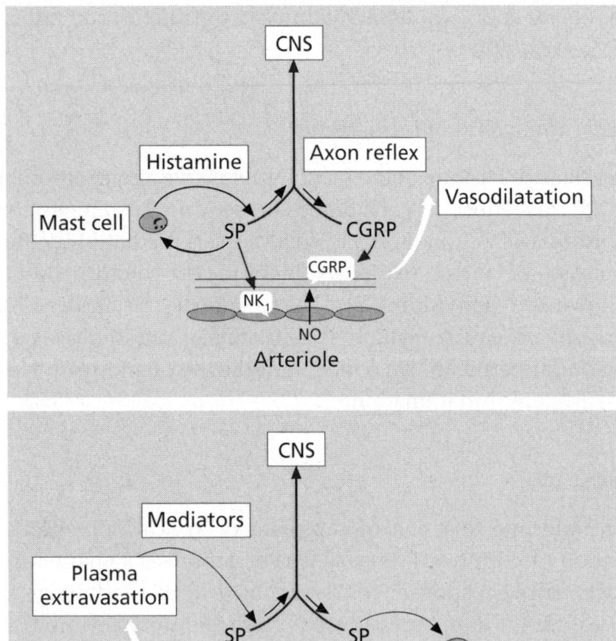

Fig. 26.1 The role of neurogenic inflammation in the skin. The activation of sensory nerves innervating the skin leads to a characteristic response consisting of reddening, weal and flare. The reddening results from the release of substance P (SP) and calcitonin gene-related peptide (CGRP) from the peripheral terminals of sensory nerves which cause arteriolar vasodilatation. The effect of CGRP is mediated via specific receptors located on the smooth muscle, while that of SP involves the release of nitric oxide from the endothelium. In addition, SP may cause the release of histamine from mast cells which, together with other mediators encountered during inflammation, may in turn activate sensory nerve endings leading to the generation of an axon reflex causing peptide release from co-lateral branches. This accounts for the spread of vasodilatation far from the initial stimulus—the flare. A similar mechanism operates on post-capillary venules where SP acts on endothelial cells to increase vascular permeability, leading to oedema and weal. The release of mediators from extravasated cells may again exacerbate this response via an axon reflex.

sensory nerve endings but may cause the release of histamine from mast cells which in turn stimulates cutaneous C fibres, thereby activating axon reflexes and the spread of the flare (Fig. 26.1). Moreover, increases in blood flow and plasma extravasation evoked by antidromic nerve stimulation or mustard oil application to the skin have been shown to be reduced by antihistamines. However, it should be borne in mind that other studies have found a lack of effect of antihistamines on these vascular effects, and whilst the potency of SP in releasing histamine correlates with that in inducing plasma extravasation, it does not with its activity in evoking vasodilatation (Foreman *et al.*, 1983; Holzer, 1988). In addition, considerable evidence now exists for a primary role of CGRP, coreleased from sensory nerves with SP, in the control of blood flow in the skin, and this will be discussed in detail later.

Airways

It is likely that the vascular effects of tachykinins in the airways may be more important than their effects on smooth muscle. As mentioned earlier, vagal stimulation and capsaicin application both cause increased microvascular leak in guinea pigs and rats. This effect is inhibited by NK_1-receptor antagonists such as CP-96,345 and FK888 (Lei *et al.*, 1992; Hirayama *et al.*, 1993). Among the naturally occurring and synthetic tachykinins, SP and [Sar^9,Met(O_2)^{11}]SP are more potent than NKB, NKA or the NK_2 selective [β-Ala^8]NKA(4–10), confirming the involvement of NK_1 receptors in this response (Rogers *et al.*, 1988; Hirayama *et al.*, 1993). Plasma extravasation seen after vagal stimulation increases from the trachea to the major bronchus and this matches the pattern of response seen after injection of SP, indicating a differential distribution of NK_1 receptors on post-capillary venules (Evans *et al.*, 1989; Belvisi *et al.*, 1990a). Whether tachykinins cause microvascular leak in human airways is not yet certain due to the difficulty in measuring such a response. However, SP applied directly onto the nasal mucosa does not appear to cause plasma protein extravasation, although others have reported an increase in nasal protein output in response to SP or NKA in patients with allergic rhinitis (Braunstein *et al.*, 1991). A similar finding has been reported with capsaicin, although this response appears to be as a result of a central cholinergic reflex (Stjarne *et al.*, 1989). Nevertheless, the fact that SP causes a weal when injected into human skin does indicate that it is able to act on human post-capillary venules. Since oedema is a major symptom of inflammatory airway disease, tachykinins could therefore be candidates for contributing to this aspect in conditions such as asthma.

Tachykinins also have potent effects on airway blood flow, and both SP and NKA increase tracheal blood flow in dogs and pigs (Salonen *et al.*, 1988; Matran *et al.*, 1989b). In pigs, vagal stimulation and capsaicin also evoke an increase in bronchial blood flow mediated by the release of CGRP as well as tachykinins (Matran *et al.*, 1989a). A similar role of tachykinins has recently been demonstrated in rats where capsaicin-evoked bronchial vasodilatation was abolished by the NK_1-receptor antagonist RP67580 (Piedmonte *et al.*, 1993). However, in dogs and sheep the increase in bronchial blood flow evoked by injection of capsaicin is largely abolished by vagotomy, indicating that it is mediated predominantly by a cholinergic reflex pathway (Pisarri *et al.*, 1993). These species differences make it difficult to predict whether tachykinins would have vasodilator effects in human lower airways. However, both SP and NKA, as well as capsaicin, have been shown to increase nasal blood flow (Stjarne *et al.*, 1989). Again this effect of tachykinins, if occurring in the human airways, could be important in airway inflammatory conditions, since it causes an increased thickness of the mucosa which could therefore contribute to the observed airway obstruction, as well as increasing the flow of blood-borne mediators and inflammatory cells to the region.

Other tissues

Vascular effects of tachykinins have also been reported in other tissues, most notably joints and dura mater. In the rat and cat, knee joint vasodilatation and plasma extravasation may be evoked by antidromic sensory nerve stimulation. This effect is mimicked by NK_1-receptor agonists and blocked by the antagonist CP-96,345 (see Lam & Ferrell, 1993). Moreover, NK_1 binding sites have been localized to vascular endothelial cells in human synovial tissue (Walsh *et al.*, 1992). Again these findings could indicate a role for tachykinins in inflammatory conditions such as arthritis. Similarly, there is currently much interest in the role of neurogenic inflammation in the pathogenesis of migraine (see Moskowitz, 1992). Stimulation of the trigeminal ganglion has been shown to evoke plasma extravasation within the dura mater of rats. This effect is blocked by the NK_1-receptor antagonist RP67580 (Shepheard *et al.*, 1993), suggesting a further potential use for these antagonists in the treatment of migraine.

In general, it can be seen that the vascular effects of tachykinins, both vasodilatation and increased permeability, are mediated through NK_1 receptors. Since these are key features of neurogenic inflammation, this has in turn led to speculation on the potential use of the new generation of NK_1-receptor antagonists in inflammatory conditions. This will be discussed later in more detail.

Secretory effects of tachykinins

In terms of inflammation, the most important glandular effects of tachykinins are seen in the airways. The secretion of mucus from submucosal glands and epithelial goblet cells is primarily a protective mechanism against inhaled irritants. However, in inflammatory conditions such as asthma or bronchitis there may be an exaggerated response with hypersecretion leading to characteristic mucous plug formation. The control of mucus secretion in the airways is primarily under parasympathetic cholinergic control. However, as mentioned earlier there is also a NANC component in the secretory response to vagal stimulation in a number of species (Ramnarine & Rogers, 1994). Vagal stimulation in guinea pigs leads to goblet cell secretion that is abolished by capsaicin pretreatment (Kuo *et al.*, 1990). Tachykinins are potent secretagogues in the guinea pig and ferret trachea, with an order of potency of SP>NKA>NKB indicating NK_1-receptor involvement (Webber, 1989; Kuo *et al.*, 1990). In the ferret trachea the NK_1-receptor-selective antagonist FK888, but not the NK_2-receptor selective SR 48,968, inhibited secretion evoked by vagal stimulation and capsaicin, confirming the release of tachykinins from sensory nerves and the role of NK_1 receptors (Ramnarine *et al.*, 1994).

Airway mucus secretion is difficult to measure in humans. However, both tachykinins and capsaicin have been shown to induce mucus secretion from isolated human airway preparations (Rogers & Barnes, 1989; Rogers *et al.*, 1989), and SP binding sites have been localized to submucosal glands in human bronchi (Carstairs & Barnes, 1986). A consistent secretory response to SP administered to the nose has not been demonstrated, and the role of endogenous tachykinins in nasal secretions is still uncertain.

Tachykinins and inflammatory cells

Tachykinins may interact with a variety of inflammatory and immune cells, although the pathophysiological significance is still unclear. As mentioned earlier, SP degranulates mast cells in human and rat skin causing the release of histamine, an effect that is mediated by the basic N-terminal region of the molecule (Foreman & Jordan, 1983). This effect contributes to the weal and flare seen after cutaneous injection of SP. In contrast, SP does not release histamine from human lung mast cells or basophils (Wardlaw *et al.*, 1986) and antihistamines do not affect tachykinin-induced bronchoconstriction in human airways. Nevertheless, morphological studies have shown a close association between mast cells and sensory nerves in the airways as well as the viscera (Skofitsch *et al.*, 1985; Bienenstock *et al.*, 1988), and there is some evidence for a functional interaction between airway sensory nerves and mast cells similar to that seen in the skin. Thus, the bronchoconstrictor response to tachykinins in rats is reduced by 5-hydroxytryptamine (5-HT) receptor antagonists and the compound 48/80 which depletes mast cells of their mediators (Joos & Pauwels, 1993). In addition, antigen application has been reported to evoke an increase in NANC bronchoconstriction in isolated guinea pig bronchi taken from sensitized guinea pigs, that is blocked by H_1 antagonists (Ellis & Undem, 1992), suggesting that histamine released from mast cells excites sensory nerve endings. Others, however, have reported that histamine applied directly onto receptive fields does not excite sensory fibre endings in guinea pig airways (Fox *et al.*, 1993). In addition to mast cells, tachykinins have also been shown to degranulate guinea pig macrophages and human monocytes in culture, leading to the release of thromboxane A_2 and cytokines such as interleukin-1 (IL-1), tumour necrosis factor-α (TNF-α) and IL-6 (Lotz *et al.*, 1988; Bruneschelli *et al.*, 1990). This effect on macrophages appears to be a receptor-mediated event involving NK_1 and NK_2 receptors (Bruneschelli *et al.*, 1990). As with mast cells, however, tachykinin-evoked degranulation of eosinophils is an N-terminal-mediated event requiring relatively high concentrations of peptide (Kroegel *et al.*, 1990). There is, however, some doubt concerning the physiological significance of this N-terminal-mediated degranulating activity, since high concentrations are generally required to elicit a response. Nevertheless, it has recently been found that SP in subnanomolar concentrations produces electrophysiological responses in rat peritoneal mast cells without causing degranulation, suggesting that SP may act as a 'primer' rather than primary degranulating agent on mast cells (Janiszewski *et al.*, 1992).

An important aspect of the effect of tachykinins on immune cells is their chemotactic ability. SP has been reported to be a chemoattractant for human monocytes (Lotz *et al.*, 1988) and rabbit and mouse neutrophils (Marasco *et al.*, 1981; Perretti *et al.*, 1993). In this latter study, SP-induced neutrophil infiltration into the mouse air-pouch was mimicked by [Sar^9]-SP and blocked by the antagonists RP67580 and CP-96,345, indicating an involvement of NK_1 receptors. Moreover, IL-1-induced infiltration was inhibited to some degree by capsaicin pretreatment and also by these NK_1-receptor antagonists, suggesting the involvement of SP from sensory nerves in IL-1-induced cellular migration. Similarly, antidromic stimulation of sensory nerves induces leucocyte accumulation in rat airways (McDonald, 1988). Whether this activity of exogenous or endogenous SP reflects a direct action on leucocytes is uncertain, since it has been recently shown that SP, via NK_1-receptor activation, can release neutrophil chemotactic factors from bovine airway epithelial cells in culture (Von Essen *et al.*, 1992). SP has no chemotactic effect on human eosinophils. However, it was found that when cells were pretreated with SP the chemotactic response to platelet-activating factor (PAF) or leukotriene B_4 (LTB_4) was increased in cells taken from allergic subjects but not in those from normals (Numao & Agrawal, 1992), again suggesting a priming role for SP.

Leucocyte infiltration is a characteristic feature of inflammatory conditions, and is especially evident in the airways where eosinophils and neutrophils in particular may be seen in large numbers in the submucosa of asthmatic subjects. A key step in the migration of cells from the circulation into the tissues is adhesion to the vascular endothelium. SP has been shown to enhance neutrophil adherence to the bronchial epithelium and to the vascular endothelium, again via NK_1-receptor activation (McDonald, 1988; DeRose *et al.*, 1994). A similar infiltration of neutrophils and eosinophils has been demonstrated in response to SP in human skin, and both here and in the airways there was shown to be a concomitant increase in the expression of cellular adhesion molecules (Smith *et al.*, 1993; DeRose *et al.*, 1994). It is clear, therefore, that SP may have potent effects on inflammatory cells which could result in their infiltration to a site of inflammation or injury and their subsequent activation.

CGRP

CGRP was isolated and sequenced comparatively recently in 1982. It is a 37-amino-acid peptide that exists in two forms, α and β, in a number of species including rat and human. α-CGRP is formed by alternate splicing of the precursor mRNA coded by the calcitonin gene, and the expression of calcitonin or CGRP is tissue specific. β-CGRP is the only biologically active product of a separate gene.

Localization

Both forms of the peptide have been localized to capsaicin-sensitive primary afferent neurones where they are colocalized with SP and NKA (Ju *et al.*, 1987). Like the tachykinins, CGRP therefore has a wide distribution in the periphery and has been described in neurones of the skin, heart, joints and viscera (Gibbins *et al.*, 1987). In most cases immunoreactivity is greatly reduced after neonatal capsaicin treatment, confirming the sensory origin of the CGRP-containing nerves. CGRP has been isolated from human airways and nasal tissue (Palmer *et al.*, 1987; Baranuik *et al.*, 1990b), and in the respiratory tract of animals CGRP immunoreactivity is found in nerve fibres in smooth muscle, submucosal glands, epithelium and around blood vessels, as well as in neuroendocrine cells (Cadieux *et al.*, 1986). As with the tachykinins, ligation experiments showed that these fibres were of vagal origin with cell bodies predominantly in jugular ganglia.

Ca^{2+}-dependent release of CGRP has been demonstrated from a number of tissues both centrally and peripherally, including spinal cord, heart, skeletal muscle, bladder and lung, following antidromic nerve stimulation or capsaicin treatment (e.g. Franco-Cereceda, 1988; Del Bianco *et al.*, 1991; Hua & Yaksh, 1993). In addition, a range of inflammatory mediators such as bradykinin, 5-HT, histamine, protons and prostaglandins have been shown to evoke CGRP release (Del Bianco *et al.*, 1991; Maggi, 1991a; Hua & Yaksh, 1993). Again, such release is prevented by capsaicin pretreatment, implying a sensory origin. In contrast to the tachykinins, little information is available concerning the degradation of CGRP. It has, however, been shown to be metabolized by tryptase and chymase released from activated mast cells (Walls *et al.*, 1992) and by neutral endopeptidase (Katayama *et al.*, 1991). The rate of degradation by the latter enzyme is relatively slow, suggesting that it is not the main route for inactivation of CGRP.

Receptors

Comparatively little is as yet known of the properties of receptors for CGRP or the possible existence of multiple sub-types. The naturally occurrring forms of CGRP exhibit very similar pharmacology and so have not proved useful for receptor characterization, and in addition there are few selective high-affinity agonists and antagonists available for classification purposes. Nevertheless, two receptor sub-types for CGRP have been proposed based primarily on the activity of the antagonist $CGRP_{8-37}$, the C-terminal fragment of human α-CGRP. Thus, $CGRP_1$ receptors, typified by those found in the guinea pig atria are sensitive to this antagonist, whereas $CGRP_2$ receptors, found in the rat vas deferens, are insensitive (Dennis *et al.*, 1989). Based on this classification scheme most of the vascular effects of CGRP are described as being mediated via $CGRP_1$ receptors. Although the CGRP receptor genes have yet to be cloned, it is generally accepted that CGRP mediates its effects through the activation of G-protein-coupled receptors and the subsequent stimulation of adenylyl cyclase and increase in intracellular cyclic adenosine monophosphate (cAMP) levels.

The distribution of receptors for CGRP correlates primarily with its major vasodilator activity. Thus, high-affinity binding sites have been demonstrated in vascular tissue from a number of species including humans (Poyner, 1992), where they are localized to the smooth muscle. Autoradiographic studies have identified CGRP receptors in human and guinea pig lung, where again they predominante in blood vessels with little binding in airway smooth muscle or epithelium (Mak & Barnes, 1988). In human nasal tissue CGRP receptors are similarly most dense on arterial vessels (Baranuik *et al.*, 1990b).

Functional effects of CGRP

Effects on smooth muscle

In general, CGRP has a relaxant effect on smooth muscle, as would be expected following a rise in intracellular cAMP. As described earlier, it is a potent vasodilator in the microvasculature, and a similar effect is seen in larger blood vessels such as the aorta and intracerebral and coronary arteries. In all cases the relaxant effect is mediated via $CGRP_1$ receptors although, at least in the aorta, these receptors appear to be located on the endothelium where they mediate NO release leading to subsequent vasorelaxation (Edwards *et al.*, 1991; Gray & Marshall, 1992). Elsewhere, CGRP relaxes smooth muscle in the urogenital tract and gastrointestinal tract, both of which contain CGRP-immunoreactive nerve fibres (Giuliani *et al.*, 1992; Bartho *et al.*, 1993). In the gut CGRP may also have a contractile effect mediated through the release of neurotransmitters from intrinsic nerves. Surprisingly, in the airways CGRP has been reported to constrict human bronchi *in vitro* (Palmer *et al.*, 1987), although it has no effect on the tone of guinea pig airway preparations. Since few receptors are found on human airway smooth muscle, it appears likely that the bronchoconstrictor effect is mediated indirectly.

Vascular effects

The best established effect of CGRP is its vasodilator activity, especially in microvascular beds. After intradermal injection into the skin of several species, including humans, it causes a long-lasting flare response (Brain *et al.*, 1985), which is blocked by $CGRP_{8-37}$ and therefore mediated via $CGRP_1$ receptors (Hughes & Brain, 1991). CGRP also has a vasodilator effect in other vascular beds, causing a decrease in perfusion pressure in isolated organs such as rat mesentery and kidney, again via $CGRP_1$ receptors (Claing *et al.*, 1992). There is now considerable evidence that CGRP may be the main mediator of the vasodilatation associated with neurogenic inflammation (Fig. 26.1). Thus, vasodilatation evoked by saphenous nerve stimulation or by cutaneous capsaicin injection is inhibited by $CGRP_{8-37}$ (Escott & Brain, 1993; Hughes & Brain, 1994). Interestingly, it appears that the release of CGRP from cutaneous sensory nerves, but not its vasodilator action, may be modified by endogenous nitric oxide (NO), since the vasodilator response to capsaicin but not CGRP has been shown to be reduced by inhibitors of NO formation (Hughes & Brain, 1994). This contrasts to its mechanism of action in larger blood vessels where it causes relaxation via an endothelium and NO-dependent mechanism. CGRP also increases blood flow in the airways and joints (Matran *et al.*, 1989a; Cambridge & Brain, 1992), sites at which neurogenic inflammation may have particular pathological significance, as described earlier. Moreover, the gastroprotective effect of capsaicin has been proposed to be due to the hyperaemia produced by released CGRP (Holzer, 1988).

By contrast, CGRP has no direct effect on vascular permeability, producing no increase in plasma extravasation in the airways, skin or joints (Brain & Williams, 1985; Rogers *et al.*, 1988; Cambridge & Brain, 1992). However, it has a considerable synergistic effect with other mediators of vascular permeability. Thus, by virtue of its vasodilator activity CGRP potentiates the oedema formation evoked by mediators such as SP in skin and joints, presumably by increasing the blood delivery to sites of plasma extravastion in post-capillary venules (Brain & Williams, 1985; Cambridge & Brain, 1992). A similar synergism is not apparent in the airways when the two peptides are administered together intravenously, although it is possible that it may occur after local release from sensory nerves.

CGRP and inflammatory cells

Little is known of the interaction of CGRP with inflammatory and immune cells. Specific receptors are found on macrophages and CGRP has been described to inhibit macrophage secretion and their interaction with T lymphocytes (Nong *et al.*, 1989). Receptors have also been localized on T lymphocytes and the proliferative response of these cells to mitogens is inhibited by CGRP (Umeda & Arisawa, 1989). In contrast, CGRP potentiates neutrophil accumulation by chemotactic mediators in rabbit skin (Buckley *et al.*, 1991) and stimulates the adhesion of neutrophils to vascular endothelial cells (Sung *et al.*, 1992).

Vasoactive intestinal polypeptide

Vasoactive intestinal peptide (VIP) is a highly basic, single-chain linear polypeptide, which contains 28 amino-acid residues in its sequence (Mutt & Said, 1974). VIP and pituitary adenylate cyclase activating peptide (PACAP) are members of a large family of structurally related peptides that includes secretin, glucagon, gastric inhibitory peptide and growth hormone releasing factor (GRF). However, VIP and PACAP have distinct distributions in the central and peripheral nervous systems, where they are thought to function as neurotransmitters and may regulate neuronal survival. In addition, these peptides are also thought to act as hormones, inasmuch as VIP is thought to control prolactin secretion from the pituitary gland and inhibits mitogen-activated T-cell proliferation. In this regard, PACAP has been suggested to control the synthesis and secretion of catecholamines from the adrenal medulla.

In addition, peptide histidine isoleucine (PHI)/peptide histidine methionine (PHM), other peptides in this family, may also share many of the same biological actions as VIP, although they are often less potent (Lundberg *et al.*, 1984b). VIP was originally isolated from porcine small intestine by Said and Mutt (1970a) and derived its name from its long-acting vasodilator action on systemic administration to animals (Said & Mutt, 1970b). VIP has been demonstrated to fulfil many of the classical criteria for a role as a neurotransmitter and has a widespread distribution in the central and peripheral nervous systems. This peptide has potent effects on airway and pulmonary vascular tone and on airway secretion, suggesting that it may have an important regulatory role in the lung (Said, 1994).

Localization

VIP was originally considered to be a gut hormone until its presence was demonstrated by immunocytochemistry in neurones of the central nervous system (CNS) and in peripheral autonomic nerves (Fahrenkrug, 1993). Subsequently, most VIP research has been directed towards establishing the peptide as a neurotransmitter. VIP was among one of the first neuropeptides to be localized in the respiratory tract and is one of the most abundant neuropeptides found in the lung (Ghatei *et al.*, 1982) and nasal mucosa (Baraniuk *et al.*, 1990c). In the trachea and bronchi, VIP-containing nerve fibres are found in a subepithelial layer and in the submucosa (Fig. 26.2). In the trachea of some species there are a few VIP-immunoreactive fibres from the subepithelial plexus that penetrate the epithelial layer and these fibres may be involved in sensory transmission (Nohr & Weihe, 1988). VIP immunoreactivity is also present in ganglion cells in the proximal trachea and around intrapulmonary bronchi but diminishes in density peripherally so that few VIP-immunoreactive nerve fibres are found in bronchioles (Lundberg *et al.*, 1984b; Uddman & Sundler, 1987) (Fig. 26.3). The VIP-containing neurones seem to correlate with the distribution of cholinergic nerves in the upper airways, and the co-existence of VIP and ACh in parasympathetic ganglia supplying the respiratory tract has been confirmed (Lundberg *et al.*, 1979). At least in some species, VIP may also be localized to sympathetic nerves (Luts & Sundler, 1989). Immunohistochemical studies have localized VIP immunoreactivity in nerve fibres around blood vessels, glandular acini and within smooth muscle bundles in the lung (Uddman *et al.*, 1978; Dey *et al.*, 1981). The persistence of VIP-containing nerve fibres in extrinsically denervated human lung supports this idea that the origin of VIP-containing nerve fibres is local parasympathetic ganglia (Springall *et al.*, 1990). In regard to other cell types, VIP-like immunoreactivity is also present in rat lung mast cells and is released from rat peritoneal cells by mast cell degranulators (Cutz *et al.*, 1978). In addition, several VIP-like peptides have been chemically characterized in rat basophilic leukaemia cells which are thought to resemble mast cells (Goetzl *et al.*, 1988). Finally, VIP has also been demonstrated in eosinophils.

As mentioned earlier, VIP has also been demonstrated in the gastrointestinal tract. Intrinsic VIP nerves have been demonstrated in the circular muscle layer of the

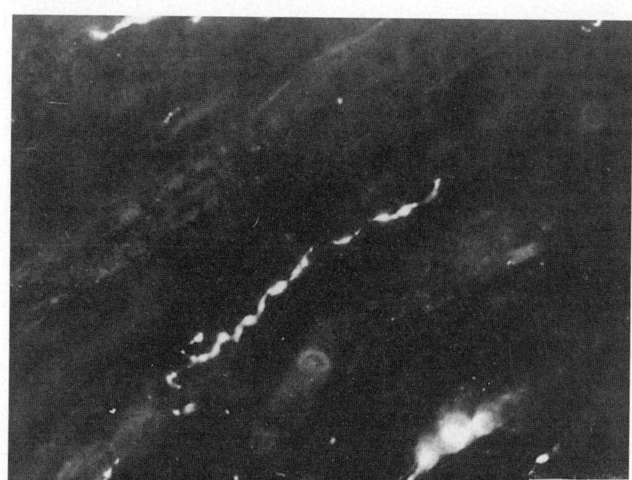
(a)

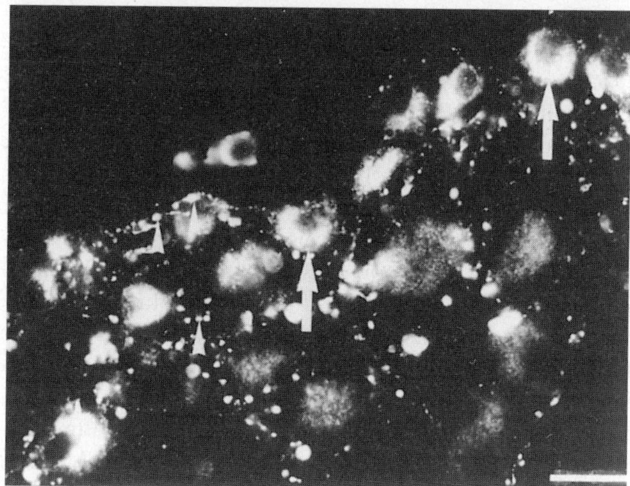
(b)

Fig. 26.2 Immunohistochemistry for vasoactive intestinal peptide (VIP) in human airways. (a) VIP-immunoreactive nerve fibres in the tracheal smooth muscle. (b) An intrinsic ganglion of a large bronchus with neurones (arrows) and nerve fibres (arrowheads) immunoreactive for VIP. (Scale bar: (a) = 20 μm; (b) = 10 μm.)

oesophageal wall and innervating the smooth-muscle layer of the stomach. Furthermore, the distribution of the VIP-containing cell bodies and nerve fibres is compatible with VIP being the transmitter of the descending inhibitory nerves. All layers of all regions of the gut contain VIP nerve fibres. The fibres are most dense in the lamina propria, where they seem to be specifically associated with blood vessels and/or lacteals and come in close contact with the surface epithelium. As in the gastrointestinal tract, VIP nerve fibres of the genital tract are intimately associated with blood vessels, non-vascular smooth muscle, and lining epithelium and glands. In the female genital tract most VIP nerve fibres are intrinsic, originating from VIP-containing ganglionic cells located in paracervical ganglia at the uterovaginal junction. In the male, neural cell bodies containing VIP occur within the proximal corpus cavernosum and in the interstitial tissue of the prostate (for a review see Fahrenkrug, 1993).

Metabolism

The actions of neuropeptides are limited or influenced by the presence of peptidase enzymes. It is now known that many different cell types contain major peptidases. For example, vascular endothelial cells contain ACE; bronchial epithelial cells and fibroblasts contain NEP. However, in addition to stationary cells, other cells that infiltrate the lung contain peptidases such as macrophages, platelets and leucocytes. The release of three enzymes from different lung cell types has been documented, including NEP, ACE and carboxypeptidase M.

Several lines of evidence suggest a major role for mast cell proteases in modulating the biological effects of many neuropeptides, including VIP, PHM and, incidentally, CGRP. However, SP, unlike VIP, is not degraded by tryptase. In fact, a combination of protease inhibitors, that are known to inhibit proteases that hydrolyse VIP, potentiated VIP-induced bronchodilatation (Tam *et al.*, 1990). Aprotonin, leupeptin and soyabean trypsin inhibitor inhibit serine and thiol proteases, including mast cell tryptase and chymase, which can be released in the proximity of airway nerves and smooth muscle and are known to inactivate VIP. These inhibitors have been demonstrated to significantly potentiate the bronchodilator response to VIP (Tam *et al.*, 1990). Therefore, this suggests that degradation by endogenous airway proteases is an important determinant of the bronchodilating potency of VIP in human airways.

Receptors

Several types of receptor that can recognize VIP or pituitary adenylate cyclase-activating polypeptide (PACAP) have been described. Type I receptors are PACAP preferring in that they recognize $PACAP_{1-27}$ and $PACAP_{1-38}$ more readily than VIP. Type II receptors are VIP-PACAP receptors as they demonstrate a similar high affinity for VIP, $PACAP_{1-27}$ and $PACAP_{1-38}$.

However, recent studies have described the cloning and expression of two distinct VIP receptors which are thought to be part of the family of G-protein-linked receptors. Firstly, a VIP receptor was cloned from a rat lung cDNA library using the secretin receptor as a probe. This receptor, termed the VIP_1 receptor, was also present in the intestine, brain and liver (Ishihara *et al.*, 1992). The human homologue of this receptor has recently been cloned from human colon carcinoma cells and is also present in the lung and kidney (Sreedharan *et al.*, 1993). A different VIP receptor, the VIP_2 receptor, was recently isolated from the rat pituitary and olfactory bulb and is found in the CNS (thalamus, hippocampus, hypothalamus) (Lutz *et al.*, 1993).

Following receptor activation, evidence points to the activation of adenylyl cyclase and the consequent rise in cAMP levels as the dominant signal transduction pathway of VIP in most cases. In fact, increased levels of cAMP appear to be involved in mediating changes in vascular and non-vascular airway smooth muscle tone, intestinal secretion, modulation of T-cell functions and stimulation of pancreatic exocrine (Said, 1994). However, there is less evidence to suggest the role of alternative secondary signalling pathways.

In conclusion, the cloning of VIP_1 and VIP_2 receptors will provide the impetus for starting research into the development of selective agonists and antagonists. This combined pharmacological and molecular biological approach will enable us to discover whether these two receptor sub-types account for all the known actions of VIP, and will allow us to investigate the involvement of different signal transduction pathways for VIP.

Functional effects of VIP

VIP as a NANC transmitter

An inhibitory non-adrenergic non-cholinergic bronchodilator (iNANC) response can be demonstrated *in vitro* by EFS in humans, guinea pig, ferret, pig, horse, cow and cat (Barnes *et al.*, 1991; Belvisi & Bai, 1995; Belvisi *et al.*, 1995). i-NANC relaxations can also be demonstrated *in situ* (Yip *et al.*, 1981) or *in vivo* by electrical stimulation of the cervical vagus nerve (Irvin *et al.*, 1980) and by reflex stimulation of the larynx (Michoud *et al.*, 1987). This relaxant response evoked by EFS *in vitro* is abolished by tetrodotoxin (TTX) and is therefore assumed to be neural in origin. In several species, both adrenergic and iNANC neural relaxant pathways co-exist, but in human airways the iNANC response is the only neural bronchodilator mechanism. Candidates for mediators of the iNANC response, such as adenosine-5′-triphosphate (ATP), VIP and NO, were considered.

The precise anatomical and neurotransmitter pathways of the iNANC innervation have not been determined and there may be species differences. Several lines of evidence have implicated VIP as a neurotransmitter of iNANC nerves in the airways. VIP produces prolonged relaxation of airway smooth muscle that is unaffected by adrenergic blockade and has a similar time-course to that of the iNANC response in terms of its relaxant ability *in vitro* and *in vivo* in several species. In addition, VIP has been shown to stimulate cAMP production in the guinea pig trachea (Frandsen *et al.*, 1978) and to be released from this tissue during relaxation induced by EFS (Matsuzaki *et al.*, 1980). cAMP metabolism by phosphodiesterases (PDE) can be inhibited by the PDE type III inhibitor SKF 94120, which potentiates the bronchodilator response to VIP and the iNANC relaxant response, suggesting that VIP may play a role in iNANC relaxation responses (Rhoden & Barnes, 1990). Furthermore, VIP can mimic the iNANC relaxant response in bovine tracheal tissue, has been found in the tracheal smooth muscle and has been detected in the effluent during stimulation of iNANC nerves in bovine trachea (Cameron *et al.*, 1983). However, the role of endogenously released VIP is uncertain, since at the time of these experiments no potent and selective antagonists were available. Two VIP antagonists have been previously described which were found to be VIP antagonists in pancreatic tissues. However, these antagonists had no effect on iNANC relaxation responses to VIP and PHI or iNANC relaxation responses in guinea pig trachea *in vitro* (Ellis & Farmer, 1989a).

Therefore, in the absence of a suitable VIP receptor antagonist, other approaches have been adopted to try to elucidate a role for VIP in neurotransmission in the airways, including using antibodies against VIP, desensitization of VIP receptors and the use of non-specific peptidases which are known to abolish the effects of endogenous VIP. Matsuzaki *et al.* (1980) found that preincubation of guinea-pig trachea with VIP antiserum reduced the iNANC response obtained. However, the specificity of the antibodies was not checked and more recently experiments performed with VIP antiserum produced a 60% reduction in the magnitude of the iNANC response (Ellis & Farmer, 1989a). Other studies have investigated the effect of specific desensitization to VIP and found that the iNANC response in guinea pig trachea was reduced by about 40% (Ellis & Farmer, 1989a). In addition, in the cat trachea VIP produced relaxation similar to the effect of inhibitory nerve stimulation and the response to nerve stimulation was reduced by prior application of several desensitizing doses of VIP (Ito & Takeda, 1982). Alternatively, in another study VIP desensitization and incubation of the tissue with specific VIP antisera did not reduce iNANC relaxation responses in the cat trachea (Fisher *et al.*, 1993). Finally, if neuropeptides are involved in iNANC neurotransmission then one may expect to find iNANC responses reduced after incubation of the tissue with a non-specific peptidase, for example α-chymotrypsin (α-CT). However, although α-CT abolishes responses to exogenous VIP in cat trachea, the iNANC relaxant response was not affected (Altiere & Diamond, 1984), suggesting that VIP, or a related peptide, is not involved in iNANC transmission in the airway smooth muscle of this species. In contrast, α-CT reduced, but did not abolish, the magnitude and the duration of the iNANC response in guinea pig trachea (Ellis & Farmer,

1989b), suggesting that the iNANC relaxant response in this species is at least partly peptidergic in nature.

VIP also has a relaxant effect on human airways *in vitro* (Palmer *et al.*, 1986; Belvisi *et al.*, 1992a) and it has been suggested that VIP may be the neurotransmitter responsible for iNANC relaxant responses. However, phosphoramidon, an inhibitor of neutral endopeptidase, significantly potentiated relaxations to low concentrations of VIP with no effect on iNANC responses (Belvisi *et al.*, 1992a). In addition, relaxations evoked by VIP were abolished by α-CT but iNANC responses were unaffected in human tracheal and bronchial smooth muscle (Belvisi *et al.*, 1992a,c). These data suggest that VIP is not involved in i-NANC relaxation responses in human airways (Fig. 26.3).

In the airways, NO synthase (NOS) inhibitors have been shown to inhibit the iNANC neural relaxation response in guinea pig trachea by between 30 and 50% (Tucker *et al.*, 1990; Li & Rand, 1991), suggesting a role for NO in neurotransmission. Similar results have been observed in humans, cat, pig and horse airways (Kannan & Johnson, 1992; Fisher *et al.*, 1993; Yu *et al.*, 1993), although, in contrast to guinea pig airways, the inhibition evoked by NOS inhibitors was almost complete (Belvisi & Bai, 1994).

In summary, the data available suggest that VIP may partially mediate the iNANC relaxant response in guinea pig airways but a role for VIP in iNANC neurotransmission has not been defined in the airways of any other species. This result exposes a marked difference in iNANC neurotransmission in guinea pig compared with human airways. This may seem surprising in view of the fact that there are a large number of VIP-IR nerves in human airway smooth muscle. Therefore, it may be that VIP is involved more in pulmonary vasodilatation than in bronchodilatation.

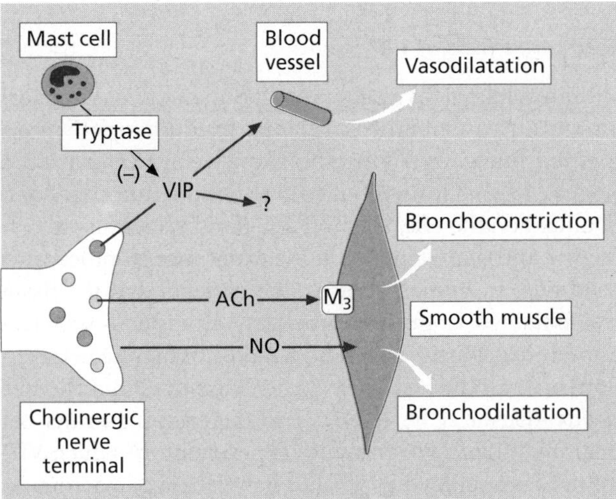

Fig. 26.3 The role of vasoactive intestinal peptide (VIP). VIP does not appear to play a role in the neural iNANC bronchodilator response in human airways, supporting the view that nitric oxide is the only demonstrable mediator/neurotransmitter to act as an endogenous 'braking' mechanism on the dominant cholinergic constrictor response in human airways. This lack of a functional effect evoked by VIP, in human airways, could be due to its enzymatic degradation by mast cell chymase and tryptase.

VIP as a neuromodulator

Exogenous VIP exerts an inhibitory effect on cholinergic neurotransmission via pre- and post-junctional mechanisms in the guinea pig trachea (Ellis & Farmer, 1989c; Stretton *et al.*, 1991; Belvisi, 1994). VIP also seems to modulate cholinergic neurotransmission at the level of the airway parasympathetic ganglia (Martin *et al.*, 1990). This action may be physiologically relevant, since VIP-IR neurones are present in local ganglia in the airways (Dey *et al.*, 1981). However, the nature of the post-junctional action of VIP is concentration dependent. At low concentrations, VIP increases the sensitivity of guinea pig trachea to methacholine, presumably owing to an increase in the affinity of the post-junctional muscarinic receptors (Ellis & Farmer, 1989c). Alternatively, at high concentrations VIP produces inhibition of contractile responses to ACh (Ellis & Farmer, 1989c; Stretton *et al.*, 1991), presumably due to functional antagonism of the contractile response at the level of the airway smooth muscle because at these concentrations VIP is a bronchodilator. VIP at low concentrations has dual effects: it enhances contractions to muscarinic agents, but inhibits cholinergic neural responses to EFS. However, the inhibitory effect is dominant, suggesting that VIP inhibits the release of ACh from cholinergic nerve endings. Similarly, VIP has an inhibitory effect on cholinergic nerve-induced contractions in feline airways (Ito & Hakoda, 1990). In summary, it appears that VIP may act as a bronchodilator or to inhibit ACh release in the airways, and thereby VIP may have a dual mechanism for combating cholinergic bronchoconstriction.

However, in species that exhibit an i-NANC neural relaxant response, which is mediated to some extent by VIP (e.g. iNANC response in guinea pig trachea), endogenously released VIP may act as a braking mechanism for cholinergic bronchoconstriction. However, the role of endogenously released VIP is uncertain, since there are no potent and selective receptor antagonists available. Nevertheless, in guinea pig and human tracheal strips α-chymotrypsin, a proteolytic enzyme, abolished relaxation responses to exogenously added VIP (Ellis & Farmer, 1989b; Belvisi *et al.*, 1992a). Furthermore, in guinea pig (Ellis & Farmer 1989b; Tucker *et al.*, 1990; Li and Rand, 1991), but not in human trachea (Belvisi *et al.*, 1992a,c), α-chymotrypsin was found to inhibit by approximately 35% the iNANC neural relaxant response evoked by EFS *in vitro*. Moreover, α-chymotrypsin enhanced cholinergic contractile responses to EFS in guinea pig trachea by a similar percentage with no effect on contractile responses to exogenous ACh (Brave *et al.*, 1991; Belvisi *et al.*, 1993). These data suggest that endogenous VIP may indeed modulate cholinergic neurotransmission via a pre-junctional action on cholinergic nerves to inhibit ACh release, or by functional antagonism of ACh at the level of the airway smooth muscle, or both. However, to directly establish whether VIP acts pre-junctionally to inhibit transmitter release from cholinergic nerves, it would be necessary to measure the effect of VIP on ACh release.

Conversely, α-chymotrypsin, at a concentration shown to inhibit VIP-induced neural responses in guinea pig trachea (Ellis & Farmer, 1989b; Tucker *et al.*, 1990; Li & Rand, 1991) and abolish responses to exogenously applied VIP in human trachea (Belvisi *et al.*, 1992a,c), had no effect on cholinergic contractile responses evoked by EFS in human airways (Ward *et al.*, 1993). This suggests that endogenous VIP does not modulate cholinergic neurotransmission in human trachea, exposing a marked difference from the guinea pig airways where endogenous VIP inhibits cholinergic contractile responses (Belvisi *et al.*, 1993a). However, this is somewhat surprising as it has been demonstrated that there are large numbers of VIP-immunoreactive nerves in human airway smooth muscle (Laitinen *et al.*, 1985); nevertheless, VIP may be more involved in pulmonary vasodilatation than in neuromodulation. Alternatively, the absence of effects of endogenously released VIP from human airways could be due to the release of tryptase, which has been shown to inhibit the bronchodilator action of VIP in airways *in vitro* (Caughey, 1989) (see above) from activated mast cells in human airways.

In addition to the modulatory action of VIP on neurotransmission, VIP has also been demonstrated to be involved in the maturation, growth and maintenance of neurones (Gozes & Brenneman, 1993).

Effects on smooth muscle

VIP relaxes airway smooth muscle from guinea pigs, rabbits, dogs and humans both *in vivo* and *in vitro*. Additionally, it also prevents bronchospasm in responses to the constrictor agents histamine, $PGF_{2\alpha}$, kallikrein, LTD_4, tachykinins and endothelin (Said, 1994). Moreover, inhaled VIP protects against the bronchoconstriction induced by histamine or $PGF_{2\alpha}$ in dogs and guinea pigs (Said, 1994). Alternatively, in humans the protective effect of aerosolized VIP in asthmatic airways or against histamine-induced challenge was negligible compared with results obtained from animal airways (Barnes & Dixon, 1984; Morice *et al.*, 1984). However, the ineffectiveness of VIP may be due to the rapid degradation of this peptide by peptidases present in the respiratory tract.

In addition to its spasmolytic action, VIP has also been shown to have effects on smooth-muscle-cell proliferation. VIP has been demonstrated to inhibit the growth and proliferation of vascular (Hultgårdh-Nilsson *et al.*, 1988) and bronchial smooth-muscle cells (Maruno & Said, 1993). This antiproliferative effect of VIP may be important in the pathogenesis of inflammatory diseases such as asthma, where a loss of VIP-immunoreactive nerves has been documented (Ollerenshaw *et al.*, 1989).

Vascular effects of VIP

VIP is also a potent vasodilator (Said, 1994) and has been shown to be 50 times more potent at dilating pulmonary blood vessels than prostacyclin. Furthermore, the pulmonary vasodilator action of VIP is not dependent on the presence of an intact endothelium (Sata *et al.*, 1986). Moreover, in the upper respiratory tract VIP dilates the vessels supplying the nose (Said, 1994).

In addition, VIP also increases airway blood flow in pigs and dogs and is more potent on tracheal rather than bronchial vessels (Matran *et al.*, 1989a). Furthermore, there is convincing evidence that VIP is the mediator of NANC vasodilatation in the trachea whereas in more peripheral airways other transmitter substances may have a role (Matran *et al.*, 1989b). The pronounced effect of VIP as a potent vasodilator, its effect on bronchial blood flow and the location of VIP-containing nerves may provide a mechanism for increasing blood flow to contracted airway smooth muscle.

Secretory effects of VIP

VIP-immunoreactive nerves are found in a dense network around airway submucosal glands. In addition, VIP receptors are found overlying the gland acini (Ramnarine & Rogers, 1994). However, it seems that the functional data obtained on the effects of VIP on gland secretion are conflicting and may depend on the experimental procedures used and, in human studies, the patients that the tissue was obtained from. Nevertheless, VIP induces secretory granule exocytosis (which is an indicator of mucous secretion) in ferret trachea *in vitro* when measured morphometrically (Gashi *et al.*, 1986). The increase in serous cell degranulation correlates with experiments in which VIP-induced secretion of [^{35}S]sulphate-labelled macromolecules by ferret trachea *in vitro* (Peatfield *et al.*, 1983; Gashi *et al.*, 1986). Measurement of lysozyme has also been employed as a marker of serous cell secretion. Conflicting results were obtained using this technique, in that VIP was found to inhibit baseline secretion of lysozyme and [^{14}C]glucosaminein-glycoconjugates (which is suggestive of serous and mucous gland cells) in bronchial explants from patients with hypersecretion (Coles *et al.*, 1981).

VIP also modulates secretory responses evoked by other agents. VIP inhibits methacholine-induced increases in mucus volume output *in vitro* in the whole ferret trachea and [^{14}C]glucosamine in human bronchi *in vitro* (Coles *et al.*, 1981; Webber & Widdicombe, 1987). These effects are thought to be due to inhibition of mucous cell discharge. However, the definitive experiments to elucidate the effect of VIP on secretion await the development of receptor-selective antagonists.

VIP and inflammatory cells

Recent data suggest that VIP has potent anti-inflammatory activity in the lung. This conclusion is based on the ability of VIP to inhibit inflammatory cell function. In rabbit platelets, VIP elevates cAMP levels and thereby inhibits aggregation and 5-HT secretion induced by PAF (Cox *et al.*, 1984). In addition, VIP inhibits the release of inflammatory mediators, including histamine, from pulmonary mast cells (Undem *et al.*, 1983). Likewise, VIP inhibits the respiratory burst in human monocytes (Wiik, 1989) and phagocytosis and superoxide radical production by rat alveolar macrophages (Litwin *et al.*, 1989). Both of these effects are associated with stimulated cAMP production. Similarly, VIP inhibits mitogen-induced T-lymphocyte proliferation and other aspects of T-lymphocyte function, including the release of cytokines, especially IL-2 (Ottaway, 1987). In addition, VIP also modulates natural killer (NK) cell activity (Rola-Pleszczynski *et al.*, 1985).

VIP-related peptides

Several peptides have now been identified that are similar in their distribution and functional effects to VIP.

PHI

PHI, and its human equivalent peptide PHM, demonstrate a marked structural similarity to VIP with approximately 50% homology. This peptide is similar to VIP in that it has 13 of the 28 amino-acid residues in the same position (Tatemoto & Mutt, 1981). Indeed, PHI and PHM are encoded by the same gene as VIP (Tatemoto, 1984). Therefore, it is not surprising that PHI has been demonstrated to have a similar immunocytochemical distribution in the lung to VIP (Christofides *et al.*, 1984). Immunostaining for PHI/PHM has also been demonstrated to be present within the sphenopalatine, otic and paratracheal ganglia.

Localization

VIP- and PHI-immunoreactive nerves supply airway smooth muscle (of the larger airways in particular), bronchial and pulmonary vessels, submucosal glands and airway ganglia (Christofides *et al.*, 1984; Lundberg *et al.*, 1984b).

Functional effects

In the airway, PHI has similar functional effects as VIP, for example, vasodilatation, and is equipotent with VIP as a bronchodilator. In human bronchi, PHM has been demonstrated to relax airway smooth muscle and is equipotent to VIP in this regard (Palmer *et al.*, 1986). In a similar manner to VIP, PHI stimulates cell-surface receptors (probably the same receptors that are activated by VIP), leading to the stimulation of adenylyl cyclase and an elevation in the intracellular concentration of cAMP. PHI and VIP potentiate cholinergic and inhibit α-adrenergic stimulation of mucus secretion *in vitro* (Webber, 1988). There are, however, some differences in the functional effects of VIP and PHI. PHI is less potent that VIP in producing pulmonary vasodilatation (Laitinen *et al.*, 1987) but more potent at evoking airway secretion (Webber, 1988). It is not yet known whether PHI/PHM can be released from nerves in the airways and, therefore, whether any of the effects of iNANC nerve stimulation are actually due to the release of PHI/PHM in addition to VIP.

Peptide histidine valine

Peptide histidine valine (PHV-42) is an N-terminally extended precursor of VIP that is also able to relax airway smooth muscle (Yiangou *et al.*, 1987). In guinea pig airways PHV relaxes airway smooth muscle *in vitro* but has no effect on airway tone when infused into asthmatic patients (Chilvers *et al.*, 1988). It has not yet been determined whether this peptide is released from nerves.

Helodermin and helospectins

Helodermin is a 35-amino-acid peptide which also has a similar structure to VIP. It was originally isolated from the salivary gland venom of the lizard *Heloderma suspectum* (Vandermeers *et al.*, 1984). Helospectin I and II are closely related peptides which were isolated from the venom of the lizard *Helodermin horridum* (Vandermeers *et al.*, 1984). Helospectin I is a 38-amino-acid peptide and helospectin II contains 37 amino-acid residues. Helospectin I and II are identical apart from one feature—helospectin II lacks serine-38. Evidence suggests that helodermin is found in endocrine-like cells in the thyroid and the lung (Luts *et al.*, 1991) and helospectin-like immunoreactivity has been demonstrated in the central and peripheral nervous systems (Absood *et al.*, 1992).

Localization

Helodermin immunoreactivity has been localized to airway nerves. Helospectin-immunoreactive nerve fibres are found in smooth-muscle bundles and close to seromucous glands and blood vessels in the tracheobronchial wall. Double immunostaining studies have demonstrated that the helospectin-IR nerve fibres make up a subpopulation of VIP-containing nerve fibres.

Functional effects

Helodermin and the helospectins, like VIP and PHI, are potent relaxants of airway smooth muscle *in vitro* (Foda & Said, 1989).

PACAP

PACAP is the latest member of the superfamily, which includes VIP, PHI/PHM, secretin, helodermin, helospectin I and II, glucagon, GIP (gastric inhibitory peptide) and GRF (growth hormone releasing peptide), to be discovered. It is a biologically active neuropeptide which seems to be active in two amidated forms: PACAP (1–27)-NH_2 ($PACAP_{1-27}$) and PACAP (1–38)-NH_2 ($PACAP_{1-38}$). Ovine $PACAP_{1-38}$ was originally extracted from the hypothalamus based on its ability to elevate cAMP in cultured rat pituitary cells (Miyata *et al.*, 1989) and ovine $PACAP_{1-27}$ was extracted later (Miyata *et al.*, 1990; Christophe, 1993).

Localization

PACAP is found by radioimmunoassay and immunocytochemistry in various parts of the brain. In addition, it has also been localized in the oesophagus, stomach, small and large intestine and a few PACAP-immunoreactive neurones are seen in the myenteric ganglia (Christophe, 1993). Nerve fibres displaying PACAP immunoreactivity were found in the respiratory tract of many species, including humans, rats, guinea pigs, ferrets, pigs, sheep and squirrel monkeys (Uddman *et al.*, 1991; Luts *et al.*, 1993). A moderate supply of PACAP-immunoreactive fibres was found in the nasal mucosa of guinea pigs (Uddman *et al.*, 1991). Few PACP-immunoreactive fibres were found in the tracheobronchial wall of rats, guinea pigs, ferrets, pigs, sheep and squirrel monkeys. The fibres were situated beneath the epithelial layer around blood vessels, seromucous glands and within smooth-muscle bundles. There is also a sparse to moderate supply of PACAP immunoreactivity in nerve cell bodies in parasympathetic and sensory ganglia. Similarly, in the lower respiratory tract of the guinea pig a moderate number of PACAP-immunoreactive fibres were seen (Cardell *et al.*, 1991). In contrast, the lower respiratory tract of humans receives a comparatively rich supply of PACAP-containing fibres (Luts *et al.*, 1993). Double immunostaining experiments have revealed that the majority of the PACAP-containing nerve fibres also contain VIP. However, some VIP-immunoreactive neurones do not demonstrate any PACAP immunoreactivity. Thus, the distribution of PACAP-containing fibres differs to some extent from that of VIP-containing fibres. This is evidenced by the rich supply of VIP-containing fibres in the upper respiratory tract compared to the more limited innervation produced by PACAP-containing fibres (Uddman *et al.*, 1978; Christiofides *et al.*, 1984). In conclusion, the presence of PACAP-immunoreactive nerves and receptors for this peptide in the respiratory tract provide a basis for a role for PACAP in neural regulation of the airways.

Receptors

Two classes of receptor for PACAP have been identified in mammalian tissues and in cell lines. Type I are PACAP-preferring receptors in that they recognize $PACAP_{1-27}$ and $PACAP_{1-38}$ more readily than VIP (500–2000 selectivity for $PACAP_{1-38}$ and $PACAP_{1-27}$ compared to VIP) and have been demonstrated in brain, adrenal gland and testis. Type I receptor activation by $PACAP_{1-27}$ and $PACAP_{1-38}$ then activates adenylyl cyclase and results in an elevation of cAMP levels within the cell. There are at least two co-existing sub-types of the type I receptor based on radioligand binding data. Experiments performed on rat brain membranes have demonstrated that $PACAP_{1A}$ receptor sub-type binds $PACAP_{1-27}$ with slightly higher affinity than $PACAP_{1-38}$ (Harmer & Lutz, 1994). Alternatively, the $PACAP_{1B}$ sub-type recognizes $PACAP_{1-38}$ with high affinity and $PACAP_{1-27}$ with low affinity (Cauvin *et al.*, 1991; Harmer & Lutz, 1994). In contrast to type II receptors, type I receptors can stimulate both adenylyl cyclase and phospholipase C (PLC) in their signal transduction pathway via the activation of G proteins of the Gs and Gq types.

Type II receptors are VIP-PACAP receptors, as they demonstrate a similar high affinity for $PACAP_{1-27}$, $PACAP_{1-38}$ and VIP and have been localized in the lung, liver, spleen, intestine and vascular smooth-muscle-cell membranes. These receptors interact, at the cellular level, almost exclusively with adenylyl cyclase.

In conclusion, it appears that there are two distinct receptors for PACAP and a third that binds VIP and PACAP with equal affinity. However, the PACAP and VIP receptors have recently been cloned, and it has now been suggested that $PACAP_{1A}$ and $PACAP_{1B}$ receptors may correspond to different affinity states of a single receptor protein, whereas two different VIP receptors with different distributions in the CNS have been cloned (Harmer & Lutz, 1994).

Functional effects

Effects on smooth muscle

Receptor binding studies have described PACAP binding sites to be located in high density in the lung (Gottshall *et al.*, 1990). $PACAP_{1-27}$ and $PACAP_{1-38}$ are equipotent at relaxing guinea-pig tracheal smooth muscle, however, $PACAP_{1-38}$ has a longer duration of action. In addition, both peptides increase cAMP levels in parallel with their relaxant action, suggesting that the elevation in cAMP is involved in their relaxant response (Araki & Takagi, 1992).

PACAP has been demonstrated to relax directly the smooth muscle of the gastrointestinal tract, probably via activation of type I receptors and apamin-sensitive K^+ channels. In contrast, VIP evokes atropine-sensitive contraction of the longitudinal muscle layer of the duodenum. This effect is probably due to activation of type II receptors on cholinergic neurones (Christophe, 1993).

Vascular effects

Skin. PACAP is a potent microvasodilator in human skin (Warren *et al.*, 1992). After intradermal injection, both VIP and PACAP cause a rapid 2–3-minute flare which becomes erythematous after 5 minutes. However, the vasodilatation induced by PACAP is longer lasting than that induced by VIP (Warren *et al.*, 1992). Therefore, it seems that PACAP may contribute to both the hyperaemia and oedema observed in the inflammatory response.

Airways. In pre-contracted segments of guinea pig pulmonary artery PACAP evokes a concentration-dependent relaxation response which was endothelium dependent. This is in contrast to relaxation responses evoked by VIP which are endothelium independent, suggesting that the two peptides relax pulmonary vascular smooth muscle via independent mechanisms (Cardell *et al.*, 1991). In addition, PACAP decreases the pulmonary lobar arterial pressure through vasodilatation in the anaesthetized cat. This effect may be mediated via activation of type I receptors, as PACAP was 10-fold more potent than VIP in dilating the pulmonary vascular bed (Minkes *et al.*, 1992).

Secretory effects of PACAP. In isolated chief cells from guinea pig stomach PACAP stimulates pepsinogen secretion through type II receptors at low concentrations and via activation of secretin receptors at higher concentrations. In addition, PACAP has been demonstrated to be an anion secretory neuropeptide on rat jejunal mucosa. Furthermore, *in vivo* it increases amylase secretion via a cholinergic mechanism in dog and glucagon release in mice (Christophe, 1993).

The question that comes immediately to mind, in view of the similar functional effects of VIP and PACAP, is whether PACAP is the physiological mediator of some of the effects originally ascribed to VIP. However, the cloning of all the receptors for VIP and PACAP and then the development of receptor-selective antagonists will help to clarify whether PACAP or VIP is the physiological mediator of these functional effects.

Neuropeptide tyrosine

Neuropeptide tyrosine (NPY) is a 36-amino-acid peptide which was first discovered in the gastrointestinal tract (Tatemoto *et al.*, 1982) and later in many neurones of the central and peripheral nervous systems (Sheppard *et al.*, 1984). NPY is usually found as a cotransmitter together with noradrenaline in adrenergic nerves but has also been described in cholinergic nerves (Luts & Sundler, 1989). NPY may therefore have a role as an autoregulator via the inhibition of noradrenaline release (Potter, 1988).

Localization

NPY-containing nerves in the respiratory tract are found in close association with blood vessels and airway smooth muscle. The distribution of NPY follows the distribution of adrenergic nerves and NPY-containing nerves predominantly innervate nasal vessels and bronchial vessels and glands, with less innervation of airway smooth muscle (Sheppard *et al.*, 1984). In some species, like the pig (Lacroix *et al.*, 1990) and the rat (Leblanc *et al.*, 1987), a population of the parasympathetic neurones in the sphenopalatine ganglion innervating exocrine elements of the nasal mucosa also contains NPY immunoreactivity. In human airways, extrinsic denervation of the lung, following heart–lung transplantation, leads to a depletion of NPY-containing nerve fibres in that tissue, suggesting that these nerves are extrinsic in origin (Springall *et al.*, 1990), in keeping with the location of NPY immunoreactivity in adrenergic nerves.

As mentioned earlier, the demonstration that NPY is released would further strengthen the case for classifying this peptide as a neurotransmitter. In fact, sympathetic stimulation, using high frequencies, is associated with extreme vascular effects and increased overflow of NPY immunoreactivity into the nasal venous effluent, suggesting that NPY has been released upon nerve stimulation (Lundblad *et al.*, 1987).

Receptors

The effector actions of this peptide are associated with the activation of several specific cell-surface receptors. Three receptors have been identified, designated Y_1, Y_2 and Y_3

according to their affinity for NPY and a related peptide, peptide tyrosine tyrosine (PYY), and analogues (Michel, 1991). The signal transduction mechanisms may differ according to which NPY receptor in activated. Therefore, it seems that pre-junctional Y_2 receptors act to inhibit adenylyl cyclase whilst post-junctional Y_1 receptors stimulate phosphoinositide hydrolysis (Håkanson & Wahlestadt, 1987). These receptors have been localized in some peripheral mammalian tissues, not including the lung, via autoradiographic techniques. However, there seems to be some problems associated with the localization of these receptors in human tissues. In future experiments it will be possible to localize these receptors using molecular biology via the technique of *in situ* hybridization using probes generated from the human and bovine NPY receptor cDNA sequences (Herzog *et al.*, 1992).

Functional effects of NPY

NPY as a neuromodulator

NPY inhibits cholinergic neurotransmission in guinea pig airways probably via an effect on ACh release, as it reduces cholinergic nerve-evoked contractile responses but has no effect on the contractile response to exogenous ACh (Grundemar *et al.*, 1988; Stretton & Barnes, 1988; Matran *et al.*, 1989c). This inhibitory effect was more pronounced at lower frequencies of stimulation. Furthermore, the inhibitory effect is unaffected by adrenergic blockade, suggesting that NPY acts at a pre-junctional NPY receptor on post-ganglionic cholinergic nerves. Alternatively, in human airways *in vitro*, NPY has no effect on cholinergic neurotransmission (C.D. Stretton & P.J. Barnes, unpublished data).

NPY also modulates excitatory NANC constrictor responses in guinea pig airways *in vitro* and *in vivo* (Giuliani *et al.*, 1989; Matran *et al.*, 1989c; Grundemar *et al.*, 1990; Stretton *et al.*, 1990). This inhibitory action of NPY is unaffected by α-adrenoceptor blockade, and NPY had no effect on bronchoconstrictor responses evoked by exogenous SP. These results suggest that the inhibitory action of NPY is likely to be mediated directly on its pre-junctional receptor on sensory nerves. The NPY receptor mediating this effect appears to be the Y_2 sub-type. Finally, the modulatory effect of NPY seems to be greater in main bronchi than in hilar bronchi, and this may relate to the distribution of adrenergic nerves (Stretton *et al.*, 1990). In summary, adrenergic nerves may therefore modulate excitatory NANC bronchoconstriction *in vivo* and *in vitro* via NPY receptors, in addition to α_2 adrenoceptors as previously described.

Effects on smooth muscle

NPY has no direct effect on airway smooth muscle of the guinea pig (Stretton & Barnes, 1988) but may evoke bronchoconstriction via the release of prostaglandins (Cadieux *et al.*, 1989).

Vasqular effects

NPY is a potent vasoconstrictor agent in the nose (Lundblad *et al.*, 1987) and in the tracheobronchial mucosa (Salonen *et al.*, 1988). However, it also has profound effects on the control of airway blood flow in. In fact NPY evokes a prolonged reduction in tracheal blood flow in anaesthetized dogs (Salonen *et al.*, 1988) but has no direct effect on canine bronchial vessels *in vitro* (McCormack *et al.*, 1989), suggesting that NPY preferentially acts on resistance vessels in the airway. Therefore, NPY may be anti-inflammatory via its constrictor action on resistance vessels, leading to a reduced mucosal blood flow and thereby a possible reduction in the perfusion of post-capillary venules and a decrease in plasma extravasation.

Effects on secretion

NPY has been reported to enhance cholinergically and adrenergically mediated mucus secretion from ferret trachea (Webber, 1988) but seems to have no direct effect on macromolecule secretion from ferret airways or human nasal mucosa *in vitro* (Baraniuk *et al.*, 1990a). On the other hand, NPY inhibits stimulated serous cell secretion (Webber, 1988).

Opioids

Together with the tachykinins, the opioid peptides are perhaps the most studied group of neuropeptides. Since the original discovery of the enkephalins (Hughes *et al.*, 1975), a large number of further opioid peptides have been discovered and this has led to the characterization of three separate families of opioids. The principal members of these families are the pentapeptides Met- and Leu-enkephalin, the 31-amino-acid β-endorphin, and the 17-amino-acid dynorphin A. Each of these peptides are derived from a separate gene and precursor protein termed pro-enkephalin, pro-opiomelanocortin (POMC) and pro-dynorphin, respectively. These precursors also encode a number of other peptides, which may be opioid or non-opioid in nature. For example, POMC also gives rise to the pituitary hormones adrenocorticotrophic hormone (ACTH) and melanocyte-stimulating hormone, whilst pro-dynorphin may also yield dynorphin$_{1-8}$ (Evans *et al.*, 1988).

Localization

All three classes of opioid are found in the CNS and spinal cord but with varying and discrete localizations. Other precursor products, particularly those derived from pro-enkephalin and pro-dynorphin, are also found in the CNS, although whether these peptides act as active opioids themselves or merely as intermediates in the processing of the precursor is uncertain (Evans *et al.*, 1988). Outside the CNS the opioids are classically found in the pituitary and adrenal glands, although in general the enkephalins and dynorphin have a wider distribution than β-endorphin. Until recently opioids were thought to be found almost exclusively in neurones. Immunohistochemistry studies have demonstrated the presence of enkephalins and dynorphin peptides in sympathetic ganglia (Shultzberg *et al.*, 1979), myenteric neurones of the gut (Costa *et al.*, 1985) and in both cell bodies and peripheral terminals of primary afferent neurones (Weihe *et al.*, 1985). This distribution is in keeping with the possible roles of opioids in the control of gut motility and in nociceptive processing. Most recently, however, it has become apparent that opioids may also be found in non-neuronal cells in the periphery, and in particular in cells of the immune system. Thus, POMC- and pro-enkephalin mRNA have been demonstrated in T cells, macrophages and mast cells from various species (Zurawski *et al.*, 1986; Martin *et al.*, 1987). Interestingly, some studies have found that inflamed but not normal tissue of rats contain cells, mainly T cells, macrophages and monocytes, which express POMC and pro-enkephalin mRNA as well as β-endorphin and Met-enkephalin (Przewlocki *et al.*, 1992). This implies a role for endogenous opioids in inflammation, and in particular in inflammatory pain (see later). In the airways, Leu-enkephalin has been localized to neuroendocrine cells (Cutz, 1982), whilst Met-enkephalin immunoreactive nerves have been described in guinea pig and rat lungs (Shimosegawa *et al.*, 1990). These nerves also contained VIP, implying a localization of enkephalin in airway parasympathetic nerves.

Receptors

The effects of opioids are mediated through an interaction with at least three different receptor types termed μ, κ and δ. As with the tachykinins, the naturally occurring opioids show some selectivity for each receptor type, with the enkephalins having higher affinity at δ-receptors, dynorphin at κ-receptors and β-endorphin at μ-receptors. It must be stressed, however, that this represents only relative affinity and all opioids will have some activity at each receptor type. The classification of opioid receptors has been confirmed with the development of receptor-selective agonists, although the development of selective antagonists has followed much more slowly. Of particular use have been the compounds [D-Ala^2,MePhe^4,Glyol^5]-enkephalin (DAMGO), U50488H and [D-Pen^2,D-Pen^5]-enkephalin (DPDPE), which are selective agonists for μ-, κ- and δ-receptors, respectively (see Zimmerman & Leander, 1990). The archetypal antagonist for all opioid receptors is naloxone. However, more recently there has been the development of the non-peptide antagonists nor-binaltorphamine and naltrindole which show selectivity for κ- and δ-receptors, respectively, as well as the δ-selective peptide antagonist ICI174864 (Takemori & Portoghese, 1992).

Each of the three receptor types appear to belong to the G-protein-coupled family of receptors and their activation leads to inhibition of adenylyl cyclase and cAMP formation. μ-Receptors have also been shown to open potassium channels whilst κ- and δ-receptors may inhibit calcium-channel function located on neurones of the CNS and in the periphery, particularly the gut (DiChiara & North, 1992); both of these effects will tend to decrease neuronal excitability. These inhibitory effects of the opioid receptors are mediated by pertussis toxin-sensitive G proteins. cDNA for the three receptor types have now been isolated and cloned and these molecular studies have confirmed that each receptor type belongs to the seven transmembrane spanning superfamily of receptors coupled to G proteins (Reisne & Bell, 1993).

Functional effects

By far the most important action of opioids is that of inhibition of neuronal function. In the periphery, opioids have been shown to inhibit neurotransmitter release from postganglionic sympathetic nerves, enteric nerves and sensory nerves, as well as having inhibitory effects on CNS neurones. Such an inhibitory effect on sensory nerves underlies, at least to a large extent, the analgesic effect of opioids. Thus, it is thought that opioids act on receptors located on primary afferent nerve terminals in the spinal cord to inhibit SP release and reduce nociceptive input. A similar inhibitory effect is seen at the peripheral terminals of sensory nerves. Here, opioids have been shown to inhibit neuronal firing of afferent fibres innervating the skin (Andreev & Dray, 1994) and joints (Russell *et al.*, 1987) and also to inhibit SP release in the joint (Yaksh, 1988). This inhibition of peripheral sensory nerve function by opioids leads to an inhibition of neurogenic inflammation (Lembeck & Donnerer, 1985).

Opioids as neuromodulators

In the airways, opioids modulate the activity of both

cholinergic and sensory nerve function. In canine and guinea pig airways, opioids inhibit cholinergic contractile responses evoked by EFS by acting on μ- and δ-receptors (Russell & Simons, 1985; Belvisi *et al.*, 1990b). These receptors appeared to be located on postganglionic nerve terminals, as the μ-opioid agonist had no effect on contractile responses to exogenously administered ACh. A similar inhibition of cholinergic transmission has been demonstrated in human airway smooth muscle (Belvisi *et al.*, 1992b), and an inhibitory effect on ACh release has recently been confirmed using neurochemical techniques in guinea pig and human airways (Belvisi *et al.*, 1993).

Opioids have also been shown to inhibit excitatory NANC bronchoconstrictor responses evoked by EFS *in vitro* and vagal stimulation *in vivo* in guinea pigs (Frossard & Barnes, 1987; Belvisi *et al.*, 1988). Again this effect was presumed to be pre-junctional, as the μ-opioid agonist had no effect on constrictor responses evoked by exogenous SP, and an inhibition of SP release from guinea pig airways by morphine has since been demonstrated. With regard to other NANC effects in the airways, morphine has been shown to inhibit neurogenic plasma extravasation evoked by vagal stimulation in anaesthetized guinea pigs in a naloxone-sensitive manner whilst having no effect on SP-induced leakage, indicating an action on opioid receptors located on sensory nerves (Belvisi *et al.*, 1989). Likewise, opioids inhibit mucus secretion from airway goblet cells in the guinea pig evoked by cigarette smoke which stimulates sensory nerves (Kuo *et al.*, 1992), and also the secretory response to capsaicin in human bronchi *in vitro* (Rogers & Barnes, 1989).

Mechanisms involved in the pre-junctional control of neurotransmitter release

The presynaptic inhibitory modulation of neurotransmitter release (by substances such as opioids) is thought to involve receptor-mediated regulation of ion channels in the nerve endings (Miller, 1990a). In the CNS, some agonists inhibit neuronal function by opening a common K^+ channel (North *et al.*, 1987). The presence of several types of K^+ channel on nerve cells has been reported, and most evidence points to an involvement of ATP-activated (K_{ATP}) and large conductance Ca^{2+}-activated (K^+_{Ca}) K^+ channels in the modulation of transmitter release from peripheral nerves, especially in the airways. For example, blockade of K^+_{Ca} using the scorpion venom toxin charybdotoxin (ChTX) (Giminez-Gallego *et al.*, 1988), reverses the pre-junctional inhibition of cholinergic responses by a μ-opioid in guinea pig and human airways (Miura *et al.*, 1992). A similar mechanism appears to operate in NANC nerves innervating the airways, such that ChTX completely blocks the modulatory action of NPY and opioids on excitatory NANC constrictor responses in guinea pig bronchi (Stretton *et al.*, 1992). Recent experiments using iberiotoxin, a more selective blocker of K^+_{Ca} (Galves *et al.*, 1990), have confirmed the involvement of K^+_{Ca} in the μ-opioid-induced pre-junctional modulation of excitatory NANC neurotransmission (Miura *et al.*, 1993). These channels could therefore be important in the regulation of neurotransmitter release by substances such as endogenous opioids. An impairment of their function, for example during inflammatory conditions, could have deleterious effects, since this would tend to potentiate neurogenic inflammation by reducing underlying inhibitory mechanisms mediated by agents such as opioids.

Gastrin-releasing peptide

Gastrin-releasing peptide (GRP) is a 27-amino-acid peptide and is the mammalian form of the amphibian peptide bombesin (14 amino-acid residues) (Miller, 1990b). GRP/bombesin share sequence homology with neuromedin C and neuromedin B. Bombesin-related peptides have been classified into three families: the bombesin family (including GRP, neuromedin C), the ranatensin family (neuromedin B) and the litorin family (no known mammalian peptides). GRP gene transcripts are processed differently in endocrine and neural tissues, suggesting that mRNA splicing may contribute to the diversity of bombesin-immunoreactive peptides.

Localization

GRP/bombesin have been identified in the nasal and tracheobronchial mucosa. In fact, GRP, together with cholecystokinin and somatostatin, have been found in nerves that were thought to be sensory in the nasal mucosa. In human nasal mucosa, GRP nerve fibres are present in the walls of arterial and venous vessels and around glandular acini (Baraniuk *et al.*, 1990d), and their distribution is similar to that of CGRP and NKA. In the airways, GRP-containing nerve fibres have been demonstrated around blood vessels and submucosal glands in the airways of several species (Uddman *et al.*, 1984). Bombesin/GRP-IR peptides are also expressed by normal human bronchial epithelial lung neuroendocrine cells in human and animal airways. In addition, bombesin can be detected in broncheolar lavage fluid of smokers (Aguayro *et al.*, 1989).

Receptors

These peptides interact with specific cell-surface receptors. Two bombesin receptor sub-types have been cloned from a human small cell lung carcinoma cell line (Corjay *et al.*, 1991). GRP receptors preferentially bind GRP, neuromedin C and bombesin, while NMB-receptors prefer neuromedin B and bombesin over GRP. Indeed, GRP binding sites have been localized to the epithelium and submucosal glands of human nasal and tracheal mucosa (Baraniuk *et al.*, 1990d).

Functional effects

In vitro, GRP induces both serous and mucous cell exocytosis from human nasal mucosa (Baraniuk *et al.*, 1990d). *In vivo*, bombesin stimulates mucous glycoconjugate and lysozyme secretion from human nasal mucosa, but does not stimulate albumin secretion, suggesting an effect on submucosal gland secretion without increases in vascular permeability. In addition, GRP and bombesin are also potent stimulants of airway mucus secretion in human and cat airways *in vitro*.

GRP mRNA in the lung is increased on the day prior to birth and then declines. Furthermore, bombesin-IR decreases with maturation and a reduction in bombesin-IR has been described in the lungs of patients who have died of fetal respiratory distress syndrome (Ghatei *et al.*, 1983). Therefore, GRP and related peptides may play a profound role in lung maturation. Bombesin is a potent mitogen and is secreted by small cell bronchial carcinomas, implying an autocrine, trophic role in tumour growth (Miller *et al.*, 1990b). It is therefore possible that it has trophic properties in the respiratory mucosa.

Bombesin is a potent bronchoconstrictor in guinea pig airways *in vivo* but does not constrict isolated airways (at each airway level) *in vitro*, suggesting that the bronchoconstrictor effect is indirect (Belvisi *et al.*, 1991). The constrictor response is not inhibited by an antihistamine, a cyclo-oxygenase inhibitor, a lipoxygenase inhibitor, a PAF antagonist or a 5-HT receptor antagonist, indicating that the release of these mediators is not involved in the bombesin-induced constrictor response. However, the bombesin-induced constrictor response is inhibited by a bombesin receptor antagonist, indicating that GRP/bombesin receptors are involved (Belvisi *et al.*, 1991).

The current data suggest that this family of peptides may be released from sensory nerves and play an important role as a serous and mucous cell secretagogue and potential growth factor in human airways and nasal mucosa.

Galanin

Galanin is a 29-amino-acid peptide originally isolated from the gut, which has a widespread distribution in the central and peripheral nervous systems (Cheung *et al.*, 1985). It is named after its N-terminal glycine and the C-terminal alanine (Tatemoto *et al.*, 1983). Galanin has been shown to contract smooth muscle of intestine, urinary bladder and uterine horn in the rat (Tatemoto *et al.*, 1983). It has also been shown to inhibit glucose-induced insulin secretion in rat and dog (Rökaeus, 1987).

Localization

Galanin has been shown by immunohistochemical methods to have a similar distribution to VIP/PHI in many species (Cheung *et al.*, 1985). In the airways, galanin is colocalized with VIP in cholinergic nerves of the airways and is present in parasympathetic ganglia (Cheung *et al.*, 1985; Dey *et al.*, 1990). However, galanin is also colocalized with SP and CGRP in sensory nerves, dorsal root, nodose and trigeminal ganglia (Ju *et al.*, 1987; Uddman & Sundler, 1987). It is found around blood vessels and submucosal glands and in the airway smooth muscle, with the highest concentration in the main bronchi. Galanin has also been identified in the nasal mucosa with the same distribution as for VIP and ACh (Cheung *et al.*, 1985).

Receptors

Comparatively little is known about the specific cell-surface receptors that are activated by galanin. However, recently a chimeric peptide called galantide made from galanin$_{1-13}$ and substance P$_{5-11}$ was described as a competitive antagonist at galanin receptors (Lindskog *et al.*, 1992). Galantide antagonizes the galanin-mediated inhibition of the glucose-induced insulin secretion from mouse pancreatic islets (Lindskog *et al.*, 1992). It also binds with high affinity to galanin binding sites in membranes from ventral hippocampus, mid-brain and spinal cord (Bartfai *et al.*, 1991). However, galantide did not antagonize the inhibitory effect of galanin on excitatory NANC constrictor responses in guinea pig bronchi (Takahashi *et al.*, 1994). Therefore, the galanin receptor in guinea pig bronchi may differ from that in pancreatic islet cells and CNS. In fact, it has been demonstrated that the anterior pituitary has a different type of galanin receptor (designated GAL-R$_2$), to which galantide does not bind, in contrast to the gut/brain receptor (designated GAL-R$_1$). Therefore, it is quite possible that the airway galanin receptors may also be different from the GAL-R$_1$ receptor.

Functional effects

Galanin seems to have no direct effect on airway tone in guinea pig airways and no effect on airway blood flow in dogs (Salonen *et al.*, 1988). However, galanin does have a role as a neuromodulator. Ekblad *et al.* (1985) demonstrated that galanin had no effect on constrictor responses evoked by electrical field stimulation in guinea pig trachea and main bronchi, although the responses to EFS were not separated into the different neural components, for example cholinergic or excitatory (e) NANC constrictor responses. However, more recently it has been demonstrated that galanin has an inhibitory effect on eNANC constrictor responses in guinea pig airways (Giuliani *et al.*, 1989; Takahashi *et al.*, 1994). Galanin, which seems to be present in cholinergic nerves (Cheung *et al.*, 1985), had no effect on the cholinergic constrictor and iNANC relaxant response to EFS in guinea pig airways (Takahashi *et al.*, 1994). Therefore, the major role for galanin in the airways is as a neuromodulator involved in the control of the release of neuropeptides from airway sensory nerves, as other functional effects remain to be elucidated.

Somatostatin

Somatostatin is a 14-amino-acid peptide which has been localized to afferent nerves (Jansco *et al.*, 1968) and has a modulatory effect on neurogenic inflammation in the rat footpad (Lembeck *et al.*, 1982). However, the concentration of somatostatin in the lung is low and somatostatin has no direct action on airway smooth muscle *in vitro*. Alternatively, in contrast to other NANC-innervated tissues somatostatin has no effect on peptidergic constrictor responses, due to stimulation of capsaicin-sensitive primary afferent nerves, in guinea pig airways (C.D. Stretton & P.J. Barnes, unpublished data) but does facilitate cholinergic neurotransmission in ferret airways *in vitro* (Sekizawa *et al.*, 1989).

Cholecystokinin

Cholecystokinin octapeptide (CCK_8) has been identified in the airways of several species (Ghatei *et al.*, 1982). CCK_8 is a potent constrictor of guinea pig and human airways *in vitro* (Stretton & Barnes, 1989). However, CCK_8 has no apparent effect on cholinergic neurotransmission, either at the level of parasympathetic ganglia or at post-ganglionic nerve terminals.

Neuropeptides and pathophysiological conditions

From the findings presented here it can be seen that many exogenous neuropeptides may have either pro- or anti-inflammatory activity. However, the evidence for their involvement in pathophysiological processes is much more scarce. Indeed, so far a pathophysiological role for only a very few neuropeptides can be proposed with any confidence, and this is outlined below. However, the rapid growth in the development of potent non-peptide receptor antagonists for several neuropeptides will undoubtedly lead to further information on their potential involvement in inflammatory conditions.

VIP

Several lines of evidence suggest that VIP is an important neurotransmitter in a number of basic physiological events, and the lack of VIP innervation in certain tissues has been linked to the pathogenesis of several disease processes. For example, in *achalasia of the oesophagus*, the loss of normal peristalsis of the oesophageal body and the failure of the lower sphincter to relax when swallowing are associated with a reduced VIP innervation of the oesophageal smooth muscle (Gridelli *et al.*, 1982). Another condition, known as Hirschsprung's disease, or congenital megacolon, is also associated with a reduction in the VIP-containing nerves within the small intestine. This reduced VIPergic innervation may be associated with the persistent contraction which is characteristic of this disease (Tsuto *et al.*, 1989).

Some inflammatory diseases of the airways are similarly associated with a decrease in VIP-immunoreactive nerves. One example of this is the significant depletion of VIP-IR nerves that has been reported in patients with severe asthma (Ollerenshaw *et al.*, 1989). In addition, reduced VIP-IR nerves are found in association with sweat glands of patients with cystic fibrosis (Heinz-Erian *et al.*, 1985), which could contribute to a decrease in VIP-induced serous cell secretion and formation of thick, mucoid secretions. Interestingly, VIP-IR nerves are markedly reduced in older animals (Geppetti *et al.*, 1988), a difference which could be relevant physiologically if the same phenomenon is observed in human airways.

Tachykinins

There is considerable evidence that neurogenic inflammation and tachykinins may be important in a number of inflammatory conditions. A whole range of pro-inflammatory mediators are now known to excite the peripheral endings of sensory nerves. Perhaps more importantly, these inflammatory mediators may also sensitize sensory fibres leading to an increased excitability of the sensory nerves and increased reflex activity. This phenomenon has been particularly well studied in the somatosensory system, where peripheral sensitization has been shown to contribute to hyperalgesia and the pain associated with arthritis (Dray *et al.*, 1994). However, as we have seen, excitation of sensory nerves may also evoke the peripheral release of tachykinins (and CGRP). Tachykinins mimic many of the symptoms, in particular the vascular effects, seen in inflammatory conditions such as asthma, arthritis and inflammatory bowel disease, and may also enhance the accumulation of immunocompetent cells to areas of tissue damage. In this way hyperactivity of sensory nerves can contribute to the pathology of such inflammatory conditions.

Asthma

SP and NKA mimic many of the key pathophysiological features of asthma, including bronchoconstriction, plasma extravasation leading to oedema, increased bronchial blood flow and mucus secretion. In asthmatic airways the epithelium is often shed which, as described earlier, will remove the primary site of metabolism leading to exaggerated effects of released tachykinins. In addition, loss of epithelium will expose sensory nerve endings such that they may be acted upon by inflammatory mediators (Fig. 26.4). Bradykinin, prostaglandins, 5-HT, histamine and protons, all of which may be formed during local inflammation in the airway, have been shown to either stimulate airway sensory nerves or to evoke the release of tachykinins from guinea pig lung tissue (Saria *et al.*, 1988; Fox *et al.*, 1993, 1995b; Satoh *et al.*, 1993). In addition, the bronchoconstriction and plasma extravasation evoked by bradykinin and acidic solutions are inhibited by NK_2 and NK_1 receptor antagonists, indicating an effect secondary to tachykinin release. Plasma extravasation evoked by antigen challenge to sensitized guinea pigs has also been shown to be inhibited by NK_1 receptor antagonists and enhanced by the NEP inhibitor phosphoramidon, indicating a role for sensory nerves in allergic reactions (Bertrand *et al.*, 1993b). This is supported by the finding that tachykinin-evoked prostanoid release from alveolar macrophages is greatly increased in cells from sensitized guinea pigs (Brunelleschi *et al.*, 1992).

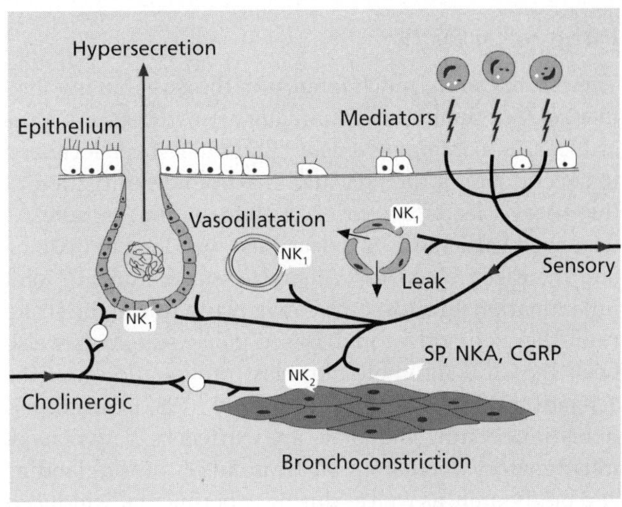

Fig. 26.4 The potential role of tachykinin-containing sensory nerves in airway inflammation. The activation of sensory nerves leads to the release of tachykinins and CGRP from peripheral endings which cause a number of effects that are characteristic features of inflammatory diseases such as asthma. These effects are mediated via NK_1 and NK_2 receptors. In addition, sensory nerve activation causes reflex bronchoconstriction, via efferent cholinergic nerves, and cough. In the normal airway these are protective reflexes serving to limit the access of inhaled irritants into the peripheral airways. However, under conditions of inflammation the epithelium is denuded leaving sensory nerve endings exposed, and inflammatory mediators released from infiltrating cells may both activate the sensory nerves and evoke sensitization such that they are hyperexcitable, leading to exaggerated effects of sensory nerve stimulation. (From Barnes *et al.*, 1993.) See text for definition of abbreviations.

Whether airway sensory nerves are sensitized during inflammation or are involved in airways hyperreactivity is still uncertain, although there is some evidence that this might occur. Thus, single-airway C fibres may be sensitized by PAF, bradykinin and some prostaglandins in the guinea pig (Fox *et al.*, 1995a), and by histamine in the dog (Lee & Morton, 1993). In addition, bradykinin-induced bronchoconstriction is increased after ozone-induced hyperresponsiveness in rats (Tsukagoshi *et al.*, 1995), and the cough reflex in guinea pigs is enhanced after chronic cigarette exposure (Karlsson *et al.*, 1991), both suggestive of sensory nerve sensitization. Finally, capsaicin pretreatment has been shown to prevent the production of airway hyperreactivity evoked by PAF and antigen challenge in guinea pigs (Matsuse *et al.*, 1991; Perretti & Manzini, 1993). It would be expected that if airway sensory nerves became sensitized then there would be enhanced central and local axon reflexes, leading to increased tachykinin release. In spite of these findings there is surprisingly little information from animal studies on this subject.

The importance of endogenous tachykinins and specifically of eNANC mechanisms in human airways is still uncertain. In the majority of studies, electrical stimulation of human airway preparations *in vitro* results in a contraction that is completely blocked by atropine (see Joos *et al.*, 1994). However, one study has reported a contractile effect of capsaicin that was potentiated by peptidase inhibitors indicating the release of endogenous peptides (Honda *et al.*, 1991), and capsaicin has also been shown to stimulate mucus secretion from human bronchi *in vitro* (Rogers & Barnes, 1989). Inhalation of capsaicin results in only a transient bronchoconstrictor response in humans which can be blocked by ipratropium bromide indicating a cholinergic reflex (Fuller *et al.*, 1985). In contrast, a recent study reported an inhibition of bradykinin-evoked bronchoconstriction by a mixed NK_1/NK_2 receptor antagonist FK224 (Ichinose *et al.*, 1992). The evidence for the endogenous release of tachykinins in humans is still therefore equivocal, although it may be that they are most important for effects such as microvascular leak which is as yet impossible to measure, or become more apparent during conditions of inflammation. In this regard it is of interest that an increase in SP-immunoreactive nerves has been reported in the airways from patients with fatal asthma, but not mild asthma (Ollerenshaw *et al.*, 1991), and NK_1 receptor expression is increased in lungs from asthmatic patients (Adcock *et al.*, 1993).

Disease of the joints

There is currently much interest in the possible involvement of tachykinins in inflammatory joint diseases such as arthritis. SP-containing sensory fibres have been localized to several joint structures and antidromic stimulation of these nerves leads to release of SP into the joint capsule. As described earlier, this SP release can then lead to oedema and increased blood flow, characteristic features of joint inflammation. In addition, SP may play a role in the structural changes evident in diseased joints, since it has also been shown to promote fibroblast proliferation and the activation of synoviocytes (Lotz *et al.*, 1987). Sensory C fibres innervating the joints are excited by a variety of inflammatory mediators such as 5-HT, prostaglandins and bradykinin, as well as during experimentally induced arthritis (McQueen *et al.*, 1991; Schepelmann *et al.*, 1992). In addition, these mediators sensitize the sensory fibres, such that they have reduced thresholds to either chemical or mechanical stimuli. Significantly, during adjuvant-induced arthritis there is a considerable hypersensitivity of these fibres with previously innocuous movements of the joint now evoking a considerable discharge. There is also evidence from such models that there is a similar hypersensitivity of spinal dorsal horn neurones during inflammation. These central and peripheral changes in the properties of the afferent fibres will obviously account for the pain associated with chronic arthritis. However, an increased excitability may also lead to increased tachykinin release into the joint, and indeed tachykinin-like immunoreactivity has been shown to be increased in the joint fluid of patients with rheumatoid arthritis (Devillier *et al.*, 1987). In addition, acute inflammation of the knee joint in rats is reduced both by capsaicin pretreatment and by an SP antagonist (Lam & Ferrell, 1989) implying a role for SP release. Such an enhanced release of SP from hyperexcitable sensory nerve endings may therefore contribute to chronic inflammation in joints through its potent effects on the vasculature and immune cells.

Other tissues

Tachykinins are implicated in inflammatory conditions involving a number of other sites, most notably the viscera. Increased levels of SP have been reported to occur in the colonic mucosa of patients with ulcerative colitis, and there is also a marked up-regulation of NK_1 receptors in gut tissue from patients suffering from ulcerative colitis or Crohn's disease (Mantye *et al.*, 1988). These receptors were located on venules, small arterioles and lymph nodes and therefore implicated in local inflammatory and immune responses. In the urinary tract, tachykinins released from capsaicin-sensitive sensory nerves are potent spasmogens of the bladder and are implicated in the control of the micturition reflex (Maggi, 1991b). They may also have a role in inflammatory processes involving hypermobility of the bladder, since NK_2 receptor antagonists have been shown to have a beneficial effect in animal models of cystitis. Finally, as mentioned earlier, SP is implicated in the pathogenesis of migraine. Cerebral blood vessels receive a rich sensory innervation and it has been suggested that local inflammation combined with abnormal vasodilatation could lead to the activation of these sensory nerve endings, leading to pain and peptide release. This SP then produces local vasodilatation and increased vascular permeability in the meninges thereby perpetuating the inflammation.

Opioids

Recent research into the analgesic activity of opioids has indicated that there may be a significant peripheral component to their mechanism of action, and has provided further evidence for interactions between the immune and sensory nervous systems (Stein, 1995). As discussed earlier the activation of peripheral opioid receptors on sensory nerve endings leads to an inhibition of firing and of transmitter release. Thus, opioids, applied locally are analgesic in models of inflammatory pain, but have little effect in normal tissue. This activity is associated with an increased axonal transport of opioid receptors and of the density of receptors in peripheral tissue after inflammation (Hassan *et al.*, 1993). Recently, the inflammatory cytokine IL-1β has been shown to cause increased axonal transport of opioid receptors in sensory nerves, and this could account for the increased efficacy of peripherally acting opioids in inflammation (Jeanjean *et al.*, 1995). Several studies have shown that immune and inflammatory cells invading inflamed tissues (e.g. after cutanous injection of Freund's adjuvant) synthesize opioid peptides, thereby providing a source of endogenous ligand for the increased receptor population (Przewlocki *et al.*, 1992). These findings suggest a potential role for peripherally acting opioids in inflammation. For example, peripherally acting opioids could be analgesic in inflammatory conditions such as arthritis without the damaging central side-effects. In addition, by providing a brake on neurogenic inflammation they could be beneficial in conditions such as asthma. It is well known that peripherally acting opioids may inhibit cough and bronchoconstriction in animals (Adcock *et al.*, 1988). However, little information is as yet available concerning the expression of opioids and their receptors in the airways during inflammation, and it would be of interest to see if the activity of exogenous opioids is enhanced during inflammation of the airways.

Therapeutic possibilities

At one time it was assumed that antagonists of tachykinins or analogues of VIP may have therapeutic application in airway diseases such as asthma. However, it is unlikely that drugs of this type would be a more effective treatment compared to the existing agents and preliminary results suggest that tachykinin antagonists have no significant effect in controlling asthma. However, in contrast tachykinin antagonists appear to improve symptoms of patients with chronic obstructive pulmonary disease (Ichinose *et al.*, 1993). VIP is a relaxant of human airways *in vitro* but it is ineffective by inhalation, probably because of the metabolizing enzymes within the airways. However, even if a stable analogue of VIP was developed it is unlikely that it would have any advantage over existing β-agonist therapy. In addition, its action as a potent vasodilator may lead to adverse side-effects. Furthermore, the absence of VIP receptors in peripheral airways may limit its bronchodilator action and that of any analogues.

In summary, TK receptor antagonists clearly have potential therapeutic usefulness in a number of inflammatory conditions, although their usefulness in the treatment of asthma is in doubt. The results of trials using newly developed non-peptide ligands in such conditions will provide the definitive answers to the pathophysiological role of these peptides.

Acknowledgements

The authors thank Drs Axel Fischer and Wolfgang Kummer for permission to reproduce Fig. 26.4. Both authors are funded by the Wellcome Trust.

References

Absood, A., Ekblad, E., Ekelund, M., Håkanson, R. & Sundler, F. (1992) Helospectin-like peptides in the gastrointestinal tract: immunocytochemical localization and immunohistochemical characterization. *Neuroscience*, **46**, 431–8.

Adcock, I.M., Peters, M., Gelder, C.M., Shirasaki, H., Brown, C.R. & Barnes, P.J. (1993) Increased tachykinin receptor gene expression in asthmatic lung and modulation by steroids. *J. Mol. Endocrinol.*, **11**, 1–7.

Adcock, J.J., Schneider, C. & Smith, T.W. (1988) Effects of codeine, morphine and a novel pentapeptide BW 443C on cough, nociception and ventilation in the unanaesthetised guinea-pig. *Brit. J. Pharmacol.*, **93**, 93–100.

Advenier, C., Naline, E., Toty, L. *et al.* (1992) Effects on the isolated human bronchus of SR 48968, a potent and selective non-peptide antagonist of the neurokinin A (NK_2) receptor. *Am. Rev. Resp. Dis.*, **146**, 1177–81.

Advenier, C., Naline, E., Drapeau, G. & Regoli, D. (1987) Relative potencies of neurokinins in guinea-pig and human bronchus. *Eur. J. Pharmacol.*, **139**, 133–7.

Aguayro, S.M., Kane, M.A., King, T.E., Schwartz, M.I., Grauer, L. & Miller, Y.E. (1989) Increased levels of bombesin-like peptides in the lower respiratory tract of asymptomatic smokers. *J. Clin. Invest.*, **84**, 1105–13.

Altiere, R.J. & Diamond, L. (1985) Effect of α-chymotrypsin on the non-adrenergic non-cholinergic inhibitory system in cat airways. *Eur. J. Pharmacol.*, **114**, 75–8.

Andreev, N. & Dray, A. (1994) Opioids supress spontaneous activity of polymodal nociceptors in rat paw skin induced by ultraviolet irradiation. *Neuroscience*, **58**, 793–8.

Araki, N. & Takagi, K. (1992) Relaxant effect of pituitary adenylate cyclase-activating polypeptide on guinea-pig tracheal smooth muscle. *Eur. J. Pharmacol.*, **216**, 113–17.

Armour, C.L., Johnson, P.R.A. & Black, J.L. (1991) Nedocromil sodium inhibits substance P-induced potentiation of cholinergic neural responses in the isolated innervated rabbit trachea. *J. Auton. Pharmacol.*, **11**, 167–72.

Baraniuk, J., Castellino, S., Lundgren, J. *et al.* (1990a) Neuropeptide Y (NPY) in human nasal mucosa. *Am. J. Respir. Cell Mol. Biol.*, **3**, L223–35.

Baraniuk, J.N., Lundgren, J.D., Goff, J. *et al.* (1990b) Calcitonin gene-related peptide (CGRP) in human nasal mucosa. *Am. J. Physiol.*, **258**, L81–8.

Baraniuk, J.N., Okayama, M., Lundgren, J.D. *et al.* (1990c) Vasoactive intestinal polypeptide (VIP) in human nasal mucosa. *J. Clin. Invest.*, **86**, 825–83.

Baraniuk, J.N., Lundgren, J.D., Goff, J. *et al.* (1990d) Gastrin releasing peptide (GRP) in human nasal mucosa. *J. Clin. Invest.*, **85**, 998–1005.

Barnes, P.J. (1986) Asthma as an axon reflex. *Lancet*, **ii**, 242–4.

Barnes, P.J., Baraniuk, J.N. & Belvisi, M.G. (1991) Neuropeptides in the respiratory tract. *Am. Rev. Resp. Dis.*, **144**, 1187–98.

Barnes, P.J., Belvisi, M.G. & Rogers, D.F. (1990) Modulation of neurogenic inflammation: novel approaches to inflammatory disease. *Trends Pharmacol. Sci.*, **11**, 185–9.

Barnes, P.J. & Dixon, C.M.S. (1984) The effect of inhaled vasoactive intestinal peptide on bronchial reactivity to histamine in humans. *Am. Rev. Resp. Dis.*, **130**, 162–6.

Bartfai, T., Bedecs, K., Land, H. *et al.* (1991) M15: high-affinity chimeric peptide that blocks the neuronal actions of galanin in the hippocampus, locus coeruleus, and spinal cord. *Proc. Nat. Acad. Sci. USA*, **88**, 10961–5.

Bartho, L., Koczan, G. & Maggi, C.A. (1993) Studies on the mechanism of the contractile action of rat calcitonin gene-related peptide and of capsaicin on the guinea-pig ileum. Effect of hCGRP(8–37) and CGRP tachyphylaxis. *Neuropeptides*, **25**, 325–9.

Belvisi, M.G. (1994) Neuropeptides and neurotransmission. In: *Neuropeptides in Respiratory Medicine* (eds M.A. Kaliner, P.J. Barnes, G.H.H. Kunkel & J.N. Baraniuk), pp. 477–500. Marcel Dekker, New York.

Belvisi, M.G. & Bai, T.R. (1994) Inhibitory non-adrenergic non-cholinergic innervation of airways smooth muscle: role of nitric oxide. In: *Airways Smooth Muscle: Structure, Innervation and Neurotransmission* (eds D. Raeburn & M.A. Giemybyez), pp. 157–87. Birkhauser Verlag, Basel.

Belvisi, M.G., Barnes, P.J. & Rogers, D.F. (1990a) Neurogenic inflammation in the airways: characterisation of electrical parameters for vagus nerve stimulation in the guinea-pig. *J. Neurosci. Methods*, **32**, 159–67,

Belvisi, M.G., Stretton, C.D. & Barnes, P.J. (1990b) Modulation of cholinergic neurotransmission in guinea-pig airways by opioids. *Brit. J. Pharmacol.*, **100**, 131–7.

Belvisi, M.G., Chung, K.F., Jackson, D.M. & Barnes, P.J. (1988) Opioid modulation of non-cholinergic neural bronchoconstriction in guinea-pig *in vivo*. *Brit. J. Pharmacol.*, **95**, 413–18.

Belvisi, M.G., Patacchini, R., Barnes, P.J. & Maggi, C.A. (1994) Facilitatory effects of selective agonists for tachykinin receptors on cholinergic neurotransmission: evidence for species differences. *Brit. J. Pharmacol.*, **111**, 103–10.

Belvisi, M.G., Rogers, D.F. & Barnes, P.J. (1989) Neurogenic plasma extravasation inhibition by morphine in guinea-pig airways *in vivo*. *J. Appl. Physiol.*, **66**, 268–72.

Belvisi, M.G., Stretton, C.D. & Barnes, P.J. (1991) Bombesin-induced bronchoconstriction in the guinea-pig: mode of action. *J. Pharmacol. Exp. Ther.*, **255**, 36–41.

Belvisi, M.G., Stretton, C.D., Miura, M. *et al.* (1992a) Inhibitory NANC nerves in human tracheal smooth muscle: a quest for the neurotransmitter. *J. Appl. Physiol.*, **73**, 2505–10.

Belvisi, M.G., Stretton, C.D., Verleden, G.M., Ledingham, S.J.L., Yacoub, M.H. & Barnes, P.J. (1992b) Inhibition of cholinergic neurotransmission in human airways by opioids. *J. Appl. Physiol.*, **72**, 1096–100.

Belvisi, M.G., Stretton, C.D., Yacoub, M.H. & Barnes, P.J. (1992c) Nitric oxide is the endogenous neurotransmitter of bronchodilator nerves in humans. *Eur. J. Pharmacol.*, **210**, 221–2.

Belvisi, M.G., Ward, J.K., Mitchell, J.A. & Barnes, P.J. (1995) Nitric oxide as a neurotransmitter in human airways. *Arch. Int. Pharmacodyn. Thér.*, **329**, 97–110.

Belvisi, M.G., Miura, M., Stretton, C.D. & Barnes, P.J. (1993a) Endogenous vasoactive intestinal peptide and nitric oxide modulate cholinergic neurotransmission in guinea-pig trachea. *Eur. J. Pharmacol.*, **231**, 97–102.

Belvisi, M.G., Ward, J.K., Patel, H.J., Tadjkarimi, S., Yacoub, M.H. & Barnes, P.J. (1993b) μ-Opioids inhibit electrically evoked acetylcholine release in human and guinea-pig trachea. *Am. Rev. Resp. Dis.*, **147**, A502.

Bertrand, C., Nadel, J., Graf, P. & Geppetti, P. (1993a) Capsaicin increases airflow resistance in guinea-pigs *in vivo* by activating both NK_2 and NK_1 tachykinin receptors. *Am. Rev. Resp. Dis.*, **148**, 909–14.

Bertrand, C., Geppetti, P., Baker, J., Yamawaki, I. & Nadel, J.A. (1993b) Role of neurogenic inflammation in antigen-induced vascular extravasation in guinea-pig trachea. *J. Immunol.*, **150**, 1497–85.

Bevan, S. & Szolcsanyi, J. (1990) Sensory neurone-specific actions of capsaicin: mechanisms and applications. *Trends Pharmacol. Sci.*, **11**, 330–3.

Bienenstock, J., Perdue, M., Blennerhassett, M. *et al.* (1988) Inflammatory cells and epithelium: mast cell/nerve interactions in lung *in vitro* and *in vivo*. *Am. Rev. Resp. Dis.*, **138**, 31–4.

Black, J.L., Johnson, P.R.A., Alouan, L. & Armour, C.L. (1990) Neurokinin A with K^+ channel blockade potentiates contraction to electrical stimulation in human bronchus. *Eur. J. Pharmacol.*, **180**, 311–17.

Brain, S.D. & Williams, T.J. (1985) Inflammatory oedema induced by synergism between calcitonin gene-related peptide (CGRP) and mediators of increased vascular permeability. *Brit. J. Pharmacol.*, **86**, 855–60.

Brain, S.D., Williams, T.J., Tippins, J.R., Morris, H.R. & MacIntyre, I. (1985) Calcitonin gene-related peptide is a potent vasodilator. *Nature*, **313**, 54–6.

Braunstein, G., Fajac, I., Lacronique, J. & Frossard, N. (1991) Clinical and inflammatory responses to exogenous tachykinins in allergic rhinitis. *Am. Rev. Resp. Dis.*, **144**, 630–5.

Brave, S.R., Hobbs, A.J., Gibson, A. & Tucker, J.F. (1991) The influence of L-N^G-nitroarginine on field stimulation induced contractions and acetylcholine release in guinea-pig isolated smooth muscle. *Biochem. Biophys. Res. Commun.*, **179**, 1017–22.

Brunelleschi, S., Parenti, A., Ceni, E., Giotti, A. & Fantozzi, R. (1992) Enhanced responsivess of ovalbumin-sensitised guinea-pig alveolar macrophages to tachykinins. *Brit. J. Pharmacol.*, **107**, 964–9.

Brunelleschi, S., Vanni, L., Ledda, F., Giotti, A., Maggi, C.A. & Fantozzi, R. (1990) Tachykinins activate guinea-pig alveolar macrophages; involvement of NK_2 and NK_1 receptors. *Brit. J. Pharmacol.*, **100**, 417–20.

Buckley, T.L., Brain, S.D., Rampart, M. & Williams, T.J. (1991) Time dependent synergistic interactions between the vasodilator neuropeptide calcitonin gene-related peptide and mediators of inflammation. *Brit. J. Pharmacol.*, **103**, 1515–19.

Burcher, E., Mussap, C.J. & Stephenson, J.A. (1994) Autoradiographic localisation of receptors in peripheral tissues. In: *The Tachykinin Receptors* (ed. S.H. Buck), pp. 125–64. Humana Press, New Jersey.

Cadieux, A., Benchekroun, M.T., St Pierre, S. & Fournier, A. (1989) Bronchoconstrictive action of neuropeptide Y (NPY) on isolated guinea-pig airways. *Neuropeptides*, **13**, 215–19.

Cadieux, A., Springall, D.R., Mulderry, P.K. *et al.* (1986) Occurrence, distribution and ontogeny of CGRP immunoreactivity in the rat lower respiratory tract: effect of capsaicin treatment and surgical denervations. *Neuroscience*, **19**, 605–27.

Cambridge, H. & Brain, S.D. (1992) Calcitonin gene-related peptide increases blood flow and potentiates plasma protein extravsation in the rat knee joint. *Brit. J. Pharmacol.*, **106**, 746–50.

Cameron, A.R., Johnston, C.F., Kirkpatrick, C.T. & Kirkpatrick, M.C.A. (1983) The quest for the inhibitory neurotransmitter in bovine tracheal smooth muscle. *Q. J. Exp. Physiol.*, **68**, 413–26.

Cardell, L.-O., Uddman, R., Luts, A. & Sundler, F. (1991) Pituitary adenylate cyclase activating peptide (PACAP) in guinea-pig lung: distribution and dilatory effects. *Regul. Pept.*, **36**, 379–90.

Carstairs, J.R. & Barnes, P.J. (1986) Autoradiographic mapping of substance P receptors in lung. *Eur. J. Pharmacol.*, **127**, 295–6.

Caughy, G.H. (1989) Roles of mast cell tryptase and chymase in airway function. *Am. J. Physiol.*, **257** (*Lung Cell Mol. Physiol.*, **1**), L39–46.

Cauvin, A., Robberecht, P., De Neef, P. *et al.* (1991) Properties and distribution of receptors for pituitary adenylate cyclase activating peptide (PACAP) in rat brain and spinal cord. *Regul. Pept.*, **35**, 161–73.

Cheung, A., Polak, J.M., Bauer, F.E. *et al.* (1985) Distribution of galanin immunoreactivity in the respiratory tract of pig, guinea-pig, rat and dog. *Thorax*, **40**, 889–96.

Chilvers, E.R., Dixon, C.M.S., Yiangou, Y., Bloom, S.R. & Ind, P.W. (1988) Effect of peptide histidine valine on cardiovascular and respiratory function in normal subjects. *Thorax*, **43**, 750–5.

Christofides, N.D., Yiangou, Y., Piper, P.J. *et al.* (1984) Distribution of peptide histidine isoleucine in the mammalian respiratory tract and some aspects on its pharmacology. *Endocrinology*, **115**, 1958–63.

Christophe, J. (1993) Type I receptors for PACAP (a neuropeptide even more important than VIP?). *Biochim. Biophys. Acta*, **1154**, 183–99.

Claing, A., Telemaque, S., Cadieux, A., Fournier, A., Regoli, D. & D'Orleans-Juste, P. (1992) Nonadrenergic and noncholinergic arterial dilatation and venoconstriction are mediated by calcitonin gene-related peptide 1 and neurokinin-1 receptors, respectively, in the mesenteric vasculature of the rat after perivascular nerve stimulation. *J. Pharmacol. Exp. Ther.*, **263**, 1226–30.

Coles, S.J., Said, S.I. & Reid, L.M. (1981) Inhibition by vasoactive intestinal peptide of glucoconjugate and lysozyme secretion by human airways *in vitro*. *Am. Rev. Resp. Dis.*, **124**, 531–6.

Corjay, M.H., Dobrzanski, D.J., Way, J.M. *et al.* (1991) Two distinct bombesin receptor subtypes are expressed and functional in human lung carcinoma cells. *J. Biol. Chem.*, **266**, 18771–9.

Costa, M., Furness, J.B. & Cuello, A.C. (1985) Separate populations of opioid containing neurons in the guinea-pig intestine. *Neuropeptides*, **5**, 445–8.

Cox, C.P., Linden, J. & Said, S.I. (1984) VIP elevates platelet cyclic AMP (cAMP) levels and inhibits *in vitro* platelet activation induced by platelet activating factor (PAF). *Peptides*, **5**, 325–8.

Cutz, E. (1982) Neuroendocrine cells of the lung — an overview of morphological characteristics and development. *Exp. Lung Res.*, **3**, 185–208.

Cutz, E., Chan, W., Track, N.S., Goth, A. & Said, S.I. (1978) Release of vasoactive intestinal polypeptide in mast cells by histamine liberators. *Nature*, **275**, 661–2.

Del Bianco, E., Santicioli, P., Tramontana, M., Maggi, C.A., Cecconi, R. & Geppetti, P. (1991) Different pathways by which extracellular Ca^{2+} promotes calcitonin gene-related peptide release from central terminals of capsaicin-sensitive afferents of guinea-pigs, effect of capsaicin, high K^+ and low pH media. *Brain Res.*, **566**, 46–53.

Dennis, T., Fournier, A., St Pierre, S. & Quirion, R. (1989) Structure activity profile of calcitonin gene-related peptide in peripheral and brain tissues. Evidence for receptor multiplicity. *J. Pharmacol. Exp. Ther.*, **251**, 718–25.

DeRose, V., Robbins, R.A., Snider, R.M. *et al.* (1994) Substance P increases neutrophil adhesion to bronchial epithelial cells. *J. Immunol.*, **152**, 1339–46.

Devillier, P., Acker, G.M., Advenier, C., Marsac, J., Regoli, D. & Frossard, N. (1992) Activation of an epithelial neurokinin NK-1 receptor induces relaxation of rat trachea through release of prostaglandin E_2. *J. Pharmacol. Exp. Ther.*, **263**, 767–72.

Devillier, P., Advenier, C., Drapeau, G., Marsac, J. & Regoli, D. (1988) Comparison of the effects of epithelium removal and of an enkephalinase inhibitor on the neurokinin-induced contractions of guinea-pig isolated trachea. *Brit. J. Pharmacol.*, **94**, 675–84.

Devillier, P., Weill, B., Renoux, M., Menkes, C. & Pradelles, P. (1987) Elevated levels of TK-LI in joint fluids from patients with rheumatic inflammatory diseases. *New Engl. J. Med.*, **314**, 1323.

Dey, R.D., Mitchell, H.W. & Coburn, R.F. (1990) Origianization and development of peptide-containing neurons in the airways. *Am. J. Respir. Cell Mol. Biol.*, **3**, 187–8.

Dey, R.D., Shannon, W.A. & Said, S.I. (1981) Localisation of VIP-immunoreactive nerves in airways and pulmonary vessels of dogs cats and human subjects. *Cell Tissue Res.*, **220**, 231–8.

DiChiara, G. & North, R.A. (1992) Neurobiology of opiate abuse. *Trends Pharmacol. Sci.*, **13**, 185–92.

Dion, S., Rouissi, N., Nantel, F. *et al.* (1990) Receptors for tachykinins in human bronchus and urinary bladder are of the NK-2 type. *Eur. J. Pharmacol.*, **178**, 215–19.

Dray, A., Urban, L. & Dickenson, T. (1994) Pharmacology of chronic pain. *Trends Pharmacol. Sci.*, **15**, 190–7.

Dusser, D.J., Umeno, E., Graf, P.D., Djokie, T., Borson, D.B. & Nadel, J.A. (1988) Airway neutral endopeptidase-like activity modulates tachykinin-induced bronchoconstriction *in vivo*. *J. Appl. Physiol.*, **65**, 2585–91.

Edwards, R.M., Stack, E.J. & Trizna, W. (1991) Calcitonin gene-related peptide stimulated adenylate cyclase and relaxes intracerebral arterioles. *J. Pharmacol. Exp. Ther.*, **257**, 1020–5.

Ekblad, E., Håkanson, R., Sundler, F. & Wahlestedt, C. (1985) Galanin: neuromodulatory and direct contractile effects on smooth muscle preparations. *Brit. J. Pharmacol.*, **86**, 241–6.

Ellis, J.L. & Farmer, S.G. (1989a) The effects of vasoactive intestinal peptide (VIP) antagonists, and VIP and peptide histidine isoleucine antisera on non-adrenergic, non-cholinergic relaxations of tracheal smooth muscle. *Brit. J. Pharmacol.*, **96**, 513–20.

Ellis, J.L. & Farmer, S.G. (1989b) Effects of peptidases on non-adrenergic, non-cholinergic inhibitory responses of tracheal smooth muscle: a comparison with effects on VIP- and PHI-induced relaxation. *Brit. J. Pharmacol.*, **96**, 521–6.

Ellis, J.L. & Farmer, S.G. (1989c) Modulation of cholinergic neurotransmission by vasoactive intestinal peptide and histidine isoleucine in guinea-pig tracheal smooth muscle. *Pulmon. Pharmacol.*, **2**, 107–12.

Ellis, J.L. & Undem, B.J. (1992) Antigen-induced enhancement of non-cholinergic contractile responses to vagus nerve and electrical field stimulation in guinea-pig isolated trachea. *J. Pharmacol. Exp. Ther.*, **262**, 646–53.

Ellis, J.L., Undem, B.J., Kays, J.S., Ghanekar, S.V., Barthlow, H.G. & Buckner, C.K. (1993) Pharmacological examination of receptors mediating contractile responses to tachykinins in airways isolated from human, guinea-pig and hamster. *J. Pharmacol. Exp. Ther.*, **267**, 95–101.

Erdös, E.G. & Skidgel, R.A. (1989) Neutral endopeptidase 24.11 (enkephalinase) and regulatory peptide hormones. *FASEB J.*, **3**, 145–51.

Escott, K.J. & Brain, S.D. (1993) Effect of a calcitonin gene-related peptide antagonist ($CGRP_{8-37}$) on skin vasodilatation and oedema induced by stimulation of the rat saphenous nerve. *Brit. J. Pharmacol.*, **110**, 772–9.

Evans, C.J., Hammond, D.C. & Friederickson, R.C.A. (1988) The opioid peptides. In: *The Opioid Receptors* (ed. G.W. Pasternak), pp. 23–71. The Human Press, New Jersey.

Evans, T.W., Rogers, D.F., Aursudkij, B., Chung, K.F. & Barnes, P.J. (1989) Regional and time-dependent effects of inflammatory mediators on airway microvascular permeability in guinea-pigs. *Clin. Sci.*, **76**, 479–85.

Fahrenkrug, J. (1993) Transmitter role of vasoactive intestinal peptide. *Pharmacol. Toxicol.*, **72**, 354–63.

Fields, H.L., Emson, P.C., Leigh, B.K., Gilbert, R.F.T. & Iversen, L.L. (1980) Multiple opiate receptor sites on primary afferent fibres. *Nature*, **284**, 351–3.

Fischer, A., Kummer, W., Couraud, J.-Y., Adler, D., Branscheid, D. & Heym, C. (1992) Immunohistochemical localisation of receptors for vasoactive intestinal peptide and substance P in human trachea. *Lab. Invest.*, **67**, 387–93.

Fisher, J.T., Anderson, J.W. & Waldron, M.A. (1993) Nonadrenergic noncholinergic neurotransmitter of feline trachealis: VIP or nitric oxide? *J. Appl. Physiol.*, **114**, 75–8.

Foda, H.D. & Said, S.I. (1989) Helodermin a C-terminally extended VIP-like peptide, evokes long-lasting tracheal relaxation. *Biomed. Res.*, **10**, 107–10.

Fong, T.M., Huang, R.R.C. & Strader, C.D. (1992) Localisation of agonist and antagonist binding domains in the human neurokinin-1 receptor. *J. Biol. Chem.*, **267**, 25664–7.

Foreman, J. & Jordan, C.C. (1983) Histamine release and vascular changes induced by neuropeptides. *Agents Actions*, **13**, 105–16.

Foreman, J.C., Jordan, C.C., Oehme, P. & Renner, H. (1983) Structure–activity relationships for some substance P-related peptides that cause wheal and flare reactions in human skin. *J. Physiol.*, **335**, 449–65.

Foulon, D.M., Champion, E., Masson, P., Rodger, I.W. & Jones, T.R. (1993) NK_1 and NK_2 receptors mediate tachykinin and resiniferatoxin-induced bronchospasm in guinea-pigs. *Am. Rev. Resp. Dis.*, **148**, 915–21.

Fox, A.J., Barnes, P.J., Urban, L. & Dray, A. (1993) An *in vitro* study of the properties of single vagal afferents innervating guinea-pig airways. *J. Physiol.*, **469**, 21–35.

Fox, A.J., Dray, A. & Barnes, P.J. (1995a) The activity of prostaglandins and platelet activating factor on single airway sensory fibres of the guinea-pig *in vitro*. *Am. J. Resp. Crit. Care Med.*, **151**, A110.

Fox, A.J., Urban, L., Barnes, P.J. & Dray, A. (1995b) The effects of capsazepine against capsaicin- and proton-evoked excitation of single airway C-fibres and vagus nerve from the guinea-pig. *Neuroscience*, **67**, 741–52.

Franco-Cereceda, A. (1988) Calcitonin gene-related peptide and tachykinins in relation to local sensory control of cardiac contractility and coronary vascular tone. *Acta Physiol. Scand.*, **569**, 1–63.

Fransden, E.K., Krishna, Y. & Said, S.I. (1978) Vasoactive intestinal peptide promotes cyclic adenosine 3′5′-monophosphate accumulation in guinea-pig trachea. *Brit. J. Pharmacol.*, **62**, 367–9.

Frossard, N. & Barnes, P.J. (1987) μ-Opioid receptors modulate noncholinergic constrictor nerves in guinea-pig airways. *Eur. J. Pharmacol.*, **141**, 519–21.

Frossard, N. & Barnes, P.J. (1991) Effect of tachykinins in small airways. *Neuropeptides*, **19**, 157–61.

Fuller, R.W., Dixon, C.M.S. & Barnes, P.J. (1985) The bronchoconstrictor response to inhaled capsaicin in humans. *J. Appl. Physiol.*, **85**, 1080–4.

Galves, A., Gimenez-Gallego, G., Reuben, J.P. *et al.* (1990) Purification and characterisation of a unique, potent, peptidyl probe for the high conductance calcium-activated potassium channel from venom of the scorpion *Buthus tamulus*. *J. Biol. Chem.*, **265**, 11083–90.

Gashi, A.A., Borson, D.B., Finkbeiner, W.E., Nadel, J.A. & Basbaum, C.B. (1986) Neuropeptides degranulate serous cells of ferret tracheal glands. *Am. J. Physiol.*, **251**, C223–9.

Geppetti, P., deRossi, M., Midne, M.C., Renzi, D. & Amenta, F. (1988) Age related changes in vasoactive intestinal peptide levels and distribution in rat lung. *J. Neurotrans.*, **74**, 1–10.

Ghatei, M.A., Sheppard, M.N., O'Shaunessy, D.J. *et al.* (1982) Regulatory peptides in the mammalian respiratory tract. *Endocrinology*, **111**, 1248–54.

Ghatei, M.A., Sheppard, M.N., Henzen-Logman, S., Blank, M.A., Polak, J.M. & Bloom, S.R. (1983) Bombesin and vasoactive intestinal peptide in the developing lung: marked changes in acute respiratory distress syndrome. *J. Clin. Endocrinol. Metab.*, **57**, 1226–32.

Gibbins, I.L., Furness, J.B., & Costa, M. (1987) Pathway-specific patterns of the co-existance of substance P, calcitonin gene-related peptide, cholecystokinin and dynorphin in neurons. Of the root ganglia of the guinea-pig. *Cell Tissue Res.*, **248**, 417–37.

Gimenez-Gallego, G., Navia, M.A., Reuben, J.P., Katz, G.M., Kaczorowski, G.M. & Garcia, M.L. (1988) Purification, sequence and model structure of charybdotoxin, a potent selective inhibitor of calcium-activated potassium channels. *Proc. Nat. Acad. Sci. USA*, **85**, 3329–33.

Giuliani, S., Amann, R., Papini, A.M., Maggi, C.A. & Meli, A. (1989) Modulatory action of galanin on responses due to antidromic activation of peripheral terminals of capsaicin-sensitive sensory nerves. *Eur. J. Pharmacol.*, **163**, 91–6.

Giuliani, S., Wimalawansa, S.J. & Maggi, C.A. (1992) Involvement of multiple receptors in the biological effects of calcitonin gene-related peptide and amylin in rat and guinea-pig preparations. *Brit. J. Pharmacol.*, **107**, 510–15.

Goetzl, E.J., Sreedharan, S.P. & Turck, S.W. (1988) Structurally distinctive vasoactive intestinal peptides from rat basophilic leukemia cells. *J. Biol. Chem.*, **263**, 9083–8.

Goldie, R.G. (1990) Receptors in asthmatic airways. *Am. Rev. Resp. Dis.*, **141**, S151–6.

Gottschall, P.E., Tatsuno, I., Miyata, A. & Arimura, A. (1990) Characterization and distribution of binding sites for the hypothalamic peptide, pituitary adenylate cyclase-activating polypeptide. *Endocrinology*, **127**, 272–7.

Gozes, I. & Brenneman, D.E. (1993) Neuropeptides as growth and differentiation factors in general and VIP in particular. *J. Mol. Neurosci.*, **4**, 1–9.

Grandordy, B.M., Frossard, N., Rhoden, K.J. & Barnes, P.J. (1988) Tachykinin-induced phosphoinositide breakdown in airway smooth muscle and epithelium: relationship to contraction. *Mol. Pharmacol.*, **33**, 515–19.

Gray, D.W. & Marshall, I. (1992) Nitric oxide synthase inhibitors attenuate calcitonin gene-related peptide endothelium-dependent relaxation in rat aorta. *Eur. J. Pharmacol.*, **212**, 37–42.

Gridelli, B., Buffa, R., Salvini, P. *et al.* (1982) Lack of VIP-immunoreactive nerves in oesophageal achalasia. *Ital. J. Gastroenterol.*, **14**, 211–6.

Grundemar, L., Grundstom, N., Johansson, I.G.M., Andersson, R.G.G. & Håkanson, R. (1990) Supression by neuropeptide Y of capsaicin-sensitive sensory nerve mediated contraction in guinea-pig airways. *Brit. J. Pharmacol.*, **99**, 473–6.

Grundemar, L., Widmark, E., Waldeck, B. & Håkanson, R. (1988) Neuropeptide Y: pre-junctional inhibition of vagally-induced contraction in the guinea-pig trachea. *Regul. Pept.*, **23**, 309–14.

Håkanson, R. & Wahlestadt, C. (1987) Neuropeptide Y acts via prejunctional (Y_2) and post-junctional (Y_1) receptors. *Neuroscience*, **22**, S679.

Hall, A.K., Barnes, P.J., Meldrum, L.A. & Maclagan, J. (1989) Facilitation by tachykinins of neurotransmission in guinea-pig pulmonary parasympathetic nerves. *Brit. J. Pharmacol.*, **97**, 274–80.

Hall, J.M. (1994) Receptor function in the periphery. In: *The Tachykinin Receptors* (ed. S.H. Buck), pp. 515–80. Humana Press, New Jersey.

Harmer, T. & Lutz, E. (1994) Multiple receptors for PACAP and VIP. *Trends Pharmacol. Sci.*, **15**, 97–9.

Hassan, A.H.S., Ableitner, A., Stein, C. & Herz, A. (1993) Inflammation of the rat paw enhances axonal transport of opioid receptors in the sciatic nerve and increases their density in the inflamed tissue. *Neuroscience*, **55**, 185–95.

Heinz-Erian, P., Dey, R.D. & Said, S.I. (1985) Deficient vasoactive intestinal peptide innervation in sweat glands of cystic fibrosis patients. *Science*, **229**, 1407–9.

Helme, R.D., Koschorke, G.M. & Zimmerman, M. (1986) Immunoreactive substance P release from skin nerves in the rat by noxious thermal stimulation. *Neurosci. Letts.*, **63**, 295–9.

Herzog, H., Hort, Y.J., Ball, H.J., Hayes, G., Shine, J. & Selbie, L.A. (1992) Cloned human neuropeptide Y receptor couples to different second messenger systems. *Proc. Nat. Acad. Sci. USA*, **89**, 5794–8.

Hirayama, Y., Lai, Y.-H., Barnes, P.J. & Rogers, D.F. (1993) Effects of two novel tachykinin antagonists, FK224 and FK888, on neurogenic airway plasma exudation, bronchoconstriction and systemic hypotension in guinea-pigs *in vivo*. *Brit. J. Pharmacol.*, **108**, 844–51.

Holzer, P. (1988) Local effector functions of capsaicin-sensitive sensory nerve endings; involvement of tachykinins, calcitonin gene-related peptide and other neuropeptides. *Neuroscience*, **24**, 739–68.

Holzer, P. (1991) Capsaicin, cellular targets, mechanisms of action, and selectivity for thin sensory neurones. *Pharmacol. Rev.*, **43**, 143–201.

Honda, I., Kohrogi, H., Yamaguchi, T., Ando, M. & Araki, S. (1991) Enkephalinase inhibitor potentiates substance P and capsaicin-induced bronchial smooth muscle contraction in humans. *Am. Rev. Resp. Dis.*, **143**, 1416–18.

Hua, X.-Y., Saria, A., Gamse, R., Theodorsson-Norheim, E., Brodin, E. & Lundberg, J.M. (1986) Capsaicin induced release of multiple tachykinins (substance P, neurokinin A and eledoisin-like material) from guinea-pig spinal cord and ureter. *Neuroscience*, **19**, 313–19.

Hua, X.-Y. & Yaksh, T.L. (1993) Pharmacology of the effects of bradykinin, serotonin and histamine on the release of cacitonin gene-related peptide from C-fiber terminals in the rat trachea. *J. Neurosci.*, **13**, 1947–53.

Hughes, J., Smith, T., Morgan, B. & Fothergill, L. (1975) Purification and properties of enkephalin—the possible endogenous ligand for the morphine receptor. *Life Sci.*, **16**, 1753–8.

Hughes, S.R. & Brain, S.D. (1991) A calcitonin gene-related peptide (CGRP) antagonist (CGRP8–37) inhibits microvascular responses induced by CGRP and capsaicin in skin. *Brit. J. Pharmacol.*, **104**, 738–42.

Hughes, S.R. & Brain, S.D. (1994) Nitric oxide dependent release of vasodilator quantities of calcitonin gene-related peptide from capsaicin-sensitive nerves in rabbit skin. *Brit. J. Pharmacol.*, **111**, 425–30.

Hultgårdh-Nilsson, A., Nilsson, J., Jonzon, B. & Dalsgaard, C.-J. (1988) Growth-inhibitory properties of vasoactive intestinal polypeptide. *Regul. Pept.*, **22**, 267–72.

Ichinose, M., Katsumata, U., Kikuchi, R. *et al.* (1993) Effect of tachykinin receptor antagonist on chronic bronchitis patients. *Am. Rev. Resp. Dis.*, **147**, A318.

Ichinose, M., Nakajima, N., Takahashi, T., Yamauchi, H., Inoue, H. & Takishima, T. (1992) Protection against bradykinin-induced bronchoconstriction in asthmatic patients by neurokinin receptor antagonist. *Lancet*, **340**, 1248–51.

Ireland, S.J., Bailey, F., Cook, A., Hagan, R.M., Jordan, C.C. & Stephens-Smith, M. (1991) Receptors mediating tachykinin-induced contractile responses in guinea-pig trachea. *Brit. J. Pharmacol.*, **103**, 1463–9.

Irvin, C.G., Boileau, R., Tremblay, J., Martin, R.R. & Macklem, P.T. (1980) Bronchodilation: non-cholinergic, non-adrenergic mediator demonstrated *in vivo* in the cat. *Science*, **207**, 791–2.

Ishihara, T., Shigemoto, R., Mori, K., Takahashi, K. & Nagata, S. (1992) Functional expression and tissue distribution of a novel receptor for vasoactive intestinal polypeptide. *Neuron*, **8**, 811–19.

Ito, Y. & Hakoda, H. (1990) Modulation of cholinergic neurotransmission by VIP, VIP-antiserum and VIP antagonists in dog and cat trachea: VIP plays a role of 'double braking' in bronchoconstriction. *Agents Actions*, **31**, 197–203.

Ito, Y. & Takeda, K. (1982) Non-adrenergic inhibitory nerves and putative transmitters in the smooth muscle of cat trachea. *J. Physiol.*, **330**, 497–511.

Jancso, N., Jancso-Gabor, A. & Szolcsanyi, J. (1968) The role of sensory nerve endings in neurogenic inflammation induced in human skin and in the eye and paw of the rat. *Brit. J. Pharmacol.*, **32**, 32–41.

Janiszewski, J., Bienenstock, J. & Blennerhassett, M.G. (1992) Mast cells show electrophysiological response to very low levels of substance P without degranulation. *FASEB J.*, **6**, A1613.

Jeanjean, A.P., Moussaoui, S.M., Maloteaux, J.-M. & Laudron, P.M. (1995) Interleukin-1β induced long-term increase of axonally transported opiate receptors and substance P. *Neuroscience*, **68**, 151–7.

Johnson, A.R., Ashton, J., Schulz, W.W. & Erdos, E.G. (1985) Neutral metalloendopeptidase in human lung tissue and cultured cells. *Am. Rev. Resp. Dis.*, **132**, 564–8.

Joos, G.F., Germonpre, P.R., Kipps, J.C., Peleman, R.A. & Pauwels, R.A. (1994) Sensory neuropeptides and the lower airways: present state and future directions. *Eur. Resp. J.*, **7**, 1161–71.

Joos, G.F. & Pauwels, R.A. (1993) The *in vivo* effect of tachykinins on airway mast cells of the rat. *Am. Rev. Resp. Dis.*, **148**, 922–6.

Joos, G.F., Pauwels, R. & Van der Straeten, M. (1987) The effect of inhaled substance P and neurokinin A on the airways of normal and asthmatic subjects. *Thorax*, **42**, 779–83.

Ju, G., Hokfelt, T., Brodin, E. *et al.* (1987) Primary sensory neurons of the rat showing calcitonin gene-related peptide immunoreactivity and their relation to substance P-, somatostatin-, vasoactive intestinal polypeptide- and cholecystokinin-immunoreactive cells. *Cell Tissue Res.*, **247**, 417–31.

Kannan, M.S. & Johnson, D.E. (1992) Nitric oxide mediates the neural non-adrenergic, non-cholinergic relaxation of pig tracheal smooth muscle. *Am. J. Physiol.*, **262**, L511–14.

Karlsson, J.-A., Zackrisson, C. & Lundberg, J.M. (1991) Hyperresponsiveness to tussive stimuli in cigarette-smoke-exposed guinea-pigs: a role for capsaicin-sensitive, calcitonin gene-related peptide-containing nerves. *Acta Physiol. Scand.*, **141**, 445–54.

Katayama, M., Nadel, J.A., Bunnett, N.W., Di Maria, G.U., Haxhiu, M. & Borson, D.B. (1991) Catabolism of calcitonin gene-related peptide and substance P by neutral endopeptidase. *Peptides*, **12**, 563–6.

Kroegel, C., Giembycz, M.A. & Barnes, P.J. (1990) Characterisation of eosinophil activation by peptides. Differential effect of substance P, melittin and f-Met-Leu-Phe. *J. Immunol.*, **145**, 2581–7.

Kummer, W., Fischer, A., Kurkowski, R. & Heym, C. (1992) The sensory and sympathetic innervation of guinea-pig lung and trachea as studied by retrograde neuronal tracing and double-labelling immunohistochemistry. *Neuroscience*, **49**, 715–37.

Kuo, H.-P., Rhode, J.A.L., Barnes, P.J. & Rogers, D.F. (1990) Capsaicin and sensory neuropeptide stimulation of goblet cell secretion in guinea-pig trachea. *J. Physiol.*, **431**, 629–41.

Kuo, H.-P., Rhode, J.A.L., Barnes, P.J. & Rogers, D.F. (1992) Opioid inhibition of neurogenic goblet cell secretion: differential effects on cigarette smoke, capsaicin and electrically induced responses in guinea-pig trachea *in vitro*. *Brit. J. Pharmacol.*, **105**, 361–6.

Kurian, S.S., Blank, M.A. & Sheppard, M.N. (1983) Vasoactive intestinal polypeptide (VIP) in vasomotor rhinitis. *Clin. Biochem.*, **11**, 425–7.

Lacroix, J.S., Änggård, A., Hökfelt, T., O'Hare, T., Fahrenkrug, J. & Lundberg, J.M. (1990) Neuropeptide Y: presence in sympathetic and parasympathetic innervation of the nasal mucosa. *Cell Tissue Res.*, **259**, 119–28.

Laitinen, A., Partanen, M., Hervonen, A., Pelto-Huikko, M. & Laitinen, L.A. (1985) VIP like immunoreactive nerves in the human respiratory tract. *Histochemistry*, **82**, 313–19.

Laitinen, L.A., Laitinen, A., Salonen, R.O. & Widdicombe, J.G. (1987) Vascular actions of airway neuropeptides. *Am. Rev. Resp. Dis.*, **136**, 59–64.

Lam, F.Y. & Ferrell, W.R. (1989) Inhibition of carageenan induced inflammation in the rat knee joint by substance P antagonist. *Ann. Rheum. Dis.*, **48**, 928–32.

Lam, F.Y. & Ferrell, W.R. (1993) Effects and interactions of naturally occurring neuropeptides on blood flow in the rat knee joint. *Brit. J. Pharmacol.*, **108**, 694–9.

Leblanc, G.G., Trimmer, B.A. & Landis, S.C. (1987) Neuropeptide Y-like immunoreactivity in rat cranial parasympathetic neurons: coexistence with vasoactive intestinal peptide and choline acetyltransferase. *Proc. Nat. Acad. Sci. USA*, **84**, 3511–17.

Lee, L.Y. & Morton, R.F. (1993) Histamine enhances vagal pulmonary C-fiber responses to capsaicin and lung inflammation. *Resp. Physiol.*, **93**, 83–96.

Lei, Y.-H., Barnes, P.J. & Rogers, D.F. (1992) Inhibition of neurogenic plasma exudation in guinea-pig airways by CP-96,345, a new non-peptide NK_1 receptor antagonist. *Brit. J. Pharmacol.*, **105**, 261–2.

Lembeck, J. & Donnerer, J. (1985) Opioid control of the function of primary afferent substance P fibres. *Eur. J. Pharmacol.*, **114**, 241–6.

Lembeck, F., Donnerer, J. & Bartho, L. (1982) Inhibition of neurogenic vasodilatation and plasma extravasation by substance P antagonists, somatostatin and (D-Met^2,Pro^5)enkephalinamide. *Eur. J. Pharmacol.*, **85**, 171–6.

Lembeck, F., Donnerer, J., Tsuchiya, M. & Nagahisa, H. (1992) The non-peptide tachykinin antagonist, CP-96,345, is a potent inhibitor of neurogenic inflammation. *Brit. J. Pharmacol.*, **105**, 527–30.

Li, C.G. & Rand, M.J. (1991) Evidence that part of the NANC relaxant response of guinea-pig trachea to electrical field stimulation is mediated by nitric oxide. *Brit. J. Pharmacol.*, **102**, 91–4.

Lindskog, S., Ahrén, B., Land, T., Langel, Ü. & Bartfai, T. (1992) The novel high-affinity antagonist, galantide, blocks the galanin-mediated inhibition of glucose mediated inhibition of glucose-induced insulin secretion. *Eur. J. Pharmacol.*, **210**, 183–8.

Litwin, D.K., Claypool, W.D., Onal, E., Foda, H.D. & Said, S.I. (1989) Vasoactive intestinal polypeptide inhibits rat alveolar macrophage phagocytosis. *Am. Rev. Resp. Dis.*, A158.

Lotvall, J.O., Skoogh, B.-E., Barnes, P.J. & Chung, K.F. (1990) Effects of aerosolised substance P on lung resistance in guinea-pigs: a comparison between inhibition of neutral endopeptidase and angiotensin-converting enzyme. *Brit. J. Pharmacol.*, **100**, 69–72.

Lotz, M., Carson, D.A. & Vaughan, J.H. (1987) Substance P activation of human synovioctyes: neural pathway in pathogenesis of arthritis. *Science*, **235**, 893–6.

Lotz, M., Vaughan, J.H. & Carson, D.A. (1988) Effect of neuropeptides on production of inflammatory cytokines by human monocytes. *Science*, **241**, 1218–20.

Lou, Y.-P., Lee, L.-Y., Satoh, H. & Lundberg, J.M. (1993) Postjunctional inhibitory effect of the NK_2 receptor antagonist SR 48968 on sensory NANC bronchoconstriction in the guinea-pig. *Brit. J. Pharmacol.*, **109**, 765–73.

Lundberg, J.M., Hokfelt, T., Martling, C.R., Saria, A. & Cuello, C. (1984a) Substance P-immunoreactive sensory nerves in the lower respiratory tract of various mammals including man. *Cell Tissue Res.*, **236**, 251–6.

Lundberg, J.M., Fahrenkrug, J., Hökfelt, T. *et al.* (1984b) Co-existence of peptide HI (PHI) and VIP in nerves regulating blood flow and bronchial smooth muscle tone in various mammals including man. *Peptides*, **5**, 593–606.

Lundberg, J.M., Hökfelt, T., Schultzberg, M., Uvnäs-Wallensten, K., Köhler, C. & Said, S.I. (1979) Occurrence of vasoactive intestinal polypeptide (VIP)-like immunoreactivity in certain cholinergic neurons in the rat: evidence from combined immunohistochemical and acetylcholinesterase staining. *Neuroscience*, **4**, 1539–59.

Lundberg, J.M., Saria, A., Brodin, E., Rosell, S. & Folkers, K. (1983) A substance P antagonist inhibits vagally induced increase in vascular permeability and bronchial smooth muscle contraction in the guinea-pig. *Proc. Nat. Acad. Sci. USA*, **80**, 1120–4.

Lundblad, L., Ånggard, A., Saria, A. & Lundberg, J.M. (1987) Neuropeptide Y and non-adrenergic sympathetic vascular control of the cat nasal mucosa. *J. Auton. Nerv. Syst.*, **20**, 189–97.

Luts, A., Absood, A., Uddman, R., Håkanson, R. & Sundler, F. (1991) Chemical coding of endocrine cells of the airways: presence of helodermin-like peptides. *Cell Tissue Res.*, **265**, 425–33.

Luts, A. & Sundler, F. (1989) Peptide containing nerve fibers in the respiratory tract of the ferret. *Cell Tissue Res.*, **258**, 259–67.

Luts, A., Uddman, R., Alam, P., Basterra, J. & Sundler, F. (1993) Peptide-containing nerve fibers in human airways: distribution and coexistence pattern. *Int. Arch. Allergy Immunol.*, **101**, 52–60.

Lutz, E.M., Sheward, W.J., West, K.M., Morrow, J.A., Fink, G. & Harmer, A.J. (1993) The VIP 2 receptor: molecular characterisation of a cDNA encoding a novel receptor for vasoactive intestinal peptide. *FEBS Letts.*, **334**, 3–8.

McCormack, D.G., Salonen, R.O. & Barnes, P.J. (1989) Effect of sensory neuropeptides on canine bronchial and pulmonary vessels *in vitro*. *Life Sci.*, **45**, 2405.

McDonald, D.M. (1988) Neurogenic inflammation in the rat trachea. I. Changes in venules, leukocytes and epithelial cells. *J. Neurocytol.*, **17**, 583–603.

McQueen, D.S., Iggo, A., Birrell, G.J. & Grubb, B.D. (1991) Effects of paracetamol and aspirin on neural activity of joint mechanonociceptors in adjucant arthritis. *Brit. J. Pharmacol.*, **104**, 178–82.

Maggi, C.A. (1991a) The pharmacology of the efferent function of sensory nerves. *J. Auton. Pharmacol.*, **11**, 173–208.

Maggi, C.A. (1991b) The role of peptides in the regulation of the micturition reflex: an update. *Gen. Pharmacol.*, **22**, 1–24.

Maggi, C.A., Patacchini, R., Perretti, F. *et al.* (1990) The effect of thiorphan and epithelium removal on contractions and tachykinin release produced by activation of capsaicin-sensitive afferents in the guinea-pig isolated bronchus. *Naunyn-Schmiedeberg's Arch. Pharmacol.*, **341**, 74–9.

Maggi, C.A., Guiliani, S., Ballati, L. *et al.* (1991) *In vivo* evidence for tachykininergic transmission using a new NK-2 receptor-selective antagonists, MEN 10,376. *J. Pharmacol. Exp. Ther.*, **257**, 1172–8.

Maggi, C.A., Patacchini, R., Rovero, P. & Giachetti, A. (1993) Tachykinin receptors and tachykinin receptor antagonists. *J. Auton. Pharmacol.*, **13**, 23–93.

Mak, J.C.M. & Barnes, P.J. (1988) Autoradiographic localisation of calcitonin gene-related peptide binding sites in human and guinea-pig lung. *Peptides*, **9**, 957–64.

Mantyh, C.R., Gates, T.S., Zimmerman, R.P. *et al.* (1988) Receptor binding sites for substance P, but not substance K or neuromedin K, are expressed in high concentrations by arterioles, venules and lymph nodes in surgical specimens obtained from patients with ulcerative colitis and Crohn's disease. *Proc. Nat. Acad. Sci. USA*, **85**, 3235–9.

Manzini, S. (1992) Bronchodilatation by tachykinins and capsaicin in the mouse main bronchus. *Brit. J. Pharmacol.*, **105**, 968–72.

Marasco, W.A., Showell, H.J. & Becker, E.L. (1981) Substance P binds to formylpeptide chemotaxis receptor on the rabbit neutrophil. *Biophys. Biochem. Res. Commun.*, **99**, 1065–72.

Martin, J., Prystowski, M.B. & Angeletti, R.H. (1987) Preproenkephalin mRNA in T-cells, macrophages and mast cells. *J. Neurosci. Res.*, **18**, 82–7.

Martin, J.G., Wang, A., Zacour, M. & Biggs, D.F. (1990) The effects of vasoactive intestinal polypeptide on cholinergic neurotransmission in an isolated innervated guinea-pig tracheal preparation. *Resp. Physiol.*, **79**, 111–12,

Martling, C.R., Theodorsson-Norheim, E. & Lundberg, J.M. (1987) Occurrence and effects of multiple tachykinins: substance P, neurokinin A and neuropeptide K in human lower airways. *Life Sci.*, **40**, 1633–43.

Maruno, K. & Said, S.I. (1993) Inhibition of human airway smooth muscle cell proliferation by vasoactive intestinal peptide (VIP). *Am. Rev. Resp. Dis.*, **147**, A253.

Matran, R., Alving, K., Martling, C.-R., Lacroix, J.S. & Lundberg, J.M. (1989a) Vagally mediated vasodilatation by motor and sensory nerves in the tracheal and bronchial circulation of the pig. *Acta Physiol. Scand.*, **135**, 29–37.

Matran, R., Alving, K., Martling, C.R., Lacroix, J.S. & Lundberg, J.M. (1989b) Effects of neuropeptides and capsaicin on tracheobronchial blood flow in the pig. *Acta Physiol. Scand.*, **135**, 335–42.

Matran, R., Martling, C.-R. & Lundberg, L.M. (1989c) Inhibition of cholinergic and non-adrenergic, non-cholinergic bronchoconstriction in the guinea-pig mediated by neuropeptide Y and α_2-adrenoceptors and opiate receptors. *Eur. J. Pharmacol.*, **163**, 15–23.

Matsuse, T., Thompson, R.J., Chen, X.-R., Salari, H. & Schellenberg, R.R. (1991) Capsaicin inhibits airway hyperresponsiveness but not lipoxygenase activity or eosinophilia after repeated aerosolised antigen in guinea-pigs. *Am. Rev. Resp. Dis.*, **144**, 368–72.

Matsuzaki, Y., Hamasaki, Y. & Said, S.I. (1980) Vasoactive intestinal peptide: a possible transmitter of non-adrenergic relaxation of guinea-pig airways. *Science*, **210**, 1252–3.

Michel, M.C. (1991) Receptors for neuropeptide Y: multiple subtypes and multiple second messengers. *Trends Pharmacol. Sci.*, **12**, 389–94.

Michoud, M.C., Amyot, R., Jeanneret-Grosjean, A. & Couture, J. (1987) Reflex decrease of histamine-induced bronchoconstriction after laryngeal stimulation in humans. *Am. Rev. Resp. Dis.*, **136**, 616–22.

Miller, R.J. (1990a) Receptor-mediated regulation of calcium channels and neurotransmitter release. *FASEB J.*, **4**, 3291–9.

Miller, Y.E. (1990b) Bombesin-like peptides: from frog skin to human lung. *Am. Rev. Resp. Dis.*, **3**, 189–90.

Minkes, R.K., McMahon, T.J., Hood, J.S. *et al.* (1992) Differential effects of PACAP and VIP on the pulmonary and hindquarters vascular beds of the cat. *J. Appl. Physiol.*, **72**, 1212–17.

Miura, M., Belvisi, M.G., Stretton, C.D., Yacoub, M.H. & Barnes, P.J. (1992) Role of K^+ channels in the modulation of cholinergic neural responses in guinea-pig and human airways. *J. Physiol.*, **445**, 1–15.

Miura, M., Belvisi, M.G., Ward, J.K. & Barnes, P.J. (1993) Role of Ca^{2+}-activated K^+ channels in opioid-induced pre-junctional modulation of airway sensory nerves. *Am. Rev. Resp. Dis.*, **147**, A815.

Miyata, A., Arimura, A., Dahl, R.R. *et al.* (1989) Isolation of a novel PACAP-38 residue hypothalamic polypeptide which stimulates adenylate cyclase in pituitary cells. *Biochem. Biophys., Res. Commun.*, **164**, 567–74.

Miyata, A., Jiang, L., Dahl, R.D. *et al.* (1990) Isolation of a neuropeptide corresponding to the N-terminal 27 residues of the pituitary adenylate cyclase activating polypeptide with 38 residues (PACAP38). *Biochem. Biophys. Res. Commun.*, **170**, 643–8.

Miyayasu, K., Mak, J.C.W., Nishikawa, M. & Barnes, P.J. (1993) Characterisation of guinea-pig pulmonary neurokinin type 1 receptors using a novel antagonist ligand, [^{3}H]FK888. *Mol. Pharmacol.*, **44**, 539–44.

Morice, A.H., Unwin, R.J. & Sever, P.S. (1984) Vasoactive intestinal peptide as a bronchodilator in asthmatic subjects. *Peptides*, **5**, 439–40.

Moskowitz, M.A. (1992) Neurogenic versus vascular mechanisms of sumatriptan and ergot alkaloids in migraine. *Trends Pharmacol. Sci.*, **13**, 307–11.

Mutt, V. & Said, S.I. (1974) Structure of the porcine vasoactive intestinal octacosapeptide. The amino acid sequence. Use of kallikrein in its determination. *Eur. J. Biochem.*, **42**, 581–9.

Naline, E., Devillier, P., Drapeau, G. *et al.* (1989) Characterisation of neurokinin effects and receptor selectivity in human isolated bronchi. *Am. Rev. Resp. Dis.*, **140**, 679–86.

Nohr, D. & Weihe, E. (1988) Light microscopic immunohistochemistry reveals species-dependent presence of tachykinins in intrinsic neurons in the mammalian respiratory tract. *Regul. Pept.*, **22**, 425.

Nong, Y.H., Titus, R.G., Riberio, J.M. & Remold, H.G. (1989) Peptides encoded by the calcitonin gene inhibt macrophage function. *J. Immunol.*, **143**, 45–9.

North, R.A., Williams, J.T., Surprenant, A. & Christie, M.J. (1987) μ and δ receptors belong to a family of receptors that are coupled to potassium channels. *Proc. Nat. Acad. Sci. USA*, **84**, 5487–91.

Numao, T. & Agrawal, K. (1992) Neuropeptides modulate human eosinophil chemotaxis. *J. Immunol.*, **149**, 3309–15.

Ollerenshaw, S.I., Jarvis, D.L., Sullivan, C.E. & Woolcock, A.J. (1991) Substance P immunoreactive nerves in airways from asthmatics and non-asthmatics. *Eur. Resp. J.*, **4**, 673–82.

Ollerenshaw, S., Jarvis, D., Woolcock, A., Sulivan, C. & Scheibner, T. (1988) Absence of immunoreactive vasoactive intestinal polypeptide in tissue from the lungs of patients with asthma. *New Engl. J. Med.*, **320**, 1244–8.

Ottaway, C.A. (1987) Selective effects of vasoactive intestinal peptide on the mitogenic response of murine T-cells. *Immunology*, **62**, 291–7.

Palmer, J.B.D., Cuss, F.M.C. & Barnes, P.J. (1986) VIP and PHM and their role in nonadrenergic inhibitory responses in isolated human airways. *J. Appl. Physiol.*, **61**, 1322–8.

Palmer, J.B.D., Cuss, F.M.C., Mulderry, P.K. *et al.* (1987) Calcitonin gene-related peptide is localised to human airway nerves and potently constricts human airway smooth muscle. *Brit. J. Pharmacol.*, **91**, 95–101.

Peatfield, A.C., Barnes, P.J., Bratcher, C., Nadel, J.A. & Davis, B. (1983) Vasoactive intestinal peptide stimulates tracheal submucosal gland secretion in ferret. *Am. Rev. Resp. Dis.*, **128**, 89–93.

Perretti, M., Ahluwalia, A., Flower, R.J. & Manzini, S. (1993) Endogenous tachykinins play a role in IL-1-induced neutrophil accumulation: involvement of NK-1 receptors. *Immunology*, **80**, 73–7.

Perretti, F. & Manzini, S. (1993) Activation of capsaicin-sensitive sensory fibers modulates PAF-induced bronchial hyperresponsiveness in anaesthetised guinea-pigs. *Am. Rev. Resp. Dis.*, **148**, 927–31.

Piedmonte, G., Hoffman, J.L.E., Husseini, W.K., Snider, R.M., Desai, M.C. & Nadel, J.A. (1993) NK_1 receptors mediate neurogenic inflammatory increase in blood flow in rat airways. *J. Appl. Physiol.*, **74**, 2462–8.

Pisarri, T.E., Coleridge, J.C.G. & Coleridge, H.M. (1993) Capsaicin-induced bronchial vasodilation in dogs: central and peripheral mechanisms. *J. Appl. Physiol.*, **74**, 259–66.

Potter, E. (1988) Neuropeptide Y as an autonomic neurotransmitter. *Pharmacol. Ther.*, **37**, 251–73.

Poyner, D.R. (1992) Calcitonin gene-related peptide: multiple actions, multiple receptors. *Pharmacol. Ther.*, **56**, 23–51.

Przewlocki, R., Hassan, A.H.S., Lason, W., Epplen, C., Herz, A. & Stein, C. (1992) Gene expression and localisation of opioid peptides in immune cells of inflamed tissue: functional role in antinociception. *Neuroscience*, **48**, 491–500.

Ramnarine, S.I., Hirayama, Y., Barnes, P.J. & Rogers, D.F. (1994) 'Sensory-efferent' neural control of mucus secretion: characterisation using tachykinin receptor antagonists in ferret trachea *in vitro*. *Brit. J. Pharmacol.*, **113**, 1183–90.

Ramnarine, S.I. & Rogers, D.F. (1994) Non-adrenergic non-cholinergic neural control of mucus secretion in the airways. *Pulmon. Pharmacol.*, **7**, 19–33.

Reisine, T. & Bell, G.I. (1992) Molecular biology of opioid receptors. *Trends Neurosci.*, **16**, 506–10.

Rhoden, K.J. & Barnes, P.J. (1990) Potentiation of nonadrenergic neural relaxation in guinea-pig airway by a cAMP phosphodiesterase inhibitor. *J. Pharmacol. Exp. Ther.*, **252**, 396–402.

Rogers, D.F., Aursudkij, B. & Barnes, P.J. (1989) Effects of tachykinins on mucus secretion of human bronchi *in vitro*. *Eur. J. Pharmacol.*, **174**, 283–6.

Rogers, D.F., & Barnes, P.J. (1989) Opioid inhibition of neurally mediated mucous secretion into human bronchi: implications for chronic bronchitis therepy. *Lancet*, **i**, 930–2.

Rogers, D.F., Belvisi, M.G., Aursudkij, B., Evans, T.W. & Barnes, P.J. (1988) Effects of interactions of sensory neuropeptides on airway microvscular leakage in guinea-pigs. *Brit. J. Pharmacol.*, **95**, 1109–16.

Rökaeus, Å. (1987) Galanin: a newly isolated biologically active neuropeptide. *Trends Neurosci.*, **10**, 158–64.

Rola-Pleszczynski, M., Bolduc, D. & St-Pierre, M. (1985) The effects of vasoactive intestinal peptide on human natural killer cell function. *J. Immunol.*, **35**, 2569–73.

Russell, J.A. & Simons, E.J. (1985) Modulation of cholinergic neurotransmission in airways by enkephalin. *J. Appl. Physiol.*, **58**, 853–8.

Russell, N.J.W., Schaible, H.G. & Schmidt, R.F. (1987) Opiates inhibit the discharges of fine afferent units from inflamed knee joint of the cat. *Neurosci. Letts.*, **76**, 107–12.

Said, S.I. (1994) Vasoactive intestinal polypeptide in the lung. In: *Neuropeptides in Respiratory Medicine* (eds M.A. Kaliner, P.J. Barnes, G.H.H. Kunkel & J.N. Baraniuk), pp. 143–60. Marcel Dekker, New York.

Said, S.I. & Mutt, V. (1970a) Polypeptide with broad activity: isolation from small intestine. *Science*, **169**, 1217–18.

Said, S.I. & Mutt, V. (1970b) Potent peripheral and splanchnic vasodilator peptide from normal gut. *Nature*, **225**, 863–4.

Salonen, R.O., Webber, S.E. & Widdicombe, J.G. (1988) Effects of neuropeptides and capsaicin on the canine tracheal vasculature *in vivo*. *Brit. J. Pharmacol.*, **95**, 1262–70.

Sann, H., Rossler, W., Hammer, K. & Pierau, F.-K. (1992) Substance P and calcitonin gene-related peptide in the ureter of the chicken and guinea-pig: distribution, binding sites and possible functions. *Neuroscience*, **49**, 699–713.

Saria, A., Martling, C.-R., Yan, Z., Theodorsson-Norheim, E., Gamse, R. & Lundberg, J.M. (1988) Release of multiple tachykinins from capsaicin-sensitive sensory nerves in the lung by bradykinin, histamine dimethylphenylpiperazinium and vagal stimulation. *Am. Rev. Resp. Dis.*, **137**, 1330–5.

Sata, T., Misra, H.P., Kubota, E. & Said, S.I. (1986) Vasoactive intestinal polypeptide relaxes pulmonary artery by an endothelium-independent mechanism. *Peptides*, **7**, 225–72.

Satoh, H., Lou, Y.-P. & Lundberg, J.M. (1993) Inhibitory effects of capsazepine and SR 48968 on citric acid-induced bronchoconstriction in guinea-pigs. *Eur. J. Pharmacol.*, **236**, 367–72.

Schepelmann, K., Meßlinger, K., Schaible, H.-G. & Schmidt, R.F. (1992) Inflammatory mediators and nociception in the joint: excitation and sensitisation of slowly conducting afferent fibres of cat's knee by prostaglandin I_2. *Neuroscience*, **50**, 237–47.

Schultzberg, M., Hokfelt, T., Nillsson, G. *et al.* (1979) Enkephalin immunoreactive nerve fibres and cell bodies in sympathetic ganglia of the guinea-pig and rat. *Neuroscience*, **4**, 249–70.

Sekizawa, K., Graf, P. & Nadel, J.A. (1989) Somatostatin potentiates cholinergic neurotransmission in ferret trachea. *J. Appl. Physiol.*, **67**, 2397–400.

Shepheard, R.J., Williamson, D.J., Hill, R.G. & Hargreaves, J.M. (1993) The non-peptide neurokinin$_1$ receptor antagonist RP67580 blocks neurogenic plasma extravasation in the dura mater of rats. *Brit. J. Pharmacol.*, **108**, 11–12.

Sheppard, M.N., Polak, J.M., Allen, A.M. & Bloom, S.R. (1984) Neuropeptide tyrosine (NPY): a newly discovered peptide is present in the mammalian respiratory tract. *Thorax*, **39**, 326–30.

Shimosegawa, T., Foda, H.D. & Said, S.I. (1990) [Met]enkephalin-Arg^6-Gly^7-Leu^8-immunoreactive nerves in guinea-pig and rat lungs: distribution, origin, and coexistence with vasoactive intestinal polypeptide immunoreactivity. *Neuroscience*, **36**, 737–50.

Skofitsch, G., Savitt, J. & Jacobwitz, D.M. (1985) Suggestive evidence for a functional unit between mast cells and substance P fibres in rat diaphragm and mesentery. *Histochemistry*, **82**, 5–8.

Smith, C.H., Barker, J.N.W.N., Morris, R.W., McDonald, D.M. & Lee, T.H. (1993) Neuropeptides induce rapid expression of endothelial cell adhesion molecules and elicit granulocytic infiltration in human skin. *J. Immunol.*, **151**, 3274–82.

Springall, D.R., Polak, J.M., Howard, J.M. *et al.* (1990) Persistence of intrinsic neurones and possible phenotypic changes after extrinsic denervation of human respiratory tract by heart-lung transplantation. *Am. Rev. Resp. Dis.*, **141**, 1538–46.

Sreedharan, S.P., Patel, D.R., Huang, J.-X. & Goetzl, E.J. (1993) Cloning and functional expression of a human neuroendocrine vasoactive intestinal peptide receptor. *Biochem. Biophys. Res. Commun.*, **193**, 546–53.

Stein, C. (1995) The control of pain in peripheral tissue by opioids. *New Engl. J. Med.*, **332**, 1685–90.

Stjarne, P., Lundblad, L., Lundberg, J.M. & Anggard, A. (1989) Capsaicin and nicotine sensitive afferent neurones and nasal secretion in healthy human volunteers and in patients with vasomotor rhinitis. *Brit. J. Pharmacol.*, **96**, 693–701.

Stretton, C.D. & Barnes, P.J. (1988) Modulation of cholinergic neurotransmission in guinea-pig trachea by neuropeptide Y. *Brit. J. Pharmacol.*, **93**, 675–82.

Stretton, C.D. & Barnes, P.J. (1989) Cholecystokinin octapeptide constricts guinea-pig and human airways. *Brit. J. Pharmacol.*, **97**, 675.

Stretton, C.D., Belvisi, M.G. & Barnes, P.J. (1990) Neuropeptide Y modulates non-adrenergic non-cholinergic neural bronchoconstriction *in vivo* and *in vitro*. *Neuropeptides*, **17**, 163.

Stretton, C.D., Belvisi, M.G. & Barnes, P.J. (1991) Modulation of neural bronchoconstrictor responses in the guinea-pig respiratory tract by vasoactive intestinal peptide. *Neuropeptides*, **18**, 149–57.

Stretton, C.D., Miura, M., Belvisi, M.G. & Barnes, P.J. (1992) Calcium-activated potassium channels mediate pre-junctional inhibition of peripheral sensory nerves. *Proc. Nat. Acad. Sci. USA*, **89**, 1325–9.

Sung, C.P., Arleth, A.J., Aiyar, N., Bhatnabar, P.K., Lysko, P.G. & Feuerstein, G. (1992) CGRP stimulates the adhesion of leukocytes to vascular endothelial cells. *Peptides*, **13**, 429–34.

Szolcsanyi, J., Anton, F., Reeh, P.W. & Handwerker, H.O. (1988) Selective activation by capsaicin of mechano-heat sensitive nociceptors in rat skin. *Brain Res.*, **446**, 262–8.

Takahashi, T., Belvisi, M.G. & Barnes, P.J. (1994) Modulation of neurotransmission in guinea-pig airways by galanin and the effect of a new antagonist Galantide. *Neuropeptides*, **26**, 245–51.

Takemori, A.E. & Portoghese, P.S. (1992) Selective naltrexone-derived opioid receptor antagonists. *Ann. Rev. Pharmacol. Toxicol.*, **32**, 239–70.

Tam, E.K., Franconi, G.M., Nadel, J.A. & Caughey, G.H. (1990) Protease inhibitors potentiate smooth muscle relaxation induced by vasoactive intestinal peptide in isolated human bronchi. *Am. J. Respir. Cell Mol. Biol.*, **2**, 449–52.

Tanaka, D.T. & Grundstein, N.M. (1986) Effect of substance P on neurally-mediated contraction of rabbit airway smooth muscle. *J. Appl. Physiol.*, **60**, 458–63.

Tatemoto, K. (1984) PHI—a new brain-gut peptide. *Peptides*, **5**, 151–4.

Tatemoto, K., Carlquist, M. & Mutt, V. (1982) Neuropeptide Y: a novel brain peptide with structural similarities to peptide YY and pancreatic polypeptide. *Nature*, **296**, 659–60.

Tatemoto, K. & Mutt, V. (1981) Isolation and characterization of the intestinal peptide porcine PHI (PHI-27), a new member of the glucagon-secretin family. *Proc. Nat. Acad. Sci.*, **78**, 6603–7.

Tatemoto, K., Rökaeus, Å., Jörnall, H., McDonald, T.J. & Mutt, V. (1983) Galanin—a novel biologically active peptide from porcine intestine. *FEBS Letts.*, **164**, 124–8.

Tsukagoshi, H., Haddad, E-B., Sun, J., Barnes, P.J. & Chung, K.-F. (1995) Ozone-induced airway hyperresponsiveness: role of superoxide anions, neutral endopeptidase and bradykinin receptors. *J. Appl. Physiol.* (in press).

Tsuto, T., Obata-Tsuto, H.L., Iwai, N., Takahashi, T. & Ibata, Y. (1989) Fine structure of neurons synthesising vasoactive intestinal peptide in the human colon from patients with Hirschsprung's disease. *Histochemistry*, **93**, 1–8.

Tucker, J.F., Brave, S.R., Charalambous, L., Hobbs, A. & Gibson, A.J. (1990) L-N^G-nitro arginine inhibits nonadrenergic, noncholinergic relaxations of guinea-pig tracheal smooth muscle. *Brit. J. Pharmacol.*, **100**, 663–4.

Uddman, R., Alumets, J., Densert, O., Håkanson, R. & Sundler, F. (1978) Occurrence and distribution of VIP nerves in the nasal mucosa and tracheobronchial wall. *Acta Otolaryngol.*, **86**, 443–8.

Uddman, R., Luts, A., Arimura, A. & Sundler, F. (1991) Pituitary adenylate cyclase-activating peptide (PACAP), a new vasoactive intestinal peptide (VIP)-like peptide in the respiratory tract. *Cell Tissue Res.*, **265**, 197–201.

Uddman, R., Moghimzadeh, E. & Sundler, F. (1984) Occurrence and distribution of GRP-immunoreactive nerve fibres in the respiratory tract. *Arch. Otorhinolaryngol.*, **239**, 145–51.

Uddman, R. & Sundler, F. (1987) Neuropeptides in the airways: a review. *Am. Rev. Resp. Dis.*, **136**, S3–8.

Umeda, Y. & Arisawa, H. (1989) Characterisation of the calcitonin gene-related peptide receptor in mouse lymphocytes. *Neuropeptides*, **14**, 237–42.

Undem, B.J., Dick, E.C. & Buckner, C.K. (1983) Inhibition by vasoactive intestinal peptide of antigen-induced histamine release from guinea-pig minced lung. *Eur. J. Pharmacol.*, **88**, 247–50.

Vandermeers, A., Vandermeers-Piret, M.-C., Robberecht, P. *et al.* (1984) Purification of a novel pancreatic secretory factor (PSF) with VIP- and secretin-like properties ((helodermin) from glia monster venom. *FEBS Letts.*, **166**, 273–6.

Von Essen, S.G., Rennard, S.I., O'Neil, D. *et al.* (1992) Bronchial epithelial cells release neutrophil chemotactic activity in response to tachykinins. *Am. J. Physiol.*, **263**, L226–31.

Walls, A.F., Brain, S.D., Desai, A. *et al.* (1992) Human mast cell tryptase attenuates the vasodilator activity of calcitonon gene-related peptide. *Biochem. Pharmacol.*, **43**, 1243–8.

Walsh, D., Mapp, P.I., Wharton, J. *et al.* (1992) Localisation and characterisation of substance P binding to human synovial tissue in rheumatoid arthritis. *Ann. Rheumatol. Dis.*, **51**, 313–17.

Walsh, D.A., Salmon, M., Featherstone, R., Wharton, J., Church, M.K. & Polak, J.M. (1994) Differences in the distribution and characteristics of tachykinin NK_1 binding sites between human and guinea-pig lung. *Brit. J. Pharmacol.*, **113**, 1407–15.

Ward, J.K., Belvisi, M.G., Fox, A.J. *et al.* (1993) Modulation of cholinergic bronchoconstrictor responses by endogenous nitric oxide and vasoactive intestinal peptide in human airways *in vitro*. *J. Clin. Invest.*, **92**, 736–42.

Wardlaw, A.J., Cromwell, A., Celestino, D. *et al.* (1986) Morphological and secretory properties of bronchoalveolar mast cells in respiratory disease. *Clin. Allergy*, **16**, 167–87.

Warren, J.B., Cockcroft, J.R., Larkin, S.R. *et al.* (1992) Pituitary adenylate cyclase activating polypeptide is a potent vasodilator in humans. *J. Cardiovasc. Pharmacol.*, **20**, 83–7.

Watson, N., Maclagan, J. & Barnes, P.J. (1993) Endogenous tachykinins facilitate transmission through parasympathetic ganglia in guinea-pig trachea. *Brit. J. Pharmacol.*, **109**, 751–9.

Webber, S.E. (1988) The effects of peptide histidine isoleucine and neuropeptide Y on mucous volume output from ferret trachea. *Brit. J. Pharmacol.*, **55**, 40–54.

Webber, S.E. (1989) Receptors mediating the effects of substance P and neurokinin A on mucous secretion and smooth muscle tone of ferret trachea: potentiation by an enkephalinase inhibitor. *Brit. J. Pharmacol.*, **98**, 1197–206.

Webber, S.E. & Widdicombe, J.G. (1987) The effect of vasoactive intestinal peptide on smooth muscle tone and mucus volume output from ferret trachea. *Brit. J. Pharmacol.*, **91**, 139–48.

Weihe, E., Hartschuch, W. & Weber, E. (1985) Prodynorphin peptides in small somatosensory primary afferents of the guinea-pig. *Neurosci. Lett.*, **58**, 347–52.

Widdicombe, J.G. (1954) Respiratory reflexes from the trachea and bronchi of the cat. *J. Physiol.*, **123**, 55–70.

Widdicombe, J.G. (1991) Neural control of airway vasculature and edema. *Am. Rev. Resp. Dis.*, **143**, S18–S21.

Wiik, P. (1989) Vasoactive intestinal peptide inhibits the respiratory burst in human monocytes by a cyclic AMP-mediated mechanism. *Regul. Pept.*, **25**, 187–97.

Yaksh, T.L. (1988) Substance P release from knee joint afferents terminals: modulation by opioids. *Brain Res.* **458**, 319–24.

Yau, W.M. & Youther, M.L. (1982) Direct evidence for a release of acetylcholine from the myenteric plexus of guinea-pig small intestine by substance P. *Eur. J. Pharmacol.*, **81**, 665–8.

Yiangou, Y., DiMarzo, V., Spokes, R.A., Panico, M., Morris, H.R. & Bloom, S.R. (1987) Isolation, characterization, and pharmacological actions of peptide histidine valine 42, a novel prepro-vasoactive intestinal peptide derived peptide. *J. Biol. Chem.*, **262**, 14010–13.

Yip, P., Palambini, B. & Coburn, R.E. (1981) Inhibitory innervation of the guinea-pig trachealis muscle. *J. Appl. Physiol.*, **50**, 373–82.

Yonehara, N., Chen Ji-Qiang, Imai, Y. & Inoki, R. (1992) Involvement of substance P present in primary afferent neurones in modulation of cutaneous blood flow in the instep of rat hind paw. *Brit. J. Pharmacol.*, **106**, 256–62.

Yu, M., Robinson, N.E. & Wang, Z. (1993) Regional distribution of nitroxidergic and adrenergic nerves in equine airway smooth muscle. *Am. Rev. Resp. Dis.*, **147**, A286.

Zimmerman, D.M. & Leander, J.D. (1990) Selective opioid receptor agonists and antagonists: research tools and potential therapeutic agents. *J. Med. Chem.*, **33**, 895–902.

Zurawski, G., Benedik, M., Kamp, B.J., Abrams, J.S., Zurawski, S.M. & Lee, F.D. (1986) Activation of mouse T-helper cells induces abundant preproenkephalin mRNA synthesis. *Science*, **232**, 772–5.

CHAPTER 27

The Autonomic Nervous System in Asthma and Rhinitis*

S.J. Smart & T.B. Casale

Introduction

Asthma is a common lung disease defined by reversible airway obstruction, airway inflammation and increased airway responsiveness to a wide variety of stimuli. Neural mechanisms are known to play a role in each of the characteristic components of asthma, including bronchospasm, hypersecretion of mucus, airway-wall oedema and airway inflammation. Likewise, rhinitis is characterized by mucus secretion, vasodilatation and mucosal oedema, all of which are influenced by neural mechanisms.

Afferent sensory and efferent parasympathetic and sympathetic† nerves regulate epithelial, vascular, glandular and smooth-muscle functions that normally protect airways from injury due to inhaled factors and microbes (Baraniuk, 1991; Barnes *et al.*, 1991a,b; Baraniuk *et al.*, 1994). Sensory nerves sense the conditions of the mucosal microenvironment, and relay signals to the central nervous system, local cholinergic ganglia and local axon response mechanisms. These nerves recruit systemic cholinergic and adrenergic reflexes, local cholinergic responses and local 'axon reflexes', respectively. Depending upon the stimulus, these responses have important physiological or pathophysiological consequences on epithelial cells, mucus secretion, mucosal oedema and airway smooth muscle. An illustration of the basic 'wiring' of these systems is shown in Fig. 27.1.

Each population of sensory, cholinergic and adrenergic nerves contains a unique combination of both classical neurotransmitters, such as acetylcholine (ACh) and noradrenaline, and various neuropeptides. Evidence suggests that cholinergic nerves contain both ACh and vasoactive intestinal peptide (VIP); adrenergic nerves contain noradrenaline and neuropeptide Y (NPY); and afferent sensory C fibres contain substance P (SP), neurokinin A (NKA), calcitonin gene-related peptide (CGRP) and gastrin-releasing peptide (GRP) (Lundberg *et al.*, 1987). Thus, stimulation of a nerve can result in corelease of neuropeptides and classic neurotransmitters with different biological actions. The net biological effect depends upon the relative quantities of individual transmitters and the environment into which they are released. Coreleased neurotransmitters may have synergistic, antagonistic or autoregulatory effects. Therefore, the net effect of nerve discharge is more complicated than that attributable to any individual neurotransmitter. Lastly, circulating adrenaline secreted by the adrenal medulla also provides important adrenergic receptor stimulation.

In attempting to understand the pathophysiology of asthma, abnormalities have been proposed within adrenergic, cholinergic and non-adrenergic non-cholinergic (NANC) pathways. In asthmatic lungs, the normal homeostatic balance between pro-asthmatic and anti-asthmatic

*The opinions expressed in this manuscript are those of the authors and do not necessarily represent those of the United States Air Force or the Department of Defense.

† The terms 'parasympathetic' and 'sympathetic' refer to the two major autonomic systems, often with opposing effects. The terms 'cholinergic' and 'adrenergic' more specifically refer to neurones containing acetylcholine (ACh) and catecholamines, respectively. These terms are often used interchangeably, but the reader is cautioned that they are not always equivalent. For example, preganglionic sympathetic neurones and postganglionic sympathetic neurones innervating sweat glands utilize ACh as a neurotransmitter, and can therefore be considered 'cholinergic'.

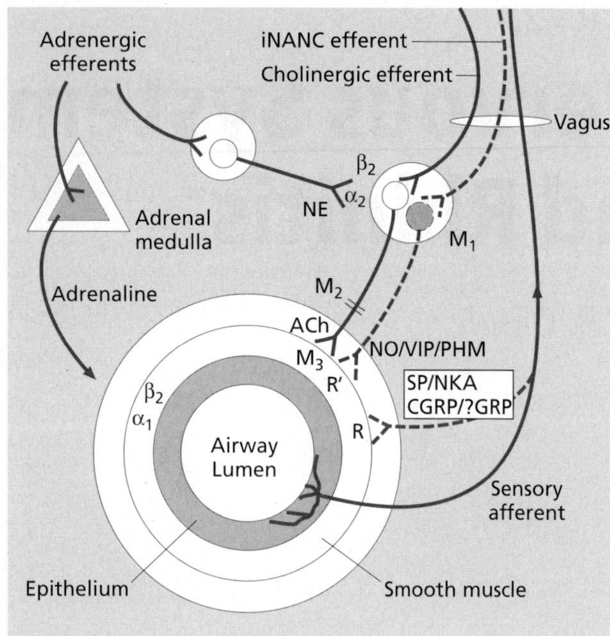

Fig. 27.1 Innervation of human airway smooth muscle illustrating the adrenergic and cholinergic nervous systems (solid lines) and the non-adrenergic non-cholinergic (NANC) nervous systems (dashed lines). Release of the neurotransmitters noradrenaline, adrenaline and acetylcholine stimulate specific α_1, β_2, and muscarinic m_3 receptors on airway smooth muscle. At the level of ganglia, cholinergic neurotransmission can be facilitated via muscarinic m_1 receptors. Conversely, both cholinergic and non-cholinergic excitatory neurotransmission can be impeded via α_2 and β_2 receptors. Non-adrenergic inhibitory nerves running in the vagus are likely to release VIP, PHM and NO. VIP and PHM act via specific airway receptors (R). Stimulation of collateral branches of sensory afferent nerves causes the antidromic relase of SP, NKA, CGRP and, possibly, GRP, which also stimulate specific airway receptors (R). (From Casale, 1993a). See text for definition of abbreviations.

forces is felt to be perturbed in favour of disease. In keeping with this paradigm, this chapter has been structured into two large parts: the adrenergic and 'inhibitory' NANC system (anti-asthmatic) and the cholinergic and 'excitatory' NANC system (pro-asthmatic). In each, the innervation, neurotransmitters, receptors and putative abnormalities in disease states, such as asthma and rhinitis, will be reviewed.

Much of the data supporting particular abnormalities, however, are indirect, and the discernment of cause vs. effect is often difficult. Moreover, much of the data are from animal models and many findings now appear to be species specific. This dictates substantial caution in extrapolating animal data to humans. Finally, neural mechanisms do not operate in isolation. Substantial evidence exists suggesting that neurotransmission both influences and is influenced by inflammatory cells and their mediators. Therefore, normal physiology, potential autonomic abnormalities and neuroimmune interactions will be considered here. These factors have important implications for both the pathogenesis and treatment of asthma and rhinitis.

Adrenergic and inhibitory NANC nervous system

The first half of this chapter will address the adrenergic system and the inhibitory non-adrenergic non-cholinergic nervous systems (iNANC). These systems are both 'inhibitory', since they generally have anti-asthmatic effects.

Adrenergic system

Innervation

The preganglionic sympathetic nerve fibres which innervate the respiratory system originate in the thoracic spinal cord and synapse in the superior cervical ganglion, en route to the nose, and the second through fourth thoracic ganglia, en route to the lung (Snell, 1992). Postganglionic fibres enter the nose accompanying branches of the carotid artery, and enter the lungs accompanying vagal nerve fibres (Dodd & Role, 1991). Airway smooth muscle itself lacks any significant direct sympathetic innervation, although evidence supports sparse innervation of submucosal glands, airway ganglia and bronchial arteries (Barnes, 1986a). Stimulation of sympathetic reflexes leads to vasoconstriction in respiratory mucosa and may stimulate glandular secretion in the trachea and bronchi. Consistent with the lack of innervation, however, sympathetic reflexes do not stimulate bronchodilatation in humans (Barnes, 1992).

As a generalization, the sympathetic system is active at all times, has fibres that ramify greatly, and is thereby capable of diffuse discharge in an 'all-or-nothing' effect. This contrasts with the parasympathetic system, which is organized mainly for discrete and localized discharge (Weiner & Taylor, 1985).

Neurotransmitters and their effects

Adrenergic nerves contain either noradrenaline, or noradrenaline plus neuropeptide Y (NPY) (Potter, 1988; Lacroix, 1989; Baraniuk *et al.*, 1990a; Lacroix *et al.*, 1990). Both noradrenaline and NPY are potent vasoconstrictors. Indeed, α_1- and α_2-adrenergic receptor agonists are popular 'nasal decongestants' that effectively reduce mucosal thickness. NPY, which accompanies noradrenaline in a subset of nerves, induces vasoconstriction which is slower in onset, but longer in duration, than noradrenaline. The walls of nasal arterioles and arteriovenous anastomoses are densely innervated by NPY nerve fibres (Uddman & Sundler, 1986; Baraniuk *et al.*, 1992b). Exogenous administration of NPY to the human nasal mucosa *in vivo* reduces nasal airway resistance and albumin exudation, without stimulating submucosal gland secretion (Laurenzi *et al.*, 1989). This suggests that NPY agonists may be useful for the treatment of diseases which are characterized by vasodilatation, vascular permeability and plasma exudation, such as rhinitis. Because NPY is a long-acting vasoconstrictor, NPY agonists may offer advantages over shorter-acting α-agonists for the treatment of chronic vascular congestion.

Noradrenaline is a very weak bronchoconstrictor, and NPY has no direct effect on tracheobronchial smooth-muscle contraction (Stretton & Barnes, 1988; Li & Rand, 1991). Indeed, due to the sparse direct innervation of human lung, circulating adrenaline secreted by the adrenal medulla probably plays a more important role than noradrenaline or NPY in lower airway functions. This postulate is supported by the potent bronchodilatation induced by physiological concentrations of adrenaline in both normal and asthmatic subjects (Berkin *et al.*, 1986). Therefore, it is not surprising that β_2-adrenergic agonists are the mainstay of effective bronchodilator therapy in asthmatic patients.

Catecholamines stimulate several other important biological responses in airway epithelium, vascular endothelium and airway smooth muscle. Catecholamines binding to β-receptors on airway epithelial cells initiate a variety of important cellular responses. These include stimulation of ciliary beating, mucus and chloride secretion, release of relaxant factors and epithelial cell proliferation (Nijkamp *et al.*, 1992). These effects are likely to be mediated through the β_2-receptor sub-type. In the rabbit, a common model for bronchial hyperreactivity and airway inflammation, the β_2-receptor sub-type predominates on both basal and columnar tracheobronchial epithelium (Kelsen *et al.*, 1994).

In contrast to α-stimulation, β-stimulation produces vasodilatation and can increase blood flow. Nonetheless, the net effect of β-stimulation is to decrease the plasma leakage caused by many inflammatory mediators, including histamine, platelet-activating factor (PAF), bradykinin, SP and allergen. Baluk and McDonald have recently provided direct *in vivo* evidence that this is true. The selective β_2-agonist formoterol reduced plasma leakage in rat trachea that was stimulated by either vagal activity or SP. They also showed that this reduced plasma extravasation was due to a 68% reduction in the number, but not size, of endothelial gaps (Baluk & McDonald, 1994). Hence, β_2-agonists appear capable of limiting airway oedema by reducing the number of endothelial gaps which are stimulated by inflammatory mediators.

In addition to effects on airway smooth-muscle tone, adrenergic stimulation also regulates other functions. For example, airway smooth-muscle hyperplasia associated with asthma may, in part, be regulated by adrenergic input. Recent studies suggest that α- and β-receptors exert opposing actions on airway smooth-muscle proliferation, with α_1-agonists inducing airway smooth-muscle-cell mitogenesis, and β-agonists causing growth inhibition (Noverall & Grunstein, 1994). The net proliferative effect of adrenergic stimulation *in vivo* remains to be discerned, however.

Adrenergic receptors

Despite minimal sympathetic innervation of airway smooth muscle, there are significant numbers of both α- and β-receptors in the human lung. Quantitatively, there is a much higher density of β-receptors than α-receptors. This is consistent with the proven efficacy of β-agonists in the treatment of asthma. β_2-receptors outnumber β_1-receptors by approximately three to one, with airway smooth muscle, epithelial cells and mast cells having exclusively β_2-receptors (Carstairs *et al.*, 1985; Spina *et al.*, 1989a). Moreover, researchers have found that the adrenergic receptor system is much more complex than previously thought. Multiple α_1-receptors ($\alpha_{1a/d}$, α_{1b}, α_{1c}), α_2-receptors (α_{2c10}, α_{2c2}, α_{2c4}) and β-receptors (β_1, β_2, β_3) have been cloned (Bylund *et al.*, 1994), but the specific receptor mRNA expressed in the respiratory tract are still being defined.

Adrenergic role in asthma

Several potential abnormalities in the adrenergic control of asthmatic lungs have been proposed. These include abnormalities in β-receptors, α-receptors and in catecholamine secretion (Table 27.1).

β-Adrenergic abnormalities

The beneficial effects of β-agonists and detrimental effects of β-antagonists have justifiably suggested a role for β-adrenergic dysfunction in bronchial asthma. Well-known effects of β_2-receptor stimulation include bronchodilatation, decreased mast cell degranulation, and increased mucus and water secretion (Casale, 1993a). Furthermore, stimulation of β_2-receptors inhibits both cholinergic and non-cholinergic excitatory neurotransmission, and blockade of these receptors may mediate β-antagonist-induced bronchospasm in asthmatics (Grieco & Pierson, 1971; Rhoden *et al.*, 1988; Ind *et al.*, 1989).

The β-adrenergic theory of asthma was first proposed by Szentivanyi over 30 years ago, and a comprehensive theory was published in 1968. Szentivanyi's theory was

Table 27.1 Potential adrenergic abnormalities in asthma.

Reduced β_2-mediated effects
Decreased density or affinity of β_2-receptors on
Parasympathetic ganglia or post-ganglionic nerves
Pre-junctional non-cholinergic excitatory nerves
Airway smooth muscle
Mast cells
Decreased post-receptor responses (cAMP generation) by
Altered G proteins
Protein kinase C activation
Autoantibodies to β_2-receptors
Increased α_1-mediated excitatory effects on
Submucosal glands
Bronchial vasculature
Airway smooth muscle
Decreased α_2-mediated inhibitory effects on
Cholinergic activity via
Parasympathetic ganglia
Postganglionic nerves
Non-cholinergic excitatory activity
α_1-Adrenergic excitatory activity
Relative catecholamine deficiency
Reduced adrenaline secretion from adrenal medulla
Increased adrenaline metabolism

based in part on a model involving injection of living or killed *Bordetella pertussis* organisms into certain strains of rodents, which led to features reminiscent of human asthma. These features included hypersensitivity to mediators, such as histamine and bradykinin, hypersensitivity to non-specific stimuli, such as cold air and respiratory irritants, and hyposensitivity to catecholamines with a reversal of normal adrenergic metabolic activity. Enhanced reagin-like antibody production and marked eosinophilia were also associated with these abnormalities. Szentivanyi felt that adrenergic abnormalities, similar to those associated with the pertussis-induced hypersensitive state, might account for both the pharmacological and immunological abnormalities associated with human asthma (Szentivanyi, 1968).

Early support for Szentivanyi's theory came from *in vivo* observations demonstrating a decreased rise in blood sugar, lactate, pyruvate, cyclic adenosine monophosphate (cAMP) and pulse pressure in response to β-adrenergic stimulation in allergic asthmatic patients compared to normal individuals. Moreover, the β-antagonist propranolol caused acute bronchoconstriction in asthmatic subjects, whereas it had no effect on airway responses in normal subjects (Casale, 1983). Subsequent *in vivo* studies by Kaliner *et al.* (1982) measuring pulse pressure and AMP responses to isoproterenol concluded that intrinsic β-adrenergic hyporeactivity exists in asthmatic subjects unrelated to previous adrenergic drug administration. Interestingly, a comparable degree of β-adrenergic hyporesponsiveness was observed in non-asthmatic allergic subjects as well.

Spina *et al.* (1989a) have recently compared the distribution, density and function of β-receptors in post-mortem lung samples from asthmatic and normal subjects. Although they found attenuated *in vitro* responsiveness to β-agonists, there was no reduction in β-receptor density in asthmatic lung samples.

Unfortunately, the analysis of lung β-receptors in living subjects has not been possible. As a surrogate, many investigators have pursued studies of β-receptor function on peripheral blood leucocytes. Several groups have reported that asthmatic patients have a lower density of β-receptors on lymphocytes (Brooks *et al.*, 1979; Kariman, 1980) and that the lymphocytes of asthmatics generate less AMP in response to β-agonists (Parker & Smith, 1973; Davis *et al.*, 1986; Sato *et al.*, 1990). Others, however, have found reduced leucocyte β-receptor number and AMP generation only after continuous treatment with β-agonists (Conolly & Greenacre, 1976; Galant *et al.*, 1980). Still others have found lower β-receptor density in mononuclear cells, but not polymorphonuclear leucocytes, of asthmatics not taking medications (Sano *et al.*, 1983).

Interpretation of these studies is difficult, because drug use can clearly affect β-receptor density on peripheral blood leucocytes. β-agonists can decrease, while corticosteroids can increase β-receptor density (Brodde *et al.*, 1988; Stern & Kunos, 1988). Furthermore, the results may differ depending on whether mononuclear or polymorphonuclear cells are studied. Lastly, a recent study found that treatment with terbutaline had no effect on human lung β-receptors, whereas a 57% decline was measured in the number of β-receptors on peripheral mononuclear cells of the same patients (Böhm *et al.*, 1991). Thus, it is very difficult to extrapolate results from studies of circulating leucocytes to the assessment of pulmonary β-receptors.

In vitro autoradiography has not substantiated a decrease in β-receptor density in the airways of asthmatics. Furthermore, neither β-antagonists nor adrenalectomy cause asthma in normal subjects. Thus, it is unlikely that a fundamental defect in the β-receptor system is solely responsible for the development of asthma and bronchial hyperreactivity.

Abnormalities that have been found in many of these studies may actually represent the consequence of the active disease state. Meurs *et al.* (1982) found a reduction in human lymphocyte β-receptor density and responsiveness only after an allergen-induced asthmatic reaction. They also demonstrated a disparity between a 20% reduction in β-receptor density and a 40% loss of agonist-induced adenylate cyclase activity. They postulated that this discrepancy may indicate an 'uncoupling' of the receptor from the adenylate cyclase complex. It has been suggested that such post-receptor mechanisms include alteration of G proteins or possibly an activation of protein kinase C (Meurs *et al.*, 1987).

Airway inflammation may lead to β-adrenergic dysfunction. Busse *et al.* (1990) have demonstrated that viral respiratory infections can lead to airway inflammation, airway hyperreactivity and concomitant neutrophil β-adrenergic hyporesponsiveness. *In vitro* incubation of neutrophils with rhinovirus-16 leads to a significantly decreased response to isoproterenol (Busse *et al.*, 1980). Release of inflammatory mediators such as PAF may contribute to β-adrenergic hyporesponsiveness. Several inflammatory cells which are felt to play a role in the pathogenesis of asthma, including mast cells and eosinophils, produce PAF. PAF, in turn, has been shown to decrease β-adrenergic responses of human lung tissue *in vitro* through a down-regulation of β-receptors (Agrawal & Townley, 1987). Moreover, activation of phospholipase A_2, in addition to initiating PAF synthesis, may also directly cause a decrease in the number of β-adrenergic receptors coincident with an increase in α_1-receptors (Hayashi *et al.*, 1988).

Lastly, some investigators have proposed that autoantibodies to β-receptors may explain a reduction in asthmatic β-receptor function (Venter, 1982). Such autoantibodies are reported to be present in 10–15% of allergic individuals and 5% of asthmatic children (Blecher *et al.*, 1984). However, since they are also found in a similar percentage of normal individuals, β-receptor autoantibodies are of doubtful pathogenic significance (Harrison *et al.*, 1982).

In summary, although there is ample evidence of β-adrenergic dysfunction in asthmatics, it remains unclear whether this is a primary abnormality, secondary to therapy, or a consequence of inflammatory processes. The latter two possibilities are most tenable. Furthermore, since most asthmatics respond very well to β-agonists and normal subjects do not become asthmatic while taking β-antagonists, any abnormality is likely to play a minor role in asthma pathogenesis.

α-Adrenergic abnormalities

In comparison to β-receptors, there are relatively few α-receptors in the lung, and their role in regulating airway function has not been definitively elucidated. α-Receptor sub-types include post-junctional excitatory α_1-receptors and pre-junctional inhibitory α_2-receptors. The sub-types of α_1- and α_2-receptors involved have not been identified.

Stimulation of α_1-receptors produces airway constriction, increased mucus production and enhanced mast cell degranulation (Casale, 1993a). Moreover, by decreasing bronchial blood flow, α_1-receptor stimulation may indirectly contribute to bronchoconstriction by facilitating airway cooling (Barnes, 1986a).

Conversely, α_2-receptors may play a protective role in asthma. Stimulation of α_2-receptors, presumably on parasympathetic ganglia and/or postganglionic fibres, has been shown to inhibit both cholinergic and non-cholinergic excitatory transmission (Grundström *et al.*, 1984; Grundström & Andersson, 1985). The role of pre-junctional α_2-receptors on airway sympathetic nerves, however, has not been defined because the airway effects mediated by sympathetic nerves, such as bronchial blood flow and mucus secretion, are more difficult to measure (Barnes, 1992). Nonetheless, abnormalities of the α-adrenergic system, such as up-regulation of α_1-mediated vasoconstriction or down-regulation of α_2-mediated effects, might be expected to contribute to the pathogenesis of asthma.

Early *in vivo* studies by Kaliner *et al.* (1982) suggested generalized α_1-adrenergic hyperresponsiveness in asthmatics. α-Adrenergic responsivity, as measured by pupillary dilation and reduction in cutaneous blood flow in response to phenylephrine, was significantly greater in allergic asthmatics compared to both normal controls and allergic rhinitics. Subsequent studies by Davis (1986) both confirmed these results and correlated pupillary responses with airway reactivity as measured by methacholine challenge.

Using a guinea pig model of asthma, Barnes *et al.* (1980) reported a doubling in the numbers of α_1-receptors of lung homogenates of sensitized animals chronically exposed to ovalbumin aerosol. The number of β-receptors was marginally decreased, such that the ratio of α- : β-receptors nearly tripled. This alteration in the ratio of α- : β-receptors was proposed as an explanation for altered adrenergic sensitivity in asthma. Other investigators, however, failed to detect a change in α_1-receptor density 24 hours after aeroallergen challenge of sensitized guinea pigs, despite a decrease in β-receptor density and exaggerated airway responsiveness to histamine (Motojima *et al.*, 1989).

In contrast, asthmatic and normal human lung from post-mortem samples revealed very low levels of α_1-receptors. Consistent with these findings, phenylephrine failed to induce significant increases in bronchial tone in tissue isolated from either asthmatic or normal human lung (Spina *et al.*, 1989b). Likewise, phenylephrine was unable to induce bronchoconstriction in asthmatic subjects (Thomson *et al.*, 1982). Finally, in a study of nine asthmatics, inhaled prazosin, a potent and selective α_1-antagonist, failed to improve spirometric measurements compared with placebo (Barnes *et al.*, 1981b).

Nonetheless, the inhalation of the non-specific α-agonist methoxamine did cause bronchoconstriction in asthmatic, but not normal human subjects (Snashall *et al.*, 1978). Moreover, α-antagonists have also been shown to partially inhibit both histamine- and exercise-induced bronchoconstriction in asthmatic subjects (Beil & De Kock, 1978; Jenkins *et al.*, 1985). Several *in vitro* studies have also suggested that α-adrenergically mediated airway constriction may only occur in inflamed lung tissue (Casale, 1987).

In summary, there is no direct sympathetic innervation of airway smooth muscle and the effects of α-agonists and α_1-antagonists on bronchoconstriction and bronchodilatation, respectively, are weak. Therefore, it is doubtful that airway smooth-muscle α_1-receptors play a significant role in airway hyperreactivity. It remains possible, however, that α_1-mediated decreases in bronchial blood flow may partially contribute to exercise-induced asthma (Barnes, 1986a).

It is also possible that dysfunction of inhibitory α_2-receptors might predispose subjects toward bronchospasm. As previously mentioned, stimulation of α_2-receptors can inhibit both cholinergic and excitatory NANC neurotransmission. A recent study showed that selective α_2-agonists could attenuate excitatory NANC neurotransmission in a dose-dependent manner (Jacobsson *et al.*, 1991). Inhaled clonidine, an α_2-agonist, can block aeroallergen-induced bronchoconstriction in allergic asthmatics (Lindgren *et al.*, 1986). Oral clonidine, however, increased bronchial hyperreactivity to histamine (Xuan *et al.*, 1988). These results may be explained by the reduction in overall sympathetic tone caused by α_2-stimulation in the central nervous system (CNS). Overall, it appears that α-adrenergic function has minimal effects on normal and asthmatic lung, but the exact contribution of α-receptors to asthma pathogenesis remains to be determined.

Circulating catecholamines

In human airways, electrical field stimulation shows no evidence of adrenergic bronchodilator responses *in vitro* (Barnes, 1992). However, since β-antagonists precipitate bronchospasm in many asthmatics, this nonetheless suggests an increase in adrenergic drive. Circulating catecholamines are probably responsible for this increased adrenergic drive. Although noradrenaline is normally present in the highest concentrations, noradrenaline infusions have no effect on airway calibre in asthmatics (Berkin *et al.*, 1986). Adrenaline, however, is a potent bronchodilator, even at low doses. Since the adrenal medulla is the sole source of adrenaline, and surgical adrenalectomy can potentiate histamine-induced bronchoconstriction, the increased adrenergic drive of asthmatics is most likely provided by circulating adrenaline (Barnes, 1986b).

Although plasma catecholamine levels are similar in stable asthmatics and normal subjects, there is evidence of a blunted rise in both adrenaline and cAMP during exercise-induced bronchoconstriction (Barnes *et al.*, 1981a; Hartley *et al.*, 1981). Therefore, an abnormality in either adrenaline secretion or clearance may be present in some asthmatic patients. Since clearance of adrenaline does not appear to be increased, these patients may well have a defect in adrenaline secretion. This defect appears to be selective for exercise-induced bronchoconstriction, however, since both insulin-induced hypoglycaemia and histamine infusion stimulate a normal rise in plasma adrenaline in asthmatics. Although this potential abnormality in catecholamine response may potentiate bronchoconstriction, it is unlikely to be a primary defect, since neither adrenalectomy nor chronic β-antagonist therapy cause asthma in normal subjects (Barnes, 1986b).

The iNANAC nervous system

Introduction

When adrenergic and cholinergic receptors are blocked, electrical field stimulation of human airway smooth muscle results in relaxation which can be blocked by tetrodotoxin, indicating that it is mediated by postganglionic nerves (Richardson & Béland, 1976). This inhibitory non-adrenergic nervous system is the only known *neural* bronchodilatory pathway in human lung (Laitinen & Laitinen, 1987). In the absence of specific antagonists, the neurotransmitters of this system are not known with absolute certainty, but they most likely include vasoactive intestinal peptide (VIP), the related peptide histidine methionine (PHM) and nitric oxide (NO) (Palmer *et al.*, 1986; Li & Rand, 1991).

Peptide neurotransmitters and their effects

VIP and PHM are predominantly colocalized with ACh in efferent cholinergic nerves in both the lung and nose (Dey *et al.*, 1981; Laitinen *et al.*, 1985; Baraniuk *et al.*, 1990d). VIP receptors have been identified in human pulmonary vascular smooth muscle, large airway smooth muscle, airway epithelium, submucosal glands and alveolar walls (Carstairs & Barnes, 1986a). VIP receptor density appears to decrease as airways become smaller, consistent with the decrease in cholinergic innervation in smaller airways. In the nose, VIP binding sites were also found on epithelium, glands and vessels (Baraniuk *et al.*, 1990d).

Both VIP and PHM are potent large airway relaxants (Lundberg *et al.*, 1984a). *In vitro*, VIP is approximately 50 times more potent than isoproterenol (Palmer *et al.*, 1986). Thus, both the localization and physiological effects of VIP and PHM on larger airways suggest that these neuropeptides antagonize the bronchoconstrictor effects of ACh. The mechanism of this antagonism appears to involve direct bronchodilatory effects on airway smooth muscle, and cholinergic inhibition at the level of both ganglia and ACh release (Sekizawa *et al.*, 1988; Martin *et al.*, 1990; Stretton *et al.*, 1991).

In nasal mucosa, VIP dilates both resistance and capacitance vessels (Malm *et al.*, 1980). VIP also stimulated serous cell secretion of lactoferrin and mucinous material from human nasal mucosal explants (Mullol *et al.*, 1992b), although VIP and ACh did not have additive effects in this system. Likewise, VIP increased mucus secretion from cat trachea (Shimura *et al.*, 1988), and epithelial cell secretion from dog and ferret trachea (Richardson & Webber, 1987). In stark contrast, VIP may inhibit mucus secretion from human bronchial explants (Coles *et al.*, 1981). VIP also inhibited mucous glycoprotein secretion by both cultured human tracheal explants and respiratory epithelium (Lundgren & Shelhamer, 1990). Anti-VIP antibodies have also been suggested to play a pathological role in the bronchorrhea of chronic bronchitis (Marom & Goswami, 1991). *In vivo*, atropine blocks essentially all glandular secretion but only partially blocks neurogenically induced blood flow (Malm *et al.*, 1980; Lundberg *et al.*, 1981; Larsson *et al.*, 1986). Thus, VIP may be more active as a vasodilator than as a modulator of mucus secretion. The relative roles of ACh and VIP in neurogenically mediated secretion in human airways will be discerned only when stable and specific VIP agonists and antagonists are developed.

VIP also has a variety of anti-inflammatory actions. VIP inhibits natural killer (NK) cell activity, lymphocyte traffic and proliferation, interleukin-2 (IL-2) release and mast cell degranulation (Undem *et al.*, 1983; Casale, 1993a). Moreover, VIP may act as a free (IL-2) radical scavenger (Said, 1991). Conversely, mast cell-mediators, such as tryptase and chymase, are capable of degrading VIP (Caughey *et al.*, 1988; Franconi *et al.*, 1989). Indeed, the limited bronchodilatory potency of VIP in several human *in vivo* studies may be related to rapid enzymatic degradation of the peptide (Barnes & Dixon, 1984; Morice & Sever, 1986; Tam *et al.*, 1990). Thus, interactions between VIP and inflammatory cells may significantly affect lung function as well.

NO

Increasing evidence suggests NO may also be an important iNANC neurotransmitter in human airways (Belvisi *et al.*, 1991; Li & Rand, 1991). In fact, one recent study suggests that in human tracheal segments, the neural bronchodilator response is mediated only by NO, without functional evidence supporting a role for VIP (Belvisi *et al.*, 1992). These observations are similar to those defined in porcine and equine airways, but stand in contrast to studies with guinea pig airways, in which both NO and VIP appear to mediate NANC relaxations (Yu *et al.*, 1994). Moreover, inhalation of NO by both animals and healthy humans rapidly increased specific airway conductance following methacholine-induced bronchoconstriction. Although significant, the bronchodilatory effects of NO in humans (at the concentrations studied) are relatively modest and less than that reported after inhalation of β-agonist drugs by asthmatics (Hogman *et al.*, 1993; Sanna *et al.*, 1994). Finally, inhibition of NO synthesis in both human and guinea pig trachea blocks non-adrenergic bronchodilatation and enhances cholinergic neurotransmission (Tucker *et al.*, 1990; Belvisi *et al.*, 1991). Thus, like VIP, NO may act as both a direct bronchodilator and antagonist of cholinergic responses.

NO may have anti-inflammatory effects as well. One recent study found that exogenous NO attenuated leucocyte adhesion to endothelium via P-selectin in a splanchnic ischaemia-reperfusion model (Gauthier *et al.*, 1994). In light of the recognized role of inflammation in the pathogenesis of asthma, processes such as this may ultimately prove to be equally as important as bronchodilatory effects.

The iNANC system's role in asthma

In summary, the iNANC system, via bronchodilatation, cholinergic antagonism, decreased mucus secretion and anti-inflammatory actions, appears to play an anti-asthmatic role. Abnormalities of this system have been postulated to contribute to the development of bronchial hyperreactivity, asthma and other chronic lung diseases. Although supporting data are sparse, these abnormalities may include a deficiency in iNANC neurone density, altered release or corelease of neurotransmitters, receptor deficiencies and depressed post-receptor responses (Table 27.2). Preliminary data, for example, suggests that airway VIP receptor numbers may be reduced in cystic fibrosis, but not in asthma (Sharma & Jeffery, 1990). Most important, however, may be the effect of inflammatory mediators, such as mast cell tryptase and chymase on degradation of VIP, and superoxide on degradation of NO. For example, pretreatment with a protease inhibitor abolished antigen-induced dysfunction of iNANC activity in a cat model (Miura *et al.*, 1992). A loss of VIP from human pulmonary nerve fibres has also been demonstrated in asthmatics in some, but not all studies examining this issue. In a study reported by Ollerenshaw *et al.* (1989), immunoreactive VIP was not seen within any lung sections from asthmatics, but was identified within nerves in more than 92% of lung sections from non-asthmatics, including smokers. Loss of actual neurones, reduced synthesis within neurones, or excessive degradation by proteases are all explanations. Whether the absence of VIP-immunoreactive nerves is a primary event or secondary to the active disease process remains unknown.

Table 27.2 Potential non-adrenergic inhibitory abnormalities in asthma.

Loss of non-adrenergic inhibitory neurones
Inhibition of neurotransmitter synthesis/release VIP/PHM Nitric oxide
Increased degradation of neurotransmitters VIP/PHM by tryptase, chymase Nitric oxide by superoxide
Decreased NPY synthesis/release
Decreased density and/or affinity of receptors
Decreased post-receptor responses

See text for definition of abbreviations.

With regard to NO, potential abnormalities are speculative at this time.

Summary of adrenergic and iNANC systems

Thus, adrenergic and iNANC mechanisms appear to attenuate cholinergic and non-cholinergic excitatory activity in addition to their direct effects on airway smooth muscle, mast cells, submucosal glands, and bronchial vasculature. Despite the sparsity of direct adrenergic lung innervation, numerous studies have implicated abnormal adrenergic activity in the pathogenesis of asthma. Most attention has focused on mechanisms of reduced β_2-mediated effects and these may, in part, be secondary to inflammation and/or medications rather than primary abnormalities. Current knowledge suggests only a minor role for α_1-mediated effects in normal or diseased lung, although decreased α_2-mediated inhibitory effects on both cholinergic and non-cholinergic excitatory activity may be important. Likewise, although a defect in adrenaline secretion may partially contribute to exercise-induced bronchoconstriction, this is unlikely to represent a fundamental abnormality in chronic asthma.

The influence of the α-adrenergic system on nasal physiology and rhinitis is more apparent, however. The potent vasoconstricting effects of α-agonists account for their popular use as nasal decongestants. NPY agonists may play an analogous therapeutic role in the future.

Although the existence of an iNANC system has been well demonstrated, the relative importance of VIP vs. NO in human airways remains open to debate. Similarly, putative abnormalities in this system are appealing, but currently rest on minimal firm evidence.

Cholinergic (parasympathetic) and excitatory NANC system

The second part of this chapter will address the cholinergic nervous system and the excitatory non-adrenergic non-cholinergic (eNANC) nervous system. These systems are considered 'excitatory' because they are generally pro-asthmatic in their effects on the lungs. Included in these tightly connected systems are the cholinergic nerves supplied by the vagus and the many unmyelinated C fibres which serve the role of afferent sensory nerves. These afferent sensory nerves trigger both central vagal reflexes and local 'axon reflexes', the latter by virtue of the antidromic release of neuropeptides.

Cholinergic system

Innervation

Preganglionic efferent parasympathetic nerve fibres which innervate the nasal mucosa, sinuses and nasopharynx originate in the superior salivatory nucleus (pons), travel down the facial nerve and synapse in the sphenopalatine ganglion (Carpenter, 1991). Likewise, preganglionic fibres destined for the larynx and lung originate in the nucleus ambiguus and dorsal motor nucleus and pass down the vagus nerve to synapse in terminal parasympathetic ganglia within these organs. Short postganglionic fibres travel from these ganglia to innervate glands and vessels in the nasal, pharyngeal, laryngeal and tracheobronchial mucosa, as well as airway smooth muscle. Additional glossopharyngeal, vagal and spinal accessory motor neurones innervate pharyngeal, laryngeal and upper oesophageal striated muscle and participate in the gag reflex that serves to protect and clear obstructions from the airway.

Afferent sensory nerve stimulation in the mucosa of both upper and lower airways leads to central recruitment of parasympathetic reflexes. In contrast to the classical 'all-or-nothing' response of the sympathetic nervous system, the brain-stem parasympathetic nuclei appear capable of regulating nasal, laryngeal and tracheobronchial efferent responses to irritant nerve stimulation independently (Weiner & Taylor, 1985). This may actually be the most important function of the sensory nerves in the human respiratory tract.

Neurotransmitters

Preganglionic parasympathetic nerves release ACh and possibly other neurotransmitters that act upon nicotinic receptors on postganglionic neurones within the ganglia residing in airway walls. Postganglionic neurones may act as electrical 'filters' by assessing various stimulatory and inhibitory inputs before being triggered to depolarize. Stimulation of excitatory autoreceptors by SP or other tachykinins may increase the likelihood of postganglionic cell depolarization (Barnes, 1992), while stimulation of inhibitory autoreceptors may decrease postganglionic cell depolarization. An impressive list of these inhibitory receptors includes muscarinic m_2, NPY, γ-aminobutyric acid $(GABA)_B$, histaminic H_3, α_2- and β_2-adrenergic, and μ-opioid receptors (Rogers & Barnes, 1989).

Postganglionic parasympathetic secretory neurones release ACh, VIP (Barnes, 1992), other VIP-related peptides (Uddman & Sundler, 1986) and probably NO (Belvisi *et al.*, 1992). As discussed in the first half of this chapter, VIP, related peptides and NO found in postganglionic parasympathetic nerves are actually considered part of the 'inhibitory' non-adrenergic nervous system. They all functionally antagonize the effects of ACh. Thus, the net effect of nerve discharge depends upon the relative release of several neurotransmitters with opposing effects. This, in turn, may vary with the rate of nerve depolarization (Hokfelt *et al.*, 1987). At low rates, ACh is released, while at high rates, ACh plus VIP are released. Feedback inhibition of VIP release may also occur as a way of conserving stored peptide. Unlike other neurotransmitters, such as ACh, there are no re-uptake mechanisms for neuropeptides. They can only be re-supplied by axonal transport from the neuronal cell body. Overall, the cholinergic component of parasympathetic reflexes, mediated by ACh, is the predominant stimulus for mucus secretion in allergic rhinitis (Lundgren & Shelhamer, 1990), is responsible for maintaining resting bronchial tone, and in large part, mediates acute bronchospastic responses.

NPY, although primarily colocalized with noradrenaline in a subset of sympathetic nerves, may also be found in some cholinergic neurones (Sheppard *et al.*, 1984; Lacroix *et al.*, 1990; Lehmann, 1990) and a small population of VIP-ergic sphenopalatine neurones that innervate nasal glands (Lacroix *et al.*, 1990). The functions of colocalized neuropeptides such as NPY and VIP are difficult to predict, since complex synergistic and antagonistic interactions are expected (Khalil *et al.*, 1988).

Muscarinic receptors

There are three pharmacologically defined muscarinic receptor sub-types (m_1, m_2 and m_3) which have been identified in the lung. However, since at least five muscarinic receptor genes (m_1 to m_5) have been cloned (Levine *et al.*, 1991), it is not known with absolute certainty which of these receptor sub-types mediates the action of ACh *in vivo* (Barnes, 1989b; Dorje *et al.*, 1991). The m_3 receptor appears to be the pre-eminent functional sub-type in both human nasal and bronchial mucosa, and is responsible for smooth-muscle contraction and glandular secretion (Mak & Barnes, 1990; Okayama *et al.*, 1993).

In nasal mucosa, about 55% of the muscarinic receptors are of the m_3 type, while the remainder are m_1 (Okayama *et al.*, 1993). Binding sites for are present on epithelium and submucosal glands. Receptors m_1 and m_3 mRNA have been identified by autoradiography and *in situ* hybridization (Baraniuk *et al.*, 1992a), respectively, on nasal epithelium, submucosal glands and endothelium. Binding sites for m_2 are not present in human nasal mucosa and m_4 sites have not been examined.

Autoradiographic studies have revealed dense muscarinic receptor labelling of submucosal glands and airway ganglia, in addition to moderate labelling of airway smooth muscle in humans (Mak & Barnes, 1990). The density of muscarinic receptors is greatest in larger proximal airways and least in the smaller peripheral airways, consistent with the pattern of vagal-mediated airway constriction (Barnes *et al.*, 1983). Vagal-mediated bronchoconstriction is blocked by atropine and potentiated by acetylcoholinesterase inhibitors, indicating that the effect is, in fact, produced by ACh acting on muscarinic receptors (Casale, 1987). The muscarinic receptors of human airway smooth muscle were entirely of the m_3 sub-type while bronchial submucosal glands contained both m_3 and m_1 receptors in a 2:1 ratio. These findings were confirmed by *in situ* hybridization techniques (Mak *et al.*, 1992). Airway parasympathetic ganglia are believed to contain predominantly m_1 receptors which act to facilitate vagal transmission which classically occurs through nicotinic receptors. The m_2-receptor sub-type is felt to be a presynaptic inhibitory autoreceptor on cholinergic nerves, although mRNA for m_2 receptors has also been described in airway smooth muscle. If also expressed, m_2-receptor stimulation might be expected to promote bronchoconstriction by inhibiting adenylate cyclase activity and cAMP formation (Eglen *et al.*, 1994). Airway smooth-muscle contraction, mucus secretion and vasodilatation are mediated predominantly by m_3 receptors, however.

Sensory nerve stimulation and parasympathetic reflexes are likely to contribute to the pathology of inflammatory conditions such as allergic rhinitis, vasomotor rhinitis, viral rhinitis (common cold), acute and chronic bronchitis, and asthma (Baraniuk, 1991). The roles of cholinergic mechanisms and anticholinergic therapy in rhinitis and asthma are discussed below.

Role of the cholinergic system in rhinitis

Parasympathetic input is the predominant stimulus for submucosal gland secretion in human nasal mucosa (Raphael *et al.*, 1991; van Megen *et al.*, 1991; Okayama *et al.*, 1993). Methacholine stimulates both serous and mucous cell exocytosis, an effect that is inhibited by m_3 antagonists, and weakly inhibited by m_1 antagonists (Mullol *et al.*, 1992a). *In vivo*, cholinergic reflexes act upon resistance vessels to increase superficial blood flow, but there is little effect on the capacitance vessels (sinusoids) that control mucosal thickness or post-capillary venules that are the site of vascular permeability.

Stimulation of nasal afferent sensory nerves by cold dry air, capsaicin, histamine, bradykinin or allergic reactions recruits parasympathetic reflexes (Naclerio, 1991; Raphael *et al.*, 1991; Stjarne *et al.*, 1991). These reflexes appear to be the most important mechanism regulating glandular serous and mucous cell exocytosis. This finding has been clearly demonstrated in unilateral provocation models. For example, unilateral histamine challenge causes direct activation of vascular H_1 receptors, stimulating arterial dilatation, sinusoidal engorgement and vascular permeability, leading to oedema fluid enriched with albumin, immunoglobuli G (IgG) and other plasma proteins. Afferent sensory nerves are also stimulated, to transmit sensations of itch and trigger protective reflexes such as sneezing. In contrast, bilateral cholinergic stimulation causes glandular secretion of mucous cell mucoglycoproteins and serous cell lysozyme, lactoferrin, secretory IgA and other enzymes (Raphael *et al.*, 1991).

Consistent with these models, the muscarinic antagonists atropine and ipratropium bromide effectively reduce glandular secretion and 'dry' the mucosa, but have no effect on sneezing or vascular congestion (Mygind & Borum, 1990). Clinically, ipratropium effectively reduces cold-induced rhinorrhea and has been used with partial success in other forms of rhinitis (Spector, 1992). In the future, selective m_3-receptor antagonists may have more clinical utility in rhinitis where glandular secretion is a significant cause of patient discomfort. However, marked reductions in glandular secretion may prove counterproductive by reducing the amount of serous cell-derived antimicrobial and lubricating proteins on the mucosal surface, and by leading to drying, irritation and possible sensory nerve stimulation.

Role of the cholinergic system in asthma

Because the cholinergic system plays an important role in maintaining resting smooth muscle tone, producing airway smooth muscle contraction and regulating airway mucous secretion, there are many potential abnormalities of this important system which may contribute to asthma pathophysiology. These abnormalities would be expected to either increase acetylcholine release from cholinergic nerve terminals or increase the responsiveness of target tissues. Potential mechanisms include enhanced vagal output from the CNS, enhanced cholinergic reflex activity, increased acetylcholine release, alterations in muscarinic receptors and enhanced airway smooth-muscle responsiveness (Table 27.3). Importantly, airway inflammation and inflammatory mediators may actively contribute to many of these mechanisms.

Enhanced vagal output from the CNS

Psychogenic factors have long been suspected to play some role in precipitating asthma attacks. Evidence does exist that psychogenic factors can influence airway tone through vagal efferent pathways. For example, in response to inhaled saline, McFadden *et al.* (1969) demonstrated a decrease in specific airways conductance in asthmatics who were led to believe they were inhaling bronchospastic agents. Furthermore, this effect was inhibited by atropine, suggesting that cholinergic pathways were involved. Moreover, enhanced vagal cardiac tone has been demonstrated in asthmatics, which indirectly suggests that asthmatics have an increase in central vagal drive. An increase in sinus arrhythmia gap corresponding to nocturnal bronchoconstriction has also been demonstrated (Postma *et al.*, 1985). Thus, enhanced vagal output from the CNS may partially contribute to asthmatic bronchoconstriction.

Enhanced cholinergic reflex activity

Enhanced cholinergic reflex activity was initially postu-

Table 27.3 Potential cholinergic abnormalities in asthma.

Enhanced vagal output from central nervous system
Enhanced cholinergic reflex activity by
Inflammatory mediators
Exogenous stimuli
Increased acetylcholine release via
Inflammatory mediator effects on:
Parasympathetic ganglia
Postganglionic nerves
Inhibitory α- and β-adrenergic receptor dysfunction
Inhibitiory m_2-receptor dysfunction
Alterations in muscarinic receptors
Enhanced m_1-mediated ganglionic transmission
Increased m_3-receptor density and/or affinity on airway smooth muscle
m_2-Autoreceptor dysfunction as result of:
Neuraminidase
Oxygen-derived free radicals
Major basic protein
NSAIDs
Ozone
Enhanced airway smooth-muscle responsiveness
Enhanced signal transduction
Decreased load or resistance to contraction

NSAIDs, non-steroidal anti-inflammatory drugs.

lated as a mechanism for bronchial hyperresponsiveness because it was observed that many stimuli which produce bronchoconstriction in asthmatics, such as sulphur dioxide and histamine, also stimulate afferent sensory nerve endings. Furthermore, cholinergic antagonists can inhibit the bronchoconstrictive responses to these same stimuli (Simonsson *et al.*, 1967). In addition, other inflammatory mediators, such as serotonin, prostaglandin $F_{2\alpha}$ ($PGF_{2\alpha}$), and bradykinin, may stimulate afferent sensory nerves, leading to bronchoconstriction (Barnes, 1992). Airway epithelial damage probably increases the exposure of these sensory nerve endings, thereby enhancing reflex activity due to any stimulus. This may trigger not only a reflex increase in efferent cholinergic activity, but also the antidromic release of tachykinins and CGRP via a 'short-circuited' local reflex loop (Barnes, 1986c), referred to as the 'axon reflex'. This axon reflex is considered in greater detail later in this chapter.

Increased AC release

Efferent discharge of ACh may be modulated at the level of postganglionic nerves or ganglia. Inflammatory mediators, such as serotonin, SP, $PGF_{2\alpha}$, thromboxane A_2 (TXA_2) and PAF (in the presence of platelets), may augment ACh release by pre-junctional mechanisms (Daniel & O'Byrne, 1991; Ito, 1991). Other mediators, such as PGE_2, PGI_2 and, surprisingly, histamine, have the opposite effect. Although histamine can inhibit vagally mediated airway contraction via H_3 receptors, its effect is relatively weak (Ichinose *et al.*, 1989; Ichinose & Barnes, 1990). Evidence suggests that both β_2-agonists and α_2-agonists can also inhibit cholinergic neurotransmission. Furthermore, feedback inhibition of cholinergic neurotransmission occurs by ACh acting on m_2 autoreceptors. Lung parasympathetic ganglia, which are located in airway walls and are surrounded by mast cells, may also be a site of neuromodulation by inflammatory mediators (Barnes, 1992). Once released, reduced degradation by acetylcholinesterase could potentially increase local ACh concentrations, but there is no direct evidence that this occurs. Thus, modulation of cholinergic neurotransmission and ACh release is complex and involves both inflammatory mediators and neural mechanisms (Fig. 27.2). Since many inflammatory mediators postulated to be important in asthma can increase ACh release, the inflammatory response characteristic of asthma might contribute to airway hyperresponsiveness via effects on vagal pathways.

Alterations in muscarinic receptors

Three pharmacologically defined muscarinic receptor sub-types have been identified in the lung. As discussed, airway smooth-muscle contraction, mucus secretion and vasodilatation appear to be mediated predominantly by m_3 receptors, while m_2 receptors are primarily autoinhibitory. Furthermore, m_1-receptor stimulation facilitates ganglionic vagal transmission. Therefore, increases (m_1, m_3) or decreases (m_2) in numbers and/or affinity of muscarinic receptors have been postulated to contribute to asthma pathophysiology.

Lammers *et al.* (1989) have shown that pirenzepine, a specific m_1-receptor antagonist, inhibits reflex bronchoconstriction due to sulphur dioxide inhalation in humans. Therefore, they hypothesized that abnormally responsive m_1 receptors in ganglia may enhance vagal reflexes in asthma by facilitating nicotinic ganglionic neurotransmission. Using non-specific ligands, numbers of muscarinic receptors have been shown to increase slightly in guinea pigs following prolonged sensitization to ovalbumin (Mita *et al.*, 1983). However, Casale (1993b) has recently found no changes in muscarinic receptor number or agonist/antagonist affinity following *in vitro* human lung anaphylaxis. Therefore, there does not appear to be generalized qualitative or quantitative muscarinic receptor alterations in acute allergic lung responses, although changes accompanying chronic allergic inflammation cannot be ruled out.

However, there are data to support down-regulation of inhibitory m_2 autoreceptors in asthmatics. For example, low doses of ipratropium can potentiate, rather than block, vagally induced bronchoconstriction in guinea pigs (Fryer & Maclagan, 1987). Fryer and colleagues subsequently showed that antigen challenge of sensitized guinea pigs, parainfluenza virus infection and ozone exposure all alter neuronal m_2 receptors so that they no longer function to inhibit ACh release (Fryer & Jacoby, 1991; Fryer & Wills-Karp, 1991; Schultheis *et al.*, 1994). Elwood *et al.* (1993), however, have been unable to demonstrate enhanced parasympathetic mechanisms using a rat model of allergen-induced airway hyperresponsiveness. Although dysfunction of m_2 receptors during acute parainfluenza infection was confirmed in a different rat model, the persistent airway hyperresponsiveness several weeks post-infection was independent of m_2-receptor function (Sorkness *et al.*, 1994).

Nonetheless, human data also indirectly support a role for m_2-receptor dysfunction in asthma. Minette *et al.* (1989) found that, in normals, pilocarpine (an m_2 agonist) inhibited cholinergic reflex bronchoconstriction induced by inhaled sulphur dioxide. Similarly, Ayala and Ahmed (1989) showed that methacholine pretreatment suppressed histamine-induced bronchoconstriction in normals. In both studies, however, asthmatic subjects were not protected by such cholinergic agonists. These studies clearly suggest the possibility of m_2-receptor dysfunction in asthma. Barnes has suggested that such a defect might explain the paradoxical bronchoconstriction seen with low doses of anticholinergics, as well as contribute to β-antagonist-induced asthma. The loss of m_2-receptor function, coupled with drug-induced blockade of β-mediated inhibitory activity, might allow unchecked cholinergic responses in asthmatics (Barnes, 1989a).

m_2-Autoreceptor dysfunction may be related to airway inflammation. Fryer suggested that neuraminidase released from inflammatory cells may cleave critical sialic acid residues from m_2 receptors and thereby weaken agonist binding (Fryer & Wills-Karp, 1991). The same mechanism might account for post-viral airway hyperreactivity. In allergic inflammation, eosinophil-derived major basic protein may also bind to and inhibit m_2 receptors. Furthermore, oxygen-derived free radicals generated by inflammatory cells may have a similar effect (Barnes, 1992). Interestingly, m_2 receptors in guinea pig lungs were also inhibited by indomethacin, suggesting that loss of m_2-receptor function may also contribute to aspirin-sensitive asthma (ASA)-induced airway hyperresponsiveness (Fryer & Okanlami, 1993).

Enhanced airway smooth-muscle responsiveness

Bai (1990) found that tracheal smooth muscle obtained from asthmatics who died during severe asthma attacks had increased *in vitro* cholinergic- and histamine-induced responsiveness. Others, however, have failed to show increased airway smooth-muscle responsiveness to cholinergic agonists *in vitro* (Goldie *et al.*, 1986). Thus, it remains unclear whether or not enhanced airway smooth-muscle responsiveness contributes to asthma pathogenesis.

There are other potential mechanisms of bronchial hyperresponsiveness, however. These include decreases in either internal or external loads on airway smooth muscle. For example, Stephens *et al.* (1991) have demonstrated that an internal resistance to shortening is markedly decreased in the airway smooth muscle of allergic dogs. Moreover, *in vivo*, geometric factors related to airway thickening and oedema may uncouple airway–parenchyma interdependence and result in exaggerated airway narrowing in response to any particular stimulus (Macklem, 1991). Therefore, compared to normals, the airways of asthmatics may narrow proportionately more in response to equivalent bronchoconstricting stimuli.

Summary of cholinergic role in asthma

Thus, by a variety of mechanisms, most notably increased cholinergic reflex activity, increased ACh release and m_2-autoreceptor dysfunction, cholinergic abnormalities might contribute to the pathogenesis of asthma and airway hyperreactivity. This has been suggested in a variety of models investigating the effects of allergens, ozone, viral infections and non-steroidal anti-inflammatory drugs. Moreover, many of these abnormalities are likely to reflect the effects of numerous inflammatory mediators on vagal pathways. Therapeutically, selective muscarinic receptor agents may prove more efficacious (and free of side-effects) than currently used anticholinergics in modulating cholinergically mediated pro-asthma effects. Indeed, knowledge about the modulatory effects of various neurotransmitters, mediators and drugs on cholinergic neutrotransmission in the lung (Fig. 27.2) are likely to provide fruitful avenues for novel therapeutic approaches.

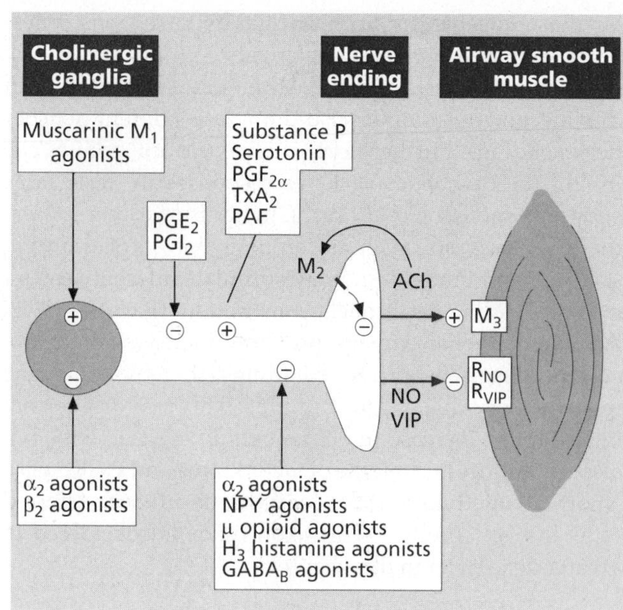

Fig. 27.2 Modulation of cholinergic neurotransmission in the lung. Corelease of acetylcholine (ACh) with nitric oxide (NO) and vasoactive intestinal peptide (VIP) is shown. NO and VIP antagonize the effects of ACh on airway smooth muscle and are felt to function as a 'braking' mechanism on cholinergic effects. Release of ACh can either be inhibited or stimulated by numerous neurotransmitters, mediators and drugs, as shown. Data support ganglionic modulation by m_1-, α_2- and β_2-receptor stimulation and inhibitory presynaptic postganglionic modulation by m_2-, α_2-, NPY-, μ-opioid, H_3- and $GABA_B$-receptor stimulation. Inflammatory mediators and substance P have negative and positive modulatory effects at unknown sites. Shown specifically is feedback inhibition by ACh via presynapthic m_2 autoreceptors. R_{NO} and R_{VIP} represent receptors for NO and VIP, respectively. See text for definition of abbreviations.

The eNANC system

Non-cholinergic excitatory pathways have been described in both animal and human lung. Current evidence suggests that these pathways consist of non-myelinated parasympathetic afferent fibres with nerve endings in the airway epithelium (Lundberg & Saria, 1982; Lundberg *et al.*, 1983a, 1984b). Mechanical irritation, cigarette smoke, sulphur dioxide, and allergic and post-viral inflammation through inflammatory mediators, such as histamine and bradykinin, can all stimulate these nerve endings to cause antidromic release of neuropeptides (Lungberg & Saria, 1983; Saria *et al.*, 1983, 1988). In human lung, the putative neurotransmitters for this system are the tachykinins, including SP and NKA, and CGRP. Relevant biological actions of these neuropeptides include vasodilatation, increased vascular permeability, increased mucus secretion, bronchoconstriction and immune/inflammatory cell activation. Thus, in addition to stimulating a reflex increase in efferent cholinergic activity, the antidromic release of neuropeptides SP, NKA and CGRP may also contribute to the pathogenesis of asthma (Fig. 27.3).

Innervation

Nasal sensory nerves originate in the trigeminal ganglion and innervate the nose via ethmoidal and posterior nasal nerves (Uddman & Sundler, 1986; Raphael *et al.*, 1991). Vagal sensory nerves have cell bodies in the small superior or nodose vagal ganglia and innervate the lower

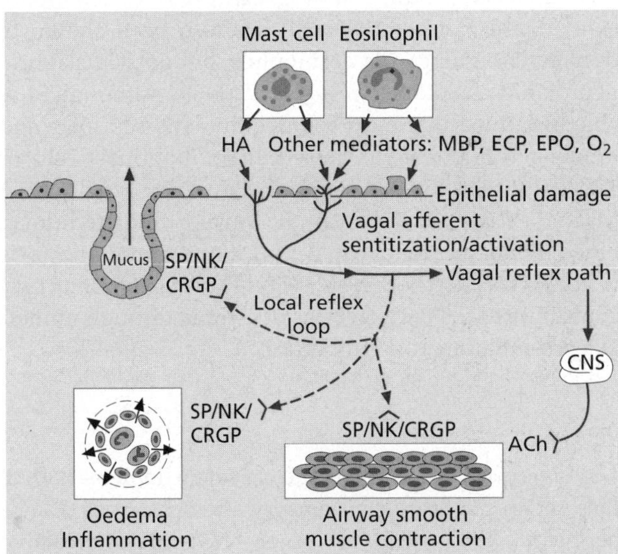

Fig. 27.3 Axon reflex mechanism as proposed by Barnes (1986c). Non-specific irritants and inflammatory cell mediators can sensitize and stimulate vagal afferent nerve endings exposed by epithelial damage. Stimulation of vagal afferents results in vagal reflex path activation, including activation of a local reflex path (dashed lines) with antidromic release of substance P (SP), neurokinin A (NKA) and calcitonin gene-related peptide (CGRP). These neuropeptides, in concert with other mediators, can then cause airway smooth-muscle contraction, oedema, inflammation and mucus production. See text for abbreviation definitions. (From Casale, 1993a.)

pharynx, epiglottis, larynx (recurrent laryngeal nerve), trachea, main stem and subsegmental bronchi, and oesophagus. These highly branched neurones innervate vessels, glands, and the epithelium where they extend between basal cells. Some endings have fine terminal extensions that reach up between epithelial cells to the region of the tight junctions. Sensory nerve stimulation and central reception of afferent nerve impulses in the brain stem and higher centres leads to the appreciation of sensations of itch, burning and congestion, and the initiation of important central reflexes such as sneeze, cough and parasympathetic secretory reflexes (Raphael *et al.*, 1991).

The afferent sensory nerves are non-myelinated type C fibres that do not have specialized sensory organs such as olfactory bulbs. C fibres have bare neural endings that are chemosensitive and mechanothermal sensitive. They can be stimulated by inflammatory mediators such as histamine, bradykinin, serotonin, K^+ and H^+, that are released following mucosal injury or mast cell degranulation after allergen exposure (Baraniuk, 1991; Casale, 1993a). Other mediators, such as prostaglandins and sulphidopeptide leukotrienes, modulate sensory nerve function by decreasing the threshold to depolarization (Martins *et al.*, 1991). Inhaled agents, such as sulphur dioxide, ozone, formaldehyde, nicotine, cigarette smoke and capsaicin, can also stimulate these nerves.

Depolarization of a peripheral sensory nerve ending generates a wave of depolarization that extends throughout the entire length of the nerve axon and all of the extensively branched rami. This wave of depolarization releases colocalized neuropeptides from neurosecretory swellings (varicosities) that are found near glands and vessels. The varicosities are strung like beads on a string along the extensively branched peripheral sensory nerve. The neuropeptides include the tachykinins SP and NKA, CGRP, GRP and possibly others (Baraniuk, 1991; Barnes *et al.*, 1991a,b; Casale, 1993a; Baraniuk *et al.*, 1994). The same combination of neuropeptides is packaged within vesicles of all the varicosities, and is released from all the central and peripheral varicosities of a single neurone (Dale Principle) (Dale, 1935; Eccles, 1986). Sensory neuropeptides act upon specific receptors on target cells to initiate and amplify inflammatory responses to mucosal injury. This 'axon response' mechanism mediates cutaneous weal-and-flare reactions in the skin (Baraniuk *et al.*, 1990b), and in the respiratory tract causes local mucosal vasodilatation, vascular permeability, glandular secretion and may facilitate vascular wall leucocyte adhesion (Holzer, 1988; McDonald, 1988).

Excitatory neuropeptides and their receptors

Although neuropeptides are addressed in detail in the

previous chapter, a comprehensive review would be incomplete without discussing the specific role of peptidergic neurones in the overall autonomic control of the airways. In human upper and lower airways, the putative neurotransmitters of this system are the tachykinins, including SP and NKA, CGRP and GRP.

SP

SP is an 11-amino-acid peptide synthesized in the cell bodies of primary sensory neurones in parasympathetic ganglia and transported down vagal nerve fibres (Sundler *et al.*, 1985). There are at least three high-affinity-tachykinin receptor sub-types (Carstairs & Barnes, 1986b; Drapeau *et al.*, 1987; Regoli *et al.*, 1989; Frossard & Advenier, 1991). The NK_1 sub-type has greatest affinity for SP and is predominantly located within lung epithelium, submucosal glands and post-capillary venules. In humans, there is dense [^{125}I]SP binding over submucosal glands and sparse binding over airway smooth muscle, suggesting a more important role for SP in secretory rather than spasmogenic processes (Goldie, 1990).

SP stimulates airway smooth-muscle contraction, submucosal gland and goblet cell secretion, and increased vascular permeability (Lundberg *et al.*, 1983b; Tokuyama *et al.*, 1990; Shimura *et al.*, 1991). SP may also increase cholinergic neural responses by potentiating postganglionic parasmpathetic activity (Barnes *et al.*, 1987; Hall *et al.*, 1989).

In normal and mildly asthmatic humans, however, neither intravenous nor inhaled SP cause significant bronchoconstriction (Fuller *et al.*, 1987; Joos *et al.*, 1987). Degradation of SP by angiotensin-converting enzyme (ACE) or neutral endopeptidase (NEP), respectively, may explain this lack of effect. In more severe asthmatics, inhaled SP did cause a dose-related decrease in forced expiratory volume in 1 second (FEV_1) which was blocked by nedocromil (Crimi *et al.*, 1988). Either increased non-specific bronchial hyperreactivity or a relative deficiency of NEP due to the increased airway epithelial damage associated with moderate-to-severe asthma may explain these findings. The latter hypothesis is supported by animal studies, which showed enhanced SP-induced airway contraction and mucus secretion with use of specific NEP inhibitors or epithelial stripping (Nadel & Borson, 1991).

Probably more important than bronchoconstriction is the effect of SP on bronchovascular permeability and blood flow. SP and, to a lesser extent, NKA, are potent inducers of bronchovascular permeability (Lundberg *et al.*, 1983b). In addition, SP, NKA and CGRP all cause vasodilatation and thereby may increase fluid exudation by increasing bronchial blood flow (Fuller *et al.*, 1987; Laitinen *et al.*, 1987).

In explants from human nasal mucosa, SP induces serous and mucous glandular secretion (Baraniuk *et al.*, 1991a). In pig nasal mucosa, SP also increases nasal blood flow and the thickness of the mucosa (Stjarne *et al.*, 1991). SP-immunoreactive material can be measured in nasal (Mosimann *et al.*, 1993) and bronchoalveolar lavage fluid (Nieber *et al.*, 1992) from allergic subjects after allergen challenge, suggesting that SP is released during this process. It is most likely that afferent sensory nerves are the source of this SP, although other sources such as inflammatory cells have been suggested in the past (Payan *et al.*, 1984). Nasal provocation with SP apparently has minimal effects in normal subjects, but induces albumin secretion and nasal airway obstruction in allergic rhinitics (Devillier *et al.*, 1988; Braunstein *et al.*, 1991). Responses appear to be greater in subjects with established inflammatory syndromes, such as allergic rhinitis or asthma, possibly due to the loss of NEP. The effects of NEP on tachykinins and neurogenic inflammation are discussed later.

Lastly, SP can directly modulate the functions of immune/inflammatory cells. SP causes T-lymphocyte proliferation (Payan *et al.*, 1983), activation of macrophages (Hartung *et al.*, 1986), enhanced macrophage and neutrophil phagocytosis (Bar-Shavit *et al.*, 1980), chemotaxis (Marasco *et al.*, 1981; Carolan & Casale, 1993) and enhanced production of IgA and IgM by B lymphocytes (Stanisz *et al.*, 1986). SP has also been shown to degranulate guinea pig eosinophils, but not via classical neurokinin receptors (Kroegel *et al.*, 1989). Although SP is able to induce skin mast cell degranulation in mice and humans, it is unable to cause human lung mast cells or basophils to release histamine (Lawrence *et al.*, 1987; Matsuda *et al.*, 1989). SP can, however, stimulate human blood monocytes to release IL-1, IL-6 and tumour necrosis factor-α (TNF-α) (Lotz *et al.*, 1988). Thus, tachykinins may contribute to the pathogenesis of asthma through numerous pro-inflammatory properties.

NKA

NKA is colocalized with SP, and capsaicin depletes both of these neuropeptides from sensory afferent nerves (Lundberg *et al.*, 1985, 1987). However, NKA-immunoreactive nerves are more prominently localized to bronchial smooth muscle (Uchida *et al.*, 1987). Moreover, while SP has a greater affinity for NK_1 receptors, NKA has a greater affinity for NK_2 receptors. Although both SP and NKA mediate non-cholinergic bronchoconstriction, the relative contribution of NK_2 receptors is greater than that of NK_1 receptors (Maggi *et al.*, 1991). NKA- and NK_2-receptor-mediated airway actions are likely to result from both direct effects on airway smooth muscle and facilitated postganglionic cholinergic activity (Hall *et al.*, 1989). NK_2

receptors are felt to be located on small airway smooth muscle, cholinergic neurones and ganglia, and on inflammatory cells. Consistent with the localization of NKA-immunoreactive nerves, NKA is a potent bronchoconstrictor, both *in vitro* and *in vivo* (Uchida *et al.*, 1987; Naline *et al.*, 1989). Unlike SP, both intravenous and inhaled NKA caused dose-dependent bronchoconstriction in mild asthmatics (Joos *et al.*, 1987). This supports a more important role for NKA in regulating airway tone.

Interestingly, tachykinin receptors belong to the same seven-transmembrane-spanning rhodopsin receptor superfamily as β-receptors (Venter *et al.*, 1988), yet stimulation of tachykinin and β-receptors have opposite effects. This suggests that differential utilization of specific G-protein pools may determine the outcome of this functional antagonism.

CGRP

CGRP is also colocalized with tachykinins in sensory afferent nerves and is released by similar stimuli (Lundberg *et al.*, 1985, 1987). *In vitro*, biological effects of CGRP include bronchoconstriction, vasodilatation and mucus secretion. These effects appear to be mediated by specific receptors linked to adenylate cyclase (Barnes *et al.*, 1991a). Although CGRP-immunoreactive nerves are found near ganglia, blood vessels, trancheobronchial smooth muscle and respiratory epithelium, CGRP receptors are localized predominantly to airway blood vessels (Mak & Barnes, 1988; Shimosegawa & Said, 1991). Therefore, in concert with SP and NKA, CGRP may contribute to airway oedema through potent and prolonged vasodilatation and increased blood flow (Salonen *et al.*, 1988). Moreover, both CGRP and SP may contribute to increased airway secretions via effects on submucosal glands, glycoprotein secretion, goblet cells, and epithelial ion transport (Rangachari & McWade, 1985; Rogers *et al.*, 1989; Barnes *et al.*, 1990b; Tokuyama *et al.*, 1990). Indirect evidence supporting a role for CGRP in airway diseases includes increased levels of tissue CGRP after aeroallergen challenge and chronic smoke exposure (Lundberg *et al.*, 1991).

CGRP and its degradation products may be chemotactic for eosinophils (Haynes & Manley, 1988). In contrast to SP, however, CGRP may also have anti-inflammatory properties, such as inhibition of hydrogen peroxide production and antigen presentation by macrophages (Daniele *et al.*, 1992).

GRP

GRP is a 27-amino-acid peptide that is related to the 14-amino-acid amphibian peptide bombesin (Sunday *et al.*, 1988). Bombesin-immunoreactive peptides are expressed by normal human bronchial epithelial neuroendocrine cells (Tsutsumi, 1988) and can be detected in bronchoalveolar lavage fluids (Aguayo *et al.*, 1989). Three receptors have been cloned for bombesin-family peptides (Battey *et al.*, 1991; Corjay *et al.*, 1991; Wada *et al.*, 1991; Fathi *et al.*, 1993), but the distributions of each receptor sub-type in normal respiratory mucosa have not been fully determined.

In human nasal mucosa, GRP nerve fibres are present in the walls of arterial and venous vessels, and around glandular acini (Baraniuk *et al.*, 1990d). Their distribution is very similar to that of CGRP and NKA, and suggests that GRP may be colocalized in the same sensory neurones. [^{125}I]GRP binding sites are localized to the epithelium and submucosal glands of human nasal and tracheal mucosa (Baraniuk *et al.*, 1990c). *In vitro*, GRP induces both serous and mucous cell exocytosis from human nasal mucosa. *In vivo*, bombesin stimulates mucous glycoconjugate and lysozyme secretion from human nasal mucosa, but does not stimulate albumin secretion (Baraniuk *et al.*, 1992c), suggesting an effect on submucosal (and possibly goblet cell) secretion without increases in vascular permeability.

Bombesin is also a bronchoconstrictor in guinea pig tracheal smooth muscle *in vitro* and *in vivo* (Belvisi *et al.*, 1991). GRP-containing neuroendocrine cells are rare in normal, non-smoking human adults, but as much as 10 times more common in cigarette smokers and in hamsters exposed to cigarette smoke (Aguayo *et al.*, 1989). GRP and its receptors are present in small cell carcinoma, and GRP and related peptides are proliferation factors for these cells (Gazdar & Carbone, 1994). GRP and related peptides may also stimulate proliferation of non-neoplastic cells in inflammatory conditions such as asthma and bronchopulmonary dysplasia, suggesting that autocrine release of GRP may play a role in many bronchial disorders.

These varied effects suggest that GRP or related peptides may be released from afferent sensory nerves and bronchial neuroendocrine cells and may act as serous and mucous cell secretagogues, bronchoconstrictors and growth factors in human respiratory mucosa.

Excitatory neuropeptide degradation

Once released, neuropeptides are subject to local hydrolysis by peptidases such as NEP (Nadel, 1990; Borson, 1991). NEP is a membrane-associated metallopeptidase that is predominantly localized to airway epithelium and serves to limit tachykinin-mediated effects (Honda *et al.*, 1991; Nadel & Borson, 1991). It is thought, however, that all cells bearing peptide receptors also express NEP. *In situ* hybridization of NEP mRNA, and immunohistochemistry of NEP-immunoreactive material have revealed NEP in epithelium, glands and vessels of human nasal mucosa (Baraniuk *et al.*, 1993), as well as tracheobronchial smooth-muscle cells (Baraniuk *et al.*, 1991b).

NEP is active upon SP, NKA, CGRP, GRP, bradykinin and many other peptides. Inhibition of NEP potentiates inflammation and bronchial smooth muscle contraction induced by substance P, capsaicin and vagal nerve stimulation. This suggests that tachykinins and/or other NEP substrates do cause neurogenic inflammation and that their effects are regulated by NEP (Umeno *et al.*, 1989; Honda *et al.*, 1991). Destruction of NEP activity may lead to prolonged, unopposed inflammatory effects of neuropeptides, and may contribute to respiratory hyperresponsiveness that can develop in some inflammatory rhinitic conditions and asthma.

Neuropeptide actions are also limited by ACE, an exopeptidase that is concentrated on the luminal side of vascular endothelium (Ohkubo *et al.*, 1994). When used as antihypertensives, ACE inhibitors have been found to produce a cough that may be associated with increased airway hyperreactivity (Bucknall *et al.*, 1988; Lindgren *et al.*, 1989b). It has been postulated that the cough and airway hyperreactivity associated with the use of ACE inhibitors are mediated by kinins. However, the role of kinins has not been clearly defined (Dixon *et al.*, 1987). ACE inhibitors have also been shown to augment both spontaneous and antigen-induced histamine release from lung and skin and to potentiate antigen-induced cutaneous responses (Lindgren *et al.*, 1989a). These data suggest that ACE inhibitors might also contribute to neurogenic inflammation.

Role of the excitatory NANC system in airway disease

As with the other autonomic systems, a variety of altered non-cholinergic excitatory nerve mechanisms have been proposed in asthmatics. Potential abnormalities include: an increase in afferent nerve density and/or accessibility to stimuli; increased synthesis/release of tachykinins, CGRP and GRP; decreased local proteolytic degradation; increased receptor density and/or affinity; and increased post-receptor responses (Table 27.4). Despite the data discussed, direct evidence supporting these putative abnormalities is lacking. Moreover, since inhaled capsaicin caused equal bronchonconstriction in asthmatic and normal subjects, a fundamental abnormality in non-cholinergic excitatory activity in asthmatics is unlikely (Fuller *et al.*, 1985).

The simplest mechanism for increasing non-cholinergic excitatory activity is increased stimulation of sensory afferent nerves. For example, allergic inflammation involves release of mast cell mediators, such as histamine and bradykinin, which are known to activate sensory nerves. Certain inflammatory mediators may also 'sensitize' afferent nerve endings, leading to 'hyperalgesia' of inflamed airways (Daniele *et al.*, 1992). Furthermore, the epithelial damage characteristic of asthma and allergic rhinitis would be expected to increase accessibility of sensory nerve endings to both inhaled stimuli and locally released mediators. A recent report by Ollerenshaw *et al.* (1991) also describes an increase in SP-immunoreactive nerves in asthmatic vs. non-asthmatic airways. Although chronic inflammation may lead to structural changes in innervation, these results may also be explained by increased neuropeptide synthesis. Alterations in local production or release of nerve growth factor may impact upon both of these possibilities (Lindsay & Harmar, 1989). Whether or not antigenic stimulation or airway inflammation can alter neuropeptide gene transcription awaits the development of specific antagonists and molecular studies (Daniele *et al.*, 1992).

Table 27.4 Potential non-cholinergic excitatory abnormalities in asthma.

Increase in non-cholinergic excitatory neurones
Increased synthesis of tachykinins, CGRP and GRP
Sensitization and stimulation of sensory nerve endings by Inflammatory mediators Exogenous stimuli
Effects of epithelial damage Increased exposure of sensory nerve endings Reduced breakdown of tachykinins due to loss of neutral endopeptidase
Increased receptor density and/or affinity
Increased post-receptor responses

Evidence suggests that reduced degradation of tachykinins by NEP may also lead to increased non-cholinergic excitatory activity, presumably by increasing local concentrations and prolonging the half-life of these neuropeptides. For example, inhibitors of NEP, such as phosphoramidon, have been shown in guinea pigs to augment airway responsiveness to both SP and capsaicin, but not ACh (Thompson & Sheppard, 1988). Neurogenic inflammation in rat trachea is also enhanced after treatment with NEP inhibitors (Umeno *et al.*, 1989). Sheppard and co-workers (1988) found that toluene diisocyanate-induced bronchoconstriction in guinea pigs occurs largely through inhibition of airway NEP. Cigarette smoke and viral infections have also been shown to decrease NEP activity while increasing airway hyperresponsiveness (Jacoby *et al.*, 1988; Dusser *et al.*, 1989). *In vitro*, removal of airway epithelium exaggerates responses to tachykinins (Naline *et al.*, 1989). Therefore, loss of NEP as a consequence of the *in vivo* epithelial denudation seen in asthma and viral infections is likely to facilitate tachykinin-induced effects. Although alterations of NEP activity or expression in human diseases have yet to be demonstrated *in vivo*, inhalation of thiorphan, another NEP inhibitor, allows inhaled NKA to exert a mild bronchoconstrictor effect in non-asthmatics who otherwise do not respond to inhaled NKA (Cheung *et al.*, 1992). This suggests that tonic neuropeptide and NEP activities exist in the normal airway, and that the balance between these two factors can be altered to produce bronchoconstriction.

On the other hand, glucocorticoid treatment has been shown to increase NEP mRNA and enzyme activity in an SV-40-transformed human epithelial cell line (Borson & Gruenert, 1991) and in Calu-1 cells (human lung epidermoid carcinoma cell line) (Lang & Murlas, 1992). This enhancement of NEP expression may explain the beneficial effects of glucocorticoids on neurogenic plasma extravasation in virus-infected rat trachea (Piedemonte *et al.*, 1990). Glucocorticoid treatment also alters the size of NEP mRNA transcripts (Borson & Gruenert 1991), suggesting complex regulation at the level of mRNA transcription and/or post-transcriptional processing. Enhanced NEP expression may represent yet another beneficial effect of glucocorticoid therapy in rhinitis and asthma.

Conclusions

Many hypotheses regarding abnormal autonomic control of the airways have been proposed. These have included abnormalities in adrenergic, cholinergic and NANC pathways. In diseased lungs, the normal homeostatic balance between pro-asthmatic and anti-asthmatic forces is tipped in favour of asthma (Fig. 27.4). There are clearly complex interactions, both between neural pathways themselves, and between neural and inflammatory processes. Unfortunately, much of the data supporting specific abnormalities are indirect. Moreover, many of the studies to date have involved animal models and differences between species are often pronounced.

Despite patchy data regarding human lung, current knowledge supports a few generalizations. Cholinergic innervation provides the main bronchoconstrictor and glandular secretory pathways. Increased cholinergic responses probably result from both pre-junctional facilitation of ACh release and vagal reflex stimulation by inflammatory mediators. Furthermore, dysfunctional m_2 autoreceptors, possibly occurring as a consequence of inflammation, may contribute to enhanced cholinergic activity. Although β-receptor abnormalities have been demonstrated, they could be secondary to chronic inflammation and/or therapy. Moreover, the importance of α-adrenergic abnormalities appears minimal.

Substantial evidence supports the existence of NANC pathways in human lung. VIP and NO are probably inhibitory, while SP, NKA, CGRP and possibly GRP, are probably excitatory NANC neurotransmitters. Bronchoconstrictor effects appear to be mediated primarily by

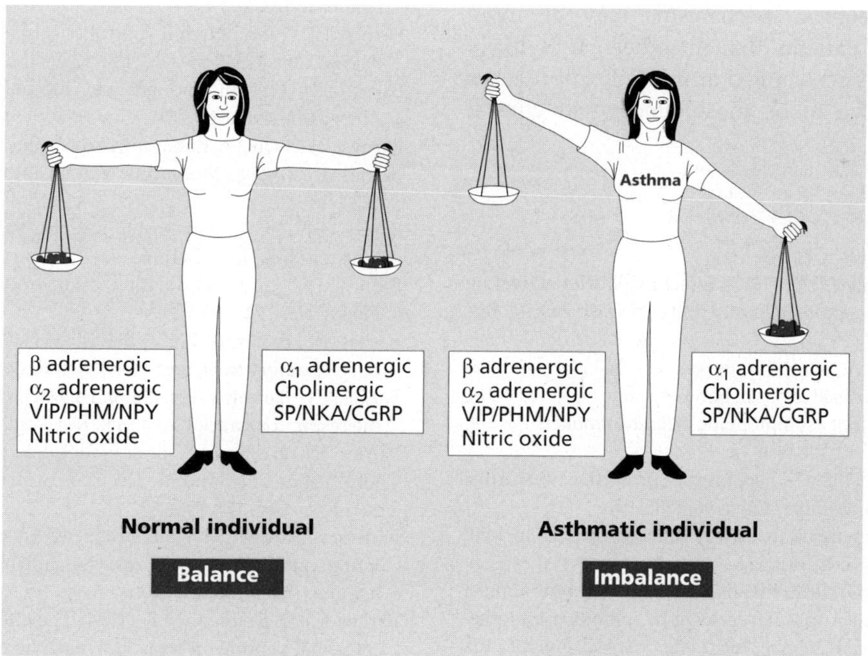

Fig. 27.4 Autonomic nervous system balance in normal and asthmatic individuals. The excitatory nervous system is evenly balanced by the inhibitory nervous system in normal individuals. Individuals with asthma potentially have either an increase in excitatory and/or a decrease in inhibitory nervous system activity that results in an imbalance in the normal autonomic nervous system regulation. See text for definition of abbreviations.

NKA, while mucus hypersecretion and airway oedema are mediated primarily by SP, CGRP and GRP. In addition, inflammation is probably the major contributing factor to defects of these pathways. Both increased degradation of VIP and NO, secondary to proteases and oxygen radicals, and decreased degradation of tachykinins, secondary to loss of epithelial-associated NEP, are likely to contribute to asthma pathogenesis. Indeed, initial lung inflammatory responses may lead to neurogenic inflammation, setting in motion a vicious cycle.

In the nose, allergens, cold dry air and other inhaled irritants and gases stimulate sensory nerves to recruit both central parasympathetic reflexes and a local axon reflex. In addition to mucus secretion and oedema formation, important protective reflexes, such as sneezing, are stimulated. The vasodilating and secretory effects of cholinergic innervation and eNANC peptides are normally balanced by the vasoconstricting and antisecretory effects of adrenergic and iNANC innervation. As in the lung, scenarios involving interactions between mucosal inflammation and opposing neural pathways appear to contribute to upper airway diseases, including allergic, infectious and other forms of rhinitis.

Hopefully, further understanding of these complex mechanisms will lead to more specific asthma and rhinitis therapy. Possibilities for future therapy include m_3-specific anticholinergics, NPY agonists, tachykinin antagonists and other neuromodulators, in addition to novel anti-inflammatory agents. Different limbs of proposed pathophysiological mechanisms may be more important in some patients than in others. It is likely that therapeutic regimens aimed at multiple approaches will ultimately prove to be most effective in clinical management.

References

Agrawal, D.K. & Townley, R.G. (1987) Effect of platelet-activating factor on beta-adrenoceptors in human lung. *Biochem. Biophy. Res. Commun.*, **143**, 1–6.

Aguayo, S.M., Kane, M.A., King, T.E. Jr, Schwarz, M.I., Graver, L. & Miller, Y.E. (1989) Increased levels of bombesin-like peptides in the lower respiratory tract of asymptomatic cigarette smokers. *J. Clin. Invest.*, **84**, 1105–13.

Ayala, L.E. & Ahmed, T. (1989) Is there loss of a protective muscarinic receptor mechanism in asthma? *Chest*, **96**, 1285–91.

Bai, T.R. (1990) Abnormalities in airway smooth muscle in fatal asthma. *Am. Rev. Resp. Dis.*, **141**, 552–7.

Baluk, P. & McDonald, D. (1994) The β_2-adrenergic receptor agonist formoterol reduces microvascular leakage by inhibiting endothelial gap formation. *Am. J. Physiol.*, **266** (*Lung Cell. Mol. Physiol.*, **10**), L461–8.

Baraniuk, J.N. (1991) Neural control of human nasal secretion. *Pulmon. Pharmacol.*, **4**, 20–31.

Baraniuk, J.N., Castellino, S., Lundgren, J.D. *et al.* (1990a) Neuropeptide Y (NPY) in human nasal mucosa. *Am. J. Respir. Cell Mol. Biol.*, **3**, 165–73.

Baraniuk, J.N., Kowalski, M. & Kaliner, M. (1990b) Neuropeptides in the skin. In: *Skin Immune System (SIS)* (ed. J.B. Bos), p. 307. CRC Press, Baton Rouge, Louisiana.

Baraniuk, J.N., Lundgren, J.D., Goff, J. *et al.* (1990c) Gastrin releasing peptide (GRP) in human nasal mucosa. *J. Clin. Invest.*, **85**, 998–1005.

Baraniuk, J.N., Lundgren, J.D., Okayama, M. *et al.* (1990d) Vasoactive intestinal peptide (VIP) in human nasal mucosa. *J. Clin. Invest.*, **86**, 825–31.

Baraniuk, J.N., Lundgren, J.D., Okayama, M. *et al.* (1991a) Substance P and neurokinin A (NKA) in human nasal mucosa. *Am. J. Respir. Cell Mol. Biol.*, **4**, 228–36.

Baraniuk, J.N., Mak, J., Letarte, M., Davies, R., Twort, C. & Barnes, P.J. (1991b) Neutral endopeptidase mRNA expression. *Am. Rev. Resp. Dis.*, **143**, A40.

Baraniuk, J.N., Kaliner, M. & Barnes, P.J. (1992a) Muscarinic M3 receptor mRNA *in situ* hybridization in human nasal mucosa. *Am. J. Rhinol.*, **6**, 145–8.

Baraniuk, J.N., Silver, P.B., Kaliner, M.A. & Barnes, P.M. (1992b) Neuropeptide Y (NPY) is a vasoconstrictor in human nasal mucosa. *J. Appl. Physiol.*, **73**, 1867–72.

Baraniuk, J.N., Silver, P.B., Lundgren, J.D., Cole, P., Kaliner, M.A. & Barnes, P.J. (1992c) Bombesin stimulates mucous cell and serous cell secretion in human nasal provocation tests. *Am. J. Physiol.*, **262** (*Lung Cell. Mol. Physiol.*), L48–52.

Baraniuk, J.N., Ohkubo, K., Kwon, O.J., Mak, J., Rohde, J. & Kaliner, M.A. (1993) Identification of neutral endopeptidase mRNA in human nasal mucosa. *J. Appl. Physiol.*, **74**, 272–9.

Baraniuk, J.N., Silver, P.B., Kaliner, M.A. & Barnes, P.J. (1994) Perennial rhinitis subjects have altered vascular, glandular, and neural responses to bradykinin nasal provocation. *Int. Arch. Allergy Appl. Immunol.*, **103**, 202–8.

Barnes, P.J. (1986a) Neural control of human airways in health and disease. *Am. Rev. Resp. Dis.*, **134**, 1289–314.

Barnes, P.J. (1986b) Endogenous catecholamines and asthma. *J. Allergy Clin. Immunol.*, **77**, 791–5.

Barnes, P.J. (1986c) Asthma as an axon reflex. *Lancet*, **i**, 242–5.

Barnes, P.J. (1989a) Muscarinic autoreceptors in airways. *Chest*, **96**, 1220–1.

Barnes, P.J. (1989b) Muscarinic receptor subtypes: implications for lung disease. *Thorax*, **44**, 161–7.

Barnes, P.J. (1992) Modulation of neurotransmission in airways. *Physiol. Rev.*, **72**, 699–729.

Barnes, P.J., Baraniuk, J.N. & Belvisi, M.G. (1991a) Neuropeptides in the respiratory tract. Part 1. *Am. Rev. Resp. Dis.*, **144**, 1187–98.

Barnes, P.J., Baraniuk, J.N. & Belvisi, M.G. (1991b) Neuropeptides in the respiratory tract. Part 2. *Am. Rev. Resp. Dis.*, **144**, 1391–9.

Barnes, P.J., Basbaum, C.B. & Nadel, J.A. (1983) Autoradiographic localization of autonomic receptors in airway smooth muscle. *Am. Rev. Resp. Dis.*, **127**, 758–62.

Barnes, P.J., Brown, M.J., Silverman, M. & Dollery, C.T. (1981a) Circulating catecholamines in exercise and hyperventilation induced asthma. *Thorax*, **36**, 435–40.

Barnes, P.J. & Dixon, C.M.S. (1984) The effect of inhaled vasoactive intestinal peptide on bronchial reactivity to histamine in humans. *Am. Rev. Resp. Dis.*, **130**, 162–6.

Barnes, P.J., Dollery, C.T. & MacDermot, J. (1980) Increased pulmonary α-adrenergic and reduced β-adrenergic receptors in experimental asthma. *Nature*, **285**, 569–71.

Barnes, P.J., Ind, P.W. & Dollery, C.T. (1981b) Inhaled prazosin in asthma. *Thorax*, **36**, 378–81.

Barnes, P.J., Kuo, H.P., Rogers, D.F., Rohde, J.A. & Tokuyama, K. (1990a) Effect of vagus nerve stimulation on goblet-cell secretion in guinea-pig trachea *in vivo*. *J. Physiol.*, **422**, 99P.

Barnes, P.J., Kuo, H.P., Rogers, D.F., Rohde, J.A. & Tokuyama, K. (1990b) Effects of sensory neuropeptides on goblet-cell secretion in guinea-pig trachea *in vivo*. *J. Physiol.*, **422**, 100P.

Barnes, P.J., Maclagan, J. & Meldrum, L.A. (1987) Effects of tachykinins on cholinergic neural responses in guinea-pig trachea. *Br. Med. J.*, **90**, 138P.

Bar-Shavit, Z., Goldman, R., Stabinsky, Y. *et al.* (1980) Enhancement of phagocytosis—a newly found activity of substance P residing in its N-terminal tetrapeptide sequence. *Biochem. Biophys. Res. Commun.*, **94**, 1445–51.

Battey, J.F., Way, J.M., Corjay, M.H. *et al.* (1991) Molecular cloning of the bombesin/gastrin releasing peptide receptor from Swiss 3T3 cells. *Proc. Nat. Acad. Sci. USA*, **88**, 395–9.

Beil, M. & de Kock, M.A. (1978) Role of alpha-adrenergic receptors in exercise-induced bronchoconstriction. In: *Respiration* (ed. H. Herzog), pp. 78–86. S. Karger, Basel.

Belvisi, M.G., Stretton, C.D., Miura, M. *et al.* (1992) Inhibitory NANC nerves in human tracheal smooth muscle: a quest for a neurotransmitter. *J. Appl. Physiol.*, **73**, 2505–10.

Belvisi, M.G., Stretton, D. & Barnes, P.J. (1991) Nitric oxide as an endogenous modulator of cholinergic neurotransmission in guinea-pig airways. *Eur. J. Pharmacol.*, **198**, 219–21.

Berkin, K.E., Inglis, G.C., Ball, S.G. & Thomson, N.C. (1986) Effect of low dose adrenaline and noradrenaline infusions on airway calibre in asthmatic patients. *Clin. Sci.*, **70**, 347–52.

Blecher, M., Lewis, S., Hicks, J.M. & Josephs, S. (1984) Beta-blocking autoantibodies in pediatric bronchial asthma. *J. Allergy Clin. Immunol.*, **74**, 246–51.

Böhm, M., Gengenbach, S., Hauck, R.W., Sunder-Plassmann, L. & Erdmann, E. (1991) Beta-adrenergic receptors and m-cholinergic receptors in human lung: findings following *in vivo* and *in vitro* exposure to the β-adrenergic receptor agonist, terbutaline. *Chest*, **100**, 1246–53.

Borson, D.B. (1991) Roles of neutral endopeptidase in airways. *Am. J. Physiol.*, **260** (*Lung Cell. Mol. Physiol.*, **4**), L212–25.

Borson, D.B. & Gruenert, D.C. (1991) Glucocorticoids induce neutral endopeptidase in transformed human trachea epithelial cells. *Am. J. Physiol.* **260** (*Lung Cell. Mol. Physiol.*, **4**), L83–9.

Braunstein, G., Fajac, I., Lacronique, J. & Frossard, N. (1991) Clinical and inflammatory responses to exogenous tachykinins in allergic rhinitis. *Am. Rev. Resp. Dis.*, **144**, 630–5.

Brodde, O.E., Howell, U., Egerszegi, S., Kometzko, M. & Michel, M.C. (1988) Effect of prednisone and ketotifen on β_2-bronchodilators. *Eur. J. Clin. Pharmacol.*, **34**, 145–50.

Brooks, S.M., McGowan, K., Bernstein, I.L., Altenau, P. & Peagler, J. (1979) Relationship between numbers of beta adrenergic receptors in lymphocytes and disease severity in asthma. *J. Allergy Clin. Immunol.*, **63**, 401–6.

Bucknall, C.E., Neilly, J.B., Carter, R., Stevenson, R.D. & Semple, P.F. (1988) Bronchial hyperreactivity in patients who cough after receiving angiotensin converting enzyme inhibitors. *Brit. Med. J.*, **296**, 86–8.

Busse, W.W. (1990) Respiratory infections: their role in airway responsiveness and the pathogenesis of asthma. *J. Allergy Clin. Immunol.*, **85**, 671–83.

Busse, W.W., Anderson, C.L., Dick, E.C. & Warshauer, D. (1980) Reduced granulocyte response to isoproterenol, histamine, and prostaglandin E, after *in vitro* incubation with rhinovirus 16. *Am. Rev. Resp. Dis.*, **122**, 641–6.

Bylund, D.B., Eikenberg, D.C., Hieble, J.P. *et al.* (1994) International union of pharmacology nomenclature of adrenoreceptors. *Pharmacol. Rev.*, **46**, 121–36.

Carolan, E.J. & Casale, T.B. (1993) Effects of neuropeptides on neutrophil migration through noncellular and endothelial barriers. *J. Allergy Clin. Immunol.*, **92**, 589–98.

Carpenter, M.B. (1991) *Core Textbook of Neuroanatomy*, 4th edn, p. 171. Williams & Wilkins, Baltimore.

Carstairs, J.R. & Barnes, P.J. (1986a) Visualization of vasoactive intestinal peptide receptors in human and guinea pig lung. *J. Pharmacol. Exp. Ther.*, **239**, 249–55.

Carstairs, J.R. & Barnes, P.J. (1986b) Autoradiographic mapping of substance P receptors in lung. *Eur. J. Pharmacol.*, **127**, 295–6.

Carstairs, J.R., Nimmo, A.J. & Barnes, P.J. (1985) Autoradiographic visualization of beta-adrenoceptor subtypes in human lung. *Am. Rev. Resp. Dis.*, **132**, 541–7.

Casale, T.B. (1983) The role of the autonomic nervous system in allergic disease. *Ann. Allergy*, **51**, 423–9.

Casale, T.B. (1987) Neuromechanisms of asthma. *Ann. Allergy*, **59**, 391–9.

Casale, T.B. (1993a) Neurogenic control of inflammation and airway function. In: *Principles and Practice* (eds E. Middleton C.E. Jr, Reed, E.F. Ellis, N.F. Adkinson & J.W. Yunginger), 4th edn, pp. 650–71. Mosby-Yearbook, St Louis, Missouri.

Casale, T.B. (1993b) Acute effects of *in vitro* mast cell degranulation on human lung muscarinic receptors. *Am. Rev. Resp. Dis.*, **147**, 940–5.

Caughey, G.H., Leidig, F., Viro, N.F. & Nadel, J.A. (1988) Substance P and vasoactive intestinal peptide degradation by mast cell tryptase and chymase. *J. Pharmacol. Exp. Ther.*, **244**, 133–7.

Cheung, D., Bel, E.H., Den Hartigh, J., Dijkman, J.H. & Sterk, P.M. (1992) The effect of an inhaled neutral endopeptidase inhibitor, thiorphan, on airway responsiveness to neurokinin A in normal humans *in vivo*. *Am. Rev. Resp. Dis.*, **145**, 1275–80.

Coles, S.J., Said, S.I. & Reid, L.M. (1981) Inhibition by vasoactive intestinal peptides of glycoconjugate and lysozyme secretion by human airways *in vitro*. *Am. Rev. Resp. Dis.*, **124**, 531–6.

Conolly, M.E. & Greenacre, J.K. (1976) The lymphocyte β-adrenoceptor in normal subjects and patients with bronchial asthma. *J. Clin. Invest.*, **58**, 1307–16.

Corjay, M.H., Dobrzanski, D.J., Way, J.M. *et al.* (1991) Two distinct bombesin receptor subtypes are expressed and functional in human lung carcinoma cells. *J. Biol. Chem.*, **266**, 18771–9.

Crimi, N., Palermo, F., Oliveri, R. *et al.* (1988) Effect of nedocromil on bronchospasm induced by inhalation of substance P in asthmatic subjects. *Clin. Allergy*, **18**, 375–82.

Dale, H.H. (1935) Pharmacology and nerve endings. *Proc. Roy. Soc. Med.*, **68**, 319–24.

Daniel, E.E. & O'Byrne, P. (1991) Autonomic nerves and airway smooth muscle: effect of inflammatory mediators on airway nerves and muscle. *Am. Rev. Resp. Dis.*, **143**, S3–5.

Daniele, R.P., Barnes, P.J., Goetzl, E.J. *et al.* (1992) Neuroimmune interactions in the lung. *Am. Rev. Resp. Dis.*, **145**, 1230–5.

Davis, P.B. (1986) Pupillary responses and airway reactivity in asthma. *J. Allergy Clin. Immunol.*, **77**, 667–2.

Davis, P.B., Simpson, D.M., Paget, G.L. & Turi, V. (1986) Beta-adrenergic responses in drug-free subjects with asthma. *J. Allergy Clin. Immunol.*, **77**, 871–9.

Devillier, P., Dessanges, J.F., Rakatosihanaka, J. *et al.* (1988) Nasal response to substance P and methacholine in subjects with and without allergic rhinitis. *Eur. Resp. J.*, **1**, 356–61.

Dey, R.D., Shannon A. Jr, Said, S.I. (1981) Localization of VIP-immunoreactive nerves in airways and pulmonary vessels of dogs, cats, and human subjects. *Cell Tissue Res.*, **220**, 231–8.

Dixon, C.M.S., Fuller, R.W. & Barnes, P.J. (1987) The effect of an angiotensin coverting enzyme inhibitor, ramipril, on bronchial responses to inhaled histamine and bradykinin in asthmatic subjects. *Brit. J. Clin. Pharmacol.*, **23**, 91–3.

Dodd, J. & Role, L.W. (1991) the autonomic nervous system. In: *Principles of Neural Science* (eds E.R. Kandel, J.H. Schwartz & J.M. Jessell), 3rd edn, p. 764. Elsevier Science, New York.

Dorje, F., Wess, J., Lambrecht, G., Tacke, R., Mutschler, E. & Broan, M.R. (1991) Antagonist binding profiles of five cloned human muscarinic receptor subtypes. *J. Pharmacol. Exp. Ther.*, **256**, 727–33.

Drapeau, G., D'Orleans-Juste, P., Dion, S., Rhaleb, N.E., Rouissi, N.E. & Regoli, D. (1987) Selective agonists for substance P and neurokinin receptors. *Neuropeptides*, **10**, 43–54.

Dupuy, P.M., Shore, S.A., Drazen, J.M., Frostell, C., Hill, W.A. & Zapol, W.M. (1992) Bronchodilator action of inhaled nitric oxide in guinea pigs. *J. Clin. Invest.*, **90**, 421–8.

Dusser, D.J., Djokic, T.D., Borson, D.B. & Nadel, J.A. (1989) Cigarette smoke induces bronchoconstrictor hyperresponsiveness to substance P and inactivates airway neutral endopeptidase in the guinea pig. *J. Clin. Invest.*, **84**, 900–6.

Eccles, J.C. (1986) Chemical transmission and Dale's principle. *Prog. Brain Res.*, **68**, 3014–20.

Eglen, R.M., Reddy, H., Watson, N. & Challiss, R.A. (1994) Muscarinic acetylcholine receptor subtypes in smooth muscle. *Trends Pharm. Sci.*, **15**, 114–19.

Elwood, W., Sakamoto, T., Barnes, P.J. & Chung, K.F. (1993) Allergen-induced airway hyperresponsiveness in Brown-Norway rat: role of parasympathetic mechanisms. *J. Appl. Physiol.*, **75**, 279–84.

Fathi, Z., Corjay, M.H., Shapira, H. *et al.* (1993) BRS-3: a novel bombesin receptor subtype selectively expressed in testis and lung carcinoma cells. *J. Biol. Chem.*, **268**, 5979–84.

Franconi, G.M., Graf, P.D., Lazarus, S.C., Nadel, J.A. & Caughey, G.H. (1989) Mast cell tryptase and chymase reverse airway smooth muscle relaxation induced by vasoactive intestinal peptide in the ferret. *J. Pharm. Exp. Ther.*, **248**, 947–51.

Frossard, N. & Advenier, C. (1991) Tachykinin receptors and the airways. *Life Sci.*, **49**, 1941–53.

Fryer, A.D. & Jacoby, D.B. (1991) Parainfluenza virus infection damages inhibitory M_2 muscarinic receptors on pulmonary parasympathetic nerves in the guinea-pig. *Brit. J. Pharmacol.*, **102**, 267–71.

Fryer, A.D. & Maclagan, J. (1987) Ipratropium bromide potentiates bronchoconstriction induced by vagal nerve stimulation in the guinea-pig. *Eur. J. Pharmacol.*, **139**, 187–91.

Fryer, A.D. & Okanlami, O.A. (1993) Neuronal M_2 muscarinic receptor function in guinea-pig lungs is inhibited by indomethacin. *Am. Rev. Resp. Dis.*, **147**, 559–64.

Fryer, A.D. & Wills-Karp, M. (1991) Dysfunction of M_2-muscarinc receptors in pulmonary parasympathetic nerves after antigen challenge. *J. Appl. Physiol.*, **71**, 2255–61.

Fuller, R.W., Dixon, C.M.S. & Barnes, P.J. (1985) Bronchoconstrictor response to inhaled capsaicin in humans. *J. Appl. Physiol.*, **58**, 1080–4.

Fuller, R.W., Maxwell, D.L., Dixon, C.M.S. *et al.* (1987) Effect of substance P on cardiovascular and respiratory function in subjects. *J. Appl. Physiol.*, **62**, 1473–9.

Galant, S.P., Duriseti, L., Underwood, S., Allred, S. & Insel, P.A. (1980) Beta adrenergic receptors of polymorphonuclear particulates in bronchial asthma. *J. Clin. Invest.*, **65**, 577–85.

Gaston, B., Drazen, J.M., Loscalzo, J. & Stamler, J.S. (1994) The biology of nitrogen oxides in the airways. *Am. J. Resp. Crit. Care Med.*, **149**, 538–51.

Gauthier, T.W., Davenpeck, K.L. & Lefer, A.M. (1994) Nitric oxide attenuates leukocyte–endothelial interaction via P-selectin in splanchnic ischemia-reperfusion. *Am. J. Physiol.*, **267** (*Gastrointest. Liver Physiol.*, **30**), G562–8.

Gazdar, A.F. & Carbone, D.P. (1994) *The Biology and Molecular Genetics of Lung Cancer*, pp. 1–142. R.G. Landes, Austin, Texas.

Goldie, R.G. (1990) Receptors in asthmatic airways. *Am. Rev. Resp. Dis.*, **141**, S151–6.

Goldie, R.G., Spina, D., Henry, P.J. & Lulich, K.M. (1986) *In vitro* responsiveness of human asthmatic bronchus to carbachol, histamine, β-adrenoceptor agonists, and theophylline. *Br. J. Clin. Pharmacol.*, **22**, 669–76.

Grieco, M.H. & Pierson R.N. Jr, (1971) Mechanism of bronchoconstriction due to beta adrenergic blockade. *J. Allergy Clin. Immunol.*, **48**, 143–52.

Grundström, N. & Andersson, R.G.G. (1985) Inhibition of the cholinergic neurotransmission in human airways via prejunctional α_2-adrenoceptors. *Acta Physiol. Scand.*, **125**, 513–17.

Grundström, N., Andersson, R.G.G. & Wikberg, J.E.S. (1984) Inhibition of the excitatory nonadrenergic, noncholinergic neurotransmission in the guinea pig tracheo-bronchial tree mediated by α_2-adrenoceptors. *Acta Pharmacol. Toxicol.*, **54**, 8–14.

Hall, A.K., Barnes, P.J., Meldrum, L.A. & Maclagan, J. (1989) Facilitation by tachykinins of neurotransmission in guinea-pig pulmonary parasympathetic nerves. *Brit. J. Pharmacol.*, **97**, 274–80.

Harrison, L.C., Callaghan, J., Venter, J.C., Fraser, C.M. & Kaliner, M.L. (1982) Atopy, autonomic function and β-adrenergic receptor autoantibodies. In: *Receptors, Antibodies, and Disease* (*Ciba Foundation Symposium*), pp. 248–62. Pitman, London.

Hartley, J.P.R., Davies, C.J., Charles, T.J., Monie, R.D.H., Nogrady, S.G. & Winson, M.D. (1981) Plasma cyclic nucleotide levels in exercise-induced asthma. *Thorax*, **36**, 823–7.

Hartung, H.P., Wolters, K. & Toyka, K.V. (1986) Substance P: binding properties and studies on cellular responses in guinea pig and macrophages. *J. Immunol.*, **136**, 3856–63.

Hayashi, K., Taki, F., Sugiyama, S., Takagi, K., Satake, T. & Ozawa, T. (1988) Mechanism responsible for alterations in numbers of autonomic nerve receptors in experimental asthma. *Int. Arch. Allergy Appl. Immunol.*, **86**, 170–5.

Haynes, L.W. & Manley, C. (1988) Chemotactic responses of guinea-pig eosinophil polymorphonucleocytes *in vitro* to rat calcitonin gene-related peptide (rCGRP-I) and proteolytic fragments. *J. Physiol.*, **422**, 79.

Hogman, M., Frostell, C., Arnberg, H. & Hedenstierna, G. (1993) Inhalation of nitric oxide modulates methacholine-induced bronchoconstriction in the rabbit. *Eur. Resp. J.*, **6**, 177–80.

Hokfelt, T., Fuxe, K. & Pernow, B. (1987) Coexistence of neuronal messengers: a new principle in chemical transmission. *Prog. Brain Res.*, **68**, 1–37.

Holzer, P. (1988) Local effector functions of capsaicin-sensitive sensory nerve endings: involvement of tachykinins, calcitonin gene related peptide and other neuropeptides. *Neuroscience*, **24**, 739–68.

Honda, I., Kohrogi, H., Yamaguchi, T., Ando, M. & Araki, S. (1991) Enkephalinase inhibitor potentiates substance P- and capasicininduced bronchial smooth muscle contractions in humans. *Am. Rev. Resp. Dis.*, **143**, 1416–18.

Ichinose, M. & Barnes, P.J. (1990) Histamine H_3 receptors modulate antigen-induced bronchoconstriction in guinea pigs. *J. Allergy Clin. Immunol.*, **86**, 491–5.

Ichinose, M., Stretton, C.D., Schwartz, J.C. & Barnes, P.J. (1989) Histamine H_3-receptors inhibit cholinergic neurotransmission in guinea-pig airways. *Brit. J. Pharmacol.*, **97**, 13–15.

Ind, P.W., Dixon, C.M.S., Fuller, R.W. & Barnes, P.J. (1989) Anticholinergic blockade of beta-blocker-induced bronchoconstriction. *Am. Rev. Resp. Dis.*, **193**, 1390–4.

Ito, Y. (1991) Prejunctional control of excitatory neuroeffector transmission by prostaglandins in the airway smooth muscle tissue. *Am. Rev. Resp. Dis.*, **143**, S6–10.

Jacobsson, L., Grundström, N. & Andersson, R.G.G. (1991) Influence of some α_2-receptor agonists and antagonists on the excitatory nonadrenergic, noncholinergic neurotransmission in the airways of guinea-pigs *in vivo*. *Acta Physiol. Scand.*, **142**, 91–6.

Jacoby, D.B., Tamaoki, J., Borson, D.B. & Nadel, J.A. (1988) Influenza infection causes airway hyperresponsiveness by decreasing enkephalinase. *J. Appl. Physiol.*, **64**, 2653–8.

Jenkins, C., Breslin, A.B.X. & Marlin, G.E. (1985) The role of alpha and beta adrenoceptors in airway hyperresponsiveness to histamine. *J. Allergy Clin. Immunol.*, **75**, 364–72.

Joos, G., Pauwels, R. & Van Der Streaten, M. (1987) Effect of inhaled substance P and neurokinin A on the airways of normal and asthmatic subjects. *Thorax*, **42**, 779–83.

Kaliner, M., Shelhamer, J.H., Davis, P.B., Smith, L.J. & Venter, J.C. (1982) Autonomic nervous system abnormalities and allergy. *Ann. Int. Med.*, **96**, 349–57.

Kariman, K. (1980) β-adrenergic receptor binding in lymphocytes from patients with asthma. *Lung*, **158**, 41–51.

Kelsen, S.G., Zhou, S., Anakwe, O., Mardini, I., Higgins, N. & Benovic, J.L. (1994) Expression of the β-adrenergic receptor-adenylylcyclase system in basal and columnar airway epithelial cells. *Am. J. Physiol.*, **267** (*Lung Cell. Mol. Physiol.*, **11**), L456–63.

Khalil, Z., Andrews, P.V. & Helme, R.D. (1988) VIP modulates substance P induced plasma extravasation *in vivo*. *Eur. J. Pharmacol.*, **151**, 281–7.

Kroegel, C., Yukawa, T. & Barnes, P.J. (1989) Substance P induces degranulation of eosinophils. *Am. Rev. Resp. Dis.*, **139**, A238.

Lacroix, J.S. (1989) Adrenergic and non-adrenergic mechanisms in sympathetic vascular control of the nasal mucosa. *Acta Physiol. Scand.*, **136** (Suppl. 581), 1–49.

Lacroix, J.S., Änggård, A., Hökfelt, T., O'Hare, M.M.T., Fahrenkrug, J. & Lundberg, J.M. (1990) Neuropeptide Y: presence in sympathetic and parasympathetic innervation of the nasal mucosa. *Cell Tissue Res.*, **259**, 119–28.

Laitinen, L.A. & Laitinen, A. (1987) Innervation of airway smooth muscle. *Am. Rev. Resp. Dis.*, **136**, S38–57.

Laitinen, L.A., Laitinen, A., Salonen, R.O. & Widdicombe, J.G. (1987) Vascular actions of airway neuropeptides. *Am. Rev. Resp. Dis.*, **136**, S59–64.

Laitinen, A., Partanen, M., Hervonen, A., Pelto-Huikko, M. & Laitinen, L.A. (1985) VIP like immunoreactive nerves in human respiratory tract: light and electron microscopic study. *Histochemistry*, **82**, 313–19.

Lammers, J.W.J., Minettte, P., McCusker, M. & Barnes, P.J. (1989) The role of pirenzepine-sensitive (M_1) muscarinic receptors in vagally mediated bronchoconstriction in humans. *Am. Rev. Resp. Dis.*, **139**, 446–9.

Lang, Z. & Murlas, C.G. (1992) Neutral endopeptidase of a human airway epithelial cell line recovers after hypochlorous acid exposure: dexamethasone accelerates this by stimulating neutral endopeptidase mRNA synthesis. *Am. J. Respir. Cell Mol. Biol.*, **7**, 300–6.

Larsson, O., Duner-Engstrom, M., Lundberg, J.M., Freholm, B.B. & Anggard, A. (1986) Effects of VIP, PHM and substance P on blood vessels and secretory elements of the human submandibular gland. *Regul. Pept.*, **13**, 319–26.

Laurenzi, M.A., Persson, M.A., Dalsgaard, C.J. & Ringd'en, O. (1989) Stimulation of human B lymphocyte differentiation by the neuropeptides substance P and neurokinin A. *Scand. J. Immunol.*, **30**, 695–701.

Lawrence, I.D., Warne, J.A., Coha, V.L., Hubbar, W.C., Kagey-Sobotk, A. & Lichtenstein, L.M. (1987) Purification and characterization of human skin mast cells: evidence for human mast cell heterogeneity. *J. Immunol.*, **139**, 3062–9.

Lehmann, J. (1990) Neuropeptide Y: an overview. *Drug Dev. Resp.*, **19**, 329–51.

Levine, R.R., Bridsall, N.J.M., North, R.A., Holman, M., Watanabe, A. & Iverson, L.L. (1991) Subtypes of muscarinic receptors III. *Trends Pharmacol. Sci.*, **9** (Suppl. 1), 1–93.

Li, C.G. & Rand, M.J. (1991) Evidence that part of the NANC relaxant response of guinea-pig trachea to electrical field stimulation is mediated by nitric oxide. *Br. J. Pharmacol.*, **102**, 91–4.

Lindgren, B.R., Ekström, T. & Andersson, R.G.G. (1986) The effect of inhaled clonidine in patients with asthma. *Am. Rev. Resp. Dis.*, **134**, 266–9.

Lindgren, B.R., Persson, K., Kihlström, J.-E. & Andersson, R.G. (1989a) ACE-inhibitor-induced enhancement of spontaneous and IgE-mediated histamine release from mast cells and basophilic leukocytes and the modulatory effect of capsaicin sensitive nerves. *Pharmacol. Toxicol.*, **64**, 159–64.

Lindgren, B.R., Rosenquist, U., Ekström, T., Gronneberg, R., Karlberg, B.E. & Anderson, R.G. (1989b) Increased bronchial reactivity and potentiated skin responses in hypertensive subjects suffering from coughs during ACE-inhibitor therapy. *Chest*, **95**, 1225–30.

Lindsay, R.M. & Harmar, A.J. (1989) Nerve growth factor regulates expression of neuropeptide genes in adult sensory neurons. *Nature*, **337**, 362–4.

Lotz, M., Vaughan, J.H. & Carson, D.A. (1988) Effect of neuropeptides on production of inflammatory cytokines by human monocytes. *Science*, **241**, 1218–21.

Lundberg, J.M., Alving, K., Karlsson, J.A., Matran, R. & Nilsson, G. (1991) Sensory neuropeptide involvement in animal models of airway irritation and of allergen-evoked asthma. *Am. Rev. Resp. Dis.*, **143**, 1429–31.

Lundberg, J.M., Anggard, A. & Fahrenkrug, J. (1981) Complementary role of vasoactive intestinal peptide (VIP) and acetylcholine for cat submandibular gland blood flow and secretion. *Acta Physiol. Scand.*, **113**, 329–36.

Lundberg, J.M., Brodin, E. & Saria, A. (1983a) Effects and distribution of vagal capsaicin-sensitive substance P neurons with special reference to the trachea and lungs. *Acta Physiol. Scand.*, **119**, 243–52.

Lundberg, J.M., Saria, A., Brodin, E., Rosell, S. & Folkers, K. (1983b) A substance P antagonist inhibits vagally induced increase in vascular permeability and bronchial smooth muscle contraction in the guinea pig. *Proc. Nat. Acad. Sci.*, **80**, 1120–4.

Lundberg, J.M., Fahrenkrug, J., Hökfelt, T. *et al.* (1984a) Co-existence of peptide HI (PHI) and VIP in nerves regulating blood flow and bronchial smooth muscle tone in various mammals including man. *Peptides*, **5**, 593–606.

Lundberg, J.M., Hökfelt, T., Martling, C.R., Saria, A. & Cuello, C. (1984b) Substance P-immunoreactive sensory nerves in the lower respiratory tract of various mammals including man. *Cell Tissue Res.*, **235**, 251–61.

Lundberg, J.M., Lundblad, L., Martling, C.R., Saria, A., St Jårne, P. & Änggård, A. (1987) Coexistence of multiple peptides and classic transmitters in airway neurons: functional and pathophysiologic aspects. *Am. Rev. Resp. Dis.*, 136, S16–22.

Lundberg, J.M. & Saria, A. (1982) Bronchial smooth muscle contraction induced by stimulation of capsaicin-sensitive sensory neurons. *Acta Physiol. Scand.*, **116**, 473–6.

Lundberg, J.M. & Saria, A. (1983) Capsaicin-induced desensitization of airway mucosa to cigarette smoke, mechanical, and chemical irritants. *Nature*, **302**, 251–3.

Lundberg, J.M., Saria, A., Theodorsson-Norheim, E. *et al.* (1985) Multiple tachykinins in capsaicin-sensitive afferents: occurrence, release, and biological effects with special reference to irritation of the airways. In: *Tachykinin Antagonists* (eds R. Håkanson & F. Sundler), pp. 159–70. Elsevier Science Publishers BV (Biomedical Division), Amsterdam.

Lundgren, J.D. & Shelhamer, J.H. (1990) Pathogenesis of airway mucus hypersecretion. *J. Allergy Clin. Immunol.*, **85**, 399–419.

McDonald, D.M. (1988) Neurogenic inflammation in the rat trachea. I. Changes in venules, leukocytes and epithelial cells. *J. Neurocytol.*, **17**, 605–28.

McFadden E.R. Jr, Luparello, T., Lyons, H.A. & Bleecker, E. (1969) The mechanism of action of suggestion in the induction of acute asthma attacks. *Psychosomol. Med.*, **31**, 134–43.

Macklem, P.T. (1991) Factors determining bronchial smooth muscle shortening. *Am. Rev. Resp. Dis.*, **143**, S47–8.

Maggi, C.A., Patacchini, R., Rovero, P. & Santicioli, P. (1991) Tachykinin receptors and noncholinergic bronchoconstriction in the guinea-pig isolated bronchi. *Am. Rev. Resp. Dis.*, **144**, 363–7.

Mak, J.C., Baraniuk, J.N. & Barnes, P.J. (1992) Localization of muscarinic receptor subtype mRNAs in human lung. *Am. J. Respir. Cell Mol. Biol.*, **7**, 344–8.

Mak, J.C. & Barnes, P.J. (1990) Autoradiographic visualization of muscarinic receptor subtypes in human and guinea pig lung. *Am. Rev. Resp. Dis.*, **141**, 1559–68.

Mak, J.C.W. & Barnes, P.J. (1988) Autoradiographic localization of calcitonin gene-related peptide (CGRP) binding sites in human and guinea pig lung. *Peptides*, **9**, 957–63.

Malm, L., Sundler, F. & Uddman, R. (1980) Effects of vasoactive intestinal peptide (VIP) on resistance and capacitance vessels in nasal mucosa. *Acta Otolaryngol. (Stockh.)*, **90**, 304–8.

Marasco, W.A., Showell, H.J. & Becker, E.L. (1981) Substance P binds to the formylpeptide chemotaxis receptor on the rabbit neutrophil. Biochem. *Biophys. Res. Commun.*, **99**, 1065–72.

Marom, Z. & Goswami, S.K. (1991) Respiratory mucus hypersecretion (bronchorrhea): a case discussion—possible mechanism(s) and treatment. *J. Allergy Clin. Immunol.*, **87**, 1050–5.

Martin, J.G., Wang, A., Zacour, M. & Biggs, D.F. (1990) The effects of vasoactive intestinal polypeptide on cholinergic neurotransmission in an isolated innervated guinea pig tracheal preparation. *Resp. Physiol.*, **79**, 111–22.

Martins, M.A., Shore, S.A. & Drazen, J.M. (1991) Release of tachykinins by histamine, methacholine, PAF, LTD4, and substance P from guinea pig lungs. *Am. J. Physiol.*, **261** (*Lung Cell. Mol. Physiol.*, **5**), L449–55.

Matsuda, H., Kawakita, K., Kiso, Y., Nakano, T. & Kitamura, Y. (1989) Substance P induces granulocyte infiltration through degranulation of mast cells. *J. Immunol.*, **142**, 927–31.

Meurs, H., Kauffman, H.F., Koëter, G.H., Timmermans, A. & de Vries, K. (1987) Regulation of the beta-receptor-adenylate cyclase system in lymphocytes of allergic patients with asthma: possible role for protein kinase C in allergen-induced nonspecific refractoriness of adenylate cyclase. *J. Allergy Clin. Immunol.*, **80**, 326–39.

Meurs, H., Koëter, G.H., de Vriesk, K. & Kauffman, H.F. (1982) The beta-adrenergic system and allergic bronchial asthma: changes in lymphocyte beta-adrenergic receptor number and adenylate cyclase activity after an allergen-induced asthmatic attack. *J. Allergy Clin. Immunol.*, **70**, 272–80.

Minette, P.A.H., Lammers, J.W.J., Dixon, C.M.S., McCusker, M.T. & Barnes, P.J. (1989) A muscarinic agonist inhibits reflex bronchoconstriction in normal but not in asthmatic subjects. *J. Appl. Physiol.*, **67**, 2461–5.

Mita, H., Yui, Y., Yasueda, H. & Shida, T. (1983) Changes of alpha$_1$- and beta-adrenergic and cholinergic muscarinic receptors in guinea pig lung sensitized with ovalbumin. *Int. Arch. Allergy Appl. Immunol.*, **70**, 225–30.

Miura, M., Ichinose, M., Kimura, K., Katsumata, U., Takahashi, T., Inoue, H. & Takishima, T. (1992) Dysfunction of nonadrenergic noncholinergic inhibitory system after antigen inhalation in actively sensitized cat airways. *Am. Rev. Resp. Dis.*, **145**, 70–4.

Morice, A.H. & Sever, P.S. (1986) Vasoactive intestinal peptide as a bronchodilator in severe asthma. *Peptides*, **7**, 279–80.

Mosimann, B.L., White, M.V., Hohman, R.J., Goldrich, M.S., Kaulback, H.C. & Kaliner, M.A. (1993) Substance P, calcitonin gene related peptide, and vasoactive intestinal peptide increase in nasal secretions after allergen challenge in atopic patients. *J Allergy Clin. Immunol.*, **92**, 95–104.

Motojima, S., Yukawa, T., Fukuda, T. & Makino, S. (1989) Changes in airway responsiveness and β- and α-1-adrenergic receptors in the lungs of guinea pigs with experimental asthma. *Allergy*, **44**, 66–74.

Mullol, J., Baraniuk, J.N., Logun, C. *et al.* (1992a) M1 and M3 muscarinic antagonists inhibit human nasal glandular secretion *in vitro*. *J. Appl. Physiol.*, **73**, 2069–73.

Mullol, J., Rieves, R.D., Lundgren, J.D. *et al.* (1992b) The effects of neuropeptides on mucous glycoprotein secretion from human nasal mucosa *in vitro*. *Neuropeptides*, **21**, 231–8.

Mygind, N. & Borum, P. (1990) Anticholinergic treatment of watery rhinorrhea. *Am. J. Rhinol.*, **4**, 1–5.

Naclerio, R.M. (1991) Allergic rhinitis. *New Engl. J. Med.*, **325**, 860–9.

Nadel, J.A. (1990) Decreased neutral endopeptidases: possible role in inflammatory diseases of airways. *Lung*, **123** (Suppl.), 123–7.

Nadel, J.A. & Borson, D.B. (1991) Modulation of neurogenic inflammation by neutral endopeptidase. *Am. Rev. Resp. Dis.*, **143**, S33–6.

Naline, E., Devillier, P., Drapeau, G. *et al.* (1989) Characterization of neurokinin effects and receptor selectivity in human isolated bronchi. *Am. Rev. Resp. Dis.*, **140**, 679–86.

Nieber, K., Baumgartern, C.R., Rathsack, R., Furkert, J., Oehme, P. & Kunkel, G. (1992) Substance P and β-endorphin-like immunoreactivity in lavage fluids of subjects with and without allergic asthma. *J. Allergy Clin. Immunol.*, **90**, 646–52.

Nijkamp, F.P., Engels, F., Henricks, P.A. & Man-Oosterhout, V.A.J. (1992) Mechanisms of β-adrenergic receptor regulation in lungs and its implications for physiological responses. *Physiol. Rev.*, **72**, 323–66.

Noverall, J.P. & Grunstein, M.M. (1994) Adrenergic receptor-mediated regulation of cultured rabbit airway smooth muscle cell proliferation. *Am. J. Physiol.*, **267** (*Lung Cell. Mol. Physiol.*, **11**), L291–9.

Ohkubo, K., Lee, C.H., Baraniuk, J.N., Merida, M., Hausfeld, J.N. & Kaliner, M.A. (1994) Angiotensin converting enzyme (ACE) in human nasal mucosa. *Am. J. Respir. Cell Mol. Biol.*, **11**, 173–80.

Okayama, M., Mullol, J., Baraniuk, J.N. *et al.* (1993) Muscarinic receptor subtypes in human nasal mucosa: characterization, autoradiographic localization, and function *in vitro*. *Am. J. Respir. Cell Mol. Biol.*, **8**, 176–87.

Ollerenshaw, S., Jarvis, D., Woolcock, A., Sullivan, C. & Scheibner, T. (1989) Absence of immunoreactive vasoactive intestinal polypeptide in tissue from the lungs of patients with asthma. *New Engl. J. Med.*, **320**, 1244–8.

Ollerenshaw, S.L., Jarvis, D.L., Woolcock, A.J., Scheibner, T. & Sullivan, C.E. (1991) Substance P immunoreactive nerve fibres in airways from asthmatics and nonasthmatics. *Eur. Resp. J.*, **4**, 673–82.

Palmer, J.B., Cuss, F.M.C. & Barnes, P.J. (1986) VIP and PHM and their role in nonadrenergic inhibitory responses in isolated human airways. *J. Appl. Physiol.*, **61**, 1322–8.

Parker, C. & Smith, J.W. (1973) Alterations in cyclic adenosine monophosphate metabolism in human bronchial asthma. I. Leukocyte responsiveness to beta-adrenergic agents. *J. Clin. Invest.*, **52**, 48–59.

Payan, D.G., Brewster, D.R. & Goetzl, E.J. (1983) Specific stimulation of human T lymphocytes by substance P. *J. Immunol.*, **131**, 1613–15.

Payan, D.G., Levine, J.D. & Goetzl, E.J. (1984) Modulation of immunity and hypersensitivity by sensory neuropeptides. *J. Immunol.*, **132**, 1601–4.

Piedemonte, G., McDonald, D.M. & Nadel, J.A. (1990) Glucocorticoids inhibit neurogenic plasma extravasation and prevent viruspotentiated extravasation in the rat trachea. *J. Clin. Invest.*, **86**, 1409–15.

Postma, D.S., Keyzer, J.J., Koeter, G.A., Sluiter, H.J. & DeVries, K. (1985) Influence of the parasympathetic and sympathetic nervous systems on nocturnal bronchial obstruction. *Clin. Sci.*, **69**, 251–8.

Potter, E.K. (1988) Neuropeptide Y as an autonomic neurotransmitter. *Pharmacol. Ther.*, **37**, 251–73.

Rangachari, P.K. & McWade, D. (1985) Effects of tachykinins on the electrical activity of isolated canine tracheal epithelium: an exploratory study. *Regul. Pept.*, **12**, 9–19.

Raphael, G.D., Baraniuk, J.N. & Kaliner, M.A. (1991) How and why the nose runs. *J. Allergy Clin. Immunol.*, **87**, 457–67.

Regoli, D., Drapeau, G., Dion, S. & D'Orléans-Juste, P. (1989) Receptors for substance P and related neurokinins. *Pharmacology*, **38**, 1–15.

Rhoden, K.J., Meldrum, L.A. & Barnes, P.J. (1988) Inhibition of cholinergic neurotransmission in human airways by β_2-adrenoceptors. *J. Appl. Physiol.*, **65**, 700–5.

Richardson, J. & Béland, J. (1976) Nonadrenergic inhibitory nervous system in human airways. *J. Appl. Physiol.*, **41**, 764–71.

Richardson, P.S. & Webber, S.E. (1987) The control of mucous secretion in the airways by peptidergic mechanisms. *Am. Rev. Resp. Dis.*, **136**, S72–7.

Rogers, D.F., Aursudkij, B. & Barnes, P.J. (1989) Effects of tachykinins on mucus secretion in human bronchi *in vitro*. *Eur. J. Pharmacol.*, **174**, 283–6.

Rogers, D.R. & Barnes, P.J. (1989) Opioid inhibitions of neurally mediated mucus secretion in human bronchi. *Lancet*, **i**, 930–2.

Said, S.I. (1991) Neuropeptides (VIP and tachykinins): VIP as a modulator of lung inflamation and airway constriction. *Am. Rev. Resp. Dis.*, **143**, S22–4.

Salonen, R.O., Webber, S.E. & Widdicombe, J.G. (1988) Effects of neuropeptides and capsaicin on the canine tracheal vasculature *in vivo*. *Brit. J. Pharmacol.*, **95**, 1262–70.

Sanna, A., Kurtansky, A., Veriter, C. & Stanescu, D. (1994) Bronchodilator effect of inhaled nitric oxide in healthy men. *Am. J. Resp. Crit. Care Med.*, **150**, 1702–4.

Sano, Y., Watt, G. & Townley, R.G. (1983) Decreased mononuclear cell beta-adrenergic receptors in bronchial asthma: parallel studies of lymphocyte and granulocyte desensitization. *J. Allergy Clin. Immunol.*, **72**, 495–503.

Saria, A., Lundberg, J.M., Skofitsch, G. & Lembeck, F. (1983) Vascular protein leakage in various tissues induced by substance P, capsaicin, bradykinin, serotonin, histamine, and by antigen challenge. *Naunyn-Schmiedeberg's Arch. Pharmacol.*, **324**, 212–18.

Saria, A., Martling, C.R., Yan, Z., Theodorsson-Norheim, E., Gamse, R. & Lundberg, J.M. (1988) Release of multiple tachykinins from capsaicin-sensitive sensory nerves in the lung by bradykinin, histamine, dimethylphenol piperazinium, and vagal nerve stimulation. *Am. Rev. Resp. Dis.*, **137**, 1330–5.

Sato, T., Bewtra, A.K., Hopp, R.J., Nair, N. & Townley, R.G. (1990) Alpha- and beta-adrenergic-receptor systems in bronchial asthma and in subjects without asthma: reduced mononuclear cell betareceptors in bronchial asthma. *J. Allergy Clin. Immunol.*, **86**, 839–50.

Schultheis, A.H., Bassett, D.J. & Fryer, A.D. (1994) Ozone-induced airway hyperresponsiveness and loss of neuronal M_2 muscarinic receptor function. *J. Appl. Physiol.*, **76**, 1088–97.

Sekizawa, K., Tamaoki, J., Graf, P. & Nadel, J.A. (1988) Modulation of cholinergic transmssion by vasoactive intestinal peptide in ferret trachea. *J. Appl. Physiol.*, **69**, 2433–7.

Sharma, R.K. & Jeffery, P.K. (1990) Airway VIP receptor number is reduced in cystic fibrosis but not asthma. *Am. Rev. Resp. Dis.*, **141**, A726.

Sheppard, D., Thompson, J.E., Scypinski, L., Dusser, D., Nadel, J.A. & Borson, D.B. (1988) Toluene diisocyanate increases airway responsiveness to substance P and decreases airway neutral endopeptidase. *J. Clin. Invest.*, **81**, 1111–15.

Sheppard, M.N., Polak, J.M., Allen, J.M. & Bloom, S.R. (1984) Neuropeptide tyrosine (NPY): a newly discovered peptide is present in the mammalian respiratory tract. *Thorax*, **39**, 326–30.

Shimosegawa, T. & Said, S.I. (1991) Pulmonary calcitonin generelated peptide immunoreactivity: nerve–endocrine cell interrelationships. *Am. J. Respir. Cell Biol.*, **4**, 126–34.

Shimura, S., Sasaki, T., Ikeda, K., Ishihara, H., Sato, M. & Sasaki, H. (1991) Neuropeptides and airway submucosal gland secretion. *Am. Rev. Resp. Dis.*, **143**, S25–7.

Shimura, S., Sasaki, T., Ikeda, K., Sasaki, K. & Takishima, T. (1988) VIP augments cholinergic-induced glycoconjugate secretion in tracheal submucosal glands. *J. Appl. Physiol.*, **65**, 2537–44.

Simonsson, B.G., Jacobs, F.M. & Nadel, J.A. (1967) Role of the autonomic nervous system and the cough reflex in the increased responsiveness of airways in patients with obstructive airway disease. *J. Clin. Invest.*, **46**, 1812–18.

Snashall, P.D., Boother, F.A. & Sterling, G.M. (1978) The effect of α-adrenoreceptor stimulation on the airways of normal and asthmatic man. *Clin. Sci. Mol. Med.*, **54**, 283–9.

Snell, R.S. (1992) *Clinical Neuroanatomy for Medical Students*, 3rd edn, p. 501. Little Brown & Company, Boston.

Sorkness, R., Clough, J.J., Castleman, W.L. & Lemanske, R.F. (1994) Virus-induced airway obstruction and parasympathetic responsiveness in adult rats. *Am. J. Resp. Crit. Care Med.*, **150**, 28–34.

Spector, S.L. (1992) Intranasal anticholinergic treatment of nasal disorders. *J. Allergy Clin. Immunol.*, **90** (Suppl.), 1041–86.

Spina, D., Rigby, P.J., Paterson, J.W. & Goldie, R.G. (1989a) Autoradiographic localization of beta-adrenoceptors in asthmatic human lung. *Am. Rev. Resp. Dis.*, **140**, 1410–15.

Spina, D., Rigby, P.J., Paterson, J.W. & Goldie, R.G. (1989b) α_1-adrenoceptor function and autoradiographic distribution in human asthmatic lung. *Brit. J. Pharmacol.*, **97**, 701–8.

Stanisz, A.M., Befus, D. & Bienestock, J. (1986) Differential effects of vasoactive intestinal peptide, substance P, and somatostatin on immunoglobulin synthesis and proliferations by lymphocytes from Peyer's patches, mesenteric lymph nodes, and spleen. *J. Immunol.*, **136**, 152–6.

Stephens, N.L., Seow, C.Y. & Kong, S.K. (1991) Mechanical properties of sensitized airway smooth muscle. *Am. Rev. Resp. Dis.*, **143**, S13–14.

Stern, L. & Kunos, G. (1988) Synergistic regulation of pulmonary β-adrenergic receptors by glucocorticoids and interleukin-1. *J. Biol. Chem.*, **263**, 15876–9.

Stjarne, P., Lacroix, J.S., Anggard, A. & Lundberg, J.M. (1991) Compartment analysis of vascular effects of neuropeptides and capsaicin in the pig nasal mucosa. *Acta Physiol. Scand.*, **141**, 335–42.

Stretton, C.D. & Barnes, P.J. (1988) Modulation of cholinergic neurotransmission in guinea-pig trachea by neuropeptide Y. *Brit. J. Pharmacol.*, **93**, 672–8.

Stretton, C.D., Belvisi, M.G. & Barnes, P.J. (1991) Modulation of neural bronchoconstrictor responses in the guinea-pig respiratory tract by vasoactive intestinal peptide. *Neuropeptides*, **18**, 149–57.

Sunday, M.E., Kaplan, L.M., Motoymam, E., Chin, W.W. & Spindel, E.R. (1988) Gastrin releasing peptide (mammalian bombesin) gene expression in health and disease. *Lab. Invest.*, **59**, 5–24.

Sundler, F., Brodin, E., Ekblad, E., Hakanson, R. & Uddman, R. (1985) Sensory nerve fibers: distribution of substance P, neurokinin A, and calcitonin gene-related peptide. In: *Tachykinin Antagonists* (eds R. Håkanson & F. Sundler), pp. 3–14. Elsevier Science Publishers BV (Biomedical Division), Amsterdam.

Szentivanyi, A. (1968) The beta adrenergic theory of the atopic abnormality in bronchial asthma. *J. Allergy*, **42**, 203–25.

Tam, E.K., Franconi, G.M., Nadel, J.A. & Caughey, G.H. (1990) Protease inhibitors potentiate smooth muscle relaxation induced by vasoactive intestinal peptide in isolated human bronchi. *Am. J. Respir. Cell Mol. Biol.*, **2**, 449–52.

Thomson, N.C., Daniel, E.E. & Hargreave, F.E. (1982) Role of smooth muscle alpha$_1$-receptors in nonspecific bronchial responsiveness in asthma. *Am. Rev. Resp. Dis.*, **126**, 521–5.

Thompson, J.E. & Sheppard, D. (1988) Phosphoramidon potentiates the increase in lung resistance mediated by tachykinins in guinea pigs. *Am. Rev. Resp. Dis.*, **137**, 337–40.

Tokuyama, K., Kuo, H.P., Rohde, J.A.L., Barnes, P.J. & Rogers, D.F. (1990) Neural control of goblet cell secretion in guinea pig airways. *Am. J. Physiol.*, **259** (*Lung Cell. Mol. Physiol.*, **3**), L108–15.

Tsutsumi, Y. (1988) Immunohistochemical localization of gastrin releasing peptided in normal and diseased human lung. *Ann. NY Acad. Sci.*, **547**, 336–50.

Tucker, J.F., Brave, S.R., Charalmabous, L., Hobbs, A.J. & Gibson, A. (1990) L-N^G-nitro arginine inhibits nonadrenergic, noncholinergic relaxations of guinea-pig isolated tracheal smooth muscle. *Brit. J. Pharmacol.*, **100**, 663–4.

Uchida, Y., Nomura, A., Ohtsuka, M. *et al.* (1987) Neurokinin A as a potent bronchoconstrictor. *Am. Rev. Resp. Dis.*, **136**, 718–21.

Uddman, R. & Sundler, F. (1986) Innervation of the upper airways. *Clin. Chest Med.*, **7**, 201–9.

Undem, B.J., Dick, E.C. & Buckner, C.K. (1983) Inhibition by vasoactive intestinal peptide of antigen-induced histamine release from guinea-pig minced lung. *Eur. J. Pharmacol.*, **88**, 247–50.

Umeno, E., Nadel, J.A., Huang, H.T. & McDonald, D.M. (1989) Inhibition of neutral endopeptidase potentiates neurogenic inflammation in the rat trachea. *J. Appl. Physiol.*, **66**, 2647–52.

van Megen, Y.J.B., Klaassen, A.B.M., Rodrigues de Miranda, J.F., van Ginneken, C.A. & Wentges, B.T. (1991) Alterations of adreno receptors in the nasal mucosa of allergic patients in comparison with nonallergic individuals. *J. Allergy Clin. Immunol.*, **87**, 530–40.

Venter, J.C., Di Porzio, U., Robinson, D.A. *et al.* (1988) Evolution of neurotransmitter receptor systems. *Prog. Neurobiol.*, **30**, 105–69.

Venter, S.C. (1982) Autoantibodies to the beta-adrenergic receptor. *Ann. Intern. Med.*, **96**, 349–57.

Wada, E., Way, J., Shapira, H. *et al.* (1991) cDNA cloning, characterization and brain region-specific expression of a neuromedin-β-preferring bombesin receptor. *Neuron*, **6**, 421–30.

Weiner, N. & Taylor, P. (1985) Neurohumoral transmission: the autonomic and somatic motor nervous systems. In: *The Pharmacologic Basis of Therapeutics*, 7th edn (eds A.G. Gilman, L.S. Goodman, T.W. Rall & F. Murad), pp. 66–99. MacMillan, New York.

Wharton, J., Polak, J.M., Bloom, S.R., Will, J.A., Brown, M.R. & Pearse, G.E. (1979) Substance P-like immunoreactive nerves in mammalian lung. *Invest. Cell. Pathol.*, **2**, 3–10.

Xuan, A.T.D., Regnard, J., Matran, R., Mantrand, P., Advenier, C. & Lockhart, A. (1988) Effects of clonidine on bronchial responses to histamine in normal and asthmatic subjects. *Eur. Resp. J.*, **1**, 345–50.

Yu, M., Wang, Z., Robinson, N.E. & LeBlanc, P.H. (1994) Inhibitory nerve distribution and mediation of NANC relaxation by nitric oxide in horse airways. *J. Appl. Physiol.*, **76**, 339–44.

CHAPTER 28
Neuropharmacology

A.D. Watkins

Introduction

Over the last 15 years, modern molecular biological techniques, such as the polymerase chain reaction, immunohistochemistry and *in situ* hybridization, have considerably increased our understanding of airway inflammation. Studies in asthmatics and in animal models of allergic inflammation have provided substantial evidence to suggest that asthma is an inflammatory disease of the lungs, involving almost all the cells included in immunity and hypersensitivity. During this time, overwhelming evidence has also accumulated to suggest that cellular and humoral immunity can be modulated by the autonomic nervous system and neuroendocrine steroids produced by the central nervous system (CNS). Although the involvement of neural mechanisms in the pathophysiology of allergic inflammation has been suspected for some time (Willis, 1679), until recently the implications of this neuroimmunomodulation (NIM) for asthma have been largely overlooked (Busse *et al.*, 1995). This chapter will review the evidence for 'neuroimmune' communication and try to reintroduce the idea that the brain plays a pivotal role in regulating the inflammatory immune response that underlies much of the pathophysiology seen in asthma, and thereby demonstrate how the interaction between the CNS, immunity and hypersensitivity might affect the morbidity and mortality of this common disease.

Autonomic innervation and regulation of the airways

There are two main efferent pathways by which the CNS regulates immunity, namely autonomic and neuroendocrine (Ader *et al.*, 1991). Autonomic NIM may be the result of catecholamine release from the adrenal medulla, or alternatively may occur via the well-established innervation of lymphoid tissue (Felten *et al.*, 1992). Assessment of the impact of autonomic innervation on allergic inflammation must not be restricted to the study of sympathetic, parasympathetic and non-adrenergic non-cholinergic (NANC) innervation of the airways (Barnes, 1986). It must include the rich innervation of the bone marrow and thymus, where lymphocytes develop (Calvo, 1968; Williams *et al.*, 1980). For example, developing thymocytes possess β-adrenoreceptors and alter their expression of T-cell surface antigens in response to catecholamines. In fact, some authors have suggested that the development and the senescence of the thymus and the sympathetic nervous system are related (Bellinger *et al.*, 1988; Ackerman *et al.*, 1989). In addition, the role of the autonomic nervous system in asthma must take into account the finding that autonomic nerves irrigate fields of lymphocytes in regional lymph nodes, where respiratory antigens are presented, modulating lymphocyte maturity and activation (Felten *et al.*, 1987). For example, the ability of Langerhans cells to present antigen is inhibited by calcitonin gene-related peptide (CGRP) released by NANC nerves (Hosoi *et al.*, 1993).

Theories of autonomic dysfunction in asthma

The importance of autonomic innervation in airway inflammation has been repeatedly contested, largely because of the failure of all-embracing theories of autonomic imbalance to explain the pathophysiology seen in the majority of the asthmatics. For example, over the years, the potent effect of β-agonists on airway calibre have provoked theories of β-adrenoreceptor hypofunction or α-adrenoreceptor hyperfunction. But, despite vigorous attempts to prove either theory, the evidence has been consistently contradictory (Casale, 1987). This is hardly surprising, in view of the diverse cellular distribution of β-adrenergic receptors in the airways (Barnes, 1986) and the widely differing metabolism of β-receptors in asthmatic individuals (Bai *et al.*, 1992). In addition, there is a wide variability of β-receptor function within one individual, according to the severity of the asthma, with signal transduction failing when asthmatic inflammation is more severe. Similarly, a great deal of research directed at trying to prove an excessive cholinergic drive in asthmatics failed to find any direct evidence for increased vagal tone or cholinergic reflexes. The results from animal models of allergic inflammation are equally contradictory, with some studies suggesting increased cholinergic sensitivity (Sorkness *et al.*, 1994), while others conclude that airway hyperresponsiveness does not involve parasympathetic mechanisms (Elwood *et al.*, 1993).

Neural networks in the airways

Despite the failure of these grand theories, there remains a significant amount of data suggesting that autonomic nerves are capable of regulating almost all the cells involved in allergic inflammation. For example, smooth-muscle contraction, mucus hypersecretion, vasodilatation and increased vascular permeability, in addition to activation of mast cells, B cells, T cells and macrophages and chemoattraction of eosinophils and neutrophils , are all subject to regulation by autonomic nerves (Barnes, 1986, 1994; Joos *et al.*, 1994). A greater understanding of the complex nature of the interaction between the autonomic neural networks and the cells involved in airway inflammation, in all three lymphoid compartments, is required before we will be able to determine the importance of autonomic innervation in asthma.

This complexity is already being unravelled. For example, it is now clear that, rather than there being a discrete population of NANC nerves, NANC neuropeptides are released from classical autonomic nerves. Thus, the inhibitory NANC neuropeptides, nitric oxide and vasoactive intestinal polypeptide (VIP), which promote airway smooth-muscle relaxation, are colocalized with bronchoconstricting acetylcholine in parasympathetic nerves. Similarly, the normally bronchodilating sympathetic nerves can release the vasoconstrictive neuropeptide Y. The situation is further complicated by the finding that a single population of nerves is not only capable of storing and coreleasing several neuropeptides, but the same neuropeptide may be released from sympathetic, parasympathetic or NANC nerves. The factors controlling whether classical transmitters or neuropeptides are released from autonomic nerves, and therefore whether neural transmission is pro- or anti-inflammatory, are unknown. These data start to bring into question the wisdom of defining a nerve as purely cholinergic or adrenergic, when the effects of impulse transmission may be either bronchodilating or bronchoconstricting depending on the transmitter released. Therefore, studies questioning the importance of a particular neuropeptide in asthma, based on the inability to demonstrate significant immunohistochemical staining in asthmatic biopsies (Howarth *et al.*, 1995), may be underestimating the role for that neuropeptide. In addition to the variability in transmitter release, the pattern of autonomic innervation may vary depending on the chronicity of the inflammatory process (McKay & Bienerstock, 1994).

Whether the neural networks promote bronchoconstriction or bronchodilatation depends, largely, on the target tissue of the transmitters and neuropeptides released. For example, excitatory NANC tachykinins may have a direct bronchoconstricting effect or, alternatively, may promote bronchoconstriction indirectly by suppressing the bronchodilating effects of inhibitory NANC nerves. Similarly β-adrenoreceptor agonists may produce a direct bronchodilating effect or alternatively promote bronchodilatation by inhibiting NANC bronchoconstriction (Verleden *et al.*, 1993). In addition, the *in vivo* metabolism of these autonomic transmitters may be important in determining airway calibre. Thus, the inhibition of adrenergic transmission by tachykinins can be blocked by substances that metabolize tachykinins, such as capsaicin, and thereby promote bronchodilatation (Van Ranst & Lauweryns, 1990; Matsuse *et al.*, 1991).

Lymphocyte migration

Although circulating levels of catecholamines are not elevated in asthmatics, there is very good evidence to suggest that the migration of lymphocytes into lymphoid tissue is finely controlled by the autonomic nervous system. This may be due to the effects of sympathetic innervation on lymphocyte–endothelial interaction or the direct effects on vascular tone (Ottaway & Husband, 1994). It is unknown whether catecholamines can explicitly alter the expression of adhesion molecules; however, they may alter the sensitivity of endothelial cells to interferon-γ (IFN-γ), which in turn may alter the expression of adhesion molecules (Bourdoulous *et al.*, 1993). Conversely, recent evidence has demonstrated that the NANC neuropeptides, VIP, substance P (SP) and CGRP can produce an early up-regulation of P-selectin followed by a later up-regulation of E-selectin in human cutaneous vascular endothelium, resulting in a rapid and sustained influx of neutrophils and eosinophils (Smith *et al.*, 1993).

Bidirectional communication

A further layer of complexity in the autonomic control of airway calibre is provided by the finding that within each lymphoid compartment there is a complex bidirectional interaction between the autonomic networks and the cells involved in inflammation. This has been most clearly demonstrated in the intestine by the interaction between mucosal mast cells and enteric nerves, although similar relationships may also exist for B cells and eosinophils (Stead *et al.*, 1987, 1991). Thus, SP can promote the degranulation of mucosal mast cells (Shanahan *et al.*, 1985), and subthreshold amounts of SP can prime mast cells to degranulate to other stimuli (Janiszewski *et al.*, 1994). This is despite a lack of SP receptors on the mast cell surface (Mousli *et al.*, 1990). Conversely, mast cell mediators can affect neuronal function (Wood, 1992). Similarly, VIP, which can inhibit mast cell mediator release, can be degraded by mast cell tryptase (Joos & Pauwels, 1993). In addition, respiratory pathogens, such as viruses and mycoplasma, and irritants, such as cigarette smoke, may promote airway inflammation by inhibiting the metabolism of tachykinins by neutral endopeptidases (Bellinger *et al.*, 1988).

Functional studies

Although this work is gradually deciphering the complex effects of autonomic innervation on the cells involved in allergic inflammation, functional studies investigating the *in vivo* effects of autonomic innervation on airway immune function have been lacking. The functional studies that have been conducted have focused on the effects of chemical sympathectomy on primary and secondary lymphoid organs (Madden *et al.*, 1994). In contrast, two recent reports have examined the influence of the cervical sympathetic trunk on the late-phase pulmonary response to antigen challenge. The first of these studies demonstrated that surgical denervation of the superior cervical ganglion by decentralization or bilateral ganglioectomy not only reduced anaphylactic death induced by intravenous administration of helminth antigen by 68%, but also attenuated the increase in bronchoalveolar lavage fluid (BALF) immunoglobulin M (IgM), IgA and IgG levels, while serum Ig levels remained unchanged. There was a similar attenuation in the BALF and peritoneal histamine levels in decentralized animals despite no change in the numbers of peritoneal mast cells. In addition, decentralization significantly reduced the pulmonary and BALF neutrophilia but had no effect on BALF eosinophilia (Ramaswamy *et al.*, 1990). These findings could not be attributed to alterations in pulmonary haemodynamics or respiratory function. This work was subsequently extended to show that the attenuation of the late-phase pulmonary inflammation following limited surgical sympathectomy was also associated with reduced neutrophil activity and macrophage lipopolysaccharide (LPS)-stimulated production of tumour necrosis factor-α (TNF-α) (Mathison *et al.*, 1994a). Since the superior cervical ganglion does not directly innervate the airways, it has been suggested that these effects may be mediated through its innervation of the thymus or, alternatively, they may be mediated by modulating the cytokine and nerve growth factor production by the submandibular gland (Mathison *et al.*, 1994b).

Efferent neuroendocrine regulation of the airways

The second efferent pathway by which the CNS regulates the immune system is via the production of neuroendocrine steroids and peptides (Fig. 28.1). Again, discussion of the effects of neurosteroids and neuropeptides on airway inflammation should not be restricted to local effects within the bronchial mucosa, but should incorporate the effects of these molecules on the primary and secondary lymphoid organs, since these molecules can have a profound effect on T-cell differentiation, proliferation and function in the thymus or regional lymph nodes (Dardenne *et al.*, 1994; Moreno *et al.*, 1994). Substantial evidence to suggest that a wide range of leucocyte functions can be inhibited or stimulated by neuropeptides and neuroendocrine steroids produced by the CNS has now accumulated. Thus, growth hormone (GH), thyrotrophin-

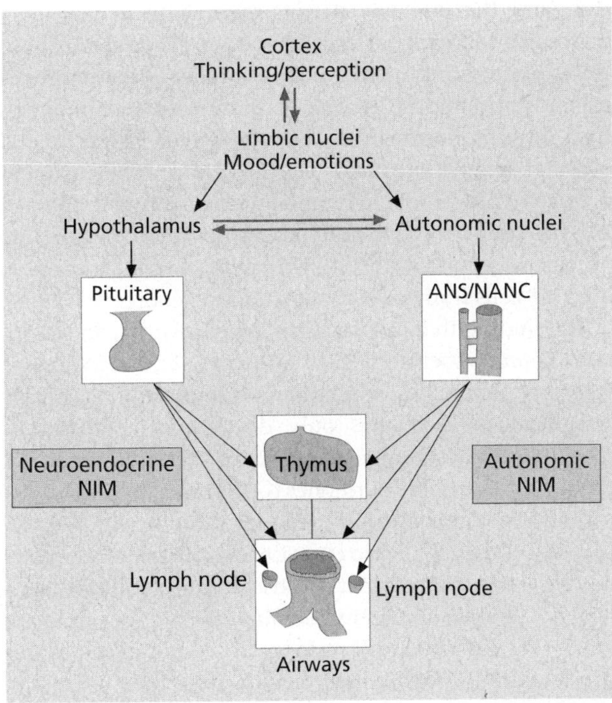

Fig. 28.1 Neuroimmunomodulatory pathways affecting airway inflammation. See text for definition of abbreviations.

releasing hormone (TRH), thyroid-stimulating hormone (TSH), prolactin (PRL), androgens, gonadotrophin-releasing hormone, human chorionic gonadotrophin, calcitriol and arginine vasopressin are all capable of immunoregulation (Mousli *et al.*, 1990; Reichlin, 1993; Blalock, 1994a). For example, painting calcitrol on to the skin can shift the immune response in local draining lymph nodes towards a T-helper 2 (Th2) response (Daynes & Araneo, 1994). Also, opiates produced following expression of the pro-opiomelanocortin gene (α-, β- and γ-endorphin, enkephalins and adrenocorticotrophic hormone (ACTH)) have been shown to have pervasive effects on the cells involved in allergic inflammation. For example, opiates may modulate cholinergic transmission, mucus secretion, neurogenic microvascular leakage, T-cell IFN-γ production, human cutaneous mast cell degranulation *in vitro*, T-lymphocyte-dependent antibody production and the expression of high-affinity interleukin-2 (IL-2) receptors (Johnson *et al.*, 1982; Casale *et al.*, 1984; Brown & Van Epps, 1986; Kavelaars *et al.*, 1992; Verleden *et al.*, 1993).

Leucocyte neuroendocrine receptors

Circulating leucocytes, particularly lymphocytes and macrophages, have high- and low-affinity receptors for most of the neuroendocrine steroids and peptides (Ader *et al.*, 1990). For example, fluorescence-activated cell sorting (FACS) has demonstrated the presence of a PRL receptor on more than 90% of thymic and bone marrow cells. In addition, more than 75% of CD4+ cells express PRL receptors, and the intensity of this expression is markedly increased following T-cell activation (Dardenne *et al.*, 1994). Interestingly, there is a higher percentage of somatostatin and SP receptors on mucosal lymphocytes than on lymphocytes found in the spleen or peripheral blood (Payan *et al.*, 1986). This suggests that neuropeptides may play a role in lymphocyte recruitment. Indeed, VIP has been shown to inhibit lymphocyte migration into murine mucosal tissue (Ottaway, 1984) and the migration of CD4+ cells from sheep lymph nodes (Moore *et al.*, 1988).

The finding that autonomic NIM pathways can modulate neuroendocrine NIM pathways and vice versa suggests that CNS regulation of immunity is highly complicated. Thus, not only does the hypothalamus receive a rich autonomic innervation, which may promote the release of trophic hormones (O'Flynn *et al.*, 1991), but it can also synthesize catecholamines (Vale *et al.*, 1983; Al-Damluji *et al.*, 1987; Terao *et al.*, 1993). Additionally, several studies have shown that electrical stimulation or electrolytic lesions of the hypothalamus, hippocampus or amygdala can profoundly affect peripheral catecholamine production and subsequent cellular immunity (Cross *et al.*, 1980; Rozman *et al.*, 1985), an effect mediated by neuroendocrine hormones other than corticosterone (Rozman & Brooks, 1985). Conversely, neuroendocrine output can have a profound effect on autonomic function (Mason *et al.*, 1976). Similarly, cytokine-induced corticotrophin-releasing factor (CRF) synthesis is lost following the destruction of hypothalamic autonomic innervation using 6-hydroxy dopamine or after adrenalectomy, and in T-cell-deficient mice (Besedovsky, 1993; Chover-Gonzalez *et al.*, 1993). Studies in chick embryos suggest that the complex communication between the brain and the immune system is functional early on during embryogenesis (Madden *et al.*, 1994).

Afferent signals from the immune system to the CNS

Following the discovery that centrally derived hormone levels are altered after an antigenic challenge (Besedovsky *et al.*, 1975), and that this is associated with an increase in the firing rates of neurones in the ventromedial hypothalamic nuclei (Besedovsky & Sorkin, 1977), it became apparent that there were a number of afferent immunoneuromodulatory pathways by which the immune system was communicating with the brain. Of these, the most thoroughly investigated is the modulation of hypothalamic and pituitary function by various leucocyte-derived cytokines. For example, it has been shown that IL-1 can activate the hypothalamic–pituitary–adrenocortical (HPAC) axis and promote ACTH release, either via a direct effect on pituitary cells, sensitized by endogenous or exogenous CRF (Payne *et al.*, 1994), or by promoting the release of CRF from the paraventricular nucleus (PVN) of the hypothalamus (Ju *et al.*, 1991). A number of other leucocyte-derived cytokines, such as IL-6 and TNF-α (Besedovsky *et al.*, 1991), have also been shown to possess immunoneuroregulatory properties, although some of these may act indirectly through IL-1. Not only may cytokine-induced activation of the HPAC axis occur through production of CRF by the PVN, but some cytokines also preferentially promote hypothalamic vasopressin release, which then stimulates ACTH production (Gillies *et al.*, 1982; Whitnall *et al.*, 1992). Cytokines may, in fact, be more potent than endogenous CRF with regard to eliciting ACTH release (Hu *et al.*, 1992). IL-1 is also capable of modulating the central production of GH, PRL and TSH (Rettori *et al.*, 1987). The importance of cytokines in regulating neuroendocrine steroid production is further supported by the demonstration of receptors for IL-1, IL-2, IL-3 and IL-6 in the hypothalamus, pituitary and a number of other sites within the brain (Blalock, 1994b).

In addition to their direct effects on hypothalamic nuclei, cytokines may also have an indirect effect on hypothalamic CRF production, either by modulating PVN innervation, or by altering neuronal or endothelial expression of nitric oxide synthetase (NOS). Nitric oxide has been implicated in the regulation of CRF production, although its exact role remains unclear. Recently it has been demonstrated that the nitric oxide precursor L-arginine and the synthetic nitrate molsidomine inhibits IL-1-induced CRF production (Costa *et al.*, 1993), whereas NG-monomethyl-L-arginine, a competitive inhibitor of NOS, completely suppresses IL-2-induced CRF release (Karanth *et al.*, 1993). A variety of neuropeptides and other limbic nuclei and thymic hormones are also capable of modulating hypothalamic CRF production (Gibbs & Vale, 1983; Malaise *et al.*, 1987; Herman *et al.*, 1989; Tizabi & Calogero, 1992).

Leucocyte-derived cytokines may not only modulate neuroendocrine hormone production, but also have a profound effect on central noradrenergic activity (Besedovsky *et al.*, 1979, 1983). The synthesis of hypothalamic noradrenaline is blocked by pretreatment with a cyclo-oxygenase inhibitor, implicating prostaglandins in the transduction of the peripheral cytokine signal into the CNS (Johnson *et al.*, 1982).

Transduction of leucocyte-derived cytokine signals into the CNS

Exactly how cytokines gain access to the hypothalamus is unclear. Four theories have been advanced. Firstly, they may utilize a cytokine-specific uptake mechanism, although the evidence for this remains unsubstantiated (Banks *et al.*, 1991). Secondly, cytokines may cross the blood–brain barrier at points of increased permeability in the circumventricular organs, and this permeability may be further increased by endogenous steroids (Long & Holaday, 1985; Katsuura *et al.*, 1990). Recently, prostaglandins have been incriminated in the transduction of the peripheral cytokine signal into the CNS, since cytokine-induced modulation of CRF production is blocked by epoxygenase and phospholipase A2 inhibitors (Lyson & McCann, 1992). Thus, at these points of increased permeability, leucocyte-derived cytokines may promote a prostaglandin-dependent production of cytokine by the microglia, resulting in a modulation of CRF synthesis. Some authors have suggested that prostaglandin $F_{2\alpha}$ ($PGF_{2\alpha}$) or PGE_2 may alter the IL-1-induced up-regulation of CRF directly (Watanabe *et al.*, 1990; Cambronero *et al.*, 1992). It is not yet clear whether the microglial production of cytokines is necessary for the modulation of CRF by leucocyte-derived cytokines. Certainly there is an increase in IL-1, IL-6 and TNF-α in the hypothalamus and hippocampus following a peripheral immune challenge with intraperitoneal (ip) LPS, and microglial-derived cytokines are capable of modulating neurosteroid production (Vankelecom *et al.*, 1989; Koenig *et al.*, 1990; Romero *et al.*, 1991).

The third mechanism by which leucocyte-derived cytokines might gain access to the CNS is via peripheral leucocytes themselves, entering at points of increased permeability. More recently, a fourth potential pathway by which peripheral cytokines can affect hypothalamic neuroendocrine steroid production has been described. Thus, leucocyte-derived cytokines may signal CNS centres via vagal afferents. For example, LPS administered by ip injection stimulates liver macrophages to produce IL-1. This IL-1 then binds to IL-1 receptors on paraganglia which synapse with the vagus. As a result, IL-1 elicits illness behaviour and hyperalgesia. Sectioning vagal afferents abolishes this LPS-induced illness behaviour. Similar results are found when peripheral IL-1 receptor antagonists are administered. Thus, leucocyte-derived cytokines may stimulate the vagus, modulating the afferent signal to tractus solitarius, which then promotes cytokine release by the microglia (Bluthe *et al.*, 1994; Watkins *et al.*, 1994).

Which of these four pathways is employed to transduce the peripheral immune signal into the CNS probably depends on the type of immune response occurring, the major cytokine driving the response as well as the lymphoid compartment involved. However, it is clear that cytokines directly affect neuroendocrine or autonomic efferent pathways.

Leucocyte-derived steroids

There is now a large body of evidence demonstrating that leucocytes are capable of synthesizing a wide range of the neuroendocrine peptides and steroids normally elaborated by the CNS. These leucocyte-derived neuropeptides and steroids may be either identical to those produced by the brain, unique structural and functional variants or cleaved subunits of the total molecule (Goetzl, 1990). Whether sufficient plasma levels of these leucocyte-derived hormones are produced to effect an endocrine function is controversial (Munck *et al.*, 1984; Olsen *et al.*, 1992). Leucocytes produce much less hormones, cell for cell, than do pituitary cells; however, since leucocytes can deposit hormones locally and there are considerably more leucocytes than pituitary cells, a massive plasma level may not be required in order to modulate other endocrine organs.

In contrast, leucocyte-derived hormones do serve a paracrine function. For example, lymphocytes spontaneously produce GH in culture, and, if this synthesis is blocked, lymphocyte DNA synthesis is inhibited (Weigent *et al.*, 1991). Similarly, depleting PRL from lymphocye cultures inhibits IL-2-stimulated T-cell proliferation (Hartman *et al.*, 1989) and *in vivo* inhibition of PRL release reduces macrophage and T-cell activation (Bernton *et al.*, 1988). Leucocyte-derived CRH, TRH and TSH have all been shown to have paracrine activity (Mason *et al.*, 1976), and this paracrine function is not limited to effects on neighbouring leucocytes. Thus, in an animal model of joint inflammation, leucocyte-derived opiates produced an analgesic effect by acting on peripheral sensory nerves (Przewlocki *et al.*, 1992). This gives rise to the startling possibility that leucocytes may modulate sensation.

The factors controlling hormone production by leucocytes differ from the feedback mechanisms normally seen in the neuroendocrine system. Leucocyte steroids are produced in direct response to powerful stimulants such as *superantigens* or viruses (Blalock, 1989), or as an indirect response to CRH-induced IL-1 release from macrophages (Kavelaars *et al.*, 1989). The role of these leucocyte-derived hormones in specific inflammatory diseases is unknown. Since they have to be synthesized *de novo* and are not preformed, they are more likely to be involved in the modulation of chronic inflammation and fine-tuning of local inflammatory responses than serving an endocrine effect.

Higher cortical centres and asthma

It is clear from the preceding discussion that autonomic activity and neuroendocrine output are capable of modulating all aspects of the immune response in primary, secondary and tertiary lymphoid tissue, including the airways. Even more intriguing, perhaps, is the volume of data suggesting that cognitive and limbic emotional centres can profoundly affect immunity by activating both hypothalamic and autonomic efferent NIM pathways. This research cuts across the fields of immunology, neurobiology and psychiatry and provides a persuasive argument for re-examining the idea that cognitive factors may play a role in asthma (Busse *et al.*, 1995). Four main areas of this research will be briefly discussed here.

Stress and immunity—animal studies

Some of the most powerful evidence supporting the importance of cognitive centres for immunity comes from the rich and extensive animal literature on the immune effects of stressful environmental events (Solomon *et al.*, 1974; Coe, 1993). Animal studies afford a much greater scope for investigating the immune response and controlling and manipulating the environment than human studies. One of the major findings to come out of this work is the remarkably consistent immunosuppressive effect of a stressful environment, across different animal populations and different kinds of events. For example, isolation, separation, overcrowding, disrupted dominance hierarchy, introduction of an aggressive intruder, restraint, cold, noise and inescapable foot shock can all produce immunosuppression in a variety of models (Justice, 1985; Moynihan *et al.*, 1990).

The processing of environmental information is complex. Following its inital perception by the cortex, the information is evaluated by the limbic system by comparing it with known information in the memory stores, and an assessment of congruency is made (Gilad, 1987). If what is observed differs markedly from what is known or expected, the mismatch produces behavioural inhibition while incoming data are checked. If the incongruency is validated, then two things occur. Firstly, a new behavioural strategy is devised to minimize the conflict caused by the uncertainty, and, secondly, the environment is judged to be stressful and this assessment is communicated to the hypothalamus (Sacher, 1975), resulting in an alteration in gene expression. For example, the genes for CRF, preproenkephalin and vasopressin are expressed after just 5 minutes of restraint stress, resulting in increased circulating levels of ACTH and corticosterone (Al-Damluji *et al.*, 1987). This change in hypothalamic neuroendocrine activity is rapidly communicated to the immune system via the hypothalamic and autonomic efferent NIM pathways (Watanabe *et al.*, 1990), resulting in an immunological change, behavioural inhibition and reproductive quiescence (Dunn *et al.*, 1991).

The vast majority of animal studies on the effects of stress on immunity have employed *in vitro* assessments of lymphocyte function, such as mitogen proliferation, cytokine production and cellular cytotoxicity, or have used gross, *in vivo* assessments of immunity, such as antibody production (Glaser *et al.*, 1986; Khansari *et al.*, 1990). There are far fewer functional studies evaluating the effects of stress on the development and progression of animal models of disease, particularly pulmonary diseases. In an exception to this trend, a recent study evaluated the effects of restraint stress on the pulmonary response to influenza virus. The authors found that restraint stress virtually abolished the viral-induced mononuclear lung infiltration and consolidation and significantly reduced the IL-2 production by cells in the mediastinal lymph nodes. In addition, restraint reduced the virus-specific cell-mediated immunity, while the humoral response remained unaltered (Sheridan *et al.*, 1991). These effects were attributed to the rise in corticosteroid levels following restraint. Subsequent studies with this model suggested that the rise in corticosteroid levels could not explain the increased survival, following restraint, of DBA/2 mice infected with influenza virus (Hermann *et al.*, 1994a). Rather, this was due to the combined effect of catecholamines and neuroendocrine steroids, with the increased corticosteroid levels modulating cell trafficking and the increased catecholamine levels limiting the activation of virus-specific effector cells (Hermann *et al.*, 1994b). These results were in agreement with earlier work suggesting that corticosteroid and catecholamine mechanisms are both important in restraint-induced inhibition of virus-specific cytotoxic T-cell response (Dobbs *et al.*, 1993). Other groups have reported the same effect using foot shock (Kusnecov *et al.*, 1992).

It has been suggested that stress may play a crucial role in driving the immune system towards a Th2-dominated response (Rook *et al.*, 1994). Support for this idea was recently provided by the report that housing conditions could influence the production of Th1 and Th2 cytokine. Thus, housing mice individually significantly increased the amount of IL-4 but not IL-2 produced by Balb/c mice in response to keyhole limpet haemocyanin (KLH). Similarly, C57BL/6 mice produced significantly more IL-2 but not IL-4 in response to KLH when housed alone compared with four mice per cage. The authors suggest that this may be due to the greater stress of group housing (Karp *et al.*, 1994). Similarly, stress odour can enhance the production of IL-4 in Balb/c mice and this effect is blocked by the administration of glucocorticoid receptor antagonists (Moynihan *et al.*, 1994).

Stress and immunity—human studies

This animal research is mirrored by an extensive literature on the immune effects of stress in humans (Herbert & Cohen, 1993). A wide variety of acute and chronic stressors have been shown to be immunosuppressive in prospective and retrospective studies, and this immunosuppression has been attributed to neuroendocrine dysfunction (Karp *et al.*, 1994). The majority of these data employed *in vitro* assessment of immune function and were not directly related to airway disease, although some research may be indirectly related to the airways in that the stressors used may promote a Th2 response (Sheridan *et al.*, 1991). For example, severe stress may reduce the level of the testosterone precursor, dihydroepiandrosterone sulphate (DHEAS), and promote a Th1 response (Daynes & Araneo, 1992). Similarly, calcitriol may serve a crucial immunomodulatory role in promoting a Th2 response (Moreno *et al.*, 1994). Despite the fact that psychological factors are commonly perceived to play a signifcant role in asthma (Thompson & Thompson, 1985), when the role of psychological factors in asthma have been examined directly the studies have been small scale and utilized questionable psychological assessments (Hollaender & Florin, 1983; Wistuba, 1986; Michel, 1994). A notable exception to the lack of functional studies on the effects of stress on pulmonary pathology was the highly publicized finding that subjects reporting higher levels of stress were much more likely to develop an upper respiratory tract infection, on exposure to five commonly encountered viruses, than subjects experiencing less stress (Cohen *et al.*, 1991).

Unfortunately, much of the human data on the effects of stress on the immune system has been confounded by the inter-individual variability in the response to stress. The importance of this variability was highlighted by the recent finding that individuals who exhibit the largest catecholamine responses to stress also produce the most dramatic alterations in cellular immunity to the same stress (Manuck *et al.*, 1991). In contrast to the paucity of functional studies, there is quite a rich literature on the effects of behavioural interventions in allergic disease (Watkins, 1994).

Depression immunity and asthma

There are a large number of heterogeneous studies investigating the effects of mood on immunity. Generally these data suggest that depression of the immune system may follow biological depression, particularly in the older, more severely depressed patients (Denney *et al.*, 1988; Stein *et al.*, 1991). But whether depression can affect a subject's asthma or vice versa, or whether a depressive mood predisposes an individual to asthma has received little attention from the scientific research community. The studies that have been performed have utilized a wide variety of psychological assessments, with the majority (Lyketsos *et al.*, 1984; Strunk *et al.*, 1985; Lyketsos *et al.*, 1987; Yellowless *et al.*, 1988; Rubin, 1993; Badoux & Levy, 1994), but not all (Janson *et al.*, 1994), reporting an increase in the association between anxiety or depression and asthma. One study suggested that up to 25% of school-age children admitted for severe asthma were depressed, and 33% were coping poorly (Klinnert *et al.*, 1985). Poor control of asthmatic symptoms has been associated with emotional or behavioural deviance (Norrish *et al.*, 1977). The potential role of mood in asthma was suggested by the finding that antidepressants have been shown to improve asthma (Meares *et al.*, 1971), with up to 62% of all asthmatics and 79% of asthmatic children reporting improved symptoms following tricyclic antidepressant medication (Sugihara *et al.*, 1965). However, this phenomenological research has not addressed the issue of how the observed psychological morbidity interacts with the physiological disruption that is common to this disease. In an exception to this trend, a recent paper suggested that the increased activation of central cholinergic pathways seen in depression might be a factor in asthmatic death. There are two patterns of asthmatic death: sudden, over a few hours, and subacute, which occurs more gradually over a few days. The authors suggested that the autonomic imbalance that may occur in depression may precipitate the sudden deterioration and subsequent death seen in some asthmatics (Miller, 1987). This provocative possibility warrants further investigation, particularly since the incidence of death from asthma remains unchanged, despite our vastly increased understanding of the pathophysiology of this disease.

Not only does a depressed mood affect autonomic function but there is good evidence to show that it also affects the HPAC axis (Charlton & Ferrier, 1989). Thus, many patients with a depressive illness have a disturbance of the central control of CRF. This can be measured as hypercortisolaemia, increased levels of CRF in their cerebrospinal fluid (CSF), a blunted ACTH response to CRF or non-suppression of cortisol following administration of dexamethasone (Sachar, 1982; Gold *et al.*, 1984, 1988). Altered hypothalamic function may interact with the autonomic dysfunction (Roy *et al.*, 1988), to produce the immune disruption seen in these patients (Kronful & House, 1984; Dorian & Garfinkel, 1987). Thus, mood may affect airway inflammation via both autonomic and neuroendocrine pathways.

Personality

Because of the wide inter-individual variability in literature on stress and particularly depression, a number of researchers have tried to define personality characteristics that can be used to identify asthmatics that are particularly 'at risk' from their asthma. These studies have revealed a complex number of behavioural traits and coping strategies associated with poorer asthmatic control. A denial of their condition (Dirks & Kinsman, 1982), associated with a repressed hostility (Lyketsos, 1984), depressive withdrawal, emotional dependence (Santiago & Klaustermeyer, 1980) and a 'negative parental aura' (Pinkerton, 1972), is characteristic. However, all these studies are uncontrolled. In the only case-controlled study to date, 21 children who died from asthma following hospital discharge were matched for age, sex, race and severity of disease with 21 children who were alive at follow-up. Hospital records were evaluated for 57 physiological and psychological variables. A stepwise discriminate analysis revealed 14 variables which could distinguish the group of children that died from the control group. Ten of these differentiating characteristics reflected the psychological adaptation of the child or their family to the situation. The authors concluded that the psychological features that characterized the children who died were more than just a consequence of severe disease, and may be important in identifying children at high risk of dying and also in developing treatment plans to prevent death (Stein *et al.*, 1991).

Conditioning immunity

Some of the most compelling evidence for the influence of higher cortical centres on the immune system comes from work showing that the immune system can be classically conditioned (Ader & Cohen, 1991). Thus, inert physiological stimuli, such as saccharine-flavoured water, can be paired with powerful immunosuppressants, and, when the inert stimuli are later presented alone, they can elicit an immunosuppression. Thus, animals can literally learn to suppress or, more dramatically, enhance their T-cell, B-cell, cytotoxic cell and natural killer cell function in a wide variety of animal models *in vivo* and *ex vivo* (Bovbjerg *et al.*, 1987; Husband *et al.*, 1987; Solvason *et al.*, 1988; Moynihan *et al.*, 1989; Klosterhalfen & Klosterhalfen, 1990). Similarly, mast cells, which are being increasingly implicated in the initiation of airway inflammation during an acute asthmatic attack, can also be conditioned in animals (Dark *et al.*, 1987; MacQueen *et al.*, 1989) and humans. Animals can also 'learn' to control the immune response to antigen and the neuroendocrine response to cytokines, utilizing the conditioning paradigm.

Neuropharmacology

The pharmaceutical industry has not been slow to see the potential of a new class of immunomodulators that may significantly change the course of inflammation by altering these brain–immune feedback loops. The race to develop novel compounds, be they neuropeptides, modulators of neuropeptide metabolism, cytokines, soluble cytokine receptors or their antagonists, has already begun (Anon., 1993). These compounds may fundamentally alter the balance between pro- and anti-inflammatory forces and may therefore be applicable to airway inflammation as well as a wide variety of other conditions in which inflammation is central. For example, a highly selective neurokinin-1 (NK_1) antagonist has recently been developed which is very effective at blocking the effects of exogenous SP on airway microvascular leakage without affecting the bronchoconstrictor response to tachykinins (an NK_2 effect) (Lei *et al.*, 1992). Similarly, potent NK_2 and CGRP antagonists have also been developed (Hughes & Brain, 1991; Emons-Alt *et al.*, 1992; Lou *et al.*, 1993).

Compounds, such as steroids, which increase the ability of neutral endopeptidases to catabolize tachykinins may provide an alternative approach to promoting bronchodilatation. Similarly, the administration of recombinant human endopeptidase to guinea pigs has been shown to inhibit tachykinin-induced cough (Kohrogi *et al.*, 1989). However, initial data suggest that endopeptidase inhibitors may be less important in humans, at least in mild asthma (Cheung *et al.*, 1992), although it may have a greater role in more severe disease (Joos *et al.*, 1994). Numerous other potential compounds that may modulate NIM pathways are at present under investigation (Anon., 1993; Barnes, 1994).

Implications for allergic inflammation

Considerable advances have been achieved in our understanding of the immunological basis of inflammation. The modern tools of molecular biology have enabled us to dissect in great detail the recruitment, activation and function of all the cells involved in allergic inflammation of the airways. The same tools have also provided an overwhelming amount of evidence to suggest that virtually every aspect of airway function is under the control of neuroendocrine steroids and the autonomic nervous system. Although the exact pathophysiological significance of these neuroimmunomodulatory pathways in allergic inflammation is not yet clear, the complexity of the interaction between the brain and the immune system, the rapidity of information sharing and the fact that disruption of the pathways connecting the two systems may have dramatic consequences for immunity (Watkins, 1995) strongly suggest that the brain may well be exerting a subtle control over the direction of the immune response.

The unravelling of the highly complex and subtle nature of NIM is forcing us to re-evaluate some of our fundamental views on how the immune system works. For example, cytokines can no longer be seen as merely leucocyte-derived pro- or anti-inflammatory signals. It is clear that they have a much wider role and are involved in behaviour and neuroendocrine steroid production and possibily critically involved in neuronal embryogenesis and senescence. Similarly, lymphocytes may have endocrine functions and under certain circumstances may alter pain perception.

It is still early days in our understanding of brain–immune interactions, but there can be little doubt that research into how the the autonomic nervous system and neuroendocrine steroids regulate the immune system will have a significant impact on our understanding of allergic inflammation of the airways and open up a number of new therapeutic possibilities. In fact, research into the function of autonomic innervation of mucosal tissue has already spawned compounds that may potentially modulate airway inflammation. In addition, the identification of neuroendocrine peptides and steroids, other than corticosteroid, that may shape the immune response provides a wide variety of points for potential therapeutic intervention either peripherally or centrally. To ignore the importance of these neuroimmunomodulatory pathways in the airways and to study individual cellular mechanisms in isolation runs the risk of obtaining biologically irrelevant data. What is now required is a multidisciplinary research effort (Vitkovic & Koslow, 1994; Busse *et al.*, 1995), prepared to ask searching questions in complex functional studies and methodically dissect the variables using sophisticated technology. It is only through such effort that we will be able to establish which of all these potential neuroimmunomodulatory pathways are important in allergic inflammation of the airways.

Finally, it is impossible to be familiar with this literature without wondering whether we must rethink our views on the importance of the differences between individuals, be they humans or animals. To date we have tended to ignore or average out individual differences. This has led to the loss of important information. For example, when differences in immune response between animals was the focus of the research, it was shown that the genetic heterogeneity in hypothalamic corticosteroid tone determined the susceptibility to and recovery from inflammatory diseases (Levine *et al.*, 1980; Chelmicka-Schorr *et al.*, 1988). Similarly, when sophisticated computer technology was utilized to analyse autonomic tone, it became apparent that individual differences, which had previously been ignored, were, in fact, vital and could predict morbidity and mortality with a high degree of specificity from a wide range of diseases (Ori *et al.*, 1992). This technology has yet to be applied to asthma. A greater understanding of the highly complex communication between the brain and the immune system and the importance of individual differences in these pathways may not only enable us to predict who will respond to a particular therapuetic intervention, but may also enable us to design individualized treatment with a much higher chance of producing therapeutic benefit in the clinically heterogeneous conditions of allergic inflammation.

References

Ackerman, K.D., Felten, S.Y., Dijkstra, C.D., Livnat, S. & Felten, D.L. (1989) Parallel development of noradrenergic sympathetic innervation and cellular compartmentalisation in the rat spleen. *Exp. Neurol.*, **103**, 239–55.

Ader, R. & Cohen, N. (1991) Conditioning the immune response. *Neth. J. Med.*, **39**, 263–73.

Ader, R., Felten, D. & Cohen, N. (1990) Interactions between the brain and the immune system. *Ann. Rev. Pharmacol. Toxicol.*, **30**, 561–602.

Ader, R., Felten, D.L. & Cohen, N. (eds) (1991) *Psychoneuroimmunology*, 2nd edn. Academic Press, San Diego, CA.

Al-Damluji, S., Perry, L., Tomlin, S. *et al.* (1987) Alpha-adrenergic stimulation of corticotropin secretion by a specific central mechanism in man. *Neuroendocrinology*, **45**, 68–76.

Anon. *Drug News Perspectives*, **6** (1), 48.

Badoux, A. & Levy, D.A. (1994) Psychological symptoms in asthma and chronic urticaria. *Ann. Allergy.*, **72**, 229–33.

Bai, T.R., Mak, J.C.W. & Barnes, P.J. (1992) A comparison of beta-adrenergic receptors and *in vitro* relaxant responses to isoproterenol in asthmatic airway smooth muscle. *Am. J. Respir. Cell Mol. Biol.*, **6**, 647–51.

Banks, W.A., Ortiz, L., Plotkin, S.R. & Kastin, A.J. (1991) Human interleukin (IL) 1α, murine IL-1α and murine IL-1β are transported from blood to brain in the mouse by a shared saturable mechanism. *J. Pharmacol.*, **259**, 988–96.

Barnes, P.J. (1986) State of art: neural control of human airways in health and disease. *Am. Rev. Resp. Dis.*, **134**, 1289–314.

Barnes, P.J. (1994) Airway neuropeptides. In: *Asthma and Rhinitis* (eds S.T. Holgate & W. Busse), pp. 667–85. Blackwell Science, Oxford.

Bellinger, D.L., Felten, S.Y. & Felten, D.L. (1988) Maintenance of noradrenergic sympathetic innervation in the involuted thymus of the aged Fischer 344 rat. *Brain Behav. Immunity*, **2**, 133–50.

Bernton, E.W., Meltzer, M.S. & Holaday, J.W. (1988) Suppression of macrophage activation and T-lymphocyte function in hypoprolactinemic mice. *Science*, **239**, 401–4.

Besedovsky, H. (1993) *Integrative role of cytokines in immuno-neuro-endocrine interactions*. Paper presented to the First Annual Congress of BSI, Brighton, UK, 6 December.

Besedovsky, H. & Sorkin, E. (1977) Network of immune–neuroendocrine interactions. *Clin. Exp. Immunol.*, **27**, 1–12.

Besedovsky, H., Sorkin, E., Keller, M. & Muller, J. (1975) Changes in blood hormone levels during the immune response. *Proc. Soc. Exp. Biol.*, **150**, 466–70.

Besedovsky, H., del Ray, A., Sorkin, E., Da Prada, M. & Keller, H. (1979) Immunoregulation mediated by the sympathetic nervous system. *Cell. Immunol.*, **48**, 346–55.

Besedovsky, H., del Ray, A., Sorkin, E., Da Prada, M., Burri, M. & Honegger, C. (1983) The immune response evokes changes in brain noradrenergic neurons. *Science*, **221**, 564–6.

Besedovsky, H.O., del Ray, A., Klusman, I., Furukawa, H., Monge-Arditi, G. & Kabiersch, A. (1991) Cytokines as modulators of the hypothalamus–pituitary adrenal axis. *J. Steroid Biochem. Mol. Biol.*, **40**, 613–18.

Blalock, J.E. (1989) A molecular basis for bidirectional communication between the immune and neuroendocrine systems. *Physiol. Rev.*, **69**, 1–32.

Blalock, J.E. (1994a) The immune system: our sixth sense. *Immunologist*, **2**, 8–15.

Blalock, J.E. (1994b) The syntax of immune–neuroendocrine communication. *Immunol. Today*, **15** (11), 504–11.

Bluthe, R.M., Pawlowski, M., Suarez, S. *et al.* (1994) Synergy between interferon-alpha and interleukin-1 in the induction of sickness behaviour in mice. *Psychoneuroendocrinology*, **19** (2), 197–207.

Bourdoulous, S., Durieu-Trautmann, O., Strosberg, A.D. & Conraud, P.O. (1993) Catecholamines stimulate MHC class I, class II and invariant chain gene expression in brain endothelium though different mechanisms. *J. Immunol.*, **150**, 1486–95.

Bovbjerg, D., Cohen, N. & Ader, R. (1987) Behaviourally conditioned enhancement of delayed-type hypersensitivity in the mouse. *Brain Behav. Immunity*, **1**, 64–71.

Brown, S.L. & Van Epps, D.E. (1986) Opioid peptides modulate production of interferon-γ by human mononuclear cells. *Cell. Immunol.*, **103**, 19–28.

Busse, W.W., Kielcolt-Glaser, J.K., Coe, C., Martin, R.J., Scott, T.W. & Parker, S.R. (1995) Stress and asthma: NHBLI Workshop Report. *Am. J. Resp. Crit. Care Med.*, **151**, 249–52.

Calvo, W. (1968) Innervation of the bone marrow in laboratory animals. *Am. J. Anat.*, **123**, 315–28.

Cambronero, J.C., Rivas, F.J., Borrell, J. & Guaza, C. (1992) Role of arachidonic acid metabolism on corticotropin-releasing factor (CRF)-release induced by interleukin-1 from superfused rat hypothalami. *J. Neuroimmunol.*, **39**, 57–66.

Casale, T.B. (1987) Neuromechanisms of asthma. *Ann. Allergy* **59** (6), 391–8.

Casale, J.B., Bowman, S. & Kaliner, M. (1984) Induction of human cutaneous mast cell degranulation by opiates and endogeous opioid peptides: evidence for opiate and non opiate receptor participation. *J. Allergy Clin. Immunol.*, **73**, 775–81.

Charlton, B.G. & Ferrier, I.N. (1989) Hypothalamo-pituitary–adrenal axis abnormalities in depression: a review and a model. *Psychosom. Med.*, **19**, 331–6.

Chelmicka-Schorr, E., Checinski, M. & Arnason, B.G.W. (1988) Chemical sympathectomy augments the severity of experimental allergic encephalomyelitis. *J. Neuroimmunol.*, **17**, 347–50.

Cheung, D., Timmers, M.C., Bel, E.H. *et al.* (1992) An inhaled neutral endopeptidase inhibitor, thiorphan, enhances airways narrowing to neurokinin A in asthmatic subjects *in vivo*. *Am. Rev. Resp. Dis.*, **145**, A682.

Chover-Gonzalez, A.J., Harbuz, M.S. & Lightman, S.L. (1993) Effect of adrenalectomy and stress on interleukin-1 beta-mediated activation of hypothalamic corticotropin-releasing factor mRNA. *J. Neuroimmunol.*, **42**, 155–60.

Coe, C.L. (1993) Psychosocial factors and immunity in nonhuman primates: a review. *Psychosom. Med.*, **55**, 298–308.

Cohen, S., Tyrrell, D.A. & Smith, A.P. (1991) Psychological stress and susceptibility to the common cold. *New Engl. J. Med.*, **325**, 606–12.

Costa, A., Trainer, P., Besser, M. & Grossman, A. (1993) Nitric oxide modulates the release of corticotrophin-releasing hormone from the rat hypothalamus *in vitro*. *Brain Res.*, **605**, 187–92.

Cross, R.J., Markesbury, W.R., Brooks, W.H. & Rozman, T.L. (1980) Hypothalamic–immune interactions I. The acute effects of anterior hypothalamic lesions on the immune response. *Brain Res.*, **196**, 79.

Dardenne, M. & Savino, W. (1994) Control of thymus physiology by peptidic hormones and neuropeptides. *Immunol. Today*, **15** (11), 518–23.

Dardenne, M., de Moraes, M.C., Kelley, P.A. & Gagnerault, M.C. (1994) Prolactin receptor expression in human haematopoietic tissue analysed by flow cytofluorometry. *Endocrinology*, **134**, 2108–14.

Dark, K., Peeke, H.V.S., Ellman, G. & Salfi, M. (1987) Behaviourally conditioned histamine release. *Ann. NY Acad. Sci.*, **496**, 578–82.

Daynes, R.A. & Araneo, B.A. (1992) Programming of lymphocyte responses to activation: extrinsic factors, provided microenvironmentally, confer flexibility and compartmentalisation to T-cell function. *Chem. Immunol.*, **54**, 1–20.

Daynes, R.A. & Araneo, B.A. (1994) The development of effective vaccine adjuvants employing natural regulators of T-cell lymphokine production *in vivo*. *Ann. NY Acad. Sci.*, **730**, 144–61.

Denney, D.R., Stephenson, L.A., Penick, E.C. & Weller, R.A. (1988) Lymphocyte subclasses and depression. *J. Abnorm. Psychol.*, **97**, 499–502.

Dirks, J. & Kinsman, R. (1982) Death in asthma: a psychosomatic autopsy. *J. Asthma*, **19**, 177–87.

Dobbs, C.M., Vasquez, M., Glaser, R. & Sheridan, J.F. (1993) Mechanisms of stress-induced modulation of viral pathogenesis and immunity. *J. Neuroimmunol.*, **48** (2), 151–60.

Dorian, B. & Garfinkel, P. (1987) Stress, immunity, and illness — a review. *Psychol. Med.*, **17**, 393–407.

Dunn, A.J., Antoon, M. & Chapman, Y. (1991) Reduction of exploratory behavior by intraperitoneal injection of interleukin-1 involves brain corticotropin-releasing factor. *Brain Res. Bull.*, **26**, 539–42.

Elwood, W., Sakamoto, T., Barnes, P.J. & Chung, K.F. (1993) Allergen-induced airway hyperresponsiveness in Brown Norway rat: role of parasympathetic mechanisms. *J. Appl. Physiol.*, **75** (1), 279–84.

Emons-Alt, X., Vilain, P., Goulaouic, P. *et al.* (1992) A potent and non-selective peptide antagonist of the neurokinin A (NK_2) receptor. *Life Sci.*, **50**, 101–9.

Felten, D.L., Felten, S.Y., Bellinger, D.L. *et al.* (1987) Noradrenergic sympathetic neural interactions with the immune system: structure and function. *Immunol. Rev.*, **100**, 225–60.

Felten, S.Y., Felten, D.L. & Olschowka, J.A. (1992) Noradrenergic and peptidergic innervation of lymphoid organs. *Chem. Immunol.*, **52**,

25–48.

Gibbs, D.M. & Vale, W. (1983) Effect of the serotonin reuptake inhibitor fluoxetine on corticotrophin-releasing factor and vasopressin secretion into hypophysial portal blood. *Brain Res.*, **280**, 176–9.

Gilad, G.M. (1987) The stress-induced response of the septohippocampal cholinergic system. A vectorial outcome of psychoneuroendocrinological interactions. *Psychoneuroendocrinology*, **12**, 167–84.

Gillies, G.E., Linton, E.A. & Lowry, P.J. (1982) Corticotrophin releasing activity of the new CRF is potentiated several times by vasopressin. *Nature*, **299**, 355–7.

Glaser, R., Rice, J., Speicher, C.E., Stout, J.C. & Kielcolt-Glaser, J.K. (1986) Stress depresses interferon production by leukocytes concomitant with a decrease in natural killer cell activity. *Behav. Neurosci.*, **100**, 675–8.

Goetzl, E.J. (1990) *Neuropeptides of the immune system.* Paper presented to the American Academy of Allergy and Immunology, 46th Annual Meeting, 23–28 March 1990.

Gold, P.W., Chrousos, G., Kellner, C. *et al.* (1984) Psychiatric implications of basic and clinical studies with cortico-trophin releasing factor. *Am. J. Psych.*, **141**, 619–27.

Gold, P.W., Goodwin, F.K. & Chrousos, G.P. (1988) Clinical and biochemical manifestations of depression: relation to the neurobiolgy of stress. *New Engl. J. Med.*, **319**, 413–20.

Hartman, D.P., Holaday, J.W. & Berntan, E.W. (1989) Inhibition of lymphocyte proliferation by antibodies to prolactin. *FASEB J.*, **3**, 2194–2022.

Herbert, T.B. & Cohen, S. (1993) Stress and immunity in humans: a metanalytic review *Psychosom. Med.*, **55**, 364–79.

Herman, J.P., Schafer, M.K., Young, E.A. *et al.* (1989) Evidence for hippocampal regulation of neuroenocrine neurons of the hypothalamo-pituitary–adrenocortical axis. *J. Neurosci.*, **9**, 3072–82.

Hermann, G., Tovar, C.A., Beck, F.M. & Sheridan, J.F. (1994a) Kinetics of glucocorticoid response to restraint stress and/or experimental influenza viral infection in two inbred strains of mice. *J. Neuroimmunol.*, **49** (1–2), 25–33.

Hermann, G., Beck, F.M., Tovar, C.A., Malarkey, W.B., Allen, C. & Sheridan, J.F. (1994b) Stress-induced changes attributable to the sympathetic nervous system during experimental influenza viral infection in DBA/2 inbred mouse strain. *J. Neuroimmunol.*, **53** (2), 173–80.

Hollaender, J. & Florin, I. (1983) Expressed emotion and airway conductance in children with bronchial asthma. *J. Psychosom. Res.*, **27** (4), 307–11.

Hosoi, J. Murphy, G.E., Egan, C.I. *et al.* (1993) Regulation of Langerhans cell function by nerves containing calcitonin gene-related peptide. *Nature*, **363**, 159–63.

Howarth, P.H., Djukanovic, R., Reddington, T., Holgate, S.T., Springall, D.R. & Polak, J.M. (1995) Neuropeptide-containing nerves in endobronchial biopsies from asthmatic and nonasthmatic subjects. *Am. J. Resp. Cell Mol. Biol.* **13**, 288–96.

Hu, S.B., Tannahill, L.A. & Lightman, S.L. (1992) Interleukin-1 beta induces corticotropin-releasing factor-41 release from cultured hypothalamic cells through protein kinase C and cAMP-dependent protein kinase pathways. *J. Neuroimmunol.*, **40**, 49–55.

Hughes, S.R. & Brain, S.D. (1991) A calcitonin gene-related peptide (CGRP) antagonist ($CGRP_{8-37}$) inhibits microvascular responses induced by CGRP and capsaicin in skin. *Brit. J. Pharmacol.*, **104**, 738–42.

Husband, A.J., King, M.G. & Brown, R. (1987) Behaviorally conditioned modification of T cell subset ratios in the rat. *Immunol. Letts.*, **14**, 91–4.

Janiszewski, J., Bienenstock, J. & Blennerhasset, M.B. (1994) Picomolar doses of substance P trigger electrical responses to mast cells without degranulation. *Am. J. Physiol.*, **264**, C138–C145.

Janson, C., Bjornsson, E., Hetta, J. & Boman, G. (1994) Anxiety and depression in relation to respiratory symptoms and asthma. *Am. J. Resp. Crit. Care Med.*, **149** (4), 930–4.

Johnson, H.M., Smith, E.M., Torres, B.A. & Blalock, J.E. (1982) Regulation of the *in vitro* antibody response by neuroendocrine hormones. *Proc. Nat. Acad. Sci. USA*, **79**, 4171–4.

Joos, G. & Pauwels, R. (1993) The *in vivo* effect of tachykinins on airway mast cells of the rat. *Am. Rev. Resp. Dis.*, **148**, 922–6.

Joos, G.F., Kips, J.C. & Pauwels, R.A. (1994) A role for neutral endopeptidases in asthma? *Clin. Exp. Allergy*, **24**, 91–3.

Ju, G., Zhang, X., Jin, B.O. & Huang, C.S. (1991) Activation of corticotropin-releasing factor containing neurons in the paraventricular nucleus of the hypothalamus by interleukin-1 in the rat. *Neurosci. Letts.*, **132**, 151–4.

Justice, A. (1985) Review of the effects of stress on cancer in laboratory animals: importance of time of stress application and type of tumour. *Psychol. Bull.*, **1**, 108–38.

Karanth, S., Lyson, K. & McCann, S.M. (1993) Role of nitric oxide in interleukin 2-induced corticotropin-releasing factor release from incubated hypothalamus. *Proc. Nat. Acad. Sci. USA*, **90**, 3383–7.

Karp, J.D., Cohen, N. & Moynihan, J.A. (1994) Quantitative differences in interleukin-2 and interleukin-4 production by antigen-stimulated splenocytes from individually- and group-housed mice. *Life Sci.*, **55** (10), 789–95.

Katsuura, G., Arimura, A., Koves, K. & Gottschall, P.E. (1990) Involvement of organum vasculosum of lamina terminalis and preoptic area in interleukin 1β-induced ACTH release. *Am. J. Physiol.*, **258**, E163–71.

Kavelaars, A., Ballieux, R.E. & Heijnen, C.J. (1989) The role of IL-1 in the corticotropin-releasing factor and arginine-vasopressin-induced secretion of immunoreactive beta-endorphin by human peripheral blood mononuclear cells. *J. Immunol.*, **142**, 2338–42.

Kavelaars, A., Beetsma, A., Von Frijtag Drabbe Kunzel, J. & Heijnen, C.J. (1992) β-Endorphin 1–17 modulates high affinity IL2 receptor expression on human T cells. *Ann. NY Acad. Sci.* **650**, 234–8.

Khansari, D.N., Murgo, A.J. & Faith, R.E. (1990) Effects of stress on the immune system. *Immunol. Today*, **11**, 17–175.

Klinnert, M., Miller, B., LaBrecque, J., Strunck, R. & Mrazek, D. (1985) *Psychological and social problems in severely asthmatic children.* Paper presented at the 32nd Annual Meeting of the American Academy of Child Psychiatry, Vol. 1, pp. 37–8.

Klosterhalfen, S. & Klosterhalfen, W. (1990) Conditioned cyclosporine effects but not conditioned taste aversion in immunised rats. *Behav. Neurosci.*, **104**, 716–24.

Koenig, J.I., Snow, K., Clark, B.D. *et al.* (1990) Intrinsic pituitary interleukin-1 beta is induced by bacterial lipopolysaccharide. *Endocrinology*, **126**, 3053–8. [Erratum, *Endocrinology* (1990), **127**, 657.]

Kohrogi, H., Nadel, J.A., Malfroy, B. *et al.* (1989) Recombinant human enkephalinase (neutral endopeptidase) prevents cough induced by tachykinins in awake guinea pigs. *J. Clin. Invest.*, **84**, 781–6.

Kronful, A. & House, J.D. (1984) Depression, cortisol and immune function. *Lancet*, **i**, 1026–7.

Kusnecov, A.V., Grota, L.J., Schmidt, S.G. *et al.* (1992) Decreased herpes simplex viral immunity and enhanced pathogenesis following stressor administration in mice. *J. Neuroimmunol.*, **38**, 129–38.

Lei, Y.-H., Barnes, P.J. & Rogers, D.F. (1992) Inhibition of neurogenic plasma exudation in guinea pig airways by CP-96,345, a new non-peptide NK_1 receptor antagonist. *Brit. J. Pharmacol.*, **105**, 261–2.

Levine, S., Sowinski, R. & Steinetz, B. (1980) Effects of experimental allergic encephalomyelitis on thymus and adrenal: relation to remission and relapse. *Proc. Soc. Exp. Biol. Med.*, **165**, 218–24.

Long, J.B. & Holaday, J.W. (1985) Blood brain barrier: endogenous modulation by adrenal-cortical function. *Science*, **227**, 580.

Lou, Y.P., Lee, L.Y., Satoh, H. & Lundberg, J.M. (1993) Postjunctional inhibitory effect of the NK2 receptor antagonist SR 48968, on sensory NANC bronchoconstriction in the guinea pig airway. *Brit. J. Pharmacol.*, **109** (3), 765–73.

Lyketsos, C.G., Lyketsos, G.C., Richardson, S.C. & Beis, A. (1987) Dysthymic states and depression syndrome in physical conditions of presumably psychological origin. *Acta Psychiatr. Scand.*, **76**, 529–34.

Lyketsos, G.C., Karabetsos, A., Jordanoglou, J., Liokis, T., Armagianidis, A. & Lyketsos, C.G. (1984) Personality characteristics and dysthymic states in bronchial asthma. *Psychother. Psychosom.*, **41**, 177–85.

Lyson, K. & McCann, S.M. (1992) Involvement of arachidonic acid cascade pathways in interleukin-6-stimulated corticotropin-releasing factor release *in vitro*. *Neuroendocrinology.*, **55**, 708–13.

McKay, D.M. & Bienenstock, J. (1994) The interaction between mast cells and nerves in the gastrointestinal tract. *Immunol. Today*, **15** (11), 533–8.

MacQueen, G., Marshall, J., Perdue, M., Siegel, S. & Bienenstock, J. (1989) Pavlovian conditioning of rat mucosal mast cells to secrete rat mast cell protease II. *Science*, **243**, 83–5.

Madden, K.S., Felten, S.Y., Felten, D.L., Hardy, C.A. & Livnat, S. (1994) Sympathetic nervous system modulation of the immune system. II. Induction of lymphocyte proliferation and migration *in vivo* by chemical sympathectomy. *J. Neuroimmunol.*, **49** (1–2), 67–75.

Malaise, M.G., Hazee-Hagelstein, M.T., Reuter, A.M. *et al.* (1987) Thymopoietin and thymopentin enhance the levels of ACTH, beta-endorphin and beta-lipotropin from rat pituitary cells *in vitro*. *Acta Endocrinol.*, **115**, 455–9.

Manuck, S.B., Cohen, S., Rabin, B.S., Muldoon, M.F. & Bachen, E.A. (1991) Individual differences in cellular immune responses to stress. *Psychol. Sci.*, **2**, 111–15.

Mason, J.W., Maher, J.T., Hartley, L.H., Mougey, E.H., Perlow, M.J. & Jones, L.G. (1976) In: *Psychopathology of Human Adaption* (ed. G. Serban), pp. 147–71. Plenum, New York.

Mathison, R., Carter, L., Mowat, C., Bissonnette, E., Davison, J.S. & Befus, A.D. (1994a) Temporal analysis of the anti-inflammatory effects of decentralisation of the rat superior cervical ganglia. *Am. J. Physiol.*, **266**, R1537–43.

Mathison, R., Davison, J.S., Befus, A.D. (1994b) Neuroendocrine regulation of inflammation and tissue repair by submandibular gland factors. *Immunol. Today*, **15** (11), 527–32.

Matsuse, T., Thomson, R.J., Chen, X.R., Salari, H. & Schellenberg, R.R. (1991) Capsaicin inhibits airway hyperresponsiveness, but not airway lipoxygenase activity nor eosinophilia following repeated aerosolized antigen in guinea pigs. *Am. Rev. Resp. Dis.*, **144**, 368–72.

Meares, R., Mills, J. & Horvath, T. (1971) Amitryptaline and asthma. *Med. J. Aust.*, **2**, 25–8.

Michel, F.B. (1994) Psychology of the allergic patient. *Allergy*, **49** (18 Suppl.), 28–30.

Miller, B.D. (1987) Depression and asthma: a potentially lethal mixture. *J. Allergy Clin. Immunol.*, **80** (3), 481–6.

Moore, T., Spruck, C. & Said, S. (1988) Depression of lymphocyte traffic in sheep by vasoactive intestinal peptide (VIP). *Immunology*, **64**, 475–8.

Moreno, J., Vincente, A., Heijnen, I. & Zapata, A.G. (1994) Prolactin and early T-cell development in embryonic chicken. *Immunol. Today*, **15** (11), 524–6.

Mousli, M., Bueb, J.L., Bronner, C., Rouot, B. & Landry, Y. (1990) G protein activation: a receptor-independent mode of action for cationic amphiphilic neuropeptides and venom peptides. *Trends Pharmacol. Sci.*, **11**, 358–62.

Moynihan, J., Koota, D., Brenner, G., Cohen, N. & Ader, R. (1989) Repeated intraperitoneal injections of saline attenuate the antibody response to a subsequent intraperitoneal injection of antigen. *Brain Behav. Immunity*, **3**, 90–6.

Moynihan, J.A., Ader, R., Grota, L.J., Schachtman, T.R. & Cohen, N. (1990) The effects of stress on the development of immunological memory following low dose antigen priming in mice. *Brain Behav. Immunity*, **4**, 1–12.

Moynihan, J.A., Karp, J.D., Cohen, N. & Cocke, R. (1994) Alterations in IL-4 and antibody production following pheromone exposure: role for glucocorticoids. *J. Neuroimmunol.*, **54**, 51–8.

Munck, A., Guyre, P.M. & Holbrook, N.J. (1984) Physiological functions of glucocorticoids in stress and their relation to pharmacological actions. *Endocr. Rev.*, **5**, 25–44.

Norrish, M., Tooley, M. & Godfrey, S. (1977) Clinical and psychological study of asthmatic children attending a hospital clinic. *Arch. Dis. Child.*, **52**, 912–17.

O'Flynn, K., O'Keane, V., Lucey, J.V. & Dinan, T.G. (1991) Effect of fluoxetine on noradrenergic mediated growth hormone release: a double blind, placebo controlled study. *Biol. Psych.*, **30** (4), 377–82.

Olsen, N.J., Nicholson, W.E., DeBold, C.R. & Orth, D.N. (1992) Lymphocyte-derived adrenocorticotrophin is insufficient to stimulate adrenal steroidogenesis in hypophysectomised rats. *Endocrinology*, **130**, 2113–19.

Ori, Z., Monir, G., Weiss, J., Sayhouni, X. & Singer, D.H. (1992) Heart rate variability: frequency domain analysis. *Cardiol. Clin.*, **10** (3), 499–537.

Ottaway, C.A. (1984) *In vitro* activation of receptors for VIP changes the *in vivo* localisation of mouse T cells. *J. Exp. Med.*, **160**, 510–12.

Ottaway, C.A. & Husband, A.J. (1994) The influence of neuroendocrine pathways on lymphocyte migration. *Immunol. Today*, **15** (11), 511–17.

Payan, D.G., McGillis, J.P. & Goetzl, E.J. (1986) Neuroimmunology. In: *Advances in Immunology* (eds F.J. Dixon, K.F. Austen, L. Hood & J.W. Uhr), pp. 299–32. Academic Press, New York.

Payne, L.C., Weigent, D.A. & Blalock, J.E. (1994) Induction of pituitary sensitivity to interleukin-1: a new function for corticotropin-releasing hormone. *Biochem. Biophys. Res. Commun.*, **198**, 480–4.

Pinkerton, P. (1972) Depression v. denial in childhood asthma: equivalent fatal hazards. In: *Depressive States in Childhood and Adolescence*, pp. 187–92. Almquist & Wiskell, Stockholm.

Przewlocki, R., Hassan, A.H.S., Lason, W., Epplen, C., Herz, A. & Stein, C. (1992) Gene expression and localisation of opiod peptides in immune cells of inflamed tissue: functional role in antinociception. *Neuroscience*, **48**, 491–500.

Ramaswamy, K., Mathison, R., Carter, L. *et al.* (1990) Marked antiinflammatory effects of decentralisation of the superior cervical ganglia. *J. Exp. Med.*, **172**, 1819–30.

Reichlin, S. (1993) Neuroendocrine–immune interactions. *New Engl. J. Med.*, **329**, 1246–53.

Rettori, V., Jurcovicova, J. & McCann, S.M. (1987) Central action of interleukin 1 in altering the release of TSH, GH, and prolactin in the male rat. *J. Neurosci. Res.*, **18**, 179–83.

Romero, L.I., Lechan, R.M., Clark, B.D., Dinarello, C.A. & Reichlin, S. (1991) IL-1 receptor antagonist inhibits h IL-1 beta but not bacterial lipopolysaccharide (LPS) stimulated IL-6 secretion by rat anterior pituitary cells. In: *Program and Abstracts of 73rd Annual Meeting of the Endocrine Society*, Washington DC, 19–22 June 1991, abstract 150. Endocrine Society, Bethesda, Maryland.

Rook, G.A.W., Hernandez-Pando, R. & Lightman, S.L. (1994) Hormones, peripherally activated prohormones and regulation of the Th1/Th2 balance. *Immunol. Today*, **15** (7), 301–3.

Roy, A., Linnoila, M., Karoum, F. & Pickar, D. (1988) Urinary free cortisol in depressed patients and controls: relationship to urinary indices of noradrenergic function. *Psychol. Med.*, **18**, 93–8.

Rozman, T.L. & Brooks, W.H. (1985) Neural modulation of immune function. *J. Neuroimmunol.*, **10**, 59–69.

Rozman, T.L., Cross, R.J., Brooks, W.H. & Markesbury, W.R. (1985) Neuroimmunomodulation: effects of neural lesions on cellular immunity. In: *Neural Modulation of Immunity* (eds R. Guillemin & T. Melnechuk), p. 95. Raven Press, New York.

Rubin, N.J. (1993) Severe asthma and depression. *Arch. Fam. Med.*, **2** (4), 433–40.

Sachar, E.J. (1975) Hormonal changes in stress and mental illness. *Hosp. Pract.*, **10**, 49–55.

Sachar, E.J. (1982) Endocrine abnormalities in depression. In: *Handbook of Affective Disorders* (ed. E.S. Paykel), pp. 191–201. Guildford, New York.

Santiago, S. & Klaustermeyer, W. (1980) Mortality in status asthmaticus: a nine year experience in a respiratory intensive care unit. *J. Asthma Res.*, **17**, 75–9.

Shanahan, F., Denburg, J., Fox, J., Bienenstock, J. & Befus, A.D. (1985) Mast cell heterogeneity: effects of neuroenteric peptides on histamine release. *J. Immunol.*, **135**, 1331–7.

Sheridan, J.F., Feng, N., Bonneau, R.H., Allen, C.M., Huneycutt, B.S. & Glaser, R. (1991) Restraint stress differentially affects anti-viral cellular and humoral immune responses in mice. *J. Neuroimmunol.*, **31**, 245–55.

Smith, C.H., Barker, J.N.W.N., Morris, R.W., MacDonald, D.M. & Lee, T.H. (1993) Neuropeptides induce rapid expression of endothelial cell adhesion molecules and elicit granulocytic infiltration in human skin. *J. Immunol.*, **151**, 3274–82.

Solomon, G.F., Amkraut, A.A. & Kasper, P. (1974) Immunity, emotions, and stress: with special reference to the mechanism of stress effects on the immune system. *Ann. Clin. Res.*, **6**, 313–22.

Solvason, H.B., Ghanta, V.K. & Hiramoto, R.N. (1988) Conditioned augmentation of natural killer cell activity: independence from nociceptive effects and dependence on interferon-β. *J. Immunol.*, **140**, 661–5.

Sorkness, R., Clough, J.J., Castleman, W.L. & Lemanske, R.F. Jr (1994) Virus induced airway obstruction and parasympathetic hyperresponsiveness in adult rats. *Am. J. Resp. Crit. Care Med.*, **150** (1), 28–34.

Stead, R.H., Tomioka, M., Quinonez, G. *et al.* (1987) Intestinal mucosal mast cells in normal and nematode-infected rat intestines are in intimate contact with peptidergic nerves. *Proc. Nat. Acad. Sci. USA*, **84**, 2975–9.

Stead, R.H., Tomioka, M., Pezzati, P. *et al.* (1991) Interaction of mucosal and peripheral nervous system. In: *Psychoneuroimmunology* (ed. R. Ader), pp. 177–207. Academic Press, San Diego, CA.

Stein, M., Miller, A.H. & Trestman, R.L. (1991) Depression and the immune system. In: *Psychoneuroimmunology* (eds R. Ader, D.L. Felten & N. Cohen), 2nd edn, pp. 897–931. Academic Press, San Diego, CA.

Strunk, R.C., Mrazek, D.A., Fuhrmann, G.S. & LaBrecque, J.F. (1985) Physiologic and psychological characteristics associated with deaths due to asthma in childhood: a case-controlled study. *JAMA*, **254** (9), 1193–8.

Sugihara, H., Ishihara, K. & Noguchi, H. (1965) Clinical experience with amitryptaline (tryptanol) in the treatment of bronchial asthma. *Ann. Allergy*, **23**, 422–9.

Terao, A., Oikawa, M. & Saito, M. (1993) Cytokine induced changes in hypothalamic norepinephrine turnover: involvement of corticotrophin-releasing hormone and prostaglandins. *Brain Res.*, **622**, 257–61.

Thompson, W.L. & Thompson, T.L. (1985) Psychiatric aspects of asthma in adults. *Adv. Psychosom. Med.*, **14**, 33–47.

Tizabi, Y. & Calogero, A.E. Effect of various neurotransmitters and neuropeptides on the release of corticotropin-releasing hormone from the rat cortex *in vitro*. *Synapse*, **10**, 341–8.

Vale, W., Rivier, C., Brown, M.R. *et al.* (1983) Chemical and biological characterization of corticotropin releasing factor. *Recent Prog. Horm. Res.*, **39**, 245–70.

Vankelecom, H., Carmeliet, P., Van Damme, J., Billiau, A. & Denef, C. (1989) Production of interleukin-6 by folliculo-stellate cells of the anterior pituitary gland in a histiotypic cell aggregate culture system. *Neuroendocrinology*, **49**, 102–6.

Van Ranst, L. & Lauweryns, J.M. (1990) Effects of long-term sensory vs. sympathetic denervation of the distribution of calcitonin gene-related peptide and tyrosine hydroxylase immunoreactivity in the rat lung. *J. Neuroimmunol.*, **29**, 131–8.

Verleden, G.M., Belvisi, M.G., Rabe, K.F., Miura, M. & Barnes, P.J. (1993) Beta 2-adrenoreceptor agonists inhibit NANC neural bronchoconstrictor responses *in vitro*. *J. Appl. Physiol.*, **74** (3), 1195–9.

Vitkovic, L. & Koslow, S.H. (eds) (1994) *Neuroimmunology and Mental Health: a Report on Neuroimmunology Research*. National Institute of Mental Health Publication No. (NIH) 94-3774, Washington.

Watanabe, T., Morimoto, A., Sakata, Y. & Murakami, N. (1990) ACTH response induced by interleukin-1 is mediated by CRF secretion stimulated by hypothalamic PGE. *Experientia*, **46**, 481–4.

Watkins, A.D. (1994) The role of alternative therapy in allergic disease. *Clin. Exp. Allergy.*, **24**, 813–25.

Watkins, A.D. (1995) Perceptions, emotions and immunity: an integrated homoeostatic network. *Q. J. Med.*, **88**, 283–94.

Watkins, L.R., Wiertelak, E.P., Goehler, L.E. *et al.* (1994) Neurocircuitry of illness-induced hyperalgesia. *Brain Res.*, **639**, 283–99.

Weigent, D., Blalock, J.E. & LeBoeuf, R.D. (1991) An antisense oligodeoxynucleotide to growth hormone messenger ribonucleic acid inhibits lymphocyte proliferation. *Endocrinology*, **128**, 2053–7.

Whitnall, M.H., Perlstein, R.S., Mougey, E.H. & Neta, R. (1992) Effects of interleukin-1 on the stress-responsive and -nonresponsive subtypes of corticotropin-releasing hormone neurosecretory axons. *Endocrinology*, **131**, 37–44.

Williams, J.W., Peterson, R.G., Shea, P.A., Schmedtje, J.F., Bauer, D.C. & Felten, D.L. (1980) Sympathetic innervation of mouse thymus and spleen: evidence for a functional link between nervous and immune systems. *Brain Res. Bull.*, **6**, 83–94.

Willis, T. (1679) *Pharmaceutice Rationalis*, Vol. 2. Dring, Harper, Leigh, London.

Wistuba, F. (1986) Significance of allergy in asthma from a behavioral medicine viewpoint. *Psychother. Psychosom.*, **45** (4), 186–94.

Wood, J.C. (1992) *Ann. NY Acad. Sci.*, **664**, 275–84.

Yellowless, P.M., Haynes, S., Potts, N. & Ruffin, R.E. (1988) Psychiatric morbidity in patients with life-threatening asthma: initial report of a controlled study. *Med. J. Aust.*, **149**, 246–9.

CHAPTER 29

Endothelin and Nitric Oxide

D.R. Springall & J.M. Polak

Introduction

Endothelin (ET) and nitric oxide (NO) are two powerful biological mediators originally discovered through their respective vasoactive roles as endothelium-derived constricting and relaxing factors. Following the discovery of these mediators, it became apparent that both have many actions beyond their vasoactivity and a distribution that is not just endothelial but bordering on ubiquitous. They are of interlinked interest as their actions are almost diametrically opposed, and yet they share similar methods of regulation and are both involved in the control of a wide variety of normal and pathological processes in many higher and lower species. Thus, they are both old in phylogenetic terms, NO being a very primitive molecule and found in species such as the horseshoe crab (*Limulus polyphenus*), and ET being closely related to the sarafatoxins that are found in the venom of primitive snakes such as the burrowing asp.

The molecules and their synthesis

The two molecules have different modes of formation: ET by gene expression and post-translational processing, NO by enzymatic synthesis from the amino acid L-arginine.

ET was the first of the two to be identified and cloned, by Yanagisawa *et al.* in 1988, following the work of Rubanyi and Vanhoutte (1985) showing vasoconstriction by a factor produced in the endothelium. It was shown to be a peptide of 21 amino acids, produced, like many peptides, from a large precursor molecule but via an intermediate form of 39 residues, called 'big ET', by several metalloproteases (Yanagisawa *et al.*, 1988) to yield the mature peptide ET1–21 (Fig. 29.1). It was subsequently found that endothelin is in fact a family of three main peptides, ET-1, ET-2 and ET-3, although a fourth, called vasoactive intestinal contractor (VIC), was isolated from gut (Inoue *et al.*, 1989). These isoforms have variations in structure (Fig. 29.2), receptor binding and actions.

Although there was awareness of NO as a possible biological mediator at around the time of the discovery of ET, and it was known that vascular endothelial cells were able to synthesize NO, an inorganic free-radical gas, from the amino acid L-arginine (Palmer *et al.*, 1988), the first isolation of the enzyme (NO synthetase) was reported in 1990 (Bredt & Snyder, 1990). NO is secreted by a variety of different cell types in many vertebrate and invertebrate animal species, and effects a multitude of physiological

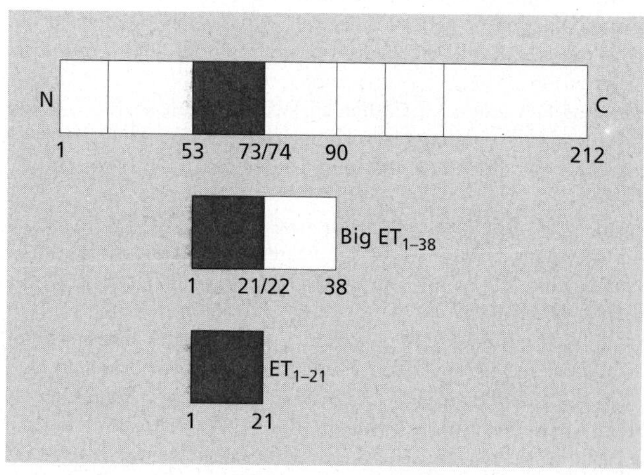

Fig. 29.1 Diagram of the formation of ET from pro-ET.

ET-1	CYS-SER-CYS-SER-SER-LEU-MET-ASP-LYS-GLU-CYS-VAL-TYR-PHE-CYS-HIS-LEU-ASP-ILE-ILE-TRP
ET-2	CYS-SER-CYS - SER - SER- TRP-LEU-ASP-LYS-GLU-CYS-VAL-TYR-PHE-CYS-HIS-LEU-ASP-ILE-ILE-TRP
ET-3	CYS-THR-CYS-PHE-THR-TYR-LYS-ASP-LYS-GLU-CYS-VAL-TYR-TYR-CYS-HIS-LEU-ASP-ILE-ILE-TRP

Fig. 29.2 Amino acid sequence of the three major forms of ET. Differences of the sequences from that of ET-1 are highlighted.

processes (Moncada *et al.*, 1991). The small size and lipophilic nature of this molecule enable it to traverse cell membranes freely and therefore ideally suit it to a role in cell–cell communication.

NO is produced by the oxidation of one or more guanidino nitrogen atoms of the substrate L-arginine in a reaction which utilizes molecular oxygen and also yields L-citrulline (Moncada *et al.*, 1991) (Fig. 29.3). This reaction is enantiomerically specific, since D-arginine is not a substrate, and it can also be inhibited, with varying degrees of affinity, by arginine analogues such as NG-monomethyl-L-arginine (L-NMMA), NG-nitro-L-arginine (L-NNA) and NG-amino-L-arginine (Moncada *et al.*, 1991).

To date, three distinct isoforms of NO synthetase have been described. Sequence analysis of molecular clones, their biochemistry and their pharmacology show that NO synthetases form a closely related family of proteins, although they are the product of separate genes (Fig. 29.4) (Nathan & Xie, 1994). They are homodimeric haemoproteins dependent on several cofactors for full activity, including reduced nicotinamide adenine dinucleotide phosphate (NADPH), flavin adenine dinucleotide (FAD), flavin mononucleotide (FMN), 6(R)-5,6,7,8-tetrahydrobiopterin (BH_4) and the Ca^{2+} binding protein, calmodulin (Fig. 29.5) (Forstermann *et al.*, 1993; Nathan & Xie, 1994). All three isoforms contain phosphorylation sites, which are known to be important determinants of their activity (Nathan & Xie, 1994).

Two of the isoforms are constitutive, wholly dependent on elevation of intracellular Ca^{2+} levels for activity, and

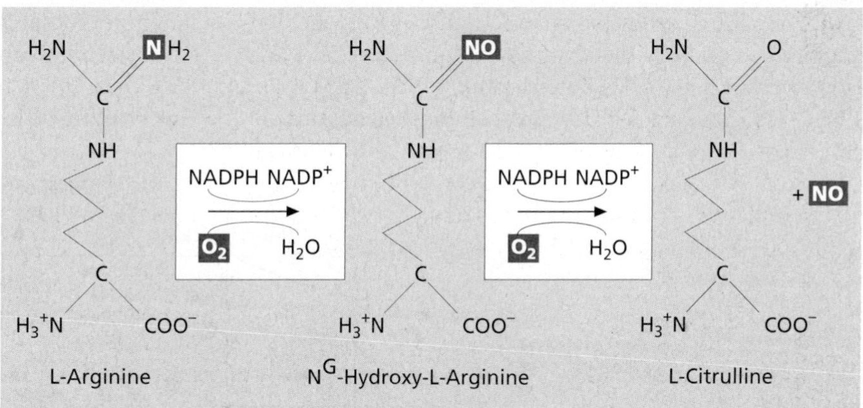

Fig. 29.3 Diagram showing the formation of NO from L-arginine with the consumption of oxygen and NADPH.

Isoform	Species	mRNA (kb)	Mr (subunit kDa)	Amino acid identity (%) sp	Amino acid identity (%) isoforms		Quaternary (active) structure (kDa)	Subcellular localization	Activity [^{3}H]arg-[^{3}H]cit (μmol/mg/min^{-1})
nNOS	Rat	10.5	160.5	93			Dimer (≈280)	Cytosolic	≈1
	Human	10	161		57				
eNOS	Bovine	4.8	133	94		94	Unknown	Particulate	≈1
	Human	4.7	133		51				
iNOS	Mouse/rat	4.0–4.4	130.6	81			Dimer (≈250)	Cytosolic	≈1.6
	Human	4.4	131.2						

Fig. 29.4 Diagram showing the sequence identity between the three isoforms of NOs, their structure and activity.

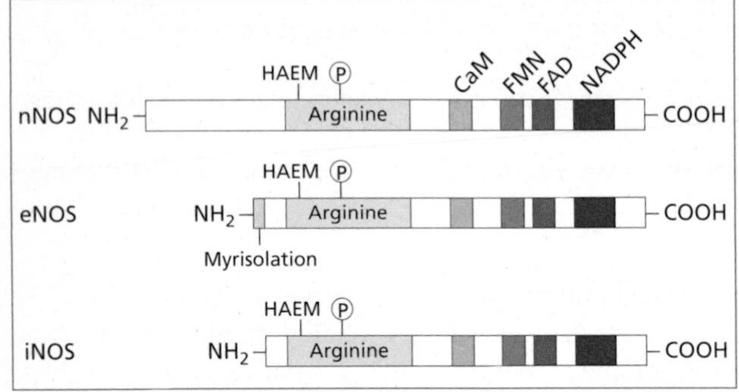

Fig. 29.5 The structure of NOs showing the position of binding sites for cofactors.

they generate low levels of NO over several minutes following activation. The first constitutive isoform to be characterized was isolated from rat brain (Bredt & Snyder, 1990) and on denaturing sodium dodecyl sulphate (SDS)-polyacrylamide gels has an observed monomeric M_r of 155 kDa. This so-called neural NO synthetase (nNOS) has now been described in a diffuse population of neurones within the central nervous system and in the non-adrenergic non-cholinergic (NANC) nerves of the peripheral nervous system, specifically supplying muscle layers of the gastrointestinal tract, airways, urogenital tract and some large blood vessels (Moncada *et al.*, 1991; Forstermann *et al.*, 1994; Buttery *et al.*, 1995a; Ward *et al.*, 1995). This isoform is also present in skeletal muscle (Forstermann *et al.*, 1994), in macula densa (Wilcox *et al.*, 1992) and in epithelial cells of lung and kidney (Asano *et al.*, 1994; Forstermann *et al.*, 1994).

The second constitutive isoform was originally isolated from bovine aortic endothelial cells (Pollock *et al.*, 1991) and subsequently from human endothelial cells (Lamas *et al.*, 1992), and has an M_r of 135 kDa on Western blots. The endothelial NO synthetase (eNOS) is unique among the NO synthetases in containing an N-terminal consensus myristolation site (Busconi & Michel, 1992), which anchors the enzyme to cellular membranes and explains why almost all eNOS activity is detected in the particulate fraction of tissue homogenates. eNOS is primarily localized to the endothelia of macro- and microvascular beds of both arterial and venous circulations (Pollock *et al.*, 1993), although more recently eNOS has also been localized to other cell types such as the syncytiotrophoblast of placenta (Buttery *et al.*, 1994a) and certain epithelial cells (Forstermann *et al.*, 1994; Shaul *et al.*, 1994).

The third isoform is not normally present but can be induced in many different types of cell in response to infection, inflammation or tissue injury and, once activated, generates large amounts of NO over many hours (Fig. 29.6) (Moncada *et al.*, 1991). This has prompted the suggestion that the inducible enzyme represents a primitive and relatively rapid immune effector system (Nussler & Billiar, 1993). Several inflammatory cytokines, notably interleukin-1 (IL-1), tumour necrosis factor-α (TNF-α) and

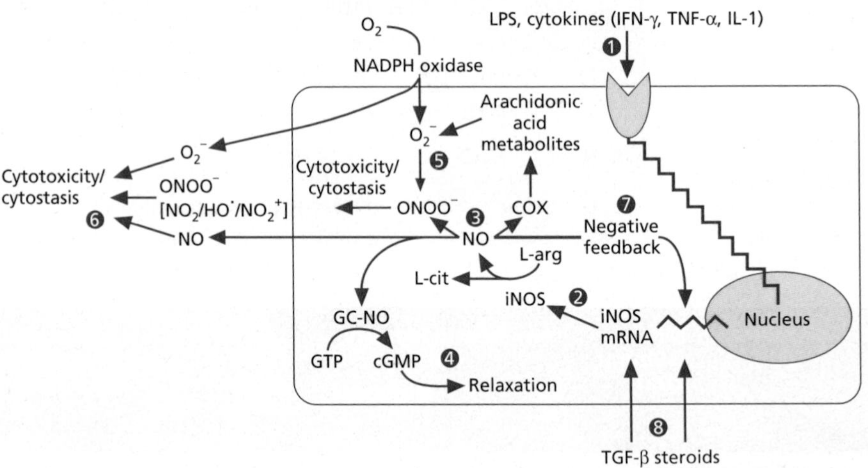

Fig. 29.6 Stimulated synthesis and actions of iNOS. (1) Bacterial toxins and pro-inflammatory cytokines activate the transcription of a number of inducible genes including iNOS. The activity of iNOS is largely independent of the ambient Ca^{2+} concentration and generates large amounts of NO over prolonged periods. High-output synthesis can augment activity of other inflammatory response proteins such as COX-2. (4) Smooth-muscle cells exposed to high concentrations of NO lead to prolonged NO-stimulated relaxation, which may contribute to the hypotension seen in conditions like sepsis. (5) Inflammation may also stimulate the activity of NADPH oxidase, which increases the generation of reactive oxygen intermediates, in particular superoxide anion, promoting the formation of peroxynitrite. (6) High levels of NO, NO-derived oxidants like peroxynitrite and its decomposition products are cytotoxic/cytostatic and indiscriminately contribute to the killing of pathogens and host tissue damage. (7) & (8) Because the activity of iNOS is potentially detrimental to the host's well-being, iNOS activity can be regulated by endogenous factors, including NO itself, which may bind to and directly inhibit the activity of the enzyme or may inactivate other factors involved in transcription. In addition, the cytokine TGF-β reduces iNOS expression by decreasing the half-life of iNOS mRNA, whereas steroids prevent transcriptional activation of the enzyme. See text for definition of abbreviations.

interferon-γ (IFN-γ), as well as bacterial lipopolysaccharide (LPS) are capable of stimulating the transcriptional induction of inducible NO synthetase (iNOS) (Geller *et al.*, 1993a; Nussler & Billiar, 1993). While each of these factors can, on its own, stimulate the production of iNOS, specific combinations synergize to augment the level of enzyme expression and activity (Geller *et al.*, 1993a; Nussler & Billiar, 1993). Originally isolated from cytokine-activated murine macrophages (Xie *et al.*, 1992), iNOS has an M_r of 130 kDa. It differs from the constitutive enzymes in being largely independent of Ca^{2+} for activity, but still requires calmodulin, which remains tightly bound to the enzyme. Once stimulated, the activity of iNOS appears to be limited only by substrate and cofactor availability, at least in cell culture systems, although it is known that tumour growth factor-β (TGF-β) can down-regulate iNOS expression (Nathan & Xie, 1994). In addition, high levels of corticosteroids can prevent *de novo* protein synthesis and are therefore able to limit or even prevent the induction of iNOS (Moncada *et al.*, 1991).

iNOS has now been isolated and characterized from rodent macrophages (Xie *et al.*, 1992), smooth muscle (Nunkawa *et al.*, 1993) and liver (Wood *et al.*, 1993) and from human hepatocytes (Geller *et al.*, 1993b) and chondrocytes (Charles *et al.*, 1993). Unlike the constitutive enzymes, which both demonstrate high conservation between species (around 95%), a comparison of rodent and human iNOS revealed a slightly lower degree of conservation, sharing approximately 80% identity. The significance of this difference, if any, is not clear, although it may help explain why expression of human iNOS in some cells, in particular leucocytes (which are a prominent site of expression of iNOS in rodents), has been difficult to demonstrate. Evidence is now emerging that iNOS and iNOS activity are present in human monocytes/macrophages (Anon., 1994) and neutrophils (Goode *et al.*, 1994), but it appears that in some instances, notably in monocytes (Anon., 1994), different types of cytokine stimuli from those described in rodents may be required.

Biological actions

Unlike NO, which freely diffuses between cells, ET signalling is more tightly controlled and the molecule acts via cell-surface receptors. The receptors are broadly of two types, although three were originally postulated (Clozel *et al.*, 1989). The receptors vary in their specificity for the different ETs: one (ETA) binds principally ET-1 with high affinity (Traish *et al.*, 1991), while the other (ETB) binds all three ET types but with a lower affinity (Urade *et al.*, 1992). The ETA receptor has a standard seven transmembrane domain conformation and is coupled to a G protein that activates phospholipase C and protein kinase C (Lee *et al.*, 1989; Reynolds *et al.*, 1989; Hayzer *et al.*, 1992). The resultant protein phosphorylation leads to actions that are dependent on the cell type and include contraction and proliferation. In some cells the ETA receptor causes uptake of Ca^{2+} and activates phospholipase A_2 (Goto *et al.*, 1989; Resink *et al.*, 1989), which can lead to triggering of the arachidonic acid pathway, or activates phospholipase D, thereby activating protein kinase C without increased intracellular Ca^{2+} (Ambar & Sokolovsky, 1993). The ETB receptor uses similar signal transduction sytems but is less specific. These pathways also lead to the activation of transcription factors and their translocation to the nucleus to increase *jun/fos* transcription and activator protein-1 (AP-1), leading to cell proliferation (Pribnow *et al.*, 1992).

Being a short-lived molecule, the principal action of NO is on target effector cells close to its site of synthesis, where it activates the soluble guanylate cyclase by binding to the haem moiety of the enzyme (Knowles *et al.*, 1989; Ignarro, 1991). NO-activated soluble guanylate cyclase stimulates intracellular elevation of cyclic guanosine monophosphate (cGMP), which initiates specific cellular functions such as relaxation of vascular smooth muscle, inhibition of platelet adhesion and aggregation and regulation of neurotransmitter release from neighbouring neurones. However, in the absence of any recognized transporter for delivery of NO to specific targets, like the soluble guanylate cyclase, NO is also capable of effecting other cellular mechanisms that are independent of the soluble guanylate cyclase–cGMP second-messenger system.

NO is a cellular cytotoxic and cytostatic agent (Hibbs *et al.*, 1988), particularly when produced in large quantities, as by iNOS, and serves as part of the body's immune defence system, contributing to the killing of bacteria and other pathogens (Hibbs *et al.*, 1988; Nathan & Hibbs, 1991) and also tumour cells (Farias-Eisner *et al.*, 1994). Cytostasis or cytotoxicity effected by NO relies on the high affinity of NO for iron or iron–sulphur-containing proteins, binding specifically to iron in both haem and non-haem proteins, and has thus been shown to inhibit enzymes involved in mitochondrial respiration and DNA synthesis (Stuehr & Nathan, 1989). NO synthetases themselves contain a haem prosthetic group and it has been shown that NO can thereby bind to either the enzyme which synthesized it or to other NO synthetase isoforms, inactivating the enzyme, and thus NO may actually modulate its own synthesis.

Alternatively, NO can exert its damaging effects indirectly, through formation or activation of other cell-damaging molecules or pathways. In many instances the damaging side of NO production is modulated by alterations in the environment into which NO is generated, particularly if reactive oxygen intermediates, such as superoxide, are present. NO and superoxide anion demonstrate an affinity for each other, reacting to form peroxynitrite anion (Beckman *et al.*, 1990; Freeman, 1994;

White *et al.*, 1994). This reaction also results in the abrogation of NO activity, since peroxynitrite is far less efficient than NO as a signalling agent, but, perhaps more significantly, peroxynitrite, itself a powerful oxidant, can contribute directly to cytotoxicity/cytostasis. NO or NO species damage DNA by base deamination and as a direct result activate the enzyme poly (adenosine diphosphate (ADP)-ribose) synthetase (PARS) (Zhang *et al.*, 1994). PARS is a nuclear enzyme that is thought to facilitate DNA repair, utilizing nicotinamide adenine dinucleotide (NAD) and adenosine triphosphate (ATP) in the process. However, prolonged activation of PARS and in particular the continued consumption of NAD and ATP can lead to rapid energy depletion, ultimately resulting in cell death.

Detection of ET and NO

ET is relatively easily detected by means of standard immunoassay techniques, such as radioimmunoassay or enzyme-linked immunosorbent assay (ELISA), in tissue homogenates and biological fluids. If linked with chromatography, it is also possible thus to distinguish big ET and degradation products from the mature peptide. However, the estimation of NO is more difficult and several methods are available (Archer, 1993). Assays for NO activity are often performed on tissue homogenates or supernatants and require meticulous monitoring of the assay conditions, in particular controlling substrate and cofactor availability, which can have substantial influence on the accuracy of the assay. Addition or depletion of Ca^{2+}, arginine analogues and also inhibitors of protein synthesis can be used to discriminate between constitutive and inducible NO synthetase activity.

Direct detection of NO itself is difficult and relies on more indirect methods to detect its oxidation products or its interaction with other molecules, and there are several different types of assay currently available. NO reacts with the haem group of reduced haemoglobin to form methaemoglobin and nitrate, and this is readily detectable by dual wavelength spectroscopy. The high affinity of NO for reduced haemoglobin or nitroso compounds forms the basis of the NO 'trapping' technique, by which the relatively unstable NO free radical reacts to form more stable compounds, the resultant reorientation of the electron spin of the radical then being detectable by electron paramagnetic resonance spectroscopy. The most commonly used and easily accessible technique is measurement of the accumulation of nitrite and nitrate, the stable oxidation products of NO, using the Greiss reaction, which relies on the reduction of nitrate to nitrite after the addition of the enzyme nitrite reductase or a metallic catalyst to the sample, the resultant colour change then being detectable spectroscopically. Chemiluminescence is the only method that detects authentic NO; it relies on the detection of light generated in reaction between NO and ozone, the amount of light being directly proportional to NO levels. Stimulation of soluble guanylate cyclase and the detection of accumulation of cGMP by radioimmunoassay or ELISA in a reporter cell has also been used as a method of detecting NO activity. An alternative to measuring NO itself is to determine NO synthetase activity, which is usually performed by estimating the formation of radiolabelled citrulline from a known amount of radiolabelled L-arginine, using a simple ion-exchange column for separation of substrate and product. This also provides useful enzyme kinetic data.

While these techniques do provide useful information on the relative levels of ET and the activity of NO synthetase, none necessarily provides an accurate account of which cell type is synthesizing ET or NO, a knowledge of which is vitally important in considering their contribution to normal physiological function and disease.

Localization of ET and NO synthetase

The isolation, purification and molecular cloning of the ET and NO synthetases have permitted the development of highly specific probes. Using immunocytochemical and *in situ* hybridization techniques, these have permitted the detailed investigation of the morphological localization of ET and NO synthetases in numerous tissues and species and also provide a means for quantifying the relative amounts of mRNA encoding them within different cells. More recently, radiolabelled arginine analogues have been used to detect the substrate binding site of NO synthetases (Hevel & Marletta, 1994), providing further information on the quantitative morphological localization and characterization of the enzyme by macro- and micro-autoradiography. The histochemical NADPH-diaphorase technique has also been described as a marker for NO synthetases (Schmidt *et al.*, 1992). However, there are many inconsistencies in the validity of NADPH-diaphorase staining, primarily due to the lack of standardization of incubation conditions and methods of tissue preservation. Many other enzymes also demonstrate NADPH-diaphorase activity, and the technique should not be used as an absolute marker for NO synthetase without confirmation by other morphological techniques such as immunocytochemistry.

Both ET and NO seem to be ubiquitously distributed throughout the mammalian body. They often share a very similar localization in the various organ systems and are increasingly recognized as having an important role in many disease processes, particularly those that involve inflammation. Both are produced by endothelium in most vascular beds (Plate 29.1, opposite page 524) by cells of the monocyte/macrophage lineage and other leucocytes, epithelia, neurones of the central and peripheral nervous system and glial cells. Two particular organs will be considered here: the cardiovascular and respiratory systems.

Cardiovascular system

In the heart, ET is produced principally by vascular endothelial cells and endocardium (Hemsen *et al.*, 1990). ET production is found mainly in large coronary arteries but not in the microvasculature unless stimulated, for example by TGF-β (Nishida *et al.*, 1993). Particular effects of ET in the heart are either direct or indirect, acting through other mediators. Direct actions include alteration of contractility of cardiomyocytes (Suzuki *et al.*, 1991), where ETA and ETB receptors are present (Galron *et al.*, 1990), leading to positive inotropy (Takanashi & Endoh, 1991), and coronary artery tone (Hemsen *et al.*, 1990); indirect effects include the activation of neutrophils and their products (Lopez Farre *et al.*, 1993) and the stimulation of catecholamines and angiotensin II (Simonson & Dunn, 1990). ET may also be an angiogenic factor, either directly or by modulating fibroblast growth factor, vascular endothelial growth factor, TGF-β or IL-8 (Pepper *et al.*, 1992).

The presence of eNOS has been described in the endothelia of a number of different vascular beds (Moncada *et al.*, 1991; Pollock *et al.*, 1993). NO is fundamental to vascular homoeostasis, contributing to the regulation of vascular tone, inhibition of aggregation and adherence of platelets and monocytes, and also modulates growth of vascular smooth muscle (Moncada *et al.*, 1991; Forstermann *et al.*, 1994; Nathan & Xie, 1994). Endothelium-derived NO is released in response to physical stimuli, such as shear stress caused by local variations in blood flow, and also by chemical stimuli, including acetylcholine, ATP, substance P, bradykinin, ET and oestrogen (Moncada *et al.*, 1991; Forstermann *et al.*, 1994; Nathan & Xie, 1994). The importance of NO in the control of vascular homeostasis is emphasized from observations that disruption to the production of NO, resulting in an increase or a decrease in the amount of NO generated, elicits profound effects on vascular pathology.

NO activity is evident in the endocardial cells, which line all chambers of the heart and which are congruous with vascular endothelial cells (Henderson *et al.*, 1992). NO derived from this site is likely to contribute to both the function of the underlying myocardial tissue and modulation of endocardium–blood-cell interactions. In addition, myocytes themselves also demonstrate NO synthetase activity (Balligand *et al.*, 1993), most probably the eNOS, where it contributes to the control of myocardial contractility, having a negative inotropic effect. This effect may be exacerbated as a consequence of induction of iNOS within myocytes (Finkel *et al.*, 1992), following immunological activation of heart tissue, with the resultant increased production of NO contributing directly to the cardiac dysfunction seen in conditions such as endotoxin shock. Indeed, functional studies on isolated myocytes from endotoxin-treated animals have demonstrated that impaired myocyte contractility can be improved through addition of inhibitors of NO synthesis (Brady *et al.*, 1992).

The involvement of NO in human heart pathology is less clear, although it has been shown that iNOS activity is evident in specific heart muscle disorders like dilated cardiomyopathy (DCM) (de Belder *et al.*, 1993) and this is likely to be an important feature of the impaired cardiac performance associated with these conditions. It is not known in which cells iNOS is present, although our own preliminary studies on isolated myocytes stimulated with cytokines confirm that human myocytes do produce iNOS.

Basal and agonist-induced endothelium-dependent release of NO is impaired in isolated human atherosclerotic arteries, and also in vessels from animal models of atherosclerosis (Sayakody *et al.*, 1988; Chester *et al.*, 1990). This loss of vascular NO activity is potentially one of the most significant determinants of both vascular function and the progression of vascular diseases like atherosclerosis. Indeed, based on the vascular activities in the control of blood-vessel tone, platelet– and monocyte–endothelium interactions and regulation of smooth-muscle growth, NO has all the attributes for filling the role as an 'anti-atherogenic' molecule (Moncada *et al.*, 1991; Forstermann *et al.*, 1994; Nathan & Xie, 1994). This is certainly compounded by the observations that administration of nitrates, which have formed the basis of the treatment of angina, are now known to work by releasing NO (Moncada *et al.*, 1991). Further, exogenous infusion of L-arginine into atherosclerotic beds *in vivo* can restore, at least in part, the loss of endothelium-dependent relaxation (Drexler *et al.*, 1991). While prolonged infusion of L-arginine in animal models of atherosclerosis can limit the development of intimal lesions (Hamon *et al.*, 1994). Taken together, such observations suggest that, while the 'machinery' through which NO exerts its actions remains operational, the diseased vessel has an overall reduced capacity to generate NO.

The reduced vascular NO activity observed in atherosclerosis appears to be the result of a combination of a number of factors associated with the development of the lesion. Neo-intimal thickening effectively increases the distance between the site of elaboration of vascular NO and its principal site of action in the smooth muscle. The presence of reactive oxygen intermediates (Beckman *et al.*, 1990; Freeman, 1994; White *et al.*, 1994) and low-density lipoprotein (Tanner *et al.*, 1991) are capable of reacting with NO and effectively reduce its vascular signalling activity. In addition, so-called 'traditional' atherosclerotic risk factors, in particular smoking, can also affect NO production, which is amply demonstrated by monitoring the time-dependent increases in NO vascular activity in patients following cessation of smoking (Higman *et al.*, 1994).

Our own observations in atherosclerotic vessels, using quantitative immunocytochemistry, suggest that there is a significant focal reduction in the relative quantity of eNOS, specifically at atherosclerotic sites, and this may help to account for the overall reduction in the activity of the endothelial L-arginine–NO system reported in such vessels. Detection of reduced amounts of eNOS present in atherosclerotic vessels is corroborated by observations of endothelial cells *in vitro*, in which down-regulation of eNOS expression can be induced by the cytokine TNF-α (Yoshizumi *et al.*, 1993) and, as such, has connotations for a similar mechanism *in vivo*, involving activated macrophages, which are often associated with intimal lesions and which are also a major source of TNF-α.

Activated macrophages are also the primary source of superoxide anion, which is capable of inactivating NO both at the site of the lesion and in smaller vessels distally. Abrogation of vascular NO activity by superoxide anion not only limits the cell signalling activity but, perhaps more significantly, as a result of the formation of peroxynitrite may exacerbate endothelial/intimal damage associated with atherosclerotic lesions (Beckman *et al.*, 1990; Freeman, 1994; White *et al.*, 1994).

Interestingly, while eNOS activity is clearly compromised in atherosclerosis, there is now evidence to suggest that the various inflammatory factors associated with atherosclerotic lesions can also lead to the production of iNOS. Transient induction of iNOS activity has been reported in the vessel wall following balloon angioplasty (Douglas *et al.*, 1994), possibly reflecting a protective mechanism to counter the loss of, or damage to, endothelial-derived NO production. Our own observations have also illustrated the presence of iNOS in both smooth muscle and macrophages, specific to atherosclerotic sites (Buttery *et al.*, 1995b). At present, the time-course of induction of iNOS in atherosclerosis is not known and, more importantly, nor is its function, but it seems likely, based on the broad-ranging vascular activities of NO, that this enzyme will have both beneficial and detrimental actions on vascular tone, growth and damage.

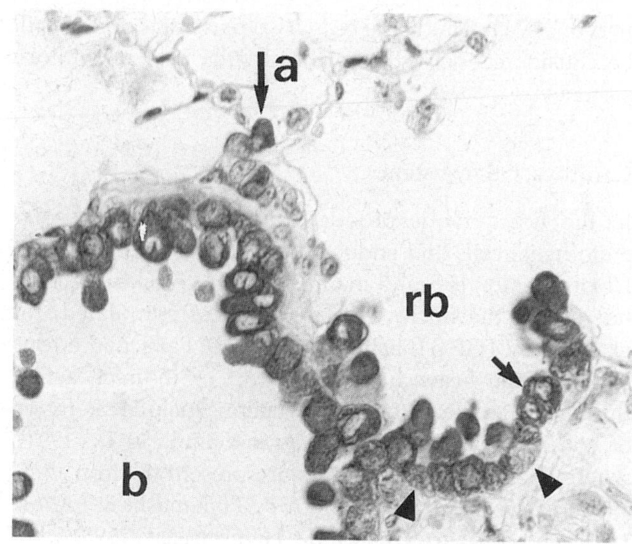

Fig. 29.7 Immunoreactivity for ET in bronchiolar epithelium of rat. b, bronchiole; rb, respiratory bronchiole; a, alveolar pneumocyte.

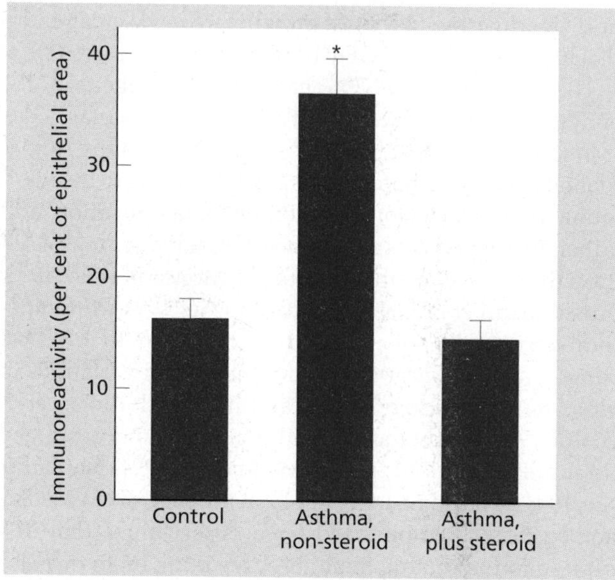

Fig. 29.8 The proportion of airway epithelial area showing staining for ET as in Plate 29.2 (opposite page 524) for a series of asthmatic patients and controls ($n = 10$ each), showing the effects of steroid treatment in reducing ET levels.

Respiratory tract

Both ET and NO are significant factors in lung physiology and pathophysiology. They are involved in broncho- and vasomotor tone, inflammation, cell damage, growth and remodelling.

The lung is one of the major sites of ET synthesis. It is found in the lung vascular endothelium, in airway epithelium and in endocrine cells (Giaid *et al.*, 1991). The demonstration of ET synthesis by airway epithelium was one of the first observations of production in a non-endothelial site (Fig. 29.7), and it was obtained in dog and rodent cells *in vitro* and *in vivo* (Black *et al.*, 1989; Rozengurt *et al.*, 1990). Subsequently, it was found that synthesis was also detectable in human airway epithelium but was associated with asthma (Plate 29.2, opposite page 524; Fig. 29.8) (Springall *et al.*, 1991) and other inflammatory diseases, such as emphysema (Springall *et al.*, 1995c). This induction is presumably due to cytokines produced by the inflammatory cells, in a manner analogous to that of iNOS

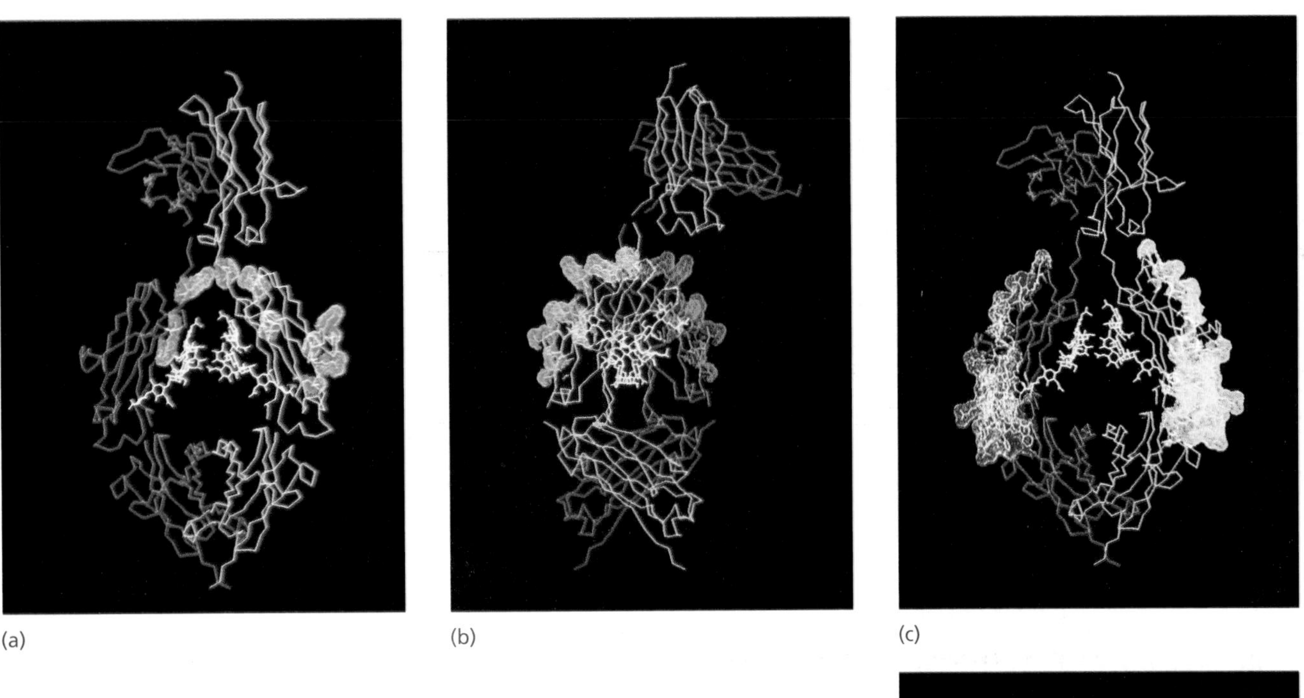

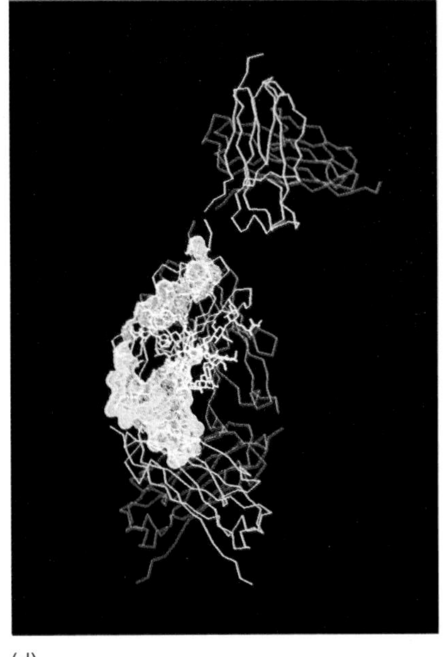

Plate 5.1 The locations of the binding sites for the high-affinity receptor (FcεRI) and low-affinity receptor (FcεRII) in IgE Fc. The two ε-chains are shown in light and dark blue as α-carbon atom traces. The pair of Cε2 domains are at the top, and the Cε4 domains are at the bottom; the conserved N-linked oligosaccharide chains attached at Asn394 are shown (light blue) between the two Cε3 domains in the centre of the Fc. The three-dimensional structure is modelled upon the crystal structure of IgG Fc, and the bend between the Cε2 and Cε3 domain pairs is based upon solution X-ray scattering data. Residues implicated in receptor binding are displayed with coloured surface areas. (a) Residues that constitute the binding site for FcεRI (green) identified by mutagenesis experiments. The site spans both Cε3 domains. (b) In this orthogonal view, the two potential binding sites for FcεRI, related by the twofold symmetry of the Cε3 domains, can be seen (green and red). The bend of the Cε2 domains occludes one site (red), leaving the other accessible (green). (c) Regions of the Fc implicated in FcεRII binding. Two symmetry-related sites (magenta and yellow) can be seen on either side of the molecule. (d) In this orthogonal view it can be seen that the bend of the Cε2 domains does not affect the accessibility of either FcεRII binding site. (See Chapter 5 for full explanation.)

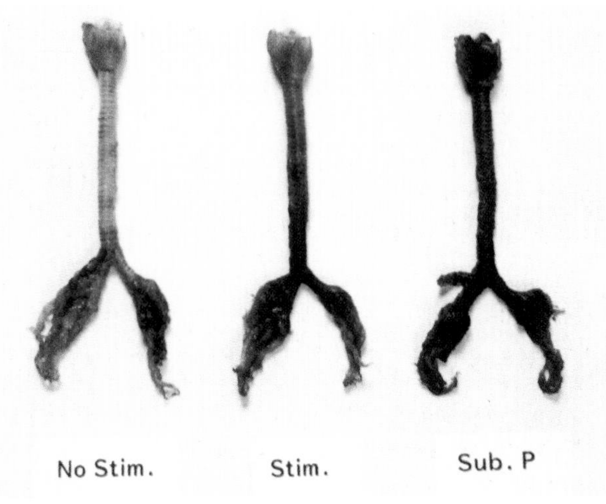

Plate 26.1 Neurogenic plasma extravasation. Guinea pigs were anaesthetized with urethane and pretreated with atropine and propranolol. Evans' blue dye was injected intravenously as a marker of plasma extravasation. Both cervical vagus nerves were stimulated electrically (Stim.), given a sham procedure (No Stim.) or given authentic substance P (Sub. P) and the animal was perfused of intravascular dye. This photograph shows dorsal view of the larynx, trachea, main bronchi and intrapulmonary airways, exposed by scraping away the parenchymal tissue. (From Belvisi *et al.*, 1989.)

(a) 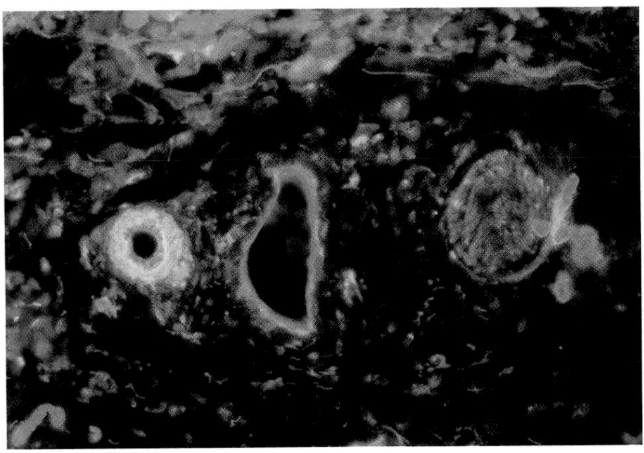

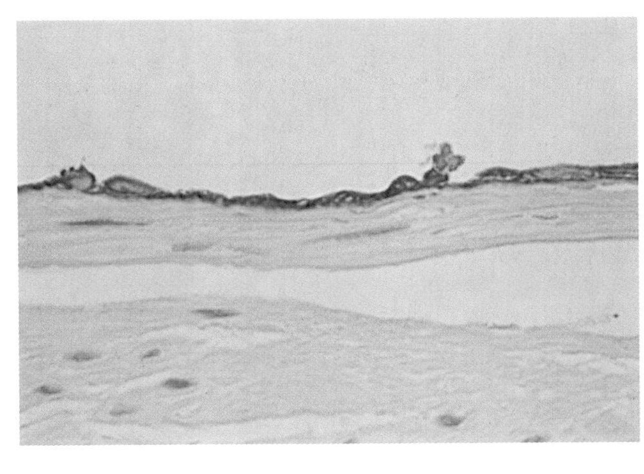 (b)

Plate 29.1 Immunohistochemical staining for (a) endothelin in an artery and a vein in the adventitia of aorta and (b) inducible nitric oxide synthetase in the endothelium of human umbilical vein.

(a) 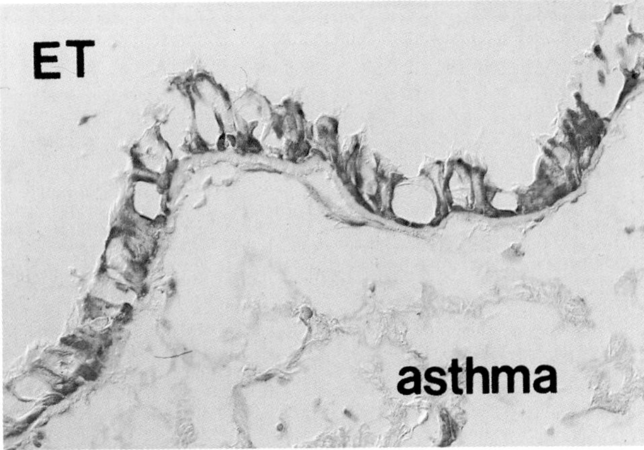

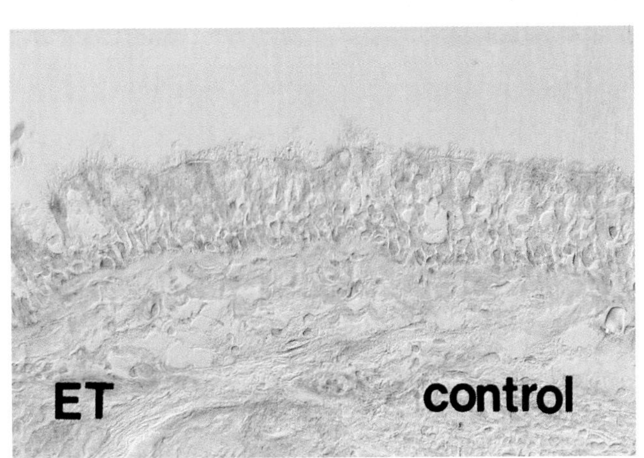 (b)

Plate 29.2 Immunoreactivity for endothelin (ET) in the airway epithelium of a biopsy obtained from an asthmatic patient (a). No staining is seen in the control biopsy from a non-asthmatic (b).

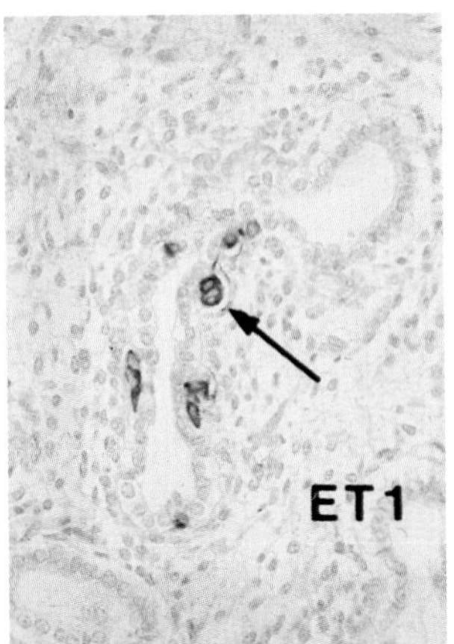

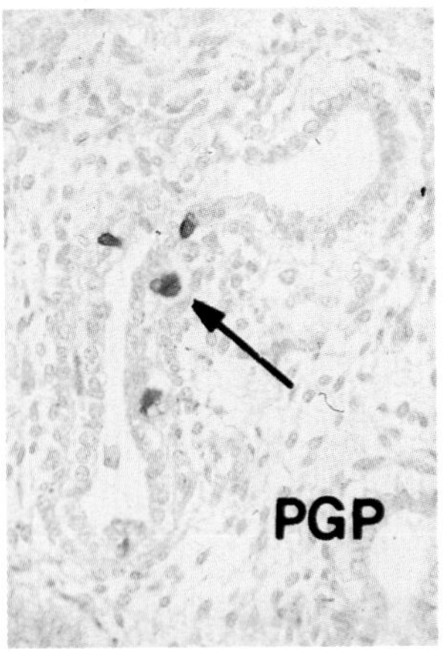

Plate 29.3 Endocrine cells in human fetal lung marked by staining for the general neuroendocrine marker PGP 9.5 and, in a serial section, showing immunoreactivity for endothelin (ET) (identical cells marked by arrows).

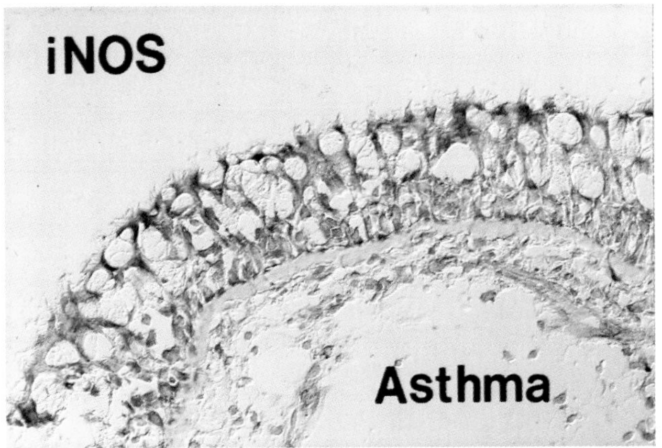

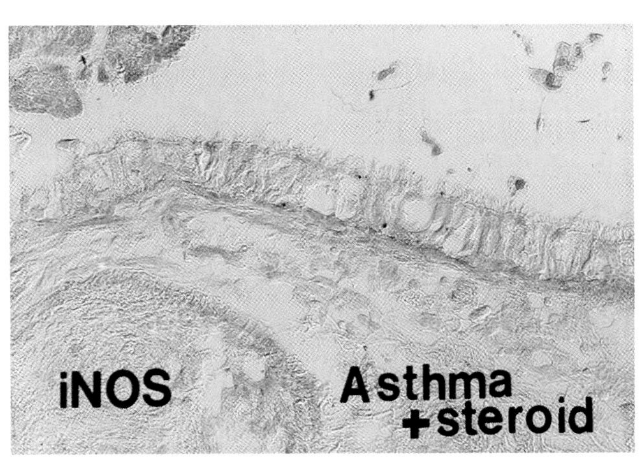

(b)

Plate 29.4 (a) Immunoreactivity for inducible nitric oxide synthetase (iNOS) in the airway epithelium of a biopsy obtained from an asthmatic patient. (b) No staining is seen in non-asthmatic controls or in the biopsy from a steroid-treated asthmatic. ET, endothelin.

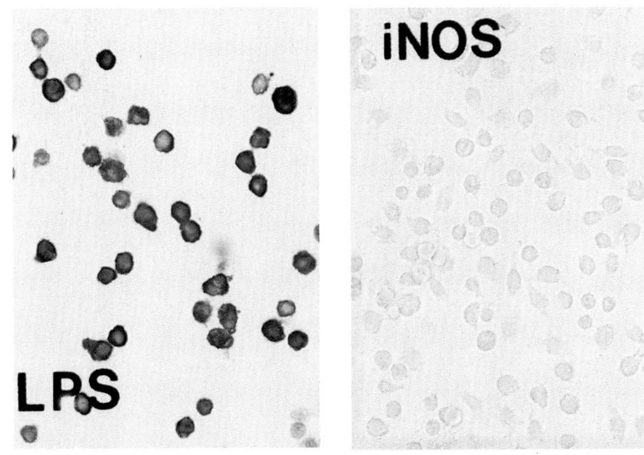

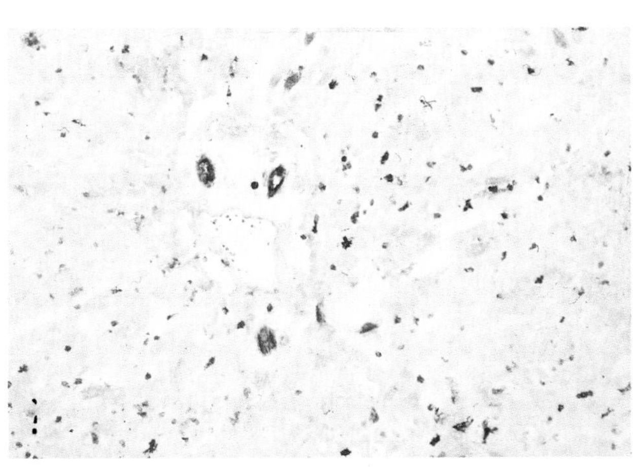

(b)

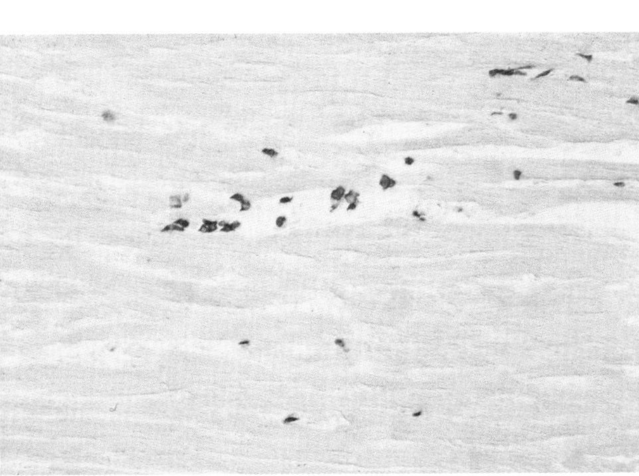

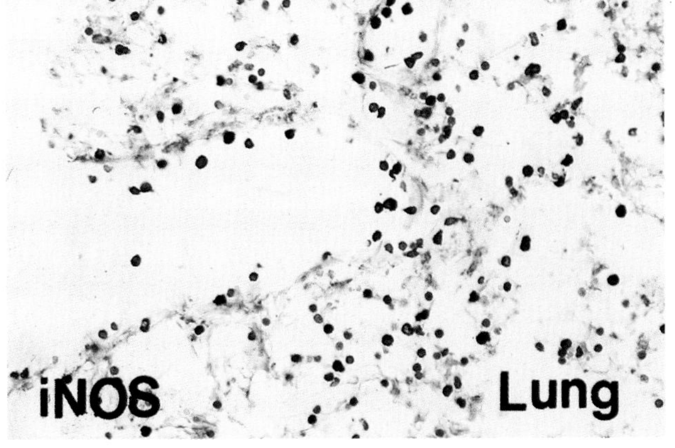

(d)

Plate 29.5 Immunoreactivity for inducible nitric oxide synthetase (iNOS) in (a) macrophages unstimulated or stimulated with lipopolysaccharide (LPS) and in tissues from endotoxin-treated rat's (b) liver; (c) heart; and (d) lung. Staining in the tissues is predominantly in macrophages.

(see below), as it is blocked by corticosteroid treatment in asthma (Springall *et al.*, 1995b). That the increased immunoreactivity for ET is not just due to decreased release is demonstrated by the increased levels of secreted ET found in bronchoalveolar lavage fluids obtained from asthmatics (Redington *et al.*, 1995). The released ET could be involved in a number of effects in the asthmatic airways, including bronchoconstriction and the growth of epithelium, smooth muscle (Hirata *et al.*, 1989) and fibroblasts (Takuwa *et al.*, 1989). Growth and differentiation of tissues in the developing lung are also probably the major role of ET from endocrine cells in the epithelium (Plate 29.3, opposite page 524). The cells produce other known growth factors, such as bombesin or gastrin-releasing peptide, and are present most abundantly in early fetal stages and then gradually decline in density towards birth (Giaid *et al.*, 1991).

Sites of NO synthesis in the lung are similar to those of ET except that NO has not been shown in endocrine cells and is also produced by nerves. The airway smooth muscle of several mammalian species, including humans, possesses an inhibitory NANC (iNANC) innervation (Richardson & Beland, 1976), effecting decreases in bronchomotor tone, and there is clear evidence that NO contributes, either fully (Belvisi *et al.*, 1992) or in part (Li & Rand, 1991), to this response. This is corroborated by the localization of nNOS to intrinsic ganglia and discrete fibres which can be seen to supply both tracheobronchial and vascular smooth muscle in several mammalian species, including humans (Kobzik *et al.*, 1993), where, in keeping with their functional effects, the number of nerves are seen to decrease down the bronchial tree (Figs 29.9 & 29.10).

In addition to nNOS, the presence and activity of eNOS have also been demonstrated in the endothelium of bronchial and pulmonary vessels, where they are of vital importance to lung tissue perfusion, as amply illustrated by the observation that administration of inhibitors of NO synthesis causes marked pulmonary vasoconstriction (Sprague *et al.*, 1992). In this context it is interesting that in pulmonary hypertension eNOS is reported to be reduced in the lung vasculature (Giaid & Saleh, 1995), whereas ET

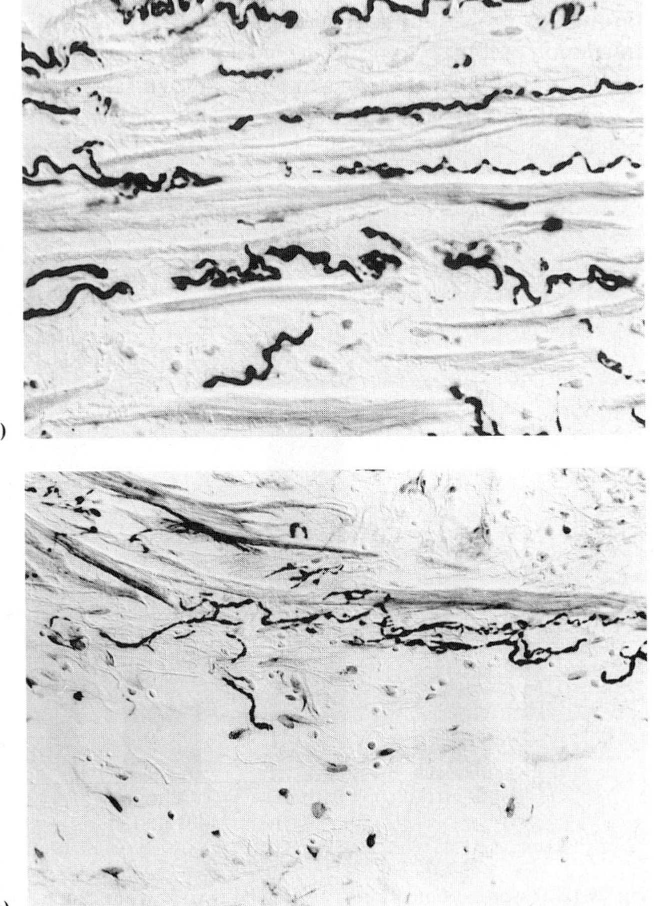

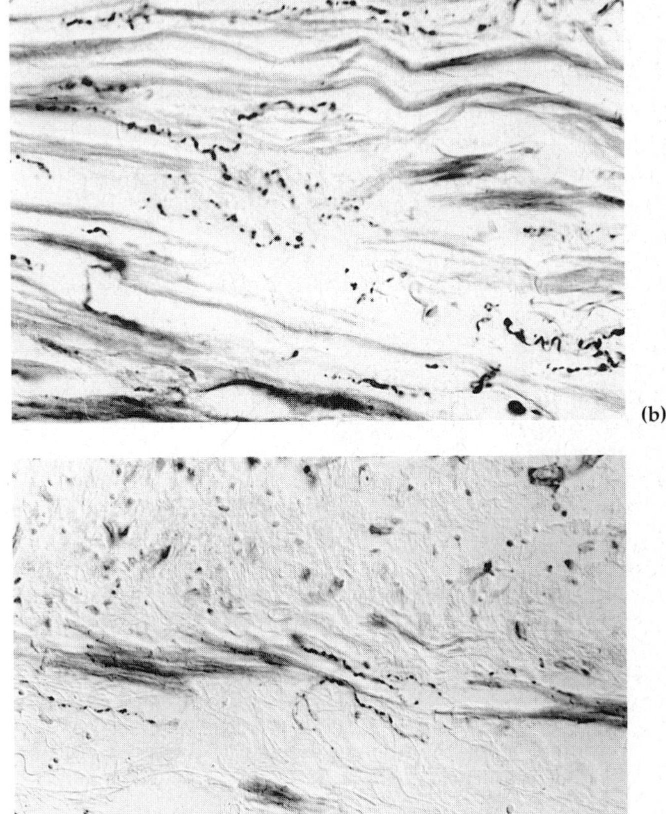

Fig. 29.9 Nerves in human tracheal smooth muscle (a,b) and a bronchiole (c,d) immunoreactive for (a,c) the general neural marker PGP 9.5 to show total nerves, and (b,d) the neural form of NO synthetase. Fewer nerves are seen in the smooth muscle of the bronchiole.

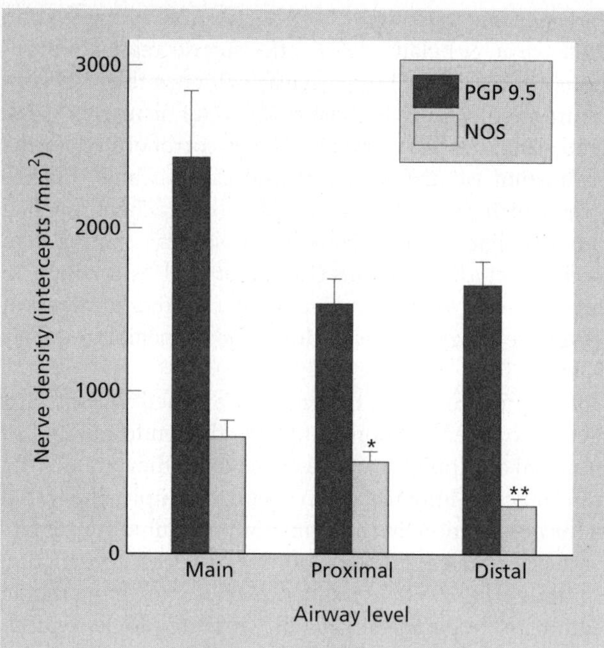

Fig. 29.10 The density of innervation in human airway smooth muscle as shown in Fig. 29.9, estimated by intercept counting in large, medium and small airways.

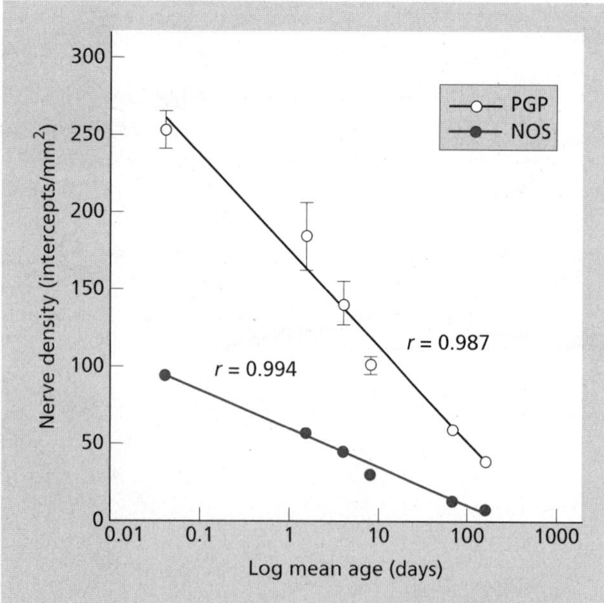

Fig. 29.11 Nerves in airways of pig lung quantified by intercept counting as in Fig. 29.10, showing the postnatal decrease, which is logarithmic with time.

synthesis is increased (Giaid *et al.*, 1993). However, these initial reports have not been confirmed and the decrease in eNOS has been contradicted (Xue & Johns, 1995).

Based on the potent vaso- and bronchodilatory actions of NO, it seemed likely that it may be involved in the physiological adaptation of the neonatal lung, which essentially has made the transition from a hypoxic, vasoconstricted state *in utero* to a normoxic, vasodilated state at birth. Indeed, expression of both message and protein for eNOS and nNOS is developmentally regulated in the rat (North *et al.*, 1994), peaking at the time of birth. Similarly, in the pig we have demonstrated that the relative abundance of nNOS-containing nerves and also the amounts of eNOS present in pulmonary and bronchial blood vessels are elevated at the time of birth, subsequently declining in a matter of days to levels observed in adults (Fig. 29.11) (Buttery *et al.*, 1995a; Hislop *et al.*, 1995). Thus, increased expression of NO synthetases, coinciding specifically with the time of birth, indicates that these enzymes may be significant in the physiological adaptation of the lung (and possibly other organs) to extrauterine life.

Alterations in the synthesis of NO are known to have profound effects on lung physiology. Indeed, reduced pulmonary activity had been postulated to be the principal underlying mechanism contributing to hypoxic pulmonary vasoconstriction and this is now supported by the finding that pulmonary hypertension can be reversed through controlled inhalation of NO (Frostell *et al.*, 1991). Inhalation of low concentrations of NO (< 80 ppm) is currently attracting great medical interest, since it selectively decreases pulmonary vascular resistance and induces potent and rapid bronchodilatation, with no apparent

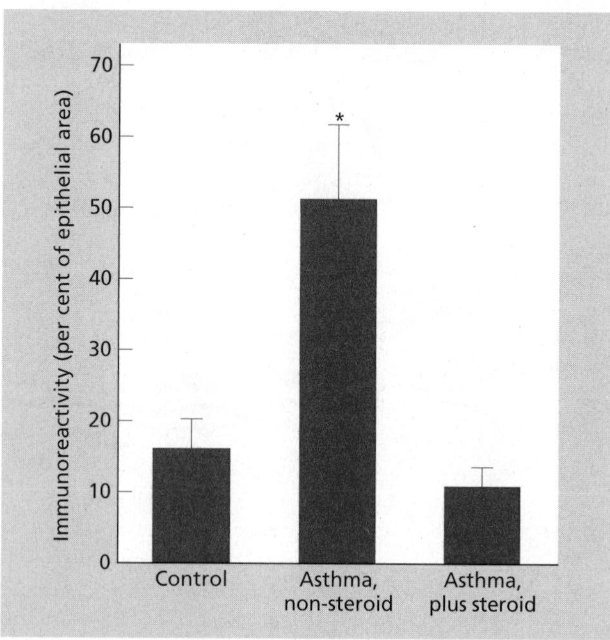

Fig. 29.12 The proportion of airway epithelial area showing staining for iNOS as in Plate 29.4, opposite page 524, for a series of asthmatic patients and controls ($n = 10$ each), showing the effects of steroid treatment in reducing iNOS levels.

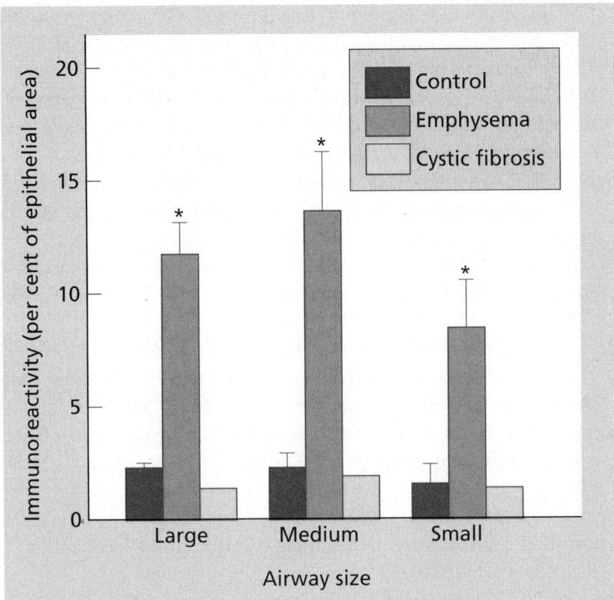

Fig. 29.13 iNOS levels in the epithelium of large, medium and small airways from patients with emphysema or cystic fibrosis compared with normal controls, measured as in Fig. 29.12.

effects on the systemic circulation (Frostell *et al.*, 1991). As such, inhaled NO may prove to be a valuable therapeutic strategy in the treatment of pulmonary hypertension associated with conditions like persistent pulmonary hypertension of the newborn and the adult respiratory distress syndrome (Frostell *et al.*, 1991; Rossaint *et al.*, 1993).

A corollary to the administration of inhaled NO to alleviate pulmonary hypertension, where pulmonary NO synthesis is apparently compromised, is the detection of increased levels of exhaled NO in the breath of subjects suffering from inflammatory lung diseases, like asthma (Persson *et al.*, 1994). Examination of bronchial biopsies from asthmatics has revealed the presence of high levels of iNOS in the airway epithelial cells, which was reduced/absent in asthmatics treated by steroids (Plate 29.4, opposite page 524; Fig. 29.12) or in control, non-asthmatic subjects (Hamid *et al.*, 1993). Similarly, we have also demonstrated that human bronchial epithelial cell primary cultures and the epithelial cell line A549 also express iNOS following stimulation with a combination of inflammatory cytokines and which could be prevented by co-incubation with glucocorticoids (Robbins *et al.*, 1994). High-output inducible NO production by airway epithelial cells is the likely source of the elevated levels of exhaled NO in asthmatics and may well form a predictive parameter of pulmonary disease or inflammation. Further, increased local NO production may mediate local bronchodilatation, although high levels of NO are potentially damaging and it could therefore also contribute to the epithelial cell damage and stripping associated with the disease. Like ET, iNOS may also be involved in other inflammatory lung diseases, being evident in the airways epithelium of subjects with emphysema, but apparently absent from subjects with cystic fibrosis (Fig. 29.13) (Springall *et al.*, 1995). The reasons for this apparent differential, disease-specific induction of iNOS remain unclear, although it may very well be related to the type/nature of the inflammatory cells present and the factors they secrete.

Inflammation

The precise roles of ET and NO in inflammation are not fully clear. However, some mention has already been made of their involvement in inflammatory processes such as atherosclerosis and asthma.

Another inflammatory condition in which NO has been demonstrated to play a role is endotoxin shock, a profound hypotensive state which is generally refractile to vasoconstrictor agents/drugs. Expression of iNOS in the vasculature, particularly in the smooth muscle, and the large quantities of NO which this enzyme is capable of producing have been implicated as the major contributory factor in mediating prolonged vasodilatation and the resultant hypotension (Moncada *et al.*, 1991). Indeed, circulating nitrite/nitrate levels are markedly elevated in patients and in animal models with endotoxin shock (Moncada *et al.*, 1991). Further, blockade of NO synthesis through administration of L-NMMA has proved effective in limiting or even reversing hypotension (Wright *et al.*, 1992). However, 'blanket' inhibition of systemic NO synthesis affecting both constitutive and inducible enzymes can be deleterious, undermining the positive effects of constitutive NO production to vascular homoeostasis, and may even potentiate the extent of organ/tissue damage (Wright *et al.*, 1992). As a consequence, therapeutic intervention to reverse NO-induced hypotension has focused on the development of iNOS selective inhibitors (Marletta, 1994), although administration of 'conventional' inhibitors of NO synthesis together with NO donors, in an attempt to protect the patient from the adverse effects of total inhibition of systemic NO synthesis, has proved to be a useful strategy (Wright *et al.*, 1992).

Localization of iNOS (Buttery *et al.*, 1994b) in animal models of endotoxin shock has now revealed its widespread distribution and, in addition, has also produced information in apparent conflict with functional observations. Most notable was the apparent failure to detect iNOS in the vasculature, in spite of the clear clinical indications for the animals having endotoxin shock and also the fact that the enzyme was readily detectable in cytokine-stimulated vascular cells in culture. In addition, we have recently found iNOS staining and activity in the vascular smooth muscle of cytokine-stimulated human internal mammary artery *ex vivo*. The apparent failure to detect iNOS after *in vivo* stimulation remains unresolved. However, it is conceivable that in conditions like endotoxin shock, where there is broad-spectrum systemic induction, the enzyme may only need to be expressed at very low levels in the vasculature, possibly beyond the immunocytochemical detection limit. This would not be unreasonable since the enzyme would be expressed at sites where it is known to have a very powerful effect. In contrast, iNOS is abundantly evident in many other cells, in particular in large numbers of macrophages distributed in many different organs (Plate 29.5, opposite page 524) as well as in mesangial cells, hepatocytes, airway and biliary epithelia and also perivascular nerves supplying mesenteric blood-vessels. These observations clearly illustrate the widespread induction of NO synthetase in endotoxin shock. It is also significant that high-output, inducible NO production from such a vast number of different cells will not only have potent local actions but is also likely to have broad systemic effects, contributing to the overall collapse of the vascular system. This is substantiated by the finding that a 'long-lived' macrophage-derived NO adduct can effect prolonged relaxation of isolated blood vessels (Uchizumi *et al.*, 1993).

Summary

Although it has been a relatively short time since the discovery of ET and NO, they have stimulated much research work and established their importance in biological control in many systems in health and disease. Both have been shown to be critically involved in inflammatory processes, but their precise roles are still being defined. Nonetheless, they have attracted much attention for the possibility of therapeutic intervention, and specific antagonists or inhibitors are under development and trial. These promise to be valuable in many diseases, but continued work is needed to establish the beneficial or detrimental effects of ET and NO production in biological tissues.

References

Ambar, I. & Sokolovsky, M. (1993) Endothelin receptors stimulate both phospholipase C and phospholipase D activities in different cell lines. *Eur. J. Pharmacol.*, **245**, 31–41.

Anon. (1994) Heterogeneous spontaneous and interleukin-4-induced nitric oxide production by human monocytes. *J. Leuc. Biol.*, **56**, 15–20.

Archer, S. (1993) Measurement of nitric oxide in biological models. *FASEB J.*, **7**, 349–60.

Asano, K., Chee, C.B., Gaston, B. *et al.* (1994) Constitutive and inducible nitric oxide synthase gene expression, regulation, and activity in human lung epithelial cells. *Proc. Nat. Acad. Sci. USA*, **91**, 10089–93.

Balligand, J.C., Kelly, R.A., Marsden, P.A., Smith, T.W. & Michel, T. (1993) Control of cardiac muscle cell function by exogenous nitric oxide signalling system. *Proc. Nat. Acad. Sci. USA*, **90**, 347–51.

Beckman, J.S., Beckman, T.W., Chen, J., Marshall, P.A. & Freeman, B.A. (1990) Apparent hydroxyl radical production by peroxynitrite: implications for endothelial injury from nitric oxide and superoxide. *Proc. Nat. Acad. Sci. USA*, **87**, 1620–4.

Belvisi, M.G., Stretton, C.D. & Barnes, P.J. (1992) Nitric oxide is the endogenous neurotransmitter of bronchodilator nerves in humans. *Eur. J. Pharmacol.*, **210**, 221–2.

Black, P.N., Ghatei, M.A., Takahashi, K. *et al.* (1989) Formation of endothelin by cultured airway epithelial cells. *FEBS Letts.*, **255**, 129–32.

Brady, A.J.B., Poole-Wilson, P.A., Harding, J.E. & Warren, J.B. (1992) Nitric oxide production within cardiac myocytes reduces their contractility in endotoxaemia. *Am. J. Physiol.*, **263**, H1963–6.

Bredt, D.S. & Snyder, S.H. (1990) Isolation of nitric oxide synthase, a calmodulin requiring enzyme. *Proc. Nat. Acad. Sci. USA*, **87**, 822–5.

Busconi, L. & Michel, T. (1992) Endothelial nitric oxide synthase: N-terminal myristolation determines its subcellular localization. *J. Biol. Chem.*, **268**, 8410–13.

Buttery, L.D.K., McCarthy, A., Springall, D.R. *et al.* (1994a) Endothelial nitric oxide synthase in the human placenta: regional distribution and proposed regulatory role at the feto-maternal interface. *Placenta*, **15**, 257–65.

Buttery, L.D.K., Evans, T.J., Springall, D.R., Carpenter, A., Cohen, J. & Polak, J.M. (1994b) Immunochemical localization of inducible nitric oxide synthase in endotoxin-treated rats. *Lab. Invest.*, **71**, 755–64.

Buttery, L.D.K., Springall, D.R., da Costa, F.A.M. *et al.* (1995a) Early abundance of NO-synthase-containing nerves in the airways of newborn pigs and subsequent decrease with age. *Neurosci. Letts.*, **201**, 219–22.

Buttery, L.D.K., Springall, D.R., Chester, A. *et al.* (1995b) Reduced expression of endothelial nitric oxide synthase in explanted vein grafts is associated with graft atherosclerosis. *J. Pathol.*, **175** (Suppl.), 105A.

Charles, I.G., Palmer, R.M.J., Hickery, M.S. *et al.* (1993) Cloning, characterization, and expression of cDNA encoding an inducible nitric oxide synthase from human chondrocytes. *Proc. Nat. Acad. Sci. USA*, **90**, 11419–23.

Chester, A.H., O'Neil, G.S., Moncada, S., Tadjkarimi, S. & Yacoub, M.H. (1990) Low basal and stimulated release of nitric oxide in atherosclerotic epicardial coronary arteries. *Lancet*, **336**, 897–900.

Clozel, M., Fischli, W. & Guilly, C. (1989) Specific binding of endothelin on human vascular smooth muscle cells in culture. *J. Clin. Invest.*, **83**, 1758–61.

de Belder, A., Radomski, M.W., Why, H.J.F. *et al.* (1993) Nitric oxide synthase activities in human myocardium. *Lancet*, **341**, 84–5.

Douglas, S.A., Vickery-Clark, L.M. & Ohlstein, E.H. (1994) Functional evidence that balloon angioplasty results in transient nitric oxide synthase induction. *Eur. J. Pharmacol.*, **255**, 81–9.

Drexler, H., Zeiher, A.M., Meinzer, K. & Just, H. (1991) Correction of endothelial dysfunction in coronary microcirculation of hypercholesterolaemic patients by L-arginine. *Lancet*, **338**, 1546–50.

Farias-Eisner, R., Sherman, M.P., Aeberland, E. & Chaudhuri, G. (1994) Nitric oxide is an important mediator for tumoricidal activity *in vivo*. *Proc. Nat. Acad. Sci. USA*, **91**, 9407–11.

Finkel, M.S., Oddis, L.U., Jacob, T.D., Watkins, S.C., Hattler, B.G. & Simmons, P.L. (1992) Negative inotropic effects of cytokines on heart mediated by nitric oxide. *Science*, **257**, 387–9.

Forstermann, U., Nakane, M., Tracey, W.R. & Pollock, J.S. (1993) Isoforms of nitric oxide synthase: functions in the cardiovascular system. *Eur. Heart J.*, **14** (S1), 10–15.

Forstermann, U., Closs, E.I., Pollock, J.S. *et al.* (1994) Nitric oxide synthase isoenzymes characterization, molecular cloning and functions. *Hypertension*, **23**, 1121–31.

Freeman, B. (1994) Free radical chemistry of nitric oxide. *Chest*, **105** (3), 79S–84S.

Frostell, C.G., Fratacci, M.D., Wain, J.C. & Zapol, W.M. (1991) Inhaled nitric oxide: a selective pulmonary vasodilator reversing hypoxic pulmonary vasoconstriction. *Circulation*, **83**, 2038–47.

Galron, R., Bdolah, A., Kloog, Y. & Sokolovsky, M. (1990) Endothelin/sarafotoxin receptor induced phosphoinositide turnover: effects of pertussis and cholera toxins and of phorbol ester. *Biochem. Biophys. Res. Commun.*, **171**, 949–54.

Geller, D.A., Nussler, A.K., Di Silvio, M. *et al.* (1993a) Cytokines, endotoxin and glucocorticoids regulate the expression of inducible nitric oxide synthase in hepatocytes. *Proc. Nat. Acad. Sci. USA*, **90**, 522–6.

Geller, D.A., Lowenstein, C.J., Shapiro, R.A. *et al.* (1993b) Molecular cloning and expression of inducible nitric oxide synthase from human hepatocytes. *Proc. Nat. Acad. Sci. USA*, **90**, 3491–5.

Giaid, A. & Saleh, D. (1995) Reduced expression of endothelial nitric oxide synthase in the lungs of patients with pulmonary hypertension. *New Engl. J. Med.*, **333**, 214–21.

Giaid, A., Polak, J.M., Gaitonde, V. *et al.* (1991) Distribution of endothelin-like immunoreactivity and mRNA in the developing and adult human lung. *Am. J. Respir. Cell Mol. Biol.*, **4**, 50–8.

Giaid, A., Yanagisawa, M., Langleben, D. *et al.* (1993) Expression of endothelin-1 in the lungs of patients with pulmonary hypertension. *New Engl. J. Med.*, **328**, 1732–9.

Goode, H.F., Webster, N.R., Howdle, P.D. & Walker, B.E. (1994) Nitric oxide production by human peripheral blood polymorphonuclear leucocytes. *Clin. Sci.*, **86**, 411–15.

Goto, K., Kasuya, Y., Matsuki, N. *et al.* (1989) Endothelin activates the dihydropyridine-sensitive, voltage-dependent Ca^{2+} channel in vascular smooth muscle. *Proc. Nat. Acad. Sci. USA*, **86**, 3915–18.

Hamid Q., Springall, D.R., Riveros-Moreno, V. *et al.* (1993) Induction of nitric oxide synthase in asthmatics patients: an immunocytochemical study of bronchial biopsies. *Lancet*, **324**, 1510–13.

Hamon M., Vallet B., Bautere C. *et al.* (1994) Long-term oral administration of L-arginine reduces intimal thickening and enhances neoendothelium-dependent acetylcholine-induced relaxation after arterial injury. *Circulation*, **90**, 1357–62.

Hayzer, D.J., Rose, P.M., Lynch, J.S. *et al.* (1992) Cloning and expression of a human endothelin receptor: subtype A. *Am. J. Med. Sci.*, **304**, 231–8.

Hemsen, A., Franco-Cereceda, A., Matran, R., Rudehill, A. & Lundberg, J.M. (1990) Occurrence, specific binding sites and functional effects of endothelin in human cardiopulmonary tissue. *Eur. J. Pharmacol.*, **191**, 319–28.

Henderson, A.H., Lewis, M.J., Shah, A.M. & Smith, J.A. (1992) Endothelium, endocardium and cardiac contraction. *Cardiovasc. Res.*, **26**, 305–8.

Hevel, J.A. & Marletta, M.A. (1994) Nitric oxide synthase assays. *Methods Enzymol.*, **233**, 250–9.

Hibbs, J.B., Taintor, R.R., Vavrin, Z. & Rachlin, E.M. (1988) Nitric oxide: a cytotoxic activated macrophage effector molecule. *Biochem. Biophys. Res. Commun.*, **157**, 87–94.

Higman, D.J., Strachan, A.M.J. & Powell, J.T. (1994) Reversibility of smoking-induced endothelial dysfunction. *Brit. J. Surg.*, **81**, 977–8.

Hirata, Y., Takagi, Y., Fukuda, Y. & Marumo, F. (1989) Endothelin is a potent mitogen for rat vascular smooth muscle cells. *Atherosclerosis*, **78**, 225–8.

Hislop, A.A., Springall, D.R., Pollock, J.S., Polak, J.M. & Haworth, S.G. (1995) Abundance of endothelial nitric oxide synthase in newborn intrapulmonary arteries. *Arch. Dis. Child.*, **73**, F17–F21.

Ignarro, L.J. (1991) Haem-dependent activation of guanylate cyclase by nitric oxide: a novel signal transduction mechanism. *Blood Vessels*, **28**, 67–73.

Inoue, A., Yanagisawa, M., Kimura, S. *et al.* (1989) The human endothelin family: three structurally and pharmacologically distinct isopeptides predicted by three separate genes. *Proc. Nat. Acad. Sci. USA*, **86**, 2863–7.

Jayakody, L., Kappagod, T., Senaratne, M.P.J. & Thomson, A.B.R. (1988) Impairment of endothelium-dependent relaxation: an early marker for atherosclerosis in the rabbit. *Brit. J. Pharmacol.*, **94**, 335–46.

Knowles, R.G., Palacios, M., Plamer, R.M.J. & Moncada, S. (1989) Formation of nitric oxide from L-arginine in the central nervous system: a transduction mechanism for stimulation of soluble guanylate cyclase. *Proc. Nat. Acad. Sci. USA*, **86**, 5159–62.

Kobzik, L., Bredt, D.S., Lowenstein, C.J. *et al.* (1993) Nitric oxide synthase in human and rat lung: immunocytochemical and histochemical localization. *Am. J. Respir. Cell Mol. Biol.*, **9**, 371–7.

Lamas, S., Marsden, P.A., Li, G.K., Tempst, P. & Michel, T. (1992) Endothelial nitric oxide synthase: molecular cloning and characterization of a distinct constitutive isoform. *Proc. Nat. Acad. Sci. USA*, **89**, 6348–52.

Lee, T.S., Chao, T., Hu, K.Q. & King, G.L. (1989) Endothelin stimulates a sustained 1,2-diacylglycerol increase and protein kinase C activation in bovine aortic smooth muscle cells. *Biochem. Biophys. Res. Commun.*, **162**, 381–6.

Li, C.G. & Rand, M.J. (1991) Evidence that part of the NANC response of guinea pig trachea to electrical field stimulation is mediated by nitric oxide. *Brit. J. Pharmacol.*, **102**, 91–4.

Lopez Farre, A., Riesco, A., Espinosa, G. *et al.* (1993) Effect of endothelin-1 on neutrophil adhesion to endothelial cells and perfused heart. *Circulation*, **88**, 1166–71.

Marletta, M.A. (1994) Approaches to selective inhibition of nitric oxide synthase. *J. Med. Chem.*, **37**, 1899–907.

Moncada, S., Palmer, R.M.J. & Higgs, E.A. (1991) Nitric oxide: physiology, pathophysiology and pharmacology. *Pharmacol. Rev.*, **48**, 109–42.

Nathan, C.F. & Hibbs, J.B. (1991) Role of nitric oxide synthesis in macrophage anti-microbial activity. *Curr. Opin. Immunol.*, **3**, 65–70.

Nathan, C. & Xie, Q.W. (1994) Regulation of biosynthesis of nitric oxide. *J. Biol. Chem.*, **269**, 13722–8.

Nishida, M., Springhorn, J.P., Kelly, R.A. & Smith, T.W. (1993) Cell–cell signaling between adult rat ventricular myocytes and cardiac microvascular endothelial cells in heterotypic primary culture. *J. Clin. Invest.*, **91**, 1934–41.

North, A.J., Star, R.A., Brannon, T.S. *et al.* (1994) Nitric oxide type I and type III gene expression are developmentally regulated in rat lung. *Am. J. Physiol.*, **266**, L635–L641.

Nunkawa, Y., Ishida, N. & Tanaka, S. (1993) Cloning of inducible nitric oxide synthase in rat vascular smooth muscle cells. *Biochem. Biophys. Res. Commun.*, **191**, 89–94.

Nussler, A.K. & Billiar, T.R. (1993) Inflammation, immunoregulation and inducible nitric oxide synthase. *J. Leuc. Biol.*, **54**, 171–8.

Palmer, R.M.J., Ashton, D.S. & Moncada, S. (1988) Vascular endothelial cells synthesize nitric oxide from L-arginine. *Nature*, **333**, 664–6.

Pepper, M.S., Ferrara, N., Orci, L. & Montesano, R. (1992) Potent synergism between vascular endothelial growth factor and basic fibroblast growth factor in the induction of angiogenesis *in vitro*. *Biochem. Biophys. Res. Commun.*, **189**, 824–31.

Persson, M.G., Zetterstrom, O., Arenius, V., Ihre, E. & Gustafsson, L.E. (1994) Single-breath measurements of nitric oxide: increased concentration in asthmatics, and reduction in smokers. *Lancet*, **343**, 146–7.

Pollock, J.S., Forstermann, U., Mitchel, J.A. *et al.* (1991) Purification and characterization of particulate endothelium-derived relaxing factor synthase from cultured and native bovine aortic endothelial cells. *Proc. Nat. Acad. Sci. USA*, **88**, 10480–4.

Pollock, J.S., Nakane, M., Buttery, L.D.K. *et al.* (1993) Immunochemical characterization of endothelial nitric oxide synthase using specific monoclonal antibodies. *Am. J. Physiol.*, **265**, C1379–C1387.

Pribnow, D., Muldoon, L.L., Fajardo, M., Theodor, L., Chen, L.Y. & Magun, B.E. (1992) Endothelin induces transcription of *fos/jun* family genes: a prominent role for calcium ion. *Mol. Endocrinol.*, **6**, 1003–12.

Redington, A.E., Springall, D.R., Ghatei, M.A. *et al.* (1995) Endothelin in bronchoalveolar lavage fluid and its relation to airflow obstruction in asthma. *Am. J. Resp. Crit. Care Med.*, **151**, 1034–9.

Resink, T.J., Scott Burden, T. & Buhler, F.R. (1989) Activation of phospholipase A2 by endothelin in cultured vascular smooth muscle cells. *Biochem. Biophys. Res. Commun.*, **158**, 279–86.

Reynolds, E.E., Mok, L.L. & Kurokawa, S. (1989) Phorbol ester dissociates endothelin-stimulated phosphoinositide hydrolysis and arachidonic acid release in vascular smooth muscle cells. *Biochem. Biophys. Res. Commun.*, **160**, 868–73.

Richardson, J.B. & Beland, J. (1976) Non adrenergic inhibitory nervous system in human airways. *J. Appl. Physiol.*, **41**, 746–71.

Robbins, R.A., Barnes, P.J., Springall, D.R. *et al.* (1994) Expression of inducible nitric oxide in human lung epithelial cells. *Biochem. Biophys. Res. Commun.*, **203**, 209–18.

Rossaint, R., Falke, K.S., Lopez, F., Slama, K., Pison, U. & Zapol, W.M. (1993) Inhaled nitric oxide for the adult respiratory distress syndrome. *New Engl. J. Med.*, **328**, 399–405.

Rozengurt, N., Springall, D.R. & Polak, J.M. (1990) Localization of endothelin-like immunoreactivity in airway epithelium of rats and mice. *J. Pathol.*, **160**, 5–8.

Rubanyi, G.M. & Vanhoutte, P.M. (1985) Hypoxia releases a vasoconstrictor substance from the canine vascular endothelium. *J. Physiol. Lond.*, **364**, 45–56.

Schmidt, H.H.H.W., Gagne, G.D., Nakane, M., Pollock, J.S., Muller, M. & Murad, F. (1992) Mapping of neural nitric oxide synthase in rat suggests frequent co-localization with NADPH-diaphorase but not with soluble guanylyl cyclase, and novel paraneural functions for nitrinergic signal transduction. *J. Histochem. Cytochem.*, **40**, 1439–56.

Shaul, P.W., North, A.J., Wu, L.C. *et al.* (1994) Endothelial nitric oxide synthase is expressed in cultured human bronchiolar epithelium. *J. Clin. Invest.*, **94**, 2231–6.

Simonson, M.S. & Dunn, M.J. (1990) Cellular signaling by peptides of the endothelin gene family. *FASEB J.*, **4**, 2989–3000.

Sprague, R., Thiemermann, C. & Vane, J.R. (1992) Endogenous endothelium-derived relaxing factor opposes hypoxic pulmonary vasoconstriction and supports blood flow to hypoxic alveoli in anaesthetized rabbits. *Proc. Nat. Acad. Sci. USA*, **89**, 8711–15.

Springall, D.R., Howarth, P.H., Counihan, H., Djukanovic, R., Holgate, S.T. & Polak, J.M. (1991) Endothelin immunoreactivity of airway epithelium in asthmatic patients. *Lancet*, **337**, 697–701.

Springall, D.R., Meng, Q.-H., Buttery, L.D.K. *et al.* (1995a) Upregulation of inducible nitric oxide synthase in airway epithelium in emphysema. *Am. J. Resp. Crit. Care Med.*, **151**, A342.

Springall, D.R., Meng, Q.-H., Redington, A., Howarth, P.H., Evans, T.J. & Polak, J.M. (1995b) Inducible nitric oxide synthase in asthmatic airway epithelium is reduced by corticosteroid therapy. *Am. J. Resp. Crit. Care Med.*, **151**, A833.

Springall, D.R., Meng, Q.-H., Buttery, L.D.K. *et al.* (1995c) Human airway epithelium expresses inducible nitric oxide synthase in emphysema. *J. Pathol.*, **175**, 105A.

Stuehr, D.J. & Nathan, C.F. (1989) Nitric oxide: a macrophage product responsible for cytostasis and respiratory inhibition in tumour target cells. *J. Exp. Med.*, **169**, 1543–55.

Suzuki, T., Hoshi, H., Sasaki, H. & Mitsui, Y. (1991) Endothelin-1 stimulates hypertrophy and contractility of neonatal rat cardiac myocytes in a serum-free medium. II. *J. Cardiovasc. Pharmacol.*, **17**, S182–S186.

Takanashi, M. & Endoh, M. (1991) Characterization of positive inotropic effect of endothelin on mammalian ventricular myocardium. *Am. J. Physiol.*, **261**, H611–H619.

Takuwa, N., Takuwa, Y., Yanagisawa, M., Yamashita, K. & Masaki, T. (1989) A novel vasoactive peptide endothelin stimulates mitogenesis through inositol lipid turnover in Swiss 3T3 fibroblasts. *J. Biol. Chem.*, **264**, 7856–61.

Tanner, F.C., Noll, G., Boulanger, C.M. & Luscher, T.F. (1991) Oxidized low density lipoproteins inhibit relaxations in porcine arteries: role of scavenger receptor and endothelium-derived nitric oxide. *Circulation*, **83**, 2012–20.

Traish, A.M., Moran, E. & Saenz de Tejada, I. (1991) Physicochemical characterization and solubilization of endothelin receptors. *Receptor*, **1**, 229–42.

Uchizumi, H., Hattori, R., Sase, K. *et al.* (1993) A stable L-arginine-dependent relaxing factor released from cytotoxic-activated macrophages. *Am. J. Physiol.*, **264**, H1472–H1477.

Urade, Y., Fujitani, Y., Oda, K. *et al.* (1992) An endothelin B receptor-selective antagonist: IRL 1038, [Cys11-Cys15]-endothelin-1(11–21). *FEBS Letts.*, **311**, 12–16.

Ward, J.K., Barnes, P.J., Springall, D.R. *et al.* (1995) Human i-NANC bronchodilation and nitric oxide immunoreactive nerves are reduced in distal airways. *Am. J. Respir. Cell Mol. Biol.*, **13**, 175–84.

White, C.R., Brock, T.A., Chang, L.-Y. *et al.* (1994) Superoxide and peroxynitrite in atherosclerosis. *Proc. Nat. Acad. Sci. USA*, **91**, 1044–8.

Wilcox, C.S., Welch, W.J., Murad, F. *et al.* (1992) Nitric oxide synthase in macula densa regulates glomerular pressure. *Proc. Nat. Acad. Sci. USA*, **89**, 11993–7.

Wood, E.R., Berger, H. Jr, Sherman, P.A. & Lapetina, E.G. (1993) Hepatocytes and macrophages express an identical nitric oxide synthase gene. *Biochem. Biophys. Res. Commun.*, **191**, 767–78.

Wright, C.L., Rees, D.D. & Moncada, S. (1992) Protective and pathophysiological roles of nitric oxide in endotoxin shock. *Cardiovasc. Res.*, **26**, 48–57.

Xie, Q.-W., Cho, H.J., Calaycay, J. *et al.* (1992) Cloning and characterization of inducible nitric oxide synthase from mouse macrophages. *Science*, **256**, 225–8.

Xue, C. & Johns, R.A. (1995) Endothelial nitric oxide synthase in the lungs of patients with pulmonary hypertension. *New Engl. J. Med.*, **333**, 1462–4.

Yanagisawa, M., Kurihara, H., Kimura, S. *et al.* (1988) A novel potent vasoconstrictor peptide produced by vascular endothelial cells. *Nature*, **332**, 411–15.

Yoshizumi, M., Perella, M.A., Burnett, J.C. Jr & Lee, M.E. (1993) Tumour necrosis factor alpha downregulates endothelial nitric oxide synthase mRNA by shortening its half-life. *Circ. Res.*, **73**, 205–9.

Zhang, J., Dawson, V.L., Dawson, T.M. & Snyder, S.H. (1994) Nitric oxide activation of poly(ADP-ribose) synthetase in neurotoxicity. *Science*, **263**, 687–9.

CHAPTER 30

Theophylline and Isoenzyme-Selective Phosphodiesterase Inhibitors

M.A. Giembycz, G. Dent & J.E. Souness

Introduction

According to recent figures, the cost associated with the diagnosis and treatment of allergic diseases is alarming (Geha, 1993). In the USA, for example, it has been estimated that money spent on over-the-counter antihistamines far exceeds the entire annual budget for the National Institutes of Health (Geha, 1993).

Allergic diseases, including all of those listed in Table 30.1, affect 20% of the population and represent a highly significant cause of morbidity and mortality. Taking allergic asthma as a specific example, recent epidemiological studies indicate that the prevalence and severity of this disease are increasing (Fleming & Crombie, 1987), together with the number of reported cases of fatal asthma (Sly, 1984; Barnes, 1988). These statistics are of particular concern, given the marked increase in the prescribing of various anti-asthma therapies (Keating *et al.*, 1983; Hay & Higenbottam, 1987).

Although the last 5 years have seen significant advances in our understanding of the pathogenesis of many allergic disorders, the aetiology of allergy is still incompletely understood. However, as described in Chapters 2, 5 and 6, the likely participation of immunoglobulin E (IgE)-driven mechanisms in many allergic diseases, including those cited in Table 30.1, has been identified and recognized by the World Health Organization (Thompson & Stewart, 1991). Since the incidence of allergy has reached epidemic proportions, it is only too clear that drugs which can prevent the overt and covert manifestations of allergic reactions and, ideally, suppress or even prevent the process of host sensitization could have a profound clinical and economic impact on the control of these diseases.

While glucocorticosteroids are currently considered the most effective anti-allergic/anti-inflammatory drugs available, they are non-selective in action and not without adverse effects (see Chapter 35). New drugs with enhanced selectivity and improved side-effect profiles are clearly required. One group of drugs which, from a theoretical perspective, may exhibit powerful anti-inflammatory and immunomodulatory activity are inhibitors of the cyclic nucleotide phosphodiesterase (PDE) isoenzymes (Torphy & Undem, 1991; Giembycz, 1992; Giembycz & Dent, 1992; Raeburn *et al.*, 1993; Nicholson & Shahid, 1994; Torphy *et al.*, 1994; Dent & Giembycz, 1995; Giembycz & Souness, 1996). The prototype PDE inhibitors which have been used in the treatment of asthma for many years are the alkylxanthines, of which theophylline is the most widely prescribed. The main beneficial activity of theophylline was originally attributed to its weak bronchodilator action. However, evidence accumulated in the early 1990s points to an anti-inflammatory action of these compounds at sub-bronchodilator doses (Ward *et al.*, 1993; Sullivan *et al.*, 1994; Djukanovic *et al.*, 1995), which has provoked a remarkable resurgence of interest in theophylline and so-called 'second-generation' PDE inhibitors not only as smooth-muscle relaxants but as potential anti-allergic and/or anti-inflammatory agents (Torphy *et al.*, 1994; Dent & Giembycz, 1995; Giembycz & Souness, 1995).

The rationale for developing new PDE inhibitors has stemmed primarily from the realization that PDE isoenzymes represent a highly heterogeneous group (seven families have thus far been identified) that are differentially expressed between different cell types and which may regulate specific functional responses (Nicholson *et al.*, 1991). Accordingly, it was rapidly appreciated that drugs which selectively suppress the activity of a particular PDE isoenzyme may result in a discrete functional alteration of cells which express a PDE variant and, theoretically, specific functional responses within the same cell. Given the prevalence of allergic diseases as a whole, it is only too apparent that the potential clinical (and financial) reward of developing a class of steroid-sparing drugs of general utility in a variety of allergic disorders is enormous and explains why many of the world's major pharmaceutical companies have an active PDE research programme and have developed highly selective PDE inhibitors, many of which are currently undergoing clinical trials for asthma and other allergic disorders (Table 30.2).

It is the purpose of this chapter to describe, very briefly, the cellular and molecular mechanisms that are currently believed to underlie the genesis of allergic disease and, this foundation having been laid, to describe the multiplicity of mammalian PDE isoenzymes, the tissue distribution of PDE expressed in cells which participate in allergic reactions, the differences in the complement of PDE in normal vs. allergic pro-inflammatory and immune cells, and the potential sites where theophylline and selective PDE inhibitors could act to alleviate the acute and chronic manifestations of allergic disease. Given that inhibitors of the PDE4, and to some extent PDE3, isoenzyme family show the most promising pharmacology with respect to suppressing various indices of allergic inflammation, they will form the basis of this chapter. The airway smooth-muscle effects of theophylline and PDE inhibitors which are relevant to allergic diseases such as asthma are not discussed here and interested readers should consult recent reviews of this subject (Giembycz & Dent, 1992; Souness & Giembycz, 1994; Torphy *et al.*, 1994; Dent & Giembycz, 1995).

Table 30.1 Allergic diseases in which IgE-driven mechanisms have been implicated.

Asthma
Atopic and contact dermatitis
Rhinitis
Eczema
Sinusitis
Hypersensitivity pneumonitis
Extrinsic alveolitis
Angioedema and anaphylaxis
Certain forms of migraine and gastrointestinal disorders
Urticaria

IgE-dependent and independent mechanisms in the pathogenesis of allergic inflammation

A primary concern with respect to drug development is the mechanism by which susceptible individuals become sensitized to foreign substances and the subsequent pathogenesis of inflammation that generally ensues when that sensitized individual re-encounters the same allergen. Although a complete understanding of host sensiti-

Table 30.2 Representative cyclic AMP phosphodiesterase inhibitors for allergic disorders.

Company	Drug	Isoenzyme selectivity	Indication	Development stage
Almirall	LAS 31025	4	Asthma	Phase III
Byk-Gulden	Tolafentrine	3/4	Asthma	Discontinued
Byk-Gulden	Zardaverine	3/4	Asthma	Discontinued
Celltech/Merck	CDP 480	4	Asthma	Phase II
Eli-Lilly	Tibenelast	4	Asthma	Phase III
Kyorin	Ibudilast	NS	Asthma	Marketed
Organon	Org 20241	3/4	Asthma	Phase I
Otsuka	Cilostazol	3	Heart failure, asthma?	Marketed
Pfizer	CP 80,633	4	Asthma and atopic dermatitis	Phase II
Rhône–Poulenc Rover	RP 73401	4	Asthma	Phase II
Sandoz	Benafentrine	3/4	Asthma	Discontinued
Sandoz	SDZ MKS 492	3	Asthma	Phase I
SmithKline–Beecham	BRL 1063	4	Asthma	Phase I
SmithKline–Beecham	SR 207,499	4	Asthma	Phase I
Syntex	RS 23355	4	Asthma	Preclinical
Troponwerke	Nitraquazone	4	Inflammation	Discontinued
Wyeth–Ayerst	WAY PDE 641	4	Asthma	Phase 1

NS, non-selective.

zation is lacking, the generation of IgE by B lymphocytes is believed to play a central role in this process and is primarily responsible for the acute consequences that follow allergen exposure. This is discussed in detail in Chapters 5–8. It is important to emphasize that, while there is unanimity of opinion that IgE-driven mechanisms are responsible for the immediate short-term exacerbations of many allergic diseases which follow allergen provocation in atopic individuals, the extent to which IgE-mediated mechanisms play a role in late-phase reactions is currently unclear. Indeed, it is likely that IgE represents only one of several, highly complex, components that regulate the chronic ongoing inflammatory responses that characterize many allergic diseases (see Chapters 2, 3 and 90).

Figure 30.1 depicts a working schema that may explain, at least in part, antigen-mediated allergic inflammation. Also shown are foci in this proposed sequence of events amenable to therapeutic intervention with theophylline and isoenzyme-selective PDE inhibitors. The paradigm proposes that two pathways operate in tandem, culminating in the acute and chronic manifestations of allergic inflammation that follow antigen provocation in sensitized individuals. The first involves the activation of granulocytes which express surface-bound Fc receptors for IgE, such as mast cells, basophils and eosinophils, with the resultant release of mediators, including histamine, prostaglandins and platelet-activating factor (PAF) (see Chapters 9 and 10). These molecules give rise to the immediate overt responses that follow allergen exposure and may be responsible for acute exacerbations of allergic symptoms in atopic individuals (see Chapters 22 and 23). In the second pathway, allergen may be presented to CD4+ T lymphocytes of the T-helper 2 (Th2) phenotype by antigen-presenting cells, including epithelial cells, macrophages and dendritic cells, resulting in their activation and elaboration of a number of pro-inflammatory cytokines, including interleukin-3 (IL-3), IL-4, IL-5, tumour necrosis factor-α (TNF-α) and granulocyte macrophage colony-stimulating factor (GM-CSF) (see Chapters 3 and 7). One major action of these so-called chronic pro-inflammatory mediators is the attraction of eosinophils to and their subsequent activation in sites of allergen entry. Through their ability to release highly basic proteins and lipid mediators, together with the generation of certain cytokines and reactive oxygen species, the chronic aspects of certain allergic diseases, including

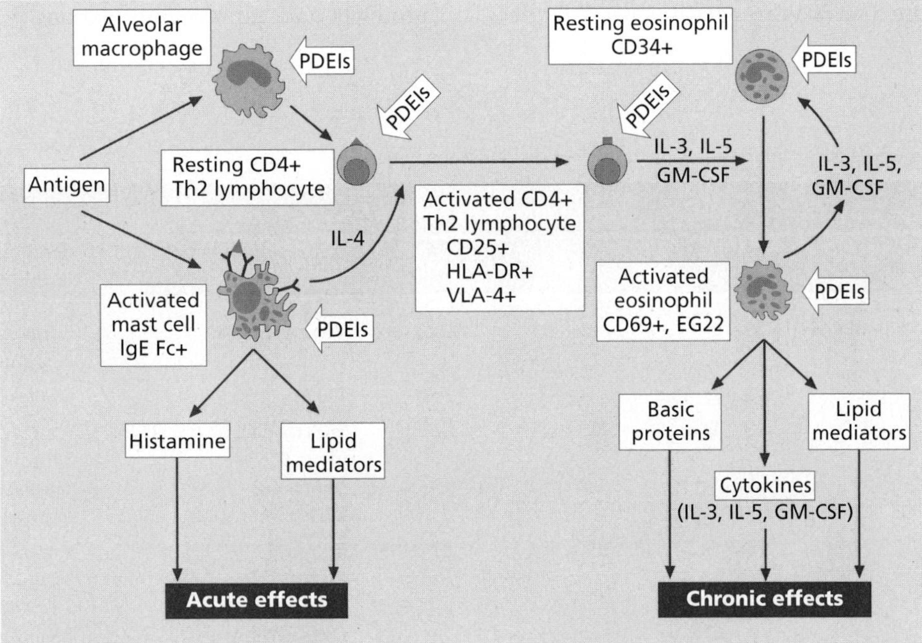

Fig. 30.1 Schema outlining a current hypothesis underlying allergen-mediated allergic inflammation and sites at which phosphodiesterase (PDE) inhibitors and theophylline may act to prevent this pathogenesis. In its simplest form, two pathways operate in parallel to give rise to the acute and chronic manifestations of inflammation. The acute effects are a consequence of the activation of mast cells bearing allergen-specific IgE which secrete lipid mediators and bioactive autacoids such as histamine. The more chronic reaction involves the activation of CD4+ T lymphocytes of the T-helper 2 (Th2) phenotype and the resultant liberation of cytokines, including interleukin-3 (IL-3), IL-5 and granulocyte macrophage colony-stimulating factor (GM-CSF), which attract other pro-inflammatory cells, in particular eosinophils, to sites of allergen entry. Here they release further cyokines, which may have an autocrine function, and basic proteins and lipid mediators, which precipitate and perpetuate chronic inflammation. See text for further details.

atopic dermatitis (Leung, 1992), asthma (Corrigan & Kay, 1992) and rhinitis (Varney *et al.*, 1992), may, at least in part, be manifested and perpetuated. It is significant that activation of this second pathway need not involve the participation of allergen-specific IgE. Indeed, while allergic disorders and atopy are closely related, the disease process can occur (apparently) in the absence of local IgE production or the excessive elaboration of IL-4. IgE-mediated mechanisms are, therefore, neither necessary nor sufficient for the development of allergy. This tempts speculation that these apparently IgE-independent disorders are antigen-driven, cell-mediated phenomena dependent upon the elaboration of pro-inflammatory cytokines.

Cyclic nucleotide PDE

The cyclic nucleotide PDEs (EC 3.1.4.17; EC 3.1.4.35) comprise a large group of enzymes whose sole function is to hydrolyse and thereby inactivate the biologically active cyclic purines, cyclic adenosine monophosphate (cAMP) and cyclic guanosine monophosphate (cGMP), and the pyrimidine, cyclic cytosine monophosphate (cCMP). A cyclic nucleotide PDE that hydrolysed the 3′-ribose phosphate bond of cAMP to the catalytically inactive 5′-AMP was identified more than 30 years ago (Butcher & Sutherland, 1962). Since then, families and, indeed, subfamilies of PDE which selectively act on cAMP and cGMP have been identified (see Beavo, 1988; Beavo & Reifsnyder, 1990; Bentley & Beavo, 1992; Giembycz & Kelly, 1994; Loughney & Ferguson, 1994, for reviews). PDEs which act on cyclic pyrimidine monophosphates have also been described (Newton *et al.*, 1990), although investigators have tended to focus, almost exclusively, on the PDE which hydrolyse cyclic purine nucleotides for which functionally important second-messenger roles have been unequivocally established.

Currently, the PDEs which metabolize cyclic purines comprise at least seven distinct families which can be distinguished by a number of criteria. In particular, these isoenzymes differ in substrate specificity, in kinetic properties, in responsiveness to endogenous allosteric regulators (calmodulin, cGMP), in susceptibility to inhibition by various compounds and in primary amino acid sequence (Table 30.3). These families are designated by the Arabic numerals 1, 2, 3, 4, 5, 6 and 7 and correspond to the Ca^{2+}/calmodulin-dependent, cGMP-stimulated, cGMP-inhibited, cAMP-specific, cGMP-specific, photoreceptor- and rolipram-insensitive, cAMP-specific isoenzymes, respectively (Table 30.3). Molecular biological studies have discovered that many PDE are separate gene products and express multivariant regulatory domains

Table 30.3 Properties and selective inhibitors of cyclic nucleotide PDE isoenzymes.

PDE family	Subunit size (kDa)	K_m (μmol/l) cAMP	K_m (μmol/l) cGMP	Representative inhibitors	Reference
1 Ca^{2+}/calmodulin-stimulated	59–75	2–70	2–20	Vinpocetine,	Souness *et al.* (1989)
				KS-505a	Nakanishi *et al.* (1992)
2 cGMP-stimulated	102–106	30–100	10–30	EHNA	Müller & Nennstiel (1992)
3 cGMP-inhibited	63–135	0.1–0.5	0.1–0.5	Siguazodan, SK&F 94120	Murray *et al.* (1990)
				SK&F 95654	Murray *et al.* (1992)
				Milrinone	Harrison *et al.* (1986)
				Enoximone	Kariya and Dage (1988)
4 cAMP-specific	60–93	0.5–18	>50	Rolipram	Reeves *et al.* (1987)
				Ro 20-1724	Nemoz *et al.* (1989)
				Nitraquazone	Glaser & Traber (1984)
				Denbufylline	Nicholson *et al.* (1989)
				RP 73401	Souness *et al.* (1995)
5 cGMP-specific	90–100	>40	1.5	Zaprinast	Souness *et al.* (1989)
				SK&F 96231	Murray (1993)
				MY5445	Hagiwara *et al.* (1984)
6 Photoreceptor	84–99	>500	17–20	Zaprinast	Gillespie and Beavo (1989)
7 Rolipram-insensitive, cAMP-specific	—	0.2	—	None	

EHNA, erythro-9-(2-hydroxy-3-nonyl)-adenine. See text for definition of other abbreviations.

linked to highly conserved (>60% amino acid identity) homologous catalytic sequences located near the carboxyl-terminus of the protein. Members of one family share 20–25% sequence homology with members of another family. Furthermore, at least five out of the seven gene families can be divided into subfamilies that are 70–90% homologous and which are derived from similar but distinct genes or, in some cases, from the same gene through alternate mRNA splicing or from differences in the initiation start sites for the transcription of the protein. At the time of writing, 16 genes were unequivocally identified which encode for more than 33 distinct PDE enzymes (Table 30.4). For further information on the molecular genetics of PDE isoenzymes, interested readers are directed towards a number of comprehensive reviews (Beavo & Reifsnyder, 1990; Torphy & Livi, 1993; Beavo *et al.*, 1994; Giembycz & Kelly, 1994; Loughney & Ferguson, 1994).

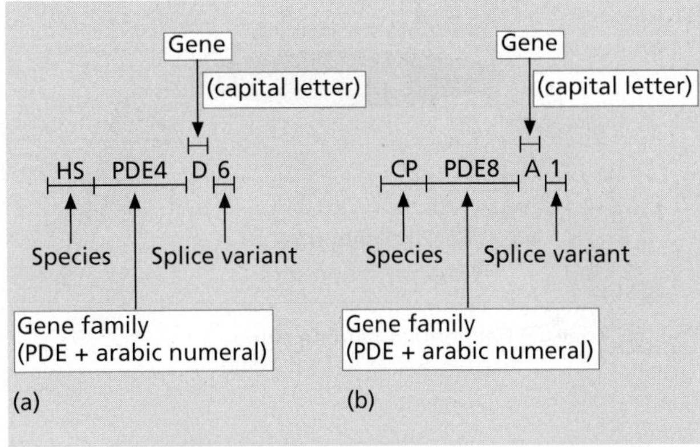

Fig. 30.2 GenBank nomenclature for the classification of cyclic purine PDE. The first two letters represent the species, the next three letters plus an arabic numeral denote the gene family and the final letter and numeral refer to the gene product within the PDE family and the spliced variant (if appropriate). See text for further details.

Nomenclature

Although several attempts at classifying PDE have been made, a new standardized 'GenBank' nomenclature for existing and newly discovered PDE was recently introduced (Beavo *et al.*, 1994). The taxonomy is novel as it is based not only on traditional biochemical criteria but also on protein sequencing and analyses of partial and full-length complementary DNA (cDNA) clones. Consider two hypothetical PDEs, CPPDE8A1 and HSPDE4D6 (Fig. 30.2). The first two letters refer to the species (CP for *Cavia porcellus*, HS for *Homo sapiens*). The next three letters plus an Arabic numeral correspond to the PDE gene family (i.e. PDE8, PDE4), while the next letter and Arabic numeral (i.e. A1, D6) denote the gene product and spliced variant (if appropriate). This nomenclature will be used throughout this chapter.

Table 30.4 Phosphodiesterase isoenzyme families.

Family	Characteristics	Genes	Gene products*
1	Calcium and calmodulin dependent; variable affinity for cAMP and cGMP	3	9+
2	cGMP stimulated; low affinity for cAMP and cGMP	1	2
3	cGMP inhibited; high affinity for cAMP and cGMP	2	2+
4	cAMP specific; high affinity for cAMP	4	15+
5	cGMP specific	1	2
6	cGMP specific; photoreceptor phosphodiesterase family	1	2
7	cAMP specific; high affinity for cAMP; differentiated from family 4 by insensitivity to rolipram and Ro-20-1724	1	1

* Including spliced variants.

Structure, properties and general characteristics

A diagrammatic representation of the primary structure of cyclic purine PDE is shown in Fig. 30.3. There is now compelling evidence that all of the well-studied mammalian PDE share essentially the same structure: there is a central core, located close to the carboxyl-terminus of the protein, that shares greater than 60% homology between isoenzyme families and which features a highly conserved domain of some 270 to 300 amino acids. Within this region, 10 sequences containing invariant histidine, threonine and serine residues have been identified which may play important, although as yet undefined, functional roles in the PDE protein (Conti *et al.*, 1991). Studies performed in a number of laboratories suggest that the highly conserved domain within this central core represents the catalytic site of the enzyme (Tucker *et al.*, 1981; Kincaid *et al.*, 1985; Stroop *et al.*, 1989).

The central core of mammalian PDE is linked, via so-called hinge regions, to carboxyl- and amino-terminal extensions (Fig. 30.3) which show little sequence homol-

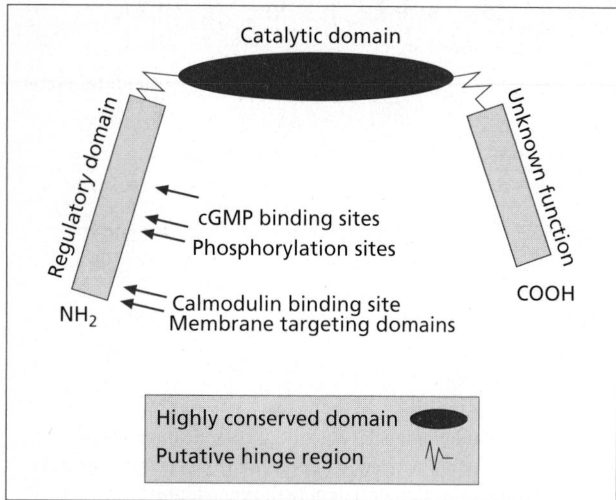

Fig. 30.3 Proposed structure of mammalian cyclic purine PDEs. Limited proteolysis and protein sequencing suggest that all mammalian PDE so far examined contain a conserved central core that features the catalytic site. This region of PDE proteins is flanked, through putative hinge regions, by highly heterologous carboxyl and amino termini, which are believed to express regulatory domains and sequence information, which determine the subcellular localization of PDE. See text for further details.

ogy between PDE families (Conti *et al.*, 1991). This finding has led to the view that the non-conserved domains subserve regulatory functions of the protein. Indeed, studies performed with members of the PDE1 and PDE2 isoenzyme families, for example, have convincingly demonstrated that the amino termini of these proteins feature allosteric domains for calmodulin (Bentley *et al.*, 1992) and cyclic GMP (Stroop *et al.*, 1989), respectively. Furthermore, studies by Houslay and colleagues have shown that a short, 25 amino acid sequence, at the amino terminus of *Rattus norvegicus* (RN)PDE4A1, an intrinsic plasma membrane-associated PDE in rat brain, confers membrane targeting (Shakur *et al.*, 1993; Scotland & Houslay, 1995). Indeed, selective deletion of these residues yields a truncated enzyme that is rendered soluble but unaltered with respect to substrate specificity and inhibitor sensitivity (Shakur *et al.*, 1993). Similar data have been described by other investigators (Pillai *et al.*, 1994; Kasuya *et al.*, 1995). Thus, in addition to regulating cyclic nucleotide hydrolysis, the amino terminus of PDEs can apparently determine the subcellular localization of the enzyme.

PDE1 isoenzyme family

Members of the PDE1 isoenzyme family are dependent upon calmodulin for catalytic activity. This phenomenon was originally documented in the early 1970s (Cheung, 1970, 1971; Kakiuchi & Yamazaki, 1970) and it is now known that PDE1 comprises a family of more than nine closely related proteins encoded by at least three genes. In each case, catalytic activity is markedly increased (five- to 20-fold) by calmodulin in the presence of micromolar concentrations of Ca^{2+} (Sharma & Wang, 1982, 1986). Detailed kinetic analyses indicate that calmodulin modulates PDE1 activity allosterically by substantially increasing the maximum velocity (V_{max}) of the reaction, while reducing, albeit to a relatively modest extent, the affinity (Michaelis constant (K_m)) of the substrate for the enzyme (Sharma & Wang, 1982, 1986).

Evidence for PDE1 multiplicity was originally provided by the immunological studies of Hansen and Beavo (1982), which effectively discriminated two bovine isoforms: a 61-kDa enzyme in brain and a 59-kDa variant in heart. Sequence analysis has revealed that the 59-kDa and the 61-kDa isoenzymes (BTPDE1A1 and BTPDE1A2 respectively) are alternatively spliced variants of the same gene (Charbonneau *et al.*, 1991; Novack *et al.*, 1991). Similar studies, subsequently reported by Sharma *et al.*, (1984), identified a 63-kDa isoenzyme in bovine brain that is immunologically distinct from BTPDE1A2 and represents a different gene product (BTPDE1B1). This enzyme was recently cloned from bovine and rat brain cDNA libraries (Repaske *et al.*, 1992). Several other putative PDE1 sub-types have also been purified and partially characterized from a number of tissues but no sequence data are yet available (see Giembycz & Kelly, 1994).

Based upon biochemical characterization of PDE1 activities in various cell types, two major forms of the enzyme can be classified: those that preferentially hydrolyse cGMP (K_m ~ 3 μmol/l) over cAMP (K_m ~ 40 μmol/l), which include the bovine brain (Sharma & Wang, 1986) and lung (Sharma *et al.*, 1980) enzymes, and those which do not display substrate selectivity for either cyclic nucleotide, which include the PDE1 in mouse testis (Rossi *et al.*, 1988) and canine trachealis (Torphy & Cieslinski, 1990).

Tissue distribution, selective inhibitors and therapeutic implications

Of those pro-inflammatory and immunocompetent cells implicated in human inflammatory and allergic diseases, only alveolar macrophages (Tenor *et al.*, 1995b) and epithelial cells (Rousseau *et al.*, 1994) express PDE1 in quantity, although trace amounts of this isoenzyme are present in CD4+ and CD8+ T lymphocytes, platelets and possibly neutrophils (Hidaka *et al.*, 1984; Engerson *et al.*, 1986; Simpson *et al.*, 1988; Tenor *et al.*, 1995a) (Table 30.5). At the present time, the functional role of PDE1 in these cells and the potential therapeutic implications of suppressing the activity of this enzyme family are obscure due to a lack of selective inhibitors. For example, while

Table 30.5 PDE Isoenzyme profiles in pro-inflammatory and immunocompetent cells implicated in allergic disorders.

Cell type	Species and source	PDE isoenzyme(s) present	Comments	Reference
Mast cell	Murine—bone cleaved	1, 4		Torphy & Undem (1992)
	Rat peritoneal mast cells	2, 3, 4		Bergstrand *et al.* (1978)
	Rat peritoneal mast cells	5 (?)	Enzyme studies not reported. Zaprinast inhibits antigen-induced histamine release	Frossard *et al.* (1981)
Basophil	Human peripheral blood	3, 4, 5		Peachell *et al.* (1992)
Eosinophil	Guinea pig peritoneal	4	Tightly membrane-bound enzyme displaying non-linear kinetics	Souness *et al.* (1991) Dent *et al.* (1991)
	Human peripheral Blood	4	Membrane-bound enzyme displaying non-linear kinetics	Dent *et al.* (1994)
	Human peripheral blood	4	Enzyme reported to be ~70% soluble	Hatzelmann *et al.* (1995)
Neutrophil	Human peripheral blood	4	Membrane-bound enzyme displaying non-linear kinetics	Wright *et al.* (1990)
	Human peripheral blood	4	Enzyme apparently soluble	Nielson *et al.* (1990) Schudt *et al.* (1991)
	Human peripheral blood	1, 4	Evidence for PDE1 provided but not universally corroborated	Engerson *et al.* (1986) Grady & Thomas (1986)
Monocyte	Human peripheral blood	4		White *et al.* (1990) Thompson *et al.* (1976)
	Human peripheral blood	1, 4, 3 (?)		Seldon *et al.* (1995) Verghese *et al.* (1995)
Macrophage	Guinea pig peritoneal macrophage	1, 4	PDE4 membrane-bound	Turner *et al.* (1993)
	Murine peritoneal macrophage	2, 3, 4		Okonogi *et al.* (1991)
	Human alveolar macrophage	1, 3, 4, 5	Major activity is PDE1 PDE3 predominantly particulate PDE4 predominantly soluble	Tenor *et al.* (1995) Dentt *et al.* (1993)
B Lymphocyte		Not known		
T lymphocyte	Rat T cells	2, 3, 4		Valette *et al.* (1990)
	Rat T cells	2, 3, 4, 5		Marcoz *et al.* (1993)
	Human peripheral blood	4	PDE3 exclusively particulate	Epstein & Hachisu (1984)
	Human peripheral blood	3, 4	PDE4 cytosolic and particulate	Robiscek *et al.* (1991, 1989)
	Human T-cell clones (HUT 78)	4, 7	Enzyme with characteristics similar to the recently cloned PDE 7 identified in T-cell lines PDE7 mRNA detected in HUT 78	Ichimura & Kase (1993) Bloom & Beavo (1994)
	Human peripheral blood CD4+ Human peripheral blood CD8+	2, 3, 4, 5, 7 2, 3, 4, 5, 7	PDE3 predominantly particulate PDE4 predominantly soluble PDE7 predominantly soluble	Tenor *et al.* (1995a) Giembycz *et al.* (1995)
Platelet	Human peripheral blood	1, 2, 3, 5		Murray *et al.* (1990) Hidaka *et al.* (1984) Hagiwara *et al.* (1984) MacPhee *et al.* (1986) Simpson *et al.* (1988)
Endothelial cell	Bovine aorta Porcine aorta	2, 3, 4	PDE profile in the microvasculature has not been determined. However, inhibitory effects of rolipram on microvascular leakage suggest presence of PDE4 in endothelial cells of microvascular beds	Souness *et al.* (1990) Lugnier & Schini (1990) Raeburn *et al.* (1994) Suttorp *et al.* (1993)
	Fetal bovine aorta	2, 4, 5		Kishi *et al.* (1992)
Epithelial cell	Bovine trachea	1, 2, 3, 4, 5	Epithelial layer strips removed. Possible contamination with smooth muscle?	Rousseau *et al.* (1994)

vinpocetine selectively inhibits PDE1 from rat (Souness *et al.*, 1989) and rabbit aorta (Hagiwara *et al.*, 1984a), it is essentially inactive upon the PDE1 variants in airway smooth muscle and cannot be used as a general investigational tool. Similarly, the alkylxanthine, 3-isobutyl-1-methyl-8-(methylamino)-xanthine, has been used as a PDE1 inhibitor but its selectivity and specificity are questionable. Of considerable interest is the recent demonstration that a heterocyclic molecule isolated from the bacterium *Streptomyces argenteolus* is a potent and highly selective inhibitor of PDE1 (Nakanishi *et al.*, 1992; Kase *et al.*, 1993). This compound, designated KS 505a, is unique inasmuch as it shows considerable selectivity not only for PDE1 over other isoenzyme families but specifically for the 61 kDa isoform, PDE1A2. Indeed, KS 505a is approximately 80-fold more potent against PDE1A2 from bovine brain (IC_{50} ~ 170 nmol/l (concentration of drug giving 50% inhibition)) than of PDE1A1 from bovine heart (Kase *et al.*, 1993). These are fascinating findings. Not only do they identify KS 505a as a selective inhibitor of PDE1, but they demonstrate that compounds can discriminate between two highly homologous proteins that are derived from the same gene by alternate splicing. Perhaps the most exciting prospect that arises from these data is the likelihood that third-generation PDE inhibitors can be synthesized for all PDE families, which would allow the selective targeting of specific enzymes encoded by the same gene. The therapeutic implications of such molecules are potentially enormous.

PDE2 isoenzyme family

The first description of what is now termed a PDE2 isoenzyme was reported in the early 1970s following the observation that cAMP hydrolysis in rat liver supernatant was stimulated by micromolar concentrations of cGMP (Beavo *et al.*, 1971). Since then, many reports have documented the presence of cGMP-stimulated PDE in a number of cells and tissues (Beavo, 1987) and the PDE2 in bovine adrenal glands, heart and liver has been purified to apparent homogeneity (Martins *et al.*, 1992; Yamamoto *et al.*, 1983).

PDE2 isoenzymes do not readily discriminate between cAMP (K_m = 30 μmol/l to 100 μmol/l) and cGMP (K_m = 10 μmol/l to 30 μmol/l), exhibit positive homotropic co-operative behaviour with respect to both substrates (n_H = 1.3 to 2) and feature a high-affinity (K_d ~ 0.1 μmol/l), non-catalytic, allosteric binding site for cGMP (Moss *et al.*, 1977; Martins *et al.*, 1992; Yamamoto *et al.*, 1983; Stroop & Beavo, 1992). An interesting property of these enzymes is that low concentrations (1–5 μmol/l) of cGMP enhance the degradation of cAMP by a mechanism which may require occupancy of the non-catalytic cGMP-binding domain (Yamamoto *et al.*, 1983; Stroop & Beavo, 1992). In contrast, cAMP does not detectably stimulate PDE2-catalysed cGMP hydrolysis (Stroop & Beavo, 1992).

Only a single gene (from the cow) has thus far been identified which encodes PDE2, although the existence of other genes is likely (Beavo & Reifsnyder, 1990; Bentley & Beavo, 1992; Beavo *et al.*, 1994). Transcription of this gene can give rise, theoretically, to two spliced variants, BTPDE2A1 and BTPDE2A2 (Le Trong *et al.*, 1990; Bentley & Beavo, 1992), of deduced molecular weight, taken from the largest open reading frame of the corresponding cDNA, of 103.2 and 105.6 kDa, respectively (Bentley & Beavo, 1992). Like many other cyclic nucleotide PDE, the native structure of PDE2 is homodimeric and of molecular weight 210 kDa (Stroop & Beavo, 1992).

The complete amino acid sequence of the PDE2 from bovine heart has been published (Le Trong *et al.*, 1990) and a cDNA which encodes an adrenal cortex PDE2 has been cloned and expressed in purified protein derivative (PPD)-S49 cells (Sonnenburg *et al.*, 1991). These two enzymes are almost identical and represent PDE2A1 isoenzymes. A membrane-associated PDE2 is also present in bovine brain (Murashima *et al.*, 1990). However, while this enzyme is structurally similar to, and kinetically indistinguishable from, PDE2A1, ribonuclease (RNase) protection assays indicate that this protein is a product of an alternatively spliced gene (Murashima *et al.*, 1990) and probably represents a PDE2A2 isoenzyme. Indeed, although the mRNA sequence encoding the catalytic and cGMP-regulatory domains is identical, significant differences exist at the amino terminus of the molecule, which is believed to feature sequence information for membrane insertion (Shakur *et al.*, 1993; Scotland & Houslay, 1995).

Tissue distribution, selective inhibitors and therapeutic implications

Northern analyses suggest that PDE2A is localized to anatomically distinct areas of the brain (hippocampus, cerebral cortex, basal ganglia) and kidney (outer red medulla, papillae), with lower levels present in trachea and lung (Sonnenburg *et al.*, 1991). Representatives of the PDE2 isoenzyme family are not ubiquitously distributed in cells and tissues relevant to the pathogenesis of allergic disease (Table 30.4). Although present in airway smooth muscle (Souness & Giembycz, 1994), platelets (Simpson *et al.*, 1988), epithelial (Rousseau *et al.*, 1994) and endothelial cells (Lugnier *et al.*, 1990; Souness *et al.*, 1990; Kishi *et al.*, 1992; Suttorp *et al.*, 1993), PDE2 has not been detected in eosinophils or neutrophils (Nielson *et al.*, 1990; Wright *et al.*, 1990; Dent *et al.*, 1991, 1994; Souness *et al.*, 1991) and only very low levels are expressed in T lymphocytes and alveolar macrophages (Tenor *et al.*, 1995a,b).

No inhibitors have been identified and fully characterized which selectively inhibit any member of the PDE2 isoenzyme family. A preliminary report, however, suggests that erythro-9-(2-hydroxy-3-nonyl)-adenine (EHNA) is a selective inhibitor of PDE2A1 in human and porcine heart. The compound has an IC_{50} value of ~1 μmol/l against these enzymes and is approximately 100-fold less potent against the other PDE expressed in these tissues (Müller & Nennstiel, 1992; Podzuweit *et al.*, 1993). EHNA apparently does not inhibit cAMP hydrolysis catalysed by the PDE2 variant expressed in human trachealis, which may indicate that it can distinguish between different PDE2 isoforms.

Currently, there is little evidence that PDE2 plays a significant role in those pro-inflammatory and immune cells where it has been detected, although PDE2 may regulate vascular endothelial cell function (Beavo *et al.*, 1994). It remains uncertain, therefore, what effect selective inhibition of the PDE2 isoenzyme family would have on cell types implicated in the pathogenesis of allergy and inflammation.

PDE3 isoenzyme family

Currently, three genetically distinct cAMP-specific PDE families have been described and, to some extent, characterized (Beavo, 1987; Beavo & Reifsnyder, 1990; Bentley & Beavo, 1992; Beavo *et al.*, 1994; Michaeli *et al.*, 1994). One of these, PDE3, is selectively inhibited by micromolar concentrations of cGMP and was originally classified as the cGMP-inhibited, cAMP PDE.

Possibly the first clear demonstrations of a cGMP-inhibited, cAMP PDE was reported in 1982 by Weber and Appleman. Since then, a PDE3 isoenzyme has been highly purified and characterized from a number of tissues, including human platelets (Grant & Coleman, 1984), bovine heart (Harrison *et al.*, 1986), rat liver (Pyne *et al.*, 1987) and rat adipocytes (Degerman *et al.*, 1987). Generally, members of this isoenzyme family hydrolyse cAMP (K_m = 0.1 to 0.5 μmol/l) and cGMP (K_m = 0.1 to 8 μmol/l) with high affinity, but the apparent V_{max} when cGMP is substrate is only about 10% of that achieved when cAMP is used (Grant & Coleman, 1984; Manganiello *et al.*, 1992). For this reason, cGMP behaves as a potent and competitive inhibitor of cAMP hydrolysis (inhibition constant (K_i) ~ 0.1 μmol/l). It is noteworthy, however, that not all PDE3 preparations hydrolyse cGMP with a low V_{max} (Torphy & Cieslinski, 1990; Manangiello *et al.*, 1992; Torphy *et al.*, 1993b). This is especially true for the PDE3 in human trachealis, where less than a twofold difference in maximum velocity is evident (Torphy *et al.*, 1993b).

Classical biochemical techniques suggest that the molecular weight of the native enzyme in the heart, platelet and adipocyte is approximately 230 kDa and is composed of two identical 110-kDa subunits (Harrison *et al.*, 1986; Macphee *et al.*, 1986). A so-called 'dense-vesicle' PDE3 in rat liver appears to be smaller (~63 kDa) and may represent a different gene product (Pyne *et al.*, 1987).

A PDE3 isoenzyme has been cloned from a human heart cDNA library and a partial clone, encoding a truncated 54 kDa form of the enzyme (which contains the conserved domain), has been expressed as a fusion protein in *Escherichia coli* (Meacci *et al.*, 1992). The open reading frame predicts that the cardiac PDE3 has a molecular weight of ~125 kDa, which is similar in size to the partially purified PDE3 from human cardiac sarcoplasmic reticulum (130 kDa). The expressed enzyme is inhibited by cGMP and by the cilostamide derivative, OPC 3911, is unaffected by rolipram, and has been designated HSPDE3A1. In addition, two distinct, but related, PDE3 cDNAs have been cloned from rat adipose tissue cDNA libraries (Taira *et al.*, 1993). One of these, rat cGMP-inhibited phosphodiesterase 2 (RcGIP2), is highly homologous to the human heart PDE3 and may be derived from vascular elements within adipose tissue. It is likely, therefore, that it represents the rat homologue of PDE3A1. The other isoenzyme, RcGIP1, may be the hormone-stimulated adipocyte PDE3 and is probably transcribed from a distinct gene, since the nucleotide differences between RcGIP1 and RcGIP2 eliminate the possibility that these proteins arise from alternative mRNA splicing (Taira *et al.*, 1993). The adipocyte PDE3 has been tentatively designated a PDE3B1 isoenzyme and has a molecular weight, calculated from the deduced amino acid sequence, of 123.1 kDa (Taira *et al.*, 1993). Neither RcGIP1 nor RcGIP2 cDNAs strongly hybridize to total RNA extracted from rat liver (a rich source of the hormone-sensitive 'dense-vesicle' PDE3), which, as mentioned above, may indicate the presence of the third PDE3 isoform.

Transcripts for at least two different forms of human PDE3A1 have been described which are transcribed from different start codons. One form encodes a membrane-bound protein of 125 kDa for which cGMP has high affinity, while the other is considerably smaller (80 kDa) since it lacks a large portion at the N terminus. This truncated enzyme is soluble in nature for which cGMP has relatively low affinity (Kasuya *et al.*, 1995).

A PDE3 is expressed by the K30a mutant of murine S49 lymphoma cells that is related to, but not identical with, the PDE3 isoform in heart (Beavo, 1987). At the present time, it is not clear if this enzyme is a mutant form of PDE3A1 or represents a spliced variant of the PDE3A subfamily (Beavo & Reifsnyder, 1990).

Regulation of PDE3 by cGMP and phosphorylation

Theoretically, stimulation of guanylyl cyclase in cell types that express a PDE3 isoenzyme could inhibit cAMP hydrolysis and so potentiate cAMP-mediated functional responses. Evidence to support this possibility is available from studies performed with human platelets (Levin *et al.*, 1982; Maurice & Haslam, 1990), vascular smooth muscle (Shimokawa *et al.*, 1988; Maurice *et al.*, 1991) and, more recently, thymocytes (Marcos *et al.*, 1993) and airways smooth muscle (Turner *et al.*, 1993). In the latter tissue, sodium nitroprusside (SNP) markedly potentiates relaxation of guinea-pig trachea by the PDE4 inhibitor, rolipram, a finding consistent with the ability of SNP to increase cAMP in this tissue.

There is both direct and indirect evidence that PDE3 activity is regulated by reversible cAMP-dependent phosphorylation. Gettys *et al.* (1988) noted that the rate of hydrolysis of 8-parachlorothiophenyl cAMP (a cell-permeant analogue that is a substrate for PDE3) in rat hepatocytes was significantly enhanced by glucagon. Similarly, prostaglandin E_1 (PGE_1), prostacyclin and forskolin stimulate cAMP hydrolysis in human and rat platelets by a mechanism postulated to involve activation of protein kinase A (PKA) and subsequent phosphorylation of PDE3 (Alvarez *et al.*, 1981; Hamet *et al.*, 1983). A direct demonstration that PDE3 is a substrate for PKA and that phosphorylation can inhibit cAMP hydrolysis was documented by Grant *et al.* (1988), using human platelets. This constitutes a universal mechanism of PDE3 regulation and has been reported for the membrane-bound enzymes in adipocytes and hepatocytes (Pyne *et al.*, 1987; Manganiello *et al.*, 1992).

The ability of cGMP and PKA to significantly alter the activity of PDE3 in a number of tissues constitutes an important short-term regulatory mechanism. In the context of allergic diseases, it is likely that either mechanism could exert a profound functional influence upon pro-inflammatory and immunocompetent cells that express PDE3. Specific examples are discussed in the isoenzyme-selective PDE inhibitor sections under 'Mast cells and basophils' and 'T lymphocytes and B lymphocytes'.

Tissue distribution and selective inhibitors

Representative inhibitors of the PDE3 isoenzyme family are widely expressed in immune and pro-inflammatory cells (Table 30.5), including the platelet (Hidaka *et al.*, 1984; Macphee *et al.*, 1986), basophil (Peachell *et al.*, 1992), mast cell (Bergstrand *et al.*, 1978), alveolar macrophage (Tenor *et al.*, 1995b), T lymphocyte (Giembycz *et al.*, 1995; Tenor *et al.*, 1995a) and epithelial and endothelial cell (Lugnier & Schnini, 1990; Souness *et al.*, 1990; Rousseau *et al.*, 1994). PDE3 is apparently not present in eosinophils (Dent *et al.*, 1994; Hatzelmann *et al.*, 1995) or neutrophils (Nielson *et al.*, 1990; Wright *et al.*, 1990; Schudt *et al.*, 1991a).

Selective inhibitors of the PDE3 isoenzyme family were developed primarily for the treatment of congestive heart failure with the hope that a greater therapeutic index could be achieved over cardiac glycosides (Fischer *et al.*, 1992). Many PDE3 inhibitors have been synthesized (Table 30.6), some of which are currently used in the clinic. Interestingly, one of these inhibitors, vesnarinone, is able to discriminate between PDE3 isoenzymes isolated from tissues within the same species (Masuoka *et al.*, 1993). Thus, the PDE3 prepared from human heart and kidney is 10- to 50-fold more sensitive to the inhibitory effects of vesnarinone than the enzyme extracted from aortic smooth muscle and platelets under conditions where cGMP and another isoenzyme-selective PDE3 inhibitor, enoximone, are equipotent. This is the first evidence that individual members of the PDE3 isoenzyme family can be distinguished pharmacologically and endorses the concept that third-generation, subfamily-selective, PDE inhibitors can be synthesized.

PDE4 isoenzyme family

With the exception of the recently identified PDE7, the enzymes which comprise the PDE4 isoenzyme family are the most poorly understood. This is somewhat ironic, given that preclinical data, discussed in detail in the sections 'Effect of theophylline and isoenzyme-selective phosphodiesterase inhibitors . . . ? and 'Anti-inflammatory effects of phosphodiesterase inhibitors *in vivo*', indicate that selective inhibitors of these enzymes may possess anti-inflammatory activity and could exert a steroid-sparing influence in humans. If true, then a number of allergic diseases, including atopic dermatitis and bronchial asthma, may be more effectively managed (Torphy & Undem, 1991; Giembycz, 1992; Torphy *et*

Table 30.6 Isoenzyme selectivity of PDE inhibitors.

Selectivity	Inhibitors
Non-selective	Enprofylline, ibudilast, 3-isobutyl-1-methylxanthine, pentoxifylline, theophylline
1	KS-505a, 3-isobutyl-8-methoxymethyl-1-methylxanthine, vinpocetine, zaprinast
2	Erythro-9-(2-hydroxy-3-nonyl)adenine
3	Amrinone, CI-930, cilostamide, imazodan, milrinone, motapizone, Org 9935, siguazodan, SDZ-MKS-492, SK&F 94120, SK&F 95654, sulmazole
Mixed 3/4	Benafentrine, Org 20241, Org 30029, tolafentrine, zardaverine
4	BRL-1063, CDP-840, denbufylline, LAS-31025, Ro 20-1724, rolipram, RP-73401, RS-23355, SB-207499, tibenelast, WAY-PDA-641
5	Dipyridamole, MY-5445, SK&F 96231, zaprinast
6	Dipyridamole, MY-5445, SK&F 96231, zaprinast
7	None reported

al., 1994; Dent & Giembycz, 1995; Giembycz & Souness, 1996).

Given the therapeutic implications of selective inhibitors of PDE4, it is not surprising that this isoenzyme family is the most rapidly expanding family of PDE. Four mammalian cDNA homologues (Colicelli *et al.*, 1989; Davis *et al.*, 1989; Swinnen *et al.*, 1989a,b) of the *Drosophila melanogaster* 'dunce' cAMP PDE (Chen *et al.*, 1986) have been identified and cloned, establishing a molecular basis for the observed heterogeneity of gene products within this PDE family. These clones, originally denoted rat PDE1–4, represent transcripts of four different genes and have been reclassified according to the nomenclature proposed by Beavo *et al.* (1994). Thus, rat PDE1, PDE2, PDE3 and PDE4 are now known as RNPDE4C, RNPDE4A, RNPDE4D and RNPDE4B, respectively. An astonishing finding that emerged from the molecular cloning of PDE4 isoenzymes is the presence of mRNA transcripts of different sizes for each of the four variants (the potential for more than 15 has been unequivocally identified at the time of writing), which are differentially expressed between tissues (Colicelli *et al.*, 1989; Davis *et al.*, 1989; Swinnen *et al.*, 1989a,b, 1991; Conti *et al.*, 1992; Welsh *et al.*, 1992). An example of this multiplicity is exemplified in germ cells, where five different mRNA transcripts derived from both the RNPDE4A and RNPDE4C gene have been identified (Welsh *et al.*, 1992). Furthermore, mRNA transcripts corresponding to RNPDE4A are present in brain, heart and testis but not in liver or kidney, whereas RNPDE4C mRNA transcripts are localized to the liver and testis only (Conti *et al.*, 1992). Similarly, two forms of RNPDE4B mRNA and three forms of RNPDE4D mRNA are co-expressed in rat Sertoli cells (Monaco *et al.*, 1994). The basis for this profound heterogeneity of PDE4 isoenzymes is attributable not only to alternative mRNA splicing but also to the fact that the PDE4 genes express multiple promoter regions and therefore provide several potential start codons for the translation of the protein (Monaco *et al.*, 1994).

Evidence was recently provided for the existence of at least four human genes that encode PDE4 isoenzymes (Livi *et al.*, 1990; Bolger *et al.*, 1993; McLaughlin *et al.*, 1993; Obernolte *et al.*, 1993; Sullivan *et al.*, 1994; Baecker *et al.*, 1995; Engels *et al.*, 1995). Like their rat counterparts, there is a restricted localization of mRNA transcripts between tissues (Livi *et al.*, 1990; McLaughlin *et al.*, 1993).

Characteristics and properties

A cAMP-specific PDE that was inhibited by the alkoxybenzyl-substituted imidazolidone, Ro 20,1724, but largely unaffected by cGMP (K_i > 200 μmol/l) was originally purified from canine kidney (Thompson *et al.*, 1979; Epstein *et al.*, 1982). It is now appreciated that this was the first report of a PDE4 isoenzyme. Since the original description, PDE4s have been purified and partially characterized from a number of sources, including rat cerebrum and heart (Nemoz *et al.*, 1989), human monocytes (Torphy *et al.*, 1993) and human leucocytes (Truong & Muller, 1994). Apparently without exception, PDE4 isoenzymes are acidic proteins (isoelectric point (pI) = 4 to 6) that preferentially or even exclusively hydrolyse cAMP (K_m = 1 to 20 μmol/l) (Conti & Swinnen, 1990; Bolger *et al.*, 1993). There has been a substantial divergence of opinion regarding the monomeric size of PDE4. However, the recent appreciation of marked heterogeneity among PDE4 isoenzymes may explain the reported differences. Unlike the other PDE isoenzymes, the quaternary structure of PDE4 is currently unclear.

Short-term regulation

A rapid increase in PDE4 activity occurs in many cells and tissues and is not dependent upon new protein synthesis. Recent data suggest that, like other PDE families, the catalytic activity of PDE4 is regulated by protein phosphorylation (Luther *et al.*, 1996; Sette *et al.*, 1994a,b). In the rat thyroid follicular cell line (FRTL-5), for example, thyroid-stimulating hormone evokes a rapid increase in cAMP hydrolysis, which is due to the phosphorylation and subsequent activation of PDE4 (Sette *et al.*, 1994a). Other short-term regulatory mechanisms may include phosphorylation of PDE4 by PKC (Chan *et al.*, 1986) and additional complex post-translational processes that are still to be defined (see Koga *et al.*, 1995).

Long-term regulation

It is well established that a prolonged elevation of intracellular cAMP results in the induction of PDE4 (Schwartz & Passoneau, 1974; Valette *et al.*, 1990; Okonogi *et al.*, 1991; Swinnen *et al.*, 1991; Torphy *et al.*, 1992c). Indeed, this phenomenon represents a common homoeostatic mechanism of cyclic nucleotide regulation. Recent studies have shown that incubating U937 cells with salbutamol and rolipram for up to 24 hours results in a time-dependent increase in the amount of a rolipram-sensitive PDE activity (Torphy *et al.*, 1992c). This phenomenon is dependent upon cAMP accumulation and PKA activation and is slowly reversible after agonist removal. Moreover, the induction involves protein and mRNA synthesis for it is abolished in cells treated with actinomycin D and cycloheximide (Torphy *et al.*, 1992c). Comparable results are obtained when salbutamol is used alone (although the induction is not as marked) and after treatment of the cells with PGE_2 and 8-bromo cAMP (Torphy *et al.*, 1992c).

Similar findings are documented in rat Sertoli cells, where an elevation in the intracellular cAMP concentration by gonadotrophin follicle-stimulating hormone initiates the transcription of two genes which encode two PDE4 sub-types, PDE4D and PDE4B (Swinnen *et al.*, 1991). An increase in PDE4 in inflammatory and immunocompetent cells in response to a variety of stimuli has also been reported (Valette *et al.*, 1990; Okonogi *et al.*, 1991). In concanavalin A-stimulated T lymphocytes (Valette *et al.*, 1990) and lipopolysaccharide-activated macrophages (Okonogi *et al.*, 1991), for example, the increase in PDE4 activity is apparent within an hour. Hanifin and colleagues (Holden *et al.*, 1989; Chan & Hanifin, 1993; Chan *et al.*, 1993a) have also described the appearance of a PDE4-like enzyme in monocytes harvested from subjects with atopic dermatitis. This is discussed in detail in the section 'cAMP PDE activity in allergic diseases'.

Tissue distribution and selective inhibitors

With the possible exception of the platelet, a high-affinity cAMP PDE4 is present in essentially all cell types that have been implicated in allergic disease (Table 30.5). Given the recent molecular biological data on PDE4 heterogeneity, it is not surprising that the complement of PDE4 isogene products is expressed differentially across cells and tissues, including those which comprise the immune system (Table 30.7).

As stated in the introduction, many of the major pharmaceutical companies have invested heavily in PDE research over the last few years. This has resulted in an increase in the number of more potent and isoenzyme-selective inhibitors with which to probe both the molecular and pharmacological role of PDE4 inhibition (Table 30.6). Table 30.2 shows some of the compounds that have been evaluated or are currently undergoing clinical assessment for allergic diseases.

Table 30.7 PDE4 sub-types identified by RT-PCR in respiratory tissues and pro-inflammatory and immunocompetent cells.

Cell tissue	PDE4A	PDE4B	PDE4C	PDE4D
Human lung	++	++	++	++
Human trachea	++	++	++	++
Human eosinophils	++	++	–	++
Guinea pig eosinophils	–	–	–	++
Human neutrophils	±	++	–	±
Human T lymphocytes	++	++	?	++
Human CD4+ T lymphocyte	++	++	–	++
Human CD8+ T lymphocyte	++	++	–	++
Jurkat (T-cell-like)	++	–	–	–
HL-60 cells	++	++	–	–
Namalwa (B-cell-like)	++	++	–	–
Human monocytes	++	++	–	++
Guinea pig macrophage	–	±	–	++
U-937	++	++	–	++

± and – represent weak and no mRNA expression, respectively; ++ represents strong expression.

PDE5 isoenzyme family

Two major cyclic nucleotide PDE families have been described which preferentially or almost exclusively hydrolyse cGMP. One of these is the PDE6 or photoreceptor family and is briefly discussed below. The other family comprises a group of cGMP-specific PDE, which have been isolated and studied primarily from peripheral tissues and are collectively known as PDE5 isoenzymes. These proteins exist as homodimers and display marked selectivity for cGMP (K_m = 3–6 µmol/l) over cAMP (K_m >> 20 µmol/l) (Francis *et al.*, 1990; Thomas *et al.*, 1990a).

PDE5 was first identified in lung (Coquil *et al.*, 1980; Francis *et al.*, 1980) and platelets (Coquil *et al.*, 1985) and has since been purified to homogeneity from a number of tissues (Francis *et al.*, 1980; Thomas, 1990a; Robichon, 1991). At the present time, only a single gene has been identified which encodes a PDE5 (Thomas *et al.*, 1990; Bentley & Beavo, 1992), although the presence of others is likely. Transcription of this gene can give rise to two PDE5 isoenzymes (PDE5A1 and PDE5A2) through alternative mRNA splicing (Thomas *et al.*, 1990a), the former protein having a deduced molecular weight, derived from the largest opening reading frame of the corresponding cDNA, of 97.6 kDa (Thomas *et al.*, 1990a).

PDE5 is a substrate for cyclic nucleotide-dependent protein kinases. Both the bovine lung and platelet isoenzymes are phosphorylated by PKG and, to a lesser extent, PKA (Francis *et al.*, 1990; Thomas *et al.*, 1990b; Robichon, 1991). Incubation of partially purified PDE5 from guinea pig lung with the catalytic subunit of PKA in the presence of adenosine triphosphate (ATP) stimulates cGMP degradation by increasing the V_{max} of the reaction (Burns *et al.*, 1992). Significantly, this effect is associated with a decrease in the potency of the selective PDE5 inhibitor, zaprinast (Burns *et al.*, 1992).

Tissue distribution, selective inhibitors and therapeutic implications

PDE5 isoenzymes are widely distributed (Table 30.5). Significant amounts are present in airway smooth muscle (Souness & Giembycz, 1994), platelets (Hidaka *et al.*, 1984) and airway epithelial cells (Rousseau *et al.*, 1994), and traces of this enzyme have been detected in mast cells, alveolar macrophages, neutrophils, basophils (Peachell *et al.*, 1992) and vascular endothelial cells (Souness *et al.*, 1990; Torphy & Undem, 1991; Giembycz, 1992; Suttorp *et al.*, 1993; Schudt & Tenor, 1994). Despite this apparent ubiquity, drugs which selectively inhibit PDE5, such as zaprinast, SK&F 96231 and MY 5445 (Tables 30.3 & 30.6) are generally, inactive or only weakly active at suppressing functional responses in these cell types. The reason for this is unclear but may relate to a low basal guanylyl cyclase activity, which would render PDE5 inhibitors unable to increase the cGMP content to a biochemically active concentration (Souness & Giembycz, 1994). Alternatively, some of these compounds may not readily permeate cells. Indeed, the finding that zaprinast, the only selective inhibitor of the PDE5 isoenzyme family that has been extensively characterized (Murray, 1993), is ionized at physiological pH supports this contention. It is also possible that PDE5 may exist predominantly in a phosphorylated form, for which zaprinast-like inhibitors have significantly less affinity (Burns *et al.*, 1992).

From a therapeutic standpoint, selective inhibitors of the PDE5 isoenzyme family are unlikely to have any major impact upon inflammatory reactions, although a modest degree of bronchodilatation may be elicited and afford some benefit in disease states characterized by reversible air-flow limitation such as allergic asthma (Giembycz, 1992; Murray, 1993). However, the concept of hybrid PDE inhibitors which act selectively on both the PDE4 and PDE5 isoenzyme families is attractive from the point of view of asthma therapy. Indeed, the rationale for adopting a mixed inhibitor approach would be to provide optimal anti-inflammatory (PDE4-mediated) and bronchodilator (PDE5-mediated) activity within the same molecule, while reducing potential cardiovascular complications that are predicted with dual PDE3/PDE4-selective inhibitors (see section on PDE3 and PDE4 inhibitors under 'Side-effects and potential limitations . . .').

PDE6 isoenzyme family

cGMP-specific PDEs are present in high concentrations in the outer segments of both the cones and the rods of the eye, where they are believed to be intimately involved in visual phototransduction (Stryer, 1986; Hurley, 1987; Stryer & Bourne, 1988). In the dark, these enzymes are essentially inert. However, following the absorption of light by the photopigments of the retina, light-dependent cGMP hydrolysis occurs, which is a requisite for the normal processes of phototransduction.

Originally, the photoreceptor PDEs were categorized as PDE5 isoenzymes. However, primary sequence analyses have identified marked differences between the PDEs of the retina and the PDE5 isoenzymes described above. Accordingly, the cGMP-specific PDEs in the cone and rod photoreceptors are now referred to as members of the PDE6 isoenzyme family.

Although it is likely that PDE6 is expressed in cells and tissues other than the retina, calmodulin-independent, cGMP hydrolytic activity is not common in immune and pro-inflammatory cells. The characteristics and properties of PDE6 are, therefore, not discussed here. For further information, interested readers are directed towards comprehensive critiques of this subject (Stryer, 1986; Hurley, 1987; Stryer & Bourne, 1988).

PDE7 isoenzyme family

In 1993, a gene isolated from a human glioblastoma cDNA library was expressed in a cAMP PDE-deficient strain of the yeast, *Saccharomyces cerevisiae* (Michaeli *et al.*, 1993). This novel gene, named high-affinity, cAMP-specific phosphodiesterase 1 gene (*HCP 1*) encodes a high-affinity (K_m = 0.2 µmol/l) cAMP-specific PDE which is insensitive to cGMP and inhibitors of the PDE3 and PDE4 isoenzyme families and does not hydrolyse cGMP (Michaeli *et al.*, 1993). Furthermore, although *HCP 1* shares sequence identity with the catalytic domain of all cyclic nucleotide PDE, it does not share extensive homology with the *Drosophila* dunce cAMP PDE (i.e. PDE4) and therefore appears to represent a member of a previously unrecognized PDE family, which has been designated PDE7 (Michaeli *et al.*, 1993).

Tissue distribution, selective inhibitors and therapeutic implications

Northern blot analyses have identified an abundance of PDE7 mRNA transcripts in human skeletal muscle. In addition, transcripts of identical size are present in human heart and kidney (Michaeli *et al.*, 1993). In the context of allergic diseases, an enzyme, termed JK-21, is expressed in several T-cell lines, including Jurkat, MOLT-4, HPB-ALL and HUT-78 (Ichimura & Kase, 1993), and shares several notable similarities with the *HCP 1* gene product expressed in *S. cerevisiae*. The possibility that this represents a PDE7 is suggested by Bloom and Beavo (1994), who have identified high levels of PDE7 mRNA in HUT-78 cells. More recently, evidence has emerged that PDE7 mRNA is ubiquitously expressed throughout mammalian tissues, including human peripheral blood CD4+ and CD8+ T lymphocytes (Giembycz *et al.*, 1996).

cAMP PDE activity in allergic diseases

cAMP PDE activity in leucocytes from atopic individuals

cAMP PDE activity is significantly elevated in mononuclear leucocytes (MNL) harvested from individuals with atopic disorders, including dermatitis, allergic rhinitis and asthma (Grewe *et al.*, 1982; Bachelet *et al.*, 1991; Townley, 1993; Goldberg *et al.*, 1994). Similar observations have also been made in MNL from patients with urticaria pigmentosa (Holden, 1990). This phenomenon is most prominent in blood monocytes (Holden *et al.*, 1986) but is also observed to a lesser extent in other immunocompetent cells, such as T lymphocytes (Chan & Hanifin, 1993) and neutrophils (Goldberg *et al.*, 1994). Curiously, the influence of atopy on cAMP PDE levels may be limited to bone marrow-derived cells since there is no apparent difference in the cAMP PDE activities in keratinocytes from normal and atopic individuals (Wright *et al.*, 1991).

Two immunochemically distinct cAMP PDE apparently exist in monocytes harvested from patients with atopic dermatitis, whereas only one form is expressed in monocytes purified from normal subjects under identical experimental conditions (Chan *et al.*, 1993a); in all cases these activities are sensitive to Ro-20-1424 and rolipram, suggesting that they represent PDE4 isoenzymes. Intriguingly, however, the Ro-20-1724-sensitive cAMP PDE unique to monocytes from atopic subjects is difficult to categorize as a PDE4 since it is stimulated by calcium and calmodulin (Holden *et al.*, 1989; Chan & Hanifin, 1993; Chan *et al.*, 1993a). Furthermore, the 'atopic' monocyte PDE is more potently inhibited by rolipram and other PDE4 inhibitors than the cAMP PDE obtained from non-atopic volunteers and displays distinct kinetic characteristics (Chan & Hanifin, 1993). Of particular interest is that theophylline exhibits an IC_{50} value of 27 μmol/l against the 'atopic' isoenzyme (Chan & Hanifin, 1993), which is approximately 20-fold lower than for the human monocyte enzyme from normal individuals.

Possible causes for increased cAMP PDE in mononuclear leucocytes from atopic individuals

Primary gene defect

The cause of the elevated cAMP PDE activity expressed by atopic MNL is uncertain. A primary gene defect may be responsible, which, if correct, might implicate increased cAMP PDE as an important factor in the aetiology of allergic disorders. The apparent novel properties of the atopic cAMP PDE may point to such a conclusion. Further evidence to support this contention is the finding that MNL taken from the cord blood of children born to atopic parents exhibits elevated cAMP PDE activity, suggesting that the defect might be inherited (Heskel *et al.*, 1984), although not all studies have demonstrated elevated MNL cAMP PDE in young children with atopic dermatitis (Coulson *et al.*, 1989). Furthermore, cAMP PDE activity remains high in individuals with atopic dermatitis whose disease is in complete remission following steroid therapy (Holden & Yuen, 1989), indicating that the phenomenon is not a consequence of inflammation. However, the strength of this latter evidence is questionable in view of the results from another study showing that prolonged steroid therapy results in restoration of normal cAMP PDE levels (Holden *et al.*, 1989). Finally, the genetic hypothesis is further supported by the demonstration of increased MNL cAMP PDE in a Basenji greyhound model of asthma and eczema (Chan *et al.*, 1985). In these dogs, MNL cAMP PDE is elevated in both unsensitized and sensitized dogs (Chan *et al.*, 1985).

Atopy and inflammation

The increase in cAMP PDE activity could also be a consequence of the atopy or of the associated inflammatory processes. Various studies have demonstrated that cAMP PDE can be induced by a number of agents which increase the intracellular concentration of cAMP (see above). Similarly, substances released during inflammatory reactions, such as cytokines and mediators, are known to influence cAMP PDE activity in bone marrow-derived cells. For example, histamine increases cAMP PDE activity in normal monocytes to levels seen in cells purified from atopic individuals, possibly by elevating intracellular cAMP (Holden *et al.*, 1987). A greater elevation of monocyte cAMP PDE is observed when mixed MNL are exposed to histamine compared to exposure of purified monocytes (Holden *et al.*, 1987). It is conceivable that, in atopy, unrestrained mediator release occurs in the skin and the mucosal surfaces of the lung and gut in response to neurohumoral and antigenic stimuli, which leads to increased MNL cAMP PDE activity, which may initiate the clinically observable signs of atopy (Hanifin *et al.*, 1985). Monocyte cAMP PDE activity is also increased following a 1 hour exposure of cells to interferon-γ (IFN-γ) (Li *et al.*, 1992, 1993), an effect enhanced by IL-4 (Li *et al.*, 1992). This only occurs in cells from normal subjects, since IFN-γ does not influence the already elevated cAMP PDE activity in monocytes from patients with atopic dermatitis (Li *et al.*, 1993).

Possible consequences of elevated mononuclear leucocyte cAMP PDE activity in atopic individuals

Decreased responsiveness to agents that stimulate cAMP synthesis, such as histamine, PGE_1 and β-adrenoceptor agonists, has been observed in MNL from atopic humans and Basenji greyhounds (Safko *et al.*, 1981; Chan *et al.*, 1982, 1985; Grewe *et al.*, 1982). Ro-20-1724 restores the responsiveness to β-adrenoceptor agonists (Chan *et al.*, 1985), suggesting that accelerated intracellular cAMP hydrolysis is responsible for this defect in atopic MNL. The contribution that alternative down-regulatory processes make to the hyporesponsiveness of the cAMP cascade in atopy is uncertain. Heterologous down-regulation of adenylyl cyclase responses can be induced by inflammatory cytokines (Beckner & Farrar, 1986; van Oosterhout *et al.*, 1992). Furthermore, agents that stimulate cAMP synthesis can induce tolerance in inflammatory cells by homologous and heterologous down-regulation of adenylyl-cyclase-linked receptors (Lefkowitz *et al.*, 1990; Chuang *et al.*, 1992).

Elevated cAMP PDE activity has been correlated with the increased histamine release (Butler *et al.*, 1983) and hyper-IgE synthesis (Cooper *et al.*, 1985) which are characteristic of atopic MNL. The suppression of histamine and IgE production from atopic MNL by Ro-20-1724 (Butler *et al.*, 1983; Cooper *et al.*, 1985) indicates a causal link between accelerated cAMP hydrolysis and these functional defects.

It has been speculated (Chan *et al.*, 1993b) that the increased cAMP PDE in monocytes from atopics results in lowered intracellular cAMP and enhanced PGE_2 generation, which, in turn, inhibits IFN-γ production from Th1 cells. Since IFN-γ inhibits cytokine release from Th2 cells, it was proposed that inhibition of its release would disinhibit the generation of IL-4, causing B-lymphocyte antibody class switching and the production of IgE (Chan *et al.*, 1993b,c). High levels of PGE_2 are released from atopic monocytes and a highly significant negative correlation exists between PGE_2 and IFN-γ levels in supernatants of atopic MNL in culture (Chan *et al.*, 1993b,c). Furthermore, the increase in IL-4 production evoked by anti-CD3 by atopic MNL correlates with elevated cAMP PDE and a relatively low concentration (1 μmol/l) of Ro-20-1724 inhibits the release of this cytokine, apparently via an action on monocytes (Chan *et al.*, 1993c).

The observations detailed above are intriguing, given that cAMP PDE inhibitors (Rott *et al.*, 1993), like other agents which elevate cAMP (Munoz *et al.*, 1990; Novak & Rothenberg, 1990; Betz & Fox, 1991), are considered to be much more effective inhibitors of cytokine production from Th1 cells than from Th2 cells. These apparently paradoxical findings show that the effects of cAMP on T lymphocytes in a mixed MNL population are difficult to predict from studies on their counterparts in purified populations. Furthermore, cAMP responses in atopic T lymphocytes may differ substantially from those reported in animal or human Th sub-type clones.

Theophylline

Theophylline was originally identified by Kossel in Berlin in 1888 and subsequently synthesized 12 years later by Boehringer. However, more than two decades elapsed before the bronchodilator activity of theophylline in humans was realized (Schultz-Werninghaus & Seier-Sydow, 1982). Since then, theophylline, and related alkylxanthines, have occupied a position of superiority in the treatment of asthma and are the most widely prescribed anti-asthma medications in the world. Despite the long history of theophylline, controversy still surrounds the molecular mechanisms responsible for its therapeutic activity, and several possibilities have been advanced that are not necessarily mutually exclusive (Fig. 30.4). With the exception of PDE inhibition, which forms the subject of this chapter, these are discussed elsewhere, along with the chemistry, pharmacokinetics and pharmacodynamics of this group of compounds (see Barnes & Pauwels, 1994; Barnes, 1995, and references therein).

PDE isoenzyme distribution in cells implicated in allergic diseases

The distribution of PDE isoenzymes in cell types implicated in allergic and inflammatory reactions is summarized in Table 30.5. It is important to emphasize that the predominant isoenzyme family represented in these cells is PDE4; PDE3 isoenzymes are also found in certain immune cells, but their distribution is less widespread. Representatives of the PDE1, PDE2, PDE5 and PDE7 families have also been identified in certain pro-inflammatory and immunocompetent cells, but their function is unclear at present.

Effect of PDE inhibitors on cells implicated in the pathogenesis of allergic diseases

The vast majority of information on the effects of theophylline and isoenzyme-selective PDE inhibitors on cell types implicated in allergic diseases and inflammation derives from studies on cells harvested from normal

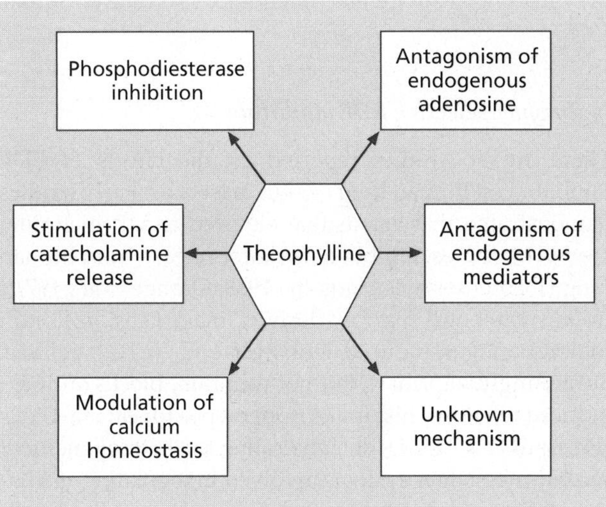

Fig. 30.4 Mechanisms postulated to account for the therapeutic efficacy of theophylline in asthma.

subjects or laboratory animals (Table 30.8). Given the evidence indicating that inflammatory and immunocompetent cells from atopic subjects may be defective (see the section 'cAMP PDE activity in allergic diseases'), the relevance of experiments conducted on 'normal' cells is questionable. In addition, to extrapolate findings obtained using isolated cells to the *in vivo* or pathological situation must also be viewed with caution. It is likely, for example, that individual immunocompetent and inflammatory cells which are highly dependent on other leucocytes for their functional responses behave entirely differently in whole blood or mixed leucocyte preparations than when in isolation. Nevertheless, preliminary evidence accrued from studies conducted in isolated cells and in *in vivo* models indicate that selective inhibitors of the PDE4 isoenzyme family show considerable therapeutic potential.

Mast cells and basophils

Theophylline

It has been established for more than 30 years that theophylline suppresses the release of histamine from mast cells and basophils (Orange *et al.*, 1971; Pearce *et al.*, 1982; Louis & Radermecker, 1990). However, the relevance of this action in the *in vivo* situation is likely to be insignificant, since these effects are seen in concentrations of theophylline far in excess of those used therapeutically. Intriguingly, theophylline inhibits the enhancement of antigen-induced histamine release from the lung parenchyma of sensitized guinea pigs at plasma concentrations achieved clinically (Welton & Simko, 1980), which has prompted the suggestion that some of the beneficial effects of theophylline are attributable to antagonizing the effects of endogenous adenosine (Welton & Simko, 1980).

Isoenzyme-selective PDE inhibitors

There are no studies reported on the effects of PDE inhibitors on human lung or skin mast cells. Early studies demonstrated that agents that elevated cAMP, including methylxanthines, inhibited mediator release from human lung (Lichtenstein & Margolis, 1968; Orange *et al.*, 1971). In murine bone marrow-derived mast cells, rolipram inhibits antigen-induced leukotriene C_4 (LTC_4) release. Surprisingly, zaprinast, but not rolipram, blocks antigen-induced release of histamine from rat peritoneal mast cells (Frossard *et al.*, 1981), demonstrating the heterogeneity of second-messenger systems involved in regulating mediator release from different populations of mast cells.

Rolipram inhibits antigen- and anti-IgE-induced mediator (histamine, LTC_4) liberation from human basophils (Frossard *et al.*, 1981; Peachell *et al.*, 1992), which is potentiated by the PDE3 inhibitors, siguazodan and SK&F 95654 (Peachell *et al.*, 1992). Although zaprinast, surprisingly, increases the cAMP content in these cells, it does not inhibit mediator release (Peachell *et al.*, 1992).

T lymphocytes and B lymphocytes

Theophylline

The direct *in vitro* effects of theophylline on T-lymphocyte function are limited to inhibition of E-rosette formation (index of maturation), proliferation and the generation of IL-2 in a mixed population of T lymphocytes in response to mitogenic stimuli (Limatibul *et al.*, 1978; Bruserud, 1984; Mary, 1987) and antigen (Scordamaglia *et al.*, 1988). Theophylline also suppresses IFN-γ-induced IL-2 biosynthesis in a cultured T-cell line (Hancock *et al.*, 1988). These actions may account, at least in part, for the ability of theophylline to suppress pro-inflammatory cell infiltration to sites of allergen entry, especially the lung. Coskey *et al.* (1993) recently reported that theophylline suppresses the activity of natural killer cells at concentrations used clinically. No information is available on the effects of theophylline in B lymphocytes.

Isoenzyme-selective PDE inhibitors

Inhibitors of PDE4 and, to a modest extent, PDE3, suppress phytohaemagglutinin (PHA)-induced blastogenesis of a mixed population of human purified T lymphocytes (Robicsek *et al.*, 1991). Only partial (50–70%) inhibition is observed when inhibitors are tested individually, but a combination of a PDE3 and PDE4 inhibitor, or the addition of a mixed-type inhibitor, elicits a much greater effect (Robicsek *et al.*, 1991). Similar results are obtained when highly purified preparations of human CD4+ and CD8+ T cells are used (Giembycz *et al.*, 1996) and in a human Th2 clone established from aeroallergen-specific T cells obtained from atopic donors (Crocker *et al.*, 1994). In the latter study, the selective PDE4 inhibitor, WAY PDA-641, and theophylline suppressed the generation of IL-4 induced by anti-CD3. Inhibition of IL-2 generation may be one mechanism by which cAMP PDE inhibitors exert their antiproliferative effects (Averill *et al.*, 1988; Thanhauser *et al.*, 1993; Giembycz *et al.*, 1994). Indeed, rolipram potently inhibits the generation of IFN-γ and IL-2 in CD4+ and CD8+ T cells stimulated with PHA under conditions where the PDE3 inhibitor, SK&F 95654, is inactive (Giembycz *et al.*, 1996). This conclusion may have to be reinterpreted, however, given that rolipram and CI-930 inhibit concanavalin A-induced murine splenocyte proliferation at concentrations below those required to suppress IL-2 generation (Lewis *et al.*, 1993), suggesting that

Table 30.8 *In vitro* effects of PDE inhibitors upon cells implicated in allergic/inflammatory diseases.

Cell type	Functional effect of PDE inhibitor	Comments	Reference
Mast cells	Inhibitor of histamine and LTC_4 release (H,M)	PDE5 but not PDE4 inhibitors suppress mediator release from rat peritoneal mast cells	Torphy and Undem (1991) Frossard *et al.* (1981)
Basophils	Inhibition of mediator release (H)	PDE3 inhibitors enhance the actions of PDE4 inhibitors	Peachell *et al.* (1992)
T lymphocytes (mixed population)	Inhibition of proliferation (H)	PDE3 inhibitors enhance the actions of PDE4 inhibitors	Robicsek *et al.* (1991) Averill *et al.* (1988)
	Inhibition of IL-2 expression (H)		Averill *et al.* (1988) Lewis *et al.* (1993)
CD4+ T lymphocytes CD8+ T lymphocytes	Inhibition of proliferation and the secretion of IL-2 and IFN-γ (H)	PDE3 inhibitors enhance the actions of PDE4 inhibitors	Giembycz *et al.* (1995)
B lymphocytes	Inhibition of IgE biosynthesis (H?)	Non-specific PDE inhibitors suppress proliferation and either increase or decrease IgE production	Kammer (1988) Cooper *et al.* (1985)
Monocytes	*Inhibition of:*		
	Arachidonic acid breakdown (H)		Godfrey *et al.* (1987)
	Phagocytosis (H)		Bessler *et al.* (1986)
	Superoxide generation (H)		Bessler *et al.* (1986)
	TNF-α release (H)	PDE inhibitors only weakly suppress IL-1β release	Semmler *et al.* (1993b) Molnar-Kimber *et al.* (1993) Hartman *et al.* (1993) Verghese *et al.* (1995) Seldon *et al.* (1995)
Eosinophils	*Inhibition of:*		
	Superoxide generation (H/GP)		Dent *et al.* (1991, 1994); Souness *et al.* (1991)
	Thromboxane release (GP)		Souness *et al.* (1994, 1995)
	Chemotaxis (GP)		Cohan *et al.* (1992)
	Degranulation (H/GP)	Effect observed with IBMX	Kita *et al.* (1991) Souness *et al.* (1995)
Neutrophils	*Inhibition of:*		
	Superoxide generation (H)		Nielson *et al.* (1990) Wright *et al.* (1990) Schudt *et al.* (1991c) Ho *et al.* (1990)
	Chemotaxis (H)		Harvath *et al.* (1991)
	Phagocytosis (H)		Bessler *et al.* (1986)
	Mediator release (H)		Fonteh *et al.* (1993)
	Degranulation (H)		Wright *et al.* (1990) cf. Busse and Anderson (1981)
Endothelial cells	Reduction of permeability of monolayers (P)	PDE3 and PDE4 inhibitors reduce permeability of pulmonary artery endothelial cells	Suttorp *et al.* (1993)
Macrophages	*Inhibition of:*		
	Hydrogen peroxide generation	Effect of PDE3 and PDE4 inhibitors weak	Dent *et al.* (1993)
	Superoxide generation (GP)		Lim *et al.* (1983); Turner *et al.* (1993)
	Mediator release (M)		Schade and Schudt (1993)
	TNF-α release (M)		Okonogi *et al.* (1991) Schade and Schudt (1993)
Platelets	*Inhibition of:*		
	Calcium mobilization (H)		Simpson *et al.* (1988)
	Aggregation (H)		Muggli *et al.* (1985)
	Mediator (ATP, 5-HT, β-thromboglobulin) release (H)		Seiler *et al.* (1987)
Epithelial cells	Inhibition of PGE_2 generation (H)	Effect observed with IBMX	Rabe *et al.* (1994)

GP, guinea pig; H, human; M, mouse; P, pig; see text for definition of other abbreviations.

their antiproliferative effects are independent of IL-2 gene transcription (Lewis *et al.*, 1993). This conclusion is supported by the finding that, in Jurkat cells, neither rolipram nor CI-930 affect steady-state levels of IL-2 mRNA (Lewis *et al.*, 1993). It is also worthy of consideration that PDE inhibitors may exert their effects by blocking mitogenic signal transduction systems (van Tits *et al.*, 1991; Anastassiou *et al.*, 1992). Indeed, agents that elevate cAMP inhibit anti-CD3-induced tyrosine phosphorylation of a 100 kDa protein implicated in T-cell activation, as well as decreasing IL-2 biosynthesis and IL-2 receptor expression (Anastassiou *et al.*, 1992). The decrease in IL-2 evoked by cAMP-elevating agents may relate to an effect on IL-2 gene transcription and a decrease in the half-life ($t\frac{1}{2}$) for IL-2 mRNA degradation (Anastassiou *et al.*, 1992).

Few studies, to date, have compared the actions of PDE inhibitors on Th1 and Th2 CD4+ T-lymphocyte functions. The weak, non-selective PDE inhibitor, pentoxifylline, is more effective at inhibiting the release of IL-2 (Th1-derived) than IL-4 (Th2-derived) (Rott *et al.*, 1993), a finding consistent with a wide body of evidence demonstrating that cAMP is more effective in suppressing the release of IL-2 and IFN-γ than of IL-4 and IL-5 (Munoz *et al.*, 1990; Novak & Rothenberg, 1990; Betz & Fox, 1991; van der Poow-Kraan *et al.*, 1992; Lee *et al.*, 1993; Tsuruta *et al.*, 1995). Indeed, under certain conditions, cAMP activates transcription of the IL-4 and IL-5 genes (Lee *et al.*, 1993; Watanabe *et al.*, 1994; Tsuruta *et al.*, 1995). In sensitized BALB/c mice, however, rolipram inhibits the appearance of IL-4 and IL-5 in bronchoalveolar lavage fluid (BALF) and in spleen cells following allergen challenge (Foissier *et al.*, 1995; Lonchampt *et al.*, 1995). Similarly, rolipram, but not siguazodan and zaprinast, more effectively blocks tetanus toxoid (Th1)- than ragweed (Th2)-driven proliferation of peripheral blood MNL (Essayan *et al.*, 1994). Reverse transcription–polymerase chain reaction revealed that rolipram attenuates IL-5 and IFN-γ, but not IL-4, gene transcription following allergen provocation (Essayan *et al.*, 1994). Furthermore, the Th1-like Jurkat cell line expresses a low level of mRNA for PDE4A (human monocyte enzyme (Livi *et al.*, 1990)) but no detectable message for PDE4B (human brain enzyme (McLaughlin *et al.*, 1993)). In contrast, the ragweed-specific oligoclonal Th2 cell line expresses mRNA for both PDE4 variants (Essayan *et al.*, 1994). Based upon these results, it is possible that the ability of rolipram to suppress Th2 T-cell proliferation may be dictated by the selective expression of PDE4 isoenzymes in Th2 cells (Essayan *et al.*, 1994).

The inhibition of Th2-derived cytokines by cAMP PDE inhibitors is observed only in a mixed population of atopic MNL and not in purified T cells. This effect is apparently mediated indirectly via monocytes and demonstrates that the effects of these inhibitors on isolated inflammatory and immunocompetent cells may be a poor indicator of their actions in whole blood or *in vivo*.

The effect of PDE inhibitors on B-lymphocyte function is poorly studied. Agents that elevate cAMP either decrease or increase antibody production and may be dependent on the time of drug addition (Kammer, 1988). Proliferation of B lymphocytes is inhibited by cAMP (Kammer, 1988). Since reduction of proliferation is associated with differentiation, it is of interest that recent studies (Lycke *et al.*, 1990; Phipps *et al.*, 1990; Roper *et al.*, 1990; Lycke, 1993; Paul-Eugene *et al.*, 1993) indicate that cAMP can, paradoxically, induce antibody class switching in B lymphocytes, leading to production of IgG1 and IgE. In spite of this, the only report, to the authors' knowledge, on the effects of PDE inhibitors on antibody production shows that in MNL from patients with atopic dermatitis Ro-20-1724 inhibits spontaneous IgE release (Cooper *et al.*, 1985). This inhibition is not observed in monocyte-depleted cells, demonstrating that the effect is indirect (Cooper *et al.*, 1985) and may be due to the suppression of IL-4 release (Chan *et al.*, 1993c). An action of PDE4 inhibitors on T cells may also contribute to the effects of cAMP on antibody production. IL-2 can contribute to the production of IgE in a mixed population of human leucocytes (Phipps *et al.*, 1990). Inhibition of IL-2 release may explain why PGE_2 mildly inhibits IgE synthesis in MNL composed of B and T lymphocytes as well as monocytes (Phipps *et al.*, 1990).

Monocytes and macrophages

Theophylline

In human alveolar macrophages purified from BALF of non-asthmatic individuals undergoing diagnostic bronchoscopy, theophylline suppresses the release of reactive oxygen species (Calhoun *et al.*, 1991; Dent *et al.*, 1994). This effect apparently involves PDE inhibition, for it is reversed in the presence of Rp 8-bromo adenosine 3′,5′-monophosphorothioate, an inhibitor of cAMP-dependent protein kinase (Dent *et al.*, 1994). Significantly, macrophages isolated from individuals who are taking theophylline are significantly less active than 'normal' cells, indicating that the plasma concentration achieved is therapeutically relevant (O'Neill *et al.*, 1986).

In human peripheral blood monocytes, micromolar concentrations of theophylline effectively inhibit the induction of TNF-α and, to a lesser extent, IL-1β by lipopolysaccharide (LPS) and IL-1α, respectively (Ghezzi & Dinarello, 1988; Endres *et al.*, 1991; Semmler *et al.*, 1993b). Low concentrations of theophylline also inhibit the generation of LTB_4 in these cells (Juergens *et al.*, 1993).

Isoenzyme-selective PDE inhibitors

PDE inhibitors suppress several functions of monocytes, including arachidonic acid breakdown (Godfrey *et al.*, 1987), phagocytosis (Bessler *et al.*, 1986) and superoxide formation (Bessler *et al.*, 1986). Inhibitors of PDE4 are particularly effective in suppressing LPS-induced TNF-α release from human monocytes (Molnar-Kimber *et al.*, 1992; Semmler *et al.*, 1993a; Seldon *et al.*, 1995; Verghese *et al.*, 1995) and alveolar macrophages (Schudt *et al.*, 1992), primarily through an effect on gene transcription (Verghese *et al.*, 1995). Inhibitors of PDE3 elicit only a weak inhibitory effect and PDE1 inhibitors are inactive, while PDE5 inhibitors are either inactive (Seldon *et al.*, 1995) or augment the LPS-induced release of TNF-α (Molnar-Kimber *et al.*, 1992). Although some early reports suggested that cAMP post-transcriptionally inhibits IL-1β release (Knudsen *et al.*, 1986), the effect of PDE4 inhibition is weak in comparison with the suppression of TNF-α generation (Molnar-Kimber *et al.*, 1992). The PDE3 inhibitor, CI-930, and vinpocetine (PDE1 inhibitor) exert little influence on monocyte IL-1β generation; consistent with its effect on TNF-α generation, zaprinast augments the LPS response (Molnar-Kimber *et al.*, 1992). The inhibitory effects of PDE4 inhibitors on LPS-induced TNF-α generation have also been reported in whole blood (Hartman *et al.*, 1993) and *in vivo* (Ochalski *et al.*, 1993).

The generation of superoxide and LTC_4 by guinea pig, mouse and human macrophages is inhibited by PDE4 inhibitors (Lim *et al.*, 1983; Dent *et al.*, 1993; Schade & Schudt, 1993; Turner *et al.*, 1993). As in monocytes, LPS-induced TNF-α generation in macrophages is exquisitely sensitive to the inhibitory effects of PDE4 inhibitors and much lower concentrations are required for suppression of this cytokine than are required for the inhibition of prostanoid generation (Schade & Schudt, 1993). Expression of major histocompatibility complex (MHC) class II molecules is inhibited by agents that elevate cAMP, including PDE inhibitors (Snyder *et al.*, 1982), which may have implications for the presentation of antigen to T cells in atopic disorders.

Eosinophils and neutrophils

Theophylline

The respiratory burst evoked by serum-opsonized zymosan (SOZ) in guinea pig and human eosinophils is suppressed by theophylline (Yukawa *et al.*, 1989) at concentrations that attenuate cAMP hydrolysis in washed membranes and elevate the cAMP content in intact cells (Dent *et al.*, 1991; Souness *et al.*, 1991). 8-Phenyltheophylline, a structural analogue that is not a PDE inhibitor, does not inhibit oxidative metabolism in these cells even when high concentrations are used, providing support for the idea that theophylline exerts its effect by inhibition of PDE (Yukawa *et al.*, 1989).

Paradoxically, at plasma concentrations of theophylline achieved therapeutically, SOZ-induced respiratory burst is augmented (~40%) by theophylline due to the antagonism of endogenously released adenosine. Indeed, the application of exogenous adenosine inhibits SOZ-evoked superoxide anion generation and an increase in oxidative metabolism is also seen with 8-phenyltheophylline, which is a more potent adenosine receptor antagonist than theophylline (Yukawa *et al.*, 1989). Pharmacological experiments have determined that an A_2 receptor sub-type probably mediates the inhibitory influence of adenosine on superoxide formation as 5′-*N*-ethylcarboximide adenosine has a greater inhibitory effect than R-*N*-phenylisopropyl adenosine (Yukawa *et al.*, 1989).

Endogenously released adenosine thus appears to exert an inhibitory effect on the nicotinamide adenine dinucleotide phosphate (NADPH) oxidase in eosinophils under normal conditions and that at therapeutic concentrations theophylline antagonizes this protective effect. This phenomenon has been documented in other leucocytes (Schrier & Imrie, 1986) and may have important therapeutic implications, as theophylline could theoretically exacerbate rather than ameliorate certain leucocyte-driven inflammatory reactions by enhancing the production of reactive oxygen-derived free radicals.

In apparent contrast, low concentrations of theophylline, which enhance SOZ-induced respiratory burst, effectively suppress prostanoid formation and degranulation evoked by LTB_4 and Ig-coated Sepharose beads, respectively (Kita *et al.*, 1991; Giembycz, 1992). A preliminary report also documents that theophylline promotes a programmed cell death or apoptosis of eosinophils maintained in culture with IL-5 (Ohta *et al.*, 1994).

Although neutrophils have an uncertain role in atopic disorders, their sensitivity to theophylline and selective PDE inhibitors has been evaluated. In studies performed by Nielson *et al.* (1986, 1988), therapeutic concentrations of theophylline suppressed the generation of reactive oxygen metabolites and potentiated the inhibitory action of isoprenaline. Paradoxically, other reports suggest that theophylline augments respiratory burst activity in neutrophils (Schrier & Imrie, 1986; Kaneko *et al.*, 1990). The reason for this discrepancy has not been investigated but could be due to the concentration of stimulus employed or to the antagonism of endogenous adenosine as reported in human eosinophils (see above). Inhibitors of PDE4 but not PDE3 reduce the adhesion of human neutrophils to human umbilical vein endothelial cells in response to formyl-methionyl-leucyl-phenylalanine (f-MLP). This effect was apparently due to a down-regulation of the β2 integrin CD11b/CD18 on the endothelial cells (Derian *et al.*, 1995). Interestingly, the inhibitory effect of PDE4 inhibitors was prevented by adenosine deaminase, implicating endogenous adenosine in this phenomenon (Derian *et al.*, 1995).

Isoenzyme-selective PDE inhibitors

PDE4 inhibitors, as well as mixed PDE3/4 inhibitors, suppress superoxide anion and H_2O_2 generation from guinea pig and human eosinophils in response to particulate and soluble stimuli (Dent *et al.*, 1991, 1994; Souness *et al.*, 1991, 1995; Maruo *et al.*, 1994; Barnette *et al.*, 1995; Hatzelmann *et al.*, 1995; Nicholson *et al.*, 1995). PDE4 inhibitors also reduce LTB_4-induced thromboxane biosynthesis (Souness *et al.*, 1994, 1995; Nicholson *et al.*, 1995), the exocytosis of eosinophil cationic protein and major basic protein (Souness *et al.*, 1995), IgG- and secretory IgA-induced degranulation (Kita *et al.*, 1991) and hrC5a-, PAF- and f-MLP-induced eosinophil chemotaxis (Cohan *et al.*, 1994; Tanimoto *et al.*, 1994). In contrast to theophylline, the selective PDE4 inhibitor, rolipram, does not promote apoptosis in eosinophils cultured in the presence of GM-CSF (Hallsworth *et al.*, 1996).

In human neutrophils, PDE inhibitors suppress the biosynthesis of both PAF and LTB_4 in response to f-MLP and the Ca^{2+} ionophore, calcimycin (Fonteh *et al.*, 1993), reduce neutrophil chemotaxis evoked by butanol-extracted *E. coli* (Rivkin & Neutze, 1977), f-MLP and LTB_4 (Harvath *et al.*, 1987) and inhibit degranulation (Zurier *et al.*, 1974; Nourshargh & Hoult, 1986) and phagocytosis (Bessler *et al.*, 1986). Activation of the respiratory burst oxidase by f-MLP is similarly sensitive to PDE4 inhibitors, such as rolipram, Ro-20-1724 and tibenelast (Ho *et al.*, 1990; Nielson *et al.*, 1990; Wright *et al.*, 1990), but is unaffected by cilostamide, amrinone or zaprinast (Nielson *et al.*, 1990; Wright *et al.*, 1990). In contrast, when opsonized zymosan (OZ) is used as the stimulus, neutrophils are reported to be resistant to the inhibitory actions of PDE4 inhibitors (Nielson *et al.*, 1990; Wright *et al.*, 1990). The reason for this apparent stimulus-specific effect is obscure, but may relate to functional antagonism in light of a study from Schudt *et al.* (1991b), who reported that rolipram and Ro-20-1724 are effective at attenuating OZ-induced superoxide generation.

Platelets

Theophylline

A preliminary investigation by Thompson *et al.* (1984) has established that theophylline inhibits platelet activation *in vitro*.

Isoenzyme-selective PDE inhibitors

Platelets have been implicated in the pathophysiology of certain allergic diseases, including asthma, providing a potential target for drug therapy (see Chapter 12). Selective inhibitors of the PDE3 isoenzyme family reduce aggregation, inhibit Ca^{2+} mobilization and suppress the secretion of 5-hydroxytryptamine (5-HT), β-thromboglobulin, ATP and thromboxane (Muggli *et al.*, 1985; Seiler *et al.*, 1987; Murray *et al.*, 1990, 1992; Simpson *et al.*, 1990; Jeremy *et al.*, 1993). These findings are thus consistent with the predominance of PDE3 in platelets. cGMP-elevating drugs similarly suppress activation of platelets, although the PDE5 inhibitor, zaprinast, is essentially inactive but potentiates nitric oxide-induced aggregation (Radomski *et al.*, 1987) and adhesion (Radomski *et al.*, 1987b).

Endothelial and epithelial cells

Isoenzyme-selective PDE inhibitors

The functions of endothelial cells, which play an important role in regulating plasma fluid and protein leakage out of blood vessels and cell recruitment into inflamed tissues, are regulated by cAMP. Agents that elevate endothelial cell cAMP levels, including PDE inhibitors, reduce albumin flux across endothelial monolayers (Casnocha *et al.*, 1989; Minnear *et al.*, 1989; Stelzner *et al.*, 1989; Suttorp *et al.*, 1992), suppress the adhesion of monocytes to human umbilical vein endothelial cells (Sung *et al.*, 1991) and inhibit TNF-α-induced expression of the surface adhesion molecules, endothelial leucocyte adhesion molecule-1 (ELAM-1) and vascular adhesion molecule-1 (VCAM-1) (Pober *et al.*, 1993).

Little has been reported on the effects of PDE inhibitors on epithelial cells. Bicarbonate secretion by airway epithelium is stimulated by IBMX (Smith & Welsh, 1992) and other agents that increase cAMP synthesis, as well as cAMP analogues, protect bronchial epithelial cells from the cytotoxic effects of endotoxin (Koyoma *et al.*, 1991). Such a cytoprotective effect may be of relevance to asthma therapy since sloughing of the epithelium is a prominent feature of the disease (Djukanovic *et al.*, 1990). Bradykinin stimulates the production of PGE_2 from human cultured bronchial basal epithelial cells, which is inhibited by IBMX (Rabe *et al.*, 1994), but the action of theophylline and selective PDE inhibitors is currently unknown.

Anti-inflammatory effects of PDE inhibitors *in vivo*

Comparatively little is known of the actions of isoenzyme-selective PDE inhibitors upon either the acute (IgE-mediated) or chronic (pro-inflammatory/immunocompetent cell-mediated) consequences of allergen provocation *in vivo*. The studies that have been performed are restricted to passive cutaneous anaphylaxis (PCA), cell infiltration into sites of inflammation and microvascular leakage.

IgE-mediated processes

It is currently unknown if PDE inhibitors are able to reduce the levels of IgE *in vivo*. The only compound that has been assessed in humans, ibudilast, which is an essentially non-selective inhibitor of PDE4 (Souness *et al.*, 1994), does not affect IgE levels in asthmatic individuals (Kawasaki *et al.*, 1992). In contrast, PDE3 and PDE4 inhibitors exhibit efficacy at reducing PCA reactions in rats, mice and guinea pigs (Davies & Evans, 1973; Broughton *et al.*, 1975). Furthermore, rolipram, but not zaprinast or SK&F 94120, is effective at reducing the infiltration of indium-labelled eosinophils into the skin of guinea pigs following a PCA reaction (Teixeira *et al.*, 1994). Collectively, these data imply that PDE4 inhibitors can suppress the degranulation of IgE-bearing leucocytes and therefore allergen-induced mediator release. Further support for this proposal derives from studies in sensitized guinea pigs where rolipram, administered intravenously, inhibits antigen- but not LTD_4-induced bronchoconstriction (Howell *et al.*, 1993). Thus, rolipram preferentially exerts an inhibitory influence at the level of mast cells and basophils rather than exerting a direct anti-spasmogenic action at the level of airway smooth muscle. In contrast, the PDE3 inhibitor, CI-930, inhibited both allergen- and LTD_4-induced bronchoconstriction under identical conditions, indicating a direct smooth-muscle effect of this compound (Howell *et al.*, 1993).

Pro-inflammatory cell infiltration

Theophylline

Intravenous injection of a low dose of theophylline into a guinea pig model of allergic asthma immediately prior to antigen prevents both the immediate bronchoconstriction and the late-phase reaction (LPR) (Andersson *et al.*, 1985). Qualitatively identical results were obtained in an allergic sheep and rabbit model (Perruchoud *et al.*, 1984; Ali *et al.*, 1992). Independent experiments conducted with sensitized guinea pigs and rats have demonstrated that theophylline suppresses pulmonary eosinophil and, in the case of the rat, also neutrophil recruitment, which is believed to be intimately associated with the development of the LPR (Gristwood *et al.*, 1991; Taraye *et al.*, 1991a,b, 1992; Sanjar *et al.*, 1992; Manzini *et al.*, 1993; Lagente *et al.*, 1994). In many of these studies, however, theophylline was administered acutely as a single dose that is significantly higher than that used therapeutically, indicating that the observed effects may not be relevant to the clinical situation. In contrast, chronic dosing of guinea pigs for 7 days with theophylline effectively prevents PAF and allergen-induced eosinophil recruitment at therapeutically relevant concentrations (Sanjar *et al.*, 1990a,b).

In another study, administration of LPS to rats evokes a non-allergic TNF-α-dependent inflammatory response that is characterized by hyperresponsiveness of the airways and pulmonary neutrophilia. This effect is significantly attenuated in animals given theophylline at plasma concentrations considered to be therapeutic (Pauwels, 1989a,b; Pauwels *et al.*, 1990) by a mechanism that apparently does not involve suppressing the elaboration of TNF-α (Kips *et al.*, 1992).

Isoenzyme-selective PDE inhibitors

A number of studies have evaluated the effect of PDE inhibitors upon the infiltration of pro-inflammatory cells into the airway lumen, skin and eye of guinea pigs, rats and monkeys in responses to PAF, bacterial LPS and allergen (Sanjar *et al.*, 1989, 1990a,b; Kings *et al.*, 1990; Sturm *et al.*, 1990; Schudt *et al.*, 1991a; Kips *et al.*, 1993; Underwood *et al.*, 1993; Lagente *et al.*, 1994; Turner *et al.*, 1994; Banner & Page, 1995; Elwood *et al.*, 1995). Schudt *et al.* (1991a) reported that pretreatment of sensitized guinea pigs with zardaverine, a mixed PDE3/4 inhibitor, markedly suppressed allergen-induced infiltration of eosinophils, macrophages and neutrophils into the BALF to a level achieved with dexamethasone. Qualitatively identical data have been reported for the PDE3/4 inhibitor, benafentrine, on PAF- (Sanjar *et al.*, 1989, 1990a) and allergen-induced (Sanjar *et al.*, 1991b) pulmonary eosinophil recruitment in guinea pigs after chronic (6 days) dosing. Studies conducted more recently with rolipram have provided results which corroborate these data. Thus, intragastric administration of rolipram to conscious guinea pigs selectively attenuated allergen-induced pulmonary eosinophil influx into the BALF and tissue (Underwood *et al.*, 1993). Similarly, the introduction of rolipram directly into the airways of guinea pigs as a micronized dry powder almost completely prevented the appearance of pro-inflammatory leucocytes into the BALF in response to allergen provocation (Raeburn *et al.*, 1993).

Treatment of sensitized *Cynomolgus* monkeys with rolipram does not block the immediate increase in airway resistance that follows acute antigen provocation (Turner *et al.*, 1994) but does abrogate the pulmonary neutrophilia and eosinophilia and airway hyperresponsiveness after multiple exposures to the antigen. Thus, these data are consistent with the findings of Howell *et al.* (1993) that PDE4 inhibitors may be anti-inflammatory and act primarily to prevent the activation of immune cells in the lung rather than by exerting an antispasmogenic or spasmolytic effect at the level of airway smooth muscle.

Other models of inflammation are also sensitive to PDE4 inhibitors. For example, allergen-induced lung eosinophilia in Brown Norway (BN) rats, an IgE-producing, steroid-sensitive species that exhibits both early-phase reaction (EPR) and LPR, is abolished by rolipram and the hybrid PDE3/4 inhibitor, Org-20241 (Elwood *et al.*, 1995). Similarly, in a guinea pig eye model of tissue eosinophilia, rolipram, when administered by gavage, significantly inhibited the number of eosinophils that appeared in the conjunctival epithelium in response to histamine and a combination of LTB_4 and LTD_4 (Newsholm & Schwartz, 1993). In another study, Griswold *et al.* (1993) reported that oral administration of mice with rolipram inhibited arachidonate-induced inflammatory cell accumulation and activation assessed by myeloperoxidase activity in the inflammatory exudate. Rolipram was also active at suppressing neutrophil accumulation into the peritoneum evoked by urate crystals and LTB_4. Zaprinast was inactive in these functional assays.

Systemic administration of rolipram, but not zaprinast or SK&F 94120, to guinea pigs suppresses the accumulation of indium-labelled eosinophils into the skin in response to zymosan-activated plasma, PAF and histamine (Teixeira *et al.*, 1994). In this model, however, the accumulation of indium-labelled neutrophils was unaffected by rolipram under identical experimental conditions, which may relate to the fact that guinea pig neutrophil function is less sensitive to inhibition by rolipram than human cells (Boucheron *et al.*, 1991), due, possibly, to a lower basal adenylyl cyclase activity. Locally injected rolipram had little effect on eosinophil accumulation (Teixeira *et al.*, 1994).

Although pro-inflammatory mediators such as PAF, histamine and LTB_4 elicit pulmonary eosinophil recruitment, it has been emphasized that the eosinophil count in the airway lumen is considerably less than that seen following antigen provocation (Aoki *et al.*, 1988). This observation, together with the finding that selective antagonists of these mediators do not abrogate eosinophil recruitment following antigen challenge, implicates mediators other than PAF, histamine and LTB_4 in eosinophil accumulation in the lung. It is now recognized that a number of so-called chronic pro-inflammatory eotaxin chemokines, including IL-3, IL-5, GM-CSF, RANTES, eotaxin, TNF-α and macrophage inflammatory protein-1α (MIP-1α) can elicit the pulmonary accumulation and activation of eosinophils. Indeed, Kings *et al.* (1990) documented the ability of human recombinant IL-3 and GM-CSF, and mouse TNF-α to selectively attract eosinophils into the lungs of guinea pigs. Significantly, pretreatment of the animals with the PDE3/4 inhibitor benafentrine effectively suppressed this response (Kings *et al.*, 1990). Comparable data are also available for the actions of zardaverine upon endotoxin-induced pulmonary neutrophil recruitment in rats (Kips *et al.*, 1993), which is partly mediated by the release of TNF-α. In that study, zardaverine also inhibited the elaboration of TNF-α in the BALF following endotoxin. Collectively, these are important observations, since they imply that selective PDE inhibitors are effective at blocking the deleterious actions of both acute (PAF, histamine, LTB_4) and chronic (cytokine) mediators of allergic inflammation.

There are no reports of the effects of selective PDE inhibitors upon eosinophil numbers in humans. However, Kawasaki *et al.* (1992) have reported that the non-selective PDE inhibitor, ibudilast, does not reduce the circulating eosinophil count in asthmatic subjects.

Microvascular leakage and oedema

It is now widely recognized that the microcirculation plays an important role in inflammatory reactions. Under normal conditions, the endothelium lining the post-capillary microvenules in the skin and bronchial circulation (capillaries in the pulmonary vasculature) is largely impermeable to blood cells and to macromolecules but, following a pro-inflammatory insult, localized arteriolar vasodilatation occurs, with a consequent increase in blood flow. This effect is induced by the liberation of pro-inflammatory mediators such as histamine and tachykinins. An increase in capillary and microvenular pressure then ensues, together with the liberation of other mediators, such as PAF and LTD_4, which directly contract the microvenular endothelial cells. Together, these effects, by increasing microvenular permeability, permit the loss of plasma proteins from the vascular compartment. Furthermore, the resulting increase in osmotic pressure due to loss of solute from the circulation leads to marked fluid exudation and to oedema.

Theophylline and isoenzyme-selective PDE inhibitors

Relatively few studies have documented the effects of theophylline and isoenzyme-selective PDE inhibitors upon plasma protein extravasation. In guinea pigs, theophylline reduces plasma exudation into the trachea, bronchi and BALF, but its efficacy may depend upon the nature and strength of the leak-evoking stimulus

(Boschetto *et al.*, 1989; Erjefalt & Persson, 1991; Raeburn *et al.*, 1991).

With respect to selective drugs, intravenous, oral and intratracheal administration of representative inhibitors of the PDE4 and PDE5 isoenzyme families markedly attenuate PAF-induced microvascular leakage in both small and large airways and in the BALF of anaesthetized guinea pigs (Ortiz *et al.*, 1992; Raeburn & Karlsson, 1993; Raeburn *et al.*, 1994). Rolipram is also effective against allergen-induced microvascular leakage in sensitized guinea pigs (Raeburn *et al.*, 1991). The finding that rolipram and zaprinast were active when given directly into the airways indicates an important local action in the lung and highlights that systemic administration is not necessary for these compounds to exert an anti-inflammatory influence. This is an important observation since the administration of PDE inhibitors by the inhaled route should reduce untoward side-effects while maintaining efficacy. Drugs which inhibit PDE1 and PDE3 do not inhibit PAF-induced microvascular leakage in guinea pig airways (Ortiz *et al.*, 1992; Raeburn *et al.*, 1993). This latter finding is curious, given that a PDE3 isoenzyme has been identified in endothelial cells and that a selective PDE3 inhibitor, motapizone, blocks the increase in permeability elicited by hydrogen peroxide *in vitro* (Suttorp *et al.*, 1993). It is likely, however, that this discrepancy is due to a difference in species, in the leak-evoking stimulus or in vessel type. In keeping with this latter possibility, Teixeira *et al.* (1994) have reported that rolipram does not inhibit oedema formation in guinea pig skin in response to histamine, zymosan-activated plasma and PAF (cf. guinea pig lung). It is tempting to speculate that the complement of PDE isoenzymes and/or the regulation of endothelial cell contractility by cyclic nucleotides varies significantly between vessels of the pulmonary and systemic vascular beds.

Svensjo *et al.* (1992) reported that PDE4 and PDE3/4 inhibitors attenuate the increase in microvascular permeability evoked by bradykinin in the hamster cheek pouch. Qualitatively identical results are obtained for the effect of rolipram and denbufylline upon arachidonate-induced rat ear (Raeburn *et al.*, 1993) and mouse ear (Crummey *et al.*, 1987) oedema, respectively.

Using [^{3}H]adenine-prelabelled, isolated rat lungs, perfused via the pulmonary circulation, rolipram markedly increases the level of radiolabelled cAMP in the perfusate after the addition of the β-adrenoceptor agonist, isoprenaline (Barnard *et al.*, 1994). This observation implicates PDE4 in cells of the pulmonary circulation but cannot with certainty be localized to the vascular endothelium or, indeed, extrapolated to the tracheobronchial microcirculation.

Clinical pharmacology

Theophylline

Until relatively recently, the therapeutic efficacy of theophylline in asthma was attributed to its weak bronchodilator activity. However, there is now increasing evidence that theophylline exerts an immunomodulatory action at plasma concentrations that do not affect airway smooth-muscle tone. Several lines of investigation have led to this conclusion. In essentially all studies that have been conducted, theophylline protects against the late asthmatic response following allergen provocation, implying that the emigration of pro-inflammatory and immunocompetent cells from the circulation into the lung and/or their subsequent activation is suppressed. In a study by Ward *et al.* (1993), theophylline, at a mean plasma concentration of 7.8 µg/ml, inhibited the LPR in asthmatics in response to allergen and the typical increase in CD4+ and CD8+ T lymphocytes. Pardi *et al.* (1984) also reported that a single infusion of theophylline into normal subjects reduced the peripheral blood T-cell count. In contrast, chronic administration of theophylline paradoxically increases CD8+ (suppressor) T-cell number in the peripheral blood of asthmatic subjects and impairs the graft vs. host reaction of these cells (Shohat *et al.*, 1983; Zocchi *et al.*, 1985; Fink *et al.*, 1987; Scordamalglia *et al.*, 1988).

In asthmatic children the number of CD8+ T lymphocytes in the peripheral blood was suppressed compared with normal individuals and the degree to which this occurs correlates with the severity of the disease (LaHat *et al.*, 1985; Shohat *et al.*, 1993). Significantly, treatment of those children for 1 month with theophylline restored the T-cell count to the level found in the control group.

Controlled withdrawal of theophylline from patients treated chronically with this medication and inhaled high-dose steroid results in a clinical deterioration and reduction of lung function (Brenner *et al.*, 1988; Kidney *et al.*, 1993, 1994). This is associated with a reduction in activated CD4+ and CD8+ T lymphocytes in the peripheral blood and a commensurate increase in the number of these cells in the lung as evinced by bronchial biopsies (Kidney *et al.*, 1993, 1994).

In addition to T lymphocytes, theophylline also modulates other pro-inflammatory and immune cells. In asthmatic children treated chronically for 10 days with theophylline, both neutrophil and macrophage activity (chemotaxis, superoxide generation, bactericidal killing) assessed *ex vivo* is suppressed, the degree of which positively correlates with the concentration of theophylline measured in the BALF (O'Neill *et al.*, 1986; Condino-Neto *et al.*, 1991). Similar experiments have demonstrated that the number of EG2+ eosinophils and CD4+ T cells are reduced in allergic subjects given low-dose theophylline (mean plasma concentration 6.6 μg/ml) for 6 weeks (Sullivan *et al.*, 1993; Jaffar *et al.*, 1994). In individuals with allergic rhinitis, theophylline inhibits nasal plasma exudation (Naclerio *et al.*, 1986), indicating a possible effect on endothelial cell permeability.

The mechanism by which theophylline exerts its immunomodulatory actions is far from clear. It has been reported, however, that oral administration of theophylline (mean level 10.9 μg/ml) to moderately severe atopic asthmatics reduced the number of cells (mostly mast cells) staining for IL-4 and IL-5, implying that theophylline may act, at least in part, to repress transcription of the IL-4 and IL-5 genes (Djukanovic *et al.*, 1995).

Isoenzyme-selective PDE inhibitors

Although a preliminary study has documented the effect of a selective PDE4 inhibitor, tibenelast, in asthma (Israel *et al.*, 1987), in which oral administration caused modest bronchodilatation, no information is available on the potential anti-inflammatory action of PDE4 inhibitors. The airway smooth-muscle action reflects a class-specific effect, as responses of generally equivalent magnitude are also produced with the mixed PDE3/PDE4 inhibitors, benafentrine and zardaverine (Brunnee *et al.*, 1992; Foster *et al.*, 1992; Ukena *et al.*, 1995), and with the PDE3-selective compounds, enoximone and cilostazol (Leeman *et al.*, 1987; Fujimura *et al.*, 1995). These drugs appear equally active in normal individuals and subjects with asthma and chronic obstructive pulmonary disease.

A PDE5 inhibitor, zaprinast, has also been evaluated in humans. Curiously, while this compound affords some protection against exercise-induced asthma in adults (Rudd *et al.*, 1983), it is apparently inactive in children (Reiser *et al.*, 1986). Moreover, the mechanism of action of zaprinast does not appear to be at the level of airway smooth muscle since it does not reverse histamine-induced bronchoconstriction (Rudd *et al.*, 1983). Further details on the airway effect of PDE inhibitors are presented elsewhere (Giembycz & Dent, 1992; Souness & Giembycz, 1994; Torphy *et al.*, 1994; Dent & Giembycz, 1995).

Like asthma, there are only a paucity of data relating to the clinical effects of PDE inhibitors in skin disorders. Results from a study reported by Baer (1985) indicate that papaverine, a non-selective PDE inhibitor, is effective at decreasing pruritus in patients with atopic dermatitis. Similarly, caffeine, which also displays weak PDE inhibitory activity, when used as a 30% cream with 0.5% hydrocortisone, was more effective than the steroid alone in treating atopic dermatitis (Kaplan *et al.*, 1978). Despite these reports, the efficacy of these weak and non-selective drugs in the treatment of atopic dermatitis has been disputed (Rasmussen, 1989). Thus, while the use of cAMP PDE inhibitors for the treatment of atopic dermatitis has been vigorously championed (Hanifin, 1986), no clinical studies have been reported which unequivocally demonstrate clinical efficacy, although Ro-20-1724 has been tested successfully in patients with psoriasis (Sawiski *et al.*, 1979).

Side-effects and potential limitations of theophylline and selective inhibitors of PDE 3 and 4

Theophylline

The adverse effects reported for theophylline generally occur at plasma concentrations above 20 μg/ml and include headache, nausea, vomiting, abdominal discomfort, diarrhoea, restlessness, irritability and insomnia. It has been documented, however, that lower concentrations may precipitate behavioural changes and lead to learning difficulties in children (Furukawa *et al.*, 1984, 1988; Rachelefsky *et al.*, 1986), although this was not confirmed in a more recent study (Lindgren *et al.*, 1992). Concentrations in excess of 30 μg/ml can evoke more serious side-effects, such as cardiac arrhythmias, gastric acid secretion, diuresis, hypokalaemia, hyperglycaemia and hypotension. Even higher concentrations can lead to seizures, brain damage and death.

It is noteworthy that many of the more common adverse effects associated with theophylline can be minimized by gradually increasing the dose until the desired therapeutic level is achieved (Hendeles & Weinberger, 1983; Weinberger & Hendeles, 1983; Hendeles *et al.*, 1984; Weinberger, 1984; Williamson *et al.*, 1988). However, it is significant that side-effects are unlikely to be a major problem if the immunomodulatory actions of theophylline are confirmed, as these effects are apparently achieved at low (sub-bronchodilator) plasma concentrations.

PDE 3 and 4 inhibitors

Selective inhibitors of the PDE3 isoenzyme family were originally developed for the therapy of congestive heart failure and therefore certain predictions can be made regarding the side-effect profile of these drugs. Of particular concern is their potential arrhythmogenic activity (Naccarelli & Goldstein, 1989) and their vasodilator action and positive inotropic and chronotropic effects on the heart (Wood & Hess, 1989). Although this would not necessarily preclude the use of PDE3 inhibitors administered directly into the airways or directly on to the skin as a topical formulation, their limited anti-inflammatory action on isolated cells and in *in vivo* models of inflammation suggests that this class of compound does not exhibit the required pharmacology to effectively treat allergic diseases. Similarly, the use of mixed inhibitors which act equally on both PDE3 and PDE4 would be subject to the same cardiovascular limitations.

Perhaps the most recognized adverse action of PDE4 inhibitors is their propensity to cause nausea (Zeller *et al.*, 1984; Brunnee *et al.*, 1992) and vomiting (Horowski *et al.*, 1985). This is likely to be a consequence of PDE4 inhibition, since emesis in laboratory animals evoked by a range of xanthine derivatives correlates with their ability to inhibit cAMP hydrolysis (Howell & Meuhsam, 1990). It is conceivable that the emetic response evoked by PDE4 inhibitors is mediated via a specific PDE4 gene product or spliced variant thereof, which could allow the development of subfamily-selective drugs. Indeed, it is known that the archetypal PDE4 inhibitor, rolipram, is approximately 100-fold less potent against PDE4C than the other isoforms. Another possibility that requires further investigation is that the conformation of PDE4 in the cell or tissue of interest can dictate the functional response evoked by an inhibitor (Barnette *et al.*, 1995a,b).

Like theophylline, PDE4 inhibitors enhance gastric acid secretion from parietal cells in the stomach (Black *et al.*, 1988) and pancreatic juice secretion from pancreatic exocrine glands (Iwatsuki *et al.*, 1991). Rolipram also evokes a dramatic, albeit transient, change in plasma osmolality (Sturgess & Searle, 1990), which may relate to the predominance of PDE4 in the kidney.

A final consideration and potential limitation of PDE4 inhibitors is that certain PDE4 isoenzymes are induced by cAMP-elevating, resulting in a heterologous desensitization of all adenylyl cyclase-coupled receptors (see section on long-term regulation under 'PDE4 isoenzyme family'). In allergic asthma, this finding could theoretically contribute to the deterioration of asthma symptoms and, indeed, mortality noted in patients receiving chronic β-adrenoceptor agonist therapy (Sears *et al.*, 1990; van Schayck *et al.*, 1990). An obvious concern for the pharmaceutical industry is whether PDE4 inhibitors will similarly render airway smooth muscle and, in particular, pro-inflammatory cells refractory to cAMP-elevating drugs after prolonged administration.

Discussion

As illustrated in Table 30.2, many of the world's major pharmaceutical companies have developed potent and novel PDE inhibitors for the treatment of a number of allergic disorders. By the end of the 1990s, it is likely that results from clinical trials will reveal whether the initial optimism for the therapeutic potential of this class of compounds was justified. The major impetus for the development of selective inhibitors of the PDE4 isoenzyme family is their anti-inflammatory and therefore steroid-sparing potential. In a number of animal models, PDE4 inhibitors effectively suppress antigen-driven responses, which points to efficacy in treating the major pathological components of allergic inflammation. However, one must be cautious of this interpretation since only the acute effects of PDE4 inhibitors in animals have been demonstrated and whether they translate into useful therapy for chronic human allergic diseases remains to be determined.

With respect to allergic asthma and atopic dermatitis, few trials on selective PDE inhibitors have been published thus far and in none of them was their anti-allergic or anti-inflammatory actions evaluated. However, one compound, which has been marketed in Japan and whose therapeutic efficacy may, at least in part, be a consequence of PDE4 inhibition, is ibudilast (Kawasaki *et al.*, 1992; Souness *et al.*, 1994). Clinically, however, this drug does not affect blood IgE levels or eosinophil numbers (Kawakasi *et al.*, 1992). Moreover, unlike more potent PDE4 inhibitors, ibudilast does not suppress antigen-induced pulmonary eosinophilia in animal models (Sanjar *et al.*, 1989). Whether PDE4 inhibitors will, as previously postulated, display a therapeutic profile similar to theophylline but with fewer side-effects again remains to be seen. Indeed, controversy still surrounds the mechanism by which theophylline exerts its anti-inflammatory effects (Barnes & Pauwels, 1994).

An explanation for the elevated cAMP PDE activity in MNL of atopic individuals remains elusive. Although this phenomenon may be a consequence of atopy, the increase in PDE is not secondary to tissue inflammation *per se*, since levels of the enzyme are normal in patients with allergic (type IV) contact dermatitis (Grewe *et al.*, 1982; Hanifin, 1986). If a genetic abnormality underlies this effect, then the expression of this cAMP PDE may be of major importance in the aetiology of allergic diseases. While the *in vivo* consequences of elevated cAMP PDE are unclear, *in vitro* data predict that the increased rate of cAMP hydrolysis in atopic MNL would have a major impact on the elaboration of pro-inflammatory allergic mediators and cytokines. Although primary sequence data are lacking, recent reports suggest the existence of a novel cAMP PDE in atopic MNL. Conceivably, this enzyme may be responsible for the abnormal functional responses of atopic MNL and may represent an important target for future therapeutic intervention in allergic diseases.

Past experience with isoenzyme-selective PDE inhibitors for the treatment of allergic disorders has been disappointing. This can be illustrated with reference to the PDE5 inhibitor, zaprinast, which has been tested in the clinic with unconvincing results (Reiser *et al.*, 1986). In retrospect, it is not surprising that this compound, which arose from the misconceived 'mast cell stabilizer' approach, failed to exhibit the anticipated activity in the clinic since the evidence that zaprinast exhibited anti-allergic activity was derived solely from inhibitory effects on rat mast cell mediator release (Frossard *et al.*, 1981) and in PCA (Broughton *et al.*, 1975). The current optimism regarding the therapeutic potential of PDE4 inhibitors is based on much firmer evidence, with the real possibility of developing a new generation of steroid-sparing, anti-inflammatory drugs.

Acknowledgements

The authors gratefully acknowledge the financial support of the Medical Research Council (UK), the National Asthma Campaign (UK) and the British Lung Foundation.

References

Ali, S., Mustafa, S.J. & Metzger, W.J. (1992) Modification of allergen-induced airway obstruction and bronchial hyper-responsiveness in the allergic rabbit by theophylline aerosol. *Agents Actions*, **37**, 165–73.

Alvarez, R., Taylor, A., Fazzari, J.J. & Jacobs, J.R. (1981) Regulation of cyclic AMP metabolism in human platelets: sequential activation of adenylate cyclase and cyclic AMP phosphodiesterase by prostaglandins. *Mol. Pharmacol.*, **20**, 302–9.

Anastassiou, E.D., Paliogianni, F., Balow, J.P., Yamada, H. & Boumpas, D.T. (1992) Prostaglandin E_2 and other cyclic AMP-elevating agents modulate IL-2 and IL-2R gene expression at multiple levels. *J. Immunol.*, **148**, 2845–52.

Andersson, P., Brange, C., Sonmark, B. *et al.* (1985) Anti-anaphylactic and anti-inflammatory effects of xanthines in the lung. In: *Anti-asthma Xanthines and Adenosine* (eds K.E. Andersson & C.G.A. Persson), pp. 187–92. Expcerpta Medica, Amsterdam.

Aoki, S., Boubekeur, K., Kristersson, A., Morley, J. & Sanjar, S. (1988) Is allergic airway hyperreactivity of the guinea-pig dependent on eosinophil accumulation in the lung? *Brit. J. Pharmacol.*, **94**, 365P.

Averill, L.E., Stein, R.L. & Kammer, G.M. (1988) Control of human T-lymphocyte interleukin-2 production by a cyclic AMP-dependent pathway. *Cell. Immunol.*, **115**, 88–99.

Baecker, P.A., Obernolte, R., Bach, C., Yee, C. & Shelton, E.R. (1995) Isolation of cDNA encoding a human rolipram-sensitive cyclic AMP phosphodiesterase (PDE IVD). *Gene*, **138**, 253–6.

Baer, R.L. (1985) Papaverine therapy in atopic dermatitis. *J. Am. Acad. Dermatol.*, **13**, 806–8.

Banner, K.H. & Page, C.P. (1995) Acute versus chronic administration of phosphodiesterase inhibitors on allergen-induced pulmonary cell influx in sensitized guinea-pigs. *Brit. J. Pharmacol.*, **114**, 93–8.

Barnard, J.W., Seibert, A.F., Prasad, V.R. *et al.* (1994) Reversal of pulmonary capillary ischemia–reperfusion injury by rolipram, a cAMP phosphodiesterase inhitor. *J. Appl. Physiol.*, **77**, 774–81.

Barnes, P.J. (1988) Asthma deaths: a continuing problem. In: *Advanced Medicine*, Vol. 24 (ed. M. Sheppard), pp. 53–61. Baillière Tindall, London.

Barnes, P.J. (1995) Methylxanthines and phosphodiesterase inhibitors. In: *Asthma and Rhinitis* (eds W.W. Busse & S.T. Holgate), pp. 1267–77. Blackwell Science, Oxford.

Barnes, P.J. & Pauwels, R.A. (1994) Theophylline in the management of asthma: time for reappraisal? *Eur. Resp. J.*, **7**, 579–91.

Barnette, M.S., Manning, C.D., Cieslinski, L.B., Burman, M., Christensen, S.B. & Torphy, T.J. (1995a) The ability of phosphodiesterase IV inhibitors to suppress superoxide production in guinea-pig eosinophils is correlated with inhibition of phosphodiesterase IV catalytic activity. *J. Pharmacol. Exp. Ther.*, **273**, 674–9.

Barnette, M.S., Grous, M., Cislinski, L.B., Burman, M., Christensen, S.B. & Torphy, T.J. (1995b) Inhibitors of phosphodiesterase IV (PDE IV) increase acid secretion in rabbit isolated gastric glands: correlation between function and interaction with a high affinity rolipram site. *J. Pharmacol. Exp. Ther.*, **273**, 1396–402.

Beavo, J.A. (1988) Multiple isozymes of cyclic nucleotide phosphodiesterase. *Adv. Sec. Mess. Phosphoprot. Res.*, **22**, 1–38.

Beavo, J.A., Hardman, J.G. & Sutherland, E.W. (1971) Stimulation of adenosine 3′,5′-monophosphate hydrolysis by guanosine 3′,5′-monophosphate. *J. Biol. Chem.*, **246**, 3841–6.

Beavo, J.A. & Reifsnyder, D.H. (1990) Primary sequence of cyclic nucleotide phosphodiesterase isozymes and the design of selective inhibitors. *Trends Pharmacol. Sci.*, **11**, 150–5.

Beavo, J.A., Conti, M. & Heaslip, R.J. (1994) Multiple cyclic nucleotide phosphodiesterases. *Mol. Pharmacol.*, **46**, 399–405.

Beckner, S.K. & Farrar, W.L. (1986) Interleukin 2 modulation of adenylate cyclase: potential role of protein kinase C. *J. Biol. Chem.*, **261**, 3043–7.

Bentley, J.K. & Beavo, J.A. (1992) Regulation and function of cyclic nucleotides. *Curr. Opin. Cell Biol.*, **4**, 233–40.

Bentley, J.K., Kadlecek, A., Sherbert, C.H. *et al.* (1992) Molecular cloning of cDNA encoding a '63' kDa calmodulin-stimulated phosphodiesterase from bovine brain. *J. Biol. Chem.*, **267**, 18676–82.

Bergstrand, H., Lundqvist, B. & Schurman, A. (1978) Rat mast cell high affinity cyclic nucleotide phosphodiesterases: separation and inhibitory effects of two anti-allergic agents. *Mol. Pharmacol.*, **14**, 848–55.

Bessler, H., Gilgal, R., Djaldatti, M. & Zahavi, I. (1986) Effect of pentoxifylline on the phagocytic activity, cyclic AMP levels, and superoxide anion production by monocytes and polymorphonuclear cells. *J. Leuc. Biol.*, **40**, 747–54.

Betz, M. & Fox, B.S. (1991) Prostaglandin E_2 inhibits production of Th1 lymphokines but not of Th2 lymphokines. *J. Immunol.*, **146**, 108–13.

Black, E.W., Strada, S.J. & Thomson, W.J. (1988) Relationships between secretagogue-induced cAMP accumulation and acid secretion in elutriated rat gastric parietal cells. *J. Pharmacol. Meth.*, **20**, 57–78.

Bloom, T.J. & Beavo, J.A. (1994) Identification of PDE VII in HUT 78 T-lymphocyte cells. *FASEB J.*, **8**, A372.

Bolger, G., Michaeli, T., Martins, T. *et al.* (1993) A family of human phosphodiesterase homologous to the dunce learning and memory gene products of *Drosophila melanogaster* are potential targets for antidepressant drugs. *Mol. Cell. Biol.*, **13**, 6558–71.

Boschetto, P., Roberts, N.M., Rogers, D.F. & Barnes, P.J. (1989) The effect of anti-asthma drugs on microvascular leak in guinea-pig airways. *Am. Rev. Resp. Dis.*, **139**, 416–21.

Boucheron, J.A., Verghese, M.W., Irsula, O. & Stacy, L. (1991) Species differences in neutrophil superoxide modulation by cyclic nucleotide phosphodiesterase inhibitors. *FASEB J.*, **5**, A510.

Brenner, M., Berkowitz, R., Marshall, N. & Strunk, R.C. (1988) Need for theophylline in severe steroid-requiring asthmatics. *Clin. Allergy*, **18**, 143–50.

Broughton, B.J., Chaplen, P., Knowles, P. *et al.* (1975) Antiallergic activity of 2-phenyl-8-azapurin-6-ones. *J. Med. Chem.*, **18**, 1117–22.

Brunnee, T., Engelstätter, R., Steinijans, V.W. & Kunkel, G. (1992)

Bronchodilatory effect of inhaled zardaverine, a phosphodiesterase III and IV inhibitor, in patients with asthma. *Eur. Resp. J.*, **5**, 982–5.

Bruserud, O. (1984) The effect of theophylline on T-lymphocyte activation *in vitro*. *Clin. Immunol. Immunopathol.*, **32**, 111–18.

Burns, F., Rodger, I.W. & Pyne, N.J. (1992) The catalytic subunit of protein kinase A triggers activation of the type V cyclic GMP-specific phosphodiesterase from guinea-pig lung. *Biochem. J.*, **283**, 487–91.

Busse, W.W. & Anderson, C.L. (1981) The granulocyte response to the phosphodiesterase inhibitor RO 20-1724 in asthma. *J. Allergy Clin. Immunol.*, **67**, 7–74.

Butcher, R.W. & Sutherland, E.W. (1962) Adenosine 3′,5′-phosphate in biological materials. *J. Biol. Chem.*, **237**, 1244–50.

Butler, J.M., Chan, S.C., Stevens, S. & Hanifin, J.M. (1983) Increased leukocyte histamine release with elevated cyclic AMP-phosphodiesterase activity in atopic dermatitis. *J. Allergy Clin. Immunol.*, **71**, 490–7.

Calhoun, W.J., Stevens, C.A. & Lambert, S.B. (1991) Modulation of superoxide production of alveolar macrophages and peripheral blood mononuclear cells by beta-agonists and theophylline. *J. Lab. Clin. Med.*, **117**, 514–22.

Casnocha, S.A., Eskin, S.G., Hall, E.R. & McIntire, L.V. (1989) Permeability of human endothelial monolayers: effect of vasoactive agonists and cyclic AMP. *J. Appl. Physiol.*, **67**, 1997–2005.

Chan, S.C. & Hanifin, J.M. (1993) Differential inhibitor effects on cyclic adenosine monophosphate-phosphodiesterase isoforms in atopic and normal leukocytes. *J. Lab. Clin. Med.*, **121**, 44–51.

Chan, S.C., Grewe, S.R., Stevens, S.R. & Hanifin, J.M. (1982) Functional desensitization due to stimulation of cyclic AMP phosphodiesterase in human mononuclear leukocytes. *J. Cyc. Nucl. Res.*, **8**, 211–24.

Chan, S.C., Hanifin, J.M., Holden, C.A., Thompson, W.J. & Hirshman, C.A. (1985) Elevated leukocyte phosphodiesterase as a basis for depressed cyclic adenosine monophosphate responses in the Basenji greyhound dog model of asthma. *J. Allergy Clin. Immunol.*, **76**, 148–58.

Chan, S.C., Trask, D.M., Sherman, S.C. & Hanifin, J.M. (1986) Histamine agonist stimulated protein kinase C phosphorylation of a 61K monocyte protein with characteristics of atopic cyclic AMP phosphodiesterase. *J. Invest. Dermatol.*, **86**, 468 [abstract].

Chan, S.C., Reifsnyder, D., Beavo, J.A. & Hanifin, M.D. (1993a) Immunochemical characterization of the distinct monocyte cyclic AMP-phosphodiesterase from patients with atopic dermatitis. *J. Allergy Clin. Immunol.*, **91**, 1179–88.

Chan, S.C., Kim, J.-W., Henderson, W.R. & Hanifin, J.M. (1993b) Altered prostaglandin E_2 regulation of cytokine production in atopic dermatitis. *J. Immunol.*, **151**, 3345–52.

Chan, S.C., Li, S.-H. & Hanifin, J.M. (1993c) Increased interleukin-4 production by atopic mononuclear leukocytes correlates with increased cyclic adenosine monophosphate-phosphodiesterase activity and is reversible by phosphodiesterase inhibition. *J. Invest. Dermatol.*, **100**, 681–4.

Charbonneau, H., Kumar, S., Novack, J.P. *et al.* (1991) Evidence for domain organization within the 61 kDa calmodulin-dependent cyclic nucleotide phosphodiesterase from bovine brain. *Biochemistry*, **30**, 7931–40.

Chen, C.N., Denome, S. & Davis, R.L. (1986) Molecular analysis of cDNA clones and the corresponding genomic coding sequences of the *Drosophila* dunce gene$^+$, the structural gene for cAMP phosphodiesterase. *Proc. Nat. Acad. Sci. USA*, **83**, 9313–17.

Cheung, W.Y. (1970) Cyclic 3′,5′-nucleotide phosphodiesterase: demonstration of an activator. *Biochem. Biophys. Res. Commun.*, **38**, 533–8.

Cheung, W.Y. (1971) Cyclic 3′,5′-nucleotide phosphodiesterase: evidence for and properties of a protein activator. *J. Biol. Chem.*, 246, 2859–69.

Chuang, T.T., Sallese, M., Ambrosini, G., Parruti, G. & De Blasi, A. (1992) A high expression of β-adrenergic receptor kinase in human peripheral blood leukocytes. *J. Biol. Chem.*, **267**, 6886–92.

Cohan, V.L., Johnson, K.L., Breslow, R., Cheng, J.B. & Showell, H.J. (1992) PDE IV is the predominant PDE isozyme regulating chemotactic factor-mediated guinea-pig eosinophil functions *in vitro*. *J. Allergy Clin. Immunol.*, **89**, 663.

Colicelli, J., Birchmeier, C., Michaeli, T., O'Neill, K., Riggs, M. & Wigler, M. (1989) Isolation and characterisation of a mammalian gene encoding a high affinity cAMP phosphodiesterase. *Proc. Nat. Acad. Sci. USA*, **86**, 3599–603.

Condino-Neto, A., Vilela, M.M., Cambiucci, E.C. *et al.* (1991) Theophylline therapy inhibits neutrophil and mononuclear cell chemotaxis from chronic asthmatic children. *Brit. J. Clin. Pharmacol.*, **32**, 557–61.

Conti, M. & Swinnen, J.V. (1990) Structure and function of the rolipram-sensitive, low Km cyclic AMP phosphodiesterase: a family of highly related enzymes. In: *Molecular Pharmacology of Cell Regulation: Cyclic Nucleotide Phosphodiesterase Structure, Regulation and Drug Action* (eds M.D. Houslay & J.A. Beavo), pp. 243–66. Wiley, New York.

Conti, M., Jin, S.L.C., Monaco, L., Repaske, D.R. & Swinnen, J.V. (1991) Hormonal regulation of cyclic nucleotide phosphodiesterases. *Endocr. Rev.*, **12**, 218–34.

Conti, M., Swinnen, J.V., Tsikalas, K.E. & Jin, S.-L.C. (1992) Structure and regulation of the rat high affinity cyclic AMP phosphodiesterase. *Adv. Sec. Mess. Prot. Phosphoryl. Res.*, **25**, 87–99.

Cooper, K.D., Kang, K., Chan, S.C. & Hanifin, J.M. (1985) Phosphodiesterase inhibition by Ro 20-1724 reduces hyper-IgE synthesis by atopic dermatitis cells *in vitro*. *J. Invest. Dermatol.*, **84**, 477–82.

Coquil, J.F., Franks, D.J., Wells, J.N., Dupuis, M. & Hamet, P. (1980) Characteristics of a new binding protein distinct from the kinase for guanosine 3′,5′-monophosphate in rat platelets. *Biochim. Biophys. Acta*, **631**, 148–65.

Coquil, J.F., Brunelle, G. & Guedon, J. (1985) Occurrence of the methylisobutylxanthine-stimulated cyclic GMP-binding protein in various rat tissues. *Biochem. Biophys. Res. Commun.*, **127**, 226–30.

Corrigan, C.J. & Kay, A.B. (1992) T cells and eosinophils in the pathogenesis of asthma. *Immunol. Today*, **13**, 501–7.

Coskey, L.A., Bitting, J. & Roth, M.D. (1993) Inhibition of natural killer cell activity by therapeutic concentrations of theophylline. *Am. J. Respir. Cell Mol. Biol.*, **9**, 659–65.

Coulson, I.H., Duncan, S.N. & Holden, C.A. (1989) Peripheral blood mononuclear leukocyte cyclic adenosine monophosphate specific phosphodiesterase activity in atopic dermatitis. *Brit. J. Dermatol.*, **120**, 607–12.

Crocker, I.C., Townley, R.G. & Khan, M.M. (1994) Phosphodiesterase inhibitors modulate cytokine secretion and proliferation. *J. Allergy Clin. Immunol.*, **93**, 286.

Crummey, A., Harper, G.P., Boyle, E.A. & Mangan, F.R. (1987) Inhibition of arachidonic acid-induced ear oedema as a model for assessing topical anti-inflammatory compounds. *Agents Actions*, **20**, 69–76.

Davies, G.E. & Evans, D.P. (1973) Studies with two new phosphodiesterase inhibitors (ICI 58, 301 and ICI 63, 197) on anaphylaxis in guinea-pigs, mice and rats. *Int. Arch. Allergy Appl. Immunol.*, **45**, 467–78.

Davis, R.L., Tadayasu, H., Eberwine, M. & Myers, J. (1989) Cloning and characterization of mammalian homologues of the *Drosophila* dunce+ gene. *Proc. Nat. Acad. Sci. USA*, **86**, 3604–8.

Degerman, E., Belfrage, P., Newman, A.H., Rice, K.C. & Manganiello, V.C. (1987) Purification of the putative hormone-sensitive cyclic AMP phosphodiesterase from rat adipose tissue using a derivative of cilostamide as a novel affinity ligand. *J. Biol. Chem.*, **262**, 5797–807.

Dent, G. & Giembycz, M.A. (1995) Selective phosphodiesterase inhibitors in the therapy of asthma. *Clin. Immunother.*, **3**, 423–37.

Dent, G., Giembycz, M.A., Rabe, K.F. & Barnes, P.J. (1991) Inhibition of eosinophil cyclic nucleotide PDE activity and opsonised zymosan-induced respiratory burst by 'type IV'-selective PDE inhibitors. *Brit. J. Pharmacol.*, **103**, 1339–46.

Dent, G., Giembycz, M.A., Rabe, K.F., Barnes, P.J. & Magnussen, H. (1993) Effects of selective phosphodiesterase inhibitors on human alveolar macrophage cyclic nucleotide hydrolysis and respiratory burst. *Brit. J. Pharmacol.*, **111**, 74P.

Dent, G., Giembycz, M.A., Rabe, K.F., Wolf, B., Barnes, P.J. & Magnussen, H. (1994) Theophylline suppresses human alveolar macrophage respiratory burst through phosphodiesterase inhibition. *Am. J. Respir. Cell Mol. Biol.*, **10**, 565–72.

Derian, C.K., Santulli, R.J., Rao, P.E., Soloman, H.F. & Barrett, J.A. (1995) Inhibition of chemotactic peptide-induced neutrophil adhesion to vascular endothelium by cAMP modulators. *J. Immunol.*, **154**, 308–17.

Djukanović, R., Roche, W.R., Wilson, J.W. *et al.* (1990) Mucosal inflammation and asthma. *Am. Rev. Resp. Dis.*, 142, 434–57.

Djukanović, R., Finnerty, J.P., Lee, C., Wilson, S., Madden, J. & Holgate, S.T. (1995) The effect of theophylline on mucosal inflammation in asthmatic airways: biopsy results. *Eur. Resp. J.*, **8**, 831–3.

Elwood, W., Sun, J., Barnes, P.J., Giembycz, M.A. & Chung, K.F. (1995) Inhibition of allergen-induced lung eosinophilia by type-IV and combined type III- and IV-selective phosphodiesterase inhibitors in Brown Norway rats. *Inflamm. Res.*, **44**, 83–6.

Endres, S., Fulle, H.-J., Sinha, B. *et al.* (1991) Cyclic nucleotides differentially regulate the synthesis of tumor necrosis factor-α and interleukin-1β by human mononuclear cells. *Immunology*, **72**, 56–60.

Engels, P., Sullivan, M., Muller, T. & Lubbert, H. (1995) Molecular cloning and functional expression in yeast on a human cAMP-specific phosphodiesterase subtype (PDE IV-C). *FEBS Letts.*, **358**, 305–10.

Engerson, T., Legendre, J.L. & Jones, H.P. (1986) Calmodulin-dependency of human neutrophil phosphodiesterase. *Inflammation*, **10**, 31–5.

Epstein, P.M. & Hachisu, R. (1984) Cyclic nucleotide phosphodiesterase in normal and leukemic human lymphocytes and lymphoblasts. *Adv. Cyc. Nucl. Prot. Phosphory. Res.*, **16**, 303–24.

Epstein, P.M., Strada, S.J., Sarada, K. & Thompson, W.J. (1982) Catalytic and kinetic properties of purified high affinity cyclic AMP phosphodiesterase from dog kidney. *Arch. Biochem. Biophys.*, **218**, 119–33.

Erjefalt, I. & Persson, C.G.A. (1991) Pharmacologic control of plasma exudation into tracheobronchial airways. *Am. Rev. Resp. Dis.*, **143**, 1008–14.

Essayan, D.M., Huang, S.-K., Undem, B.J., Kagey-Sobotka, A. & Lichtenstein, L.M. (1994) Modulation of antigen- and mitogen-induced proliferative responses of peripheral blood mononuclear cells by non-selective and isozyme-selective cyclic nucleotide phosphodiesterase inhibitors. *J. Immunol.*, **153**, 3408–16.1

Fink, G., Mittelman, M., Shohat, B. & Spitzer, S.A. (1987) Theophylline-induced alterations in cellular immunity in asthmatic patients. *Clin. Allergy*, **17**, 316–21.

Fischer, T.A., Erbel, R. & Treese, N. (1992) Current status of phosphodiesterase inhibitors in the treatment of congestive heart failure. *Drugs*, **44**, 928–45.

Fleming, D.M. & Crombie, D.L. (1987) Prevalence of asthma and hay fever in England and Wales. *Brit. Med. J.*, **294**, 279–83.

Foissier, M., Longchampt, F., Coge, E. & Canet, E. (1995) *In vitro* effect of cAMP-modulating agents on antigen-induced interleukin-4 (IL-4) and IL-5 mRNA expression and protein production by spleen cells from BALB/c mice. *Am. J. Resp. Crit. Care Med.*, **151**, A827.

Fonteh, A.N., Winkler, J.D., Torphy, T.J., Heravi, J., Undem, B.J. & Chilton, F.H. (1993) Influence of isoproterenol and phosphodiesterase inhibitors on platelet-activating factor biosynthesis in the human neutrophil. *J. Immunol.*, **151**, 339–50.

Foster, R.W., Rakshu, K., Carpenter, J.R. & Small, R.C. (1992) Trials of the bronchodilator activity of the isoenzyme phosphodiesterase inhibitor AH 21-132 in healthy volunteers during a methacholine challenge. *Brit. J. Clin. Pharmacol.*, **34**, 527–34.

Francis, S.H., Lincoln, T.M. & Corbin, J.D. (1980) Characterization of a novel cGMP-binding protein phosphodiesterase from rat lung. *J. Biol. Chem.*, **255**, 620–6.

Francis, S.H., Thomas, M.K. & Corbin, J.D. (1990) Cyclic GMP-binding cyclic GMP-specific phosphodiesterase from lung. In: *Cyclic Nucleotide Phosphodiesterases: Structure, Regulation and Drug Action* (eds J.A. Beavo & M.D. Houslay), pp. 117–40. Wiley, New York.

Frossard, N., Landry, Y., Pauli, G. & Ruckstuhl, M. (1981) Effects of cyclic AMP- and cyclic GMP-phosphodiesterase inhibitors on immunological release of histamine and on lung contractions. *Brit. J. Pharmacol.*, **73**, 933–8.

Fujimura, M., Kamio, Y., Saito, M., Hashimoto, T. & Matsuda, T. (1995) Bronchodilator and bronchoprotective effects of cilostazol in humans *in vivo*. *Am. Rev. Resp. Crit. Care Med.*, **151**, 222–5.

Furukawa, C.T., Shapiro, C.G., Duhamel, T., Weimer, L., Pierson, W.E. & Bierman, C.W. (1984) Learning and behaviour problems associated with theophylline. *Lancet*, **i**, 621.

Furukawa, C.T., Duhamel, T., Weimer, L., Shapiro, C.G., Pierson, W.E. & Bierman, C.W. (1988) Cognitive and behavioural findings in children taking theophylline. *J. Allergy Clin. Immunol.*, **81**, 83–8.

Geha, R.S. (1993) Atopic allergy and other hypersensitivities: understanding the allergic response as a step towards its eradication. *Curr. Opin. Immunol.*, **5**, 935–6.

Gettys, T.W., Vine, A.J., Simonds, M.F. & Corbin, J.D. (1988) Activation of the particulate low *Km* phosphodiesterase of adipocytes by addition of cyclic AMP-dependent protein kinase. *J. Biol. Chem.*, **263**, 10359–63.

Ghezzi, P. & Dinarello, C.A. (1988) IL-1 induces IL-1. III. Specific inhibition of IL-1 production by IFN-γ. *J. Immunol.*, **140**, 4238–44.

Giembycz, M.A. (1992) Could isoenzyme-selective phosphodiesterase inhibitors render bronchodilator therapy redundant in the treatment of bronchial asthma? *Biochem. Pharmacol.*, **43**, 2041–51.

Giembycz, M.A. & Dent G. (1992) Prospects for selective cyclic nucleotide phosphodiesterase inhibitors in the treatment of bronchial asthma. *Clin. Exp. Allergy*, **22**, 337–44.

Giembycz, M.A. & Kelly, J.J. (1994) Current status of cyclic nucleotide phosphodiesterase isoenzymes. In: *Methylxanthines and Phosphodiesterase Inhibitors and the Treatment of Respiratory Disease* (eds P.J.

Piper & J. Costello), pp. 27–80. Parthenon Publishing, London.

Giembycz, M.A., Corrigan, C.J., Kay, A.B. & Barnes, P.J. (1994) Inhibition of CD4 and CD8 T-lymphocytes (T-LC) proliferation and cytokine secretion by isoenzyme-selective phosphodiesterase (PDE) inhibitors: correlation with intracellular cyclic AMP (cAMP) concentrations. *J. Allergy Clin. Immunol.*, **93**, 167.

Giembycz, M.A. Seybold, J., Barnes, P.J. & Corrigan, C.J. (1995) Identification of cyclic AMP phosphodiesterases 3, 4, and 7 in human CD4+ and CD8+ T-lymphocytes: role in regulating proliferation and the induction of interleukin-2 and interferon-γ. Brit. J. Pharmacol. (in press).

Giembycz, M.A. & Souness, J.E. (1996) Phosphodiesterase IV inhibitors as potential therapeutic agents in allergic disease. In: Immunopharmacology of Allergic Disease (eds R.G. Townley & D.K. Agarwal). New York, Dekker.

Gillespie, P.G. & Beavo, J.A. (1989) Inhibition and stimulation of photoreceptor phosphodiesterase by dipyridamole and M&B 22,948. *Mol. Pharmacol.*, **36**, 773–81.

Glaser, T. & Traber, J. (1984) TVX 2706 — a new phosphodiesterase inhibitor with anti-inflammatory action: biochemical characterization. *Agents Actions*, **15**, 341–8.

Godfrey, R.W., Manzi, R.M., Gennaro, D.E. & Hoffstein, S.T. (1987) Phospholipid and arachidonic acid metabolism in zymosan-stimulated human monocytes: modulation by cyclic AMP. *J. Cell. Physiol.*, 131, 384–92.

Goldberg, B.J., Lad, P.M. & Ghekiere, L. (1994) Phosphodiesterase activity and superoxide production in normal and asthmatic neutrophils. *J. Allergy Clin. Immunol.*, **93**, 166.

Grady, P.G. & Thomas, L.L. (1986) Characterization of cyclic-nucleotide phosphodiesterase activities in resting and *N*-formyl-methionyl-leucyl-phenylalanine-stimulated human neutrophils. *Biochim. Biophys. Acta*, **855**, 282–93.

Grant, P.G. & Coleman, R.W. (1984) Purification of a human platelet cyclic nucleotide phosphodiesterase. *Biochemistry*, **23**, 1801–7.

Grant, P.G., Mannarino, A.F. & Coleman, R.W. (1988) cAMP-mediated phosphorylation of the low-K_m cAMP phosphodiesterase markedly stimulates its catalytic activity. *Proc. Nat. Acad. Sci. USA*, **85**, 9071–5.

Grewe, S., Chan, S.C. & Hanifin, J.M. (1982) Elevated leukocyte cyclic AMP-phosphodiesterase in atopic disease. *J. Allergy Clin. Immunol.*, **70**, 452–7.

Gristwood, R.W., Llupia, J., Fernandez, A.G. & Berga, P. (1991) Effect of theophylline compared with prednisolone on late phase airway leukocyte infiltration in guinea-pigs. *Int. Arch. Allergy Appl. Immunol.*, **94**, 293–4.

Griswold, D.E., Webb, E.F., Breton, J., White, J.R., Marshall, P.J. & Torphy, T.J. (1993) Effect of selective phosphodiesterase type IV inhibitor, rolipram, on fluid and cellular phases of inflammatory responses. *Inflammation*, **17**, 333–44.

Hagiwara, M., Endo, T. & Hidaka, H. (1984a) Effects of vinpocetine on cyclic nucleotide metabolism in vascular smooth muscle. *Biochem. Pharmacol.*, **33**, 453–7.

Hagiwara, M., Endo, T., Kanayama, T. & Hidaka, H. (1984b) Effect of 1-(3-chloroanilino)-4-phenylphthalazine (MY 5445), a specific inhibitor of cyclic GMP phosphodiesterase on human platelet aggregation. *J. Pharmacol. Exp. Ther.*, **228**, 467–71.

Hallsworth, M.P., Giembycz, M.A., Barnes, P.J. & Lee, T.H. (1996) Inhibition of GM-CSF-induced eosinophil survival by cyclic AMP-elevating agents. *Brit. J. Pharmacol*, **117**, 79–86.

Hamet, P., Franks, D.J., Tremblay, J. & Coquil, J.F. (1983) Rapid activation of cyclic AMP phosphodiesterase in rats platelets. *Can. J. Biochem. Cell Biol.*, **61**, 1158–65.

Hancock, W.W., Pleau, M.E. & Kobzik, L. (1988) Recombinant granulocyte–macrophage colony-stimulating factor down-regulates expression of IL-2 receptors on human mononuclear phagocytes by induction of prostaglandins. *J. Immunol.*, **140**, 3021–5.

Hanifin, J.M. (1986) Pharmacophysiology of atopic dermatitis. *Clin. Rev. Allergy*, **4**, 43–65.

Hanifin, J.M., Butler, J.M. & Chan, S.C. (1985) Immunopharmacology of the atopic diseases. *J. Invest. Dermatol.*, **85**, 161s–164s.

Hansen, R.S. & Beavo, J.A. (1982) Purification of two calcium/calmodulin dependent forms of cyclic nucleotide phosphodiesterase by using conformation-specific monoclonal antibody chromatography. *Proc. Nat. Acad. Sci. USA*, **79**, 2788–92.

Harrison, S.A., Reifsnyder, D.H., Gallis, B., Cadd, G.G. & Beavo, J.A. (1986) Isolation and characterization of bovine cardiac muscle cyclic GMP-inhibited phosphodiesterase: a receptor for new cardiotonic drugs. *Mol. Pharmacol.*, **29**, 506–14.

Hartman, D.A., Ochalski, S.J. & Carlson, R.P. (1993) The effects of anti-inflammatory and antiallergic drugs on the release of IL-1β and TNF-α in the human whole blood assay. *Agents Actions*, **39**, C70–C72.

Harvath, L., Robbins, J.D., Russell, A.A. & Seaman, K.B. (1991) Cyclic AMP and human neutrophil chemotaxis: elevation of cyclic AMP differentially affects chemotactic responsiveness. *J. Immunol.*, **146**, 224–32.

Hatzelmann, A., Tenor, H. & Schudt, C. (1995) Differential effects of non-selective and selective phosphodiesterase inhibitors on human eosinophil functions. *Brit. J. Pharmacol.*, **114**, 821–31.

Hay, I.F.C. & Higenbottam, T.W. (1987) Has the management of asthma improved? *Lancet*, **ii**, 609–11.

Hendeles, L. & Weinberger, M. (1983) Theophylline: a state of the art review. *Pharmacotherapy*, **3**, 2–44.

Hendeles, L., Amarshi, N. & Weinberger, M. (1984) A clinical and pharmacokinetic basis for the selection and use of slow release theophylline products. *Clin. Pharmacokinet.*, **9**, 95–135.

Heskel, N.S., Chan, S.C., Thiel, M.L., Stevens, S.R., Casperson, L.S. & Hanifin, J.M. (1984) Elevated umbilical cord blood leukocyte cyclic adenosine monophosphate-phosphodiesterase activity in children with atopic parents. *J. Am. Acad. Dermatol.*, **11**, 422–6.

Hidaka, H., Teraka, T. & Itoh, H. (1984) Selective inhibitors of three forms of cyclic nucleotide phosphodiesterases. *Trends Pharmacol. Sci.*, **5**, 237–9.

Ho, P.P.K., Wang, L.Y., Towner, R.D. *et al.* (1990) Cardiovascular effect and stimulus-dependent inhibition of superoxide generation from human neutrophils by tibenelast 5,6-diethoxybenzo(*b*)thiophene 2-carboxylic acid, sodium salt (LY 186655). *Biochem. Pharmacol.*, **40**, 2085–92.

Holden, C.A. (1990) Atopic dermatitis: a defect of intracellular secondary messenger systems? *Clin. Exp. Allergy*, **20**, 131–6.

Holden, C.A. & Yuen, C.-T. (1989) Response of mononuclear leukocyte cyclic adenosine monophosphate-phosphodiesterase activity to treatment with topical fluorinated steroid ointment in atopic dermatitis. *J. Am. Acad. Dermatol.*, **21**, 69–74.

Holden, C.A., Chan, S.C. & Hanifin, J.M. (1986) Monocyte localization of elevated cyclic AMP phosphodiesterase activity in atopic dermatitis. *J. Invest. Dermatol.*, **87**, 372–6.

Holden, C.A., Chan, S.C., Norris, S. & Hanifin, J.M. (1987) Histamine-induced elevation of cyclic AMP phosphodiesterase activity in human monocytes. *Agents Actions*, **22**, 36–42.

Holden, C.A., Yuen, C.-T. & Coulson, I.H. (1989) The effect of *in vitro* exposure to histamine on mononuclear leukocyte phosphodiesterase activity in atopic dermatitis. *Clin. Exp. Dermatol.*, **14**, 186–90.

Horowski, R. & Sastre-Y-Hernandez, M. (1985) Clinical effects of the neurotropic selective cAMP phosphodiesterase inhibitor rolipram in depressed patients: global evaluation of the preliminary reports. *Curr. Ther. Res.*, **38**, 23–9.

Howell, R.E. & Meuhsam, W.T. (1990) Mechanism for the emetic side-effect of xanthine bronchodilators. *Life Sci.*, **46**, 563–8.

Howell, R.E., Sickles, B.D. & Woeppel, S.L. (1993) Pulmonary antiallergic and bronchodilator effects of isozyme-selective phosphodiesterase inhibitors in guinea-pigs. *J. Pharmacol. Exp. Ther.*, **264**, 609–15.

Hurley, J.B. (1987) Molecular properties of the cGMP cascade of vertebrate photoreceptors. *Ann. Rev. Physiol.*, **49**, 793–812.

Ichimura, M. & Kase, H. (1993) A new cyclic nucleotide phosphodiesterase isozyme expressed in the T-lymphocyte cell lines. *Biochem. Biophys. Res. Commun.*, **193**, 985–90.

Israel, E., Mathur, P.N., Tachkin, D. & Drazen, J.M. (1987) LY 186655 prevents bronchospasm in asthma of moderate severity. *Chest*, **91**, 71S.

Iwatsuki, K., Horiuchi, A., Ren, L.M. & Chiba, S. (1991) Effects of the cyclic nucleotide phosphodiesterase inhibitor, rolipram 3-isobutyl-1-methylxanthine, amrinone and zaprinast, on pancreatic exocrine secretion in dogs. *Eur. J. Pharmacol.*, **209**, 63–8.

Jaffar, Z., Sullivan, P., Page, C.P. & Costello, J. (1994) Modulation of T-lymphocyte activity in atopic asthmatics by low dose theophylline therapy. *Eur. Resp. J.*, **7**, 160S.

Juergens, U.R., Overlack, A. & Vetter, H. (1993) Theophylline inhibits the formation of leukotriene B_4 (LTB_4) by enhancement of cyclic-AMP and prostaglandin E_2 (PGE_2) production in normal monocytes *in vitro*. *Eur. Resp. J.*, **6** (Suppl. 17), 3685.

Kakiuchi, S. & Yamazaki, R. (1970) Calcium-dependent phosphodiesterase activity and its activating factor (PAF) from brain: studies on cyclic 3′,5′-nucleotide phosphodiesterase (III). *Biochem. Biophys. Res. Commun.*, **41**, 1104–10.

Kammer, G.M. (1988) The adenylate cyclase–cyclic AMP–protein kinase A pathway and regulation of the immune response. *Immunol. Today*, **9**, 222–9.

Kaneko, M., Suzuki, K., Furui, H., Takagi, K. & Satake, T. (1990) Comparison of theophylline and enprofylline effects of human neutrophil superoxide production. *Clin. Exp. Physiol. Pharmacol.*, **17**, 849–59.

Kaplan, H.J., Deman, L., Rosenberg, E.W. & Feigenbaum, S. (1978) Topical use of caffeine with hydrocortisone in the treatment of atopic dermatitis. *Arch. Dermatol.*, **114**, 60–2.

Kariya, T. & Dage, R.C. (1988) Tissue distribution and selective inhibition of subtypes of high affinity phosphodiesterase. *Biochem. Pharmacol.*, **37**, 3267–70.

Kase, H., Yoshizaki, R., Shiozaki, M. & Ichimura, M. (1993) KS 505a, an isoform-selective inhibitor of calmodulin-dependent cyclic nucleotide phosphodiesterase. *Brit. J. Pharmacol.*, **108**, 300P.

Kasuya, J., Goko, H. & Fujita-Yamaguchi, Y. (1995) Multiple transcripts for the human cardiac form of the cGMP-inhibited cAMP phosphodiesterase. *J. Biol. Chem.*, **270**, 14305–12.

Kawasaki, A., Hoshino, K., Osaki, R., Mizushima, Y. & Yano, S. (1992) Effect of ibudilast, a novel anti-asthmatic agent on airway hypersensitivity in bronchial asthma. *J. Asthma*, **29**, 245–52.

Keating, G., Mitchell, E.A., Jackson, R., Beaglehole, R. & Rea, H. (1983) Trends in the sales of drugs for asthma in New Zealand, Australia and the United Kingdom. *Brit. Med. J.*, **289**, 348–51.

Kidney, J.C., Dominguez, M., Rose, M., Aikman, S., Chung, K.F. & Barnes, P.J. (1993) Immune modulation by theophylline: the effect of withdrawal of chronic treatment. *Am. Rev. Resp. Dis.*, **147**, A772.

Kidney, J.C., Dominguez, M., Taylar, P., Rose, M., Chung, K.F. & Barnes, P.J. (1994) Withdrawal of chronic theophylline treatment increases airway lymphocytes. *Thorax*, **49**, 396P.

Kincaid, R.L., Stith-Coleman, I.E. & Vaughan, M. (1985) Proteolytic activation of calmodulin-dependent phosphodiesterase. *J. Biol. Chem.*, **260**, 9009–15.

Kings, M.A., Chapman, I., Kristersson, A., Sanjar, S. & Morley, J. (1990) Human recombinant lymphokines and cytokines induce pulmonary eosinophilia in the guinea-pig which is inhibited by ketotifen and AH 21-132. *Int. Arch. Allergy Appl. Immunol.*, **91**, 354–61.

Kips, J.C., Tavernier, J. & Pauwels, R. (1992) Tumor necrosis factor (TNF) causes bronchial hyper-responsiveness in rats. *Am. Rev. Resp. Dis.*, **145**, 332–6.

Kips, J.C., Joos, G.F., Peleman, R.A. & Pauwels, R.A. (1993) The effect of zardaverine, an inhibitor of phosphodiesterase isoenzymes III and IV, on endotoxin-induced airway changes in rats. *Clin. Exp. Allergy*, **23**, 518–23.

Kishi, Y., Ashikaya, T. & Numano, F. (1992) Phosphodiesterases in vascular endothelial cells. *Adv. Sec. Mess. Phosphoprot. Res.*, **25**, 201–13.

Kita, H., Abu-Ghazaleh, R.I., Gleich, G.J. & Abraham, R.T. (1991) Regulation of Ig-induced eosinophil degranulation by adenosine 3′,5′-cyclic monophosphate. *J. Immunol.*, **146**, 2712–18.

Knudsen, P.J., Dinarello, C.A. & Strom, T.B. (1986) Prostaglandins posttranscriptionally inhibit monocyte expression of interleukin 1 activity by increasing intracellular cyclic adenosine monophosphate. *J. Immunol.*, **137**, 3189–94.

Koga, S., Morris, S., Ogawa, S. *et al.* (1995) TNF modulates endothelial properties by decreasing cAMP. *Am. J. Physiol.*, **268**, C1104–C1113.

Koyoma, S., Rennard, S.I., Claessen, L. & Robbins, R.A. (1991) Dibutyryl cyclic AMP, prostaglandin E_2, and antioxidants protect cultured bovine epithelial cells from endotoxin. *Am. J. Physiol.*, **261**, L126–L132.

Lagente, V., Moodley, I., Perrin, S., Mottin, G. & Junien, J.-L. (1994) Effect of isoenzyme-selective phosphodiesterase inhibitors on eosinophil infiltration in the guinea-pig lung. *Eur. J. Pharmacol.*, **255**, 253–6.

LaHat, N., Nir, E., Horenstein, L. & Colin, A.A. (1985) Effect of theophylline on the proportion and function of T-suppressor cells in asthmatic children. *Allergy*, **40**, 453–7.

Lee, H.J., Koyano-Nakagawa, N., Naito, Y. *et al.* (1993) Cyclic AMP activates the IL-5 promoter synergistically with phorbol ester through the signaling pathway involving protein kinase A in mouse thymoma line EL-4. *J. Immunol.*, **151**, 6135–42.

Leeman, M., Lejeune, P., Melot, C. & Naeije, R. (1987) Reduction in pulmonary hypertension and in airway resistance by enoximone (MDL 17,043) in decompensated COPD. *Chest*, **91**, 662–6.

Lefkowitz, R.J., Hausdorff, W.P. & Caron, M.G. (1990) Role of phosphorylation in desensitization of the β-adrenergic receptor. *Trends Pharmacol. Sci.*, **11**, 190–4.

Le Trong, H., Beier, N., Sonnenburg, B. *et al.* (1990) Amino acid sequence of the cyclic GMP-stimulated cyclic nucleotide phosphodiesterase from bovine heart. *Biochemistry*, **29**, 10280–8.

Leung, D.Y.M. (1992) Immunopathology of atopic dermatitis. *Springer Semin. Immunopathol.*, **13**, 427–40.

Levin, R.I., Weksler, B.B. & Jaffe, E.A. (1982) The interaction of sodium nitroprusside with human endothelial cells and platelets: nitroprusside and prostacyclin synergistically inhibit function. *Circulation*, **66**, 1299–307.

Lewis, G.M., Caccese, R.G., Heaslip, R.L. & Bansbach, C.C. (1993) Effects of rolipram and CI-930 on IL-2 mRNA transcription in human Jurkat cells. *Agents Actions*, **39**, C89–C92.

Li, S.-H., Chan, S.C., Toshitani, A., Leung, D.Y.M. & Hanifin, J.M. (1992) Synergistic effects of interleukin 4 and interferon-gamma on monocyte phosphodiesterase activity. *J. Invest. Dermatol.*, **99**, 65–70.

Li, S.-H., Chan, S.C., Kramer, S.M. & Hanifin, J.M. (1993) Modulation of leukocyte cyclic AMP phosphodiesterase activity by recombinant interferon-γ: evidence for a differential effect on atopic monocytes. *J. Interferon Res.*, **13**, 197–202.

Lichtenstein, L.M. & Margolis, S. (1968) Histamine release *in vitro*: inhibition by catecholamines and methylxanthines. *Science*, **161**, 902–3.

Lim, L.K., Hunt, N.H. & Widemann, M.J. (1983) Reactive oxygen production, arachidonate metabolism and cyclic AMP in macrophages. *Biochim. Biophys. Acta*, **114**, 549–55.

Limatibul, S., Shore, A., Rorsch, H.M. & Gelfand, E. (1978) Theophylline modulation of E-rosette formation: an indicator of T-cell maturation. *Clin. Exp. Allergy*, **33**, 503–13.

Lindgren, S., Lokshin, B., Stromqvist, A. *et al.* (1992) Does asthma or treatment with theophylline limit children's academic performance? *New Engl. J. Med.*, **327**, 926–30.

Livi, G.P., Kmetz, P., McHale, M.M. *et al.* (1990) Cloning and expression for a human low-K_m, rolipram sensitive cyclic AMP phosphodiesterase. *Mol. Cell. Biol.*, **10**, 2678–86.

Lonchampt, M., Pennel, L. & Canet, E. (1995) *In vivo* effect of rolipram on antigen-induced interleukin-4 (IL-4) and interleukin-5 (IL-5) production in bronchoalveolar lavage of sensitised BALB/c mice. *Am. J. Resp. Crit. Care Med.*, **151**, A827.

Loughney, K. & Ferguson, K.M. (1994) The human cyclic nucleotide phosphodiesterases. In: *Methylxanthines and Phosphodiesterase Inhibitors and the Treatment of Respiratory Disease* (eds P.J. Piper & J. Costello), pp. 81–100. Parthenon Publishing, London.

Louis, R.E. & Radermecker, M.F. (1990) Substance P-induced histamine release from human basophils, skin and lung fragments: effect of nedocromil sodium and theophylline. *Int. Arch. Allergy Appl. Immunol.*, **92**, 329–33.

Lugnier, C. & Schini, V.B. (1990) Characterization of cyclic nucleotide phosphodiesterases from cultured bovine aortic endothelial cells. *Biochem. Pharmacol.*, **39**, 75–84.

Luther, M., Holmes, B., Kassal, D. *et al.* (1994) Identification and functional characterization of various phosphorylated forms of human recombinant, rolipram-sensitive cAMP-specific type IV phosphodiesterase. *FASEB J.*, **8**, 2141 [abstract 370].

Lycke, N.Y. (1993) Cholera toxin promotes B cell isotype switching by two different mechanisms. *J. Immunol.*, **150**, 4810–21.

Lycke, N., Severinson, E. & Strober, W. (1990) Cholera toxin acts synergistically with IL-4 to promote IgG1 switch differentiation. *J. Immunol.*, **145**, 3316–24.

McLaughlin, M.M., Cieslinski, L.B., Burman, M., Torphy, T.J. & Livi, G.P. (1993) A low-K_m, rolipram-sensitive, cAMP phosphodiesterase from human brain: cloning and expression of cDNA, biochemical characterization of recombinant protein, and tissue distribution of mRNA. *J. Biol. Chem.*, **268**, 6470–6.

Macphee, C.H., Harrison, S.A. & Beavo, J.A. (1986) Immunological identification of the major platelet low K_m cAMP phosphodiesterase: probable target for antithrombotic agents. *Proc. Nat. Acad. Sci. USA*, **83**, 6660–3.

Manganiello, V.C., Degerman, E., Smith, C.J., Vasta, V., Tornqvist, H. & Belfrage, P. (1992) Mechanisms for activation of the rat adipocyte particulate cyclic GMP-inhibited cyclic AMP phosphodiesterase and its importance in the antilipolytic action of insulin. *Adv. Sec. Mess. Phosphoprot. Res.*, **25**, 147–64.

Manzini, S., Perretti, F., Abelli, L., Evangelista, S., Seeds, E.A.M. & Page, C.P. (1993) Isbufylline, a new xanthine derivative, inhibits airways hyperresponsiveness and airways inflammation in guinea-pigs. *Eur. J. Pharmacol.*, **249**, 251–7.

Marcos, P., Prigent, A.F., Lagarde, M. & Nemoz, G. (1993) Modulation of rat thymocyte proliferative response through the inhibition of different cyclic nucleotide phosphodiesterase isoforms by means of selective inhibitors of cGMP-elevating agents. *Mol. Pharmacol.*, **44**, 1027–35.

Martins, T.J., Mumby, M.C. & Beavo, J.A. (1982) Purification and characterization of cyclic GMP-stimulated cyclic nucleotide phosphodiesterase from bovine tissues. *J. Biol., Chem.*, **257**, 1973–9.

Maruo, H., Tanimoto, Y., Bewtra, A.K. & Townley, R.G. (1994) Effect of phosphodiesterase IV inhibitor (WAY-PDE-641) on PAF-induced superoxide generation from human eosinophils. *J. Allergy Clin. Immunol.*, **93**, 257.

Mary, D., Aussel, C., Ferrua, B. & Fehlmann, M. (1987) Regulation of interleukin-2 synthesis by cyclic AMP in human T-cells. *J. Immunol.*, **139**, 1179–84.

Masuoka, H., Ito, M., Sugioka, M. *et al.* (1993) Two isoforms of cGMP-inhibited cyclic nucleotide phosphodiesterases in human tissues distinguished by their responses to vesnarinone, a new cardiotonic agent. *Biochem. Biophys. Res. Commun.*, **190**, 412–17.

Maurice, D.H. & Haslam, R.J. (1990) Molecular basis of the synergistic inhibition of platelet function by nitrovasodilators and activators of adenylate cyclase: inhibition of cyclic AMP breakdown by cyclic GMP. *Mol. Pharmacol.*, **37**, 671–81.

Maurice, D.H., Crankshaw, D. & Haslam, R.J. (1991) Synergistic actions of nitrovasodilators and isoprenaline on rat aortic smooth muscle. *Eur. J. Pharmacol.*, **192**, 235–42.

Meacci, E., Taira, M., Moos, M. *et al.* (1992) Molecular cloning and expression of human myocardial cGMP-inhibited cAMP phosphodiesterase. *Proc. Nat. Acad. Sci. USA*, **89**, 3721–5.

Michaeli, T., Bloom, T.J., Martins, T. *et al.* (1993) Isolation and characterization of a previously undetected human cyclic AMP phosphodiesterase by complementation of cyclic AMP phosphodiesterase-deficient *Saccharomyces cerevisiae*. *J. Biol. Chem.*, **268**, 12925–32.

Minnear, F.L., DeMichele, M.A., Moon, D.G., Rieder, C.L. & Fenton, J.W. (1989) Isoproterenol reduces thrombin-induced pulmonary endothelial permeability *in vitro*. *Am. J. Physiol.*, **257**, H1613–H1623.

Molnar-Kimber, K.L., Yonno, L., Heaslip, R.J. & Weichman, B.M. (1993) Differential regulation of TNF-α and IL-1β production from endotoxin stimulated human monocytes by phosphodiesterase inhibitors. *Mediat. Inflamm.*, **1**, 411–17.

Monaco, L., Vicini, E. & Conti, M. (1994) Structure of two rat genes coding for closely related rolipram-sensitive cAMP phosphodiesterases: multiple mRNA variants originate from alternative splicing and multiple start sites. *J. Biol. Chem.*, **269**, 347–57.

Moss, J., Manganiello, V.C. & Vaughan, M. (1977) Substrate and effector specificity of a guanosine 3′:5′-monophosphate phosphodiesterase from rat liver. *J. Biol. Chem.*, **252**, 5211–15.

Muggli, R., Tschopp, T.B., Mittelholzer, E. & Baumgartner, H.R.

(1985) 7-Bromo-1,5-dihydro-3,6-dimethylimidazo [2,1-b] quinazolin-2 (3H)-one (Ro 15-2041), a potent anti-thrombotic agent that selectively inhibits platelet cyclic AMP phosphodiesterase. *J. Pharmacol. Exp. Ther.*, **235**, 212–19.

Müller, A. & Nennstiel, P. (1992) Selective inhibition of the cyclic GMP-stimulated cyclic nucleotide phosphodiesterase from pig and human myocardium. *J. Mol. Cell. Cardiol.*, **24** (Suppl. V), S102.

Munoz, E., Zubiaga, A.M., Merrow, M., Sauter, N.P. & Huber, B.T. (1990) Cholera toxin discriminates between T helper 1 and 2 cell receptor-mediated activation: role of cyclic AMP in T cell proliferation. *J. Exp. Med.*, **172**, 95–103.

Murashima, S., Tanaka, T., Hockman, S. & Manganiello, V.C. (1990) Characterization of particulate cyclic nucleotide phosphodiesterase from bovine brain: purification of a distinct cGMP-stimulated enzyme. *Biochemistry*, **29**, 5285–92.

Murray, K.J. (1993) Phosphodiesterase V_A inhibitors. *Drugs News Perspect.*, **6**, 150–6.

Murray, K.J., England, P.J., Hallam, T.J. *et al.* (1990) The effects of siguazodan, a selective phosphodiesterase inhibitor, on human platelet function. *Brit. J. Pharmacol.*, **99**, 612–16.

Murray, K.J., Eden, R.J., Dolan, J.S. *et al.* (1992) The effect of SK&F 95654, a novel phosphodiesterase inhibitor, on cardiovascular, respiratory and platelet function. *Brit. J. Pharmacol.*, **107**, 463–70.

Naccarelli, G.V. & Goldstein, R.A. (1989) Electrophysiology of phosphodiesterase inhibitors. *Am. J. Cardiol.*, **63**, 35A–40A.

Naclerio, R.M., Bertenfelder, D., Proud, D. *et al.* (1986) Theophylline reduces histamine release during pollen-induced rhinitis. *J. Allergy Clin. Immunol.*, **78**, 874–6.

Nakanishi, S., Osawa, K., Saito, Y., Kawamoto, I., Kuroda, K. & Kase, H. (1992) KS-505a, a novel inhibitor of bovine brain Ca^{2+} and calmodulin-dependent cyclic nucleotide phosphodiesterase from *Streptomyces argenteolus*. *J. Antibiot.*, **45**, 341–7.

Némoz, G., Mouequit, M., Prigent, A.-F. & Pacheco, H. (1989) Isolation of similar rolipram-inhibitable cyclic AMP-specific phosphodiesterases from rat brain and heart. *Eur. J. Biochem.*, **184**, 511–20.

Newsholme, S.J. & Schwartz, L. (1993) cAMP-specific phosphodiesterase inhibitor, rolipram, reduces eosinophil infiltration evoked by leukotrienes or by histamine in guinea-pig conjunctiva. *Inflammation*, **17**, 25–31.

Newton, R.P., Sabih, S.G. & Khan, J.A. (1990) Cyclic CMP-specific phosphodiesterase activity. In: *Cyclic Nucleotide Phosphodiesterases: Structure, Regulation and Drug Action* (eds J.A. Beavo & M.D. Houslay), pp. 141–59. Wiley, Chichester.

Nicholson, C.D., Jackman, S.A. & Wilke, R. (1989) The ability of denbufylline to inhibit cyclic nucleotide phosphodiesterase and its affinity for adenosine receptors and the adenosine re-uptake site. *Brit. J. Pharmacol.*, **97**, 889–97.

Nicholson, C.D., Challiss, R.A.J. & Shahid, M. (1991) Differential modulation of tissue function and therapeutic potential of selective inhibitors of cyclic nucleotide phosphodiesterase isoenzymes. *Trends Pharmacol. Sci.*, **2**, 19–27.

Nicholson, CD & Shahid, M. (1994) Inhibitors of cyclic nucleotide phosphodiesterase isoenzymes — their potential utility in the therapy of asthma. *Pulmonary Pharmacol.*, **7**, 1–17.

Nicholson, C.D., Shahid, M., Bruin, J. *et al.* (1995) Characterization of ORG 20241, a combined phosphodiesterase IV/III inhibitor for asthma. *J. Pharmacol. Exp. Ther*, **274**, 678–87.

Nielson, C.P., Crawley, J.J., Cusak, B.J. & Vestal, R.E. (1986) Therapeutic concentrations of theophylline and enprophylline potentiate catecholamine effects and inhibit leukocyte activation. *J. Allergy Clin. Immunol.*, **78**, 660–7.

Nielson, C.P., Crawley, J.J., Morgan, M.E. & Vestal, R.E. (1988) Polymorphonuclear leukocyte inhibition by therapeutic concentrations of theophylline is mediated by cyclic 3′,5′-adenosine monophosphate. *Am. Rev. Resp. Dis.*, **137**, 25–30.

Nielson, C.P., Vestal, R.E., Sturm, R.J. & Heaslip, R. (1990) Effects of selective phosphodiesterase inhibitors on the polymorphonuclear leukocyte respiratory burst. *J. Allergy. Clin. Immunol.*, **86**, 801–8.

Nourshargh, S. & Hoult, J.R.S. (1986) Inhibition of human neutrophil degranulation by forskolin in the presence of phosphodiesterase inhibitors. *Eur. J. Pharmacol.*, **122**, 205–12.

Novack, J.P., Charbonneau, H., Bentley, J.K., Walsh, K.A. & Beavo, J.A. (1991) Sequence comparison of the 63-, 61-, and 59-kDa calmodulin-dependent cyclic nucleotide phosphodiesterases. *Biochemistry*, **30**, 7940–7.

Novak, T.J. & Rothenberg, E.V. (1990) Cyclic AMP inhibits induction of interleukin 2 but not of interleukin 4 in T cells. *Proc. Nat. Acad. Sci. USA*, **87**, 9353–7.

Obernolte, R., Bhakta, S., Alvarez, R. *et al.* (1993) The cDNA of a human lymphocyte cyclic-AMP phosphodiesterase (PDE IV) reveals a multigene family. *Gene*, **129**, 239–47.

Ochalski, S.J., Hartman, D.A., Belfast, M.T., Walter, T.L., Glaser, K.B. & Carlson, R.P. (1993) Inhibition of endotoxin-induced hypothermia and serum TNF-α levels in CD-1 mice by various pharmacological agents. *Agents Actions*, **39**, C52–C54.

Ohta, K., Sawamoto, S., Nakajima, M. *et al.* (1994) Theophylline induces apoptosis in eosinophils surviving with interleukin-5 *in vitro*. *J. Allergy Clin. Immunol.*, **93**, 200.

Okonogi, K., Gettys, T.W., Uhing, R.J., Tarry, C., Adams, P.O. & Prpic, V. (1991) Inhibition of prostaglandin E_2-stimulated cAMP accumulation by lipopolysaccharide in murine peritoneal macrophages. *J. Biol. Chem.*, **266**, 10305–12.

O'Neill, S.J., Sitar, D.S., Klass, D.J., Taraska, V.A., Kepron, W. & Mitenko, P.A. (1986) The pulmonary disposition of theophylline and its influence on human macrophage bactericidal function. *Am. Rev. Resp. Dis.*, **134**, 1225–8.

Orange, R.P., Kaliner, M.A., Laraia, P.J. & Austin, K.F. (1971) Immunological release of histamine and slow reacting substance of anaphylaxis from human lung. II. Influence of cellular levels of cyclic AMP. *Fed. Proc.*, **30**, 1725–9.

Ortiz, J.L., Cortijo, J., Valles, J.M., Bou, J. & Morcillo, E.J. (1992) Rolipram inhibits PAF-induced airway microvascular leakage in guinea-pig: a comparison with milrinone and theophylline. *Fund. Clin. Pharmacol.*, **6**, 247–9.

Pardi, R., Zocchi, M., Ferrero, E., Ciboddo, G.F., Inverardi, L. & Rugarli, C. (1984) *In vivo* effects of a single infusion of theophylline on human peripheral blood lymphocytes. *Clin. Exp. Immunol.*, **57**, 722–8.

Paul-Eugene, N., Kolb, J.P., Calenda, A. *et al.* (1993) Functional interaction between β_2-adrenoceptor agonists and interleukin-4 in the regulation of CD23 expression and release and IgE production in human. *Mol. Immunol.*, **30**, 157–64.

Pauwels, R. (1989a) The relationship between airway inflammation and bronchial hyper-responsiveness. *Clin. Exp. Allergy*, **19**, 395–8.

Pauwels, R. (1989b) New aspects of the therapeutic potential of theophylline in asthma. *J. Allergy Clin. Immunol.*, **83**, 548–53.

Pauwels, R., Kips, J.C., Peleman, R.A. & van der Straeten, M.E. (1990) The effect of endotoxin inhalation on airway responsiveness and cellular influx in rats. *Am. Rev. Resp. Dis.*, **141**, 540–5.

Peachell, P.T., Undem, B.J., Schleimer, R.P. *et al.* (1992) Preliminary identification and role of phosphodiesterase isozymes in human basophils. *J. Immunol.*, **148**, 2503–10.

Pearce, F.L., Befus, A.D., Gauldie, J. & Bienenstock, J. (1982) Effect of anti-allergic compounds on histamine secretion by isolated mast cells. *J. Immunol.*, **128**, 2481–6.

Perruchoud, A.P., Yerger, L. & Abraham, W.M. (1984) Differential effects of aminophylline on the early and late antigen-induced bronchial obstruction in allergic sheep. *Respiration*, **46**, 44.

Phipps, R.P., Roper, R.L. & Stein, S.H. (1990) Regulation of B-cell tolerance and triggering by macrophages and lymphoid dendritic cells. *Immunol. Rev.*, **117**, 135–58.

Pillai, R., Fluckiger-Staub, S. & Colicelli, J. (1994) Mutational mapping of kinetic and pharmacological proerties of a human cardiac cAMP phosphodiesterase. *J. Biol. Chem.*, **269**, 30676–81.

Pober, J.S., Slowik, M.R., De Luca, L.G. & Ritchie, A.J. (1993) Elevated cyclic AMP inhibits endothelial cell synthesis and expression of TNF-induced endothelial leukocyte adhesion molecule-1, and vascular cell adhesion molecule-1, but not intercellular adhesion molecule-1. *J. Immunol.*, **150**, 5114–23.

Podzuweit, T., Muller A, & Opie, L.H. (1993) Anti-arrhythmic effects of selective inhibition of myocardial phosphodiesterase II. *Lancet*, 341, 760.

Pyne, N.J., Cooper, M.E. & Houslay, M.D. (1987) The insulin- and glucagon-stimulated 'dense vesicle' high affinity cyclic AMP phosphodiesterase from rat liver: purification, characterization and inhibitor sensitivity. *Biochem. J.*, **242**, 33–42.

Rabe, K.F., Tenor, H., Spaethe, S.M. *et al.* (1994) Identification of the PDE isoenzymes in human bronchial epithelial cells and the effect of PDE inhibition on PGE_2 secretion. *Am. J. Resp. Crit. Care Med.*, **149**, A986.

Rachelefsky, G.S., Wo, J., Adelson, J. *et al.* (1986) Behavioural abnormalities and poor school performance due to oral theophylline use. *Pediatrics*, **78**, 1113–38.

Radomski, M.W., Palmer, R.M.J. & Moncada, S. (1987a) Comparative pharmacology of endothelium-derived relaxing factor, nitric oxide and prostacyclin in platelets. *Brit. J. Pharmacol.*, **92**, 181–7.

Radomski, M.W., Palmer, R.M.J. & Moncada, S. (1987b) The role of nitric oxide and cyclic GMP in platelet adhesion to vascular endothelium. *Biochem. Biophy. Res. Commun.*, **148**, 1482–9.

Raeburn, D. & Karlsson, J.-A. (1991) Effects of isoenzyme-selective inhibitors of cyclic nucleotide phosphodiesterase on microvascular leak in guinea-pig airways. *J. Pharmacol. Exp. Ther.*, **267**, 1147–52.

Raeburn, D., Woodman, V., Buckley, G. & Karlsson, J.-A. (1993) Inhibition of PAF-induced microvascular leakage in the guinea-pig *in vivo*: the effects of rolipram and theophylline. *Eur. Resp. J.*, **4** (Suppl. 14), 590S.

Raeburn, D., Souness, J.E., Tomkinson, A. & Karlsson, J.-A. (1993) Isozyme-selective cyclic nucleotide phosphodiesterase inhibitors: biochemistry, pharmacology and therapeutic potential in asthma. *Prog. Drugs Res.*, **40**, 9–31.

Raeburn, D., Underwood, S.L., Lewis, S.A. *et al.* (1994) Anti-inflammatory and bronchodilator properties of RP 73401, a novel and selective phosphodiesterase IV inhibitor. *Brit. J. Pharmacol.*, **113**, 1423–31.

Rasmussen, J.E. (1989) Advances in nondietary management of children with atopic dermatitis. *Ped. Dermatol.*, **6**, 210–15.

Reeves, M.L., Leigh, B.K. & England, P.J. (1987) The identification of a new cyclic nucleotide phosphodiesterase activity in human and guinea-pig cardiac ventricle. *Biochem. J.*, **241**, 535–41.

Reiser, J., Yeang, Y. & Warner, J.O. (1986) The effect of zaprinast, an orally absorbed mast cell stabiliser, on exercise-induced asthma in children. *Brit. J. Dis. Chest*, **80**, 157–63.

Repaske, D.R., Swinnen, J.V., Jin, S.L.-C., Vam Wyk, J.J. & Conti, M. (1992) A polymerase chain reaction strategy to identify and clone cyclic nucleotide phosphodiesterase cDNAs: molecular cloning of the cDNA encoding the 63 kDa calmodulin-dependent phosphodiesterase. *J. Biol. Chem.*, **267**, 18683–8.

Rivkin, I. & Neutze, J.A. (1977) Influence of cyclic nucleotides and a phosphodiesterase inhibitor on *in vitro* human blood neutrophil chemotaxis. *Arch. Int. Pharmacodyn. Thér.*, **228**, 196–204.

Robichon, A. (1991) A new cyclic GMP phosphodiesterase isolated from bovine platelets is a substrate for cyclic AMP- and cyclic GMP-dependent protein kinases: evidence for a key role in the process of platelet activation. *J. Cell. Biochem.*, **47**, 147–57.

Robicsek, S.A., Krzanowski, J.J., Szentivanyi, A. & Polson, J.B. (1989) High pressure liquid chromatography of cyclic AMP phosphodiesterase from purified human T-lymphocytes. *Biochem. Biophys. Res. Commun.*, **163**, 554–60.

Robicsek, S.A., Blanchard, D.K., Djeu, J.Y., Krzanowski, J.J., Szentivanyi, A. & Polson, J.B. (1991) Multiple high-affinity cyclic AMP phosphodiesterases in human T-lymphocytes. *Biochem. Pharmacol.*, **42**, 869–77.

Roper, R.L., Conrad, D.H., Brown, D.M., Warner, C.L. & Phipps, R.P. (1990) Prostaglandin E_2 promotes IL-4-induced IgE and IgG_1 synthesis. *J. Immunol.*, **145**, 2644–51.

Rossi, P., Giorgi, M., Geremia, R. & Kincaid, R.L. (1988) Testis-specific calmodulin-dependent phosphodiesterase: a distinct high-affinity isozyme immunologically related to brain calmodulin-dependent cyclic GMP phosphodiesterase. *J. Biol. Chem.*, **263**, 15521–7.

Rott, O., Cash, E. & Fleischer, B. (1993) Phosphodiesterase inhibitor pentoxifylline, a selective suppressor of T-helper type 1- but not type 2-associated lymphokine production, prevents induction of experimental autoimmune encephalomyelitis in Lewis rats. *Eur. J. Immunol.*, **23**, 1745–51.

Rousseau, E., Gagnon, J. & Lugnier, C. (1994) Biochemical and pharmacological characterization of cyclic nucleotide phosphodiesterase in airway epithelium. *Mol. Cell. Biochem.*, **140**, 171–5.

Rudd, R.M., Gellert, A.R., Studdy, P.R. & Geddes, D.M. (1983) Inhibition of exercise-induced asthma by an orally absorbed mast cell stabilizer (M&B 22,948). *Brit. J. Dis. Chest*, **80**, 78–86.

Safko, M.J., Chan, S-C., Cooper, K.D. & Hanifin, J.M. (1981) Heterologous desensitization of leukocytes: a possible mechanism of beta-adrenoceptor blockade in atopic dermatitis. *J. Allergy Clin. Immunol.*, **68**, 218–25.

Sanjar, S., Aoki, S., Boubekeur, K. *et al.* (1989) Inhibition of PAF-induced eosinophil accumulation in pulmonary airways of guinea-pigs by anti-asthma drugs. *Jpn. J. Pharmacol.*, **51**, 167–72.

Sanjar, S., Aoki, S., Boubekeur, K. *et al.* (1990a) Eosinophil accumulation in pulmonary airways of guinea-pigs induced by exposure to an aerosol of platelet activating factor: effect of anti-asthma drugs. *Brit. J. Pharmacol.*, **99**, 267–72.

Sanjar, S., Aoki, S., Kristersson, A., Smith, D. & Morley, J. (1990b) Antigen challenge induces pulmonary airway eosinophil accumulation and airway hyperreactivity in sensitised guinea-pigs: the effect of anti-asthma drugs. *Brit. J. Pharmacol.*, **99**, 679–86.

Sawiski, M.A., Rusin, L.J., Burns, T.L., Weinstein, G.D. & Voorhees, J.J. (1979) Ro 20-1724: an agent that significantly improves psoriatic lesions in double-blind clinical trials. *J. Invest. Dermatol.*, **73**, 261–3.

Schade, F.U. & Schudt, C. (1993) The specific type III and IV phosphodiesterase inhibitor zardaverine suppresses formation of tumour necrosis factor by macrophages. *Eur. J. Pharmacol.*, **230**, 9–14.

Schmidt, J., Fleissner, S., Heimann-Weitschat, I., Lindstaedt, R. & Szelenyi, I. (1994) Histamine increases anti-CD3 induced IL-5 production of TH2-type T cells via histamine H_2-receptors. *Agents Actions*, **42**, 81–5.

Schrier, D.J. & Imrie, R.M. (1986) The effect of adenosine antagonists on human neutrophil function. *J. Immunol.*, **137**, 3284–9.

Schudt, C. & Tenor, H. (1994) PDE isoenzyme patterns in human inflammatory cells. In: *Phosphodiesterase: A Key Enzyme in Regulation of Smooth Muscle and Inflammation?* (eds A. Keller, H. Tenor & C. Schudt), pp. 19–27. Byk-Gulden, Konstanz, Germany.

Schudt, C., Winder, S., Litze, M., Kilian, U. & Beume, R. (1991a) Zardaverine: a cyclic AMP specific PDE III/IV inhibitor. *Agents Actions*, **34**, 161–77.

Schudt, C., Winder, S., Muller, B. & Ukena, D. (1991b) Zardaverine as a selective inhibitor of phosphodiesterase isozymes. *Biochem. Pharmacol.*, **42**, 153–62.

Schudt, C., Winder, S., Forderkunz, S., Hatzelmann, A. & Ullrich, V. (1991c) Influence of selective phosphodiesterase inhibitors on human neutrophil functions and levels of cAMP and Ca_i. *Naunyn Schmiedeberg's Arch. Pharmacol.*, **344**, 682–90.

Schudt, C., Tenor, H., Wendel, A. *et al.* (1992) Effect of selective phosphodesterase (PDE) inhibitors on activation af human macrophages and lymphocytes. *Naunyn Schmiedeberg's Arch. Pharmacol.*, **345**, R69.

Schultz-Werninghaus, G. & Meier-Sydow (1982) The clinical and pharmacological history of theophylline. *Clin. Allergy.*, **12**, 211–15.

Schwartz, J.P. & Passoneau, J.V. (1974) Cyclic AMP-mediated induction of the cyclic AMP phosphodiesterase of C-6 glioma cells. *Proc. Nat. Acad. Sci. USA*, **71**, 3844–8.

Scordamaglia, A., Ciprandis, G., Ruffoni, S. *et al.* (1988) Theophylline and the immune response: *in vitro* and *in vivo* effects. *Clin. Immunol. Immunopathol.*, **48**, 238–46.

Scotland, G. & Houslay, M.D. (1995) Chimeric constructs show that the unique N-terminal domain of the cyclic AMP phosphodiesterase RD1 (RNPDE4A1A; rPDE-IV_{A1}) can confer membrane association upon the normally cytosolic protein chloramphenicol acetyltransferase. *Biochem. J.*, **308**, 673–81.

Sears, M.R., Taylor, D.R., Print, C.G., Lake, D.C., Herbson, G.P. & Flannery, E.M. (1990) Regular inhaled β-agonist treatment in bronchial asthma. *Lancet*, **336**, 1391–6.

Seiler, S., Arnold, A.J., Grove, R.I., Fifer, C.A., Keely, S.L. & Stanton, H.C. (1987) Effects of anagrelide on platelet cAMP levels, cAMP-dependent protein kinase and thrombin-induced Ca^{2+} fluxes. *J. Pharmacol. Exp. Ther.*, **243**, 767–73.

Seldon, P.M., Barnes, P.J., Meja, K. & Giembycz, M.A. (1995) Suppression of lipopolysaccharide-induced tumor necrosis factor-α generation from human peripheral blood monocytes by inhibitors of phosphodiesterase 4: interaction with stimulants of adenylyl cyclase. *Mol. Pharmacol*, **48**, 747–57.

Semmler, J., Wachtel, H. & Endres, S. (1993a) The selective type IV phosphodiesterase inhibitor rolipram suppresses tumour necrosis factor-α production by human mononuclear cells. *Int. J. Immunopharmacol.*, **15**, 409–13.

Semmler, J., Gerbert, U., Eisenhut, T. *et al.* (1993b) Xanthine derivatives: comparison between suppression of tumour necrosis factor-α production and inhibition of cAMP phosphodiesterase activity. *Immunology*, **78**, 520–5.

Sette, C., Iona, S. & Conti, M. (1994a) The short term activation of a rolipram-sensitive, cAMP-specific phosphodiesterase by thyroid-stimulating hormone in thyroid FRTL-5 cells is mediated by a cAMP-dependent phosphorylation. *J. Biol. Chem.*, **269**, 9245–52.

Sette, C., Vicini, E. & Conti, M. (1994b) The rat PDE3/IVd phosphodiesterase gene codes for multiple proteins differentially activated by cAMP-dependent protein kinase. *J. Biol. Chem.*, **269**, 18271–4.

Shakur, Y., Pryde, J.G. & Houslay, M.D. (1993) Engineered deletion of the unique N-terminal domain of the cyclic AMP-specific phosphodiesterase RD1 prevents plasmamembrane association and the attainment of enhanced thermostability without altering its sensitivity to inhibition by rolipram. *Biochem. J.*, **292**, 677–86.

Sharma, R.K. & Wang, J.H. (1982) Regulation of cAMP concentration by calmodulin-dependent cyclic nucleotide phosphodiesterase. *Biochem. Cell Biol.*, **64**, 1072–80.

Sharma, R.K. & Wang, J.H. (1986) Purification and characterization of bovine lung calmodulin-dependent cyclic nucleotide phosphodiesterase: an enzyme containing calmodulin as a subunit. *J. Biol. Chem.*, **261**, 14160–6.

Sharma, R.K., Wang, T.H., Wirch, E. & Wang, J.H. (1980) Purification and properties of bovine brain calmodulin-dependent cyclic nucleotide phosphodiesterase. *J. Biol. Chem.*, **255**, 5916–23.

Sharma, R.K., Adachi, A.M., Adachi, K. & Wang, J.H. (1984) Demonstration of bovine brain calmodulin-dependent cyclic nucleotide phosphodiesterase isozymes by monoclonal antibodies. *J. Biol. Chem.*, **259**, 9248–54.

Shimokawa, H., Flavahan, N.A., Lorenz, R.R. & Vanhoutte, P.M. (1988) Prostacyclin releases endothelium-derived relaxing factor and potentiates its action in coronary arteries of the pig. *Brit. J. Pharmacol.*, **95**, 1197–203.

Shohat, B., Volovitz, B. & Varsano, I. (1983) Induction of suppressor T-cells in asthmatic children by theophylline treatment. *Clin. Allergy*, **13**, 487–93.

Simpson, A.W.M., Reeves, M.L. & Rink, T.J. (1988) Effects of SK&F 94120, an inhibitor of cyclic nucleotide phosphodiesterase type III, on human platelets. *Biochem. Pharmacol.*, **37**, 2315–20.

Sly, R.M. (1984) Increases in death from asthma. *Ann. Allergy*, **53**, 2–25.

Smith, J.J. & Welsh, M.J. (1992) Cyclic AMP stimulates bicarbonate secretion across normal, but not cystic fibrosis airway epithelia. *J. Clin. Invest.*, **89**, 1148–53.

Snyder, D.S., Beller, D.I. & Unanue, E.R. (1982) Prostaglandins modulate macrophage Ia expression. *Nature*, **299**, 163–5.

Sonnenburg, W.K., Mullaney, P.J. & Beavo, J.A. (1991) Molecular cloning of a cyclic GMP-stimulated cyclic nucleotide phosphodiesterase cDNA: identification and distribution of isozyme variants. *J. Biol. Chem.*, **266**, 17655–61.

Souness, J.E. & Giembycz, M.A. (1994) Cyclic nucleotide phosphodiesterases in airways smooth muscle. In: *Airways Smooth Muscle: Biochemical Control of Contraction and Relaxation* (eds D. Raeburn & M.A. Giembycz), pp. 271–308. Birkhauser Verlag, Basle, Switzerland.

Souness, J.E., Brazdil, R., Diocee, B.K. & Jordan, R. (1989) Role of selective cyclic GMP phosphodiesterase inhibition in the myorelaxant actions of M&B 22,948, MY 5445, vinpocetine and 1-methyl-3-isobutyl-8-(methylamino)xanthine. *Brit. J. Pharmacol.*, **98**, 725–34.

Souness, J.E., Diocee, B.K., Martin, W. & Moodie, S.A. (1990) Pig aortic endothelial cell cyclic nucleotide phosphodiesterase: use of phosphodiesterase inhibitors to evaluate their roles in regulating cyclic nucleotide levels in intact cells. *Biochem. J.*, **266**, 127–32.

Souness, J.E., Carter, C.M., Diocee, B.K., Hassall, G.A., Wood, L.J. & Turner, N.C. (1991) Characterization of guinea-pig eosinophil phosphodiesterase activity: assessment of its involvement in regulating superoxide generation. *Biochem. Pharmacol.*, **42**, 937–45.

Souness, J.E., Villamil, M.E., Scott, L.C., Tomkinson, A., Giembycz, M.A. & Raeburn, D. (1994) Possible role of cyclic AMP phosphodiesterase in the actions of ibudilast on eosinophil thromboxane generation and airways smooth muscle tone. *Brit. J. Pharmacol.*, **111**, 1081–8.

Souness, J.E., Maslen, C., Webber, S. *et al.* (1995) Suppression of eosinophil function by RP 73401, a potent and selective inhibitor of cyclic AMP-specific phosphodiesterase: comparison with rolipram. *Brit. J. Pharmacol.*, **115**, 39–46.

Stelzner, T.J., Weil, J.V. & O'Brien, R.F. (1989) Role of cyclic adenosine monophosphate in the induction of endothelial barrier properties. *J. Cell. Physiol.*, **139**, 157–66.

Stroop, S.D. & Beavo, J.A. (1992) Sequence homology and structure–function studies of the bovine cyclic GMP-stimulated and retinal phosphodiesterases. *Adv. Sec. Mess. Phosphorprot. Res.*, **25**, 55–71.

Stroop, S.D., Charbonneau, H. & Beavo, J.A. (1989) Direct photolabeling of the cGMP-stimulated cyclic nucleotide-stimulated phosphodiesterase. *J. Biol. Chem.*, **264**, 13718–25.

Stryer, L. (1986) Cyclic GMP cascade of vision. *Ann. Rev. Neurosci.*, **9**, 89–199.

Stryer, L. & Bourne, H.R. (1988) G-protein: a family of signal transducers. *Ann. Rev. Cell Biol.*, **2**, 391–419.

Sturgess, I. & Searle, G.F. (1990) The acute effect of the phosphodiesterase inhibitor rolipram on plasma osmolality. *J. Clin. Pharmacol.*, **29**, 369–70.

Sturm, R.J., Osborne, M.C. & Heaslip, R.J. (1990) The effect of phosphodiesterase inhibitors on pulmonary inflammatory cell influx in ovalbumin-sensitized guinea-pigs. *J. Cell. Biochem.*, **14**, 337.

Sullivan, M., Egerton, M., Shakur, Y., Marquardsen, A. & Houslay, M. (1994) Molecular cloning and expression, in both COS-1 cells and *S. cerevisiae*, of a human cytosolic type-IVA, cyclic AMP specific phosphodiesterase (hPDE-IVA-h6.1). *Cell. Signal.*, **6**, 793–812.

Sullivan, P.J., Bekir, S., Jaffar, Z., Page, C.P., Jeffery, P.K. & Costello, J. (1993) The effects of low dose theophylline on the bronchial wall infiltrate after antigen challenge. *Lancet*, **343**, 1006–8.

Sullivan, P.J., Bekir, S., Jaffar, Z., Page, C.P., Jefery, P.K. & Costello, J. (1994) The effect of low dose theophylline on the bronchial wall infiltrate after antigen challenge. *Lancet*, **343**, 1006–8.

Sung, C.-P., Arieth, A.J., Storer, B. & Feuerstein, G.Z. (1991) Modulation of U937 cell adhesion to vascular endothelial cells by cyclic AMP. *Life Sci.*, **49**, 375–82.

Suttorp, N., Weber, U., Welsch, T. & Schudt, C. (1993) Role of phosphodiesterases in the regulation of endothelial permeability *in vitro*. *J. Clin. Invest.*, **91**, 1421–8.

Svensjo, E., Andersson, K.E., Bouskela, E., Cyrino, F.Z.G.A. & Lindgren, S. (1992) Effects of two vasodilatory phosphodiesterase inhibitors on bradykinin induced permeability increase in the hamster. *Int. J. Microcirc.*, **11**, A179.

Swinnen, J.V., Joseph, D.R. & Conti, M. (1989a) Molecular cloning of rat homologues of the *Drosophila melanogaster*, dunce cAMP phosphodiesterase: evidence for a family of genes. *Proc. Nat. Acad. Sci. USA*, **86**, 5325–9.

Swinnen, J.V., Joseph, D.R. & Conti, M. (1989b) The mRNA encoding a high affinity cAMP phosphodiesterase is regulated by hormones and cAMP. *Proc. Nat. Acad. Sci. USA*, **86**, 8197–201.

Swinnen, J.V., Tsikalas, K.E. & Conti, M. (1991) Properties and hormonal regulation of two structurally related cAMP phosphodiesterases from rat Sertoli cells. *J. Biol. Chem.*, **266**, 18370–7.

Taira, M., Hockman, S.C., Calvo, J.C., Taira, M., Belfrage, P. & Manganiello, V.C. (1993) Molecular cloning of the rat adipocyte hormone-sensitive cyclic GMP-inhibited cyclic nucleotide phosphodiesterase. *J. Biol. Chem.*, **268**, 18573–9.

Tanimoto, Y., Maruo, H., Bewtra, A.K. & Townley, R.G. (1994) Effects of phosphodiesterase IV inhibitor (WAY-PDE-641) on human eosinophil and neutrophil migration *in vitro*. *J. Allergy Clin. Immunol.*, **93**, 257.

Taraye, J.P., Aliaga, M., Barbara, M., Tisseyre, N., Vieu, S. & Tisne-Versaille, J. (1991a) Pharmacological modulation of a model of bronchial inflammation after aerosol-induced active anaphylactic shock in conscious guinea-pigs. *Int. J. Immunopharmacol.*, **13**, 349–56.

Tarayre, J.P., Aliaga, M., Barbara, M., Malfetes, N., Vieu, S. & Tisne-Versaille, J. (1991b) Theophylline reduces pulmonary eosinophilia after various types of active anaphylactic shock in guinea-pigs. *J. Pharm. Pharmacol.*, **43**, 877–9.

Tarayre, J.P., Aliaga, M., Barbara, M., Tisseyre, N., Vieu, S. & Tisne-Versaille, J. (1992) Model of bronchial allergic inflammation in the Brown Norway rat: pharmacological modulation. *Int. J. Immunopharmacol.*, **14**, 847–55.

Teixeira, M.M., Rossi, A.G., Williams, T.J. & Hellewell, P.G. (1994) Effects of phosphodiesterase isoenzyme inhibitors on cutaneous inflammation in the guinea-pig. *Brit. J. Pharmacol.*, **112**, 332–40.

Tenor, H., Stanciu, L., Schudt, C. *et al.* (1995a) Cyclic nucleotide phosphodiesterases from purified human $CD4^+$ and $CD8^+$ T-lymphocytes. *Clin. Exp. Allergy*, **25**, 616–24.

Tenor, H., Hatzelmann, A., Kupferschmidt, R. *et al.* (1995b) Cyclic nucleotide phosphodiesterase isoenzyme activities in human alveolar macrophages. *Clin. Exp. Allergy*, **25**, 625–33.

Thanhauser, A., Reiling, N., Bohle, A. *et al.* (1993) Pentoxifylline: a potent inhibitor of IL-2 and IFNγ biosynthesis and BCG-induced cytotoxicity. *Immunology*, **80**, 151–6.

Thomas, M.K., Francis, S.H. & Corbin, J.D. (1990a) Characterization of a purified bovine lung cGMP-binding phosphodiesterase. *J. Biol. Chem.*, **265**, 14964–70.

Thomas, M.K., Francis, S.H. & Corbin, J.D. (1990b) Substrate- and kinase-directed regulation of phosphorylation of a cGMP binding phosphodiesterase by cGMP. *J. Biol. Chem.*, **265**, 14971–8.

Thompson, P.J. & Stewart, G.A. (1991) Allergens. In: *Allergy* (eds S.T. Holgate & M.K. Church), pp. 1.1–1.14. Raven Press, London.

Thompson, P.J., Hanson, J.M., Turner-Warwick, M. & Morley, J. (1984) Platelets, platelet activating factor and asthma. *Am. Rev. Resp. Dis.*, **129**, A3.

Thompson, W.J., Ross, C.P., Pledger, W.J., Strada, S.J., Bannewr, R.L. & Hersh, E.M. (1976) Cyclic adenosine 3′:5′-monophosphate phosphodiesterase: distinct forms in human lymphocytes and monocytes. *J. Biol. Chem.*, **251**, 4922–9.

Thompson, W.J., Epstein, P.M. & Strada, S.J. (1979) Purification and characterization of a high affinity cyclic adenosine monophosphate phosphodiesterase from dog kidney. *Biochemistry*, **18**, 5228–37.

Torphy, T.J. & Cieslinski, L.B. (1990) Characterisation and selective inhibition of cyclic nucleotide phosphodiesterase isozymes in canine tracheal smooth muscle. *Mol. Pharmacol.*, **37**, 206–14.

Torphy, T.J. & Livi, G.P. (1993) Phosphodiesterase isozymes in airways. In: *Pharmacology of the Respiratory Tract: Experimental and Clinical Research — Lung Biology in Health and Disease*, Vol. 67 (eds K.F. Chung & P.J. Barnes), pp. 177–222. Marcel Dekker, New York.

Torphy, T.J. & Undem, B.J. (1991) Phosphodiesterase inhibitors: new opportunities for the treatment of asthma. *Thorax*, **46**, 512–23.

Torphy, T.J., Livi, G.P., Balcarek, J.M., White, J.R. & Undem, B.D. (1992a) Therapeutic potential of isozyme-selective phosphodiesterase inhibitors in the treatment of asthma. *Adv. Sec. Mess. Phosphoprot. Res.*, **25**, 289–305.

Torphy, T.J., Stadel, J.M., Burman, M. *et al.* (1992b) Coexpression of human cyclic AMP-specific phosphodiesterase activity and high-affinity rolipram binding in yeast. *J. Biol. Chem.*, **267**, 1798–804.

Torphy, T.J., Zhou, H.-L. & Cieslinski, L.B. (1992c) Stimulation of beta adrenoceptors in a human monocyte cell line (U937) up-regulates cyclic AMP-specific phosphodiesterase activity. *J. Pharmacol. Exp. Ther.*, **263**, 1195–1205.

Torphy, T.J., De Wolf, W.E., Green, D.W. & Livi, G.P. (1993a) Biochemical characteristics and cellular regulation of phosphodiesterase IV. *Agents Actions*, **43** (Suppl.), 51–71.

Torphy, T.J., Undem, B.J., Cieslinski, L.B., Luttmann, M.A., Reeves, M.L. & Hay, D.W.P. (1993b) Identification, characterization and functional role of phosphodiesterase isozymes in human airway smooth muscle. *J. Pharmacol. Exp. Ther.*, **265**, 1213–23.

Torphy, T.J., Murray, K.J. & Arch, J.R.S. (1994) Selective phosphodiesterase isozyme inhibitors. In: *Drugs and the Lung* (eds C.P. Page & W.J. Metzger), pp. 397–447. Raven Press, New York.

Townley, R.G. (1993) Elevated cyclic AMP-phosphodiesterase in atopic disease: cause of effect? *J. Lab. Clin. Med.*, **121**, 15–17.

Tsurata, L., Lee, H.-J., Masuda, E.S. *et al.* (1995) Cyclic AMP inhibits expression of the IL-2 gene through the nuclear factor of activated T-cells (NF-AT) site, and transfection of NF-AT cDNAs abrogates the sensitivity of EL-4 cells to cyclic AMP. *J. Immunol.*, **154**, 5255–64.

Tucker, M.M., Robinson, J.B. & Stellwagen, E. (1981) The effect of proteolysis on the calmodulin activation of cyclic nucleotide phosphodiesterase. *J. Biol. Chem.*, **256**, 9051–8.

Turner, C.D., Andreson, C.J., Smith, W.B. & Watson, J.W. (1994) Effects of rolipram on responses to acute and chronic antigen exposure in monkeys. *Am. J. Resp. Crit. Care Med.*, **149**, 1153–9.

Turner, N.C., Wood, L.J., Burns, F.M., Gueremy, T. & Souness, J.E. (1993) The effect of cyclic AMP and cyclic GMP phosphodiesterase inhibitors on the superoxide burst of guinea-pig peritoneal macrophages. *Brit. J. Pharmacol.*, **108**, 876–83.

Turner, N.C., Lamb, J., Worby, A. & Murray, K.J. (1994) Relaxation of guinea-pig trachea by cyclic AMP phosphodiesterase inhibitors and their enhancement by sodium nitroprusside. *Brit. J. Pharmacol.*, **111**, 1047–52.

Ukena, D., Rentz, K., Reiber, C. & Sybrecht, G.W. (1995) Effects of the mixed phosphodiesterase III/IV inhibitor, zardaverine, on airway function in patients with chronic airflow obstruction. *Resp. Med.*, **89**, 441–4.

Underwood, D.C., Osborn, R.R., Novak, L.B. *et al.* (1993) Inhibition of antigen-induced bronchoconstriction and eosinophil infiltration in the guinea-pig by the cyclic AMP-specific phosphodiesterase inhibitor, rolipram. *J. Pharmacol. Exp. Ther.*, **266**, 306–13.

Valette, L., Prigent, A.F., Nemoz, G., Anker, G., Macovschi, O. & Lagarde, M. (1990) Concanavalin A stimulates the rolipram-sensitive isoforms of cyclic nucleotide phosphodiesterase in rat thymic lymphocytes. *Biochem. Biophys. Res. Commun.*, **169**, 864–72.

van der Poow-Kraan, T., Van Kooten, C., Rensink, I. & Aarden, L. (1992) Interleukin (IL)-4 production by human T cells: differential regulation of IL-4 vs IL-2 production. *Eur. J. Immunol.*, **22**, 1237–41.

van Oosterhout, A.J.M., Stamm, W.B., Vanderschueren, R.G.J.R.A. & Nijkamp, F.P. (1992) Effects of cytokines on β-adrenoceptor function of human peripheral blood mononuclear cells and guinea-pig trachea. *Clin. Immunol.*, **90**, 340–8.

van Schayck, C.P., Graafsma, S.J., Visch, M.B., Dompeling, E., van Weel, C. & van Harwaarden, C.L. (1990) Increased bronchial hyperresponsiveness after inhaling salbutamol during one year is not caused by subsensitisation to salbutamol. *J. Allergy Clin. Immunol.*, **86**, 793–800.

van Tits, L.J.H., Michel, M.C., Motulsky, H.J., Maisel, A.S. & Brodde, O.-E. (1991) Cyclic AMP counteracts mitogen-induced inositol phosphate generation and increases in intracellular Ca^{2+} concentrations in human lymphocytes. *Brit. J. Pharmacol.*, **103**, 1288–94.

Varney, V.A., Jacobson, M.R., Sudderick, R.M. *et al.* (1992) Immunohistology of the nasal mucosa following antigen-induced rhinitis. *Am. Rev. Resp. Dis.*, **146**, 170–6.

Verghese, M.W., McConnell, R.T., Strickland, A.B. *et al.* (1995) Differential regulation of human monocyte-derived TNFα and IL-1α by type IV cAMP-phosphodiesterase (cAMP-PDE) inhibitors. *J. Pharmacol. Exp. Ther.*, **272**, 1313–20.

Ward, A.J.M., McKenniff, M., Evans, J.M., Page, C.P. & Costello, J.F. (1993) Theophylline—an immunomodulatory role in asthma. *Am. Rev. Resp. Dis.*, **147**, 518–23.

Watanabe, S., Yssel, H., Harada, Y. & Arai, K. (1994) Effect of prostaglandin E2 on Th0-type T cell clones: modulation of functions of nuclear proteins involved in cytokine production. *Int. Immunol.*, **6**, 523–32.

Weber, H.W. & Appleman, M.M. (1982) Insulin-dependent and insulin-independent low K_m cyclic AMP phosphodiesterase. *J. Biol. Chem.*, **257**, 5339–41.

Weinberger, M. (1984) The pharmacology and therapeutic use of theophylline. *J. Allergy Clin. Immunol.*, **73**, 525–40.

Weinberger, M. & Hendeles, L. (1983) Slow release theophylline: rationale and basis for product selection. *New Engl. J. Med.*, **308**, 760–4.

Welsh, J.E., Swinnen, J.V., O'Brien, D.A., Eddy, E.M. & Conti, M. (1992) Unique adenosine 3′,5′ cyclic monophosphate phosphodiesterase messenger ribonucleic acids in rat spermatogenic cells: evidence for differential gene expression during spermatogenesis. *Biol. Reprod.*, **46**, 1027–33.

Welton, A.K. & Simko, B.A. (1980) Regulatory role of adenosine in antigen-induced histamine release from the ling tissue of actively sensitized guinea-pigs. *Biochem. Pharmacol.*, **29**, 1085–92.

White, J.R., Torphy, T.J., Christensen, S.B., Lee, J.A. & Mong, S (1990) Purification and characterization of the rolipram sensitive, low-Km phosphodiesterase from human monocytes. *FASEB J.*, **4**, A1987.

Williamson, B.H., Milligan, C., Griffiths, K., Sparta, S., Tribe, A.C. & Thompson, P.J. (1988) An assessment of major and minor side effects of theophylline. *Aust. NZ. J. Med.*, **19**, 539–45.

Wood, M.A. & Hess, M.L. (1989) Long term therapy of congestive heart failure with phosphodiesterase inhibitors. *Am. J. Med. Sci.*, **297**, 105–13.

Wright, C.D., Kuipers, P.J., Kobylarz-Singer, D., Devall, L.J., Klinkefus, B.A. & Weishaar, R.E. (1990) Differential inhibition of neutrophil functions: role of cyclic AMP-specific, cyclic GMP-insensitive phosphodiesterase. *Biochem. Pharmacol.*, **40**, 699–707.

Wright, S., Navsaria, H. & Leigh, I.M. (1991) Cyclic adenosine monophosphate-phosphodiesterase activity in cultured keratinocytes from patients with atopic eczema. *J. Dermatol. Sci.*, **2**, 263–7.

Yamamoto, T., Manganiello, V.C. & Vaughan, M. (1983) Purification and characterization of cyclic GMP-stimulated cyclic nucleotide phosphodiesterase from calf liver: effects of divalent cations on activity. *J. Biol. Chem.*, **258**, 12526–33.

Yukawa, T., Kroegel, C., Dent, G., Chanez, P., Ukena, D. & Barnes, P.J. (1989) Effect of theophylline and adenosine on eosinophil function. *Am. Rev. Resp. Dis.*, **140**, 327–33.

Zeller, E., Stief, H.J., Pfung, B. & Sastre-Y-Hernandez, M. (1984) Results of a phase II study of the antidepressant effect of rolipram. *Pharmacopsychiatry*, **17**, 180–90.

Zocchi, M.R., Pardi, R., Gromo, G. *et al.* (1985) Theophylline induced non-specific suppressor cell activity by therapeutic concentrations of theophylline. *J. Immunopharmacol.*, **7**, 217–34.

Zurier, R.B., Weishmann, G., Hoffstein, S., Kemmerman, S. & Tai, H.H. (1974) Mechanisms of lysosomal enzyme release from human leukocytes. II. Effects of cAMP and cGMP, autonomic agonists, and agents which affect microtubule function. *J. Clin. Invest.*, **53**, 297–309.

CHAPTER 31

Adrenergic Agonists and Antagonists

T.R. Bai

Introduction

Long before Langley (1905) and Dale (1906) developed the concept that the specific biological effects of hormones, neurotransmitters and drugs result from high-affinity, stereospecific interactions with tissues, the English physician, Henry Salter, reported in 1859 what is probably the first account in modern times of the therapeutic effects of activation of adrenergic receptors (adrenoceptors) when he wrote that 'asthma is immediately cured in situations of either sudden alarm or violent fleeting excitements' (Persson, 1985). Endogenous levels of circulating catecholamines, in particular adrenaline (epinephrine), are now known to influence airway calibre in asthmatic patients, and it is likely that Salter was describing sympatho-adrenal release of adrenaline following emotional triggers. At the turn of the century, the vasodilator hypothesis of asthma had considerable support in both Germany and the USA. This hypothesis stated that airway obstruction was caused by swelling of the bronchial mucosa secondary to vasodilatation. The other major hypothesis at that time was that asthma was due to 'the spasm of the circular muscles of the bronchi'. Thus, in 1900, Solis-Cohen, encouraged by reports that adrenal extracts caused vasoconstriction, gave large oral doses of desiccated adrenal glands to asthmatic subjects with success, which he interpreted to be consistent with his view that asthma was a 'vasomotor ataxia of the relaxing variety' (Solis-Cohen, 1900). However, it is unlikely that the adrenaline content of the adrenals could have survived the oral route as an active drug and, indeed, the slow onset of action of the extract treatment reported in his paper is now thought more likely to be the demonstration of the beneficial effects of glucocorticosteroids (Persson, 1989). Soon after this, adrenaline became available as a pure substance and in 1903 Bullowa and Kaplan successfully gave injections of it to asthmatic patients. They too thought this success was consistent with the vascular hypothesis of asthma, but in 1907 adrenaline was shown to relax airway smooth muscle (Kahn, 1907). Although it is possible in some asthmatics that the α-adrenoceptor agonist (α-agonist) effect of adrenaline contributes to increased airway calibre, it is probable that the β-adrenoceptor agonist (β-agonist) effect dominates (Barnes, 1986a). In 1924, ephedrine was introduced to western medicine, although the plant from which it is derived has been used for more than 5000 years in China for respiratory and other allergic conditions. Ephedrine, an α-agonist with a weak β-agonist activity, and adrenaline were widely used over the ensuing decades in the treatment of asthma, rhinitis and anaphylaxis. Konzett (1941) isolated isoprenaline (isoproterenol), the first β-adrenoceptor agonist devoid of α-adrenergic effect. Subsequently, Ahlquist (1948) used isoprenaline to partition sympathomimetic effects into α (mainly excitatory) and β (mainly inhibitory), based on physiological responses in isolated tissues.

Adrenoceptor localization

The receptor population mediating α effects is characterized by a rank order of potency of adrenaline > noradrenaline > isoprenaline and β effects by an order of isoprenaline > adrenaline > noradrenaline (Table 31.1).

Prior to 1974, the adrenergic receptors were known only indirectly as entities that responded to drugs in a selective manner to mediate a variety of physiologically important responses. Then a variety of high-affinity ^{125}I-labelled radioligands selective for these receptors were developed, which led to experiments utilizing direct binding assays to establish the biochemical properties of the receptor proteins. These techniques, when coupled with efficient methods for detergent solubilization, formed the basis of receptor purification using affinity chromatography, and when coupled with autoradiographic methods led to the cellular localization and quantification of adrenergic receptors on thin sections of tissues (Stadel & Lefkowitz, 1991).

β-Adrenoceptors

Evaluation of a large volume of data generated in the study of β-adrenergic pharmacology enabled Lands *et al.* in 1967 to suggest a further division of the β-adrenoceptor response into sub-types termed β_1 and β_2. Again, this distinction was based on the relative potency of the naturally occurring catecholamines, adrenaline and noradrenaline. The β_1 responses are equally sensitive to these two agonists; β_2 responses are more potently stimulated by adrenaline. Generally, but not invariably, β_1 responses appear to be initiated by the neurotransmitter, noradrenaline, in innervated tissues, whereas β_2 responses are triggered by the circulating hormone adrenaline (O'Donnell & Worstall, 1987). Subsequently, a third sub-type of β-adrenocepter, β_3, was defined (Emorine *et al.*, 1989). The β-adrenoceptors are, in general, low-abundance receptors (500–5000 sites/cell).

Tissue distributions of both α- and β-adrenoceptors are summarized in Table 31.1.

Heart

In the ventricle 40% and in the atrium up to 55% of the β-adrenoceptors are of the β_2 sub-type (Bristow & Ginsburg, 1986). The remainder are β_1 sub-type.

Table 31.1 Tissue distribution of adrenoceptor sub-types.

Site	α	β
Airways	α_1	β_2
Lung parenchyma		β_1
Nose	α_1, α_2	β_2
Heart	α_1, α_2	β_1, β_2
Blood vessels	α_1	β_2
Inflammatory cells	α_2	β_2
Gut, kidney, liver, pancrease, spleen	α_1, α_2	β_2
Uterus		β_2
Adipose tissue		β_3
Noradrenergic and cholinergic nerve terminals	α_2	β_2
Brain	α_1, α_2	β_1, β_2

Vasculature

On vascular smooth muscle, β_2-adrenoceptors predominate.

Nose

A homogenous population of β_2-adrenoceptors has been noted in several studies (van Megan *et al.*, 1991).

Lung

Organ bath and autoradiographic studies (Fig. 31.1) have demonstrated that the airway smooth-muscle relaxant effect of β-agonists is largely via β_2-adrenoceptors directly on the muscle surface (Nadel & Barnes, 1984; Carstairs *et al.*, 1985; Barnes, 1986a; Bai *et al.*, 1989). This is not unexpected, given that β_1-adrenoceptors are found at sites of sympathetic innervation responding to noradrenaline release and there is no direct sympathetic innervation of human airway smooth muscle (Barnes, 1986b). Similarly, the adrenoceptors on mucous and serous glands and inflammatory cells are largely of the β_2 type (Basbaum *et al.*, 1990). β_2-Adrenoceptors also predominate on bronchial epithelium, type I and II pneumocytes and pulmonary vascular smooth muscle, so that they make up 70% of the β-adrenoceptors in the human lung, the other 30% being β_1 on alveolar walls. The density of β_2-adrenoceptors increases from the large to small airways and is much greater on alveolar walls than on other structures in the lung (Carstairs *et al.*, 1985).

Other sites

Functional and gene expression studies suggest that adipocytes contain β_1- and β_3-adrenoceptors.

α-Adrenoceptors

At least seven α-adrenoceptor sub-types — α_{1A-C} and α_{2A-C} — have been proposed based on pharmacological experiments and gene cloning. However, the classification is still controversial. For example, α_{1A} and α_{1C} sub-types have very similar pharmacological properties (Hieble & Bond, 1994). The α_1 sub-types are located on smooth-muscle membranes of most sympathetically innervated tissues, mediating contraction. α_1-Adrenoceptors are found on arterioles in skin, mucosa, viscera and resistance vessels in the kidney, as well as in all veins. The α_2-adrenoceptors are primarily presynaptic, inhibiting traffic through autonomic ganglia and other nerve terminals.

Table 31.2 α_2-Receptor sub-types.

Sub-type	Localization	Pharmacological properties
α_{1A}	Brain, vas deferens, kidney, heart, spleen	Noradrenaline > adrenaline > phenylephrine
α_{1B}	Lung, brain, heart, liver, kidney, spleen	Oxymetazoline > adrenaline > noradrenaline
α_{1C}	Brain and kidney	Noradrenaline > adrenaline > phenylephrine
α_{2A}	Brain and platelets	*p*-Aminoclonidine > adrenaline
α_{2B}	Kidney, neonatal lung	Clonidine > noradrenaline > oxymetazoline
α_{2C}	Kidney	Oxymetazoline > noradrenaline
α_{2D}	Brain, kidney, salivary gland	Oxymetazoline > adrenaline > noradrenaline

The localization and pharmacological properties of α_1 and α_2 sub-types are summarized in Table 31.2.

In the nasal vasculature, both α_1- and α_2-adrenoceptors are present (Lacroix, 1989; van Megen *et al.*, 1991). In the nasal capacitance vessels, α_2-adrenoceptors dominate over α_1-adrenoceptors.

Adrenoceptor biology

Molecular structure

Improvements in receptor isolation techniques in the first half of the last decade led to the availability of substantial amounts of purified β_2-adrenoceptor, which allowed determination of the molecular mass and amino acid sequence of part of the receptor. This was the first adrenergic receptor isolated. This new information in turn led to the production of polynucleotide probes and eventually to cloning of the receptor gene and determination of the complete primary sequence of the receptor protein

(a)

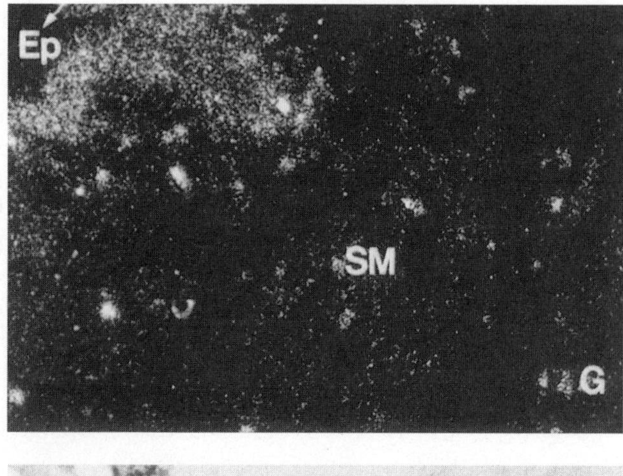

(b)

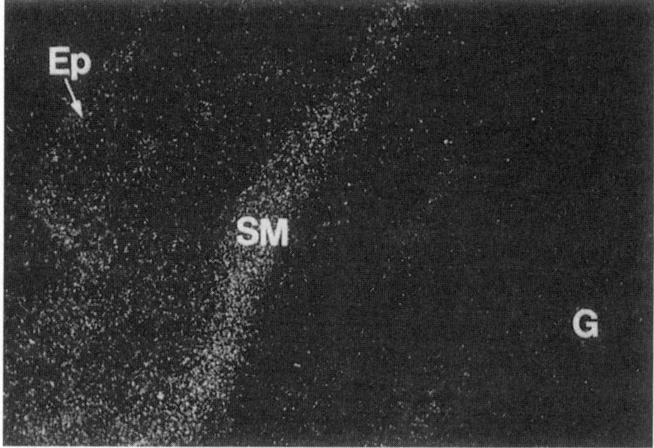

(c)

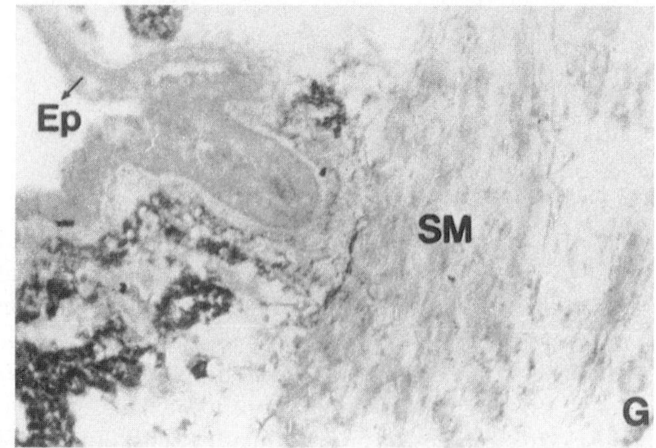

(d)

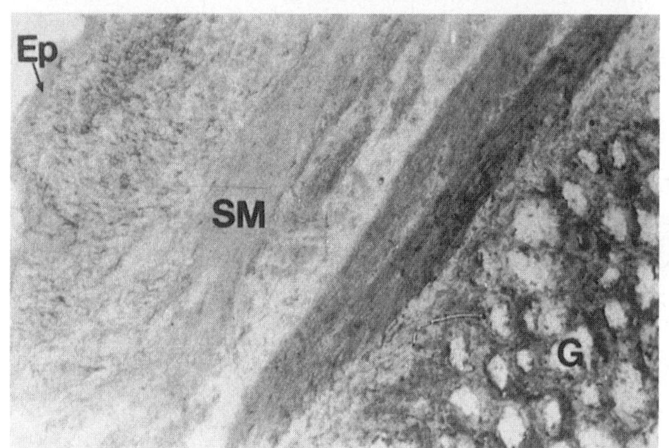

Fig. 31.1 Distribution of β-adrenoceptors in human normal and asthmatic bronchi. Panels (a) and (b) are dark-field photomicrographs of sections showing the distribution of autoradiographic grains after incubation with 25 pmol/l I^{125}-iodocyanopindolol. Panels (c) and (d) are bright-field photomicrographs of adjacent sections showing the epithelium (Ep), smooth muscle (SM) and submucosal glands (G) after staining with 1% cresyl fast violet. The epithelium is partially shed in the asthmatic sections. (Reproduced from Bai *et al.*, 1992, with permission.)

(Strader *et al.*, 1989; Fraser & Venter, 1990; Stadel & Lefkowitz, 1991). The β_2-adrenoceptor gene maps to chromosome 5 and encodes a protein of 413 amino acids, only 54% of which are shared with β_1-adrenoceptors (Emorine *et al.*, 1987; Strader *et al.*, 1989). α-Adrenoceptors were cloned using similar techniques and show many homologies to β-adrenoceptors (Fraser & Venter, 1990).

Adrenoceptors belong to the G-protein-linked rhodopsin-related receptor superfamily, one of at least three cell-membrane receptor superfamilies. Current models of the adrenoceptors show seven transmembrane segments connected by alternating intracellular and extracellular loops (Fig. 31.2). Homology among all the members of the seven transmembrane region (serpentine) receptor family is greatest in the transmembrane-spanning domains. Genetic and biochemical manipulation of the β_2-adrenoceptor has identified that the ligand-binding domain is a pocket buried within the membrane bilayer, with agonists interacting with transmembrane helices III and V (Strader *et al.*, 1989; Fraser & Venter, 1990). Three residues are of critical importance, namely the aspartate residue 113, positioned on the third domain, and two serine residues, 204 and 207, on the fifth domain. Aspartate binds to the nitrogen of the β_2-agonist molecule, while the two serine residues interact with the hydroxyl groups on the phenyl rings. Antagonists do not bind with the same amino acids. Thus, β-antagonists bind to aspartate 113 and a residue in the seventh domain rather than with serine residues in the fifth domain (Tota *et al.*, 1991).

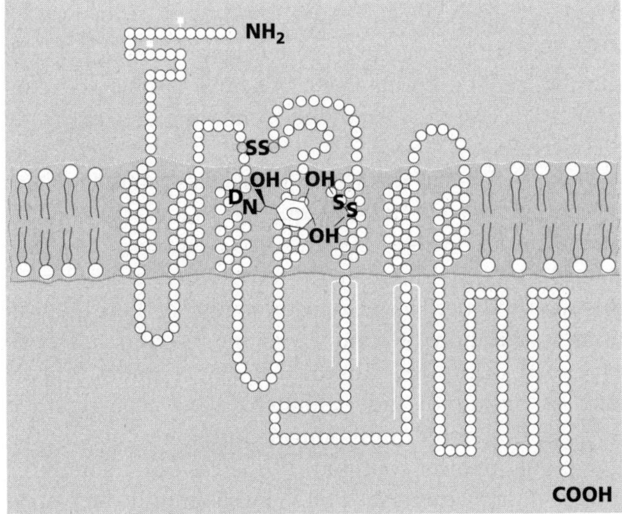

Fig. 31.2 Structural model of the β_2-adrenoceptor. The 418 amino acid residues are shown as white circles with noradrenaline shown in the proposed agonist ligand-binding pocket. The cytoplasmic regions predicted to be required for G-protein coupling are shown enclosed in cylinders. (Reproduced from Strader *et al.*, 1989, with permission.)

Studies of the regulation of adrenergic receptor gene transcription are incomplete but in both cell culture and homogenized human lung, glucocorticoids increase β_2-adrenoceptor mRNA levels and receptor protein by increasing the rate of gene transcription, and isoprenaline decreases mRNA levels by decreasing stability of the mature mRNA (Collins *et al.*, 1988; Hadcock & Malbon, 1988; Bai *et al.*, 1993; Mak *et al.*, 1995). Hamid *et al.* (1991) have reported the distribution of β_2-adrenoceptor mRNA in human lung by *in situ* hybridization and correlated this with receptor autoradiographic distribution. They report qualitative differences between the density of labelling with the two techniques in different cell types. Pulmonary vascular and airway smooth muscle showed a high intensity of mRNA but only a low density of adrenoceptors, and the converse was reported for the alveolar epithelium. These differences may be due to either a rapid rate of β_2-adrenoceptor synthesis or high stability of mRNA in the airways and may explain the difficulty in demonstrating desensitization in airway smooth muscle (Hasegawa & Townley, 1983; Whicker & Black, 1991).

G proteins are membrane-associated heterotrimers composed of α-, β- and γ-subunits. Interaction with a receptor causes the release of guanosine diphosphate (GDP) from the α-subunit of the G protein, allowing guanosine triphosphate (GTP) to bind and leading to the dissociation of the activated α-subunit from the receptor and from the βγ-complex. Various G proteins activate or inhibit different effector enzymes, modulating the levels of intracellular second messengers. In the case of the β_2-adrenoceptor, which is coupled to the stimulatory guanine nucleotide binding protein, G_s, binding of an agonist to the receptors catalyses the release of GDP from the α-subunit of the G protein (α_s), allowing the binding of GTP; this in turn leads to the direct activation of adenylyl cyclase by α_s-GTP. Adenylyl cyclase catalyses the formation of the classical second-messenger cyclic adenosine monophosphate (cAMP) so that levels of cAMP up to 400-fold over basal can occur within minutes of agonist exposure (Malbon 1989; Strader *et al.*, 1989; Fraser & Venter, 1990; Hausdorff *et al.*, 1990; Stadel & Lefkowitz, 1991). Upon removal of agonist, the activation of adenylyl cyclase persists until the intrinsic guanosine triphosphatase (GTPase) activity of α_s hydrolyses the bound nucleotide (Fraser & Venter, 1990; Hausdorff *et al.*, 1990).

Mechanisms of adrenoceptor agonist action

The contractile state of smooth muscle, the primary therapeutic target of most adrenergic agonists, is determined by cytoplasmic Ca^{2+} concentrations. The cell membrane is negative with respect to the extracellular space and more positive potentials (depolarization) open voltage-gated Ca^{2+} channels, causing Ca^{2+} influx to increase cytoplasmic

Table 31.3 Mechanisms of smooth-muscle relaxation by β_2-agonists.

Stimulation of cAMP and subsequent reduction of MLCK activity
cAMP inhibition of PLC with reduction of IP_3 formation
Stimulation of Ca^{2+} extrusion pumps
Stimulation of a Ca^{2+}-activated potassium channel
Inhibition of acetylcholine release from cholinergic nerve terminals

See text for definition of abbreviations.

Ca^{2+} and trigger contraction. The effect of adrenergic agonists on smooth muscle are complex and vary from one site to the next. For example, α-agonists relax intestinal smooth muscle and contract vascular smooth muscle by different and now well-understood mechanisms, involving coupling of G proteins with different second-messenger pathways. Thus, the contractile response to α_1-agonists is determined by activation of G-protein-linked adrenoceptors that activate phospholipase C (PLC), releasing inositol 1,4,5-triphosphate (IP_3) and increasing intracellular Ca^{2+}. α_2-Agonists inhibit adenylyl cyclase activity and decrease cAMP level (Exton, 1982; Brown, 1992).

A number of other mechanisms, apart from increases in cAMP, have been shown to be involved in the smooth-muscle relaxation induced by β-agonists (Bai, 1992) (Table 31.3). Relaxation is primarily determined by generation of cAMP and activation of cAMP-dependent kinases, which have several actions, including shifting myosin light-chain kinase (MLCK) to a less active form. The rise in cAMP also leads to Ca^{2+} re-uptake into the sarcoplasmic reticulum and organelles and Ca^{2+} extrusion from the cell. cAMP also causes suppression of IP_3 formation. β-Agonists also reduce acetylcholine release from smooth-muscle cholinergic nerve terminals and thus inhibit contraction (Barnes, 1986b; Bai *et al*., 1989). Finally, activation of β_2-adrenoceptors stimulates a Ca^{2+}-activated potassium channel in the cell membrane, which leads to hyperpolarization of the membrane and cell relaxation (Jones, 1990).

β-Adrenoceptor agonists

Structure and metabolism

The structures of commonly used agonists and the natural catecholamines from which they are derived are shown in Fig. 31.3. The term catecholamine refers to all compounds with a catechol nucleus (benzene plus two adjacent hydroxyl groups) and an amine group. The three principal naturally occurring catecholamines are dopamine (dihydroxyphenylethylamine) and the metabolic products of dopamine, noradrenaline and adrenaline. Monoamine oxidase, predominantly an intraneuronal enzyme, and catechol-*O*-methyltransferase, predominantly an extraneuronal enzyme, are the two enzymes primarily responsible for degradation of catecholamines. Ligand receptor interactions are stereospecific. All the commonly used β-agonists exist in racemic mixtures of optical isomers, referred to as R and S (or (–) and (+)) enantiomers. The agonist activity lies predominantly in the R enantiomer. There has been speculation that the S enantiomers possess adverse effects in clinical usage, but this remains unclear (Chapman *et al*., 1992). There are, as yet, no preparations of R enantiomers alone available for commercial usage.

Isoprenaline is a catecholamine like adrenaline and this class of compounds is both chemically and metabolically unstable. The resorcinol analogue orciprenaline (metaproterenol) is structurally closely related to isoprenaline, and thus shares the non-selective actions of isoprenaline, but is more stable. Both salbutamol and terbutaline, the first of the current generation of 'short-acting', relatively β_2-adrenoceptor-specific agonists used in the treatment of asthma, were synthesized and characterized before the report of Lands *et al*. (1967) sub-typing β-adrenoceptors. Since the 1960s, a number of other β_2-agonists have been developed as therapeutic agents. The key substitutions to the β-phenylethylamine parent have been to the catechol ring, or related structure, to make the compounds resistant to metabolism by endogenous methyl transferases and monoamine oxidase, and addition of an ethanolamine side chain of varying length (Fig. 31.3). Such alterations prolong the half-life and increase the selectivity of these agents for β_2-adrenoceptors. In clinical research, a short-acting, β_2-selective compound still metabolized by endogenous enzymes is desirable and rimiterol is one such compound, although only modestly β_2-selective.

The prototypal short-acting β_2-agonists salbutamol and terbutaline, despite the subsequent development of many other compounds, such as fenoterol, clenbuterol and procaterol (Table 31.4), remain the most widely prescribed of this class of drug. The major shortcoming of these medications is duration of action, and much effort has been expended to prolong duration beyond 4 hours. Agents such as pirbuterol and clenbuterol have been reported to possess a significantly longer duration of action, but this is marginal at best and, in the case of clenbuterol, only after oral administration. A more recently developed compound, bambuterol, does have a more extended duration of action, but this drug is a pro-drug of terbutaline and is effective only after oral administration, the least preferred route of administration because of systemic side-effects.

Two compounds in advanced clinical study or in use,

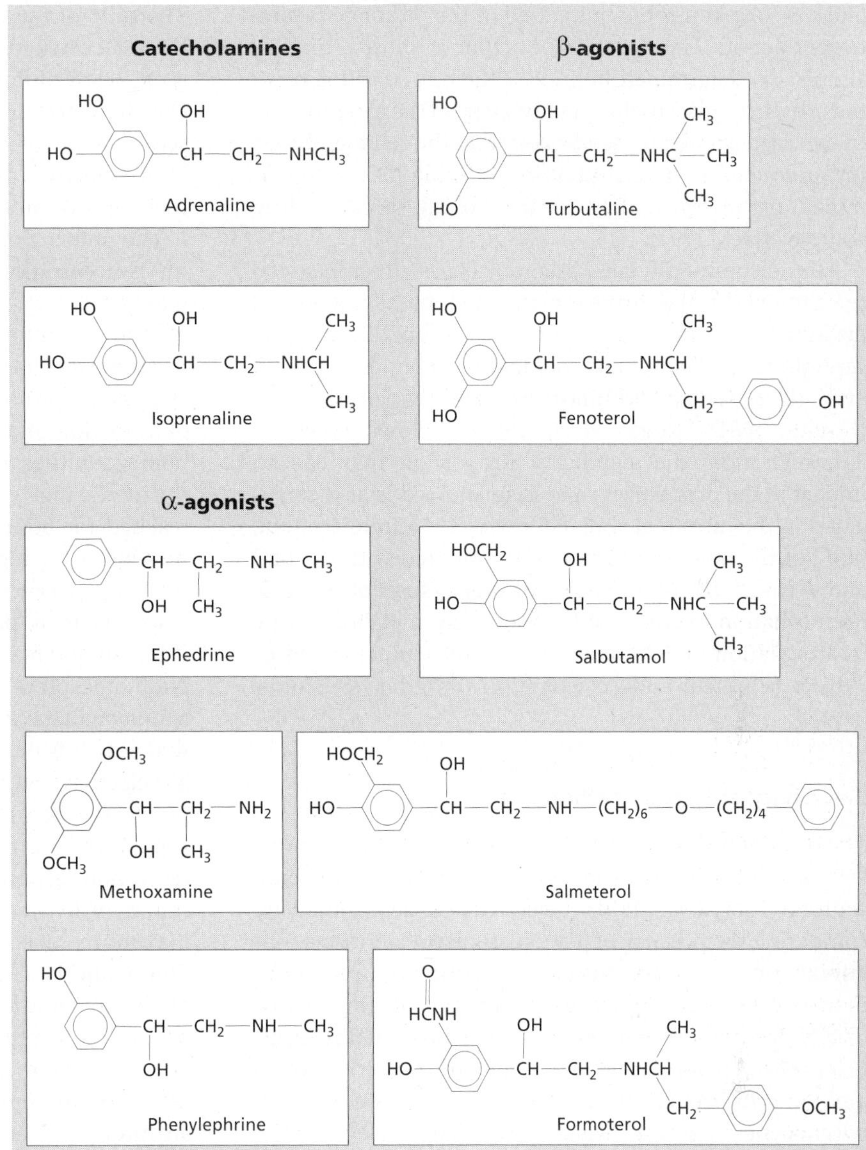

Fig. 31.3 Representative catecholamines and selective α- and β-adrenoceptor agonists.

Table 31.4 β-Agonists in clinical use.

Short-acting (β_2-selective)	Long-acting (β_2-selective)
Salbutamol	Salmeterol
Terbutaline	Formoterol
Fenoterol	
Orciprenaline (metaproterenol)	*Catecholamines*
Clenbuterol	Adrenaline (epinephrine)
Pirbuterol	Isoprenaline (isoproterenol)
Bitolterol	Isoetharine
Procaterol	

formoterol and salmeterol, have been shown to have therapeutically significant increased duration of action by inhalation. Formoterol was developed by investigating β-agonist analogues with increasing affinity for the β_2-adrenoceptor itself. In contrast, salmeterol was designed to introduce large lipophilic N-substituents into saligenin ethanolamines to facilitate binding in hydrophobic regions of the cell membrane or to non-polar amino acid residues in the β_2-adrenoceptor protein (Jack, 1991). These differences in design lead to important differences between these two long-acting β_2-adrenoceptor agonists. Both are moderately lipophilic compared with salbutamol and terbutaline, which are hydrophilic in nature; this property leads to greater persistence in the cell membrane and may explain some but not all of the prolonged duration of action. The duration of action of short-acting β_2-agonists is determined in part by the rate of diffusion of these hydrophilic compounds away from the receptor site. In contrast, salmeterol seems bound to the cell membrane for prolonged periods and offset of action may be determined by internalization of the bound receptor–drug complex (Jack, 1991).

All the commonly used β_2-agonists are either excreted unchanged in the urine or excreted in a conjugated fashion. For example, salbutamol and terbutaline are susceptible to 4-O′-sulphate conjugation in intestinal wall and liver (when administered by the oral route) (Davies, 1984; Morgan *et al.*, 1986). Following aerosol administration, the significant proportion that has an impact in the oropharynx and is swallowed is also conjugated in the intestinal wall. Following i.v. administration, more of the free drug is excreted compared with the oral and aerosolized route. Fenoterol is also susceptible to 5-O′-sulphation. Salmeterol is extensively metabolized by hydroxylation and formoterol is excreted unchanged or subject to glucuronide conjugation (Brogden & Faulds, 1991).

Selectivity, affinity and efficacy

The basis of β_1/β_2-adrenoceptor selectivity may be in differences in the amino acid sequences of the two adrenoceptors (Tota *et al.*, 1991). Selectivity is determined by comparing the potency of β-agonists on preparations containing primarily β_1-adrenoceptors (for example, atrial inotropic responses) vs. preparations containing primarily β_2-adrenoceptors (for example, bronchial relaxant responses). In this situation, agents are ranked in comparison with the effect of a completely non-selective β-adrenoceptor agonist, usually isoprenaline (Table 31.5).

Table 31.5 Potency, selectivity and intrinsic activity of commonly used β-adrenoceptor agonists. (Data from O'Donnell & Wanstall (1978); Decker *et al.* (1982); Bai *et al.* (1989); and Johnson (1991).)

Agonist	β_1	β_2	Selectivity ratio (β_1:β_1)	Airway smooth-muscle intrinsic activity
Isoprenaline	1.0	1.0	1.0	1.0
Salbutamol	0.0004	0.48	1375	0.91
Terbutaline	0.003	0.08	267	0.83
Fenoterol	0.005	0.9	180	0.99
Salmeterol	0.001	8.5	85 000	0.70
Formoterol	0.05	25	100	0.94

Data are relative to response to isoprenaline. Intrinsic activity is a measure of efficacy.

The ratio of the relative potencies at β_2 vs. β_1 sites gives the selectivity ratio (O'Donnell & Wanstall, 1978; Decker *et al.*, 1982; Johnson *et al.*, 1993). Using these criteria, the long-acting agent, salmeterol, is the most β_2-selective agent in common use and fenoterol is the least selective. Formoterol is not very selective using these approaches.

The potency of a given agonist is usually measured as the concentration of the drug required to cause 50% of maximum response to that agonist. Potency is a function of both receptor affinity and receptor efficacy and of tissue-related factors, such as receptor density and efficiency of G-protein coupling. Affinity describes the degree of attraction of a ligand for a receptor, as determined by binding studies. A radiolabelled version of agonist is used in increasing concentrations until the maximum is reached for bound label compared with labelling in the presence of a high concentration of unlabelled agonist. Efficacy describes the ability of an agonist to induce a response in a particular tissue (Stephenson, 1956). β-Agonists and β-antagonists may share similar affinities for β-adrenoceptors but have different efficacies. A full agonist will have a high efficacy while the pure antagonist will have low or zero efficacy. The majority of short-acting β_2-selective agonists have intermittent efficacy and potency compared with isoprenaline (Table 31.5).

β_2-Agonist efficacy is usually assessed by examining relaxation responses in the presence of contracted preparations of airway smooth muscle. Again, one compares the maximum relaxant response with that of isoprenaline. This value is called the intrinsic activity and is a ratio of the maximum response of a given β-agonist to the maximum response of isoprenaline. Using these criteria, none of the synthetic β-agonists has higher intrinsic activity than isoprenaline. Agents with equivalent efficacy are procaterol and formoterol, whereas most saligenins and resorcinols are of moderate efficacy (65–85% of isoprenaline). The efficacy of β-agonists at extrapulmonary sites may be of clinical relevance. Fenoterol and formoterol have the same efficacy as isoprenaline at cardiac β_1-adrenoceptors, despite being less potent, whereas albutamol and salmeterol have very low efficacy (Table 31.5). In contrast to efficacy, lung β_2-adrenoceptor potency can be greater than that of isoprenaline. For example, salmeterol is five times more potent than isoprenaline, formoterol 25-fold more potent and procaterol 24-fold more potent. Neither intermediate intrinsic activity (efficacy) nor intermediate potency negates the clinical value of a given β-agonist as a bronchodilator drug. Rather, the adverse consequences of prolonged use of these drugs may be influenced by whether they are partial or full agonists. The rate of desensitization is one phenomenon that could be influenced by full vs. partial agonist activity (see later).

Physiological effects

Lung cells

Although *in vivo* the most obvious and therapeutic pulmonary effect of β-adrenergic stimulation is bronchodilatation mediated by airway smooth-muscle relaxation, a number of other effects also occur (Table 31.6). β-Agonists promote secretion from serous cells and, to a lesser extent, mucous cells, in mucous glands. Serous cell stimulation produces antibacterial proteins, such as lysosomes and lactoferrin. This effect has been demonstrated convincingly *in vitro* only, using human tracheal explants at relatively high concentrations of β-agonists (Basbaum *et al.*, 1990). However, theoretical calculations of luminal β_2-agonist concentrations following inhalation indicate that such levels may be achieved *in vivo* (Kerrebijn, 1991). Furthermore, β_2-agonists increase chloride iron transport through apical membranes of epithelial cells via an increase in cAMP. Sodium follows passively via paracellular channels and water by osmosis. The net effect is to increase periciliary fluid (Wanner, 1988; Widdicombe, 1989). The combined effects of stimulation of mucous glands and chloride channels, together with an increase in ciliary beat frequency (Wanner, 1988), are to increase mucociliary clearance. Increased clearance has been demonstrated *in vivo* using radiotracer methods, although the clinical relevance of this enhancement in patients with asthma is unknown (Wanner, 1988). β_2-Agonists also stimulate the secretion of surfactant from alveolar type II cells *in vitro*, although the magnitude of the effect is modest (Mason & Williams, 1991). In animal models of inflammation, mediators increase microvascular permeability by contracting post-capillary venular endothelial cells so that spaces form between the cells. In such models, β_2-agonists relax endothelial cells and therefore reduce permeability (Persson & Svensjo, 1985). However, β_2-agonists also increase bronchial blood flow by acting as vasodilators of bronchial arterioles (Kelly *et al.*, 1992). The net effect of these two opposing effects on exudation or transudation of fluid into the lumen and wall of inflamed human airways is unclear. A report that nebulized adrenaline was no more effective in producing bronchodilatation in acute asthma than a nebulized β-agonist which lacked an α-adrenergic vasoconstrictor effect suggests that potential alterations in bronchial blood flow induced by β_2-agonists do not adversely affect fluid shifts across the lumen wall (Coupe *et al.*, 1986). Moreover, the lack of additational benefit by adrenaline suggests that the potential decrease in lumen area produced by mucosal bronchodilation induced by β-agonists is not an important component of air-flow resistance in asthma.

Table 31.6 Physiological effects of β_2-adrenoceptor stimulation in human lung.

Airway smooth-muscle relaxation
Prejunctional inhibition of acetylcholine release from parasympathetic neurones in airway smooth muscle
Stimulation of mucous and serous cell secretion
Stimulation of chloride ion secretion across the apical membrane of airway epithelial cells
Increase in ciliary beat freqeuncy
Stimulation of surfactant secretion from alveolar type II cells
Inhibition of mediator release from lung mast cells and neutrophils
? Reduction in microvascular permeability (animal models)
? Increase in bronchial blood flow (animal models)

β-Adrenoceptors are present in peribronchial parasympathetic ganglia, which receive direct sympathetic innervation (Barnes, 1986b). β_2-Adrenoceptors are also present on cholinergic nerve terminals in airway smooth muscle and act here to inhibit acetylcholine release (pre-junctional inhibition), thereby reducing the cholinergic component of bronchoconstriction (Rhoden *et al.*, 1988; Bai *et al.*, 1989). It is possible that β-antagonists such as propranolol induce asthma exacerbations not only by reducing the tonic bronchodilator effect of circulating adrenaline on airway smooth muscle in maintaining airway patency, but also by blocking the effect of adrenaline on cholinergic nerve terminals leading to the exuberant release of acetylcholine. The observation by Grieco and Pierson (1971) that cholinergic antagonists partially reverse propranolol-induced bronchoconstriction provides some support for this hypothesis.

Inflammatory cells

β_2-Adrenoceptors are present on a variety of inflammatory cells, including lymphocytes, granulocytes, mast cells and macrophages. Circulating lymphocytes and neutrophils have low numbers of adrenoceptors which appear to be relatively poorly coupled to second-messenger pathways in that they are easily down-regulated (Insel, 1991). Human neutrophils possess approximately 900–1800 β_2-adrenoceptors per intact cell and mediator release is inhibited in a dose-dependent manner by isoprenaline (Busse & Sosman, 1984). Studies employing circulating lymphocytes or neutrophils as a marker of pulmonary β-adrenoceptor function can therefore be misleading (see below). However, one report showed a strong relationship between β_2-adrenoceptor densities on circulating mononuclear leucocytes and in lung tissue obtained at thoracotomy (Liggett *et al.*, 1988). The effect of β-agonists on lymphocyte cytokine production is unknown. Human alveolar macrophages contain 5000 β_2-adrenoceptors per cell (Liggett, 1989), but short-acting β_2-agonists do not prevent mediator release from activated human alveolar macrophages (Fuller *et al.*, 1988), although high concentrations of salmeterol may (Baker *et al.*, 1991). There is evidence that β-agonists reduce the release of histamine from mast cells. β-Agonist-mediated inhibition of mast cell mediator release is probably one mechanism of action of adrenaline in reducing symptoms of anaphylaxis, such as itch and oedema. In addition, inhibition of mast cell mediator release is part of the mechanism of action of β-agonists in abating the early response to allergic bronchial challenge. β-Agonists are also functional antagonists of the airway smooth-muscle contraction induced by release of mediators (Butchers *et al.*, 1980; Howarth *et al.*, 1985; Church & Hiroi, 1987). β-Agonists may also inhibit mediator release from basophils (Barnes, 1986a). Mediator release from the human eosinophil, although possessing a greater density and affinity of β_2-adrenoceptors (5000 sites per cell) than neutrophils, is not inhibited by isoprenaline (Yukawa *et al.*, 1990). Both alveolar macrophages and eosinophils are thought to be important effector cells in the pathogenesis of asthma, and the lack of influence of short-acting β-agonists on these cell types may explain in part the poor efficacy of these agents as monotherapy in asthma (see below).

Cardiovascular

The cardiovascular effects of β-agonists have been reviewed by Lipworth and McDevitt (1992). β-Agonists increase the force and rate of cardiac contraction and thus cause an increase in systolic blood pressure. Increases in inotropic responses are predominantly mediated via β_1-adrenoceptors, although β_2-adrenoceptors also contribute. In contrast, chronotropic responses are predominantly β_2-mediated (Fig. 31.4). β_2-Agonists are also vasodilators via β_2-adrenoceptors on vascular smooth muscle, which leads to a slight fall in diastolic blood pressure. The role of baroreceptor-mediated reflex withdrawal of cardiac vagal tone, in response to peripheral vasodilatation, in determining heart-rate increases seems less important than direct cardiac effects of β-agonists. β-Agonists cause a dose-dependent increase in Q–Tc interval, which has been reported to be correlated with the degree of hypokalaemia induced by these agents (Fig. 31.4) (Crane *et al.*, 1989). However, isoprenaline, which causes minimal hypokalaemia, prolongs the Q–Tc interval to a similar degree to salbutamol, suggesting a direct cardiac β-adrenoceptor-mediated effect (Lipworth & McDevitt, 1992).

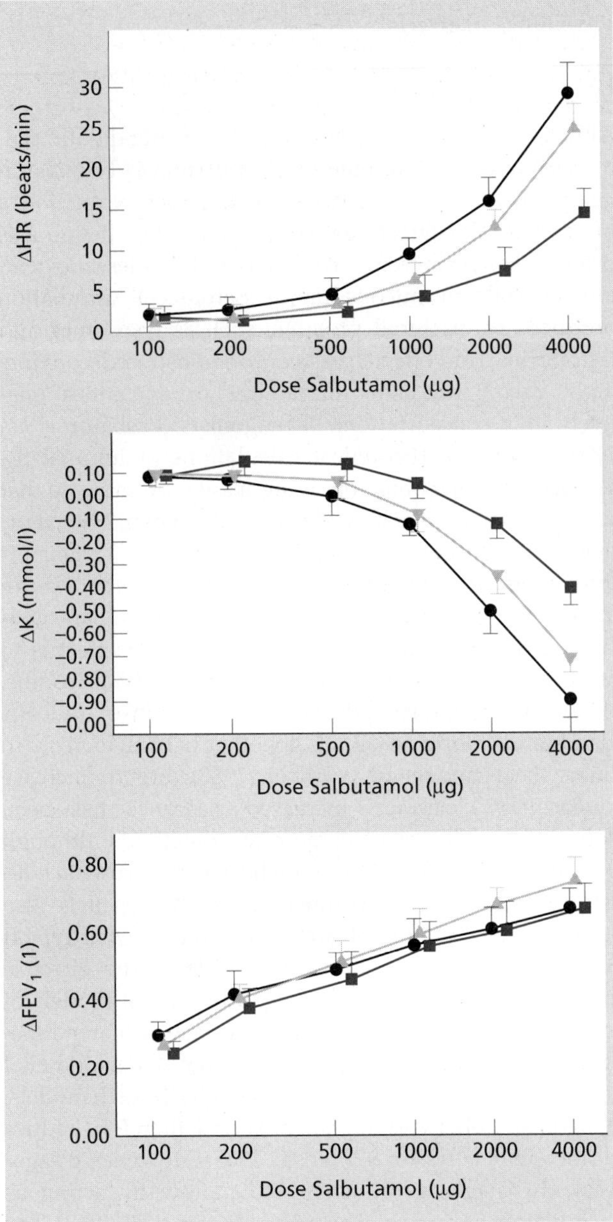

Fig. 31.4 Changes in heart rate (upper panel), plasma potassium (middle panel) and forced expiratory volume in 1 second (FEV_1) (lower panel) in response to cumulative doubling doses of inhaled salbutamol from pressurized metered-dose inhalers in 12 mild asthmatic patients. Subjects were studied after 2 weeks pretreatment with placebo (circles), low-dose regular salbutamol (800 μg/day) (triangles) or high-dose regular salbutamol (4000 μg/day) (squares). Randomized crossover design. Note that significant tolerance to the systemic but not bronchodilator effects of the β-agonist develop with regular use. (Redrawn from Lipworth *et al.*, 1989, with permission.)

Pharmacokinetics of β-adrenoceptor agonists

Oral administration

After administration of an oral or parenteral β-agonist, the bronchodilator effect is closely dependent on serum levels (Morgan *et al.*, 1986). Orally administered β-agonists are incompletely absorbed and the greater proportion is metabolized by sulphate conjugation in the gut epithelium and liver. For example, oral terbutaline absorption varies from 30 to 65% and, of this, only 25% remains unconjugated in the urine (Davies, 1984). Net bioavailability is thus 10–15%. Protein binding of terbutaline varies from 14 to 25%. Salbutamol is more completely absorbed, with peak levels within 1 hour of administration when the subject is fasting (Morgan *et al.*, 1986). Sixty per cent of the absorbed dose is conjugated. Sustained-release preparations of salbutamol and terbutaline are available in various formations and may be particularly valuable in asthmatics with marked nocturnal symptoms, although long-acting inhaled β_2-agonists such as salmeterol may supersede such preparations.

Parenteral administration

Subcutaneous, intramuscular or intravenous injection of terbutaline, salbutamol or adrenaline provides almost immediate action and assured delivery. Following subcutaneous terbutaline 0.5 mg, significant levels are present within a few minutes and peak at 20 minutes (Vanden Berg, 1984). Adrenaline has a slightly shorter duration of action, although a slow-release form is available in some countries. In an intensive-care setting, intravenous infusion is sometimes used when patients are moribund or responding poorly to intermittent administration of β-agonists by other routes. Both terbutaline and salbutamol have been quite widely used, with a loading dose followed by a continuous infusion of 10–20% of the loading dose. Intravenous isoprenaline has little advantage, apart from quicker onset of action, and has greater side-effects, including possibly myocardial toxicity, and use is not recommended.

Aerosol administration

This is the preferred method of administration of all β-agonists, as there is an effect on airway calibre within seconds, with the effect of short-acting β-agonists such as salbutamol reaching 80% of maximum in 5 minutes (Figs 31.4 & 31.5). Compared with parenteral or oral administration, following aerosolization a given degree of bronchodilatation is achieved, with significantly fewer adverse effects, such as tremor or palpitations. Short-acting β_2-agonists achieve peak effects within 30–60 minutes and bronchodilatation slowly reduces over a variable time after this, in part dependent on the severity of asthma, but airway calibre is back to baseline within 4–5 hours. There are no important clinical differences between commonly availible short-acting β_2-agonists in terms of bronchodilatation or duration of action. The effects of catecholamine aerosols such as rimiterol or adrenaline peak earlier and bronchodilatation persists for only 30 minutes to 2 hours.

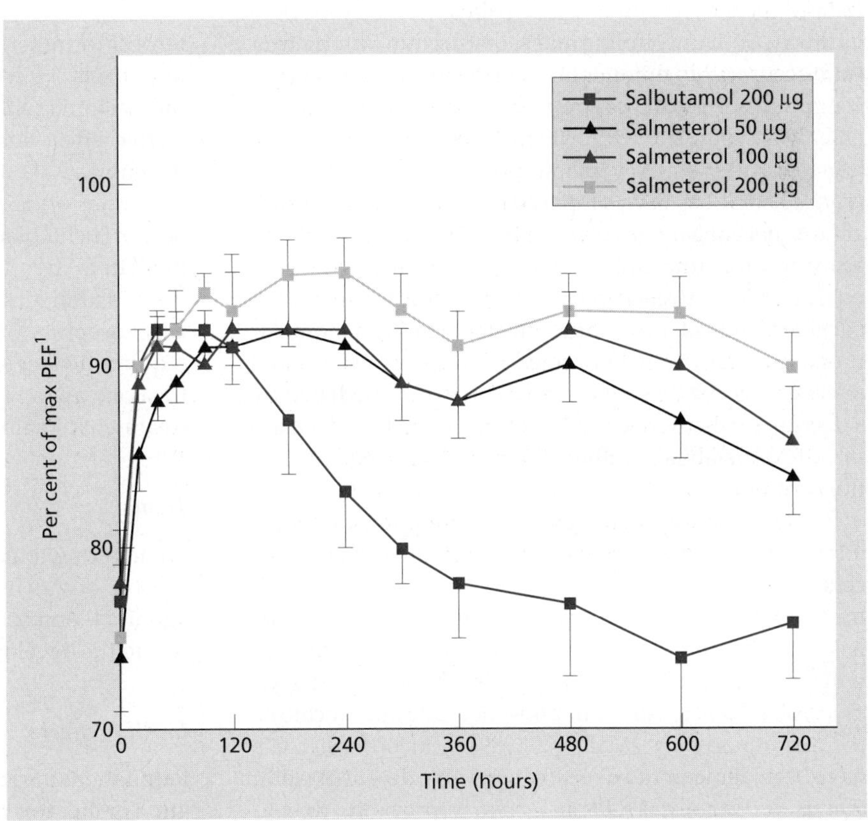

Fig. 31.5 Time-course of bronchodilator response to standard short- and long-acting β-agonists. Peak expiratory flow (PEF) after inhalation of salbutamol or salmeterol. (From Ullman & Svedmyr, 1988.)

Serum levels are very low after inhaled administration and do not correlate with bronchodilatation. The effects of different aerosol delivery devices on intrapulmonary β-agonist deposition will be discussed in a subsequent chapter.

Adverse effects

Desensitization

β-Adrenoceptor desensitization, that is, waning of the response in the face of continuous or repeated agonist exposure, can occur by several mechanisms (Hausdorff *et al.*, 1990). Rapid desensitization is mediated by an alteration in the function of the β-adrenoceptor, in that it becomes uncoupled from the stimulatory G protein, G_s. This uncoupling phenomenon involves phosphorylation of the receptor in its terminal intracellular segment by at least two different kinases, protein kinase A and a β-adrenoceptor-associated kinase (β-ARK), which are activated under different desensitization conditions. The decreased efficiency of coupling of the β-adrenoceptor to G_s leads to decreased adenylyl cyclase activity and hence decreased cAMP levels. Desensitization can also occur by intracellular sequestration of the receptor complex or by 'down-regulation', which refers to an agonist-induced decrease in receptor number. Down-regulation occurs upon prolonged exposure to agonists and results in degradation of the receptor, presumably via a lysozymal pathway. Both uncoupling and sequestration (internalization) occur within minutes of exposure to micromolar concentrations of β-adrenoceptor agonists and the process is essentially complete within 30 minutes. Down-regulation is evident after only several hours of exposure (Hausdorff *et al.*, 1990). It has been proposed that the rapid desensitization mechanisms involving phosphorylation of the β-adrenoceptor (uncoupling) may be operative mainly for non-neural β_2-adrenoceptors that respond to circulating concentrations of adrenaline, which are in the nanomolar range (Barnes, 1986b; O'Donnell & Worstall, 1987; Stadel & Lefkowitz, 1991). Down-regulation is also mediated by a decrease in β-adrenoceptor mRNA, caused by a decrease in mRNA stability rather than a decreased rate of transcription.

Phosphorylation and therefore uncoupling of the β-adrenoceptor can also be induced by stimulation of adjacent receptors ('receptor crosstalk'), such as cholinergic muscarinic receptors. Activation of muscarinic receptors leads to stimulation of phosphatidylinositol pathways with secondary activation of protein kinase C by diacylglycerol, which, in turn, can phosphorylate and uncouple the β-adrenoceptor (Malbon, 1989). Glucorticosteroids have been demonstrated *in vitro* to reverse desensitization (Davis & Conolly, 1980) and this is probably due to increased β_2-adrenoceptor gene transcription (Mak *et al.*, 1995), and possibily increased coupling, and may be an important mechanism of action of glucocorticosteroids in the treatment of asthma. Relatively large numbers of β-adrenoceptors on human airway smooth muscle or rapid turnover of adrenoceptors may explain why this tissue is relatively resistant to desensitization (Hamid *et al.*, 1991; Hall *et al.*, 1993).

There have been many clinical studies of desensitization following regular short-acting β-agonist use (reviewed by Nelson *et al.*, 1990). There is evidence in some studies (Weber *et al.*, 1982), but not others (Harvey *et al.*, 1981), of a small decrease in peak bronchodilator effect and duration of action in stable mild asthma but not in peak bronchodilator effect in more severely asthmatic patients (Lipworth *et al.*, 1989; Fig. 31.4). The majority of positive reports have used oral β-agonists. Most investigators have examined only peak bronchodilator effects and, if duration of action is important, as has been suggested, then further research is required. In contrast to studies in asthmatics, normal subjects readily demonstrate densensitization both in the lung and in non-pulmonary β-adrenergic systems (Harvey *et al.*, 1981).

Small increases in airway responsiveness have been detected following cessation of regular short-acting β-agonists. One explanation of these findings is desensitization of airway smooth muscle β-adrenoceptors (Kraan *et al.*, 1985; Vathenen *et al.*, 1988). There is no evidence that long-term use of long-acting β_2-agonists such as salmeterol or formoterol leads to tolerance to their bronchodilating effects. However, regular treatment of patients with mild asthma with salmeterol leads to tolerance to its protective effect against *in vivo* bronchoconstrictor stimuli (Cheung *et al.*, 1992; Ramage *et al.*, 1994). In addition, O'Connor *et al.* (1992) have demonstrated tolerance to non-bronchodilator effects of terbutaline (effects possibly mediated by lung mast cell β_2-adrenoceptors) in mild asthmatics. The effect of desensitization of β-adrenoceptors on cell types other than smooth muscle requires further study. Overall, the importance of desensitization as a clinically relevant effect of β-agonist treatment remains unclear.

Tremor

Tremor, due to activation of β_2-adrenoceptors in skeletal muscle, occurs in up to 20% of patients at initiation of β_2-agonist therapy. Tremor usually abates with regular use due to the development of desensitization.

Cardiac effects

Palpitations are reported by up to 5% of asthmatics at initiation of therapy, more so with agents which are full rather than partial agonists at β_2-adrenoceptors. Desensitization develops with regular therapy (Fig. 31.4). Despite concern that tachyarrhythmias could develop secondary to effects of β-agonists on the Q–Tc interval and potassium in hypoxaemic patients, serious cardiovascular events are extremely rare. However, caution should be exercised in individuals with unstable ischaemic heart disease receiving high doses of nebulized β-agonists, as angina has been precipitated in this situation.

Hypokalaemia and other metabolic effects

Hypokalaemia is seen following both inhaled or systemic administration of β-agonists due to stimulation of Na^+/K^+ adenosine triphosphatase (ATPase) activity and stimulation of insulin secretion (Fig. 31.4). When high cumulative inhaled doses of salbutamol and fenoterol (1200 µg) were given to normal subjects, decreases of 0.67 and 1.13 mmol/l, respectively, were observed. Again desensitization is observed to this effect with chronic use of β agonists (Fig. 31.4). Glyconeolysis also occurs secondary to β_2-adrenoreceptor activation; the changes induced are small and of uncertain significance in patients with diabetes mellitus. Lipolysis is activated by β-agonists via β_1-, β_2- and possibly β_3-adrenoceptors and results in the mobilization of free fatty acids from adipose tissue.

Hypoxaemia

All β-agonists, including adrenaline, can reduce arterial oxygen tension. These changes are apparent 5 minutes after administration of inhaled β-agonists and return to normal values by 30 minutes. These changes are secondary to an increase in pulmonary blood flow in poorly ventilated regions of the lung, hence worsening ventilation perfusion inequality. The increase in blood flow may be secondary to pulmonary vasodilatation via stimulation of β_2-adrenoceptors on vascular smooth muscle in the lung and also to increases in cardiac output following cardiac adrenoceptor stimulation. The reduction in arterial oxygen tension is small and unlikely to be clinically significant.

Potential adverse effects of regular β-adrenergic agonist therapy

β-Agonists have been widely used for many years in asthma treatment but recent reports have raised the possibility that regular β-agonist use is hazardous (Kraan *et al.*, 1985; Vathenen *et al.*, 1988; Pearce *et al.*, 1990; Sears *et al.*, 1990; Grainger *et al.*, 1991; Spitzer *et al.*, 1992). Although some studies have suggested that adverse effects are limited to specific agents such as fenoterol and isoprenaline (Grainger *et al.*, 1991), more recent evidence supports a class effect (Spitzer *et al.*, 1992). A number of speculations and hypotheses have been advanced to explain these findings (Table 31.7). One explanation is that excessive reliance on potent bronchodilators leads to delay in presentation for more effective therapy such as corticosteroids and oxygen and hence more severe or even fatal asthma attacks. This is a well-recognized risk of β-agonist use (Sears & Rea, 1987). A second hypothesis is that prolonged bronchodilatation resulting from regular β-agonist use leads to an increase in the amount of antigen or irritant inhaled into the lung. Normally, bronchoconstriction serves as a protective reaction to restrict entry of noxious materials into the airways. Furthermore, the bronchodilatation can mask the usual warning signs of an attack (the immediate allergic response) so that the usual avoidance measures are not taken. Although there is little direct evidence for this possibility, it may be an important mechanism whereby asthma can worsen (Lai *et al.*, 1989). The third possibility that excessive β-agonist use leads to clinically significant desensitization of β-adrenoceptors has been extensively investigated (see above). A fourth hypothesis, which could increase mortality but not morbidity, is that stimulation of cardiac β-adrenoceptors, by increasing heart rate and inotropy in the setting of the hypokalaemia induced by β-agonists and hypoxaemia, gives rise to fatal cardiac arrhythmias. There is little direct evidence to support this hypothesis (Crane *et al.*, 1989; Wong *et al.*, 1990). Additional speculations include: (i) inhibition of mast cell mediator release by β-agonists gives rise to an abnormal prolongation of inflammation by preventing the release of natural anti-inflammatory substances, such as heparin and other proteoglycans, which are normally released along with other mediators following mast cell activation (Page, 1991); (ii) promotion of airway secretions by β-agonists leads to worsening airflow obstruction (Williams *et al.*, 1981; Sears *et al.*, 1990);

Table 31.7 Potential mechanisms of adverse effects of β-adrenoceptor agonist treatment.

Excess reliance on bronchodilators leads to delay in seeking more appropriate care
Bronchodilatation increases allergen/irritant load
Regular use leads to desensitization of adrenoceptors and rebound airway hyperresponsiveness
Stimulation of cardiac β-adrenoceptors, in the setting of hypoxaemia and hypokalaemia, causes cardiac arrhythmias
Inhibition of mast cell mediator release prevents release of anti-inflammatory autocoids
Regular use promotes airway secretions, exacerbating air-flow obstruction
Dilation of the bronchial vasculature worsens obstruction by thickening airway walls
S enantiomers in racemic mixtures possess harmful properties
Regular use increases airway smooth-muscle contractility

(iii) dilatation of the bronchial vasculature induced by β-agonists worsens obstruction, by causing vascular engorgement and thickening of airway walls (Wang *et al.*, 1995); (iv) S enantiomers in racemic mixtures possess harmful properties (Chapman *et al.*, 1992); and (v) regular use of β-agonists increases airway smooth-muscle contractility (Wang *et al.*, 1995). Overall, much of the data suggesting that β-agonist therapy is hazardous can be explained by such treatment modifying patient behaviour so as to place him or her at greater risk of illness by both inducing delay in obtaining more appropriate treatment and suppressing the early asthmatic response.

β-Adrenoceptor antagonists

Propranolol was the first β-antagonist developed for clinical use and remains the prototypic agent (Van Zwieten, 1985). It is a non-selective, competitive antagonist without agonist activity. Nadolol, timolol, pindolol and sotalol are other examples of this group. Although selectivity is not absolute, metoprolol, atenolol, acebutolol and esmolol are relatively β_1-adrenoceptor selective. Labetalol represents a class of drugs that act as competitive antagonists at both α_1- and β-adrenoceptors, with greater potency for the latter, as well as some partial agonist activity at β_2-adrenoceptors. Pindolol and acebutolol also have partial agonist activity ('intrinsic sympathomimetic activity') at β_1-adrenoceptors. Esmolol is a very short-acting β-antagonist useful intravenously when short-duration β-blockade is desired.

None of these antagonists can be safely used in asthmatics, even by topical application, and should be used with great caution in patients with chronic air-flow obstruction. The use of β-antagonists, predictably, also increases the severity and resistance to treatment of anaphylaxis (Schellenberg *et al.*, 1991).

α-Adrenoceptor agonists

Most of these compounds are drugs with mixed effects, i.e. they both displace noradrenaline from storage sites within the neurone and have direct α-adrenoceptor-stimulating effects. As for β-agonists, the receptor subtype specificity and potency is determined by chemical structure (Fig. 31.1). Ephedrine is the classic compound in this category. Ephedrine is an alkaloid derived from mahuang (*Ephedra equisetina*) and exists in four enantiomers: (+) and (–) ephedrine and (+) and (–) pseudoephedrine. The most potent form in relation to sympathomimetic activity is (–)-ephedrine; this compound is used clinically, as is (–)-pseudoephedrine. Ephedrine produces a prompt rise in blood pressure, causes coronary vessel vasodilatation and increases heart rate. The other commonly used oral α-agonist is phenylpropanolamine. Ephedrine and phenylpropanolamine possess both α_1- and α_2-agonist activity and are both commonly used as nasal and sinus decongestants. In the nasal vasculature, stimulation of the α_1- and α_2-adrenoceptors on resistance blood-vessels regulates blood flow. In the capacitance vessels, regulating blood volume changes (Lacroix, 1989), α_2-adrenoceptor response predominate over α_1-adrenoceptors. Phenylpropanolamine and pseudoephedrine are well absorbed, with a half-life of 4 hours. Slow-release preparations enable twice-daily dosage. Direct effects of ephedrine on airway β_2-adrenoceptors result in bronchodilatation.

Both α_1- and α_2-agonists reduce vascular engorgement and therefore improve nasal patency (Bende & Loth, 1986). There may be advantages to using selective α_1-agonists, as α_2-agonists reduce mucosal blood flow by 30–40%, which may impair long-term mucosal (i.e. nasal epithelium) health. Phenylephrine is a selective α_1-agonist used clinically that is chemically closely related to adrenaline but is less potent and has a longer duration of action. It has little effect on α_2-adrenoceptors. It is a useful agent as a topical nasal decongestant but is poorly absorbed orally. Methoxamine is also an effective α_1-agonist, sometimes used to reduce airway narrowing when the latter is due to the dilation of bronchial mucosal vessels secondary to left heart failure ('cardiac asthma'). Selective α_1-agonists have a short duration of action and the predominantly α_2-agonist imidazole derivatives, oxymetazoline and xylometazoline, are useful sympathomimetic agents with a longer duration of action. Use of α-agonists causes rebound vasodilatation in the nose following onset of action, and prolonged use may lead to rhinitis medicamentosa.

Other selective α_2-agonists include clonidine and α-methyldopa, which are widely used in hypertension and in conditions of 'sympathetic overactivity'. These compounds stimulate presynaptic α_2-adrenoceptors present on both adrenergic and cholinergic neurones. They inhibit noradrenaline release and they also inhibit, in some circumstances, acetylcholine release.

α-Adrenoceptor antagonists

Currently there are no specific indications for α-adrenergic antagonists in the management of allergic diseases. Dale (1906) reported that the pressor effects of large doses of adrenaline could be reversed to cause a fall in blood pressure by certain ergot preparations now known to have α-adrenoceptor-blocking properties. Large numbers of drugs with the ability to antagonize the effects of α-adrenoceptor stimulation have been synthesized. They are classified into reversible, non-competitive antagonists, for example phenoxybenzamine, and reversible competitive antagonists, such as phentolamine and prazosin. Phentolamine and phenoxybenzamine are non-selective antagonists, whereas prazosin selectively blocks α_1-adrenoceptors. Yohimbine is a plant alkaloid with selective α_2-antagonist action. Interest has continued in the possibility of using α-adrenergic antagonists in the treatment of asthma as, in some patients, the administration of an α-agonist such as methoxamine provokes airway narrowing (Black *et al.*, 1984). There is also the long-standing observation of increased α-adrenergic responsiveness in patients with allergic disorders. Overall, the response to α-adrenergic antagonists in clinical trials has been disappointing (Barnes, 1986a), although the possibility of individual responses to α-adrenergic antagonists still exists.

Acknowledgements

This work was supported by the British Columbia (BC) Health Research Foundation, the BC Lung Association and the Medical Research Council of Canada.

References

Ahlquist, R.P. (1948) A study of the adrenotrophic receptor. *Am. J. Physiol.*, **153**, 586–99.

Bai, T.R. (1992) β_2 adrenergic receptors in asthma: a current perspective. *Lancet*, **170**, 125–41.

Bai, T.R., Lam, R. & Prasad, F.Y.F. (1989) Effects of adrenergic agonists and adenosine on cholinergic neurotransmission in human tracheal smooth muscle. *Pulm. Pharmacol.*, **1**, 193–9.

Bai, T.R., Mak, J.C. & Barnes, P.J. (1992) A comparison of β-adrenoceptors and *in vitro* relaxant responses to isoproterenol in asthmatic airway smooth muscle. *Am. J. Respir. Cell Mol. Biol.*, **6**, 647–51.

Bai, T.R., Zhou, D., Aubert, J.-D., Lizee, G., Hayashi, S. & Bondy, G.P. (1993) Expression of β_2-adrenergic receptor mRNA in peripheral lung in asthma and chronic obstructive pulmonary disease. *Am. J. Respir. Cell Mol. Biol.*, **8**, 325–33.

Baker, A.J. & Fuller, R.W. (1991) Comparison of the anti-inflammatory effects of salmeterol on human airway macrophages with those on peripheral monocytes. *Eur. Resp. J.*, **4** (Suppl. 14), 426 [abstract].

Barnes, P.J. (1986a) Endogenous catecholamines and asthma. *J. Allergy Clin. Immunol.*, **77**, 791–5.

Barnes, P.J. (1986b) Neural control of human airways in health and disease. *Am. Rev. Resp. Dis.*, **134**, 1289–314.

Basbaum, C.B., Madison, J.M., Sommerhoff, C.P., Brown, J.K. & Finkbeiner, W.E. (1990) Adrenoceptors on airway gland cells. *Am. Rev. Resp. Dis.*, **141**, S141–S144.

Bende, M. & Loth, S. (1986) Vascular effects of topical oxymetazoline on human nasal mucosa. *J. Laryngology Otology*, **100**(3), 285–8.

Black, J.L., Salome, C., Yan, K. *et al.* (1984) The action of prazosin and proplylene glycol on methoxamine-induced bronchoconstriction in asthmatic subjects. *Brit. J. Clin. Pharmacol.*, **18**, 349.

Bristow, M.R., & Ginsberg, R. (1986) Beta-2 receptors on myocardial cells in human ventricular myocardium. *Am. J. Cardiol.*, **57**, 3F–6F.

Brogden, R.N. & Faulds, D. (1991) Salmeterol xinafoate: a review of its pharmacological properties and therapeutic potential in reversible obstructive airways disease. *Drugs*, **42**, 893–912.

Brown, O.M. (1992) Adrenergic drugs. In: *Textbook of Pharmacology* (eds C.M. Smith & A.M. Reynard), pp. 141–67. W.B. Saunders, Philadelphia.

Bullowa, J.G.M. & Kaplan, D.M. (1903) On the hypodermatic use of adrenalin chloride in the treatment of asthmatic attacks. *Med. News*, **83**, 787–90.

Busse, W.W. & Sosman, J.M. (1984) Isoproterenol inhibition of isolated human neutrophil function. *J. Allergy Clin. Immunol.*, **73**, 404–10.

Butchers, P.R., Skidmore, F., Vardey, C.J. & Wheeldon, A.M. (1980) Characterization of the receptor mediating the anti-anaphylactic effects of β-adrenoceptor agonists in human lung tissue *in vitro*. *Brit. J. Pharmacol.*, **71**, 663–7.

Carstairs, J.R., Nimmo, A.J. & Barnes, P.J. (1985) Autoradiographic visualization of β-adrenoceptor subtypes in human lung. *Am. Rev. Resp. Dis.*, **132**, 541–7.

Chapman, I.D., Buchhkit, K.H., Morley, P. & Morley, J. (1992) Active enantiomers may cause adverse effects in asthma. *Trends Pharmacol. Sci.*, **13**, 231–2.

Cheung, D., Timmers, M.C., Zwinderman, A.H., Bel, E.H., Dijkman, J.H. & Sterk, P.J. (1992) Long-term effects of long-acting β_2-adrenoceptor agonist, salmeterol, on airway hyperresponsiveness in patients with mild asthma. *New Engl. J. Med.*, **327**, 1198–203.

Church, M.K. & Hiroi, J. (1987) Inhibition of IgE-dependent histamine release from human dispersed lung mast cells by anti-allergic drugs and salbutamol. *Brit. J. Pharmacol.*, **90**, 421–9.

Collins, S., Caron, M.G. & Lefkowitz, R.J. (1988) B_2-adrenergic adrenoceptors in hamster smooth muscle cells are transcriptionally regulated by glucocorticoids. *J. Biol. Chem.*, **263**, 9067–70.

Coupe, M.O., Guly, U. & Barnes, P.J. (1986) Comparison of nebulized adrenaline and salbutamol in acute severe asthma. *Clin. Sci.*, **71**, 80–1.

Crane, J., Burgess, C. & Beasley, R. (1989) Cardiovascular and hypokalemic effects of inhaled salbutanol, fenoterol and isoprenaline. *Thorax*, **44**, 136–40.

Dale, H.H. (1906) On some physiological actions of ergot. *J. Physiol.*, **34**, 165–206.

Davies, D.S. (1984) The fate of inhaled terbutaline. *Eur. J. Resp. Dis.*, **65** (Suppl. 134), 141.

Davis, C. & Conolly, M.E. (1980) Tachyphylaxis to B-adrenoceptor agonists in human bronchial smooth muscle: studies *in vitro*. *Brit. J. Clin. Pharmacol.*, **10**, 417–21.

Decker, N. (1982) Effects of N-atalkyl substitution of β-agonists on α and β-adrenoreceptor subtypes: pharmacological studies and binding assays. *J. Pharm. Pharmacol.*, **34**, 107–12.

Emorine, L.J., Marullo, S., Delavier-Klutchko, C., Kaveri, S.V., Durien-Trantmann, O. & Strosberg, A.D. (1987) Human β_2-adrenergic receptor: expression and promotor characterization. *Proc. Nat. Acad. Sci. USA*, **84**, 6995–9.

Emorine, L.J., Marullo, S., Briend-Sutren, M.-M. *et al.* (1989) Molecular characterization of the human β_3-adrenergic receptor. *Science*, **245**, 1118–21.

Exton, J.H. (1982) Molecular mechanisms involved in alpha-adrenoceptor responses. *Trends Pharmacol. Sci.*, **3**, 111.

Fraser, C.M. & Venter, J.C. (1990) β adrenoceptors — relationship of primary structure, receptor function and regulation. *Am. Rev. Resp. Dis.*, **141**, S22–S30.

Fuller, R.W., O'Malley, G., Baker, A.J. & MacDermot, J. (1988) Human alveolar macrophage activation: inhibition by forskolin but not β adrenoceptor stimulation or phosphodiesterase inhibition. *Pulm. Pharmacol.*, **1**, 101–6.

Grainger, J., Woodman, K., Pearce, N. *et al.* (1991) Prescribed fenoterol and death from asthma in New Zealand 1981–87: a further case–control study. *Thorax*, **46**, 105–11.

Grieco, M.H. & Pierson, R.N. (1971) Mechanisms of bronchoconstriction due to β-adrenergic blockage. *J. Allergy Clin. Immunol.*, **48**, 143–52.

Hadcock, J.R. & Malbon, C.C. (1988) Down-regulation of β-adrenergic adrenoceptors: agonist-induced reduction in receptor mRNA levels. *Proc. Nat. Acad. Sci. USA*, **85**, 5021–5.

Hall, I.P., Daykin, K. & Widdop, S. (1993) β_2-adrenoceptor desensitization in cultured human airway smooth muscle. *Clin. Sci.*, **84**, 151–7.

Hamid, Q.A., Mak, J.C.W., Sheppard, M.N., Corrin, B., Ventor, J.C. & Barnes, P.J. (1991) Localization of β_2-adrenoceptor messenger RNA in human and rat lung using *in situ* hybridization: correlation with receptor autoradiography. *Eur. J. Pharmacol. (Mol. Pharmacol.)*, **206**, 133–8.

Harvey, J.E., Baldwin, C.J., Wood, P.J., Alberti, K.G. & Tattersfield, A.E. (1981) Airway and metabolic responsiveness to intraveneous salbutamol in asthma: effect of regular inhaled salbutamol. *Clin. Sci.*, **60**, 579–85.

Hasegawa, M. & Townley, R.G. (1983) Difference between lung and spleen susceptibility of β-adrenergic adrenoceptors to desensitization by terbutaline. *J. Allergy Clin. Immunol.*, **71**, 230–5.

Hausdorff, W.P., Caron, M.C. & Lefkowitz, R.J. (1990) Turning off the signal: desensitization of β-adrenergic receptor function. *FASEB J.*, **4**, 2881–9.

Hieble, J.P. & Bond, R.A. (1994) New directions in adrenoceptor pharmacology. *Trends Pharmacol.*, **15**, 397–9.

Howarth, P.H., Durham, S.R., Lee, T.H., Kay, A.B., Church, M.K. & Holgate, S.T. (1985) Influence of albuterol, cromolyn sodium and ipratropium bromide on the airway and circulating mediator responses to allergen bronchial provocation in asthma. *Am. Rev. Resp. Dis.*, **132**, 986–92.

Insel, P.A. (1991) B-adrenergic adrenoceptors in pathophysiologic states and in clinical medicine. In: *The B-Adrenergic Adrenoceptors* (ed. J.P. Perkins), pp. 294–343. Humana Press, Clifton, NJ.

Jack, D. (1991) A way of looking at agonism and antagonism: lessons from salbutamol, salmeterol and other β-adrenocepter agonists. *Brit. J. Clin. Pharmacol.*, **31**, 501–14.

Johnson, M., Butchers, P.R., Coleman, R.A. *et al.* (1993) The pharmacology of salmeterol. *Life Sci.*, **26**, 2131–43.

Jones, T.R., Charette, L., Garcia, M.L. & Kaczorowski, G.I. (1990) Selective inhibition of relaxation of guinea pig trachea by charybdotoxin, a potent Ca^{2+} activated potassium channel inhibitor. *J. Pharmacol. Exp. Ther.*, **255**, 697–706.

Kahn, R.H. (1907) Zur Physiologie der Trachea. *Arch. Physiol.*, 398–426.

Kelly, W.T., Baile, E.M., Brancatisano, A., Paré, P.D. & Engel, L.A. (1992) The effects of inspiratory resistance, inhaled β agonist and histamine on canine tracheal blood flow. *Eur. Resp. J.*, **5**, 1206–14.

Kerrebijn, K.F. (1991) B agonists. In: *Asthma: Its Pathology and Treatment*, Vol. 49, *Lung Biology in Health and Disease* (eds M.A. Kaliner, P.J. Barnes & C.G.A. Persson), p. 526. Marcel Dekker, New York.

Konzett, H. (1941) Neue broncholytische Hochwirk same Korper der Adrenalinreihe. *NS Arch. Exp. Pathol. Pharmakol.*, **197**, 27–32.

Kraan, J., Koeter, G.H., Vandermark, T.W. *et al.* (1985) Changes in bronchial hyperreactivity induced by four weeks of treatment with anti-asthmatic drugs in patients with allergic asthma: a comparison between budesonide and terbutaline. *J. Allergy Clin. Immunol.*, **76**, 628–36.

Lacroix, J.S. (1989) Adrenergic and non-adrenergic mechanisms in sympathetic vascular control of the nasal mucosa. *Acta Physiol. Scand.*, **581**, 1–63.

Lai, C.K., Twentyman, O.P. & Holgate, S.T. (1989) The effect of an increase in inhaled allergen dose after rimiterol hydrobromide on the occurrence and magnitude of the late asthmatic response and the associated change in non-specific bronchial responsiveness. *Am. Rev. Resp. Dis.*, **140**, 917–23.

Lands, A.M., Arnold, A., McAuliffe, J.P., Ludnena, F.P. & Brown, T.G. (1967) Differentiation of receptor systems activated by sympathomimetic amines. *Nature*, **214**, 597–9.

Langley, J.N. (1905) On the reaction of cells and nerve endings to certain poisons, in regards to the reaction of striated muscle to nicotine and curari. *J. Physiol.*, **33**, 374–413.

Liggett, S.B. (1989) Identification and characterization of a homogenous population of β_2-adrenergic adrenoceptors on human alveolar macrophages. *Am. Rev. Resp. Dis.*, **139**, 552–5.

Liggett, S.B., Marker, J.C., Shah, S.D., Roper, C.L. & Cryer, P.E. (1988) Direct relationship between mononuclear leukocyte and lung β-adrenergic adrenoceptors and apparent reciprocal regulation of extravascular, but not intravascular α and β-adrenergic adrenoceptors by the sympathochromaffin system in humans. *J. Clin. Invest.*, **82**, 48–56.

Lipworth, B.J. & McDevitt, D.G. (1992) Inhaled β_2-adrenoceptor agonists in asthma: help or hindrance? *Brit. J. Clin. Pharmacol.*, **33**, 129–38.

Lipworth, B.J., Struthers, A.D. & McDevitt, D.G. (1989) Tachyphylaxis to systemic but not to airway responses during prolonged therapy with high dose inhaled salbutamol in asthmatics. *Am. Rev. Resp. Dis.*, **140**, 586–92.

Mak, J.C.W., Nishikawa, M. & Barnes, P.J. (1995) Glucocorticosteroids increase β_2-adrenergic receptor transcription in human lung. *Am. J. Physiol. Lung Cell. Mol. Physiol.*, **12**, L41–L46.

Malbon, C. (1989) Physiological regulation of transmembrane signalling elements. *Am. J. Cell. Mol. Biol.*, **1**, 449–50.

Mason, R.J. & Williams, M.C. (1991) Alveolar type II cells. In: *The Lung: Scientific Foundations*, Vol. 1 (eds R.G. Crystal & J.B. West), pp. 235–46. Raven Press, New York.

Morgan, D.J., Paull, J.D., Richmond, B.H., Wison-Evered, E. & Ziccone, S.P. (1986) Pharmacokinetics of intravenous and oral salbutamol and its sulphate conjugate. *Brit. J. Clin. Pharmacol.*, **22**, 587–93.

Nadel, J.A. & Barnes, P.J. (1984) Autonomic regulation of the airways. *Ann. Rev. Med.*, **35**, 451–67.

Nelson, H.S., Szefler, S.J. & Martin, R.J. (1990) Regular inhaled β-adrenergic agonists in the treatment of bronchial asthma: beneficial or detrimental. *Am. Rev. Resp. Dis.*, **144**, 249–50.

O'Connor, B.J., Aikman, S.L. & Barnes, P.J. (1992) Tolerance to the nonbronchodilator effects of inhaled β_2-agonists in asthma. *New Engl. J. Med.*, **327**, 1204–8.

O'Donnell, S.R. & Wanstall, J.C. (1978) Functional evidence for differential regulation of B-adrenoceptor subtypes. *Trends Pharmacol. Sci.*, **8**, 265–8.

Page, C.P. (1991) Hypothesis. One explanation of the asthma paradox: inhibition of natural anti-inflammatory mechanism by β_2-agonists. *Lancet*, **337**, 717–20.

Pearce, N., Grainger, J., Atkinson, M. *et al.* (1990) Case–control study of prescribed fenoterol and death from asthma in New Zealand, 1977–81. *Thorax*, **45**, 170–5.

Persson, C.G.A. (1985) On the medical history of xanthines and other remedies for asthma: a tribute to H.H. Salter. *Thorax*, **40**, 881–6.

Persson, C.G.A. (1989) Glucocorticoids for asthma—early contributions. *Pulm. Pharmacol.*, **2**, 163–6.

Persson, C.G.A. & Svensjo, E. (1985) Vascular responses and their suppression: drugs interfering with venular permeability. In: *Handbook of Inflammation*, Vol. 5 (eds I.L. Banta, M.A. Bray & M.J. Parnham), pp. 61–81. Elsevier, Amsterdam.

Phipps, R.J., Williams, I.P., Richardson, P.S., Pell, J., Pack, R.J. & Wright, N. (1992) Sympathomimetic drugs stimulate the output of secretory glycoproteins from human bronchi *in vitro*. *Clin. Sci.*, **63**, 23–8.

Ramage, L., Lipworth, B.J., Ingram, C.G., Cree, I.A. & Dhillon, D.P. (1994) Reduced protection against exercise induced bronchoconstriction after chronic dosing with salmeterol. *Resp. Med.*, **88**, 363–8.

Rhoden, K.J., Meldrum, L.A. & Barnes, P.J. (1988) Inhibition of cholinergic neurotransmission in human airways by β_2 adrenoceptors. *J. Appl. Physiol.*, **65**, 700–5.

Schellenberg, R.R., Ohtaka, H., Paddon, H.B., Bramble, S.E. & Rangno, R.E. (1991) Catecholamine responses to histamine infusion in man. *J. Allergy Clin. Immunol.*, **87** (2), 499–504.

Sears, M.R. & Rea, H.H. (1987) Patients at risk of dying of asthma: New Zealand experience. *J. Allergy Clin. Immunol.*, **80**, 477–81.

Sears, M.R., Taylor, D.R. & Print, C.G. (1990) Regular inhaled β-agonist treatment in bronchial asthma. *Lancet*, **336**, 1391–6.

Solis-Cohen, S. (1900) The use of adrenal substance in the treatment of asthma. *JAMA*, **34**, 1164–6.

Spitzer, W.O., Suissa, S., Ernst, P. *et al.* (1992) Asthma death and near-fatal asthma in relation to β-agonist use. *New Engl. J. Med.*, **326**, 501–6.

Stadel, J.M. & Lefkowitz, R.J. (1991) β-Adrenergic adrenoceptors: identification and characterization by radioligand binding studies. In: *B-adrenergic Adrenoceptors* (ed. J.P. Perkins), pp. 1–41. Humana Press, Clifton, NJ.

Stephenson, R.P. (1956) Modification of receptor therapy. *Brit. J. Pharmacol.*, **11**, 379–93.

Strader, C.D., Sigal, I.S. & Dixon, R.A. (1989) Mapping the functional domains of the β-adrenergic receptor. *Am. J. Cell. Mol. Biol.*, **1**, 81–6.

Tota, M.R., Candelore, M.R., Dixon, R.A.F. & Strader, C.D. (1991) Biophysical and genetic analysis of the ligand-binding site of the beta-adrenoceptor. *Trends Pharmacol. Sci.*, **12**, 4–6.

Ullman, A. & Svedmyr, N. (1988) Salmeterol, a new long-acting inhaled β_2 adrenoceptor agonist: comparison with salbutamol in adult asthmatic patients. *Thorax*, **43**, 674.

van den Berg, W., Leferink, J.G., Maes, R.A., Fokkens, J.K., Kreukniet, J. & Bruynzeel, P.L. (1984) The effects of oral and subcutaneous terbutaline in asthmatic patients. *Eur. J. Resp. Dis.*, **65** (Suppl. 134), 181–93.

van Megen, Y.J.B., Klaassen, A.B.M., de Miranda, J.F.R., van Ginneken, C.A.M. & Wentges, B.T.R. (1991) Alterations of adrenoceptors in the nasal mucosa of allergic patients in comparison with nonallergic individuals. *J. Allergy Clin. Immunol.*, **87**, 530–40.

van Zwieten, P.A. (1988) Antihypertensive drugs interacting with alpha- and beta-adrenoceptors: a review of basic pharmacology. *Pharmacology*, **37**, 115–24.

Vathenen, A.S., Knox, A.J., Higgins, B.G., Britton, J.R. & Tatterfield, A.E. (1988) Rebound increase in bronchial responsiveness after treatment with inhaled terbutaline. *Lancet*, **1**, 554–8.

Wang, Z.L., Walker, B.A.M., Weir, T. *et al.* (1995) Effect of chronic antigen and β_2 agonist exposure on airway remodelling in guinea pigs. *Am. J. Resp. Crit. Care Med.*, **152**, 2097–104.

Wanner, A. (1988) Autonomic control of mucociliary function. In: *The Airways: Neural Control in Health and Disease* (eds M.A. Kaliner & P.J. Barnes), pp. 551–74. Marcel Dekker, New York.

Weber, R.W., Smith, J.A. & Nelson, H.S. (1982) Aerosolized terbutaline in asthmatics: development of subsensitivity with long-term administration. *J. Allergy Clin. Immunol.*, **70**, 417–22.

Whicker, S.D. & Black, J.L. (1991) β-Receptor desensitization in human airway tissue preparations. *Am. Rev. Resp. Dis.*, **143** (4), A429.

Widdicombe, J.G. (1989) Airway mucus. *Eur. Resp. J.*, **2**, 107–15.

Wong, C.S., Pavord, I.D., Williams, J., Britton, J.R. & Tattersfield, A.E. (1990) Bronchodilator, cardiovascular, and hypokalaemic effects of fenoterol, salbutamol, and terbutaline in asthma. *Lancet*, **336**, 1396–9.

Yukawa, T., Ukena, D., Kroegel, C. *et al.* (1990) β_2-adrenergic adrenoceptors on eosinophils—binding and functional studies. *Am. Rev. Resp. Dis.*, **141**, 1446–52.

CHAPTER 32

Nedocromil Sodium and Sodium Cromoglycate: Pharmacology and Putative Modes of Action

R.P. Eady & A.A. Norris

Introduction

Asthma is now recognized as a condition of the airways in which the underlying pathophysiology is inflammation. Cytokine mediators, such as interleukin-3 (IL-3), IL-4 and IL-5 and granulocyte macrophage colony-stimulating factor (GM-CSF), are produced by the inflammatory cells and are likely to perpetuate a vicious circle in which the activity of key effector cells such as mast cells and sensory nerves is enhanced. This might be expected to result in an increased frequency of symptoms such as bronchospasm, wheeze and cough. According to the International Guidelines for the Treatment of Asthma (International Concensus Report on Treatment of Asthma, 1992), use of anti-inflammatory agents such as glucocorticoids and the non-steroidal agents, nedocromil sodium and sodium cromoglycate (Fig. 32.1), is warranted in the presence of continuing symptoms or if there is a requirement for regular bronchodilator therapy and all have been shown to reduce symptoms in therapeutic studies. This position is consistent with a reduction in the activation status or numbers of inflammatory cells in the bronchial lumen or mucosa following treatment with these agents.

Background

Sodium cromoglycate was discovered in the 1960s by Dr Roger Altounyan, who showed initially that the compound prevented antigen-induced bronchospasm when inhaled before challenge (Altounyan, 1967). Following the launch of this compound, many companies attempted to find improved versions, using the structure sodium cromoglycate as the chemical starting-point. Most of these attempts failed and only one new compound, nedocromil sodium, which was discovered using a conventional medicinal chemistry and biological approach, demonstrated clinical efficacy (Eady, 1986). Early studies on immunoglobulin E (IgE)-mediated, mast cell-dependent reactions indicated that nedocromil sodium and sodium cromoglycate had similar potencies (Table 32.1). In contrast, marked differences between the two compounds were demonstrated when studies were carried out in a primate model of lung inflammation which was induced by infecting macaques with the pig nematode *Ascaris suum* (Eady, 1986) (Table 32.1). Bronchoalveolar lavage (BAL) cells containing up to 20% of mast cells release histamine, prostaglandin D_2 (PGD_2) and leukotriene C_4 (LTC_4) when stimulated with *Ascaris* antigen or antibody to human IgE. Addition of nedocromil sodium to the cells prior to challenge suppressed the release of mediators, although sodium cromoglycate was inactive. Inhibition by nedocromil sodium was dose-related, with IC_{30} values (concentrations of drug giving 30% inhibition) of approximately 2 μmol/l for inhibition of both newly formed lipid and preformed mediators. The differential effects of nedocromil sodium and sodium cromoglycate were confirmed *in vivo* using anaesthetized infected monkeys challenged by aerosolized *Ascaris* antigen.

Immediate bronchospasm (measured as an increase in lung resistance) was inhibited by pretreating animals with an aerosol of 2% nedocromil sodium. In a comparative study, sodium cromoglycate had no significant effects. These findings were considered sufficiently valuable and novel to support a full development of nedocromil sodium, leading to the launch of Tilade in the UK in 1986 and in the USA in 1992.

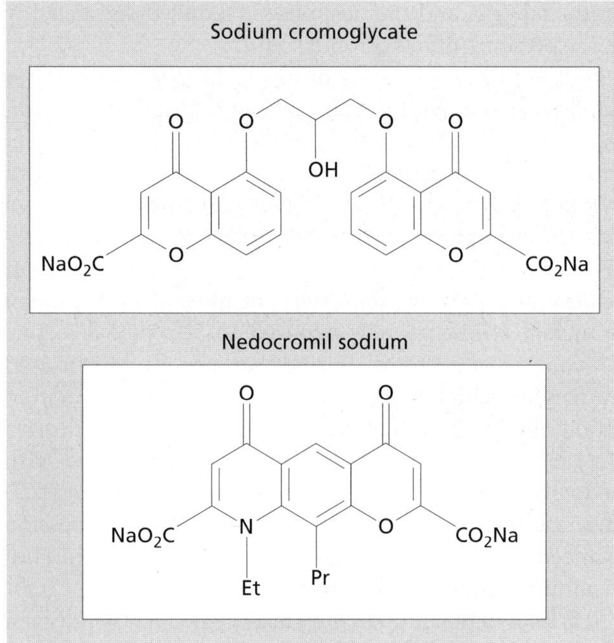

Fig. 32.1 Structures of nedocromil sodium and sodium cromoglycate.

This review discusses the recent biology of nedocromil sodium and sodium cromoglycate and their putative mechanisms of action.

Effects on cells and mediators involved in asthmatic inflammation

Considerable attention has been paid to the role of eosinophils in asthma since deMonchy *et al.* (1985) demonstrated that these cells increase in the lung at the time of the late reaction following antigen challenge, and Bousquet *et al.* (1990) showed a significant correlation between the numbers of eosinophils in peripheral blood and in bronchial lavage fluid and clinical severity of asthma. The technique of fibreoptic bronchoscopy allows lavage of the bronchial lumen and biopsy of the bronchial mucosa to be carried out routinely in asthmatics, and studies have shown that nedocromil sodium is capable of reducing eosinophil numbers in lavage fluid (Calhoun *et al.*, 1993) and the number of activated eosinophils (EG2+ staining cells) in the bronchial submucosa (Trigg *et al.*, 1993).

Nedocromil sodium inhibits the release of both preformed (granule-associated) (Spry *et al.*, 1986) and newly generated eicosanoid mediators (Bruijnzeel *et al.*, 1989a)

Table 32.1 Comparison of effects of nedocromil sodium and sodium cromoglycate in allergic models based on different mast cell subgroups (connective-tissue (CTMC) and mucosal (MMC)).

Laboratory model	Nedocromil sodium	Sodium cromoglycate	Reference
Rat CTMC			Eady, 1986
Histamine release from peritoneal mast cells (IC_{30})	1.1×10^{-6} mol/l	6.0×10^{-7} mol/l	
Passive cutaneous anaphylactic test (ID_{50})	2.2 mg/kg	1.3 mg/kg	
Passive lung anaphylactic test (ID_{50})	0.9 mg/kg	1.5 mg/kg	
Monkey MMC			Eady, 1986
Antigen-induced release from BAL cells (IC_{30})			
Histamine	2.1×10^{-6} mol/l	$>10^{-3}$ mol/l	
LTC_4	2.3×10^{-6} mol/l	$>10^{-4}$ mol/l	
PGD_2	1.9×10^{-6} mol/l	$>10^{-4}$ mol/l	
Anti-IgE-induced release from BAL cells (IC_{30})			
Histamine	5.2×10^{-6} mol/l	9.9×10^{-4} mol/l	
LTC_4	1.3×10^{-6} mol/l	$>10^{-4}$ mol/l	
PGD_2	1.3×10^{-6} mol/l	$>10^{-4}$ mol/l	
Antigen-induced bronchoconstriction (%I with 50 breaths 2% aerosol)			
Increase in resistance	85% ($P < 0.05$)	35% (NS)	
Decrease in compliance	55% ($P < 0.05$)	36% (NS)	
Human mast cells			Leung *et al.*, 1988
Anti-IgE-induced release of histamine—lung (IC_{30})			
BAL cells	0.5×10^{-6} mol/l	7×10^{-6} mol/l	
Parenchymal cells	6×10^{-6} mol/l	$>10^{-4}$ mol/l	

I, inhibition; NS, not significant. See text for definition of other abbreviations.

from activated eosinophils and prevents the decrease in cell density which occurs during short-term culture (Sedgewick *et al.*, 1992). The chemotactic response of eosinophils to platelet-activating factor (PAF) and LTB_4 is also blocked by nedocromil sodium, whereas sodium cromoglycate selectively inhibits the response to zymosan-activated serum (Bruijnzeel *et al.*, 1989b). Both agents are known to block the activation of human blood eosinophils when measured by their ability to inhibit expression of complement and IgG (Fc) rosettes (Kay *et al.*, 1987; Moqbel *et al.*, 1988). IL-5 has been detected in lung lavage fluid accompanied by an eosinophilia in the late response (Sedgewick *et al.*, 1991) and is known to exert a number of effects on eosinophils, including an increase in the survival time of cells in culture (Stern *et al.*, 1992). Using an *in vitro* culture model, the increased survival of eosinophils in the presence of IL-5 is blocked by nedocromil sodium (Resler *et al.*, 1992), and this may also represent an important activity of the compound in regulating the numbers of these cells, as shown in the *in vivo* studies. The functional consequences for the inhibitory effects of nedocromil sodium on eosinophil activation may include the marked inhibition of the late reaction when the compound was administered as three doses of 2 mg over a 90-minute period prior to the predicted onset of the late response in asthmatic patients (Knottnerus & Pelikan, 1993). It is the accumulation of inflammatory cells during the late asthmatic response which is thought to be responsible for the bronchial hyperreactivity which ensues, at least in an experimental situation.

Nedocromil sodium also inhibited bronchial hyperreactivity at both 3 and 24 hours after challenge when given before antigen (Aalburs *et al.*, 1991), although airway eosinophils were not measured in this study.

Incubation of human blood eosinophils with nedocromil sodium and an activating stimulus (phorbol myristate acetate or opsonized latex beads) inhibits their ability to impair the normal ciliary beat frequency of cultured airway epithelial cells *in vitro*, and this effect is associated with an inhibition of release of eosinophil cationic protein (ECP) from eosinophils (Devalia *et al.*, 1992). The clearance of particulate matter from the airways is dependent on an intact mechanism of ciliary beat activity, and nedocromil sodium might therefore be expected to maintain the functions of this key primary host defence response *in vivo* in the presence of asthmatic inflammation.

Epithelial cells act as a barrier between the external environment and the body and are subject to constant stimulation by many airborne agents. One such agent, toluene diisocyanate, which is a causative factor in occupational asthma (Fabbri *et al.*, 1987), has been shown by Mattoli *et al.* (1990) to induce the release of 15-hydroxyeicosatetraenoic acid (15-HETE) from cultured bronchial epithelial cells and this response is reduced significantly in the presence of nedocromil sodium.

Pollutant gases such as nitrogen dioxide and sulphur dioxide are known to increase airway reactivity in asthmatic subjects (Devalia *et al.*, 1994a) and are potent activators of bronchial epithelial cells, resulting in the release of cytokines (Devalia *et al.*, 1993). *In vitro* studies have shown nedocromil sodium to reduce the release of tumour necrosis factor-α (TNF-α), IL-8 and the soluble intercellular adhesion molecule (ICAM-1) from cultured human bronchial epithelial cells exposed to 50 p.p.b. of ozone (Devalia *et al.*, 1994b). Further studies using cultured human bronchial epithelial cells have also shown an inhibition of GM-CSF (Marini *et al.*, 1992) and IL-8 (Vittori *et al.*, 1992) production when the cells are pretreated with nedocromil sodium prior to challenge with IL-1 (Fig. 32.2) and an inhibition of cell-surface ICAM-1 expression induced by challenge of epithelial cells with 1 μmol/l of histamine (Vignola *et al.*, 1993).

It is known that human lung mast cells can also release a number of pro-inflammatory cytokines, such as IL-4, IL-5 and TNF-α (Bradding *et al.*, 1992), which are capable of contributing to the inflammatory response in asthma. Inhibition of TNF-α release (Bissonnette & Befus, 1993) by

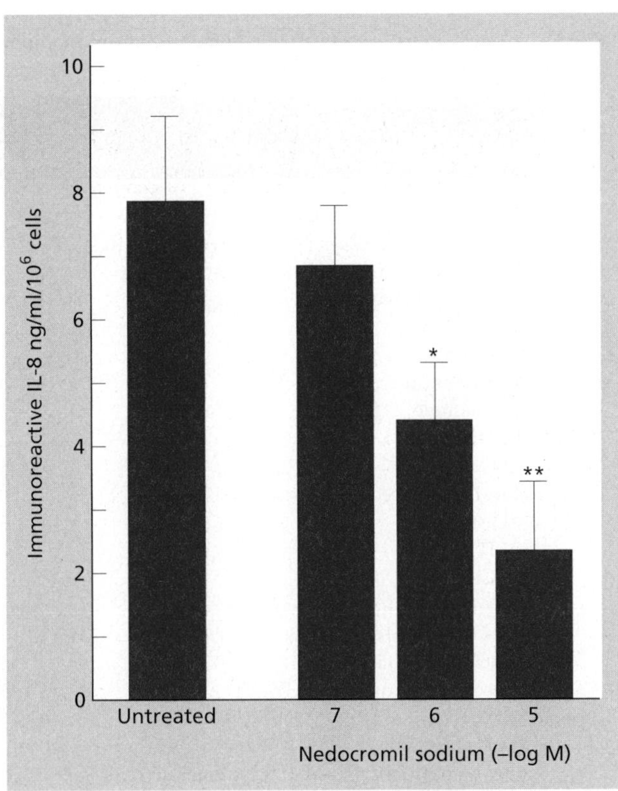

Fig. 32.2 Inhibition by nedocromil sodium of immunoreactive IL-8 release from human bronchial epithelial cells. (From Vittori *et al.*, 1992, with kind permission.)

sodium cromoglycate and nedocromil sodium may in part explain the anti-inflammatory effects of both compounds in asthma. An inhibitory effect of nedocromil sodium on IL-6 production from human airway macrophages following challenge with specific antigen or with anti-IgE over a 16-hour time-scale has been described by Borish *et al.* (1992) and may also represent an activity with significant clinical consequences. Using anti-IgE to stimulate lysosomal enzyme release from human alveolar macrophages and oxygen radical release from human monocytes, it was also possible to demonstrate an inhibitory effect on these responses with nedocromil sodium (Thorel *et al.*, 1988).

Aspirin-sensitive asthma (ASA) is a distinct disease, which can affect up to 20% of adult asthmatic patients, and involves an intolerance to aspirin and to other non-steroidal anti-inflammatory drugs (NSAID) (Szczeklik, 1983). The disease is characterized by nasal polyposis, and the bronchospasm induced by oral administration of such agents is likely to be mediated in part by the activation of blood platelets. The release of cytotoxic mediators from platelets taken from individuals with ASA can be readily shown *in vitro*, and this response is inhibited by inhalation of 4 mg nedocromil sodium but not by sodium cromoglycate (5 or 20 mg) (Marquette *et al.*, 1990). Furthermore, nedocromil sodium can inhibit IgE-mediated activation of passively sensitized human blood platelets following exposure to *Schistosoma* antigen (Thorel *et al.*, 1988) and the generation of thromboxane B_2 and intracellular messengers (e.g. inositol 1,4,5-trisphosphate (IP_3)) from thrombin-stimulated platelets (Roth *et al.*, 1993).

Although a less prominent role is played by neutrophils in asthma, nedocromil sodium and sodium cromoglycate have been shown to inhibit activation (Moqbel *et al.*, 1988), chemotaxis (Bruijnzeel *et al.*, 1989b, 1990) and mediator release (Rubin, 1991; White & Kaliner, 1991) from these cells.

A comparison of the activities of nedocromil sodium and sodium cromoglycate on a range of inflammatory cell types is shown in Table 32.2.

Effect on cells and mediators responsible for causing symptoms of asthma

Studies on mast cells from a variety of species, including humans, have shown that both compounds inhibit histamine release (Wells *et al.*, 1986; Leung *et al.*, 1988) and that nedocromil sodium inhibits the release of slow-reacting substance of anaphylaxis (Napier *et al.*, 1990). These activities are considered compatible (Broide *et al.*, 1991) with an inhibitory effect of the compounds on antigen-induced bronchoconstriction (Cockcroft & Murdock, 1987; Aalburs

Table 32.2 Comparison of effects of nedocromil sodium and sodium cromoglycate on inflammatory cells *in vitro*.

Cell type	Response inhibited	Nedocromil sodium	Sodium cromoglycate	Reference
Human alveolar macrophage	IgE-dependent enzyme production	+++	++ and −−−	Thorel *et al.*, 1998; Fuller & Mac Dermott, 1986
Human blood platelet (ASA)	Aspirin-induced cytotoxic mediator release (*ex vivo*)	+++	−−−	Marquette *et al.*, 1990
Human blood eosinophil/ neutrophil	F-MLP-induced activation	+++ +++	++ ++	Moqbel *et al.*, 1986, 1988
Human blood neutrophil/ eosinophil	Chemotaxis induced by:			
	$ZAS/PAF/f\text{-}MLP/LTB_4$	+++	+++	Bruijnzeel *et al.*, 1989
	ZAS	−−−	+++	
	PAF/LTB_4	+++	−−−	Bruijnzeel *et al.*, 1990
Rabbit peritoneal neutrophil	Enzyme secretion induced by:			
	f-MLP	+	+	Rubin, 1991
	PDBu	++	−−−	
Human blood basophil activated by human blood eosinophil	Anti-IgE/ECP-induced basophil degranulation	−−−	−−−	Beauvais *et al.*, 1989
	Indirect inhibition by blocking IgG4-induced ECP release from eosinophil	+++	++	Beauvais *et al.*, 1989

Scoring system: +, slightly active; ++, moderately active; +++, very active; −−−, no activity.
PDBu, phorbol dibutyrate; ZAS, zymosan activated serum. See text for definition of other abbreviations.

et al., 1991) and it has been possible to demonstrate a reduction in histamine content of lavage fluid in asthmatics after inhalation of nedocromil sodium prior to challenge with antigen (Calhoun *et al.*, 1993) or hypertonic saline (Maxwell *et al.*, 1993).

Although neurogenic mechanisms are unlikely to be involved in the initiation of inflammation in asthma (Barnes, 1986), it is possible that they act to amplify the response through the release of pro-inflammatory neuropeptides from sensory nerves and may contribute to the symptoms of asthma, such as cough and wheeze. It has been recognized for many years that sodium cromoglycate can modulate reflex bronchoconstriction and this effect may be a result of its ability to inhibit sensory C (non-myelinated) fibre activation in response to stimulation with capsaicin, as demonstrated in dogs by Dixon *et al.* (1980). Recent findings have shown sodium cromoglycate to inhibit angiotensin-converting enzyme inhibitor-induced cough in patients receiving enalopril or captopril to control hypertension (Hargreaves & Benson, 1995).

In these subjects, it is likely that the cough reflex is initiated by stimulation of laryngeal C fibres by the release (and/or prevention of breakdown) of bradykinin and this study demonstrates the potential value of the drug in non-asthmatic cough through an effect on neuronal mechanisms.

Altounyan (1969) reported that atopic asthmatics were relatively insensitive to the bronchodilator effects of atropine but the response could be enhanced markedly following a short (1- to 3-week) course of treatment with sodium cromoglycate. It is possible therefore that cholinergic reflexes are greatly up-regulated in allergic asthma, either directly or indirectly by sensory nerve activation, as suggested by Hall *et al.* (1989), and that sodium cromoglycate acting through suppressing sensory nerves allows atropine to exert its effects.

Nedocromil sodium has been shown also to possess neuromodulatory activity, including the ability to inhibit substance-P-induced histamine release from human lung mast cells (Louis & Radermecker, 1990) and substance-P-induced potentiation of contraction of the isolated innervated rabbit trachea preparation, when stimulated preganglionically (Armour *et al.*, 1991). It also inhibits non-adrenergic, non-cholinergic contraction of the isolated guinea pig bronchus (Verleden *et al.*, 1991) through an effect which is purported to be due to inhibition of neuropeptide release rather than by end-organ antagonism (Fig. 32.3).

Such findings may explain the ability of nedocromil sodium to suppress bronchoconstriction to agents such as sodium metabisulphite (Wright *et al.*, 1990) and bradykinin (Dixon & Barnes, 1989) and to reduce asthma symptoms such as cough within 3 days, in therapeutic studies (Cherniak *et al.*, 1990). Alternatively, it has been suggested by Jackson *et al.* (1989) that the ability of nedocromil sodium to activate a population of bronchial C fibres in the dog lung may also contribute to its ability to inhibit reflex responses such as cough, which is mediated largely by myelinated Aδ fibres, by interfering with or blocking neuronal transmission associated with tussive agents. Altounyan *et al.* (1986) showed that the effects of nedocromil sodium at suppressing responses which are likely to consist of a neuronal component are usually greater than those of sodium cromoglycate.

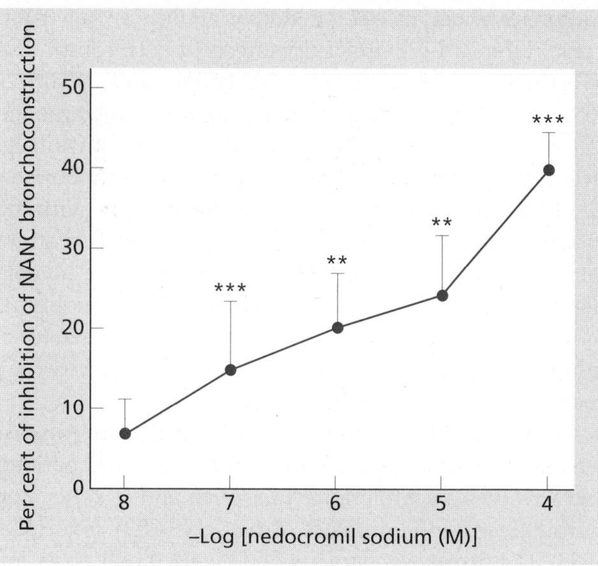

Fig. 32.3 Inhibition by nedocromil sodium of non-adrenergic, non-cholinergic contraction of the guinea-pig bronchus. (From Verleden *et al.*, 1991, with kind permission.)

Effects on cells and mediators involved in the development of the atopic state

It is likely that one of the initial events in the development of the allergic condition is the differentiation of T-helper (Th) cells under the influence of IL-4 into a Th2-like cell phenotype characterized by its ability to release cytokines such as IL-3, IL-4, IL-5 and IL-10 (Wierenga *et al.*, 1990). IL-4 is also a key factor in supporting IgE production by B cells (Vercelli *et al.*, 1989), and this cytokine can be produced by mast cells (Bradding *et al.*, 1992) and basophils (Brunner *et al.*, 1993), as well as by Th2-like cells (Mosmann & Coffman, 1989).

As a result, it is likely that non-T-cell sources of IL-4 may be crucial for both initiation and amplification of Th2-mediated responses and it has been shown already that mast cells and basophils can influence IgE production by B cells in the absence of T cells (Gauchat *et al.*, 1993).

Both sodium cromoglycate and nedocromil sodium have been shown by Kimata *et al.* (1991, 1993) to exert an inhibitory effect on IgE antibody formation by mixed mononuclear cells isolated from the tonsils of non-asthmatic individuals and incubated with IL-4 (Fig. 32.4). The mechanism of this response has been elucidated further by Loh *et al.* (1994a,b) and shown to occur by inhibiting the production of mRNA for IgE from purified B cells which were stimulated with IL-4 and B-cell-activating agents such as T cells, a monoclonal antibody to the B-cell antigen, CD40 or hydrocortisone. These agents are responsible for a deletional Sμ to Sε switch recombination, expression of mature ε transcripts and IgE synthesis and release. It is noteworthy that both drugs inhibited switch recombination in IL-4-treated cells and had no effect on the induction of ε germ-line transcripts by IL-4. No inhibitory effects were observed on IgM or IgA formation by B cells, although IgG4 production was also suppressed. The finding that both compounds inhibit IgE isotype switching but have no effect on B cells which have already undergone switching, such as in those obtained from patients with hyper-IgE syndrome, suggests that these compounds may be able to affect the development of atopy but would not be expected to reverse the atopic state.

However, Diaz *et al.* (1984) showed a reduction from elevated baseline levels in antigen (house dust mite)-specific IgE in the bronchial lavage fluid after 4 weeks' treatment with sodium cromoglycate. Although these data appear at variance to the *in vitro* studies described above, they may be explained perhaps in terms of an effect on naïve B cells which are recruited to the process of antigen-specific IgE production during the trial period. A significant reduction in eosinophils in BAL fluid and in clinical symptoms was also recorded in this trial. Similar studies have yet to be carried out with nedocromil sodium.

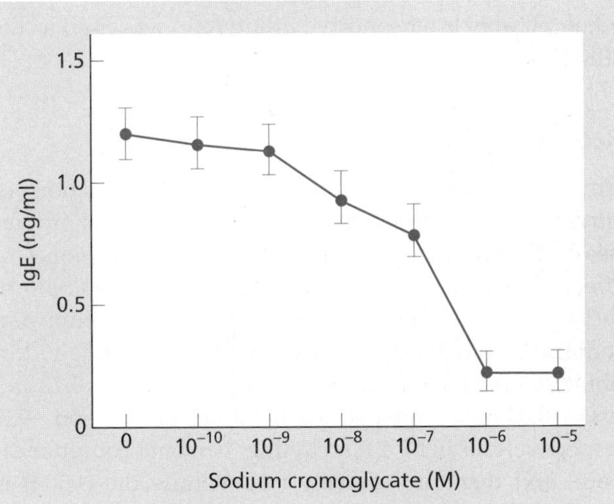

Fig. 32.4 Inhibition by sodium cromoglycate of IL-4-induced IgE production by mixed mononuclear cells from non-atopic subjects. (From Kimata *et al.*, 1991, with kind permission.)

Although reports exist to suggest that both drugs are capable of inhibiting allergen- and mitogen-induced proliferation of T cells (Holen *et al.*, 1992; Mekori *et al.*, 1993), these findings are refuted by the studies of O'Hehir and Moqbel (1989), who showed that no inhibitory effects were observed with nedocromil sodium or sodium cromoglycate on allergen or IL-2-induced proliferation of human CD4+ house dust mite-specific T cells. It is unlikely that T cells are a major target for these compounds, thus distinguishing them markedly from steroids, which are known to inhibit potently the activation of lymphocytes (O'Hehir & Moqbel, 1989).

Mechanism of action

The inhibitory effects against bronchospasm caused by such a range of stimuli would imply that both compounds are affecting a number of cell types in the asthmatic airways — as shown previously from *in vitro* studies — including mast cells, eosinophils, epithelial cells and sensory nerves (Rainey, 1992; Edwards, 1994). Any explanation of the mode of action of the chromones should therefore consider their wide range of effects in a unifying fashion. Since both compounds are relatively selective for the treatment of asthma, it is possible that an understanding of their mechanism of action could shed light on the biochemical defect responsible for causing the disease.

Many studies have been performed to determine the molecular mechanism by which chromones inhibit the activation of cells. Initial studies used the mast cells as the target cell but, with the recognition that these compounds, particularly nedocromil sodium, affect a variety of cells, it has been assumed that a common mechanism must exist, whether through a specific receptor or by modulation of a second-messenger signal.

Effects on second-messenger systems

Studies on the mast cell implicated Ca^{2+} as the target for sodium cromoglycate (Foreman *et al.*, 1977), but this was challenged by the work of Pearce's group, who showed that sodium cromoglycate could inhibit activation of connective-tissue mast cells in the presence of Ca^{2+}-chelating agents (Ennis *et al.*, 1980). As indicated later in this section, chromones may affect Ca^{2+} mobilization indirectly (Sagi-Eisenberg *et al.*, 1984).

Theoharides *et al.* (1980) demonstrated that immunological activation of rat peritoneal mast cell leads to the phosphorylation of four proteins. One of these proteins, of molecular weight 78 000 (78 kDa), was produced several minutes after the others and appeared to be associated with the termination of histamine release.

In separate experiments sodium cromoglycate in the absence of releasing agent was shown to rapidly phosphorylate the same 78-kDa protein (Theoharides *et al.*, 1980; Wells & Mann, 1983). Similar findings have been reported subsequently for nedocromil sodium (Wells *et al.*, 1986) (Fig. 32.5). In the studies carried out by Wells and Mann (1983), it was shown that cyclic guanosine monophosphate (cGMP) caused an identical phosphorylation reaction to sodium cromoglycate, indicating that the 78-kDa protein may be a substrate for cGMP-dependent phosphorylation.

Recent studies have also shown a cross-tachyphlaxis to exist between the inhibitory effects of sodium cromoglycate and cGMP on histamine release from rat peritoneal mast cells (Mackay & Pearce, 1993). However, the significance of these findings has not been investigated further. As already indicated, sodium cromoglycate and nedocromil sodium produce differential effects in primate cells and we had hoped this difference would have been reflected at the level of protein phosphorylation. Unfortunately, macaque BAL mast cells stimulated with anti-human IgE did not produce a phosphorylated protein analogous to the 78-kDa molecule (S.T. Harper, personal communication) and no further studies were carried out on this cell type.

Several groups have suggested that protein kinase C is the molecular target for sodium cromoglycate. Sagi-Eisenberg *et al.* (1984) supported the earlier work of Foreman *et al.* (1977) by demonstrating that sodium cromoglycate appeared to interfere with the Ca^{2+}-gating mechanism in rat basophil leukaemia (RBL) cells. These

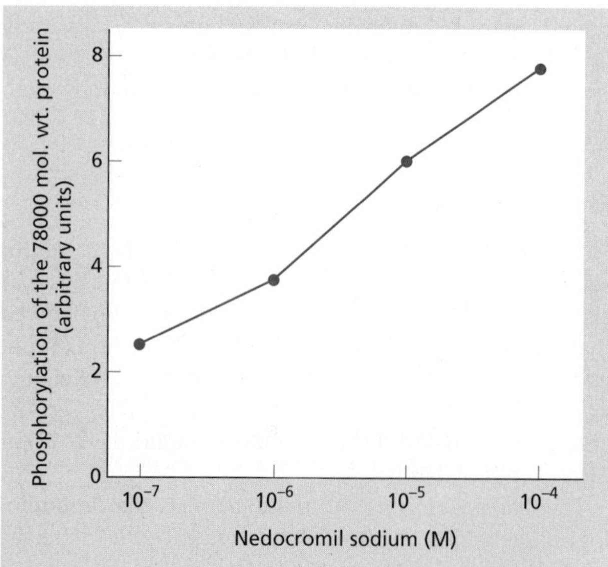

Fig. 32.5 Phosphorylation by nedocromil sodium of a 78-kDa protein in rat peritoneal mast cells. (From Wells *et al.*, 1986, with kind permission.)

authors pointed out that mediator release from mast cells was associated with a rise in phosphoinositol turnover and speculated that phosphorylation and activation of protein kinase C were linked. In a subsequent publication, Sagi-Eisenberg (1987) reported that sodium cromoglycate inhibited the phosphorylation of endogenous substrate proteins which comigrate with protein kinase C isolated from RBL cells. It should be noted that in our hands chromones have no effect on the immunological activation of RBL cells (S.T. Harper, personal communication).

However, it is of interest that in a totally different system nedocromil sodium and sodium cromoglycate have been reported to inhibit the activation of protein kinase C. Pigment dispersion in the melanophores of the lizard *Anolis carolinenis* can be induced by α-melanin-stimulating hormone (α-MSH) through an effect on G-protein activation and an elevation of cyclic adenosine monophosphate (cAMP) (Lucus & Shuster, 1987), although the receptor can be bypassed using the phorbol ester TPA (tetradecanoyl phorbol acetate). Nedocromil sodium (5–50 μmol/l) inhibited the α-MSH response in a dose-related manner.

Control studies excluded the possibility that nedocromil sodium was interfering at the level of the α-MSH receptor, α_2-receptor or Ca^{2+} mobilization. However, nedocromil sodium also inhibited the TPA-potentiated α-MSH response, implicating protein kinase C as the target for this chromone. Similar results were obtained with sodium cromoglycate. Finally, it has been demonstrated that nedocromil sodium and sodium cromoglycate at high concentrations (10 μmol/l) inhibited lysozyme secretion from rabbit neutrophils stimulated with formyl-methionyl-leucyl-phenylalanine (f-MLP) (Bradford & Rubin, 1986; Rubin, 1991). However, nedocromil sodium but not sodium cromoglycate suppressed the response when phorbol ester (phorbol dibutyrate) was used as the stimulus.

Receptor-binding studies

Any consideration of the mechanism of action of chromones should take into account the physical properties of the compounds. The ability of the chromones to affect intracellular targets directly are, in the opinion of the authors, unlikely, as both nedocromil sodium and sodium cromoglycate are extremely polar and hydrophilic, having pK_{a2} isonization constants of 1.99 ± 0.12 and 1.93 ± 0.03 and estimated log D values of –9.1 and –9.7, respectively, at pH 7.4 (D. Payling, personal communication), and therefore unlikely to penetrate the cell. It is assumed, therefore, that these compounds must operate on a receptor and modulate intracellular events as a result of acting as agonists. The search for a specific receptor for these molecules has attracted the attention of a number of workers, including ourselves. In 1980, Mazurek *et al.* reported specific binding to RBL and mast cells by fluorescent beads covalently bound with sodium cromoglycate and the binding was shown to be Ca^{2+} and cell specific. Using RBL-2H3 cells and immunoprecipitation techniques with sodium cromoglycate conjugated to bovine serum albumin, a 'binding protein' of molecular weight 50–60 kDa was isolated. A similar material was isolated using affinity chromatography with cromoglycate-immobilized polyacrylhydrazido-agarose beads. In subsequent studies, Mazurek *et al.* (1983) described variants of the RBL-2H3 cell which lacked the binding protein for sodium cromoglycate.

These cells failed to release mediators on activation with immunological stimuli, but this response was restored in cells transfected with the 'sodium cromoglycate-binding protein'. Results from the measurement of conductance changes in artificial lipid membrane implanted with the 'sodium cromoglycate-binding protein' have indicated that this protein may indeed be involved in Ca^{2+} mobilization (Mazurek *et al.*, 1984).

It is of some concern that the binding protein for sodium cromoglycate has only been identified in RBL cells, which in our hands are insensitive to chromones. Furthermore, it is disappointing that other groups have not confirmed these findings. We have continued to search for the receptor of nedocromil sodium and sodium cromoglycate. In our studies we have used a radiolabelled chromone ligand (FPL 61369), which is three orders of magnitude more potent than sodium cromoglycate on rat peritoneal mast cells. Results have been equivocal because, although binding of the label to several cell types (RBL-2H3 rat peritoneal mast cells, Chinese hamster ovary (CHO) cells) and tissues (monkey and guinea pig lung) was observed, the binding could be displaced with sodium cromoglycate but was not saturable (S. Harper and C. Hallam, unpublished observations). In separate experiments using FPL 61369 bound to an affinity matrix, several proteins could be isolated following elution with sodium cromoglycate, although, to date, identification of any of these proteins as the chromone binding protein has not been possible.

Modulation of chloride channel activity

Since sodium cromoglycate and nedocromil sodium are believed not to interfere with Ca^{2+} channels but have been shown previously to reduce Ca^{2+} influx into cells (Foreman *et al.*, 1977), it is necessary to invoke other mechanisms to explain their ability to prevent degranulation. Electrophysiological studies on rat peritoneal mast cells have demonstrated that degranulation is dependent on a sustained elevation of intracellular Ca^{2+}; following a transient IP_3-induced increase in Ca^{2+} due to the release of Ca^{2+} from intracellular stores (Beavan *et al.*, 1984). The second phase consists of the sustained elevation of $[Ca^{2+}]_i$ due to Ca^{2+} influx, and has been shown to be mediated by two pathways (Penner *et al.*, 1988). A large-conductance (~50 pS), non-specific cation channel which can be activated by antigen or by compound 48/80 and regulated by internal messengers, such as guanosiese triphosphate-γ-S (GTP-γ-S), allows divalent cations to enter the cell but is unlikely to produce sufficient Ca^{2+} influx to influence degranulation. Penner *et al.* (1988) also described a small-conductance but highly specific Ca^{2+} channel which could be activated by intracellular application of IP_3 and which required membrane hyperpolarization to support Ca^{2+} influx. However, it was shown that a small-conductance chloride channel (0.5–1 pS) in rat peritoneal mast cells activated by secretagogues and by intracellular application of cAMP and high $[Ca^{2+}]_i$ could provide the negative membrane potential or hyperpolarization necessary to maintain Ca^{2+} influx and its sustained elevation, leading to degranulation.

Hoth and Penner (1992) have subsequently identified the Ca^{2+} current which is activated by this mechanism and described it as I_{CRAC} (Ca^{2+} release-activated Ca^{2+}) at it is likely to be responsible ultimately for refilling depleted intracellular calcium stores. Furthermore, pharmacological studies by Friis *et al.* (1994) have also demonstrated that antigen-stimulated histamine secretion from rat peritoneal mast cells was inhibited when extracellular chloride ions were replaced by either isethionate or gluconate anions, although some histamine secretion still occurred. In light of these findings, it is significant that sodium cromoglycate has been shown to block intermediate-conductance chloride channels which are activated following immunological stimulation of patches of cultured mucosa-like mast cells (RBL-2H3) (IC_{50} 15 μmol/l) (Romanin *et al.*, 1991) (Fig. 32.6) and of colonic carcinoma HT29 epithelial cells (IC_{50} 19 μmol/l) (Reinsprecht *et al.*, 1992) when applied to the cytoplasmic side. In the experiments carried out with RBL cells, it was shown that a parallel inhibition of both serotonin release and chloride channel activity occurred when either sodium cromoglycate or the classical, non-specific chloride channel blocking agent 5-nitro-2-(3-phenylpropylamino)-benzoic acid (NPPB) was applied to the patches. This finding led these investigators to believe that chloride channels play a functional role in mediator release from mast cells. It follows that, by preventing chloride channel activation, sodium cromoglycate would be expected to maintain cells in a normal resting physiological state and this is also associated with a lack of side-effects of the compound.

Recent studies have further evaluated the ability of these compounds to modulate a chloride channel in mouse 3T3 fibroblasts, which is likely to be a major channel involved in cell volume regulation. This channel may be identical to a previously reported chloride channel

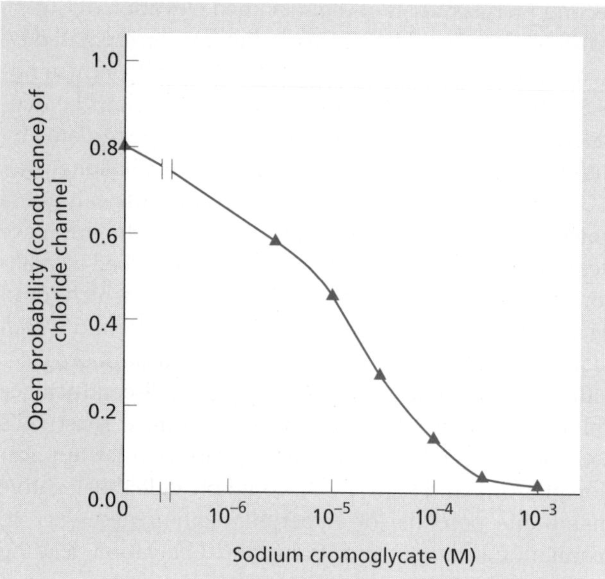

Fig. 32.6 Inhibition of intermediate-conductance chloride channels in inside-out membrane patches of RBL-2H3 cells. (From Romanin *et al.*, 1991, with kind permission.)

which was characterized following expression cloning, using Madin Darby canine kidney (MDCK) epithelial cells as the source of mRNA (Paulmichl *et al.*, 1992). The chloride (Cl^-) channel which carried the current (I) was characterized as outwardly rectifying, Ca^{2+}-insensitive and blocked by nucleotides (n) and was defined therefore as the ICln channel.

Electrophysiological recordings of chloride current were carried out in mouse 3T3 fibroblasts, using a two-electrode voltage clamp. Voltage steps (800 milliseconds) were made from –80 mV to +40 mV and amplitudes of the currents were measured 50 milliseconds after stepping to the different voltages. Both nedocromil sodium and sodium cromoglycate blocked the ICln after the voltage clamp step to +40 mV. Nedocromil sodium was more efficacious and more potent than sodium cromoglycate at blocking this channel. These findings have shown both sodium cromoglycate and nedocromil sodium to inhibit hypotonic saline-induced activation of a chloride channel in mouse 3T3 fibroblasts (Paulmichl *et al.*, 1995).

It is well known that changes in osmolarity of the periciliary fluid are capable of increasing airway resistance and this can provoke an attack of asthma (Allegra & Bianco, 1980).

The inhibitory effects of nedocromil sodium and sodium cromoglycate on bronchoconstriction (fall in forced expiratory volume in 1 second (FEV_1)) induced by aerosol challenge with hypotonic or hypertonic saline (Robuschi *et al.*, 1987; Rodwell *et al.*, 1992) might be accounted for by the ability of both drugs to modulate chloride ion flux and thus cell volume changes, which may activate sensory nerve endings. It is interesting that loop diuretics such as frusemide, which possess chloride channel-blocking activity in addition to inhibitory effects on the $Na^+/K^+/2Cl^-$ cotransporter mechanism, also block bronchoconstriction and cough in asthmatics induced by aerosols of low chloride solution, as well as by antigen (Bianco *et al.*, 1989; Ventresca *et al.*, 1990). In a study carried out to compare the effects of a single dose of sodium cromoglycate (40 mg) given before hypertonic saline (4.5%) challenge to allergic asthmatics with those of a 3- to 8-week course of inhaled budesonide (1000 μg), it was found that equivalent inhibitory effects on the PC_{20} (concentration causing 20% inhibition) value were observed (Anderson *et al.*, 1994). Additive effects were demonstrated when the treatments were combined, and only sodium cromoglycate showed the ability to cause a plateau in the dose–response curve to hypertonic saline challenge.

As discussed in a previous section, the inhibitory effects of sodium cromoglycate and nedocromil sodium on reflex bronchoconstriction induced by irritants and agonists such as ultrasonically nebulized distilled water, sulphur dioxide, sodium metabisulphite and bradykinin could be due to a direct effect of the drug on neuronal pathways, and this is supported by *in vitro* studies. It has been shown that nedocromil sodium induces a slow depolarization of the rabbit vagus nerve, which is prevented by removal of chloride ions from the bathing solution (Jackson *et al.*, 1992). The nerve preparation which contains predominantly C or non-myelinated sensory fibres is then unresponsive to further exposure to nedocromil sodium. These findings may represent an initial opening of a chloride channel followed by a longer-lasting block of channel activity. Interestingly, in the same preparation, sodium cromoglycate did not depolarize the nerve but was capable of preventing the response to nedocromil sodium. These findings which demonstrate a direct action of the compounds on nerve fibres may explain some of the biological effects described above.

The inhibitory effects of sodium cromoglycate and nedocromil sodium on the underlying inflammation and on symptoms such as wheeze and cough may derive from the ability of the drugs to prevent the activation of different cell types, including mast cells, eosinophils and nerves. Thus, a common mechanism of action, perhaps involving chloride channel modulation, as described above, may serve as a unifying hypothesis to explain the effects of these compounds on a diverse range of cells.

References

Aalburs, R., Kauffman, H.K., Groen, H., Koeter, G.H. & de Monchy, J.G.R. (1991) The effect of nedocromil sodium on the early and late reaction and allergen-induced bronchial hyperresponsiveness. *J.*

Allergy Clin. Immunol., **87**, 993–1001.

Allegra, L. & Bianco, S. (1980) Non-specific bronchoreactivity obtained with an ultrasonic aerosol of distilled water. *Eur. J. Resp. Dis.*, **61**, 41–9.

Altounyan, R.E.C. (1967) Inhibition of experimental asthma by a new compound, disodium cromoglycate 'INTAL'. *Acta Allergol.*, **22**, 487–9.

Altounyan, R.E.C. (1969) Changes in histamine and atropine responsiveness as a guide to diagnosis and evaluation of therapy in obstructive airways disease. In: *Disodium Cromoglycate in Allergic Airways Disease: Proceedings of the Royal Society of Medicine Symposium* 1969 (eds J. Pepys & A.W. Frankland), pp. 47–53. Butterworth, London.

Altounyan, R.E.C., Cole, M. & Lee, T.B. (1986) Inhibition of sulphur dioxide induced bronchoconstriction by nedocromil sodium and sodium cromoglycate in non-asthmatic, atopic subjects. *Eur. J. Resp. Dis.*, **69** (Suppl. 147), 274–6.

Anderson, S.D., du Toit, J.I., Rodwell, L.T. & Jenkins, C.R. (1994) Acute effect of sodium cromoglycate on airway narrowing induced by 4.5% saline aerosol. *Chest*, **105**, 673–80.

Armour, C.L., Johnson, P.R.A. & Black, J.L. (1991) Nedocromil sodium inhibits substance P-induced potentiation of the cholinergic neural responses in the isolated innervated rabbit trachea. *J. Auton. Pharmacol.*, **11**, 167–72.

Barnes, P.J. (1986) Asthma as an axon reflex. *Lancet*, **i**, 242–5.

Beauvais, F., Hieblot, C. & Benveniste, J. (1989) Effect of sodium cromoglycate and nedocromil sodium on anti-IgE-induced and anti-IgG_4-induced basophil degranulation. *Drugs*, **37** (Suppl. 1), 4–8.

Beaven, M.A., Rogers, J., Moore, J.P., Hesketh, T.R., Smith, G.A. & Metcalfe, J.C. (1984) The mechanism of the calcium signal and correlation with histamine release in 2H3 cells. *J. Biol. Chem.*, **259**, 7129–36.

Bianco, S., Pieroni, M.G., Refini, R.M., Rattloi, L. & Sestini, P. (1989) Protective effect of inhaled frusemide on allergen induced early and late asthmatic reactions. *New Engl. J. Med.*, **321**, 1069–73.

Bissonnette, E.Y. & Befus, A.D. (1993) Modulation of mast cell function in the GI tract. In: *Handbook of Immunopharmacology: Gastrointestinal System* (ed. J.L. Wallace). Academic Press, New York.

Borish, L., Williams, J., Johnson, S., Mascali, J.J., Miller, R.P. & Rosenwasser, L.J. (1992) Anti-inflammatory effects of nedocromil sodium: inhibition of alveolar macrophage function. *Clin. Exp. Allergy*, **22**, 984–90.

Bousquet, J., Chanez, P., Lacoste, J.Y. *et al.* (1990) Eosinophilc inflammation in asthma. *New Engl. J. Med.*, **323**, 1033–9.

Bradding, P., Feather, I.H., Howarth, P.H. *et al.* (1992) Interleukin 4 is localised to and released from human mast cells. *J. Exp. Med.*, **176**, 1381–6.

Bradford, P.G. & Rubin, R.P. (1986) The differential effects of nedocromil sodium and sodium cromoglycate on the secretory response of rabbit peritoneal neutrophils. *Eur. J. Resp. Dis.*, **69** (Suppl. 147), 238–40.

Broide, D.H., Gleich, G.J., Cuomo, A.J. *et al.* (1991) Evidence of ongoing mast cell and eosinophil degranulation in symptomatic asthma airway. *J. Allergy Clin. Immunol.*, **88**, 637–48.

Bruijnzeel, P.L.B., Hamelink, M.L., Kok, P.T.M. & Kreukniet, J. (1989a) Nedocromil sodium inhibits the A23187- and opsonised zymosan-induced leukotriene formation by human eosinophils but not by human neutrophils. *Brit. J. Pharmacol.*, **96**, 631–6.

Bruijnzeel, P.L.B., Warringa, R.A.J. & Kok, P.T.M. (1989b) Inhibition of platelet-activating factor- and zymosan-activated serum-induced chemotaxis of human neutrophils by nedocromil sodium, BN 52021 and sodium cromoglycate. *Brit. J. Pharmacol.*, **97**, 1251–7.

Bruijnzeel, P.L.B., Warringa, R.A.J., Kok, P.T.M. & Kreukniet, J. (1990) Inhibition of neutrophil and eosinophil induced chemotaxis by nedocromil sodium and sodium cromoglycate. *Brit. J. Pharmacol.*, **99**, 798–802.

Brunner, T., Heusser, C.H. & Dahinden, C.A. (1993) Human peripheral blood basophils primed by interleukin 3 (IL-3) produce IL-4 in response to immunoglobulin E receptor stimulation. *J. Exp. Med.*, **177**, 605–11.

Calhoun, W.J., Sedgwick, J.B., Jariour, N., Swenson, C.A. & Busse, W.W. (1993) The effect of mast cell activation on eosinophil recruitment to the airways after antigen challenge. *Am. Rev. Resp. Dis.*, **147**, A241.

Cherniack, R.M., Wasserman, S.I., Ramsdell, J.W. *et al.* (1990) A double-blind multicenter group comparative study of the efficacy and safety of nedocromil sodium in the management of asthma. *Chest*, **97**, 1299–306.

Cockcroft, D.W. & Murdock, K.W. (1987) Comparative effects of inhaled salbutamol, sodium cromoglycate and beclomethasone on allergen-induced early asthmatic responses and increased bronchial responsiveness to histamine. *J. Allergy Clin. Immunol.*, **79**, 734–40.

deMonchy, J.G.R., Kauffman, H.F., Venge, P. *et al.* (1985) Bronchoalveolar eosinophilia during allergen-induced late asthmatic reactions. *Am. Rev. Resp. Dis.*, **181**, 373–6.

Devalia, J.L., Sapsford, R.J., Rusznak, C. & Davies, R.J. (1992) The effect of human eosinophils on cultured human nasal epithelial cell activity and the influence of nedocromil sodium. *Am. J. Respir. Cell Mol. Biol.*, **7**, 270–7.

Devalia J.L., Campbell, A.M., Sapsford, R.J. *et al.* (1993) Effect of nitrogen dioxide on synthesis of inflammatory cytokines expressed by human epithelial cells *in vitro*. *Am. J. Respir. Cell Mol. Biol.*, **9**, 271–8.

Devalia, J.L., Ruznak, C., Herdman, M.J., Trigg, C.J., Tarraf, H. & Davies, R.J. (1994a) Effect of nitrogen dioxide and sulphur dioxide on airway response of mild asthmatic patients to allergen inhalation. *Lancet*, **344**, 1668–71.

Devalia, J.L., Rusznak, C., Calderon, M., Sapsford, R.J. & Davies, R.J. (1994b) The effect of nedocromil sodium on ozone-induced synthesis of cytokines by human bronchial epithelial cell cultures *in vitro*. *Am. J. Resp. Crit. Care Med.*, **149**, A317.

Diaz, P., Galleguillos, F.R., Gonzalez, M.C., Pantin, C.F.A. & Kay, A.B. (1984) Bronchoalveolar lavage in asthma: the effect of disodium cromoglycate (cromolyn) on leukocyte counts, immunoglobulins and complement. *J. Allergy Clin. Immunol.*, **74**, 41–8.

Dixon, C.M.S. & Barnes, P.J. (1989) Bradykinin-induced bronchoconstriction: inhibition by nedocromil sodium and sodium cromoglycate. *Brit. J. Clin. Pharmacol.*, **27**, 831–6.

Dixon, M., Jackson, D.M. & Richards, I.M. (1980) The action of sodium cromoglycate on 'C' fibre endings in the dog lung. *Brit. J. Pharmacol.*, **70**, 11–13.

Eady, R.P. (1986) The pharmacology of nedocromil sodium. *Eur. J. Resp. Dis.*, **69**, 112–19.

Edwards, A. (1994) Sodium cromoglycate (Intal) as an anti-inflammatory agent for the treatment of chronic asthma. *Clin. Exp. Allergy*, **24**, 612–23.

Ennis, M., Atkinson, S. & Pearce, F.L. (1980) Inhibition of histamine release induced by Compound 48/80 and peptide 401 in the presence and absence of calcium: implications for the mode of action of anti-allergic compounds. *Agents Actions*, **10**, 222–8.

Fabbri, L.M., Boschetto, P., Zocca, E. *et al.* (1987) Bronchoalveolar neutrophilia during late asthmatic reactions induced by toluene diisocyanate. *Am. Rev. Resp. Dis.*, **136**, 36–42.

Foreman, J.C., Hallett, M.B. & Monger, J.L. (1977) The relationship between histamine secretion and [45]calcium uptake by mast cells. *J. Physiol.*, **271**, 193–214.

Friis, U., Johansen, T., Hayes, N. & Foreman, J. (1994) IgE-receptor activated chloride uptake in relation to histamine secretion from rat mast cells. *Brit. J. Pharmacol.*, **111**, 1179–83.

Fuller, R. & MacDermot, J. (1986) Stimulation of IgE-sensitized human alveolar macrophages by anti-IgE is unaffected by sodium cromoglycate. *Clin. Allergy*, **16**, 523–6.

Gauchat, J.-F., Henchoz, S., Mazzei, G. *et al.* (1993) Induction of human IgE synthesis in B cells by mast cells and basophils. *Nature*, **365**, 340–3.

Hall, A.K., Barnes, P.J., Meldrum, L.A. & Maclagan, J. (1989) Facilitation by tachykinins of neurotransmission in guinea-pig pulmonary parasympathetic nerves. *Brit. J. Pharmacol.*, **97**, 274–80.

Hargreaves, M.R. & Benson, M.K. (1995) Inhaled sodium cromoglycate in angiotensin-converting enzyme inhibitor cough. *Lancet*, **345**, 13–16.

Holen, E., Bruserud, O. & Elsayed, S. (1992) The effect of disodium cromoglycate on *in vitro* proliferation of peripheral blood mononuclear cells from allergic and healthy donors. *Scand. J. Immunol.*, **36**, 721–31.

Hoth, M. & Penner, R. (1992) Depletion of intracellular calcium stores activates a calcium current in mast cells. *Nature*, **355**, 353–5.

International Consensus Report on Treatment of Asthma (1992) International Asthma Management Project. *Clin. Exp. Allergy*, **22** (Suppl. 1).

Jackson, D.M., Norris, A.A. & Eady, R.P. (1989) Nedocromil sodium and sensory nerves in the dog lung. *Pulm. Pharmacol.*, **2**, 179–84.

Jackson, D.M., Pollard, C.E. & Roberts, S.M. (1992) The effect of nedocromil sodium on the isolated rabbit vagus nerve. *Eur. J. Pharmacol.*, **221**, 175–7.

Kay, A.B., Walsh, G.M., Moqbel, R. *et al.* (1987) Disodium cromoglycate inhibits activation of human inflammatory cells *in vitro*. *J. Allergy Clin. Immunol.*, **80**, 1–8.

Kimata, H. & Mikawa, H. (1993) Nedocromil sodium selectively inhibits IgE and IgG_4 production in human B cells stimulated with IL-4. *J. Immunol.*, **151**, 6723–32.

Kimata, H., Yoshida, A., Ishioka, C. & Mikawa, H. (1991) Disodium cromoglycate (DSCG) selectively inhibits IgE production and enhances IgG_4 production by human B cells *in vitro*. *Clin. Exp. Immunol.*, **84**, 395–9.

Knottnerus, I.G. & Pelikan, Z. (1993) Inhibition of the late allergic response by nedocromil sodium administered more than two hours after allergen challenge. *J. Allergy Clin. Immunol.*, **92**, 19–28.

Leung, K.B.P., Flint, K.C., Brostoff, J. *et al.* (1988) Effects of sodium cromoglycate and nedocromil sodium on histamine secretion from human lung mast cells. *Thorax*, **43**, 756–61.

Locus, A.M. & Shunter, S. (1987) Cromolyn inhibition of protein kinase C activity. *Biochem. Pharmacol.*, **36**, 562–5.

Loh, R.K.S., Jabara, H.H. & Geha, R.S. (1994a) Cromolyn sodium and nedocromil sodium inhibit $S\mu \rightarrow S\varepsilon$ deletional switch recombination and IgE synthesis in human B cells. *J. Allergy Clin. Immunol.*, **93**, 219.

Loh, R.K.S., Jabara, H.H. & Geha, R.S. (1994b) Disodium cromoglycate inhibits $S\mu \rightarrow S\varepsilon$ deletional switch recombination and IgE synthesis in human B cells. *J. Exp. Med.*, **180**, 663–71.

Louis, R.E. & Radermecker, M.F. (1990) Substance P-induced histamine release from human basophils, skin and lung fragments: effect of nedocromil sodium and theophylline. *Int. Arch. Allergy Appl. Immunol.*, **92**, 329–33.

Mackay, G. & Pearce, F. (1993) Extracellular cGMP has a spectrum of activity in rodent isolated mast cells similar to that of sodium cromoglycate. *Brit. J. Pharmacol.*, **109**, 65P.

Marini, M., Soloperto, M., Zheng, Y., Mezzetti, M. & Mattoli, S. (1992) Protective effect of nedocromil sodium on the IL1-induced release of GM-CSF from cultured human bronchial epithelial cells. *Pulm. Pharmacol.*, **5**, 61–5.

Marquette, C.H., Joseph M., Tonnel, A.B. *et al.* (1990) The abnormal *in vitro* response to aspirin of platelets from aspirin-sensitive asthmatics is inhibited after inhalation of nedocromil sodium but not of sodium cromoglycate. *Brit. J. Clin. Pharmacol.*, **29**, 525–31.

Mattoli, S., Mezzetti, M., Fasoli, A., Patalano, F. & Allegra, L. (1990) Nedocromil sodium prevents the release of 15-hydroxyeicosatetraenoic acid from human bronchial epithelial cells exposed to toluene diisocyanate *in vitro*. *Int. Arch. Allergy Appl. Immunol.*, **92**, 16–22.

Maxwell, D.L., Hawksworth, R.J. & Lee, T.H. (1993) Inhaled nedocromil sodium reduces histamine release from isolated large airway segments of asthmatic subjects *in vivo*. *Eur. Resp. J.*, **6**, 1145–50.

Mazurek, N., Berger, G. & Pecht, I. (1980) A binding site on mast cells and basophils for the anti-allergic drug cromolyn. *Nature*, **286**, 722–3.

Mazurek, N., Bashkin, P., Loyter, A. & Pecht, I. (1983) Restoration of Ca^{2+} influx and degranulation capacity of variant RBL-2H3 cells upon implantation of isolated cromolyn binding protein. *Proc. Nat. Acad. Sci. USA*, **80**, 6014–18.

Mazurek, N., Schindler, H., Schurholz Th. & Pecht, I. (1984) The cromolyn binding protein constitutes the Ca^{2+} channel of basophils opening upon immunological stimulus. *Proc. Nat. Acad. Sci. USA*, **81**, 6841–5.

Mekori, Y.A., Baam, D., Goldberg, A., Hershkoviz, R., Reshef, T. & Sredni, D. (1993) Nedocromil sodium inhibits T cell function *in vitro* and *in vivo*. *J. Allergy Clin. Immunol.*, **91**, 817–24.

Moqbel, R., Walsh, G.M., MacDonald, A.J. & Kay, A.B. (1986) The effect of disodium cromoglycate on activation of human eosinophils and neutrophils following reversed (anti-IgE) anaphylaxis. *Clin. Allergy*, **16**, 73–84.

Moqbel, R., Cromwell, O., Walsh, G.M., Wardlow, A.J., Kurlak, L. & Kay, A.B. (1988) Effects of nedocromil sodium (Tilade) on the activation of human eosinophils and neutrophils and the release of histamine from mast cells. *Allergy*, **43**, 268–76.

Mosmann, T.R. & Coffman, R.L. (1989) Th1 and Th2 cells: different patterns of lymphokine secretion lead to different functional properties. *Ann. Rev. Immunol.*, **7**, 145–73.

Napier, F.E., Shearer, M.A. & Temple, D.A. (1990) Nedocromil sodium inhibits antigen-induced contraction of human lung parenchymal and bronchial strips, and the release of sulphidopeptide-leukotrienes and histamine from human lung fragments. *Brit. J. Pharmacol.*, **100**, 247–50.

O'Hehir, R.E. & Moqbel, R. (1989) Action of nedocromil sodium and sodium cromoglycate on cloned human allergen-specific CD4+ T lymphocytes. *Drugs*, **37** (Suppl. 1), 23–5.

Paulmichl, M., Li, Y., Wickman, K., Ackerman, M., Peralta, E. & Clapham, D. (1992) New mammalian chloride channel identified by expression cloning. *Nature*, **356**, 238–41.

Paulmichl, M., Norris, A.A. & Rainey, D.K. (1995) Role of chloride channel modulation in the mechanism of action of nedocromil sodium. *Int. Arch, Allergy Appl. Immunol.*, **107**, 416.

Penner, R., Matthews, G. & Neher, E. (1988) Regulation of calcium influx by second messengers in rat mast cells. *Nature*, **334**, 499–504.

Rainey, D.K. (1992) Evidence for the anti-inflammatory activity of nedocromil sodium. *Clin. Exp. Allergy*, **22**, 976–9.

Reinsprecht, M., Pecht, I., Schindler, H. & Romanin, C. (1992) Potent block of Cl^- channels by anti-allergic drugs. *Biochem. Biophys. Res. Commun.*, **188**, 57–963.

Resler, B., Sedgwick, J.B. & Busse, W.W. (1992) Inhibition of interleukin-5 effects on human eosinophils by nedocromil sodium. *J. Allergy Clin. Immunol.*, **89**, 235.

Robuschi, M., Vaghi, A., Simone, P. & Bianco, S. (1987) Prevention of fog-induced bronchospasm by nedocromil sodium. *Clin. Allergy*, **17**, 69–74.

Rodwell, L.T., Anderson, S.D., Du Toit, J. & Seale, J.P. (1992) Nedocromil sodium inhibits the airway response to hyperosomolar challenge in patients with asthma. *Am. Rev. Resp. Dis.*, **146**, 1149–55.

Romanin, C., Reinsprecht, M., Pecht, I. & Schindler, H. (1991) Immunologically activated chloride channels involved in degranulation of rat mucosal mast cells. *EMBO J.*, **10**, 3606–8.

Roth, M., Soler, M., Lefkowitz, H. *et al.* (1993) Inhibition of receptor-mediated platelet activation by nedocromil sodium. *J. Allergy Clin. Immunol.*, **91**, 1217–25.

Rubin, R.P. (1991) On the mode of action of the anti-asthmatic drug nedocromil sodium on neutrophil function. *Einstein Q. J. Biol. Med.*, **9**, 4–9.

Sagi-Eisenberg, R. (1987) The role of protein kinase C in histamine secretion: implications for the mode of action of the antiasthmatic drug cromoglycate. *Curr. Topics Pulm. Pharmacol. Toxicol.*, **2**, 24–42.

Sagi-Eisenberg, R., Mazurek, N. & Pecht, I. (1984) Ca^{2+} fluxes and protein phosphorylation in stimulus–secretion coupling of basophils. *Mol. Immunol.*, **21**, 175–81.

Sedgewick, J.B., Calhoun, W.J., Gleich, G.J. *et al.* (1991) Immediate and late airway response of allergic rhinitis patients to segmental antigen challenge. *Am. Rev. Resp. Dis.*, **144**, 1274–81.

Sedgewick, J.B., Bjornsdottir, U., Geiger, K.M. & Busse, W.W. (1992) Inhibition of eosinophil density change and leukotriene C_4 generation by nedocromil sodium. *J. Allergy Clin. Immunol.*, **90**, 202–9.

Spry, C.J.F., Kumaraswami, V. & Tai, P.C. (1986) The effect of nedocromil sodium on secretion from human eosinophils. *Eur. J. Resp. Dis.*, **69**, 241–3.

Stern, M., Meagher, L., Savill, J. & Haslett, C. (1992) Apoptosis in human eosinophils. *J. Immunol.*, **148**, 3543–9.

Szczeklik, A. (1983) Analgesics and nonsteroidal anti-inflammatory drugs. In: *Handbook of Experimental Pharmacology*, Vol. 63, *Allergic Reactions to Drugs* (eds A.L. deWeck & H. Bundgard). Springer Verlag, Berlin.

Theoharides, T.C., Sieghart, W., Greengard, P. & Douglas, W.W. (1980) Antiallergic drug cromolyn may inhibit histamine secretion by regulating phosphorylation of a mast cell protein. *Science*, **207**, 80–2.

Thorel, T., Joseph, M., Tsicopoulos, A., Tonnel, A.B. & Capron, A. (1988) Inhibition by nedocromil sodium of IgE-mediated activation of human mononuclear phagocytes and platelets in allergy. *Int. Arch. Allergy Appl. Immunol.*, **85**, 232–7.

Trigg, C., Manolitsas, N., McAulay, A., Norton, A., Wang, J. & Davies, R.J. (1993) A pilot comparative study of the effects of inhaled nedocromil sodium and albuterol on bronchial biopsies is asthma. *Am. Rev. Resp. Dis.*, **147**, A522.

Ventresca, P.G., Nichol, G.M., Barnes, P.J. & Chung, K.F. (1990) Inhaled frusemide inhibits cough induced by low chloride content solutions but not by capsaicin. *Am. Rev. Resp. Dis.*, **142**, 143–6.

Vercelli, D., Jabbara, H.H., Arai, K. & Geha, R.S. (1989) Induction of human IgE synthesis requires interleukin 4 and T/B cell interactions involving the T cell receptor/CD3 complex and MHC class II antigens. *J. Exp. Med.*, **169**, 1295–307.

Verleden, G.M., Belvisi, M.G., Stretton, C.D. & Barnes, P.J. (1991) Nedocromil sodium modulates nonadrenergic, noncholinergic bronchoconstrictor nerves in guinea pig airways *in vitro*. *Am. Rev. Resp. Dis.*, **143**, 114–18.

Vignola, A.M., Chanez, P., Lacoste, P. *et al.* (1993) Nedocromil modulates the histamine induced expression of ICAM-1 and HLA DR molecules on bronchial epithelial cells. *Am. Rev. Resp. Dis.*, **147**, A45.

Vittori, E., Sciacca, F., Colotta, F, Mantovani, A. & Mattoli, S. (1992) Protective effect of nedocromil sodium on the interleukin-1 induced production of interleukin-8 in human bronchial epithelial cells. *J. Allergy Clin. Immunol.*, **90**, 76–84.

Wells, E. & Mann, J. (1983) Phosphorylation of a mast cell protein in response to treatment with anti-allergic compounds. *Biochem. Pharmacol.*, **32**, 837–42.

Wells, E., Jackson, C.G., Harper, S.T., Mann, J. & Eady, R.P. (1986) Characterisation of primate bronchoalveolar mast cells II. Inhibition of histamine, LTC_4 and PGD_2 release from primate bronchoalveolar mast cells and a comparison with rat peritoneal mast cells. *J. Immunol.*, **137**, 3941–5.

White, M.V., Phillips, R.L. & Kaliner, M.A. (1991) Neutrophils and mast cells: nedocromil sodium inhibits the generation of neutrophil-derived histamine-releasing activity. *J. Allergy Clin. Immunol.*, **87**, 812–20.

Wierenga, E.A., Snoek, M., de Groot, C. *et al.* (1990) Evidence for compartmentalization of functional subsets of CD2+ T lymphocytes in atopic patients. *J. Immunol.*, **144**, 4651–6.

Wright, W., Zhang, Y.G., Salome, C.M. & Woolcock, A.J. (1990) Effect of inhaled preservatives on asthmatic subjects. 1 Sodium metabisulfite. *Am. Rev. Resp. Dis.*, **141**, 1400–4.

CHAPTER 33

Cholinergic Antagonists

N.J. Gross

Introduction

The airways, like most hollow organs, are under extensive autonomic control, which provides tonic and phasic alterations in airway calibre and secretions. In humans, the cholinergic, parasympathetic branch of the autonomic system accounts for a substantial portion of this control in both normal and abnormal airways. Cholinergic antagonists therefore offer a pharmacological avenue that can be exploited for clinical purposes.

Anatomy of the cholinergic system in the lungs

There are both afferent and efferent branches, both of which travel through the vagus nerves (Richardson, 1979) (Fig. 33.1). Efferent nerves arise in the vagal nuclei of the brain stem and enter the lungs at the hila, travelling with the airways and branching with them. These preganglionic fibres terminate in peribronchial ganglia, which are found on the posterior walls of the central airways, few penetrating further into the lungs. Within the ganglia the preganglionic fibres synapse with the postganglionic nerves, whose fibres, in turn, travel short distances to structures within the airway wall, which they supply with parasympathetic activity. The structures are the smooth muscles, mucus glands and possibly ciliated epithelial cells of the airway wall and the pulmonary and bronchial vasculature. The postganglionic terminals are not typical of efferent terminals in other organs; rather, they form a string of varicosities which contain and release preformed mediator, acetylcholine, adjacent to the airway structures they innervate. The effect of mediator release is to cause contraction of smooth muscle, release of mucus from submucosal glands and augmentation of ciliary activity (Barnes, 1986), and anticholinergic agents inhibit these effects. (The effects of the cholinergic system on the pulmonary and bronchial vasculature are relatively small.) As peribronchial ganglia and muscarinic receptors are mainly concentrated in the central airways (Richardson, 1979; Barnes *et al.*, 1983; Barnes, 1986), one expects cholinergic activity to be exerted mainly on these airways. Indeed, physiological evidence tends to suggest that this is so (Ingram *et al.*, 1977).

Although the preponderance of efferent autonomic fibres in human lungs are branches of the vagus, and therefore parasympathetic, there are important interactions between this and other branches of the autonomic nervous system in the lungs (Fig. 33.2). Fibres of the sympathetic nervous system also enter the lungs at the hila and travel into the lungs along the airways. Although β-adrenergic endings are not found close to airway smooth-muscle cells, they appear to innervate the peribronchial ganglia, where they are believed to inhibit transmission of cholinergic traffic, thus opposing parasympathetic drive. In addition, β-adrenergic receptors are found on smooth-muscle cells of both airways and vasculature, where they presumably respond to circulating catecholamines and exogenous β-adrenergic therapy. Additional opposition to cholinergic activity comes from the third nervous system, also known as the non-adrenergic non-cholinergic (NANC) system (Barnes, 1984). A separate anatomical system has not been described for this system; instead, it appears to use the same fibres as the cholinergic system because its mediators, vasoactive intestinal peptide (VIP), peptide histidine methionine and possibly other peptides, are located in secretory vesicles in the varicosities of the

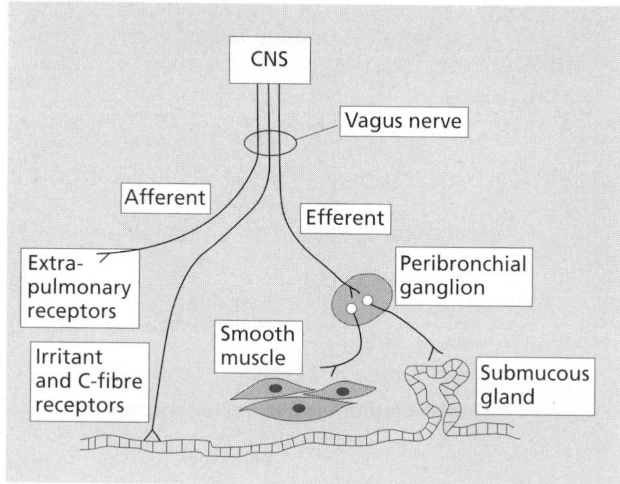

Fig. 33.1 Diagrammatic representation of vagal afferent and efferent pathways in the lungs.

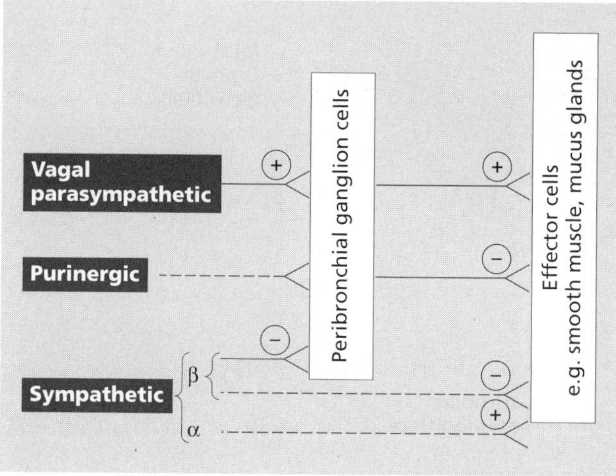

Fig. 33.2 Diagrammatic scheme of efferent autonomic innervation of human airways. +, Excitatory; −, inhibitory; dashed line, existence doubtful. (Redrawn from Gross & Skorodin, 1984a, with permission.)

parasympathetic postganglionic fibres. (Presumably the release of acetylcholine and NANC mediators is under different control mechanisms.) Nitric oxide is released from the same varicosities, but whether it is a principal mediator of the NANC system (Ward *et al.*, 1993) or whether its generation is stimulated by VIP (Lilly *et al.*, 1993) is unclear.

The afferent nerves of the vagus are derived from intrapulmonary and extrapulmonary sources. The sensory endings are the irritant receptors and C fibres located within the airway walls close to the mucosal surface. Extrapulmonary sources that also probably participate in autonomic regulation of the airways are derived from sensory endings in the oesophagus and carotid structures.

Physiology of the cholinergic system

The activity of the parasympathetic system in the lungs can be seen as a continuous low level of tonic activity upon which phasic augmentation is superimposed by a variety of stimuli. Tonic cholinergic activity is known in animals from the detection of electrical activity in pulmonary efferents under resting conditions. Its presence in humans is inferred from the fact that anticholinergic agents result in a modest amount of bronchodilatation even in normal subjects in the absence of bronchoconstricting stimuli (Ingram *et al.*, 1977). Cholinergic bronchomotor tone may be increased in subjects with airway disease because anticholinergic agents result in greater bronchodilatation in these patients (Gross *et al.*, 1989a). The physiological function of bronchomotor tone is unknown (Macklem & Engel, 1975).

Phasic activity—acute increases in cholinergic drive—is mediated through a neural reflex arc, which originates in the receptors described above and is transmitted through afferent branches of the vagus through the brain stem to vagal efferents (Fig. 33.1). A wide variety of agents that stimulate these receptors produce almost immediate bronchoconstriction and mucus hypersecretion via this arc. The stimuli (reviewed in Gross & Skorodin, 1984; Barnes, 1987; Gross, 1988b) include physical agents, dusts, irritant aerosols and gases, cold dry air, exercise, a variety of inflammatory mediators, such as histamine and prostaglandin $F_{2\alpha}$ ($PGF_{2\alpha}$), and allergens. Although the evidence that these agents can produce acute increases in airway resistance through cholinergic neural reflexes is quite strong, their contribution to the totality of airway obstruction in human airway disease is variable and at most only partial, because blocking muscarinic receptors with anticholinergic agents rarely completely inhibits the bronchoconstriction they cause.

Muscarinic receptor sub-types in lungs

Atropine and related agents have anticholinergic effects because they compete with the cholinergic mediator, acetylcholine, at muscarinic receptors. Molecular biology techniques have revealed the presence of at least five probable genes for separate muscarinic receptor subtypes, three of which are known to be expressed in the lungs. These are known as M_1, M_2 and M_3 receptor subtypes (Wess, 1993). The deduced sequence of the muscarinic receptor proteins shows them to belong to a superfamily of receptors whose intracellular actions are coupled to G proteins, and which includes β-adrenergic receptors, rhodopsin and many other receptors. Activation of M_1 and M_3 receptors results in phosphoinositide hydrolysis and release of Ca^{2+} ions, which promotes smooth-muscle contraction, while activation of M_2 receptors inhibits adenyl cyclase activity, counteracting the effects of adrenergic activity. A tentative scheme of the location and physiology of muscarinic receptor sub-types in the airways has been described (Gross & Barnes, 1988) and is shown in Fig. 33.3. M_1 receptors are found in peribronchial ganglia, where they may serve to amplify the cholinergic signal by collateral activation of adjacent postganglionic neurones. M_2 receptors are believed to be present on postganglionic neurones, where they serve an 'autoreceptor' function, inhibiting the release of acetylcholine from the terminals and varicosities of the same nerves in a feedback–inhibition manner. M_3 receptors are those on the effector organs, smooth muscles and submucous glands. According to this scheme, activation of M_1 and M_3 receptors would promote bronchoconstriction and release of mucus, while activation of M_2 autoreceptors would limit these effects. Conversely, selective inactivation of M_2 receptors would tend to promote cholinergic bronchoconstriction. None of the currently available anticholinergic agents is selective for receptor sub-types.

Evidence has recently been obtained that parainfluenza virus infection may selectively damage M_2 autoreceptors (Fryer *et al.*, 1990; Fryer & Jacoby, 1991). Human eosinophilic major basic protein (Jacoby *et al.*, 1993) and other inflammatory mediators (Fryer & Jacoby, 1993) may also impair M_2 receptor function. These findings may help to explain, in part, the transient bronchoconstriction of children during acute viral respiratory tract infections and that due to airway inflammation in patients with asthma. They also argue for the development of anticholinergic agents that do not inhibit M_2 receptors.

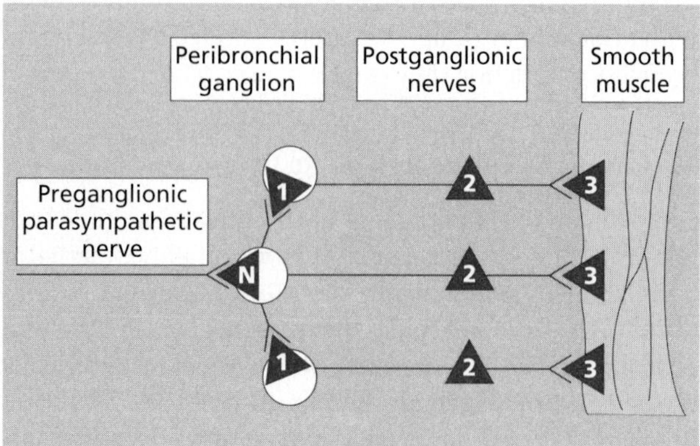

Fig. 33.3 Postulated location of acetylcholine receptors (triangles) in the airways. The receptor labelled N is a nicotinic receptor, those labelled 1, 2 and 3 represent M_1, M_2 and M_3 muscarinic receptor sub-types, respectively. The precise location of M_1 receptors within the peribronchial ganglion is speculative.

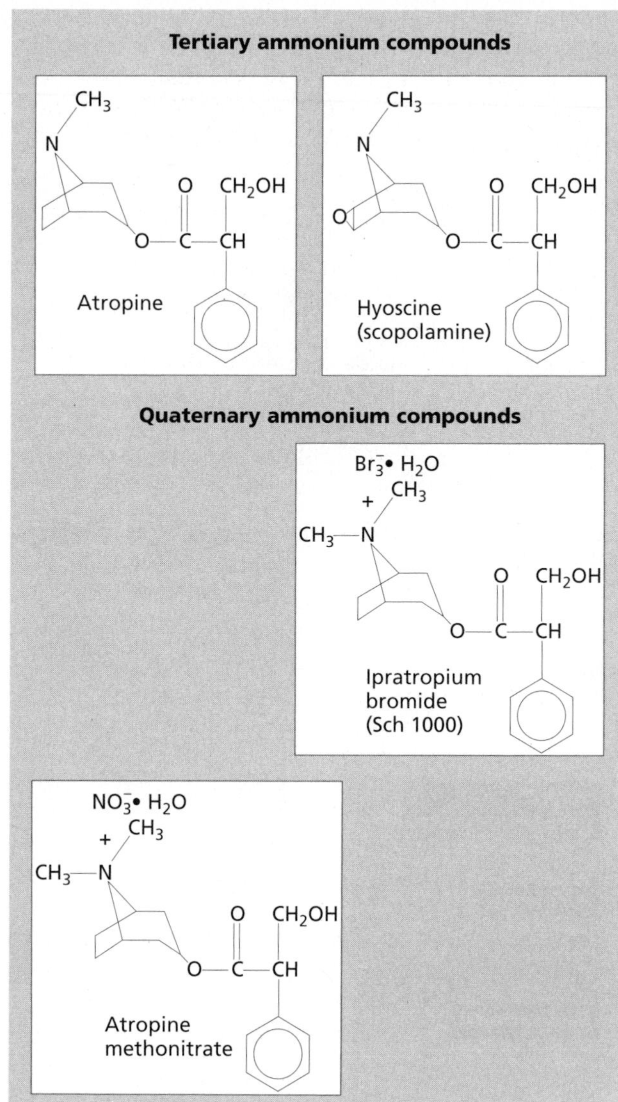

Fig. 33.4 Structural formulae of some anticholinergic agents.

Available anticholinergic agents

The type example of anticholinergic agents is atropine, which is highly selective for muscarinic receptors but not selective among muscarinic receptor sub-types. Atropine, together with its congeners scopolamine, hyoscine and others, is a naturally occurring alkaloid found in high concentration in the leaves, seeds, stems and roots of the *Datura* genus of plants. All natural agents of this class are tertiary ammonium compounds, by reference to the 3-valent nitrogen atom in the tropine ring (Fig. 33.4). Herbal forms of atropine have been widely used for respiratory and other purposes for centuries (Gandevia, 1975) and were the only effective bronchodilators available in western medicine until the discovery of adrenaline (epinephrine) in the 1920s and methylxanthines in the next decade. They are all freely absorbable from mucosal surface and widely distributed throughout the body, including the central nervous system (CNS), where they counteract all the 'housekeeping' functions of the parasympathetic system. This results in many side-effects, which limit their usefulness. To avoid this drawback, pharmaceutical chemists developed a series of synthetic quaternary ammonium congeners, whose tropine nitrogen atom is 5-valent and carries a charge. This minor chemical change results in major pharmacological and clinical effects, almost all of which are due to the fact that the quaternary ammonium compounds are very poorly absorbed while retaining their local anticholinergic actions. Of these synthetic agents, ipratropium bromide (Atrovent) and oxitropium bromide (Oxivent) have been the most extensively studied, although other synthetic quaternary agents such as glycopyrrolate (Robinul) which are only distantly related chemically share similar clinical properties.

Pharmacology of anticholinergic agents

Pharmacokinetics and pharmacodynamics

The pharmacological properties of atropine and related tertiary ammonium alkaloids (which are quite similar) have been known for more than a century. As they are well described in standard texts (Reynolds, 1989; Brown, 1990), they will be only briefly summarized here. Atropine is well absorbed from mucosal surfaces and, to some extent, from the skin. Blood levels are detectable within a few minutes and reach a peak within about an hour. The half-life in the circulation is of the order of 3–4 hours. Atropine causes relaxation of smooth muscle in the airways (mainly central) and in the gastrointestinal and biliary tracts, iris, peripheral vasculature, bladder and ureters; however, it inhibits relaxation of the urinary sphincter. It causes mild bradycardia in small doses and tachycardia in higher doses. It reduces the rate of apocrine and salivary secretions and inhibits mucociliary clearance in the airways. It crosses the blood–brain barrier and can cause mild central stimulation—excitement and restlessness. All of these effects are dose related and can occur in normal doses, 0.035 mg/kg, but are usually well tolerated by patients, except possibly with repeated long-term use. The bronchodilator effect of atropine (0.02 mg/kg) following intravenous administration returns to baseline at 3–4 hours (Gal & Suratt, 1981). The therapeutic margin is very small, and doses only slightly above usual are associated with intensification of the above effects and toxicity (see below).

Ipratropium (Gross, 1988a) and oxitropium (Calverley, 1992), in contrast, are very poorly absorbed and blood levels can only be estimated reliably using radiolabeliled drug. The half-life in the circulation is about an hour longer than that of atropine and clearance is mainly through the biliary tract and gut and, to a lesser extent, as metabolites in the urine. They have local anticholinergic effects at the site of delivery but are not significantly absorbed from these sites. Thus, ipratropium dilates the pupil when delivered to the conjunctiva, and dilates the airways when delivered by inhalation; however, in each case no systemic effects occur, even after doses up to 100 times the recommended amount. When delivered parenterally (for experimental purposes), ipratropium causes systemic anticholinergic effects similar to those of atropine, indicating that a high degree of organ specificity can be obtained by choosing the site of delivery. However, even when delivered parenterally, these agents fail to cross the blood–brain barrier. In contrast to the natural tertiary agents, quaternary agents tend to have longer durations of action. This can be partly explained by the fact that tertiary agents are removed from the site of action by absorption, while quaternary agents are not absorbed and presumably remain longer at the site of deposition. Thus, the bronchodilator effect of ipratropium in conventional dosage lasts for 5–6 hours (Gross, 1988a) and that of oxitropium persists for up to 8 hours (Skorodin *et al.*, 1986). Tiotropium and glycopyrrolate (Walker *et al.*, 1987) remain active for 8–12 hours.

Dose–response

Atropine and its congeners occur in nature in two isomeric forms, only one of which is pharmacologically active. Some quaternary congeners, e.g. atropine methonitrate, are synthesized from plant sources of atropine and are thus a mixture of both isomers. Newer agents, such as ipratropium and oxitropium, are synthesized *de novo* in the active isomeric form, making them approximately twice as potent as naturally derived agents for this reason alone.

The dose of atropine conventionally used for bronchodilatation is 0.15–0.4 mg/kg in both children and adults. This is usually given as a nebulized solution for inhalation, although it has been given parenterally. Although this dose is probably not optimal, side-effects are a certainty at higher dosage.

Dose–response studies of ipratropium by metered dose inhaler (MDI) suggest maximal response following 40–80 μg (Gross, 1975; Storms *et al.*, 1975; Yeager *et al.*, 1976; Allen & Campbell, 1980a; Gomm *et al.*, 1983). However, these studies were performed in subjects with only mild airway obstruction. It is now recognized that penetration of aerosols into the airways is a function of airway patency and is limited in subjects with severe airway disease (Dolovich *et al.*, 1976; Pavia *et al.*, 1977), so higher doses are almost certainly required in these. In patients with moderate to severe chronic obstructive pulmonary disease (COPD), an optimal dose of 160 μg by MDI was suggested (Gross *et al.*, 1989). As this would require eight puffs of the conventional MDI, a more potent form (Atrovent forte), which delivers twice the amount per puff, is widely used in Europe, and seems rational. An uncontrolled 6-month study of 160 μg ipratropium four times daily suggests that this dose is safe (Leak & O'Connor, 1988). The optimal dose of oxitropium by MDI in patients with COPD is 100–200 μg (Skorodin *et al.*, 1986) and this is the dose that is conventionally used.

The optimal dose of ipratropium nebulized solution varies widely among studies, presumably reflecting wide differences in performance between nebulizers as well as patient populations. The optimal dose is in the region of 400 μg (Gross *et al.*, 1989), although other studies report lower optimal doses, patients with more severe airway obstruction again requiring larger doses for optimal effect. The figure of 400 μg is in keeping with the fact that the dose of an agent delivered by wet nebulization is between two and 10 times that delivered by an MDI for equivalent effect (Weber *et al.*, 1979). The currently recommended dose of ipratropium by this route is 500 μg in adults. In children, doses of 100–250 μg ipratropium have been found to be optimal (Davis *et al.*, 1984; Friberg & Graff-Lonnevig, 1989). The optimal dose of atropine methonitrate by nebulized solution has been reported to be 1500 μg (Allen & Campbell, 1980b). The optimal dose of glycopyrrolate nebulized solution is 100–200 μg (Walker *et al.*, 1987).

Clinical efficacy

The efficacy of anticholinergic agents has been studied in three main settings: as protectants against common stimuli and known mediators of bronchoconstriction in the laboratory, as bronchodilators in stable asthma or COPD and as bronchodilators in the acute setting. These will be considered in turn.

Against stimulated bronchoconstriction

The results of some of these studies are shown in Table 33.1 (Gross & Skorodin, 1984a). As would be expected, anticholinergic agents are very effective in preventing the bronchoconstriction resulting from the inhalation of cholinergic agonists such as methacholine, acetylcholine or carbachol. Against a variety of inflammatory mediators such as histamine, bradykinin, $PGF_{2\alpha}$, serotonin and leukotrienes, they were partially effective at best. Their protective effect against non-specific agents, such as irritant gases, irritant aerosols, cigarette smoke, exercise and cold dry air, and allergens, varied from none to partial, suggesting that the bronchoconstriction these agents produce is only partially and variably due to vagal reflexes. Similarly, they were only partially effective against nocturnal bronchospasm (Cox *et al.*, 1984; Coe & Barnes, 1986). Thus, for many of the bronchospastic stimuli thought to be important in clinical airway disease, anticholinergic agents provide protection that is only partial at best. In only two clinical situations are anticholinergic agents felt to provide better protection than alternative agents—that due to psychogenic bronchospasm (McFadden *et al.*, 1969; Rebuck & Marcus, 1979; Nield & Cameron, 1985) and the bronchospasm that can result from administration of a β_2-adrenergic-blocking agent (Grieco & Pierson, 1971; Ind *et al.*, 1989).

In stable asthma

The very large number of studies on this use of ipratropium have been reviewed elsewhere (Gross & Skorodin, 1984a; Gross, 1988a, 1992; Sterling, 1987). As the results are quite consistent, we will summarize them. The typical short-term response is exemplified in Fig. 33.5 (Ruffin *et*

Table 33.1 Summary of efficacy of anticholinergic agents against specific bronchospastic stimuli. (From Gross & Sicorodin, 1984a, with permission.)

Stimulus	Efficacy of anticholinergic agents	Efficacy of adrenergic agents relative to anticholinergic agents
Cholinergic agents	Fully protective	Less effective
Histamine	Partially protective	More effective
Mediators, prostaglandin $F_{2\alpha}$, serotonin	Partially protective	More effective
β-Blockade	Protective	Ineffective
Gases, dusts, irritants	Usually protective	—
Antigens	Variable	More effective
Exercise, hyperventilation	Modestly protective	More effective
Psychogenic factors	Good protection	Less effective

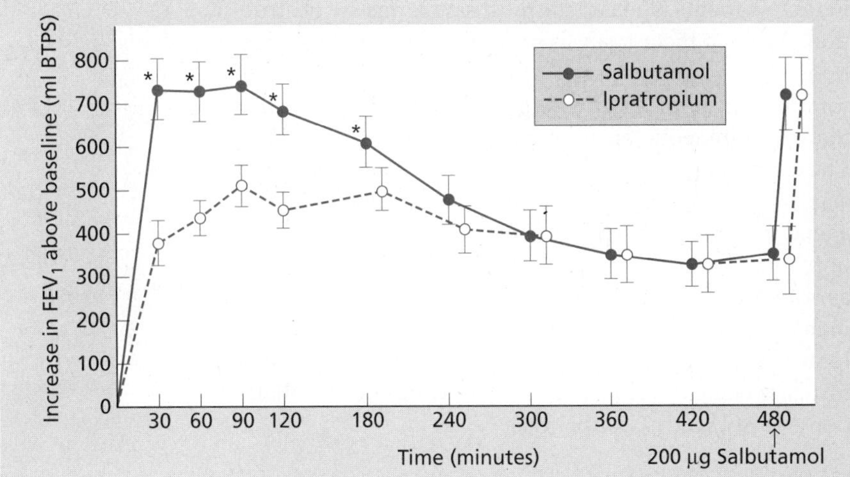

Fig. 33.5 Responses of 25 asthmatic subjects to inhaled salbutamol (200 μg by MDI) and ipratropium bromide (40 μg by MDI). All subjects received additional salbutamol at 480 minutes. *, Significant difference between agents at $P < 0.05$. (From Ruffin *et al.*, 1977, with permission.)

al., 1977). After administration of the usual dose of ipratropium, the onset of bronchodilatation occurs within minutes; however, it develops more slowly than following a conventional (i.e. not long-acting) β_2-adrenergic agent, reaching peak effect between 1 and 2 hours later. At peak effect, it is consistently less potent than a β_2-adrenergic agent, although individual differences among patients are large. Attempts have been made to identify subgroups of asthmatics who may respond better, but with limited success. In general, subjects with intrinsic asthma or asthma of longer duration (Jolobe, 1984) and older asthmatics—those above 40 years of age (Ullah *et al.*, 1981)—tend to respond better, although children can sometimes respond well (see below). An individual trial is probably the only reliable way to identify the patient who will respond well to an anticholinergic bronchodilator (Brown *et al.*, 1984).

For these reasons, anticholinergics are not regarded as first-line treatment in stable chronic asthma. They may be sufficient to control symptoms of mild asthma in subjects who cannot tolerate the side-effects of an adrenergic bronchodilator, and in very severe asthma their addition to all other therapy may provide an increment of bronchodilatation that permits better control or that avoids oral steroid therapy.

In acute severe asthma

A few small studies have compared the efficacy of ipratropium alone with a β_2-adrenergic agent alone in acute asthma and these have been reviewed (Ward, 1993). The results have been mixed. The one large multicentre study on this question (Rebuck *et al.*, 1987) showed the adrenergic agent to be more effective, but not significantly so (Fig. 33.6). However, a recent meta-analysis of six double-blind controlled studies shows that an adrenergic agent was significantly more effective overall (Ward, 1993). Because of the potential for fatality in this condition and the urgent need for immediate relief of airway obstruction, most clinicians would now consider it inappropriate to treat acute asthma with an anticholinergic agent as the sole bronchodilator.

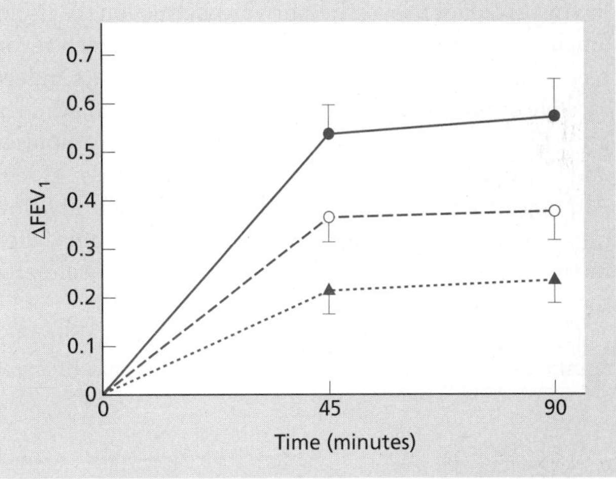

Fig. 33.6 Bronchodilator treatment of acute severe asthma in 148 patients. Patients received either ipratropium 0.5 mg, fenoterol 1.25 mg or the combination by wet nebulization as the sole initial bronchodilator. Bars are ± SE. Differences between the combination and single agents were significant at $P < 0.05$. (From Rebuck *et al.*, 1987, with permission.)

However, there has also been debate whether an anticholinergic agent should be added to an adrenergic in the early management of acute asthma. The study of Rebuck *et al.* (1987) shows that the combination of fenoterol 1.25 mg plus ipratropium 0.5 mg was significantly more effective than the same dose of fenoterol alone (Fig. 33.6). Moreover, the advantage of the combination was greatest in those patients who had the most severe airway obstruction. Again, a meta-analysis of nine studies on this question shows quite clearly that the combination of ipratropium with an adrenergic agent is more effective than an adrenergic agent alone (Ward, 1993) (Fig. 33.7). The conclusion is that the bronchodilator management of acute severe asthma should include an anticholinergic agent, together with a β_2-adrenergic agent. Combinations of fenoterol and ipratropium (Berodual, Duovent), either as solutions for nebulization or as MDI, are available in many countries, and a combination of salbutamol and ipratropium (Combivent), in both solution and MDI forms, is being developed in the USA (Combivent Inhalation Aerosol Study Group, 1994).

In stable COPD

Patients with COPD have been traditionally regarded as having 'fixed' or irreversible airway obstruction that is not amenable to bronchodilators. However, this view is incorrect. It has been amply documented that they are indeed capable of bronchodilatation in response to both adrenergic and anticholinergic agents, as shown by Anthonisen and Wright (1986) and reviewed by Gross (1986). Although they are rarely capable of as much absolute improvement in air flow as patients with asthma, their increase in air flow is based on a much lower baseline, so the symptomatic relief they experience is as great.

The short- and long-term effects of anticholinergic agents vs. adrenergic agents in this group of patients have

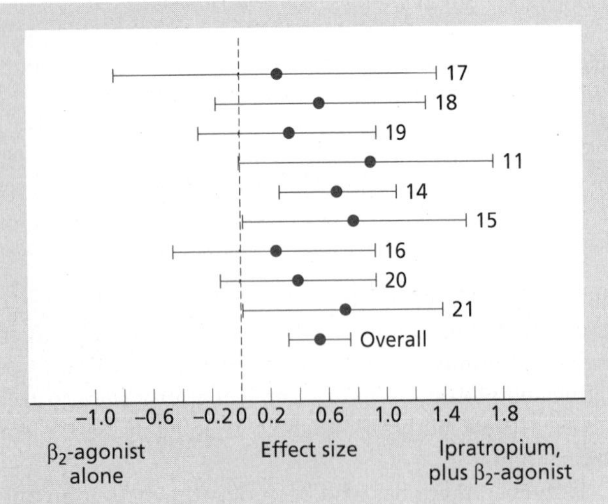

Fig. 33.7 Meta-analysis of nine studies comparing the effect of a β_2-agonist alone with that of a β_2-agonist plus ipratropium in acute severe asthma. Bars show 95% confidence limits. The pooled result, 'overall', is shown. Numbers adjacent to bars refer to individual studies in the original publication. (From Ward, 1993, with permission.)

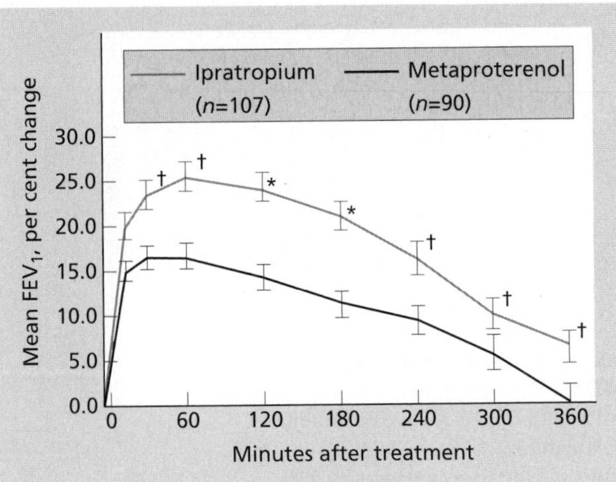

Fig. 33.8 Bronchodilator response in stable COPD. Patients received 36 μg ipratropium or 1.5 mg metaproterenol by MDI. Symbols denote significant differences between treatments. (From Tashkin *et al.*, 1986, with permission.)

been studied in several hundred studies, which have been reviewed (Gross & Skorodin, 1984a; Sterling, 1987; Gross, 1988a, 1992). Again, the results have been quite uniform and will be summarized. All but a few studies show that in this patient population an anticholinergic agent provides more improvement in air flow than other bronchodilators, whether compared with metaproterenol, e.g. Fig. 33.8 (Tashkin *et al.*, 1986), salbutamol (Braun *et al.*, 1990) or a methylxanthine (Bleecker & Britt, 1991). Most such studies have compared recommended doses of each agent, rather than optimal doses, which may be higher, as stated above. However, when optimal doses of each class of agent have been used, the result has been similar (Douglas *et al.*, 1979, Gross & Skorodin, 1984b). In particular, both studies show that the bronchodilatation achieved by cumulative and maximal doses of an adrenergic agent could be augmented by subsequent administration of an anticholinergic agent; in reverse order, an adrenergic agent did not augment the bronchodilatation achieved by cumulative doses of an anticholinergic agent. These studies support the notion that anticholinergic bronchodilators are more effective than adrenergic agents in COPD.

As this conclusion is the reverse of that generally found in patients with asthma, it can be re-examined in the few studies that have compared the bronchodilator responses of patients with either asthma or COPD to each class of agent in side-by-side comparisons (Marlin *et al.*, 1978; Lefcoe *et al.*, 1982). These again show a consistent result, an example of which is shown in Fig. 33.9, from which some conclusions can be drawn. The responses of both groups of patients to ipratropium were similar; however, the asthmatic patients responded very well to the adrener-

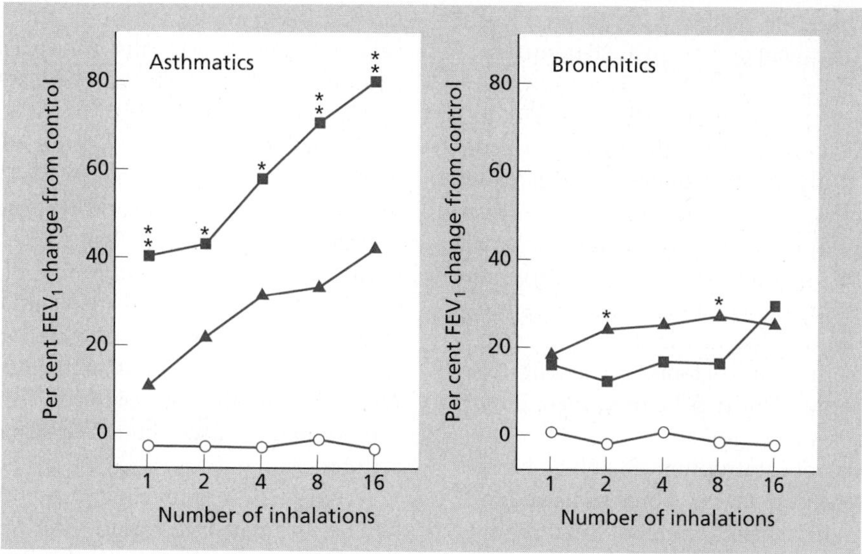

Fig. 33.9 Response of six patients with asthma and six with chronic bronchitis to cumulative inhalations of fenoterol (200 μg per inhalation, squares) vs. ipratropium (20 μg per inhalation, triangles), vs. placebo. Baseline forced expiratory volume in 1 second (FEV_1) values were comparable in the two groups. Significant differences between active agents are indicated by a single asterisk ($P < 0.05$) or double asterisk ($P < 0.01$). (From Marlin *et al.*, 1978, with permission.)

gic agent while the bronchitic patients responded poorly to this agent. Mainly because of the difference in response to the adrenergic agent, the asthmatic patients responded better to the adrenergic agent while the bronchitic patients responded better to the anticholinergic agent. The reasons for this difference in response, although unknown, have been considered (Gross & Skorodin, 1987; Gross, 1988b). The airway obstruction in asthma has a multitude of mechanisms, including airway inflammation, mucosal oedema and mucus hypersecretion, cellular desquamation and exudate in the airway lumen, none of which is amenable to anticholinergic actions but which are partly amenable to adrenergic activity. In COPD, airway obstruction is due mostly to structural changes in and around airway walls, leaving the reversal of bronchomotor tone as the only bronchoconstrictive factor amenable to pharmacotherapy. As bronchomotor tone is largely due to vagal, cholinergic mechanisms, anticholinergic agents are more effective in COPD. Whatever the explanation, the clinical implication is clear. Patients with asthma are more likely to achieve better bronchodilatation with an adrenergic agent, while patients with COPD are more likely to achieve better bronchodilatation with an anticholinergic agent.

In acute exacerbations of COPD

The role of anticholinergic agents in acute exacerbations of COPD has been studied less often (Lloberes *et al.*, 1988; O'Driscoll *et al.*, 1989; Karpel *et al.*, 1990; Karpel, 1991). The response to any bronchodilator tends to be less than in non-acute situations. Rebuck *et al.* (1987) found no difference in the improvement in air flow, regardless of whether ipratropium or fenoterol or their combination was used, and Karpel (1991) found no difference between ipratropium and metaproterenol. The only difference is the potential for adrenergic agents to reduce the partial pressure of arterial oxygen ($Pa{O_2}$) (Karpel *et al.*, 1990), which was not seen following an anticholinergic agent. One concludes that it makes little difference which class of bronchodilator is used in acute COPD.

In paediatric airway disease

The role of ipratropium in the management of acute asthma in children has been examined in two important studies from Canada. Beck *et al.* (1985) compared salbutamol alone with salbutamol plus ipratropium, both by nebulizer solution, in children aged 5–15 whose initial forced expiratory volume in 1 second (FEV_1) was less than 50% of predicted. All patients received salbutamol inhalations each 20 minutes for 2 hours. One group received ipratropium by nebulization at 1 hour in addition to salbutamol, the other received placebo inhalation at the same time in addition to salbutamol. The responses of both groups were identical during the first hour; in the second hour, the group that received ipratropium experienced further bronchodilatation, which was significantly greater than that of the control group. In the second study (Reisman *et al.*, 1988), a similar protocol was adopted except that ipratropium (or placebo) treatments were given at the onset of treatment and again at 40 minutes in addition to salbutamol every 20 minutes. The group that received ipratropium achieved significantly greater bronchodilatation from 20 minutes after the first treatment until the end of the study at 150 minutes. In both these studies, ipratropium was well tolerated. These two studies strongly suggest, therefore, that, despite optimal administration of a potent adrenergic agent, ipratropium significantly augments bronchodilatation in acute asthma in children—similar to the findings in adults reviewed above. However, two other studies found no benefit from the addition of ipratropium (Storr & Lenney, 1986; Boner *et al.*, 1987).

The evidence for use of ipratropium in stable chronic childhood asthma is less convincing. Three trials suggest that ipratropium adds little benefit to an optimal regime with adrenergic agents (Mann & Hiller, 1982; Sly *et al.*, 1987; Freeman & Landau, 1989). In two consensus reports from North America (Warner *et al.*, 1989; Hargreave *et al.*, 1990), the view was expressed that ipratropium probably had a minor, adjunctive role in the management of chronic paediatric asthma, and that it was safe in these patients, but that it was, at best, only mildly effective.

Although there are reports of ipratropium use in a variety of other paediatric conditions, including cystic fibrosis, viral bronchiolitis, exercise-induced bronchospasm and bronchopulmonary dysplasia, the sparsity of such reports and the lack of strong evidence of benefit do not permit firm conclusions about its role in these conditions.

Side-effects and toxicity

The side-effects of anticholinergic agents are almost entirely due to effects that result from absorption and systemic distribution. As tertiary and quaternary agents differ markedly in their absorbability, their propensity to produce side-effects is similarly different.

Tertiary ammonium compounds

The side-effects of atropine and its naturally occurring congeners have been well known for many years and are fully described in standard texts (Reynolds, 1989; Brown, 1990) and will be only briefly discussed. Agents of this group are more or less quantitatively absorbed from mucosal surfaces and widely distributed in the body, including the CNS. Side-effects occur at therapeutic dose levels and are mostly dose related. The therapeutic margin of these agents is thus small.

Hotness and flushing of the skin and dryness of the mouth are common following usual doses of atropine but are rarely troublesome, although dysphagia and dysphonia can occur in higher doses. In the respiratory tract, atropine inhalation results in impairment of mucociliary clearance at doses equal to or only slightly above those that produce bronchodilatation (Lopez-Vidriero *et al.*, 1975; Sackner *et al.*, 1977; Berger *et al.*, 1978; Foster & Bergofsky, 1986; Groth *et al.*, 1991). This is partly due to a reduction in the volume and water content of secretions (Sturgess & Reid, 1972; Boat & Kleinerman, 1975) and partly due to a reduction in ciliary beat frequency (Corssen & Allen, 1959; Yeates *et al.*, 1975). These findings raise concern, as retention of secretions and mucous plugging of airways is a consistent finding in fatal asthma. They suggest that atropine and its tertiary congeners should not be used in the treatment of acute severe asthma.

Tertiary ammonium compounds cross the blood–brain barrier and cause a variety of CNS effects, from mild excitement, irritability or restlessness in usual doses, to disorientation, hallucinations and coma in higher doses. Acute psychosis following usual doses has been reported in adults (Bergman *et al.*, 1980) and children (Herschman *et al.*, 1991). These agents can also cause acute ocular hypertension in subjects susceptible to narrow-angle glaucoma, but not in wide-angle glaucoma. They cause minor effects in the cardiovascular system, including tachycardia, atrial arrhythmias and atrioventricular (AV) dissociation in higher doses. They may cause relaxation of the lower oesophageal sphincter and promote reflux (Cotton & Smith, 1981; Hey *et al.*, 1983), inhibit gastric motility and delay gastric emptying (Botts *et al.*, 1985). Urinary symptoms are important in the older, COPD, male population, in whom urinary retention may be a problem. Atropine can cause acute urinary retention in usual doses.

Quaternary ammonium compounds

Because of their limited absorption when taken by inhalation, ipratropium, oxitropium, atropine methonitrate and glycopyrrolate have a relatively wide therapeutic margin. The side-effects of ipratropium and oxitropium have been extensively examined. In the upper respiratory tract (nasal passages), ipratropium causes a significant reduction in stimulated secretion of mucus, but has no effect on basal secretory rates (Borum, 1987; Meltzer, 1991). In the lower respiratory tract, ipratropium has been reported to have negligible effects on mucociliary clearance (Francis *et al.*, 1977; Sackner *et al.*, 1977; Ruffin *et al.*, 1978; Pavia *et al.*, 1980; Wanner, 1986) or mucus composition (Chervinsky, 1977). After 7 weeks of continuous treatment with ipratropium, a small decrease in sputum volume was found in one study (Ghafouri *et al.*, 1984). After 4 weeks' treatment with oxitropium in either asthmatic or bronchitic subjects, no significant changes were found in sputum production, mucociliary clearance rates or sputum viscosity (Pavia *et al.*, 1989). The lack of effects on the mucociliary apparatus in the face of relaxation of smooth muscles which are adjacent to the mucous glands is surprising and unexplained.

In the eye, ipratropium by inhalation causes no changes in intraocular tension, pupil diameter or accommodation, in both normal subjects and patients with glaucoma, even when taken in larger than recommended doses (Ruffin *et al.*, 1978; Scheuffler, 1975; Thumm, 1975). However, prolonged pupillary dilatation and blurred vision have been reported following inadvertent administration directly into the eye (Samaniego & Newman, 1986), an effect that can apparently be intensified by co-administration with salbutamol (Kalra & Bone, 1988; Shah *et al.*, 1992). Care should be taken that the MDI is not directed towards the eye. When ipratropium solution is administered by face mask, the upper portion of the mask should fit tightly.

In the genitourinary system, no effects on urinary flow characteristics were found when ipratropium was given to men 50–70 years of age, and therefore presumably at risk for prostatic hypertrophy (Molkenboer & Lardenoye, 1979).

In contrast to adrenergic agents, ipratropium had relatively minor effects on the cardiovascular system (Chapman *et al.*, 1985; Anderson, 1986), even when given in eightfold excess of the recommended dose (Sackner *et al.*, 1977).

With regard to gas exchange, atropine methonitrate has no tendency to reduce acutely the $Pa\text{O}_2$ in either normal subjects (Field, 1967) or patients with COPD and hypoxaemia at rest (Gross & Bankwala, 1987). Nor did ipratropium adversely affect $Pa\text{O}_2$ in acute exacerbations of COPD (Karpel *et al.*, 1990).

Paradoxical bronchoconstriction to ipratropium has been reported in a handful of publications from the UK. This unusual reaction takes the form of an increase in bronchospasm and a fall in air flow shortly after receiving ipratropium, usually by nebulized solution (Connolly, 1982). Variously attributed to hypotonicity of the nebulizer solution (Mann *et al.*, 1984), hypersensitivity to bromide (Patel & Tullett, 1983) and preservatives in the solution (Miszkiel *et al.*, 1988; Rafferty *et al.*, 1988), its cause has not been definitively identified. Correction of these possible causes has apparently not eliminated its occasional occurrence (O'Callaghan *et al.*, 1989; Yuksel *et al.*, 1991). The possibility remains that it is an idiosyncratic reaction to the drug itself. There are anecdotal accounts of paradoxical bronchoconstriction following oxitropium use as well; however, these have not been published. Although apparently rare and never fatal, to our knowledge, the possibility of paradoxical bronchoconstriction to any anticholinergic agent should be borne in mind and the drug promptly withdrawn in the event of an adverse response.

One other rare but important side-effect is the occurrence of ileus in a patient with cystic fibrosis who received ipratropium (Mulherin & Fitzgerald, 1990). The presumption is that ipratropium swallowed by the patient resulted in a meconium ileus-equivalent syndrome.

The very large clinical experience obtained since ipratropium was released for general use in the middle 1970s and oxitropium in the late 1980s suggests that these agents are remarkably well tolerated by the majority of patients.

Management of anticholinergic toxicity

The side-effects of atropine can be readily reversed, if their severity warrants, by parenteral administration of an anticholinesterase, e.g. physostigmine 1–2 mg. This should be administered with caution, however, because the removal of inhibition of cholinergic activity can result in a return of bronchospasm. On the other hand, anticholinesterases are rapidly metabolized and additional doses may be needed to prevent the return of anticholinergic toxicity. For ocular toxicity, topical neostigmine or physostigmine can be used.

Phenothiazines should be avoided as they have some intrinsic anticholinergic activity.

Clinical considerations

The major use of anticholinergic bronchodilators is in the management of stable COPD, in which condition they are appropriate first-line therapy. They are probably best used on a regular basis, three or four times daily, because their relatively slow onset of action makes them unsuitable for the rapid relief of symptoms. If the recommended dose of ipratropium, 40 µg by MDI, does not provide control of symptoms, the more potent form, Atrovent forte, should be used. Alternatively, oxitropium 200 µg by MDI can be tried. Their benefit in acute exacerbations of COPD is not extensively documented.

The role of anticholinergics in asthma is mainly as adjunctive treatment. In acute severe asthma they should not be used as the sole bronchodilator. However, they clearly add to the bronchodilatation achieved with an adrenergic agent, and combinations of the two classes of bronchodilator should be used in severe attacks, at least initially, in both adults and children. In general, they are relatively ineffective in stable asthma, although large individual differences occur. They are worth a trial in patients who, despite all other therapy, are not well controlled.

Anticholinergic bronchodilators are the treatment of choice in counteracting the bronchospasm induced by the inadvertent administration of a β-blocking agent. However, they are only marginally effective in preventing exercise-induced bronchospasm and that produced by similar bronchospastic stimuli.

With the advent of quaternary agents in many useful forms that are all well tolerated, there is probably no role for the use of atropine and other tertiary ammonium compounds in the management of airway obstruction.

References

Allen, C.J. & Campbell, A.H. (1980a) Dose response of ipratropium bromide assessed by two methods. *Thorax*, **35**, 137–9.

Allen, C.J. & Campbell, A.H. (1980b) Comparison of inhaled atropine sulphate and atropine methonitrate. *Thorax*, **35**, 932–5.

Anderson, W.M. (1986) Hemodynamic and non-bronchial effects of ipratropium bromide. *Am. J. Med.*, **81** (Suppl. 5A), 45–52.

Anthonisen, N.R. & Wright, E.C. (1986) Bronchodilator response in COPD. *Am. Rev. Resp. Dis.*, **133**, 814–19.

Barnes, P.J. (1984) The third nervous system in the lungs: physiology and clinical perspectives. *Thorax*, **39**, 561–7.

Barnes, P.J. (1986) Neural control of human airways in health and disease. *Am. Rev. Resp. Dis.*, **134**, 1289–314.

Barnes, P.J. (1987) Cholinergic control of airway smooth muscle. *Am. Rev. Resp. Dis.*, **136**, 542–5.

Barnes, P.J., Basbaum, C.B. & Nadel, J.A. (1983) Autoradiographic localization of autonomic receptors in airway smooth muscle: marked differences between large and small airways. *Am. Rev. Resp. Dis.*, **127**, 758–62.

Beck, R., Robertson, C., Galdes-Sebaldt, M. & Levison, H. (1985) Combined salbutamol and ipratropium bromide by inhalation in the treatment of severe acute asthma. *J. Pediatr.*, **107**, 605–8.

Berger, J., Albert, R.E., Sanborn, K. & Lippman, M. (1978) Effects of atropine and methacholine on deposition and clearance of inhaled particles in the donkey. *J. Toxicol. Environ. Health*, **4**, 587–604.

Bergman, K.R., Pearson, C., Waltz, G.W. & Evans, R. (1980) Atropine-induced psychosis, an unusual complication of therapy with inhaled atropine sulfate. *Chest*, **78**, 891–3.

Bleecker, E.R. & Britt, E.J. (1991) Acute bronchodilating effects of ipratropium bromide and theophylline in chronic obstructive pulmonary disease. *Am. J. Med.*, **91**, 24S–27S.

Boat, T.F. & Kleinerman, J.I. (1975) Human respiratory tract secretions. 2 Effect of cholinergic and adrenergic agents on *in vitro* release of protein and mucous glycoproteins. *Chest*, **67** (Suppl.), 32–4.

Boner, A.L., De Stefano, G., Niero, E., Vallone, G. & Gaburro, D. (1987) Salbutamol and ipratropium bromide solution in the treatment of bronchospasm in asthmatic children. *Ann. Allergy*, **58**, 54–8.

Borum, P. (1987) Nasal disorders and anticholinergic therapy. *Postgrad. Med. J.*, **63** (Suppl. 1), 61–8.

Botts, L.D., Pingleton, S.K., Schroeder, C.E., Robinson, R.G. & Hurwitz, A. (1985) Prolongation of gastric emptying by aerosolized atropine. *Am. Rev. Resp. Dis.*, **131**, 725–6.

Braun S.R., McKenzie, W.N., Copeland, C., Knight, L. & Ellersieck, M. (1990) A comparison of the effect of ipratropium and albuterol in the treatment of chronic obstructive airway disease. *Arch. Intern. Med.*, **149**, 544–7.

Brown, I.G., Chan, C.S., Kelley, C.A., Dent, A.G. & Zimmerman, P.V. (1984) Assessment of the clinical usefulness of nebulized ipratropium bromide in patients with chronic airflow limitation. *Thorax*, **39**, 272–6.

Brown, J.H. (1990) Atropine, scopolamine, and related antimuscarinic drugs. In: *Goodman and Gilman's The Pharmacologic Basis of Therapeutics*, 8th edn. (eds A.G. Gilman, T.W. Rall, A.S. Nies & P. Taylor), pp. 150–65. Pergamon Press, New York.

Calverley, P.M.A. (1992) The clinical efficacy of oxitropium bromide. *Rev. Contemp. Pharmacother.*, **3**, 189–96.

Chapman, K.R., Smith, D.L., Rebuck, A.S. & Leenen, F.H. (1985) Hemodynamic effects of inhaled ipratropium bromide, alone and combined with an inhaled beta2-agonist. *Am. Rev. Resp. Dis.*, **132**, 845–7.

Chervinsky, P. (1977) Double-blind study of ipratropium bromide, a new anticholinergic bronchodilator. *J. Allergy Clin. Immunol.*, **59**, 22–30.

Coe, C.I. & Barnes, P.J. (1986) Reduction in nocturnal asthma by an inhaled anticholinergic drug. *Chest*, **90**, 485–8.

Combivent Inhalation Aerosol Study Group (1994) In chronic obstructive pulmonary disease, a combination of ipratropium and albuterol is more effective than either agent alone, an 85-day multicenter trial. *Chest*, **105**, 1411–19.

Connolly, C.K. (1982) Adverse reaction to ipratropium bromide. *Brit. Med. J.*, **285**, 934–5.

Corssen, G. & Allen, C.R. (1959) Acetylcholine: its significance in controlling ciliary activity of human respiratory epithelium *in vitro*. *J. Appl. Physiol.*, **14**, 901–4.

Cotton, B.R. & Smith, G. (1981) Single and combined effects of atropine and metaclopramide on the lower oesophageal sphincter pressure. *Brit. J. Anaesth.*, **53**, 869–74.

Cox, I.D., Hughes, D.T.D. & McDonnell, K.A. (1984) Ipratropium bromide in patients with nocturnal asthma. *Postgrad. Med. J.*, **60**, 526–8.

Davis, A., Vickerson, F., Worsley, G., Mindorff, L.C., Kazim, F. & Levison, H. (1984) Determination of dose–response relationship for ipratropium in asthmatic children. *J. Pediatr.*, **105**, 1002–5.

Dolovich, M.B., Sanchis, J., Rossman, C. & Newhouse, M.T. (1976) Aerosol penetrance: a sensitive index of peripheral airways obstruction. *J. Appl. Physiol.*, **40**, 468–71.

Douglas, N.J., Davidson, I., Sudlow, M.F. & Flenley, D.C. (1979) Bronchodilatation and the site of airway resistance in severe chronic bronchitis. *Thorax*, **34**, 51–6.

Field, G.B. (1967) The effects of posture, oxygen, isoproterenol, and atropine on ventilation–perfusion relationships in the lung in asthma. *Clin. Sci.*, **32**, 279–88.

Foster, W.M. & Bergofsky, E.H. (1986) Airway mucus membrane: effects of beta-adrenergic and anticholinergic stimulation. *Am. J. Med.*, **81** (Suppl. 5A), 28–35.

Francis, R.A., Thomson, M.L., Pavia, D. & Douglas, R.B. (1977) Ipratropium bromide: mucociliary clearance rate and airway resistance in normal subjects. *Brit. J. Dis. Chest*, **71**, 173–8.

Freeman, J. & Landau, L.I. (1989) The effects of ipratropium bromide and fenoterol nebulizer solutions in children with asthma. *Clin. Pediatr.*, **28**, 556–60.

Friberg, S. & Graff-Lonnevig, V. (1989) Ipratropium bromide (Atrovent) in childhood asthma: a cumulative dose–response study. *Ann. Allergy*, **62**, 131–4.

Fryer, A.D. & Jacoby, D.B. (1991) Parainfluenza virus infection damages inhibitory M2-muscarinic receptors on pulmonary parasympathetic nerves in the guinea pig. *Brit. J. Pharmacol.*, **102**, 267–71.

Fryer, A.D. & Jacoby, D.B. (1993) Effect of inflammatory cell mediators on M2 muscarinic receptors in the lungs. *Life Sci.*, **52**, 529–36.

Fryer, A.D., Fakahany, E.E. & Jacoby, D.B. (1990) Parainfluenza virus type I reduces the affinity of agonists for muscarinic receptors in guinea-pig lung and heart. *Eur. J. Pharmacol.*, **181**, 51–8.

Gal, T.J. & Suratt, P.M. (1981) Atropine and glycopyrrolate effects on lung mechanics in normal man. *Anesth. Analg.*, **60**, 85–90.

Gandevia, B. (1975) Historical review of the use of parasympatholytic agents in the treatment of respiratory disorders. *Postgrad. Med. J.*, **51** (Suppl. 7), 13–20.

Ghafouri, M.A., Patil, K.D. & Kass, I. (1984) Sputum changes associated with use of ipratropium bromide. *Chest*, **86**, 387–93.

Gomm, S.A., Keaney, N.P., Hunt, L.P., Allen, S.C. & Stretton, T.B. (1933) Dose–response comparison of ipratropium bromide from a metered-dose inhaler and by jet nebulization. *Thorax*, **38**, 297–301.

Grieco, M.H. & Pierson, R.N. Jr (1971) Mechanism of bronchoconstriction due to beta-adrenergic blockade. *J. Allergy Clin. Immunol.*, **48**, 143–52.

Gross, N.J. (1975) Sch 1000: a new anticholinergic bronchodilator. *Am. Rev. Resp. Dis.*, **112**, 823–8.

Gross, N.J. (1986) COPD, a disease of reversible airways obstruction. *Am. Rev. Resp. Dis.*, **133**, 725–6.

Gross, N.J. (1988a) Ipratropium bromide. *New Engl. J. Med.*, **319**, 486–94.

Gross, N.J. (1988b) Cholinergic control. In: *Asthma: Basic Mechanisms and Clinical Management* (eds P.J. Barnes, I.W. Rodger & N.C. Thomson), pp. 381–93. Academic Press, New York.

Gross, N.J. (1992) Anticholinergic bronchodilators. In: *Asthma: Basic Mechanisms and Clinical Management*, 2nd edn. (eds P.J. Bames, I.W. Roger & N.C. Thomson), pp. 555–67. Academic Press, New York.

Gross, N.J. & Bankwala, Z. (1987) Effects of an anticholinergic bronchodilator on arterial blood gases of hypoxemic patients with chronic obstructive pulmonary disease. *Am. Rev. Resp. Dis.*, **136**, 1091–4.

Gross, N.J. & Barnes, P.J. (1988) A short tour around the muscarinic receptor. *Am. Rev. Resp. Dis.*, **138**, 765–7.

Gross, N.J. & Skorodin, M.S. (1984a) Anticholinergic, antimuscarinic bronchodilators. *Am. Rev. Resp. Dis.*, **129**, 856–70.

Gross, N.J. & Skorodin, M.S. (1984b) Role of the parasympathetic in airway obstruction due to emphysema. *New Engl. J. Med.*, **311**, 421–5.

Gross, N.J. & Skorodin, M.S. (1987) Anticholinergic agents. In: *Drug Therapy for Asthma: Research and Clinical Practice* (eds J.W. Jenne & S. Murphy), pp. 615–68. Marcel Dekker, New York.

Gross, N.J., Co, E. & Skorodin, M.S. (1989a) Cholinergic bronchomotor tone in COPD: estimates of its amount in comparison to normal. *Chest*, **96**, 984–7.

Gross, N.J., Petty, T.L., Friedman, M., Skorodin, M.S., Silvers, G.W & Donohue, J.F. (1989b) Dose–response to ipratropium nebulized solution in COPD, a 3-center study. *Am. Rev. Resp. Dis.*, **139**, 1188–91.

Groth, M.L., Langenback, E.G. & Foster, W.M. (1991) Influence of inhaled atropine on lung mucociliary function in humans. *Am. Rev. Resp. Dis.*, **144**, 1042–7.

Hargreave, F.E., Dolovich, J. & Newhouse, M.T. (1990) The assessment and treatment of asthma: a conference report. *J. Allergy Clin. Immunol.*, **85**, 1098–112.

Herschman, Z.J., Silverstein, J., Blumberg, G. & Lehrfield, A. (1991) Central nervous system toxicity from nebulized atropine sulfate. *J. Toxicol. Clin. Toxicol.*, **29**, 273–7.

Hey, V.M.F., Phillips, K. & Woods, I. (1983) Pethidine, atropine, metaclopramide and the lower oesophageal sphincter. *Anaesthesia*, **38**, 650–3.

Ind, P.W., Dixon, C.M., Fuller, R.W. & Barnes, P.J. (1989) Anticholinergic blockade of beta-blocker-induced bronchoconstriction. *Am. Rev. Resp. Dis.*, **139**, 1390–4.

Ingram, R.H., Wellman, J.J., McFadden, E.R. & Mead, J. (1977) Relative contribution of large and small airways to flow limitation in normal subjects before and after atropine and isoproterenol. *J. Clin. Invest.*, **59**, 696–703.

Jacoby, D.B., Gleich, G.J. & Fryer, A.D. (1993) Human eosinophil major basic protein is an endogenous allosteric antagonist at the inhibitory muscarinic M2 receptor. *J. Clin. Invest.*, **91**, 1314–18.

Jolobe, O.M.P. (1984) Asthma versus non-specific reversible airflow obstruction, clinical features and responsiveness to anticholinergic drugs. *Respiration*, **45**, 237–42.

Kalra, L. & Bone, M. (1988) The effect of nebulized bonchodilator therapy on intraocular pressure in patients with glaucoma. *Chest*, **93**, 739–41.

Karpel, J.P. (1991) Bronchodilator responses to anticholinergic and beta-adrenergic agents in acute and stable COPD. *Chest*, **99**, 871–6.

Karpel, J.P., Pesin, J., Greenberg, D. & Gentry, E. (1990) A comparison of the effects of ipratropium bromide and metaproterenol sulfate in acute exacerbations of COPD. *Chest*, **98**, 835–9.

Leak, A. & O'Connor, T. (1988) High dose ipratropium, is it safe? *Practitioner*, **232**, 9–10.

Lefcoe, N.M., Toogood, J.H., Blennerhassett, G., Baskerville, J. & Patterson, N.A.M. (1982) The addition of an aerosol anticholinergic to an oral beta agonist plus theophylline in asthma and bronchitis: a double-blind single dose study. *Chest*, **82**, 300–5.

Lilly, C.M., Stamler, J.S., Gaston, B., Meckel, C., Loscalzo, J. & Drazen, J.M. (1993) Modulation of vasoactive intestinal peptide pulmonary relaxation by NO in tracheally perfused guinea pig lungs. *Am. J. Physiol.*, **265**, L410–15.

Lloberes, P., Ramis, L., Montserrat, J.M., Serra, J., Campistol, J. & Picado, C. (1988) Effect of 3 different bronchodilators during an exacerbation of chronic obstructive pulmonary disease. *Eur. Resp. J.*, **1**, 536–9.

Lopez-Vidriero, M.T., Costello, J., Clark, T.J.H., Das, I., Keal, E.E. & Reid, L. (1975) Effect of atropine on sputum production. *Thorax*, **30**, 543–7.

McFadden, E.R. Jr, Luparello, T., Lyons, H.A. & Bleecker, E. (1969) The mechanism of action of suggestion in the induction of acute asthma attacks. *J. Psychosom. Med.*, **31**, 134–43.

Macklem, P.T. & Engel, L.A. (1975) The physiological implications of airways smooth muscle constriction. *Postgrad. Med. J.*, **51** (Suppl. 7), 45–50.

Mann, J.S., Howarth, P.H. & Holgate, S.T. (1984) Bronchoconstriction induced by ipratropium bromide in asthma: relation to hypotonicity. *Brit. Med. J.*, **289**, 469.

Mann, N.P. & Hiller, E.J. (1982) Ipratropium bromide in children with asthma. *Thorax*, **37**, 72–4.

Marlin, G.E., Bush, D.E. & Berend, N. (1978) Comparison of ipratropium bromide and fenoterol in asthma and chronic bronchitis. *Brit. J. Pharmacol.*, **6**, 547–9.

Meltzer, E.O. (1991) Anticholinergic treatment of nasal disorders. *Immunol. Allergy Clin. N. Am.*, **11**, 31–44.

Miszkiel, K.A., Beasley, R. & Holgate, S.T. (1988) The influence of ipratropium bromide and sodium cromoglycate on benzalkonium-induced bronchoconstriction in asthma. *Brit. J. Clin. Pharmacol.*, **26**, 295–301.

Molkenboer, J.F.W.M. & Lardenoye, J.G. (1979) The effect of Atrovent on micturition function, double-blind cross-over study. *Scand. J. Resp. Dis.*, **103** (Suppl.), 154–8.

Mulherin, D. & Fitzgerald, M.X. (1990) Meconium ileus equivalent in association with nebulized ipratropium bromide in cystic fibrosis. *Lancet*, **335**, 552.

Nield, J.E. & Cameron, I.R. (1985) Bronchoconstriction in response to suggestion, its prevention by an inhaled anticholinergic agent. *Brit. Med. J.*, **290**, 674.

O'Callaghan, C., Milner, A.D. & Swarbrick A. (1989) Paradoxical bronchoconstriction in wheezing infants after nebulized preservative free iso-osmolar ipratropium bromide. *Brit. Med. J.*, **299**, 1433–4.

O'Driscoll, B.R., Taylor, R.J., Horsley, M.G., Chambers, D.K. & Bernstein, A. (1989) Nebulized salbutamol with and without ipratropium bromide in acute airflow obstruction. *Lancet*, **i**, 1418–20.

Patel, K.R. & Tullett, W.M. (1983) Bronchoconstriction in response to ipratropium bromide. *Brit. Med. J.*, **286**, 1318.

Pavia, D., Thomson, M.L., Clark, S.W. & Shannon, H.S. (1977) Effect of lung function and mode of inhalation on penetration of aerosol into the human lung. *Thorax*, **32**, 194–7.

Pavia, D., Bateman, J.R., Sheahan, N.F. & Clarke, S.W. (1980) Clearance of lung secretions in patients with chronic bronchitis: effect of terbutaline and ipratropium bromide aerosols. *Eur. J. Resp. Dis.*, **61**, 245–53.

Pavia, D., Lopez-Vidriero, M.T., Agnew, J.E., Taylor, R.G., Eyre-Brook, A. & Lawton, W.A. (1989) Effect of four-week treatment with oxitropium on lung mucociliary clearance in patients with chronic bronchitis or asthma. *Respiration*, **55**, 33–43.

Rafferty, P., Beasley, R. & Holgate, S.T. (1988) Comparison of the efficacy of preservative free ipratropium bromide and Atrovent nebulizer solution. *Thorax*, **43**, 446–50.

Rebuck, A.S. & Marcus, H.I. (1979) SCH 1000 in psychogenic asthma. *Scand. J. Resp. Dis.*, **103** (Suppl.), 186–91.

Rebuck, A.S., Chapman, K.R., Abboud, R. *et al.* (1987) Nebulized anticholinergic and sympathomimetic treatment of asthma and chronic obstructive airways disease in the emergency room. *Am. J. Med.*, **82**, 59–64.

Reisman, J., Galdes-Sebaldt, M., Kazim, F., Canny, G. & Levison, H. (1988) Frequent administration by inhalation of salbutamol and ipratropium bromide in the initial management of severe acute asthma in children. *J. Allergy Clin. Immunol.*, **81**, 16–20.

Reynolds, J.E.F. (1989) Antimuscarinic agents. In: *The Extra Pharmacopoeia*, 29th edn. (ed. Martindale), pp. 522–45. Pharmaceutical Press, London.

Richardson, J.B. (1979) Nerve supply to the lungs. *Am. Rev. Resp. Dis.*, **119**, 785–802.

Ruffin, R.E., Fitzgerald, J.D. & Rebuck, A.S. (1977) A comparison of the bronchodilator activity of Sch1000 and salbutamol. *J. Allergy Clin. Immunol.*, **59**, 136–41.

Ruffin, R.E., Wolff, R.K., Dolovich, M.B., Rossman, C.M., Fitzgerald, J.D. & Newhouse, M.T. (1978) Aerosol therapy with Sch 1000: short-term mucociliary clearance in normal and bronchitic subjects and toxicology in normal subjects. *Chest*, **73**, 510–506.

Sackner, M.A., Chapman, G.A. & Dougherty, R.D. (1977a) Effects of nebulized ipratropium bromide and atropine sulfate on tracheal mucus velocity and lung mechanics in anesthetized dogs. *Respiration*, **34**, 181–5.

Sackner, M.A., Friedman, M., Silva, G. & Fernandez, R. (1977b) The pulmonary hemodynamic effects of aerosols of isoproterenol and ipratropium in normal subjects and patients with reversible airways obstruction. *Am. Rev. Resp. Dis.*, **116**, 1013–22.

Samaniego, F. & Newman, L.S. (1986) Migratory anisocoria: a novel clinical entity. *Am. Rev. Resp. Dis.*, **143**, 844.

Scheuffler, G. (1975) Ophthalmotonometry, pupil diameter and visual accommodation following repeated administration of Sch1000 MDI in patients with glaucoma. *Postgrad. Med. J.*, **51** (Suppl. 7), 132 [abstract].

Shah, P., Dhurjon, L., Metcalfe, T. & Gibson, J.M. (1992) Acute angle closure glaucoma associated with nebulized ipratropium bromide and salbutamol. *Brit. Med. J.*, **304**, 40–1.

Skorodin, M.S., Gross, N.J., Moritz, T. *et al.* (1986) Oxitropium bromide: a new anticholinergic bronchodilator. *Ann. Allergy*, **56**, 229–32.

Sly, P.D., Landau, L.I. & Olinsky, A. (1987) Failure of ipratropium bromide to modify diurnal variation of asthma in asthmatic children. *Thorax*, **42**, 357–60.

Sterling, G.M. (1987) Anticholinergic therapy in chronic asthma. *Postgrad. Med. J.*, **63** (Suppl. 1), 41–6.

Storms, W.W., DoPico, G.A. & Reed, C.E. (1975) Aerosol Sch 1000: an anticholinergic bronchodilator. *Am. Rev. Resp. Dis.*, **111**, 419–22.

Storr, J. & Lenney, W. (1986) Nebulized ipratropium and salbutamol in asthma. *Arch. Dis. Child.*, **61**, 602–3.

Sturgess, J. & Reid, L. (1972) An organ culture study of the effect of drugs on the secretory activity of the human bronchial submucosal gland. *Clin. Sci.*, **43**, 533–43.

Tashkin, D.P., Ashutosh, K., Bleecker, E. *et al.* (1986) Comparison of the anticholinergic ipratropium bromide with metaproterenol in chronic obstructive pulmonary disease, a 90-day multicenter study. *Am. J. Med.*, **81** (Suppl. 5A), 81–6.

Thumm, H.W. (1975) Ophthalmic effects of high doses of Sch 1000 MDI in healthy volunteers and patients with glaucoma. *Postgrad. Med. J.*, **51** (Suppl. 7), 132–3 [abstract].

Ullah, M.I., Newman, G.B. & Saunders, K.B. (1981) Influence of age on ipratropium and salbutamol in asthma. *Thorax*, **36**, 523–9.

Walker, F.B., Kaiser, D.L., Kowal, M.B. & Suratt, P.M. (1987) Prolonged effect of inhaled glycopyrrolate in asthma. *Chest*, **91**, 49–51.

Wanner, A. (1986) Effect of ipratropium on airway mucociliary function. *Am. J. Med.*, **81** (Suppl. 5A), 23–7.

Ward, J.K., Belvisi, M.G., Fox, A.J. *et al.* (1993) Modulation of cholinergic neural bronchoconstriction by endogenous nitric oxide and vasoactive intestinal peptide in human airways *in vitro*. *J. Clin. Invest.*, **92**, 736–42.

Ward, M.J. (1993) The role of anticholinergic agents in acute asthma. In: *Anticholinergic Therapy in Obstructive Airways Disease* (ed. N.J. Gross), pp. 155–62. Franklin Scientific Publications, London.

Warner, J.O., Getz, M., Landau, L.I. *et al.* (1989) Management of asthma: a consensus statement. *Arch. Dis. Child.*, **64**, 1065–79.

Weber, R.W., Petty, T.L. & Nelson, H.S. (1979) Aerosolized terbutaline in asthmatics: comparison of dosage strength, schedule, and method of administration. *J. Allergy Clin. Immunol.*, **63**, 116–21.

Wess, J. (1993) Molecular basis of muscarinic acetylcholine receptor function. *Trends Pharmacol. Sci.*, **141**, 308–13.

Yeager, H. Jr, Weinberg, R.M., Kaufman, L.V. & Katz, S. (1976) Asthma: comparative bronchodilator effects of ipratropium bromide and isoproterenol. *J. Clin. Pharmacol.*, **16**, 198–204.

Yeates, D.B., Aspin, N., Levison, H., Jones, M.T. & Bryan, A.C. (1975) Mucociliary tracheal transport rates in man. *J. Appl. Physiol.*, **39**, 487–95.

Yuksel, B., Greenough, A. & Green, S. (1991) Paradoxical response to nebulized ipratropium bromide in preterm infants asymptomatic at follow up. *Resp. Med.*, **85**, 189–94.

CHAPTER 34

Potassium Channel Openers as Anti-Asthma Drugs

R.C. Small & R.W. Foster

Introduction

The agonists at β-adrenoceptors (β-agonists) currently form the mainstay of bronchodilator therapy in the treatment of bronchial asthma. There is a wealth of evidence to suggest that these substances promote the opening of large-conductance, Ca^{2+}-dependent K^+ channels (BK_{Ca}) in the plasmalemma of airway smooth muscle cells. However, the relaxant actions of the β-agonists do not crucially depend on BK_{Ca} channel opening (Small *et al.*, 1993; Black *et al.*, 1994) and this review will focus on a group of agents that open a plasmalemmal, adenosine triphosphate (ATP)-sensitive K^+ channel (K_{ATP}; see below) of relatively small unitary conductance.

Cromakalim may be regarded as the type substance of this latter group of agents and they have collectively come to be known as the K^+ channel openers (KCOs). They may be classified into benzopyran, cyanoguanidine, pyridine or thioformamide families (Edwards & Weston, 1994). The benzopyran derivatives include cromakalim (BRL 34915), its active enantiomer, levcromakalim (BRL 38227), BRL 55834, SDZ PCO 400, Ro 31-6930, bimakalim, rilmakalim (HOE 234), KC 128 and KC 399. Pinacidil is a member of the cyanoguanidine family. The pyridine family includes nicorandil and YM 934. The thioformamide family includes RP 49356 and its active enantiomer, aprikalim (Fig. 34.1).

The therapeutic potential of the KCOs has yet to become fully clear. However, pinacidil is marketed in Belgium as an antihypertensive agent. It finds similar use in Denmark and Ireland, although, in these two countries, the drug is regarded as being of second-line status. Nicorandil has recently been licensed in the UK for the management of angina pectoris. Other KCO are currently being evaluated as chemotherapy for conditions such as cardiac dysrhythmias, essential hypertension, the irritable bladder syndrome and bronchial asthma.

The action of cromakalim-like drugs on airway smooth-muscle cells

KCOs suppress the spontaneous tone of guinea pig trachealis (Allen *et al.*, 1986; Bray *et al.*, 1987; Arch *et al.*, 1988; Nielsen-Kudsk *et al.*, 1988; Paciorek *et al.*, 1990; Berry *et al.*, 1991; Raeburn & Brown, 1991; Chapman *et al.*, 1992; Englert *et al.*, 1992; Small *et al.*, 1992a,b; Imagama *et al.*, 1993) and human bronchial smooth muscle (Taylor *et al.*, 1988; Black *et al.*, 1990, 1994; Chapman *et al.*, 1992; Imagama *et al.*, 1993; Miura *et al.*, 1993), although their maximal effects may be only 60–100% of those of isoprenaline or theophylline. The KCOs are also effective against the contraction of airway smooth muscle induced by exogenous spasmogens but, in this case, the relaxant potency of the KCOs is reduced to an extent that depends upon the concentration and identity of the spasmogen used (Allen *et al.*, 1986; Taylor *et al.*, 1988, 1992a; Black *et al.*, 1990; Raeburn & Brown, 1991; Chapman *et al.*, 1992; Englert *et al.*, 1992; Miura *et al.*, 1993).

Several observations suggest that the relaxant action of the cromakalim-like drugs in airway smooth muscle is associated with the opening of plasmalemmal K^+ channels. For example, these agents hyperpolarize tracheal and bronchial smooth muscle so that the membrane potential moves towards the potassium equilibrium potential (Allen *et al.*, 1986; Murray *et al.*, 1989; Berry *et al.*, 1991; Longmore *et al.*, 1991; Shieh *et al.*, 1992; Small *et al.*,

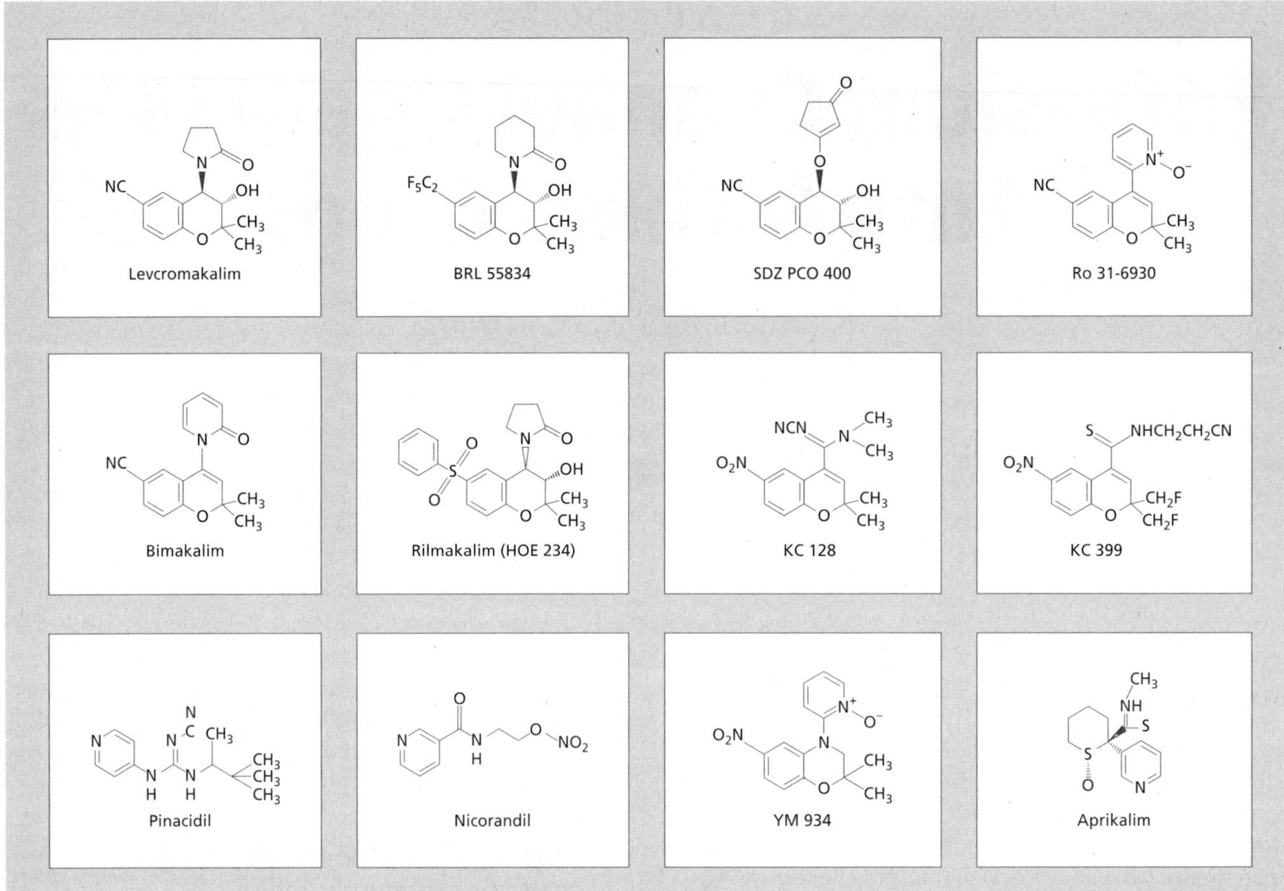

Fig. 34.1 The chemical structures of some potassium channel openers.

1992a,b; Kamei *et al.*, 1994a,b). The cromakalim-like drugs also promote the efflux of $^{42}K^+$ or $^{86}Rb^+$ (a marker for the movement of K^+) from airway smooth muscle cells preloaded with these radiotracers (Allen *et al.*, 1986; Foster, 1989; Gater, 1989; Berry *et al.*, 1992; Foster *et al.*, 1992; Small *et al.*, 1992a; Buckle *et al.*, 1993; Kamei *et al.*, 1994b). Furthermore, the cromakalim-like drugs can be antagonized by agents such as 4-aminopyridine, bretylium, glibenclamide, guanethidine, phentolamine, procaine and tetraethylammonium (Allen *et al.*, 1986; Gater, 1989; Murray *et al.*, 1989; McPherson & Angus, 1990; Nielsen-Kudsk *et al.*, 1990; Berry *et al.*, 1991, 1992; Longmore *et al.*, 1991; Raeburn & Brown, 1991; Bang & Nielsen-Kudsk, 1992; Small *et al.*, 1992a; Buckle *et al.*, 1993; Imagama *et al.*, 1993; Miura *et al.*, 1993; Kamei *et al.*, 1994a,b). Each of these antagonists is suspected, or known, to inhibit the opening of plasmalemmal K^+ channels.

The failure of KCOs to suppress contraction of airway smooth muscle induced by a K^+-rich (>40 mmol/l) medium (Allen *et al.*, 1986; Bray *et al.*, 1987; Taylor *et al.*, 1988; Gater, 1989; Raeburn & Brown, 1991; Small *et al.*, 1992b) has also been assumed to indicate that the relaxant action of these agents depends upon K^+ channel opening. This assumption is based on the reasoning that, when $[K^+]_o$ is raised above 40 mmol/l, the potassium equilibrium potential assumes a reduced value very close to the membrane potential of the cell. In this circumstance K^+ channel opening will result in so little cellular hyperpolarization that the opening of L-type voltage-dependent Ca^{2+} channels (VOCs) will not be inhibited. In the presence of the K^+-rich medium, therefore, cromakalim-like drugs cannot inhibit Ca^{2+} influx through the VOCs. However, since the K^+-rich medium itself promotes Ca^{2+} influx, it is likely to cause functional antagonism of many different types of relaxant drug. Recent data (Cook *et al.*, 1995; Fig. 34.2) suggest that, in identifying drugs whose action depends on K^+ channel opening, the discriminatory power of the K^+-rich medium can be increased by the addition of an inhibitor of VOCs, such as nifedipine.

Patch clamp experimentation has shown that glibenclamide and phentolamine both inhibit the K_{ATP} of the

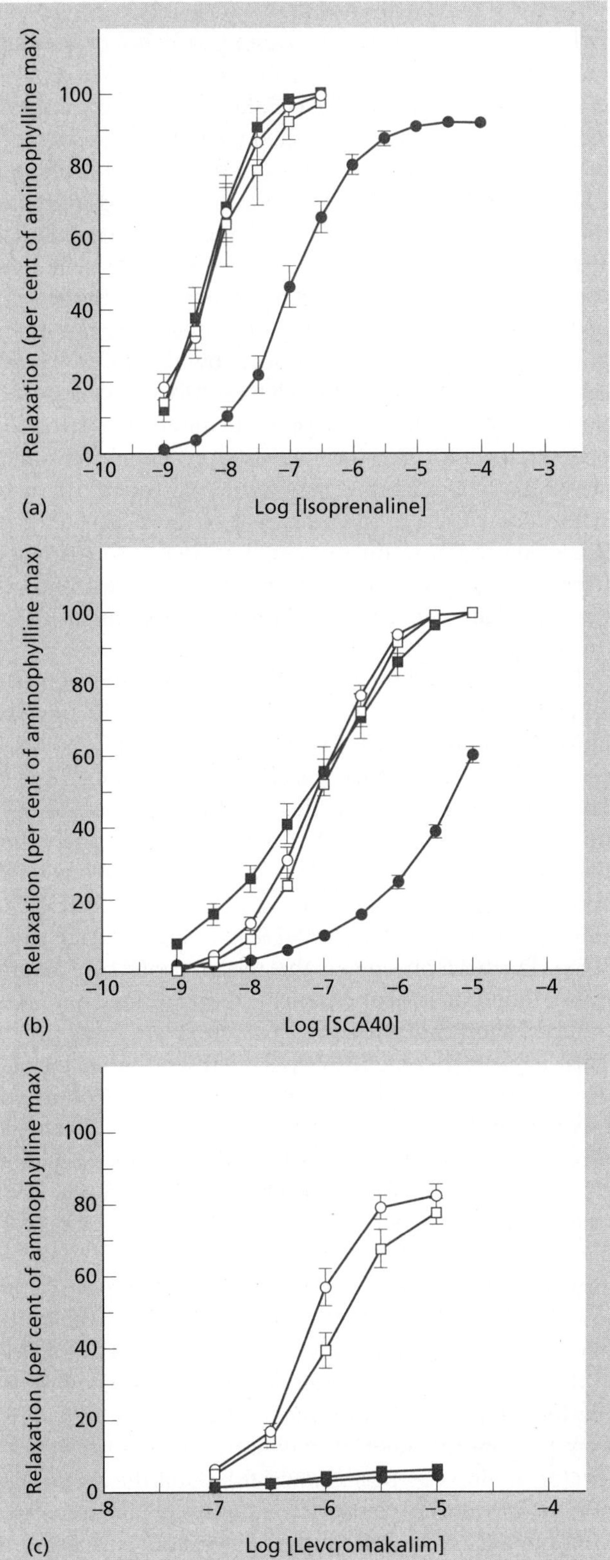

pancreatic β-cell (Schmid-Antomarchi *et al.*, 1987; Sturgess *et al.*, 1988; Plant & Henquin, 1990). Since glibenclamide and phentolamine each selectively inhibit the relaxant actions of KCOs in smooth muscle, the belief has grown that K_{ATP} is expressed in the smooth-muscle cell membrane and represents the site of the relaxant action of the KCOs. However, the concentration of glibenclamide required to antagonize KCOs acting on smooth muscle is much greater than that required to inhibit K_{ATP} in the pancreatic β-cell. It therefore seems likely that K_{ATP} of smooth muscle is analogous to, but not identical with, that seen in insulin-secreting cells.

Preliminary patch clamp studies (Collier *et al.*, 1991) have shown that K_{ATP} of airway smooth muscle may be of relatively small (30–39 pS) conductance. The opening of the channel is only weakly voltage dependent and the open-state probability is normally low (less than 0.2). Channel opening is promoted by levcromakalim and is inhibited either by glibenclamide or by the application of ATP (2 mmol/l) to the inner surface of the plasmalemmal patch.

Hitherto, the assumption has often been made that the opening of K_{ATP} in smooth muscle, as in pancreatic β-cells, is primarily regulated by the cytosolic concentration of ATP ($[ATP]_i$), an increase in $[ATP]_i$ promoting channel closure. However, recent studies in vascular smooth muscle (Beech *et al.*, 1993; Zhang & Bolton, 1995) suggest that the opening of this channel is more importantly controlled by nucleoside diphosphates, such as uridine diphosphate and guanidine diphosphate. These nucleoside diphosphates have been shown not only to be necessary for channel opening to occur but also to exert a permissive role in the action of ATP in promoting channel closure (Beech *et al.*, 1993).

Patch clamp studies of vascular smooth muscle and insulinoma cells (Edwards & Weston, 1993; Edwards *et al.*, 1993; Ibbotson *et al.*, 1993) led Weston and coworkers to suggest that K_{ATP} may not be a discrete type of channel in its own right but may simply represent a dephosphory-

Fig. 34.2 Guinea pig isolated trachealis muscle: the effects of nifedipine (1 μmol/l) on the ability of an isosmolar K^+-rich (80 mmol/l) medium to inhibit the relaxant actions of isoprenaline, SCA40 and levcromakalim. Abscissae: $\log_{10}$ molar concentration of isoprenaline (A), SCA40 (B) or levcromakalim (C). Ordinates: relaxation expressed as a percentage of the maximal relaxation induced by aminophylline. In each panel, (○) indicates the log concentration–effect curve for the relaxant as observed in normal Krebs' solution, (●) the curve obtained in K^+-rich (80 mmol/l) Krebs' solution, (□) the curve obtained in the presence of nifedipine (1 μmol/l) and (■) the curve obtained in the presence of a combination of the K^+-rich (80 mmol/l) medium and nifedipine (1 μmol/l). Data points are the means of values from at least six tissues. Vertical lines show standard error (SE) mean. (From Cook *et al.* (1995) by kind permission of the *British Journal of Pharmacology*.)

lated state of the delayed rectifier channel (K_{dr}). This suggestion was prompted by the observation that the unitary conductance of K_{ATP} is similar to that of K_{dr}. Furthermore, dephosphorylating conditions or exposure to KCOs evokes a decrease in current carried by K_{dr} that parallels the increase in current presumed to be carried by K_{ATP}.

Irrespective of whether K_{ATP} is a dephosphorylated version of K_{dr} or a discrete entity, its importance to the physiology of the airway smooth muscle cell remains to be clarified. If it can be assumed that glibenclamide and phentolamine are inhibitors of K_{ATP}, then the failure of these two agents significantly to depolarize guinea pig trachealis muscle (Murray *et al.*, 1989) suggests that few of the plasmalemmal K_{ATP} channels are open under resting conditions. Furthermore, the failure of these two putative inhibitors of K_{ATP} to convert the spontaneous electrical slow waves of guinea pig trachealis muscle into regenerative action potentials (Murray *et al.*, 1989) suggests that K_{ATP} does not exert a powerful regulatory effect on the changes in plasmalemmal Ca^{2+} conductance that are assumed to underlie the depolarizing phase of the slow wave. Furthermore, in guinea pig isolated trachealis muscle, glibenclamide does not potentiate carbachol, histamine or KCl (Isaac & Small, 1994). This indicates that, under normal conditions, K_{ATP} does not act to modulate the sensitivity or responsiveness of airway smooth muscle to spasmogenic substances.

Role of plasmalemmal K^+ channel opening in mediating the relaxant effects of KCO acting on airway smooth muscle

The tension generated by an airway smooth-muscle cell is related, albeit in a complex way, to the cytosolic concentration of free Ca^{2+} ($[Ca^{2+}]_i$) (Rodger & Small, 1991). In general terms, however, a decrease in $[Ca^{2+}]_i$ leads to decreased tension development. That cromakalim can lower $[Ca^{2+}]_i$ in airway smooth muscle has been demonstrated by Shieh *et al.* (1992). These workers measured $[Ca^{2+}]_i$ in porcine trachealis muscle by using the fluorophore fura-2. They demonstrated that cromakalim (10 μmol/l) was able to reduce the early, transient rise in $[Ca^{2+}]_i$ induced by a low (0.1 μmol/l) concentration of acetylcholine. However, no such effect was observed at higher concentrations of the muscarinic agonist. The secondary, smaller, but more sustained rise in $[Ca^{2+}]_i$ induced by acetylcholine was also reduced by cromakalim and, here, the KCO was effective against a much broader range of acetylcholine concentrations. Shieh *et al.* (1992) attributed these cromakalim-induced changes in $[Ca^{2+}]_i$ to the ability of the KCO to evoke plasmalemmal hyperpolarization.

The cellular hyperpolarization induced by a KCO might reduce $[Ca^{2+}]_i$, and thereby evoke relaxation, in several different ways. As discussed above, membrane hyperpolarization would inhibit the opening of VOCs in the plasmalemma and hence reduce the cellular influx of Ca^{2+} through such channels. The cellular loss of K^+ induced by the KCO would also be expected to stimulate the activity of plasmalemmal Na^+/K^+ adenosine triphosphatase (ATPase). The activity of this enzyme is linked to that of the plasmalemmal Ca^{2+}/Na^+ exchanger (Rodger & Small, 1991). However, the activity of the Ca^{2+}/Na^+ exchanger would not only be stimulated by an increase in the activity of Na^+/K^+ ATPase but also, more directly, by the membrane hyperpolarization induced by the KCO. Hence there are two pathways by which a KCO may stimulate the Ca^{2+}/Na^+ exchanger to promote the cellular extrusion of Ca^{2+}. In addition, the increased potential difference across the cell membrane may result in greater binding of intracellular Ca^{2+} to the inner leaf of the plasmalemma. Reduced cellular influx of Ca^{2+}, increased Ca^{2+} extrusion from the cell and increased intracellular sequestration of Ca^{2+} could all therefore contribute to a reduction in $[Ca^{2+}]_i$ caused by a KCO (Quast, 1993).

The roles played by each of these mechanisms in mediating the relaxant actions of the KCOs is still unclear. However, inhibition of Ca^{2+} influx through L-type VOC cannot be the primary mechanism of KCO-induced relaxation. In contrast to the KCOs, inhibitors of Ca^{2+} influx through L-type VOCs (e.g. nifedipine and verapamil) have relatively little relaxant effect against the spontaneous tone of guinea pig trachealis (Foster *et al.*, 1984; Ahmed *et al.*, 1985; Small & Foster, 1986; Arch *et al.*, 1988). Furthermore, when the relaxant effect of a Ca^{2+} influx inhibitor is near-maximal, the addition of a KCO induces significant further relaxation (Black *et al.*, 1990). This suggests that the KCOs induce relaxation by mechanisms additional to the inhibition of Ca^{2+} influx through L-type VOCs.

Several groups of workers (Allen *et al.*, 1986; Taylor *et al.*, 1988, 1992a; Black *et al.*, 1990; Raeburn & Brown, 1991; Chapman *et al.*, 1992; Englert *et al.*, 1992; Miura *et al.*, 1993) have shown that KCOs can reduce the contraction of airway smooth muscle evoked by agonists that use an intracellular rather than an extracellular source of activator Ca^{2+}. There is some evidence to suggest that this action of the KCOs may reflect their ability to interfere with the production of inositol phosphate second messengers. For example, pretreatment of bovine trachealis muscle with levcromakalim has been shown to inhibit the accumulation of [^{3}H]-inositol phosphate induced by histamine and low (1 μmol/l) concentrations of carbachol. Furthermore, the inhibitory effect of levcromakalim against histamine-induced [^{3}H]-inositol phosphate accumulation was ablated when $[K^+]_o$ was raised to 65 mmol/l (Challiss *et al.*, 1992). This is consistent with the notion that levcromakalim-induced hyperpolarization, by reducing $[Ca^{2+}]_i$, inhibits phosphoinositidase C, an enzyme whose activity is known to be Ca^{2+}-dependent. When the activity of phosphoinositidase C falls, so does the synthesis of inositol 1,4,5-trisphosphate (IP_3) and *sn*-1,2-diacylglycerol (DAG). Reduced production of IP_3 would reduce agonist-induced Ca^{2+} release from the endoplasmic reticulum and may help to explain the ability of KCOs to inhibit contraction of airway smooth muscle induced by agents utilizing an intracellular source of activator Ca^{2+}. Furthermore, reduced production of DAG would reduce the Ca^{2+} sensitivity of the contractile proteins (Rodger & Small, 1991).

Quast (1993) has proposed that the smooth-muscle relaxant actions of the KCOs are not entirely explicable in terms of their ability to promote plasmalemmal K^+ channel opening and, hence, cellular hyperpolarization. The results of several studies on airway smooth muscle lend weight to this proposal. For example, Foster *et al.*, (1992) performed experiments with guinea pig trachealis muscle in which the K^+ content of the physiological salt solution was entirely replaced by Rb^+. The Rb^+-containing medium prevented cromakalim from promoting $^{42}K^+$ or $^{43}K^+$ efflux from tissue preloaded with the radiotracer, suggesting that the KCO was no longer able to promote the opening of plasmalemmal K^+ channels. Despite this, cromakalim retained some relaxant activity. The relaxant response to cromakalim in the Rb^+-containing medium was smaller and quite transient compared with that observed in the K^+-containing medium. However, this relaxant response was inhibited by glibenclamide. These findings could indicate that a part of cromakalim's relaxant action is independent of membrane hyperpolarization. The studies of Chopra *et al.* (1992) using digitonin-permeabilized rabbit trachealis muscle lend support to this idea. Chopra *et al.* (1992) showed that levcromakalim could cause concentration-dependent inhibition of Ca^{2+} uptake by the permeabilized cells, an action inhibited by glibenclamide. This action of levcromakalim on permeabilized airway smooth muscle cells indicates that KCO may inhibit the loading of the intracellular Ca^{2+} store in a manner that is independent of the potential difference across the cell membrane.

The antibronchoconstrictor effects of KCOs observed *in vivo*

The oral or inhalational administration of KCOs to conscious guinea pigs protects against the bronchoconstrictor effects of histamine or (in sensitized animals) ovalbumin (Arch *et al.*, 1988; Ho *et al.*, 1990; Paciorek *et al.*, 1990; Bowring *et al.*, 1991). Similar results have been obtained with the oral, inhalational or intravenous administration of KCO in anaesthetized animals (Arch *et al.*, 1988; De Souza *et al.*, 1989; Ho *et al.*, 1990; Paciorek *et al.*, 1990; Chapman *et al.*, 1992; Englert *et al.*, 1992; Taylor *et al.*, 1992a; Bowring *et al.*, 1993; Buckle *et al.*, 1993). In the latter type of study (where homoeostatic cardiovascular reflexes are inhibited by the anaesthetic agent) the orally or intravenously administered KCO also caused some reduction in blood pressure (Arch *et al.*, 1988; De Souza *et al.*, 1989; Bowring *et al.*, 1993; Buckle *et al.*, 1993). Administered intravenously to anaesthetized dogs, levcromakalim reduced the increases in peripheral airway resistance, evoked either by hypercapnia or by the inhalation of dry air, without attenuating the bronchoconstrictor response to an aerosol of acetylcholine (Lindeman & Freed, 1993). The antibronchoconstrictor action of levcromakalim in this model was inhibited by glibenclamide but, again, was accompanied by a fall in mean arterial blood pressure. However, there is some evidence to suggest that the selectivity of KCO for the airways can be improved by their selective administration. In experiments where levcromakalim was administered by inhalation, bronchodilatation could be achieved at doses that did not reduce mean arterial blood pressure (Bowring *et al.*, 1991).

Working with anaesthetized guinea pigs, Bowring *et al.* (1993) administered levcromakalim and BRL 55834 by intravenous injection. Compared with levcromakalim, the benzopyran BRL 55834 was relatively more potent in producing antibronchoconstrictor effects than in lowering mean arterial blood pressure (Bowring *et al.*, 1993). This seems to indicate that, *in vivo*, BRL 55834 exhibits some selectivity for the airways as opposed to the vascular system.

Does the smooth muscle relaxant effect of the KCO explain their anti-asthma activity?

Williams *et al.* (1990a) showed that an oral dose of 0.25 mg of cromakalim was effective in the treatment of nocturnal asthma. The data of Gill *et al.* (1989) suggest that the peak plasma concentration of levcromakalim (the active enantiomer) following such treatment is about 0.024 μmol/l. This represents the threshold concentration of levcromakalim in producing relaxation of human bronchial smooth muscle *in vitro* (Black *et al.*, 1990, 1994). There may be several explanations for the clinical efficacy of such low concentrations of the active enantiomer of cromakalim. For example, *in vivo*, cromakalim may be selectively distributed to, or accumulated in, airway smooth muscle. The potency of cromakalim as a relaxant of human airway smooth muscle may be greater under *in vivo* conditions than under *in vitro* conditions. Alternatively, it is possible that the anti-asthma action of cromakalim depends not on its direct relaxation of airway smooth muscle but, instead, on an effect on other cell types within the lung. Such cells could include those involved in the expression of neurogenic inflammation or airway hyperreactivity.

Although *in vitro* and *in vivo* studies indicate that cromakalim can inhibit the process of cholinergic neuroeffector transmission in the lung (Hall & Maclagan, 1988; McCaig & De Jonckheere, 1989; Ichinose & Barnes, 1990; Burka *et al.*, 1991), the concentrations or doses of cromakalim required for this effect are similar to those that directly relax airway smooth muscle (Hall & Maclagan, 1988; Ichinose & Barnes, 1990; Burka *et al.*, 1991; Gater *et al.*, 1993). However, Wessler *et al.* (1993) have demonstrated that levcromakalim can inhibit the release of [^{3}H]-acetylcholine from parasympathetic nerves in rat trachea in concentrations below 0.1 μmol/l. This suggests that inhibition of neurotransmitter output can contribute to the action of cromakalim in suppressing cholinergic neuroeffector transmission in the airways.

The KCOs can also inhibit non-adrenergic, non-cholinergic (NANC) excitatory neuroeffector transmission (Ichinose & Barnes, 1990; Lewis & Raeburn, 1990; Burka *et al.*, 1991; Good *et al.*, 1992; Lei *et al.*, 1993; Saitoh *et al.*, 1994). This effect against NANC excitatory neuroeffector transmission in the airways is observed at concentrations or doses slightly lower than those causing relaxation of airway smooth muscle, suggesting that the KCO can act pre-junctionally to inhibit the release of the peptidergic excitatory neurotransmitter. The effect of KCO against cholinergic and NANC excitatory neuroeffector transmission is sensitive to antagonism by glibenclamide (Ichinose & Barnes, 1990; Burka *et al.*, 1991; Good *et al.*, 1992; Lei *et al.*, 1993), suggesting a role for K_{ATP} in modulating transmitter output from nerve fibres.

The activation of NANC excitatory neurones may evoke inflammatory responses in the airways, including promotion of plasma exudation from microvessels. Lei *et al.* (1993) studied the *in vivo* effect of levcromakalim on plasma exudation into guinea pig main bronchus. The plasma exudation was induced by stimuli such as inhalation of cigarette smoke and, after pretreatment of the animals with atropine and propranolol, vagal stimulation. The intravenous administration of levcromakalim inhibited the plasma exudation induced by either of the two stimuli without affecting plasma exudation produced by substance P. These findings led Lei *et al.* (1993) to conclude that inhibition of neural mechanisms promoting plasma exudation could form an important feature of the anti-asthma actions of KCOs of this type.

The mechanisms underlying airway hyperreactivity are poorly understood, but some forms of hyperreactivity seem to have a neurogenic basis. For example, Kristersson *et al.* (1989) have reported that the intravenous injection of preformed immune complexes (bovine gammaglobulin + antibovine gammaglobulin serum) in guinea pigs induces airway hyperreactivity to histamine. This effect is not observed in animals that have been bilaterally vagotomized. Using this animal model, Chapman *et al.* (1992) showed that the intravenous injection of SDZ PCO 400 could suppress airway hyperreactivity to histamine at doses that did not attenuate bronchoconstrictor responses to the same agent in normoreactive, control animals. This could suggest that the site of action of KCO in suppressing airway hyperreactivity is at the level of excitatory neurone terminals rather than the plasmalemma of airway smooth-muscle cells. However, SDZ PCO 400 also suppressed the hyperreactivity of guinea pig airways to bombesin induced by platelet-activating factor (PAF) (Chapman *et al.*, 1992) and YM 934 suppressed PAF-induced hyperreactivity to histamine (Saitoh *et al.*, 1994). In the guinea pig, PAF-induced airway hyperreactivity to bombesin or histamine is known to be independent of vagal integrity (Mazzoni *et al.*, 1985). The importance of neural effects of KCOs in modulating the development of airway hyperreactivity therefore remains unclear.

There is currently little evidence to suggest that KCOs inhibit the release of allergic mediators from mast cells or inhibit allergen-induced leucocyte accumulation in the lung. Nagai *et al.* (1991) found that cromakalim, pinacidil and nicorandil (each in concentration up to 10 μmol/l) were unable to inhibit allergen-induced histamine release from sensitized guinea pig lung tissue. Working with sensitized guinea pigs, Chapman *et al.* (1992) observed that SDZ PCO 400 reduced the bronchospasm induced by an ovalbumin aerosol. However, SDZ PCO 400 did not suppress the spasm of sensitized trachealis muscle evoked by ovalbumin under *in vitro* conditions. These findings led Chapman *et al.* (1992) to suggest that SDZ PCO 400 and other KCOs do not have potent effects in inhibiting the release of allergic mediators from mast cells. Furthermore, the same authors were unable to detect any inhibitory effect of SDZ PCO 400 against ovalbumin-induced accumulation of eosinophils and neutrophils in the airway lumen of sensitized guinea pigs. This may suggest that, in the lung, the KCO do not interfere with the leucocyte accumulation induced by exposure to allergen.

Will the KCO prove to be drugs useful in the treatment of bronchial asthma?

A clinical trial in patients with nocturnal asthma (Williams *et al.*, 1990a) showed that a single oral dose of 0.25 mg or 0.5 mg of cromakalim attenuated the dip in forced expiratory volume in 1 second (FEV_1) measured at 0600 hours the following morning. However, when the dose of cromakalim was raised to 1.5 mg, no significant improvement in the morning value of FEV_1 was observed. The authors of this study suggested that the ineffectiveness of the 1.5 mg dose of cromakalim was due to a high incidence of headache, which prevented the subjects from properly performing the manoeuvre necessary to measure

FEV_1 (Williams *et al.*, 1990a). Similar problems have been encountered in clinical trials of levcromakalim.

In a randomized, double-blind, parallel-group, placebo-controlled study, levcromakalim (0.125–0.75 mg once daily) was given orally for 28 days to patients with reversible bronchoconstriction. A small improvement in FEV_1 was recorded at 4 hours post-dose in the levcromakalim-treated patients but no significant effect was observed 16 hours after the final dose. Thus, in these patients, levcromakalim induced a modest but short-lived improvement in FEV_1. However, a high incidence of headache was reported (Williams, 1992). A further trial of levcromakalim was performed in asthmatic subjects by Kidney *et al.* (1991). In this study, FEV_1 and the concentration of histamine causing a 20% reduction in FEV_1 were measured before and 5 hours after the oral administration of 0.125, 0.25 or 0.5 mg levcromakalim on each of 4 study days. In a separate part of this study, the effects of similar doses of levcromakalim were tested against a bronchoconstrictor challenge with methacholine. The levcromakalim treatment provided no significant protection against histamine- or methacholine-induced bronchospasm, and ingestion of the 0.5 mg dose of levcromakalim was associated with a high incidence of headache. Collectively, these findings suggest that, in the oral dose ranges so far studied, the bronchodilator effects of cromakalim and its active enantiomer are relatively small. Furthermore, the dose range available for inducing bronchodilatation is limited by the incidence of unwanted effects on the cardiovascular system.

The unwanted cardiovascular effects of β-agonist bronchodilators have classically been minimized by their administration by the inhalational rather than the oral route. Can inhalational administration improve the ratio of bronchodilator to vasodilator activity for KCO? Williams *et al.* (1990b) have reported that, in healthy volunteers, cromakalim may be inhaled in doses as high as 1 mg without causing changes in pulse rate or systolic or diastolic blood pressure. However, the commercial development of cromakalim and levcromakalim as anti-asthma chemotherapy has now been abandoned. The same is true of Ro 31-6930 (which entered phase 2 clinical trials as a bronchodilator) and SDZ PCO 400. We are therefore unlikely to learn whether, in asthmatic subjects, these substances would have yielded useful bronchodilator effects by the inhalational route of administration.

This route of administration has, however, been used in a clinical trial of bimakalim (Faurschou *et al.*, 1994). In this prospective, double-blind, placebo-controlled, crossover study the effects of doses (10, 25, 40 and 100 μg cumulatively inhaled) of bimakalim were examined in 12 adult patients with chronic mild to moderate non-allergic asthma. No cardiovascular disturbances were promoted by the 175 μg cumulative dose of bimakalim but nor were any beneficial effects on FEV_1 observed. The reasons for the lack of beneficial effect of bimakalim are unclear. However, it may have been that the doses of bimakalim employed were too small to evoke bronchodilatation or were not adquately delivered to the patients' airways by the nebulization process.

At present, therefore, it is still unclear whether the administration of KCOs by the inhaled route can produce useful bronchodilatation in asthmatic subjects without causing unacceptable vasodilatation. In order to render a KCO clinically useful as a bronchodilator, it may be that the degree of distributional selectivity demanded cannot be achieved by selective administration (inhalation) alone and that reinforcement by other distributional mechanisms of achieving selectivity (e.g. prevention of the escape of active drug from the lung) will be required.

While distributional methods of achieving airway-selective actions of the KCO have not yet been fully explored or exploited, the alternative approach is to develop compounds whose selectivity for the airways has a pharmacodynamic rather than a distributional basis. However, attempts to produce KCOs that, under *in vitro* conditions, selectively relax airway smooth muscle rather than vascular smooth muscle have so far met with only limited success. The benzopyran derivative KC 128 has been reported (Koga *et al.*, 1993) to suppress the spontaneous tone of guinea pig trachea at concentrations much smaller than those required to relax rat aorta precontracted with KCl. At present, it is unclear whether such a potency difference represents true pharmacodynamic selectivity of the compound for airway smooth muscle, an interspecies difference in tissue sensitivity to the KCO or non-equivalence of the background contractile stimuli in the two tissues. In any event, commercial development of this compound (and its analogue KC 399) as an anti-asthma drug has ceased and no data are available to indicate whether it can, in the intact animal, produce bronchodilatation without change in blood pressure or heart rate.

Tested on guinea pig portal vein precontracted with KCl (30 mmol/l), the relaxant potency of BRL 55834 was similar to that observed in guinea pig trachea either under spontaneous tone or under tone induced by one of a variety of different spasmogens (Taylor *et al.*, 1992). This suggests that BRL 55834 does not exhibit pharmacodynamic selectivity for airways as opposed to vascular smooth muscle. As mentioned above, when BRL 55834 was tested in anaesthetized guinea pigs or rats, its anti-bronchoconstrictor dose–response curve lay significantly to the left of and/or above the corresponding dose–response curve for the reduction of blood pressure (Bowring *et al.*, 1993). The basis of this *in vivo* airway selectivity of BRL 55834 remains to be established. However, this compound is currently in the final stages of phase 1 clinical trials and the outcome of such trials is awaited with interest.

Whether a cromakalim-like opener of K_{ATP} will eventually find clinical use as an anti-asthma drug remains to be seen. It is the authors' understanding that several pharmaceutical companies have recently terminated their research programmes in this area. Others are giving more attention to the modulation of BK_{Ca}. Recent reports (Laurent *et al.*, 1993; Michel *et al.*, 1993) have suggested that the pyrazine derivative, SCA 40, might relax airway smooth muscle by promoting the opening of BK_{Ca}. However, further studies of this compound (Cook *et al.*, 1995) have indicated, instead, that it may act as a selective inhibitor of the isoenzyme types III and IV of cyclic nucleotide phosphodiesterase.

References

Ahmed, F., Foster, R.W. & Small, R.C. (1985) Some effects of nifedipine in guinea-pig isolated trachealis. *Brit. J. Pharmacol.*, **84**, 861–9.

Allen, S.L., Boyle, J.P., Cortijo, J., Foster, R.W., Morgan, G.P. & Small, R.C. (1986) Electrical and mechanical effects of BRL 34915 in guinea-pig isolated trachealis. *Brit. J. Pharmacol.*, **89**, 395–405.

Arch, J.R.S., Buckle, D.R., Bumstead, J., Clarke, G.D., Taylor, J.F. & Taylor, S.G. (1988) Evaluation of the potassium channel activator cromakalim, BRL 34915, as a bronchodilator in the guinea-pig: comparison with nifedipine. *Brit. J. Pharmacol.*, **95**, 763–70.

Bang, L. & Nielsen-Kudsk, J.E. (1992) Smooth muscle relaxation and inhibition of responses to pinacidil and cromakalim induced by phentolamine in guinea-pig isolated trachea. *Eur. J. Pharmacol.*, **211**, 235–41.

Beech, D.J., Zhang, H., Nakao, K. & Bolton, T.B. (1993) K channel activation by nucleoside diphosphates and its inhibition by glibenclamide in vascular smooth muscle. *Brit. J. Pharmacol.*, **110**, 573–82.

Berry, J.L., Elliott, K.R.F., Foster, R.W., Green, K.A., Murray, M.A. & Small, R.C. (1991) Mechanical, biochemical and electrophysiological studies of RP 49356 and cromakalim in guinea-pig and bovine trachealis muscle. *Pulm. Pharmacol.*, **4**, 91–8.

Berry, J.L., Small, R.C. & Foster, R.W. (1992) Tracheal relaxation induced by potassium channel opening drugs: its antagonism by adrenergic neurone blocking agents. *Brit. J. Pharmacol.*, **106**, 813–18.

Black, J.L., Armour, C.L., Johnson, P.R.A., Alouan, L.A. & Barnes, P.J. (1990) The action of a potassium channel activator BRL 38227, lemakalim, on human airway smooth muscle. *Am. Rev. Resp. Dis.*, **142**, 1384–9.

Black, J.L., Johnson, P.R.A., McKay, K.O., Carey, D. & Armour, C.L. (1994) Levcromakalim- and isoprenaline-induced relaxation of human isolated airways—role of the epithelium and of K+-channel activation. *Pulm. Pharmacol.*, **7**, 195–203.

Bowring, N.E., Buckle, D.R., Clarke, G.D., Taylor, J.F. & Arch, J.R.S. (1991) Evaluation of the potassium channel activator BRL 38227 as an inhaled bronchodilator in the guinea-pig: contrast with nifedipine and salbutamol. *Pulm. Pharmacol.*, **4**, 99–105.

Bowring, N.E., Arch, J.R.S., Buckle, D.R. & Taylor, J.F. (1993) Comparison of the airways relaxant and hypotensive potencies of the potassium channel activators BRL 55834 and levcromakalim (BRL 38227) *in vivo* in guinea-pigs and rats. *Brit. J. Pharmacol.*, **109**, 1133–9.

Bray, K.M., Newgreen, D.T., Small, R.C. *et al.* (1987) Evidence that the mechanism of the inhibitory action of pinacidil in rat and guinea-pig smooth muscle differs from that of glyceryl trinitrate. *Brit. J. Pharmacol.*, **91**, 421–9.

Buckle, D.R., Arch, J.R.S., Bowring, N.E. *et al.* (1993) Relaxant effects of the potassium channel activators BRL 38227 and pinacidil on guinea-pig and human airway smooth muscle and blockade of their effects by glibenclamide and BRL 31660. *Pulm. Pharmacol.*, **6**, 77–86.

Burka, J.F., Berry, J.L., Foster, R.W., Small, R.C. & Watt, A.J. (1991) Effects of cromakalim on neurally-mediated responses of guinea-pig tracheal smooth muscle. *Brit. J. Pharmacol.*, **104**, 263–9.

Challiss, R.A.J., Patel, N. & Arch, J.R.S. (1992) Comparative effects of BRL 38227, nitrendipine and isoprenaline on carbachol- and histamine-stimulated phosphoinositide metabolism in bovine airway smooth muscle. *Brit. J. Pharmacol.*, **105**, 997–1003.

Chapman, I.D., Kristersson, A., Mathelin, G. *et al.* (1992) Effects of a potassium channel opener (SDZ PCO 400) on guinea-pig and human pulmonary airways. *Brit. J. Pharmacol.*, **106**, 423–9.

Chopra, L.C., Twort, C.H.C. & Ward, J.P.T. (1992) Direct action of BRL 38227 and glibenclamide on intracellular calcium stores in cultured airway smooth muscle of rabbit. *Brit. J. Pharmacol.*, **105**, 259–60.

Collier, M.L., Twort, C.H.C. & Ward, J.P.T. (1991) ATP-dependent potassium channels in rabbit and bovine airway smooth muscle. *Biophys. J.*, **59**, 16a.

Cook, S.J., Archer, K., Martin, A. *et al.* (1995) Further analysis of the mechanisms underlying the tracheal relaxant action of SCA40. *Brit. J. Pharmacol.*, **114**, 143–51.

De Souza, R.N., Gater, P.R. & Alabaster, V.A. (1989) Bronchodilator and tracheal relaxant effects of potassium channel openers in the guinea-pig. *Brit. J. Pharmacol.*, **98**, 803P.

Edwards, G. & Weston, A.H. (1993) Induction of a glibenclamide-sensitive K current by modification of a delayed rectifier channel in rat portal vein and insulinoma cells. *Brit. J. Pharmacol.*, **110**, 1280–1.

Edwards, G. & Weston, A.H. (1994) Effect of potassium channel modulating drugs on isolated smooth muscle. In: *Handbook of Experimental Pharmacology*, Vol. III (eds L. Szekeres & J.Gy. Papp), pp. 469–531. Springer-Verlag, Heidelberg.

Edwards, G., Ibbotson, T. & Weston, A.H. (1993) Levcromakalim may induce a voltage-independent K-current in rat portal veins by modifying the gating properties of the delayed rectifier. *Brit. J. Pharmacol.*, **110**, 1037–48.

Englert, H.C., Wirth, K., Gehring, D. *et al.* (1992) Airway pharmacology of the potassium channel opener, HOE 234, in guinea-pigs: *in vitro* and *in vivo* studies. *Eur. J. Pharmacol.*, **210**, 69–75.

Faurschou, P., Mikkelsen, K.L., Steffensen, I., & Franke, B. (1994) The bronchodilating effect and the short-term safety of cumulative single doses of an inhaled potassium channel opener (bimakalim) in adult patients with mild to moderate bronchial asthma: a prospective double-blind, placebo-controlled cross-over study. *Eur. Resp. J.*, **7** (Suppl. 18), P1187.

Foster, K.A. (1989) Cromakalim activation of potassium channels in guinea-pig trachea: effects of extracellular rubidium. *Brit. J. Pharmacol.*, **96**, 233P.

Foster, K.A., Arch, J.R.S., Newson, P., Shaw, D. & Taylor, S.G. (1992) Effect of Rb^+ on cromakalim-induced relaxation and ion fluxes in guinea-pig trachea. *Eur. J. Pharmacol.*, **222**, 143–51.

Foster, R.W., Okpalugo, B.I. & Small, R.C. (1984) Antagonism of Ca^{2+} and other actions of verapamil in guinea-pig isolated trachealis. *Brit. J. Pharmacol.*, **81**, 499–507.

Gater, P.R. (1989) Effects of K^+-channel openers on bovine tracheal smooth muscle. *Brit. J. Pharmacol.*, **98**, 660P.

Gater, P.R., Paciorek, P.M., McKean, J.C., Wilson, K., Brewster, M. & Waterfall, J.F. (1993) The inhibitory effects of Ro 31-6930 and BRL 38227 on cholinergically-mediated bonchoconstriction in the guinea-pig. *Eur. J. Pharmacol.*, **238**, 59–64.

Gill, T.S., Karran, M.A., Davies, B.E., Allen, G.D. & Tasker, T.C.G. (1989) Lack of an effect of atenolol on the stereochemical pharmacokinetics of cromakalim in healthy male subjects. *Brit. J. Clin. Pharmacol.*, **27**, 112P.

Good, D.M., Clapham, J.C. & Hamilton, T.C. (1992) Effects of BRL 38227 on neurally-mediated responses in the guinea-pig isolated bronchus. *Brit. J. Pharmacol.*, **105**, 933–40.

Hall, A.K. & Maclagan, J. (1988) Effect of cromakalim on cholinergic neurotransmission in the guinea-pig trachea. *Brit. J. Pharmacol.*, **95**, 792P.

Ho, P.P.K., Towner, R.D., Esterman, M. & Bertsch, B. (1990) Pinacidil, *N′*-cyano-*N*-4-pyridinyl-*N′*-(1,2,2-trimethylpropyl) guanidine, is a potent bronchodilator. *Eur. J. Pharmacol.*, **183**, 2132–3.

Ibbotson, T., Edwards, G. & Weston, A.H. (1993) Antagonism of levcromakalim by imidazole- and guanidine-derivatives in rat portal vein cells: involvement of the delayed rectifier. *Brit. J. Pharmacol.*, **110**, 1556–64.

Ichinose, M. & Barnes, P.J. (1990) A potassium channel activator modulates both excitatory noncholinergic and cholinergic neurotransmission in guinea-pig airways. *J. Pharmacol. Exp. Ther.*, **252**, 1207–12.

Imagama, J.-I., Yoshida, S., Koga, T., Kamei, K. & Nabata, H. (1993) The effect of a novel benzopyran derivative, KC 399, on the isolated guinea-pig trachealis and human bronchi. *Gen. Pharmacol.*, **24**, 1505–12.

Isaac, L. & Small, R.C. (1994) The effects of some K^+-channel inhibitors on the actions of spasmogens in guinea-pig isolated trachealis muscle. *Brit. J. Pharmacol.*, **112**, 535P.

Kamei, K., Nabata, H. & Kuriyama, H. (1994a) Effects of KC 399, a novel ATP-sensitive K^+-channel opener, on electrical and mechanical responses in dog tracheal smooth muscle. *J. Pharmacol. Exp. Ther.*, **268**, 319–27.

Kamei, K., Shoshin, Y., Imagawa, J., Nabata, H. & Kuriyama, H. (1994b) Regional and species differences in glyburide-sensitive K^+-channels in airway smooth muscles as estimated from actions of KC 128 and levcromakalim. *Brit. J. Pharmacol.*, **113**, 889–97.

Kidney, J.C., Worsdell, Y.M., Lavender, E.A., Chung, K.F. & Barnes, P.J. (1991) The effect of an ATP-dependent potassium channel activator, BRL 38227, in asthmatics. *Am. Rev. Resp. Dis.*, **143**, A423.

Koga, H., Sato, H., Ishizawa, T. *et al.* (1993) *N,N*-Disubstituted benzopyran-4-(*N′*-cyano)-carboxamidines: cromakalim analogues with selective activity for guinea-pig trachealis. *Bio-org. Med. Chem. Letts.*, **3**, 1111–14.

Kristersson, A., Smith, D., Sanjar, S., Newth, C. & Morley, J. (1989) Characterisation of airway hyperreactivity induced by intravenous injection of immune complexes in the guinea-pig. *Am. Rev. Resp. Dis.*, **139**, A592.

Laurent, F., Michel, A., Bonnet, P.A., Chapat, J.P. & Boucard, M. (1993) Evaluation of the relaxant effects of SCA40, a novel charybdotoxin-sensitive potassium channel opener, in guinea-pig isolated trachealis. *Brit. J. Pharmacol.*, **108**, 622–6.

Lei, Y.H., Barnes, P.J. & Rogers, D.F. (1993) Inhibition of neurogenic plasma exudation and bronchoconstriction by a K^+-channel activator, BRL 38227, in guinea-pig airways *in vivo*. *Eur. J. Pharmacol.* **239**, 257–9.

Lewis, S.A. & Raeburn, D. (1990) Preferential pre-junctional site of inhibition of non-cholinergic bronchospasm by potassium channel openers (KCOs). *Brit. J. Pharmacol.*, **100**, 474P.

Lindeman, K.S. & Freed, A.N. (1993) Lemakalim attenuates hypocapnia- and dry air-induced bronchoconstriction in canine peripheral airways. *J. Appl. Physiol.*, **75**, 86–92.

Longmore, J., Bray, K.M., & Weston, A.H. (1991) The contribution of Rb-permeable potassium channels to the relaxant and membrane hyperpolarizing actions of cromakalim, RP 49356 and diazoxide in bovine tracheal smooth muscle. *Brit. J. Pharmacol.*, **102**, 979–85.

McCaig, D.J. & De Jonckheere, B. (1989) Effect of cromakalim on bronchoconstriction evoked by cholinergic nerve stimulation in guinea-pig isolated trachea. *Brit. J. Pharmacol.*, **98**, 662–8.

McPherson, G.A. & Angus, J.A. (1990) Characterization of responses to cromakalim and pinacidil in smooth and cardiac muscle by use of selective antagonists. *Brit. J. Pharmacol.*, **100**, 201–6.

Mazzoni, L., Morley, J., Page, C.P. & Sanjar, S. (1985) Induction of hyperreactivity by platelet activating factor in the guinea-pig. *J. Physiol.*, **365**, 107P.

Michel, A., Laurent, F., Bompart, J. *et al.* (1993) Cardiovascular effects of SCA40, a novel potassium channel opener, in rats. *Brit. J. Pharmacol.*, **110**, 1031–6.

Miura, M., Belvisi, M.G., Ward, J.K., Tadjkarimi, S., Yacoub, M.H. & Barnes, P.J. (1993) Bronchodilating effects of the novel potassium channel opener HOE 234 in human airways *in vitro*. *Brit. J. Clin. Pharmacol.*, **35**, 318–20.

Murray, M.A., Boyle, J.P. & Small, R.C. (1989) Cromakalim-induced relaxation of guinea-pig isolated trachealis: antagonism by glibenclamide and by phentolamine. *Brit. J. Pharmacol.*, **98**, 865–74.

Nagai, H., Kitagaki, K., Goto, S., Suda, H. & Koda, A. (1991) Effect of three novel K^+-channel openers, cromakalim, pinacidil and nicorandil on allergic reaction and experimental asthma. *Jpn. J. Pharmacol.*, **56**, 13–21.

Nielsen-Kudsk, J.E., Mellemkjaer, S., Siggaard, C. & Nielsen, C.B. (1988) Effects of pinacidil on guinea-pig airway smooth muscle contracted by asthma mediators. *Eur. J. Pharmacol.*, **157**, 221–6.

Nielsen-Kudsk, J.E., Bang, L. & Bronsgaard, A.M. (1990) Glibenclamide blocks the relaxant action of pinacidil and cromakalim in airway smooth muscle. *Eur. J. Pharmacol.*, **180**, 291–6.

Paciorek, P.M., Cowlrick, I.S., Perkins, R.S., Taylor, J.C., Wilkinson, G.F. & Waterfall, J.F. (1990) Evaluation of the bronchodilator properties of Ro 31-6930, a novel potassium channel opener, in the guinea-pig. *Brit. J. Pharmacol.*, **100**, 289–94.

Plant, T.D. & Henquin, J.C. (1990) Phentolamine and yohimbine inhibit ATP-sensitive K^+-channels in mouse pancreatic β-cells. *Brit. J. Pharmacol.*, **101**, 115–20.

Quast, U. (1993) Do the K^+-channel openers relax smooth muscle by opening K^+-channels? *Trends Pharmacol. Sci.*, **14**, 332–7.

Raeburn, D.M. & Brown, T.J. (1991) RP 49356 and cromakalim relax airway smooth muscle *in vitro* by opening a sulphonylurea-sensitive K^+-channel: a comparison with nifedipine. *J. Pharmacol. Exp. Ther.*, **256**, 492–9.

Rodger, I.W. & Small, R.C. (1991) Pharmacology of airway smooth muscle. In: *Handbook of Experimental Pharmacology*, Vol. 98. *Pharmacology of Asthma* (eds C.P. Page & P.J. Barnes), pp. 107–41. Springer-Verlag, Berlin.

Saitoh, C., Ishikawa, J. & Asano, M. (1994) Anti-asthma effects of YM934, a novel K^+-channel opener in guinea-pigs. *Can. J. Physiol. Pharmacol.* **72** (Suppl. 1), P16.1.034.

Schmid-Antomarchi, H., Deweille, J., Fosset, M. & Lazdunski, M. (1987) The receptor for antidiabetic sulphonylureas controls the activity of the ATP-modulated K^+-channel in insulin-secreting cells. *J. Biol. Chem.*, **262**, 15840–4.

Shieh, C.C., Petrini, M.F., Dwyer, T.M. & Farley, J.M. (1992) Cromakalim effects on acetylcholine-induced changes in cytosolic calcium and tension in swine trachealis. *J. Pharmacol. Exp. Ther.*, **260**, 261–8.

Small, R.C. & Foster, R.W. (1986) Airways smooth muscle: an overview of morphology, electrophysiology and aspects of the pharmacology of contraction and relaxation. In: *Asthma: Clinical Pharmacology and Therapeutic Progress* (ed. A.B. Kay), pp. 101–13. Blackwell Scientific Publications, Oxford.

Small, R.C., Berry, J.L., Foster, R.W., Blarer, S. & Quast, U. (1992a) Analysis of the relaxant action of SDZ PCO 400 in airway smooth muscle from the ox and guinea-pig. *Eur. J. Pharmacol.*, **219**, 81–8.

Small, R.C., Berry, J.L., Foster, R.W., Green, K.A. & Murray, M.A. (1992b) The pharmacology of potassium-channel modulators in airways smooth muscle: relevance to airways disease. In: *Potassium Channel Modulators: Pharmacological, Molecular and Clinical Aspects* (eds A.H. Weston & T.C. Hamilton), pp. 424–63. Blackwell Scientific Publications, Oxford.

Small, R.C., Chiu, P., Cook, S.J., Foster, R.W. & Isaac, L. (1993) β-Adrenoceptor agonists in bronchial asthma: role of K^+-channel opening in mediating their bronchodilator effects. *Clin. Exp. Allergy*, **23**, 802–11.

Sturgess, N.C., Kozlowski, R.Z. Carrington, C.A., Hales, C.N. & Ashford, M.L.J. (1988) Effects of sulphonylureas and diazoxide on insulin secretion and nucleotide-sensitive channels in an insulin-secreting cell line. *Brit. J. Pharmacol.*, **95**, 83–94.

Taylor, S.G., Bumstead, J., Morris, J.E.J., Shaw, D.J. & Taylor, J.F. (1988) Cromakalim inhibits cholinergic-mediated responses in human isolated bronchioles but not in guinea-pig airways. *Brit. J. Pharmacol.*, **95**, 795P.

Taylor, S.G., Arch, J.R.S., Bond, J. *et al.* (1992a) The inhibitory effects of cromakalim and its active enantiomer, BRL 38227, against various agonists in guinea-pig and human airways: comparison with pinacidil and verapamil. *J. Pharmacol. Exp. Ther.*, **261**, 429–37.

Taylor, S.G., Buckle, D.R., Shaw, D.J., Ward, J.S. & Arch, J.R.S. (1992b) An investigation into the selectivities of BRL 55834 and BRL 38227 as relaxants of guinea-pig tracheal spirals relative to portal vein. *Brit. J. Pharmacol.*, **105**, 242P.

Wessler, I., Holz, C., Maclagan, J., Pohan, D., Reinheimer, T. & Racke, K. (1993) Cromakalim inhibits electrically-evoked [^{3}H]-acetylcholine release from a tube preparation of the rat isolated trachea by an epithelium-dependent mechanism. *Naunyn Schmiedeberg's Arch. Pharmacol.*, **34**, 14–20.

Williams, A.J. (1992) Potassium channel modulators: clinical aspects. In: *Potassium Channel Modulators: Pharmacological, Molecular and Clinical Aspects* (eds A.H. Weston & T.C. Hamilton), pp. 486–501. Blackwell Scientific Publications, Oxford.

Williams, A.J., Lee, T.H., Cochrane, G.M. *et al.* (1990a) Attenuation of nocturnal asthma by cromakalim. *Lancet*, **336**, 334–6.

Williams, A.J., Verden, P. & Lavender, E. (1990b) Inhalation of a potassium channel activator, cromakalim, is well tolerated in healthy volunteers. *Eur. J. Pharmacol.*, **183**, 1045–6.

Zhang, H. & Bolton, T.B. (1995) Activation by intracellular GDP, metabolic inhibition and pinacidil of a glibenclamide-sensitive K-channel in smooth muscle cells of rat mesenteric artery. *Brit. J. Pharmacol.*, **114**, 662–72.

CHAPTER 35

Glucocorticosteroids

P.J. Barnes

Introduction

Glucocorticosteroids (also known as corticosteroids or steroids) are the most effective therapy in the treatment of asthma, and asthma may be defined clinically as airway obstruction which improves with steroids. Oral steroids are still very useful for the control of asthma exacerbations but their chronic use in the control of asthma has sharply declined with the introduction of inhaled steroids. Inhaled steroids give effective control of asthma and are largely free of the side-effects associated with maintenance treatment with oral steroids. Inhaled steroids have now become the mainstay of chronic asthma treatment in many countries (Barnes, 1995). The recognition that airway inflammation is present even in the mildest of asthmatic patients has led to the introduction of inhaled steroids at a much earlier stage in therapy. Inhaled steroids are effective in all types of asthma and at all ages. The only limitation to their use is side-effects, but recent evidence suggests that this is not a problem for most patients.

This chapter discusses new advances in understanding the mechanism of action of steroids in asthma, the clinical use of oral and inhaled steroids in asthma and assessment of their side-effects.

Mechanism of action

Although steroids are the most effective therapy known for asthma, their precise mechanism of action is not yet understood. Important advances have been made in elucidating some of the molecular and cellular actions of steroids that are relevant to their anti-asthma effects (Barnes & Adcock, 1993; Taylor & Shaw, 1993). There have recently been important advances in understanding the molecular mechanisms of steroid action, largely through the application of molecular biology techniques (Miesfield, 1990; Gronemeyer, 1992).

Glucocorticoid receptors

Glucocorticoids exert their effects by binding to a single glucocorticoid receptor (GR), which is predominantly localized to the cytoplasm of target cells, and only on binding of the glucocorticoid does it move into the nuclear compartment (Fig. 35.1). The affinity of cortisol binding to GR is approximately 30 nmol/l, which falls within the normal range for plasma concentrations of free hormone. There is a single class of GR with no evidence for sub-types of differing affinity in different tissues, and its structure has been elucidated using site-directed mutagenesis, which has revealed distinct domains (Muller & Renkawitz, 1991). The glucocorticoid-binding domain is at the C-terminal end of the molecule and in the middle of the molecule are two finger-like projections that interact with DNA. Each of these 'zinc fingers' is formed by a zinc molecule bound to four cysteine residues. An N-terminal domain (τ_1) is involved in transcriptional *trans*-activation of genes once binding to DNA occurs and this region may also be involved in binding to other transcription factors. This is the least conserved part of the molecule. Deletion analysis has demonstrated a 41 amino acid core at the C-terminal end of the τ_1 domain that is critical for *trans*-activation. In human GR there is another *trans*-acting domain (τ_2) adjacent to the steroid-binding domain, and this region is also important for the nuclear translocation of

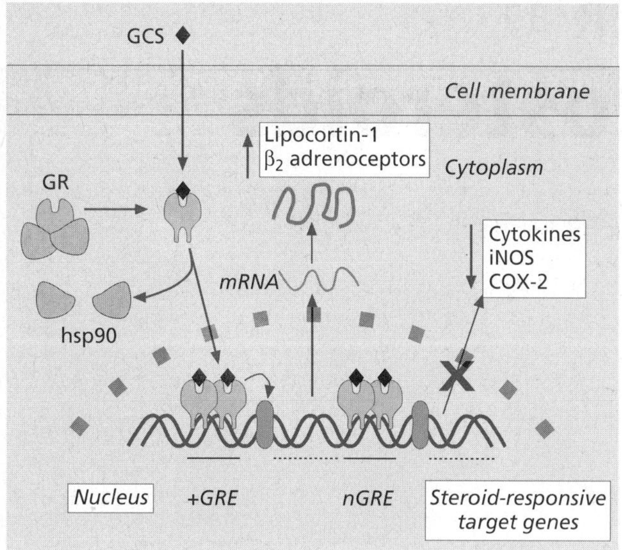

Fig. 35.1 Classical model of glucocorticoid action. The glucocorticoid enters the cell and binds to a cytoplasmic glucocorticoid receptor (GR), which is complexed with two molecules of a 90 kDa heat-shock protein (hsp 90). GR translocates to the nucleus, where, as a dimer, it binds to a glucocorticoid recognition sequence (glucocorticoid response element (GRE)) on the 5′-upstream promoter sequence of steroid-responsive genes. GRE may increase transcription and negative GRE (nGRE) may decrease transcription, resulting in increased or decreased mRNA and protein synthesis.

the receptor. GR is phosphorylated (predominantly on serine residues at the N terminus), but the role of phosphorylation in steroid actions is not yet certain (Muller & Renkawitz, 1991).

The inactivated GR is bound to a protein complex (≈ 300 kDa) that includes two molecules of 90-kDa heat-shock protein (hsp 90), a 59-kDa immunophilin protein and various other inhibitory proteins. The hsp 90 molecules act as a 'molecular chaperon', preventing the unoccupied GR localizing to the nuclear compartment. Once the glucocorticoid binds to GR, hsp 90 dissociates, thus allowing the nuclear localization of the activated GR–steroid complex and its binding to DNA.

Effect on gene transcription

Glucocorticoids produce their effect on responsive cells by activating GR to directly or indirectly regulate the transcription of certain target genes (Gronemeyer, 1992). The number of genes per cell directly regulated by steroids is estimated to be between 10 and 100, but many genes are indirectly regulated through an interaction with other transcription factors (see below). Upon activation, GR forms a dimer, which binds to DNA at consensus sites termed glucocorticoid response elements (GRE) in the 5′-upstream promoter region of steroid-responsive genes. This interaction changes the rate of transcription, resulting in either induction or repression of the gene. The consensus sequence for GRE binding is the palindromic 15-bp sequence GGTACA*nnn*TGTTCT (where *n* is any nucleotide), although for repression of transcription the negative GRE (nGRE) has a more variable sequence (ATYAC*nn*T*n*TGATC*n*). Crystallographic studies indicate that the zinc finger binding to DNA occurs within the major groove of DNA, with each finger interacting with one half of the palindrome. In contrast to these simple GRE, there are 'composite' GRE that do not share these GRE sequences, but depend on the presence of other transcription factors binding to DNA. Interaction with other transcription factors may also be important in determining differential steroid responsiveness in different cell types. Other transcription factors binding in the vicinity of GRE may have a powerful influence on steroid inducibility, and the relative abundance of different transcription factors may contribute to the steroid responsiveness of a particular cell type. GR may also inhibit protein synthesis by reducing the stability of mRNA via enhanced transcription of specific ribonucleases that break down mRNA containing constitutive AU-rich sequences in the untranslated 3′ region, thus shortening the turnover time of mRNA.

Interaction of the GR with other transcription factors

GR may interact directly with other transcription factors, which bind to each other via so-called leucine zipper interactions (Ponta *et al.*, 1992). This could be an important determinant of steroid responsiveness and is a key mechanism whereby glucocorticoids exert their anti-inflammatory actions (Barnes & Adcock, 1993). This interaction was first demonstrated for the collagenase gene, which is induced by the transcription factor activator protein-1 (AP-1), which is a heterodimer of Fos and Jun oncoproteins. AP-1 binds to a specific DNA binding site (TRE or TPA response element, TGACTCA). Steroids are potent inhibitors of collagenase gene transcription induced by tumour necrosis factor-α (TNF-α) and phorbol esters which activate AP-1. AP-1 forms a protein–protein complex with activated GR, and this prevents GR interacting with DNA and thereby reduces steroid responsiveness (Fig. 35.2).

In human lung, TNF-α and phorbol esters increase AP-1 binding to DNA and this is inhibited by glucocorticoids (Adcock *et al.*, 1994c, 1995a). GR may interact with other transcription factors that are activated by inflammatory signals, including nuclear factor-κB (NF-κB) in a similar manner (Adcock *et al.*, 1994c, 1995a; Ray & Prefontaine, 1994). There is evidence that β-agonists, via cyclic adenosine monophosphate (cAMP) formation and activation of protein kinase A, result in the activation of the transcrip-

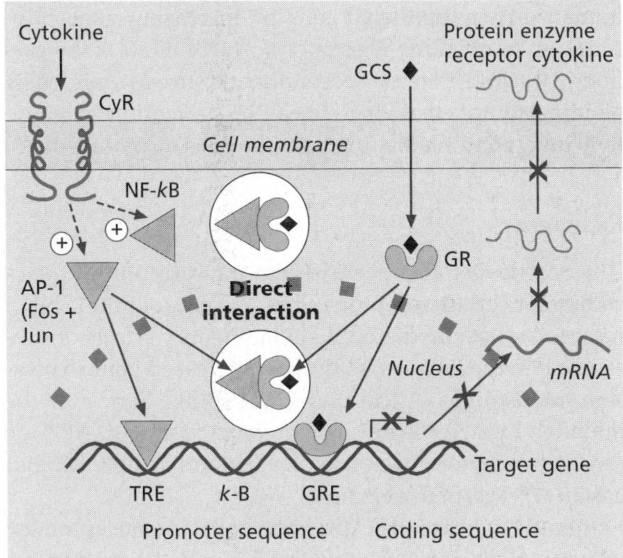

Fig. 35.2 Direct interaction between the transcription factors activator protein-1 (AP-1) and nuclear factor-κB (NF-κB) and the glucocorticoid receptor (GR) may result in mutual repression. In this way steroids may counteract the chronic inflammatory effects of cytokines that activate these transcription factors.

tion factor (CREB) that binds to a cAMP-responsive element (CRE) on genes. A direct interaction between CREB and GR has been demonstrated (Imai *et al.*, 1993). β-Agonists increase CRE binding in human lung *in vitro* and at the same time reduce GRE binding, suggesting that there may be a protein–protein interaction between CREB and GR within the nucleus (Peters *et al.*, 1993a, 1995). Similar interactions have also been described in human pulmonary epithelial cells (Stevens *et al.*, 1995). These interactions between activated GR and transcription factors occur within the nucleus, but recent observations suggest that these protein–protein interactions may also occur in the cytoplasm (Adcock & Barnes, 1995).

Target genes in asthma therapy

Corticosteroids may be effective in controlling asthma by inhibiting several aspects of the inflammatory process through increasing or decreasing gene transcription (Barnes & Adcock, 1993) (Table 35.1).

Cytokines

Although it is not yet possible to be certain of the most critical aspects of steroid action in asthma, it is likely that their inhibitory effects on cytokine synthesis are of particular relevance. Steroids inhibit the transcription of several cytokines that are relevant in asthma, including interleukin-1 (IL-1), TNF-α, granulocyte macrophage colony-stimulating factor (GM-CSF), IL-3, IL-4, IL-5, IL-6 and IL-8. These effects may be mediated directly via interaction of GR with an nGRE in the upstream promoter sequence of the cytokine gene, resulting in reduced gene transcription.

Surprisingly, there is no apparent nGRE consensus sequence in the upstream promoter region of many cytokines, suggesting that glucocorticoids inhibit transcription indirectly. Thus the 5′-promoter sequence of the human IL-2 gene has no GRE consensus sequences, and yet glucocorticoids are potent inhibitors of IL-2 gene transcription in T lymphocytes. Transcription of the IL-2 gene is predominantly regulated by a cell-specific transcription factor, nuclear factor of activated T cells (NF-AT), which is activated in the cytoplasm on T-cell receptor stimulation via calcineurin. A nuclear factor is also necessary for increased activation and this factor appears to be AP-1, which binds directly to NF-AT to form a transcriptional complex (Northrop *et al.*, 1993). Glucocorticoids therefore inhibit IL-2 gene transcription indirectly by binding to AP-1, thus preventing increased transcription due to NF-AT (Paliogianni *et al.*, 1993). Other examples of cytokine genes negatively regulated by glucocorticoids that do not have a GRE in their promoter region include IL-8, which is regulated predominantly via NF-κB (Mukaido *et al.*, 1994), and RANTES, which is regulated by NF-κB and AP-1 (Nelson, P.J. *et al.*, 1993). There may be marked differences in the response of different cells and of different cytokines to the inhibitory action of glucocorticoids and this may be dependent on the relative abundance of transcription factors. Thus, in alveolar macrophages and peripheral blood monocytes, GM-CSF secretion is more potently inhibited by glucocorticoids than IL-1β or IL-6 secretion.

Table 35.1 Effect of glucocorticoids on transcription of genes relevant to asthma.

Increased transcription
Lipocortin-1
β_2-Adrenoceptor
Endonucleases
Secretory leucocyte inhibitory protein
Decreased transcription
Cytokines (IL-1, IL-2, IL-3, IL-4, IL-5, IL-6, IL-8, IL-11, IL-12, IL-13, TNF-α, GM-CSF, RANTES, MIP-1α, SCF)
Inducible nitric oxide synthetase (iNOS)
Inducible cyclo-oxygenase (COX-2)
Inducible phospholipase A_2 ($cPLA_2$)
Endothelin-1
NK_2 receptors
Adhesion molecules (ICAM-1)

See text for definition of abbreviations.

Enzymes

Nitric oxide (NO) synthetase (NOS) may be induced by various cytokines, resulting in increased NO production. NO may increase airway blood flow and plasma exudation and may amplify the proliferation of T-helper 2 (Th2) lymphocytes, which orchestrate eosinophilic inflammation in the airways (Barnes & Liew, 1995). The induction of the inducible form of NOS (iNOS) is potently inhibited by glucocorticoids. In cultured human pulmonary epithelial cells, pro-inflammatory cytokines result in increased expression of iNOS and increased NO formation (Robbins *et al.*, 1994). This is due to increased transcription of the iNOS gene and is inhibited by glucocorticoids. There is no obvious nGRE in the promoter sequence of the iNOS gene, but NF-κB appears to be the most important transcription factor in regulating iNOS gene transcription (Xie *et al.*, 1994). Since TNF-α and oxidants may activate NF-κB in airway epithelial cells, this may account for their activation of iNOS expression (Adcock *et al.*, 1994a). Glucocorticoids may therefore prevent induction of iNOS by inactivating NF-κB, thereby inhibiting transcription.

Glucocorticoids inhibit the synthesis of several inflammatory mediators implicated in asthma through an inhibitory effect on enzyme induction. Glucocorticoids inhibit the induction of the gene coding for inducible cyclo-oxygenase (COX-2) in monocytes and epithelial cells, and this also appears to be via NF-κB activation (Mitchell *et al.*, 1994; Newton *et al.*, 1995). Glucocorticoids also inhibit the gene transcription of a form of phospholipase A_2 (PLA_2) induced by cytokines. Whether steroids also modulate expression of the 5-lipoxygenase has not yet been established, but studies of cysteinyl-leukotriene formation in asthmatic patients *in vivo* indicate that doses of oral glucocorticoids that are effective clinically do not significantly reduce the excretion of leukotriene E_4 (LTE_4), the major metabolite of LTD_4 (Dworski *et al.*, 1994).

Steroids also inhibit the synthesis of endothelin-1 in lung and airway epithelial cells, and this effect may also be via inhibition of transcription factors.

Inhibitory proteins

Glucocorticoids may have an inhibitory effect on inflammation by increasing the synthesis of anti-inflammatory proteins. Steroids increase the synthesis of lipocortin-1, a 37 kDa protein that has an inhibitory effect on PLA_2, and therefore may inhibit the production of lipid mediators. Steroids induce the formation of lipocortin-1 in several cells, and recombinant lipocortin 1 has acute anti-inflammatory properties (Flower & Rothwell, 1994). However, glucocorticoids do not induce lipocortin-1 expression in all cells and this may be only one of many genes regulated by glucocorticoids. Glucocorticoids also increase the synthesis of secretory leucocyte protease inhibitor (SLPI) in human airway epithelial cells by increasing gene transcription (Abbinante-Nissen *et al.*, 1995). SLPI is the predominant antiprotease in conducting airways and may be important in reducing airway inflammation by counteracting inflammatory enzymes, such as tryptase.

Receptors

Glucocorticoids also decrease the transcription of genes coding for certain receptors. Thus, the neurokinin 1 (NK_1) receptor, which mediates the inflammatory effects of substance P in the airways, may show increased gene expression in asthma (Adcock *et al.*, 1993b). This may be inhibited by steroids through an interaction with AP-1, as the NK_1 receptor gene promoter region has no GRE, but has an AP-1 response element.

Steroids increase the expression of β_2-adrenoceptors by increasing the rate of transcription, and the human β_2-receptor gene has three potential GRE. Steroids increase β-receptor gene transcription in human lung *in vitro* (Mak *et al.*, 1995). This may be relevant in asthma as it may prevent down-regulation in response to prolonged treatment with β_2-agonists. In rats glucocorticoids prevent the down-regulation and reduced transcription of β_2-receptors in response to chronic β-agonist exposure (Nishikawa *et al.*, 1993).

IL-1 acts on two types of surface receptor designated IL-1 RI and IL-1 RII. The inflammatory effects of IL-1β are mediated exclusively via IL-1 RI, whereas IL-1 RII has no signalling activity, but binds IL-1 and therefore acts as a molecular trap that interferes with the actions of IL-1. Glucocorticoids are potent inducers of this decoy IL-1 receptor and result in release of a soluble form of the receptor, thus reducing the functional activity of IL-1 (Colotta *et al.*, 1993).

Cell survival

Steroids markedly reduce the survival of certain inflammatory cells, such as eosinophils. Eosinophil survival is dependent on the presence of certain cytokines, such as IL-5 and GM-CSF. Exposure to steroids blocks the effects of these cytokines and leads to programmed cell death or apoptosis (Owens *et al.*, 1991). This may involve the increased expression of specific endonucleases. Steroids may increase the transcription of specific endonucleases and this may be relevant to the action of steroids on eosinophil and mast cell survival in the airways of asthmatic patients.

Adhesion molecules

Adhesion molecules play a key role in the trafficking of inflammatory cells to sites of inflammation. The expression of many adhesion molecules on endothelial cells is induced by cytokines and steroids and may lead indirectly to a reduced expression via their inhibitory effects on cytokines, such as IL-1β and TNF-α. Steroids may also have a direct inhibitory effect on the expression of adhesion molecules, such as intercellular adhesion molecule-1 (ICAM-1) and E-selectin, at the level of gene transcription (Cronstein *et al.*, 1992). ICAM-1 expression in bronchial epithelial cell lines and monocytes is inhibited by glucocorticoids (Van De Stolpe *et al.*, 1993).

Other effects

Steroids exert a number of other anti-inflammatory effects which are not yet understood at a molecular level. Steroids have a direct inhibitory effect on plasma exudation from post-capillary venules at inflammatory sites. The onset of effect is delayed, suggesting that gene transcription and protein synthesis are involved. The mechanism for this antipermeability effect has not been fully elucidated, but there is evidence that synthesis of a 100 kDa protein distinct from lipocortin-1 termed vasocortin may be involved (Carnuccio *et al.*, 1987).

Effect on inflammatory and airway cells

Steroids may have direct inhibitory actions on several inflammatory cells implicated in asthma (Schleimer, 1990) (Fig. 35.3). Steroids inhibit the release of inflammatory mediators and cytokines from alveolar macrophages *in vitro*. Oral prednisone inhibits the increased gene expression of IL-1β in alveolar macrophages obtained by bronchoalveolar lavage from asthmatic patients. Steroids have a direct inhibitory effect on mediator release from eosinophils, although they are only weakly effective in inhibiting secretion of reactive oxygen species and eosinophil basic proteins. Steroids appear to inhibit the permissive action of cytokines such as GM-CSF and IL-5 on eosinophil survival, presumably by activation of an endonuclease that leads to programmed cell death. One of the best described actions of steroids in asthma is a reduction in circulating eosinophils, which may reflect an action on eosinophil production in the bone marrow. After inhaled steroids, there is a marked reduction in the number of low-density eosinophils, presumably reflecting inhibition of cytokine production in the airways. An important target cell in asthma may be the T lymphocyte, since steroids are very effective in inhibition of activation of these cells and in blocking the release of cytokines which are likely to play an important role in the recruitment and survival of several inflammatory cells involved in asthmatic inflammation.

While steroids do not appear to have a direct inhibitory effect on mediator release from lung mast cells (Schleimer, 1990), chronic steroid treatment is associated with a marked reduction in mucosal mast cell number. This may

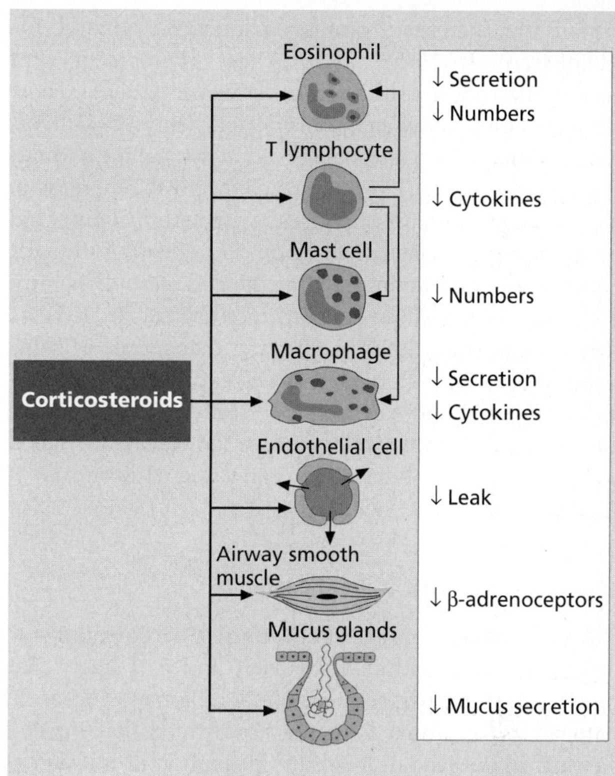

Fig. 35.3 Cellular effects of glucocorticoids in asthma.

be linked to a reduction in IL-3 or stem-cell factor (SCF) production, which appear to be necessary for mast cell expression in tissues. Mast cells also secrete various cytokines, but whether this is inhibited by steroids is not yet certain.

Steroids do not appear to directly inhibit the expression of adhesion molecules, although they may inhibit cell adhesion indirectly by suppression of cytokines involved in the regulation of adhesion molecule expression (Schleimer, 1990). Steroids may have an inhibitory action on airway microvascular leakage induced by inflammatory mediators (Boschetto *et al.*, 1991). This appears to be a direct effect on post-capillary venular epithelial cells. The mechanism for this antipermeability effect has not been fully elucidated, but induction of vasocortin may be involved (Carnuccio *et al.*, 1987). Although there have been no direct measurements of the effects of steroids on airway microvascular leakage in asthmatic airways, regular treatment with inhaled steroids decreases the elevated plasma proteins found in bronchoalveolar lavage fluid of patients with stable asthma.

Epithelial cells may be one of the most important targets for inhaled glucocorticoids in asthma. Steroids inhibit the increased transcription of the IL-8 gene induced by TNF-α in cultured human airway epithelial cells *in vitro* (Kwon *et al.*, 1994) and the transcription of the RANTES gene in an epithelial cell line (Kwon *et al.*, 1995). Inhaled steroids inhibit the increased expression of GM-CSF and the chemokine RANTES (which is chemotactic for eosinophils) in the epithelium of asthmatic patients. There is expression of iNOS in the airway epithelium of patients with asthma, which is not observed in normal individuals (Hamid *et al.*, 1993). This may account for the increase in NO in the exhaled air of patients with asthma compared with normal subjects (Kharitonov *et al.*, 1994). Asthmatic patients who are taking regular inhaled steroid therapy, however, do not show such an increase in exhaled NO (Kharitonov *et al.*, 1994), suggesting that glucocorticoids have suppressed epithelial iNOS expression. Furthermore, double-blind randomized studies show that oral and inhaled glucocorticoids reduce the elevated exhaled NO in asthmatic patients to normal values (Kharitonov *et al.*, 1995; Yates *et al.*, 1995).

Effects on asthmatic inflammation

Glucocorticoids are remarkably effective in controlling the inflammation in asthmatic airways and it is likely that they have multiple cellular effects. Biopsy studies in patients with asthma have now confirmed that inhaled steroids reduce the number and activation of inflammatory cells in the airway (Burke *et al.*, 1992; Djukanovic *et al.*, 1992; Jeffery *et al.*, 1992; Laitinen *et al.*, 1992; Trigg *et al.*, 1994). Similar results have been reported in bronchoalveolar lavage of asthmatic patients, with a reduction in both eosinophil number and eosinophil cationic protein concentrations, a marker of eosinophil degranulation, after inhaled budesonide (Ädelroth *et al.*, 1990). These effects may be due to inhibition of cytokine synthesis in T lymphocytes and other inflammatory and structural cells. There is also a reduction in activated CD4+ T cells (CD4+/CD25+) in bronchoalveolar lavage fluid after inhaled glucocorticoids (Wilson *et al.*, 1994). The disrupted epithelium is restored and the ciliated to goblet cell ratio is normalized after 3 months of therapy with inhaled steroids (Laitinen *et al.*, 1993). There is also some evidence for a reduction in the thickness of the basement membrane (Trigg *et al.*, 1994), although in asthmatic patients taking inhaled steroids for over 10 years the characteristic thickening of the basement membrane was still present (Lungren *et al.*, 1988). A surprising finding is an apparent increase in the number of fibroblasts in the airway after steroid treatment (Laitinen *et al.*, 1992), possibly related to the fact that steroids increase the production of platelet-derived growth factor, a fibroblast mitogen, from alveolar macrophages (Haynes & Shaw, 1992).

Effects on airway hyperresponsiveness

Asthma is characterized by airway hyperresponsiveness (AHR) to many stimuli and this is related to airway inflammation. By reducing airway inflammation, inhaled steroids consistently reduce AHR in asthmatic adults and children (Barnes, 1990). Chronic treatment with inhaled steroids reduces responsiveness to histamine, cholinergic agonists, allergen (early and late responses), exercise, fog, cold air, bradykinin, adenosine and irritants (such as sulphur dioxide and metabisulphite). The reduction in AHR takes place over several weeks and may not be maximal until after several months of therapy. The magnitude of reduction is variable between patients, being in the order of one to two doubling dilutions for most challenges, and often fails to return to the normal range. This may reflect suppression of the inflammation but persistence of structural changes, which cannot be reversed by steroids. Inhaled steroids not only make the airways less sensitive to spasmogens, but also limit the maximal airway narrowing in response to a spasmogen (Bel *et al.*, 1991).

Clinical efficacy of inhaled steroids

Inhaled steroids are very effective in controlling asthma symptoms in asthmatic patients of all ages and severity (Konig, 1988; Barnes, 1993, 1995; Barnes & Pedersen, 1993).

Studies in adults

Inhaled steroids were first introduced to reduce the requirement for oral steroids in patients with severe asthma and many studies have confirmed that the majority of patients can be weaned off oral steroids (Reed, 1990). As experience has been gained with inhaled steroids, they have been introduced in patients with milder asthma, with the recognition that inflammation is present even in patients with mild asthma (Barnes, 1989). Inhaled anti-inflammatory drugs have now become first-line therapy in any patient who needs to use a β_2-agonist inhaler more than once a day, and this is reflected in national and international guidelines for the management of chronic asthma (Sheffer, 1991, 1992; British Thoracic Society, 1993). In patients with newly diagnosed asthma, inhaled steroids (budesonide 600 μg twice daily) reduced symptoms and β_2-agonist inhaler usage and improved peak expiratory flows. These effects persisted over the 2 years of the study, whereas in a parallel group treated with inhaled β_2-agonists alone there was no significant change in symptoms or lung function (Haahtela *et al.*, 1991). In another study, patients with mild asthma treated with a low dose of inhaled steroid (budesonide 200 μg twice daily) showed fewer symptoms and a progressive improvement in lung function over several months and many patients became completely asymptomatic (Juniper *et al.*, 1990). Similarly, inhaled beclomethasone dipropionate (BDP, 400 μg twice daily) improved asthma symptoms and lung function and this was maintained over the $2\frac{1}{2}$ years of the study (Kerrebijn *et al.*, 1987). There was also a significant reduction in the number of exacerbations. Although the effects of inhaled steroids on AHR may take several months to reach a plateau, the reduction in asthma symptoms occurs more rapidly (Vathenen *et al.*, 1991).

High-dose inhaled steroids have now been introduced in many countries for the control of more severe asthma. This markedly reduces the need for maintenance oral steroids and has revolutionized the management of more severe and unstable asthma (Salmeron *et al.*, 1989; Toogood, 1989; Lacronique *et al.*, 1991). Inhaled steroids are the treatment of choice in nocturnal asthma, which is a manifestation of inflamed airways (Barnes, 1988), reducing night-time awakening and reducing the diurnal variation in airway function (Dahl *et al.*, 1989; Wempe *et al.*, 1992).

Inhaled steroids effectively control asthmatic inflammation but must be taken regularly. When inhaled steroids are discontinued, there is usually a gradual increase in symptoms and airway responsiveness back to pretreatment values (Vathenen *et al.*, 1991), although in patients with mild asthma who have been treated with inhaled steroids for a long time symptoms may not recur in some patients (Juniper *et al.*, 1991).

Studies in children

Inhaled steroids are equally effective in children. In an extensive study of children aged 7–17 years, there was a significant improvement in symptoms, peak flow variability and lung function, compared with a regular inhaled β_2-agonist which was maintained over the 22 months of the study (van Essen-Zandvliet *et al.*, 1992), but asthma deteriorated when the inhaled steroids were withdrawn (Waalkens *et al.*, 1993). There was a high proportion of drop-outs (45%) in the group treated with inhaled β_2-agonist alone. Inhaled steroids are also effective in younger children. Nebulized budesonide reduced the need for oral steroids and also improved lung function in children under the age of 3 (Ilangovan *et al.*, 1993). Inhaled steroids given via a large-volume spacer improved asthma symptoms and reduced the number of exacerbations in preschool children and in infants (Gleeson & Price, 1988; Bisgard *et al.*, 1990).

Prevention of irreversible changes

Some patients with asthma develop an element of irreversible air-flow obstruction, but the pathophysiological basis of these changes is not yet understood. It is likely that they are the result of chronic airway inflammation and that they may be prevented by treatment with inhaled steroids. There is some evidence that the annual decline in lung function may be slowed by the introduction of inhaled steroids (Dompeling *et al.*, 1992). Recent evidence also suggests that delay in starting inhaled steroids may result in less overall improvement in lung function in both adults and children (Agertoft & Pedersen, 1994; Haahtela *et al.*, 1994; Selroos *et al.*, 1994).

Reduction in mortality

Whether inhaled steroids may reduce the mortality from asthma is not yet established, as prospective studies are almost impossible to conduct. In a retrospective review of the risk of mortality and prescribed anti-asthma medication, there was a significant apparent protection provided by regular inhaled BDP therapy (adjusted odds ratio of 0.1), although numbers were small (Ernst *et al.*, 1992).

Effects in chronic obstructive pulmonary disease

While the beneficial effects of inhaled steroids in asthma are now well documented, their role in the management of chronic obstructive pulmonary disease (COPD) is less clear. The failure of a short course (2–4 weeks) of an oral steroid to improve airway obstruction discriminates COPD from asthma. Inhaled steroids over 3 months fail to improve lung function or airway responsiveness in patients with mild to moderate COPD (Watson *et al.*, 1992), although with longer duration of treatment some beneficial effect may be apparent (Kertjens *et al.*, 1992). Larger studies of the effects of long-term treatment with inhaled steroids on the progression of airway obstruction in patients with COPD are currently under way (Pauwels *et al.*, 1992).

Comparison between inhaled steroids

Several inhaled steroids are currently prescribable in asthma, although their availability varies between countries (Fig. 35.4). There have been relatively few studies comparing efficacy of the different inhaled steroids, and it is important to take into account the delivery system and the type of patient under investigation when such comparisons are made. In the UK, BDP, betamethasone valerate, budesonide and fluticasone proprionate are available, whereas in the USA, BDP, flunisolide and triamcinolone are available. There are few studies comparing different doses of inhaled steroids in asthmatic patients. Budesonide has been compared with BDP and in adults and children appears to have comparable anti-asthma effects at equal doses (Ebden *et al.*, 1986; Baran, 1987). There do appear to be some differences between inhaled steroids in terms of their systemic effects at comparable anti-asthma doses, however.

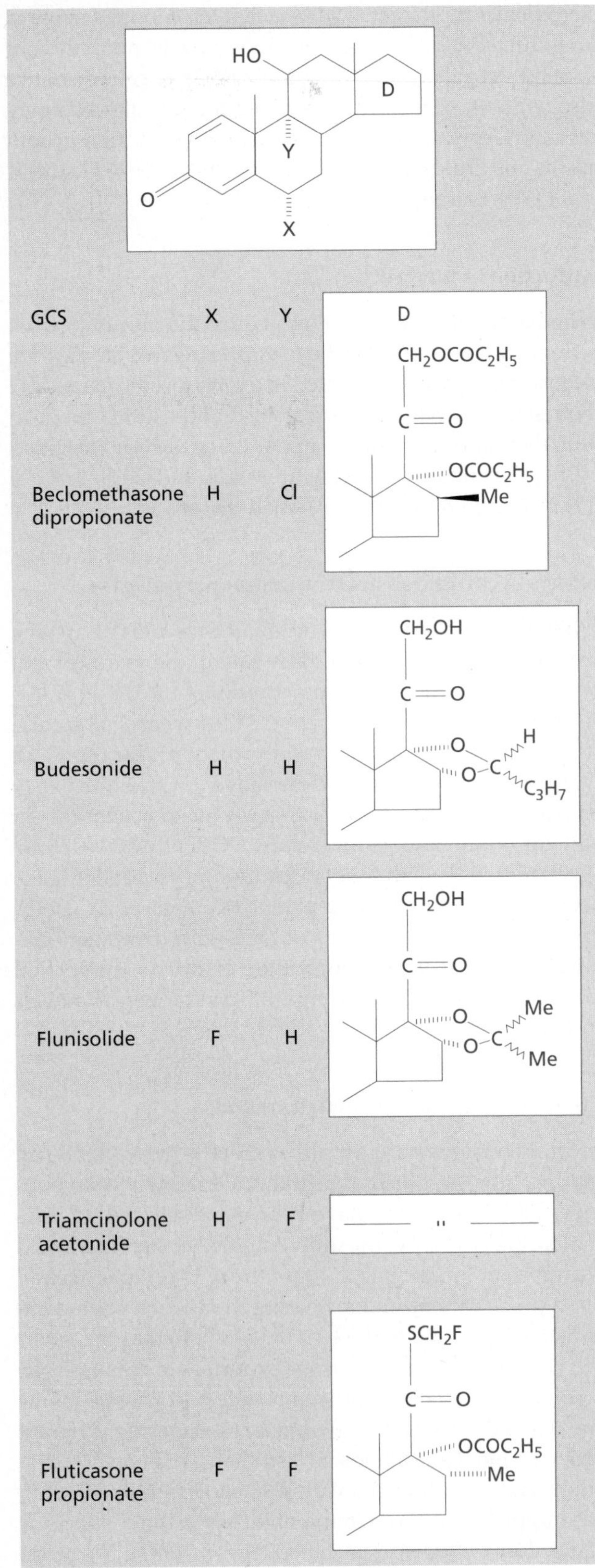

Fig. 35.4 Structure of currently available inhaled glucocorticosteroids.

Pharmacokinetics

The pharmacokinetics of inhaled steroids is important in determining the concentration of drug reaching target cells in the airways and in the fraction of drug reaching the systemic circulation and therefore causing side-effects (Szefler, 1991; Barnes, 1995). Beneficial properties in an inhaled steroid are a high topical potency, a low systemic bio-availability of the swallowed portion of the dose and rapid metabolic clearance of any steroid reaching the systemic circulation. After inhalation, a large proportion of the inhaled dose (80–90%) is deposited on the oropharynx and is then swallowed and therefore available for absorption via the liver into the systemic circulation (Fig. 35.5). This fraction is markedly reduced by using a large-volume spacer device with a metered dose inhaler (MDI) or by mouth washing and discarding the washing with dry powder inhalers. Between 10 and 20% of inhaled drug enters the respiratory tract, where it is deposited in the airways, and this fraction is available for absorption into the systemic circulation. Most of the studies on the distribution of inhaled steroids have been conducted in healthy volunteers, and it is not certain what effect inflammatory disease, airway obstruction, age of the patient or concomitant medication may have on the disposition of the inhaled dose. There may be important differences in the metabolism of different inhaled steroids. BDP is metabolized to its more active metabolite beclomethasone monopropionate in many tissues, including lung (Wurthwein & Rohdewald, 1990), but there is no information about its absorption or the metabolism of this metabolite in humans. Flunisolide and budesonide are subject to extensive first-pass metabolism in the liver so that less reaches the systemic circulation (Chaplin *et al.*, 1980; Ryrfeldt *et al.*, 1982). Little is known about the distribution of triamcinolone (Mollman *et al.*, 1985). Fluticasone propionate has a low oral bio-availability which reduces systemic effects (Harding, 1990).

Frequency of administration

When inhaled steroids were first introduced, it was recommended that they should be given four times daily, but several studies have now demonstrated that twice-daily administration gives comparable control (Toogood *et al.*, 1982; Meltzer *et al.*, 1985), although administration four times daily may be preferable in patients with more severe asthma (Malo *et al.*, 1989). However, patients may find it difficult to comply with such frequent administration unless they have troublesome symptoms. For patients with mild asthma, once-daily therapy may be sufficient (Jones *et al.*, 1993).

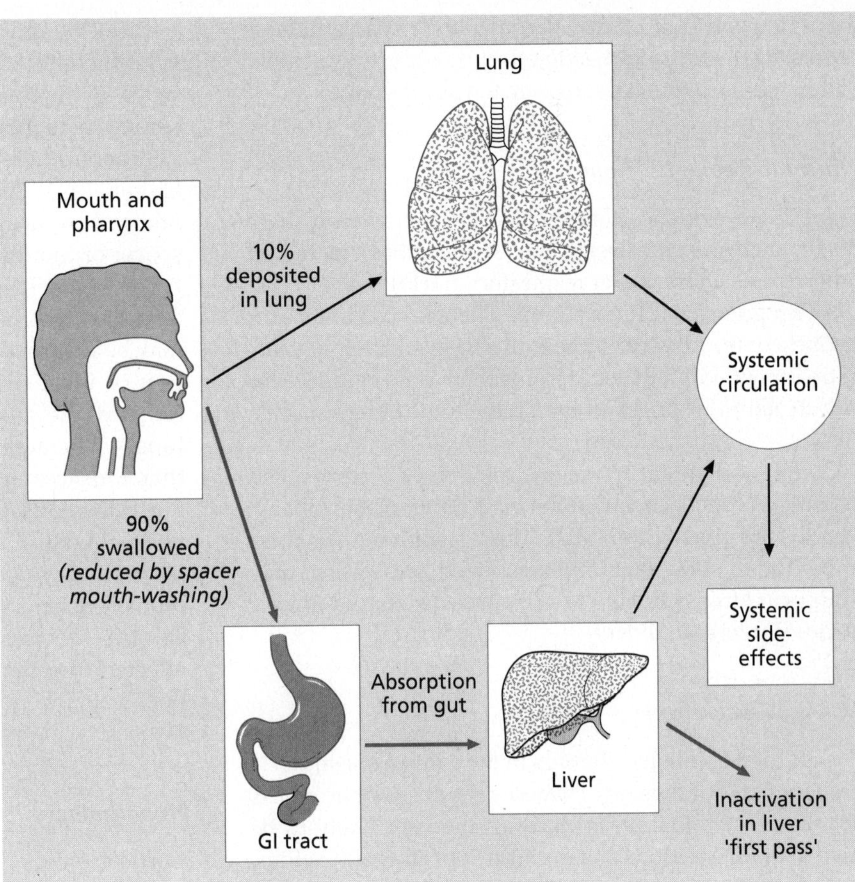

Fig. 35.5 Pharmacokinetics of inhaled steroids. The amount of inhaled steroid reaching the systemic circulation (and therefore exerting systemic effects) is derived from the swallowed fraction, absorbed from the gastrointestinal (GI) tract via the hepatic circulation, and the inhaled fraction.

Side-effects of inhaled steroids

The efficacy of inhaled steroids is now established in short- and long-term studies in adults and children, but there are still concerns about side-effects, particularly in children and when high inhaled doses are needed. Several side-effects have been recognized (Table 35.2).

Local side-effects

Side-effects due to the local deposition of the inhaled steroid in the oropharynx may occur with inhaled steroids, but the frequency of complaints depends on the dose and frequency of administration and on the delivery system used.

Dysphonia

The commonest complaint is of hoarseness of the voice (dysphonia) and may occur in over one-third of patients (Toogood *et al.*, 1980). Dysphonia may be due to myopathy of laryngeal muscles and is reversible when treatment is withdrawn (Williams *et al.*, 1983). For most patients it is not troublesome but it may be disabling in singers.

Oropharyngeal candidiasis

Oropharyngeal candidiasis (thrush) may be a problem in some patients, particularly in the elderly, with concomitant oral steroids and more than twice-daily administra-

Table 35.2 Side-effects of inhaled steroids.

Local side-effects
Dysphonia
Oropharyngeal candidiasis
Local irritation (cough, bronchoconstriction)
Systemic side-effects
Hypothalamic–pituitary–adrenal suppression
Increased bone turnover (increased breakdown, reduced formation, reduced density)
Impaired growth
Connective tissue effects (skin thinning, easy bruising)
Cataracts (postcapsular)
Metabolic disturbance (impaired insulin tolerance, increased glucose, hyperlipidaemia)
Haematological changes (decreased eosinophils, monocytes, increased neutrophils)
Psychiatric disturbance

tion (Toogood *et al.*, 1980). Large-volume spacer devices protect against this local side-effect by reducing the dose of inhaled steroid that deposits in the oropharynx.

Other local complications

There is no evidence that inhaled steroid, even in high doses, increases the frequency of infections, including tuberculosis, in the lower respiratory tract (Brogden *et al.*, 1984; Brogden & McTavish, 1992). There is no evidence for atrophy of the airway epithelium and even after 10 years of treatment with inhaled steroids there is no evidence for any structural changes in the epithelium (Lungren *et al.*, 1988).

Cough and throat irritation, sometimes accompanied by reflex bronchoconstriction, may occur when inhaled steroids are given via an MDI. These symptoms are likely to be due to surfactants in pressurized aerosols, as they disappear after switching to a dry-powder steroid inhaler device (Engel *et al.*, 1989).

Systemic side-effects

The efficacy of inhaled steroids in the control of asthma is undisputed, but there are concerns about systemic effects of inhaled steroids, particularly as they are likely to be used over long periods and in children of all ages (Geddes, 1992; Boner & Piacentini, 1993; Monson, 1993). The safety of inhaled steroids has been extensively investigated since their introduction almost 30 years ago. One of the major problems is to decide whether a measurable systemic effect has any significant clinical consequence and this will require careful long-term follow-up studies. As biochemical markers of systemic steroid effects become more sensitive, then systemic effects may be seen more often, but this does not mean that these effects are clinically relevant. There are several case reports of adverse systemic effects of inhaled steroids, and these are often idiosyncratic reactions, which may be due to abnormal pharmacokinetic handling of the inhaled steroid. The systemic effect of an inhaled steroid will depend on several factors, including the dose delivered to the patient, the site of delivery (gastrointestinal tract and lung), the delivery system used and individual differences in the patient's response to the steroid.

Effect of delivery systems

The systemic effect of an inhaled steroid is dependent on the amoung of drug absorbed into systemic circulation. As discussed above, approximately 90% of the inhaled dose from an MDI deposits in the oropharynx and is swallowed and subsequently absorbed from the gastrointestinal tract. Use of a large-volume spacer device markedly reduces the oropharyngeal deposition, and therefore the systemic effects of inhaled steroids (Brown *et al.*, 1990, 1993a; Selroos & Halme, 1991). For dry-powder inhalers, similar reductions in systemic effects may be achieved with mouth washing and discarding the fluid (Selroos & Halme, 1991). All patients using a daily dose of 800 μg or more of an inhaled steroid should therefore use either a spacer or mouth washing to reduce systemic absorption. Approximately 10% of an MDI enters the lung and this fraction (which presumably exerts therapeutic effect) may be absorbed into the systemic circulation. As the fraction of inhaled steroid deposited in the oropharynx is reduced, the proportion of the inhaled dose entering the lungs is increased. More efficient delivery to the lungs is therefore accompanied by increased systemic absorption, but this is offset by a reduction in the dose needed for optimal control of airway inflammation. For example, a multiple dry-powder delivery system, the Turbuhaler, delivers approximately twice as much steroid to the lungs as other devices, and therefore has increased systemic effects. However, this is compensated for by the fact that only half the dose is required (Thorsson & Edsbäcker, 1993).

Hypothalamic–pituitary–adrenal axis

Corticosteroids may cause hypothalamic–pituitary–adrenal (HPA) axis suppression by reducing corticotrophin (adrenocorticotrophic hormone (ACTH)) production, which reduces cortisol secretion by the adrenal gland. The degree of HPA suppression is dependent on dose, duration, frequency and timing of steroid administration. The clinical significance of HPA axis suppression is twofold. Firstly, prolonged adrenal suppression may lead to reduced adrenal response to stress. There is no evidence that cortisol responses to the stress of an asthma exacerbation or insulin-induced hypoglycaemia are impaired, even with high doses of inhaled steroids (Brown *et al.*, 1992). Secondly, measurement of HPA axis function provides evidence for systemic effects of an inhaled steroid. Basal adrenal cortisol secretion may be measured by a morning plasma cortisol, a 24-hour urinary cortisol or a plasma cortisol profile over 24 hours (Holt *et al.*, 1990). Other tests measure the HPA response following stimulation with tetracosactrin (which measures adrenal reserve) or stimulation with metyrapone and insulin (which measure the response to stress).

There are many studies of HPA axis function in asthmatic patients with inhaled steroids, but the results are inconsistent, as they have often been uncontrolled and patients have also been taking courses of oral steroids (which may affect the HPA axis for weeks) (Barnes & Pedersen, 1993). Both BDP and budesonide at high doses by conventional MDI (> 1600 μg daily) give a dose-related decrease in morning serum cortisol levels and 24-hour urinary cortisol, although values still lie well within the normal range (Pedersen & Fuglsang, 1988; Löfdahl *et al.*, 1989). However, when a large-volume spacer is used, doses of 2000 μg daily of BDP or budesonide have no effect on 24-hour urinary cortisol excretion (Brown *et al.*, 1993b). Studies with inhaled flunisolide and triamcrinolone in children show no effect on 24-hour cortisol excretion at doses of up to 1000 μg daily (Sly *et al.*, 1978; Placcentini *et al.*, 1990). Stimulation tests of HPA axis function show no consistent effects of doses of 1500 μg or less of inhaled steroid. At high doses (> 1500 μg daily) budesonide and fluticasone have less effect than BDP on HPA axis function (Pedersen & Fuglsang, 1988; Fabbri *et al.*, 1993). In children, no suppression of urinary cortisol is seen with doses of BDP of 800 μg or less (Bisgaard *et al.*, 1988; Prahl, 1991; Volovitz *et al.*, 1993). In studies where plasma cortisol has been measured at frequent intervals, there was a significant reduction in cortisol peaks with doses of inhaled BDP as low as 400 μg daily (Law *et al.*, 1986), although this does not appear to be dose-related in the range 400–1000 μg (Tabacknik & Zadik, 1991; Philip *et al.*, 1992). The clinical significance of these effects is not certain, however.

Overall, the studies which are not confounded by concomitant treatment with oral steroids have consistently shown that there are no significant suppressive effects on HPA axis function at doses of ≤ 1500 μg in adults and ≤ 400 μg in children.

Effects on bone metabolism

Steroids lead to a reduction in bone mass by direct effects on bone formation and resorption, and indirectly by suppression of the pituitary–gonadal and HPA axes, with effects on intestinal Ca^{2+} absorption and on renal tubular Ca^{2+} reabsorption and secondary hyperparathyroidism (Hosking, 1993). The effects of oral steroids on osteoporosis and increased risk of vertebral and rib fractures are well known, but there are no reports suggesting that long-term treatment with inhaled steroids is associated with an increased risk of fractures. Bone densitometry has been used to assess the effect of inhaled steroids on bone mass. Although there is evidence that bone density is less in patients taking high-dose inhaled steroids, interpretation is confounded by the fact that these patients are also taking intermittent courses of oral steroids (Packe *et al.*, 1992).

Changes in bone mass occur very slowly and several biochemical indices have been used to assess the short-term effects of inhaled steroids on bone metabolism. Bone formation has been measured by plasma concentrations of bone-specific alkaline phosphatase or serum osteocalcin, a non-collagenous 49-amino-acid peptide secreted by osteoblasts. Bone resorption may be assessed by urinary hydroxyproline after a 12-hour fast, urinary Ca^{2+} excretion and pyridinium cross-link excretion. It is important to consider the age, diet, time of day and physical activity of the patient in interpreting any abnormalities. It is also necessary to choose appropriate control groups, as asthma itself may have an effect on some of the measurements, such as osteocalcin (König *et al.*, 1993). Inhaled steroids, even at doses up to 2000 μg daily, have no significant effect on Ca^{2+} excretion, but acute and reversible dose-related suppression of serum osteocalcin has been reported with BDP and budesonide when given by conventional MDI in several studies (Barnes & Pedersen, 1993). Budesonide consistently has less effect than BDP at equivalent doses and only BDP increases urinary hydroxyproline at high doses (Ali *et al.*, 1991). With a large-volume spacer, even doses of 2000 μg daily of either BDP or budesonide are without effect on plasma osteocalcin concentrations, however (Brown *et al.*, 1993b). Urinary pyridinium and deoxypyridinoline cross-links, which are a more accurate and stable measurement of bone and collagen degradation, are not increased with inhaled steroids (BDP > 1000 μg daily), even with intermittent courses of oral steroids (Packe *et al.*, 1992).

There has been particular concern about the effect of inhaled steroids on bone metabolism in growing children. A very low dose of oral steroids (prednisolone 2.5 mg) causes significant changes in serum osteocalcin and urinary hydroxyproline excretion, whereas daily BDP and budesonide at doses up to 800 μg daily have no effect (König *et al.*, 1993; Wolthers & Pedersen, 1993a).

It is important to recognize that the changes in biochemical indices of bone metabolism are less than those seen with even low doses of oral steroids. This suggests that even high doses of inhaled steroids, particularly when used with a spacer device, are unlikely to have any long-term effect on bone structure. Careful long-term follow-up studies in patients with asthma are needed.

Effects on connective tissue

Oral and topical steroids cause thinning of the skin, telangiectasiae and easy bruising, probably as a result of loss of extracellular ground substance within the dermis, due to an inhibitory effect on dermal fibroblasts. There are reports of increased skin bruising and purpura in patients using high doses of inhaled BDP, but the amount of intermittent oral steroids in these patients is not known (Capewell *et al.*, 1990; Mak *et al.*, 1992). Easy bruising in association with inhaled steroids is more frequent in elderly patients and there are no reports of this problem in children. Long-term prospective studies with objective measurements of skin thickness are needed with different inhaled steroids.

Cataracts

Long-term treatment with oral steroids increases the risk of posterior subcapsular cataracts and there are several case reports describing cataracts in individual patients taking inhaled steroids (Barnes & Pedersen, 1993). In a study of 48 patients who were exposed to oral and/or high-dose inhaled steroids, the prevalence of posterior subcapsular cataracts (27%) correlated with the daily dose and duration of oral steroids, but not with the dose and duration of inhaled steroids (Toogood *et al.*, 1993). In a recent cross-sectional study in patients aged 5–25 years taking either inhaled BDP or budesonide, no cataracts were found on slit-lamp examination, even in patients taking 2000 μg daily for over 10 years (Simons *et al.*, 1993).

Growth

There has been particular concern that inhaled steroids may cause stunting of growth and several studies have addressed this issue. Asthma itself (as with other chronic diseases) may have an effect on the growth pattern and has been associated with delayed onset of puberty and deceleration of growth velocity, which is more pronounced with more severe disease (Russell, 1993). However, asthmatic children appear to grow for longer, so that their final height is normal. The effect of asthma on growth makes it difficult to assess the effects of inhaled steroids on growth in cross-sectional studies, particularly as courses of oral steroids are a confounding factor. Longitudinal studies have demonstrated that there is no significant effect of inhaled steroids on statural growth in doses of up to 800 μg daily and for up to 5 years of treatment (Balfour-Lynn, 1986; Ninan & Russell, 1992; van Essen-Zandvliet *et al.*, 1992; Barnes & Pedersen, 1993; Boner & Piacentini, 1993). A prospective study of inhaled BDP (400 μg daily) vs. theophylline in children with mild to moderate asthma showed no effect on height, although there was some reduction in growth velocity compared with children treated with theophylline (Tinkelman *et al.*, 1993). However, it is not possible to relate changes in growth velocity to final height, as other studies have demonstrated that there is a 'catch-up' period. A longitudinal study in children aged 2–7 years with severe asthma, budesonide 200 μg daily had no effect on growth over 3–5 years (Volovitz *et al.*, 1993). A meta-analysis of 21 studies, including over 800 children, showed no effect of inhaled BDP on statural height, even with higher doses and long duration of therapy (Allen *et al.*, 1993).

Short-term growth measurements (knemometry) have demonstrated that even a low dose of an oral steroid (prednisolone 2.5 mg) is sufficient to give complete suppression of lower leg growth. However, inhaled budesonide up to 400 μg is without effect, although some suppression is seen with 800 μg and with 400 μg BDP (Wolthers & Pedersen, 1993b,c). The relationship between knemometry measurements and final height is uncertain, since low doses of oral steroid that have no effect on final height cause profound suppression.

Metabolic effects

Several metabolic effects have been reported after inhaled steroids, but there is no evidence that these are clinically relevant at therapeutic doses. In adults, fasting glucose and insulin are unchanged after doses of BDP up to 2000 μg daily (Ebden *et al.*, 1986) and in children with inhaled budesonide up to 800 μg daily (Turpeinen *et al.*, 1991). In normal individuals high-dose inhaled BDP may slightly increase resistance to insulin (Kruszynska *et al.*, 1987). However, in patients with poorly controlled asthma a high-dose BDP and budesonide paradoxically decrease insulin resistance and improve glucose tolerance, suggesting that the disease itself may lead to abnormalities in carbohydrate metabolism (Kiviranta & Turpeinen, 1993). Neither BDP 2000 μg daily in adults nor budesonide 800 μg daily in children has any effect on plasma cholesterol or triglycerides (Ebden *et al.*, 1986; Turpeinen *et al.*, 1991).

Haematological effects

Inhaled steroids may reduce the numbers of circulating eosinophils in asthmatic patients (Evans *et al.*, 1993), possibly due to an effect on local cytokine generation in the airways. Inhaled steroids may cause a small increase in circulating neutrophil counts (Toogood *et al.*, 1984; Brown *et al.*, 1993b).

Central nervous system effects

There are various reports of psychiatric disturbance, including emotional lability, euphoria, depression, aggressiveness and insomnia, after inhaled steroids. Only eight such patients have so far been reported, suggesting that this is very infrequent, and a causal link with inhaled steroids has usually not been established (Barnes & Pedersen, 1993).

Safety in pregnancy

Based on extensive clinical experience, inhaled steroids appear to be safe in pregnancy, although no controlled studies have been performed. There is no evidence for any adverse effects of inhaled steroids on the pregnancy, the delivery or the fetus (Barnes & Pedersen, 1993). It is important to recognize that poorly controlled asthma may increase the incidence of perinatal mortality and retard intrauterine growth, so that more effective control of asthma with inhaled steroids may reduce these problems.

Clinical use of inhaled steroids

Inhaled steroids are now recommended as first-line therapy for all but the mildest of asthmatic patients (Barnes, 1989, 1995). Inhaled steroids should be started in any patient who needs to use a β-agonist inhaler for symptom control more than once daily (or possibly three times weekly). It is conventional to start with a low dose of inhaled steroid and to increase the dose until asthma control is achieved. However, this may take time and a preferable approach is to start with a dose of steroids in the middle of the dose range (400 μg twice daily) to establish control of asthma more rapidly. Once control is achieved (defined as normal or best possible lung function and infrequent need to use an inhaled β_2-agonist), the dose of inhaled steroid should be reduced in a stepwise manner to the lowest dose needed for optimal control. It may take as long as 3 months to reach a plateau in response and any changes in dose should be made at intervals of 3 months or more. When doses of ≤800 μg daily are needed, a large-volume spacer device should be used with an MDI and mouth washing with a dry powder inhaler in order to reduce local and systemic side-effects. Inhaled steroids are usually give as a twice-daily dose in order to increase compliance. When asthma is more unstable, four-times-daily dosage is preferable (Malo *et al.*, 1989). For patients who require ≤400 μg daily, once-daily dosing appears to be as effective as twice-daily dosing, at least for budesonide (Jones *et al.*, 1993).

The dose of inhaled steroid should be increased to 2000 μg daily if necessary, but higher doses may result in systemic effects and it may be preferable to add an oral steroid, since higher doses of inhaled steroids are expensive and have a high incidence of local side-effects. Nebulized budesonide has been advocated in order to give an increased dose of inhaled steroid and to reduce the requirement for oral steroids (Otulana *et al.*, 1992), but this treatment is expensive and may achieve its effects largely via systemic absorption.

Most of the guidelines for asthma treatment suggest that additional bronchodilators (slow-release theophylline preparations, inhaled and oral long-acting β_2-agonists and inhaled anticholinergics) should be introduced after increasing the dose of inhaled steroid to 1600–2000 μg daily. However, an alternative approach is to introduce these treatments when patients are taking 800–1000 μg inhaled steroid daily. Carefully designed clinical trials of long duration are needed to determine the optimal approach.

Systemic steroids

Oral or intravenous steroids may be indicated in several situations. Prednisolone, rather than prednisone, is the preferred oral steroid, as prednisone has to be converted in the liver to the active prednisolone. In pregnant patients, prednisone may be preferable, as it is not converted to prednisolone in the fetal liver, thus diminishing the exposure of the fetus to glucocorticosteroids. Enteric-coated preparations of prednisolone are used to reduce side-effects (particularly gastric side-effects) and give delayed and reduced peak plasma concentrations, although the bio-availability and therapeutic efficacy of these preparations is similar to those of uncoated tablets. Prednisolone and prednisone are preferable to dexamethasone, betamethasone or triamcinolone, which have longer plasma half-lives and therefore an increased frequency of adverse effects.

Short courses of oral steroids (30–40 mg prednisolone daily for 1–2 weeks or until the peak flow values return to best attainable) are indicated for exacerbations of asthma, and the dose may be tailed off over 1 week once the exacerbation is resolved. The tail-off period is not strictly necessary (O'Driscoll *et al.*, 1993), but some patients find it reassuring.

Maintenance oral steroids are only needed in a small proportion of asthmatic patients with the most severe asthma, which cannot be controlled with maximal doses of inhaled steroids (2000 μg daily) and additional bronchodilators. The minimal dose of oral steroid needed for control should be used, and reductions in the dose should be made slowly in patients who have been on oral steroids for long periods (e.g. by 2.5 mg per month for doses down to 10 mg daily and thereafter by 1 mg per month). Oral steroids are usually given as a single morning dose, as this reduces the risk of adverse effects since it coincides with the peak diurnal concentrations. There is some evidence that administration in the afternoon may be optimal for some patients who have severe nocturnal asthma (Beam *et al.*, 1992). Alternate-day administration may also reduce adverse effects, but control of asthma may not be as good on the day when the oral dose is omitted in some patients.

Intramuscular triamcinolone acetonide (80 mg monthly) has been advocated in patients with severe asthma as an alternative to oral steroids (McLeod *et al.*, 1985; Ogirala *et al.*, 1991). This may be considered in patients in whom compliance is a particular problem, but the major concern is the high frequency of proximal myopathy associated with this fluorinated steroid. Some patients who do not respond well to prednisolone are reported to respond to oral betamethasone, presumably because of pharmacokinetic handling problems with prednisolone (Grandordy *et al.*, 1987).

Steroid-sparing therapy

In patients who have serious side-effects with maintenance steroid therapy, there are several treatments which have been shown to reduce the requirement for oral steroids. These treatments are commonly termed steroid-sparing, although this is a misleading decription that could be applied to any additional asthma therapy (including bronchodilators). The amount of steroid sparing with these therapies is not impressive.

Several immunosuppressive agents have been shown to have steroid effects, including methotrexate (Mullarkey *et al.*, 1988; Mullarkey *et al.*, 1990; Shiner *et al.*, 1990), oral gold (Klaustermeyer *et al.*, 1987; Nierop *et al.*, 1992) and cyclosporin A (Szczfklik *et al.*, 1991; Alexander *et al.*, 1992). These therapies all have side-effects that may be more troublesome than those of oral steroids and are therefore only indicated as an additional therapy to reduce the requirement of oral steroids. None of these treatments is very effective, but there are occasional patients who appear to show a particularly good response. Because of side-effects these treatments cannot be considered as a way to reduce the requirement for inhaled steroids. Side-effects are a problem with these immunosuppressive drugs and include nausea, vomiting, hepatic dysfunction, hepatic fibrosis, pulmonary fibrosis and increased infections for methotrexate and renal dysfunction for cyclosporin and oral gold. Several other therapies, including azathioprine, dapsone and hydroxychloroquine have not been found to be beneficial. The macrolide antibiotic troleandomycin is also reported to have steroid-sparing effects, but this is only seen with methylprednisolone and is due to reduced metabolism of this steroid, so that there is little therapeutic gain (Nelson, H.S. *et al.*, 1993).

Acute severe asthma

Intravenous hydrocortisone is given in acute severe asthma. The recommended dose is 200 mg i.v. (British Thoracic Society, 1993). While the value of corticosteroids in acute severe asthma has been questioned, others have found that they speed the resolution of attacks (Engel & Heinig, 1991). There is no apparent advantage in giving very high doses of intravenous steroids (such as methylprednisolone 1 g). Indeed, intravenous steroids have occasionally been associated with an acute severe myopathy (Decramer *et al.*, 1995). In a recent study, no difference in recovery from acute severe asthma was seen, whether i.v. hydocortisone in doses of 50, 200 or 500 mg 6-hourly was used (Bowler *et al.*, 1992), and another placebo-controlled study showed no beneficial effect of i.v. steroids (Morell *et al.*, 1992). Intravenous steroids are indicated in acute asthma if lung function is $<30\%$ predicted and in whom there is no significant improvement with nebulized β_2-agonist. Intravenous therapy is usually given until a satisfactory response is obtained and then oral prednisolone may be substituted.

Oral prednisolone (40–60 mg) has a similar effect to that of intravenous hydrocortisone and is easier to administer (Harrison *et al.*, 1986; Engel & Heinig, 1991). Oral prednisolone is the preferred treatment for acute severe asthma, providing there are no contraindications to oral therapy (British Thoracic Society, 1993).

Steroid-resistant asthma

Although most patients with asthma respond to steroids, there is a small minority of patients who appear to be resistant to steroid therapy. Steroid resistance is defined by a lack of response to oral steroids (usually 40 mg prednisolone daily for 2 weeks) (Carmichael *et al.*, 1981; Cypcar & Busse, 1993; Barnes & Adcock, 1995). Other patients require very high doses of oral steroids for control and these patients should be considered as part of the steroid-resistant asthma spectrum (Woolcock, 1993). It is important before diagnosing steroid-resistant asthma to ensure that the patient has asthma, that there are no problems with compliance and that absorption of the oral steroid is normal (Woolcock, 1993). There are no epidemiological surveys of true steroid-resistant asthma, but as strictly defined above this may only occur in 1 : 1000 to 1 : 10 000 asthmatics. There is a tendency for these patients to have more severe asthma of a longer duration and with nocturnal exacerbations. There is often a family history of asthma. Steroid resistance does not appear to be explained by pharmacokinetic problems, such as impaired absorption or rapid elimination of oral steroids (Corrigan *et al.*, 1991; Lane & Lee, 1991; Alvarez *et al.*, 1992). The inhibitory effect of steroids on phytohaemagglutinin-stimulated growth of cultured blood monocytes is reduced in steroid-resistant patients compared with steroid-sensitive controls (Poznansky *et al.*, 1984; Alvarez *et al.*, 1992), suggesting that there is a cellular defect in steroid responsiveness. Steroids also fail to suppress the release of cytokines from monocytes of resistant patients (Wilkinson *et al.*, 1989). This defect is not confined to monocytes, but is also seen in peripheral T lymphocytes (Corrigan *et al.*, 1991), and a defect in the skin blanching response to topical steroids has also been described in such patients (Brown *et al.*, 1991).

Molecular mechanisms

The precise mechanism of steroid resistance is not certain. There is no significant defect in binding of steroids to GR in monocytes or lymphocytes from these patients and no defect in nuclear transcription of GR (Corrigan *et al.*, 1991; Lane & Lee, 1991). Chemical mutational analysis shows that there is no apparent abnormality in the structure of GR (Lane *et al.*, 1994). This is in contrast to the rare patients with familial glucocorticoid resistance, who may have marked abnormalities in steroid receptor-binding parameters and an abnormality in GR sequence (Lamberts *et al.*, 1992; Malchoff *et al.*, 1993). There is no evidence for lipocortin-1 autoantibodies in patients with steroid-resistant asthma (Wilkinson *et al.*, 1990; Chung *et al.*, 1991), as has been described in patients with steroid-resistant arthritis (Hirata *et al.*, 1981; Goulding *et al.*, 1989).

A recent study has suggested that there is impaired binding of GR to GRE and also a defect in the inhibitory effect of AP-1 activation on GRE binding in peripheral-blood mononuclear cells of resistant compared with sensitive patients (Adcock *et al.*, 1993a, 1995b). There is also an increase in basal AP-1 activity in these cells and this may result in a reduced number of GR available for DNA binding or for binding to other activated transcription factors (Fig. 35.6). This would explain why resistance to the anti-inflammatory effects of steroids is seen in these patients, and yet circulating cortisol levels, adrenal suppression in response to steroids and metabolic actions of steroids are apparently normal.

Resistance to steroids is not confined to asthma, but is also described in other conditions where steroids are required for disease control, including rheumatoid arthritis, leukaemias and transplant rejection (Cypcar & Busse, 1993; Barnes & Adcock, 1995). Although patients with resistance to steroids may be an extreme, there may be a spectrum of steroid responsiveness. Down-regulation of steroid receptors after exposure to steroids *in vitro* is well described (Rosewicz *et al.*, 1988; Okret *et al.*, 1991), and there is some evidence that this can occur in circulating lymphocytes *in vivo* after oral steroid treatment. Reduction in GR mRNA has been described in human lung *in vitro* after exposure to high-dose steroids (Adcock *et al.*, 1991), but whether this is important in asthmatic patients exposed to high-dose inhaled steroids is not known. Another possibility is that inflammation itself may counteract the anti-inflammatory effects of steroids through the direct interaction between GR and AP-1 (activated by exposure to pro-inflammatory cytokines) (Schüle & Evans, 1991; Barnes & Adcock, 1993) or with the transcription factor CREB activated by exposure to high-dose β-agonists (Peters *et al.*, 1995).

Secondary steroid resistance

Although complete steroid resistance is uncommon, there may be a spectrum of steroid responsiveness in inflammatory diseases. This may reflect several mechanisms that are secondary either to disease activity itself or to the effects of therapy (Fig. 35.7).

Several pro-inflammatory cytokines, including IL-1β, IL-6 and TNF-α, activate AP-1 and NF-κB in human lung (Adcock *et al.*, 1994b,c). As all these cytokines are known to be secreted in asthmatic inflammation, this suggests that these transcription factors will be activated in the cells of asthmatic airways. These activated transcription factors may then form protein–protein complexes with activated GR, both in the cytoplasm and within the nucleus, thus reducing the number of effective GR and thereby decreasing steroid responsiveness (Barnes & Adcock, 1993). In a model *in vitro* system, increased expression of c-Fos or c-Jun oncoproteins prevents the activation of mouse mammary tumour virus promoter by GR, thus creating a model of steroid resistance (Yang-Yen *et al.*, 1990). Addition of recombinant c-Jun or c-Fos proteins to partially purified GR results in inhibition of DNA binding (Yang-Yen *et al.*, 1990). Phorbol esters, which activate AP-1, result

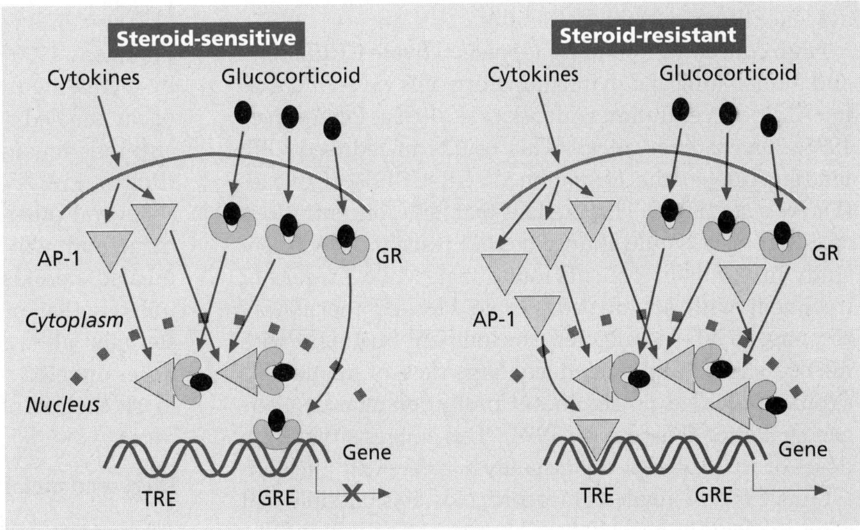

Fig. 35.6 Possible mechanism of primary steroid resistance in asthma. Increased activation of activator protein-1 (AP-1) results in the complexing of glucocorticoid receptors (GR), thus preventing the anti-inflammatory action of steroids.

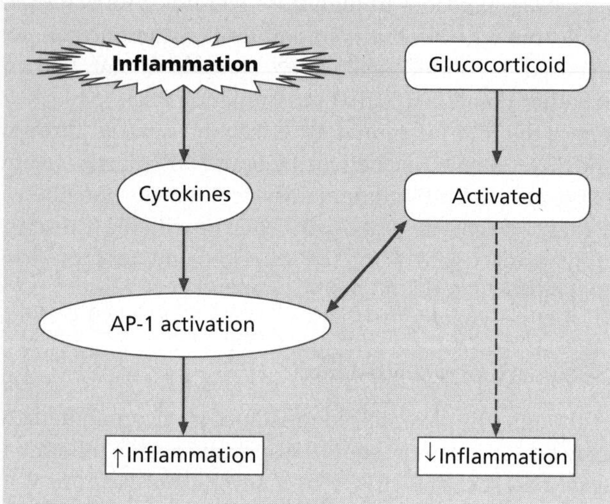

Fig. 35.7 Secondary steroid resistance caused by the effects of pro-inflammatory cytokines on AP-1.

in attenuation of glucocorticoid-mediated gene activation (Vacca *et al.*, 1989). Any reduction in glucocorticoid responsiveness would be greater as the intensity of asthmatic inflammation increased and may contribute, for example, to the failure of oral or intravenous glucocorticoids to control acute exacerbations of asthma. Once the inflamation is brought under control with large doses of oral glucocorticoids, steroid responsiveness increases again so that lower doses of inhaled or oral glucocorticoids are needed to control asthmatic inflammation.

Increased resistance may also be due to the effects of cytokines on GR receptor function, since high concentrations of IL-2 and IL-4 have been shown to reduce GR affinity in T lymphocytes *in vitro* (Kam *et al.*, 1993). This effect would only be seen in mucosal T cells of patients with severe asthma and it is therefore difficult to obtain evidence to support this possibility.

High concentrations of β_2-agonists activate CREB in rat and human lung and in inflammatory cells via an increase in cAMP concentration (Adcock *et al.*, 1995a; Peters *et al.*, 1995; Stevens *et al.*, 1995). This results in reduced GRE binding due to the formation of GR–CREB complexes (Peters *et al.*, 1993a). This predicts that high concentrations of β_2-agonists would induce steroid resistance. A recent study in asthmatic patients found that, while 3 weeks of treatment with an inhaled steroid blocked the airway response to inhaled allergen, concomitant treatment with inhaled steroid and a relatively large dose of inhaled β_2-agonist provided no significant protection against allergen challenge (Wong *et al.*, 1994). This suggests that high doses of an inhaled β_2-agonist may interfere with the anti-asthma effect of inhaled glucocorticoids. It is possible that some patients who use very high doses of inhaled β_2-agonists (over two canisters per month of MDI or regular nebulized doses) may develop a degree of steroid resistance, which is overcome by increasing the dose of inhaled or oral glucocorticoid. This may account for some of the deleterious effects of high-dose β-agonists on asthma mortality and morbidity (Barnes & Chung, 1992; Taylor *et al.*, 1993; Suissa *et al.*, 1994). The use of high doses of nebulized β_2-agonists in the treatment of acute exacerbations of asthma may result in resistance to the effects of high-dose intravenous glucocorticoids in the treatment of these exacerbations. Steroid responsiveness might be restored by reducing the dose of inhaled β_2-agonists. In an uncontrolled study in steroid-dependent patients with severe asthma, gradual withdrawal of nebulized β_2-agonists resulted in a reduced requirement for oral prednisolone (Peters *et al.*, 1993b).

Future developments

Because inhaled steroids are the most effective therapy currently available for asthma, perhaps the most useful advances in asthma therapy in the future may be the improvement of inhaled steroids so that systemic and local adverse effects are less likely. The use of new delivery devices has partly achieved the desired reduction in local and systemic effects, but novel types of steroid for inhalation or the development of non-steroidal drugs that mimic the essential anti-asthma effects of steroids are also a possibility. It is clear that there is a single type of GR (Muller & Renkawitz, 1991) and therefore it is not possible to develop novel steroids that have a greater selectivity. Improvements in inhaled steroids must therefore be based on pharmacokinetic differences. Inhaled steroids exert their anti-asthmatic effects topically in the airways rather than via a systemic effect. This is demonstrated by a recent study in which a systemic dose of budesonide given to mimic the small systemic effect of inhaled budesonide (400 μg daily) was without anti-asthma effect (Toogood & Frankism, 1990). New inhaled steroids may be developed by increasing the inactivation of the systemic component of the inhaled steroid and/or by potentiating the topical anti-inflammatory action of steroids in the airways (Brattsand & Axelsson, 1992).

Several other anti-asthma drugs are now in development and will eventually have to be compared with inhaled steroids as a 'gold standard' (Barnes, 1992). It is unlikely that any of these treatments will replace inhaled steroids, although they may reduce the need for high doses. Inhaled steroids are here to stay and it is important to use them as effectively as possible.

Increased metabolism

The fraction of inhaled steroid deposited in the oropharynynx and swallowed is available for absorption from the gastrointestinal tract. First-pass metabolism in the liver is therefore important in limiting the systemic effect of inhaled steroids. Budesonide has a very efficient first-pass metabolism (90%). The swallowed fraction of inhaled steroids is also markedly reduced by the use of a large-volume spacer device or by mouth washing. However, the major component of inhaled steroid which reaches the systemic circulation is derived from the respiratory tract. It can be calculated that, for a steroid with 90% first-pass hepatic metabolism, approximately 75% of the total systemic availability originates from the lung-absorbed fraction, and that mouth rinsing after inhalation can enhance this figure to approximately 90% (Brattsand & Axelsson, 1992). This calculation has recently been supported by *in vivo* experiments in human volunteers, where the oral absorption was completely blocked by administration of charcoal by mouth (Thorsson & Edsbäcker, 1993). The large lung-absorbed fraction could be reduced by the development of inhaled steroids that are inactivated in the lung or in the circulation by esterases. Examples of such steroids are fluocortinbutyl ester (hydrolysed in tissue and blood) and tixocortol pivalate (inactivated in blood by S-methyltransferases) (Brattsand & Axelsson, 1992). However, the same properties reduce the topical potency of these steroids, resulting in local metabolism in the airways, and neither of these steroids has useful anti-asthma effects. It is possible that steroids with a higher receptor affinity could be developed to exert a topical action before metabolism occurs.

Increased binding

Currently effective inhaled steroids derived from lipophilic substitution in the 17α, 17β positions of the glucocorticoid structure have a high affinity for GR and also have a high mucosal uptake and retention in airways and lung (Ryrfeldt *et al.*, 1989; Brattsand & Axelsson, 1992; Miller-Larsson *et al.*, 1992). However, increasing the local tissue retention time carries the risk of more troublesome local effects in the oropharynx. More selective targeting of the inhaled steroid to the key target cells may be another approach in the future, although it is likely that several target cells are involved in asthma. One possibility is to target airway macrophages by the use of liposomes coated with surface receptors that trigger phagocytosis (Brattsand & Axelsson, 1992).

Genomic selectivity

Steroids exert their anti-inflammatory and immunomodulatory effect by regulating gene transcription via several different mechanisms, as discussed above. By the use of site-directed mutagenesis of GR it is possible to differentiate some of these mechanisms so that some receptor mutants may more selectively mediate a particular type of genomic mechanism. It is possible that different types of steroid might be developed in the future which may cause conformational changes in the receptor to lead to more selective genomic effects.

Conclusions

Glucocorticosteroids are by far the most effective anti-asthma therapy currently available. The problem of side-effects encountered with oral steroid has largely been avoided by the development of potent inhaled steroids. Inhaled steroids are very effective in controlling asthma symptoms and in reducing asthma exacerbations. There is also preliminary evidence that they may prevent irreversible airway changes and may reduce asthma mortality. An important consideration is their risk–benefit ratio, and inhaled steroids have now been studied more extensively than any other drug in both adults and children. These studies, conducted in normal volunteers and asthmatic patients of varying severity, have demonstrated that, irrespective of the inhaled steroid, there are minimal systemic effects, even using the most sensitive indicators, at doses of ≤400 μg in children or ≤800 μg in adults. At higher doses, there is some evidence for systemic effects, although this is less noticeable with budesonide and fluticasone than with BDP. Even at high doses (up to 2000 μg daily), there is little evidence of any adverse effects, although occasional patients may have idiosyncratic responses. The small risk of adverse effects at high doses of inhaled steroids has to be offset against the risks of not adequately controlling severe asthma. The risk of systemic absorption is markedly reduced by the use of spacer devices with MDI and by mouth washing with dry-powder inhalers and these should be used whenever doses of ≥800 μg daily are needed for asthma control. More detailed dose–response curves for beneficial and adverse effects of different inhaled steroids are needed. Additional long-term studies of the effects of inhaled steroids in adults and children are needed, taking into account long-term benefits, adverse effects and costs. It is also important that other anti-asthma treatments, including new therapies, such as leukotriene antagonists and selective phosphodiesterase inhibitors, are compared with inhaled steroids in long-term studies.

References

Abbinante-Nissen, J.M., Simpson, L.G. & Leikauf, G.D. (1995) Corticosteroids increase secretory leukocyte protease inhibitor transcript levels in airway epithelial cells. *Am. J. Physiol.*, **12**, 601–6.

Adcock, I.M. & Barnes, P.J. (1995) Actions of the glucocorticoid receptor on transcription factors within the cytoplasma. *Am. J. Resp. Crit. Care Med.*, **151**, A159.

Adcock, I.M., Brönnegård, M. & Barnes, P.J. (1991) Glucocorticoid receptor mRNA localization and expression in human lung. *Am. Rev. Resp. Dis.*, **143**, A628.

Adcock, I.M., Brown, C.R., Virdee, H. *et al.* (1993a) DNA binding of glucocorticoid receptor from peripheral blood monocytes of steroid resistance and resistant patients. *Am. Rev. Resp. Dis.*, **147**, A244.

Adcock, I.M., Peters, M., Gelder, C., Shirasaki, H., Brown, C.R. & Barnes, P.J. (1993b) Increased tachykinin receptor gene expression in asthmatic lung and its modulation by steroids. *J. Mol. Endocrinol.*, **11**, 1–7.

Adcock, I.M., Brown, C.R., Kwon, O.J. & Barnes, P.J. (1994a) Oxidative stress induces NF-κB DNA binding and inducible NOS mRNA in human epithelial cells. *Biochem. Biophys. Res. Commun.*, **199**, 1518–24.

Adcock, I.M., Brown, C.R., Shirasaki, H. & Barnes, P.J. (1994b) Effects of dexamethasone on cytokine and phorbol ester stimulated c-Fos and c-Jun DNA binding and gene expression in human lung. *Eur. Resp. J.*, **7**, 2117–23.

Adcock, I.M., Shirasaki, H., Gelder, C.M., Peters, M.J., Brown, C.R. & Barnes, P.J. (1994c) The effects of glucocorticoids on phorbol ester and cytokine stimulated transcription factor activation in human lung. *Life Sci.*, **55**, 1147–53.

Adcock, I.M., Brown, C.R., Gelder, C.M., Shirasaki, H., Peters, M.J. & Barnes, P.J. (1995a) The effects of glucocorticoids on transcription factor activation in human peripheral blood monoclucear cells. *Am. J. Physiol.*, **37**, C331–8.

Adcock, I.M., Lane, S.J., Brown, C.A., Peters, M.J., Lee, T.H. & Barnes, P.J. (1995b) Differences in binding of glucocorticoid receptor to DNA in steroid-resistant asthma. *J. Immunol.*, **154**, 3500–5.

Ädelroth, E., Rosenhall, L., Johansson, S.-A., Linden, M. & Venge, P. (1990) Inflammatory cells and eosinophilic activity in asthmatics investigated by bronchoalveolar lavage. *Am. Rev. Resp. Dis.*, **142**, 91–9.

Agertoft, L. & Pedersen, S. (1994) Effects of long-term treatment with an inhaled corticosteroid on growth and pulmonary function in asthmatic children. *Resp. Med.*, **5**, 369–72.

Alexander, A.G., Barnes, N.C. & Kay, A.B. (1992) Trial of cyclosporin in corticosteroid-dependent chronic severe asthma. *Lancet*, **339**, 324–8.

Ali, N.J., Capewell, S. & Ward, M.J. (1991) Bone turnover during high dose inhaled corticosteroid treatment. *Thorax*, **46**, 160–4.

Allen, D.B., Mullen, M. & Mullen, B. (1993) A meta-analysis of the effects of oral and inhaled corticosteroids on growth. *J. Allergy Clin. Immunol.*, **93**, 967–76.

Alvarez, J., Surs, W., Leung, D.Y., Ikle, D., Gelfand, E.W. & Szefler, S.J. (1992) Steroid-resistant asthma: immunologic and pharmacologic features. *J. Allergy Clin. Immunol.*, **89**, 714–21.

Balfour-Lynn, L. (1986) Growth and childhood asthma. *Arch. Dis. Child.*, **61**, 1049–55.

Baran, D. (1987) A comparison of inhaled budesonide and beclomethasone diproprionate in childhood asthma. *Brit. J. Dis. Chest*, **81**, 170–5.

Barnes, P.J. (1988) Inflammatory mechanisms and nocturnal asthma. *Am. J. Med.*, **85** (Suppl. 1B), 64–70.

Barnes, P.J. (1989) A new approach to asthma therapy. *New Engl. J. Med.*, **321**, 1517–27.

Barnes, P.J. (1990) Effect of corticosteroids on airway hyperresponsiveness. *Am. Rev. Resp. Dis.*, **141**, S70–S76.

Barnes, P.J. (1992) New drugs for asthma. *Eur. Resp. J.*, **5**, 1126–36.

Barnes, P.J. (1993) Antiinflammatory therapy in asthma. *Ann. Rev. Med.*, **44**, 229–49.

Barnes, P.J. (1995) Inhaled glucocorticoids for asthma. *New Engl. J. Med.*, **332**, 868–75.

Barnes, P.J. & Adcock, I.M. (1993) Anti-inflammatory actions of steroids: molecular mechanisms. *Trends Pharmacol. Sci.*, **14**, 436–41.

Barnes, P.J. & Adcock, I.M. (1995) Steroid resistant asthma. *Quart. J. Med.*, **88**, 455–68.

Barnes, P.J. & Chung, K.F. (1992) Questions about inhaled β_2-agonists in asthma. *Trends Pharmacol. Sci.*, **13**, 20–3.

Barnes, P.J. & Liew, F.Y. (1995) Nitric oxide and asthmatic inflammation. *Immunol. Today*, **16**, 128–30.

Barnes, P.J. & Pedersen, S. (1993) Efficacy and safety of inhaled steroids in asthma. *Am. Rev. Resp. Dis.*, **148**, S1–S26.

Beam, W.R., Ballard, R.D. & Martin, R.J. (1992) Spectrum of corticosteroid sensitivity in nocturnal asthma. *Am. Rev. Resp. Dis.*, **145**, 1082–6.

Bel, E.H., Timers, M.C., Zwinderman, A.H., Dijkman, J.H. & Sterk, P.J. (1991) The effect of inhaled corticosteroids on the maximal degree of airway narrowing to methacholine. *Am. Rev. Resp. Dis.*, **143**, 109–13.

Bisgaard, H., Damkjaer Nielsen, M. & Andersen, B. (1988) Adrenal function in children with bronchial asthma treated with beclomethasone diproprionate or budesonide. *J. Allergy Clin. Immunol.*, **81**, 1088–95.

Bisgaard, H., Munck, S.L., Nielsen, J.P., Peterson, W. & Ohlsson, S.V. (1990) Inhaled budesonide for treatment of recurrent wheezing in early childhood. *Lancet*, **336**, 649–51.

Boner, A.L. & Piacentini, G.L. (1993) Inhaled corticosteroids in children: is there a 'safe' dosage? *Drug Safety*, **9**, 9–20.

Boschetto, P., Rogers, D.F., Fabbri, L.M. & Barnes, P.J. (1991) Corticosteroid inhibition of airway microvascular leakage. *Am. Rev. Resp. Dis.*, **143**, 605–9.

Bowler, S.D., Mitchell, C.A. & Armstrong, J.G. (1992) Corticosteroids in acute severe asthma: effectiveness of low doses. *Thorax*, **47**, 584–7.

Brattsand, R. & Axelsson, B. (1992) New inhaled glucocorticosteroids. In: *New Drugs for Asthma*, Vol. 2 (ed. P.J. Barnes), pp. 192–207. IBC Technical Services, London.

British Thoracic Society (1993) Guidelines on the management of asthma. *Thorax*, **48** (Suppl.), S1–S24.

Brogden, R.N. & McTavish, D. (1992) Budesonide: an updated review of its pharmacological properties and therapeutic efficacy in asthma and rhinitis. *Drugs*, **44**, 375–407.

Brogden, R.N., Heel, R.C., Speight, T.M. & Avery, G.S. (1984) Beclomethasone diproprionate: a reappraisal of its pharmacodynamic properties and therapeutic efficacy after a decade of use in asthma and rhinitis. *Drugs*, **28**, 99–126.

Brown, P.H., Blundell, G., Greening, A.P. & Crompton, G.K. (1990) Do large volume spacer devices reduce the systemic effects of high dose inhaled corticosteroids? *Thorax*, **95**, 736–9.

Brown, P.H., Teelucksingh, S., Matusiewicz, S.P., Greening, A.P., Crompton, G.K. & Edwards, C.R.W. (1991) Cutaneous vasoconstrictor responses to glucocorticoids in asthma. *Lancet*, **337**, 576–80.

Brown, P.H., Blundell, G., Greening, A.P. & Crompton, G.K. (1992) High dose inhaled corticosteroids and the cortisol induced response to acute severe asthma. *Resp. Med.*, **86**, 495–7.

Brown, P.H., Greening, A.P. & Crompton, G.K. (1993a) Large volume spacer devices and the influence of high dose beclomethasone diproprionate on hypothalamo-pituitary-adrenal axis function. *Thorax*, **48**, 233–8.

Brown, P.H., Matusiewicz, S.P., Shearing, C., Tibi, L., Greening, A.P. & Crompton, G.K. (1993b) Systemic effects of high dose inhaled steroids: comparison of beclomethasone diproprionate and budesonide in healthy subjects. *Thorax*, **48**, 967–73.

Burke, C., Power, C.K., Norris, A., Condez, A., Schmekel, B. & Poulter, L.W. (1992) Lung function and immunopathological changes after inhaled corticosteroid therapy in asthma. *Eur. Resp. J.*, **5**, 73–9.

Capewell, S., Reynolds, S., Shuttleworth, D., Edwards, C. & Finlay, A.Y. (1990) Purpura and dermal thinning associated with high dose inhaled corticosteroids. *Brit. Med. J.*, **300**, 1548–51.

Carmichael, J., Paterson, I.C., Diaz, P., Crompton, G.K., Kay, A.B. & Grant, I.W.B. (1981) Corticosteroid resistance in chronic asthma. *Brit. Med. J.*, **282**, 1419–22.

Carnuccio, R., Di Rosa, M., Guerrasio, B., Iuvone, T. & Satebin, L. (1987) Vasocortin: a novel glucocorticoid-induced anti-inflammatory protein. *Brit. J. Pharmacol.*, **90**, 443–5.

Chaplin, M.D., Rooks, W., Svenson, E.W., Couper, W.C., Nerenberg, C. & Chu, N.I. (1980) Flunisotide metabolism and dynamics of a metabolite. *Clin. Pharmacol. Ther.*, **27**, 402–13.

Chung, K.F., Podgorski, M.R., Goulding, N.J. *et al.* (1991) Circulating autoantibodies to recombinant lipocortin-1 in asthma. *Resp. Med.*, **95**, 121–4.

Colotta, F., Re, F., Muzio, M. *et al.* (1993) Interleukin-1 type II receptor: a decoy target for IL-1 that is regulated by IL-4. *Science*, **261**, 472–5.

Corrigan, C., Brown, P.H., Barnes, N.C. *et al.* (1991) Glucocorticoid resistance in chronic asthma. *Am. Rev. Resp. Dis.*, **144**, 1016–25.

Cronstein, B.N., Kimmel, S.C., Levin, R.I., Martiniuk, F. & Weissmann, G. (1992) A mechanism for the antiinflammatory effects of corticosteroids: the glucocorticoid receptor regulates leukocyte adhesion to endothelial cells and expression of endothelial-leukocyte adhesion molecule 1 and intercellular adhesion molecule 1. *Proc. Nat. Acad. Sci. USA*, **89**, 9991–5.

Cypcar, D. & Busse, W.W. (1993) Steroid-resistant asthma. *J. Allergy Clin. Immunol.*, **92**, 362–72.

Dahl, R., Pedersen, B. & Hägglöf, B. (1989) Nocturnal asthma: effect of treatment with oral sustained-release terbutaline, inhaled budesonide and the two in combination. *J. Allergy Clin. Immunol.*, **83**, 811–15.

Decramer, M., Lacquet, L.M., Fagard, R. & Rogiers, P. (1995) Corticosteroids contribute to muscle weakness in chronic airflow obstruction. *Am. J. Resp. Crit. Care Med.*, **150**, 11–16.

Djukanovic, R., Wilson, J.W., Britten, Y.M. *et al.* (1992) Effect of an inhaled corticosteroid on airway inflammation and symptoms of asthma. *Am. Rev. Resp. Dis.*, **145**, 699–674.

Dompeling, E., Van Schayck, C.P., Molema, J., Folgering, H., van Grusven, P.M. & van Weel, C. (1992) Inhaled beclomethasone improves the course of asthma and COPD. *Eur. Resp. J.*, **5**, 945–52.

Dworski, R., Fitzgerald, G.A., Oates, J.A. & Sheller, J.R. (1994) Effect of oral prednisone on airway inflammatory mediators in atopic asthma. *Am. J. Resp. Crit. Care Med.*, **149**, 953–9.

Ebden, P., Jenkins, A., Houston, G. & Davies, B.H. (1986) Comparison of two high-dose corticosteroid aerosol treatments, beclomethasone diproprionate (1500 mcg/day) and budesonide (1600 mcg/day) for chronic asthma. *Thorax*, **41**, 869–74.

Engel, T. & Heinig, J.H. (1991) Glucocorticoid therapy in acute severe asthma—a critical review. *Eur. Resp. J.*, **4**, 881–9.

Engel, T., Heinig, J.H., Malling, H.-J., Scharing, B., Nikander, K. & Masden, F. (1989) Clinical comparison of inhaled budesonide delivered either by pressurized metered dose inhaler or Turbuhaler. *Allergy*, **44**, 220–5.

Ernst, P., Spitzer, W.D., Suissa, S. *et al.* (1992) Risk of fatal and near fatal asthma in relation to inhaled corticosteroid use. *JAMA*, **268**, 3462–4.

Evans, P.M., O'Connor, B.J., Fuller, R.W., Barnes, P.J. & Chung, K.F. (1993) Effect of inhaled corticosteroids on peripheral eosinophil counts and density profiles in asthma. *J. Allergy Clin. Immunol.*, **91**, 643–9.

Fabbri, L., Burge, P.S., Croonenburgh, L. *et al.* (1993) Comparison of fluticasone proprionate with beclomethasone diproprionate in moderate to severe asthma treated for one year. *Thorax*, **48**, 817–23.

Flower, R.J. & Rothwell, N.J. (1994) Lipocortin-1: cellular mechanisms and clinical relevance. *Trends Pharmacol. Sci.*, **15**, 71–6.

Geddes, D.M. (1992) Inhaled corticosteroids: benefits and risks. *Thorax*, **47**, 404–7.

Gleeson, J.G.A. & Price, J.E. (1988) Controlled trial of budesonide given by Nebuhaler in preschool children with asthma. *Br. Med. J.*, **297**, 163–6.

Goulding, N.J., Podgorski, M.R., Hall, N.D. *et al.* (1989) Autoantibodies to recombinant liportin-1 in rheumatoid arthritis and systemic lupus erythematosus. *Ann. Rheum. Dis.*, **48**, 843–50.

Grandordy, B., Beilmatoug, N., Morelle, A., De Lauture, D. & Marac, J. (1987) Effect of betamethasone on airway obstruction and bronchial response to salbutamol in prednisolone resistant asthma. *Thorax*, **42**, 65–71.

Gronemeyer, H. (1992) Control of transcription activation by steroid hormone receptors. *FASEB J.*, **6**, 2524–9.

Haahtela, T., Järvinen, M., Kava, T. *et al.* (1991) Comparison of a β_2-agonist terbutaline with an inhaled steroid in newly detected asthma. *New Engl. J. Med.*, **325**, 388–92.

Haahtela, T., Järvinen, M., Kava, T. (1994) Effects of reducing or discontinuing inhaled budesonide in patients with mild asthma. *New Engl. J. Med.*, **331**, 700–5.

Hamid, O., Springall, D.R., Riveros-Moreno, V. *et al.* (1993) Induction of nitric oxide synthase in asthma. *Lancet*, **342**, 1510–13.

Harding, S.M. (1990) The human pharmacology of fluticasone diproprionate. *Resp. Med.*, **84** (Suppl. A), 25–9.

Harrison, B.D.N., Stokes, T.C., Hart, G.J., Vaughan, D.A., Ali, N.J. & Robinson, A.A. (1986) Need for intravenous hydrocortisone in addition to oral prednisolone in patients admitted to hospital with severe asthma without ventilatory failure. *Lancet*, **i**, 181–4.

Haynes, A.R. & Shaw, R.J. (1992) Dexamethasone-induced increase in platelet-derived growth factor (B) mRNA in human alveolar macrophages and myelomonocytic HL60 macrophage-like cells. *Am. J. Respir. Cell Mol. Biol.*, **7**, 198–206.

Hirata, F., del Carmine, R., Nelson, C.A. *et al.* (1981) Presence of autoantibody for phospholipase inhibitory protein, lipomodulin, in patients with rheumatic diseases. *Proc. Nat. Acad. Sci. USA*, **78**, 3190–4.

Holt, P.R., Lowndes, D.W., Smithies, E. & Dixon, G.T. (1990) The effect of an inhaled steroid on the hypothalamic–pituitary–adrenal axis: which tests should be used? *Clin. Exp. Allergy*, **20**, 145–9.

Hosking, D.J. (1993) Effect of corticosteroids on bone turnover. *Resp. Med.*, **87** (Suppl. A), 15–21.

Ilangovan, P., Pedersen, S., Godfrey, S., Nikander, K., Novisky, N. & Warner, J.O. (1993) Nebulised budesonide suspension in severe steroid-dependent preschool asthma. *Arch. Dis. Child.*, **68**, 356–9.

Imai, F., Minger, J.N., Mitchell, J.A., Yamamoto, K.R. & Granner, D.K. (1993) Glucocorticoid receptor–cAMP response element-binding protein interaction and the response of the phosphoenolpyruvate carboxykinase gene to glucocorticoids. *J. Biol. Chem.*, **268**, 5353–6.

Jeffery, P.K., Godfrey, R.W., Ädelroth, E., Nelson, F., Rogers, A. & Johansson, S.-A. (1992) Effects of treatment on airway inflammation and thickening of basement membrane reticular collagen in asthma. *Am. Rev. Resp. Dis.*, **145**, 890–9.

Jones, A.H., Langdon, C.G. & Lee, P.S. (1993) Pulmicort Turbuhaler once daily as initial prophylactic therapy for asthma. *Resp. Med.*, **88**, 293–9.

Juniper, E.F., Kline, P.A., Vanzieleghem, M.A., Ramsdale, E.H., O'Byrne, P.M. & Hargreave, F.E. (1990) Effect of long-term treatment with an inhaled corticosteroid (budesonide) on airway hyperresponsiveness and clinical asthma in nonsteroid-dependent asthmatics. *Am. Rev. Resp. Dis.*, **142**, 832–6.

Juniper, E.F., Kline, P.A., Vanzielegmem, M.A. & Hargreave, F.E. (1991) Reduction of budesonide after a year of increased use: a randomized controlled trial to evaluate whether improvements in airway responsiveness and clinical asthma are maintained. *J. Allergy Clin. Immunol.*, **87**, 483–9.

Kam, J.C., Szefler, S.J., Surs, W., Sher, F.R. & Leung, D.Y.M. (1993) Combination IL-2 and IL-4 reduces glucocorticoid–receptor binding affinity and T cell response to glucocorticoids. *J. Immunol.*, **151**, 3460–6.

Kerrebijn, K.F., Von Essen-Zandvliet, E.E.M. & Neijens, H.J. (1987) Effect of long-term treatment with inhaled corticosteroids and beta-agonists on bronchial responsiveness in asthmatic children. *J. Allergy Clin. Immunol.*, **79**, 653–9.

Kertjens, H.A.M., Brand, P.L.P., Hughes, M.D. *et al.* (1992) A comparison of bronchodilator therapy with or without inhaled corticosteroid therapy for obstructive airways disease. *New Engl. J. Med.*, **327**, 1413–19.

Kharitonov, S.A., Yates, D., Robbins, R.A., Logan-Sinclair, R., Shinebourne, E. & Barnes, P.J. (1994) Increased nitric oxide in exhaled air of asthmatic patients. *Lancet*, **343**, 133–5.

Kharitonov, S.A., Yates, D.H. & Barnes, P.J. (1995) Regular inhaled budesonide decreases nitric oxide concentration in the exhaled air of asthmatic patients. *Am. J. Resp. Crit. Care Med.*, **153**, 454–7.

Kiviranta, K. & Turpeinen, M. (1993) Effect of eight months of inhaled beclomethasone diproprionate and budesonide on carbohydrate metabolism in adults with asthma. *Thorax*, **48**, 974–8.

Klaustermeyer, W.B., Noritake, D.T. & Kwong, F.K. (1987) Chrysotherapy in the treatment of corticosteroid-dependent asthma. *J. Allergy Clin. Immunol.*, **79**, 720–5.

König, P. (1988) Inhaled corticosteroids—their present and future role in the management of asthma. *J. Allergy Clin. Immunol.*, **82**, 297–306.

König, P., Hillman, L. & Cervantes, C.I. (1993) Bone metabolism in children with asthma treated with inhaled beclomethasone diproprionate. *J. Pediatr.*, **122**, 219–26.

Kruszynska, Y.T., Greenstone, M. & Home, P.D. (1987) Effect of high dose inhaled beclomethasone diproprionate on carbohydrate and lipid metabolism in normal subjects. *Thorax*, **42**, 881–4.

Kwon, O.J., Au, B.T., Collins, P.D. *et al.* (1994) Tumor necrosis factor-induced interleukin 8 expression in cultured human epithelial cells. *Am. J. Physiol.*, **11**, L398–L405.

Kwon, O.J., Jose, P.J., Robbins, R.A., Schall, T.J., Williams, T.J. & Barnes, P.J. (1995) Glucocorticoid inhibition of RANTES expression in human lung epithelial cells. *Am. J. Respir. Cell Mol. Biol.*, **12**, 488–96.

Lacronique, J., Renon, D., Georges, D., Henry-Amar, M. & Marsac, J. (1991) High-dose beclomethasone: oral steroid-sparing effect in severe asthmatic patients. *Eur. Resp. J.*, **4**, 807–12.

Laitinen, L.A., Laitinen, A. & Haahtela, T. (1992) A comparative study of the effects of an inhaled corticosteroid, budesonide, and of a β_2-agonist, terbutaline, on airway inflammation in newly diagnosed asthma. *J. Allergy Clin. Immunol.*, **90**, 32–42.

Lamberts, S.W.J., Kioper, J.W. & de Jong, F.H. (1992) Familial and iatrogenic cortisol receptor resistance. *J. Steroid Biochem. Mol. Biol.*, **43**, 385–8.

Lane, S.J. & Lee, T.H. (1991) Glucocorticoid receptor characteristics in monocytes of patients with corticosteroid-resistant bronchial astham. *Am. Rev. Resp. Dis.*, **143**, 1020–4.

Lane, S.J., Arm, J.P., Staynov, D.Z. & Lee, T.H. (1994) Chemical mutational analysis of the human glucocortiocoid receptor cDNA in glucocorticoid-resistant bronchial asthma. *Am. J. Respir. Cell Mol. Biol.*, **11**, 42–8.

Law, C.M., Honour, J.W., Marchant, J.L., Preece, M.A. & Warner, J.O. (1986) Nocturnal adrenal suppression in asthmatic children taking inhaled beclomethasone dipropionate. *Lancet*, **i**, 942–4.

Löfdahl, C.G., Mellstrand, T. & Svedmyr, N. (1989) Glucocorticosteroids and asthma—studies of resistance and systemic effects of glucocorticosteroids. *Eur. J. Resp. Dis.*, **65** (Suppl. 130), 69–79.

Lungren, R., Soderberg, M., Horstedt, P. & Stenling, R. (1988) Morphological studies on bronchial mucosal biopsies from asthmatics before and after ten years treatment with inhaled steroids. *Eur. Resp. J.*, **1**, 883–9.

McLeod, D.T., Capewell, S.J., Law, J., MacLaren, W. & Seaton, A. (1985) Intramuscular triamcinolone acetamide in chronic severe asthma. *Thorax*, **40**, 840–5.

Mak, J.C.W., Nishikawa, M. & Barnes, P.J. (1995) Glucocorticosteroids increase β2-adrenergic receptor transcription in human lung. *Am. J. Physiol.*, **12**, L41–L46.

Mak, V.H.F., Melchor, R. & Spiro, S. (1992) Easy bruising as a side-effect of inhaled corticosteroids. *Eur. Resp. J.*, **5**, 1068–74.

Malchoff, D.M., Brufsky, A., McDermott, P. *et al.* (1993) A mutation of the glucocorticoid receptor in primary cortisol resistance. *J. Clin. Invest.*, **91**, 1918–25.

Malo, J.-L., Cartier, A., Merland, N. *et al.* (1989) Four-times-a-day dosing frequency is better than twice-a-day regimen in subjects requiring a high-dose inhaled steroid, budesonide, to control moderate to severe asthma. *Am. Rev. Resp. Dis.*, **140**, 624–8.

Meltzer, E.O., Kemp, J.P., Welch, M.J. & Orgel, H.A. (1985) Effect of dosing schedule on efficacy of beclomethasone diproprionate aerosol in chronic asthma. *Am. Rev. Resp. Dis.*, **131**, 732–6.

Miesfield, R.L. (1990) Molecular genetics of corticosteroid action. *Am. Rev. Resp. Dis.*, **141**, S11–S17.

Miller-Larsson, A., Lundin, P. & Brattsand, R. (1992) Affinity for airway tissue of topical corticosteroid budesonide, but not hydrocortisone — study in a rat tracheal model in situ. *Eur. Resp. J.*, **5** (Suppl. 15), 364S.

Mitchell, J.A., Belvisi, M.G., Akarasereemom, P. *et al.* (1994) Induction of cyclo-oxygenase-2 by cytokines in human pulmonary epithelial cells: regulation by dexamethasone. *Brit. J. Pharmacol.*, **113**, 1008–14.

Mollman, H., Rohdewald, P., Schmidt, E.W., Salomon, V. & Derendorf, H. (1985) Pharmacokinetics of triamcinolone acetonide and its phosphate ester. *Eur. J. Clin. Pharmacol.*, **29**, 85–9.

Monson, J.P. (1993) Systemic effects of inhaled steroids. *Thorax*, **48**, 955–6.

Morell, F., Orkiols, R., de Gracia, J., Curul, V. & Pujol, A. (1992) Controlled trial of intravenous corticosteroids in severe acute asthma. *Thorax*, **47**, 588–91.

Mukaido, N., Morita, M., Ishikawa, Y. *et al.* (1994) Novel mechanisms of glucocorticoid-mediated gene repression: NFRB is target for glucocorticoid-mediated IL-8 gene expression. *J. Biol. Chem.*, **269**, 13289–95.

Mullarkey, M.F., Blumenstein, B.A., Mandrade, W.P., Bailey, G.A., Olason, I. & Wetzel, C.E. (1988) Methotrexate in the treatment of corticosteroid-dependent asthma. *New Engl. J. Med.*, **318**, 683–7.

Mullarkey, M.F., Lammert, J.K. & Blumenstein, B.A. (1990) Long-term methotrexate treatment in corticosteroid-dependent asthma. *Ann. Intern. Med.*, **112**, 577–81.

Muller, M. & Renkawitz, R. (1991) The glucocorticoid receptor. *Biochim. Biophys. Acta*, **1088**, 171–82.

Nelson, H.S., Hamilos, D.L., Corsello, P.R., Levesque, N.V., Buchameier, A.D. & Bucher, B.L. (1993) A double-blind study of troleandamycin and methylprednisolone in asthmatic patients who require daily corticosteroids. *Am. Rev. Resp. Dis.*, **147**, 398–404.

Nelson, P.J., Kim, H.T., Manning, W.C., Goralski, T.J. & Krensky, A.M. (1993) Genomic organisation and transcriptional regulation of the RANTES chemokine gene. *J. Immunol.*, **151**, 2601–12.

Newton, R., Adcock, I.M. & Barnes, P.J. (1995) Stimulation of COX-2 message by cytokines or phorbol ester is preceded by a massive and rapid induction of NF-κB binding activity. *Am. J. Resp. Crit. Care Med.*, **151**, A165.

Nierop, G., Gijzel, W.P., Bel, E.H., Zwinderman, A.H. & Dijkman, J.H. (1992) Auranofin in the treatment of steroid dependent asthma: a double blind study. *Thorax*, **47**, 349–54.

Ninan, T. & Russell, G. (1992) Asthma, inhaled corticosteroid treatment and growth. *Arch. Dis. Child.*, **67**, 703–5.

Nishikawa, M., Shirasaki, M., Mak, J.W. & Barnes, P.J. (1993) Protective effects of dexamethasone on isoproterenol-induced down-regulation of pulmonary β_2-receptors in rat. *Am. Rev. Resp. Dis.*, **147**, A275.

Northrop, J.P., Ullman, K.S. & Crabtree, G.R. (1993) Characterization of the nuclear and cytoplasmic components of the lymphoid-specific nuclear factor of activated T cells (NF-AT). *J. Biol. Chem.*, **268**, 2917–23.

O'Driscoll, B.R., Kalra, S., Wilson, M., Pickering, C.A.C., Caroll, K.B. & Woodcocok, A.A. (1993) Double blind trial of steroid tapering in acute asthma. *Lancet*, **341**, 324–7.

Ogirala, R.G., Aldrich, T.K., Prezant, D.J., Sinnett, M.J., Enden, J.B. & Williams, M.H. (1991) High dose intramuscular triamcinolone in severe life-threatening asthma. *New Engl. J. Med.*, **329**, 585–9.

Okret, S., Dong, Y., Brönnegård, M. & Gustafsson, J.Å. (1991) Regulation of glucocorticoid receptor expression. *Biochimie*, **73**, 51–9.

Otulana, B.A., Varma, N., Bullock, A. & Higenbottam, T. (1992) High dose nebulized steroid in the treatment of chronic steroid-dependent asthma. *Resp. Med.*, **86**, 105–8.

Owens, G.P., Hahn, W.E. & Cohen, J.J. (1991) Identification of mRNAs associated with programmed cell death in immature thymocytes. *Mol. Cell. Biol.*, **11**, 4177–88.

Packe, G.E., Douglas, J.G., MacDonald, A.F., Robins, S.P. & Reid, D.M. (1992) Bone density in asthmatic patients taking high dose inhaled beclomethasone diproprionate and intermittent systemic steroids. *Thorax*, **47**, 414–17.

Paliogianni, F., Raptis, A., Ahuja, S.S., Najjar, S.M. & Boumpas, D.T. (1993) Negative transcriptional regulation of human interleukin 2 (IL-2) gene by glucocorticoids through interference with nuclear transcription factors AP-1 and NF-AT. *J. Clin. Invest.*, **91**, 1481–9.

Pauwels, R.A., Löfdahl, C.-G., Pride, N.B., Postma, D.S., Laitinen, L.A. & Ohlsson, S.V. (1992) European Respiratory Society study on chronic obstructive pulmonary disease (EUROSCOP): hypothesis and design. *Eur. Resp. J.*, **5**, 1254–61.

Pedersen, S. & Fuglsang, G. (1988) Urine cortisol excretion in children treated with high doses of inhaled corticosteroids: a comparison of budesonide and beclomethasone. *Eur. Resp. J.*, **1**, 433–5.

Peters, M.J., Adcock, I.M., Brown, C.R. & Barnes, P.J. (1993a) β-Agonist inhibition of steroid-receptor DNA binding activity in human lung. *Am. Rev. Resp. Dis.*, **147**, A772.

Peters, M.J., Yates, D.H., Chung, K.F. & Barnes, P.J. (1993b) β_2-Agonist dose reduction: strategy and early results. *Thorax*, **48**, 1066.

Peters, M.J., Adcock, I.M., Brown, C.R. & Barnes, P.J. (1995) β-Adrenoceptor agonists interfere with glucocorticoid receptor DNA binding in rat lung. *Eur. J. Pharmacol. (Mol. Section)*, **289**, 275–81.

Philip, M., Aviram, M., Lieberman, E. *et al.* (1992) Integrated plasma cortisol concentration in children with asthma receiving long-term inhaled corticosteroids. *Pediatr. Pulmonol.*, **12**, 84–9.

Placcentini, G., Sette, L., Peroni, D.G., Bonizatto, C., Bonetti, S. & Boner, A.L. (1990) Double blind evaluation of effectiveness and safety of flunisolide aerosol for treatment of bronchial asthma in children. *Allergy*, **45**, 612–16.

Ponta, H., Cato, A.C.B. & Herrlick, P. (1992) Interference of specific transcription factors. *Biochim. Biophys. Acta*, **1129**, 255–61.

Poznansky, M.C., Gordon, A.C.H., Douglas, J.G., Krajewski, A.S., Wyllie, A.H. & Grant, I.W.B. (1984) Resistance to methylprednisolone in cultures of blood mononuclear cells from glucocorticoid-resistant asthmatic patients. *Clin. Sci.*, **67**, 639–45.

Prahl, P. (1991) Adrenocortical suppression following treatment with beclomethasone and budesonide. *Clin. Exp. Allergy*, **21**, 145–6.

Ray, A. & Prefontaine, K.E. (1994) Physical association and functional antagonism between the p65 subunit of transcription factor NF-κB and the glucocorticoid receptor. *Proc. Nat. Acad. Sci. USA*, **91**, 752–6.

Reed, C.E. (1990) Aerosol glucocorticoid treatment of asthma: adults. *Am. Rev. Resp. Dis.*, **140**, S82–S88.

Robbins, R.A., Barnes, P.J., Springall, D.R. *et al.* (1994) Expression of inducible nitric oxide synthase in human bronchial epithelial cells. *Biochem. Biophys. Res. Commun.*, **203**, 209–18.

Rosewicz, S., McDonald, A.R., Maddux, B.A., Godfine, I.D., Miesfeld, R.L. & Logsden, C.D. (1988) Mechanism of glucocorticoid receptor down-regulation by glucocorticoids. *J. Biol. Chem.*, **263**, 2581–4.

Russell, G. (1993) Asthma and growth. *Arch. Dis. Child.*, **69**, 695–8.

Ryrfeldt, Å., Andersson, P., Edsbacker, S., Tonnesson, M., Davies, D. & Pauwels, R. (1982) Pharmacokinetics and metabolism of budesonide, a selective glucocorticoid. *Eur. J. Resp. Dis.*, **63** (Suppl. 122), 86–95.

Ryrfeldt, Å., Persson, G. & Nilsson, E. (1989) Pulmonary deposition of the potent glucocorticoid budesonide evaluated in an isolated perfused rat lung model. *Biochem. Pharmacol.*, **38**, 17–22.

Salmeron, S., Guerin, J.-C., Godard, P. *et al.* (1989) High doses of inhaled corticosteroids in unstable chronic asthma. *Am. Rev. Resp. Dis.*, **140**, 167–71.

Schleimer, R.P. (1990) Effects of glucocorticoids on inflammatory cells relevant to their therapeutic application in asthma. *Am. Rev. Resp. Dis.*, **141**, S59–S69.

Schüle, R. & Evans, R.M. (1991) Cross-coupling of signal transduction pathways: zinc finger meets leucine zipper. *Trends Genet.*, **7**, 377–81.

Selroos, O. & Halme, M. (1991) Effect of a Volumatic spacer and mouth rinsing on systemic absorption of inhaled corticosteroids from a metered-dose inhaler and dry powder inhaler. *Thorax*, **46**, 891–4.

Selroos, O., Backman, R., Forsen, K.-O. *et al.* (1994) When to start treatment of asthma with inhaled steroids. *Eur. Resp. J.*, **7** (Suppl. 18), 151S.

Sheffer, A.L. (1991) National Heart Lung and Blood Institute National Asthma Education Programme Expert Panel Report: guidelines for the diagnosis and management of asthma. *J. Allergy Clin. Immunol.*, **88**, 425–534.

Sheffer, A.L. (1991) International Consensus Report on Diagnosis and Management of Asthma. *Clin. Exp. Allergy*, **22** (Suppl. 1), 1–72.

Shiner, R.J., Nunn, A.J., Chung, K.F. & Geddes, D.M. (1990) Randomized, double-blind, placebo-controlled trial of methotrexate in steroid-dependent asthma. *Lancet*, **336**, 137–40.

Simons, F.E.R., Persaud, M.P., Gillespie, C.A., Cheang, M. & Shuckett, E.P. (1993) Absence of posterior subcapsular cataracts in young patients treated with inhaled glucocorticoids. *Lancet*, **342**, 736–8.

Sly, R.M., Imseis, M., Frazer, M. *et al.* (1978) Treatment of asthma in children with triamcinolone acetonide aerosol. *J. Allergy Clin. Immunol.*, **62**, 76–82.

Stevens, D.A., Barnes, P.J. & Adcock, I.M. (1995) β-Agonists inhibit DNA binding of glucocorticoid receptors in human pulmonary and bronchial epithelial cells. *Am. J. Resp. Crit. Care Med.*, **151**, A195.

Suissa, S., Ernst, P., Boivin, J.-F. *et al.* (1994) A cohort analysis of excess mortality in asthma and the use of inhaled β-agonists. *Am. J. Resp. Crit. Care Med.*, **149**, 604–10.

Szczeklik, A., Nizankoska, E., Dworski, R., Domagala, B. & Pinis, G. (1991) Cyclosporin for steroid-dependent asthma. *Allergy*, **46**, 312–15.

Szefler, S. (1991) Glucocorticoid therapy for asthma: clinical pharmacology. *J. Allergy Clin. Immunol.*, **88**, 147–5.

Tabacknik, E. & Zadik, Z. (1991) Diurnal cortisol secretion during therapy with inhaled beclomethasone diproprionate in children with asthma. *J. Pediatr.*, **118**, 294–7.

Taylor, D.R., Sears, M.R., Herbison, G.P. *et al.* (1993) Regular inhaled β-agonist in asthma: effects on exacerbation and lung function. *Thorax*, **48**, 134–8.

Taylor, I.K. & Shaw, R.J. (1993) The mechanism of action of corticosteroids in asthma. *Resp. Med.*, **4**, 261–78.

Thorsson, L. & Edsbäcker, S. (1993) Lung deposition of budesonide from Turbuhaler is twice that from a pressurized metered dose inhaler. *Thorax*.

Tinkelman, D.G., Reed, C.E., Nelson, H.S. & Offord, K.P. (1993) Aerosol beclomethasone diprionate compared with theophylline as primary treatment of chronic, mild to moderately severe asthma in children. *Pediatrics*, **92**, 64–77.

Toogood, J.H. & Frankism, C.W. (1990) A study of the antiasthma action of inhaled budesonide. *J. Allergy Clin. Immunol.*, **85**, 872–80.

Toogood, J.H., Jennings, B., Greenway, R.W. & Chung, L. (1980) Candidiasis and dysphonia complicating beclomethasone treatment of asthma. *J. Allergy Clin. Immunol.*, **65**, 145–53.

Toogood, J.H. (1989) High dose inhaled steroid therapy for asthma. *J. Allergy Clin. Immunol.*, **83**, 528–36.

Toogood, J.H., Baskerville, J.C., Jennings, B., Lefcoe, N.M. & Johansson, S.A. (1982) Influence of dosing frequency and schedule on the response of chronic asthmatics to the aerosol steroid budesonide. *J. Allergy Clin. Immunol.*, **70**, 288–98.

Toogood, J.H., Baskerville, J. & Jennings, B. (1984) Use of spacers to facilitate inhaled corticosteroid treatment of asthma. *Am. Rev. Resp. Dis.*, **129**, 723–9.

Toogood, J.H., Markov, A.E., Baskerville, J. & Dyson, C. (1993) Association of ocular cataracts with inhaled and oral steroid therapy during long term treatment for asthma. *J. Allergy Clin. Immunol.*, **91**, 571–9.

Trigg, C.J., Manolistas, N.D., Wang, J. *et al.* (1994) Placebo-controlled immunopathological study of four months inhaled corticosteroids in asthma. *Am. J. Resp. Crit. Care Med.*, **150**, 17–22.

Turpeinen, M., Sorva, R. & Juntungen-Backman, K. (1991) Changes in carbohydrate and lipid metabolism in children with asthma inhaling budesonide. *J. Allergy Clin. Immunol.*, **88**, 384–9.

Vacca, A., Screpanati, I., Maroder, M., Petrangeli, E., Frati, L. & Guline, A. (1989) Tumor promoting phorbol ester and raw oncogene expression inhibit the glucocorticoid-dependent transcription from the mouse mammary tumor virus long terminal repeat. *Mol. Endocrinol.*, **3**, 1659–65.

Van De Stolpe, A., Caldenhoven, E., Raaijmakers, J.A.M., Van Der Saag, P.T. & Koendorman, L. (1993) Glucocorticoid-mediated repression of intercellular adhesion molecule-1 expression in human monocytic and bronchial epithelial cell lines. *Am. J. Respir. Cell Mol. Biol.*, **8**, 340–7.

van Essen-Zandvliet, E.E., Hughes, M.D., Waalkens, H.J., Duiverman, E.J., Pocock, S.J. & Kerrebijn, K.F. (1992) Effects of 22 months of treatment with inhaled corticosteroids and/or beta$_2$-agonists on lung function, airway responsiveness and symptoms in children with asthma. *Am. Rev. Resp. Dis.*, **146**, 547–54.

Vathenen, A.S., Knox, A.J., Wisniewski, A. & Tattersfield, A.E. (1991) Time course of change in bronchial reactivity with an inhaled corticosteroid in asthma. *Am. Rev. Resp. Dis.*, **143**, 1317–21.

Volovitz, B., Amir, J., Malik, H., Kauschansky, A. & Varsano, I. (1993) Growth and pituitary-adrenal function in children with severe asthma treated with inhaled budesonide. *New Engl. J. Med.*, **329**, 1703–8.

Waalkens, H.J., van Essen-Zandvliet, E.E., Hughes, M.D. *et al.* (1993) Cessation of long-term treatment with inhaled corticosteroids (budesonide) in children with asthma results in deterioration. *Am. Rev. Resp. Dis.*, **148**, 1252–7.

Watson, A., Lim, T.K., Joyce, H. & Pride, N.B. (1992) Failure of inhaled corticosteroids to modify bronchoconstrictor or bronchodilator responses in middle-aged smokers with mild airflow obstruction. *Chest*, **101**, 350–5.

Wempe, J.B., Tammeling, E.P., Postma, D.S., Auffarth, B., Teengs, J.P. & Koëter, G.H. (1992) Effects of budesonide and bambuterol on circadian variation of airway responsiveness and nocturnal asthma symptoms of asthma. *J. Allergy Clin. Immunol.*, **90**, 349–57.

Wilkinson, J.R.W., Crea, A.E.G., Clark, T.J.H. & Lee, T.H. (1989) Identification and characterization of a monocyte-derived neutrophil-activating factor in corticosteroid-resistant bronchial asthma. *J. Clin. Invest.*, **84**, 1930–41.

Wilkinson, J.R.W., Podgorski, M.R., Godolphin, J.L., Goulding, N.J. & Lee, T.H. (1990) Bronchial asthma is not associated with autoantibodies to lipocortin-1. *Clin. Exp. Allergy*, **20**, 189–92.

Williams, A.J., Baghat, M.S., Stableforth, D.E., Cryton, R.M., Shenos, P.M. & Skinner, C. (1983) Dysphonia caused by inhaled steroids: recognition of a characteristic laryngeal abnormality. *Thorax*, **38**, 813–21.

Wilson, J.W., Djukanovic, R., Howarth, P.H. & Holgate, S.T. (1994) Inhaled beclomethasone diproprionate downregulates airway lymphocyte activation in atopic asthma. *Am. J. Resp. Crit. Care Med.*, **149**, 86–90.

Wolthers, O.D. & Pedersen, S. (1993a) Bone turnover in asthmatic children treated with oral prednisolone or inhaled budesonide. *Paediatr. Pulmonol.*, **16**, 341–6.

Wolthers, O.D. & Pedersen, S. (1993b) Growth in asthmatic children treated with budesonide. *Pediatrics*, **90**, 517–18.

Wolthers, O. & Pedersen, S. (1993c) Short term growth during treatment with inhaled fluticasone diproprionate and beclomethasone diproprionate. *Arch. Dis. Child.*, **68**, 673–6.

Wong, C.S., Wamedna, I., Pavord, I.D. & Tattersfield, A.E. (1994) Effect of regular terbutaline and budesonide on bronchial reactivity to allergen challenge. *Am. J. Resp. Crit. Care Med.*, **150**, 1268–78.

Woolcock, A.J. (1993) Steroid resistant asthma: what is the clinical definition? *Eur. Resp. J.*, **6**, 743–7.

Wurthwein, G. & Rohdewald, P. (1990) Activation of beclomethasone diproprionate by hydrolysis to beclomethasone-17-monophosphate. *Biopharmaceut. Drug Dispos.*, **11**, 381–94.

Xie, Q.-W., Kashiwarbara, Y. & Nathan, C. (1994) Role of transcription factor NF-αB/Rel in induction of nitric oxide synthase. *J. Biol. Chem.*, **269**, 4705–8.

Yang-Yen, H.-F., Chambard, J.-C., Sun, Y.-L. *et al.* (1990) Transcriptional interference between c-Jun and the glucocorticoid receptor: mutual inhibition of DNA binding due to direct protein–protein interaction. *Cell*, **62**, 1205–15.

Yates, D.H., Kharitonov, S.A., Robbins, R.A., Thomas, P.S. & Barnes, P.J. (1995) Effect of a nitric oxide synthase inhibitor and a glucocorticosteroid on exhaled nitric oxide. *Am. J. Resp. Crit. Care Med.*, **152**, 892–6.

CHAPTER 36

Immunosuppressants (Drugs and Monoclonal Antibodies)

C.A. Bonham & A.W. Thomson

Introduction

As our understanding of the cellular and molecular events that underlie immune responses has expanded in recent years, it has become apparent that many allergic diseases have a component of chronic cell-mediated hypersensitivity. Many cells involved in the allergic response play key roles in this pathological process. These include, but are not limited to, lymphocytes, eosinophils and mast cells. Corticosteroids, first shown to be effective immunosuppressants in the early 1950s, have demonstrated efficacy in both the treatment and the prophylaxis of the more chronic or severe allergic diseases. However, patients with more debilitating disorders not infrequently develop manifestations of toxicity from prolonged or high-dose steroid use. In addition, a subgroup of patients do not respond to conventional therapies for allergic diseases, including high-dose steroids.

Immunosuppressive drugs are widely used in solid organ and bone marrow transplantation. In the past 25 years, the development of more powerful and more selective immunosuppressive agents has revolutionized the field of transplantation. These agents also provide powerful tools for the investigation of the molecular mechanisms involved in immune responses. More recently, as experience has been gained in their clinical use, immunosuppressants have been employed in a number of autoimmune diseases with encouraging results in some disorders. As new agents with broader therapeutic windows are developed, it is very likely that the indications for use of these drugs will be liberalized. Thus, the treatment of allergic diseases with immunosuppressants may allow the reduction or elimination of steroids, and may prove effective in steroid-resistant patients.

The cellular and molecular events of the immune response have been described in earlier chapters, and will be reviewed here only in relation to immunosuppressive therapy. Likewise, the pathophysiology of allergic diseases is presented elsewhere, and will not be discussed. The actions of immunosuppressive drugs will be reviewed, with particular reference to the most recent developments. The clinical uses of these agents will be highlighted. Corticosteroids are covered in a separate chapter of this book. We also briefly review aspects of the use of monoclonal antibodies (mAb), fusion proteins and gene targeting as approaches to therapeutic immunosuppression.

Immunosuppressive drugs

Mechanisms of action

Our understanding of the key events occurring during immune cell activation has advanced enormously in recent years. The immunosuppressive drugs act at distinct sites involved in this activation process. Significantly, the actions of these agents have shed light on the biochemical phenomena crucial for immune function. The molecular events affected by immunosuppressants, as outlined in Table 36.1, can be grouped into several potential sites of drug action: alteration of gene expression, inhibition or interference with cytokine action, inhibition of DNA synthesis and interference with cell maturation, differentiation and function (reviewed by Thomson & Starzl, 1993; Thomson *et al.*, 1993b). As illustrated in Fig. 36.1, these differing modes of action have an impact on the immune response at distinct sites. The specific phase of the cell cycle affected by these drugs differs, as noted in Table 36.2. The role of mAb in immunosuppressive therapy will be addressed later in this chapter.

Alteration of gene expression (cyclosporin and tacrolimus)

The prototypal immunosuppressive agent altering gene expression, known for its ability to selectively inhibit cytokine gene expression in CD4+ T-helper (Th) lymphocytes, is cyclosporin A (CsA). The molecular mode of

Table 36.1 Modes of action of immunosuppressive drugs.

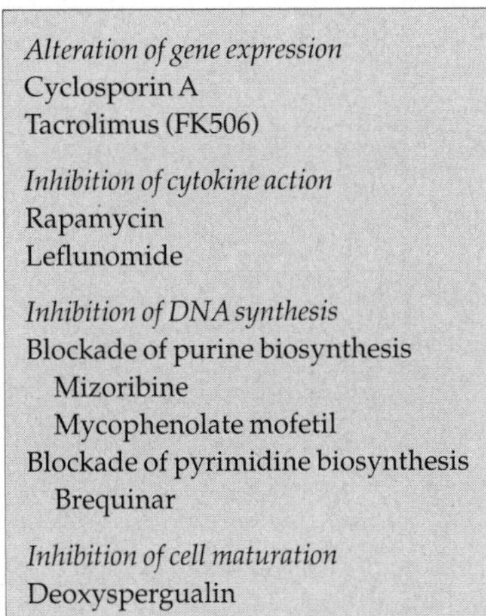

Alteration of gene expression
Cyclosporin A
Tacrolimus (FK506)

Inhibition of cytokine action
Rapamycin
Leflunomide

Inhibition of DNA synthesis
Blockade of purine biosynthesis
  Mizoribine
  Mycophenolate mofetil
Blockade of pyrimidine biosynthesis
  Brequinar

Inhibition of cell maturation
Deoxyspergualin

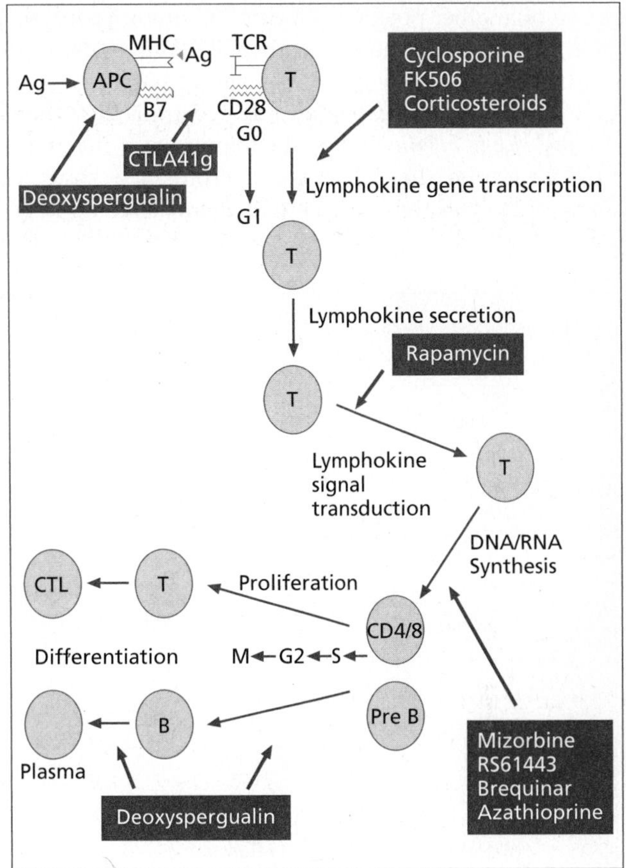

Fig. 36.1 Schematic representation of the sites of action of immunosuppressive drugs. (From Tepper, 1993.)

Table 36.2 Differential effects of immunosuppressive agents on cell signalling in the rejection response. (After Keown, 1994.)

Agent	APC function	Phase of cell cycle affected G0	G1(E)	G1(L)	S	Immune amplification
OKT3		+				
ALG		+				
Anti-ICAM		+				
Anti-CD28		+				
Cyclosporin A	(+)		+			(+)
Tacrolimus			+			(+)
Rapamycin	(+)			+		
Leflunomide				+		
Anti-IL-2R				+		
Antisense nucleotides				+		
Azathioprine					+	
Mycophenolate mofetil					+	
Mizoribine					+	
Brequinar					+	

+, Principal effect; (+), secondary effect, often dose-dependent; (E), early; (L), late; see text for definition of other abbreviations.

action of another potent T-cell-directed immunosuppressant, tacrolimus (formerly known as FK506), closely parallels that of CsA, and will also be reviewed in this section. CsA is a cyclic undecapeptide isolated from the fungus *Tolypocladium inflatum gams*. Tacrolimus is a macrolide produced from the fermentation broth of a strain of *Streptomyces tsukubaensis*. The two agents have no structural homology (Fig. 36.2), but closely share biological activities.

CsA and tacrolimus bind specifically to cellular proteins termed immunophilins — cyclophilin and FK506 binding protein (FKBP), respectively (Schreiber, 1991; Thomson, 1993; Thomson & Starzl, 1993; Thomson *et al.*, 1993b; Wiederrecht *et al.*, 1993; Fruman *et al.*, 1994). Table 36.3 lists

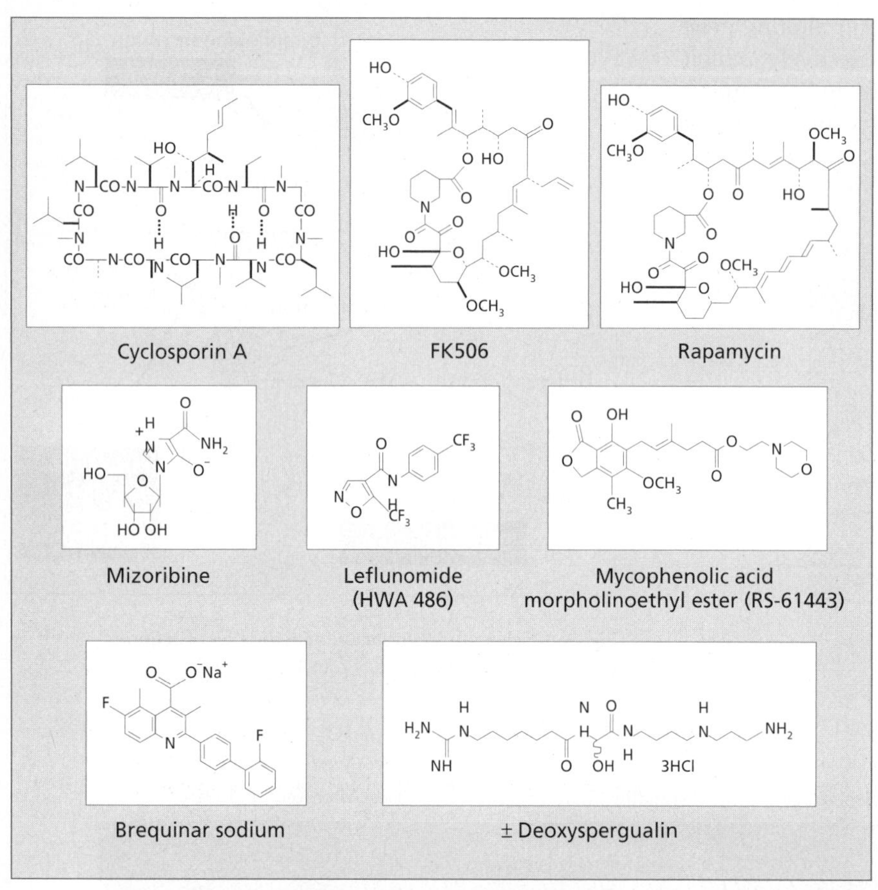

Fig. 36.2 Chemical structures of immunosuppressive drugs.

Table 36.3 Cloned human immunophilins (cyclophilins and FKBP). (From Fruman *et al.*, 1994.)

Immunophilin	Size (kDa)	Drug affinity (nmol/l)		Subcellular location
Cyclophilin				
CyPA	17.7	2.6 (K_i)		Cytosol, nucleus
CyPB	21*	6.9 (K_i)		Secretory pathway
CyPC†	22.8*			?Secretory pathway
CyPD	18*	10 (K_i)		?Mitochondria
FKBP		Tacrolimus	Rapamycin	
FKBP12	11.8	0.4 (K_d)	0.2 (K_d)	Cytosol
FKBP13	13.2*			Endoplasmic reticulum
FKBP25	25.4	160 (K_i)	0.9 (K_i)	Nucleus
FKBP52	51.8	10 (K_i)	8 (K_i)	Cytosol

* Sizes shown refer to the molecular masses of the mature proteins after cleavage of N-terminal extensions.
† Only the murine CyPC complementary DNA sequence has been reported.

the known immunophilins bound by these drugs. These proteins have peptidyl-prolyl *cis–trans* isomerase, or rotamase activity, and are postulated to accelerate protein folding. However, inhibition of this rotamase activity is not responsible for the immunosuppressant effects of these drugs. Rather, intracellular complexes formed between each drug and its respective immunophilin interact with additional intracellular molecules; modulation of the function of these molecular targets is responsible for the biological activity of the immunosuppressant. A principal target of the drug–immunophilin complexes is calcineurin, or phosphatase 2B (Fig. 36.3) (Liu *et al.*, 1991; Clipstone & Crabtree, 1993; Thomson, 1993; Thomson & Starzl, 1993; Wiederrecht *et al.*, 1993; Fruman *et al.*, 1994). Calcineurin is a heterodimeric serine-threonine phosphatase, the enzymatic activity of which is greatly enhanced by Ca^{2+} and calmodulin. This suggests that calcineurin plays a role in Ca^{2+}-dependent signalling processes. Its significance in immunological responses is outlined in Table 36.4.

One substrate of calcineurin is a phosphoprotein, the nuclear factor of activated T cells, cytoplasmic component ($NF\text{-}AT_c$) (Flanagan *et al.*, 1991; Clipstone & Crabtree, 1993; Thomson, 1993; Thomson & Starzl, 1993; Wiederrecht *et al.*, 1993; Fruman *et al.*, 1994). This is one of several transcription factors associated with the interleukin-2 (IL-2) promoter/enhancer (shown in Fig. 36.4). The DNA region regulating transcription of the IL-2 gene extends approximately 300 bp upstream of the transcription start site. The binding site for NF-AT is found in this region. NF-AT is present only in activated lymphocytes, but a number of other transcription factors found in a variety of cell types also have binding sites in this region of DNA. These other factors include Oct-1, nuclear factor-κB (NF-κB) and activator protein-1 (AP-1). In response to Ca^{2+}-dependent cell activation, $NF\text{-}AT_c$ is dephosphorylated and translocates to the nucleus where it combines with a nuclear component ($NF\text{-}AT_n$), the synthesis of which is induced by stimuli that activate protein kinase C (PKC). The complex binds to DNA to drive transcription of the IL-2 gene. By inhibiting the phosphatase activity of

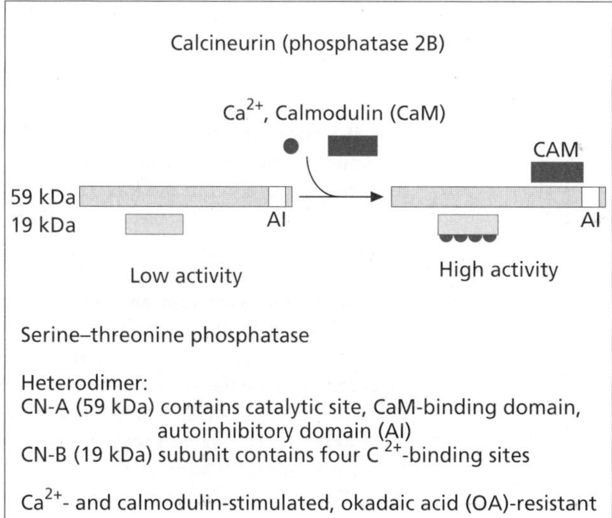

Fig. 36.3 Schematic representation of calcineurin structure and enzymatic activity. This serine-threonine phosphatase is most active in the presence of Ca^{2+} ions and calmodulin. Calmodulin binding appears to interfere with the function of a C-terminal autoinhibitory (AI) domain originally defined by limited proteolytic studies. (From Fruman *et al.*, 1994.)

Table 36.4 The immunological significance of calcineurin.

Calcineurin is a key rate-limiting enzyme in T-cell signal transduction and mediator of Ca^{2+}-dependent events
IL-2 production in T cells activated via the TcR/CD3 complex correlates closely with the level of calcineurin activity
Cells expressing low levels of calcineurin (e.g. T cells) are most sensitive to CsA/FK506
Overexpression of calcineurin overcomes the CsA/FK506-mediated inhibition of NF-AT-dependent cytokine gene transcription
Immunosuppressive activity of cyclosporin analogues correlates with inhibition of calcineurin phosphatase activity
Calcineurin is involved in signalling events that lead to degranulation of cytotoxic T cells
Calcineurin activity plays a key role in TcR/CD3-mediated induction of apoptosis in T-cell hybridomas

See text for definition of abbreviations.
For further details the reader is referred to the following papers and reviews (Schreiber & Crabtree, 1992; Clipstone & Crabtree 1992, 1993; Fruman *et al.*, 1993).

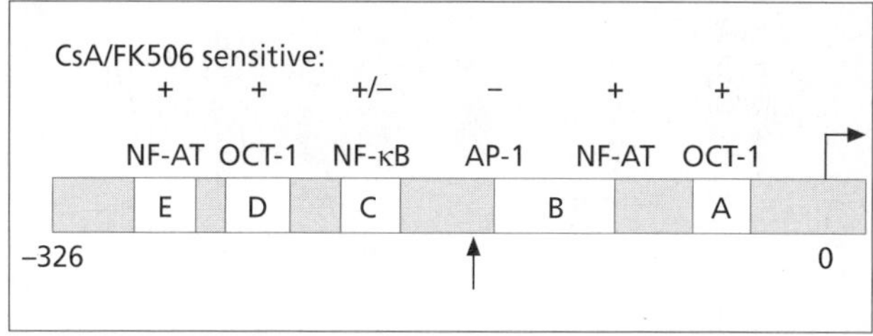

Fig. 36.4 Diagram of the upstream regulatory region of the human IL-2 gene. Five regions important for gene induction were originally defined by deletional analysis and termed the IL-2A, IL-2B, IL-2C, IL-2D and IL-2E sites, based on their proximity to the start site of transcription. Factors which bind to these sites are shown above the DNA segment, and those whose activity is modulated by CsA and FK506 are indicated with a '+' sign. Although two binding sites exist for both NF-AT and NF-IL-2A–Oct-1 factors, the distal NF-AT site (IL-2E) and the proximal Oct-1 site (IL-2A) have been studied most extensively. The arrow indicates a site, termed CD28RE, which appears to bind a factor induced specifically by ligation of the CD28 surface receptor. See text for definition of abbreviations. (From Fruman *et al.*, 1994.)

calcineurin, CsA and tacrolimus each inhibit the translocation of NF-AT_c from the cytoplasm to the nucleus, as shown in Fig. 36.5, while NF-AT_n generation is unaffected. These drugs also inhibit transcriptional activation driven by multimers of Oct-1-binding protein sites (termed NF-IL-2A). NF-κB activity induced by Ca^{2+}-dependent stimuli is also drug sensitive. AP-1 activity, in contrast, is completely drug resistant.

Calcineurin has been implicated in activation of the ubiquitous transcription factor cyclic adenosine monophosphate (cAMP)-responsive element binding protein (CREB) (Schwaninger *et al.*, 1993), which modulates transcription of a wide variety of genes through the cAMP-responsive element (CRE). Interference with CRE-mediated gene transcription represents a novel mechanism of CsA/tacrolimus action, which may underlie the pharmacological effects and toxic manifestations of these drugs.

By inhibiting calcineurin-catalysed dephosphorylation of candidate substrates, CsA and tacrolimus can affect not only cytokine gene transcription, but also apoptosis and cell degranulation (Thomson, 1993; Thomson & Starzl, 1993; Thomson *et al.*, 1993b; Fruman *et al.*, 1994). Calcineurin may also regulate the activity of other enzymes. Thus, it has been demonstrated that regulatory subumits of phosphatase 1 and cAMP-dependent protein kinase

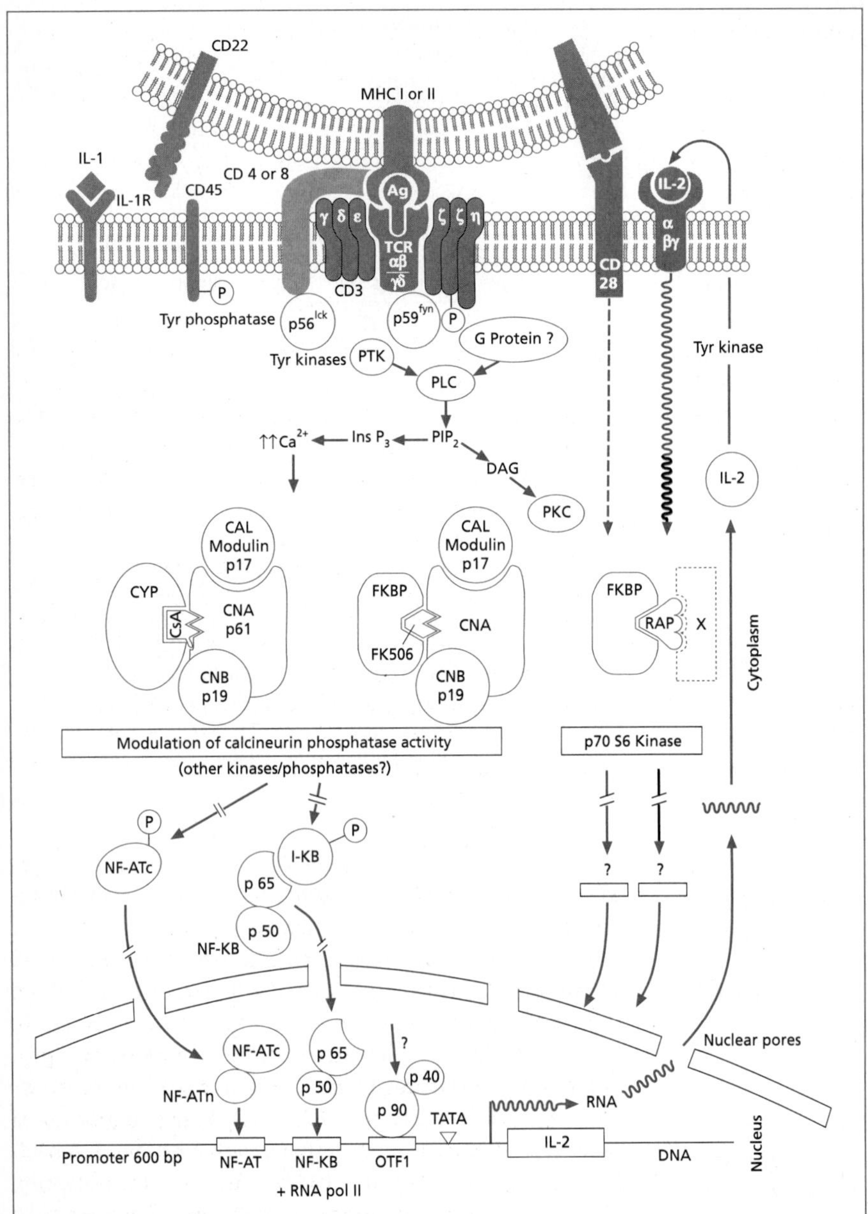

Fig. 36.5 Signal transduction in activated T cells and the sites (centre of figure) at which CsA, tacrolimus (FK506) and RAP are believed to act. CsA or FK506 bound to their respective immunophilins CYP or FK506 binding protein (FKBP) form pentameric complexes with calmodulin and calcineurin A (CNA) and B. Inhibition of the phosphatase activity of calcineurin is believed to inhibit translocation to the nucleus of the cytoplasmic component of the nuclear factor of activated T cells (NF-AT_c), which is required for activation of the IL-2 gene. RAP, which also binds to FKBP, inhibits phosphorylation and activation of a 70 kDa ribosomal S6 protein kinase (p70S6), which normally occur within minutes of cell activation via cytokine receptors. RAP also targets other kinases (not shown) that are essential for cell cycle progression. See text for definition of abbreviations. (From Shreirer *et al.*, 1993.)

are both calcineurin substrates (Fruman *et al.*, 1994). Moreover, CsA inhibits induction of the enzyme nitric oxide synthetase by IL-1 (Muhl *et al.*, 1993). Tacrolimus inhibits the enzyme by blocking its dephosphorylation by calcineurin (Dawson *et al.*, 1993; Oyanagui, 1994). CsA inhibits induction of the intracellular activation signal, activator of DNA replication (ADR) (Kimball *et al.*, 1993a,b). ADR is a constituent of the PKC phosphoregulatory cascade essential for cell cycle progression in activated lymphocytes. Inhibition of ADR induction correlates directly with CsA proliferation inhibition.

Immunophilins of the FKBP class have been identified in association with the glucocorticoid and progesterone receptors (GR and PR, respectively) (Ning & Sanchez, 1993; Oyanagui, 1994; Renoir *et al.*, 1994; Tai *et al.*, 1994). Steroid receptor-associated heat-shock protein 56 (hsp 56) binds tacrolimus. This complex probably protects the GR from dephosphorylation and inactivation by calcineurin. In the presence of tacrolimus, GR translocation to the nucleus is enhanced, with resultant potentiation of GR binding to the GR response element (Fig. 36.6). Binding of this complex may block IL-2 gene transcription and enhance transcription of other genes. Similarly, tacrolimus binds to FKBP59. This complex, in association with hsp 70 and hsp 90, protects PR from calcineurin-dependent dephosphorylation. PR-mediated gene expression is enhanced.

Both CsA and tacrolimus clearly inhibit activation of certain genes encoding growth-promoting cytokines (e.g. IL-2, IL-3, granulocyte macrophage colony-stimulating factor (GM-CSF), proto-oncogenes (e.g. *H-ras*, *c-myc*, *c-rel*)

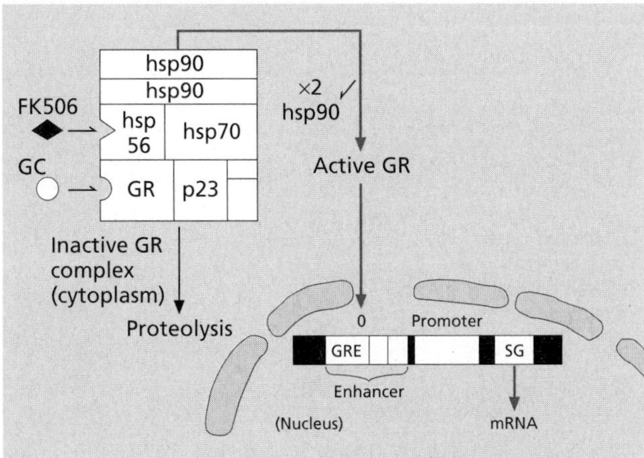

Fig. 36.6 A hypothetical schematic representation of the interaction between tacrolimus (FK506) and the GR. Tacrolimus may bind to heat-shock protein 56 (hsp 56), protecting the GR from dephosphorylation. The GR complex is thus stabilized, and after translocation to the nucleus, binds to the GRE, leading to increased production of anti-inflammatory proteins.

and receptors for specific cytokines (e.g. the IL-2 receptor (IL-2R)) (Thomson, 1993; Thomson & Starzl, 1993; Thomson *et al.*, 1993b, 1994; Fruman *et al.*, 1994; Hess, 1994; Zheng *et al.*, 1994; Venkataraman *et al.*, 1995). Table 36.5 documents the effects of CsA on cytokine production. Recently, CsA has been found to promote the transcription and production *in vitro* by T cells of transforming growth factor-β (TGF-β), a potent inhibitor of T-cell proliferation (Sharma *et al.*, 1994; Khanna *et al.*, 1995). This observation has implicated TGF-β in both the immunoregulatory and the toxic effects of CsA administration. Whether CsA enhances TGF-β expression *in vivo*, however, has not been ascertained.

Inhibition of the rotamase activity of FKBP by tacrolimus was felt to contribute little to the immunosuppressive effect of the drug. Recent studies, however, impart a more substantial role for the rotamase activity of FKBP. FKBP12, one of the four described FKBP, modulates gating of intracellular Ca^{2+} release channels of the sarcoplasmic and endoplasmic reticula. By inhibiting FKBP activity, tacrolimus destabilizes these effects (Brillantes *et al.*, 1994). This may affect Ca^{2+}-dependent events within the cell.

Cellular effects of CsA and tacrolimus

CsA and tacrolimus exhibit potent inhibitory effects on resting T lymphocytes, as illustrated in Fig. 36.7. Human T-cell antigen-presenting cell (APC) interactions appear to exhibit differential sensitivity to these agents *in vitro*, the most sensitive being the CD4+ Th-self-APC, followed by the CD8+ Th-allo-APC and the CD4+ Th-allo-APC interactions (Clerici & Shearer, 1990; Thomson, 1993; Hess, 1994, Thomson *et al.*, 1994). Stimulation of T cells through the T-cell receptor (TcR)/CD3 complex is drug sensitive, as is activation via the CD2 pathway. Both CsA and tacrolimus are much less effective in suppressing activated T cells.

Expression of the genes encoding IL-2, IL-3, IL-4, IL-6, tumour necrosis factor-α (TNF-α), interferon-γ (IFN-γ), GM-CSF, *c-myc*, IL-2R and IL-4R in response to TcR/CD3 ligation is inhibited by CsA and tacrolimus (for reviews see Thomson, 1993; Thomson & Starzl, 1993; Thomson *et al.*, 1993b, 1994; Fruman *et al.*, 1994; Hess, 1994; Zheng *et al.*, 1994). On the other hand, there is evidence that transcription of the IL-10 gene by cloned Th2 cells is spared, as depicted in Fig. 36.8. This differential effect of CsA (IL-10 cross-regulates the activity of Th1 cells) may contribute to the immunosuppressive action of the drug. In T lymphocytes, activation of the genes for IL-2 and its receptor determines the progression of the cell from the G0 to the G1 phase of the cell cycle. G1 to S phase progression is then regulated by IL-2. CsA and tacrolimus directly interfere with the first step and, by inhibiting IL-2 production, also block the second step in the cell cycle. The autocrine

Table 36.5 Effects of CsA on cytokine production.

Cytokine	Cellular source	Activity	Effect of CsA
IL-1α	Monocytes	Pleiotropic effect on T lymphocytes and fibroblasts (cytokine release, growth)	–
IL-1β	Monocytes		–
IL-2	T cells	Proliferation of activated T cells	↓
IL-3	Monocytes, T cells	Proliferation of haemopoietic multipotential stem cells	↓
IL-4	T cells	Proliferation T cells	↓
IL-5	T cells	Differentiation of eosinophils	↓
IL-6	T cells, monocytes, fibroblasts	Pleiotropic effects, production of acute-phase proteins by hepatocytes, MHC class I expression on fibroblasts	↓
IL-7	Bone marrow stromal cells	Haemopoietic factor; B- and T-cell growth factor	–
IL-8	Leucocytes, fibroblasts, endothelial cells	Neutrophil chemotaxis and activation	↓
IL-10	T and B cells, macrophages	Inhibition of macrophages, NK cells, Th1 cells; stimulation of B cells, mast cells	↓, ↑*
IL-12	Stimulated B cells and macrophages	Enhances activity of activated NK and Th1 cells	?
IFN-γ	T cells	Expression of MHC class II on endothelial cells and fibroblasts; antimicrobial and tumoricidal activity	↓
TNF-α	Mononuclear phagocytes	Pleiotropic effects on most cells	↓
TNF-β	Activated lymphocytes	Pleiotropic effects on most cells	↓
GM-CSF	Activated macrophages	Haemopoietic growth factor	↓
G-CSF	Activated macrophages, endothelial cells	Haemopoietic growth factor	?
M-CSF	Mononuclear phagocytes, endothelial cells, fibroblasts	Haemopoietic growth factor	?
TGF-β	Leucocytes, fibroblasts	Proliferation of mesenchymal cells; inhibition of immune cells	↑

* Differential effect depending on nature of stimulus.
–, No effect; ↓, decreases; ↑, Increases.
G-CSF, granulocyte colony-stimulating factor; M-CSF, macrophage colony-stimulating factor; MHC, major histocompatibility complex; see text for definition of other abbreviations.

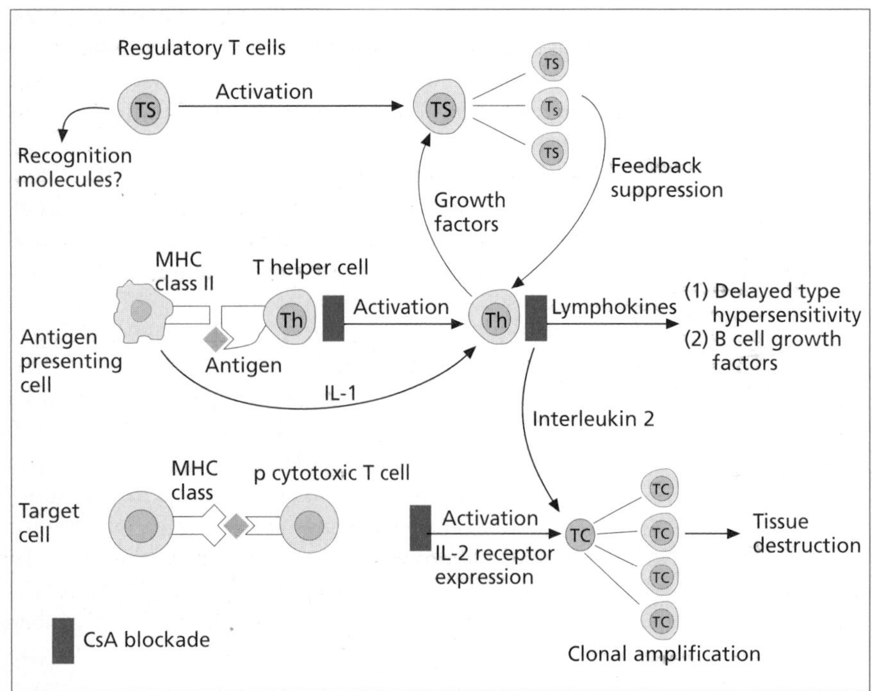

Fig. 36.7 Effect of CsA on the cells of the immune response. (From Hess, 1994.)

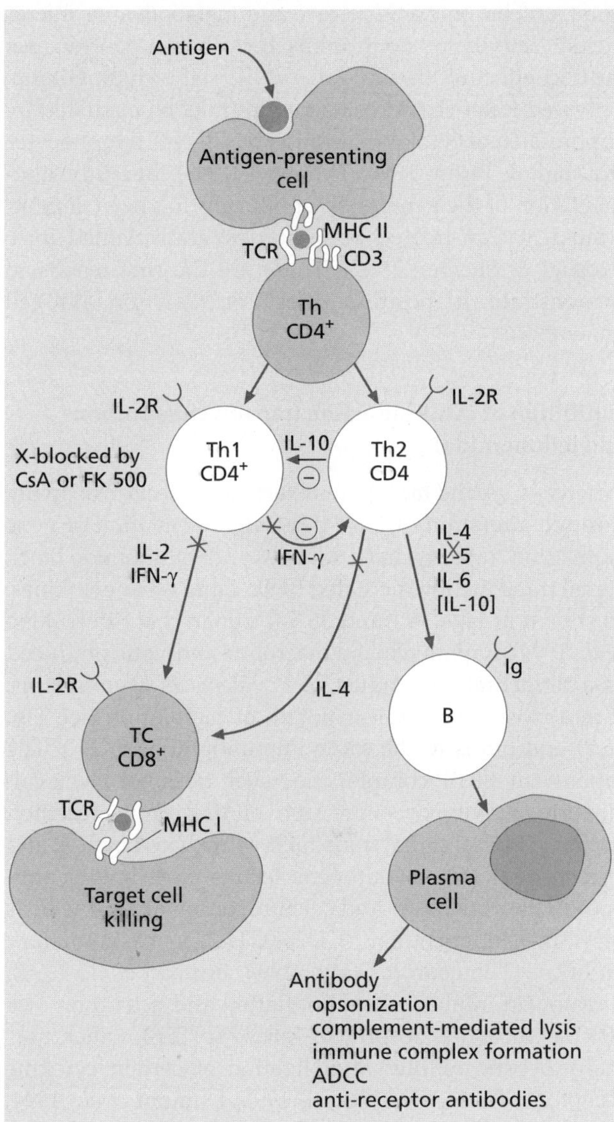

Fig. 36.8 T-helper (CD4+) cells can be divided into functionally distinct subsets (Th1 and Th2) based on their cytokine secretion profiles. Cytokines secreted by Th1 cells play a key role in cell-mediated hypersensitivity, whereas those produced by Th2 cells are important in B-cell stimulation and antibody production. An important feature of the Th1/Th2 cell paradigm is that cross-regulation of function between Th1 and Th2 cells occurs. Thus, for example, IFN-γ stimulates Th2 cells, whereas IL-10 inhibits Th1 cells. Cyclosporin and tacrolimus (FK506) are potent inhibitors of IL-2 and IFN-γ production by Th1 cells. There is evidence, however, that they may spare IL-10 (cytokine synthesis inhibitory factor) production by Th2 cells. See text for definition of abbreviations.

and paracrine stimulation and proliferation of Th cells is thus inhibited.

In vitro, CsA and tacrolimus also inhibit the expression of T-cell-mediated cytotoxicity (Thomson, 1993; Thomson *et al.*, 1993b, 1994; Hess, 1994). Clearly, proliferation and maturation of CD8+ cytotoxic T lymphocytes (CTL) are prevented by blocking the induction of cytokine secretion by CD4+ Th cells (see Fig. 36.7) (Thomson, 1993; Hess, 1994). Moreover, both drugs partially reduce the induction of mRNA for serine esterase and perforin by IL-2 in human CD8+ T cells. Granule exocytosis stimulated by Ca^{2+}-dependent signals is profoundly inhibited. Table 36.6 outlines the effects of CsA on T cells *in vivo*.

A contributory mechanism to the inhibitory effects of CsA and tacrolimus on immune responses may be the sparing of the generation of CD8+ T-suppressor (Ts) cells (Thomson, 1993; Hess, 1994) (see Fig. 36.7), which is dependent on CD4+ Th cells and requires IL-2. High drug concentrations, however, appear to inhibit Ts-cell induction. The proliferative response and production of cytokines by antigen-dependent, IL-2-dependent Th and CTL clones are very sensitive to the drugs. Maximal inhibition is dependent on the presence of the drug at the initiation of cultures. Tacrolimus exhibits similar potency at concentrations 100 times lower than those of CsA.

The immunosuppressive efficacy of CsA and tacrolimus may be due, in part, to indirect effects on non-T-cell components of the immune system, resulting from inhibition of cytokine production. In addition, there is considerable evidence that these agents can directly affect certain other cells. Activation of B lymphocytes is blocked by a mechanism similar to that observed in T cells. Typically, proliferative responses to anti-immunoglobulin (Ig) (which are Ca^{2+} dependent) are CsA sensitive, while lipopolysaccharide (LPS)-stimulated B-cell proliferation (which is Ca^{2+} independent) is only affected by high concentrations of the drug (Table 36.7) (Hornung *et al.*, 1993; Thomson, 1993; Thomson *et al.*, 1993b; Hess, 1994). Specific primary IgM and IgG antibody responses to thymic-dependent antigens are suppressed by CsA, but secondary responses are unaffected (Chang *et al.*, 1993; Thomson, 1993; Hess, 1994; Yoshimura *et al.*, 1994).

Early work examining the influence of CsA on macrophage functions indicated that these cells were insensitive to drug concentrations which markedly

Table 36.6 Effects of CsA on T cells *in vivo* consistent with its immunosuppressive properties.

Interference with thymocyte maturation
Reductions in T-dependent areas of spleen
Reductions in CD4 : CD8 ratio
Reduction in expression of T-cell activation markers (e.g. IL-2R)
Generation of suppressor cells
Reduced lymphoproliferative and lymphokine-secreting capacity
Inhibition of cytotoxic T-cell generation
Capacity to adoptively transfer transplantation tolerance (rat)
Interference with cell migration

Table 36.7 Influence of CsA on murine B cells.

Stimulus	Ca^{2+} mobilization	Sensitivity to CsA
Anti-IgM	+++	High
Con-A	++	High
Ca^{2+} ionophore	+++	High
LPS	–	Low
PMA	–	Low
IL-4	–	Low
IL-5	–	High
Ca^{2+} ionophore plus PMA	+++	High
IL-4 plus anti-IgM	++	High

LPS, *Escherichia coli* lipopolysaccharide; PMA, phorbol myristate acetate.
– to +++ denotes relative degree of Ca^{2+} mobilization.

affected T-cell function. CsA does not impair antigen uptake and metabolism, oxidative burst or bactericidal activity (Thomson, 1993; Hess, 1994). Conflicting reports exist on the effect of CsA on antigen presentation. Studies demonstrating a reduction of major histocompatibility complex (MHC) class II antigen expression on mononuclear phagocytes by CsA treatment are subject to criticism for possible drug 'carry-over' to the indicator system. CsA may indirectly decrease MHC expression on various cells by blocking T-cell cytokine secretion (i.e. IFN-γ), thus indirectly altering antigen presentation.

Inhibition of extracellular Ca^{2+} uptake by CsA or tacrolimus may relate directly to the inhibition of mast cell activation by these drugs (Hatfield *et al.*, 1992; Paulis *et al.*, 1992; Thomson, 1993; Hess, 1994; Thomson *et al.*, 1994). Physiologically relevant concentrations of these drugs inhibit histamine release from mast cells stimulated by Ca^{2+} ionophore, compound 48/80, and concanavalin A (Con-A) plus phosphatidylserine (Thomson, 1993). CsA also inhibits the release of *de novo* synthesized mediators (prostaglandin D_2) from activated human lung mast cells. The drug blocks IgE receptor-mediated exocytosis in rat basophils and histamine release from human peripheral-blood basophils challenged with anti-IgE (Thomson, 1993). Since CsA is active when added after anti-IgE stimulation, inhibition probably occurs at the post-transcriptional level, unlike its mode of action in T lymphocytes. Tacrolimus similarly inhibits IgE activation-induced cytokine transcripts in murine mast cells expressing FKBP12 (Fruman *et al.*, 1994). CsA and tacrolimus treatment can lead to depletion of mucosal mast cells, probably by inhibiting T-cell production of IL-3, and tacrolimus inhibits mast cell proliferation (Hultsch *et al.*, 1992).

Eosinophilia is T-cell-dependent and is highly sensitive to both agents (Thomson, 1993; Fruman *et al.*, 1994; Thomson *et al.*, 1994). No effects on chemotaxis, oxidative burst, arachidonic acid release and metabolism or microbicidal activity of neutrophils have been reported. An indirect effect on natural killer (NK) cell or lymphokine-activated killer (LAK) cell activities may be mediated by suppression of cytokine secretion by CD4+ T lymphocytes (Kasaian & Biron, 1990; Thomson, 1993). Recently, augmentation of the generation of NK cells has been demonstrated in CsA-treated bone marrow-transplanted mice (Kosugi & Shearer, 1991). These are the first results to demonstrate a positive effect of CsA on NK-cell generation.

Inhibition of cytokine action (rapamycin/sirolimus and leflunomide)

Whereas CsA and tacrolimus exert their effects principally through alteration of Ca^{2+}-dependent activation of gene expression, rapamycin (sirolimus) and leflunomide block signal transduction mediated by IL-2 and other cytokines, as shown in Figs 36.1 and 36.5 (Fruman *et al.*, 1994; Xiao *et al.*, 1994). Rapamycin is a macrolide antibiotic produced as a fermentation product of *Streptomyces hygroscopicus*. It is a close structural analogue of tacrolimus (see Fig. 36.2) and binds to the same immunophilin (FKBP). The rapamycin–FKBP complex, however, does not block calcineurin activity or expression of IL-2 or its receptor. Rather, it blocks signal transduction mediated by IL-2 and other growth factors, mitogenic lectins, cross-linking antibodies, phorbol esters and calcium ionophores, as well as the Ca^{2+}-independent CD28/CTLA-4 costimulatory pathway (Thomson & Starzl, 1993; Fruman *et al.*, 1994). Rapamycin inhibits phosphorylation and activation of a 70 kDa ribosomal S6 protein kinase (p70S6), which normally occurs minutes after ligation of certain cytokine receptors (Thomson & Starzl, 1993; Dumont *et al.*, 1994; Fruman *et al.*, 1994). Although this finding has implicated p70S6 kinase activation as important in Ca^{2+}-independent signalling leading to cell proliferation, there is no evidence that p70S6 kinase is involved directly in S-phase entry. Rapamycin inhibits association of cyclin D with cyclin-dependent kinases (cdk) recognized by histone H_1 kinase, that is cdc2, cdk2 and cdk3 (Albers *et al.*, 1993a,b; Flanagan & Crabtree, 1993; Morice *et al.*, 1993; Brown *et al.*, 1994). Normally, association of a cyclin with its respective cdk leads to activation of the kinase. The cyclin D/cdk complex activates cyclin E/cdk2 complex. This complex, in turn, hyperphosphorylates the retinoblastoma (Rb) protein, which releases the E2F transcription factor necessary for further cdc2, cyclin A and *c-myb* gene expression (Fig. 36.9). Cyclin A/cdc2 complexes subsequently form. These complexes are essential for progression of the cell cycle. Rapamycin blocks activation of the cascade of cyclin/cdk complexes. The drug thus targets a pathway late in G1, preventing resting cells from entering the cell

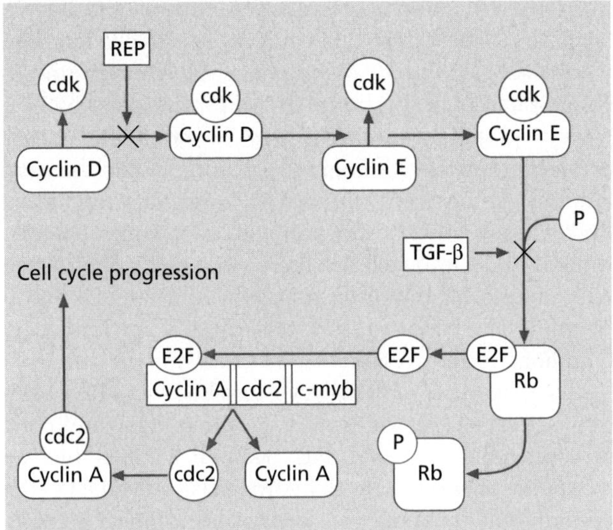

Fig. 36.9 Effect of rapamycin on T-cell activation in G1–S phase progression. REP, rapamycin effector protein. An as yet unidentified effector protein targeted by the rapamycin/FKBP complex interferes with the association of cyclin D with its respective cdk. This blocks the cascade of events leading to cell cycle progression. TGF-β, as illustrated, prevents the phosphorylation of the retinoblastoma protein (Rb), blocking subsequent release of the transcription factor E2F. Expression of the genes for cyclin A, cdc2 and c-myb, normally driven by E2F, is inhibited. Thus, TGF-β appears to block the cell cycle in the same phase as rapamycin. See text for definition of abbreviations.

cycle, but not directly arresting cell cycle progression once cells have entered the cycle.

Rapamycin has also been shown to inhibit phytohaemagglutinin (PHA)-induced *c-jun* expression (Shan *et al.*, 1993) and induction of ADR by PKC (Kimball *et al.*, 1993a,b). The drug destabilizes IL-2 and GM-CSF mRNA (Hanke *et al.*, 1992). Whether these actions are mediated directly by drug–immunophilin complexes or result from actions on other enzymes remains to be determined. Since tacrolimus and rapamycin compete for a common immunophilin ligand, they have antagonistic immunosuppressive effects. CsA and rapamycin, on the other hand, act synergistically (Thomson & Starzl, 1993; Boyle & Kahan, 1994; Fruman *et al.*, 1994). In rats, for example, subtherapeutic or minimally effective doses of each drug act in combination to induce donor-specific tolerance to organ allografts (Boyle & Kahan, 1994). The synergistic activity of CsA and rapamycin holds promise of clinical application.

Leflunomide is an isoxazole derivative developed as an anti-rheumatic drug (see Fig. 36.2). Its activity resembles that of rapamycin in that both agents suppress T-cell proliferation principally by inhibition of T-cell responsiveness to IL-2. Leflunomide appears to function as a protein tyrosine kinase (PTK) inhibitor (Bartlett *et al.*, 1991; Xiao *et al.*, 1994). PTK activation is an initial step in the signal transduction pathway of many receptors, as seen in Fig. 36.5. Leflunomide inhibits this activity in response to IL-2 and IL-4, as well as in response to platelet-derived growth factor and epidermal growth factor. With its distinct mechanism of action, it behaves synergistically with CsA and tacrolimus.

Rapamycin and leflunomide both inhibit T-cell responses to IL-2 by disrupting signal transduction (Bartlett *et al.*, 1991; Thomson & Starzl, 1993; Fruman *et al.*, 1994; Xiao *et al.*, 1994). IL-2R expression is not affected. T-cell stimulation via the CD28 pathway, while insensitive to CsA and tacrolimus, is blocked by rapamycin and leflunomide (Thomson & Starzl, 1993; Fruman *et al.*, 1994; Sharma *et al.*, 1994). Rapamycin spares Th2-specific IL-10 mRNA, while inhibiting IL-8 mRNA expression (Wieder *et al.*, 1993; Ferraresso *et al.*, 1994). It inhibits T-lymphocyte proliferation, even when added as late as 12 hours after stimulation (Flanagan & Crabtree, 1993; Fruman *et al.*, 1994; Luo *et al.*, 1994). It has no effect on several early responses, such as lymphokine gene activation, that are sensitive to CsA and tacrolimus. B-cell proliferation in response to numerous stimuli, including Ca^{2+}-independent signals, is rapamycin-sensitive (Aagard-Tillery & Jelinek, 1994), as are *c-kit* ligand (stem-cell factor (SCF))-dependent and IL-3-dependent proliferation in mast cells (Hultsch *et al.*, 1992; Tsai *et al.*, 1993). Furthermore, IgM and IgG production by pre-activated human B cells is inhibited (Kim *et al.*, 1994). Primary alloantibody and xenoantibody synthesis is potently suppressed (Luo *et al.*, 1992; Propper *et al.*, 1992; Thomson & Starzl, 1993; Thomson *et al.*, 1993a; Fruman *et al.*, 1994; Schmidbauer *et al.*, 1994). Rapamycin decreases the ability of IL-5 to maintain survival of eosinophils in culture (Hom & Estridge, 1993). Significantly, rapamycin blocks *in vitro* responses to haematopoietic cytokines and inhibits recovering but not steady-state haematopoiesis *in vivo* (Quesniaux *et al.*, 1994).

Leflunomide blocks B- and T-lymphocyte proliferation and partially inhibits IL-2 production by activated T cells (Bartlett *et al.*, 1991; Xiao *et al.*, 1994). It is a more potent inhibitor of B-cell proliferation than of T-cell proliferation. It probably produces effects similar to those of rapamycin on other cells of the immune system.

Inhibition of DNA synthesis

Antiproliferative agents inhibit the full expression of the immune response by preventing the differentiation and division of immunocompetent lymphocytes after their encounter with antigen (for a review see Marino & Doyle, 1994). They either structurally resemble essential metabolites or combine with certain cellular components and thereby interfere with cellular function.

Methotrexate inhibits the enzyme dihydrofolate reductase, and prevents the conversion of folic acid to tetrahydrofolic acid. This step is necessary for the synthesis of DNA, RNA and certain coenzymes. The low therapeutic ratio of immunosuppression to toxicity has not justified the use of methotrexate in most clinical settings apart from oncology and bone marrow transplantation.

Cyclophosphamide belongs to the class of alkylating agents. These agents have highly reactive rings, which combine with electron-rich nucleophilic groups, such as the tertiary nitrogens in purines and pyrimidines. The alkylating agents combine with these constituents to form stable covalent bonds. Alkylation of DNA strands, if not repaired, results in faulty chromosomal replication. Cyclophosphamide acts on both the humoral and the cellular immune responses. B lymphocytes appear to be more susceptible than T lymphocytes. The drug is a potent inhibitor of antibody formation. Its usefulness is limited by its toxicity.

Azathioprine was the most widely used immunosuppressive drug until the introduction of CsA in 1979. It interferes with the synthesis of DNA. Several other agents have since been developed which selectively interfere with DNA synthesis in lymphocytes. Azathioprine is cleaved to 6-mercaptopurine (6-MP), principally by erythrocyte glutathione. 6-MP is then converted into a series of mercaptopurine-containing nucleotides which interfere with the synthesis of DNA and polyadenylate-containing RNA. The synthesis and action of coenzymes are disrupted, and chromosomal breaks occur. By interfering with mitosis, azathioprine affects the division of T and B lymphocytes. Unfortunately, this effect is not limited to lymphocytes and accounts for the toxicity of the drug.

Mycophenolate mofetil (MM), also known as RS-61443, is a semisynthetic derivative of the fungal antibiotic mycophenolic acid (see Fig. 36.2). It inhibits inosine monophosphate (IMP) dehydrogenase (IMPDH), the rate-limiting enzyme in guanosine monophosphate (GMP) synthesis (Fig. 36.10) (Allison & Eugui, 1993, 1994; Allison *et al.*, 1993). Lymphocyte proliferation is dependent on *de novo* purine biosynthesis. Specifically, adequate levels of guanosine and deoxyguanosine nucleotides are

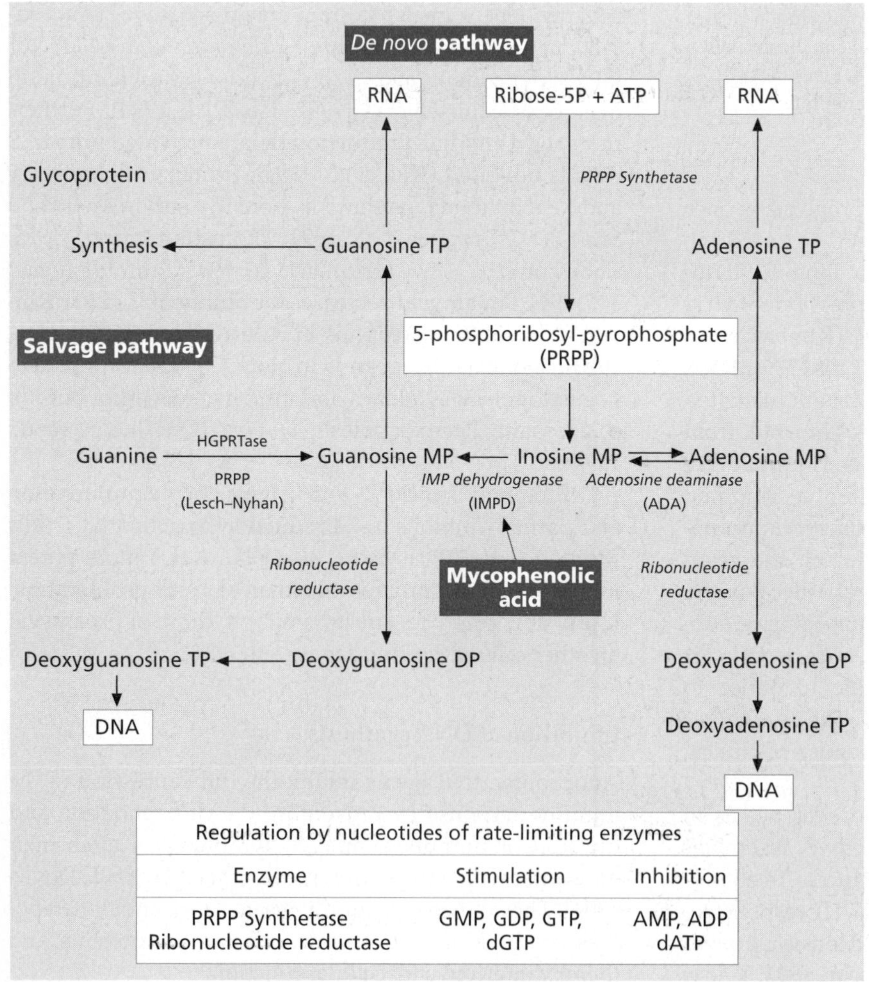

Regulation by nucleotides of rate-limiting enzymes		
Enzyme	Stimulation	Inhibition
PRPP Synthetase Ribonucleotide reductase	GMP, GDP, GTP, dGTP	AMP, ADP dATP

Fig. 36.10 Pathways of purine biosynthesis, showing the central position of IMP. MPA inhibits IMP dehydrogenase, thereby depleting GMP, GTP and dGTP. Two rate-limiting enzymes in lymphocytes are activated by guanosine ribonucleotides and dGTP, but inhibited by AMP, ADP and dATP, respectively. See text for definition of abbreviations. (From Allison & Eugui, 1994.)

required for lymphocyte proliferation, whereas an excess of adenosine or deoxyadenosine nucleotides inhibits proliferation. This is mediated by allosteric inhibition of ribonucleotide reductase. By inhibiting IMPDH, guanosine nucleotides are depleted. Lymphocytes do not contain the enzymes of the salvage pathway to compensate for this depletion. With subsequent reduction of ribonucleotide reductase activity, DNA synthesis is suppressed.

MM has certain advantages over nucleoside analogues. Nucleoside analogues can inhibit DNA repair enzymes and produce chromosomal breaks, both of which are mutagenic effects. MM inhibits an enzyme involved in purine biosynthesis and has no direct effects on DNA.

MM does not inhibit gene expression or signal transduction. MM-mediated depletion of guanosine triphosphate (GTP) inhibits the transfer of fucose and mannose to glycoproteins, some of which are adhesion molecules (Allison *et al.*, 1993; Allison & Eugui, 1994). By this mechanism, cell–cell interactions could be affected. Some G proteins may be sensitive to GTP depletion. This mechanism may account for the near-complete inhibition of B-cell antibody formation by MM (Allison *et al.*, 1993; Chang *et al.*, 1993; Allison & Eugui, 1994).

Mizoribine (Bredinin; MZ) is an antibiotic substance isolated from culture filtrates of *Eupenicillium brefeldianum* (see Fig. 36.2). It exerts strong suppressive activity on lymphocyte growth (Thomson *et al.*, 1993b; Amemiya & Itoh, 1994; Dayton & Turka, 1994). MZ is metabolized into an active form, mizoribine-5′-monophosphate (MZ-5-P) by adenosine kinase. This product inhibits GMP synthesis from IMP. IMPDH and, to a lesser extent, GMP synthetase are targeted by MZ-5-P, resulting in almost complete inhibition of guanine nucleotide synthesis and subsequent DNA synthesis. MZ-5-P is dephosphorylated intracellularly, and leaves cells when the extracellular concentration falls. Consequently, the action of MZ is dependent on its continued presence within the cell. MZ inhibits the passage of cells from the G1 to the S phase of the cell cycle. T- and B-lymphocyte proliferation is suppressed, although the effects of MZ are not limited to these cells. In addition, MZ-5-P can inhibit DNA repair mechanisms, which explains the presence of chromosome breaks in cells treated with MZ. The agent exhibits considerable synergism with CsA and tacrolimus, and greater safety than azathioprine (Amemiya & Itoh, 1994).

Brequinar sodium (BQR) (see Fig. 36.2) was originally developed as an antimetabolite for cancer chemotherapy. It acts by its ability to non-competitively inhibit the activity of the enzyme dihydro-orotate dehydrogenase (Simon *et al.*, 1993; Thomson *et al.*, 1993b; Makowka & Cramer, 1994). This enzyme catalyses the conversion of dihydro-orotate to orotate in the *de novo* pyrimidine synthesis pathway (Fig. 36.11). As for the purine pathway, lymphocytes cannot utilize the salvage pathway for pyrimidine biosynthesis. In the presence of BQR, the nucleotide precursors uridine triphosphate (UTP) and cytosine triphosphate (CTP) are depleted, and DNA and RNA synthesis are inhibited. Recently it has been noted that BQR may inhibit cytidine deaminase, which converts cytidine to uridine. Cytidine, when combined with BQR, complements the antimetabolic effects of the drug (Woo *et al.*, 1993). Cells are most sensitive to BQR during the active, proliferative phase of an immune response, when DNA and RNA synthesis are at high levels. BQR inhibits IL-6-induced differentiation of human B cells into IgM-secreting plasma cells (Tamura *et al.*, 1993). Like MZ and MM, BQR exhibits synergism with CsA. It carries some toxicity, as its effects are not limited to lymphocytes (Makowka & Cramer, 1994).

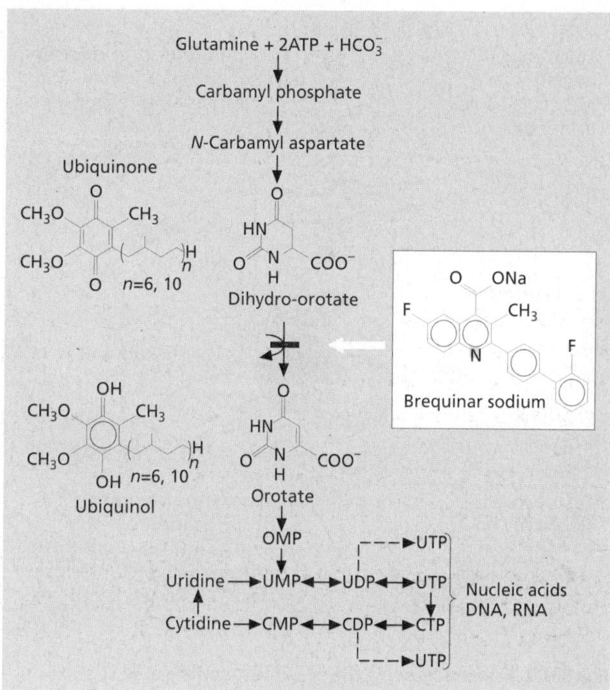

Fig. 36.11 The chemical stucture and mechanism of action of BQR. (From Makowka & Cramer, 1994.)

The purine and pyrimidine biosynthesis inhibitors exhibit antiproliferative effects on T and B lymphocytes at therapeutic concentrations. Antibody formation by polyclonally activated human B lymphocytes is almost completely inhibited by MM. Secondary responses of human spleen cells to tetanus toxoid are similarly affected. MM is a potent inhibitor of the proliferation of monocytic lineage cells and an inducer of differentiation, as shown by the acquisition of surface molecules (Fcγ receptor (FcγR), C3R), production of lysozyme and expression of IL-1R antagonist after treatment with this agent. MM does not deplete GTP in neutrophils, and consequently does not

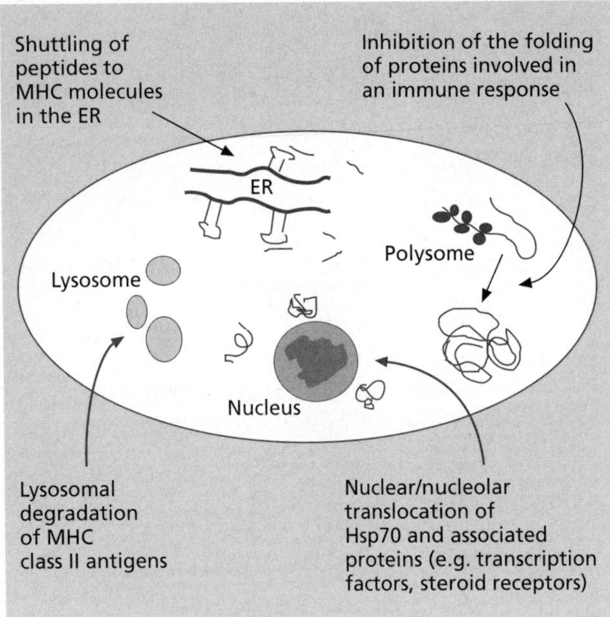

Fig. 36.12 Scheme showing the possible functions of heat-shock proteins, which may be targets for inhibition by the binding of DSG. (From Thomas *et al.*, 1993.)

affect the growth or responses of these cells to chemoattractants or their capacity to produce superoxide and kill bacteria (Allison & Eugui, 1993, 1994; Allison *et al.*, 1993). MZ and BQR probably exhibit a similar range of cellular effects.

Interference with cell maturation and differentiation

The drugs reviewed thus far act at the molecular level by altering gene activation, signal transduction or DNA synthesis and repair. The mechanism of action of 15-deoxyspergualin (DSG), a synthetic analogue of the antitumour antibiotic spergualin (see Fig. 36.2), is not so clearly defined. DSG appears to exert a cytostatic effect on precursor cells, preventing cell differentiation. It also impairs antigen processing and presentation (Tepper, 1993; Thomas *et al.*, 1993; Amemiya, 1994; Suzuki, 1994). Multiple substances are targeted by DSG. It inhibits the enzymes spermine synthetase, spermidine synthetase, polyamine oxidase, spermidine/spermine *N*′-acetyltransferase and ornithine decarboxylase (Thomas *et al.*, 1993). The resulting depletion of polyamides prevents synthesis of cellular macromolecules necessary for normal differentiation and function.

DSG binds to Hsc 70, a constitutively expressed member of the heat-shock protein (hsp) 70 family (Nadler *et al.*, 1992; Mazzucco *et al.*, 1993; Tepper, 1993; Thomas *et al.*, 1993; Nadeau *et al.*, 1994). Hsp may be involved in numerous cellular functions, as depicted in Fig. 36.12. They contain peptide-binding grooves similar to those of MHC molecules, and may play a role in the binding and intracellular transport of antigenic peptides in APC. This may account for the impairment of antigen presentation to T cells by monocytes exposed to DSG. Hsp 70 and hsp 90 complex with GR and possibly cyclophilins, and are involved in translocation of proteins to the nucleus. Interference with the normal function of these substances may account for the additional effects of this agent.

DSG inhibits proliferation and differentiation of CTL, probably by preventing IL-2R expression (Tepper, 1993). It blocks the ability of mature CTL to lyse target cells (Fujii *et al.*, 1992; Tepper, 1993). Th cell functions are not affected. DSG does not affect mitogen responses or the early stage of the mixed lymphocyte response (MLR). IL-2 release from T lymphocytes and IL-1 release from macrophages are not impaired (Tepper, 1993; Suzuki, 1994). The drug inhibits the mitogenic stage of B cells. Primary and secondary antibody responses are inhibited, as well as production of xenophile antibodies (Tepper, 1993; Amemiya, 1994; Suzuki, 1994). DSG suppresses the differentiation of human B cells into plasma cells (Morikawa *et al.*, 1992). It suppresses the production of macrophage-activating factor (MAF) by murine cells stimulated with antigens. DSG impairs superoxide production in cells of the monocyte/macrophage lineage, as well as decreasing MHC class II expression and IL-1 production in these cells. Antigen presentation by monocytes is inhibited. DSG inhibits LAK cell activity (Thomas *et al.*, 1992) and induces lymphocytopenia, granulocytopenia and anaemia.

Monoclonal antibodies

The ultimate goals of immunosuppressive therapy are to narrow the target cell population and to induce antigen-specific tolerance with minimal untoward side-effects. mAb (Table 36.8) are uniquely suited for the realization of these goals because of their remarkable specificity. Thus far, the major emphasis in improving mAb selectivity has been in identifying suitable molecular targets expressed on the surface of responding T cells (Marshall &

Table 36.8 mAb that induce antigen-specific tolerance in experimental animals.

mAb
Anti-CD45
Anti-CD3
Anti-CD4
Anti-IL-2R
Anti-LFA-1
Anti-ICAM-1
Anti-CD52

See text for definition of abbreviations.

Waldmann, 1994). Anti-T-lymphocyte mAb are examples of this approach.

Certain anti-CD4 and anti-CD8 mAb selectively deplete CD4+ and CD8+ T lymphocytes, respectively. Anti-CD4 mAb have demonstrated the capacity to prolong allograft survival and induce transplantation tolerance in rodents and to inhibit allograft rejection in non-human primates (Wee *et al.*, 1992; Marshall & Waldmann, 1994; Olive & Mawas, 1993). Both antibodies selectively deplete their target cells in renal allograft recipients. The anti-CD3 mAb OKT3 reacts with the TcR complex. It is used to treat established episodes of acute rejection in kidney, liver, heart and heart–lung transplant patients (Marshall & Waldmann, 1994). By engaging the TcR/CD3 complex, OKT3 blocks the function of cytotoxic T cells and prevents activation of naïve T cells. The major limitation to its use is the development of neutralizing antibodies to the immunogenic mAb.

A more selective approach targets only activated immune cells. The α-chain of the IL-2R (also designated CD25) is present only on activated T cells and a subset of activated B cells and APC. Anti-CD25 mAb therapy targets these cells and has been shown to prolong allograft survival in laboratory animals (Marshall & Waldmann, 1994; Shapiro *et al.*, 1992; Strom *et al.*, 1994). In recent clinical trials, the anti-CD25 mAb 'anti-Tac' decreased the number of early rejection episodes and delayed the time to first rejection in human kidney transplant recipients (Kirkman *et al.*, 1991; Shapiro *et al.*, 1992). As with OKT3, a limitation of these mAb has been the development of neutralizing antibodies to immunogenic epitopes of the mAb.

Another useful group of mAb are those that block cellular adhesion molecules, such as lymphocyte function-associated antigen-1 (LFA-1), very late appearing antigen-4 (VLA-4), vascular cell adhesion molecule-1 (VCAM-1) and intercellular adhesion molecule-1 (ICAM-1). These molecules are involved in the homing of T cells to areas of immune reactivity. LFA-1–ICAM-1 interaction provides a costimulatory signal for T-cell activation that is synergistic to the signal delivered via the TcR/CD3 complex. Anti-ICAM-1 mAb has been shown to enhance 6-month graft survival in a group of high-risk cadaveric renal allograft recipients (Haug *et al.*, 1993).

Anti-IgE mAb can block B-lymphocyte maturation (Heusser *et al.*, 1989). Similar mAb can bind to mast cells, inhibiting degranulation induced by allergens (Stadler *et al.*, 1991). Other target molecules for mAb therapy include CD28 and its structural homologue CTLA-4. These molecules are involved in the costimulatory pathway of T-lymphocyte activation, and interact with the B7 family of proteins expressed on APC (see Fig. 36.1). Fusion proteins have been developed which interact with these molecules (Steele, 1994). Fusion proteins are the translational products of fusion of the genes encoding separate protein elements. The impetus to develop these agents for immunosuppressive therapy stemmed from the failure of 'standard' mAb to deliver on their potential advantages. The ubiquitous human anti-mouse xenoantibody response limits the usefulness of standard therapeutic murine mAb. After a period of time, the murine mAb are neutralized by human anti-mouse antibodies (HAMA). Xenoantibodies are also poor recruiters of human effector mechanisms. By fusing the antigen-binding region of a murine mAb to a human Ig constant-region scaffold, bioavailability is improved, as is recruitment of effector responses. Table 36.9 presents a list of chimeric mAb and immunoligands that are under development for immunosuppressive therapy. One such fusion protein, CTLA-4Ig, has been used to induce antigen-specific hyporesponsiveness in rodent allograft models (Lin *et al.*, 1993; Steele, 1994). Another, IL-2/Fcγ2a, prolonged the survival of islet-cell allografts in a murine model (Steele, 1994). In addition, humanized anti-Tac (anti-Tac-H) prolonged cardiac allograft survival in monkeys, and was noted to have a longer half-life than its murine counterpart (Brown *et al.*, 1991; Steele, 1994). Anaphylaxis occurred less frequently in the animals treated with the chimeric mAb.

Conjugates between mAb and specific toxins or radionuclides (immunotoxins) can be used to deliver a lethal 'package' to specific target cells. ^{90}Y-labelled murine anti-Tac, for example, is effective in prolonging primate allografts (Parenteau *et al.*, 1992) and xenografts (Cooper *et al.*, 1990), and anti-CD5 ricin α-chain immunotoxin has efficacy in steroid-resistant graft-vs.-host disease (Filipovich *et al.*, 1992). Anticytokine mAb, such as anti-TNF-α and anti-TNF-β, have been shown to enhance allograft survival in experimental systems (Imagawa *et al.*, 1991; Lin *et al.*, 1992). A marked response has been observed with chimeric mAb to TNF-α in rheumatoid arthritis.

Table 36.9 Fusion proteins (chimeric mAb and immunoligands) for immunosuppression.

Name	Target
Humanized mAb	
OKT3 (humanized)	CD3ε
Anti-Tac-H	IL-2R
CAMPATH-1H	CD52
Immunoligands	
IL-2/Ig	IL-2R
IL-10/Fc	IL-10R
CTLA-4/Ig	B7-1
CD2/Ig	LFA-3

See text for definition of abbreviations.

Antisense oligonucleotides

A new experimental approach to immunosuppressive therapy is selective gene-targeted treatment. Recently, the use of antisense technology has been used to prolong organ allograft survival in mice. ICAM-1 antisense oligonucleotides inhibited rejection of murine cardiac allografts and, in combination with anti-LFA-1 mAb, induced donor-specific tolerance (Stepkowski *et al.*, 1994). The oligonucleotides exhibited no toxic side-effects and did not produce an immunogenic response. It has also been shown that antisense DNA can effectively block the synthesis of soluble FcεRII and proliferation of B lymphocytes (Bhatti *et al.*, 1992).

Clinical use of immunosuppressants

Virtually all of the immunosuppressive drugs discussed in this chapter have demonstrated efficacy in clinical trials, and many of them are used routinely in the prevention and treatment of allograft rejection in transplant recipients. Azathioprine, CsA and, more recently, tacrolimus have been utilized successfully in kidney, heart, heart–lung, liver, pancreas, small bowel and multivisceral transplants. All the drugs have been used to reverse episodes of acute rejection. Tacrolimus, DSG, MM, rapamycin and leflunomide have been useful in the treatment of refractory rejection. Chronic rejection may respond to rapamycin, leflunomide and MM. Antibody-mediated rejection is sensitive to DSG, BQR, MZ, MM and rapamycin. In addition, combination therapy with agents with different mechanisms of action provides more effective, less toxic and possibly more specific immunosuppression. The success of immunosuppressants in the field of transplantation has led to a number of clinical trials of these agents in autoimmune diseases. There is experimental and clinical evidence that several of these drugs (e.g. CsA, tacrolimus) can be effective in certain immune-mediated disease states refractory to conventional treatments. Table 36.10 outlines a number of autoimmune diseases that have shown responsiveness to immunosuppressive therapy, in either animals or humans.

Immunosuppressive agents in experimental models of allergic disease

Immunosuppressants have been studied extensively in models of asthma. Recently, accumulated data have demonstrated that many cases of asthma have a component of chronic inflammation. Corticosteroids interrupt the development of airway inflammation, have a prophylactic and suppressive action and are currently the most effective anti-inflammatory agents used in the management of asthma. However, there is substantial morbidity associated with the prolonged use of steroids. Table 36.11 documents the many side-effects of prolonged or high-dose use. A small subset of patients develop resistance to steroids.

There is now abundant evidence that T-lymphocyte infiltration is a feature of asthma and that activated Th lymphocytes play a vital role in the pathogenesis of the disease. The view that T-cell-directed immunosuppressive drugs may be therapeutic in bronchial asthma derives in part from these observations.

Table 36.10 Autoimmune diseases which have shown responsiveness to immunosuppressants, either experimentally or clinically.

Autoimmune disease	Immunosuppressants
Rheumatoid arthritis	CsA, FK, Rapa, MTX, AZA, MM, DSG
Lupus	CsA, FK, Rapa, Lef, MZ, DSG
Nephritis, glomerulonephritis	CsA, FK, Lef, MZ, DSG
Psoriasis	CsA, FK, MTX
Diabetes mellitus	CsA, FK, AZA, Rapa, MM, DSG
Uveoretinitis, Behçet's disease	CsA, FK, AZA, Rapa, MM
Myasthenia gravis	AZA, DSG
Experimental autoimmune encephalomyelitis	CsA, FK, Rapa, DSG
Autoimmune thyroiditis	CsA, FK, DSG
Autoimmune hepatitis	AZA, CsA, FK
Primary biliary cirrhosis	MTX, CsA, FK
Goodpasture's syndrome	DSG
Idiopathic thrombocytopenic purpura	AZA
Crohn's disease	CsA, FK
Pemphigus, bullous pemphigoid	AZA

MTX, methotrexate; Rapa, rapamycin; Lef, leflunomide; AZA, azathioprine; See text for definition of other abbreviations.

Table 36.11 Complications related to corticosteroid therapy.

Bone disease
Cataract
Colon perforation
Cushingoid habitus
Diabetes
Growth retardation
Hypertension
Infection
Psychoses
Nervous sytem disturbances
Obesity
Peptic ulceration
Wound-healing impairment

An animal model has been developed to investigate the effect of immunosuppressive agents on asthma. In this model, guinea pigs were sensitized by exposure to aerosolized ovalbumin and then challenged with high concentrations of aerosolized antigen 6 days after sensitization. Each guinea pig received CsA, tacrolimus or olive oil by gavage every other day throughout the immunization period. A late asthmatic response developed within 3–9 hours after antigen challenge in 12 of 15 control animals. However, in the animals treated with CsA or tacrolimus, no late asthmatic responses were observed. CsA and tacrolimus also significantly blocked the decrease in the provocative concentration of acetylcholine that increases respiratory resistance to twice the baseline value 24 hours after antigen challenge. Eosinophilic infiltration in the tracheal wall at 72 hours was reduced by CsA (Arima *et al.*, 1991; Fukuda, 1994).

CsA inhibited antigen-induced eosinophil infiltration in guinea pig lung (Lagente *et al.*, 1994). More recently, inhaled tacrolimus has been shown to inhibit the development of a late asthmatic response, a subsequent increase in bronchial hyperresponsiveness and airway eosinophilia (Akutsu, 1990; Fukuda, 1994).

A similar model was developed in which guinea pigs were injected intravenously with Sephadex beads to induce lung inflammation and bronchial hyperreactivity. Rapamycin was injected intramuscularly 2 or 12 hours after Sephadex injection. In animals treated with rapamycin at 2 hours, the numbers of lymphocytes and eosinophils present in brochoalveolar lavage (BAL) samples taken after 24 hours were reduced by more than 50% compared with controls. Rapamycin administered at 12 hours after Sephadex injection decreased lymphocyte and eosinophil counts in the BAL and, in addition, reduced bronchial hyperreactivity. The increase in neutrophil numbers in the BAL caused by Sephadex bead injection was not modified by rapamycin treatment (Franchisi *et al.*, 1993a,b). In a separate study, rapamycin was noted to inhibit leucocyte migration and bronchial hyperreactivity to both histamine and acetylcholine in guinea pigs injected with Sephadex beads. Rapamycin was more effective than dexamethasone or CsA in this model (Nogueria de Franchisi *et al.*, 1993).

Candidate therapies for the future include such new immunosuppressive drugs as tacrolimus and rapamycin, and also mAb. Experimentally, mAb to IL-5 have been shown to inhibit allergic bronchial eosinophilia in guinea pigs (Chand *et al.*, 1992; Gulbenkian *et al.*, 1992), as has the IL-1R antagonist (Selig & Tocker, 1992). Direct blockade of cellular adhesion with mAb to ICAM-1 has also shown some promise (Wegner *et al.*, 1990). Less specific methods, including inhibition of phosphodiesterase type IV and inducible nitric oxide synthetase have also been proposed (Thomson & Forrester, 1994).

Clinical use of immunosuppressants in allergic disease

The greatest experience with immunosuppressants in the treatment of allergic diseases has been in patients with asthma. Corticosteroids (the subject of Chapter 35) are the mainstay of treatment for acute and chronic severe asthma. Most patients respond to inhaled or systemic steroids given for short time periods. However, there is a group of asthmatics who, to control their symptoms, require prolonged courses of high-dose steroids, which may produce debilitating complications. A more serious problem is that some patients with chronic asthma are refractory to steroids, even when given in high doses. During the 1960s and 1970s, immunosuppressive agents such as azathioprine and 6-MP were tried, with little success (Asmundsson *et al.*, 1971; Fukuda, 1994). In 1986, methotrexate used to treat psoriasis exhibited a steroid-sparing effect in an elderly patient with steroid-dependent asthma (Mullarkey *et al.*, 1986). A subsequent long-term trial in patients requiring high-dose steroids for resistant asthma showed that methotrexate treatment allowed reduction of the daily prednisolone dose from a mean of 26.9 to 6.3 mg/day. Of 25 patients, 15 required no further steroids, and only one failed to respond (Mullarkey *et al.*, 1990). More recent studies have not recognized the beneficial effects of methotrexate (Erzurum *et al.*, 1991). The drug may even induce airway hyperresponsiveness in some cases (Jones *et al.*, 1991). This, in addition

Table 36.12 Problems of long-term immunosuppression in humans.

Failure to induce tolerance
Spontaneous neoplasms
Lymphoproliferative disorders
Metabolic alterations
Growth retardation

Table 36.13 Known toxicities of specific immunosuppressants based on experimental or clinical observations.

Toxicity	CYC	MTX	AZA	CsA	FK	Rapa	LEF	MM	BQR	DSG	mAb
Haematological											
BM suppression			×				×	×	×		
↓ Leucocytes	×	×	×					×	×	×	
↓ Granulocytes									×		
↓ Platelets			×			×			×	×	
Megaloblastic anaemia			×								
Cutaneous											
Skin fragility			×								
Hair loss	×		×					×			
Hirsutism				×							
Dermatitis									×		
GI											
Stomatitis		×									
Mucositis		×					×		×		
Anorexia	×					×	×	×		×	
Nausea/vomiting	×	×	×			×	×			×	
Diarrhoea									×		
Hepatotoxicity		×	×					×			
GU											
↓ GFR				×	×						
Nephrotoxicity				×	×						
Testicular atrophy						×					
Haemmorrhagic cystitis	×										
Cardiovascular											
Hypertension				×	×						
Cardiotoxicity	×										
Vasculitis (of GI tract)					×	×					
CNS											
Headache										×	
Fatigue										×	
Seizure				×	×						
Metabolic											
Diabetes mellitus				×	×			×			
Hyperlipidaemia				×							
Hyperuricaemia				×							
↓ Cholesterol					×						
Gingival hyperplasia				×							
Facial dysmorphism				×							
Pulmonary fibrosis	×										
Cytokine release syndrome											×
Antiglobulin sensitivity											×

CYC, cyclophosphamide; MTX, methotrexate; AZA, azathioprine; Rapa, rapamycin; LEF, leflunomide; BM, bone marrow; GI, gastrointestinal; GU, genitourinary; GFR, glomerular filtration rate; CNS, central nervous system. See text for definition of other abbreviations.

to the occurrence of toxic side-effects, has prevented methotrexate from assuming a role in the therapy of steroid-dependent asthma.

T lymphocytes from patients with glucocorticoid-resistant asthma are inhibited *in vitro* by CsA or rapamycin (Haczku *et al.*, 1994). This finding and the encouraging results of experiments investigating the effects of CsA in animal models of asthma have led to several clinical trials. In one trial, oral CsA produced a mean increase over placebo of 12% in peak expiratory force (PEF) and 17.6% in forced expiratory volume in 1 second (FEV_1) in 33 patients with long-standing, steroid-dependent asthma. There was a reduction of 48% in the frequency of exacerbations. Side-effects included hypertension and a slight decrease in the glomerular filtration rate (Alexander *et al.*, 1992).

Another group of nine patients with steroid-dependent asthma demonstrated a mean increase of 18.8% in morning PEF and improved bronchial hyperresponsiveness to acetylcholine at 12 weeks. Frequency of asthma exacerbations was strikingly decreased during CsA treatment. There was a tendency, however, to develop hypertension (Fukuda, 1994). In one study of 12 patients with steroid-dependent asthma, the daily prednisolone dose was reduced from a mean of 30 to 11 mg/day without deterioration in six subjects receiving CsA (Szczeklik *et al.*, 1991).

Lock and colleagues (1996) investigated the steroid-sparing properties of cyclosporin A (CsA) over a 36-week period. After a 4-week run-in period, 39 corticosteroid-dependent asthmatic patients were randomized to receive CsA (19 patients, initial dose 5 mg/kg per day) or matched placebo (20 patients) for 36 weeks. Attempts were then made to reduce their prednisolone dosages at 14-day intervals. Three patients receiving CsA had to be withdrawn from the study before they completed 12 weeks of therapy. The remaining 16 patients achieved a statistically significant reduction in median daily prednisolone dosage of 62%, compared with a decrease of 25% in the patients taking placebo. This reduction was most pronounced during the last 12 weeks of active therapy. In addition, morning peak expiratory flow rate improved significantly in the active-treatment group but not in the placebo group. Predictable changes in renal function and blood pressure, and an increased incidence of hypertrichosis and paraesthesia, were observed in the patients treated with CsA, but these did not necessitate withdrawal from the study, and were reversed during a 4-week run-out period. Therefore, low-dose CsA therapy, as compared with placebo, allowed a significant reduction in oral corticosteroid dosages in patients with severe asthma, and also improved lung function.

Identification of patients likely to respond to CsA therapy was not possible from these studies. In addition, the incidence of undesirable side-effects appeared to be fairly high. There appears to be little justification to use CsA in the treatment of refractory asthma other than in clinical trials until its role is more clearly defined.

Systemic immunosuppression with corticosteroids has long been considered effective in the treatment of atopic dermatitis refractory to other therapies. The undesirable side-effects of steroids have led to trials of other agents in atopic dermatitis. Oral CsA at a dose of 5 mg/kg/day was highly effective in reducing disease extent and severity scores and in improving itch and sleep scores in a double-blind crossover study of atopic dermatitis (Ross & Camp, 1990; Wahlgren *et al.*, 1990; Sowden *et al.*, 1991). Additional double-blind trials have also demonstrated significant clinical efficacy of CsA even at doses as low as 2.5 mg/kg/day, although only short-term safety profiles are available so far (Salek *et al.*, 1993).

Toxicity associated with immunosuppressants

The broader use of immunosuppressive drugs is limited by their toxic side-effects. A number of well-recognized complications are inherent to immunosuppressive therapy in general. These are outlined in Table 36.12. In addition, each of the agents reviewed thus far has specific side-effects related to its mechanism of action. These are presented in Table 36.13. Well-designed clinical trials will be necessary to ascertain the place of immunosuppressants in the treatment of allergic diseases.

References

Aagard-Tillery, K.M. & Jelinek, D.F. (1994) Inhibition of human B lymphocyte cell cycle progression and differentiation by rapamycin. *Cell Immunol.*, **156**, 493–507.

Akutsu, I., Fukuda, T., Numao, T. & Makino, S. (1990) Inhibitory effect of FK 506 on the development of late asthmatic response and on the increased bronchial responsiveness. *Arerugi — Jpn. J. Allergol.*, **39** (7), 605–9.

Albers, M.W., Brown, E.J., Tanaka, A., Williams, R.T., Hall, F.L. & Schreiber, S.L. (1993a) An FKBP-rapamycin-sensitive, cyclin-dependent kinase activity that correlates with the FKBP-rapamycin-induced G1 arrest point in MG-63 cells. *Ann. NY Acad. Sci.*, **696**, 54–62.

Albers, M.W., Williams, R.T., Brown, E.J., Tanaka, A., Hall, F.L. & Schreiber, S.L. (1993b) FKBP-rapamycin inhibits a cyclin-dependent kinase activity and a cyclin D1-Cdk association in early G1 of an osteosarcoma cell line. *J. Biol. Chem.*, **268**, 22825–9.

Alexander, A.G., Barnes, N.C. & Kay, A.B. (1992) Trial of cyclosporin in corticosteroid-dependent chronic severe asthma. *Lancet*, **339**, 324–8.

Allison, A.C. & Eugui, E.M. (1993) Immunosuppressive and other effects of mycophenolic acid and an ester prodrug, mycophenolate mofetil. *Immunol. Rev.*, **136**, 5–28.

Allison, A.C. & Eugui, E.M. (1994) Mycophenolate mofetil (RS-61443): mode of action and effects on graft rejection. In: *Immunosuppressive Drugs: Developments in Anti-Rejection Therapy* (eds A.W.

Thomson & T.E. Starzl), pp. 141–59. Edward Arnold, London.

Allison, A.C., Kowalski, W.J., Muller, C.D. & Eugui, E.M. (1993) Mechanisms of action of mycophenolic acid. *Ann. NY Acad. Sci.*, **696**, 63–87.

Amemiya, H. (1994) 15-Deoxyspergualin. In: *Medical Intelligence Unit: New Immunosuppressive Modalities and Anti-rejection Approaches in Organ Transplantation* (ed. J.W. Kupiec-Weglinski), pp. 75–91. R.G. Landes, Austin.

Amemiya, H. & Itoh, H. (1994) Mizoribine (Bredinin): mode of action and effects on graft rejection. In: *Immunosuppressive Drugs: Developments in Anti-Rejection Therapy* (eds A.W. Thomson & T.E. Starzl), pp. 161–76. Edward Arnold, London.

Arima, M., Yukawa, T., Terashi, Y. & Makino, S. (1991) Cyclosporine A inhibits allergen-induced late asthmatic response and increase of airway hyperresponsiveness in guinea pigs. *Nippon Kyobu Shikkan Gakkai Zasshi—Jpn. J. Thoracic Dis.*, **29**, 1089–95.

Asmundsson, T., Kilburn, K.H., Laszlo, J. & Krock, C.J. (1971) Immunosuppressive therapy of asthma. *J. Allergy*, **47**, 136–47.

Bartlett, R.R., Dimitrijevic, M., Mattar, T. *et al.* (1991) Leflunomide (HWA 486), a novel immunomodulating compound for the treatment of autoimmune disorders and reactions leading to transplantation rejection. *Agents Actions*, **32**, 10–21.

Bhatti, L., Behle, K. & Stevens, R.H. (1992) Inhibition of B cell proliferation by antisense DNA to both alpha and beta forms of Fc epsilon R II. *Cell. Immunol.*, **144**, 117–30.

Boyle, M.J. & Kahan, B.D. (1994) Immunosuppressive role of rapamycin in allograft rejection. In: *Immunosuppressive Drugs: Developments in Anti-Rejection Therapy* (eds A.W. Thomson & T.E. Starzl), pp. 129–40. Edward Arnold, London.

Brillantes, A.B., Ondrias, K., Scott, A. *et al.* (1994) Stabilization of calcium release channel (ryanodine receptor) function by FK 506-binding protein. *Cell*, **77**, 513–23.

Brown, E.J., Albers, M.W., Shin, T.B. *et al.* (1994) A mammalian protein targeted by G1-arresting rapamycin-receptor complex. *Nature*, **369**, 756–8.

Brown, P.S. Jr, Parenteau, G.L., Dirbas, F.M. *et al.* (1991) Anti-Tac-H, a humanized antibody to the interleukin 2 receptor, prolongs primate cardiac allograft survival. *Proc. Nat. Acad. Sci. USA*, **88**, 2663–7.

Chand, N., Harrison, J.E., Rooney, S. *et al.* (1992) Anti-IL-5 monoclonal antibody inhibits allergic late phase bronchial eosinophilia in guinea pigs: a therapeutic approach. *Eur. J. Pharmacol.*, **211**, 121–3.

Chang, C.C., Aversa, G., Punnonen, J., Yssel, H. & de Vries, J.E. (1993) Brequinar sodium, mycophenolic acid, and cyclosporin A inhibit different stages of IL-4- or IL-13-induced human IgG4 and IgE production *in vitro*. *Ann. NY Acad. Sci.*, **696**, 108–22.

Clerici, M. & Shearer, G.M. (1990) Differential sensitivity of human T helper cell pathways by *in vitro* exposure to cyclosporin A. *J. Immunol.*, **144**, 2480–5.

Clipstone, N.A. & Crabtree, G.R. (1992) Identification of calcineurin as a key signalling enzyme in T-lymphocyte activation. *Nature*, **357**, 695–7.

Clipstone, N.A. & Crabtree, G.R. (1993) Calcineurin is a key signaling enzyme in T lymphocyte activation and the target of the immunosuppressive drugs cyclosporin A and FK 506. *Ann. NY Acad. Sci.*, **696**, 20–30.

Cooper, M.M., Robbins, R.C., Goldman, C.K. *et al.* (1990) Use of yttrium-90-labeled anti-Tac antibody in primate xenograft transplantation. *Transplantation*, **50**, 760–5.

Dawson, T.M., Steiner, J.P., Dawson, V.L., Dinerman, J.L., Uhl, G.R. & Snyder, S.H. (1993) Immunosuppressant FK 506 enhances phosphorylation of nitric oxide synthase and protects against glutamate neurotoxicity. *Proc. Nat. Acad. Sci. USA*, **90**, 9808–12.

Dayton, J.S. & Turka, L.A. (1994) Mizoribine. In: *Medical Intelligence Unit: New Immunosuppressive Modalities and Anti-Rejection Approaches in Organ Transplantation* (ed. J.W. Kupiec-Weglinski), pp. 31–42. R.G. Landes, Austin.

Dumont, F.J., Altmeyer, A., Kastner, C. *et al.* (1994) Relationship between multiple biologic effects of rapamycin and the inhibition of p70S6 protein kinase activity: analysis in mutant clones of a T cell lymphoma. *J. Immunol.*, **152**, 992–1003.

Erzurum, S.C., Leff, J.A., Cochran, J.E. *et al.* (1991) Lack of benefit of methotrexate in severe, steroid-dependent asthma: a double-blind, placebo-controlled study. *Ann. Intern. Med.*, **114**, 353–60.

Ferraresso, M., Tian, L., Ghobrial, R., Stepkowski, S.M. & Kahan, B.D. (1994) Rapamycin inhibits production of cytotoxic but not noncytotoxic antibodies and preferentially activates T helper 2 cells that mediate long-term survival of heart allografts in rats. *J. Immunol.*, **153**, 3307–18.

Filipovich, A.H., Shapiro, R.S., Ramsay, N.K. *et al.* (1992) Unrelated donor bone marrow transplantation for correction of lethal congenital immunodeficiencies. *Blood*, **80**, 270–6.

Flanagan, W.M. & Crabtree, G.R. (1993) Rapamycin inhibits p34cdc2 expression and arrests T lymphocyte proliferation at the G1/S transition. *Ann. NY Acad. Sci.*, **696**, 31–7.

Flanagan, W.M., Corthesy, B., Bram, R.J. & Crabtree, G.R. (1991) Nuclear association of a T-cell transcription factor blocked by FK 506 and cyclosporin A. *Nature*, **352**, 803–7.

Francischi, J.N., Conry, D.M., Cloutier, S. & Sirois, P. (1993a) Reduction of Sephadex-induced lung inflammation and bronchial hyperractivity by rapamycin. *Brazil J. Med. Biol. Res.*, **26**, 1105–10.

Francischi, J.N., Conry, D., Maghni, K. & Sirois, P. (1993b) Rapamycin inhibits airway leukocyte infiltration and hyperreactivity in guinea pigs. *Agents Actions*, **39**, C139–C141.

Fruman, D.A., Burakoff, S.J. & Bierer, B.E. (1994) Molecular actions of cyclosporin A, FK 506 and rapamycin. In: *Immunosuppressive Drugs: Developments in Anti-Rejection Therapy* (eds A.W. Thomson & T.E. Starzl), pp. 15–35. Edward Arnold, London.

Fujii, H., Takada, T., Nemoto, K. *et al.* (1992) Deoxyspergualin, a novel immunosuppressant, markedly inhibits human mixed lymphocyte reaction and cytotoxic T-lymphocyte activity *in vitro*. *Int. J. Immunopharmacol.*, **14**, 731–7.

Fukuda, T. (1994) Immunosuppressive agents and asthma. *Clin. Rev. Allergy*, **12**, 95–108.

Gulbenkian, A.R., Egan, R.W., Fernandez, X. *et al.* (1992) Interleukin-5 modulates eosinophil accumulation in allergic guinea pig lung. *Am. Rev. Resp. Dis.*, **146**, 263–6.

Haczku, A., Alexander, A., Brown, P. *et al.* (1994) The effect of dexamethasone, cyclosporine, and rapamycin on T-lymphocyte proliferation *in vitro*: comparison of cells from patients with glucocorticoid-sensitive and glucocorticoid-resistant chronic asthma. *J. Allergy Clin. Immunol.*, **93**, 510–19.

Hanke, J.H., Nichols, L.N. & Coon, M.E. (1992) FK 506 and rapamycin selectively enhance degradation of IL-2 and GM-CSF mRNA. *Lymphokine Cytokine Res.*, **11**, 221–31.

Hatfield, S.M., Mynderse, J.S. & Roehm, N.W. (1992) Rapamycin and FK 506 differentially inhibit mast cell cytokine production and cytokine-induced proliferation and act as reciprocal antagonists. *J. Pharmacol. Exp. Ther.*, **261**, 970–6.

Haug, C.E., Colvin, R.B., Delmonico, F.L. (1993) A phase I trial of immunosuppression with anti-ICAM-1 (CD54) mAb in renal allograft recipients. *Transplantation*, **55**, 766–72.

Hess, A.D. (1994) Cellular immunobiology of cyclosporin A. In: *Immunosuppressive Drugs: Developments in Anti-Rejection Therapy* (eds A.W. Thomson & T.E. Starzl), pp. 47–62. Edward Arnold, London.

Heusser, C.H., Wagner, K., Brinkmann, V., Severinson, E. & Blaser, K. (1989) Establishment of a memory *in vitro* murine IgE response to benzylpenicillin and its resistance to suppression by anti-IL-4 antibody. *Int. Arch. Allergy Appl. Immunol.*, **1**, 45–50.

Hom, J.T. & Estridge, T. (1993) FK 506 and rapamycin modulate the functional activities of human peripheral blood eosinophils. *Clin. Immunol. Immunopathol.*, **68**, 293–300.

Hornung, N., Raskova, J., Raska, K. Jr & Degiannis, D. (1993) Responsiveness of preactivated B cells to IL-2 and IL-6: effect of cyclosporine and rapamycin. *Transplantation*, **56**, 985–90.

Hultsch, T., Martin, R. & Hohman, R.J. (1992) The effect of the immunophilin ligands rapamycin and FK 506 on proliferation of mast cells and other hematopoietic cell lines. *Mol. Biol. Cell*, **3**, 981–7.

Imagawa, D.K., Millis, J.M., Seu, P. *et al.* (1991) The role of tumor necrosis factor in allograft rejection. III. Evidence that anti-TNF antibody therapy prolongs allograft survival in rats with acute rejection. *Transplantation*, **51**, 57–62.

Jones, G., Mierins, E. & Karsh, J. (1991) Methotrexate-induced asthma. *Am. Rev. Resp. Dis.*, **143**, 179–81.

Kasaian, M.T. & Biron, C.A. (1990) Cyclosporin A inhibition of interleukin 2 gene expression, but not natural killer cell proliferation, after interferon induction *in vivo*. *J. Exp. Med.*, **171**, 745–62.

Keown, P.A. (1994) Influence of cyclosporin A on graft rejection. In: *Immunosuppressive Drugs: Developments in Anti-Rejection Therapy* (eds A.W. Thomson & T.E. Starzl), pp. 63–81. Edward Arnold, London.

Khanna, A., Li, B., Sehajpal, P.K., Sharma, V.K. & Suthanthiran, M. (1995) Mechanism of action of cyclosporine: a new hypothesis implicating transforming growth factor-β. *Transplant Rev.*, **9**, 41–8.

Kim, H.S., Raskova, J., Degiannis, J.D. & Raska, K. (1994) Effects of cyclosporine and rapamycin on immunoglobulin production by preactivated human B cells. *Clin. Exp. Immunol.*, **96**, 508–12.

Kimball, P.M., Kerman, R.K., Van Buren, C.T., Lewis, R.M., Katz, S. & Kahan, B.D. (1993a) Cyclosporine and rapamycin affect protein kinase C induction of the intracellular activation signal, activator of DNA replication. *Transplantation*, **55**, 1128–32.

Kimball, P., Kerman, R.H., Williams, J. & Kahan, B.D. (1993b) Cyclosporine and rapamycin block protein kinase C-mediated induction of the activation signal, activator of DNA replication, in cell-free assay. *Transplant. Proc.*, **25**, 518–19.

Kirkman, R.L., Shapiro, M.E., Carpenter, C.B. *et al.* (1991) A randomized prospective trial of anti-Tac monoclonal antibody in human renal transplantation. *Transplantation*, **51**, 107–13.

Kosugi, A. & Shearer, G.M. (1991) Effect of cyclosporin A on lymphopoiesis. III. Augmentation of the generation of natural killer cells in bone marrow transplanted mice treated with cyclosporin A. *J. Immunol.*, **146**, 1416–21.

Lagente, V., Carre, C., Kyriacopoulos, F., Boichot, E., Mencia-Huerta, J.M. & Braquet, P. (1994) Inhibitory effect of cyclosporin A on eosinophil infiltration in the guinea-pig lung induced by antigen, platelet-activating factor and leukotriene B4. *Eur. Resp. J.*, **7**, 921–6.

Lin, H., Chensue, S.W., Strieter, R.M. *et al.* (1992) Antibodies against tumor necrosis factor prolong cardiac allograft survival in the rat. *J. Heart Lung Transplant.*, **11**, 330–5.

Lin, H., Bolling, S.F., Linsley, P.S. *et al.* (1993) Long-term acceptance of major histocompatibility complex mismatched cardiac allografts induced by CTLA4Ig plus donor-specific transfusion. *J. Exp. Med.*, **178**, 1801–6.

Liu, J., Farmer, J.D. Jr, Lane, W.S., Friedman, J., Weissman, I. & Schreiber, S.L. (1991) Calcineurin is a common target of cyclophilin-cyclosporin A and FKBP-FK 506 complexes. *Cell*, **66**, 807–15.

Lock, S.H., Kay, A.B. & Barnes, N.C. (1996) Double-blind, placebo-controlled study of cyclosporin A as a corticosteroid-sparing agent in corticosteroid-dependent asthma. *Am. J. Respir. Crit. Care Med.*, **153**, 509–14.

Luo, H., Chen, H., Daloze, P., Chang, J.Y., St-Louis, G. & Wu, J. (1992) Inhibition of *in vitro* immunoglobulin production by rapamycin. *Transplantation*, **53**, 1071–6.

Luo, H., Duguid, W., Chen, H., Maheu, M. & Wu, J. (1994) The effect of rapamycin on T cell development in mice. *Eur. J. Immunol.*, **24**, 692–701.

Makowka, L. & Cramer, D.V. (1994) Brequinar sodium: mode of action and effects on graft rejection. In: *Immunosuppressive Drugs: Developments in Anti-Rejection Therapy* (eds A.W. Thomson & T.E. Starzl), pp. 177–86. Edward Arnold, London.

Marino, I.R. & Doyle, H.R. (1994) Conventional immunosuppressive agents. In: *Immunosuppressive Drugs: Developments in Anti-Rejection Therapy* (eds A.W. Thomson & T.E. Starzl), pp. 1–14. Edward Arnold, London.

Marshall, S.E. & Waldmann, H. (1994) Monoclonal antibody therapy in clinical transplantation. In: *Medical Intelligence Unit: New Immunosuppressive Modalities and Anti-Rejection Approaches in Organ Transplantation* (ed. J.W. Kupiec-Weglinski), pp. 107–24. R.G. Landes, Austin.

Mazzucco, C.E. & Nadler, S.G. (1993) A member of the Hsp70 family of heat-shock proteins is a putative target for the immunosuppressant 15-deoxyspergualin. *Ann. NY Acad. Sci.*, **685**, 202–4.

Morice, W.G., Wiederrecht, G., Brunn, G.J., Siekierka, J.J. & Abraham, R.T. (1993) Rapamycin inhibition of interleukin-2-dependent p33cdk2 and p34cdc2 kinase activation in T lymphocytes. *J. Biol. Chem.*, **268**, 22737–45.

Morikawa, K., Oseko, F. & Morikawa, S. (1992) The suppressive effect of deoxyspergualin on the differentiation of human B lymphocytes maturing into immunoglobulin-producing cells. *Transplantation*, **54**, 526–31.

Muhl, H., Kunz, D., Rob, P. & Pfeilschifter, J. (1993) Cyclosporin derivatives inhibit interleukin 1 beta induction of nitric oxide synthase in renal mesangial cells. *Eur. J. Pharmacol.*, **249**, 95–100.

Mullarkey, M.F., Webb, D.R. & Pardee, N.E. (1986) Methotrexate in the treatment of steroid-dependent asthma. *Ann. Allergy*, **56**, 347–50.

Mullarkey, M.F., Lammert, J.K. & Blumenstein, B.A. (1990) Long-term methotrexate treatment in corticosteroid-dependent asthma. *Ann. Intern. Med.*, **112**, 577–81.

Nadeau, K., Nadler, S.G., Saulnier, M., Tepper, M.A. & Walsh, C.T. (1994) Quantitation of the interaction of the immunosuppressant deoxyspergualin and analogs with Hsp70 and Hsp90. *Biochemistry*, **33**, 2561–7.

Nadler, S.G., Tepper, M.A., Schacter, B. & Mazzucco, C.E. (1992) Interaction of the immunosuppressant deoxyspergualin with a member of the Hsp70 family of heat shock proteins. *Science*, **258**, 484–6.

Ning, Y.M. & Sanchez, E.R. (1993) Potentiation of glucocorticoid receptor-mediated gene expression by the immunophilin ligands FK 506 and rapamycin. *J. Biol. Chem.*, **268**, 6073–6.

Nogueria de Francischi, J., Conroy, D.M., Maghni, K. & Sirois, P. (1993) Inhibition by rapamycin of leukocyte migration and bronchial hyperreactivity induced by injection of Sephadex beads to guinea-pigs. *Brit. J. Pharmacol.*, **110**, 1381–6.

Olive, D. & Mawas, C. (1993) Therapeutic applications of anti-CD4 antibodies. *Crit. Rev. Ther. Drug Carrier Sys.*, **10**, 29–63.

Oyanagui, Y. (1994) Nitric oxide and hydrogen peroxide-mediated gene expression by glucocorticoids and FK 506 in histamine paw edema of mice. *Life Sci.*, **55**, PL177–PL185.

Parenteau, G.L., Dirbas, F.M., Garmestani, K. *et al.* (1992) Prolongation of graft survival in primate allograft transplantation by yttrium-90-labeled anti-Tac in conjunction with granulocyte colony-stimulating factor. *Transplantation*, **54**, 963–8.

Paulis, A., Stellato, C., Cirillo, R., Ciccarelli, A., Oriente, A. & Marone, G. (1992) Anti-inflammatory effect of FK-506 on human skin mast cells. *J. Invest. Dermatol.*, **99**, 723–8.

Propper, D.J., Woo, J., Macleod, A.M., Catto, G.R. & Thomson, A.W. (1992) The effects of rapamycin on humoral immunity *in vivo*: suppression of primary responses but not of ongoing alloantibody synthesis or memory responses. *Transplantation*, **54**, 1058–63.

Quesniaux, V.F., Wehrli, S., Steiner, C. *et al.* (1994) The immunosuppressant rapamycin blocks *in vitro* responses to hematopoietic cytokines and inhibits recovering but not steady-state hematopoiesis *in vivo*. *Blood*, **84**, 1543–52.

Renoir, J.M., Le Bihan, S., Mercier-Bodard, C. *et al.* (1994) Effects of immunosuppressants FK 506 and rapamycin on the heterooligomeric form of the progesterone receptor. *J. Steroid Biochem. Mol. Biol.*, **48**, 101–10.

Ross, J.S. & Camp, R.D. (1990) Cyclosporin A in atopic dermatitis. *Br. J. Dermatol.*, **122** (Suppl.), 41–5.

Salek, M.S., Finlay, A.Y., Luscombe, D.K. *et al.* (1993) Cyclosporin greatly improves the quality of life of adults with severe atopic dermatitis: a randomized, double-blind, placebo-controlled trial. *Brit. J. Dermatol.*, **129**, 422–30.

Schmidbauer, G., Hancock, W.W., Wasowska, B., Badger, A.M. & Kupiec-Weglinski, J.W. (1994) Abrogation by rapamycin of accelerated rejection in sensitized rats by inhibition of alloantibody responses and selective suppression of intragraft mononuclear and endothelial cell activation, cytokine production, and cell adhesion. *Transplantation*, **57**, 933–41.

Schreiber, S.L. (1991) Chemistry and biology of the immunophilins and their immunosuppressive ligands. *Science*, **251**, 283–7.

Schreiber, S.L. & Crabtree, G.R. (1992) The mechanism of action of cyclosporin A and FIC506. *Immunol. Today*, **13**, 136–42.

Schwaninger, M., Blume, R., Oetjen, E. & Knepel, W. (1993) The immunosuppressive drugs cyclosporin A and FK 506 inhibit calcineurin phosphatase activity and gene transcription mediated through the cAMP-responsive element in a nonimmune cell line. *Naunyn Schmiedeberg's Arch. Pharmacol.*, **348**, 541–5.

Selig, W. & Tocker, J. (1992) Effect of interleukin-1 receptor antagonist on antigen-induced pulmonary responses in guinea pigs. *Eur. J. Pharmacol.*, **213**, 331–6.

Shan, X., Luo, H., Chen, H., Daloze, P., St-Louis, G. & Wu, J. (1993) The effect of rapamycin on *c-jun* expression in human lymphocytes. *Clin. Immunol. Immunopathol.*, **69**, 314–17.

Shapiro, M.E., Kirkman, R.L., Kelley, V.R., Bacha, P., Nichols, J.C. & Strom, T.B. (1992) *In vivo* studies with chimeric toxins: interleukin-2 fusion toxins as immunosuppressive agents. *Targeted Diagn. Ther.*, **7**, 383–93.

Sharma, V.K., Li, B., Khanna, A., Sehajpal, P.K. & Suthanthiran, M. (1994) Which way for drug-mediated immunosuppression? *Curr. Opin. Immunol.*, **6**, 784–90.

Shreirer, M.H., Quesniausc, V.F.J., Baumann, G. *et al.* (1993) Molecular basis of immunosuppression. *Transpl. Sci.*, **3**, 185–9.

Simon, P., Townsend, R.M., Harris, R.R., Jones, E.A. & Jaffee, B.D. (1993) Brequinar sodium: inhibition of dihydroorotic acid dehydrogenase, depletion of pyrimidine pools, and consequent inhibition of immune functions *in vitro*. *Transplant. Proc.*, **25**, 77–80.

Sowden, J.M., Berth-Jones, J., Ross, J.S. *et al.* (1991) Double-blind, controlled, crossover study of cyclosporin in adults with severe refractory atopic dermatitis. *Lancet*, **338**, 137–40.

Stadler, B.M., Gang, Q., Vogel, M. *et al.* (1991) IgG anti-IgE autoantibodies in immunoregulation. *Int. Arch. Allergy Appl. Immunol.*, **94**, 83–6.

Steele, A.W. (1994) Fusion proteins. In: *Medical Intelligence Unit: New Immunosuppressive Modalities and Anti-Rejection Approaches in Organ Transplantation* (ed. J.W. Kupiec-Weglinski), pp. 135–53. R.G. Landes, Austin.

Stepkowski, S.M., Tu, Y., Condor, T.P. & Bennett, C.F. (1994) Blocking of heart allograft rejection by intercellular adhesion molecule-1 antisense oligonucleotides alone or in combination with other immunosuppressive modalities. *J. Immunol.*, **153**, 5336–46.

Strom, T.B., Kelley, V.R., Murphy, J.R., Nichols, J. & Woodworth, T.G. (1994) Interleukin-2 receptor directed therapies: antibody or cytokine based targeting molecules. In: *Medical Intelligence Unit: New Immunosuppressive Modalities and Anti-Rejection Approaches in Organ Transplantation* (ed. J.W. Kupiec-Weglinski), pp. 125–33. R.G. Landes, Austin.

Suzuki, S. (1994) Deoxyspergualin: mode of action and effects on graft rejection. In: *Immunosuppressive Drugs: Developments in Anti-Rejection Therapy* (eds A.W. Thomson & T.E. Starzl), pp. 187–202. Edward Arnold, London.

Szczeklik, A., Nizankowska, E., Dworski, R., Domagala, B. & Pinis, G. (1991) Cyclosporin for steroid-dependent asthma. *Allergy*, **46**, 312–5.

Tai, P.K., Albers, M.W., McDonnell, D.P., Chang, H., Schreiber, S.L. & Faber, L.E. (1994) Potentiation of progesterone receptor-mediated transcription by the immunosuppressant FK 506. *Biochemistry*, **33**, 10666–71.

Tamura, K., Woo, J., Bakri, M.T. & Thomson, A.W. (1993) Brequinar sodium inhibits interleukin-6-induced differentiation of a human B-cell line into IgM-secreting plasma cells. *Immunology*, **79**, 487–93.

Tepper, M.A. (1993) Deoxyspergualin: mechanism of action studies of a novel immunosuppressive drug. *Ann. NY Acad. Sci.*, **696**, 123–32.

Thomas, F., Matthews, C., Pittman, K. & Thomas, J. (1992) 15-Deoxyspergualin produces inhibition of lymphokine-activated killer cell activity. *Transplant. Proc.*, **24**, 712–13.

Thomas, F.T., Tepper, M.A., Thomas, J.M. & Haisch, C.E. (1993) 15-Deoxyspergualin: a novel immunosuppressive drug with clinical potential. *Ann. NY Acad. Sci.*, **685**, 175–92.

Thomson, A.W. (1993) Immunological effects of cyclosporin A. In: *T Cell-Directed Immunosuppression* (ed. J.-F. Bach), pp. 26–50. Blackwell Scientific Publications, Oxford.

Thomson, A.W. & Forrester, J.V. (1994) Therapeutic advances in immunosuppression. *Clin. Exp. Immunol.*, **98**, 351–7.

Thomson, A.W. & Starzl, T.E. (1993) New immunosuppressive drugs: mechanistic insights and potential therapeutic advances. *Immunol. Rev.*, **136**, 71–98.

Thomson, A.W., Propper, D.J., Woo, J., Whiting, P.H., Milton, J.I. & Macleod, A.M. (1993a) Comparative effects of rapamycin, FK 506 and cyclosporine on antibody production, lymphocyte populations and immunoglobulin isotype switching in the rat. *Immunopharmacol. Immunotoxicol.*, **15**, 355–69.

Thomson, A.W., Shapiro, R., Fung, J.J. & Starzl, T.E. (1993b) New immunosuppressive drugs: mechanisms of action and early clinical experience. In: *Immunology of Renal Transplantation* (eds A.W. Thomson & G.R.D. Catto), pp. 264–80. Edward Arnold, London, Boston.

Thomson, A.W., Woo, J. & Zeevi, A. (1994) The influence of FK 506 on lymphocyte responses *in vitro* and *in vivo*. In: *Immunosuppressive Drugs: Developments in Anti-Rejection Therapy* (eds A.W. Thomson & T.E. Starzl), pp. 95–111. Edward Arnold, London.

Tsai, M., Chen, R.H., Tam, S.Y., Blenis, J. & Galli, S.J. (1993) Activation of MAP kinases, pp90rsk and pp70-S6 kinases in mouse mast cells by signaling through the *c-kit* receptor tyrosine kinase or Fc epsilon RI: rapamycin inhibits activation of pp70-S6 kinase and proliferation in mouse mast cells. *Eur. J. Immunol.*, **23**, 3286–91.

Venkataraman, L., Burakoff, S.J. & Sen, R. (1995) FK 506 inhibits antigen receptor-mediated induction of *c-rel* in B and T lymphoid cells. *J. Exp. Med.*, **181**, 1091–9.

Wahlgren, C.F., Sheynius, A. & Hagermark, O. (1990) Antipruritic effect of oral cyclosporin A in atopic dermatitis. *Acta Dermato-Venereol.*, **70**, 323–9.

Waldmann, H. & Cobbold. S. (1993) The use of monoclonal antibodies to achieve immunological tolerance. *Trends Pharmacol. Sci.*, **14**, 143–8.

Wee, S.L., Stroka, D.M., Preffer, F.I., Jolliffee, L.K., Colvin, R.B. & Cosimi, A.B. (1992) The effects of OKT4A monoclonal antibody on cellular immunity of nonhuman primate renal allograft recipients. *Transplantation*, **53**, 501–7.

Wegner, C.D., Gundel, R.H., Reilly, P., Haynes, N., Letts, L.G. & Rothlein, R. (1990) Intercellular adhesion molecule-1 (ICAM-1) in the pathogenesis of asthma. *Science*, **247**, 456–9.

Wieder, K.J., Hancock, W.W., Schmidbauer, G. *et al.* (1993) Rapamycin treatment depresses intragraft expression of KC/MIP-2, granzyme B, and IFN-gamma in rat recipients of cardiac allografts. *J. Immunol.*, **151**, 1158–66.

Wiederrecht, G., Lam, E., Hung, S., Martin, M. & Sigal, N. (1993) The mechanism of action of FK 506 and cyclosporin A. *Ann. NY Acad. Sci.*, **696**, 9–19.

Woo, J., Lemster, B., Tamura, K., Starzl, T.E. & Thomson, A.W. (1993) The antilymphocytic activity of brequinar sodium and its potentiation by cytidine: effects on lymphocyte proliferation and cytokine production. *Transplantation*, **56**, 374–81.

Xiao, F., Chong, A.S-F., Bartlett, R.R. & Williams, J.W. (1994) Leflunomide: a promising immunosuppressant in transplantation. In: *Immunosuppressive Drugs: Developments in Anti-Rejection Therapy* (eds A.W. Thomson & T.E. Starzl), pp. 203–12. Edward Arnold, London.

Yoshimura, N., Ohmoto, Y., Yasui, H. *et al.* (1994) The direct effect of FK 506 and rapamycin on interleukin 1(beta) and immunoglobulin production *in vitro*. *Transplantation*, **57**, 1815–18.

Zheng, X.X., Strom, T.B. & Steele, A.W. (1994) Quantitative comparison of rapamycin and cyclosporine effects on cytokine gene expression studied by reverse transcriptase-competitive polymerase chain reaction. *Transplantation*, **58**, 87–92.

PART 4

Physiology

CHAPTER 37

Physiological Aspects of Airway, Pulmonary and Respiratory Muscle Function in Asthma

N.B. Pride

The pathophysiology of asthma is thought to be confined to the sublaryngeal airways, effects on pulmonary gas exchange, pulmonary circulation, control of breathing and respiratory muscles all being secondary responses to the airway obstruction. While this view ignores such systemic changes as high immunoglobulin E (IgE) levels and blood eosinophilia and such physiological aspects as central nervous system effects on airway tone, it will be followed in this chapter, which puts most emphasis on the pathophysiology of the airways, with a briefer section on mechanisms preserving adequate ventilation and gas exchange in the asthmatic crisis. Some areas of current interest are discussed, but space does not allow a comprehensive description of applied physiology in asthma.

Airway function

Factors determining airway luminal area

The concept that luminal narrowing may be due to contraction of airway smooth muscle (ASM), mucosal swelling or luminal obstruction by muco-inflammatory plugs is long established. However, this presents a static, single lung volume view of the obstructive process. Much recent work has investigated the factors which distend the airways and the ways in which airway narrowing may be restricted or amplified *in vivo* by pathophysiological factors. In particular, the response of the airway to deep inflation (DI) or to the avoidance of DI has been used to localize airway responses, as a surrogate marker of an active inflammatory response and to explain the difficulty in removing contraction of ASM in asthma. Hence, airway compliance, hitherto mainly of research interest, is now relevant to clinical investigation.

Airway compliance and transmural pressure

The distensibility or compliance of conducting airways can be studied directly *in vitro* by measuring luminal cross-sectional area (or volume) as transmural pressure is varied. Excised conducting airways have a sigmoid transmural pressure–area curve, with a plateau of maximum area at positive transmural pressures, while luminal narrowing at negative transmural pressure is often restricted by stiffening of the airway wall before complete collapse occurs.

In vivo intrathoracic but extrapulmonary airways are exposed to transpulmonary pressure (difference between airway and pleural surface pressure). During breath holding, they distend as lung volume is increased. The situation is more complex for intrapulmonary airways; for the larger intrapulmonary airways the extra-airway pressure is very similar to pleural surface pressure, but for the small intrapulmonary airways distension as lung volume increases depends on the attachment of alveolar walls, which transmit the forces distending the alveoli to the external perimeter of the airway (Mead *et al.*, 1970).

Contraction of ASM narrows the airway lumen but also stiffens the airway wall, reducing its expansion and probably its narrowing as transmural pressure varies. Apart from a direct effect on the compliance of the muscle, ASM contraction brings airway cartilage plates together in the central conducting airways, 'fortifying' their walls (Olsen *et al.*, 1967; James *et al.*, 1987); folding of the mucosa may also play a role in maintaining a patent lumen in the presence of ASM contraction. The extent of airway narrowing is also limited by extra-airway forces; when airways constrict, the immediately adjacent alveolar walls are put under tension, restricting airway narrowing. These extra-airway forces should have their greatest stabilizing effect at large lung volumes, so that a given amount of activation of ASM would lead to greater shortening at small than at large volume. Experiments in excised lobes of dogs have shown that, while methacholine can induce complete airway closure in collapsed lung, this is not possible when the lungs are inflated (Murtagh *et al.*, 1971). *In vivo*, in humans the magnitude of maximum bronchoconstriction to inhaled methacholine is also greater at small than at large lung volume and is quite sensitive to relatively small changes in volume above and below functional residual capacity (FRC) (Ding *et al.*, 1987). However, lesser degrees of airway narrowing produced by submaximal doses of methacholine appear to be unchanged by moderate changes in lung volume (Ding *et al.*, 1987; Wang *et al.*, 1990). This suggests that ASM initially may contract freely and that the restraints applied by surrounding lung chiefly act to prevent extreme narrowing or closure.

In practice, in many normal subjects (Woolcock *et al.*, 1984; Sterk *et al.*, 1985) and patients with mild asthma (Woolcock *et al.*, 1984; Bel *et al.*, 1991), there appears to be a limit to the amount of airway narrowing produced by increasing doses of histamine or methacholine aerosol, with a plateau of forced expiratory volume in 1 second (FEV_1) developing. However, this 'protective' effect is not present in all normal subjects (Fig. 37.1) or in patients with significant resting airway obstruction due to asthma. Consequently, it has been suggested that an aim of asthma treatment should be not only to restore normal baseline function but to restore a plateau of airway narrowing, preferably one developing with only a small deterioration in airway function.

Airway wall thickening is an important feature of chronic asthma and is found in all sizes of airway from <2 mm to >10 mm diameter (James *et al.*, 1989). On average, wall thickness is doubled due to broadly similar increases in the thickening of epithelial, submucosal and muscular layers, although in the smallest airways muscle is not incresed. Functionally the most obvious effect of the thickening of the airway wall internal to the muscle layer is to amplify the effects of ASM contraction in reducing the airway lumen. Moreno and colleagues (1986) in Vancouver have modelled the effects of the observed increases in airway wall thickness and concluded the associated reduction in airway lumen would cause little alteration in basal airway resistance, but would greatly enhance the response to a given amount of ASM shortening induced by challenge procedures. Hence, airway hyperresponsivess (AHR) could result from a normal amount of

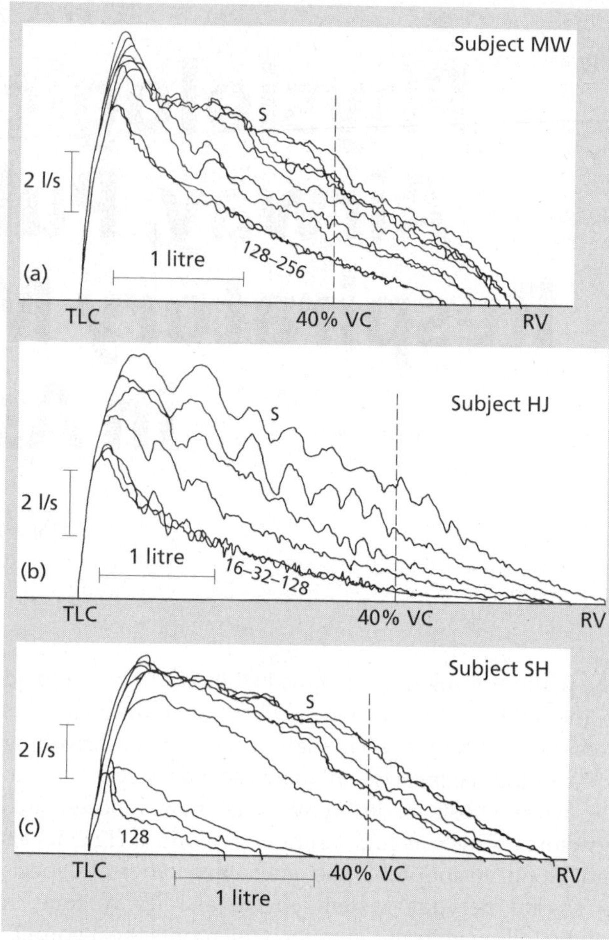

Fig. 37.1 Airway responses of three normal subjects to saline(s) and increasing concentrations (1–256 mg/ml) of aerosols of methacholine. Changes in airway function followed by sequential maximum expiratory flow–volume (MEFV) curves superimposed at full inflation (total lung capacity, TLC). (a) A normal subject who developed a plateau of airway function at 128 and 256 mg/ml of methacholine with relatively little reduction of maximum expiratory flow (final FEV_1 68% of baseline value). (b) A plateau of maximum expiratory flow develops at 16 mg/ml but with more severe reduction of flow (final FEV_1 53% of baseline value). (c) Extremely severe reduction of maximum expiratory flow, without development of plateau when the procedure was terminated, when FEV_1 was 27% of baseline value. Note dramatic increase in residual volume (RV). (Data from Pertuze *et al.*, in preparation.)

muscle shortening giving a disproportionate reduction in luminal calibre. In practice, there is also an increased mass of ASM, which further amplifies this effects.

Airway compliance is reduced whenever there is wall thickening. A further significant factor in determining airway compliance is likely to be the contractile state of ASM. The role of collagen deposition beneath the basement membrane (Roche *et al.*, 1989) is uncertain because it is not clear whether this makes a significant contribution to the compliance of the submaximally distended airway or merely determines its maximum diameter.

A more subtle effect of increased wall thickness occurs if the outer diameter of the airway is larger in asthma; in that event the immediately adjacent alveolar walls, although intact, are probably under less tension (Fig. 37.2), so the coupling between lung expansion and the forces applied to the airway perimeter is less tight. A similar partial uncoupling may occur if there is peri-airway inflammation and oedema (Macklem, 1985). Although there is no evidence that emphysema develops in chronic asthma, there is a small reduction in static transpulmonary pressure at all lung volumes, reducing the tension in all alveolar walls. Hence, extra-airway forces stabilizing airway diameter are likely to be reduced in chronic asthma.

Apart from sustained structural changes thickening the airway wall, acute thickening may occur with mucosal oedema due to inflammatory changes or with expansion of blood volume in or around the airway wall, as has been proposed to occur after exercise on isocapnic hyperventilation (see Chapter 39).

Role of ASM in determining airway wall compliance

Contraction of ASM may immediately stiffen the airway wall, either by a direct effect or by inducing mucosal folding or cartilage overlap. Recent studies have also shown an effect of volume history with time. In asthmatic subjects the extent of airway narrowing and, by implication ASM contraction, in response to inhalation of methacholine is greatly enhanced when deep inflations are avoided for several minutes (Skloot *et al.*, 1995). This time dependence may reflect ASM becoming less 'fluid' and stiffening with the absence of distension. Conversely, methacholine inhalation induces less airway narrowing when administered while tidal volume is increased as during exercise or voluntary hyperventilation (Freedman, 1992).

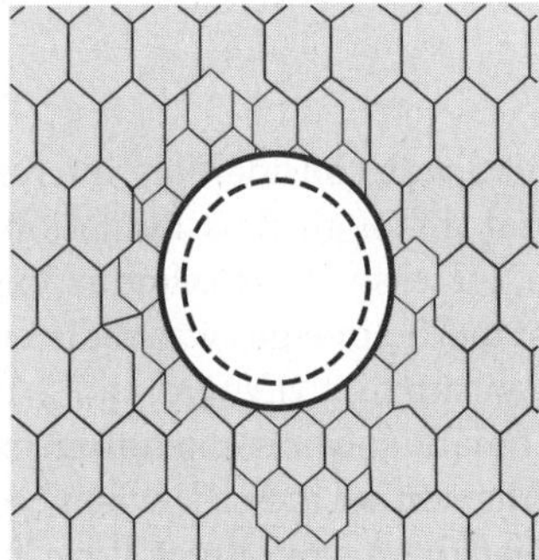

Fig. 37.2 Schematic represention of effect of an increase in outer diameter of airway (outer continuous circle) from its initial diameter (inner dashed circle) on surrounding alveoli, which are less distended than those distant from the airway wall.

Table 37.1 Factors determining effective airway compliance.

Initial luminal area
Encroachment by wall thickening or secretions
Wall stiffness
Thickening of wall (collagen deposition beneath basement membrane)
Cartilage fortification
State of airway smooth muscle
Extra-airway distending forces
Reduction in lung recoil pressure
Impaired alveolar attachments/airway perimeter coupling

In vivo *assessment of airway compliance*

Airway lumen size therefore depends on luminal factors, airway wall compliance, the state of ASM and the transmural pressure which acts across its walls, which during quiet breathing is essentially determined by extra-airway forces (Table 37.1) The airway lumen may be reduced under baseline conditions because of encroachment by wall thickening or by secretions. *In vivo* assessment using tests of overall lung function cannot distinguish these different mechanisms reducing the expansion of airways with increase in lung volume. Total airway conductance shows an abnormally small rise as lung volume is increased in asthmatic subjects (Butler *et al.*, 1960; Colebatch *et al.*, 1973). While this could be accounted for by stiffening and reduced compliance of airway walls, it could equally be caused by poor coupling between lung expansion and extra-airway distending forces or a reduced airway lumen due to partial or complete obstruction by secretions. Increase in anatomical dead space (which indicates the volume of the larger intrathoracic airways) with increase in lung volume is also reduced (Wilson *et al.*, 1993). Studies of individual central airways by imaging at different lung volumes provides more direct information but even then effective transmural pressure cannot be fully assessed.

Origins of AHR

Initially AHR was explained largely in terms of enhanced 'twitchiness' and contraction of ASM, whether due to enhanced mediator or neural stimulation of muscle contraction or an increased ASM mass or contractility. Overall it has been difficult to demonstrate increases in the *in vitro* contractility of ASM from asthmatic subjects, although this question is not completely resolved (see Chapter 42).

There is no doubt about the increased mass of ASM found in asthmatic subjects. Recent work has emphasized that enhanced reductions in luminal calibre can also occur because: (i) a normal amount of shortening of ASM can give a disproportionate reduction in luminal calibre when relatively subtle wall thickening is present; or (ii) greater muscle shortening is produced for a given stimulus to ASM because the restraining load produced by extra-airway attachments is reduced. Conceivably, therefore, AHR could be sustained purely by wall thickening in the absence of airway inflammation or abnormality of ASM. A further important factor determining AHR may be the contractile state of ASM itself and how this responds to lung volume changes. The precise role of each of these possible additional mechanisms in causing AHR remains to be elucidated.

Site of intrathoracic airway narrowing

Because so much of the airway narrowing in attacks of asthma is likely to be due to the transient mechanisms of contraction of ASM, mucosal swelling and intraluminal secretions—and may vary within the duration of an attack and between a sequence of attacks — studies of the serial site of airway narrowing have not been as conclusive as in chronic obstructive pulmonary disease (COPD).

Post-mortem studies have shown that inflammation of the airway mucosa extends throughout the tracheo-bronchial tree, indicating the potential for narrowing to develop in all sizes of airways. However, studies of regional ventilation show that airway narrowing varies greatly between parallel airways, despite the likely presence of asthmatic changes in all airways. Presumably there can be non-uniformity on a longitudinal basis also.

Direct visualization of airways, either at bronchoscopy or by external imaging (plain radiographs, bronchography, computed tomography), is inevitably confined to the larger conducting airways. Occasional reports where an asthmatic attack develops during bronchoscopy or bronchography have commented on the narrowing of the large airways. A similar limitation applies to the acoustic reflection technique, in which an acoustic pulse is generated at the airway opening to obtain a distance–total cross-sectional area function of the airways; so far useful results can only be obtained to just beyond the carina (Molfino *et al.*, 1992; Louis *et al.*, 1994). Inhalation of radio-opaque dusts to obtain a bronchogram has produced disappointingly non-uniform coating of airway walls.

Only limited information can be obtained from standard tests of lung function breathing air. In normal subjects older than about 40 years old, residual volume (RV) is known to be determined by closure of peripheral airways, so increase in RV, which is a consistent feature in an exacerbation of asthma, is sometimes considered to indicate an abnormality of small airways. While this may usually be the case, it is not inevitable. In asthma, airway closure may be enhanced by intraluminal muco-inflammatory plugs, and pathological examination suggests that even lobar or segmental airways may close as the lungs are deflated. In normal lungs, maximum flows at large volumes (such as peak expiratory flow (PEF)) are influenced particularly by the size of the central airways, but this is because of the low frictional flow resistance in the normal small airways at large lung volume, which results in the dominant airway pressure drop being due to convective acceleration in central airways. An increase in peripheral airway resistance will reduce maximum flow at all lung volumes, including PEF. In clinical remission of asthma, increases in closing volume and reductions in flow in the terminal part of the maximum expiratory flow–volume (MEFV) curve persist and may be due to mucous plugs in the peripheral airways, which have been observed in the lungs of young asthmatic subjects who have died from unrelated causes. Inevitably the MEFV curve must be affected by differences in emptying rate of differing parallel parts of the lung, as well as by the serial distribution of airway narrowing.

Another approach has been to compare values of two different tests of airway function; thus, for a given FEV_1, airway resistance tends to be higher in asthma than in emphysema, suggesting a wider distribution of airway narrowing in asthma. A comparison of changes in dead space (dominated by large airways) and in resistance (affected by all airways) has been used to evaluate the central or peripheral site of action of bronchodilators (Yanai *et al.*, 1991). However, these methods have not been very discriminatory or widely applied.

Two other indirect, non-invasive techniques have been used to define the site of airway narrowing: the response to breathing a helium–oxygen mixture and the response to a deep inflation.

Airway response to breathing a helium–oxygen mixture

MEFV curves

In the 1970s there was considerable interest in trying to localize the serial site of air-flow limitation in asthma by measuring the increase in maximum expiratory flow when density of the expired gas was reduced by breathing a helium–oxygen mixture (Despas *et al.*, 1972). In some (but not all) asthmatic subjects, maximum expiratory flow does not show the normal increase when breathing HeO_2; this suggests that the major site of flow limitation is no longer in central airways, as in normal subjects, but has moved to more peripheral airways, where flow is presumed to be laminar and independent of density (Ingram & McFadden, 1977). This change is usually attributed to increased frictional pressure losses in narrowed peripheral airways. Some asthmatic subjects consistently lose or consistently retain density dependence of maximum flow with repeated attacks, but this is not invariably the case; in general, loss of density dependence becomes more common as expiratory air-flow limitation increases in severity (Fairshter & Wilson, 1980; Partridge & Saunders, 1981) and is particularly observed in asthmatic subjects who smoke (Antic & Macklem, 1976). Reduction in density dependence of maximum expiratory flow should not be interpreted as indicating *only* peripheral airways are narrowed, even if they are the site of flow limitation.

In recent years, interest in the use of helium response on maximum expiratory flow has waned. The method analysed the changes in the airways between the alveoli and the sites of expiratory flow limitation ('choke points'), but experimental studies in dogs showed that relatively small changes in geometry and position of choke points could profoundly affect the helium response (Jadue *et al.*, 1985). There is considerable variation in size of the helium response in the normal population and in disease; changes in helium response in an individual before and after an acute intervention may be more reliable.

Pulmonary resistance

An alternative method is to study the reduction in pulmonary resistance (R_L) (measured by the oesophageal balloon technique) when switching from breathing air to a helium–oxygen mixture. A large decrease in R_L with helium breathing suggests a large component of R_L breathing air is in the central conducting airways and a small response indicates that much of the resistance breathing air is in the peripheral airways. This tidal breathing technique is probably more relevant to asthma, but is more invasive and requires more elaborate analysis. A detailed analysis using the effects of helium breathing on R_L has suggested that the extrathoracic airway is narrowed in a significant proportion of attacks of asthma (Lisboa *et al.*, 1980).

Airway response to a DI

A DI may transiently affect airway dimensions when tidal breathing is resumed. Early studies demonstrated airway widening after DI in normal subjects when narrowing had been induced by inhaled histamine or methacholine. In contrast, DI can lead to subsequent airway narrowing in subjects with acute asthma (Simonsson *et al.*, 1967). These differences between normal and asthmatic subjects exaggerate differences in airway responsiveness as assessed by conventional tests of forced expiration. To overcome problems induced by a full inflation, a forced expiration can be started from about 60% vital capacity (VC) (Bouhuys *et al.*, 1969) (Fig. 37.3). In this technique the flow at the onset of expiration (over about 10% of VC) is augmented by the expulsion of air from collapsing central intrathoracic airways as they change from their expanded dimensions at the onset of expiration to their collapsed state during forced expiration. Measurements are usually made at volumes between 30 and 40% VC, thus balancing the conflicting demands of avoiding undue lung inflation and artefactual flow at the start of expiration, while still ensuring an adequate flow signal. Initially, changes after DI were attributed to a change in bronchial muscle activity (direct or reflex) produced by stretch. An alternative hypothesis is that the relation between parenchymal and airway hysteresis explains the variable changes in airway function after DI (Ingram, 1987, 1990). When airway hysteresis exceeds that of parenchyma, DI results in temporary airway widening when tidal breathing is resumed. When parenchymal hysteresis exceeds that of the airways, DI results in airway narrowing. Equal degrees of hysteresis result in no effect of DI on resting airway calibre, as found in most normal subjects. A major interest of this idea is that it might localize the site of disease within the lung. Contraction of smooth muscle in conducting airways would be expected to increase airway hysteresis without affecting parenchymal hysteresis. Increased tone or other causes of airway narrowing in the extreme periphery of the lung (respiratory bronchioles and alveolar ducts) would be expected to increase parenchy-

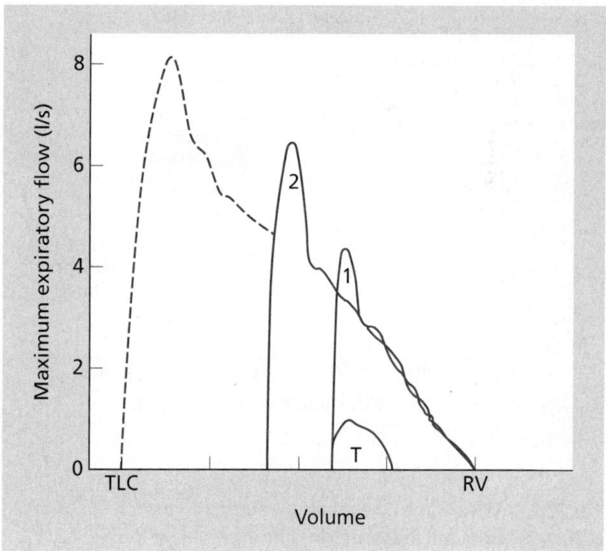

Fig. 37.3 Forced expirations started from the end of a tidal inspiration (1), about 60% VC (2), and from (TLC) (dashed curve) shown as maximum expiratory flow vs. absolute lung volume. Note the large transient of flow on curves 1 and 2. In this normal subject, maximum expiratory flow on partial curves 1 and 2 coincided with that on the maximum curve from TLC.

mal hysteresis with only a small increase in airway hysteresis.

The effects of DI can be examined by measuring the effects on airways resistance, or more simply by comparing maximal expiratory flow at 30–40% VC above RV from forced expirations begun from about 60% VC (partial curve, P) and from total lung capacity (TLC) (maximal curve, M) (Fig. 37.4a) (Ingram, 1990) and expressing results as $\dot{V}_m/\dot{V}_p$ ratios. In normal subjects under basal conditions $\dot{V}_m/\dot{V}_p$ ratios on average are a little greater than 1.0 (Berry & Fairshter, 1985). In spontaneous episodes of asthma $\dot{V}_m/\dot{V}_p$ ratios are less than 1.0 (airway function worse after DI) and tend to fall as FEV_1 (% predicted) falls (Berry & Fairshter, 1985; Lim *et al.*, 1987) (Fig. 37.4b). This suggests an important obstruction of the most peripheral airways in spontaneous asthma. In contrast, when acute obstruction is induced by challenge with inhaled short-acting drugs, $\dot{V}_m/\dot{V}_p$ ratios rise, sometimes to very high values, indicating that DI removes obstruction. This is characteristic of a conducting airway response. Similar rises in $\dot{V}_m/\dot{V}_p$ ratios have been found when airway narrowing is induced by other acute, short-lived challenges such as exercise or hyperventilation; with antigen challenge, however, rises in $\dot{V}_m/\dot{V}_p$ ratios are less pronounced for the impairment of FEV_1 in the early phase of the reaction and tend to be lower (although often still more than 1.0) in the late phase (Ingram, 1990; Pellegrino *et al.*, 1990). Thus, changes after allergen challenge are intermediate between those found with a simple pharmacological challenge and spontaneous asthma (Fig. 37.4b). The results have been interpreted as providing evidence for the presence of inflammatory changes in the peripheral airways in spontaneous asthma and, to a lesser extent, in the late response to allergen. The tendency to airway narrowing after a DI has been shown to relate to elevated concentrations of eosinophils and histamine in bronchoalveolar lavage fluid in asthmatic subjects (Pliss *et al.*, 1989). A similar response to DI to that found in spontaneous asthma is also found in smokers with air-flow obstruction, in whom the dominant role of peripheral airway changes is well established.

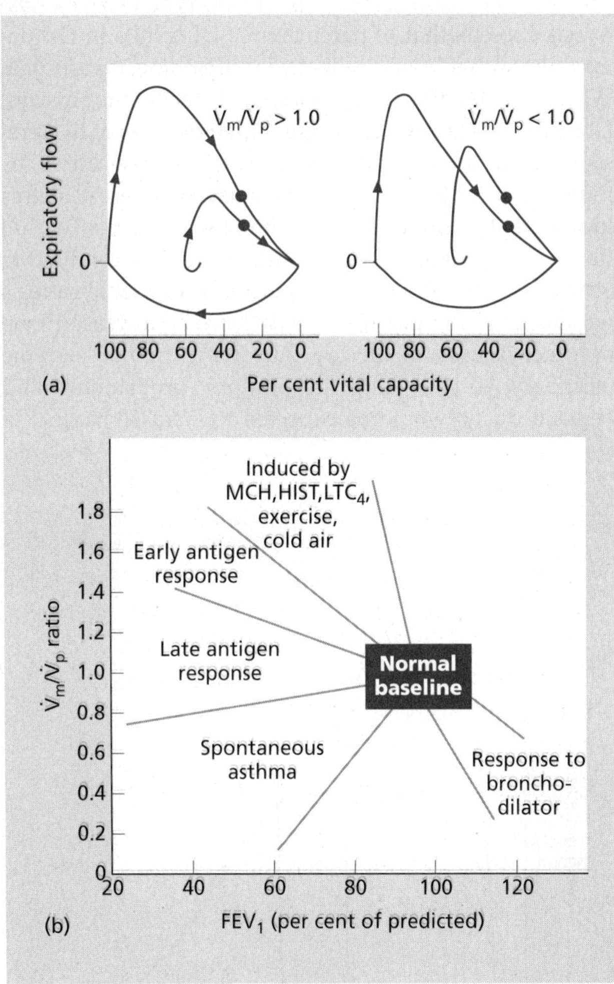

Fig. 37.4 (a) Use of forced expirations started from 60% VC (partial curve) and from full inflation (maximum curves) to derive $\dot{V}_m/\dot{V}_p$ ratios at 30% VC. For simplicity the transient overshoot of flow at the start of the partial curve (see Fig. 37.3) is not shown. (b) Scheme of typical change in $\dot{V}_m/\dot{V}_p$ ratios. In the normal subject this ratio is close to 1.0. With acute bronchoconstrictor challenges, the ratio rises as FEV_1 falls, but in spontaneous asthma $\dot{V}_m/\dot{V}_p$ ratios are < 1.0 and falls as FEV_1 falls. Changes with antigen challenge are intermediate. (From Ingram, 1990, with permission.)

These studies of DI have usually been made after 45–60 seconds of normal tidal breathing without DI. When ASM contraction is induced experimentally, its persistence depends on the timing and frequency of DI. When DI is avoided for several minutes after inhaling an aerosol of methacholine, a much greater airway narrowing is induced. In normal subjects DI still rapidly restores normal airway function, but a single DI is much less effective in removing ASM contraction in asthmatic subjects (Skloot *et al.*, 1995). In contrast, inhaling bronchoconstrictor aerosols during exercise with increased tidal volume results in much less airway narrowing than is induced by the same aerosol during tidal breathing at rest (Freedman, 1992).

Endobronchial catheter studies

While endobronchial pressure measurements are the obvious approach for defining the distribution of air-flow resistance, their invasive nature restricts their use and there are important physiological limitations. Endobronchial catheters may stimulate mucosal receptors and induce reflex bronchoconstriction and mucus production and can only be used in central airways without compromising air flow through the catheterized airway. Two different wedged-catheter techniques have been developed which measure pressure at a more peripheral site; in one, a 3 mm catheter is wedged in a right lower-lobe bronchus and lateral pressure measured proximally (Yanai *et al.*, 1992). Total lung resistance in normal subjects with this technique appears about 50% higher than without the presence of a catheter. In remission of asthma, inspiratory (but not expiratory) peripheral aiway resistance was slightly increased; in middle-aged patients with persistent air-flow obstruction due to chronic asthma, there were increases in both central and peripheral resistance (Table 37.2). Allowing for the contribution of the extrathoracic airway to total R_L, peripheral resistance accounted for about one-third of intrathoracic resistance in normal subjects and about 50% in the subjects with chronic, persistent asthma (Yanai *et al.*, 1992).

Another technique measures pressure–flow relations in the occluded lung beyond a bronchoscope wedged in a segmental bronchus; gas flow via the bronchoscope slowly inflates the occluded lung (Wagner *et al.*, 1990). In asthmatic subjects in remission with normal total airway resistance and FEV_1, a considerable increase in peripheral lung resistance has been found; this technique measures the combined resistance of peripheral airways, collateral channels and lung tissue. These results directly confirm earlier suggestions from pathological and physiological studies that there are residual changes in the peripheral airways even in remission of asthma.

Using tests of airway function to detect mucosal inflammation

Tests of airway mechanical function can only supply indirect information on the pathophysiological basis of airway narrowing; rapid changes in less than 60 seconds are said to favour a response in ASM rather than an increase or decrease in mucosal thickness.

A number of attempts have been made to distinguish airway changes in the early and late response to antigen. The usual hypothesis has been that the early response is mainly due to narrowing of conducting airways, with a large component due to contraction of ASM, and that the late response is due to inflammatory changes in more peripheral airways with a small component due to smooth muscle contraction. Indirect support for these hypotheses comes from the differences in the speed of onset and of resolution in the two phases and from the supposed lack of effect of β-adrenergic agonists in attenuating the late phase. However, when short-acting β-agonists are given at appropriate times (Eiser, 1991) or long-acting β-agonists are used (Twentyman *et al.*, 1990), it is clear that the late response can be attenuated, if not completely removed, by inhaled β-agonists. Studies using the response of maximum expiratory flow to breathing helium–oxygen have been inconclusive. Considerable use has been made of changes in the $\dot{V}_m/\dot{V}_p$ ratio. As discussed above, the acute response to a bronchoconstrictor drug, such as methacholine or histamine, is an increase in $\dot{V}_m/\dot{V}_p$ ratio above basal values of about 1.0, while severe spontaneous asthma is associated with a reduction in $\dot{V}_m/\dot{V}_p$ ratio to below 1.0. In the response to antigen, the rise in $\dot{V}_m/\dot{V}_p$ is less than with bronchoconstrictor drugs in the early response and is lower in the late than the early response, so falling in an intermediate range (Fig. 37.4). A relatively low $\dot{V}_m/\dot{V}_p$ ratio has been interpreted as indicating an airway inflammatory response, possibly in the more peripheral airways, with poor dilatation of the airways following DI, and has been found with provocation by pro-inflammatory mediators as well as by antigen (Ingram, 1990).

Although different patterns of changes in the $\dot{V}_m/\dot{V}_p$ ratio must indicate differences in mechanical behaviour of the airways in response to DI, their reliability as surrogate markers of an inflammatory response remains to be established. For instance, a DI-induced contraction of ASM by a reflex or a direct 'myogenic' response could reduce the $\dot{V}_m/\dot{V}_p$ ratio without being associated with inflammation. A more direct and exciting approach is to monitor expired nitric oxide (NO) (Kharitonov *et al.*, 1994; see Chapter 28). Conceivably in the future other analyses of the chemical composition of expired air may be useful.

Chronic asthma with persistent air-flow obstruction

In middle-aged and older patients with asthma, the best airway function after optimal treatment has been established is often below expected reference values (Brown *et*

Table 37.2 Peripheral and total pulmonary resistance in normal subjects and chronic persistent asthma. (Data from Yanai *et al.*, 1992.)

	M/F	Mean age (years)	FEV_1 (% pred.)	R_L (cmH_2O/ l/second)	R_P (cmH_2O/ l/second)	R_P/R_L (%)
Normal	5/0	56 (±6)	88 (±2)	3.1 (±0.1)	0.7 (±0.3)	23
Chronic, persistent asthma	7/3	57 (±3)	54 (±3)	9.3 (±1.9)	4.1 (±1.0)	44

Values are mean (±SE).

M/F, male/female; R_L, total pulmonary resistance, measured during tidal breathing; R_P, peripheral resistance of airways < 3 mm diameter and lung tissue.

al., 1984). This leads to difficulty in distinction from, and genuine overlap with, smoking-related COPD, although the prognosis in chronic asthma is much better than for COPD. Surprisingly little is known about the pathological basis for this loss of airway function. Conventionally, chronic asthma, at least in the absence of smoking, is not associated with the development of emphysema or loss of alveolar attachments to the airway perimeter; this is confirmed indirectly by the preservation of normal carbon monoxide (CO) transfer coefficient (CO transfer per litre of lung volume) (Keens *et al.*, 1979) and the few available studies of lung pressure–volume characteristics (Pride & Macklem, 1986). As pointed out above, airway wall thickening alone, even when quite severe, causes little increase in baseline airway resistance, despite playing a large role in enhancing the luminal narrowing that occurs with ASM contraction. It is uncertain whether laying down collagen beneath the basement membrane reduces the maximum airway diameter achieved with full distension. The increase in R_L appears to be in both central and peripheral (<3 mm diameter) airways, with the proportionate increase in peripheral airways being slightly greater (Yanai *et al.*, 1992) (Table 37.2), so that airway function resembles that in the subgroup of COPD patients whose disability is due mainly to chronic airway disease.

Practical assessment of airway function

In summary, functional abnormality of the peripheral airways is usually present in spontaneous asthma, even when in remission; the extent to which larger conducting airways are involved may vary between individuals and between attacks in an individual. Measurements before and after a DI suggest that easily reversible airway narrowing, such as that induced by histamine, methacholine or exercise, may chiefly involve central conducting airways, while the less reversible changes of spontaneous asthma and the reaction to allergens may be in more peripheral airways. In chronic, persistent asthma in middle age, narrowing involves central conducting as well as peripheral airways.

In clinical practice and many laboratory investigations, airway function is monitored by tests which require a full inflation, such as FEV_1 or PEF. Because of the varying response to a DI, there is a case for making resistance (or partial flow–volume curve) measurements in the tidal breathing range. However, in practice many studies have shown a broad correlation between changes in the two types of measurement, as an assessment both of baseline state and of response to bronchodilator or bronchoconstrictor agents. While the frequency of DI may have a profound effect on the development of airway narrowing, in practice when DI at rest is not artificially constrained or encouraged FEV_1 or PEF provides a reliable assessment of airway narrowing.

Involvement of the extrathoracic airway

Although most attention naturally has been paid to the intrathoracic airways, extrathoracic airways may also be involved.

Nose

The most obvious extrathoracic airway involvement is nasal obstruction due to rhinitis and/or polyps. In normal subjects, during tidal breathing the nose provides a resistance of about 2 cmH_2O/l/second, about 50% of the total air-flow resistance. Nasal resistance may be considerably higher in the presence of rhinitis, particularly when lying down (Table 37.3). Presumably, if nasal resistance is greatly raised, tidal breathing is divided between the oral and nasal routes, with reduction of the protective and humidifying effects of the nose.

Reflexes between the nose and intrapulmonary airways have been investigated extensively in experimental animals, but their importance in humans is uncertain. The better-established interaction is between acute nasal stimulation and transient narrowing of intrapulmonary airways, but the reverse relationship—nasal congestion following the provocation of intrapulmonary airway narrowing—has been described (Yap & Pride, 1994). Whether these interactions can lead to sustained airway narrowing or nasal congestion and whether they are exaggerated by chronic nasal or bronchial disease is unknown.

Trachea, glottis and pharynx

Important narrowing of the glottis and extrathoracic airway occurs in some attacks of asthma. Even in normal subjects, inhaled or intravenous histamine results in some narrowing of the glottis; this narrowing is more pronounced in asthmatic subjects. Detailed studies of resistance during air and helium–oxygen breathing suggest involvement of the glottis and/or extrathoracic trachea in a significant proportion of asthmatic attacks (Lisboa *et al.*, 1980). Expiratory narrowing of the supraglottic airway has also been demonstrated (Collett *et al.*, 1983, 1986). How often extrathoracic narrowing plays an important role in attacks of asthma is unknown. The airway obstruction of asthma has to be distinguished from structural or functional obstruction of the extrathoracic airways. Structural narrowing results in distinctive changes in maximum expiratory and inspiratory flow–volume curves (Miller & Hyatt, 1973). Functional obstruction may mimic acute asthma and because of its variability be more difficult to diagnose. Symptoms caused by disease of the

Table 37.3 Contributions of nasal resistance to total respiratory resistance during tidal breathing. (Data from Duggan *et al.*, in preparation.)

	Total respiratory resistance (cmH_2O/l/second)		Nasal airway resistance (cmH_2O/l/second)
	Mouth breathing	Nose breathing	
Normal subjects (*n* = 10)			
Sitting	2.2 (0.1)	4.2 (0.4)	2.1
Supine	3.0 (0.1)	5.7 (0.4)	2.7
Asthma alone (*n* = 8)			
Sitting	4.6 (0.8)	7.1 (0.6)	2.5
Supine	5.3 (0.9)	8.8 (0.6)	3.4
Asthma with nasal symptoms (*n* = 10)			
Sitting	3.7 (0.2)	7.6 (1.4)	3.9
Supine	5.4 (0.3)	11.2 (1.9)	5.8

Values are mean (SE). Resistance was measured by forced oscillation at 6 Hz at the airway opening.

extrathoracic airway may overlap with those of asthma (Bucca *et al.*, 1995).

Involvement of lung parenchyma

Conventionally, asthma is regarded as a disease of the airways without significant changes in the lung tissue or air spaces. Emphysema is believed not to develop in never smokers who develop persistent air-flow obstruction due to chronic asthma; this is supported by the consistent preservation of a normal or even increased value of the CO transfer coefficient (Keens *et al.*, 1979). Nevertheless, there is a modest loss of lung recoil pressure (Pride & Macklem, 1986), and, as discussed above, expansion of the airway outer diameter and peri-airway inflammation may reduce the distension of the smaller airways produced by alveolar attachments to the perimeter.

A more controversial area is involvement of lung tissue in the constrictor response. In animals, changes in lung tissue resistance have accounted for a large part of the increase in R_L after bronchoconstrictor aerosols, sometimes exceeding the contribution of narrowing of the conducting airways (Ludwig *et al.*, 1989). The origins of the increased lung tissue resistance are uncertain; possibilities are contractile elements in the lung periphery, such as smooth muscle in alveolar ducts, small pulmonary vessels or contractile interstitial (Kapanci) cells. Alternatively, contracted conducting airways may act as struts within the lung parenchyma, directly impeding its expansion. A very comprehensive study of the effects of inhaled methacholine in humans with asthma failed to show any increase in lung tissue resistance—but showed a considerable increase in resistance of the conducting airways (Kariya *et al.*, 1989); however, a further study using inhaled histamine in humans has found some peripheral lung effects (Pellegrino *et al.*, 1993). Further studies are required, because it seems possible that animal models of asthma involve very different sites of increase in resistance from those found in humans.

Response to increasing severity of airway obstruction

As airway obstruction becomes more severe, there is increasing difficulty in sustaining ventilation and gas exchange. Minute ventilation (and probably cardiac output) have to be increased and hyperinflation places an additional burden on the inspiratory muscles. In fatal cases, the degree of overinflation and airway blockage by muco-inflammatory plugs is so gross that it is difficult to conceive how air flow could have been sustained shortly before. While there is no intrinsic abnormality of the gas-exchanging part of the lungs, pulmonary circulation, control of breathing and respiratory muscles in asthma are all stressed by severe obstruction.

Progression of acute severe asthma

The progression of changes is reasonably clear, although such obvious measurements as minute ventilation, the degree of hyperinflation and the intrathoracic pressures generated during tidal breathing have only been made on rare occasions in severe asthma.

As airway obstruction becomes more severe, airways close off at larger and larger volumes on expiration, increasing RV and reducing VC. In addition, maximum expiratory flows in the lower part of the VC are reduced, so that there may be expiratory flow limitation during tidal breathing. To achieve adequate ventilation, it is necessary to breathe at large lung volume, so that large distending forces are put on the airways, minimizing the narrowing. Adequate expiratory flow rates to meet the demand for total ventilation (increased because of increased oxygen consumption and by increase in physiological dead space) can only be obtained over a relatively small range of volumes, close to the position of full inflation; typically there is a small tidal volume and rapid frequency of respiration.

The limited studies of the intrathoracic pressure generated during severe asthmatic attacks emphasize the very negative pressures generated on inspiration, with only small positive pressures generated on expiration (Hedstrand, 1971). Optimum expiratory pressures to generate maximum expiratory flow are lower in attacks of asthma than during remission. At this optimum pressure, there will be little dynamic narrowing of central airways and therefore expiratory wheezing may not be pronounced. When excessive expiratory pressures are generated, there is no increase in ventilation but work done by the respiratory muscles will be increased and wheezing more pronounced. Thus, increased total ventilation, hyperinflation, small tidal volumes and fast respiratory frequency are all appropriate adaptations to the air-flow obstruction, and expiratory wheezing will bear a variable relation to the severity of the obstruction.

A vigorous drive to breathing is essential to overcome the mechanical and gas-exchange inefficiency and prevent severe hypoxaemia and carbon dioxide retention. In most patients, the arterial P_{O_2}(Pa_{O_2}) is only moderately reduced (McFadden & Lyons, 1968), usually being above 50 mmHg (6.7 kPa), even when FEV_1 is <25% predicted values. The arterial P_{CO_2} (Pa_{CO_2}) remains in or slightly below the normal range (McFadden & Lyons, 1968) until a late stage in the majority of patients, but a significant minority develop hypercapnia and tend to present with a similar Pa_{CO_2} in each episode (Mountain & Sahn, 1988), suggesting a role for relative hyporesponsiveness to carbon dioxide (Rebuck & Read, 1971). If respiratory efforts are strenuous and yet mild elevation of Pa_{CO_2} is present when breathing air, the implication is that the severity of ventilation–blood flow imbalance, coupled with the impaired bellows performance, is such that compensatory hyperventilation is stretched to the limit, and any further deterioration in either ventilation–blood flow balance or airway function could be followed by a precipitous rise in Pa_{CO_2}. If carbon dioxide retention develops, there will be a respiratory acidosis and acidaemia, as the acute changes will precede the renal retention of bicarbonate. In general, at least in adults, metabolic acidosis is not present until a very late stage. Although there are tachycardia and increased resistance in the pulmonary circulation, particularly during expiration, overt cardiac abnormalities are uncommon. Pulsus paradoxus is related to the increased pleural pressure swings during breathing.

Pulmonary gas exchange and oxygenation

The standard description of pulmonary gas exchange in asthma established 25 years ago has been little modified in recent years. There is grossly uneven ventilation between lung regions, which can be visualized on regional ventilation scans, but this is also found within small regions of lung. This leads to inequality of ventilation–perfusion ($\dot{V}/\dot{Q}$) ratios and reduction in Pa_{O_2}. Increase in total minute ventilation usually results in Pa_{CO_2} levels below normal until airway obstruction becomes very severe and attenuates, but does not eliminate, the fall in Pa_{O_2}. Small increases in inspired O_2 concentration restore Pa_{O_2} to normal values. These findings emphasize two aspects which have received recent detailed study—analysis of the precise $\dot{V}/\dot{Q}$ abnormality, using the multiple inert-gas elimination technique (MIGET), and the importance of the ventilatory (and possibly also the circulatory) response in maintaining oxygenation.

The MIGET technique has been used to study $\dot{V}/\dot{Q}$ abnormality over a wide range of severity of asthma (Fig. 37.5; Rodriguez-Roisin & Roca, 1994). In asymptomatic asthmatic subjects the distribution of $\dot{V}/\dot{Q}$ ratios is often as narrow as in normal subjects, although occasional patients show increased dispersion of ventilation or perfusion. No anatomical shunt ($\dot{V}/\dot{Q}$ ratio = 0) has been demonstrated. Subsequent studies have shown less abnormality in $\dot{V}/\dot{Q}$ dispersion in asymptomatic patients than found in the initial report (Wagner *et al.*, 1978).

In chronic, symptomatic asthma, the distribution of $\dot{V}/\dot{Q}$ ratios becomes broader, but without very low ratios or anatomical shunt, despite the expected presence of many severely obstructed airways (Corte & Young, 1985; Ballester *et al.*, 1990). These results suggest considerable compensatory reductions in perfusion to poorly ventilated areas, diminishing any fall in Pa_{O_2}; patients with similar airway obstruction due to COPD have more pronounced chronic hypoxaemia. In acute attacks requiring emergency admission, there is a much wider dispersion of $\dot{V}/\dot{Q}$ ratios, which is often bimodal with alveolar units with low $\dot{V}/\dot{Q}$ ratios (and so still ventilated), but again without significant increase in shunt (Rodriguez-Roisin *et al.*, 1989). In none of these studies was there an increase in alveolar units with continuing ventilation but completely without blood flow ($\dot{V}/\dot{Q} = \infty$). However, the increased dispersion of $\dot{V}/\dot{Q}$ ratios includes an increase in alveolar units with higher $\dot{V}/\dot{Q}$ ratios, so that physiological dead space is increased and the ventilatory efficiency for excreting CO_2 is decreased. Only in the most severe asthma, requiring mechanical ventilation, was there a significant anatomical shunt, averaging 8% of the cardiac output.

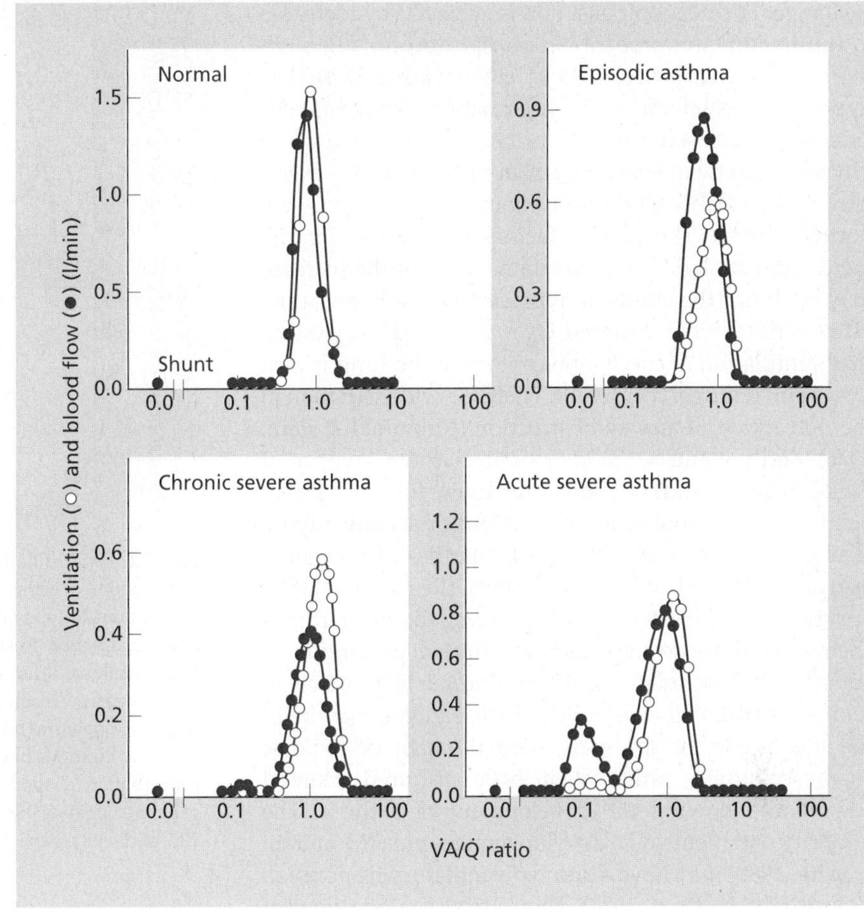

Fig. 37.5 Different patterns of $\dot{V}_A/\dot{Q}$ ratio distributions (ventilation (○) and blood flow (●) plotted against a $\dot{V}_A/\dot{Q}$ ratio on a log scale. Healthy young individuals have narrowly unimodal distributions centred around 1.0; in contrast, patients with episodic or chronic severe asthma have broader unimodal distributions and an increase in units with high $\dot{V}_A/\dot{Q}$ ratios; those with acute severe asthma in addition develop a bimodal pattern of blood-flow distribution. Shunt (left-hand ●) is absent. Note different scaling of axes. (From Rodriguez-Roisin & Roca, 1994, with permission.)

Pathological studies in fatal cases of asthma show multiple occlusions of airways by muco-inflammatory plugs, sometimes extending into major segmental or even lobar airways. Presumably main airways are occluded by plugs in less severe attacks, and yet obvious atelectasis on the chest radiograph is unusual. The most attractive explanation of the absence of shunt is that low $\dot{V}/\dot{Q}$ units receive some collateral ventilation, whose efficiency may depend on the accompanying hyperinflation. An important consequence is that small increases in inspired O_2 correct hypoxaemia.

These studies have provided other important information (Rodriguez-Roisin & Roca, 1994). Thus, in individual patients, there is a relatively poor correlation between abnormality of $\dot{V}/\dot{Q}$ ratios, $Pa{O_2}$ and FEV_1, and full recovery of normal pulmonary gas exchange may lag behind recovery of a normal FEV_1 after an acute attack of asthma. Secondly, except in the most severe asthma, abnormalities of $\dot{V}/\dot{Q}$ ratios could entirely account for the measured $Pa{O_2}$, so there was no evidence of any abnormality of diffusion. This is confirmed by the preservation of a normal or even increased value of single-breath CO transfer coefficient (Keens *et al.*, 1979). A possible explanation for increased values is that there is a more even distribution of blood flow to the lungs in asthma at rest. Measuring CO transfer is useful in the initial assessment of chronic, persistent asthma, because reduced values are found in many patients with smoking-related COPD. Thirdly, there appears to be an efficient compensatory reduction in blood flow to poorly ventilated areas. Breathing increased concentrations of inspired O_2 broadens the dispersion of blood flow, and breathing 100% O_2 may result in the development of atelectasis and anatomical shunt (Corte & Young, 1985; Rodriguez-Roisin *et al.*, 1989). These changes may follow removal of hypoxic pulmonary vasoconstriction in poorly ventilated areas. In clinical practice, of course, there is never any indication for giving high concentrations of inspired O_2. Bronchodilators, particularly when given intravenously, may also remove pulmonary vasoconstriction by a direct effect on pulmonary vascular smooth muscle and so increase abnormality of $\dot{V}/\dot{Q}$ ratios, and sometimes reduce $Pa{O_2}$ (Rodriguez-Roisin & Roca, 1994).

The efficiency of collateral ventilation and of pulmonary vasoconstriction considerably reduces the effects of the widespread airway narrowing on pulmonary gas exchange. Further compensation is achieved by increases in ventilation (and probably in cardiac output), although there are few measurements of either (Table 37.4). The hypocapnia usually found in severe asthma suggests considerably increased ventilation, because an increase in physiological dead space results in inefficient CO_2 excretion, and probably CO_2 output is increased above usual normal values. The precise factors responsible for the increased ventilation are uncertain. Some of the increase may be due to the effects of hypoxaemia, but hypocapnia often persists when inspired O_2 is increased, suggesting that stimulation of mechanoreceptors in the lung is also important (Hudgel *et al.*, 1979). There is a wide variation in the perception of airway obstruction (Rubinfeld & Pain, 1976), and patients who do not perceive the severity of the obstruction and/or show a relatively low increase in ventilation in response to obstruction (or accompanying changes in blood gases) are at particular risk of a repeated near-fatal or fatal attacks of asthma (Rea *et al.*, 1986). Survivors of near-fatal attacks have shown reduced chemosensitivity to hypoxia and blunted perception of added loads to breathing when studied later when in remission (Kikuchi *et al.*, 1994). Such patients may lie in the lower part of the wide normal range of hypoxic chemosensitivity, rather than have acquired blunted responses following the development of asthma. The minority of patients who develop hypercapnia (Mountain & Sahn, 1988) may have a blunted ventilatory response to CO_2 (Rebuck & Read, 1971). There are also suggestions of differences in personality and possibly even in the ability to achieve and sustain maximum voluntary activation of the respiratory muscles in such survivors.

Table 37.4 Factors minimizing fall in arterial $P\text{O}_2$ in severe asthma.

Collateral ventilation, preventing atelectasis and shunt
Local pulmonary vasoconstriction in poorly ventilated areas of lung
Increased ventilation, increasing alveolar $P\text{O}_2$
Increased circulation, increasing mixed venous $P\text{O}_2$

Table 37.5 Hyperinflation.

Advantages	Disadvantages
Widens airways, reducing resistive work and improving flow capacity	Increases elastic work of breathing
Improves collateral ventilation, preventing shunt and improving response to increase in inspired O_2 concentration	Shortens initial length of inspiratory muscles, decreasing their capacity to generate force

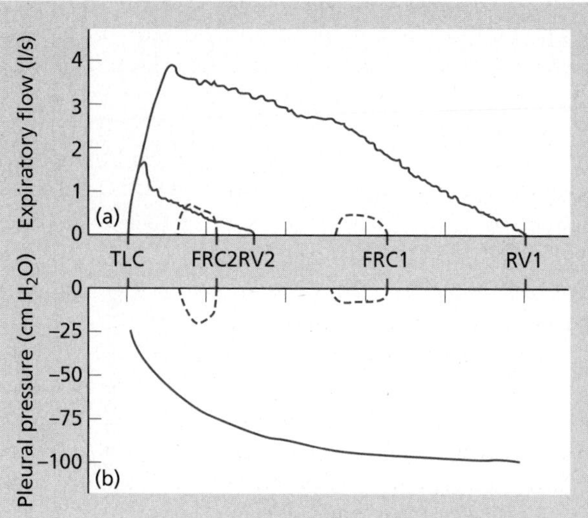

Fig. 37.6 Hyperinflation and expiratory flow limitation in exacerbation of asthma. (a) Tidal (dashed lines) and maximum (continuous lines) expiratory flow–volume curves during remission and exacerbation. Residual volume in exacerbation (RV_2) is larger than functional residual capacity (FRC_1) during remission. Tidal expiratory flow reaches maximum values during exacerbation. (b) Inspiratory pleural pressure during maximum inspiratory efforts (lower continuous line) and during tidal breathing in remission and exacerbation (dashed lines). The ability of inspiratory muscles to generate negative pleural pressures declines rapidly in the upper 20% of the vital capacity.

Hyperinflation and respiratory muscle function (Table 37.5)

End-tidal volume (FRC) consistently rises during an attack of asthma. In the normal subject, FRC is the volume at which the inward recoil of the lungs is equal to the opposing outward recoil of the chest cage; at this relaxation volume alveolar pressure equals atmospheric pressure. During a passive expiration, expiratory flow ceases at this volume. In an asthmatic attack, the end-expired volume is larger than the relaxed volume of the chest. Several different mechanisms contribute to this increase in end-expired volume. Firstly, there is usually a large increase in RV, presumably due to enhanced airway closure or near-closure; RV may sometimes be larger than the control FRC (Fig. 37.6). Additional dynamic mechanisms maintain end-expired volume above that dictated by airway closure. Thus, if there is expiratory flow limitation during tidal expiration, expiration may then be terminated by the initiation of the following inspiration rather than by the cessation of passive expiratory flow. But, even in the absence of expiratory flow limitation, a large end-expiratory volume may be maintained by persistent inspiratory muscle activity throughout expiration. At such an increased end-expired volume, the passive effect of respiratory system recoil generates an intrinsic positive end-expiratory pressure (intrinsic PEEP) in the alveoli, which has to be overcome before inspiratory air flow begins. Although hyperinflation is relatively well maintained when awake in the supine posture, this depends on appropriate respiratory muscle activity. Hyperinflation reduces during sleep and particularly during rapid-eye-movement sleep, and this must contribute to the worsening of pulmonary function that occurs at night (Ballard *et al.*, 1990). Probably much of the discomfort in severe asthmatic attacks arises from the stress on the inspiratory muscles, which may ultimately lead to fatigue. The inspiratory muscles have to generate larger pressures to overcome the airway narrowing, and total ventilation is increased. Breathing at large lung volume stresses the inspiratory muscles in three additional ways: firstly, by greatly increasing the work required to overcome elastic recoil of the lungs and chest wall; secondly, because hyperinflation shortens the initial length of the inspiratory muscles, reducing their capacity to reduce pleural pressure; and, thirdly, when dynamic hyperinflation is severe, by the need to overcome intrinsic PEEP before inspiratory flow commences.

As airway size enlarges with increase in lung volume, breathing at a larger lung volume partially overcomes the effects of airway narrowing and allows ventilation to be sustained or increased. A further favourable effect is probably improving collateral ventilation, avoiding atelectasis and further decrease in oxygenation. The physiological factors determining the extent of hyperinflation are not well understood. Recent studies with experimental bronchoconstriction suggest that the degree of hyperinflation may be adjusted to minimize the total work of breathing and to avoid expiratory flow limitation during tidal breathing. When moderate bronchoconstriction is induced by histamine, spontaneous hyperinflation reduces the total work of breathing, a slight increase in total inspiratory work (the increase in elastic work outweighing the decrease in resistive work) above that at the original FRC being offset by a larger reduction in expiratory flow-resistive work (Wheatley *et al.*, 1990). However, with severe spontaneous asthma, hyperinflation is less likely to reduce airway resistance sufficiently to prevent a considerable increase in total inspiratory work and to avoid expiratory flow limitation during tidal breathing.

Twenty or more years ago, many measurements were made of FRC and TLC during crises of asthma, and it was suggested that improvement in symptoms could be due to a fall in FRC without accompanying improvement in spirometry or PEF and that TLC could acutely increase in a crisis (Woolcock & Read, 1966; Woolcock *et al.*, 1971). Usually, however, with bronchodilators or spontaneous improvement, there is both improvement in spirometry and a fall in FRC. Most recent studies, using body plethysmography, have failed to show an increase in TLC when airway narrowing is induced in asthma (Kirby *et al.*, 1986); older results probably overestimated TLC in the presence of airway obstruction, due to lack of equilibration of mouth with alveolar pressure during panting (Stanescu *et al.*, 1982). A simple means of measuring hyperinflation would greatly amplify the assessment of lung mechanics during the asthmatic crisis.

Most studies suggest that respiratory muscle strength is normal in younger asthmatic subjects during remission. However, skeletal muscle strength is known to decline with age and is less in women than men at all ages; other important factors influencing respiratory muscle performance are the degree of hyperinflation and any weakness induced by corticosteroid treatment or loss of muscle bulk. Gross inspiratory muscle weakness has been demonstrated in a few obese women with asthma who had been on chronic high doses of oral corticosteroids (Melzer & Souhrada, 1980). Smaller doses have not been shown to have a definite effect. A careful study comparing 34 middle-aged patients with asthma who were taking an average prednisolone dose of 12 mg a day and 34 matched control patients who had never been on continuous steroid treatment found no differences in respiratory and shoulder muscle strength, which appeared normal in both groups of patients (Picado *et al.*, 1990). A recent study of patients with chronic airway obstruction, studied on the 10th day after hospital admission while on treatment with corticosteroids, found that mean oral corticosteroid dosage during the preceding 6 months was inversely related to maximum inspiratory pressure and, more strongly, to quadriceps force (Decramer *et al.*, 1994). However, most of these patients received methylprednisolone or triamcinolone, which are believed to have greater deleterious effects on muscle bulk and strength than the prednisolone generally used for booster courses in the UK, and further studies of larger numbers of patients suggest that the effect is not found in chronic asthma but is confined to patients with COPD. Acute loss of skeletal muscle mass can be important after prolonged episodes of acute severe asthma which require large doses of corticosteroids (Williams *et al.*, 1988) and may grossly restrict physical activity, but is not obvious in the chronic stable state, in contrast to patients with severe emphysema.

Overall, most studies that have taken account of the hyperinflation of the chest wall have concluded that the strength of both inspiratory and expiratory muscles is well preserved. Indeed, it has been suggested that endurance of the respiratory muscles is better in asthmatic than in control subjects (McKenzie & Gandevia, 1986; Gorman *et al.*, 1992). A weakness of existing studies is that almost all the patients were young adults, with only modest hyperinflation and airway obstruction. Eventually, in the most severe attacks the load is so great that fatigue must occur, even in fit young subjects; elderly, female and obese subjects are likely to be at greater risk. Unfortunately, no techniques have yet been developed for simply detecting muscle fatigue in the presence of severe airway obstruction, and the need for pressure support or positive-pressure ventilation still has to be determined on clinical assessment.

References

Antic, R. & Macklem, P.T. (1976) The influence of clinical factors on site of airway obstruction in asthma. *Am. Rev. Resp. Dis.*, **114**, 851–9.

Ballard, R.D., Irvin, C.G., Martin, R.J., Pak, J., Pandey, R. & White, D.P. (1990) Influence of sleep on lung volume in asthmatic patients and normal subjects. *J. Appl. Physiol.*, **68**, 2034–41.

Ballester, E., Roca, J., Ramis, L.I., Wagner, P.D., Rodriguez-Roisin, R. (1990) Pulmonary gas exchange in chronic asthma. Response to 100% oxygen and salbutamol. *Am. Rev. Resp. Dis.*, **141**, 558–62.

Bel, E.H., Timmers, M.C., Zwinderman, A.H., Dijkman, J.H. & Sterk, P.J. (1991) The effect of inhaled corticosteroids on the maximal degree of airway narrowing to methacholine in asthmatic subjects. *Am. Rev. Resp. Dis.*, **143**, 109–13.

Berry, R.B. & Fairshter, R.D. (1985) Partial and maximal flow–volume curves in normal and asthmatic subjects before and after inhalation of metaproterenol. *Chest*, **88**, 697–702.

Bouhuys, A., Hunt, V.R., Kim, B.M. & Zapletal, A. (1969) Maximum expiratory flow rates in induced bronchoconstriction in man. *J. Clin. Invest.*, **48**, 1159–68.

Brown, P.J. Greville, H.W. & Finucane, K.E. (1984) Asthma and irreversible airflow obstruction. *Thorax*, **39**, 131–6.

Bucca, C., Rolla, G., Brussino, L., De Rose, V. & Bugiani, M. (1995) Are asthma-like symptoms due to bronchial or extrathoracic airway dysfunction? *Lancet*, **346**, 791–5.

Butler, J., Caro, C.G., Alcala, R. & DuBois, A.B. (1960) Physiological factors affecting airway resistance in normal subjects and in patients with obstructive respiratory disease. *J. Clin. Invest.*, **39**, 584–91.

Colebatch, H.J.H., Finucane, K.E. & Smith, M.M. (1973) Pulmonary conductance and elastic recoil relationship in asthma and emphysema. *J. Appl. Physiol.*, **34**, 143–53.

Collett, P.W., Brancatisano, T. & Engel, L.A. (1983) Changes in the glottic aperture during bronchial asthma. *Am. Rev. Resp. Dis.*, **128**, 719–23.

Collett, P.W., Brancatisano, A.P. & Engel, L.A. (1986) Upper airway dimensions and movements in bronchial asthma. *Am. Rev. Resp. Dis.*, **133**, 1143–9.

Corte, P. & Young, I.H. (1985) Ventilation–perfusion relationships in symptomatic asthma: response to oxygen and clemastine. *Chest*, **88**, 167–75.

Decramer, M., Lacquet, L.M., Fagard, R. & Rogiers, P. (1994) Corticosteroids contribute to muscle weakness in chronic airflow obstruction. *Am. J. Resp. Crit. Care Med.*, **150**, 11–16.

Despas, P.J., Leroux, M. & Macklem, P.T. (1972) Site of airway obstruction in asthma as determined by measuring maximal expiratory flow breathing air and helium–oxygen mixture. *J. Clin. Invest.*, **51**, 3235–43.

Ding, D.J., Martin, J.G. & Macklem, P.T. (1987) The effects of lung volume on maximal methacholine-induced bronchoconstriction in normal humans. *J. Appl. Physiol*, **62**, 1324–30.

Eiser, N. (1991) The effect of a β_2-adrenergic agonist and a histamine H_1-receptor antagonist on the late asthmatic response to inhaled antigen. *Resp. Med.*, **85**, 393–9.

Fairshter, R.D. & Wilson, A.F. (1980) Relationship between the site of airflow limitation and localization of the bronchodilator response in asthma. *Am. Rev. Resp. Dis.*, **122**, 27–32.

Freedman, S. (1992) Exercise as a bronchodilator. *Clin. Sci.*, **83**, 383–9.

Gorman, R.B., McKenzie, D.K., Gandevia, S.C. & Plassman, B.L. (1992) Inspiratory muscle strength and endurance during hyperinflation and histamine induced bronchoconstriction. *Thorax*, **47**, 922–7.

Hedstrand, U. (1971) Ventilation, gas exchange, mechanisms of breathing and respiratory work in acute bronchial asthma. *Acta Soc. Med. Ups.*, **76**, 248–70.

Hudgel, D.W., Capehart, M. & Hirsch, J.E. (1979) Ventilation response and drive during hypoxia in adult patients with asthma. *Chest*, **76**, 294–9.

Ingram, R.H. Jr (1987) Site and mechanism of obstruction and hyperresponsiveness in asthma. *Am. Rev. Resp. Dis.*, **136**, S62–4.

Ingram, R.H. Jr (1990) Physiological assessment of inflammation in the peripheral lung of asthmatic patients. *Lung*, **168**, 237–48.

Ingram, R.H. Jr & McFadden, E.R. Jr (1977) Localization and mechanisms of airway responses. *New Engl. J. Med.*, **297**, 596–600.

Jadue, C., Greville, H., Coalson, J.J. & Mink, S.N. (1985) Forced expiration and HeO_2 response in canine peripheral airway obstruction. *J. Appl. Physiol.*, **58**, 1788–801.

James, A.L., Paré, P.D., Moreno, R.H. & Hogg, J.C. (1987) Quantitative measurement of smooth muscle shortening in isolated pig trachea. *J. Appl. Physiol.*, **63**, 1360–5.

James, A.L., Paré, P.D. & Hogg, J.C. (1989) The mechanics of airway narrowing in asthma. *Am. Rev. Resp. Dis.*, **139**, 242–6.

Kariya, S.T., Thompson, L.M., Ingenito, E.P. & Ingram, R.H. (1989) Effects of lung volume, volume history, and methacholine on lung tissue viscance. *J. Appl. Physiol.*, **66**, 977–82.

Keens, T.G., Mansell, A., Krastins, I.R.B. *et al.* (1979) Evaluation of the single-breath diffusing capacity in asthma and cystic fibrosis. *Chest*, **76**, 41–4.

Kharitonov, S.A., Yates, D., Robbins, R.A., Logan-Sinclair, R., Shinebourne, E.A. & Barnes, P.J. (1994) Increased nitric oxide in exhaled air of asthmatic patients. *Lancet*, **343**, 133–5.

Kikuchi, Y., Okabe, S., Tamura, G. *et al.* (1994) Chemosensitivity and perception of dyspnea in patients with a history of near-fatal asthma. *New Engl. J. Med.*, **330**, 1329–34.

Kirby, J.G., Juniper, E.F., Hargreave, F.E. & Zamel, N. (1986) Total lung capacity does not change during methacholine-stimulated airway narrowing. *J. Appl. Physiol.*, **61**, 2144–7.

Lim, T.K., Pride, N.B. & Ingram, R.H. Jr (1987) Effects of volume history during spontaneous and acutely induced air-flow obstruction in asthma. *Am. Rev. Resp. Dis.*, **135**, 591–6.

Lisboa, C., Jardim, J., Angus, E. & Macklem, P.T. (1980) Is extrathoracic airway obstruction important in asthma? *Am. Rev. Resp. Dis.*, **122**, 115–21.

Louis, B., Glass, G.M. & Fredberg, J.J. (1994) Pulmonary airway area by the two-microphone acoustic reflection method. *J. Appl. Physiol.*, **76**, 2234–40.

Ludwig, M.S., Romero, P.V. & Bates, J.H.T. (1989) A comparison of the dose–response behaviour of canine airways and parenchyma. *J. Appl. Physiol.*, **67**, 1220–5.

McFadden, E.R. Jr & Lyons, H.A. (1968) Arterial blood gas tension in asthma. *New Engl. J. Med.*, **278**, 1027–32.

McKenzie, D.K. & Gandevia, S.C. (1986) Strength and endurance of inspiratory, expiratory and limb muscles in asthma. *Am. Rev. Resp. Dis.*, **134**, 999–1004.

Macklem, P.T. (1985) Bronchial hyporesponsiveness. *Chest*, **87**, 158S–159S.

Mead, J., Takishima, T. & Leith, D. (1970) Stress distribution in lungs: a model of pulmonary elasticity. *J. Appl. Physiol.*, **28**, 596–608.

Melzer, E. & Souhrada, J.F. (1980) Decrease of respiratory muscle strength and static lung volumes in obese asthmatics. *Am. Rev. Resp. Dis.*, **121**, 17–22.

Miller, R.D. & Hyatt, R.E. (1973) Evaluation of obstructive lesions of the trachea and larynx by flow–volume loops. *Am. Rev. Resp. Dis.*, **108**, 475–81.

Molfino, N.A., Slutsky, A.S., Hoffstein, V. *et al.* (1992) Changes in cross-sectional airway areas induced by methacholine, histamine and LTC_4 in asthmatic subjects. *Am. Rev. Resp. Dis.*, **146**, 577–80.

Moreno, R.H., Hogg, J.C. & Paré, P.D. (1986) Mechanics of airway narrowing. *Am. Rev. Resp. Dis.*, **133**, 1171–80.

Mountain, R.D. & Sahn, S.A. (1988) Clinical features and outcome in patients with acute asthma presenting with hypercapnia. *Am. Rev. Resp. Dis.*, **138**, 535–9.

Murtagh, P.S., Proctor, D.F., Permutt, S., Kelly, B. & Evering, S. (1971) Bronchial closure with mecholyl in excised dog lobes. *J. Appl. Physiol.*, **31**, 409–15.

Olsen, C.R., Stevens, A.E., Pride, N.B. & Staub, N.C. (1967) Structural basis for decreased compressibility of constricted trachea and bronchi. *J. Appl. Physiol.*, **23**, 35–9.

Partridge, M.R. & Saunders, K.B. (1981) The site of airflow limitation in asthma: the effect of time, acute exacerbations of disease and clinical features. *Brit. J. Dis. Chest*, **75**, 263–72.

Pellegrino, R., Violante, B., Crimi, E. & Brusasco, V. (1990) Effects of deep inhalation during early and late asthmatic reactions to allergen. *Am. Rev. Resp. Dis.*, **143**, 822–5.

Pellegrino, R., Violante, B., Crimi, E. & Brusasco, V. (1993) Effects of aerosol methacholine and histamine on airways and lung parenchyma in healthy humans. *J. Appl. Physiol.*, **74**, 2681–6.

Picado, C., Fiz, J.A., Montserrat, J.M. *et al.* (1990) Respiratory and skeletal muscle function in steroid-dependent bronchial asthma. *Am. Rev. Resp. Dis.*, **141**, 14–21.

Pliss, I.B., Ingenito, E.P. & Ingram, R.H. Jr (1989) Responsiveness, inflammation, and effects of deep breaths on obstruction in mild asthma. *J. Appl. Physiol.*, **66**, 2298–304.

Pride, N.B. & Macklem, P.T. (1986) Lung mechanics in disease. In: *Handbook of Physiology: Respiratory System*, Vol. III. *Mechanics of Breathing* (ed. P. Macklem & J. Mead), pp. 678–9. American Physiological Society, Bethesda, MD.

Rea, H.H., Scragg, R., Jackson, R., Beaglehole, R., Fenwick, J. & Sutherland, D.C. (1986) A case–control study of deaths from asthma. *Thorax*, **41**, 833–9.

Rebuck, A.S. & Read, J. (1971) Patterns of ventilatory response to carbon dioxide during recovery from severe asthma. *Clin. Sci.*, **41**, 13–21.

Roche, W.R., Beasley, R., Williams, J.H. & Holgate, S.T. (1989) Subepithelial fibrosis in the bronchi of asthmatics. *Lancet*, **i**, 520–4.

Rodriguez-Roisin, R., Ballester, E., Roca, J., Torres, A. & Wager, P.D. (1989) Mechanisms of hypoxemia in patients with status asthmaticus requiring mechanical ventilation. *Am. Rev. Resp. Dis.*, **139**, 732–9.

Rodriguez-Roisin, R. & Roca, J. (1994) Bronchial asthma. *Thorax*, **49**, 1027–33.

Rubinfeld, A.R. & Pain, M.C.F. (1976) Perception of asthma. *Lancet*, **i**, 882–4.

Simonsson, B.G., Jacobs, F.M. & Nadel, J.A. (1967) Role of autonomic nervous system and the cough reflex in the increased responsiveness of airways in patients with obstructive airway disease. *J. Clin. Invest.*, **46**, 1812–18.

Skloot, G., Permutt, S. & Togias, A. (1995) Airway hyperresponsiveness in asthma: a problem of limited smooth muscle relaxation with inspiration. *J. Clin. Invest.*, **96**, 2393–403.

Stanescu, D.C., Rodenstein, D., Cauberghs, M. & Van de Woestijne, K.P. (1982) Failure of body plethysmography in bronchial asthma. *J. Appl. Physiol. Resp. Environ. Exercise Physiol.*, **52**, 939–48.

Sterk, P.J., Daniel, E.E., Zamel, N. & Hargreave, F.E. (1985) Limited bronchoconstriction to methacholine using partial flow–volume curves in non-asthmatic subjects. *Am. Rev. Resp. Dis.*, **132**, 272–7.

Twentyman, O.P., Finnerty, J.P., Harris, A., Palmer, J. & Holgate, S.T. (1990) Protection against allergen-induced asthma by salmeterol. *Lancet*, **336**, 1338–42.

Wagner, E.M., Liu, M.C., Weinmann, G.G., Permutt, S. & Bleecker, E.R. (1990) Peripheral lung resistance in normal and asthmatic subjects. *Am. Rev. Resp. Dis.*, **141**, 584–8.

Wagner, P.D., Dantzker, D.R., Iacovoni, V.E., Tomlin, W.C. & West, J.B. (1978) Ventilation–perfusion inequality in asymptomatic asthma. *Am. Rev. Resp. Dis.*, **118**, 511–24.

Wang, Y.T., Coe, C.I. & Pride, N.B. (1990) The effect of reducing airway dimensions by altering posture on histamine responsiveness. *Thorax*, **45**, 530–5.

Wheatley, J.R., West, S., Cala, S.J. & Engel, L.A. (1990) The effect of hyperinflation on respiratory muscle work in acute induced asthma. *Eur. Resp. J.*, **3**, 625–32.

Williams, T.J., O'Hehir, R.E., Czarny, D., Horne, M. & Bowes, G. (1988) Acute myopathy in severe acute asthma treated with intravenously administered corticosteroids. *Am. Rev. Resp. Dis.*, **137**, 460–3.

Wilson, J.W., Li, X. & Pain, M.C.F. (1993) The lack of distensibility of asthmatic airways. *Am. Rev. Resp. Dis.*, **148**, 806–9.

Woolcock, A.J. & Read, J. (1966) Lung volumes in exacerbations of asthma. *Am. J. Med.*, **41**, 259–73.

Woolcock, A.J., Rebuck, A.S., Cade, J.F. & Read, J. (1971) Lung volume changes in asthma measured concurrently by two methods. *Am. Rev. Resp. Dis.*, **104**, 703–9.

Woolcock, A.J., Salome, C.M. & Yan, K. (1984) The shape of the dose–response curve to histamine in asthmatic and normal subjects. *Am. Rev. Resp. Dis.*, **130**, 71–5.

Yanai, M., Ohrui, T., Sekizawa, K., Shimizu, Y., Sasaki, H. & Takishima, T. (1991) Effective site of bronchodilation by antiasthma drugs in subjects with asthma. *J. Allergy Clin. Immunol.*, **87**, 1080–7.

Yanai, M., Sekizawa, K., Ohrui, T., Sasaki, H. & Takishima, T. (1992) Site of airway obstruction in pulmonary disease: direct measurement of intrabronchial pressure. *J. Appl. Physiol.*, **72**, 1016–23.

Yap, J.C.H. & Pride, N.B. (1994) Effect of induced bronchoconstriction on nasal airflow resistance in patients with asthma. *Clin. Sci.*, **86**, 55–8.

CHAPTER 38

Bronchial Hyperresponsiveness

R. Pauwels

Introduction

Bronchial hyperresponsiveness (BHR) is an important physiopathological characteristic of bronchial asthma that can explain many of the clinical features of this airway disease. The development of methods to demonstrate and quantify BHR has greatly contributed to the understanding of the pathogenesis of asthma and its diagnosis and treatment. Studies on BHR have also highlighted the complexity of the mechanisms involved in the increased airway responses in asthma. BHR is also observed in diseases other than asthma and in some apparently healthy subjects.

The aim of this chapter is to review the pathogenesis and pathophysiology of BHR in asthma and the effect of therapeutic interventions on BHR.

Historical background

The first recognition that patients with asthma have hyperresponsive airways to certain bronchoconstrictory substances dates back to the observation by Alexander and Paddock (1921) that asthmatic subjects developed asthma-like symptoms following the subcutaneous injection of pilocarpine, while healthy subjects did not. Weiss *et al.* (1932) showed that asthmatic subjects developed bronchoconstriction following the intravenous administration of histamine. Curry and Lowell (1948) quantified the response to histamine by measuring lung function and demonstrated that the most responsive subjects had the most severe asthma. Curry (1947) also administered histamine by inhalation and observed an increased bronchial response in asthmatics. The concept of a dose–response curve and defining the bronchial responsiveness as a dose that causes a predetermined change in airway calibre (*dose liminaire* or threshold dose) was developed by Tiffeneau (1957). Chai *et al.* (1975) recommended that bronchial responsiveness to agonists should be defined by the use of *in vivo* cumulative dose–response curves. The clinical significance of BHR was further explored and methods were refined both for clinical and epidemiological investigations (de Vries *et al.*, 1968; Hargreave *et al.*, 1981; Woolcock *et al.*, 1984). The number of stimuli that were demonstrated to cause an increased bronchial response in asthma compared with healthy subjects gradually enlarged, as well as the understanding that the mechanisms involved in BHR to these different stimuli were multiple and complex (Pauwels *et al.*, 1988) (Fig. 38.1).

Definition

The increased understanding of the complexity of the enhanced bronchial response to different agonists and of the measured parameters of airway function has made a simple definition of BHR rather difficult. Bronchial or airway hyperresponsiveness is an abnormal increase in air-flow limitation following the exposure to a stimulus. In this definition the word 'abnormal' refers to a comparison with the airway response to the same agonist, using the same method to measure the air-flow limitation, in a group of healthy subjects. The wording 'air-flow limitation' is chosen because it encompasses the different mechanisms that can lead to a decrease in the parameters of air flow that are used in studies on BHR, such as the forced expiratory volume in 1 second (FEV_1) or the airway resistance (R_{aw}). A decrease in FEV_1 or R_{aw} following exposure

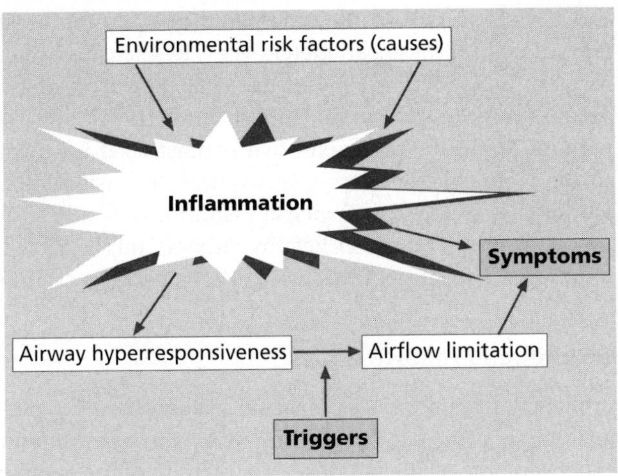

Fig. 38.1 Mechanisms underlying asthma symptoms.

to a stimulus can reflect constriction of airway smooth muscle, oedema of the airway wall, increased amounts of fluid or sputum in the airway wall or a decrease in the elastic recoil pressure on the airways.

Methods for measuring bronchial responsiveness

The optimal way to measure bronchial responsiveness to one or another agonist is to perform a dose–response curve to the selected agonist and to quantify the response. It has become clear that several agonists can be used to study bronchial responsiveness and that the mechanisms involved in the bronchial response differ from agonist to agonist. Measuring bronchial responsiveness with one agonist therefore gives different information from the measurement of bronchial responsiveness with another agonist. The term non-specific BHR has been introduced to differentiate the bronchial response to agonists such as histamine, methacholine, etc. from the bronchial response to an allergen. However, it is now evident that the term 'non-specific' is a misnomer, since the mechanisms involved in the bronchial response to these agonists are indeed very specific for each agonist. The term 'non-allergenic bronchial responsiveness' seems therefore more appropriate if there is a need for a general term that covers all the different ways of measuring bronchial responsiveness.

In order to highlight the heterogeneity of the airway response to the different stimuli and to better understand the effect of treatment on BHR, the stimuli have been divided into direct and indirect stimuli (Pauwels *et al.*, 1988). Direct stimuli cause air-flow limitation by a direct action on the effector cells involved in the air-flow limitation, such as airway smooth-muscle (ASM) cells, bronchial vascular endothelial cells and mucus-producing cells. Indirect stimuli cause air-flow limitation by an action on cells other than the effector cells (Fig. 38.2). These other cells then interact with the above-mentioned effector cells. Examples of cells that act as an intermediary between the indirect stimuli and the effector cells are inflammatory cells, such as mast cells and neuronal cells. Table 38.1 lists a number of stimuli that have been used to demonstrate BHR in asthma. The stimuli have been classified according to the dominant mechanism of air-flow limitation in response to the stimulus. Indeed, some stimuli have both direct and indirect activity. An appropriate way to see if a stimulus acts indirectly is to investigate the effects of drugs that are neither a specific antagonist of the stimulus nor a functional antagonist of the airway response to the stimulus, e.g. the effect of an anticholinergic drug on the airway response to metabisulphite or the effect of cromoglycate or nedocromil on the same stimulus.

The fact that a mediator antagonist blocks a large part of the airway response to an indirect stimulus has sometimes been interpreted as proof of the dominant role of that mediator in the airway response. However, this inter-

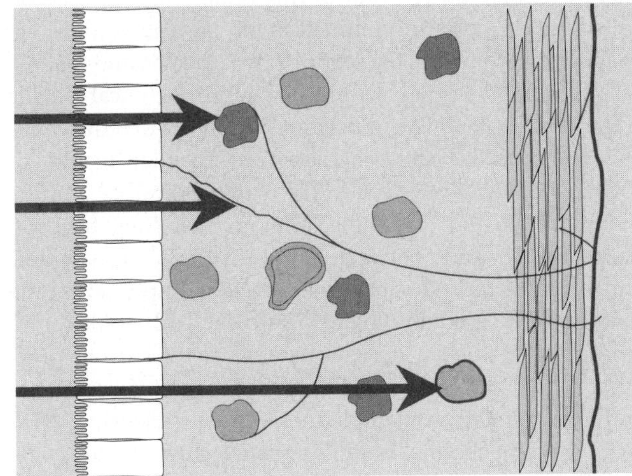

Fig. 38.2 Indirect bronchial responsiveness.

Table 38.1 Stimuli for measuring bronchial responsiveness.

Direct	Indirect
Histamine	Adenosine
Methacholine	Bradykinin
Carbachol	SO_2/Metabisulphite
Acetylcholine	Exercise
KCl	Hypertonic/hypotonic solutions
PGD_2	Cold/dry air
$PGF_{2\alpha}$	Propranolol
LTC_4, LTD_4, LTE_4	Neurokinin A
	Substance P

PG, prostaglandin; LT, leukotriene.

pretation does not take into consideration the possible synergism between different mediators. If there is indeed a significant synergism between two mediators involved in an airway response, then inhibition of either one of the two mediators will greatly reduce the airway response.

Methods of delivering the stimulus

Various routes of delivery of stimuli have been used to demonstrate BHR in patients with asthma, including intravenous, subcutaneous and oral administration, but most stimuli used in studies on BHR have been given via inhalation for reasons of safety and specificity. The essential characteristics of a good method of delivery are a reproducible and preferably quantifiable delivery of the stimulus into the airways. The site of deposition in the airways is another important issue when studying the airway response to a stimulus. Many stimuli used to measure BHR are soluble and can therefore be administered with nebulizers. Standardization of the droplet size and the flow characteristics and output of the nebulizers are all relevant to this issue, but a discussion of these important parameters of administration via nebulizers is outside the scope of this chapter, and readers are referred to other sources for more technical details (Sterk *et al.*, 1993). The important message is that the nebulizer should be well characterized so that results of bronchial challenges with the same stimulus can be compared within the same laboratory or lung function department and between investigations. This inter-investigator reproducibility is especially important in the settings of epidemiological studies and multicentre therapeutic studies. A rigorous analysis of current practice shows that reproducibility between different laboratories of relatively simple methods of measuring BHR, e.g. to methacholine, is still not satisfactory (Bailey *et al.*, 1994).

Much more difficult to standardize are challenges with stimuli that cannot be brought into a solution, such as fog, cold air and exercise. However, serious efforts have also been made here to increase inter-laboratory reproducibility.

Methods for measuring the airway response

Many different methods have been used to measure the airway response in studies on BHR. These include FEV_1, R_{aw}, specific R_{aw}, specific conductance of the airways (sG_{aw}), peak expiratory flow rate (PEFR) and flow rates at different levels of the maximal or partial expiratory flow–volume curve. The choice of which parameter to use is almost always a trade-off between the reproducibility and the sensitivity of the parameter. FEV_1 is the most reproducible of these parameters but is less sensitive than sG_{aw} or V_P30 (flow at 30% of the vital capacity using a partial flow–volume curve) (Enright *et al.*, 1994). FEV_1 is without doubt the parameter that is most used for measuring bronchial hyperresponsiveness in asthmatics. Studies using weak or expensive stimuli or studies on airway responsiveness in healthy subjects might choose more sensitive parameters, such as V_P30 or sG_{aw}.

Quantification of BHR

Bronchial responsiveness is usually quantified by performing a dose–response study with the agonist and expressing the result as a dose or a quantity of the agonist that causes a predetermined change in the measured airway parameter. The most frequently used measures are the PC_{20}-FEV_1 or the PD_{20}-FEV_1, respectively the concentration and the dose of the agonist that cause a fall in FEV_1 or 20% from baseline. To determine the PC_{20} or PD_{20}, the dose–response curve is plotted on a semilogarithmic scale and the PC_{20} or PD_{20} is calculated by interpolation. Similar procedures can be used for other parameters, such as the PC_{35}- or PD_{35}-sG_{aw} (concentration or dose that decreases the sG_{aw} by 35% from baseline) or the PC_{100}- or PD_{100}-R_{aw} (concentration or dose that doubles the airway resistance).

This method of quantifying the airway responsiveness is only applicable for agonists where a proper dose–response curve can be performed. With agonists such as exercise, a dose–response curve is not possible due to the tachyphylaxis that occurs after the challenge. The responsiveness will then be expressed as the percentage change of the measured airway parameter following a standardized challenge.

A dose–response curve to histamine or methacholine is characterized by its slope and by the maximal bronchoconstriction that can be reached. Normal individuals have a limited bronchoconstriction even if the amount of histamine or methacholine that is administered is further increased (Sterk *et al.*, 1985). This plateau level is not observed in moderate to severe asthmatics.

Mechanisms involved in BHR and relationship to symptoms in asthma

The phenomenon of BHR can only be understood if the mechanisms involved in the airway response to different agonists and the mechanisms of air-flow limitation caused by these stimuli are known. Differences in these mechanisms may be the cause of BHR in asthma and other diseases.

Mechanisms involved in airway response to different stimuli

Direct stimuli

Histamine

Histamine causes bronchoconstriction by binding to H_1 receptors on ASM cells (Levy & Seabury, 1947; Nogrady & Bevan, 1978; White *et al.*, 1987). The possibility cannot be excluded that part of the air-flow limitation caused by inhalation of histamine may be caused by vasodilatation of the bronchial vessels and that H_2 receptors may be involved, but studies on the effect of H_2 antagonists on the bronchial response to histamine have not been conclusive (Nathan *et al.*, 1979; Thomson & Kerr, 1980; Eiser *et al.*, 1981; Schacter *et al.*, 1982).

Cholinergic agonists

Acetylcholine and the synthetic cholinergic agonists carbachol and methacholine have all been used for the assessment of bronchial responsiveness. Methacholine is currently preferred because of its higher solubility and duration of action. Cholinergic agonists cause bronchoconstriction by directly acting on the ASM cell via the M_3 muscarinic receptor (Roffel *et al.*, 1990).

Leukotrienes

The inhalation of leukotriene C_4 (LTC_4), LTD_4 or LTE_4 causes airway narrowing via interaction with a specific leukotriene receptor, now called $cysLT_1$ (LTD_4) receptor (Drazen, 1986). Patients with asthma have a relatively increased bronchial responsiveness to LTE_4 compared with their responsiveness to LTC_4 and LTD_4, and this has been used as evidence to suggest that patients with asthma might have a specific LTE_4 receptor on their ASM (Arm *et al.*, 1990). Final evidence for this mechanism of enhanced airway responsiveness to LTE_4 in asthma has not yet been provided.

Indirect stimuli

Exercise

Exercise of sufficient intensity and duration causes airway narrowing in subjects with asthma (Jones *et al.*, 1963; Anderson *et al.*, 1975). The airway narrowing following exercise can be completely prevented when warm, fully saturated air is inhaled during the exercise. The mechanisms of exercise-induced airway narrowing are therefore triggered by water loss, and maybe also some heat loss at the level of the airway mucosa (Deal *et al.*, 1979; Anderson, 1984, 1985; Anderson *et al.*, 1985; McFadden *et al.*, 1986; McFadden, 1987). There is still a debate about the precise contribution of different mechanisms but the most plausible explanation is that the water loss causes hyperosmolarity at the level of the airway mucosa and thereby activates the inflammatory cells that are present, resulting in the release of histamine, leukotrienes, etc. (Wiebicke *et al.*, 1988; Manning *et al.*, 1990). These mediators then cause ASM constriction. The relative contribution of vasodilatation, extravasation and oedema formation to the airway narrowing is not known (McFadden, 1990).

Hypo- and hypertonic aerosols

Hypo- and hypertonic solutions cause airway narrowing in asthma (de Vries *et al.*, 1968; Anderson *et al.*, 1983). Both the tonicity and the duration of exposure are important factors for the airway response. The mechanism involved is very similar to that of exercise-induced asthma and is related to changes in the osmolarity of the airway mucosa, leading to activation of inflammatory cells and the release of bronchoconstrictory mediators (Finney *et al.*, 1990).

Cold- and dry-air hyperventilation

Hyperventilation can induce asthma (Herxheimer, 1946). The studies on the mechanisms involved in exercise-induced asthma have led to a standardization of the challenge with cold- and dry-air hyperventilation. The mechanisms involved are very similar to those involved in exercise- and hypo- and hypertonic solution-induced airway narrowing, i.e. change in the osmolarity and temperature of the airway mucosa, resulting in activation of inflammatory cells in the airway mucosa, release of bronchoconstrictory and vasoactive mediators and ASM constriction (O'Byrne *et al.*, 1982; Fischer *et al.*, 1995). The role of an activation of sensory nerve endings with the release of neuropeptides in these challenges cannot be studied, due to the lack of active neuropeptide antagonists that can be used in humans.

Adenosine

Adenosine and the more soluble adenosine monophosphate (AMP) have been used to measure bronchial responsiveness (Cushley *et al.*, 1983). AMP causes bronchoconstriction by direct action on ASM but mainly by the activation of airway mast cells and the release of bronchoconstrictor vasoactive mediators from these cells (Phillips *et al.*, 1989; Polosa *et al.*, 1989, 1991). Histamine and leukotrienes are released upon inhalation of AMP.

Tachykinins

The inhalation of substance P and neurokinin A causes airway narrowing (Joos *et al.*, 1987; Crimi *et al.*, 1990). The mechanisms involved in the human airway response to these tachykinins are not fully elucidated but probably involve both direct activation of ASM and the activation of mast cells (Joos *et al.*, 1994). Nedocromil sodium significantly inhibits the airway response to tachykinins (Joos *et al.*, 1989). The role of the activation of the vagal nerve by these tachykinins is also not clear (Joos *et al.*, 1988).

Sulphur dioxide/metabisulphite

The inhalation of sulphur dioxide or metabisulphite causes bronchoconstriction in asthmatic patients (Nichol *et al.*, 1989). The reaction is not inhibited by H_1 antagonists, suggesting that mast cell activation plays no significant role in this bronchial reaction (Dixon & Ind, 1988). Anticholinergic agents, sodium cromoglycate and nedocromil sodium clearly inhibit the bronchial response to sulphur dioxide or metabisulphite, supporting the hypothesis that the activation of vagal and possibly other neurones plays an essential role (Altounyan *et al.*, 1985; Wright *et al.*, 1990).

Propranolol

The inhalation of propranolol causes bronchoconstriction in patients with asthma, not via the anticipated blocking of the bronchodilating effect of the circulating catecholamines but via the activation of the vagal nerve (de Vries *et al.*, 1968; Ind *et al.*, 1985, 1989).

Bradykinin

The bronchial response to inhaled bradykinin is partially inhibited by an anticholinergic agent and by a rather weak neurokinin antagonist (Fuller *et al.*, 1987; Ichinose *et al.*, 1992). A selective H_1 antagonist or a potent inhibitor of cyclo-oxygenase had no influence on the reaction (Polosa *et al.*, 1990; Rajakulasingam *et al.*, 1993). Both sodium cromoglycate and nedocromil significantly inhibit the bradykinin-induced bronchoconstriction (Dixon & Barnes, 1989). Taken together, these data suggest that bradykinin causes airway narrowing via interaction with the autonomous nervous system in the airways.

Airway inflammation, BHR and symptoms

BHR in asthma is caused by the interaction between the baseline bronchial responsiveness and the airway changes due to the inflammatory process in asthma. There are a number of arguments that suggest that the baseline bronchial responsiveness might differ from individual to individual and that genetic factors might control this baseline hyperresponsiveness (Townley *et al.*, 1986; Postma *et al.*, 1995). However, the largest part of the BHR in asthma is probably acquired and related to the airway inflammation that is present, as outlined in Fig. 38.2 (Global Initiative for Asthma, 1995).

Airway inflammation can enhance the airway responsiveness in different ways (Elwood *et al.*, 1983; James *et al.*, 1989; Wiggs *et al.*, 1990; Lambert *et al.*, 1993).

- Oedema of the airway wall and loss of elastic recoil of the airway wall. Both mechanisms will result in an increased narrowing of the airway for the same degree of ASM activation.
- Hypertrophy and hyperplasia of the ASM.
- Change in ASM contractility.
- Presence of inflammatory mediators that can act synergistically with the inhaled agonist on the ASM.
- Increase in activation or number of inflammatory cells involved in the indirect airway responsiveness.
- Decrease in the production of inhibitory factors (epithelial-derived relaxing factors?)

The relative contribution of each of these mechanisms is currently unclear.

The fact that usually no good correlation can be found between BHR and symptoms in asthma can easily be explained by the complexity of the mechanisms involved in the BHR, the variable air-flow obstruction and the role of inflammation in directly causing symptoms (Hargreave *et al.*, 1981; Josephs *et al.*, 1989, 1992).

Long-term avoidance of the causal allergen or long-term treatment with inhaled steroids does not result in a complete disappearance of BHR in the majority of patients with asthma (Platts-Mills *et al.*, 1982; Van Essen-Zandvliet *et al.*, 1992). This suggests either that a part of the inflammation is no longer responsive to treatment or that irreversible changes have occurred in the airway tissues.

BHR in diseases other than asthma

BHR has been demonstrated in a number of diseases other than asthma. The difficulty in the interpretation of these findings is that the bronchial response is related to the initial airway calibre and that, for the same degree of shortening of the ASM, the change in airway calibre will be greater if the initial airway calibre was smaller. Therefore, an increased bronchial response in diseases with a decreased baseline airway calibre might not have the same meaning as an increased response in subjects with a normal baseline.

Chronic obstructive pulmonary disease

Chronic obstructive pulmonary disease (COPD) is characterized by the development of a progressive, largely irreversible air-flow limitation. The most important cause is cigarette smoking. Not all smokers develop such an air-flow limitation and BHR is considered to be a risk factor (Sluiter *et al.*, 1991). Many patients with COPD have an increased bronchial responsiveness to histamine or methacholine (Yan *et al.*, 1985; Ramsdale & Hargreave, 1990). The correlation with the baseline FEV_1 is good and it is therefore very difficult to differentiate between cause and effect. The BHR in patients with COPD is less than in asthma for a comparable degree of baseline air-flow limitation. Patients with asthma also differ from patients with COPD with regard to their responsiveness to indirect stimuli. No response was found in patients with COPD after challenge with propranolol, methoxamine, cold-air hyperventilation, polymyxin B or sulphur dioxide (Ramsdale & Hargreave, 1990). Challenge with AMP, another indirect agonist, caused airway narrowing in the majority of patients with COPD, especially if they were smokers (Oosterhoff *et al.*, 1993). Further studies to investigate differences and similarities in the BHR between asthma and COPD are clearly needed to understand the mechanisms involved in both diseases.

Other diseases

An increased frequency of BHR to histamine or methacholine has been observed in subjects with rhinitis without asthmatic symptoms (Hargreave *et al.*, 1981), patients with cystic fibrosis (Van Asperen *et al.*, 1981), patients with sarcoidosis (Manresa *et al.*, 1986) and patients with bronchiectasis (Pang *et al.*, 1989). The significance of these findings and the relationship with pathological changes in the airways is not yet understood.

Effect of therapeutic interventions

Non-pharmacological therapy

Allergen avoidance

If the hypothesis about the role of airway inflammation in BHR in asthma is correct (Fig. 38.1), then avoidance of the causal factor should result in a decrease in the BHR. This has indeed been shown in a number of studies. Avoidance of house dust mite (HDM) allergen by staying in a hospital environment results in a progressive decrease in bronchial responsiveness to histamine (Platts-Mills *et al.*, 1982; Murray & Ferguson, 1983). The decrease is progressive over several months. Similar findings were observed in a study on the effect of dust-free bedrooms on asthma. The result of avoidance of occupational agents is less predictable, and some subjects with occupational asthma remain hyperresponsive despite complete avoidance of the causal agent (Chan-Yeung *et al.*, 1988; Saetta *et al.*, 1992). It seems that these individuals with persistent BHR have developed persistent airway inflammation. The risk of developing persistent BHR is dependent on the duration of exposure to the causal agent, the severity of the occupational asthma and the duration of the asthmatic symptoms before removal (Chan-Yeung & Malo, 1995).

Allergen immunotherapy

The role of immunotherapy in asthma is still controversial (Bousquet *et al.*, 1990). A meta-analysis of clinical trials of allergen immunotherapy in asthma showed that this form of therapy significantly reduced non-allergenic BHR (Abramson *et al.*, 1995). The odds for reduction in BHR were 6.8 (95% confidence interval (CI) 3.8 to 12.0).

Pharmacological therapy

When discussing the effect of pharmacological treatment on bronchial responsiveness, it is important to make a difference between the immediate effect of a drug on the airway response to an agonist and the long-term effects of this drug on the bronchial responsiveness to the agonist. This difference is quite easy to make when the drug is not a specific or functional antagonist of the agonist that is used, but the interpretation becomes extremely difficult when the drug is a functional antagonist. Long-term effects on bronchial responsiveness are then often assessed after stopping the drug for a certain time, so that the short-term functional antagonism is no longer present at the moment of the measurement of the bronchial responsiveness. This approach, however, does not exclude possible interference by rebound phenomena.

Glucocorticosteroids

Treatment with inhaled steroids results in a progressive decrease of the non-allergenic BHR (Haahtela *et al.*, 1991; Djukanovic *et al.*, 1992; Jeffery *et al.*, 1992; Van Essen-Zandvliet *et al.*, 1992). The effect is dose dependent and takes several months to achieve a plateau (Kraan *et al.*, 1985; Kerstjens *et al.*, 1992; Van Essen-Zandvliet *et al.*, 1992). Many subjects with asthma, however, do not return to a completely a normal level of bronchial responsiveness, despite long-term treatment with inhaled steroids. Inhaled steroids also inhibit the increase in BHR following allergen challenge and during the pollen season in sensitive subjects (Hargreave *et al.*, 1990). Stopping the chronic treatment with inhaled steroids results in an increase in BHR, together with a recurrence of the asthmatic symptoms (Waalkens *et al.*, 1993; Haahtela *et al.*, 1994).

Sodium cromoglycate and nedocromil sodium

Neither sodium cromoglycate nor nedocromil inhibits the bronchial response to direct agonists when administered immediately before the challenge. Both drugs are potent inhibitors of the bronchial response to all indirect agonists, such as exercise, hyper- and hypotonic solutions, adenosine, tachykinins, bradykinin, sulphur dioxide, etc. (Busse *et al.*, 1989). Sodium cromoglycate and nedocromil sodium also inhibit the increase in non-allergenic bronchial responsiveness following allergen challenge and during the pollen season (Lowhagen & Rak, 1985; Busse *et al.*, 1989). Long-term treatment with sodium cromoglycate or nedocromil sodium results in a decrease of the non-allergenic BHR in patients with asthma (Petty *et al.*, 1989; De Jong *et al.*, 1994).

Theophylline

Several studies have shown a small protective effect of theophylline upon non-allergenic challenges such as histamine, methacholine, distilled water and exercise (Barnes & Pauwels, 1994). The protective effect upon adenosine challenge is regarded as a specific antagonistic effect at the level of the adenosine receptor (Mann & Holgate, 1985). Long-term treatment with theophylline failed to show any significant effect on the histamine bronchial responsiveness in a group of patients with relatively severe asthma (Dutoit *et al.*, 1987). The effects of theophylline on the allergen-induced increase in BHR have been difficult to demonstrate, but this might be a type II error since in a larger study theophylline significantly inhibited this increase (Barnes & Pauwels, 1994; Hendeles *et al.*, 1995).

β-Agonists

β_2-Agonists are potent functional antagonists and therefore inhibit the bronchial response to all agonists when administered immediately before the challenge. The long-term effects on BHR have been studied after stopping the treatment for one or two dosings. It is clear that long-term treatment with short-acting β_2-agonists does not modify the BHR significantly, except maybe for a short rebound increase after stopping the treatment (Kraan *et al.*, 1985; Haahtela *et al.*, 1991). Long-term treatment with long-acting inhaled sympathomimetics results in a decrease of the protective effect of these drugs (Cheung *et al.*, 1992).

Short-acting inhaled sympathomimetics do not protect against allergen-induced increase in BHR (Cockcroft & Murdock, 1987). The effect of the long-acting inhaled sympathomimetics on allergen-induced changes in BHR is difficult to interpret in view of the long-lasting functional antagonistic activities of these drugs (Twentyman *et al.*, 1990).

Anticholinergics

Inhaled anticholinergics have, of course, a pronounced inhibitory effect on the bronchial response to cholinergic agonists, but, apart from this, these drugs are rather poor functional antagonists and chronic treatment does not modulate non-allergenic BHR (Britton *et al.*, 1988).

Conclusions

BHR is a physiopathological characteristic of asthma. The methods to measure it have evolved greatly and have revealed the complexity of the airway response in patients with asthma. The interaction between asthmatic airway inflammation and BHR can be explained by many different mechanisms, and further studies are needed to determine their relative importance. The effects of anti-asthma medication on BHR help us to understand both the mechanisms of BHR and the mode of action of these drugs.

References

Abramson, M.J., Puy, R.M. & Weiner, J.M. (1995) Is allergen immunotherapy effective in asthma? A meta-analysis of randomized controlled trials. *Am. J. Resp. Crit. Care Med.*, **151**, 969–74.

Alexander, H.L. & Paddock, R. (1921) Bronchial asthma: response to pilocarpine and epineprine. *Arch. Intern. Med.*, **27**, 184–91.

Altounyan, R.E.C., Cole, M. & Lee, T.B. (1985) Inhibition of sulphur dioxide induced bronchoconstriction by nedocromil sodium in non-asthmatic atopic subjects. *Ann. Allergy*, **55**, A689.

Anderson, S.D. (1984) Is there a unifying hypothesis for exercise-induced asthma? *J. Allergy Clin. Immunol.*, **73**, 660–5.

Anderson, S.D. (1985) Issues in exercise induced asthma. *J. Allergy Clin. Immunol.*, **76**, 763–72.

Anderson, S.D., Silverman, M., Godfrey, S. & Konig, P. (1975) Exercise-induced asthma: a review. *Brit. J. Dis. Chest*, **69**, 1–39.

Anderson, S.D., Schoeffel, R.E. & Finney, M. (1983) Evaluation of ultrasonically nebulised solutions as a provocation in patients with asthma. *Thorax*, **38**, 284–91.

Anderson, S.D., Schoeffel, R.E., Black, J.L. & Daviskas, E. (1985) Airway cooling as the stimulus to exercise induced asthma: a re-evaluation. *Eur. J. Resp. Dis.*, **67**, 20–30.

Arm, J.P., O'Hickey, S.P., Hawkesworth, R.J. *et al.* (1990) Asthmatic airways have a disproportionate hyperresponsiveness to LTE4 as compared to normal airways, but not to LTC4, LTD4, methacholine and histamine. *Am. Rev. Resp. Dis.*, **142**, 1112–18.

Bailey, W.C., Wilson, S.R., Weiss, K.B., Windsor, R.A. & Wolle, J.M. (1994) Measures for use in asthma clinical research: overview of a NIH workshop. *Am. J. Resp. Crit. Care Med.*, **149**, S1–S8.

Barnes, P.J. & Pauwels, R.A. (1994) Theophylline in the management of asthma—time for reappraisal. *Eur. Resp. J.*, **7**, 579–91.

Bousquet, J., Hejjaoue, A. & Michel, F.B. (1990) Specific immunotherapy in asthma. *J. Allergy Clin. Immunol.*, **86**, 292–306.

Britton, J.R., Hanley, S.P., Garrett, H.V., Hadfield, J.W. & Tattersfield, A.E. (1988) Dose related effects of salbutamol and ipratropium bromide on airway calibre and reactivity in subjects with asthma. *Thorax*, **43**, 300–5.

Busse, W.W., Orr, T.S.C. & Pauwels, R. (1989) International symposium on nedocromil sodium. *Drugs*, **37**, 1–137.

Chai, H., Farr, R.S., Froehilch, L.A. *et al.* (1975) Standardisation of bronchial inhalation procedures. *J. Allergy Clin. Immunol.*, **56**, 323–7.

Chan-Yeung, M., Leriche, J., Maclean, L. & Lam, S. (1988) Comparison of cellular and protein changes in bronchial lavage fluid of symptomatic and asymptomatic patients with red cedar asthma on follow-up examination. *Clin. Allergy*, **18**, 359–65.

Chan-Yeung, M. & Malo, J.L. (1995) Current concepts: occupational asthma. *New Engl. J. Med.*, **333**, 107–12.

Cheung, D., Timmers, M.C., Zwinderman, A.H., Bel, E.H., Dijkman, J.H. & Sterk, P.J. (1992) Long-term effects of a long-acting beta 2-adrenoceptor agonist, salmeterol, on airway hyperresponsiveness in patients with mild asthma. *New Engl. J. Med.*, **327**, 1198–203.

Cockcroft, D.W. & Murdock, K.Y. (1987) Comparative effects of inhaled salbutamol, sodium cromoglycate and beclomethasone dipropionate on allergen-induced early asthmatic response, late asthmatic responses and increased bronchial responsiveness to histamine. *J. Allergy Clin. Immunol.*, **79**, 734–40.

Crimi, N., Palermo, F., Oliveri, R. *et al.* (1990) Influence of antihistamine (astemizole) and anticholinergic drugs (ipratropium bromide) on bronchoconstriction induced by substance P. *Ann. Allergy*, **65**, 115–20.

Curry, J.J. (1947) Comparative action of acetyl-beta-methylcholine and histamine on the respiratory tract in normals, patients with hay fever and subjects with bronchial asthma. *J. Clin. Invest.*, **26**, 430–8.

Curry, J.J. & Lowell, F.C. (1948) Measurement of vital capacity in asthmatic subjects receiving histamine and acetyl-methylcholine. *J. Allergy Clin. Med.*, **19**, 9–18.

Cushley, M.J., Tattersfield, A.E. & Holgate, S.T. (1983) Inhaled adenosine and guanosine on airway resistance in normal and asthmatic subjects. *Brit. J. Clin. Pharmacol.*, **15**, 161–5.

Deal, E.W., McFadden, E.R., Ingram, R.H., Strauss, R.H. & Jaeger, J.J. (1979) Role of respiratory heat exchange in production of excercise induced asthma. *J. Appl. Physiol.*, **46**, 467–75.

De Jong, J.W., Teengs, J.P., Postma, D.S., Van der Mark, T.W., Koeter, G.H. & de Monchy, J.G. (1994) Nedocromil sodium versus albuterol in the management of allergic asthma. *Am. J. Resp. Crit. Care Med.*, **149**, 91–7.

de Vries, K., Booij-Noord, H., van der Lende, R., Van Lookeren-Campagne, J.G. & Orie, N.G.M. (1968) Reactivity of the bronchial tree to different stimuli. *Bronches*, **18**, 439–542.

Dixon, C.M.S. & Barnes, P.J. (1989) Bradykinin induced bronchoconstriction: inhibition by nedocromil sodium and sodium cromoglycate. *Brit. J. Clin. Pharmacol.*, **270**, 8310–60.

Dixon, C.M.S. & Ind, P.W. (1988) Metabisulfite-induced bronchoconstriction: mechanisms. *Am. Rev. Resp. Dis.*, **137**, 238A.

Djukanovic, R., Wilson, J.W., Britten, K.M. *et al.* (1992) Effect of an inhaled corticosteroid on airway inflammation and symptoms in asthma. *Am. Rev. Resp. Dis.*, **145**, 669–74.

Drazen, J.M. (1986) Inhalation challenge of humans with sulfidopeptide leukotrienes. *Chest*, **89**, 414–19.

Dutoit, J., Salome, C.M. & Woolcock, A.J. (1987) Inhaled corticosteroids reduce the severity of bronchial hyperresponsiveness in asthma but oral theophylline does not. *Am. Rev. Resp. Dis.*, **136**, 1174–8.

Eiser, N., Mills, J., Snashall, P. & Guz, A. (1981) The role of histamine receptors in asthma. *Clin. Sci.*, **60**, 363–70.

Elwood, R.K., Kennedy, S., Belzberg, A., Hogg, J.C. & Pare, P.D. (1983) Respiratory mucosal permeability in asthma. *Am. Rev. Resp. Dis.*, **128**, 523–7.

Enright, P., Lebowitz, M.D. & Cockcroft, D.W. (1994) Physiologic measures: pulmonary function tests. *Am. J. Resp. Crit. Care Med.*, **149**, S9–S18.

Finney, M.J.B., Anderson, S.D. & Black, J.L. (1990) Terfenadine modifies airway narrowing induced by the inhalation of non-isotonic aerosols in subjects with asthma. *Am. Rev. Resp. Dis.*, **141**, 1151–7.

Fischer, A.R., Mcfadden, C.A., Frantz, R. *et al.* (1995) Effect of chronic 5-lipoxygenase inhibition on airway hyperresponsiveness in asthmatic subjects. *Am. J. Resp. Crit. Care Med.*, **152**, 1203–7.

Fuller, R.W., Dixon, C.M.S., Cuss, F.M.C. & Barnes, P.J. (1987) Bradykinin induced bronchoconstriction in man: mode of action. *Am. Rev. Resp. Dis.*, **135**, 176–80.

Global Initiative for Asthma (1995) *Global Strategy for Asthma Management and Prevention: NHLBI/WHO Workshop Report*. National Institutes of Health, National Heart, Lung and Blood Institute, Washington.

Haahtela, T., Jarvinen, M., Kava, T. *et al.* (1991) Comparison of a beta2-agonist, terbutaline, with an inhaled corticosteroid, budesonide, in newly detected asthma. *New Engl. J. Med.*, **325**, 388–92.

Haahtela, T., Jarvinen, M., Kava, T. *et al.* (1994) Effects of reducing or discontinuing inhaled budesonide in patients with mild asthma. *New Engl. J. Med.*, **331**, 700–5.

Hargreave, F.E., Ryan, G., Thomson, N.G. *et al.* (1981) Bronchial responsiveness to histamine or methacholine in asthma: measurement and clinical significance. *J. Allergy Clin. Immunol.*, **68**, 347–55.

Hargreave, F.E., Dolovich, J. & Newhouse, M.T. (1990) The assessment and treatment of asthma: a conference report. *J. Allergy Clin. Immunol.*, **85**, 1098–111.

Hendeles, L., Harman, E., Huang, D., Obrien, R., Blake, K. & Delafuente, J. (1995) Theophylline attenuation of airway responses to allergen: comparison with cromolyn metered-dose inhaler. *J. Allergy Clin. Immunol.*, **95**, 505–14.

Herxheimer, H. (1946) Hyperventilation asthma. *Lancet*, **i**, 83–7.

Ichinose, M., Nakajima, N., Takahashi, T., Yamauchi, H., Inoue, H. & Takishima, T. (1992) Protection against bradykinin-induced bronchoconstriction in asthmatic patients by neurokinin receptor antagonist. *Lancet*, **340**, 1248–51.

Ind, P.W., Barnes, P.J., Brown, M.J. & Dollery, C.T. (1985) Plasma histamine concentration during propranolol-induced bronchoconstriction. *Thorax*, **40**, 903–9.

Ind, P.W., Dixon, C.M.S., Fuller, R.W. & Barnes, P.J. (1989) Anticholinergic blockade of β-blocker induced bronchoconstriction. *Am. Rev. Resp. Dis.*, **139**, 1390–4.

James, A.L., Paré, P.D. & Hogg, J.C. (1989) The mechanics of airway narrowing in asthma. *Am. Rev. Resp. Dis.*, **139**, 242–6.

Jeffery, P.K., Godrey, R.W., Adelroth, E. *et al.* (1992) Effects of treatment on airway inflammation and thickening of basement membrane reticular collagen in asthma. *Am. Rev. Resp. Dis.*, **145**, 890–9.

Jones, R.S., Wharton, M.J. & Buston, M.H. (1963) The place of physical exercise and bronchodilator drugs in the assessment of the asthmatic child. *Arch. Dis. Child.*, **38**, 539–45.

Joos, G.F., Pauwels, R. & Van Der Straeten, M. (1987) Effect of inhaled substance P and neurokinin A in the airways of normal and asthmatic subjects. *Thorax*, **42**, 779–83.

Joos, G.F., Pauwels, R.A. & Van Der Straeten, M.E. (1988) The effect of oxitropium bromide on neurokinin A-induced bronchoconstriction in asthmatics. *Pulm. Pharmacol.*, **1**, 41–5.

Joos, G.F., Pauwels, R.A. & Van Der Straeten, M.E. (1989) The effect of nedocromil sodium on the bronchoconstrictor effect of neurokinin A in subjects with asthma. *J. Allergy Clin. Immunol.*, **83**, 663–8.

Joos, G.F., Germonpre, P.R., Kips, J.C., Peleman, R.A. & Pauwels, R.A. (1994) Sensory neuropeptides and the human lower airways—present state and future directions. *Eur. Resp. J.*, **7**, 1161–71.

Josephs, L.K., Gregg, I., Mullee, M.A. & Holgate, S.T. (1989) Non-specific bronchial reactivity and its relationship to the clinical expression of asthma. *Am. Rev. Resp. Dis.*, **140**, 350–7.

Josephs, L.K., Gregg, I., Mullee, M.A., Campbell, M.J. & Holgate, S.T. (1992) A longitudinal study of baseline FEV_1 and bronchial responsiveness in patients with asthma. *Eur. Resp. J.*, **5**, 32–9.

Kerstjens, H.A.M., Brand, P.L.P., Hughes, M.D. *et al.* (1992) A comparison of bronchodilator therapy with or without inhaled corticosteroid therapy for obstructive airways disease. *New Engl. J. Med.*, **327**, 1413–19.

Kraan, J., Koeter, G.H., van de Mark, T.W., Sluiter, H.J. & de Vries, K. (1985) Changes in bronchial hyperreactivity induced by 4 weeks of treatment with antiasthmatic drugs in patients with allergic asthma: a comparison between budesonide and terbutaline. *J. Allergy Clin. Immunol.*, **76**, 628–36.

Lambert, R.K., Wiggs, B.R., Kuwano, K., Hogg, J.C. & Paré, P.D. (1993) Functional significance of increased airway smooth muscle in asthma and COPD. *J. Appl. Physiol.*, **74**, 2771–81.

Levy, L. & Seabury, J. (1947) Spirometric evaluation of benadryl in asthma. *J. Allergy*, **18**, 244–50.

Lowhagen, O. & Rak, S. (1985) Modification of bronchial hyperreactivity after treatment with sodium cromoglycate during pollen season. *J. Allergy Clin. Immunol.*, **75**, 460–7.

McFadden, E.R. (1987) Exercise induced asthma: assessment of current etiologic concepts. *Chest*, **91**, 151S–157S.

McFadden, E.R. (1990) Hypothesis: exercise-induced asthma as a vascular phenomenon. *Lancet*, **335**, 880–3.

McFadden, E.R., Lenner, K.A. & Strohl, K.P. (1986) Postexertional airway rewarming and thermally induced asthma: new insights into pathophysiology and possible pathogenesis. *J. Clin. Invest.*, **78**, 18–25.

Mann, J.S. & Holgate, S.T. (1985) Specific antagonism of adenosine induced bronchoconstriction in asthma by oral theophylline. *Brit. J. Clin. Pharmacol.*, **19**, 685–92.

Manning, P.J., Watson R.M., Margolskee, D.J., Williams, V.C., Schwartz, J.I. & O'Byrne, P.M. (1990) Inhibition of exercise-induced bronchoconstriction by MK-571, a potent leukotriene D4-receptor antagonist. *New Engl. J. Med.*, **323**, 1736–9.

Manresa, P.F., Romero, C.P. & Rodriguez, S.B. (1986) Bronchial hyperreactivity in fresh stage I sarcoidosis. *Ann. NY Acad. Sci.*, **465**, 523–9.

Murray, A.B. & Ferguson, A.C. (1983) Dust free bedrooms in the treatment of asthmatic children with house dust or house dust mite allergy: a controlled trial. *Pediatrics*, **71**, 418–22.

Nathan, R., Segall, N., Glover, G. & Schocket, A. (1979) The effects of H1 and H2 antihistamines on histamine inhalation challenges in asthmatic patients. *Am. Rev. Resp. Dis.*, **120**, 1251–8.

Nichol, G.M., Nix, A., Chung, K.F. & Barnes, P.J. (1989) Characterisation of bronchoconstrictor responses to sodium metabisulphite aerosol in atopic asthmatic and non-asthmatic subjects. *Thorax*, **44**, 1009–14.

Nogrady, S. & Bevan, C. (1978) Inhaled antihistamines—bronchodilatation and effects on histamine- and methacholine-induced bronchoconstriction. *Thorax*, **33**, 700–4.

O'Byrne, P.M., Ryan, G., Morris, M. (1982) Asthma induced by cold air and its relation to nonspecific bronchial responsiveness to methacholine. *Am. Rev. Resp. Dis.*, **125**, 281–5.

Oosterhoff, Y., Dejong, J.W., Jansen, M.A.M., Koeter, G.H. & Postma, D.S. (1993) Airway responsiveness to adenosine 5′-monophosphate in chronic obstructive pulmonary disease is determined by smoking. *Am. Rev. Resp. Dis.*, **147**, 553–8.

Pang, J., Chan, H.S. & Sung, J.Y. (1989) Prevalence of asthma, atopy and bronchial hyperreactivity in bronchiectasis: a controlled study. *Thorax*, **44**, 948–51.

Pauwels, R., Joos, G. & Van Der Straeten, M. (1988) Bronchial hyperresponsiveness is not bronchial hyperresponsiveness is not bronchial asthma. *Clin. Allergy*, **18**, 317–21.

Petty, T.L., Rollins, D.R., Christopher, K., Good, J.T. & Oakley, R. (1989) Cromolyn sodium is effective in adult chronic asthmatics. *Am. Rev. Resp. Dis.*, **139**, 694–701.

Phillips, G.D., Polosa, R. & Holgate, S.T. (1989) The effect of histamine-H1 receptor antagonism with terfenadine on concentration-related AMP-induced bronchoconstriction in asthma. *Clin. Exp. Allergy*, **19**, 405–9.

Platts-Mills, T.A.E., Mitchell, E.B., Nock, P., Tovey, E.R., Moszoro, H. & Wilkins, S.R. (1982) Reduction of bronchial hyperreactivity during prolonged allergen avoidance. *Lancet*, **ii**, 675–8.

Polosa, R., Holgate, S.T. & Church, M.K. (1989) Adenosine as a proinflammatory mediator in asthma. *Pulm. Pharmacol.*, **2**, 21–6.

Polosa, R., Phillips, G.D., Lai, C.K.W. & Holgate, S.T. (1990) Contribution of histamine and prostanoids to bronchoconstriction provoked by inhaled bradykinin in atopic asthma. *Allergy*, **45**, 174–82.

Polosa, R., Phillips, G.D., Rajakulasingam, K. & Holgate, S.T. (1991) The effect of inhaled ipratropium bromide alone and in combination with oral terfenadine on bronchoconstriction provoked by adenosine 5′-monophosphate and histamine in asthma. *J. Allergy Clin. Immunol.*, **87**, 939–47.

Postma, D.S., Bleecker, E.R., Amelung, P.J. *et al.* (1995) Genetic susceptibility to asthma — bronchial hyperresponsiveness coinherited with a major gene for atopy. *New Engl. J. Med.*, **333**, 894–900.

Rajakulasingam, K., Church, M.K., Howarth, P.H. & Holgate, S.T. (1993) Factors determining bradykinin bronchial responsiveness and refractoriness in asthma. *J. Allergy Clin. Immunol.*, **92**, 140–2.

Ramsdale, E.H. & Hargreave, F.E. (1990) Differences in airway responsiveness in asthma and chronic airflow obstruction. *Med. Clin. N. Am.*, **74**, 741–51.

Roffel, A.F., Elzinga, C.R.S. & Zaagsma, J. (1990) Muscarinic M3 receptors mediate contraction of human central and peripheral airway smooth muscle. *Pulm. Pharmacol.*, **3**, 47–51.

Saetta, M., Maestrelli, P., Di Stefano, A. *et al.* (1992) Effect of cessation of exposure to toluene diisocyanate (TDI) on bronchial mucosa of subjects with TDI-induced asthma. *Am. Rev. Resp. Dis.*, **145**, 169–74.

Schacter, E., Brown, S., Lach, E. & Gertenhaber, B. (1982) Histamine blocking agents in healthy and asthmatic subjects. *Chest*, **82**, 143–7.

Sluiter, H.J., Koeter, G.H., de Monchy, J.G.R., Postma, D.S., de Vries, K. & Orie, N.G.M. (1991) The Dutch hypothesis (chronic nonspecific lung disease) revisited. *Eur. Resp. J.*, **4**, 479–89.

Sterk, P.J., Daniel, E.E., Zamel, N. & Hargreave, F.E. (1985) Limited maximal airway narrowing in non-asthmatic subjects: role of neural control and prostaglandin release. *Am. Rev. Resp. Dis.*, **132**, 865–70.

Sterk, P.J., Fabbri, L.M., Quanjer, P.H. *et al.* (1993) Airway responsiveness: standardized challenge testing with pharmacological, physical and sensitizing stimuli in adults. *Eur. Resp. J.*, **6** (Suppl. 16), 53–83.

Thomson, N. & Kerr, J. (1980) Effect of inhaled H1 and H2 receptor antagonists in normal and asthmatic subjects. *Thorax*, **35**, 428–34.

Tiffeneau, R. (1957) *Examen pulmonaire de l'asthmatique. Déductions diagnostiques, prognostiques et thérapeutiques.* Masson, Paris.

Townley, R.G., Bewtra, A.K., Wilson A.F. *et al.* (1986) Segregation analysis of bronchial response to methacholine inhalation challenge in families with and without asthma. *J. Allergy Clin. Immunol.*, **77**, 101–7.

Twentyman, O.P., Finnerty, J.P., Harris, A., Palmer, J. & Holgate, S.T. (1990) Protection against allergen induced asthma by salmeterol. *Lancet*, **336**, 1338–42.

Van Asperen, P., Mellis, C.M., South, R.T. & Simpson, S.J. (1981) Bronchial reactivity in cystic fibrosis with normal pulmonary function. *Am. J. Dis. Child.*, **135**, 815–19.

Van Essen-Zandvliet, E.E., Hughes, M.D., Waalkens, H.J., Duiverman, E.J., Pocock, S.J. & Kerrebijn, K.F. (1992) Effects of 22 months of treatment with inhaled corticosteroids and/or beta-2-agonists on lung function, airway responsiveness, and symptoms in children with asthma. *Am. Rev. Resp. Dis.*, **146**, 547–54.

Waalkens, H.J., Van Essen-Zandvliet, E.E., Hughes, M.D. *et al.* (1993) Cessation of long-term treatment with inhaled corticosteroid (budesonide) in children with asthma results in deterioration. *Am. Rev. Resp. Dis.*, **148**, 1252–7.

Weiss, S., Robb, G.P. & Ellis, L.B. (1932) The systemic effects of histamine in man with special reference to the cardiovascular system. *Arch. Intern. Med.*, **49**, 360–9.

White, M.V., Slater, J.E. & Kaliner, M.A. (1987) Histamine and asthma. *Am. Rev. Resp. Dis.*, **135**, 1165–76.

Wiebicke, W., Poynter, A., Montgomery, M., Chernick, V. & Pasterkamp, H. (1988) Effect of terfenadine on the response to exercise and cold air in asthma. *Ped. Pulmonol.*, **4**, 225–9.

Wiggs, B.R., Moreno, R., Hogg, J.C., Hilliam, C. & Pare, P.D. (1990) A model of the mechanics of airway narrowing. *J. Appl. Physiol.*, **69**, 849–60.

Woolcock, A.J., Salome, C.M. & Yan, K. (1984) The shape of the dose–response curve to histamine in asthmatic and normal subjects. *Am. Rev. Resp. Dis.*, **130**, 71–5.

Wright, W., Zhang, Y.G., Salome, C.M. & Woolcock, A.J. (1990) Effect of inhaled preservatives on asthmatic subjects. I. Sodium metabisulfite. *Am. Rev. Resp. Dis.*, **141**, 1400–4.

Yan, K., Salome, C.M. & Woolcock, A.J. (1985) Prevalence and nature of bronchial hyperresponsiveness in subjects with chronic obstructive pulmonary disease. *Am. Rev. Resp. Dis.*, **132**, 25–9.

CHAPTER 39

Exercise-Induced Asthma

S.D. Anderson

Introduction

Exercise-induced asthma (EIA) is the name used to describe the transitory increase in airway resistance which follows vigorous exercise (Anderson *et al.*, 1988a). EIA most commonly occurs in people with clinically recognized asthma, but in the last 10 years there have been many reports of EIA occurring in asymptomatic 'healthy people', in particular, schoolchildren, élite athletes, skiers, skaters and defence force recruits (Barry *et al.*, 1991; Nish & Schweitz, 1992; Brudno *et al.*, 1994; Haby *et al.*, 1995).

The increase in airways resistance following exercise is most commonly measured indirectly by recording a fall in peak expiratory flow (PEF) or forced expiratory volume in 1 second (FEV_1) (Fig. 39.1). A fall > 15% of the pre-exercise value is generally regarded as diagnostic, but a fall > 10% is usually abnormal for healthy subjects exercising in a temperate (Burr *et al.*, 1974; Anderson *et al.*, 1975) or cold climate (O'Cain *et al.*, 1980).

The stimulus for the airways to narrow in response to exercise is the loss of water from the airways in bringing large volumes of ambient air to body conditions in a short time (Strauss *et al.*, 1978; Anderson *et al.*, 1982). The mechanism whereby water loss causes the airways to narrow is not precisely known but it is likely to relate to the osmotic (Anderson, 1984) and thermal effects (Deal *et al.*, 1979) of evaporative water loss. The potential osmotic effects include release of substances (Eggleston *et al.*, 1990) with the capacity to cause contraction of bronchial smooth muscle, an increase in vascular permeability (Umeno *et al.*, 1990) and an increase in bronchial blood flow (Smith *et al.*, 1993). The potential thermal effects include a reactive hyperaemia and vascular engorgement following airway cooling and vasoconstriction (McFadden *et al.*, 1986; Gilbert & McFadden, 1992).

In children, EIA appears to be an early manifestation of asthma (Martin *et al.*, 1980; Balfour-Lynn *et al.*, 1981; Jones & Bowen, 1994). Thus, early recognition and treatment of EIA in schoolchildren may reduce the risk of developing symptomatic asthma. While it is thought unlikely that EIA is an entity in itself, it is possible that chronic dehydration of the airway mucosa by hyperpnoea with cold and dry air leads to reduced lung functon (Schaeffer *et al.*, 1980) and inflammatory changes that predispose a person to EIA. This would explain the high frequency of EIA in élite athletes, cross-country skiers and skaters.

In recognized asthmatics, EIA is associated with active asthma, usually in the moderate to severe range, and can usually be markedly reduced with acute treatment with sodium cromoglycate, nedocromil sodium or a β_2-adrenoceptor agonist given immediately before exercise or with chronic treatment with aerosol corticosteroids (Henriksen & Dahl, 1983; Henriksen *et al.*, 1985; Waalkens *et al.*, 1994). This approach would be in keeping with the statement by the International Paediatric Consensus Group that 'the goal of treatment should be to allow children to be involved with normal activity including full participation in exercise and sport' (Warner *et al.*, 1992).

A diagnosis of EIA can often be made on history alone. If a patient complains of breathlessness or chest tightness with a dry cough that is profoundly worse after, rather than during, exercise, and this is relieved by inhaling a β_2-adrenoceptor agonist, then the history is consistent with EIA. If the breathlessness after exercise is prevented by taking a β_2-adrenoceptor agonist or sodium cromoglycate immediately before exercise, it is consistent with a diagno-

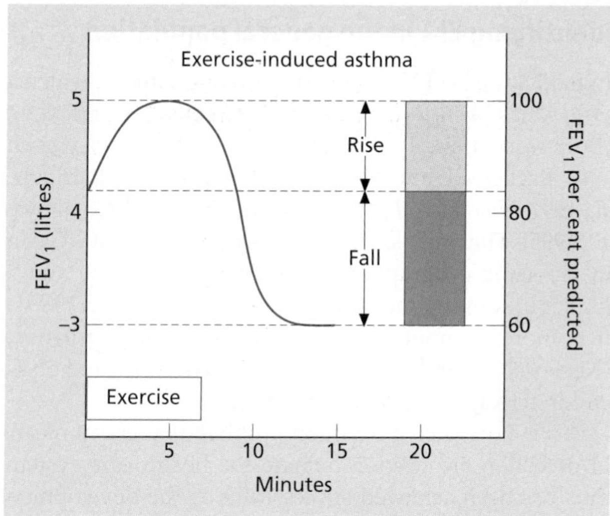

Fig. 39.1 Typical values for FEV_1 at rest during and after exercise in a non-steroid-treated young asthmatic exercising for 8 minutes. The bar graph representing the values for FEV_1 at rest (central bar), highest value during exercise (top bar) and the lowest value after exercise (bottom bar), expressed as a percentage of the predicted normal value.

sis of asthma. It should be noted that EIA is not predicted by risk factors that include positive answers relating to asthma in questionnaires—poor lung function and cough (Rupp *et al.*, 1993). Many healthy subjects, particularly regular runners, may have exercise-induced cough that is not associated with airway narrowing (Banner *et al.*, 1984). There are recent reviews and editorials on EIA covering, in detail, the history, importance and treatment of EIA (Anderson, 1993b; Carlson & Boe, 1993; Godfrey & Bar-Yishay, 1993; McFadden & Gilbert, 1994).

EIA in recognized asthmatics

Under standardized laboratory exercise conditions, EIA occurs in 70–80% of non-steroid-treated asthmatic subjects and about 55% of steroid-treated asthmatics referred to hospital clinics (Anderson *et al.*, 1975; Waalkens *et al.*, 1993). A lower prevalence of EIA has been found in field studies, particularly where the diagnosis of asthma has been made on questionnaire and when treatment was not withheld before exercise testing (Terblanche & Stewart, 1990; Bardagi *et al.*, 1993).

EIA is equally common in asthmatic adults and children. Many adult asthmatics do not give a history as they have adjusted their lifestyle to avoid vigorous exercise. The presence or severity of EIA cannot be predicted from the measurement of lung function at rest. While EIA occurs more frequently in asthmatics whose lung function is below the normal predicted values, it can still occur in asthmatics with normal lung function, particularly in those taking aerosol corticosteroids. Approximately 55% of children whose asthma was 'under control' still had demonstrable EIA in the laboratory (Waalkens *et al.*, 1993). Similarly, we have found 50% of adults to remain hyperresponsive to hyperosmolar (4.5%) saline (Anderson *et al.*, 1994), a surrogate challenge for identifying EIA (Smith & Anderson, 1990). EIA seems to be one of the earliest signs of asthma and one of the last to respond to chronic treatment with aerosol corticosteroids, thus making it important to investigate before or at least after treatment.

EIA is frequently associated with arterial hypoxaemia (Fig. 39.2) (Bye *et al.*, 1980) and hyperinflation (Anderson *et al.*, 1972). The extent of the fall in oxygen tension is related to the severity of EIA. We have rarely found hypercapnia. When an 'attack of asthma' develops during exercise, it is potentially dangerous for a person to continue to exercise, as oxygen consumption may exceed delivery, leading to rapid hypoxaemia. There have been several newspaper and physicians' reports of sudden death after exercise, of children and adults suffering from asthma. As the attack is usually the most severe within 10 minutes of ceasing exercise, it is advisable to monitor the subjects' lung function during this time and, in the absence of measurement, to observe them closely. EIA is not always accompanied by a wheeze and severe air-flow limitation can often result in a 'silent chest'.

Spontaneous recovery within 60 minutes normally occurs followng mild EIA. However, moderate to severe EIA frequently requires rescue medication with a β_2-adrenoceptor agonist (for details, see below). The physical discomfort associated with exercise often discourages asthmatics from exercising. Prescribing treatment to prevent EIA, rather than treatment to reverse an attack, can demonstrate to the patient that exercise can be a pleasurable event, not necessarily causing an attack of asthma.

EIA is followed by a period of refractoriness (Edmunds *et al.*, 1978; Schoeffel *et al.*, 1980) and approximately 50% of asthmatics will be protected from the effects of exercise for 2–3 hours. The mechanism of this appears to involve the direct or indirect effects of prostaglandins released in response to exercise (O'Byrne & Jones, 1986; Margolskee *et al.*, 1988; Wilson *et al.*, 1994).

EIA may be enhanced in some asthmatics when they are exposed to environmental pollutants such as nitrogen dioxide (Bauer *et al.*, 1986) and sulphur dioxide (Lin *et al.*, 1985). However, short-term (1 hour) exposure to ozone (Weymer *et al.*, 1994) or tobacco smoke (Magnussen *et al.*, 1993) appears to have no effect on EIA. In sensitized asthmatics, EIA is more severe during the pollen season and, for some, this may be the only time it occurs (Karjalainen *et al.*, 1989). However, a single exposure to an allergen in a laboratory (Boulet *et al.*, 1992) failed to demonstrate enhancement of EIA 48 hours later. Cold-air exposure can

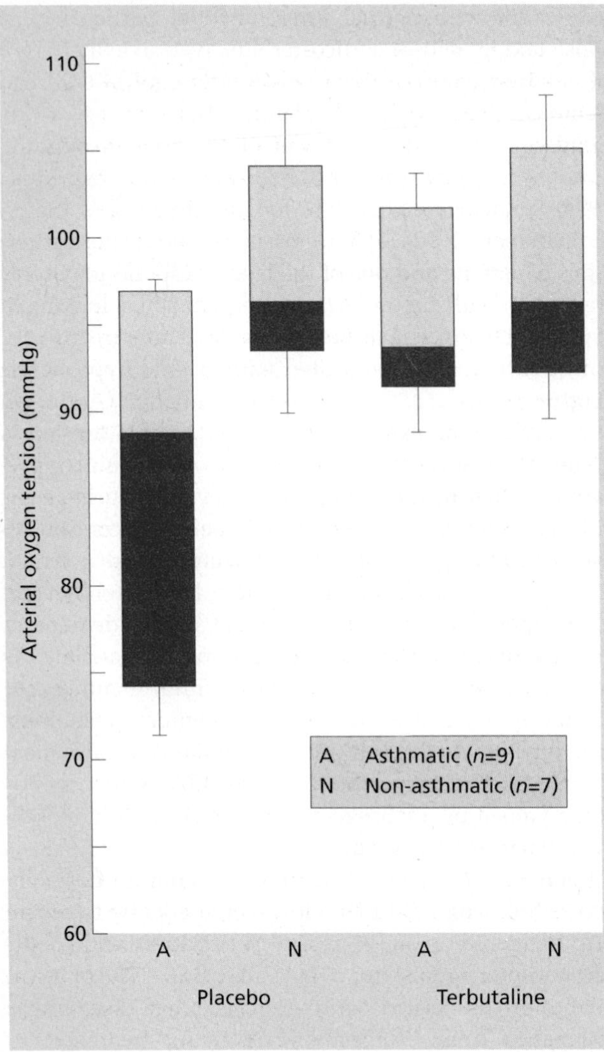

Fig. 39.2 The mean value ± 1 standard error of mean (SEM) for arterial oxygen tension (Pa_{O_2}) at rest (top of closed bar), during exercise (light green part of bar) and the lowest after cycling exercise (dark green part of bar), in nine asthmatic and seven healthy adults after placebo and after 1250 μg of terbutaline sulphate. The results demonstrate hypoxaemia after exercise with placebo in the asthmatic, but not the healthy subjects, and normalization of the arterial oxygen in the asthmatic subjects when exercise was performed in the presence of terbutaline.

also bring on EIA or make it more severe (Deal *et al.*, 1979). By far the most important determinant of severity of EIA, however, is not the temperature but the water content of the inspired air (Anderson *et al.*, 1982; Hahn *et al.*, 1984). The absolute water content air can hold decreases with temperature and subfreezing air is always 'dry'. EIA can occur in hot dry climates but is not often found in hot humid climates.

Identifying EIA in the general population

In field studies of the general population, the prevalence of EIA has been reported to be between < 1% and 18.9% (Burr *et al.*, 1974, 1989; Clough *et al.*, 1991; Keeley *et al.*, 1991; Backer & Ulrik, 1992; Auerbach *et al.*, 1993; Bardagi *et al.*, 1993; Nicolai *et al.*, 1993; O'Donnell *et al.*, 1993; Haby *et al.*, 1995). The prevalence has increased in the last 20 years in the same geographical area (Burr *et al.*, 1989) and is higher in some countries than in others (Barry *et al.*, 1991). It is more common in urban than in rural populations (Keeley *et al.*, 1991) and in developed countries and obese children (Kaplan & Montana, 1993).

EIA is now such a common problem that cheap means of detection are needed outside the health care system. This has been achieved successfully by the development of excellent protocols for identifying EIA in schoolchildren under field conditions (Haby *et al.*, 1994). When applied to a group of 802 Australian schoolchildren, 152 (18.9%) were found to have EIA defined as a fall in FEV_1 greater than 15%. Forty per cent of this group had never been given a diagnosis of asthma! Similarly, 50% of the positive responders to cold-air hyperventilation or exercise reported by Weiss *et al.* (1984) and Backer & Ulrik (1992) did not have a diagnosis of asthma.

These studies also demonstrated clearly that EIA can occur in persons who are non-responsive to pharmacological agents (Backer & Ulrik, 1992; Haby *et al.*, 1995) (Fig. 39.3). These important observations bring into question the use of pharmacological challenges to rule out airway responsiveness in recruits for the defence forces and other professions where EIA would be potentially hazardous on the job. Responsiveness to exercise but not to pharmacological agents comes as a surprise, because it is rarely the case in patients referred by doctors to lung function laboratories for testing. Thus, when assessing persons from the general population for bronchial responsiveness, it would seem appropriate to request both an indirect provocation test (exercise, hyperventilation, hyperosmolar saline, adenosine, distilled water) and a direct (histamine, methacholine) challenge to be carried out on separate days. With this approach to assessment, the presence of abnormal bronchial responsiveness is unlikely to be missed (Eliasson *et al.*, 1991). As indirect challenge tests are known to be more specific for detecting current asthma and differentiating this from chronic lung disease (Godfrey *et al.*, 1991), the additional information may determine whether treatment is required.

Identifying EIA in known asthmatic patients

In known asthmatic patients, a laboratory evaluation of EIA can be useful to assess severity, the effects of preven-

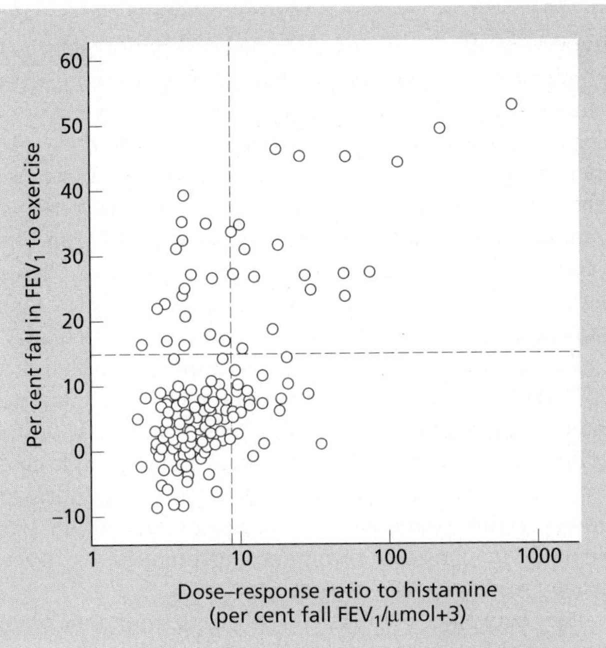

Fig. 39.3 Values for the % fall after running exercise in relation to the dose–response ratio to inhaled histamine in a group of schoolchildren. The data points above the horizontal line represent an abnormal response to exercise, and data points to the right of the vertical line represent an abnormal response to histamine. Thirty-eight children reacted to one challenge and not the other. Eighteen responded to exercise but not histamine (top left-hand quarter). (From Haby *et al.*, 1995.)

tive therapy given acutely, the duration of protection of a drug, the existence of a refractory period and the effects of long-term treatment with aerosol corticosteroids. Before referring patients for exercise tests, the medical practitioner should be aware of general guidelines for safety (Eggleston *et al.*, 1979) and screen patients suspected of having cardiovascular disease or those who may have risk factors for exercise-induced cardiac arrythmias.

The patient should be advised to withhold medications that could affect the test, as follows: antihistamines for 48 hours; sustained-release oral bronchodilators for 24 hours; and for ordinary-release preparations for 12 hours. Patients should not take sodium cromoglycate or nedocromil sodium or short-acting aerosol β_2-adrenoceptor agonists (isoprenaline, salbutamol, terbutaline, ephedrine, rimiterol) for 6 hours. They should not have taken the long-acting β_2-adrenoceptor agonists (salmeterol, formoterol) for 24 hours. Corticosteroids, either aerosol or oral, are usually withheld the morning of the study. It is best to avoid caffeine-containing drinks on the day of the study. The patient to be tested should have an FEV_1 of 75% or more of her/his normal predicted value and be able to perform spirometry reproducibly.

Identifying EIA in the laboratory

EIA is best measured by recording changes in the FEV_1 (see Fig. 39.1). There are also advantages to recording other parameters of the flow–volume curve, particularly the FEF_{25-75}, which is the flow through the mid-portion of the vital capacity (Cropp, 1979; Custovic *et al.*, 1994). As many patients have their own peak flow meters, they also like to know their peak flow rate, but FEV_1 is best and its measurement should be mandatory. The cheap and portable FEV_1 meters (Meter, Sonadyne USA, Micromedical Kent, UK) make this measurement easier to obtain than in the past.

Most accredited laboratories will have a recognized standard protocol for provoking EIA. However, it is important for the referring doctor to be assured by the laboratory that due diligence has been given to the factors that determine presence and severity of EIA (Silverman & Anderson, 1972). This becomes particularly important if the test for EIA is negative. For example, it is mandatory that a patient should not have had medications for the required time before exercise and that more than 3 hours should have passed since exercise was last performed. Information provided by the laboratory should include the intensity and duration for which the exercise was performed, the heart rate and ventilation this induced and the temperature and water content of the inspired air (< 10 mg H_2O/l, i.e. 50% relative humidity (RH) at 20°C). Compressed air which is dry is the most practical inspired air condition and is suitable for most assessments. Any enhancement of EIA that may be observed with inspiring air of subfreezing temperature can usually be observed by increasing the duration or intensity of exercise while breathing dry air of room temperature.

Different types of exercise can be used to raise the ventilation to the appropriate level, i.e. 50 ± 10% of the predicted maximum voluntary ventilation ($FEV_1 \times 35$). Bicycle exercise is commonly used, as it is safe and it is easy to measure ventilation and heart rate while cycling. Running at high speeds on a treadmill is not always practical or safe and it is difficult to make measurements of exercise intensity during running exercise. As cycling may cause the ventilation to increase more slowly than running, it is often necessary to increase the duration of cycling exercise. The ventilation level of 50% maximum voluntary ventilation (MVV) should be sustained for at least 4 minutes and preferably longer. Some laboratories only use heart rate to monitor intensity of exercise. However, in order to exclude a diagnosis of EIA, a measure of ventilation is required to ensure that the appropriate level is reached and sustained.

Quantifying the response

EIA has been traditionally expressed as the % fall in FEV_1 or PEF. The % fall index is calculated as follows:

$$\% \text{ fall } FEV_1/PEF = \frac{\begin{array}{c}100 \times \text{pre-exercise } FEV_1/PEF \\ - \text{lowest } FEV_1/PEF \text{ in} \\ 20 \text{ minutes after exercise}\end{array}}{\text{Pre-exercise } FEV_1/PEF}$$

The times for measurements have traditionally been 3, 5, 7, 10 and 15 minutes after exercise, but recent reports suggest the time should be increased to 20 or even 30 minutes (Brudno *et al.*, 1994). EIA is considered to be mild if there is a 10–25% fall in FEV_1 or PEF, moderate for 25.1–50% and severe if it causes a greater than 50% fall. In addition to the % fall index, the pre-exercise FEV_1 and the lowest FEV_1 recorded after exercise should be reported and expressed as a percentage of the predicted normal value (Fig. 39.1). Some investigators consider that it is important to use the maximum expiratory flow–volume curve to assess EIA (Haas *et al.*, 1993). A fall in FEF_{25-75} of >26% is also abnormal and in some cases this index detects EIA when the fall in EFV_1 is not abnormal (Custovic *et al.*, 1994). Unfortunately, the measurement of FEF_{25-75} is more variable than FEV_1 and its accurate measurement is dependent on a maximal forced expiration to residual volume. Such a manoeuvre may be difficult to perform on multiple occasions after exercise. However, we recommend the inclusion of FEF_{25-75} when assessing competitive athletes, the reason being that small reductions in this parameter will reduce the maximum flow that can be achieved during exercise, with consequent effects on performance. We also measure FEF_{25-75} in those intending to scuba dive, as a reduced value is more likely to be associated with gas trapping (an increase in residual volume).

When a measurement of FEV_1 is made after a bronchodilator at the end of exercise, a lability index can be calculated to express bronchial responsiveness. The lability is the difference between the highest value (after bronchodilator) and the lowest value after exercise, expressed as a percentage of the predicted value. A value of 25% or more is abnormal (Jones *et al.*, 1962). Although they do occur, responses following EIA (Iikura *et al.*, 1985; Speelberg *et al.*, 1989), are relatively uncommon (Karjalainen, 1991). Thus, there seems to be no need to follow subjects for longer than recovery to baseline lung function.

Surrogate challenges to identify EIA

Isocapnic or eucapnic hyperventilation with dry air is an excellent test for identifying EIA (Latimer *et al.*, 1983; Zach *et al.*, 1984; Phillips *et al.*, 1985; Smith *et al.*, 1988; Nicolai *et al.*, 1993). There are some definite advantages in using hyperventilation, in that a dose–response curve is obtained with a stepwise challenge and it is a more sensitive challenge test than exercise. Further, hyperventilation is quieter to perform in a laboratory setting and the equipment needed is less costly than that required for exercise. The challenge requires the person to voluntarily hyperventilate a dry gas containing 4.9% CO_2, 21% O_2 and the balance N_2. The level of ventilation is usually increased progressively. Initially the person hyperventilates for 3 minutes at 30% MVV, followed by a measurement of FEV_1 3 minutes later; this is followed by 3 minutes ventilating at 60% MVV, and a further measurement of FEV_1 3 minutes later; a final 3 minutes at MVV is performed if the test is still negative. An alternative protocol using a single challenge for 6 minutes at 60% MVV can be performed; however, this protocol should be used with caution, particularly in clinically recognized asthmatics, as severe airway narrowing can occur.

The eucapnic voluntary hyperventilation challenge appears to be very appropriate for excluding a diagnosis of EIA. The reason for this is that the level of ventilation achieved voluntarily is much higher than the level that can be achieved during exercise. Thus, for élite athletes, the high ventilation rates achieved during vigorous exercise are more likely to be reached during a hyperventilation test than they are performing an exercise on a laboratory ergometer for which the athlete may not be 'trained'. Hyperventilation is also useful for investigating the modifying effects of drugs and for determining the ventilation level below which a subject may exercise and not suffer EIA. Hyperventilation is, however, a very potent challenge and some drugs have been found to be ineffective whereas they do protect against EIA when given in the same dose (Wiebicke *et al.*, 1988). Further, hyperventilation may not necessarily simulate the environment or the physiology in which the patient gets EIA. The high cardiac output and sympathetic drive are absent during hyperventilation. These missing factors may serve to modify the severity of EIA and the refractoriness that follows.

The severity of the airway response to hyperventilation can be expressed in different ways. Probably the most useful index for athletes and those practitioners who are knowledgeable about ventilation rates and intensity of exercise is the ventilation rate required to provoke a 10, 15 and 20% fall in FEV_1 (PVE_{10}, PVE_{15}, PVE_{20}) (Fig. 39.4). An alternative way is to consider the % fall in FEV_1 after the three levels of ventilation. If it is 10–20% after MVV, it is mild, after 60% predicted MVV it is moderate, and after 30% prediced MVV it is severe. If the value of a greater than 20% fall in FEV_1 is achieved at the lower levels of ventilation, it is not necessary to proceed with the challenge. For the evaluation of drug therapy, however, it

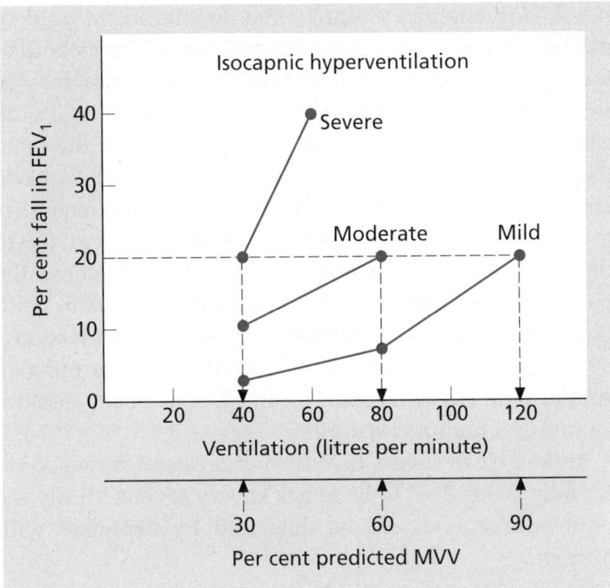

Fig. 39.4 Fall in FEV_1 expressed as a percentage of the baseline value, in relation to the ventilation rate, and the ventilation rate expressed as a percentage of the predicted maximum voluntary ventilation ($FEV_1 \times 35$). The PVE_{20} is shown for three persons, one with severe, one with moderate and one with mild bronchial responsiveness to breathing dry air (4.9% CO_2, 21% O_2, balance N_2). A fall in FEV_1 greater than 10% is usually regarded as abnormal, so that the PVE_{10} and the PVE_{15} can also be used to express severity.

is useful to document several points on the dose–response curve.

Challenge with hyperosmolar saline

In the quest to identify the mechanism whereby the evaporative water loss of hyperpnoea provoked airway narrowing, it was observed that asthmatic patients with EIA or hyperventilation-induced asthma were similarly sensitive to inhaling wet aerosols of 3.6% and 4.5% sodium chloride (Kivity *et al.*, 1986; Smith & Anderson, 1986, 1989a, 1990; Belcher *et al.*, 1989).

Thus, a standard challenge using 4.5% saline (Rodwell *et al.*, 1993; Sterk *et al.*, 1993) can be used as a surrogate for exercise. It is particularly useful for assessing the modifying effects of drugs given acutely (sodium cromoglycate, nedocromil sodium, β_2-adrenoceptor agonists) or chronically (aerosol corticosteroids) (Rodwell *et al.*, 1992a,b; Anderson *et al.*, 1994). Bronchial provocation using 4.5% saline is frequently requested to assess suitability for recreational or professional diving with self-contained underwater breathing apparatus (scuba). We have found that a positive response usually results in a voluntary abstention from scuba diving.

It has been shown that persons who have a 15% or more reduction in FEV_1 after inhaling 20 ml of 4.5% saline over 12–15 minutes are also likely to have EIA (Kivity *et al.*, 1986; Smith & Anderson, 1986, 1989, 1990; Belcher *et al.*, 1989). There have been some exceptions to this in field studies in persons with mild asthma (Riedler *et al.*, 1995), but, in general, sensitivity to 4.5% saline indicates that the person has the potential to have an attack of asthma provoked by exercise or hyperventilation. Thus, a positive test to hyperosmolar saline should lead to advice with regard to prevention and treatment of EIA. The response to 4.5% saline is said to be mild when the dose causing a fall of 15% (PD_{15}) is greater than 6 ml, 2.1–6.0 ml moderate and <2 ml severe. As the aerosol delivery is ~1.5 ml/minute, this can be a faster challenge to perform than exercise or hyperventilation when the response is positive, although it takes the same time or more when there is no response and the full dose of 22 ml needs to be delivered.

EIA as a marker for current asthma prevalence

Epidemiologists have expressed concern about the low sensitivity of exercise and hyperosmolar saline for detecting known asthmatics (Terblanche & Stewart, 1990), although it is generally acknowledged that the specificity of these challenges is >93% (Terblanche & Stewart, 1990; Haby *et al.*, 1995). The reason for the low sensitivity in part relates to the fact that many investigators have given insufficient attention to the factors that determine the presence and severity of EIA, e.g. weather conditions, intensity and duration of exercise, etc. Another reason for low sensitivity is the inclusion, in the statistical analysis, of negative tests in known asthmatics: (i) who have not been required, by the protocol, to refrain from taking acute preventive medication before the exercise challenge (Bardagi *et al.*, 1993); and (ii) whose potential for EIA has been reduced by chronic treatment with aerosol corticosteroids (Riedler *et al.*, 1995). The hyperresponsiveness provoked by hyperpnoea of dry air and by aerosols of hyperosmolar saline is markedly reduced and, in 50% of cases, is abolished in patients with mild to moderate asthma who are given 8 weeks' treatment with steroids (Anderson *et al.*, 1994; Waalkens *et al.*, 1993). Thus, 'failure' to detect asthma in treated subjects under an epidemiological survey using exercise or salt challenges leads to a low sensitivity of the test. This is misleading in that the 'failure' reflects good treatment and control of the person's asthma and demonstrates the effectivess of treatment to reduce responsiveness to these naturally occurring provocative stimuli. An analogy can be made to the use of insulin to control blood-sugar levels in diabetics. The diagnosis of diabetes would not be excluded by epidemiologists because the subject was taking insulin.

The other problem relates to specificity, i.e. the number of persons with a negative response as a percentage of those predicted to be negative by their history. In epidemiological terms, a positive test in a person with a negaive history reduces specificity. There are good reasons why a person will not report EIA spontaneously. They may simply have avoided vigorous exercise or they do not perceive their EIA, or they do not consider the breathlessness associated with vigorous exercise as an abnormal sign or symptom. These reasons provide a good argument for objective testing to detect prevalence of EIA. The likely medical outcome for an asymptomatic person with an abnormal fall in FEV_1 in response to exercise is treatment for asthma. It would be reasonable to think about positive responses to hyperpnoea and salt as being highly predictive of current asthma and negative responses as being consistent with normality or asthma of insufficient severity to require any treatment.

Airway narrowing provoked by hyperpnoea or hyperosmolar saline would seem to be a more acceptable criterion for a diagnosis of current asthma than a positive response to a pharmacological challenge. The reason for this relates to the low specificity of pharmacological challenges for identifying current asthma (Woolcock *et al.*, 1987; Cockcroft *et al.*, 1992; Haby *et al.*, 1995). Further, pharmacological challenges are not as useful as previously thought for detecting bronchial hyperresponsiveness in the general population (Backer *et al.*, 1991; Cockcroft *et al.*, 1992; Haby *et al.*, 1995). A re-evaluation of current gold standards for recognition of asthma is urgently required. For example, Backer and Ulrik (1992) and Haby *et al.* (1995) found children sensitive to exercise but not to histamine. There are cases of EIA in methacholine-negative adults being recruited for the US defence forces (O'Donnell & Fling, 1993). High specificity for the diagnosis of asthma is of vital importance to the study of the genetics of the disease.

The results of epidemiological studies clearly demonstrate that the prevalence of EIA has increased over the last 15 years (Burr *et al.*, 1989) and is now high enough to suggest that schools should have some protocol to detect EIA. It would seem appropriate to advise that those who are found to be positive should be carefully evaluated for other signs, symptoms or markers of asthma.

Treatment of EIA

A person should be advised to stop exercising immediately should they feel an attack of asthma coming on. From laboratory tests, it can be predicted that the attack will worsen on cessation of exercise, usually within the first 5 minutes after exercise but often as late as 10 minutes and in some unusual cases even later (Brudno *et al.*, 1994).

Under most circumstances, an attack of asthma provoked by exercise can be quickly reversed by inhaling a β_2-adrenoceptor agonist (terbutaline, salbutamol, rimiterol, isoprenaline, orciprenaline, fenoterol). In mild or moderate EIA, two or three inhalations of a bronchodilator with 1 to 2 minutes separating each inhalation may be required. It is best if there is a 10-second breath-hold with each inhalation of the drug. This ensures that the drug particles settle in the airways. It is not necessary to take a large inhalation, as the volume of the airways, including the mouth, is less than 400 ml. Spacing devices (Nebuhaler, Volumatic, Fisonair) are also useful because the patient requires less co-ordination and can breathe with tidal respiration. When terbutaline has been administered by a pressurized metered dose inhaler or by a Turbuhaler, similar patterns of recovery from EIA have been demonstrated (Svenonius *et al.*, 1994).

In the case of severe EIA, further doses of bronchodilator may be needed. If the attack is very severe, ideally the bronchodilator should be delivered by nebulizer with oxygen.

Prevention of EIA

Pharmacological methods

For 90% of patients with asthma, EIA may be prevented by administering, as an aerosol, a β_2-adrenoceptor agonist or sodium cromoglycate (or nedocromil sodium) either alone or in combination immediately before exercise (Figs 39.5, 39.6 & 39.7) (Anderson *et al.*, 1976, 1979, 1991; Latimer *et al.*, 1983; Tullet *et al.*, 1985; Konig *et al.*, 1987; Anderson, 1988; Woolley *et al.*, 1990; Albazzaz *et al.*, 1992; Speelberg *et al.*, 1992; Comis *et al.*, 1993). While most studies have been carried out in young adults and children, there is nothing contrary to suggest that EIA documented in an asymptomatic person or the elderly would not be prevented by the same treatment.

If the person has air-flow limitation before exercise, the use of a β_2-adrenoceptor agonist is mandatory if maximal exercise performance is to be achieved. If the air-flow limitation is not reversed and the lung function is less than 75% of the predicted value, it is probably unwise for vigorous exercise to be performed. For such patients, a trial of aerosol corticosteroids is recommended. For persons who have well-controlled asthma, few symptoms and good pre-exercise lung function, sodium cromoglycate in a dose of 10–20 mg or nedocromil sodium 4–8 mg may be all that is required to prevent EIA. However, a quick-acting β_2-adrenoceptor agonist should always be available for rescue if EIA occurs unexpectedly. In patients with moderately severe EIA, we recommend a trial with aerosol corticosteroids. If severe EIA still occurs, we recommend the use of β_2-adrenoceptor agonist and sodium cromoglycate/nedocromil sodium in combination and, if this fails, we recommend that the dose of cromoglycate or nedocromil sodium be doubled. Aerosol corticosteroids

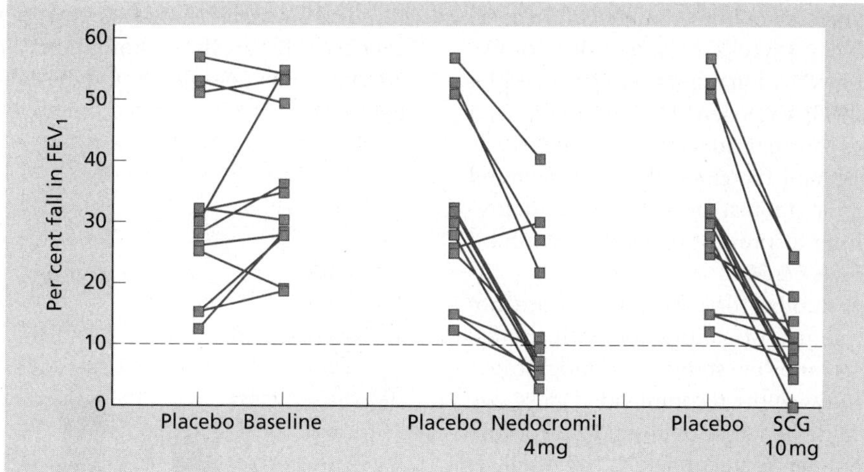

Fig. 39.5 Mean value ± 1 standard error of mean (SEM) for FEV_1 measured before and after 6 minutes of running exercise (22–25°C, 35–45% relative humidity) in a group of 12 children who inhaled either 10 mg of sodium cromoglycate, 4 mg of nedocromil sodium or the placebo 30 minutes before exercise, on 3 separate days. The children had withdrawn their steroids 1 week before the study and no β_2-adrenoceptor agonist had been taken for 12 hours.

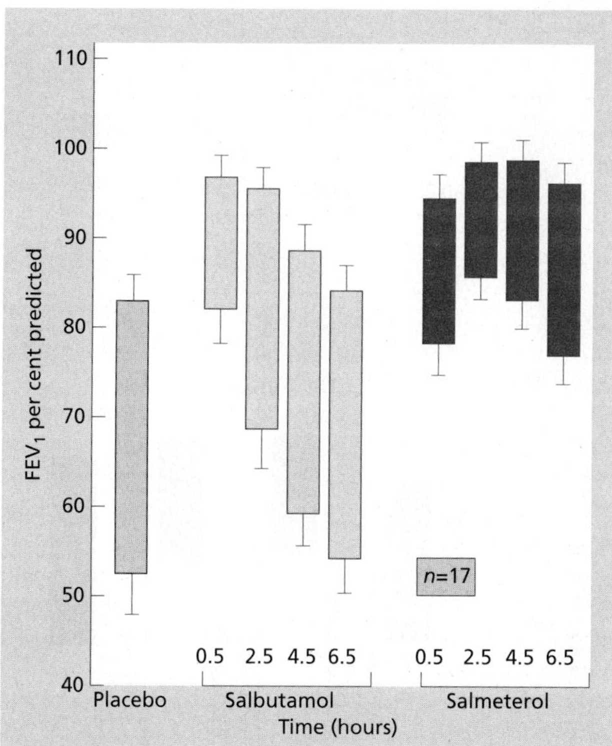

Fig. 39.6 The mean value ± 1 standard error of mean (SEM) for the pre-exercise value for FEV_1 and the lowest value after exercise, expressed as a percentage of the predicted value, in 17 asthmatic adults exercising on a bicycle ergometer while breathing compressed air at 50% of maximum voluntary ventilation. The optimal effect of 200 µg of salbutamol was observed at 0.5 hours and for 50 µg of salmeterol at 2.5 hours after administration as an aerosol. Salmeterol had a significantly longer effect compared with salbutamol. (Data redrawn from Anderson *et al.*, 1991.)

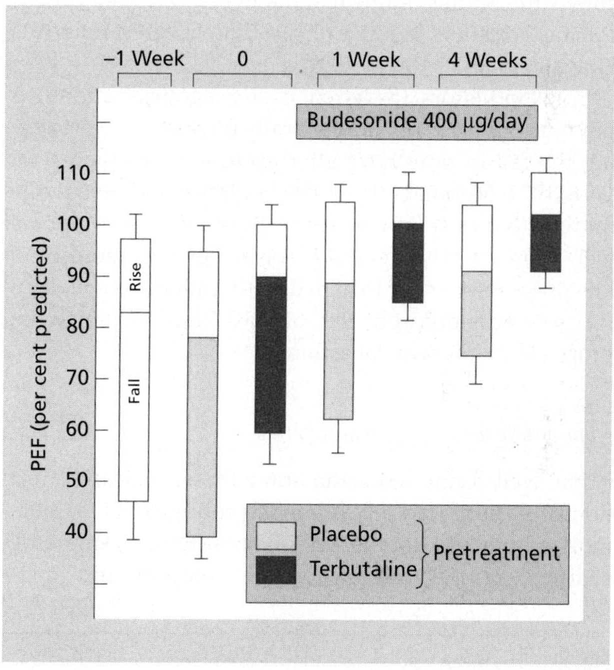

Fig. 39.7 The mean value ± 1 standard error of mean (SEM) for peak flow measured at rest (central bar), during exercise (top of bar) and lowest after running exercise (bottom of bar) in 14 asthmatic children before and during treatment with 400 µg of budesonide daily. The effect of a very small dose of terbutaline sulphate (32.5 µg) and its placebo is shown. The introduction of steroids reduced the severity of EIA and improved the inhibitory effect of terbutaline sulphate.

do not prevent EIA when taken immediately before exercise. When taken daily for 4 weeks, they do reduce or minimize the amount of medication required to prevent EIA (Henriksen & Dahl, 1983; Vathenen *et al.*, 1991). Thus, a person who achieves normal function on steroids is unlikely to need more than the clinically recommended dose of β_2-adrenoceptor agonist or sodium cromoglycate/nedocromil sodium to prevent or markedly inhibit his/her EIA (Figs 39.5, 39.7 & 39.8).

For the very small number of patients who are not controlled with chronic use of steroids or with the β_2-adrenoceptor agonists and/or sodium cromoglycate/nedocromil sodium in twice the recommended dose, we add ipratropium bromide in a dose of 80 μg. Ipratropium bromide is an anticholinergic agent which, by itself, is ineffective in preventing EIA in the majority of subjects (Anderson, 1985; Poppius *et al.*, 1986). For reasons as yet unknown, it can work well in combination with other drugs in people with moderate (Smith *et al.*, 1988) and severe EIA. Another approach to the control of severe EIA is to prescribe, in addition to the aerosol therapy described above, the antihistamine teldane to be taken in a dose of 120 mg 2–3 hours before exercise (Patel, 1984; Finnerty & Holgate, 1990).

Bronchodilators (β_2-adrenoceptor agonists and theophylline) given orally are generally ineffective in preventing the fall in flow rates after exercise (Anderson *et al.*, 1976, 1979; Merland *et al.*, 1988; Fuglsang *et al.*, 1993). The finding that very low doses of β_2-adrenoceptor agonist were more effective against EIA when given as aerosols in low doses than orally in high doses (Anderson *et al.*, 1976) focused attention on the airways for administering prophylactic therapy for asthma.

Appropriate use of aerosol medication

In the well-controlled asthmatic with normal lung function, the short-acting β_2-adrenoceptor agonists (salbutamol, terbutaline, isoprenaline, metaproteronol, rimiterol), sodium cromoglycate/nedocromil sodium and ipratropium bromide should be taken immediately before exercise. If air-flow limitation is present, the β_2-adrenoceptor agonist should be taken 5 to 10 minutes before exercise. Sodium cromoglycate and nedocromil

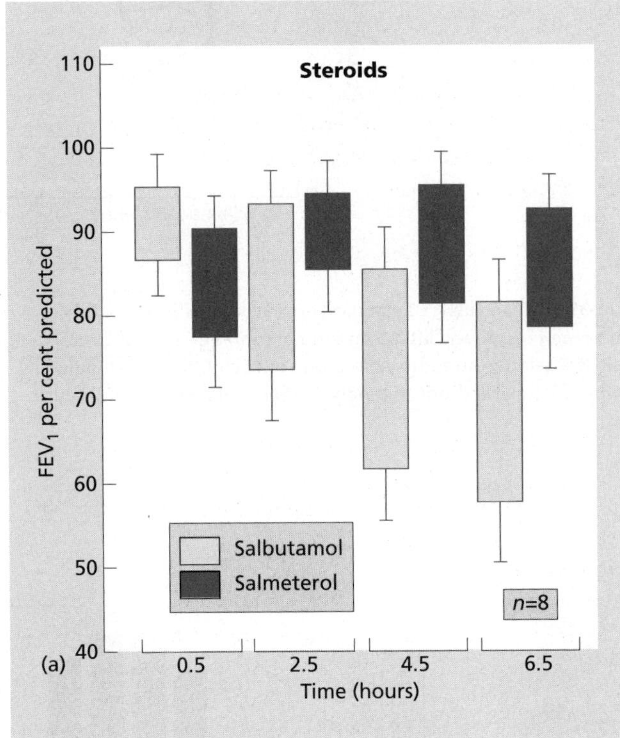

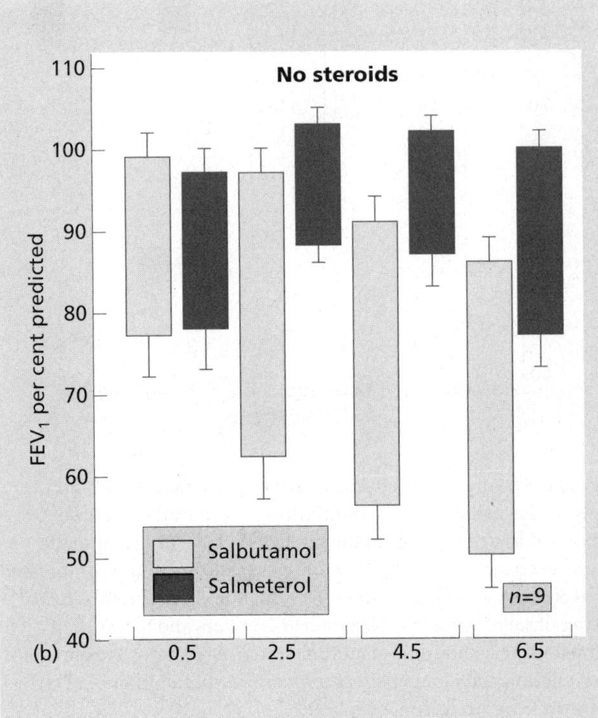

Fig. 39.8 The mean value ± 1 standard error of mean (SEM) for FEV_1 pre-exercise and the lowest value after exercise in steroid- and non-steroid-treated asthmatic subjects. Cycling exercise was performed for 8 minutes while breathing compressed air at a ventilation equivalent to 50% maximum voluntary ventilation. Salbutamol (200 μg) or salmeterol (50 μg) was given 0.5 hours before the first exercise test. The data show that, for salmeterol, the pre-exercise values for FEV_1 were high and the post-exercise values for FEV_1 were similar in the steroid and non-steroid group. In contrast, for the same subjects given salbutamol, the non-steroid group were not as well protected against EIA as the steroid group. The patients not taking steroids were better off using salmeterol to reduce the severity of EIA. No subjects had ever taken salmeterol before the study days.

sodium can be taken immediately before exercise, and no time is required for their protective action to take effect. The need to take drugs as close to performing exercise as possible relates to their short duration of action in preventing EIA (Patel & Wall, 1986; Konig *et al.*, 1987; Smith *et al.*, 1988; Woolley *et al.*, 1990; Anderson *et al.*, 1991). The duration of the protective effect of the β_2-adrenoceptor agonists is far less, by hours, than their bronchodilating effect (see Fig. 39.6). The reason for this may be that a higher concentration of the drug is needed to prevent EIA than is needed to induce bronchodilatation. The failure of the short-acting β_2-adrenoceptor agonists and sodium cromoglycate to protect for longer than 1–2 hours is probably due to their rapid clearance (Richards *et al.*, 1989; Schmekel *et al.*, 1992) from the airway by the bronchial circulation, which increases its flow during exercise.

It is this short duration of protection of drugs in EIA which has caused us to promote the use of sodium cromoglycate and nedocromil sodium in EIA. For persons who perform exercise many times in a day, e.g. children, it seems inadvisable to prescribe multiple uses of β_2-adrenoceptor agonists and they are probably best kept for rescue medication. No serious side-effects have been reported with multiple use of sodium cromoglycate (Kuzemko, 1989). Providing the person has normal lung function before exercise, 20 mg of sodium cromoglycate or 4 mg of nedocromil sodium, given by metered dose inhaler, EIA will be prevented in up to 60% of subjects. If this dose is doubled, it can improve to 80% (Schoeffel *et al.*, 1983; Tullet *et al.*, 1985; Patel & Wall, 1986; Albazzaz *et al.*, 1989).

Appropriate use of long-acting β_2-adrenoceptor agonists. The problem of short duration of protection has to some extent been overcome by the introduction of formoterol (McAlpine & Thomson, 1990; Patessio *et al.*, 1991; Henriksen *et al.*, 1992; Boner *et al.*, 1994) and more recently salmeterol (Anderson *et al.*, 1991; Green & Price, 1992; Newnham *et al.*, 1993). Both these drugs have been shown to protect against mild EIA (<25% fall) for up to 12 hours. We have found the time of protection with salmeterol to be shorter than this in adult asthmatics with moderate to severe EIA (Anderson *et al.*, 1991).

Some caution needs to be taken in prescribing these drugs in that the onset of the protective effect is slower than that of the short-acting β_2-adrenoceptor agonists. For the same reason, they are not recommended to be used as rescue medication, although in the absence of quick-acting β_2-adrenoceptor agonists they could be used. It is possible that using a combination of a long-acting β_2-adrenoceptor agonist with sodium cromoglycate or nedocromil sodium may result in day-long protection for some asthmatics.

It has been reported that twice-daily use of salmeterol (50 μg) over 4 weeks can lead to a reduction in its protective effect against EIA (Ramage *et al.*, 1994). This has important implications for the recommendation of use of this drug in EIA and more studies are urgently required to confirm or refute this finding.

Other drugs. Recently there have been a number of investigators who have shown that leukotriene antagonists given by inhalation, orally or intravenously are effective in inhibiting EIA (Israel *et al.*, 1990; Manning *et al.*, 1990; Finnerty *et al.*, 1992; Robuschi *et al.*, 1992; Makker *et al.*, 1993). The source of the leukotrienes involved in EIA is not known but presumably could include both mast cells and epithelial cells. At present, leukotriene antagonists are being used for research purposes but they should be kept in mind for trial in a patient in whom the standard therapy is failing.

There has been a research interest in identifying drugs that prevent EIA but are not used in the treatment of asthma. The objective of this research has been to obtain information regarding the mechanism of EIA, as opposed to an intention to prescribe. Thus, furosemide (Bianco *et al.*, 1988; Seidenberg *et al.*, 1992) and acetazolamide (O'Donnell *et al.*, 1992), but not amiloride (Rodwell *et al.*, 1993), have been shown to be very effective in reducing EIA. Heparin given by inhalation in a dose of 1000 units/kg has also been shown to be effective (Ahmed *et al.*, 1993). Other drugs that have a variable beneficial effect are: (i) the Ca^{2+} antagonists, and nifedipine in particular; (ii) the isorbide nitrates; and (iii) the antihistamines, particularly the non-sedating ones, taken in higher doses (summarized in Anderson, 1988a, 1993b).

The thromboxane receptor antagonists GR 32191 (Finnerty *et al.*, 1991) and BAY u 3405 (Magnussen *et al.*, 1992) have not been shown to be effective against EIA. Endogenously released opioids do not appear to be important, as naloxene and nalmefene are without effect on EIA.

Non-pharmacological methods to prevent EIA

There are a number of techniques that can be used to prevent EIA without recourse to the use of pharmacological agents. Some of these techniques are based on the knowledge that the stimulus to EIA is the loss of water from the airways. Thus, any intervention which reduces respiratory water loss or increases delivery of water to the airways may be expected to reduce the severity of EIA. EIA can be prevented or markedly reduced by inhaling air of alveolar conditions (34–37°C, 100% RH) (Chen & Horton, 1977; Strauss *et al.*, 1978; Anderson *et al.*, 1982). It was this very important observation that made investigators focus on the airway lumen being the site of the stimulus to EIA and on the mechanism being related to the effects of respiratory water loss (Anderson *et al.*, 1982; Anderson, 1984; Hahn *et al.*, 1984a; Eschenbacher & Sheppard, 1985). However, preventing heat and water loss from the airways by inhaling warm humid air during exercise is not very practical and could be dangerous, because the respiratory tract is a major route for heat loss in the body.

The knowledge that reducing respiratory water loss reduces the severity of EIA has led to the development and study of the effects of masks and mouthpieces that capture expired water and permit rebreathing (Eiken *et al.*, 1989; Nisar *et al.*, 1992). For example, one mask with low resistance at high flow rates will recover 42% of water at 16°C (Nisar *et al.*, 1992). In Australia we have found patients unwilling to use masks regularly or in public, but others report success in countries with colder climates.

Although simply breathing via the nose will reduce water loss and EIA, this may not be possible or even practical for many people. When the ventilation rate exceeds 35 l/minute, there is a natural tendency to switch from nose to mouth breathing because the resistance to breathing is less via the mouth. Breathing via the nose at high ventilation rates places a greater burden on the nasal mucosa to humidify the inspired air. This causes dehydration and can lead to nasal stuffiness from the release of mediators (Togias *et al.*, 1988; Anderson & Togias, 1994). The consequent increase in nasal resistance makes breathing by the nose impossible during exercise, even at very low levels of ventilation.

Physical training and EIA

Physical activity is often avoided by persons suffering EIA, and their exercise tolerance may be poor. With appropriate medication to prevent EIA, fitness can be improved in most asthmatics who do not exercise regularly. One study has shown that athletes with mild to moderate asthma can develop a high degree of endurance fitness and sustain a high percentage of their maximal oxygen uptake (Freeman *et al.*, 1990). There has been an increasing interest in the cardiopulmonary effects of physical training in asthmatic subjects (Cochrane & Clark, 1990; Varray *et al.*, 1993). These studies have shown a marked improvement in cardiovascular fitness in young asthmatics after aerobic training (Cochrane & Clark, 1990; Varray *et al.*, 1993). This improvement is associated with a reduction in ventilatory equivalent, that is, the amount of ventilation required per litre of oxygen consumption (Cochrane & Clark, 1990). A reduction in the ventilatory level is predicted to improve cardiac output and thus oxygen uptake in severe asthmatics who have reduced work performance at altitude (Varray *et al.*, 1993). As ventilation rate is a major determinant of the severity of EIA, it is concluded that a general increase in fitness reduces the threshould for developing EIA. However, fitness may not affect the severity of EIA if the person is tested at equivalent levels of ventilation before and after training.

While there is no argument with respect to the benefits of training on well-being, there is some controversy as to whether training *per se* reduces the severity of EIA. Some investigators have found no reduction in EIA after training programmes (Fig. 39.9) (Fitch *et al.*, 1976, 1986), even though there has been an improvement in maximum oxygen uptake (Bundgaard *et al.*, 1982). Others, however, have reported reduced severity of EIA after 6–24 weeks' training (Henriksen & Nielsen, 1983; Svenonius *et al.*,

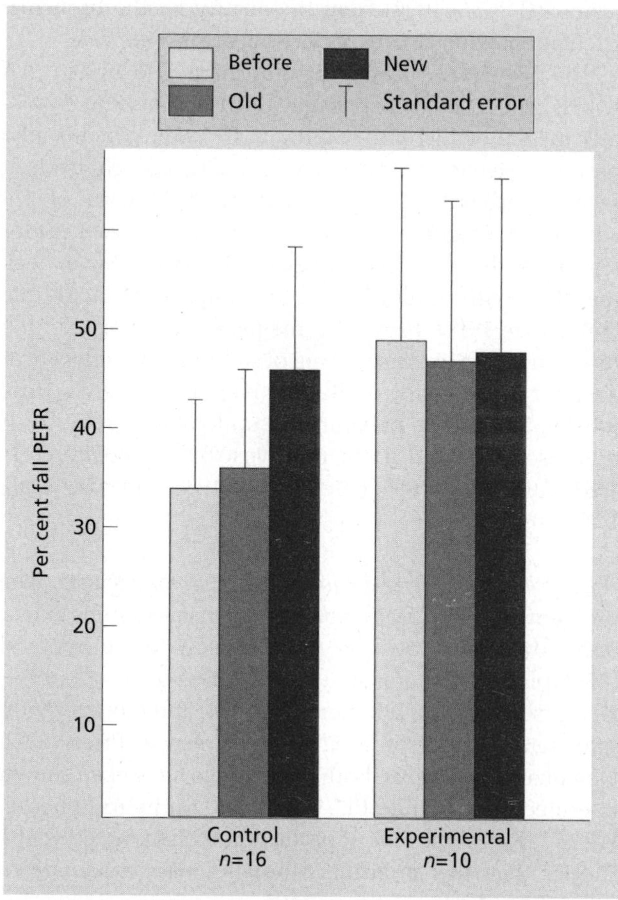

Fig. 39.9 Maximum reduction in PEFR, expressed as a percentage of the pre-exercise value in 16 children who acted as controls and 10 children who trained by running for a period of 1 hour, four times/week for 3 months. For assessment of EIA, exercise was performed by running for 8 minutes on a treadmill at 80% of the subject's previously measured maximum oxygen uptake (Before). For EIA tests after training, two levels of work were performed, one at 80% of the old maximal uptake (Old) and the second at 80% of the new maximal oxygen uptake (New). In the experimental group, there was no significant change in severity of EIA after training. (From Fitch *et al.*, 1986.)

1983; Haas *et al.*, 1987). The finding of a small, if any, reduction in EIA with training is consistent with the concept that respiratory water loss is the stimulus to EIA. It is not to be expected that respiratory water loss will be reduced with training unless the ventilation rate for the task is reduced.

Acupuncture

There are several reports on traditional acupuncture and EIA (Chow *et al.*, 1983; Fung *et al.*, 1986). In a study of 19 children, it was shown that both real and sham acupuncture, performed 20 minutes before exercise, reduced severity of EIA (Fung *et al.*, 1986). This approach to prevention of EIA would seem impractical for most sufferers. A study using laser acupuncture for 20 seconds at five sites commonly used for treatment of respiratory problems showed no effect on EIA severity (Morton *et al.*, 1993).

Using the refractory period

For a period of 1–2 hours following EIA, approximately 50% of asthmatics who spontaneously recover to their pre-exercise lung function will be refractory to the effects of an identical exercise task (Schoeffel *et al.*, 1980; Anderson, 1985) (Fig. 39.10). EIA is not necessary for refractoriness to develop (Henriksen *et al.*, 1981; Ben-Dov *et al.*, 1982; Wilson *et al.*, 1990; Johnston *et al.*, 1992), although this is not a universal finding. Severe EIA has been reported within 40 minutes of an identical exercise task which did not provoke asthma (Anderson *et al.*, 1979; Hahn *et al.*, 1985). It is of interest that the refractory period to hyperventilation is less predictable (Rakotasihanaka *et al.*, 1986; Rosenthal *et al.*, 1990).

Many persons who participate in competitive sport have recognized that they are refractory and choose to have their EIA 30–60 minutes before the 'real game' begins. The ability to become refractory is lost by taking non-steroidal anti-inflammatory agents and is well described following treatment with indomethacin for 3 days (O'Byrne *et al.*, 1986; Margolskee *et al.*, 1988; Wilson *et al.*, 1994). It has recently been proposed that exercise refractoriness is due to leukotriene-induced inhibitory prostaglandin release (Manning *et al.*, 1993).

There is cross-refractoriness between hyperosmolar saline and exercise (Belcher *et al.*, 1987) and sodium metabisulphite and exercise (Pavord *et al.*, 1994), but not between pharmacological challenges (methacholine, histamine) and exercise (Hahn *et al.*, 1984b; Magnussen *et al.*, 1986). Rather than using exercise to become refractory, a person may choose to conserve energy and provoke an attack of asthma by inhaling hyperosmolar saline.

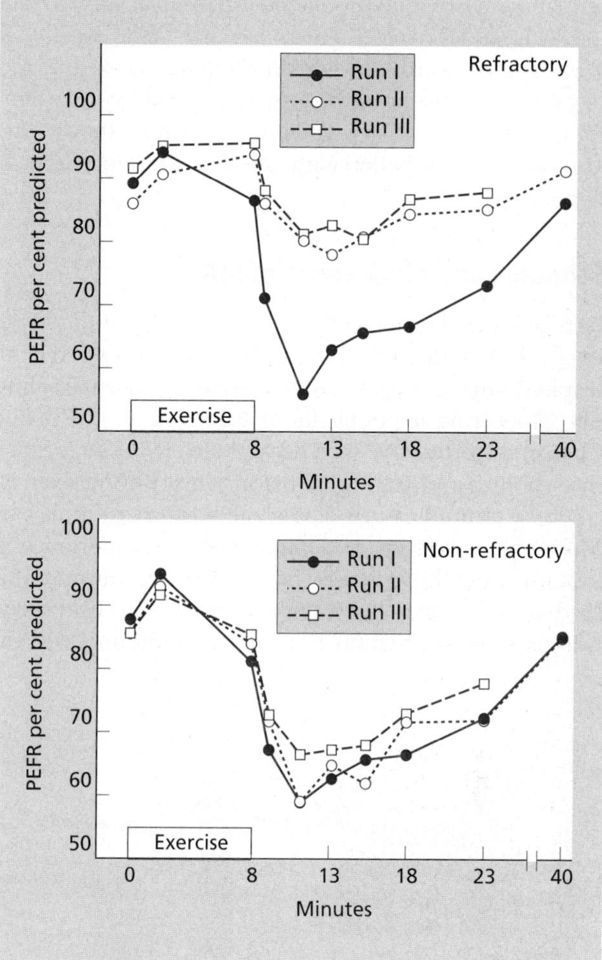

Fig. 39.10 Peak expiratory flow rate (PEFR) expressed as a percentage of the predicted normal value, before, during and after three exercise challenges in 16 asthmatic patients. A period of 40 minutes separated each challenge. Patients were selected on the basis of their recovery to within 10% of the pre-challenge lung function after each challenge. Eight patients were refractory after the initial challenge, although there was a small but reproducible fall after the second and third challenge. In the second group of eight patients, EIA was reproducible with each challenge. (From Anderson, 1988.)

Warm-up

There have been considerable differences reported over the effect of warm-up on severity of EIA. In some studies, no significant effect was found from either short-term or long-term warm-up (Morton *et al.*, 1979, 1982). However, in one study, it was found that multiple episodes of 30-second sprints performed 30 minutes before exercise could reduce the severity of EIA (Schnall & Landau, 1980). There has been renewed interest in this topic and a more recent study (Reiff *et al.*, 1989) has demonstrated a marked reduction in EIA with prolonged warm-up at submaximal load (Fig. 39.11).

Sprints or warm-ups are likely to increase the rate of delivery of water to the airway mucosa by increasing the bronchial blood flow. Thus, after warm-up the airways are able to cope better with the dehydrating effects of hyperpnoea.

Stimulus and mechanism of EIA

In 1976 Weinstein and colleagues reported that the severity of EIA could be reduced by conditioning the air inspired during exercise with an aerosol of normal saline. The pioneering experiments of Bar-Or *et al.* (1977) and Chen and Horton (1977) on heat loss led to the suggestion that cooling and drying of the airways during exercise could be stimuli to EIA. Later, the Boston group, led by McFadden, went on to demonstrate the importance of heat loss from the airways. They put forward the hypothesis that cooling of the airways, as a result of the heat lost in bringing the inspired air to alveolar conditions, was the stimulus leading to EIA (Deal *et al.*, 1979). They interpreted the beneficial effect of hot humid air in preventing EIA (Strauss *et al.*, 1979) to be due to a reduction in heat loss from the airways. An alternative to the cooling hypothesis was put forward by Anderson in 1984. This hypothesis acknowledged the importance of water loss from the airways and suggested that EIA was due to an increase in osmolarity of the periciliary fluid caused by the evaporation of water. The beneficial effect of inhaling hot humid air, it was claimed, came from preventing the osmotic change rather than a reduction in heat loss (Anderson, 1984).

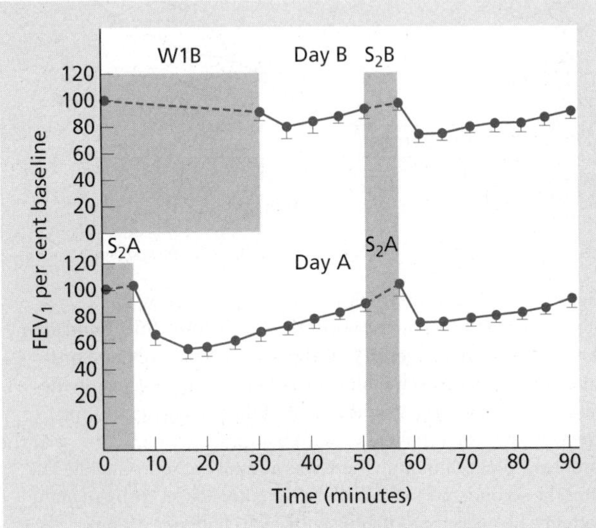

Fig. 39.11 Mean FEV$_1$, expressed as a percentage of the pre-exercise or baseline value, in a group of seven asthmatic subjects who performed four exercise tests on 2 separate days. On day A (bottom panel), the first exercise test was performed for 6 minutes at 6 km/hour up a 15% incline, and this workload provoked EIA. The second exercise test, about 40 minutes later, was performed at the same intensity, but the reduction in FEV$_1$ was less and the group demonstrated refractoriness to the repeated challenge. On day B (top panel), the first exercise test was used as a warm-up and was performed for 30 minutes (6 km/hour, 3% incline). This test did not provoke EIA. Twenty-five minutes later, a second challenge was performed at a similar intensity to that which provoked EIA on day A (6 km/hour, 15% incline). The subjects also demonstrated refractoriness to this challenge. The authors were able to conclude from these studies that warm-up exercise that does not provoke EIA may render a person refractory to EIA. (From Reiff *et al.*, 1989.)

Later, it was acknowledged by the proponents of the cooling hypothesis that a reduction in airway temperature *per se* did not account for EIA (McFadden *et al.*, 1986). The hypothesis put forward, in place of the cooling one, was rewarming of the airways by a reactive hyperaemia of the bronchial circulation (McFadden *et al.*, 1986). This was an important shift in thinking, as they proposed that the narrowing of the airways after exercise was not due to contraction of the bronchial smooth muscle. They suggested that the airway narrowing was a consequence of increased bronchial blood flow and oedema of the airway wall as a result of cooling and vasoconstriction.

The cooling and rewarming hypothesis has been evaluated and discussed in detail elsewhere (Anderson & Daviskas, 1989, 1993). Based on the experimental evidence, Anderson & Daviskas (1989, 1993) concluded that neither cooling and vasoconstriction nor rapid rewarming is a prerequisite for EIA. It was further concluded that an abnormal temperature gradient is not needed for EIA to occur and rapid rewarming of the airways does not necessarily enhance EIA (Smith *et al.*, 1989). These conclusions have recently been supported by other investigators (Argyros *et al.*, 1993).

Further, the experimental evidence in both animals (Baile *et al.*, 1987; Parsons *et al.*, 1989) and humans (Agostoni *et al.*, 1990) demonstrates that there is an increase in bronchial blood flow, rather than a decrease, in response to hyperpnoea with dry air. There is strong evidence from studies in animals to support the concept that the increase in blood flow is in response to a hyperosmotic stimulus and that this is mediated by nitric oxide (Deffebach *et al.*, 1989; Smith *et al.*, 1993). In addition to increasing flow, hyperosmolarity has been shown to increase microvascular permeability (Umeno *et al.*, 1990). It is in this area that the two seemingly opposing hypotheses for EIA may come together (Anderson & Daviskas, 1992). Thus, there is the potential for the vasculature to be involved in the events that accompany exercise, but they occur as a consequence of an osmotic stimulus rather than a cooling stimulus. This concept would serve to explain many of the inconsistencies that arise from the experimental data relating to the cooling/rewarming hypothesis.

The concept of dehydration of the airways is in keeping with the need to humidify the inspired air when patients are intubated and mechanically ventilated. Bypassing the upper airways by intubation results in a loss of water below the pharynx equivalent to the amount which would be lost breathing air of temperate conditions via the mouth at approximately 60 l/minute. Even though the net loss of water per litre of air from the intrathoracic airways has been calculated to be 3 mg or less, at high ventilation rates (40–100 l/minute) the small volume of fluid on the airway surface could be evaporated in minutes. Mathematical models, based on experimental data for intra-airway temperature, confirm the possibility that the airways can become dehydrated unless the replacement of water is instantaneous (Daviskas *et al.*, 1990, 1991), and this is unlikely (Willumsen *et al.*, 1994). The finding of a reduction in mucociliary clearance during hyperpnoea with dry air is also consistent with the concept that the periciliary fluid layer may be compromised by evaporative water loss (Daviskas *et al.*, 1995). The reason for this may relate to the increase in thickness of the basement membrane that occurs in asthmatics (Dukanovic *et al.*, 1992; Jeffrey *et al.*, 1992). The small increase in thickness of this membrane would increase the distance that water needs to travel to the epithelium.

There have not been any measurements of osmolarity in the lower airways before, during or after exercise, although increases in osmolarity have been measured after dry-air challenge in the nose (Togias *et al.*, 1988). It is hard to conceive of measuring accurately the osmolarity of a fluid layer that is predicted to be < 0.8 ml and covers 320 cm (Anderson, 1992)! Although it is technically possible to make measurements of the osmolarity of the airway surface liquid (Jorris *et al.*, 1993), it is unlikely that these will be accurate if the airways are instrumented before hyperpnoea with dry air.

Measurements of expired water concentration have shown that, during exercise, asthmatics are less able to cope with heat stress than non-asthmatics (Tabka *et al.*, 1988). The lower values for expired water concentration measured during recovery compared with normal subjects support the suggestion that the airways of asthmatics are dehydrated and hyperosmolar.

It is also known that, subsequent to the reduction in mucociliary clearance during hyperpnoea with dry air, there is an increase in clearance (Daviskas *et al.*, 1995). This increase is also consistent with hyperosmolarity of the airway surface liquid as hyperosmolar aerosols also increase mucociliary clearance (Daviskas *et al.*, 1996). It is also known that asthmatics are extremely sensitive to increases in airway osmolarity (Smith & Anderson, 1989), and their sensitivity to hyperosmolarity correlates well with their response to exercise and hyperventilation (Smith *et al.*, 1986; Smith & Anderson, 1987, 1989).

It is the current belief of the authors that, as the airway surface liquid evaporates, there is movement of water from the epithelial cell. The authors predict that the epithelial cell volume is not replaced instantaneously because the basement membrane of human epithelial cells are less permeable than the apical membrane (Willumsen *et al.*, 1994). The reduction in epithelial cell volume may be the stimulus for the release of substances that subsequently lead to regulatory volume increase (Eveloff *et al.*, 1987) and possibly to airway narrowing. The same stimulus would occur whether the water moves from the epithelial cell in response to airway drying or in response to the deposition of hyperosmolar fluids on the airway surface. Although water could move across the paracellular pathway in response to a hyperosmotic stimulus, this does not seem to occur (Willumsen *et al.*, 1994). It has been observed that the lateral spaces collapse as the epithelial cell volume decreases in response to the osmotic movement of water, and this event acts to 'zip up' the airways (Willumsen *et al.*, 1994).

If increased airway or submucosal osmolarity were the stimulus to increase bronchial blood flow, it would serve to explain a number of observations in EIA. It would explain why both intensity and duration are important and why it is not necessary to have an abnormal temperature gradient during recovery or abnormally cool airways during exercise. It would explain why drugs that affect the vasculature could modify EIA as water delivery to the airways improved.

Mediators and EIA

There has been vigorous debate as to the role of chemical mediators in EIA. The development of specific antagonists to both histamine and leukotrienes and the success of these in preventing EIA (see above) are strongly suggestive of a role for these mediators. In contrast, prostaglandins appear to play no role in EIA but are important for the development of the refractory period. Further evidence to support the involvement of mast cells comes from biopsy studies showing increased degranulation following exercise (Crimi *et al.*, 1992). The mediators themselves, however, have been hard to find. Early studies using arterial blood demonstrated significant increases in the concentration of circulating histamine (Anderson *et al.*, 1981; Hartley *et al.*, 1981). This technique had an advantage in that the sampling could be performed at the same time as the airway response and before the blood had recirculated. However, the use of venous blood, the dilution, by the systemic circulation, of the histamine generating from the airways and the possibility of rapid deactivation of histamine by diamine oxidase made interpretation of studies showing negative findings very difficult. Similar comments can be made in respect of the measurement of mediators in bronchial lavage fluid, where the dilution effect is enormous (Broide *et al.*, 1990; Jarjour *et al.*, 1992). A further disadvantage of lavage is the time difference between the release and the sampling. However, an increase in levels of leukotrienes was found with lavage following hyperventilation challenge with dry air (Pliss *et al.*, 1990). We await technology to provide us with superior techniques for harvesting and measuring small concentrations of mediators. Until then, we must conclude that the strongest evidence for implicating chemical mediators comes from the studies using the specific antagonists to inhibit the airway responses to exercise.

Conclusion

Airway narrowing following exercise, usually known as exercise-induced asthma, is a common finding both in clinically recognized asthmatics and in asymptomatic healthy subjects in the general community. EIA appears to be an early manifestation of asthma in children and studies are required to determine if this is the case in adults. It is generally accepted that EIA is due to the dehydrating effects of evaporative water loss. More studies are required to determine if EIA is simply due to the inflammatory effects of airway dehydration or if the classic inflammation of asthma is necessary for its occurrence. It is also important to determine if the EIA that occurs in asymptomatic healthy subjects is associated with the same physiological changes that occur in asthmatics, whether the responses are reproducible, as they are in asthmatics, and whether the EIA responds to the acute effects of drugs such as sodium cromoglycate and nedocromil sodium and chronic treatment with corticosteroids given as aerosols. Meanwhile, hyperpnoea with dry air should still be regarded as the provocation test of choice in patients who are suspected of having asthma and who complain of breathlessness on or after exertion. By documenting the airway response to exercise or hyperventilation, a diagnosis of EIA can be confirmed and appropriate therapy prescribed.

References

Agostoni, P., Arena, V., Doria, E. & Susini, G. (1990) Inspired gas relative humidity affects systemic to pulmonary bronchial blood flow in humans. *Chest*, **97**, 1377–80.

Ahmed, T., Garrigo, J. & Danta, I. (1993) Preventing bronchoconstriction in exercise-induced asthma with inhaled heparin. *New Engl. J. Med.*, **329**, 90–5.

Albazzaz, M.K., Neale, M.G. & Patel, K.R. (1992) Dose duration of nebulized nedocromil sodium in exercise-induced asthma. *Eur. Resp. J.*, **5**, 967–9.

Anderson, S.D. (1984) Is there a unifying hypothesis for exercise-induced asthma? *J. Allergy Clin. Immunol.*, **73**, 660–5.

Anderson, S.D. (1985) Exercise-induced asthma: the state of the art. *Chest*, **87S**, 191S–195S.

Anderson, S.D. (1988a) Exercise-induced asthma. In: *Allergy: Principles and Practice*, Vol. 2, 3rd edn (eds E. Middleton, C. Reed, E. Ellis, N.F. Adkinson & J.W. Yunginger), pp. 1156–75. C.V. Mosby, St Louis.

Anderson, S.D. (1988b) Exercise-induced asthma: stimulus, mechanism, and management. In: *Asthma: Basic Mechanisms and Clinical Management* (eds P.J. Barnes, I. Rodger & N.C. Thomson), pp. 503–22. Academic Press, London.

Anderson, S.D. (1992) Asthma provoked by exercise, hyperventilation, and the inhalation of non-isotonic aerosols. In: *Asthma: Basic Mechanisms and Clinical Management*, 2nd edn (eds P.J. Bames, I.W. Rodger & N.C. Thomson), pp. 473–90. Academic Press, London.

Anderson, S.D. (1993a) Drugs and the control of exercise-induced asthma [editorial]. *Eur. Resp. J.*, **6**, 1090–2.

Anderson, S.D. (1993b) Exercise-induced asthma. In: *Allergy: Principles and Practice*, Vol. 2 (eds E. Middleton, C. Reed, E. Ellis, N.F. Adkinson & J.W. Yunginger), pp. 1343–67. C.V. Mosby, St Louis.

Anderson, S.D. & Daviskas, E. (1992) The airway microvasculature in exercise-induced asthma. *Thorax*, **47**, 748–52.

Anderson, S.D. & Daviskas, L. (1993) An evaluation of the airway cooling and rewarming hypothesis as the mechanism for exercise induced asthma. In: *Asthma: Physiology, Immunopharmacology, and Treatment. 4th International Symposium* (eds S. Holgate, A.B. Kay, L. Lichtenstein & F. Austen), pp. 323–35.

Anderson, S.D. & Togias, A. (1994) Dry air and hyperosmolar challenge in asthma and rhinitis. In: *Asthma and Rhinitis* (eds W. Busse & S. Holgate), pp. 1178–95. Blackwell Scientific Publications, Oxford.

Anderson, S.D., Mc Evoy, J.D.S. & Bianco, S. (1972) Changes in lung volumes and airway resistance after exercise in asthmatic subjects. *Am. Rev. Resp. Dis.*, **106**, 30–7.

Anderson, S.D., Silverman, M., Godfrey, S. & Konig, P. (1975) Exercise-induced asthma: a review. *Brit. J. Dis. Chest*, **69**, 1–39.

Anderson, S.D., Seale, J.P., Rozea, P., Bandler, L., Theobald, G. & Lindsay, D.A. (1976) Inhaled and oral salbutamol in exercise-induced asthma. *Am. Rev. Resp. Dis.*, **114**, 493–500.

Anderson, S.D., Seale, J.P., Ferris, L., Schoeffel, R.E. & Lindsay, D.A. (1979) An evaluation of pharmacotherapy for exercise-induced asthma. *J. Allergy Clin. Immunol.*, **64**, 612–24.

Anderson, S.D., Bye, P.T.P., Schoeffel, R.E., Seale, J.P., Taylor, K.M. & Ferris, L. (1981) Arterial plasma histamine levels at rest, during and after exercise in patients with asthma: effects of terbutaline aerosol. *Thorax*, **36**, 259–67.

Anderson, S.D., Schoeffel, R.E., Follet , R., Perry, C.P., Daviskas, E. & Kendall, M. (1982) Sensitivity to heat and water loss at rest and during exercise in asthmatic patients. *Eur. J. Resp. Dis.*, **63**, 459–71.

Anderson, S.D., Daviskas, E. & Smith, C.M. (1989) Exercise-induced asthma: a difference in opinion regarding the stimulus. *Allergy Proc.*, **10**, 215–26.

Anderson, S.D., Rodwell, L.T., Du Toit, J. & Young, I.H. (1991) Duration of protection of inhaled salmeterol in exercise-induced asthma. *Chest*, **100**, 1254–60.

Anderson, S.D., du Toit, J.I., Rodwell, L.T. & Jenkins, C.R. (1994) Acute effect of sodium cromoglycate on airway narrowing induced by 4.5 percent saline aerosol: outcome before and during treatment with aerosol corticosteroids in patients with asthma. *Chest*, **105**, 673–80.

Argyros, G.J., Phillips, Y.Y., Rayburn, D.B., Rosenthal, R.R. & Jaeger, J.J. (1993) Water loss without heat flux in exercise-induced bronchospasm. *Am. Rev. Resp. Dis.*, **147**, 1419–24.

Auerbach, I., Springer, C. & Godfrey, S. (1993) Total population survey of the frequency and severity of asthma in 17 year old boys in an urban area in Israel. *Thorax*, **48**, 139–41.

Backer, V. & Ulrik, C.S. (1992) Bronchial responsiveness to exercise in a random sample of 494 children and adolescents from Copenhagen. *Clin. Exp. Allergy*, **22**, 741–7.

Backer, V., Dirksen, A., Bach-Mortensen, N., Hansen, K.K., Laursen, E.M. & Wendelboe, D. (1991) The distribution of bronchial responsiveness to histamine and exercise in 527 children and adolescents. *J. Allergy Clin. Immunol.*, **88**, 68–76.

Baile, E.M., Dahlby, R.W., Wiggs, B.R., Parsons, G.H. & Pare, P.D. (1987) Effect of cold and warm dry air hyperventilation on canine airway blood flow. *J. Appl. Physiol.*, **62**, 526–32.

Balfour-Lynn, L., Tooley, M. & Godfrey, S. (1981) Relationship of exercise-induced asthma to clinical asthma in childhood. *Arch. Dis. Child.*, **56**, 450–4.

Banner, A.S., Green, J. & O'Connor, M. (1984) Relation of respiratory water loss to coughing after exercise. *New Engl. J. Med.*, **311**, 883–6.

Bardagi, S., Agudo, A., Gonzalez, C.A. & Romero, P.V. (1993) Prevalence of exercise-induced airway narrowing in schoolchildren from a Mediterranean town. *Am. Rev. Resp. Dis.*, **147**, 1112–15.

Bar-Or, O., Neuman, I. & Dotan, R. (1977) Effects of dry and humid climates on exercise-induced asthma in children and preadolescents. *J. Allergy Clin. Immunol.*, **60**, 163–8.

Barry, D.M.J., Burr, M.L. & Limb, E.S. (1991) Prevalence of asthma among 12 year old children in New Zealand and South Wales: a comparative survey. *Thorax*, **46**, 405–9.

Bauer, M.A., Utell, M.J., Morrow, P.E., Speers, D.M. & Gibb, F.R. (1986) Inhalation of 0.30 ppm nitrogen dioxide potentiates exercise-induced bronchospasm in asthmatics. *Am. Rev. Resp. Dis.*, **134**, 1203–8.

Belcher, N.G., Rees, P.J., Clark, T.J.M. & Lee, T.H. (1987) A comparison of the refactory periods induced by hypertonic airway challenge and exercise in bronchial asthma. *Am. Rev. Resp. Dis.*, **135**, 822–5.

Belcher, N.G., Lee, T.H. & Rees, P.J. (1989) Airway responses to hypertonic saline, exercise and histamine challenges in bronchial asthma. *Eur. Resp. J.*, **2**, 44–8.

Ben-Dov, I., Bar-Yishay, E. & Godfrey, S. (1982) Refractory period after exercise-induced asthma unexplained by respiratory heat loss. *Am. Rev. Resp. Dis.*, **125**, 530–4.

Bianco, S., Vaghi, A., Robuschi, M. & Pasargiklian, M. (1988) Prevention of exercise-induced bronchoconstriction by inhaled frusemide. *Lancet*, July 30, 252–5.

Boner, A.L., Spezia, E., Piovesan, P., Chiocca, E. & Maiocchi, G. (1994) Inhaled formoterol in the prevention of exercise-induced bronchoconstriction in asthmatic children. *Am. J. Resp. Crit. Care Med.*, **149**, 935–8.

Boulet, L.-P., Corbeil, F. & Turcotte, H. (1992) Influence of a single antigenic challenge on the pattern of airway response to exercise in asthma. *Ann. Allergy*, **68**, 363–70.

Broide, D.H., Eisman, S., Ramsdell, J.W., Ferguson, P., Schwartz, L.B. & Wasserman, S.I. (1990) Airway levels of mast cell-derived mediators in exercise-induced asthma. *Am. Rev. Resp. Dis.*, **141**, 563–8.

Brudno, D.S., Wagner, J.M. & Rupp, N.T. (1994) Length of postexercise assessment in the determination of exercise-induced bronchospasm. *Ann. Allergy*, **73**, 227–31.

Bundgaard, A., Ingemann-Hansen, T., Schmidt, A. & Halkjaer-Kristensen, J. (1982) Effect of physical training on peak oxygen consumption rate and exercise-induced asthma in adult asthmatics. *Scand. J. Clin. Lab. Invest.*, **42**, 9–13.

Burr, M.L., Eldridge, B.A. & Borysiewicz, L.K. (1974) Peak expiratory flow rates before and after exercise in schoolchildren. *Arch. Dis. Child.*, **49**, 923–6.

Burr, M.L., Butland, B.K., King, S. & Vaughan-Williams, E. (1989) Changes in asthma prevalence: two surveys 15 years apart. *Arch. Dis. Child.*, **64**, 1452–6.

Bye, P.T.P., Anderson, S.D., Daviskas, E., Marty, J.J. & Sampson, D. (1980) Plasma cyclic AMP levels in response to exercise and terbutaline sulphate aerosol in normal and asthmatic patients. *Eur. J. Resp. Dis.*, **61**, 287–97.

Carlsen, K.-H. & Boe, J. (1993) Exercise-induced asthma in children. *Eur. Resp. J.*, **6**, 614–16.

Chen, W.Y. & Horton, D.J. (1977) Heat and water loss from the airways and exercise-induced asthma. *Respiration*, **34**, 305–13.

Chow, O.K.W., So, S.Y. & Lam, W.K. (1983) Effect of acupuncture on exercise-induced asthma. *Lung*, **161**, 321–6.

Clough, J.B., Hutchinson, S.A., Williams, J.D. & Holgate, S.T. (1991) Airway response to exercise and methacholine in children with respiratory symptoms. *Arch. Dis. Child.*, **66**, 579–83.

Cochrane, L.M. & Clark, C.J. (1990) Benefits and problems of a physical training programme for asthmatic patients. *Thorax*, **45**, 345–51.

Cockcroft, D.W., Murdock, K.Y., Berscheid, B.A. & Gore, B.P. (1992) Sensitivity and specificity of histamine PC_{20} determination in a random selection of young college students. *J. Allergy Clin. Immunol.*, **89**, 23–30.

Comis, A., Valletta, E.A., Sette, L., Andreoli, A. & Boner, A.L. (1993) Comparison of nedocromil sodium and sodium cromoglycate administered by pressurized aerosol, with and without a spacer device in exercise-induced asthma in children. *Eur. Resp. J.*, 523–6.

Crimi, E., Balbo, A., Milanese, M., Miadonna, A., Rossi, G.A. & Brusasco, V. (1992) Airway inflammation and occurrence of delayed bronchoconstriction in exercise-induced asthma. *Am. Rev. Resp. Dis.*, **146**, 507–12.

Cropp, G.J.A. (1979) The exercise bronchoprovocation test: standardization of procedures and evaluation of response. *J. Allergy Clin. Immunol.*, **64**, 627–33.

Custovic, A., Arifhodzic, N., Robinson, A. & Woodcock, A. (1994) Exercise testing revisited: the response to exercise in normal and atopic children. *Chest*, **105**, 1127–32.

Daviskas, E., Gonda, I. & Anderson, S.D. (1990) Mathematical modelling of heat and water transport in human respiratory tract. *J. Appl. Physiol.*, **69**, 362–72.

Daviskas, E., Gonda, I. & Anderson, S.D. (1991) Local airway heat and water vapour losses. *Resp. Physiol.*, **84**, 115–32.

Daviskas, E., Anderson, S.D., Gonda, I., Chan, H.K., Cook, P. & Fulton, R. (1995a) Changes in mucociliary clearance during and after isocapnic hyperventilation in asthmatic and healthy subjects. *Eur. Resp. J.*, **8**, 742–51.

Daviskas, E., Anderson, S.D., Gonda, I., *et al.* (1995b) Inhalation of hypertonic saline aerosol enhancess mucociliary clearance (MCC) in asthmatic and healthy subjects. *Eur. Resp. J.*, **9**, 725–32.

Deal, E.C., McFadden, E.R., Ingram, R.H., Strauss, R.H. & Jaeger, J.J. (1979) Role of respiratory heat exchange in production of exercise-induced asthma. *J. Appl. Physiol. Resp. Environ. Exercise Physiol.*, **46**, 467–75.

Deffebach, M.E., Salonen, R.O., Webber, S.E. & Widdicombe, J.G. (1989) Cold and hyperosmolar fluids in canine trachea: vascular and smooth muscle tone and albumin flux. *J. Appl. Physiol.*, **66** (3); 1309–15.

Djukanovic, R., Wilson, J.W., Britten, K.M. *et al.* (1992) Effect of an inhaled corticosteroid on airway inflammation and symptoms in asthma. *Am. Rev. Resp. Dis.*, **145**, 669–74.

Edmunds, A., Tooley, M. & Godfrey, S. (1978) The refractory period after exercise-induced asthma: its duration and relation to the severity of exercise. *Am. Rev. Resp. Dis.*, **117**, 247–54.

Eggleston, P.A., Rosenthal, R.R., Anderson, S.D. *et al.* (1979) Guidelines for the methodology of exercise challenge testing of asthmatics. *J. Allergy Clin. Immunol.*, **64**, 642–5.

Eggleston, P.A., Kagey-Sobotka, A., Proud, D., Franklin-Adkinson, K. & Lichtenstein, L. (1990) Disassociation of the release of histamine and arachidonic acid metabolites from osmotically activated basophils and human lung mast cells. *Am. Rev. Resp. Dis.*, **141**, 960–4.

Eiken, O., Kaiser, P., Holmer, I. & Baer, R. (1989) Physiological effects of a mouth-borne heat exchanger during heavy exercise in a cold environment. *Ergonomics*, **32**, 645–53.

Eliasson, A.H., Phillips, Y.Y. & Rajagopal, K.R. (1992) Sensitivity and specifity of bronchial provocation testing: an evaluation of four techniques in exercise-induced bronchospasm. *Chest*, **102**, 347–55.

Eschenbacher, W.L. & Sheppard, D. (1985) Respiratory heat loss is not the sole stimulus for bronchoconstriction induced by isocapnic hyperpnea with dry air. *Am. Rev. Resp. Dis.*, **131**, 894–901.

Eveloff, J.L. & Warnock, D.G. (1987) Activation of ion transport systems during cell volume regulation. *Am. J. Physiol.*, **252** (*Renal Electrolyte Phys.*, **21**), F1–F10.

Finnerty, J.P. & Holgate, S.T. (1990) Evidence for the roles of histamine and prostaglandins as mediators in exercise-induced asthma: the inhibitory effect of terfenadine and flurbiprofen alone and in combination. *Eur. Resp. J.*, **3**, 540–7.

Finnerty, J.P., Twentyman, O.P., Harris, A., Palmer, J.B.D. & Holgate, S.T. (1991) Effect of GR32191, a potent thromboxane receptor antagonist, on exercise induced bronchoconstriction in asthma. *Thorax*, **46**, 190–2.

Finnerty, J.P., Wood-Baker, R., Thomson, H., Thomson, H. & Holgate, S.T. (1992) Role of leukotrienes in exercise-induced asthma: inhibitory effect of ICI 204219, a potent leukotriene D_4 receptor antagonist. *Am. Rev. Resp. Dis.*, **145**, 746–9.

Fitch, K.D., Morton, A.R. & Blanksby, B.A. (1976) Effects of swimming training on children with asthma. *Arch. Dis. Child.*, **51**, 190–4.

Fitch, K.D., Blitvich, J.D. & Morton, A.R. (1986) The effect of running training on exercise-induced asthma. *Ann. Allergy*, **7**, 90–4.

Freeman, W., Williams, C. & Nute, M.G.L. (1990) Endurance running performance in athletes with asthma. *J. Sports Sci.*, **8**, 103–17.

Fuglsang, G., Hertz, B. & Holm, E.-B. (1993) No protection by oral terbutaline against exercise-induced asthma in children: a dose–response study. *Eur. Resp. J.*, **6**, 527–30.

Fung, K.P., Chow, O.K.W. & So, S.Y. (1986) Attenuation of exercise-induced asthma by acupuncture. *Lancet*, Dec. 20, 1419–21.

Gilbert, I.A. & McFadden, E.R. (1992) Airway cooling and rewarming: the second reaction sequence in exercise-induced asthma. *J. Clin. Invest*, **90**, 699–704.

Godfrey, S. & Bar-Yishay, E. (1993) Exercise-induced asthma revisited. *Resp. Med.*, **87**, 331–44.

Godfrey, S., Springer, C., Noviski, N., Maayan, Ch. & Avital, A. (1991) Exercise but not methacholine differentiates asthma from chronic lung disease in children. *Thorax*, **46**, 488–92.

Green, C.P. & Price, J.F. (1992) Prevention of exercise induced asthma by inhaled salmeterol zinofoate. *Arch. Dis. Child.*, **67**, 1014–17.

Haas, F., Pasierski, S., Levine, N. *et al.* (1987) Effect of aerobic training on forced expiratory airflow in exercising asthmatic humans. *J. Appl. Physiol.*, **63**, 1230–5.

Haas, F., Axen, K. & Schicchi, J.S. (1993) Use of maximum expiratory flow–volume curve parameters in the assessment of exercise-induced bronchospasm. *Chest*, **103**, 64–8.

Haby, M.M., Anderson, S.D., Peat, J.K., Mellis, C.M., Toelle, B.G. & Woolcock, A.J. (1994) An exercise challenge protocol for epidemiological studies of asthma in children: comparison with histamine challenge. *Eur. Resp. J.*, **7**, 43–9.

Haby, M.M., Peat, J.K., Mellis, C.M., Anderson, S.D. & Woolcock, A.J. (1995) An exercise challenge for epidemiological studies of childhood asthma: validity and repeatability. *Eur. Resp. J.*, **8**, 729–36.

Hahn, A., Anderson, S.D., Morton, A.R., Black, J.L. & Fitch, K.D. (1984a) A re-interpretation of the effect of temperature and water content of the inspired air in exercise-induced asthma. *Am. Rev. Resp. Dis.*, **130**, 575–9.

Hahn, A.G., Nogrady, S.G., Tumilty, D.McA., Lawrence, S.R. & Morton, A.R. (1984b) Histamine reactivity during the refractory period after exercise induced asthma. *Thorax*, **39**, 919–23.

Hartley, J.P.R., Charles, T.J., Monie, R.D.G. *et al.* (1981) Arterial plasma histamine after exercise in normal individuals and in patients with exercise induced asthma. *Clin. Sci.*, **61**, 151–7.

Henriksen, J.M. (1985) Effect of inhalation of corticosteroids on exercise induced asthma: randomised double blind crossover study of budesonide in asthmatic children. *Brit. Med. J.*, **291**, 248–9.

Henriksen, J.M. & Dahl, R. (1983) Effects of inhaled budesonide alone and in combination with low-dose terbutaline in children with exercise-induced asthma. *Am. Rev. Resp. Dis.*, **128**, 993–7.

Henriksen, J.M. & Nielsen, T.T. (1983) Effect of physical training on exercise-induced bronchoconstriction. *Acta Paediatr. Scand.*, **72**, 31–6.

Henriksen, J.M., Dahl, R. & Lundqvist, G.R. (1981) Influence of relative humidity and repeated exercise on exercise-induced bronchoconstriction. *Allergy*, **36**, 463–70.

Henriksen, J.M., Agertoft, L. & Pedersen, S. (1992) Protective effect and duration of action of inhaled formoterol and salbutamol on exercise-induced asthma in children. *J. Allergy Clin. Immunol.*, **89**, 1176–82.

Iikura, Y., Inui, H., Nagakura, T. & Lee, T.H. (1985) Factors predisposing to exercise-induced late asthmatic responses. *J. Allergy Clin. Immunol.*, **75**, 285–9.

Israel, E., Dermarkarian, R., Rosenberg, M. *et al.* (1990) The effects of a 5-lipoxygenase inhibitor on asthma induced by cold, dry air. *New Engl. J. Med.*, **323**, 1740–4.

Jarjour, N.N. & Calhoun, W.J. (1992) Exercise-induced asthma is not associated with mast cell activation or airway inflammation. *J. Allergy Clin. Immunol.*, **89**, 60–8.

Jeffrey, P.K., Godfrey, R.W., Adelroth, E., Nelson, F., Rogers, A. & Johansson, S.-A. (1992) Effect of treatment on airway inflammation and thickening of basement membrane recticular collagen in asthma: a quantitative light and electron study. *Am. Rev. Resp. Dis.*, **145**, 890–9.

Johnston, S.L., Perry, D., O'Toole, S., Summers, Q.A. & Holgate, S.T. (1992) Attenuation of exercise induced asthma by local hyperthermia. *Thorax*, **47**, 592–7.

Jones, A. & Bowen, M. (1994) Screening for childhood asthma using an exercise test. *Brit. J. Gen. Pract.*, **44**, 127–31.

Jones, R.S., Buston, M.H. & Wharton, M.W. (1962) The effect of exercise on ventilatory function in the child with asthma. *Brit. J. Dis. Chest*, **56**, 78–86.

Joris, L., Dab, I. & Quinton, P.M. (1993) Elemental composition of human airway surface fluid in health and diseased airways. *Am. Rev. Resp. Dis.*, **148**, 1633–7.

Kaplan, T.A. & Montana, E. (1993) Exercise-induced bronchospasm in nonasthmatic obese children. *Clin. Pediatr.*, **32**, 220–5.

Karjalainen, J., Lindqvist, A. & Laitenen, L.A. (1989) Seasonal variability of exercise-induced asthma especially out-doors: effect of birch pollen allergy. *Clin. Exp. Allergy*, **19**, 273–9.

Karjalainen, J. (1991) Exercise response in 404 young men with asthma: no evidence for a late asthmatic reaction. *Thorax*, **46**, 100–4.

Keeley, D.J., Neill, P. & Gallivan, S. (1991) Comparison of the prevalence of reversible airways obstruction in rural and urban Zimbabwean children. *Thorax*, **46**, 549–53.

Kivity, S., Greif, J., Reisner, B., Fireman, E. & Topilsky, M. (1986) Bronchial inhalation challenge with ultrasonically nebulized saline: comparison to exercise-induced asthma. *Ann. Allergy*, **57**, 355–8.

Konig, P., Hordvik, N.L. & Kreutz, C. (1987) The preventative effect and duration of action of nedocromil sodium and cromolyn sodium on exercise-induced asthma (EIA) in adults. *J. Allergy Clin. Immunol.*, **79**, 64–8.

Kuzemko, J.A. (1989) Twenty years of sodium cromoglycate treatment: a short review. *Resp. Med.*, **83**, 11–6.

Latimer, K.M., O'Byrne, P.M., Morris, M.M., Roberts, R. & Hargreave, F.E. (1983) Bronchoconstriction stimulated by airway cooling: better protection with combined inhalation of terbutaline sulphate and cromolyn sodium than with either alone. *Am. Rev. Resp. Dis.*, **128**, 440–3.

Lin, W.S., Shamoo, D.A., Anderson, K.R., Whynot, S.D., Avol, E.L. & Hackney, J.D. (1985) Effects of heat and humidity on the responses of exercising asthmatics to sulphur dioxide exposure. *Am. Rev. Resp. Dis.*, **131**, 221–5.

McAlpine, L.G. & Thomson, N.C. (1990) Prophylaxis of exercise-induced asthma with inhaled formoterol, a long-acting β_2-adrenergic agonist. *Resp. Med.*, **84**, 293–5.

McFadden, E.R. & Gilbert, I.A. (1994) Exercise-induced asthma. *New Engl. J. Med.*, **330**, 1362–7.

McFadden, E.R., Lenner, K.A. & Strohl, K.P. (1986) Postexertional airway rewarming and thermally induced asthma. *J. Clin. Invest.*, **78**, 18–25.

Magnussen, H., Reuss, G. & Jörres, R. (1986) Airway response to methacholine during exercise induced refractoriness in asthma. *Thorax*, **41**, 667–70.

Magnussen, H., Boerger, S., Templin, K. & Baunack, A.R. (1992) Effects of a thromboxane-receptor antagonist, BAY u3405, on prostaglandin D_2- and exercise-induced bronchoconstriction. *J. Allergy Clin. Immunol.*, **89**, 1119–26.

Magnussen, H., Lehnigk, B., Oldigs, M. & Jörres, R. (1993) Effects of acute passive smoking on exercise-induced bronchoconstriction in asthmatic children. *J. Appl. Physiol.*, **75**, 553–8.

Makker, H.K., Lau, L.C., Thomson, H.W., Binks, S.M. & Holgate, S.T. (1993) The protective effect of inhaled leukotriene D_4 receptor antagonist ICI 204 219 against exercise-induced asthma. *Am. Rev. Resp. Dis.*, **147**, 1413–18.

Manning, P.J., Watson, R.M., Margolskee, D.J., Williams, V.C., Schwartz, J.I. & O'Byrne, P.M. (1990) Inhibition of exercise-induced bronchoconstriction by MK-571, a potent leukotriene D4-receptor antagonist. *New Engl. J. Med.*, **323**, 1736–9.

Manning, P.J., Watson, R.M. & O'Byrne, P.M. (1993) Exercise-induced refractoriness in asthmatic subjects involves leukotriene and prostaglandin interdependent mechanisms. *Am. Rev. Resp. Dis.*, **148**, 950–4.

Margolskee, D.J., Bigby, B.G. & Boushey, H.A. (1988) Indomethacin blocks airway tolerance to repetitive exercise but not to eucapnic hyperpnea in asthmatic subjects. *Am. Rev. Resp. Dis.*, **137**, 842–6.

Martin, A.J., Landau, L.I. & Phelan, P.D. (1980) Lung function in young adults who had asthma in childhood. *Am. Rev. Resp. Dis.*, **122**, 609–16.

Merland, N., Cartier, A., L'Archeveque, J., Ghezzo, H. & Malo, J.-L. (1988) Theophylline minimally inhibits bronchoconstriction induced by dry cold air inhalation in asthmatic subjects. *Am. Rev. Resp. Dis.*, **137**, 1304–8.

Morton, A.R., Fitch, K.D. & Davis, T. (1979) The effect of (warm-up) on exercise-induced asthma. *Ann. Allergy*, **42**, 257–60.

Morton, A.R., Hahn, A.G. & Fitch, K.D. (1982) Continuous and intermittent running in the provocation of asthma. *Ann. Allergy*, **48**, 123–9.

Morton, A.R., Fazio, S. & Miller, D. (1993) Efficacy of laser-acupuncture in the prevention of exercise-induced asthma. *Ann. Allergy*, **70**, 295–8.

Newnham, D.M., Ingram, C.G., Earnshaw, J., Palmer, J.B.D. & Dhillon, D.P. (1993) Salmeterol provides prolonged protection against exercise-induced bronchoconstriction in a majority of subjects with mild, stable asthma. *Resp. Med.*, **87**, 439–44.

Nicolai, T., Mutius, E.V., Reitmeir, P. & Wjst, M. (1993) Reactivity to cold-air hyperventilation in normal and in asthmatic children in a survey of 5697 schoolchildren in southern Bavaria. *Am. Rev. Resp. Dis.*, **147**, 565–72.

Nisar, M., Spence, D.P.S., West, D. *et al.* (1992) A mask to modify inspired air temperature and humidity and its effect on exercise induced asthma. *Thorax*, **47**, 446–50.

Nish, W.A. & Schwietz, L.A. (1992) Underdiagnosis of asthma in young adults presenting for USAF basis training. *Ann. Allergy*, **69**, 239–42.

O'Byrne, P.M. & Jones, G.L. (1986) The effect of indomethacin on exercise-induced bronchoconstriction and refractoriness after exercise. *Am. Rev. Resp. Dis.*, **134**, 69–72.

O'Cain, C.F., Dowling, N.B., Slutsky, A.S. *et al.* (1980) Airway effects of respiratory heat loss in normal subjects. *J. Appl. Physiol. Resp. Environ. Exercise Physiol.*, **49**, 875–80.

O'Donnell, A.E. & Fling, J. (1993) Exercise-induced airflow obstruction in a healthy military population. *Chest*, **103**, 742–4.

O'Donnell, W.J., Rosenberg, M., Niven, R.W., Drazen, J.M. & Israel, E. (1992) Acetazolamine and furosemide attenuate asthma induced by hyperventilation of cold, dry air. *Am. Rev. Resp. Dis.*, **146**, 1518–23.

Parsons, G.H., Pare, P.D., White, D.A. & Baile, E.M. (1989) Airway blood flow response to eucapnic dry air hyperventilation in sheep. *J. Appl. Physiol.*, **66**, 1443–7.

Patel, K.R. (1984) Terfenadine in exercise-induced asthma. *Brit. Med. J.*, **85**, 1496–7.

Patel, K.R. & Wall, R.T. (1986) Dose–duration effect of sodium cromoglycate aerosol in exercise-induced asthma. *Eur. J. Resp. Dis.*, **69**, 256–60.

Patessio, A., Podda, A., Carone, M., Trombetta, N. & Donner, C.F. (1991) Protective effect and duration of action of formoterol aerosol on exercise-induced asthma. *Eur. Resp. J.*, **4**, 296–300.

Pavord, I., Lazarowicz, H., Inchley, D., Baldwin, D., Knox, A. & Tattersfield, A.E. (1994) Cross refractoriness between sodium metabisulphite and exercise induced asthma. *Thorax*, **49**, 245–9.

Phillips, Y.Y., Jaeger, J.J., Laube, B.L. & Rosenthal, R.R. (1985) Eucapnic voluntary hyperventilation of compressed gas mixture: a simple system for bronchial challenge by respiratory heat loss. *Am. Rev. Resp. Dis.*, **131**, 31–5.

Pliss, L.B., Ingenito, E.P., Ingram, R.H. & Pichurko, B. (1990) Assessment of bronchoalveolar cell and mediator response to isocapnic hyperpnea in asthma. *Am. Rev. Resp. Dis.*, **142**, 73–8.

Poppius, H., Sovijarvi, A.R.A. & Tammilehto, L. (1986) Lack of protective effect of high-dose ipratropium on bronchoconstriction following exercise with cold air breathing in patients with mild asthma. *Eur. J. Resp. Dis.*, **68**, 319–25.

Rakotosihanaka, F., Melamam, F., d'Athis, P., Florentin, D., Dessanges, J.F. & Lockhar, A. (1986) Refractoriness after hyperventilation-induced asthma. *Bull. Eur. Physiopathol. Resp.*, **22**, 581–7.

Ramage, L., Lipworth, B.J., Ingram, C.G., Cree, I.A. & Dhillon, D.P. (1994) Reduced protection against exercise induced bronchoconstriction after chronic dosing with salmeterol. *Resp. Med.*, **88**, 363–8.

Reiff, D.B., Choudry, N.B., Pride, N.B., & Ind, P.W. (1989) The effect of prolonged submaximal warm-up exercise on exercise-induced asthma. *Am. Rev. Resp. Dis.*, **139**, 479–84.

Richards, R., Fowler, C., Simpson, S.F., Renwick, A.G. & Holgate, S.T. (1989) Deep inspiration increases the absorption of inhaled sodium cromoglycate. *Brit. J. Clin. Pharmacol.*, **27**, 861–5.

Riedler, J., Reade, T., Daltono, M., Holst, D. & Robertson, C. (1994) Hypertonic saline challenge in an epidemiological survey of asthma in children. *Am. J. Respir. Crit. Care Med.*, **150**, 1632–9.

Robuschi, M., Riva, E., Fuccella, L.M. *et al.* (1992) Prevention of exercise-induced bronchoconstriction by a new leukotriene antagonist (SK&F 104353): a double-blind study versus disodium cromoglycate and placebo. *Am. Rev. Resp. Dis.*, **145**, 1285–8.

Rodwell, L.T., Anderson, S.D. & Seale, J.P. (1992) Inhaled steroids modify bronchial responses to hyperosmolar saline. *Eur. Resp. J.*, **5**, 953–62.

Rodwell, L.T., Anderson, S.D., du Toit, J. & Seale, J.P. (1993a) Inhaled amiloride does not protect against dry air challenge in subjects in whom protection is afforded by furosemide. *Eur. Resp. J.*, **6**, 855–61.

Rodwell, L.T., Anderson, S.D., du Toit, J. & Seale, J.P. (1993b) Nedocromil sodium inhibits the airway response to hyperosmolar challenge in patients with asthma. *Am. Rev. Resp. Dis.*, **146**, 1149–55.

Rosenthal, R.R., Laube, B.L., Hood, D.B. & Norman, P.S. (1990) Analysis of refractory period after exercise and eucapnic voluntary hyperventilation challenge. *Am. Rev. Resp. Dis.*, **141**, 368–72.

Rupp, N.T., Brudno, S. & Guill, M.F. (1993) The value of screening for risk of exercise-induced asthma in high school athletes. *Ann. Allergy*, **70**, 339–332.

Schaefer, O., Eaton, R.D.P., Timmermans, F.J.W. & Hildes, J.A. (1980) Respiratory function impairment and cardiopulmonary consequences in long-term residents of the Canadian Arctic. *Can. Med. Assoc. J.*, **123**, 997–1004.

Schmekel, B., Borgström, L. & Wollmer, P. (1992) Exercise increases the rate of pulmonary absorption of inhaled terbutaline. *Chest*, **101**, 742–5.

Schnall, R.P. & Landau, L.I. (1980) Protective effects of repeated short sprints in exercise-induced asthma. *Thorax*, **35**, 828–32.

Schoeffel, R.E., Anderson, S.D., Gillam, I. & Lindsay, D.A. (1980) Multiple exercise and histamine challenge in asthmatic patients. *Thorax*, **35**, 164–70.

Schoeffel, R.E., Anderson, S.D. & Lindsay, D.A. (1983) Sodium cromoglycate as a pressurized aerosol (Vicrom) in exercise-induced asthma. *Aust. NZ J. Med.*, **13**, 157–61.

Seidenberg, J., Dehning, J. & Von der Hardt, H. (1992) Inhaled furosemide against cold air induced bronchoconstriction in asthmatic children. *Arch. Dis. Child.*, **67**, 214–17.

Silverman, M. & Anderson, S.D. (1972) Standardization of exercise tests in asthmatic children. *Arch. Dis. Child.*, **47**, 882–9.

Smith, C.M. & Anderson, S.D. (1986) Hyperosmolarity as the stimulus to asthma induced by hyperventilation? *J. Allergy Clin. Immunol.*, **77**, 729–36.

Smith, C.M. & Anderson, S.D. (1987) An investigation of the hyperosmolar stimulus to exercise-induced asthma. *Aust. NZ J. Med.*, **17**, A513.

Smith, C.M. & Anderson, S.D. (1989a) A comparison between the airway response to isocapnic hyperventilation and hypertonic saline in subjects with asthma. *Eur. Resp. J.*, **2**, 36–43.

Smith, C.M. & Anderson, S.D. (1989b) Inhalation provocation tests using non-isotonic aerosols. *J. Allergy Clin. Immunol.*, **4**, 781–90.

Smith, C.M. & Anderson, S.D. (1990) Inhalational challenge using hypertonic saline in asthmatic subjects: a comparison with responses to hyperpnoea, methacholine and water. *Eur. Resp. J.*, **3**, 144–51.

Smith, C.M., Anderson, S.D. & Seale, J.P. (1988) The duration of the combination of fenoterol hydrobromide and iptratropium bromide in protecting against asthma provoked by hyperpnea. *Chest*, **94**, 709–17.

Smith, C.M., Anderson, S.D., Walsh, S. & McElrea, M. (1989) An investigation of the effects of heat and water exchange in the recovery period after exercise in children with asthma. *Am. Rev. Resp. Dis.*, **140**, 598–605.

Smith, T.L., Prazma, J., Coleman, C.C., Drake, A.F. & Boucher, R.C. (1993) Control of the mucosal microcirculation in the upper respiratory tract. *Otolaryngol. Head Neck Surg.*, **109**, 646–52.

Speelberg, B., van den Berg, N.J., Ooshoek, C.H.A., Verhoeff, N.P.L.G. & van den Brink, W.T.J. (1989) Immediate and late asthmatic responses induced by exercise in patients with reversible airflow limitation. *Eur. Resp. J.*, **2**, 402–8.

Speelberg, B., Verhoeff, N.P.L.G., van den Berg, N.J., Oosthoek, C.H.A., van Herwaarden, C.L.A. & Bruijnzeel, P.L.B. (1992) Nedocromil sodium inhibits the early and late asthmatic response to exercise. *Eur. Resp. J.*, **5**, 430–7.

Sterk, P.J., Fabbri, L.M., Quanjer, Ph.H. *et al.* (1993) Airway responsiveness: standardized challenge testing with pharmacological, physical and sensitizing stimuli in adults. *Eur. Resp. J.*, **6** (Suppl. 16), 53–83.

Strauss, R.H., McFadden, E.R., Ingram, R.H., Deal, E.C., Jaegar, J.J. & Stearns, D. (1978) Influence of heat and humidity on the airway obstruction induced by exercise in asthma. *J. Clin. Invest.*, **61**, 433–40.

Svenonius, E., Kautto, R. & Arborelius, M. (1983) Improvement after training of children with exercise-induced asthma. *Acta Paediatr. Scand.*, **72**, 23–30.

Svenonius, E., Arborelius, M., Wiberg, R., Stahl, E. & Svensson, M. (1994) A comparison of terbutaline inhaled by Turbuhaler and by a chlorofluorocarbon (CFC) inhaler in children with exercise-induced asthma. *Allergy*, **49** (6), 408–12.

Tabka, Z., Ben Jebria, A., Vergeret, J. & Guenard, H. (1988) Effect of dry warm air on respiratory water loss in children with exercise-induced asthma. *Chest*, **94**, 81–6.

Terblanche, E. & Stewart, R.I. (1990) The prevalence of exercise-induced bronchoconstriction in Cape Town schoolchildren. *SAMJ*, **78**, 744–7.

Togias, A.G., Proud, D., Lichenstein, L.M. *et al.* (1988) The osmolality of nasal secretions increases when inflammatory mediators are released in response to inhalation of cold, dry air. *Am. Rev. Resp. Dis.*, **137**, 625–9.

Tullett, W.M., Tan, K.M., Wall, R.T. & Patel, K.R. (1985) Dose–response effect of sodium cromoglycate pressurised aerosol in exercise induced asthma. *Thorax*, **40**, 41–4.

Umeno, E., McDonald, D.M. & Nadel, J.A. (1990) Hypertonic saline increases vascular permeability in the rat trachea by producing neurogenic inflammation. *J. Clin. Invest.*, **851**, 1905–8.

Varray, A., Mercier, J., Savy-Pacaux, A.-M. & Préfaut, C. (1993) Cardiac role in exercise limitation in asthmatic subjects with special reference to disease severity. *Eur. Resp. J.*, **6**, 1011–17.

Vathenen, A.S., Knox, A.J., Wisniewski, A. & Tattersfield, A.E. (1991) Effect of inhaled budesonide on bronchial reactivity to histamine, exercise, and eucapnic dry air hyperventilation in patients with asthma. *Thorax*, **46**, 811–16.

Waalkens, H.J., van Essen-Zandvliet, E.E.M., Gerritsen, J. *et al.* (1993) The effect of an inhaled corticosteroid (budesonide) on exercise-induced asthma in children. *Eur. Resp. J.*, **6**, 652–6.

Warner, J.O., Neijens, H. & Landau, L. (1992) Asthma: a follow up statement of an international paediatric asthma consensus group. *Arch. Dis. Child.*, **67**, 240–8.

Weinstein, R.E., Anderson, J.A., Kvale, P. & Sweet, L.C. (1976) Effects of humidification on exercise induced asthma (EIA). *J. Allergy Clin. Immunol.*, **57**, A250–A251.

Weiss, S.T., Tager, I.B., Weiss, J.W., Munoz, A., Speizer, F.E. & Ingram, R.H. (1984) Airways responsiveness in a population sample of adults and children. *Am. Rev. Resp. Dis.*, **129**, 898–902.

Weymer, A.R., Gong, J., Lyness, A. & Linn, W.S. (1994) Pre-exposure to ozone does not enhance or produce exercise-induced asthma. *Am. J. Resp. Crit. Care Med.*, **149**, 1413–19.

Wiebicke, W., Poynter, A., Montgomery, M., Chernick, V. & Pasterkamp, H. (1988) Effect of terfenadine on the response to exercise and cold air in asthma. *Pediatr. Pulm.*, **4**, 225–9.

Willumsen, J.N., Davis, C.W. & Boucher, R.C. (1994) Selective response of human airway epithelia to luminal but not serosol solution hypertonicity. *J. Clin. Invest.*, **94**, 779–87.

Wilson, B.A., Bar-Or, O. & Seed, L.G. (1990) Effects of humid air breathing during arm or treadmill exercise on exercise-induced bronchoconstriction and refractoriness. *Am. Rev. Resp. Dis.*, **142**, 349–52.

Wilson, B.A., Bar-Or, O. & O'Byrne, P.M. (1994) The effects of indomethacin on refractoriness following exercise both with and without bronchoconstriction. *Eur. Resp. J.*, **12**, 2174–8.

Woolcock, A.J., Peat, J.K., Salome, C.M. *et al.* (1987) Prevalence of bronchial hyperresponsiveness and asthma in a rural adult population. *Thorax*, **42**, 361–8.

Woolley, M., Anderson, S.D. & Quigley, B.M. (1990) Duration of protective effect of terbutaline sulfate and cromolyn sodium alone and in combination on exercise-induced asthma. *Chest*, **97**, 39–45.

Zach, M., Polgar, G., Kump, H. & Kroisel, P. (1984) Cold air challenge of airway hyperreactivity in children: practical application and theoretical aspects. *Pediatr. Res.*, **18**, 469–78.

CHAPTER 40

Mucus and Mucociliary Clearance

P.J. Wills & P.J. Cole

Introduction

The airways are subjected to formidable environmental assaults. Every day, a surface the area of a tennis-court is exposed to the volume of air contained in a small room. The need for a surface mediating efficient gas exchange results in potential vulnerability to noxious airborne substances. Even air above the ocean contains bacteria, and the air of our normal habitat is laden with substances of toxic, infective or allergenic potential (Cohen & Gold, 1975).

The anatomy of the airways is at first sight unfavourable to the maintenance of cleanliness. They derive embryologically from the primitive foregut and share part of their course with the digestive tract. Thus, there is the danger of aspirating digestive liquids which commonly occurs during sleep even in normal individuals (Huxley *et al.*, 1978). The low position of the human glottis makes this a particular risk. However, in contrast with the gut, the lungs are blind-ending. Therefore, inhaled foreign material must generally be expelled from the lungs the way it entered, with no help from gravity. In addition, the epithelium is continually being shed into the airway lumen and the cell debris also needs to be cleared.

It is therefore not surprising that respiratory complaints are so common, leading to 31% of visits to British general practitioners (Anon., 1995), or that pneumonia is by far the leading infective cause of death in western societies. In 1991 pneumonia was the immediate cause of over 28 000 deaths in England and Wales, which is more than 10 times the number of deaths caused by all other infections combined (Anon., 1993). Chronic allergic or infective upper and lower respiratory diseases remain major causes of morbidity.

The mucociliary system is the first line of host defence in maintaining lung hygiene. Two-phase flow may make a contribution to the clearance of lung mucus, and cough occurs when these systems malfunction or are overloaded. Phagocytosis deals with very small particles which escape entrapment by mucus and are deposited in the alveoli (du Bois, 1985).

The mucociliary system comprises the cilia, the periciliary fluid and mucus, which will be discussed in turn.

Cilia

Structure

The basic structure of a respiratory cilium is shown in Fig. 40.1. In cross-section, each cilium has one pair of central microtubules surrounded by nine peripheral pairs (Fawcett & Porter, 1954; Rhodin, 1966), constructed of tubulin. One of each of the peripheral tubulin doublets possesses two dynein arms projecting towards the next doublet, and a radial spoke is attached to one of the central microtubules. The dynein arms contain adenosine triphosphatase (ATPase), which converts chemical energy into a sliding motion between adjacent microtubules. The tips of respiratory cilia have projections which are presumed to interact in a claw-like way with the overlying mucus (Foliguet & Puchelle, 1986). At the base of each cilium is a foot-like structure, which defines its axis of movement (Fig. 40.2). Cilia in the central airways are approximately 6 μm long but are less than 4 μm peripherally (Serafini & Michaelson, 1977).

(a)

Outer arm
Inner arm
Dynein
Nexin link
Radial spoke
Cell membrane

(b)

Fig. 40.1 (a) Normal human nasal cilia in cross-section (×70 000) (prepared by A. Rutman and A. Dewar). (b) Diagrammatic key. (After Allen, 1968.)

Each ciliated cell contains approximately 200 cilia (Rhodin, 1966). Ciliated cells have been reported to comprise 53% of epithelial cells in the human trachea, but this proportion is lower peripherally, being 15% in the fifth generation (Serafini & Michaelson, 1977). The airways are ciliated from behind the nasal entrance to the terminal bronchioles, with the exception of the larynx and parts of the pharynx, which are covered by squamous epithelium, and the olfactory area (Sleigh *et al.*, 1988). A scanning electron micrograph of normal human nasal epithelium is shown in Fig. 40.3.

Function

The ciliary beat cycle (Fig. 40.4) comprises a recovery stroke followed by an effective stroke. The cilia appear to rest pointing in the direction of mucus movement, probably with their tips in contact with the mucus. For the recovery stroke, the cilium uncouples from the mucus, bends, and moves close to the cell surface to a position ready for the effective stroke. For the effective stroke, the cilium extends fully and moves approximately 110° in a plane perpendicular to the cell surface. Neighbouring cilia beat in a co-ordinated fashion, forming a metachronous propulsive wave, which propagates in a direction opposite ('antiplectic') to that of mucus flow (Sleigh *et al.*, 1988). Respiratory cilia appear to be continuously active, irrespective of the presence of overlying mucus. Cultured ciliated cells, however, can be stimulated to beat faster by mechanical stimulation of a single cell with a microprobe, and this increased beat frequency propagates to its neighbours, a process mediated by changes in intracellular Ca^{2+}. Inositol triphosphate appears to be the intercellular chemical messenger involved (Sanderson *et al.*, 1992).

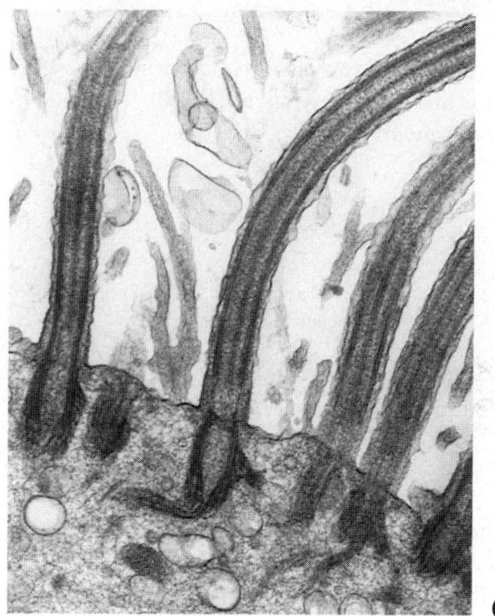

(a)

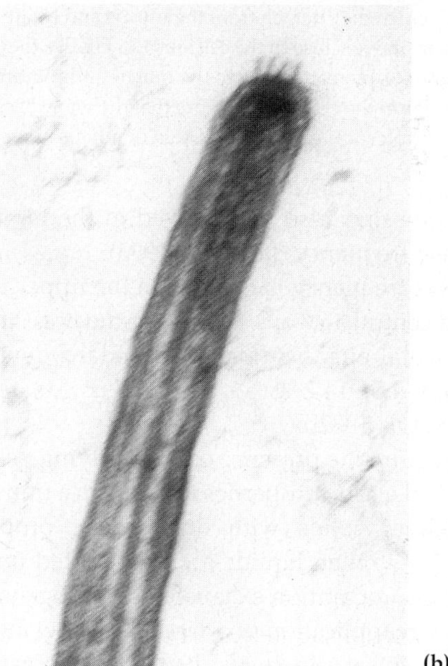

(b)

Fig. 40.2 Normal human nasal cilia in longitudinal section, showing (a) a basal foot process (×35 000) and (b) the 'crown' at the tip (×100 000). (Prepared by A. Rutman and A. Dewar.)

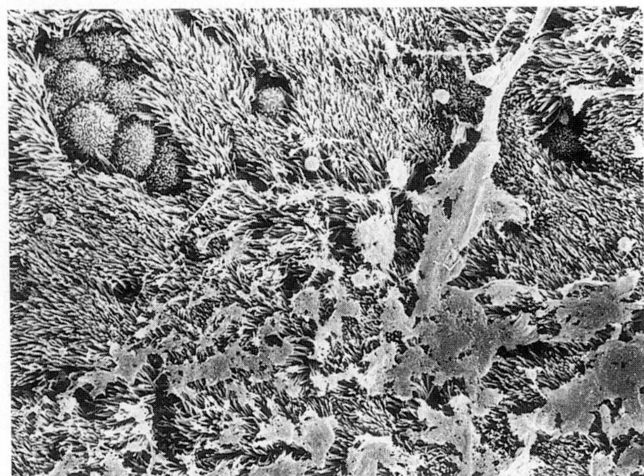

Fig. 40.3 Normal human nasal epithelial surface, illustrating the partial ciliation and overlying mucus (×1500). (Prepared by A. Rutman and A. Dewar.)

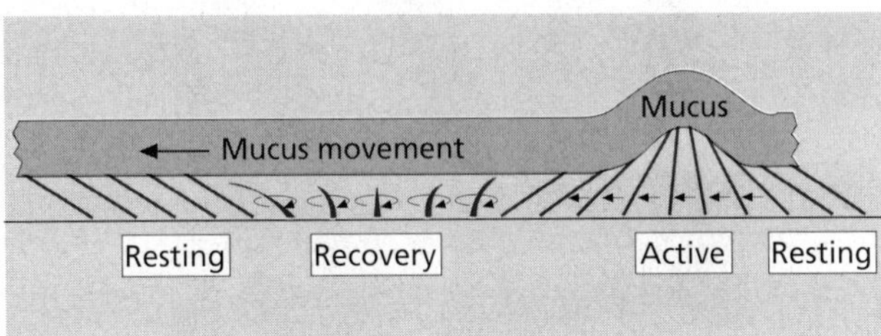

Fig. 40.4 Schematic diagram of the mucociliary interaction, viewed in a plane perpendicular to the cell surface. The ciliary beat cycle begins with the cilia in the resting phase, in contact with the mucus and pointing in the direction of mucus flow. The 'recovery' stroke follows, in which they detach from the mucus and rotate clockwise (as seen from above) close to the cell surface. Finally, they perform the active stroke, by reattaching to the mucus and rotating in a plane perpendicular to the cell surface. Note that the wave of ciliary beating is antiplectic, i.e. opposite to that of mucus movement.

Nitric oxide may also be involved in the modulation of ciliary beat frequency (Jain *et al.*, 1993).

The beat frequency is greatest in the upper respiratory tract and central airways. Values for the nose, trachea and subsegmental airways (mean ± standard deviation, Hz) are 14.0 ± 1.5, 14.2 ± 1.3 and 10.3 ± 1.0, respectively (Rutland *et al.*, 1982b).

Cilia require the presence of an overlying gel with both viscous and elastic properties to perform a transport function. Neither solids with only elastic properties nor viscous Newtonian liquids are transported on a ciliated frog palate preparation exhausted of endogenous mucus. However, reapplication of a viscoelastic gel allows transport to occur (Sadé *et al.*, 1970). The mucus-depleted bovine trachea also fails to transport small metal particles, which are, however, transported normally when carried by reapplied mucus (Wills *et al.*, 1995a).

Measurement of ciliary function

A simple, non-invasive, but reasonably accurate screening test, measuring the function of the mucociliary system as a whole, is the saccharin test, which is described in detail below. The structure and function of the cilia in isolation may be assessed in a reasonably non-invasive way by nasal brushing (Rutland & Cole, 1980). The inferior turbinate is sampled with a cytology brush and the suspension of epithelial cells so obtained examined by light microscopy, using an instrument equipped with a photoelectric device and a processor unit. The cilia remain active outside the body for many hours. Electron microscopy may need to be assessed to reveal ultrastructural defects.

The interpretation of all these tests is complicated by the fact that viral and bacterial infection can cause ciliary abnormalities that mimic a primary ciliary problem functionally and microscopically (see below). The patient should not be tested during or shortly after a viral respiratory infection, and it may be necessary to confirm an abnormal result after a period of vigorous antibacterial therapy.

Pathology

Ciliary dysfunction may be primary, or secondary to infection.

Primary ciliary dysfunction

Afzelius (1976) first described immotile cilia in association with Kartagener's syndrome of bronchiectasis, sinusitis and situs inversus. Since then, many different abnormalities of ciliary ultrastructure have been described (Barlocco *et al.*, 1991) which may not lead to complete ciliary immotility but which are associated with similar symptoms of mucus retention and consequent infections of the upper and lower respiratory tract. Some examples of ultrastructural defects are shown in Fig. 40.5. Note that these abnormalities are sometimes difficult to identify, and may not be present in all the cilia of an affected person. The diagnosis of primary ciliary dyskinesia therefore requires considerable experience in electronmicrograph interpretation. The aetiology appears to be genetic, the evidence favouring autosomal recessive inheritance (Sturgess *et al.*, 1986). A very few patients have been described with complete ciliary agenesis (DeBoeck *et al.*, 1992), and there are case reports of subjects with similar symptomatology in whom the cilia are abnormally long (15 μm) (Niggemann *et al.*, 1992) or abnormally short (2.5 μm) (Rautiainen *et al.*, 1991). Primary ciliary disorientation can also occur, in which the beat frequency may be normal but mucus propulsion is inefficient because the

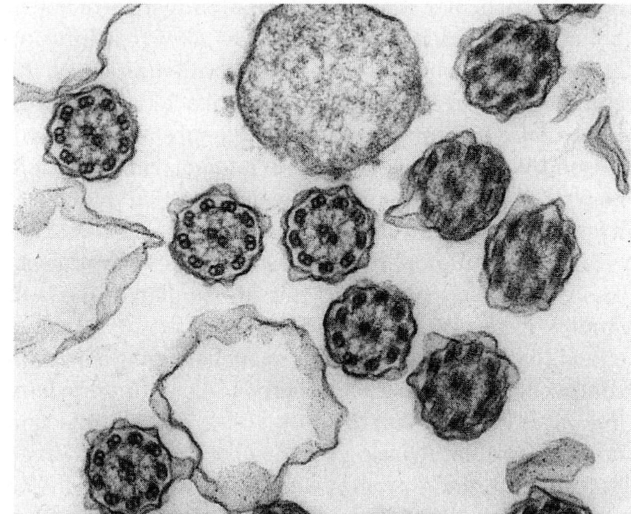
(a)

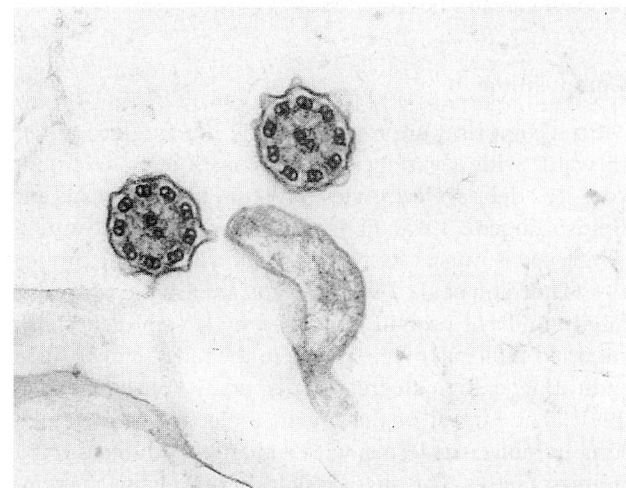
(b)

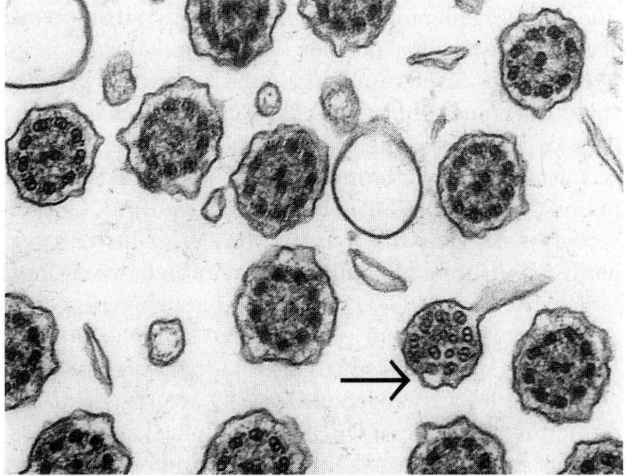
(c)

Fig. 40.5 Cross-sections of human nasal cilia showing ultrastructural defects (×70 000). (a) Absence of outer dynein arms. (b) Absence of both dynein arms. (c) Transposition of the microtubular doublet. Note that the defect is not seen in all cilia. (Prepared by A. Rutman and A. Dewar.)

cilia do not beat in the same direction. This is apparent on electron microscopy by poor alignment of the central microtubular doublet (Rayner *et al.*, 1995).

Secondary ciliary dysfunction

Cilia may be constitutionally normal but damaged because of the presence of infection. Damage to the upper respiratory ciliated epithelium is a sequel of the common cold (Pedersen *et al.*, 1983). Ciliated cells are sloughed from the nasal epithelium in the first few days of the illness. On day 4 of the cold, ciliated cells comprised less than 4% of the epithelium, compared with 25% normally. The beating frequency of the cilia was also reduced. Full recovery had not occurred even after 32 days. Such virus-induced damage is a plausible explanation for the fact that bacterial respiratory infection is often preceded by a viral infection.

Chronic bacterial sepsis may also lead to ciliary malfunction. Cell-free supernatants from cultures of *Haemophilus influenzae* and *Pseudomonas aeruginosa* are ciliotoxic *in vitro*, causing slowing of ciliary beating (Wilson *et al.*, 1985). The *P. aeruginosa* exotoxin pyocyanin slows ciliary beating in concentrations present in infected secretions *in vivo*, an effect mediated by depletion of intracellular cyclic adenosine monophosphate (Kanthakumar *et al.*, 1993). Ultrastructural studies of epithelium subjected to chronic infection often show ciliary disorientation and axonemal defects, which revert to normal when infection is controlled (Rutland *et al.*, 1982a). This is one way in which bacteria damage the structures which usually expel them, a tactic which appears to promote chronic airway sepsis.

Periciliary fluid

It is generally agreed that there exists between the mucus and the cell surface a layer of liquid without any gel-like properties (Boucher, 1994a). It must be acknowledged that there is little direct evidence for its existence in health in quantities greater than those required for a 'virtual' fluid. It is assumed that efficient ciliary beating requires that the shafts of the cilia be surrounded by a low-viscosity fluid. However, there is evidence that respiratory cilia do not actually require this: the beating frequency of a monolayer of respiratory ciliated cells changed little in response to a greater than 10-fold increase in the viscosity of periciliary fluid (Johnson *et al.*, 1991). Therefore, the efficiency of ciliary beating does not appear to depend greatly on the viscosity of the medium in which they beat.

Surface tension forces (Meyer & Silberberg, 1980), to which the microvilli contribute, are likely to ensure that an aqueous solution normally just covers the cilia, filling the interstices between them. Periciliary fluid cannot in normal circumstances bury the cilia to any depth or they would be unable to attach to the mucus and propel it. Also, any excess is likely to be removed by gravity. The alveoli appear to be equipped with the ion transport mechanisms to remove excess fluid (Barker, 1994). Attempts have been made to analyse it (Joris *et al.*, 1993), but the problems are formidable and appear insuperable with present technology. The fundamental criticism of current approaches is that the available analytical techniques cannot be used *in vivo* on the small quantities normally present, and collection methods are likely to perturb its properties in an unknown way. Mucus may also be present in any collected material. Our ignorance of its chemical and physical properties is therefore profound (Quinton, 1994).

Periciliary fluid is, however, likely to be of crucial importance in mucociliary clearance, not only because it is probably the medium in which the cilia beat, but also because it governs the composition of the mucus. Mucus is secreted in small, highly concentrated quanta which practically 'explode' in the periciliary fluid, increasing their volume by several 100-fold (Verdugo, 1991, 1995). Thus, mucus is largely the product of the periciliary liquid. Free diffusion of solutes takes place within a mucous gel, so gel composition probably reflects that of the underlying periciliary liquid (Tam & Verdugo, 1981).

It is highly probable that it is an abnormality in periciliary fluid composition that leads to the sinus and lung damage in cystic fibrosis. The only known primary defect in affected individuals is in epithelial sodium and chloride ion transport (Boucher, 1994b). How, if at all, this genetic defect affects periciliary fluid composition is unknown, but it appears that this ion transport abnormality may in some way alter mucus rheology to impede mucociliary clearance (see below), which invites bacterial infection and leads to a vicious circle of respiratory damage. Similar considerations may apply in the case of Young's syndrome, which appears to be an acquired abnormality of mucus, leading to bronchiectasis, sinusitis and male infertility, probably as a consequence of mercury poisoning (Hendry *et al.*, 1993). However, it is not known whether the primary defect in this condition is in the mucus or the periciliary fluid.

A better understanding of the nature of the periciliary fluid in health and disease would be likely to advance our understanding of mucociliary transport fundamentally.

Mucus

General

Mucus is the polymer gel which overlies the cilia. Its properties are compatible with its manifold protective functions. In particular, it has the physical properties of both a liquid and a solid. Its liquid properties allow free diffusion of water and solutes, to maintain the hydration of the epithelium, and deployment of antibacterial defences. Particulates are entrapped and soluble substances diluted. Its solid-like properties allow it to interact with the cilia to be propelled against gravity towards the pharynx, where it is eliminated by swallowing.

Normal respiratory mucus exists as a microscopic layer. The difficulties in studying this are similar to those of studying the periciliary fluid, and it must be acknowledged that we have no certain knowledge of its chemical composition or physical properties. As with periciliary fluid, it is very difficult to study *in situ*, and all collection methods are unphysiological to some degree. However, pathological mucus from several disease states is easy to obtain in quantity, and mucus produced by normal airways can also be collected.

Composition

Mucus comprises approximately 1% mucin glycoprotein in water with a variety of other constituents, including cells, cell debris, electrolytes, proteins, proteoglycans and lipids (Rogers, 1995). It is almost certainly the mucin which gives mucus its characteristic viscoelastic properties (Thornton *et al.*, 1990). Mucins are a highly glycosylated family of proteins, encoded by several genes. The reported molecular weights are in the range 3 to 32 MDa, indicating a high degree of dispersity (Sheehan *et al.*, 1991). The largest of the mucin molecules is extremely long in molecular terms, with a chain length measurable in micrometres. The oligosaccharide side chains make up over half the weight of the molecule, which is a polyanion due to the frequent presence of sialic acid and sulphated sugars at the terminal position of the side chains.

The degree of intermolecular cross-linking has been the subject of some controversy. The direct evidence favours little or no three-dimensional covalent cross-linking of mucin chains. Any intermolecular bonds that exist appear to link the chains end to end (Slayter *et al.*, 1984). The previously held view that mucins were cross-linked covalently by disulphide bonds to form a three-dimensional lattice (Roberts, 1978) has been seriously questioned (Verdugo, 1990). There was no direct evidence for this hypothesis, which rested largely on the *in vitro* mucolytic action of sulfhydryl reagents such as acetylcysteine and dithiothreitol. It does not fit easily with the fact that intracellular mucin is stored in highly condensed granules, which expand several 100-fold in milliseconds when released from the cell (Verdugo, 1991), or with the fact that separate portions of mucus readily anneal when brought together. It appears from direct electron microscopy and laser correlation spectroscopy (Verdugo *et al.*, 1983) that mucins exist as aggregates or extended threads, which diffuse into each other in a snake-like ('reptative') manner. The non-covalent interactions within and between mucin molecules are thought to contribute largely to the rheology of the resulting gel (Verdugo *et al.*, 1983). Sulfhydryl reagents may exert their mucolytic actions either by reducing mucin chain length by cleaving the end-to-end disulphide bonds, or by activating proteolysis (Houdret *et al.*, 1983).

The ionic composition of the mucus is likely to be of importance in these non-covalent interactions. We have some knowledge of the composition of mucus collected from normal lungs. An early series of thorough studies (Matthews *et al.*, 1963; Potter *et al.*, 1967) compared the mucus collected from otherwise healthy laryngectomized individuals with sputum. The mucus collected from healthy lungs contains sodium and chloride as the major ions, in concentrations (165 and 162 mmol/kg, respectively) somewhat higher than those found in plasma. Other constituents measured were potassium (13 mmol/kg), calcium (6 mmol/kg) and phosphorus (27 mmol/kg). The osmolarity of the mucus was approximately 350 milliosmolar, slightly hypertonic compared with plasma.

Other proteins are also present, in much smaller amounts than mucin. Many, such as lysozyme, lactoferrin, immunoglobulin (predominantly IgA) are part of the antibacterial defences. Proteoglycans and lipids are also present (Boat *et al.*, 1995).

Pathological mucus has been largely studied as sputum. This is likely to comprise normal mucus to which the products of inflammation and possibly some saliva have been added. There are major differences in composition between this and 'normal' mucus. Sputum is often produced in response to an allergic or infective challenge. The cellular inflammatory infiltrate, imparting a visible purulence, is the most obvious change, which results in the release of a multitude of substances designed to eliminate the insult, but some of them with pro-inflammatory potential. These include elastase, which is destructive to lung tissue, and a powerful mucus secretagogue (Schuster *et al.*, 1995), DNA and actin (Vasconcellos *et al.*, 1994), which may affect mucus rheology. Large numbers of viable bacteria may be present, with their products. Inflammation allows capillary leakage, which results in increased concentrations of albumin and other plasma proteins (Boat *et al.*, 1995).

Water content tends to be reduced in purulent secretions, and the sodium and chloride concentrations also fall, the lowest values being found in cystic fibrosis sputum. Potassium is somewhat increased. The overall osmolarity of purulent sputum is, however, similar to that of the mucus from normal lungs (Potter *et al.*, 1967), consistent with the passive movement of water (Nadel *et al.*, 1979).

Secretion

Mucus-secreting cells store mucus in highly concentrated secretory granules, surrounded by a membrane, where a low pH (3.5 to 5) and a high (0.1 mol/l) Ca^{2+} concentration shield the anionic charges of mucin to store it in a condensed dehydrated state. Exocytosis involves the formation of a channel between the contents of the granule and the extracellular environment. The influx of water and sodium and the efflux of Ca^{2+} cause a sudden phase change in the mucin, which expands explosively in milliseconds, presumably as a result of the electrostatic forces (Verdugo, 1991).

Regulation of secretion

The overall picture of the physiology of mucus production is remarkably obscure, despite a wealth of detail.

In the human lung, the cells with stainable mucus include the epithelial goblet, serous and Clara cells, and the cells of the submucosal glands (Rogers, 1995). Goblet cells are found throughout the respiratory tract, but submucosal glands are found only in the larger cartilaginous airways. It has been estimated that the ratio of gland to goblet cells is 40:1 by volume (Reid, 1954), and it is usually assumed that the submucosal glands secrete most of the mucus in human airways, but this is by no means certain, and the glands can make no contribution to the mucus of the smaller airways.

Physical stimuli and noxious agents are known to induce mucus secretion. Dust particles induce secretion in the feline trachea, and both a local mechanism and a vagally mediated reflex appear to be responsible (Peatfield & Richardson, 1983). The mucus-secreting structures of the airways are innervated and secretion can be stimulated via the parasympathetic, sympathetic and non-adrenergic non-cholinergic pathways (Rogers, 1995). Sensory fibres also innervate the airways and it is probable that afferent impulses from these cause reflex mucus secretion, as well as being able to induce cough.

Rheology

Several parameters are used to describe the rheological characteristics of mucus (King & Rubin, 1995). The parameters most studied in relation to mucociliary clearance are viscosity, elasticity and spinnability.

Viscosity describes the ratio of applied stress to resulting flow, and is a property of liquids and gases. In an ordinary ('Newtonian') fluid, all the applied stress is dissipated as deformation, and when the stress ceases to be applied no recoil occurs.

Elasticity, a characteristic property of solids, is the ratio of the stress applied, divided by the resulting deformation or strain. When the stress is withdrawn, recoil occurs. These parameters can be measured in many ways (King & Rubin, 1995), and some methods are grossly destructive of mucus, causing radical changes to the property which was to be measured. Current methods are relatively, though possibly not entirely, free of this drawback. One such method involves placing the mucus between two plates. One plate is stationary and the other rotates, making very small displacements, allowing both viscosity and elasticity to be measured. In another method, suitable for microlitre quantities, a steel ball is placed within the mucus and its motion monitored optically in response to the application of a magnetic field (King & Macklem, 1977). This, too, allows the elasticity to be measured.

Spinnability (*Spinnbarkeit, filance*) is the characteristic property of mucus which allows it to be pulled into a thread. It is usually measured as the maximum length to which it is possible to pull the mucus before it breaks (Iravani & Melville, 1976).

The essential nature of the viscoelastic properties of respiratory mucus will appear from a theoretical consideration of mucociliary transport.

A viscous non-elastic liquid would be able to trap and retain inhaled particulates, and be propelled by two-phase flow and cough. However, pulmonary mucus needs to interact favourably with the cilia. The cilia are very small in comparison with the overlying rafts of mucus, which need to be at least as large as that of the foreign body to be trapped and may cover thousands of cilia. The only way that cilia could transport such a raft of a non-elastic liquid is if the cilia in contact with the mucus beat in synchrony. The energy of any non-synchronous ciliary motion would be dissipated in a rheologically simple liquid such as water. In a rowing-boat with many oars, efficiency is poor unless all the oars in contact with the water pull at the same time. If, however, the overlying fluid has some elasticity, i.e. resembles mucus, it is not necessary that all the cilia beat together, because the motion of one wave of beating, which may only affect a small part of the mucus raft, can be stored in the mucus and the recoil can propagate in a wave-like manner through the gel to give a propulsive effect. The situation is analogous to the motion of a millipede. Its body lengthens and shortens rhythmically according to the metachronous motion of its legs. It is easy to see that, if its body were non-elastic, motion would be most inefficient. In both these systems, nature has adopted similar solutions to the problem of how to transport a relatively large object with multiple small 'legs'.

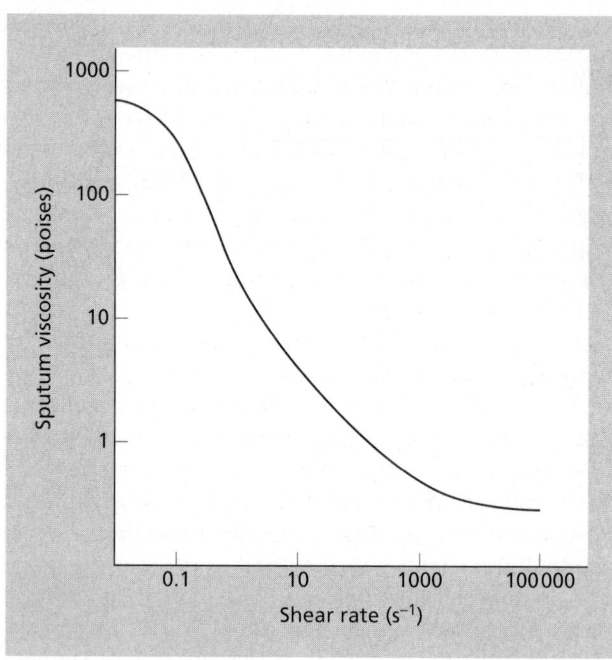

Fig. 40.6 Respiratory mucus viscosity as a function of shear rate. Note the large fall in viscosity as the shear rate increases. (Redrawn from Lopez-Vidriero & Reid, 1978, with permission.)

Respiratory mucus also possesses the remarkable property of thixotropy to an astonishing degree. This describes the fact that the viscosity of mucus is dependent on the shearing stress: at high stress (e.g. the explosive propulsive force of a cough), the viscosity is low, whereas at low stress (e.g. gravity) the viscosity is higher, by a factor of approximately 1000 (Lopez-Vidriero & Reid, 1978) (Fig. 40.6). This enormous difference is exactly what is needed to allow effective propulsion by a cough while minimizing the tendency of mucus to fall back under gravity. This property will also help the forces of normal breathing ('two-phase flow') (Clarke, 1973) to cause the net movement of lung mucus towards the pharynx. The inspiratory and expiratory phases of respiration are normally of roughly equal duration, but the airways are narrower in expiration, resulting in a faster air flow in this phase. This alone would tend to favour the expulsion of lung mucus. Moreover, the effect of this factor is amplified by mucus thixotropy: the increased shear stress of the expiratory phase acts to lower mucus viscosity and facilitate its movement with the air flow, while the lower stress in the inspiratory phase results in higher viscosity and resistance to movement. These facts probably explain the effectiveness of the forced expiratory technique of physiotherapy ('huffing') in which patients with mucus retention are now commonly instructed. The helpful effects of exercise on mucus expulsion may also have a similar basis (Wolff *et al.*, 1977).

Ex vivo ciliary transportability

Healthy mucus presumably has the rheological properties suitable for optimal ciliary transport, and this physiological property can be measured directly. The study of the ciliary transportability of mucus in isolation requires a ciliated epithelium free of endogenous mucus, which would otherwise contaminate the applied mucus that it is desired to study. Two such systems have been described, and it is fortunate that ciliary activity after death is very robust and can persist in tissues where mucus production is exhausted. The frog palate has been studied for many years, is easy to exhaust of mucus and has cilia which remain active for many days (Rubin *et al.*, 1990). The ciliated epithelium resembles mammalian respiratory epithelium microscopically (Dulfano & Adler, 1975). It is, however, an amphibian digestive system. A mucus-depleted state can also be achieved in explants of bovine trachea, without damaging the cilia (Wills *et al.*, 1995a). This system may have more relevance to the study of lung mucociliary clearance, and its larger size avoids some of the difficulties with the frog palate assay.

The relationship between the ciliary transportability and rheology measured by physical means has been assessed in a number of studies. These are complicated by the difficulty in altering one component of the rheology without affecting others. In general, there is little or no correlation between transportability and viscosity over a wide range (Dulfano & Adler, 1975; Puchelle *et al.*, 1976; Gelman & Meyer, 1979). There appears to be an optimum elasticity, but extreme values of either parameter lead to a gel which is not transported (Gelman & Meyer, 1979). Spinnability appeared to correlate positively with transportability in one study (Puchelle *et al.*, 1983) but negatively in another (App *et al.*, 1990). This rather confused picture reflects the difficulty in altering one mucus rheological parameter in isolation, but may also indicate the inadequacy of current physical measurement techniques in predicting the requirements of ciliary transportability.

Mucociliary clearance

General

In health, cough is not effective in removing small inhaled particles (Camner *et al.*, 1979; Camner, 1981), and neither gravity nor the phase of respiration has a measurable effect on tracheobronchial clearance (Isawa *et al.*, 1991). This indicates that mucociliary transport is normally entirely responsible for maintaining airway cleanliness.

Particles larger than 10 μm in diameter are effectively trapped in the upper respiratory passages, and few reach the lungs in normal nasal breathing. Therefore, the nasal passages are the site of deposition of most seasonal allergens, which are usually larger than this. It is of interest that, in persons with seasonal asthma, treatments given to the nose alleviated pulmonary symptoms. It was suggested that this restored normal nasal breathing, which protected the lungs (Welsh *et al.*, 1987). Particles smaller than 5 μm often reach the smaller airways and may be deposited there (Salvaggio, 1994). Long thin fibres such as asbestos can also penetrate deeply.

Mucus is secreted along the whole length of the tracheobronchial tree. The fact that it does not accumulate at any point along its path is probably due to a combination of several factors. Mucus probably exists in discontinuous rafts, which coalesce as it is transported centrally (Iravani & van As, 1972). Mucus-secreting cells appear to be fewer peripherally: the density of goblet cells is less, and the submucosal glands are absent. The mucociliary transport rate is also slower in the more distal airways (Asmundsson & Kilburn, 1970; Iravani & van As, 1972), and a number of factors contribute to this. The cilia peripherally are shorter, which means that each effective stroke has less propulsive effect (Serafini & Michaelson, 1977). The ciliary beat frequency is also slower peripherally (Rutland *et al.*, 1982b). The epithelium, which in the trachea is largely covered with a carpet of cilia, has a considerably patchier ciliated covering in the distal airways and this would be expected to lead to slower transport (Serafini & Michaelson, 1977). Bronchial branch points become progressively more frequent distally, which will impede mucus transport (Hilding, 1957). Finally, changing epithelial potential difference along the bronchial tree may cause water to be absorbed as the mucus progresses proximally, decreasing its volume (App *et al.*, 1993).

Measurement of mucociliary clearance

The simplest test of mucociliary function is the saccharin test (Stanley *et al.*, 1984). For this, a 1 mm cube of saccharin is placed under direct vision on the inferior turbinate of an unobstructed nostril, 1 cm behind its anterior margin. The subject sits with the head tilted slightly forwards and is instructed not to sniff, sneeze or blow the nose. The time at which the saccharin is first tasted is then noted. This is normally less than 30 minutes after placement of the saccharin. Times greater than 60 minutes usually indicate an abnormality in mucociliary clearance, unless the subject is unable to taste saccharin, which should always be checked.

A copious postnasal drip may give a falsely normal reading by washing the saccharin down, particularly if the subject was recumbent. An abnormal result may be due to ciliary dyskinesia, either primary or secondary, or to conditions with normal cilia but delayed clearance due to mucus or periciliary fluid abnormalities, such as cystic fibrosis or Young's syndrome.

Two main methodologies have been used for measuring *in vivo* tracheobronchial clearance rates. Tracheal mucus transport can be directly viewed with a bronchoscope, by measuring the speed of a small applied foreign body, such as a Teflon disc (Sackner *et al.*, 1973). This method has the advantage of directness and conceptual simplicity, but is invasive. Such discs can be made radio-opaque, allowing external monitoring of their transport rate. The other main technique is to administer a radioactive aerosol, and monitor its rate of expulsion from the lungs by external scanning (Pavia *et al.*, 1980). This method is less invasive, although the radiation dose is considerably higher than that for a plain chest radiograph. This method measures clearance in the smaller airways, but results are less easy to interpret for several reasons. An inhaled aerosol will be deposited throughout the bronchial tree, each part of which will have a different clearance rate, as discussed above. Inhaled aerosols are not deposited uniformly, but preferentially at areas of turbulent flow, e.g. at bifurcations, areas where ciliary clearance is not straightforward. The predominant site of deposition will also be crucially dependent on individual factors, such as local bronchial pathology. It is also difficult to control for non-ciliary clearance mechanisms such as cough. Considerable thought has to be given to the nature of the radioactive inhaled particle. Soluble particles such as albumin may diffuse through the mucus and dissolve in the periciliary fluid, giving a complex clearance pattern. A proportion of the aerosol will reach the alveoli and be cleared by the much slower non-ciliary mechanisms.

In the light of these considerations, it is not surprising that different results are obtained with these different methods. Using direct observation of the transport of Teflon discs, tracheal rates of 10–20 mm/minute are observed in healthy young non-smokers (Santa Cruz *et al.*, 1974; Mezey *et al.*, 1978). The clearance of a radioactive aerosol appears to be slower, at 4.7 mm/minute (Yeates *et al.*, 1995). Clearance declines with increasing age (Puchelle *et al.*, 1979).

Pathology of delayed mucociliary clearance

Lung mucociliary clearance is delayed in conditions characterized by expectoration. When measured by the Teflon disc method, dramatic reductions in tracheal clearance were observed in cases of cystic fibrosis (Wood *et al.*, 1975) and smoking-related chronic bronchitis (Santa Cruz *et al.*, 1974), at 2.6 and 1.7 mm/minute, respectively, about 10% of that of normal subjects. Other workers, however, have found a less profound impairment in chronic bronchitis sufferers (Olivieri *et al.*, 1985). Stable asthmatics with a degree of baseline airway dysfunction had moderately impaired clearance, which fell further, to 47% of baseline, 1 hour after challenge with a specific antigen. Pretreatment with cromoglycate prevented the provocation-induced fall in mucus transport rate (Mezey *et al.*, 1978). Studies using radioactive clearance techniques broadly confirm these findings, showing diminished clearance in cystic fibrosis (Regnis *et al.*, 1994), chronic bronchitis (Goodman *et al.*, 1978), bronchiectasis (Currie *et al.*, 1987) and asthma in exacerbation (Messina *et al.*, 1991) and when stable (Bateman *et al.*, 1983; O'Riordan *et al.*, 1992), although not when in complete remission (O'Riordan *et al.*, 1992). Fatal cases of asthma are characterized by marked mucous plugging (Hogg, 1993), and it is probable that both diminished clearance and mucus hypersecretion are responsible. Interestingly, histamine appears to accelerate mucociliary transport (Mussatto *et al.*, 1988; Garrard *et al.*, 1989). Acute influenza also leads to a reduction in tracheobronchial clearance (Camner *et al.*, 1973).

Nasal mucociliary clearance is, unsurprisingly, diminished in cases of primary ciliary dyskinesia (Stanley *et al.*, 1984). It is also slow in cystic fibrosis, where ciliary beat frequency is normal (Rutland & Cole, 1981). Persons with sinusitis tend to have a slow nasal mucociliary clearance time (Rutland & Cole, 1981; Ogino *et al.*, 1993), and the common cold causes a marked impairment, which lasts for weeks (Pedersen *et al.*, 1983). Persons with asthma have been reported to have normal (Ogino *et al.*, 1993) or prolonged (Kurashima *et al.*, 1992) saccharin clearance times.

The reason for the diminished clearance in these conditions is not clearly understood. In most cases a primary ciliary problem does not exist, and it seems rather unlikely that these disparate conditions all lead to a primary slowing of transport by directly slowing or disorganizing ciliary action. Particularly in the case of allergic conditions, toxic bacterial products cannot be implicated, as they have been in chronic bronchial sepsis (see below). Most probably, an abnormality of mucus causes it to be retained. One possibility is that the mucus secretagogue effects of these illnesses overload the ciliary escalator, leading to inefficient transport. Alternatively, the inflammatory products present in the pathological mucus have a toxic effect on the cilia or alter mucus rheology to make it unfavourable to mucus transport.

Using the mucus-depleted bovine trachea, the transportability of mucus collected from normal human lungs, either post-surgical or post-mortem, has been compared with sputum from patients with bronchiectasis (Wills *et al.*, 1995a). The sputum was transported at approximately one-fifth of the rate of the mucus from normal lungs, which was transported at a similar rate to that of bovine tracheal mucus. There was no detectable relation between transportability and either sputum purulence or the presence of *P. aeruginosa*. Preliminary studies with the sputum of patients with cystic fibrosis and chronic bronchitis give similar results (Wills *et al.*, 1995b). A direct ciliotoxic effect of the sputum on the cilia does not appear to explain the poor transport of sputum on this model. This suggests that there is a defect in the rheology of sputum when compared with mucus from healthy lungs.

Therefore it appears that defective mucus rheology explains, at least in part, the poor tracheobronchial clearance observed in these conditions.

Where chronic mucus retention leads to chronic bronchial sepsis, as in cystic fibrosis and bronchiectasis of other causes, many other factors act synergistically to delay clearance, leading to a vicious circle of events (Fig. 40.7). Bacteria, particularly the relatively non-virulent strains most commonly present in lung mucus, synthesize an array of exotoxins which slow ciliary beating, are directly cytotoxic, alter ion transport and stimulate mucus production (Cole & Wilson, 1989). The effect of this is to impair further the ability of the host to eliminate the pathogen. Moreover, the host inflammatory response, which has obviously failed in its primary purpose of eradicating the bacteria, appears to be subverted and to cause self-inflicted damage. Large amounts of elastase are present in such secretions (Stockley *et al.*, 1984), overwhelming the antiproteases, and this probably contributes to bronchial damage. Elastin is characteristically absent in the bronchial walls of cases of bronchiectasis (Cole, 1995).

This concept of the vicious circle goes far towards explaining how chronic bronchial sepsis may be self-perpetuating and can lead to bronchiectasis. It does not, however, shed light on how chronic sepsis is established in the first place. The matter is particularly intriguing in the case of cystic fibrosis, where the only known primary defect is in epithelial ion transport (Boucher, 1994b).

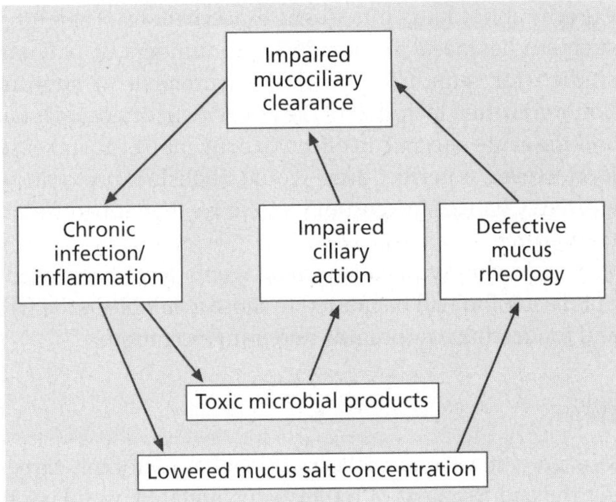

Fig. 40.7 The vicious circle of chronic mucus retention. If the host defences fail to eliminate an infective or other insult, the persistent inflammation and continued presence of bacteria will tend to exacerbate the impaired mucociliary clearance by affecting both ciliary action and mucus rheology.

Preliminary data show that sputum, which is poorly transportable on the mucus-depleted bovine trachea, is rendered rapidly transportable by the addition of either hypertonic saline solution (Wills & Cole, 1994) or solid sodium chloride (Wills & Cole, 1995). This phenomenon is seen with sputum from cases of idiopathic bronchiectasis, cystic fibrosis and chronic bronchitis. This is compatible with the fact that mucus from normal lungs has a much higher sodium chloride concentration than sputum (Matthews *et al.*, 1963), and that the aggregation of purified cystic fibrosis mucin has been shown to depend on the saline concentration (Chace *et al.*, 1989). The sodium chloride concentration of the mucus appears to exert a profound influence on its ciliary transportability.

A 'salt' hypothesis of mucus retention

The fact that sputum is transformed from a poorly transported gel into a rapidly transported gel simply by adding solid sodium chloride allows a hypothesis for the pathophysiology of mucus retention to be constructed. It is suggested that normal lung mucus has a higher salt concentration than sputum. When the airway suffers an infective or allergic insult, the products of inflammation are added to the normal mucus. Much of this exudate will contain substances which, though poorly ionized, will still exert an osmotic effect. Water transport across the airway epithelium appears to be a passive process, and osmotic equilibrium appears to be maintained in the airway fluid and mucus at the expense of saline concentration. In this respect, the situation is analogous to that in blood plasma in a hyperglycaemic state which has arisen gradually: blood osmolarity is near normal but plasma sodium and chloride are low. However, the ionic environment of mucin is critical for its structure and function, and the large reduction in the concentration of the major ions causes the rheology to alter in a way unfavourable to ciliary transport. The state of hydration of the mucus, which has so preoccupied workers in this field, is comparatively irrelevant. Indeed, pathological mucus appears to be poorly transported because it contains too much water in comparison with sodium chloride.

This model provides an explanation for the primary mucus retention in cystic fibrosis. It is logical to assume that the defect in chloride secretion and increased sodium absorption will lead to a lowering of airway surface fluid sodium chloride concentration. The ensuing rheological change in the mucus and its delayed clearance may invite infection, which leads to a vicious circle of respiratory decline (Fig. 40.7). The beneficial effects of nebulized amiloride are also easily explained on this model. The effects of aerosolized hypertonic saline, but not water, in accelerating tracheobronchial clearance would also be predicted (see below).

Therapeutic approaches

General

Impaired mucociliary clearance of the upper respiratory tract will result in nasal drip, sinusitis and middle-ear disease. Current medical treatments are directed at the underlying allergic or infective cause, rather than at the delayed clearance itself. Often, impaired clearance is manifested in a blocked sinus or Eustachian tube, which is then inaccessible to local medical therapy and requires surgical correction. The lack of interest in mucoactive treatments for upper respiratory tract ailments contrasts with the considerable literature on mucus retention in the lungs, so the discussion will therefore focus on lung clearance.

When lung mucociliary clearance is impaired, expulsion of the mucus needs to be encouraged in other ways. Postural drainage and huffing can improve lung function in states of mucus retention (Cochrane *et al.*, 1977; Hasani *et al.*, 1994). Coughing causes stepwise falls in lung radioactivity after inhalation of a radioaerosol in cases of Kartagener's syndrome and cystic fibrosis (Kollberg *et al.*, 1978). The patient with chronic bronchial sepsis should be instructed in such techniques and encouraged to practise them, particularly when exacerbations occur. The effectiveness of physical treatments on long-term prognosis has, however, not been studied; it is obviously impossible to mount placebo-controlled trials, and assessment of compliance is notoriously difficult (Currie *et al.*, 1986).

The many necessary functions of mucus indicate that its rheological properties are crucial and that deviations from the normal, in whichever direction, are likely to be detrimental. In the light of this, it is perhaps not surprising that so many mucoactive drugs have largely failed to provide much benefit. In most illnesses, we start by knowing the healthy state of the organ or system, and the way in which its pathological state differs. This allows a logical approach to designing and testing therapies. However, those working to develop mucoactive agents labour in ignorance of the properties of normal mucus. Very often the simplistic line of therapeutic attack has been to 'thin' the mucus, with little or no consideration for the needs of the ciliary escalator or for the retention of thixotropy. It is clear that there is great potential for doing harm as well as good.

The philosophy behind the development of mucoactive agents in the past has largely been to produce agents that aid expectoration. However, in the light of new evidence that sputum has a seriously impaired ability to be transported by the ciliary escalator, the goals of this research might need to be reconsidered. The ideal mucoactive agent would be one which restored the healthy state in which the ciliary escalator alone, unaided by cough, clears the mucus. Obviously, such an ideal may not be attainable where there is serious anatomical damage to the bronchial tree, as in bronchiectasis, or an overproduction of mucus which overloads the ability of the cilia to cope. Nevertheless, rationally designed mucoactive agents of the future are likely to be 'mucokinetic' rather than 'mucolytic' in nature, reflecting an appreciation of the importance of restoring mucociliary clearance.

There are considerable difficulties in assessing the efficacy of new mucoactive agents (Lurie *et al.*, 1992). Much of the patient's suffering cannot be measured objectively and is dependent on climatic factors and intercurrent infections. The most logical objective measurement to assess efficacy is probably the clearance of inhaled radioaerosol, but mounting a clinical trial with this end-point with more than a few patients is a formidable undertaking. For this reason, surrogate outcome measures have been more commonly studied, in particular lung function, radiology and rates of infective exacerbation. Lung function is a relatively crude outcome measure, because airway obstruction and mucus retention can change independently (Demedts, 1987). However, it has been successfully used in the recent trials of recombinant human deoxyribonuclease (rhDNase). Plain chest radiology is too insensitive to assess efficacy, but computed tomography (CT) scanning to assess mucous plugging may have a useful role. Infective exacerbation rates are an important measurement of the health of the lungs, but have the disadvantage that many patients, even those troubled with daily purulent expectoration, have infrequent exacerbations. Therefore, such studies need to include large numbers of patients studied for months or years. Measurement of sputum volume is often included in the assessment of a mucolytic, and the acute effect of an effective drug may be to increase it. However, a perfect drug would abolish expectoration entirely. Changes in sputum volume are therefore difficult to interpret.

A wide variety of mucoactive agents have been used, but discussion will be limited to those available in the UK and interesting compounds under investigation.

Water

Inhaled water vapour is a traditional expectorant, carrying the endorsement of the British National Formulary. It had a widespread vogue some decades ago in the treatment of cystic fibrosis, particularly in the USA. However, long-term studies failed to show a benefit and even suggested that it caused a deterioration in the expiratory flow in children undergoing regular therapy (Motoyama *et al.*,

1972; Taussig, 1974). The use of mist tents has now been virtually abandoned in this condition. However, use of humidified air as an adjunct to postural drainage and forced expiratory techniques was effective at improving the clearance of radioactive aerosol in bronchiectatic patients (Conway *et al.*, 1992). This study did not attempt to assess any effect on mucociliary clearance; it is probable that the therapeutic benefit was due to improved cough clearance. Water can induce cough and bronchoconstriction in susceptible individuals (Waltemath & Bergman, 1973; Eschenbacher *et al.*, 1984), and its effect on mucociliary clearance is doubtful (Foster *et al.*, 1976).

Saline solutions

Hypertonic (7%) saline aerosol is one of the few substances that markedly improves mucociliary clearance. This has been shown in persons with chronic bronchitis (Pavia *et al.*, 1978) and cystic fibrosis (Robinson *et al.*, 1994). It has been increasingly used to induce sputum for diagnostic purposes in persons who do not normally expectorate, for example human immunodeficiency virus (HIV)-positive individuals in whom a diagnosis of *Pneumocystic carinii* is being considered (Bigby *et al.*, 1986). It is remarkable that a large acceleration in tracheobronchial clearance also occurs in healthy volunteers, where a greater than 10-fold increase in clearance was observed (Leigh *et al.*, 1994). Twice daily nebulized 6% saline caused a significant improvement in the spirometry of cystic fibrosis patients when given for 2 weeks (Eng *et al.*, 1996).

The mechanism of its action has been a matter of some speculation. There is no evidence that increasing salinity stimulates ciliary beating frequency; on the contrary, the frequency seems to have a plateau, which extends from isotonic to 500 mosmol/l (Luk & Dulfano, 1983; Ingels *et al.*, 1991). Unpublished observations (P.J. Wills and P.J. Cole) indicate that it acts directly on mucus to alter its rheology in a way that allows more rapid transportation by the cilia. This effect is very rapid: sputum dipped in 2% saline for less than 30 seconds is transformed from a slowly transported gel to one which is rapidly transported on the mucus-depleted bovine trachea. This is probably because the cilia interact only with the very thin outer layer of a portion of mucus, the composition of which is quickly altered by a surrounding solution.

Hypertonic saline, like water, is irritant and can cause bronchospasm (Eschenbacher *et al.*, 1984). The beneficial and toxic effects of chronic administration have not been studied. It cannot therefore be recommended for long-term use until further studies are performed.

Emetics

Emetics in subemetic doses are probably the most commonly used expectorants, having been in use for generations and being generally available without prescription. There is a paucity of scientific data on their use, and much that exists is unfavourable. Their use may not, however, be entirely without scientific respectability, because vagal stimulation causes mucus secretion, as does emesis. Guaiphenesin does appear to increase the volume of respiratory tract secretions in animals (Perry & Boyd, 1941). It is, of course, another matter whether the doses employed in humans have this effect, and more doubtful still whether further mucus secretion is clinically desirable. One clearance study with guaiphenesin indicated increased clearance (Thomson *et al.*, 1973), but another did not (Pavia *et al.*, 1983). Controlled trials examining its effects on symptoms and lung function have mostly failed to demonstrate a benefit.

Iodide has a mucolytic action *in vitro*, and is concentrated in the secretions when administered orally in large doses, which are unpleasant to take. A large uncontrolled survey suggested symptomatic benefit, which seems to be due to a general secretagogue effect (Bernecker, 1969). A double-blind study of the effect of iodinated glycerol indicated that it also appeared to improve symptoms and overall health in chronic bronchitis (Repsher, 1993).

Sulfhydryl agents

These include acetylcysteine, carbocisteine and methylcysteine. Most experience has been with acetylcysteine, which has an *in vitro* mucolytic effect (Scheffner *et al.*, 1964), generally attributed to its ability to cleave disulphide bonds. It can be administered orally or as an aerosol, but the latter method has the drawback that the drug has an unpleasant smell and is irritant (Waltemath & Bergman, 1973). When taken orally, it does not reach the lung epithelial lining fluid in detectable amounts, but levels of reduced glutathione are raised there (Bridgeman *et al.*, 1991). It has been claimed to reduce infective exacerbation rates in chronic bronchitis (Boman *et al.*, 1983). Tracheobronchial clearance does not seem to be improved either by acetylcysteine (Millar *et al.*, 1984) or by carbocisteine (Clarke *et al.*, 1980).

Recently, inhaled *N*-acetylcysteine-L-lysinate, a salt of acetylcysteine, has been investigated. When administered to healthy dogs, a small non-significant increase in tracheal mucus velocity was observed, but the mucus was rendered considerably more transportable on the frog palate (Tomkiewicz *et al.*, 1994). This result suggests that the mucociliary escalator in health may not be functioning at its maximum rate possible.

It may be that the antioxidant properties of this class of drugs are as important as any mucolytic action in exerting their therapeutic effects (Heffner & Repine, 1989). Acetylcysteine appears to counteract the damaging effects of ozone (Allegra *et al.*, 1991) and to reduce the numbers of intrabronchial bacteria in chronic bronchitics (Riise *et al.*, 1994). Oxidant damage has been postulated as an important cause of the long-term decline in lung function in chronic air-flow obstruction and even in normal ageing. There is evidence that a diet with regular fresh fruit, which is rich in antioxidants, is protective against this decline (Sridhar, 1995). Therefore, the sulfhydryl agents may not be acting *in vivo* as simple mucolytics.

Corticosteroids

Beneficial effects on mucociliary clearance in asthma have been documented following treatment with prednisolone (Agnew *et al.*, 1983, 1984). The interpretation of these and similar studies is complicated by the beneficial effects of the corticosteroid on the airway obstruction, but the results were interpreted as indicating an additional benefit on mucociliary clearance.

Bronchodilators

Many studies (Santa Cruz *et al.*, 1974; Foster *et al.*, 1976; Lafortuna & Fazio, 1984; Yeates *et al.*, 1995), but not all (Pavia *et al.*, 1983; Isawa *et al.*, 1990), indicate a beneficial effect on mucociliary clearance following β-agonist administration. Aminophylline appears to accelerate tracheobronchial clearance (Serafini *et al.*, 1976; Sutton *et al.*, 1981). A large proportion of patients with mucus retention have an element of reversible airway obstruction, which will, as with corticosteroids, complicate the interpretation of these studies. Ipratropium at therapeutic doses has been reported to have no effect (Pavia *et al.*, 1983).

Deoxyribonuclease

Purulent sputum contains large amounts of DNA, released from host inflammatory cells. In a pure solution, DNA forms a highly viscous gel in the concentrations found in sputum (Conway & Butler, 1954), and catalytic quantities of deoxyribonuclease (DNase) cause liquefaction of cystic fibrosis sputum *in vitro* (Lieberman, 1968; Shak *et al.*, 1990). Nebulized extracts of bovine pancreatic DNase were used a generation ago in uncontrolled trials with apparent benefit, but the medication was withdrawn after a rare but serious allergic reaction (Raskin, 1968). Recently, rhDNase has been marketed, which appears to be free of this drawback, and has been efficacious in several outcome measures in the treatment of cystic fibrosis (Ranasinha *et al.*, 1993; Fuchs *et al.*, 1994). It was ineffective in the short term in stable chronic bronchitis (Thompson *et al.*, 1993) and in patients with bronchiectasis not due to cystic fibrosis (Wills *et al.*, in press) but it had detrimental effects when used for 6 months in patients with bronchiectasis not due to cystic fibrosis (Barker *et al.*, 1995).

Although the action of the drug is a specific one to cleave DNA, its effects on sputum appear to be more complex. Although purulent sputum contains large amounts of DNA, it is no more viscid than mucoid sputum without DNA (Picot *et al.*, 1978; Rubin *et al.*, 1994), and sputum viscosity does not correlate with DNA content (Rubin *et al.*, 1994). Nevertheless, DNase rapidly transforms purulent sputum from a gel into a pourable liquid. An explanation for this apparant paradox was provided by Lieberman (Lieberman & Kurnick, 1962, 1963). Purulent sputum contains proteases of bacterial and host origin, but the mucin is relatively protected from degradation by the DNA, which inhibits the interaction of protease with its substrate. If the DNA is removed, protease degradation of mucin is accelerated. This provides an explanation for the fact that rhDNase destroys the gel structure of purulent sputum *in vitro*, and that similar effects follow in *in vivo* administration, both viscosity and elasticity of sputum being reduced (Shah *et al.*, 1995). It also explains the increase in sputum elastase activity following rhDNase administration (Rochat *et al.*, 1994).

Ex vivo transportability of sputum from DNase-treated patients is not generally improved (Zahm *et al.*, 1995), and it does not improve mucociliary clearance *in vivo* (Laube *et al.*, 1996). Its *in vitro* actions leave open the possibility that it may actually impair mucus expulsion in some circumstances. The agent therefore falls short of the requirements for the ideal mucokinetic drug, and its use outside the context of a clinical trial should be restricted to the situations in which benefit has been shown.

Amiloride

This drug is a sodium channel blocker which, when administered systemically, acts as a diuretic. It has been given in nebulized form in several trials in cystic fibrosis, mostly with beneficial results. It has been associated with a reduced rate of decline of pulmonary function (Knowles *et al.*, 1990) and accelerated tracheobronchial and cough clearance (App *et al.*, 1990). Studies of expectorated sputum indicate improvement in certain rheological parameters, with increased sodium chloride concentrations but no measurable change in sputum hydration. The original rationale for its use was that defective chloride secretion and excessive sodium absorption in this condition lead to dehydrated secretions, and that the drug may counteract this. The studies performed to date, although generally indicating efficacy, have not supported this view of the pathophysiology of the lung secretions in cystic fibrosis, in that benefit has occurred in spite of the lack of a demonstrable change in sputum hydration (Tomkiewicz *et al.*, 1993). These results would, however, be predicted from the observed effects *in vitro* of adding sodium chloride alone to cystic fibrosis (and other) sputum (see above).

One major trial failed to show any benefit from nebulized amiloride administration, using a number of endpoints, including pulmonary function, sputum rheology, infective exacerbation rates and tracheobronchial clearance, measured by the clearance of radiolabelled polystyrene particles (Graham *et al.*, 1993). This study, however, differed from the others in that the vehicle in which amiloride was dissolved was a very dilute (0.13%) saline solution. The other studies used considerably higher concentrations of saline. Possibly this hypotonic vehicle may have counteracted the benefit of sodium channel blockade, by diluting the sodium in the mucus.

Other investigational substances

Surfactants appear to have mucokinetic properties. When Curosurf, a porcine lung preparation, was sprayed on to the canine trachea, the tracheal mucus velocity increased approximately fourfold (De Sanctis *et al.*, 1994). Lung mucus from babies with respiratory distress syndrome was changed by *in vivo* Exosurf therapy: it became more transportable on the frog palate assay, its hydration increased and its viscoelasticity decreased (Rubin *et al.*, 1992).

The nucleotide triphosphates adenosine triphosphate (ATP) and uridine triphosphate (UTP) have also been studied. ATP is the immediate source of energy for ciliary beating. It appears to increase the ciliary beat frequency of animal respiratory cilia, both when applied topically and when administered systemically (Saano *et al.*, 1992). It has also been claimed to induce active movement of the cilia from patients with immotile cilia syndrome (Forrest *et al.*, 1979). UTP and ATP stimulate chloride transport across cystic fibrosis airway epithelia in the presence of amiloride, but UTP has the advantage that it is not metabolized into bronchoconstrictor degradation products (Knowles *et al.*, 1991). Aerosolized UTP combined with amiloride has been claimed to accelerate clearance of a radioaerosol (Knowles *et al.*, 1994).

Airway cleanliness is maintained by a combination of mucociliary clearance, two-phase flow and cough. Much of the basic physiology appears to be fairly well understood, but vital gaps in our knowledge remain. In particular, the pathophysiology of mucus retention has hardly begun to be unravelled, although the mucus salt concentration probably plays a pivotal role. Cystic fibrosis remains a major challenge in our understanding of the pathophysiology of mucus retention. If the connection can be made in this disease between the genetic defect and the infected phenotype, this is likely also to cast light on the pathogenesis of other more common mucus-retaining states.

References

Afzelius, B.A. (1976) A human syndrome caused by immotile cilia. *Science*, **193**, 317–19.

Agnew, J.E., Bateman, J.R.M., Sheahan, N.F., Lennard-Jones, A.M. & Pavia, D. (1983) Effect of oral corticosteroids on mucus clearance by cough and mucociliary transport in stable asthma. *Bull. Eur. Physiopathol. Resp.*, **19**, 37–41.

Agnew, J.E., Bateman, J.R.M., Pavia, D. & Clarke, S.W. (1984) Peripheral airways mucus clearance in stable asthma is improved by oral corticosteroid therapy. *Bull. Eur. Physiopathol. Resp.*, **20**, 295–301.

Allegra, L., Moavero, N.E. & Rampoldi, C. (1991) Ozone-induced impairment of mucociliary transport and its prevention with *N*-acetylcysteine. *Am. J. Med.*, **91** (Suppl. 3C), 67S–71S.

Allen, R.D. (1968) A reinvestigation of cross-sections of cilia. *J. Cell Biol.*, **37**, 825.

Anon. (1993) Great Britain Office of Population, Censuses and Surveys. *Mortality Statistics, General, 1991*. HMSO Publications, London.

Anon. (1995) Great Britain Office of Population Censuses and Surveys. *Morbidity Statistics from General Practice 1991–92*. HMSO Publications, London.

App, E.M., King, M., Helfesrieder, R., Köhler, D. & Matthys, H. (1990) Acute and long-term amiloride inhalation in cystic fibrosis lung disease. A rational approach to cystic fibrosis therapy. *Am. Rev. Resp. Dis.*, **141**, 605–12.

App, E.M., Zayas, J.G. & King, M. (1993) Rheology of mucus and transepithelial potential difference: small airways versus trachea. *Eur. Resp. J.*, **6**, 67–75.

Asmundsson, T. & Kilburn, K.H. (1970) Mucociliary clearance rates at various levels in dog lungs. *Am. Rev. Resp. Dis.*, **102**, 388–97.

Barker, A., O'Donnell, A., Mallon, K., Fox, N.L. & Fick, R. (1995) Phase II trial of recombinant human DNase I in non-CF bronchiectasis. *Am. J. Resp. Crit. Care Med.*, **151**, A463 [abstract].

Barker, P.M. (1994) Transalveolar Na^+ absorption — a strategy to counter alveolar flooding? *Am. J. Resp. Crit. Care Med.*, **150**, 302–3.

Barlocco, E.G., Valletta, E.A., Canciani, M. *et al.* (1991) Ultrastructural ciliary defects in children with recurrent infections of the lower respiratory tract. *Pediatr. Pulmonol.*, **10**, 11–17.

Bateman, J.R.M., Pavia, D., Sheahan, N.F., Agnew, J.E. & Clarke, S.W. (1983) Impaired tracheobronchial clearance in patients with mild stable asthma. *Thorax*, **38**, 463–7.

Bernecker, C. (1969) Intermittent therapy with potassium iodide in chronic obstructive disease of the airways: a review of 10 years' experience. *Acta Allergol.*, **24**, 216–25.

Bigby, T.D., Margolskee, D., Curtis, J.L. *et al.* (1986) The usefulness of induced sputum in the diagnosis of *Pneumocystis carinii* pneumonia in patients with the acquired immunodeficiency syndrome. *Am. Rev. Resp. Dis.*, **133**, 515–18.

Boat, T.F., Cheng, P.-W. & Leigh, M.W. (1995) Biochemistry of mucus. In: *Airway Secretion* (eds T. Takishima & S. Shimura), pp. 217–82. Marcel Dekker, New York.

Boman, G., Bäcker, U., Larsson, S., Melander, B. & Wåhlander, L. (1983) Oral acetylcysteine reduces exacerbation rate in chronic bronchitis: report of a trial organised by the Swedish Society for Pulmonary Diseases. *Eur. J. Resp. Dis.*, **64**, 405–15.

Boucher, R.C. (1994a) Human airway ion transport. Part one. *Am. J. Resp. Crit. Care Med.*, **150**, 271–81.

Boucher, R.C. (1994b) Human airway ion transport. Part two. *Am. J. Resp. Crit. Care Med.*, **150**, 581–93.

Bridgeman, M.M.E., Marsden, M., MacNee, W., Flenley, D.C. & Ryle, A.P. (1991) Cysteine and glutathione concentrations in plasma and bronchoalveolar lavage fluid after treatment with *N*-acetylcysteine. *Thorax*, **46**, 39–42.

Camner, P. (1981) Studies on the removal of inhaled particles from the lungs by voluntary coughing. *Chest*, **80** (Suppl.), 824–7.

Camner, P., Jarstrand, C. & Philipson, K. (1973) Tracheobronchial clearance in patients with influenza. *Am. Rev. Resp. Dis.*, **108**, 131–5.

Camner, P., Mossberg, B., Philipson, K. & Strandberg, K. (1979) Elimination of test particles from the human tracheobronchial tract by voluntary coughing. *Scand. J. Resp. Dis.*, **60**, 56–62.

Chace, K.V., Naziruddin, B., Desai, V.C., Flux, M. & Sachdev, G.P. (1989) Physical properties of purified human respiratory mucus glycoproteins: effects of sodium chloride concentration on the aggregation properties and shape. *Exp. Lung Res.*, **15**, 721–37.

Clarke, S.W. (1973) The role of two-phase flow in bronchial clearance. *Bull. Eur. Physiopathol. Resp.*, **9**, 359–72.

Clarke, S.W., Thomson, M.L. & Pavia, D. (1980) Effect of mucolytic and expectorant drugs on tracheobronchial clearance in chronic bronchitis. *Eur. J. Resp. Dis.*, **61** (Suppl. 110), 179–91.

Cochrane, G.M., Webber, B.A. & Clarke, S.W. (1977) Effects of sputum on pulmonary function. *Brit. Med. J.*, **2**, 1181–3.

Cohen, A.B. & Gold, W.M. (1975) Defense mechanisms of the lungs. *Ann. Rev. Physiol.*, **37**, 325–49.

Cole, P. & Wilson, R. (1989) Host–microbial interrelationships in respiratory infection. *Chest*, **95**, 217S–221S.

Cole, P.J. (1995) Bronchiectasis. In: *Respiratory Medicine*, Vol. 2 (eds R.A.L. Brewis, G.J. Gibson & D.M. Geddes) pp. 1286–316. Baillière Tindall, London.

Conway, B.E. & Butler, J.A. (1954) Effect of salts on the interaction of nucleic acid particles. *J. Polym. Sci.*, **12**, 199–208.

Conway, J.H., Fleming, J.S., Perring, S. & Holgate, S.T. (1992) Humidification as an adjunct to chest physiotherapy in aiding tracheobronchial clearance in patients with bronchiectasis. *Resp. Med.*, **86**, 109–14.

Currie, D.C., Munro, C., Gaskell, D. & Cole, P.J. (1986) Practice, problems and compliance with postural drainage: a survey of chronic sputum producers. *Brit. J. Dis. Chest*, **80**, 249–53.

Currie, D.C., Pavia, D., Agnew, J.E. *et al.* (1987) Impaired tracheobronchial clearance in bronchiectasis. *Thorax*, **42**, 126–30.

DeBoeck, K., Jorissen, M., Wouters, K. *et al.* (1992) Aplasia of respiratory tract cilia. *Pediatr. Pulmonol.*, **13**, 259–65.

Demedts, M. (1987) Assessment of airway secretions by pulmonary function tests. *Eur. J. Resp. Dis.*, **71**, 330–3.

De Sanctis, G.T., Tomkiewicz, R.P., Rubin, B.K., Schürch, S. & King, M. (1994) Exogenous surfactant enhances mucociliary clearance in the anaesthetized dog. *Eur. Resp. J.*, **7**, 1616–21.

du Bois, R.M. (1985) The alveolar macrophage. *Thorax*, **40**, 321–7.

Dulfano, M.J. & Adler, K.B. (1975) Physical properties of sputum. VII. Rheologic properties and mucociliary transport. *Am. Rev. Resp. Dis.*, **112**, 341–7.

Eng, P.A., Morton, J., Douglass, J.A., Riedler, J. Wilson, J. & Robertson, C.F. (1996) Short-term efficacy of ultrasonically nebulized hypertonic saline in cystic fibrosis. *Pediatr. Pulmonol.*, **21**, 77–83.

Eschenbacher, W.L., Boushey, H.A. & Sheppard, D. (1984) Alteration in osmolarity of inhaled aerosols cause bronchoconstriction and cough, but absence of a permeant anion causes cough alone. *Am. Rev. Resp. Dis.*, **129**, 211–15.

Fawcett, D.W. & Porter, K.R. (1954) A study of the fine structure of ciliated epithelia. *J. Morphol.*, **94**, 221–81.

Foliguet, B. & Puchelle, E. (1986) Apical structure of human respiratory cilia. *Bull. Eur. Physiopathol. Resp.*, **22**, 43–7.

Forrest, J.B., Rossman, C.M., Newhouse, M.T. & Ruffin, R. (1979) Activation of nasal cilia in immotile cilia syndrome. *Am. Rev. Resp. Dis.*, **120**, 511–15.

Foster, W.M., Bergofsky, E.H., Bohning, D.E., Lippman, M. & Albert, R.E. (1976) Effect of adrenergic agents and their mode of action on mucociliary clearance in man. *J. Appl. Physiol.*, **41**, 146–52.

Fuchs, H.J., Borowitz, D.S., Christiansen, D.H. *et al.* (1994) Effect of aerosolised recombinant human DNase on exacerbations of respiratory symptoms and on pulmonary function in patients with cystic fibrosis. *New Engl. J. Med.*, **331**, 637–42.

Garrard, C.S., Mussatto, D.J. & Lourenco, R.V. (1989) Lung mucociliary transport in asymptomatic asthma: effects of inhaled histamine. *J. Lab. Clin. Med.*, **113**, 190–5.

Gelman, R.A. & Meyer, F.A. (1979) Mucociliary transference rate and mucus viscoelasticity: dependence on dynamic storage and loss modulus. *Am. Rev. Resp. Dis.*, **120**, 553–7.

Goodman, R.M., Yergin, B.M., Landa, J.F., Golinvaux, M.H. & Sackner, M.A. (1978) Relationship of smoking history and pulmonary function tests to tracheal mucus velocity in nonsmokers, young smokers, ex-smokers, and patients with chronic bronchitis. *Am. Rev. Resp. Dis.*, **117**, 205–14.

Graham, A., Haasani, A., Alton, E.W.F.W. *et al.* (1993) No added benefit from nebulised amiloride in patients with cystic fibrosis. *Eur. Resp. J.*, **6**, 1243–8.

Hasani, A., Pavia, D., Agnew, J.E. & Clarke, S.W. (1994) Regional lung clearance during cough and forced expiration technique (FET): effects of flow and viscoelasticity. *Thorax*, **49**, 557–61.

Heffner, J.E. & Repine, J.E. (1989) Pulmonary strategies of antioxidant defense. *Am. Rev. Resp. Dis.*, **140**, 531–54.

Hendry, W.F., A'Hern, R.P. & Cole, P.J. (1993) Was Young's syndrome caused by exposure to mercury in childhood? *Brit. Med. J.*, **307**, 1579–82.

Hilding, A.C. (1957) Ciliary streaming in the bronchial tree and the time element in carcinogenesis. *New Engl. J. Med.*, **256**, 634–40.

Hogg, J.C. (1993) Pathology of asthma. *J. Allergy Clin. Immunol.*, **92**, 1–5.

Houdret, N., Lamblin, G., Scharfman, A., Humbert, P. & Roussel, P. (1983) Activation of bronchial mucin proteolysis by 4-aminophenylmercuric acetate and disulphide bond reducing agents. *Biochim. Biophys. Acta*, **758**, 24–9.

Huxley, E.J., Viroslav, J., Gray, W.R. & Pierce, A.K. (1978) Pharyngeal aspiration in normal adults and patients with depressed consciousness. *Am. J. Med.*, **64**, 564–8.

Ingels, K.J.A.O., Kortmann, M.J.W., Nijziel, M.R., Graamans, K. & Huizing, E.H. (1991) Factors influencing ciliary beat measurements. *Rhinology*, **29**, 17–26.

Iravani, J. & Melville, G.N. (1976) A simple method for the determination of the thread-forming property of tracheobronchial secretions. *Respiration*, **33**, 289–93.

Iravani, J. & van As, A. (1972) Mucus transport in the tracheobronchial tree of normal and bronchitic rats. *J. Pathol.*, **106**, 81–93.

Isawa, T., Teshima, T., Hirano, T. *et al.* (1990) Does a β2-stimulator really facilitate mucociliary transport in the human lungs *in vivo*? A study with procaterol. *Am. Rev. Resp. Dis.*, **141**, 715–20.

Isawa, T., Teshima, T., Anazawa, Y., Miki, M., Shiraishi, K. &

Motomiya, M. (1991) Effect of respiratory phases and gravity on mucociliary transport in the normal lungs. *Sci. Rep. Res. Int. Tohoku Univ. (Med.)*, **38**, 43–50.

Jain, B., Rubinstein, I., Robbins, R.A., Leise, K.L. & Sisson, J.H. (1993) Modulation of airway epithelial cell ciliary beat frequency by nitric oxide. *Biochem. Biophys. Res. Commun.*, **191**, 83–8.

Johnson, N.T., Villalón, M., Royce, F.H., Hard, R. & Verdugo, P. (1991) Autoregulation of beat frequency in respiratory ciliated cells: demonstration by viscous loading. *Am. Rev. Resp. Dis.*, **144**, 1091–4.

Joris, L., Dab, I. & Quinton, P.M. (1993) Elemental composition of human airway surface fluid in healthy and diseased airways. *Am. Rev. Resp. Dis.*, **148**, 1633–7.

Kanthakumar, K., Taylor, G., Tsang, K.W.T. *et al.* (1993) Mechanisms of action of *Pseudomonas aeruginosa* pyocyanin on human ciliary beat *in vitro*. *Infect. Immun.*, **61**, 2848–53.

King, M. & Macklem, P.T. (1977) Rheological properties of microliter quantities of mucus. *J. Appl. Physiol.*, **42**, 797–802.

King, M. & Rubin, B.K. (1995) Rheology of airway mucus: relationship with clearance function. In: *Airway Secretion* (eds T. Takishima & S. Shimura), pp. 283–314. Marcel Dekker, New York.

Knowles, M.R., Church, N.L., Waltner, W.E. *et al.* (1990) A pilot study of aerosolized amiloride for the treatment of lung disease in cystic fibrosis. *New Engl. J. Med.*, **322**, 1189–94.

Knowles, M.R., Clarke, L.L. & Boucher, R.C. (1991) Activation by extracellular nucleotides of chloride secretion in the airway epithelia of patients with cystic fibrosis. *New Engl. J. Med.*, **325**, 533–8.

Knowles, M.R., Olivier, K.N., Bennett, W. *et al.* (1994) Aerosolised uridine triphosphate (UTP) ± amiloride: safety and effect on mucociliary clearance in normal subjects and CF patients. *Pediatr. Pulmonol.*, (Suppl. 10), 99.

Kollberg, H., Mossberg, B., Afzelius, B.A., Philipson, K. & Camner, P. (1978) Cystic fibrosis compared with the immotile-cilia syndrome. *Scand. J. Resp. Dis.*, **59**, 297–306.

Kurashima, K., Ogawa, H., Ohka, T., Fujimura, M. & Matsuda, T. (1992) Thromboxane A2 synthase inhibitor (OKY-046) improves abnormal mucociliary transport in asthmatic patients. *Ann. Allergy*, **68**, 53–6.

Lafortuna, C.L. & Fazio, F. (1984) Acute effect of inhaled salbutamol on mucociliary clearance in health and chronic bronchitis. *Respiration*, **45**, 111–23.

Laube, B.L., Auci, R.M., Shields, D.E. *et al.* (1996) Effect of rhDNase on airflow obstruction and mucociliary clearance in cystic fibrosis. *Am. J. Respir. Crit. Care Med.*, **153**, 752–60.

Leigh, T.R., Jones, B.E., Ryan, P. & Collins, J.V. (1994) The use of radioisotopes for measuring the effect of sputum induction on tracheobronchial clearance. *Nucl. Med. Commun.*, **15**, 156–60.

Lieberman, J. (1968) Measurement of sputum viscosity in a cone-plate viscometer II. An evaluation of mucolytic agents *in vitro*. *Am. Rev. Resp. Dis.*, **97**, 662–72.

Lieberman, J. & Kurnick, N.B. (1962) Influence of deoxyribonucleic acid content on the proteolysis of sputum and pus. *Nature*, **196**, 988–90.

Lieberman, J. & Kurnick, N.B. (1963) Proteolytic enzyme activity and the role of desoxyribose nucleic acid (DNA) in cystic fibrosis sputum. *Pediatrics*, **31**, 1028–32.

Lopez-Vidriero, M.T. & Reid, L. (1978) Bronchial mucus in health and disease. *Brit. Med. Bull.*, **34**, 63–74.

Luk, C.K.A. & Dulfano, M.J. (1983) Effect of pH, viscosity and ionic-strength changes on ciliary beating frequency of human bronchial explants. *Clin. Sci.*, **64**, 449–51.

Lurie, A., Mestiri, M., Huchon, G., Marsac, J., Lockart, A. & Straugh, G. (1992) Methods for clinical assessment of expectorants: a critical review. *Int. J. Clin. Pharmacol. Res.*, **12**, 47–52.

Matthews, L.W., Spector, S., Lemm, J. & Potter, J.L. (1963) Studies on pulmonary secretions I. The over-all chemical composition of pulmonary secretions from patients with cystic fibrosis, bronchiectasis, and laryngectomy. *Am. Rev. Resp. Dis.*, **88**, 199–204.

Messina, M.S., O'Riordan, T.G. & Smaldone, G.C. (1991) Changes in mucociliary clearance during acute exacerbations of asthma. *Am. Rev. Resp. Dis.*, **143**, 993–7.

Meyer, F.A. & Silberberg, A. (1980) The rheology and molecular organization of epithelial mucus. *Biorheology*, **17**, 163–8.

Mezey, R.J., Cohn, M.A., Fernandez, R.J., Januszkiewicz, A.J. & Wanner, A. (1978) Mucociliary transport in allergic patients with antigen-induced bronchospasm. *Am. Rev. Resp. Dis.*, **118**, 677–84.

Millar, A.B., Pavia, D., Agnew, J.E., Lopez-Vidriero, M.T., Lauque, D. & Clarke, S.W. (1984) Oral *N*-acetylcysteine has no demonstrable effect on mucus clearances in chronic bronchitis. *Thorax*, **39**, 238.

Morrell, D.C. (1971) Expressions of morbidity in general practice. *Brit. Med. J.*, **2**, 454–8.

Motoyama, E.K., Gibson, L.E. & Zigas, C.J. (1972) Evaluation of mist tent therapy in cystic fibrosis using maximum expiratory flow volume curve. *Pediatrics*, **50**, 299–306.

Mussatto, D.J., Garrard, C.S. & Lourenco, R.V. (1988) The effect of inhaled histamine on human tracheal mucus velocity and bronchial mucociliary clearance. *Am. Rev. Resp. Dis.*, **138**, 775–9.

Nadel, J.A., Davis, B. & Phipps, R.J. (1979) Control of mucous secretion and ion transport in airways. *Ann. Rev. Physiol.*, **41**, 369–81.

Niggemann, B., Müller, A., Nolte, A., Schnoy, N. & Wahn, U. (1992) Abnormal length of cilia—a cause of primary ciliary dyskinesia—a case report. *Eur. J. Pediatr.*, **151**, 73–5.

Ogino, S., Nose, M., Irifune, M., Kikumori, H. & Igarashi, T. (1993) Nasal mucociliary clearance in patients with upper and lower respiratory diseases. *J. Otorhinolaryngol. Relat. Spec.*, **55**, 352–5.

Olivieri, D., Marsico, S.A. & Del Donno, M. (1985) Improvement of mucociliary transport in smokers by mucolytics. *Eur. J. Resp. Dis.*, **66** (Suppl. 139), 142–5.

O'Riordan, T.G., Zwang, J. & Smaldone, G.C. (1992) Mucociliary clearance in adult asthma. *Am. Rev. Resp. Dis.*, **146**, 598–603.

Pavia, D., Thomson, M.L. & Clarke, S.W. (1978) Enhanced clearance of secretions from the human lung after the administration of hypertonic saline aerosol. *Am. Rev. Resp. Dis.*, **117**, 199–203.

Pavia, D., Bateman, J.R.M., Sheahan, N.F., Agnew, J.E., Newman, S.P. & Clarke, S.W. (1980) Techniques for measuring lung mucociliary clearance. *Eur. J. Resp. Dis.*, **61** (Suppl. 110), 157–68.

Pavia, D., Sutton, P.P., Lopez-Vidriero, M.T., Agnew, J.E. & Clarke, S.W. (1983) Drug effects on mucociliary function. *Eur. J. Resp. Dis.*, **64** (Suppl. 128), 304–17.

Peatfield, A.C. & Richardson, P.S. (1983) The action of dust in the airways on secretion into the trachea of the cat. *J. Physiol.*, **342**, 327–34.

Pedersen, M., Sakakura, Y., Winther, B., Brofeldt, S. & Mygind, N. (1983) Nasal mucociliary transport, number of ciliated cells, and beating pattern in naturally acquired common colds. *Eur. J. Resp. Dis.*, **64** (Suppl. 128), 355–64.

Perry, W.F. & Boyd, E.M. (1941) Method for studying expectorant action in animals by direct measurement of respiratory tract fluids. *J. Pharmacol. Exp. Ther.*, **73**, 65–77.

Picot, R., Das, I. & Reid, L. (1978) Pus, deoxyribonucleic acid, and sputum viscosity. *Thorax*, **33**, 235–42.

Potter, J.L., Matthews, L.W., Spector, S. & Lemm, J. (1967) Studies on pulmonary secretions II. Osmolality and the ionic environment of pulmonary secretions from patients with cystic fibrosis, bronchiectasis, and laryngectomy. *Am. Rev. Resp. Dis.*, **96**, 83–7.

Puchelle, E., Girard, F. & Zahm, J.M. (1976) Rheology of bronchial secretions and mucociliary transport. *Bull. Eur. Physiopathol. Resp.*, **12**, 771–9.

Puchelle, E., Zahm, J.-M. & Bertrand, A. (1979) Influence of age on bronchial mucociliary transport. *Scand. J. Resp. Dis.*, **60**, 307–13.

Puchelle, E., Zahm, J.M. & Duvivier, C. (1983) Spinnability of bronchial mucus: relationship with viscoelasticity and mucous transport properties. *Biorheology*, **20**, 239–49.

Quinton, P.M. (1994) Viscosity versus composition in airway pathology. *Am. J. Resp. Crit. Care Med.*, **149**, 6–7.

Ranasinha, C., Assoufi, B., Christiansen, D. *et al.* (1993) Efficacy and safety of short-term administration of aerosolised recombinant human DNase I in adults with stable stage cystic fibrosis. *Lancet*, **342**, 199–202.

Raskin, P. (1968) Bronchospasm after inhalation of pancreatic dornase. *Am. Rev. Resp. Dis.*, **98**, 697–8.

Rautiainen, M., Nuutinen, J. & Collan, Y. (1991) Short nasal respiratory cilia and impaired mucociliary function. *Eur. Arch. Otorhinolaryngol.*, **248**, 271–4.

Rayner, C.F.J., Rutman, A., Dewar, A., Cole, P.J. & Wilson, R. (1995) Ciliary disorientation in patients with chronic upper respiratory tract inflammation. *Am. J. Resp. Crit. Care Med.*, **151**, 800–4.

Regnis, J.A., Robinson, M., Bailey, D.L. *et al.* (1994) Mucociliary clearance in patients with cystic fibrosis and in normal subjects. *Am. J. Resp. Crit. Care Med.*, **150**, 66–71.

Reid, L. (1954) Pathology of chronic bronchitis. *Lancet.*, **i**, 275–8.

Repsher, L.H. (1993) Treatment of stable chronic bronchitis with iodinated glycerol: a double blind, placebo-controlled trial. *J. Clin. Pharmacol.*, **33**, 856–60.

Rhodin, J.A.G. (1966) Ultrastructure and function of the human tracheal mucosa. *Am. Rev. Resp. Dis.*, **93** (Suppl.), 1–15.

Riise, G.C., Larsson, S., Larsson, P., Jeansson, S. & Andersson, B.A. (1994) The intrabronchial microbial flora in chronic bronchitis patients: a target for *N*-acetylcysteine therapy? *Eur. Resp. J.*, **7**, 94–101.

Roberts, G.P. (1978) Chemical aspects of respiratory mucus. *Br. Med. Bull.*, **34**, 39–41.

Robinson, M., King, M., Tomkiewicz, R.P. *et al.* (1994) Effect of hypertonic saline, amiloride and cough on mucociliary clearance in patients with cystic fibrosis. *Am. J. Resp. Crit. Care Med.*, **149**, A669.

Rochat, T., Dayer, F., Schlegel, S. *et al.* (1994) Effect of treatment with rhDNase on leucocytic elastase activity and quantitative sputum bacteriology. *Pediatr. Pulmonol.*, Suppl. 10, 237.

Rogers, D.F. (1995) Airway submucosal gland and goblet cell secretion. In: *Pharmacology of the Respiratory Tract: Experimental and Clinical Research* (eds K.F. Chung & P.J. Barnes), pp. 583–620. Marcel Dekker, New York.

Rubin, B.K., Ramirez, O. & King, M. (1990) Mucus-depleted frog palate as a model for the study of mucociliary clearance. *J. Appl. Physiol.*, **69**, 424–9.

Rubin, B.K., Ramirez, O. & King, M. (1992) Mucus rheology and transport in neonatal respiratory distress syndrome and the effect of surfactant therapy. *Chest*, **101**, 1080–5.

Rubin, B.K., Ramirez, O., Shak, S., Toy, K.J. & Sinicropi, D. (1994) DNA concentration of CF sputum correlates with hydration and spinnability but not with viscoelasticity. *Pediatr. Pulmonol.*, (Suppl. 10), 241.

Rutland, J. & Cole, P.J. (1980) Non-invasive sampling of nasal cilia for measurement of beat frequency and study of ultrastructure. *Lancet*, **ii**, 564–5.

Rutland, J. & Cole, P.J. (1981) Nasal mucociliary clearance and ciliary beat frequency in cystic fibrosis compared with sinusitis and bronchiectasis. *Thorax*, **36**, 654–8.

Rutland, J., Cox, T., Dewar, A., Cole, P. & Warner, J.O. (1982a) Transitory ultrastructural abnormalities of cilia. *Brit. J. Dis. Chest*, **76**, 185–8.

Rutland, J., Griffin, W.M. & Cole, P.J. (1982b) Human ciliary beat frequency in epithelium from intrathoracic and extrathoracic airways. *Am. Rev. Resp. Dis.*, **125**, 100–5.

Saano, V., Virta, P., Joki, S., Nuutinen, J., Karttunen, P. & Silvasti, M. (1992) ATP induces respiratory ciliostimulation in rat and guinea pig *in vitro* and *in vivo*. *Rhinology*, **30**, 33–40.

Sackner, M.A., Rosen, M.J. & Wanner, A. (1973) Estimation of tracheal mucus velocity by bronchofiberscopy. *J. Appl. Physiol.*, **34**, 495–9.

Sadé, J., Eliezer, N., Silberberg, A. & Nevo, A.C. (1970) The role of mucus in transport by cilia. *Am. Rev. Resp. Dis.*, **102**, 48–52.

Salvaggio, J.E. (1994) Inhaled particles and respiratory disease. *J. Allergy Clin. Immunol.*, **94**, 304–9.

Sanderson, M.J., Lansley, A.B. & Dirksen, E.R. (1992) Regulation of ciliary beat frequency in respiratory tract cells. *Chest*, **101**, 69S–71S.

Santa Cruz, R., Landa, J., Hirsch, J. & Sackner, M.A. (1974) Tracheal mucous velocity in normal man and patients with obstructive lung disease: effects of terbutaline. *Am. Rev. Resp. Dis.*, **109**, 458–63.

Scheffner, A.L., Medler, E.M., Jacobs, L.W. & Sarett, H.P. (1964) The *in vitro* reduction in viscosity of human tracheobronchial secretions by acetylcysteine. *Am. Rev. Resp. Dis.*, **90**, 721–9.

Schuster, A., Fahy, J.V., Ueki, I. & Nadel, J.A. (1995) Cystic fibrosis sputum induces a secretory response from airway gland serous cells that can be prevented by neutrophil protease inhibitors. *Eur. Resp. J.*, **8**, 10–14.

Serafini, S.M. & Michaelson, E.D. (1977) Length and distribution of cilia in human and canine airways. *Bull. Eur. Physiopathol. Resp.*, **13**, 551–9.

Serafini, S.M., Wanner, A. & Michaelson, E.D. (1976) Mucociliary transport in central and intermediate size airways: effect of aminophyllin. *Bull. Eur. Physiopathol. Resp.*, **12**, 415–22.

Shah, P.L., Scott, S., Marriott, C. & Hodson, M.E. (1995) A preliminary report on *in vivo* reduction of sputum viscoelasticity in cystic fibrosis patients treated with aerosolised recombinant human DNase I. *Am. J. Resp. Crit. Care Med.*, **149**, A671.

Shak, S., Capon, D.J., Hellmiss, R., Marsters, S.A. & Baker, C.L. (1990) Recombinant human DNase I reduces the viscosity of cystic fibrosis sputum. *Proc. Nat. Acad. Sci. USA*, **87**, 9188–92.

Sheehan, J.K., Thornton, D.J., Somerville, M. & Carlstedt, I. (1991) 1. Mucin structure: the structure and heterogeneity of respiratory mucus glycoproteins. *Am. Rev. Resp. Dis.*, **144**, S4–S9.

Slayter, H.S., Lamblin, G., Le Treut, A. *et al.* (1984) Complex structure of human bronchial mucus glycoprotein. *Eur. J. Biochem.*, **142**, 209–18.

Sleigh, M.A., Blake, J.R. & Liron, N. (1988) The propulsion of mucus by cilia. *Am. Rev. Resp. Dis.*, **137**, 726–41.

Sridhar, M.K. (1995) Nutrition and lung health. *Brit. Med. J.*, **310**, 75–6.

Stanley, P., MacWilliam, L., Greenstone, M., Mackay, I. & Cole, P. (1984) Efficacy of a saccharin test for screening to detect abnormal mucociliary clearance. *Brit. J. Dis. Chest*, **78**, 62–5.

Stockley, R.A., Hill, S.L., Morrison, H.M. & Starkie, C.M. (1984) Elastolytic activity of sputum and its relation to purulence and to lung function in patients with bronchiectasis. *Thorax*, **39**, 408–13.

Sturgess, J.M., Thompson, M.W., Czegledy-Nagy, E. & Turner, J.A. (1986) Genetic aspects of immotile cilia syndrome. *Am. J. Med. Genet.*, **25**, 149–60.

Sutton, P.P., Pavia, D., Bateman, J.R.M. & Clarke, S.W. (1981) The effect of oral aminophylline on lung mucociliary clearance in man. *Chest*, **80**, 889–91.

Tam, P.Y. & Verdugo, P. (1981) Control of mucus hydration as a Donnan equilibrium process. *Nature*, **292**, 340–2.

Taussig, L.M. (1974) Mists and aerosols: new studies, new thoughts. *J. Pediatr.*, **84**, 619–22.

Thompson, A.B., Fuchs, H., Corkery, K., Pun, E., Fick, R.B. & Rennard, S.I. (1993) Phase II trial of recombinant human DNase for the therapy of chronic bronchitis. *Am. Rev. Resp. Dis.*, **147**, A318.

Thomson, M.L., Pavia, D. & McNicol, M.W. (1973) A preliminary study of the effect of guaiphenesin on mucociliary clearance from the human lung. *Thorax*, **28**, 742–7.

Thornton, D.J., Davies, J.R., Kraayenbrink, M. & Richardson, P.S. (1990) Mucus glycoproteins from 'normal' human tracheobronchial secretion. *Biochem. J.*, **265**, 179–86.

Tomkiewicz, R.P., App, E.M., Zayas, J.G. *et al.* (1993) Amiloride inhalation therapy in cystic fibrosis: influence on ion content, hydration, and rheology of sputum. *Am. Rev. Resp. Dis.*, **148**, 1002–7.

Tomkiewicz, R.P., App, E.M., Coffiner, M., Fossion, J., Mase, P. & King, M. (1994) Mucolytic treatment with *N*-acetylcysteine L-lysinate metered dose inhaler in dogs: airway epithelial function changes. *Eur. Resp. J.*, **7**, 81–7.

Vasconcellos, C.A., Allen, P.G., Wohl, M.E., Drazen, J.M., Janmey, P.A. & Stossel, T.P. (1994) Reduction in viscosity of cystic fibrosis sputum *in vitro* by gelsolin. *Science*, **263**, 969–71.

Verdugo, P. (1990) Goblet cells secretion and mucogenesis. *Ann. Rev. Physiol.*, **52**, 157–76.

Verdugo, P. (1991) Mucin exocytosis. *Am. Rev. Resp. Dis.*, **144**, S33–S37.

Verdugo, P. (1995) Molecular biophysics of mucin secretion. In: *Airway Secretion* (eds T. Takishima & S. Shimura), pp. 101–21. Marcel Dekker, New York.

Verdugo, P., Tam, P.Y. & Butler, J. (1983) Conformational structure of respiratory mucus studied by laser correlation spectroscopy. *Biorheology*, **20**, 223–30.

Waltemath, C.L. & Bergman, N.A. (1973) Increased respiratory resistance provoked by endotracheal administration of aerosols. *Am. Rev. Resp. Dis.*, **108**, 520–5.

Welsh, P.W., Stricker, W.E., Chu, C.P. *et al.* (1987) Efficacy of beclomethasone nasal solution, flunisolide, and cromolyn in relieving symptoms of ragweed allergy. *Mayo Clin. Proc.*, **62**, 125–34.

Wills, P.J. & Cole, P.J. (1994) Hypertonic saline increases the ciliary transportability of bronchiectatic sputum. *Am. J. Resp. Crit. Care Med.*, **149**, A119.

Wills, P.J. & Cole, P.J. (1995) Sodium chloride improves ciliary transportability of sputum. *Am. J. Resp. Crit. Care Med.*, **151**, A720 [abstract].

Wills, P.J., Garcia Suarez, M.J., Rutman, A., Wilson, R. & Cole, P.J. (1995a) The ciliary transportability of sputum is slow on the mucus-depleted bovine trachea. *Am. J. Resp. Crit. Care Med.*, **151**, 1255–8.

Wills, P.J., Wodehouse, T., Abdallah, S., Wilson, R. & Cole, P.J. (1995b) Sputum from bronchiectasis, chronic bronchitis and cystic fibrosis is poorly transported by cilia. *Am. J. Resp. Crit. Care Med.*, **151**, A244 [abstract].

Wills, P.J., Wodehouse, T., Corkery, K., Mallon, K., Wilson, R. & Cole, P.J. (1996) Short term reombinant human DNase in bronchiectasis: effect on clinical state and *in vitro* sputum transportability. *Am. J. Respir. Crit. Care Med.* (in press).

Wilson, R., Roberts, D. & Cole, P.J. (1985) Effect of bacterial products on human ciliary function *in vitro*. *Thorax*, **40**, 125–31.

Wolff, R.K., Dolovich, M.B., Obminski, G. & Newhouse, M.T. (1977) Effects of exercise and eucapnic hyperventilation on bronchial clearance in man. J. Appl. Physiol., **43**, 46–50.

Wood, R.E., Wanner, A., Hirsch, J. & Farrell, P.M. (1975) Tracheal mucociliary transport in patients with cystic fibrosis and its stimulation by terbutaline. *Am. Rev. Resp. Dis.*, **111**, 733–8.

Yeates, D.B., Aspin, N., Levison, H., Jones, M.T. & Bryan, A.C. (1995) Mucociliary tracheal transport rates in man. *J. Appl. Physiol.*, **39**, 487–95.

Zahm, J.M., Girod de Bentzmann, S., Deneuville, E. *et al.* (1995) Dose-dependent properties of recombinant human DNase on the transport properties of cystic fibrosis respiratory mucus. *Am. J. Resp. Crit. Care Med.*, **149**, A671.

CHAPTER 41

New Approaches in Aerosol Drug Delivery for the Treatment of Asthma

V. Knight & J.C. Waldrep

Introduction

Aerosols are dispersions in air of solid or liquid particles, of fine enough particle size, and consequent low enough settling velocities, to have relative airborne stability. In quiet air, a spherical unit density particle of 10 μm diameter would take 17 minutes to settle the height of a room (3 m). A 1 μm particle would take 24 hours to settle this distance (Knight, 1973).

Aerosols have been widely and beneficially used for many years for delivery of drugs for the treatment of asthma. The treatment nevertheless has limitations, resulting from the exceptional efficiency of the human respiratory tract to limit the penetration of inhaled particles to the lower respiratory tract and to remove particles deposited in upper respiratory sites by mucociliary action and swallowing. It is probably a manifestation of these difficulties that there are myriad devices on the market, each seeking to improve efficiency of pulmonary deposition of inhaled particles. These include the widely used metered dose inhalers (MDI) of various configurations and dry-powder inhalers (DPI). Recently, the problem has been further complicated by the requirement that the use of chlorofluorocarbon (CFC) propellants, the most widely used methodology, must be discontinued because of environmental hazard. There is a major effort now under way to develop alternative methods of aerosol treatment, but the technology by which this will be achieved has not yet emerged. In this chapter, we shall review both traditional and newly developed technologies applicable to the treatment of asthma.

General considerations of particle deposition in the respiratory tract

The advantages of aerosol delivery of drugs to the respiratory tract are that the drug is deposited on diseased lung surfaces immediately after start of treatment and the total dose required for treatment is generally much lower than that required by oral or intravenous routes. Drugs deposited in the respiratory tract are cleared by macrophages or slowly enter the circulation directly or through lymphatics. Many drugs are metabolized to some extent in the lung as well (Andersson & Ryerfeldt, 1984; Debs, 1990). When these effects are combined with the low total dose, concentrations in serum and organs other than the lung are low and high peak levels that may cause systemic toxicity are avoided. The rate of clearance from the lung is influenced by biochemical properties of the compound, such as solubility, lipophilicity and molecular size (Schanker *et al.*, 1986; Byron & Patton, 1994). Water-soluble drugs are absorbed more slowly than lipid-soluble drugs (Schanker *et al.*, 1986). Absorption is greatest in the alveolar area, which constitutes the largest absorbing surface in the respiratory tract. The clearance of both lipid-soluble and water-soluble drugs is reduced substantially by incorporation into liposomes.

A disadvantage of aerosol treatment is the loss of aerosol that is produced in excess of the patient's capacity to inhale it and the exhalation of inhaled aerosol that is not deposited. In addition, with nasal breathing, large numbers of particles deposit in the nose and are promptly cleared by mucociliary action to the pharynx where they are swallowed. Nasal deposition constitutes essentially oral dosage and may present a risk of systemic toxicity when powerful agents such as glucocorticoids (GC) are used. Drugs deposited in the tracheobronchial area are transported upward to the pharynx by mucociliary action, where they are swallowed. The larger bronchi do not constitute a large surface area and thus their burden of deposited particles is small. Larger numbers of particles deposit in the more peripheral and more extensive smaller airways. They, too, are transported upward through mucociliary action, but the process is much slower, allowing time for local drug action. The most peripheral and most extensive portion of the lungs, consisting of partially and fully alveolated airways, do not possess the mucociliary system and clearance from these sites is primarily into the circulation.

From the foregoing, it is evident that avoiding nasal deposition by using mouth breathing would be advantageous. Greater efficiency of treatment would result if aerosol could be supplied to the patient only during inspiration. This methodology is currently available and details of its use will be presented. A drawback to mouth breathing is patient discomfort when long periods of treatment are required, but this is not a problem in asthma therapy.

As the use of aerosol treatments increases with a greater variety of drugs, adjuvants of aerosol delivery, such as liposomes or other carrier particles, and the use of different kinds of devices to generate aerosols are being studied. A method that can be used to make comparisons among these potentially numerous delivery systems would be advantageous. In the past, model systems resembling the human respiratory tract have also been used successfully. There are logistic reasons, however, that discourage their widespread use.

We propose an alternative system for valuating aerosols for human treatment, namely, calculation of regional deposition of inhaled aerosol based primarily on particle size but also including quantitative deposition, so that precise comparisons among aerosol generators can be made (Lippman *et al.*, 1980; Persons *et al.*, 1987a,b). Such a method could compare the output from jet nebulizers, MDI, DPI and other devices. The experimental and theoretical basis of particle deposition is substantial, and reasonable approximations of regional deposition of aerosols are possible.

The expanding use of aerosols has also increased the need to know which pattern of pulmonary deposition is best for the treatment of particular disease entities. While the disease, asthma, is most conspicuous because of its interference with small airway function, the most efficient and effective site of aerosol treatment for it has not been clinically defined. In the following section, we shall describe a lung model which uses particle size, drug content and other variables to predict regional dosage of inhaled particles.

Calculation of drug delivery by aerosol

While the predominant sites of deposition of particles generated by propellants under pressure, as with MDI or DPI, or droplets generated from liquid suspensions by jet nebulizers is determined principally by the size of the particles or droplets, some particles throughout the size range will be deposited throughout the respiratory tract. The generalization can be made that the largest particles will deposit in nose, throat and bronchial passages and the smallest particles will deposit principally in the lung periphery.

This process can be defined more precisely by relating it to Weibel's anatomical model of the human lung (Weibel, 1963). Above the larynx, most particle deposition, by far, occurs in the nose. Figure 41.1 shows the Weibel model of the lung, in which the conducting airway generations are numbered 0–16 from the trachea to the fine bronchioles. As stated earlier, these areas are ciliated and contain mucus-secreting cells to form the mucociliary system, which propels deposited particles proximally to be eventually swallowed. Generations 17–23 are increasingly alveolated and do not contain the mucociliary apparatus, but they constitute the largest portion of the lung surface.

If nasal deposition is excluded from consideration, as is proposed for the treatment of asthma, calculated deposition of inhaled particles in the lung, with mouth breathing, according to a range of particle sizes is shown in Table 41.1. We believe that, for asthma treatment, deposition in the mouth and upper generations of the conducting airways should also be minimized, and this can be best achieved with a particle size of about 1.6 μm mass median aerodynamic diameter (MMAD). Such particles deposit principally in the alveolated lung area, but a significant amount will deposit in the 0–16 generations. We believe, also, that deposition in these lung areas will be suitable for the treatment of asthma; however, data describing other deposition patterns according to particle size are shown. Major factors which determine site of particle deposition include inertial impaction, occurring principally in the nasopharynx and upper airways, where the rate of air flow is greatest. Sedimentation in smaller airways is principally due to gravity. Particles <0.5 μm MMAD, however, deposit in terminal airways by gaseous diffusion (Brain *et al.*, 1985; Kohler & Fleisher, 1991). Obviously, the size and configuration of the respiratory tract in health and disease will further affect particle deposition. As a generalization, any process which distorts the airway or reduces its diameter will cause increased deposition of particles.

Hygroscopicity influences deposition, due to increase in size of droplets as they progress down the warm and humid passages of the respiratory tract. This effect is most

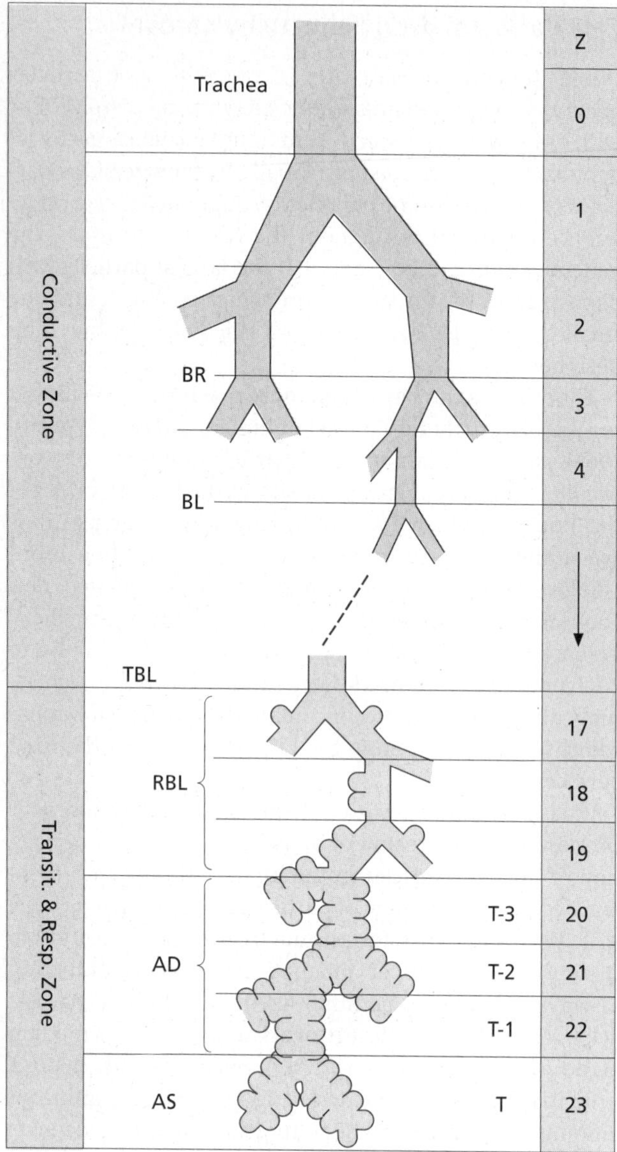

Fig. 41.1 Diagrammatic representation of the sequence of elements in the conducting and transitory zones of the airways leading to terminal alveolated lung spaces. (From Weibel, 1963.)

conspicuous with nasal breathing, during which 35–70% of inhaled hygroscopic particles of 2–6 μm MMAD will deposit in the nose (Knight, 1973). With mouth breathing, which bypasses the nose, there is little difference in deposition patterns of non-hygroscopic and a range of aerosols of increasing hygroscopicity (Table 41.2). Increasing tidal volume (Table 41.3) causes increased peripheral lung deposition, because of deeper penetration and longer residence time of particles in the lung. Breath holding (Table 41.4) is associated with an even greater effect on peripheral lung deposition. It has been found difficult, however, to employ these procedures in patients who are ill.

Asthma has a large impact on children; because of their greater need of respiratory gas exchange to provide for metabolic and growth requirements, individual dose calculations based on age are required. Table 41.5 shows that, when breathing the same aerosol over the same period of time as an adult, a 6-year-old child will deposit 1.9 times as many particles as the adult per kilogram of body

Table 41.1 Effect of particle size on regional aerosol particle deposition* (tidal volume 750 ml, geometric standard deviation (GSD) 2.0). (Data provided by Keyvan Keyhani, Department of Bioengineering, University of Pennsylvania, Philadelphia, PA.)

MMAD (μm)	Mouth (%)	0–16 (%)	17–23 (%)	Total (%)
0.8	0.2	1.7	11.6	13.5
1.6	2.0	4.6	17.6	24.3
3.2	10.6	11.0	22.7	44.3
6.4	29.8	20.0	18.1	68.0
9.6	41.9	22.3	11.7	77.3

* Regional deposition of inhaled particles according to the Weibel lung model (Weibel, 1963). Breathing characteristics assumed for an adult were functional residual capacity 3300 ml; mouth breathing, inspiration 2 seconds; expiration 2 seconds; no breath holding.

Table 41.2 Effect of salt concentration on regional aerosol particle deposition* (tidal volume 750 ml, MMAD 1.6 μm, GSD 2.0).

Salt concentration	Mouth (%)	0–16 (%)	17–23 (%)	Total (%)
Non-hygroscopic	3.8	9.3	20.7	33.8
0.0045 g/ml ($\frac{1}{2}$ normal)	2.0	4.6	17.6	24.3
0.0090 g/ml (normal)	2.1	6.2	20.9	29.1
0.0180 g/ml (2 × normal)	2.2	8.2	24.1	34.5

* Footnote as in Table 41.1

Table 41.3 Effect of tidal volume on regional aerosol particle deposition* (MMAD 1.6 μm, GSD 2.0). (Data from Keyvan Keyhani, Department of Bioengineering, University of Pennsylvania, Philadelphia, PA.)

Tidal volume (ml)	Mouth (%)	0–16 (%)	17–23 (%)	Total (%)
1000	3	4.3	20.1	28.1
750	2	4.6	17.6	24.2
500	1.2	5.5	11	17.6

* Breathing characteristics as in Table 41.1, except for tidal volumes.

Table 41.4 Effect of breath holding on regional aerosol particle deposition* (tidal volume 750 ml, MMAD 1.6 μm, GSD 2.0). (Data from Keyvan Keyhani, Department of Bioengineering, University of Pennsylvania, Philadelphia, PA.)

Breath holding time (seconds)	Mouth (%)	0–16 (%)	17–23 (%)	Total (%)
0	2.01	4.63	17.6	24.3
2	2.04	7.12	35.5	44.7
10	2.22	10.9	53.4	66.5
30	2.6	13.9	60.4	76.8

* Breathing characteristics as in Table 41.1 except for breath holding.

Table 41.5 Respiratory tract deposition of aqueous aerosol particles in intubated patients according to age (MMAD 1.4 μm, GSD 1.6).

Age (years)	0–16 (%)	17–23 (%)	Total (%)	Relative dose* (mg/kg)
6	36	19	55	1.9
8	33	21	54	1.7
12	30	22	53	1.3
16	29	24	53	1.0
25	29	24	52	1.0

* Adjusted for age-related differences in ventilation; 25 years' ventilation = 1, based on aqueous ribavirin aerosol (Knight *et al.*, 1988).

weight. This value is 1.7, 1.3 and 1.0 for children of ages 8, 12 and 16. Dosage calculations for children should take these factors into account. In contrast to total deposited dose, there is little difference in regional deposition between children and adults (Table 41.5).

Currently available drug aerosol delivery systems

MDI

In recent years, aerosol administration of asthma medications has been dominated by the widespread usage of MDI. MDI have been developed and effectively utilized with different bronchodilators (e.g. albuterol), anti-allergics (e.g. nedocromil sodium) and GC. Inhaled GC are a very effective treatment of asthma (Reed, 1991; Szefler, 1992; McFadden, 1993; Toogood, 1993). These topically active GC have minimal effects on the hypothalamic–pituitary–adrenal axis, except when daily doses of 1000 μg or more are employed. The development of topically potent GC with first-pass liver metabolism has minimized systemic side-effects (Ryrefeldt *et al.*, 1982; Andersson & Ryrefeldt, 1984; Brattsand *et al.*, 1992). However, oropharyngeal complications of candidiasis (localized inhibition of host defences by GC) and dysphonia (toxic response to CFC propellants) are more common with MDI (Toogood *et al.*, 1980; Toogood, 1993). The development of spacer extensions or holding chambers has been necessitated by these complications (Toogood *et al.*, 1984).

However, environmental concerns and the 1996 worldwide ban on CFC propellants have caused manufacturers to phase out CFC production and have necessitated the development of alternative propellants and devices (Newman, 1990; Balmes, 1991). Most of the propellants in development for current MDI devices are not compatible with existing metering valves, excipients and some manufacturing components, and the toxicology issues remain to be delineated. Complex interactions may occur between the newer propellants, surfactants and drugs (Niven, 1993). Furthermore, contribution to the greenhouse effect by the newer propellants could lead to regulated utilization (Martin *et al.*, 1994).

MDI may be unsuitable in some patients, such as infants, children, the elderly or the chronically ill (O'Doherty & Miller, 1993). Furthermore, the required coordination between actuation and inhalation may result in inadequate aerosol drug delivery from MDI in many patients (DeBlaquiere *et al.*, 1989; Manzella, 1989; Hilton, 1990). Much of the aerosolized drug from the MDI is lost in the device or deposited in the upper part of the respiratory tract. Particle sizes produced by MDI are generally large and the deposition patterns can be reasonably well predicted from data supplied in this chapter. Table 41.6 shows droplet size produced by several commercially available MDI. The average particle size is calculated at 4–5 μm MMAD with a geometric standard deviation (GSD) of > 2. By interpolation from our computer model of mouth breathing, the deposition pattern at 4.8 μm MMAD would be about 20% deposited in mouth, 15% in 0–16 generations and 21% in 17–23 generations. Some estimates, however, put the lung deposition value at approximately 10% (Newman *et al.*, 1981).

DPI

In response to the above concerns regarding MDI, alternative delivery systems, such as the DPI, have been developed. The complex design features of DPI rely on the patient's inspiratory flow to generate and deliver drug aerosols. DPI have been developed for the aerosol delivery of β_2-agonists, bronchodilators, sodium cromoglycate and some GC (Timsina *et al.*, 1994). Suitable DPI formulation requires that the powdered drug be available in a stable, bioactive form (Niven, 1993). The performance of DPI is determined, in part, by powder formulation,

Table 41.6 Aerodynamic size distribution of metered dose inhaler aerosols. (Condensed from Kim *et al.*, 1985.)

Tade name	Generic name	MMAD (90% RH) (μm)	GSD
Duo-Medihaler	Isoprenaline Phenylephrine	5.7	2.3
Medihaler ISO	Isoprenaline	4.1	2.0
Medihaler EPI	Adrenaline	5.2	2.2
Alupent	Orciprenaline	5.3	2.1
Proventil	Albuterol	2.6	2.3
Bronkometer	Isoetharine Phenylephrine	5.7	2.4
Mistometer	Isoprenaline	3.9	2.2
Beclovent	Beclomethason	4.0	2.1
Aristocort	Triamcinolone Acetonide	4.7	2.4

See text for definition of abbreviations.

including the carrier powder. The effects of formulation variables on pulmonary deposition of DPI aerosols, surface properties of the carrier, optimum carrier size, drug to carrier ratio, relative humidity, electrostatic behaviour, the use of tertiary components and process conditions are poorly characterized (Martin *et al.*, 1994; Timsina *et al.*, 1994).

Some carriers have induced irritation, coughing or bronchoconstriction (Timsina *et al.*, 1994). An important variable in DPI therapy is the required energy input during inspiration for deaggregation of drug particles from carrier. Forces between drug and carrier must be sufficient to ensure that there is no deaggregation during filling and handling, but to allow extensive detachment when subjected to the turbulent air flow generated within the device (Martin *et al.*, 1994). While DPI are clinically effective in certain types of patient, the breath-actuated output is inefficient and highly variable, delivering a pulmonary dose of about 10% (Niven, 1993). Resistance to air flow through various DPI devices is a problem in some asthmatics, children and the elderly and is dependent on age, sex, height and disease state (Martin *et al.*, 1994; Timsina *et al.*, 1994). The main advantages of DPI are drug delivery co-ordinated with inhalation, environmental safety and low cost (Martin *et al.*, 1994; Olsson & Asking, 1994).

Continuous-flow jet nebulizers

Continuous-flow jet nebulizers have been utilized in asthma for aerosol delivery of different water-soluble medications (bronchodilators, e.g. albuterol) and a few micronized GC suspension formulations (beclomethasone dipropionate (Bec) and budesonide) (Bisgaard, 1994; Wood & Knowles, 1994). Nebulizer-based aerosol therapy is on the increase worldwide, particularly in Europe. The clinical utilization of nebulizers has proved to be particularly successful for hospital and non-ambulatory settings, as well as paediatric and geriatric patients (Dalby & Tiano, 1993). More efficient, convenient, portable and disposable nebulizers and compressors will be utilized with increased regularity in the future (Dalby & Tiano, 1993). A major limitation in this form of aerosol therapy has been the paucity of suitable formulations. There are several important factors which affect therapeutic efficacy of aerosol formulations delivered by nebulizers. Nebulizer design, operating conditions (e.g. flow rate) and ancillary equipment (tubing, connectors, mouthpiece, face masks) are important variables which must be standardized (Dalby & Tiano, 1993). Nebulizer variation, either within manufactured lots or among devices, is an important variable affecting aerosol output efficiency and aerodynamic properties (O'Doherty, 1993). The composition of the aerosol preparation will also influence aerosol output efficiency and aerodynamic properties (Waldrep *et al.*, 1993, 1994c). For example, formulations of liposomes developed for intravenous or other delivery routes are generally not suitable for aerosolization, due to instability or inappropriate biophysical properties (Waldrep *et al.*, 1993, 1994a,c). To achieve the best lower-pulmonary deposition with minimized systemic delivery, aerosols should contain particles less than 5 μm MMAD (ideally between 1 and 3 μm). Many of the currently available jet nebulizers produce aerosols in this size range (Waldrep *et al.*, 1993, 1994c). The operating parameters (e.g. flow rate) must be strictly defined and tested for each device with each standardized formulation (Dalby & Tiano, 1993; Waldrep *et al.*, 1994b).

Alternative aerosol therapy for asthma: drug–liposomes

Aerosol delivery of water-insoluble, hydrophobic compounds currently available for the treatment of asthma has been limited. The recent development of liposomal formulations compatible with aerosol delivery has expanded the potential for more effective utilization with additional drugs and has many potential advantages including: aqueous compatibility, sustained pulmonary release to maintain therapeutic drug levels and facilitated intracellular delivery (particularly to alveolar macrophages) (Schrier *et al.*, 1993). The half-life of drug–liposomes in the lung is significantly longer than that of soluble formulations (Juliano & McCullough, 1980). Liposomes are retained for an even longer period; for example, 50–60% of phosphatidylcholine (PC) liposomes may be retained for 24 hours after inhalation (Morimoto & Adachi, 1982; Pettenazzo *et al.*, 1989; Vidgren *et al.*, 1994). Inhaled liposomes delivered to the terminal airspaces associate rapidly with the alveolar surfactant and enter the intracellular phospholipid pool without altering normal metabolism or macrophage activity (Mihalko *et al.*, 1988). In addition, phospholipase-mediated hydrolysis is minimal (Mihalko *et al.*, 1988). These results suggest that drug–liposome aerosols should be more effective for delivery, deposition and retention of water-insoluble, hydrophobic, lipophilic compounds, in contrast to water-soluble compounds (Niven & Schrier, 1990; Taylor *et al.*, 1990; Taylor & Farr, 1993). Drug–liposome aerosol technology is readily adaptable to conventional or alternative asthma drugs not currently available for aerosol treatment (Szefler, 1992). The highly potent, extremely lipophilic GC currently employed in MDI/DPI for aerosol-based asthma therapies are well suited for liposome aerosol formulation (Waldrep *et al.*, 1993; 1994b,c). In addition, a more innovative development is the use of cyclosporin A (CsA) liposome aerosol for the treatment of asthma (and other immunologically mediated pulmonary diseases) (Gilbert *et al.*, 1993; Waldrep *et al.*, 1993).

In general, hydrophobic drugs incorporate into liposome membranes and hydrophilic drugs are entrapped in the aqueous vesicles of liposomes (New *et al.*, 1990). Large or intermediate-sized multilamellar liposomes are best for use with hydrophilic drugs because of their greater volume; however, hydrophilic compounds are lost in appreciable amounts from liposomes as a result of nebulization (Niven *et al.*, 1990). Biophysical properties of liposomes are influenced by both drug and lipid composition. Nuclear magnetic resonance (NMR) spectroscopy has proved to be a useful tool for determining the orientation of drugs and cholesterol within the liposomal bilayers (Garcon *et al.*, 1989). GC may interact with phospholipid bilayers as its structural analogue, cholesterol. Association of other more hydrophobic drugs, like CsA, in liposomal bilayer or aqueous compartment varies with the phospholipid composition of the liposome (Stuhne-Sekalec *et al.*, 1988, 1991). With liposomal formulations of many hydrophobic drugs (like some GC and CsA), there is a stable association which withstands the shear forces generated during nebulization, reflux and recirculation within the nebulizer reservoir. However, Gilbert *et al.* (1988) and Farr *et al.* (1985) demonstrated significant size reduction in multilamellar vesicle (MLV) liposomes within the nebulizer reservoir resulting from shearing during nebulization. In aerosol it is the aqueous droplet and not the liposome that determines particle size distribution (Farr *et al.*, 1985; Niven *et al.*, 1990; Taylor *et al.*, 1990; Waldrep *et al.*, 1993).

Aerosol droplets may contain none, one or more drug–liposome particles. Aqueous droplets containing lipid particles resist reduction in MMAD in conditions of decreasing relative humidity (RH) until RH reaches about 70% from 95% (Marks *et al.*, 1983). In contrast, hygroscopic saline aerosol droplets shrink in size stepwise with reducing RH. As noted earlier, hygroscopic effects have little effect on respiratory tract deposition of aerosols inhaled through the mouth.

Characteristics of liposome aerosols produced with commercially available jet nebulizers

In a recent study, the MMAD, GSD and aerosol output of 18 commercially available jet nebulizers was determined using Bec–liposomal formulation (Waldrep *et al.*, 1994b). Figure 41.2 shows the estimated percentage regional deposition of inhaled aerosol droplets within Weibel lung generations 0–23. Nebulizers were ranked by increasing value with estimated percentage deposition approximating 25% for generation 17–23 and ranging from 5 to 8% in generations 0–16. Mouth deposition was calculated at about 5%. Thus, there is a considerable degree of uniformity of droplet distribution according to size among these randomly selected, commercially available nebulizers. Differences in output can be attributed to different flow rates employed to generate aerosols as well as design differences (Fig. 41.3). Thus, while MMAD and GSD are

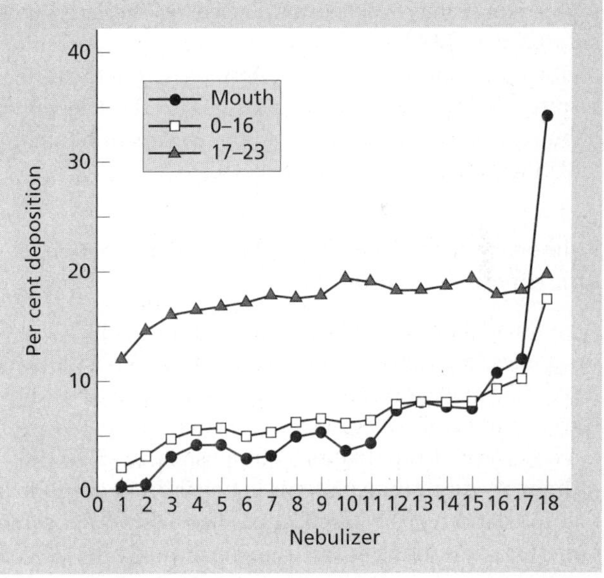

Fig. 41.2 Calculated percentage deposition from 18 nebulizers of beclomethasone dipropionate (Bec) contained in Bec–dilauroyl PC (DLPC) liposome aerosol in mouth, Weibel generations 0–16 and 17–23. The reservoir contained 0.5 mg/ml of Bec in liposomes. Nebulizers 1–18 were Up Mist, Power Mist, Hudson Hand Held, Nb Mist, Ava Neb, Respirgard, Acorn, Whisper Jet, Aqua Tower, Permanent Neb, Custom Neb, Pari-Jet, Puritan Single Jet, Raindrop 3040, SPAG, Spira and Heart. (From Waldrep *et al.*, 1994b.)

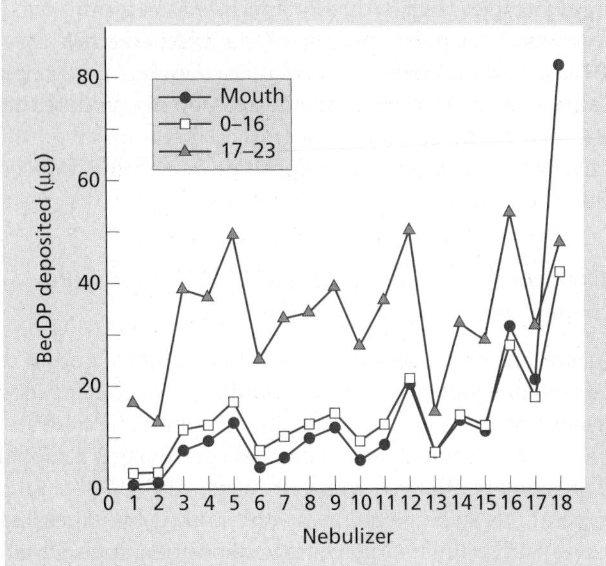

Fig. 41.3 Weight in micrograms of Bec calculated to deposit on regional sites as described in Fig. 41.2. (From Waldrep *et al.*, 1994b.)

major determinants of the site of deposition of aerosol particles within the respiratory track, the amount of drug delivered is a function of the nebulizer design and operation. The results of this study suggest that there is a wide range of operating characteristics among nebulizers, and performance may also be influenced by the substances nebulized. MMAD, GSD and the predicted percentage regional deposition of drug–liposomes within the human respiratory tract could provide a basis for the selection of nebulizers best suited for use in the treatment of asthma and other inflammatory lung diseases.

Pulmonary deposition of technetium-99m-labelled drug–liposome aerosols

A gamma-labelling method for Bec–dilauroyl PC (DLPC) liposomes has been developed to monitor deposition and mucociliary clearance of aerosolized Bec-DLPC liposomes, and this has been performed in normal volunteers (Vidgren *et al.*, 1994). Plate 41.1 (opposite page 524) shows pulmonary deposition patterns in two individuals following inhalation of ^{99m}Tc-labelled Bec–DLPC liposomes (anterior scan). Lung scans were performed after 20 consecutive inhalations from breath-actuated nebulizers: (A) using an Aerotech II nebulizer with Bec–DLPC liposome aerosol output of MMAD 1.5 µm and GSD 2.4; and (B) using a Spira nebulizer with Bec–DLPC liposome aerosol output of MMAD 3.6 µm and GSD 2.5. Pulmonary scans were performed immediately after inhalation and at 1, 2 and 3 hours post-inhalation. In the A series, scintigraphs of pulmonary radioactivity displayed both central and peripheral deposition patterns, which remained nearly constant (some loss due to decay is apparent). Some accumulation of radioactivity was noted in the stomach at 0 and 1 hours. In contrast, in B, pulmonary radioactivity was initially less, with more central deposition. Lung clearance proceeded more rapidly and activity in the stomach was substantially greater throughout the period of observation.

Figure 41.4 demonstrates pulmonary radioactivity in a similar study following inhalation of a ^{99m}Tc-labelled liposome preparation (Farr *et al.*, 1985). The size of the inhaled liposome aerosol droplets was 3.7 µm MMAD and GSD 1.5. Greatest radioactivity was localized centrally, presumably associated with the conducting airways, with much less activity detected in the periphery of the lung. This distribution resembles that in Plate 41.1B, in which the droplet size of the inhaled liposome aerosol was similar, at 3.6 µm MMAD. Observations in both of these studies are consistent with patterns of deposition predicted by our computer model for aerosols containing these droplet sizes. Although drug–liposome aerosols may be less hygroscopic than aerosols of aqueous drugs, the difference is probably not great, and it is a reasonable assumption that drug–liposome aerosol deposits within

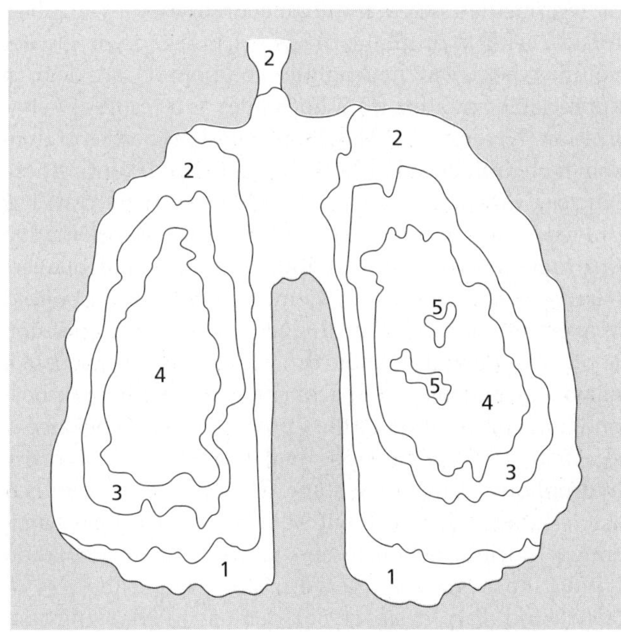

Fig. 41.4 Diagnostic representation of gamma-activity contours obtained from a typical scintigram. Posterior view immediately after inhalation of ^{99m}Tc-labelled liposomes, MMAD 3.7 µm, GSD 1.5. Areas marked 1–5 represent increasing intensity of activity. Note values of 4 and 5 in the hilar region of both lungs, an area corresponding with the first few Weibel generations of conductive airway branchings. (From Farr *et al.*, 1985.)

the lung in a manner analogous to that of 0.5 normal saline (0.0045 g/ml NaCl).

Tolerance and safety of liposome aerosols

Toxicity studies have been performed in animals and humans after inhalation of empty liposomes. Myers *et al.* (1993) exposed mice for 4 weeks to inhalations of commercially available hydrogenated soybean phosphatidylcholine (HSBPC) in concentrations approximating those that might be used for human treatment. A variety of observations, including lung histology, fatty acid analysis of lung tissue, macrophage morphology, phagocytic function, weight gain, and physical appearance, showed no untoward effects of aerosol treatment. Thomas *et al.* (1991) exposed 10 volunteers to a 1-hour aerosol treatment with HSBPC–liposomes in aerosol (15 mg/ml in the aerosol generator reservoir) and later to a 10-fold higher dose. Pulmonary function studies revealed no adverse effects and the liposome aerosol treatment was otherwise well tolerated. Knight, C.M. *et al.* (1994) exposed 10 volunteers to inhalations of DLPC–liposomes (25 mg/ml) followed by Bec–DLPC (1 mg Bec/ml plus 25 mg/ml of DLPC) for 15 minutes each on consecutive days. There were no significant changes in pulmonary function, and laboratory studies and the inhalations were well tolerated.

Liposome-encapsulated drugs have been associated with reduced toxicity *in vitro* and *in vivo* in a number of other experimental systems. Joly *et al.* (1992) cited reduced renal toxicity in rabbits and reduced renal tubular cell toxicity *in vitro* of amphotericin B liposomes. Wyde *et al.* (1988) found a greater than 10-fold reduction in toxicity to multiple cell culture lines of enviroxime in a liposomal formulation compared with the drug in the absence of liposomes. Furthermore, drug–liposomes may prevent local irritation and reduce toxicity both locally and systemically (Juliano & McCullough, 1980; Smeesters *et al.*, 1988; Aguado *et al.*, 1993; Schrier *et al.*, 1993). Increased potency with reduced toxicity is characteristic of many drug–liposomal formulations (Cullis *et al.*, 1989). It is likely that these findings will apply to aerosolized drug–liposomes; however, this remains to be determined in clinical studies.

GC–liposome aerosols

Studies from our laboratory have demonstrated that five different topically potent, hydrophobic GC, currently employed for asthma therapy with MDI/DPI, can be formulated into stable liposomes suitable for aerosol therapy (Waldrep *et al.*, 1994c). From these studies we have chosen DLPC as the most suitable for GC–liposome aerosols, although other natural or synthetic PC could be substituted, including HSBPC. It is important to employ ultrapure phospholipids to form well-defined and stable liposomes. Encapsulation of GC into liposomes increases the aerosol GC output from most jet nebulizers two to five times over that of microcrystalline GC suspensions of Becotide and Pulmicort, which nebulize with very low efficiency (Waldrep *et al.*, 1994a). GC–liposome aerosol formulations also possess another advantage over current microcrystalline suspensions, namely, particle sizes from selected nebulizers and in the 1–2 μm size range (Waldrep *et al.*, 1993), whereas Becotide particles are reported to be 3.7 μm in diameter and Pulmicort is 2.4 μm (Edman, 1994). The low aerosol output (which is nebulizer dependent) and large particle size may explain the inconsistent clinical efficacy, particularly with Becotide (Bisgaard, 1994).

By using the computer model of particle size and measured output as described, patterns of respiratory tract deposition of GC–liposome aerosols can be estimated. Table 41.7 shows the size characteristics of aerosols of five GC–DLPC liposomes. The average aerosol GC output was 21–22 μg/l of aerosol, an amount suitable for delivering a daily GC dose in 15 minutes or less (based on MDI/DPI daily dosages). The potential increased efficacy of GC–liposomes over microcrystalline GC particles deposited within the airways could lead to reduced dosages (or shorter treatment periods).

CsA–liposome aerosol

Alexander *et al.* (1992) found that oral CsA (5 mg/kg) produced clinical benefit in asthmatics. Prolonged systemic use of CsA, however, seems unacceptable, due to its systemic toxicity. The promising results of this work suggest that aerosolized CsA may prove to be an effective alternative to conventional delivery systems for the treatment of asthma. The use of CsA in aerosol with ethanol as a solvent was examined by Detwiler *et al.* (1990) in rats and

Table 41.7 Size characteristics of five hydrophobic glucocorticoid DLPC liposome aerosols*. (Modified from Waldrep, 1994c.)

Drug	MMAD† (μm)	GSD†
Budesonide	1.7	2.4
Beclomethasone dipropionate	1.6	2.1
Flunisolide	1.7	2.5
Triamcinolone acetonide	1.6	2.6
Dexamethasone	1.6	2.4

* Puritan Bennett twin jet nebulizer modified to single jet.
† Particle size and GSD were based on samples obtained in the Andersen Cascade Impactor.
See text for definition of abbreviations.

in dogs by Dowling *et al.* (1990). In the Detwiler *et al.* (1990) study, no abnormalities of lung histology were detected and CO_2 response curves were not abnormal during a 15-day study. In the Dowling *et al.* (1990) study, rejection of canine lung allografts was prevented or reduced by dosages of CsA in which 95% did not reach serum trough levels of 150 ng/ml. No histological evidence of tissue toxicity from CsA was found. In a preliminary human study in patients with severe, advanced allograft rejection, response to aerosol treatment was variable (Duncan *et al.*, 1994), possibly because of differences in delivery of drug to the allograft. Marked differences in regional deposition appeared to explain the variability, as assessed by radioaerosol technique (O'Riordan *et al.*, 1994). Airway irritation (by ethanol) caused the discontinuation of the use of this treatment.

CsA has been prepared in a liposome aerosol formulation (Gilbert *et al.*, 1993; Waldrep *et al.*, 1993). In Table 41.8, data are presented as particle size and drug output for several formulations nebulized with a modified Puritan Bennett 1600 nebulizer. Aerosol CsA output was reduced with dimyristoyl PC (DMPC), egg yolk PC (EYPC) and dipalmitoyl PC (DPPC) liposomes and is probably related to the phase transition temperature above the nebulizer operating temperature of 16°C. Thus, for best results with drug–liposome aerosols, phospholipids with lower phase transition temperature should be selected (Waldrep *et al.*, 1993). A liposome formulation containing CsA, 5 mg/ml and DLPC, 37.5 mg/ml (phase transition temperature –2.0°C) with the Aerotech II nebulizer produced an average aerosol output of 90 μg/l over a 20-minute interval with MMAD of 1.6 μm and GSD 1.9. Estimated deposition with this formulation was 13.5 mg CsA/hour of inhalation (11.25 (minimum volume in litres) × 90 μg × 22.3% (deposition in lung) × 60 minutes = 13.5 mg/hour) (Knight, V., 1994). This dosage level should be sufficient to produce beneficial clinical effects in the asthmatic lung while minimizing local and systemic toxicity.

Aerosol treatment during inspiratory flow

While the foregoing estimates of lung deposition were based on continuous-flowing aerosols, more efficient aerosol delivery can be achieved through the use of breath actuation of air flow to the nebulizer (Wolf & Niven, 1994). Co-ordination between nebulizer flow and inspiration prevents unnecessary generation of aerosol and consequent loss into the environment. Figure 41.5 illustrates the particle size and output of CsA–DLPC liposome aerosol preparation during repeated actuations using an Aerotech II nebulizer. The MMAD produced by 12 5-second actuations was 1.5 μm with a calculated GSD of 1.7. The CsA–DLPC liposome aerosol particles were thus slightly smaller than those produced by continuous flow, and this was apparently related to the smaller numbers of larger particles (>5 μm) produced. Similarly, Fig. 41.6 shows the

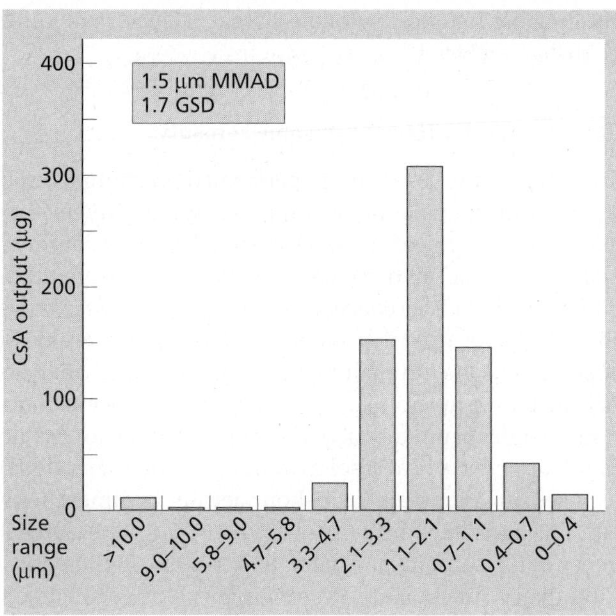

Fig. 41.5 CsA–DLPC liposome aerosol output from Aerotech II nebulizer with manual actuator valve (Pari Jet Interrupter Value System, Munich, Germany); 12 5-second pulses were sampled. Measured output was 59 μg CsA in 22 μl of liquid per actuation. Initial reservoir concentration was 5 mg CsA and 37.5 mg DLPC in combination in liposomes. (Data from J.C. Waldrep, unpublished.) See text for definition of abbreviations.

Table 41.8 Comparison of particle size and output of CsA with six different phospholipids. (From Waldrep *et al.*, 1993.)

	DOPC	DLPC	POPC	DMPC	EYPC	DPPC
MMAD (μm)	1.35	0.82	1.38	1.23	1.29	1.25
GSD	2.3*	1.7	2.8	2.7	2.2	3.6*
CsA (5 minutes operation)	654	581	503	379	371	126

* Puritan Bennett twin jet nebulizer with one liquid supply tube removed. CsA to phospholipid ratios 1 : 7.5 (by weight).
See text for definition of abbreviations.

discrete aerosol produced by actuation during inspiration with Bec–DLPC liposomes using the Aerotech II nebulizer, with a resulting MMAD of 1.2 μm and GSD of 1.7. It is thus possible to produce drug–liposome aerosols with similar properties either by actuation during inspiration or by continuous flow to provide efficient alternative methods for the treatment of asthma.

Summary

This chapter, has described aerosol-based therapy, in which aerodynamic particle size is the main determinant for predicting inhaled particle deposition and dosage. By selection of aerosol formulations and delivery systems in which the MMAD is within the range of 1–3 μm and GSD of approximately 2.0, with mouth inhalation, a rather precise targeting of aerosol to the peripheral conducting airways and the alveolated area of the lung is possible. This methodology applies to aqueous aerosols through the usual ranges of salinity and to non-hygroscopic aerosols. A review of studies indicating the feasibility of treatment of asthma with drug–liposome aerosols containing GC and CsA is presented. The authors believe that this methodology has applicability for administration of a wide range of medications for asthma and other pulmonary diseases.

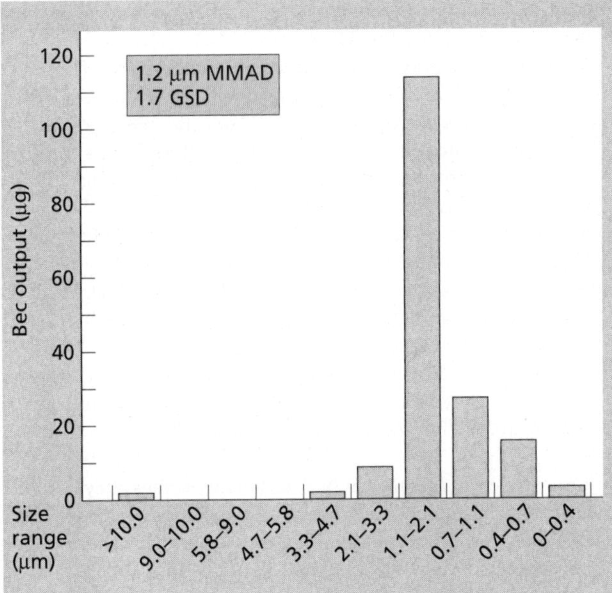

Fig. 41.6 Bec–DLPC liposome aerosol produced by 50 5-second pulses from the nebulizer. Shown is the amount of Bec recovered on the 10 stages of the Andersen Cascade Aerosol Sampler according to particle size. The actuations were controlled by the Pari Jet Interrupter valve system (Munich, Germany). Calculated output per actuation was 3 μg in 72 μl. The reservoir of the nebulizer contained 500 μg/ml of beclomethasone in liposomal formulation. See text for definition of abbreviations. (Data from J.C. Waldrep, unpublished.)

Acknowledgements

This research was supported in part by the Clayton Foundation for Research, Houston, TX, and by a State of Texas Applied Technology Program Grant #004949-054. We thank Dr Keyvan Keyhani, Department of Bioengineering, University of Pennsylvania, and Dr C.P. Yu, Department of Mechanical and Aerospace Engineering, New York State University, Buffalo, New York, for providing data on particle deposition in the respiratory tract. We thank Ms Kathy Blais for expert secretarial assistance.

References

Aguado, J.M., Hidalgo, M., Moya, I., Alcazar, J.M., Jimenez, M.J. & Noriega, A.R. (1993) Ventricular arrhythmias with conventional and liposomal amphotericin. *Lancet*, **342**, 1239.

Alexander, A.G., Barnes, N.C. & Kay, A.B. (1992) Trial of cyclosporin in corticosteroid-dependent chronic severe asthma. *Lancet*, **339**, 324–8.

Andersson, P. & Ryrefeldt, A. (1984) Biotransformation of the topical glucocorticoids budesonide and beclomethasone 17a,21-dipropionate in human liver and lung homogenate. *J. Pharm. Pharmacol.*, **36**, 763–5.

Balmes, J.R. (1991) The environmental impact of chlorofluorocarbon use in metered dose inhalers. *Chest*, **100**, 1101–2.

Bisgaard, H. (1994) Clinical efficacy of nebulized drugs. *J. Aerosol Med.*, **7**, S33–S37.

Brain, J.D., Valberg, P.A. & Sneddon, S. (1985) Mechanisms of aerosol deposition and clearance. In: *Aerosols in Medicine* (eds F. Moren, M.T. Newhouse & M.B. Dolovich), pp. 123–45. Elsevier, Amsterdam.

Brattsand, R., Thalen, A., Roempke, K., Kallstrom, L. & Gruvstad, E. (1992) Development of new glucocorticoids with a very high ratio between topical and systemic activities. *Eur. J. Resp. Dis.*, **63** (Suppl. 122), 62–73.

Byron, P.R. & Patton, J.S. (1994) Drug delivery via the respiratory tract. *J. Aerosol Med.*, **7**, 49–76.

Cullis, P.R., Mayer, L.D., Bally, M.B., Madden, T.D. & Hope, M.J. (1989) Generating and loading of liposomal systems for drug-delivery applications. *Adv. Drug Deliv. Rev.*, **3**, 267–82.

Dalby, R.N. & Tiano, S.L. (1993) Pitfalls and opportunities in the inertial sizing and output testing of nebulizers. *Pharmaceut. Technol.*, **17**, 144–56.

De Blaquiere, P., Christensen, D.B., Carter, W.B. & Martin, T.R. (1989) Use and misuse of metered-dose inhalers by patients with chronic lung disease: a controlled, randomized trial of two instruction methods. *Am. Rev. Resp. Dis.*, **140**, 910–16.

Debs, R., Brunette, E., Fuchs, H. *et al.* (1990) Biodistribution, tissue reaction, and lung retention of pentamidine aerosolized as three different salts. *Am. Rev. Resp. Dis.*, **142**, 1164–7.

Detwiler, K., Schaper, M., Burckart, G. *et al.* (1990) Evaluation of the effects of cyclosporin aerosols in rats following repeated exposure. *Toxicologist*, **10** (1), 178.

Dowling, R., Zenati, M., Burckart, G. *et al.* (1990) Aerosolized cyclosporine as single-agent immunotherapy in canine lung allografts. *Surgery*, **108**, 198–205.

Duncan, S.R., O'Riordan, T.G., Smaldone, G.C. *et al.* (1994) Aerosolized cyclosporin for the treatment of refractory chronic lung rejection: a preliminary report. *Am. J. Resp. Crit. Care Med.*,

149, A198 [abstract].

Edman, P. (1994) Pharmaceutical formulations — suspensions and solutions. *J. Aerosol Med.*, **7**, S3–S6.

Farr, S.J., Kellaway, I.W., Parry-Jones, D.R. & Woolfrey, S.G. (1985) ^{99m}Techetium as a marker of liposomal deposition and clearance in the human lung. *Int. J. Pharmaceut.*, **6**, 303–16.

Garcon, N., Six, H., Frazer, J., Hazlewood, C., Gilbert, B. & Knight, V. (1989) Liposomes of enviroxime and phosphatidylcholine: definition of the drug phospholipid interactions. *Antiviral Res.*, **11**, 89–98.

Gilbert, B., Six, H., Wilson, S., Wyde, P. & Knight, V. (1988) Small particle aerosols of enviroxime-containing liposomes. *Antiviral Res.*, **9**, 355–65.

Gilbert, B.E., Wilson, S.Z., Garcon, N.M., Wyde, P.R. & Knight, V. (1993) Characterization and administration of cyclosporine liposomes as a small-particle aerosol. *Transplantation*, **56**, 974–7.

Hilton, S. (1990) An audit of inhaler technique among patients of 34 general practitioners. *Brit. J. Gen. Pract.*, **40**, 505–6.

Joly, V., Bolard, J., Saint-Julien, L., Carbon, C. & Yeni, P. (1992) Influence of phospholipid/amphotericin B ratio and phospholipid type on *in vitro* renal cell toxicities and fungicidal activities of lipid-associated amphotericin B formulations. *Antimicrob. Agents Chemother.*, **36** (2), 262–6.

Juliano, R.L. & McCullough, H.N. (1980) Controlled delivery of an anti-tumor drug: pharmacologic studies of liposome encapsulated cytosine arabinoside administered via the respiratory system. *J. Pharmacol. Exp. Ther.*, **213**, 381–7.

Kim, C.S., Trujillo, D. & Sackner, M.A. (1985) Size aspects of metered-dose inhaler aerosols. *Am. Rev. Resp. Dis.*, **132**, 137–42.

Knight, C.M., Gilbert, B.E., Waldrep, J.C., Black, M., Knight, V. & Eschenbacher, W. (1994) Inhalation of a corticosteroid–liposome preparation by normal subjects causes no adverse effects. *Am. J. Resp. Crit. Care Med.*, **149**, A220 [abstract].

Knight, V. (1973) *Viral and mycoplasmal infections of the respiratory tract*, p. 2. Lea and Febiger, Philadelphia.

Knight, V., Yu, C.P., Gilbert, B.E. & Divine, G.W. (1988) Estimating the dosage of ribavirin aerosol according to age of patient and other variables. *J. Infect. Dis.*, **158** (2), 443–8.

Knight, V., Black, M.T. & Waldrep, J.C. (1994) Development of cyclosporin A liposome aerosol therapy for pulmonary diseases. *Am. J. Resp. Crit. Care Med.*, **149**, A1095 [abstract].

Kohler, D. & Fleisher, W. (1991) *Established Facts in Inhalation Therapy*. Arcis Verlag, Munich.

Lippmann, M., Yeates, D.B. & Albert, R.E. (1980) Deposition, retention, and clearance of inhaled particles. *Brit. J. Industr. Med.*, **37**, 337–62.

McFadden, E.R. (1993) Dosages of corticosteroids in asthma. *Am. Rev. Resp. Dis.*, **147**, 1306–10.

Manzella, B.A., Brooks, C.M., Richards, J.M., Windsor, R.A., Soong, S. & Bailey, W.C. (1989) Assessing the use of metered dose inhalers by adults with asthma. *J. Asthma*, **26**, 223–30.

Marks, L., Oberdîster, G. & Notter, R. (1983) Generation and characterization of aerosols of dispersed surface active phospholipids by ultrasonic and jet nebulization. *J. Aerosol Sci.*, **14** (5), 683–94.

Martin, G.P., Onyechi, J.O. & Marriott, C. (1994) Future prospects for pulmonary delivery of drugs. *STP Pharmaceut. Sci.*, **4**, 5–10.

Mihalko, P.J., Schreier, H. & Abra, R.M. (1988) Liposomes: a pulmonary perspective. In: *Liposomes as Drug Carriers* (ed. G. Gregoriadis), pp. 679–94. New York.

Morimoto, Y. & Adachi, Y. (1982) Pulmonary uptake of liposomal phosphatidylcholine upon intratracheal administration into rats. *Chem. Pharmaceut. Bull.*, **30**, 2248–51.

Myers, M., Thomas, D., Straub, L. *et al.* (1993) Pulmonary effects of chronic exposure to liposome aerosols in mice. *Exp. Lung Res.*, **19**, 1–19.

New, R.R.C. (1990) Characterization of liposomes. In: *Liposomes: a Practical Approach* (ed. New R.R.C.) pp. 105–61. IRL Press, Oxford.

Newman, S.P. (1990) Metered dose pressurized aerosols and ozone layer. *Eur. Resp. J.*, **3**, 3495–7.

Newman, S.P., Pavia, D., Moren, F., Sheahan, N.F. & Clarke, S.W. (1981) Deposition of pressurized aerosols in the human respiratory tract. *Thorax*, **36**, 52–5.

Niven, R.W. (1993) Delivery of biotherapeutics by inhalation aerosols. *Pharmaceut. Technol.*, **17**, 72–82.

Niven, R.W. & Schreier, H. (1990) Nebulization of liposomes. I. Effects of lipid composition. *Pharmaceut. Res.*, **7**, 1127–31.

O'Doherty, M.J. & Miller, R.F. (1993) Aerosols for therapy and diagnosis. *Eur. J. Nucl. Med.*, **20**, 1201–13.

Olsson, B. & Asking, L. (1994) Critical aspects of the function of inspiratory flow driven inhalers. *J. Aerosol Med.*, **7**, S-43–S-47.

O'Riordan, T., Iacono, A., Keenan, R. *et al.* (1994) Delivery and distribution of aerosolized cyclosporine in lung allograft recipients. *Am. J. Resp. Crit. Care Med.*, **149**, A1094 [abstract].

Persons, D.D., Hess, G.D., Muller, W.J. & Scherer, P.W. (1987a) Airway deposition of hygroscopic heterodispersed aerosols: results of a computer calculation. *J. Appl. Physiol.*, **63**, 1195–204.

Persons, D.D., Hess, G.D. & Scherer, P.W. (1987b) Maximization of pulmonary hygroscopic aerosol deposition. *J. Appl. Physiol.*, **63**, 1205–9.

Pettenazzo, A., Jobe, A., Ikegami, M., Abra, R., Hogue, E. & Mihalko, P. (1989) Clearance of phosphatidylcholine and cholesterol from liposomes, liposomes loaded with metaproterenol, and rabbit surfactant from adult rabbit lungs. *Am. Rev. Resp. Dis.*, **139**, 752–8.

Reed, C.E. (1991) Aerosol steroids as primary treatment of mild asthma. *New Engl. J. Med.*, **325**, 425–6.

Ryrefeldt, A., Andersson, P., Edsbacker, S., Tonnesson, M., Davies, D. & Pauwels, R. (1982) Pharmacokinetics and metabolism of budesonide, a selective glucocorticoid. *Eur. J. Resp. Res.*, **63**, 86–95.

Schanker, L.S., Mitchell, E.W. & Brown, R.A. (1986) Species comparison of drug absorption from the lung after aerosol inhalation or intratrachael injection. *Drug Metabol. Depos.*, **14**, 79–88.

Schrier, H., Gonzalez-Rothi, R. & Stecenko, A.A. (1993) Pulmonary delivery of liposomes. *J. Controlled Release*, **24**, 209–23.

Smeesters, C., Giroux, L., Vinet, B. *et al.* (1988) Reduced nephrotoxicity of cyclosporine A after incorporation into liposomes. *Transplant. Proc.*, **20** (3, Suppl. 3), 831–2.

Stuhne-Sekalec, L. & Stanacev, N.Z. (1988) Interaction of cyclosporine A with 1.2-dimyristoyl-*sn*-glycero-3-phosphocholine unilamellar vesicles studied by electron spin resonance. *Chem. Phys. Lipids*, **48**, 1–6.

Stuhne-Sekalec, L. & Stanacev, N.Z. (1991) Liposomes as cyclosporin A carriers: the influence of ordering of hydrocarbon chains of phosphotidylglycerol liposomes on the association with and topography of cyclosporin A. *J. Microencapsul.*, **8**, 283–94.

Szefler, S.J. (1992) Anti-inflammatory drugs in the treatment of allergic disease. *Med. Clin. North Am.*, **76**, 953–75.

Taylor, K.M.G. & Farr, S.J. (1993) Liposomes for drug delivery to the respiratory tract. *Drug Dev. Industr. Pharm.*, **19**, 123–42.

Taylor, K.M.G., Taylor, G., Kellaway, I.W. & Stevens, J. (1990) The stability of liposomes to nebulization. *Int. J. Pharmaceut.*, **58**, 57–61.

Thomas, D., Myers, M., Wichert, B., Schreier, H. & Gonzalez-Rothi, R. (1991) Acute effects of liposome aerosol inhalation on pulmonary function in healthy human volunteers. *Chest*, **99**, 1268–70.

Timsina, M.P., Martin, G.P., Marriott, C., Ganderton, D. & Yianneskis, M. (1994) Drug delivery to the respiratory tract using dry powder inhalers. *Int. J. Pharmaceut.*, **101**, 1–13.

Toogood, J.H. (1993) Making better and safer use of inhaled steroids. *J. Resp. Dis.*, **14**, 221–38.

Toogood, J.H., Jennings, B., Greenway, R.W. & Chuang, L. (1980) Candidiasis and dysphonia complicating beclomethasone treatment of asthma. *J. Allergy Clin. Immunol.*, **65**, 143–53.

Toogood, J.H., Baskerville, J., Jennings, B., Lefcoe, N.M. & Johansson, S.A. (1984) Use of spacers to facilitate inhaled glucocorticoids treatment of asthma. *Am. Rev. Resp. Dis.*, **129**, 723–9.

Vidgren, M., Waldrep, J.C., Arppe, J. *et al.* (1995) A study of ^{99m}Technetium-labelled beclomethasone dipropionate dilauroylphosphatidylcholine liposome aerosol in normal volunteers. *Int. J. Pharmaceut.*, **115**, 209–16.

Waldrep, J.C., Scherer, P.W., Keyhani, K. & Knight, V. (1993) Cyclosporin A liposome aerosol: particle size and calculated respiratory deposition. *Int. J. Pharmaceut.*, **97**, 205–12.

Waldrep, J.C., Vidgren, M.T., Palander, A., Black, M. & Knight, V. (1994a) Analysis of glucocorticoid–liposome and microcrystalline suspension aerosol formulations. *Am. J. Resp. Crit. Care Med.*, **149**, A220 [abstract].

Waldrep, J.C., Keyhani, K., Black, M. & Knight, V. (1994b) Operating characteristics of 18 different continuous-flow jet nebulizers with beclomethasone dipropionate liposome aerosol. *Chest*, **105**, 106–10.

Waldrep, J.C., Scherer, P.W., Hess, G.D., Black, M. & Knight, V. (1994c) Nebulized glucocorticoids in liposomes: aerosol characteristics and human dose estimates. *J. Aerosol Med.*, **7** (2), 135–45.

Weibel, E.R. (1963) *Morphometry of Human Lung*. Academic Press, New York.

Wolf, R.K. & Niven, R.W. (1994) Generation of aerosolized drugs. *J. Aerosol Med.*, **7**, 89–106.

Wood, R.E. & Knowles, M.R. (1994) Recent advances in aerosol therapy. *J. Aerosol Med.*, **7**, 1–11.

Wyde, P., Six, H., Wilson, S., Gilbert, B. & Knight, V. (1988) Activity against rhinoviruses, toxicity, and delivey in aerosol of enviroxime in liposomes. *Antimicrob. Agents Chemother.*, **32** (6), 890–5.

CHAPTER 42

Airway Smooth Muscle

I.W. Rodger

Introduction

Contraction of airway smooth muscle (ASM) is universally accepted as being a principal component of the acute phase of air-flow limitation that characterizes an asthmatic attack. It is also well acknowledged that the airway structure of asthmatic subjects is abnormal. The abnormality is, in all likelihood, a consequence of the profound inflammatory processes that underlie the disease state. Thus, these inflammatory events thicken the airway wall, promote transudation of mucus and oedema fluid into the airway lumen and promote emigration of leucocytes from the vascular space into the interstitium and the airway lumen. Coincident with, or consequent upon, these changes there occurs an increase in ASM mass and the muscle displays a hyperresponsiveness to a wide range of provoking stimuli. However, despite detailed knowledge of such fundamental changes in ASM structure and its contractile state, some of which have been recognized for a considerable period of time, it is only relatively recently that the complex molecular mechanisms underlying both the control and contraction of ASM have begun to be unravelled. Detailed discussion of several different aspects of this subject (e.g. ASM innervation, neuropeptide control of the airways, airway remodelling and airway hyperresponsiveness) can be found elsewhere in this textbook. The specific objective of this chapter is to provide a brief overview of the physiology of ASM. In this context, our attention will be focused on structural aspects of the cell, receptor–effector coupling mechanisms and mechanisms underlying excitation—contraction coupling in ASM cells. Given the necessary space constraints in a book of this nature, this chapter is not intended to provide an exhaustive review of the literature. Rather, it is an attempt to provide a readily comprehensible overview and, where appropriate, direct the interested reader to authoritative key references on particular aspects of the topic.

Structural aspects of ASM

In general, there are few studies concerning the structure of human ASM, especially of the small airways, which are the principal site of airway obstruction in asthma. In one of the few authoritative studies, however, it has been shown that the musculature of the first- and second-order human bronchi closely resembles that of the trachea, which is a much more extensively researched tissue (Daniel *et al.*, 1986). In contrast, that of the fourth- to seventh-order airways is substantially different in terms of the size and arrangement of the muscle bundles, number and size of gap junctions and appearance of the contractile myofilaments (Daniel *et al.*, 1986). Interestingly, mast cells also appear to be more intimately associated with the smooth muscle of these smaller airways. Furthermore, innervation of the smaller airways is much denser than that of the trachea and large bronchi. This has led to the suggestion (Daniel *et al.*, 1986) that the larger airways are adapted for myogenic control with a secondary neuromodulatory aspect, whereas the smaller bronchial airways are organized principally for control by neural elements. In general, ASM is regarded as being of the multi-unit type, in that each cell is innervated and that cell–cell communication is poor. This is the result of a paucity of gap junctions, which normally provide pathways of low resistance along which electrical signals can be transmitted. Spontaneous activity is rarely observed in such smooth-muscle types. Action potentials are nearly always absent and the response to contractile agonists is via graded depolarization. In normal ASM such a situation usually prevails. However, in asthmatic ASM pronounced action potential has been observed (Akasaka *et al.*, 1975). Such activity is indicative not of multi-unit but of single-unit-type smooth muscle. This type of smooth muscle is generally poorly innervated and relies heavily upon gap junctions to provide cell–cell communication. Thus, it has been suggested (Barnes, 1983; Thomson, 1983) that asthmatic subjects with hyperresponsive airways may possess a greater degree of electrical coupling between smooth-muscle cells due to an increased presence of gap junctions. Precisely how multi-unit ASM changes to become strongly single-unit in character is not yet known, although certain experimental observations may provide useful pointers (Kannan & Daniel, 1980; Kannan *et al.*, 1983; Agrawal & Daniel, 1986; Berry *et al.*, 1991; Green *et al.*, 1991).

In terms of contraction of ASM, two of the more important intracellular organelles are the sarcoplasmic reticulum (SR) and mitochondrion. Generally, smooth muscles are regarded as possessing a paucity of SR, especially in comparison with cardiac and skeletal muscle. Notwithstanding, that which exists is thought to play an important physiological role, in that it is capable of both sequestering and storing free Ca^{2+} ions and releasing them on demand, as so-called activator Ca^{2+}. It is these activator Ca^{2+} that initiate the biochemical events that ultimately generate contraction of ASM (see later). In sharp contrast, mitochondria are thought not to play a major role in Ca^{2+} homoeostasis, except in certain pathological conditions (Daniel *et al.*, 1983).

Contractile proteins

All smooth-muscle cells contain the contractile proteins actin, myosin, tropomyosin, caldesmon and calponin (Stull, 1980; Kamm & Stull, 1985, 1989). These contractile proteins function by forming into filaments, arranged in parallel such that they can slide past each other. Actin is a highly conserved molecule found in most eukaryotic cells and represents the major contractile protein of smooth muscle, being 10–20 times more abundant than myosin. The thin actin filaments are composed of two linear polymers of a 42 kDa globular protein, wrapped together in a helical configuration. Intertwined along its length, in the groove of the thin filament helix, lie tropomyosin, caldesmon and calponin. In contrast to the thin filaments of actin, the filaments of myosin are thick, bipolar and arranged asymmetrically in a hexameric structure. Myosin comprises one pair of heavy chains (each of 200 kDa) and two pairs of light chains (one pair of 17 kDa and the other of 20 kDa). The myosin molecule can essentially be divided into two components: a so-called 'head' section attached to a long spine or 'tail' section. The globular head section of myosin is the region of the molecule that possesses both the binding sites for attachment to actin and the enzymatic (adenosine triphosphatase (ATPase)) sites that cleave adenosine triphosphate (ATP) and so provide the energy necessary for the binding reactions to take place. The two sets of myosin light chains are also located at the head of the myosin molecule. The 20 kDa light chains of myosin are considered to be essential regulators of the contractile process (Adelstein, 1983; Allen & Walsh, 1994).

Intermediate filaments

Intermediate filaments consist of a group of relatively insoluble proteins that are considered by many to form the cytoskeleton of numerous cell types. In smooth muscle the cytoskeletal and contractile proteins are distributed in two distinct cellular domains (Small, 1985; Fürst *et al.*, 1986; Small *et al.*, 1986). The first domain consists of longitudinal intermediate filaments free of myosin but containing α-actinin, desmin, filamin and actin. The second cellular domain consists of contractile protein filaments, i.e. actin, myosin, tropomyosin and caldesmon. Elucidation of this assembly of proteins has led to the proposition that the intermediate filament domain may be responsible for the tonic phase of a smooth-muscle contractile response, with the initiation of contraction (the phasic component) being the responsibility of the contractile protein domain (Small *et al.*, 1986). A modification of this proposal has also been advanced. In this scheme, phosphorylation of different proteins (both contractile and intermediate) is responsible for the different phases of the contractile response (Rasmussen *et al.*, 1987).

Signal transduction

Transmembrane signalling from cell-surface receptors can essentially be thought of as belonging to two main categories. In the more conceptually simple of these, an agonist, on interacting with its recognition sites on the receptor protein, induces a conformational change that is transmitted throughout the macromolecular receptor complex in such a way that a transmembrane ion channel is opened. In its open state, the ion channel then permits the flow of particular ions through the membrane under their electrochemical gradient. Receptors belonging to this group initiate and transmit signals extremely rapidly. Generally speaking, this type of signalling system does not exist in smooth muscle. The second type of transmembrane signalling, which is substantially slower than the first, involves the interaction of an agonist (or first messenger) with its specific cell-surface receptor. This leads to activation (or in some instances inactivation) of a membrane-associated enzyme, or it leads to opening or closing of a membrane ion channel that is separate from the receptor complex. This type of signalling mechanism frequently involves the interplay of a guanosine triphosphate (GTP) binding protein (G protein) (Linder & Gilman, 1992; Pyne & Rodger, 1993). When activation of an enzyme occurs, one or more products known as second messengers are produced as part of an amplification system that ultimately leads to the cellular response. It is this type of signalling mechanism that exists principally in ASM cells.

G proteins possess α-, β- and γ-subunits which, in their resting state, exist as an αβγ-holomer (Fig. 42.1). In the inactive or ground state, the three subunits are combined because of the presence of guanosine diphosphate (GDP) bound to the α-subunit (Fig. 42.1). When an agonist binds to its receptor, it promotes the exchange of GDP for GTP in the α-subunit (Pyne & Rodger, 1993). The binding of GTP to the α-subunit induces a dissociation of the αβγ-holomeric assembly to provide free, activated, GTP–bound α-subunits and the βγ-dimeric assembly (Fig. 42.1). The GTP–α-subunit complex drifts through the cytosol immediately adjacent to the membrane, repeatedly colliding with and activating (or in some cases inactivating) enzyme molecules until GTP is hydrolysed. It is an intrinsic guanosine triphosphatase (GTPase) activity of the α-subunit that hydrolyses the GTP to yield GDP. With GDP now bound to the α-subunit, the latter loses its effector-activating capability and is thus able to recombine with the βγ-assembly and so return the cycle to its ground state.

Different forms of the α-, β- and γ-subunits are known to exist. This gives rise to a heterogeneity of G proteins involved in signal transduction mechanisms in different systems (Pyne & Rodger, 1993). In the context of contraction of ASM, receptors for contractile agonists are coupled to a G protein termed G_q/G_{11}, the nature and characteristics of which are still being fully elucidated (Pyne & Pyne, 1993; Pyne & Rodger, 1993; Emala *et al.*, 1994; Lee *et al.*, 1994). Activation of G_q/G_{11} stimulates phospholipase C. This enzyme is responsible for cleaving a minor membrane phospholipid, phosphatidylinositol 4,5-bisphosphate (PIP_2), thus generating inositol 1,4,5-trisphosphate (IP_3) and *sn*-1,2-diacylglycerol. These two intracellular second messengers are widely regarded as playing pivotal

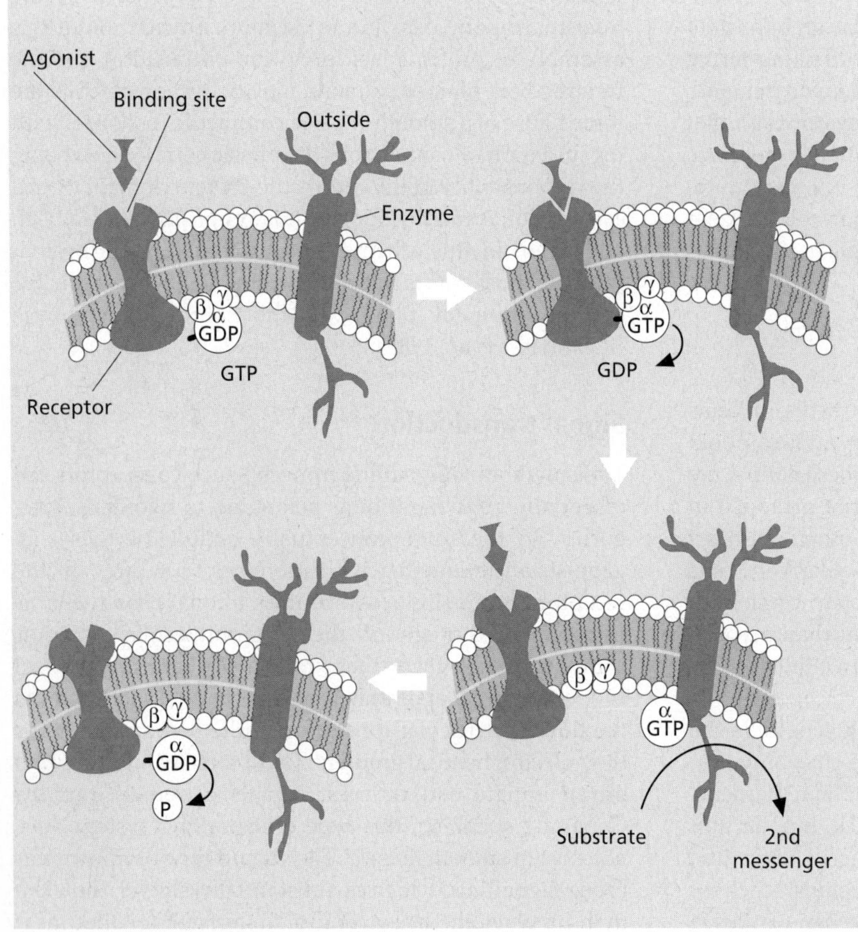

Fig. 42.1 Diagrammatic representation of the G-protein/GTP/GDP cycle, which is regarded as critical in the receptor-mediated signal transduction process. In their resting state, G proteins, which consist of α-, β- and γ-subunits, are bound by the nucleotide guanosine diphosphate (GDP) and have no contact with their receptors. When a contractile agonist binds to its receptor, the receptor causes the G protein to exchange GDP for the nucleotide guanosine triphosphate (GTP), which activates the G protein. The G protein then dissociates, after which the GTP-bound α-subunit diffuses along the membrane and binds to an effector, thus activating it. After a brief period, the α-subunit converts GTP to GDP by virtue of an intrinsic GTPase, thereby inactivating itself. The α-subunit then reassociates itself with the βγ-complex and returns the cycle to its ground state. (From Rodger, 1993.)

roles in the excitation–contraction coupling process that operates in ASM cells (see Rodger & Pyne, 1992, for references).

Involvement of Ca^{2+} in airway smooth-muscle contraction

It is now almost universally accepted that two forms of excitation–contraction coupling exist: electromechanical and pharmacomechanical. As the term suggests, electromechanical coupling depends either on electrical depolarization of the plasma membrane, which opens Ca^{2+} channels, so leading to Ca^{2+} influx from the extracellular space and a consequent increase in the intracellular concentration of free Ca^{2+}, or on a voltage-dependent release of Ca^{2+} from intracellular stores, such as the SR. In sharp contrast, the pharmacomechanical coupling mechanism is regarded as being voltage independent. Thus, it may involve either extracellular Ca^{2+} influx via ligand-gated Ca^{2+} channels or release of activator Ca^{2+} from intracellular stores. The intracellular release mechanism is executed either via ligand-generated intracellular second messengers (for example, IP_3 or cyclic adenosine diphosphate (ADP)-ribose) or via a direct action of a ligand on the intracellular SR stores.

When a contractile agonist activates its specific cell-surface receptors, the intracellular concentration of Ca^{2+} in airway smooth muscle cells rises abruptly from its resting level (<0.2 μmol/l) to between 0.5 and 3 μmol/l (Kotlikoff *et al.*, 1987; Felbel *et al.*, 1988; Taylor *et al.*, 1989; Panettieri *et al.*, 1989; Kajita & Yamaguchi, 1993; Murray *et al.*, 1993). These activator Ca^{2+} can only be derived from two sources. They may be derived from the extracellular domain, where they reside in abundance, or from intracellular stores, such as those present within the SR. The relative contribution of activator Ca^{2+} from each of these sources is wholly dependent on both the nature and the concentration of the spasmogen that is initiating contraction and the type of the contractile response that is being produced (phasic or tonic). In addition to the role that extracellular Ca^{2+} ions play in either initiating or maintaining a contractile response, they are also known to play a fundamental role in replenishing the intracellular Ca^{2+} pools, which are depleted by the action of those ligands that induce contraction via the intermediacy of either IP_3-dependent or cyclic ADP-ribose-dependent mechanisms (Galione, 1993).

The plasma membrane and Ca^{2+} channels

The resting membrane potential of ASM cells lies somewhere between −45 mV and −60 mV. Under normal circumstances, most species (guinea pig (Small & Foster, 1988) and human beings (Davis *et al.*, 1982; Honda & Tomita, 1987; Richards *et al.*, 1991; McCray, 1993) being notable exceptions) do not exhibit spontaneous oscillations of the membrane potential, i.e. the cells are electrically quiescent. A further characteristic feature is the cell membrane's remarkable propensity for outward electrical rectification consequent upon a depolarizing stimulus. This rectification behaviour is thought to be largely due to a voltage-dependent Ca^{2+}-insensitive delayed rectifier K^+ current (Kotlikoff, 1989, 1990, 1993). In addition, G-protein-regulated (both G_s and G_i), Ca^{2+}-activated K^+ channels of either low (~90 pS) or high (250–290 pS) conductance are abundant in the ASM plasma membrane (Kume & Kotlikoff, 1991; Saunders & Farley, 1991). In addition to limiting the magnitude of any depolarization, the membrane's ability to electrically rectify effectively prevents the membrane potential from attaining the threshold necessary to elicit opening of voltage-operated Ca^{2+} channels (VOC). For a fuller description of the electrophysiological characteristics of ASM, the reader is directed to Giembycz and Rodger (1987), Kotlikoff (1989) and Small and Foster (1995).

Given that the cell membrane very effectively and efficiently partitions the intracellular and extracellular domains, it is self-evident that activator Ca^{2+} originating in the extracellular domain can only gain admission to the cell once the membrane has been rendered more permeable to them. This is achieved via the opening of Ca^{2+} channels in the plasma membrane through which the Ca^{2+} ions flow down their electrochemical and concentration gradients. Two types of Ca^{2+} channels have been proposed (Bolton, 1979). These are the VOC and the receptor-operated Ca^{2+} channels (ROC) (Bolton, 1979).

Voltage-operated Ca^{2+} channels

VOC, as the term implies, possess a Ca^{2+} conductance that is directly proportional to the potential difference that exists across the plasma membrane. Thus, membrane depolarization increases both the probability of VOC opening and the duration of the open channel time. Numerous studies in many different laboratories, using both electrophysiological and pharmacological techniques, have distinguished several types of VOC. It is currently accepted that there are four main types of VOC (Spedding & Paoletti, 1992). These are defined as the L type, the T type, the N type and the P type. Of these four VOC, it is the voltage-dependent L-type Ca^{2+} channels that are the most well defined, because of the availability of high-affinity drugs with which to probe the channels and because of recent molecular genetic studies (see Spedding & Paoletti, 1992). It is the L-type Ca^{2+} channel, which is exquisitely sensitive to dihydropyridine Ca^{2+} channel antagonists, that is most abundant in the plasmalemma of ASM cells (Small & Foster, 1995).

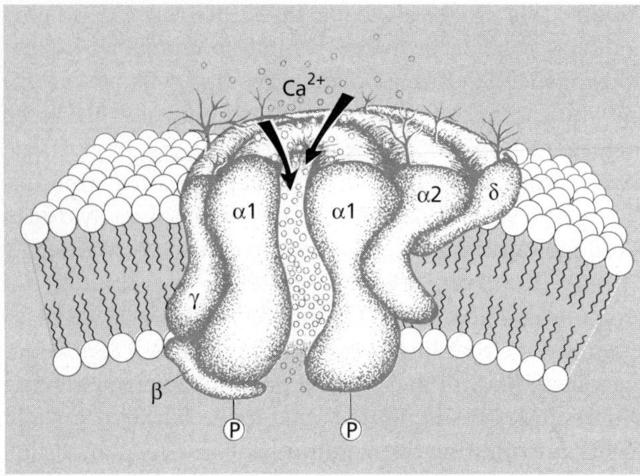

Fig. 42.2 Diagrammatic representation of the structural organization of the L-type Ca^{2+} channel. The Ca^{2+} channel is a pentameric protein complex. Each of the five different polypeptide subunits (α_1, α_2, β, γ, δ) has a different molecular mass. The α_1-subunit is depicted as the ion channel or pore. It contains the dihydropyridine and phenylalkylamine Ca^{2+} antagonist binding sites, essential regulatory (cyclic adenosine monophosphate (cAMP)-dependent) phosphorylation sites as well as the voltage sensor apparatus. Like the α_1-subunit, the β-subunit has similar phosphorylation sites for cAMP-dependent protein kinase. The α_2-, γ- and δ-subunits are involved in modulating channel conductance (see text for further details). (From Rodger, 1995a.)

Structural considerations

The VOC is a multimeric protein complex composed of five different polypeptide subunits, each with a different molecular mass (Fig. 42.2) (Spedding & Paoletti, 1992). These subunits are referred to as α_1, α_2, β, γ and δ (Fig. 42.2). The α_1-subunit, which is encoded by three different genes, appears to form the ion-selective pore. It also contains essential phosphorylation sites (it is an important characteristic of the L-type Ca^{2+} channel that, in order for it to open when the membrane is depolarized, it must first be phosphorylated), as well as binding sites for some Ca^{2+} antagonists (Armstrong & Eckert, 1987; Ellis *et al.*, 1988; Spedding & Paoletti, 1992). The α_1-subunit has been cloned from a variety of tissue types, including lung, and Northern blot analysis has revealed specific mRNA transcript sizes that are tissue specific (Spedding & Paoletti, 1992). This indicates that, in all likelihood, distinct isoforms of the L-type Ca^{2+} channel exist, most probably through alternative splicing. Comparison of the deduced amino acids from the nucleotide sequences is consistent with the existence of different isoforms. While the roles of the other subunits have not been as well characterized as that of the α_1-subunit, they do appear to exert modulatory control over the function of the α_1-subunit. Thus, for example, the α_2-subunit does not appear to possess binding sites for Ca^{2+} antagonists nor does it appear to act as a channel in itself. However, in conjunction with the δ-subunit, it is capable of increasing the flow of Ca^{2+} through the channel. For further details the interested reader is directed to Rodger (1995a).

Physiological regulation of VOC

There is a substantial literature of compelling evidence, from both electrophysiological and ion-flux/pharmacological studies, that supports the view both that the VOC are present in ASM and that they are true L-type Ca^{2+} channels (Rodger, 1987; Kotlikoff, 1988, 1990; Marthan *et al.*, 1989; Hisada *et al.*, 1990; Worley & Kotlikoff, 1990; Small & Foster, 1995). With regard to contractile events, there is overwhelming evidence demonstrating that VOC are primarily responsible for contractions elicited by depolarizing solutions and manoeuvres (for references see Rodger, 1995a). Additionally, drugs such as the dihydropyridine Ca^{2+}-channel agonists BAYK8644 and BAYR5417, which enhance the open-state probability of L-type Ca^{2+} channels, have been shown to augment unitary cation currents (conductance ~25 pS), extracellular $^{45}Ca^{2+}$ uptake and potassium chloride and Ca^{2+}-induced contractions of ASM (Allen *et al.*, 1985; Advenier *et al.*, 1986; Marthan *et al.*, 1987; Worley & Kotlikoff, 1990). It is generally agreed, therefore, that the opening of VOC in ASM cells is the principal mechanism underlying the entry of extracellular Ca^{2+} in response to a variety of depolarizing stimuli that generate smooth-muscle contraction. In sharp contrast, however, there is no real evidence to support the involvement of similar L-type, dihydropyridine-sensitive VOC in the mechanism underlying contraction initiated by a wide range of physiologically relevant agonists (Rodger, 1987, 1995a,b; Henry, 1993; Kajita & Yamaguchi, 1993). The current consensus is that such physiological agonists elicit contractions of ASM via induction of the release of Ca^{2+} from intracellular stores (see later).

While VOC may not be involved in admitting extracellular Ca^{2+} in order to initiate the sequence of contractile events, there is evidence to suggest that they may be intimately involved in the process of refilling intracellular Ca^{2+} stores (Bourreau *et al.*, 1991). It is activator Ca^{2+} from these stores, released in response to IP_3 and cADP-ribose generated by agonist–receptor stimulations, that is regarded as critical in initiating the contractile events in ASM (Rodger & Pyne, 1992). It has been shown, for example (Bourreau *et al.*, 1991), that repetitive stimulation of ASM with acetylcholine, in the continuous presence of nifedipine, resulted in a progressive loss of developed tension. This was associated with a decrease in the content of the spasmogen-sensitive intracellular Ca^{2+} stores. Similarly, agonist-sensitive internal Ca^{2+} stores were readily depleted by successive or prolonged agonist stimulation in Ca^{2+}-free medium. The refilling of the emptied Ca^{2+} stores after washout of the spasmogen required extracellular Ca^{2+}. This refilling process was decreased by nifedipine and increased by the Ca^{2+}-channel agonist BAYK8644 or by increasing the extracellular Ca^{2+} concentration. Refilling of the intracellular stores during an acetylcholine contraction in a Ca^{2+}-containing medium was similarly decreased by nifedipine and increased by BAYK8644. These results strongly suggest that replenishment of internal Ca^{2+} stores is, at least in part, dependent on the influx of extracellular Ca^{2+} via a dihydropyridine-sensitive, L-type Ca^{2+} channel.

Recently, it has been proposed that a Ca^{2+} influx factor (CIF) is generated as a consequence of the depletion of activator Ca^{2+} from intracellular Ca^{2+} stores (Clapham, 1993; Parekh *et al.*, 1993; Randriamampita & Tsien, 1993). The CIF is thought to be responsible for gating the plasmalemmal 'capacitative' Ca^{2+} refilling process. Detailed information on the CIF-activated process is not yet available, but it will be interesting to learn whether the process is sensitive to inhibition by dihydropyridine Ca^{2+} antagonists.

One final feature of the L-type VOC in ASM is their ability to be modulated by β-adrenoceptor agonists. It has been recognized for some time that the open-state probability of the cardiac L-type Ca^{2+} channel is enhanced by cyclic adenosine monophosphate (cAMP)-dependent phosphorylation mechanisms (Hartzell *et al.*, 1991) and also by the α-subunit of G_s (Imoto *et al.*, 1988). Given the extensive sequence identity between the cardiac and airway smooth-muscle L-type channel proteins, it is perhaps not surprising to find that β-adrenoceptor agonists modulate the airway L-type VOC. In the initial studies (Felbel *et al.*, 1988; Takuwa *et al.*, 1988), it was reported that isoprenaline increased the intracellular Ca^{2+} concentration, apparently via a dihydropyridine-sensitive pathway. Further examination of this phenomenon shows that isoprenaline-stimulated peak Ca^{2+} currents were not mediated via stimulation of a K^+ or Na^+ current, by a decrease in intracellular concentrations of Ca^{2+} or H^+ or by stimulation of either the Na^+–H^+ or the Na^+–Ca^{2+} exchanger (Welling *et al.*, 1992). Neither the basal nor the isoprenaline-stimulated Ca^{2+} current was affected by internal dialysis of the cell with either cAMP or analogues of cAMP or by the catalytic subunit of cAMP-dependent protein kinase. In contrast, internal dialysis of the cells with GDP-βS blocked the stimulation induced by isoprenaline, whereas dialysis with GTP-γS induced an isoprenaline-like maximal increase in the Ca^{2+} current. Thus, these results clearly illustrate that β-adrenoceptor agonists augment the L-type VOC Ca^{2+} current in isolated tracheal smooth-muscle cells. Interestingly, since this effect occurs independently of either cAMP or its dependent protein kinase, it is in all likelihood an effect mediated via a GTP/GDP-regulated protein, probably G_s. While these are interesting observations concerning a possible hormonal (adrenaline) regulatory mechanism, the precise physiological significance remains to be established.

ROC

ROC are ion channels that are opened as a consequence of the interaction of an agonist ligand with its specific receptors (Bolton, 1979). It is generally accepted that ROC are not wholly selective for Ca^{2+}, have an ionic permeability determined by the controlling receptor, can be gated by either voltage-dependent or voltage-independent events and are not readily inhibited by organic Ca^{2+} antagonists, such as nifedipine (Bolton, 1979; Murray & Kotlikoff, 1991). In contrast to the extensive molecular biology effort that has been directed at the L-type Ca^{2+} channels, there is little or no similar information concerning ROC. Indeed, the postulated existence of ROC in ASM stems largely from pharmacological evidence, which is of a more indirect nature.

It is beyond the scope of this chapter to provide a detailed discussion of the arguments for and against the existence of ROC in ASM cells. Such information can be obtained in Rodger (1995b). Notwithstanding, one or two key observations are worth highlighting. Most pharmacological agonists elicit contraction of ASM, coincident with a graded membrane depolarization (see Rodger, 1995b, for references). Furthermore, these same agonists can elicit contractions in fully depolarized airway preparations. It has proved impossible, using radiotracer techniques (e.g., the lanthanum technique), to detect extracellular Ca^{2+} influx into airway smooth-muscle cells that is associated with the contractile response elicited by spasmogens (Ahmed *et al.*, 1984; Raeburn & Rodger, 1984). Collectively, therefore, these data argue against both the existence of ROC in ASM and the involvement of VOC, to any significant extent, in the action underlying receptor stimulation by pharmacological agonists. This latter view is strengthened by the many observations that Ca^{2+} antagonists fail to inhibit contractions elicited by a wide range of spasmogens in airway preparations from several species, including human beings (see Rodger, 1995b, for references).

In the light of the above evidence, it is tempting, and in many ways not unreasonable, to dispel the notion that ROC are present in the plasma membrane of ASM cells. A critical weakness in the above data, however, is the inability to measure, using fairly crude techniques, the influx of extracellular Ca^{2+} entry into cells. It is well recognized that the lanthanum technique is ill equipped to measure small changes which are associated with Ca^{2+} entry through ion channels. Recently, however, the application of patch clamp and FURA-2 fluorescence techniques has been used to measure intracellular Ca^{2+} concentrations in both cultured human and canine ASM cells (Murray & Kotlikoff, 1991; Murray *et al.*, 1993; Yang *et al.*, 1993). Through use of these far more sensitive detection systems, it has been demonstrated that there exists a receptor-activated Ca^{2+} influx mechanism that is dihydropyridine-insensitive and which has biophysical characteristics that are inconsistent with those of VOC (Murray & Kotlikoff, 1991; Murray *et al.*, 1993). Thus, in these experiments, contractile agonists activate sustained Ca^{2+} influx, which is decreased when the cell is depolarized and is increased at more negative membrane potentials. These data are entirely consistent with the much earlier information described by Coburn (1979), in which hyperpolarization increased contractions following exposure of canine tracheal smooth muscle to acetylcholine. The cation permeability of the influx pathway described by Murray and Kotlikoff (1991) not only is distinct from that of VOC in ASM but also differs substantially from that described in non-excitable cells such as platelets and endothelial cells (Hallam & Rink, 1985; Hallam *et al.*, 1988; Merrit *et al.*, 1989). Furthermore, the fact that divalent cations block this pathway is suggestive that it is highly specific for Ca^{2+} and that a non-specific cation channel is unlikely to be involved.

Precisely how such ROC are activated and/or regulated or how important they are to the overall physiological contractile process is not yet known. In terms of activation, however, recent studies in mast cells (Penner *et al.*, 1988; Hoth & Penner, 1992) have supported the 'capacitative' entry hypothesis (Putney, 1986, 1993). Thus, emptying of the agonist/IP_3-sensitive Ca^{2+} pool in the SR can create an enhanced permeability in the plasma membrane, so permitting Ca^{2+} entry.

The compelling conclusion from the above data is that intracellular activator Ca^{2+} ions are responsible for the initiation of contraction, but the tonic or sustained phase of a contraction is associated with a low level of extracellular Ca^{2+} influx, via a mechanism that bears all the hallmarks of an ROC-mediated event. To date, there are no known inhibitors of ROC activity in excitable cells. However, the fact that the compound SKF96365, which is an inhibitor of ROC activity in non-excitable cells, has been shown to block extracellular Ca^{2+} entry in the experiments of Murray and Kotlikoff (1991) simply confirms the above conclusion. While these findings are of a very exciting nature, they clearly require substantiation. However, they may well signal for the first time not only the presence but also the active participation of ROC in the excitation–contraction coupling process in ASM cells. Unambiguous definition of such a role, through the development of more selective inhibitors of Ca^{2+} influx via these ROC, may very well lead to the development of exciting, novel, therapeutic agents for use in allergic diseases such as asthma. The precise involvement of the CIF (Clapham, 1993) in regulating these ROC, either as a means of supporting sustained contraction of ASM cells or as a means of refilling the intracellular Ca^{2+} stores, is an exciting area for further research.

Contraction of ASM: an integrated scheme

Over the past 10 years or so, there has been a dramatic advance in our understanding of both the physiological and the biochemical mechanisms underlying contraction of ASM. Inevitably with such a complicated system, there remain numerous unresolved issues that lie beyond the scope of this chapter. Notwithstanding, the account given below is an attempt to provide a simplified version of the sequence of events that is thought to occur, woven into an integrated scheme.

Contractile agonists, on combining with their specific cell-surface receptors, activate phospholipase C or phospholipase D via a G-protein linkage. As far as phospholi-

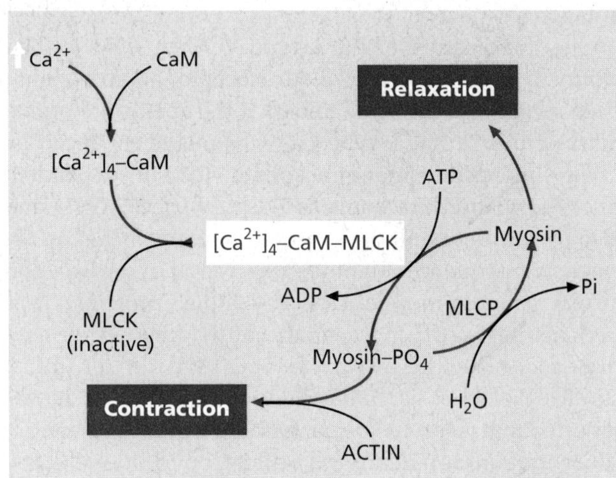

Fig. 42.3 Sequence of events involved in the regulation of myosin by Ca^{2+}. These events are widely regarded as being pivotal in mediating the rapid generation of tension following receptor stimulation by a contractile agonist. Once Ca^{2+} levels rise within the cell, the cations bind to calmodulin (CaM; four cations per molecule of CaM). This leads to a conformational change in CaM which allows the formation of a ternary complex with myosin light-chain kinase (MLCK). The $(Ca^{2+})_4$–CaM–MLCK complex catalyses the transfer of phosphate groups to each of the two 20 kDa light chains of myosin. This phosphorylation reaction triggers cross-bridge cycling between actin and myosin with consequent contraction of airway smooth muscle. This process is fuelled by energy derived from the actin-activated myosin Mg^{2+}-ATPase. Relaxation of airway smooth muscle is brought about by a lowering of intracellular activator Ca^{2+}, which, in turn, inactivates MLCK by causing dissociation of Ca^{2+} from CaM. Consequently, myosin-PO_4 is dephosphorylated by myosin light-chain phosphatase (MLCP), cross-bridge cycling ceases and the smooth muscle assumes a relaxed state.

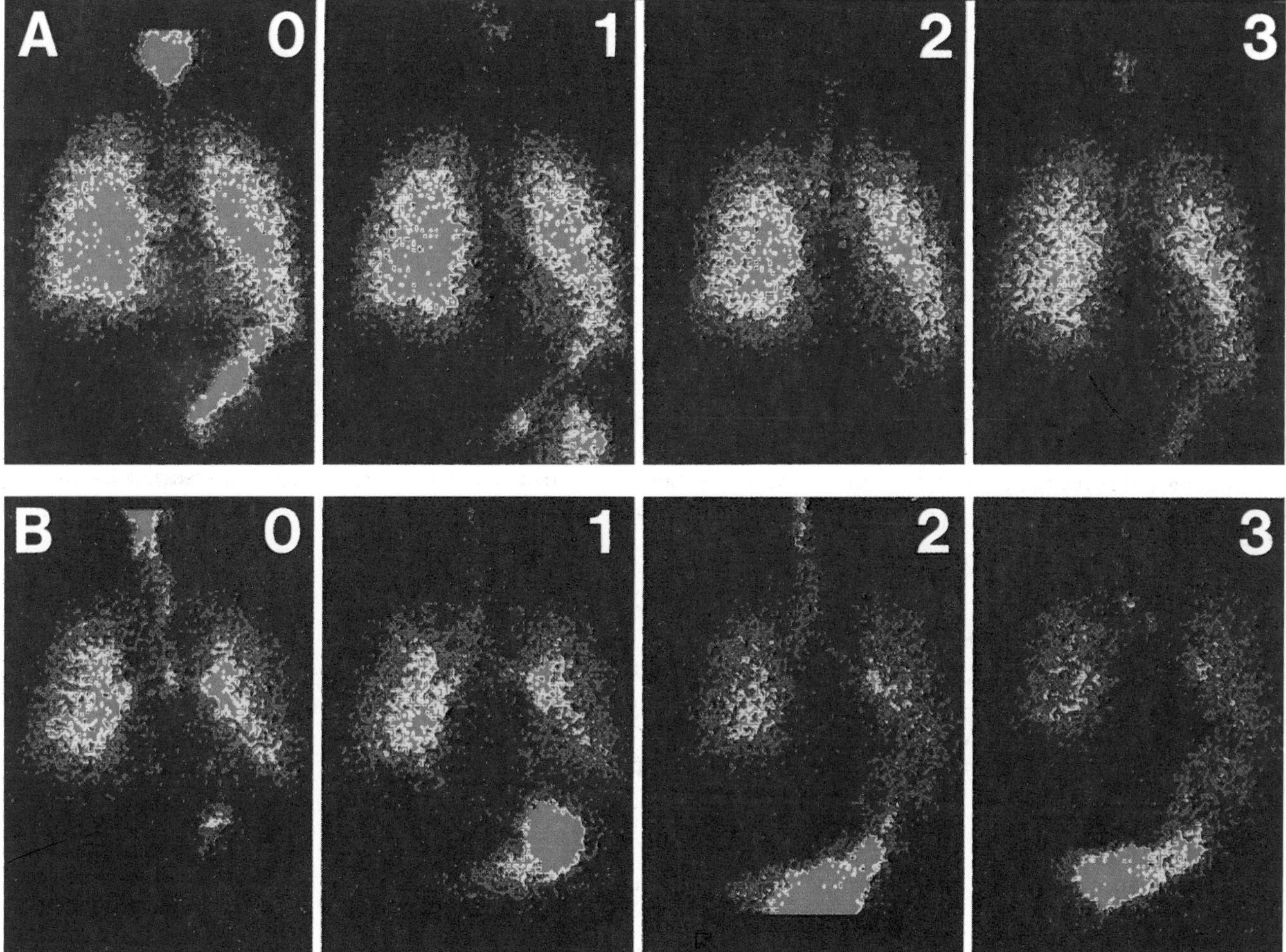

Plate 41.1 Clearance of ^{99m}Tc from two volunteers following mouth breathing of technetium-labelled Bec-DLPC aerosol. Aerosols were generated during inspiration with the Pari Jet Interrupter valve system, Munich, Germany. Scintigraphs in A & B, from left to right were taken at 0, 1, 2 and 3 hours. The nebulizer reservoir contained 2.5 ml of 0.4 normal (0.0036 gm/cc of saline). Bec-DLPC liposomes 200 μg of Bec/cc. DLPC was labelled with ^{99m}Tc stannous chloride (Vidgren *et al.*, 1994). (A) Exposure using Aerotech II nebulizer, mass median aerodynamic diameter (MMAD) 1.5 μm, geometric standard deviation (GSD) 2.4. (B) Exposure using Spira nebulizer, MMAD 3.6 μm, GSD 2.5.

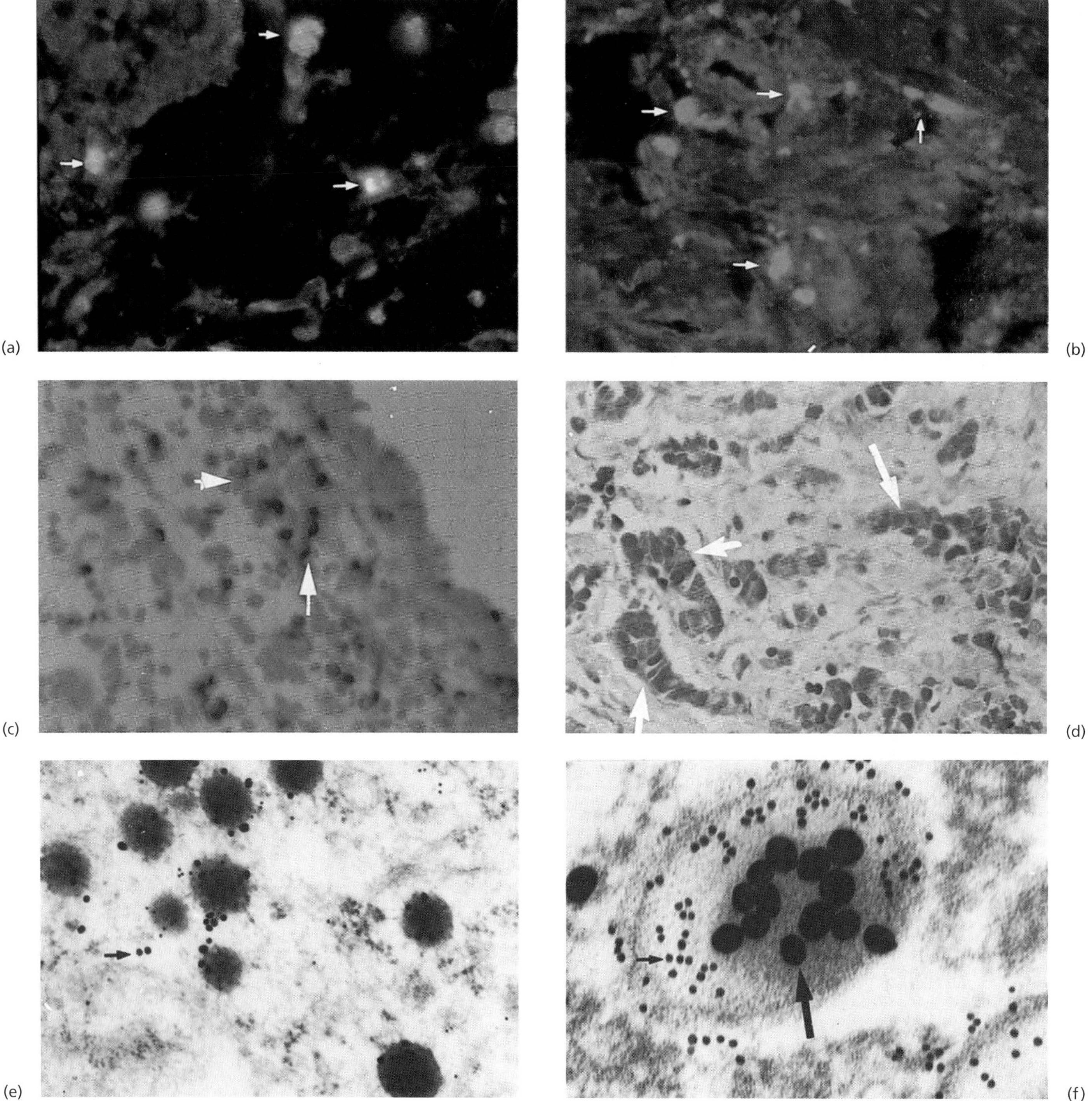

Plate 45.1 (a) Example of immunostaining using monoclonal antibody to CD3 in skin biopsy using direct immunofluorescence technique (FITC). (b) Example of immunofluorescence staining of nasal biopsy using indirect technique (Texas Red). (c) Example of immunostaining using alkaline phosphatase-anti-alkaline phosphatase (APAAP) technique with antibody to Eg2 in nasal biopsy. (d) Example of immunostaining of tumour cells using peroxidase anti-peroxidase (PAP) technique developed with DAB. (e) and (f) Single and double electron microscopy immunostaining using different size gold particles. Glucagon and GLP1 co-localization in neurosecretory granules of a pancreatic cell.

pase C is concerned, it cleaves PIP_2, creating the two second messengers IP_3 and diacylglycerol. It is the principal responsibility of IP_3 to promptly induce the release of Ca^{2+} from intracellular stores within the SR. Whenever the intracellular Ca^{2+} levels increase, these free Ca^{2+} ions combine with the Ca^{2+} binding protein calmodulin. It is generally accepted that four Ca^{2+} bind to each molecule of calmodulin, so inducing a conformational change that exposes hydrophobic sites for interaction with a number of target proteins (Allen & Walsh, 1994) (Fig. 42.3). One of these proteins is myosin light-chain kinase. The resultant tertiary complex ($(Ca^{2+})_4$-calmodulin-myosin light-chain kinase), which represents the active form of myosin light-chain kinase, catalyses the transfer of the terminal phosphoryl group of Mg^{2+}-ATP to serine 19 on each of the two 20 kDa light chains of myosin (Fig. 42.3). This simple phosphorylation reaction triggers the cycling of myosin cross-bridges along the actin filaments, with the consequent development of contractile force. The rate at which tension is then generated (the phasic component of a contraction) is determined by the rate at which the cross-bridges between actin and myosin cycle. This, in turn, is determined by the magnitude of myosin light-chain phosphorylation. It is now widely accepted that the generation of IP_3 by a contractile agonist is transient (Chilvers *et al.*, 1989, 1994; Langlands *et al.*, 1989). Consequently, the second-messenger-induced release of Ca^{2+} from the SR is thought to be discontinuous. Thus, it appears that IP_3 is adapted only to provide an initial burst of intracellular Ca^{2+} release to induce rapid cross-bridge cycling and thus tension development. (For detailed information concerning IP_3 and other inositol phosphates in ASM cells the interested reader is directed to reviews by Chilvers *et al.* (1994) and Rodger (1995b).) In the absence of further release of intracellular Ca^{2+}, the cellular level returns towards, although not precisely to, resting levels. This fall in the intracellular concentration of Ca^{2+} is a consequence of extrusion of Ca^{2+} from the cell by the sarcolemmal Ca^{2+} pump, or by an Na^+–Ca^{2+} exchanger in the cell membrane, or via pumping of Ca^{2+} into the SR by a Ca^{2+} pump sited in the SR membrane (see Rodger & Pyne, 1992). This fall in the intracellular Ca^{2+} level results in the dissociation of Ca^{2+} from calmodulin and the consequent termination of the activity of myosin light-chain kinase. Phosphorylation of the 20 kDa light chain of myosin must therefore decline and, consequently, so must the ATPase activity of myosin. Coincident with this event, myosin is dephosphorylated by a myosin light-chain phosphatase.

In the face of these events, which one might expect to uncouple the excitation–contraction coupling sequence and so promote relaxation, the developed tension of ASM cells is well maintained. It has been proposed, therefore, that such steady-state force maintenance does not require a continued myosin light-chain phosphorylation, because of an alteration in the type of attachment formed between actin and myosin. Thus, instead of rapidly cycling cross-bridges, so-called latch bridges (or dephosphorylated myosin cross-bridges), which cycle slowly or not at all, are formed (Hai & Murphy, 1989; Kamm & Stull, 1989; Murphy, 1989). The maintenance of these latch bridges is Ca^{2+} dependent, since smooth muscle in the latch state can be relaxed by removal of Ca^{2+}. This does not necessarily imply that a latch-bridge state is directly regulated by Ca^{2+}. However, it does mean that some Ca^{2+}-dependent process must be involved in the formation of latch bridges, possibly utilizing extracellular Ca^{2+} entering the cell via ROC, as discussed earlier. In view of the low intracellular Ca^{2+} levels that exist during the tonic phase of a contraction, one of the characteristic features of the latch-bridge state must be an enhanced sensitivity of the contractile apparatus Ca^{2+}. Acceptance of this assumption implies a change in the Ca^{2+} concentration requirement of Ca^{2+} binding proteins or of Ca^{2+}-dependent protein kinase activities, such as myosin light-chain kinase or Ca^{2+}-calmodulin, calponin or caldesmon. However, dissociation of force and intracellular Ca^{2+} levels might also be a consequence of increased contractile or regulatory protein phosphorylation, secondary to the activation of protein kinase C or inhibition of phosphoprotein phosphatase activities. Each of these postulated activities is now under intense scrutiny, with particular attention being devoted to the possible phosphorylation reactions that are governed by protein kinase C.

Diacylglycerol is generated from more than one source during the sustained phase of an ASM contraction following agonist receptor stimulation (Rasmussen *et al.*, 1990). Initially, arachidonic acid-rich diacylglycerol is generated from PIP_2 by phospholipase C. Subsequently, diacylglycerol can be derived from phosphatidylcholine via phosphatidylcholine-specific phospholipase C and also via the action of phospholipase D. Interestingly, it has been shown recently that bradykinin stimulates phospholipase D in primary cultures of guinea pig tracheal smooth muscle (Pyne & Pyne, 1993). The end result of these events is a sustained increase in the total levels of diacylglycerol within the ASM cell and the consequent persistent activation of various isoforms of protein kinase C. In this context, it has been proposed that phosphorylation of certain contractile proteins by protein kinase C can bring about an enhanced sensitivity to Ca^{2+} (Rodger, 1986; Rasmussen *et al.*, 1987). An alternative proposal has been advanced to explain Ca^{2+}-independent contractile responses to certain substances, such as phorbol esters and physiological agonists (Allen & Walsh, 1994). In this scheme, ligand occupancy of appropriate receptors triggers activation, via G proteins, of phosphatidylcholine-specific phospholipase C or D, producing diacylglycerol, without any concomitant change in the intracellular Ca^{2+} concentration. This is thought to lead to the specific activation of the Ca^{2+}-independent epsilon form of protein kinase C (Allen & Walsh, 1994). To date, little is known about the events following protein kinase C activation. However, both the actin-associated protein calponin and caldesmon have been implicated as direct and/or indirect downstream targets of protein kinase C.

The conclusion to be drawn from the above discussion is that two distinct, although in many respects interdependent, pathways exist to control contraction of ASM. The first, a calmodulin/Ca^{2+}/myosin light-chain kinase pathway is widely regarded as being responsible for the initial rapid development of tension in ASM cells resulting from contractile agonist stimulation. The second pathway, via protein kinase C-mediated phosphorylations, is postulated either to adapt the cell to accommodate sustained muscle contraction at minimum cost to itself, in terms of both energy expenditure and protection against the toxic consequences of prolonged intracellular Ca^{2+} overload, or to induce slowly developing contractions of smooth muscle via Ca^{2+}-independent mechanisms.

Conclusion

It is clear from the information presented in this chapter that much is known about the structure, function and physiological regulation of ASM cells and the cellular events underlying receptor activation by a contractile agonist. The advent of sophisticated molecular biological and biochemical techniques has allowed us to gain substantial insight into events such as receptor–G-protein interactions, G-protein activation/regulation of certain critical enzymes such as phospholipases C and D, the generation of second messengers such as IP_3, diacylglycerol and cADP-ribose, intracellular Ca^{2+} release mechanisms and activation and regulation of contractile proteins with respect to the initial generation of smooth-muscle tension. It is also clear, however, that the cellular events involved in the maintenance of developed tension, which equates with the sustained bronchospasm of an asthmatic attack, and those cellular events which underlie Ca^{2+}-independent contraction of ASM cells remain to be elucidated.

Acknowledgement

I am grateful to Barbara Pearce for the careful typing and preparation of the manuscript for this chapter.

References

Adelstein, R.S. (1983) Regulation of contractile proteins by phosphorylation. *J. Clin. Invest.*, **72**, 1863–6.

Advenier, C., Naline, E. & Renier, A. (1986) Effects of BAY-K 8644 on contraction of the human isolated bronchus and guinea-pig isolated trachea. *Brit. J. Pharmacol.*, **88**, 33–9.

Agrawal, R. & Daniel, E.E. (1986) Control of gap junction formation in canine trachea by arachidonic acid metabolites. *Am. J. Physiol.*, **250**, C495–C505.

Ahmed, F., Foster, R.W., Small, R.C. & Weston, A.H. (1984) Some features of the spasmogenic actions of acetylcholine and histamine in guinea-pig isolated trachealis. *Brit. J. Pharmacol.*, **83**, 227–33.

Akasaka, K., Konno, K., Ono, Y., Mue, S. & Abe, C. (1975) Electromyographic study of bronchial smooth muscle in bronchial asthma. *Tohoku J. Exp. Med.*, **117**, 55–9.

Allen, B.G. & Walsh, M.P. (1994) The biochemical basis of the regulation of smooth-muscle contraction. *Trends Biochem. Sci.*, **19**, 362–8.

Allen, S.L., Foster, R.W., Small, R.C. & Towart, R. (1985) The effects of the dihydropyridine BAY-K 8644 in guinea pig isolated trachealis. *Brit. J. Pharmacol.*, **86**, 171–80.

Armstrong, D. & Eckert, R. (1987) Voltage-activated calcium channels that must be phosphorylated to respond to membrane depolarization. *Proc. Nat. Acad. Sci. USA*, **84**, 2518–22.

Barnes, P.J. (1983) Pathogenesis of asthma: a review. *J. Roy. Soc. Med.*, **76**, 580–6.

Berry, J.L., Elliott, K.R.F., Foster, R.W., Green, K.A., Murray, M.A. & Small, R.C. (1991) Mechanical, biochemical and electrophysiological studies of RP 49356 and cromakalim in guinea-pig and bovine trachealis muscle. *Pulm. Pharmacol.*, **4**, 91–8.

Bolton, T.B. (1979) Mechanisms of action of transmitters and other substances on smooth muscle. *Physiol. Rev.*, **59**, 606–718.

Bourreau, J.-P., Abela, A.P., Kwan, C.Y. & Daniel, E.E. (1991) Acetylcholine Ca^{2+} stores refilling directly involves a dihydropyridine-sensitive channel in dog trachea. *Am. J. Physiol.*, **261**, C497–C505.

Chilvers, E.R., Challiss, R.A.J., Barnes, P.J. & Nahorski, S.R. (1989) Mass changes of inositol (1,4,5)tris-phosphate in trachealis muscle following agonist stimulation. *Eur. J. Pharmacol.*, **164**, 587–90.

Chilvers, E.R., Lynch, B.J. & Challiss, R.A.J. (1994) Phosphoinositide metabolism in airway smooth muscle. *Pharmacol. Ther.*, **62**, 221–45.

Clapham, D.E. (1993) Cellular calcium. A mysterious new influx factor? *Nature*, **364**, 763–4.

Coburn, R.F. (1979) Electromechanical coupling in canine trachealis muscle: acetylcholine contractions. *Am. J. Physiol.*, **236**, C177–C184.

Daniel, E.E., Grover, A.K. & Kwan, C.Y. (1983) Calcium. In: *Biochemistry of Smooth Muscle*, Vol. III (ed. N.L. Stephens), pp. 1–88. CRC Press, Boca Raton.

Daniel, E.E., Kannan, M., Davis, C. & Posey-Daniel, V. (1986) Ultrastructural studies on the neuromuscular control of human tracheal and bronchial muscle. *Resp. Physiol.*, **63**, 109–28.

Davis, C., Kannan, M., Jones, T. & Daniel, E. (1982) Control of human airway smooth muscle: *in vitro* studies. *J. Appl. Physiol.*, **53**, 1080–7.

Ellis, S.B., Williams, M.E., Ways, N.R. *et al.* (1988) Sequence and expression of mRNAs encoding the α_1 and α_2 subunits of a DHP-sensitive calcium channel. *Science*, **241**, 1661–4.

Emala, C.W., Yang, J., Hirschman, C.A. & Levine, M.A. (1994) G protein subunits in lung cells. *Life Sci.*, **55**, 593–602.

Felbel, J., Trockur, B., Ecker, T., Landgraf, W. & Hofmann, F. (1988) Regulation of cytosolic calcium by cAMP and cGMP in freshly isolated smooth muscle cells from bovine trachea. *J. Biol. Chem.*, **263**, 16764–71.

Fürst, D.O., Cross, R.A., De Mey, J. & Small, J.V. (1986) Caldesmon is an elongated, flexible molecule localized in the actomyosin domains of smooth muscle. *EMBO J.*, **5**, 251–7.

Galione, A. (1993) Cyclic ADP-ribose: a new way to control calcium. *Science*, **259**, 325–6.

Giembycz, M.A. & Rodger, I.W. (1987) Electrophysiological and other aspects of excitation–contraction coupling and uncoupling in mammalian airway smooth muscle. *Life Sci.*, **41**, 111–32.

Green, K.A., Foster, R.W. & Small, R.C. (1991) A patch-clamp study of K^+-channel activity in bovine isolated tracheal smooth muscle cells. *Brit. J. Pharmacol.*, **102**, 871–8.

Hai, C.-M. & Murphy, R.C. (1989) Ca^{2+}, crossbridge phosphorylation and contraction. *Ann. Rev. Physiol.*, **51**, 285–98.

Hallam, T.J. & Rink, T.J. (1985) Agonists stimulate divalent cation channels in the plasma membrane of human platelets. *FEBS Letts.*, **186**, 175–9.

Hallam, T.J., Jacob, R. & Merritt, J.E. (1988) Evidence that agonists stimulate bivalent-cation influx into human endothelial cells. *Biochem. J.*, **255**, 179–84.

Hartzell, H.C., Méry, P.-F., Fischmeister, R. & Szabo, G. (1991) Sympathetic regulation of cardiac calcium current is due exclusively to cAMP-dependent phosphorylation. *Nature*, **351**, 573–6.

Henry, P.J. (1993) Endothelin-1 (ET-1)-induced contraction in rat isolated trachea: involvement of ET_A and ET_B receptors and multiple signal transduction systems. *Brit. J. Pharmacol.*, **110**, 435–41.

Hisada, T., Kurachi, Y. & Sugimoto, T. (1990) Properties of membrane currents in isolated smooth muscle cells from guinea-pig trachea. *Pflugers Arch Eur. J. Physiol.*, **416**, 151–61.

Honda, K. & Tomita, T. (1987) Electrical activity in isolated human tracheal muscle. *Jpn. J. Physiol.*, **37**, 333–6.

Hoth, M. & Penner, R. (1992) Depletion of intracellular calcium stores activates a calcium current in mast cells. *Nature*, **355**, 353–6.

Imoto, Y., Yatani, A., Reeves, J.P., Codina, J., Birnbaumer, L. & Brown, A.M. (1988) α-Subunit of G_s directly activates cardiac calcium channels in lipid bilayers. *Am. J. Physiol.*, **255**, H722–8.

Kajita, J. & Yamaguchi, H. (1993) Calcium mobilization of muscarinic cholinergic stimulation in bovine single airway smooth muscle. *Am. J. Physiol.*, **264**, L496–L503.

Kamm, K.E. & Stull, J.T. (1985) The function of myosin and myosin light chain kinase phosphorylation in smooth muscle. *Ann. Rev. Pharmacol. Toxicol.*, **25**, 593–620.

Kamm, K.E. & Stull, J.T. (1989) Regulation of smooth muscle contractile elements by second messengers. *Ann. Rev. Physiol.*, **51**, 299–313.

Kannan, M.S. & Daniel, E.E. (1980) Structural and functional study of control of canine tracheal smooth muscle. *Am. J. Physiol.*, **238**, C27–C33.

Kannan, M.S., Jager, L.P., Daniel, E.E. & Garfield, R.E. (1983) Effects of 4-aminopyridine and tetraethyl-ammonium chloride on the electrical activity and cable properties of canine tracheal smooth muscle. *J. Pharmacol. Exp. Ther.*, **227**, 706–15.

Kotlikoff, M.I. (1988) Calcium currents in isolated canine airway smooth muscle cells. *Am. J. Physiol.*, **254**, C793–C801.

Kotlikoff, M.I. (1989) Ion channels in airway smooth muscle. In: *Airway Smooth Muscle in Health and Disease* (ed. R.F. Coburn), pp. 169–80. Plenum, New York.

Kotlikoff, M.I. (1990) Potassium currents in canine airway smooth muscle cells. *Am. J. Physiol.*, **259**, L384–L395.

Kotlikoff, M.I. (1993) Potassium channels in airway smooth muscle: a tale of two channels. *Pharmacol. Ther.*, **58**, 1–12.

Kotlikoff, M.I., Murray, R.K. & Reynolds, E.E. (1987) Histamine-induced calcium release and phorbol antagonism in cultured airway smooth muscle cells. *Am. J. Physiol.*, **253**, C561–6.

Kume, H. & Kotlikoff, M.I. (1991) Muscarinic inhibition of single K_{ca} channels in smooth muscle cells by a pertussis-sensitive G-protein. *Am. J. Physiol.*, **261**, C1204–9.

Langlands, J.M., Rodger, I.W. & Diamond, J. (1989) The effect of M&B 22948 on methacholine- and histamine-induced contraction and inositol 1,4,5-trisphosphate levels in guinea-pig tracheal tissue. *Brit. J. Pharmacol.*, **98**, 336–8.

Lee, J., Uchida, Y., Sakamoto, T., Hirata, A., Hasegawa, S. & Hirata, F. (1994) Alteration of G-protein levels in antigen-challenged guinea-pigs. *J. Pharmacol. Exp. Ther.*, **271**, 1713–20.

Linder, M.E. & Gilman, A.G. (1992) G proteins. *Sci. Am.*, **267**, 56–65.

McCray, P.B. & Joseph, T. (1993) Spontaneous contractility of human fetal airway smooth muscle. *Am. J. Respir. Cell Mol. Biol.*, **8**, 573–80.

Marthan, R., Armour, C.L., Johnson, P.R.A. & Black, J.L. (1987) The calcium channel agonist BAY-K 8644 enhances the responsiveness of human airway muscle to KCl and histamine but not to carbachol. *Am. Rev. Resp. Dis.*, **135**, 185–9.

Marthan, R., Martin, C., Amédée, T. & Mironneau, J. (1989) Calcium channel currents in isolated smooth muscle cells from human bronchus. *J. Appl. Physiol.*, **66**, 1706–14.

Merritt, J.E., Jacob, R. & Hallam, T.J. (1989) Use of manganese to discriminate between calcium influx and mobilization from internal stores in stimulated human neutrophils. *J. Biol. Chem.*, **264**, 1522–7.

Murphy, R.A. (1989) Contraction in smooth muscle cells. *Ann. Rev. Physiol.*, **51**, 275–83.

Murray, R.K. & Kotlikoff, M.I. (1991) Receptor-activated calcium influx in human airway smooth muscle cells. *J. Physiol.*, **435**, 123–44.

Murray, R.K., Fleischmann, B.K. & Kotlikoff, M.I. (1993) Receptor-activated Ca influx in human airway smooth muscle: use of Ca imaging and perforated patch-clamp techniques. *Am. J. Physiol.*, **264**, C485–C490.

Panettieri, R.A., Murray, R.K., DePalo, L.R., Yadvish, P.A. & Kotlikoff, M.I. (1989) A human airway smooth muscle cell line that retains physiological responsiveness. *Am. J. Physiol.*, **256**, C329–C335.

Parekh, A.B., Terlau, H. & Stuhmer, W. (1993) Depletion of $InsP_3$ stores activates a Ca^{2+} and K^+ current by means of a phosphatase and a diffusable messenger. *Nature*, **364**, 814–18.

Penner, R., Mathews, G. & Neher, E. (1988) Regulation of calcium influx by second messengers in rat mast cells. *Nature*, **334**, 499–504.

Putney, J.W. Jr (1986) A model for receptor-regulated calcium entry. *Cell Calcium*, **7**, 1–12.

Putney, J.W. Jr (1993) Excitement about calcium signaling in inexcitable cells. *Science*, **262**, 676–8.

Pyne, N.J. & Rodger, I.W. (1993) Guanine-nucleotide binding regulatory proteins in receptor-mediated actions. In: *Lung Biology in Health and Disease*, Vol. 67. *Pharmacology of the Respiratory Tract: Experimental and Clinical Research* (eds K.F. Chung & P.J. Barnes), pp. 47–61. Marcel Dekker, New York.

Pyne, S. & Pyne, N.J. (1993) Bradykinin stimulates phospholipase D in primary cultures of guinea-pig tracehal smooth muscle. *Biochem. Pharmacol.*, **45**, 593–603.

Raeburn, D. & Rodger, I.W. (1984) Lack of effect of leukotriene D_4 on Ca-uptake in airway smooth muscle. *Brit. J. Pharmacol.*, **83**, 499–504.

Randriamampita, C. & Tsien, R.Y. (1993) Emptying of intracellular Ca^{2+} stores releases a novel small messenger that stimulates Ca^{2+} influx. *Nature*, **364**, 809–14.

Rasmussen, H., Takuwa, Y. & Park, S. (1987) Protein kinase C in the regulation of smooth muscle contraction. *FASEB J.*, **1**, 177–85.

Rasmussen, H., Kelley, G. & Douglas, J.S. (1990) Interactions between Ca^{2+} and cAMP messenger system in regulation of airway smooth muscle contraction. *Am. J. Physiol.*, **258**, L279–L288.

Richards, I.S., Kulkarni, A. & Brooks, S.M. (1991) Human fetal tracheal smooth muscle produces spontaneous electromechanical oscillations that are Ca^{2+}-dependent and cholinergically potentiated. *Dev. Pharmacol. Ther.*, **16**, 22–8.

Rodger, I.W. (1986) Calcium ions and contraction of airways smooth muscle. In: *Asthma: Clinical Pharmacology and Therapeutic Progress* (ed. A.B. Kay), pp. 114–27. Blackwell Scientific Publications, Oxford.

Rodger, I.W. (1987) Calcium channels. *Am. Rev. Resp. Dis.*, **136**, S15–S17.

Rodger, I.W. (1993) Airway smooth muscle: Signal transduction and contractile mechanisms. In: *Asthma: Physiology, Immunopharmacology and Treatment.* (eds S.T. Holgate, K.F. Austen, L.M. Lichtenstein & A.B. Kay), pp. 243–57. Academic Press, London.

Rodger, I.W. (1995a) Voltage-dependent and receptor-operated calcium channels. In: *Airways Smooth Muscle: Ion Channels, Receptors and Signal Transduction* (eds M.A. Giembycz & D. Raeburn). Birkhauser Verlag, Basle.

Rodger, I.W. (1995b) Biochemistry of activation–contraction coupling. In: *Asthma and Rhinitis* (eds W.W. Busse & S.T. Holgate). Blackwell Science Inc., Boston, MA.

Rodger, I.W. & Pyne, N.J. (1992) Airway smooth muscle. In: *Asthma: Basic Mechanisms and Clinical Management* (eds P.J. Barnes, I.W. Rodger & N.C. Thompson), pp. 59–84. Academic Press, London.

Saunders, H.-M.H. & Farley, J.M. (1991) Spontaneous transient outward currents and Ca^{2+}-activated K^+ channels in swine tracheal smooth muscle cells. *J. Pharmacol. Exp. Ther.*, **257**, 1114–20.

Small, J.V. (1985) Geometry of actin-membrane attachments in the smooth muscle cell: the localisations of vinculin and α-actinin. *EMBO J.*, **4**, 45–9.

Small, J.V., Fürst, D.O. & De Mey, J. (1986) Localization of filamin in smooth muscle. *J. Cell Biol.*, **102**, 210–20.

Small, R.C. & Foster, R.W. (1988) Electrophysiology of the airway smooth muscle cell. In: *Asthma: Basic Mechanisms and Clinical Management* (eds P.J. Banes, I.W. Rodger & N.C. Thomson), pp. 35–56. Academic Press, London.

Small, R.C. & Foster, R.W. (1995) The electrophysiology of plasmalemmal Ca^{2+}-channels in airway smooth muscle. In: *Airway Smooth Muscle: a Reference Source*, Vol. 1 (eds M.A. Giembycz & D. Raeburn). Birkhauser Verlag, Basle.

Spedding, M. & Paoletti, R. (1992) Classification of calcium channels and the sites of action of drugs modifying channel function. *Pharmacol. Rev.*, **44**, 363–76.

Stull, J.T. (1980) Phosphorylation of contractile proteins in relation to muscle function. *Adv. Cyclic Nucleotide Res.*, **13**, 39–93.

Takuwa, Y., Takuwa, N. & Rasmussen, H. (1988) The effects of isoproterenol on intracellular calcium concentration. *J. Biol. Chem.*, **263**, 762–8.

Taylor, D.A., Bowman, B.F. & Stull, J.T. (1989) Cytoplasmic Ca^{2+} is a primary determinant for myosin phosphorylation in smooth muscle cells. *J. Biol. Chem.*, **264**, 6207–13.

Thomson, N.C. (1983) Neurogenic and myogenic mechanisms of nonspecific bronchial hyperresponsiveness. *Eur. J. Resp. Dis.*, **64** (Suppl. 128), 206–11.

Welling, A., Felbel, J., Peper, K. & Hofmann, F. (1992) Hormonal regulation of calcium current in freshly isolated airway smooth muscle cells. *Am. J. Physiol.*, **262**, L351–L359.

Worley, J.F., III & Kotlikoff, M.I. (1990) Dihydropyridine-sensitive single calcium channels in airway smooth muscle cells. *Am. J. Physiol.*, **259**, L468–L480.

Yang, C.M., Yo, Y.-L. & Wang, Y.-Y. (1993) Intracellular calcium in canine cultured tracheal smooth-muscle cells is regulated by M_3 muscarinic receptors. *Brit. J. Pharmacol.*, **110**, 983–8.

PART 5

Cellular and Molecular Techniques in the Study of Allergic Disease

CHAPTER 43
T-Cell Cloning

R.E. O'Hehir, B.A. Askonas & J.R. Lamb

Introduction

Marked heterogeneity of specificity and function occurs in the T-lymphocyte pool and has provided the scientific rationale for the isolation of monoclonal populations of immunocompetent cells. However, initially an incomplete knowledge of the physiology of T cells hampered the technical advances needed to produce T-cell clones. It was assumed that T-cell antigen receptors would parallel those of B cells in function and structural characteristics, by binding directly to native antigen in free form, and that they would be secreted into the supernatants of cultured cells. Now, however, it is well recognized that the activation of both CD4+ and CD8+ T lymphocytes and the subsequent induction of an immune response require the formation of molecular interactions between the T-cell antigen receptor and peptide fragments of antigen complexed with gene products of the major histocompatibility complex (MHC), as reviewed in Schwartz (1985) and Townsend and Bodmer (1989). Appreciation of this key difference between T-cell and B-cell antigen recognition provided a molecular explanation for the failure to isolate T cells using free native soluble antigen.

As knowledge of the different biological signals and receptors required for T-cell activation and proliferation unfolded, in particular on the critical role of antigen-non-specific lymphokines, the technical constraints on the expansion of monoclonal populations of T cells were eased. In particular, two scientific advances in knowledge facilitated the cloning of T cells. Firstly, demonstration that the interaction between T cells and antigen is MHC dependent indicated the essential role of histocompatible antigen-presenting cells (APC) for T-cell activation, proliferation and target-cell recognition. Secondly, Morgan *et al.* (1976) identified the ability of tissue-culture medium, conditioned with supernatants from mitogen-stimulated human peripheral-blood mononuclear cells (lymphocytes) (PBMC), to induce the *in vitro* proliferation of T lymphoblasts. The antigen-non-specific growth factor in the conditioned medium was identified as interleukin-2 (IL-2; Gillis & Smith, 1977), and its addition to *in vitro* cultures subsequently allowed the expansion of antigen-specific murine and human cytotoxic (Von Boehmer *et al.*, 1979; Lin & Askonas, 1981) and helper (Th) (Fathman & Hengartner, 1978; Nabholtz *et al.*, 1978; Bach *et al.*, 1979; Schreier & Tees, 1980; Sredni *et al.*, 1981; Lamb *et al.*, 1982; Spits *et al.*, 1982) T cells.

Manipulation of the IL-2 dependence of activated T cells is not the only method for the propagation of T-cell clones, and alternative techniques, including hybridization (Kappler *et al.*, 1981) and viral transformation (Finn *et al.*, 1979; Popovic *et al.*, 1983), are considered.

This chapter will be restricted to methods for the selection and maintenance of human CD4+ and CD8+ antigen-specific T-cell lines and clones, as well as the important functional assays by which they are characterized. Basic methods vary with different antigen systems and individual laboratory preferences. Therefore, we provide representative recipes which can be developed to suit specific requirements (Fig. 43.1).

Lymphocyte cultures

Culture conditions

Cultures are incubated under maximal humidification,

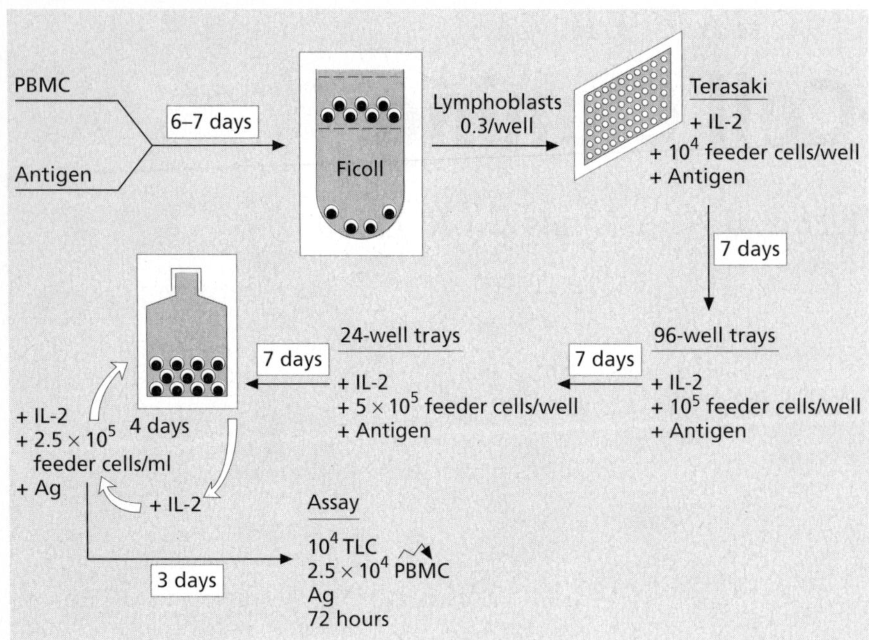

Fig. 43.1 An overview of a standard T-cell cloning procedure.

with an atmosphere of 5–6% CO_2 in air at 37°C. Fungal contamination can be minimized by using copper-lined incubators or by the addition of copper sulphate to the water trays.

Media

Commonly used tissue-culture media include RPMI-1640, Dulbecco's modified Eagle's medium (DMEM) and Iscove's modified Dulbecco's medium (IMDM). Powdered preparations or liquid media are obtainable but, if powdered media are used, it is essential that high-quality, endotoxin-free distilled water is available. Buffering, such as sodium hydrogen carbonate and/or hydroxyethylpiperazine ethanesulphonic acid (HEPES), facilitates equilibration of pH 7.4 at 5% CO_2. Antibiotic supplementation (penicillin 100 IU/ml and streptomycin 100 μg/ml or gentamicin 50 μg/ml) is usual. Routine use of antimycoplasma agents is not recommended to avoid subclinical infection but Antimycoplasma Removal Agent (Flow) or Ciproflaxacin (Bayer) have been found useful for controlling mild contamination. Routinely, commercially prepared RPMI-1640 with 2 g/l sodium bicarbonate supplemented with 2 mmol/l L-glutamine, 100 IU/ml penicillin and 100 μg/ml streptomycin is used for all lymphocyte cultures. Human cell cultures require serum supplementation with fetal calf serum (FCS) or normal human serum (preferably AB but the more readily available A+ serum is also suitable). Batch screening of sera is mandatory. Standard proliferation assays should be performed against a common recall antigen, such as influenza or tetanus, in media containing 5, 10, 15 and 20% serum with a requirement for good positive responses and low background proliferation. Sera should be heat-inactivated at 56°C for 30 minutes and then may be stored at –70°C for extended periods. Optimal concentration for cultures should be determined for each batch but is usually 5–10%. A variety of commercial serum-free media are now available (e.g. AIM V; Gibco) and may be useful in combination with RPMI-1640 for polyclonal proliferation assays, to decrease background counts, or cytokine assays, to increase sensitivity, but long-term cultured human T cells prefer human serum. Routinely, human T-cell culture media are supplemented with human AB or A serum, Epstein–Barr virus (EBV)-transformed B-cell lines (BCL) with FCS and murine L-cell cultures with FCS.

Lymphocyte preparation

Density centrifugation

PBMC are isolated from heparinized (preservative-free, 5 U/ml; Paines and Byrne Ltd, Greenford, UK) peripheral venous blood. One volume of whole blood is mixed with an equal volume of medium and layered over one volume of Ficoll Hypaque (density 1.077) or equivalent lymphocyte separation medium. Mononuclear cells are harvested from the plasma density-gradient interface after centrifugation at 1200 *g* for 20 minutes at room temperature, and washed twice (800 *g* for 15 minutes, then 400 *g* for 10 minutes). If large numbers of PBMC are present, 1% additive free heparin should also be added to the first wash. As

T cells represent 75% of PBMC, further purification is usually not required prior to growth.

Cryopreservation and thawing

For storage, cells are resuspended at the required concentration in complete medium. A chilled 15% solution of dimethylsulphoxide (DMSO) in FCS is added dropwise to an equal volume of cell suspension, mixing throughout at 4°C. One-millilitre aliquots of the final cell suspension are added to sterile cryovials and frozen slowly in a rate-controlled freezer or a polystyrene box, which is sealed and placed at –70°C overnight. Vials may then be transferred to liquid nitrogen storage (–180°C).

Frozen vials of cells are removed from –180°C storage and rapidly thawed over 1–2 minutes in a 37°C water-bath. The cell suspension is then added to a universal bottle and 1 ml of complete medium added dropwise, with continuous mixing. A further 20 ml of medium is then added to dilute the DMSO from the cells, which are spun at 300 *g* for 10 minutes. The pellet is resuspended to the required concentration in complete medium for tissue culture.

CD4+ T-cell growth *in vitro*

T-cell proliferative assays

Polyclonal responses

PBMC (5×10^4 – 1×10^5/well) are cultured with antigen over a dose range in 96-well round-bottom microtitre plates. Optimal conditions for culture are determined by incubating over a concentration range for various periods of time. Cultures are then pulsed with 1 µCi of tritiated methyl thymidine ([^{3}H]-TdR, 28 Ci/mmol specific activity) for 6–16 hours before harvesting on to glass-fibre filters. Proliferation is measured by liquid scintillation spectroscopy, using a β-counter, with results expressed as mean counts per minute (cpm) of replicate cultures (three to six replicates).

T-cell lines and clones

T cells from oligoclonal (lines) and monoclonal (clones) T-cell populations (1–2 × 10^4/well) are cultured with antigen in 96-well round-bottom microtitre plates in the presence of accessory (antigen-presenting) cells (2.5×10^4 irradiated PBMC/well or 1×10^4 irradiated EBV-transformed B cells/well). After incubation for 48 hours (soluble antigen) or 72 hours (particulate antigen), the cultures are pulsed and harvested as above. If mitomycin-C-treated murine L cells are used as accessory cells (2×10^4/well), 96-well flat-bottom microtitre plates are used with increased T-cell numbers (2×10^4/well). An overnight pulse of accessory cells with antigen prior to the addition of T cells may help to minimize background counts.

Accessory cells for antigen presentation

Because of the requirements for T-cell activation, the establishment and maintenance of long-term T-cell cultures require a source of antigen and histocompatible APC or feeders. Functional accessory activity does not require cell division, which would otherwise contaminate T-cell populations. Therefore, cells are treated by either irradiation (a γ-emitting source such as ^{60}Co or ^{137}Cs or from any X-ray source) or mitomycin-C treatment.

PBMC

Fresh or cryopreserved histocompatible PBMC (autologous or allogeneic; 0.5–1.0 × 10^6/ml) provide the best accessory cell activity. Optimally, fresh autologous irradiated PBMC (2500–3000 rad) should be used, but buffy coats provide a good PBMC supply for cryopreservation. T-cell depletion of PBMC is not necessary.

EBV-transformed B cells

Transformed B-cell lines (BCL) are useful feeders in short-term assays (McKean *et al.*, 1981; Ratcliffe *et al.*, 1984), but long-term cultures tend to be poorly supported when transformed cells provide the sole accessory cells. Relative radioresistance of transformed B cells necessitates higher radiation doses of 5000–6000 rad.

The cell line B95.8, which is derived from cotton-topped marmoset PBMC infected with EBV obtained from a cell line derived from a patient with infectious mononucleosis (Miller & Lipman, 1973), can be used to transform human B cells. The cells are grown to confluence and the culture supernatant is harvested and passed through a 0.45 µm filter. Infection of B cells is carried out by resuspending up to 10^7 PBMC, washed in serum-free complete medium, in 1 ml B95.8 culture supernatant for 1 hour at 37°C with gentle agitation. The cells are then pelleted, the supernatant is removed and the cells are cultured. Immortalized EBV-infected BCL may be obtained from infected cells seeded at 5×10^5 cells/ml in complete medium/10% FCS in 24-well plates. T-cell lysis is promoted by the addition of cyclosporin A (CsA) (Sandoz; 10 µg/ml) for the first 2–3 weeks of culture. Alternatively, phytohaemagglutinin (PHA) may be used to remove T-cell populations. Cultures are fed biweekly, with replacement of half the medium without disturbing the cell layer. Using an inverted microscope, foci of proliferating transformed B cells are usually identifiable after 1–2 weeks, although many lines may take as long as 6 weeks. As the transformed cells approach confluence (10^6 cells/ml) they should be diluted to 10^5 cells/ml.

Transfected murine fibroblasts (L cells)

As murine fibroblasts (L cells) have no endogenous MHC class II molecules, L cells expressing the products of transfected human MHC class II genes as accessory cells allow the MHC class II products to be studied in isolation. L cells are prepared in serum-free complete medium by treatment with mitomycin C (50 μg/ml for 45 minutes at 37°C), washed four times in complete medium plus serum and then used in assays (Germain & Malissen, 1986). Thorough washing is essential to avoid contamination and toxicity of T-cell cultures.

T-cell hybridization

Adaptations of technology for the propagation of B-cell hybridomas have fused normal T cells and AKR thymoma BW 5147 (e.g. Nabholz *et al.*, 1980; Kappler *et al.*, 1981) to establish monoclonal T cells. Results with human T-cell populations have been disappointing. Normal PBMC activated *in vitro* with antigen or mitogen have been fused to human T-lymphoblastoid cells by means of polyethylene glycol and stable lines cloned by limiting dilution (Okada *et al.*, 1981; Butler *et al.*, 1983). The T-cell lymphoma Jurkat line has been fused to antigen-specific IL-2-dependent T-cell lines to obtain functional antigen-specific human T-cell hybrids (De Freitas *et al.*, 1982). Attempts to develop IL-2-dependent antigen-specific cytotoxic T-cell hybridomas have been less successful. Complications associated with human hybridoma technology have been chromosomal loss with phenotypic and functional changes.

Viral transformation

Viral transformation of human T lymphocytes was achieved by cocultivation with neoplastic T-cell lines secreting the RNA retrovirus human T-cell leukaemia/lymphoma virus (HTLV-I), which is tropic for CD4 T cells (Popovic *et al.*, 1983, 1984). However, problems of dysregulation developed with induced changes in activation requirements, B-cell help and lymphokine production (Volkman *et al.*, 1985), minimizing the usefulness of this approach also for the study of normal T-cell physiology.

Sources of IL-2

Long-term T-cell cultures require a source of T-cell growth factor or IL-2 (Morgan *et al.*, 1976; Gillis & Smith, 1977).

Lectin-stimulated human T cells

PBMC cultured at 10^6/ml in complete medium with normal human serum and PHA 0.1 μg/ml (or concanavalin A 5 μg/ml) for 48 hours will elaborate lymphokines into the culture supernatants. The IL-2-containing supernatant may be harvested and stored at −20°C. Commercial preparations, such as Lymphocult-T Lectin Free (Biotest Folex, FRG) are highly effective. Optimal concentration for supplementation should be determined but is usually 5–10%.

Recombinant IL-2

Gene cloning in bacteria (Taniguchi *et al.*, 1983) has allowed the production of recombinant human IL-2 (rIL-2), which is now commercially available from several sources. Problems of lectin and mycoplasma contamination are avoided, but lack of glycosylation may decrease stability and low levels of bacterial products may be present.

Assay for IL-2

IL-2-dependent cell lines, such as Th2 (Watson, 1979) or cytotoxic T lymphocyte 1 (CTL1) (Gillis & Smith, 1977) may be used in a bioassay for IL-2 production. Test supernatants are serially diluted and cultured with cells (5×10^3/well) in 96-well round-bottom microtitre plates at a volume of 200 μl/well. Plates are pulsed with [3H]-TdR after 24 hours and harvested 6 hours later. IL-2 concentrations are read off a standard curve generated by using rIL-2 of known concentration.

Cloning techniques for human CD4+ T cells

Primary cultures

PBMC

The concentration of antigen required to produce optimal stimulation of the PBMC, assayed by the incorporation of [^{3}H]-TdR, should be previously determined, using standard proliferation-assay kinetics studies.

A bulk culture of PBMC is prepared by incubating 2–2.5 × 10^6 PBMC in complete medium/5% A+ serum with optimal antigen concentration in a volume of 2 ml in a 24-well tissue-culture plate.

Tissue sites (antigen unknown)

Skin-punch biopsy

Tissue fragment is cultured for 10–14 days in 2 ml complete medium/5% A+ serum in a 24-well plate in the presence of 10% IL-2 to expand *in vivo*-activated T cells. Teasing of the tissue with sterile needles helps to release entrapped T cells. After 4 days, if T-cell expansion is slow, activation with insolubilized anti-CD3 antibody (OKT3; 10 µg/ml) and 10% IL-2 may be used, stimulating through the T-cell receptor (TcR), with subsequent expansion in IL-2.

Synovial fluid

Mononuclear cells are isolated from heparinized aspirated synovial fluid, using the same method as for the preparation of PBMC. The *in vivo*-activated T cells are expanded in 2 ml complete medium/5% A+ serum in a 24-well megatitre plate in the presence of 10% IL-2 for 10–14 days. Anti-CD3 activation may also be used, if necessary.

Established T-cell lines

Primary culture under the optimal conditions of antigen concentration and duration of culture are established and then the T-blast cells are recovered by density centrifugation over Ficoll-Paque for 20 minutes at 1200 *g*. Blast-enriched cell suspensions at the interface are diluted to 1×10^5/ml of complete medium/5% A+ serum, supplemented with 5×10^5/ml autologous PBMC X-irradiated (2500 rad) as APC, optimal concentration of antigen and 5% IL-2. Cultures are aliquoted in 2 ml volumes in 24-well plates and incubated in humidified chambers at 37°C in 5% CO_2/air. If limited autologous or allogeneic PBMC are available for use as accessory cells, a combination of pooled irradiated allogeneic PBMC (10^6/ml; 2500–3000 rad), autologous or histocompatible, irradiated EBV-transformed BCL (10^5/ml; 6000 rad) and PHA-P (0.5 µg/ml) may be used. If the antigen is known, optimal concentration of antigen should also be added. Supplementary IL-2 (10% Lymphocult-T) should be added after 4 days, with further splitting as required. Seed vials should be frozen when T cells are resting, at least 10–14 days after the last addition of PHA.

Limiting-dilution isolation of T-cell clones

Autologous or allogeneic accessory cells

Cloning from a long-term T-cell line

Antigen-specific T-cell clones may be derived from antigen-specific T-cell lines. The T blasts are recovered by density centrifugation, washed and then resuspended in complete medium/5% A+ serum. They are then plated by limiting dilution in microtest-II trays with 0.3 blasts/well, 10^4 accessory cells and optimal antigen concentration in the presence of 10% v/v IL-2, with a total volume of 20 µl/well. Cultures are incubated for 6 days, after which the growing clones are identified, using an inverted microscope, and transferred to fresh medium (200 µl) containing 10% IL-2, accessory cells (10^5/well) and antigen in 96-well flat-bottom plates. After 7 additional days of culture, the clones are transferred to 24-well plates containing the same concentration of IL-2, accessory cells and antigen in a total volume of 2 ml.

Cloning from a primary culture

After primary culture under optimal conditions, cells are harvested by density centrifugation. Blast-enriched suspensions are diluted to 30 blasts/ml of complete medium/5% A+ serum containing 10% IL-2, 5×10^5 accessory cells/ml and antigen and added to microtest-II trays in 20 µl aliquots as above.

Autologous or histocompatible allogeneic EBV-transformed B cells combined with non-histocompatible allogeneic PBMC

When autologous or histocompatible accessory cells are unavailable, an alternative feeding suspension may be used. This should contain autologous or histocompatible EBV-transformed B cells (6000 rad; 10^5/ml), a pool of two or more non-histocompatible allogeneic PBMC (2500 rad; 10^6/ml), optimal antigen concentration and 0.5 µg/ml PHA. A feeding mixture of non-histocompatible cells in the presence of PHA induces a vigorous mixed-lymphocyte reaction with release of a cocktail of cytokines to drive T-cell growth (Spits *et al.*, 1982; Van Schooten *et al.*, 1988). Supplementation with fresh medium and 10% IL-2 is given after 4–5 days. This method is also suitable for cloning from tissue sites where the antigen is unknown, for example synovial compartment T cells. Limiting-dilution cloning using this accessory cell mixture may be carried out in microtest-II trays (20 µl/well) or 96-well round- or flat-bottom plates (200 µl/well). Clones generated in this way should not be used for assays until at least 10–14 days after the last stimulation with PHA, by which time cells should be in resting phase. Background proliferation counts should be less than 1000 cpm at this stage.

CD8+ cytotoxic T-cell lines and clones

The media, reagents and cytokines required for the culture of CD8+ T cells are the same as the ones detailed above for the culture of CD4+ T cells.

CD8+ T cells are class I MHC-restricted and have the

ability to strongly lyse target cells sharing class I MHC complexed with fragments of foreign proteins. They differ in function, cytokine production and induction requirements from CD4+ T cells. While CD4+ T cells can be primed and activated by purified proteins, infectious agents and appropriate peptide epitopes, CD8+ T cells are poorly activated by purified proteins, but respond to APC infected with live pathogens or live vectors encoding antigen genes (Bennink & Yewdell, 1990) or APC pulsed with peptide epitopes they can recognize (Deres *et al.*, 1989). Hence the most efficient antigen presentation to cytotoxic T cells (CTL) is by APC endogenously producing the antigen. Dendritic cells are particularly effective for primary antiviral CTL responses *in vitro* (e.g. Macatonia *et al.*, 1989, 1991). In addition, IL-7 has been found to enhance primary CTL responses *in vitro* (Kos & Mullbacher, 1992). Recently, synthetic peptides of tumour antigens have also been used successfully to induce anti-tumour CTL (Houbiers *et al.*, 1993; Celis *et al.*, 1994). Some purified proteins, for example influenza nucleoprotein (Wraith & Askonas, 1985) or APC with a high cytoplasmic concentration of foreign protein (Yewdell *et al.*, 1988; Carbone & Bevan, 1990), have the ability to induce low levels of CTL or stimulate secondary responses *in vitro*. Hence antigen presentation to CTL requires the recognition on the cell surface of MHC molecules complexed with short peptides derived from the antigens.

Since the findings of Townsend *et al.* in 1986 that recognition by class-I-restricted CTL of virus-infected cells can be defined by protein fragments, i.e. short peptides derived from the viral components, naturally processed peptides seen in conjunction with MHC class I have been shown to be 8–10 amino-acid residues in length (Falk *et al.*, 1991) and to vary with different MHC restriction molecules (see reviews by Rammensee *et al.*, 1993; Germain, 1994). Provided the sequence of a given antigen is known, then pools of five or six synthetic peptides can be used to define the appropriate CTL epitopes recognized in conjunction with a particular class I MHC. Recently, CTL to tumour-associated antigens were induced by stripping peptides from autologous cells and reloading the stripped cells with tumour-derived peptides (Langlande-Demoyen *et al.*, 1994). The first human virus-specific and MHC class I-restricted CTL were reported by McMichael and Askonas (1978), using secondary responses to influenza. The influenza system has been studied widely and will be used largely to illustrate techniques. It must be noted, however, that every virus or other infective agent behaves differently in tissue and cell tropism, as well as in the mode of infection and replication mechanisms; therefore the techniques to select CTL will vary and need to be adapted to each type of infection.

The generation of CTL and their culture

In general, methods for the selection of human PBMC follow the principles described below. CTL in peripheral blood from donors during or after an infection generally are not cytotoxic *per se* but have to be stimulated with antigen *in vitro* for several days to generate cytotoxic activity. An exception to this comes in some acute infections, particularly in acquired immune deficiency syndrome (AIDS), where fresh peripheral-blood lymphocytes (PBL) show strong human immunodeficiency virus (HIV)-specific and class I MHC-restricted cytolytic activity (e.g. Walker *et al.*, 1987). Presumably this can be attributed to continuous stimulation of CD8+ T cells in the circulation by infected monocytes and dendritic cells.

Human PBMC are separated from red blood cells (RBC) on Ficoll-Paque, as described above; responder white blood cells at 1.5×10^6/ml are incubated for 6–7 days in RPMI-1640 medium with antigen in an upright 50 ml plastic tissue-culture bottle (8–10 ml total volume). FCS (specifically chosen for this type of culture) is included at 10% v/v (in many instances 5% autologous serum is preferable). For stimulation with influenza virus, the cells can be incubated with 5–10 haemagglutinin units (HAU)/ml of virus; this needs to be done in the absence of serum, which prevents infectivity, and serum will then be added after 1–2 hours' incubation at 37°C. With many infective agents with high virulence or a tropism for the T cells themselves, it is necessary to stimulate with autologous APC that are pretreated with an infectious agent or pulsed with peptides before addition to the responder T cells. Stimulator cells are generally autologous PBMC or irradiated EBV-transformed BCL at 1/5 or 1/20 the number of responder T cells (Gotch *et al.*, 1987).

With human PBMC (even if the donor had been exposed to the infection), the first *in vitro* antigen stimulation often results in very low antigen-specific cytotoxicity. However, CTL lines with strong reactivity can be selected by restimulating several times with APC (irradiated and virus-infected or peptide-pulsed and then washed, as detailed above). Cultures should be fed by replacement of half the medium every 3–4 days and restimulated with antigen every 8–12 days. Three to four days after the second and any subsequent antigen stimulation, a source of IL-2 should be added (5–10 U/ml of rIL-2 or Lymphocult-T at 5–10% v/v).

Cloning techiques for CD8+ CTL

In mouse systems extensive work has been published with cloned CD8+ CTL to study the repertoire of CTL for components of viruses, bacteria or parasites, to identify the dominant peptide epitopes and to define the role of CTL effector function in infections *in vivo*. *In vivo* functional studies (i.e. the transfer of specific cytolytic T-cell clones into infected hosts to examine the course of infection and possible immunopathology) are, of course, restricted to animal models. Detailed methods have been described in many publications, relating to, for example, influenza (Lin & Askonas, 1981; Luckacher *et al.*, 1984), respiratory syncytial virus (Cannon *et al.*, 1988) and malaria (Romero *et al.*, 1989). Human CD8+ virus-specific or alloreactive T-cell clones have also been selected and numerous specificity studies have identified the dominant peptide epitopes of various pathogens and self epitopes that can be seen by CTL in donors differing in MHC class I haplotype (see, for example, the review by Rammensee *et al.*, 1993). In general, the methods used for cloning of human CTL are similar to those developed for murine cells. In early attempts to clone human CTL, overgrowth by CD4+ cells was often observed. If this becomes a problem, it is preferable to positively select for CD8+ T cells with Dynabeads or to remove CD4+ cells with beads or with antibody and complement. Cloning can be done by limiting dilution, using restimulated cultures (e.g. Gotch *et al.*, 1990); if the peptide epitope has been defined, the best selection for the desired clones is to restimulate with peptide-pulsed autologous irradiated APC or BCL, although infected stimulator cells can be used. Activated T cells are then distributed in varying numbers (e.g. 50, 10, 3 and 1/well) into 96-well plastic microtitre plates in the presence of 10^4–10^5 antigen-pulsed APC and rIL-2 or Lymphocult-T in a total volume of about 150 μl. Every few days, the wells are fed with RPMI 1640/10% FCS medium containing a source of IL-2. Once the cells grow, they are transferred to 24-well tissue-culture plates and restimulated with antigen-pulsed APC (responder/stimulator cell ratio of 1 : 1) and fed with IL-2, as detailed for the CTL lines.

Target cells for cytotoxicity assay

Target cells for CTL need to be labelled with $Na^{51}CrO_4$ and loaded with antigen, either by infection with the agent under test or by pulsing with peptides to be tested or the appropriate peptide if the epitope has been defined (Fig. 43.2). Tumour cells sharing class I MHC human leucocyte antigen (HLA) molecules with the T cells, either by expressing these molecules constitutively or following transfection, are suitable. For the assays with human cells,

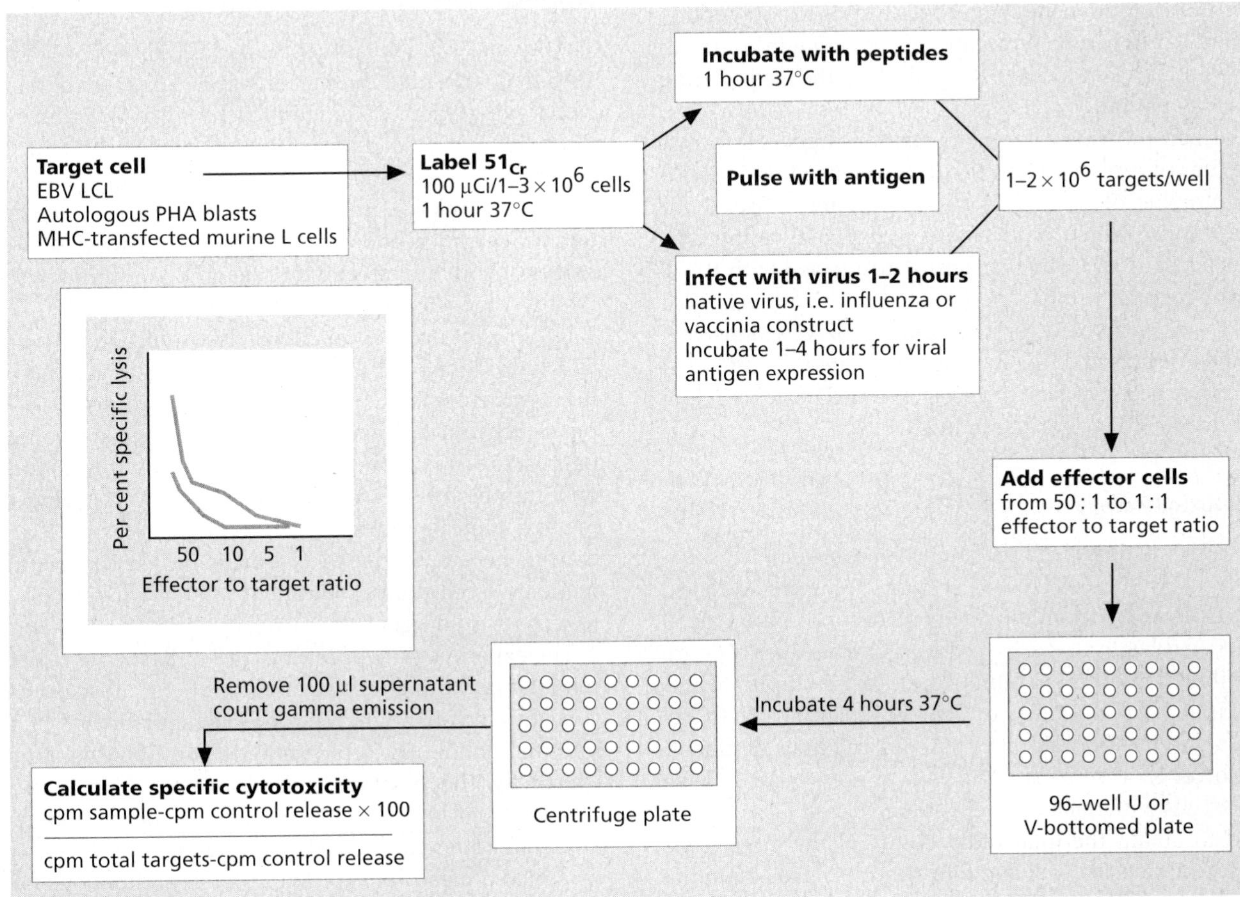

Fig. 43.2 A overview of the chromium-release cytotoxic assay procedure.

autologous EBV-transformed BCL are most widely utilized, but mouse cell lines transfected with shared HLA class I MHC molecules are also suitable (e.g. Gotch *et al.*, 1987; Bodmer *et al.*, 1989). If neither of these are available, PHA-activated autologous PBMC can serve as target cells, although they are less efficiently lysed by CTL. The target cells are washed, labelled with ^{51}Cr (100 μc/1–3 × 10^6 cells) for 1 hour at 37°C in 0.1–0.2 ml of serum-free medium, washed and then infected with about 1000 HAU influenza virus (in a very small volume of serum-free medium (0.1–0.2 ml) for 1–2 hours at 37°C. With some viruses, the radiolabelling and infection can be done at the same time. The cells are then washed three times in full medium (RPMI 1640/10% FCS), incubated for 4 hours at 37°C (for adequate expression of viral proteins), washed three times in RPMI 1640, resuspended in 1 ml RPMI 1640/10% FCS and viable cells counted for the assay.

Alternatively, target cells can be pulsed with peptide after the ^{51}Cr labelling by incubating for 1 hour at 37°C in RPMI/10% FCS with an excess of peptide (generally about 10^{-6} mmol/l, depending on the affinity or sensitivity of the peptide), washed three times and diluted to 2 × 10^5 cells/ml to be dispensed for the assay (see below). Another way to titre the peptide concentration required for CTL recognition and target cells lysis is to add peptide to the assay at various concentrations ranging from 10^{-5} to 10^{-12} mmol/l and to leave the peptide in the wells during the assay period.

Purified proteins cannot be used for target-cell formation, but recombinant vaccinia viruses encoding individual proteins of pathogens have been most useful for determining which proteins are recognized by the CTL (Gotch *et al.*, 1987). The target cells are infected with 10–20 plaque-forming units (pfu) of recombinant vaccinia virus/cell, incubated for 1–2 hours at 37°C, extensively washed in full medium and then incubated at 37°C for 4 hours for the expression of virally encoded proteins before CTL-mediated lysis is determined.

Cytotoxicity assay

The CTL and target-cell preparations are suspended separately in RPMI 1640/10% FCS. Target cells are added to 96-well round-bottom microwell plates in a volume of 50 or 100 μl (usually 1–2 × 10^4 cells/well). The killer cells are distributed in different numbers, at least in duplicate and in triplicate if possible, to achieve killer/target (K/T) ratios varying from 50 : 1 to 1 : 1. For cell lines or clones, the lower K/T ratios are sufficient. It is essential to have 8–10 wells with the target cells alone; four of these will be used to obtain the total radioactivity of the target cells seeded out in each well and four to six wells to obtain the spontaneous Cr release into the supernatant during the incubation (control release). The final volume in every well has to be the same (i.e. 200 μl) during the incubation, except for the wells destined to give us the total radioactivity of the target cells, which remain at 100 μl; at the end of the incubation time, these will be treated with 100 μl of 5% Triton X 100. The plates are centrifuged lightly (30 minutes at 500 rpm) and incubated at 37°C for 3–5 hours, depending on the particular system under test and the level of cytotoxicity. After incubation, the plates are centrifuged (5 minutes at 1000 rpm) and 100 μl of the supernatant is withdrawn into small tubes to count the released radioactivity in a γ-counter. The % specific target lysis is calculated as follows:

$$\frac{\text{cpm experimental sample} - \text{cpm control release}}{\text{cpm of total target cells} - \text{cpm control release}} \times 100$$

For smaller assays, 20 μl of supernatant can be removed on to filter-papers, which are dried and counted in scintillation fluid on a flat-bed γ/β counter (Potter *et al.*, 1987).

Not all cell types are equally susceptible to CTL-mediated lysis and normal cells generally show a much lower lysis plateau than that of established tumour cell lines. CTL cannot lyse resting small lymphocytes.

Applications of T-cell cloning

The advances in cell-culture technology between 1975 and 1985 that facilitated the isolation and expansion of monoclonal populations of antigen-reactive T cells (Fathman & Fitch, 1982) provided a wealth of reagents with which to investigate many aspects of T-cell biology that had previously been masked in polyclonal responses. The subsequent generation and analysis of a wide variety of T-cell clones of both human and murine origin have established the heterogeneity of function and specificity at the single T-cell level. As a result of T-cell clones and, in particular, T–T hybridomas for murine T cells, questions regarding the structure of T-cell antigen receptors, the physicochemical basis of T-cell antigen recognition and pathways of signalling were addressed, and these studies on a number of different antigen systems are well documented in the literature. It is not possible to review that literature here but only to comment on the contribution made by T-cell cloning to our current knowledge of T cell responses to allergens.

The experimental approaches of T-cell cloning in determining the cellular parameters of allergic disease have concentrated on the analysis of T-cell regulation of specific immunoglobulin E (IgE) synthesis and defining antigen specificity, the practical application of which is in the development of new approaches to immunotherapy. Understanding the growth requirements of T cells has provided a means of expanding T-cell populations taken from specific sites of allergic disease, including bronchial biopsy specimens, bronchoalveolar fluid, punch biopsies of skin affected by atopic dermatitis and conjunctival biopsies. In general, the cell populations obtained by this approach have had similar characteristics to the peripheral-blood T cells. This observation supports the information on the qualitative nature of T-cell responses in allergic disease, which has been based on the analysis of the peripheral-blood T-cell repertoire and are discussed below.

The combination of T-cell clones, murine fibroblasts expressing particular MHC class II molecules and synthetic peptides has facilitated the construction of T-cell epitope maps and detailed analysis of the antigen and restriction specificity of T-cell recognition for different allergens (O'Hehir *et al.*, 1991). Furthermore, synthetic peptides with single amino-acid substitutions used in functional and direct binding assays have been useful for identifying the MHC class II and TcR residues that are critical for the binding of peptides in different haplotypes and for different peptide epitopes. Recent studies with murine T-cell clones have demonstrated that peptide analogues with substitutions that affect contact with either TcR or MHC class II molecules can dissociate T-cell effector function, an observation that is particularly relevant to altering the qualitative nature of immune responses to allergens.

Monoclonal populations of human T cells were also first used to demonstrate the ability of allergen-specific CD4+ T cells isolated from an atopic subject with clinically defined allergy to support allergen-specific IgE synthesis *in vitro* from autologous B cells and to show that this was IL-4-dependent (O'Hehir *et al.*, 1989). Such T cells, with the capacity to support allergic responses, have been used to study different approaches to the down-regulation of T-cell function, using allergen-derived peptides, superantigens and antibodies reactive with accessory molecules. It was documented from these studies that allergen-derived peptides may induce T-cell anergy, characterized by a reduction in cell-surface expression of TcR and CD28 molecules and the up-regulation of CD25. The loss of T-cell proliferation and B-cell help by the anergic T cells is accompanied by selective regulation of cytokines. Hyperactivation, reflected by the enhancement of cytokine-specific mRNA, occurs during the induction phase of anergy but restimulation results in the down-regulation of IL-4 and IL-5, while interferon-γ (IFN-γ) production is maintained. The functional consequence of this modulation in cytokine release is a shift from the Th2 to Th1 pathway. While the effects of peptide-mediated desensitization of lymphokine production by human T cells can be analysed *in vitro*, there is a need to understand how peptides are handled *in vivo*, and their ability to down-regulate Th2 responses must be determined (Briner *et al.*, 1993; Hoyne *et al.*, 1993).

With respect to CTL, there has been minimal success in the isolation and characterization of allergen-specific CD8+ T-cell populations *in vitro* and their role in allergic immune responses is less clear. This may be due to the chronic allergen exposure encountered in allergic diseases, whereas CD8+ T cells are usually sensitized by infection. The contribution of CD8+ T cells in the pathogenesis or inhibition of allergic inflammatory responses remains to be looked at more systematically.

Without doubt, the ability to select and expand clonal populations of T cells has revolutionized our understanding of T-cell physiology. As technology advances and the diversity of the T-cell populations that are isolated and investigated at the clonal level increases, differences in T-cell structure and the signals regulating the growth and functions of T cells and their role in the homeostasis of the host will be resolved. This accumulated knowledge will aid the development of new therapeutic strategies for the manipulation of T cells in the prevention and control of disease.

Acknowledgement

This chapter is in part an updated version of a previously published review on T-cell cloning (O'Hehir *et al.*, 1993).

References

Bach, F.H., Inouye, H., Hank, J.A. & Alter, B.J. (1979) Human T-lymphocyte clones reactive in primed lymphocyte typing in cytotoxicity. *Nature*, **281**, 307–10.

Bennink, J.R. & Yewdell, J.W. (1990) Recombinant vaccinia viruses as vectors for studying T-lymphocyte specificity and function. *Curr. Topics Microbiol. Immunol.*, **163**, 154–84.

Bodmer, H., Gotch, F. & McMichael, A.J. (1989) Class I cross restricted T cells reveal low responder alleles due to processing of viral antigen. *Nature*, **337**, 653–5.

Briner, T.J., Kuo, M.-C., Keating, K.M., Rogers, B.L. & Greenstein, J.L. (1993) Peripheral T cell tolerance induced in naive and primed mice by subcutaneous injection of peptides from the major cat allergen *Fel d* I. *Proc. Nat. Acad. Sci. USA*, **90**, 7608–12.

Butler, J.L., Muraguchi, A., Lane, H.C. & Fauci, A.S. (1983) Development of a human T–T cell hybridoma secreting B-cell growth factor. *J. Exp. Med.*, **157**, 60–7.

Cannon, M.J., Openshaw, P.J.M. & Askonas, B.A. (1988) Cytotoxic T cells clear virus but augment lung pathology in mice infected with respiratory syncytial virus. *J. Exp. Med.*, **168**, 1163–8.

Carbone, F.R. & Bevan, M.J. (1990) Class I restricted processing and presentation of exogenous cell-associated antigen *in vivo*. *J. Exp. Med.*, **171**, 377–8.

Celis, E., Tsai, V., Crimi, C. *et al.* (1994) Induction of anti-tumour cytotoxic T lymphocytes in normal humans using primary cultures and synthetic peptide epitopes. *Proc. Nat. Acad. Sci. USA*, **91**, 2105–9.

De Freitas, E.C., Vella, S., Linnenbach, A., Zimijewski, C., Koprowski, H. & Croce, C.M. (1982) Antigen-specific human T-cell hybrids with helper activity. *Proc. Nat. Acad. Sci. USA*, **79**, 6646–50.

Deres, K., Schild, H., Wiesmuller, K.H., Jung, G. & Ramensee, H.G. (1989) *In vivo* priming of virus specific cytotoxic T lymphocytes with synthetic lipopeptide vaccine. *Nature*, **342**, 561–4.

Falk, K., Rotzschke, O., Stevanovic, S., Jung, G. & Rammensee, H.-G. (1991) Allele specific motifs revealed by sequencing of self-peptides eluted from MHC molecules. *Nature*, **351**, 290–6.

Fathman, C.G. & Fitch, F.W. (1982) *Isolation, Characterisation and Utilisation of T Lymphocyte Clones*. Academic Press, New York.

Fathman, C.G. & Hengartner, H. (1978) Clones of alloreactive T-cells. *Nature*, **272**, 617–18.

Finn, O.J., Boniver, J. & Kaplan, H.S. (1979) Induction, establishment *in vitro* and characterisation of functional, antigen-specific, carrier primed murine T-cell lymphomas. *Proc. Nat. Acad. Sci. USA*, **76**, 4033–7.

Germain, R.N. (1994) MHC-dependent antigen processing and peptide presentation: providing ligands for T lymphocyte activation. *Cell*, **76**, 287–99.

Germain, R.N. & Malissen, B. (1986) Analysis of the expression and function of class II major histocompatibility complex-encoded molecules by DNA-mediated gene transfer. *Ann. Rev. Immunol.*, **4**, 281–316.

Gillis, S. & Smith, K.A. (1977) Long term culture of tumour specific cytotoxic T-cells. *Nature*, **268**, 154–6.

Gotch, F.M., McMichael, A.J., Smith, G.L. & Moss, B. (1987) Identification of the virus molecules recognised by influenza specific human cytotoxic T lymphocytes. *J. Exp. Med.*, **165**, 408–14.

Gotch, F.M., Nixon, D.F., Alp, N., McMichael, A.J. & Borysiewicz, L.K. (1990) High frequency of memory and effector gag specific cytotoxic T cells in HIV seropositive individuals. *Int. Immunol.*, **2**, 707–12.

Houbiers, J.G.A., Nijman, H.W., van der Burgh, S.H. *et al.* (1993) *In vitro* induction of human cytotoxic T lymphocyte responses against peptides of mutant and wild-type p53. *Eur. J. Immunol.*, **23**, 2072–7.

Hoyne, G.J., O'Hehir, R.E., Wraith, D.C., Thomas, W.R. & Lamb, J.R. (1993) Inhibition of T-cell and antibody responses to house dust mite allergen by inhalation of the dominant T-cell epitope in naive and sensitised mice. *J. Exp. Med.*, **178**, 1783–8.

Kappler, J.W., Skidmore, B., White, J. & Marrac, P. (1981) Antigen-inducible, H-2 restricted, interleukin-2 producing T-cell hybridomas: lack of independent antigen and H-2 recognition. *J. Exp. Med.*, **153**, 1198–214.

Kos, F.J. & Mullbacher, A. (1992) Induction of primary anti-viral cytotoxic T cells by *in vitro* stimulation with short synthetic peptide and interleukin-7. *Eur. J. Immunol.*, **22**, 3183–8.

Lamb, J.R., Eckels, D.D., Lake, P., Johnson, A.H., Hartzman, R.J. & Woody, J.N. (1982) Antigen specific human T-lymphocyte clones; induction, antigen specificity and MHC restriction of influenza virus immune clones. *J. Immunol.*, **128**, 233–8.

Langlade-Demoyen, P., Levraud, J.-P., Kourilsky, P. & Abastsdo, J.-P. (1994) Primary T lymphocyte induction using peptide stripped autologous cells. *Int. Immunol.*, **6**, 1759–66.

Lin, Y.L. & Askonas, B.A. (1981) Biological properties of an influenza A virus-specific killer T-cell clone: inhibition of virus replication *in vivo* and induction of delayed type hypersensitivity reactions. *J. Exp. Med.*, **154**, 225–34.

Lukacher, E., Braciale, V.L. & Braciale, T.J. (1984) *In vivo* effector function of influenza virus specific cytotoxic T lymphocyte clones is highly specific. *J. Exp. Med.*, **160**, 1560–5.

Macatonia, S.E., Taylor, P.M., Knight, S.C. & Askonas, B.A. (1989) Primary stimulation by dendritic cells induces anti-viral proliferative and cytotoxic T cell responses *in vitro*. *J. Exp. Med.*, **169**, 1255–64.

Macatonia, S.E., Patterson, S. & Knight, S.C. (1991) Primary proliferative and cytotoxic T cell responses to HIV induced *in vitro* by human dendritic cells. *Immunology*, **74**, 399–406.

McKean, D., Infante, A., Nilson, A. *et al.* (1981) Major histocompatibility complex-restricted antigen presentation to antigen-reactive T-cells by B-lymphocyte tumour cells. *J. Exp. Med.*, **154**, 1419–31.

McMichael, A.J. & Askonas, B.A. (1978) Influenza virus specific cytotoxic T cells in man: induction and properties of the cytotoxic T cells. *Eur. J. Immunol.*, **8**, 705–11.

Miller, G. & Lipman, M. (1973) Release of infectious Epstein–Barr virus by transformed marmoset leukocytes. *Proc. Nat. Acad. Sci. USA*, **69**, 383–7.

Morgan, D.A., Ruscetti, F.W. & Gallo, R.C. (1976) Selective *in vitro* growth of T-lymphocytes from normal human bone marrow. *Science*, **193**, 1007–8.

Nabholtz, M., Engers, H.D., Collaro, D. & North, M. (1978) Cloned T-cell lines with specific cytolytic activity. *Curr. Topics Microbiol. Immunol.*, **81**, 176–87.

Nabholz, M., Cianfriglia, M., Acuto, O. *et al.* (1980) Cytolytically active murine T-cell hybrids. *Nature*, **287**, 437–40.

O'Hehir, R.E., Bal, V., Quint, D.J. *et al.* (1989) An *in vitro* model of allergen-dependent IgE synthesis by human B lymphocytes: comparison of the responses of an atopic and a nonatopic individual to *Dermatophagoides* spp. (house dust mite). *Immunology*, **66**, 499–504.

O'Hehir, R.E., Garman, R., Greenstein, J. & Lamb, J.R. (1991) The specificity and regulation of T-cell responsiveness to allergens. *Ann. Rev. Immunol.*, **9**, 67–95.

O'Hehir, R.E., Askonas, B.A. & Lamb, J.R. (1993) Lymphocyte clones. In: *Methods of Immunological Analysis* (ed R.F. Masseyeff, W.H. Albert & N.A. Staines), pp. 120–38. VCH Verlagsgesellschaft mbH, Weinheim, Germany.

Okada, M., Yoshimura, N., Kaieda, T., Yamamura, Y. & Kishimoto, T. (1981) Establishment and characterisation of human T-hybrid cells secreting immunoregulatory molecules. *Proc. Nat. Acad. Sci. USA*, **78**, 7717–21.

Popovic, M., Lange-Wantzin, G., Sarin, P.S., Mann, D. & Gallo, R.C. (1983) Transformation of human umbilical cord blood T-cells by human T-cell leukaemia/lymphoma virus. *Proc. Nat. Acad. Sci. USA*, **80**, 5402–6.

Popovic, M., Flomenberg, N., Volkman, D.J. *et al.* (1984) Alteration of T-cell functions by infection with HTLV-I or HTLV-II. *Science*, **226**, 459–62.

Potter, C.G., Gotch, F., Warner, G.T. & Oestrup, Y. (1987) Lymphocyte proliferation and cytotoxic assays using flat bed scintillation counting. *J. Immunol. Meth.*, **105**, 171–7.

Rammensee, H.-G., Falk, K. & Rotzsche, O. (1993) Peptides naturally presented by MHC class I molecules. *Ann. Rev. Immunol.*, **11**, 213–44.

Ratcliffe, M.J.H., Julius, M.H. & Kim, K.-J. (1984) Heterogeneity in the response of T-cells to antigens presented by B-lymphoma cells. *Cell. Immunol.*, **88**, 49–60.

Romero, P., Maryanski, J.L., Corradin, G., Nussenzweig, R.S., Nussenweig, V. & Zavala, F. (1989) Cloned cytotoxic T cells recognise an epitpoe in the circumsporozoite protein and protect against malaria. *Nature*, **341**, 323–6.

Schreier, M.H. & Tees, T. (1980) Clonal induction of helper T-cells: conversion of specific signals to non-specific signals. *Int. Arch. Allergy Appl. Immunol.*, **61**, 227–37

Schwartz, R.H. (1985) T-lymphocyte recognition of antigen in association with gene products of the major histocompatibility complex. *Ann. Rev. Immunol.*, **3**, 237–61.

Spits, H., Borst, J., Terhorst, C. & de Vries, J.E. (1982) The role of T-cell differentiation markers in antigen specific and lectin dependent cellular cytotoxicity mediated by T8+ and T4+ human cytotoxic T-cell clones directed at class I and class II MHC antigens. *J. Immunol.*, **129**, 1563–9.

Sredni, B., Yolkman, D., Schwartz, R.H. & Fauci, A.S. (1981) Antigen specific human T-cell clones: development of clones requiring HLA-DR compatible presenting cells for stimulation in the presence of antigen. *Proc. Nat. Acad. Sci. USA*, **78**, 1858–62.

Taniguchi, T., Matsui, H., Fujita, T. *et al.* (1983) Structure and expression of a cloned cDNA for human interleukin-2. *Nature*, **302**, 305–10.

Townsend, A. & Bodmer, H. (1989) Antigen recognition by class I restricted T-lymphocytes. *Ann. Rev. Immunol.*, **7**, 601–24.

Townsend, A.R.M., Rothbard, J., Gotch, F.M., Bahadur, G., Wraith, D. & McMichael, A.J. (1986) The epitopes of influenza nucleoprotein recognised by cytotoxic T lymphocytes can be defined with short synthetic peptides. *Cell*, **44**, 959–68.

Van Schooten, W.C.A., Ottenhof, T.H.M., Klatser, P.R., Thole, J., De Vries, R.R.P. & Kolk, A.H.J. (1988) T cell epitopes on the 36K and 65K *Mycobacterium leprae* antigens defined by human T cell clones. *Eur. J. Immunol.*, **18**, 849–54.

Volkman, D.J., Popovic, M., Gallo, R.C. & Fauci, A.S. (1985) Human T-cell leukaemia/lymphoma virus-infected antigen specific T-cell clones: indiscriminant helper function and lymphokine production. *J. Immunol.*, **134**, 4237–43.

Von Boehmer, H., Hengartner, H., Nabholtz, M., Lernhardt, W., Schreier, M.H. & Haas, W. (1979) Fine specificity of a continuously growing killer-cell clone specific for HY antigen. *Eur. J. Immunol.*, **9**, 592–7.

Walker, B.D., Chakraharti, S., Moss, B. *et al.* (1987) HIV-specific cytotoxic T lymphocytes in seropositive individuals. *Nature*, **328**, 345–8.

Watson, J. (1979) Continuous proliferation of murine antigen-specific helper T-lymphocytes in culture. *J. Exp. Med.*, **150**, 1510–19.

Wraith, D.C. & Askonas, B. (1985) Induction of influenza A virus cross-reactive cytotoxic T cells by a nucleoprotein/haemagglutinin preparation. *J. Gen. Virol.*, **66**, 1327–31.

Yewdell, J.W., Bennink, J.R. & Hosaka, Y. (1988) Cells process exogenous proteins for recognition by cototoxic T lymphocytes. *Science*, **239**, 637–40.

CHAPTER 44

In Situ Hybridization

Q. Hamid

Introduction

In situ hybridization (ISH) is the cellular localization of specific nucleic acid sequences (DNA or RNA), using a labelled complementary strand. DNA and RNA are found in both the nucleus and the cytoplasm, and the technical approach to the demonstration of these molecules in each anatomical situation is different.

ISH was first introduced in 1969 (Pardue & Gall, 1969) and was used primarily for the localization of DNA sequences. In more recent years, ISH has been applied to localize mRNA (Hamid *et al.*, 1987, 1990, 1991a; Hofler *et al.*, 1987). mRNA is the intermediate molecule in the transfer of genetic information from genomic DNA to functional polypeptide. The regulation of gene expression through transcriptional activation and inactivation within a cell, and hence its functional state, is reflected by the cellular content and distribution of the specific message. The demonstration of mRNA within a cell provides valuable information about gene expression and indicates possible synthesis of the corresponding protein. It can also be used for temporal studies in relation to physiological, pathological and developmental processes. In this chapter, we shall consider the principles, technique and application of mRNA ISH.

Principles of mRNA hybridization

The general principle of mRNA ISH is based on the fact that labelled single-stranded RNA or DNA containing complementary sequences (probes) are hybridized intracellularly to mRNA under appropriate conditions, thereby forming stable hybrids. These will be detected according to the type of labelling of the probe (Fig. 44.1).

Probe construction

Different types of probes are available to detect mRNA, including double- (Singer *et al.*, 1986) and single-stranded DNA probes (Herrington & McGee, 1990), oligonucleotides (Denny *et al.*, 1989) and single-stranded RNA probes (Cox *et al.*, 1984). Double-stranded DNA probes are used primarily for DNA detection (Brigati *et al.*, 1983) but have also been used in ISH for targeting RNA (Morimoto *et al.*, 1987). They most commonly consist of a bacterial plasmid into which the probe sequence has been inserted. These probes are usually labelled by nick translation or by random primer-directed synthesis (RPDS). Single-stranded DNA can be obtained from sequences cloned into the filamentous bacteriophage M13 or phagemids activated by phage superinfection. However, there is difficulty in cloning one of the two complementary strands. Strand-specific labelling is performed by random or unique primer labelling (Lawrence *et al.*, 1988). The unlabelled template remains in equimolar concentrations and probe denaturation is necessary. These probes have been used, but not widely, for RNA detection.

Oligonucleotides have been used more widely in mRNA ISH, particularly when the mRNA species is present in abundance (Thein & Wallace, 1986; Bramwell & Burns, 1988; Ochman *et al.*, 1990) — for example, immunoglobulin light-chain mRNA in plasma cells (Pringle *et al.*, 1990). These probes are short and usually labelled by addition of labelled nucleotides to either or both ends by chemical or enzymatic means. They are therefore less sen-

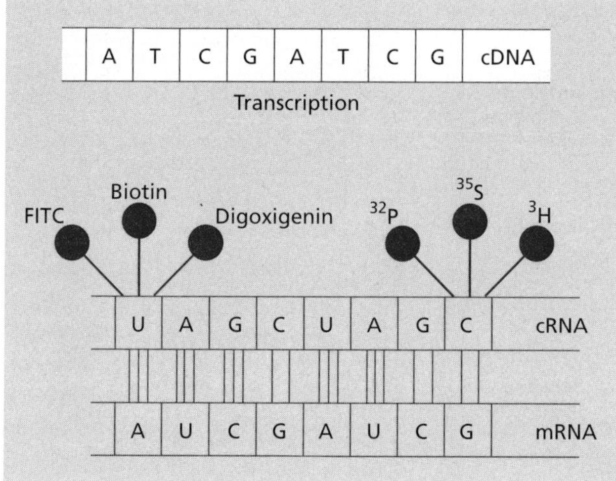

Fig. 44.1 Diagrammatic representation of the principle of mRNA hybridization using a cRNA probe.

sitive than other probes; however, an advantage of using these probes is that they can be rapidly tailor-made by automated chemical synthesis for any sequenced nucleic acid or from sequences deduced from amino-acid sequences (Herrington *et al.*, 1990a). Single-stranded RNA probes have been used extensively in recent years for the detection of mRNA by both isotopic and non-isotopic ISH (Hofler *et al.*, 1986; Broidie & Firestein, 1991; Hamid *et al.*, 1991b; Marc De Block & Debrouwer, 1993). The use of RNA probes has a number of advantages over other types of probes. These include the ability to synthesize probes of relatively constant size and with no vector sequences, the high thermal stability and affinity of RNA–RNA hybrids and the availability of ribonuclease (RNase) to remove the unhybridized probe at the washing stage of the hybridization. All these favour high specificity and sensitivity for RNA probes (Herrington *et al.*, 1990b; Hamid, 1993).

The construction of a labelled RNA probe is illustrated in Figs 44.2 and 44.3.

Subcloning of template DNA into RNA expression vectors

Generation of single-stranded, 'antisense' or complementary RNA (cRNA) probes requires the use of special transcription vectors, all of which contain one or two nucleotide sequences (promoters). These are recognized by polymerases, allowing the transcription of RNA from a subcloned specific DNA insert. The promoters are flanked (in a downstream direction) by a multiple cloning site, which allows subcloning of template DNA (see Fig. 44.2). To obtain specific cRNA, the template complementary DNA (cDNA) has to be in reverse orientation with regard to the promoter regions.

Bluescribe and pGEM vectors contain a multiple cloning site flanked by two promoters, which allow transcription of the insert in alternate directions. Consequently, from a particular insert, 'antisense' (probes complementary to mRNA) and 'sense' (with identical sequence to mRNA) RNA can be synthesized by the use of different polymerases.

Linearization of the vector

To obtain transcripts of the right size with or without only short non-specific vector sequences, the vector must be linearized immediately downstream of the insert or within the insert. Usually, an enzyme cutting in the multiple cloning region is used.

In vitro transcription and probe labelling

To synthesize a single-stranded, radiolabelled RNA probe, the cDNA, which is attached now to a promoter site, must be transcribed in the presence of labelled nucleotide and the appropriate RNA polymerase (SP6, T7 or T3 polymerase) (Fig. 44.3). Following transcription, the label probe will be extracted from the mixture, the incorporation of the label will be assessed and the probe can be used immediately or stored at –20°C for a limited time in case of radiolabelled probes and unlimited time for non-radiolabelled probes.

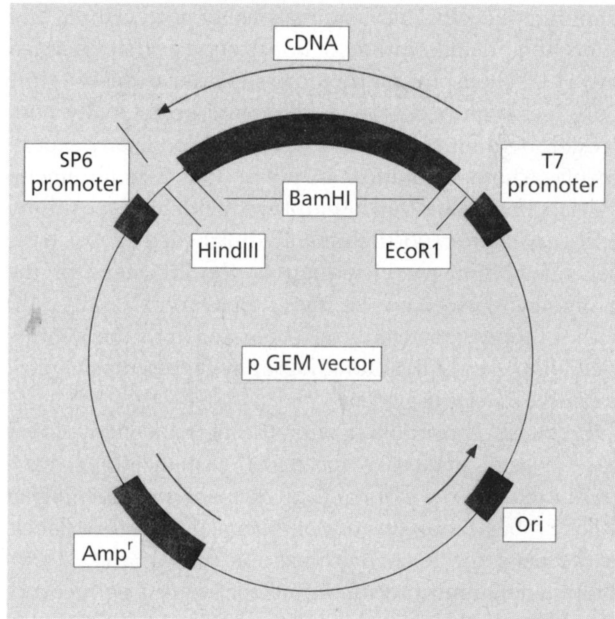

Fig. 44.2 Diagrammatic representation of cDNA subcloning into pGEM vector.

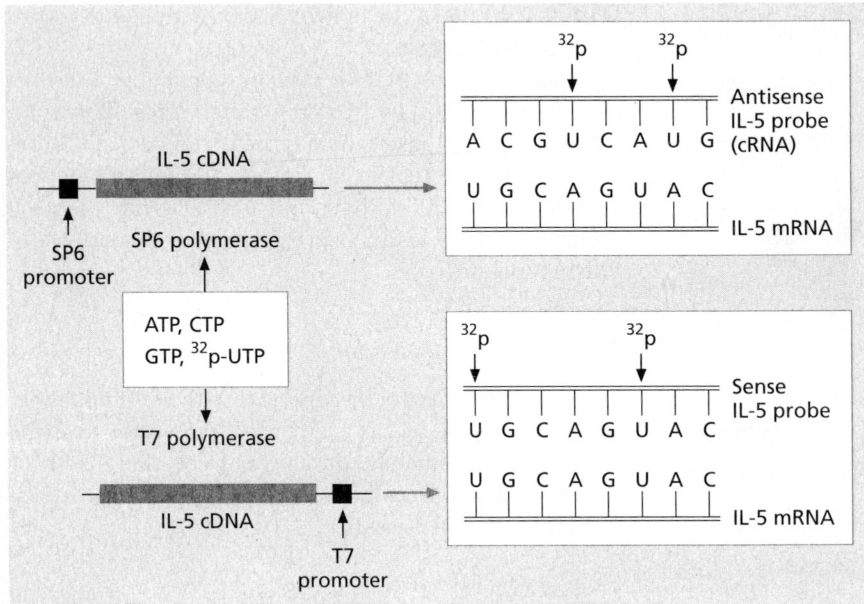

Fig. 44.3 Diagrammatic representation of *in vitro* transcription of RNA probe and synthesis of antisense and sense probes.

Choice of labels

Two types of labelling can be used for RNA probes: isotopic and non-isotopic labelling. Several types of isotopes can be employed for labelling RNA. These include ^{3}H, ^{125}I, ^{32}P, ^{35}S and ^{33}P. The hybridization signal can be detected with audioradiography using liquid emulsion or by X-ray films. The ^{3}H label produces higher cellular resolution due to its slow energy emission, but it requires long exposure times. ^{125}I is not used very frequently for ISH. ^{35}S-labelled probe has high specific activity and gives high photographic efficiency and reasonably good cellular and subcellular details, although not as good as that obtained by ^{3}H-labelled probes. It requires shorter exposure time but gives high background levels and occasionally non-specific binding, which has to be controlled in any experiment. Where resolution is not a major requirement, ^{32}P-labelled probes can be employed with high sensitivity and very short exposure time. Radiolabelled probes have several advantages including: (i) the efficiency of the probe synthesis can be monitored more easily; (ii) radioisotopes are readily incorporated into the synthesized RNA; and (iii) autoradiography represents the most sensitive detection system.

Problems encountered with the radiolabelled probes (e.g. waste disposal, speed of visualization) have prompted the development of non-isotopic labelling of RNA probes. Biotin was one of the first non-isotopic labels to be used for RNA hybridization (Giaid *et al.*, 1989). Biotin-containing precursor nucleotides can be incorporated into double-stranded DNA or RNA. Modification of the biotin probes has included the use of allylamine-uridine triphosphate (UTP) for biotin and long-chain diamino compounds conveniently linked to biotin. Other types of non-isotopic labels have also been employed, and these include fluorochrome, acetylaminofluorene, dinitrophen and sulphydryl–hapten ligands. Recently, a very sensitive and efficient label has been employed in labelling RNA probes (digoxigenin-11-UTP) (Yap *et al.*, 1992; Ying *et al.*, 1993, 1994). The RNA hybrids obtained by using non-radiolabelled probes are usually detected by immunocytochemical methods. The cellular resolution obtained with non-isotopically labelled probes is usually excellent and the signals are developed in a very short time when compared with radiolabelled probes. The major limitation of non-isotopic methods is the relatively poor sensitivity for detection of low copy numbers of mRNA.

Probe size

The diffusibility of the probe into the cell and its hybridization to the messenger sequences (associated with ribosomes and cross-linked with the cell matrix) are both influenced by the size of the probe fragment after transcription. Paraformaldehyde-fixed cells tolerate a broad range of probe sizes. This is consistent with the hypothesis that cells or tissue fixed with paraformaldehyde is less cross-linked and hence more permeable. A reasonable result can be obtained with probes of 100–400 bases. Probes of length of more that 500 bases should be digested to an average of 150–200 bases, using limited alkaline hydrolysis (Wolfl *et al.*, 1987).

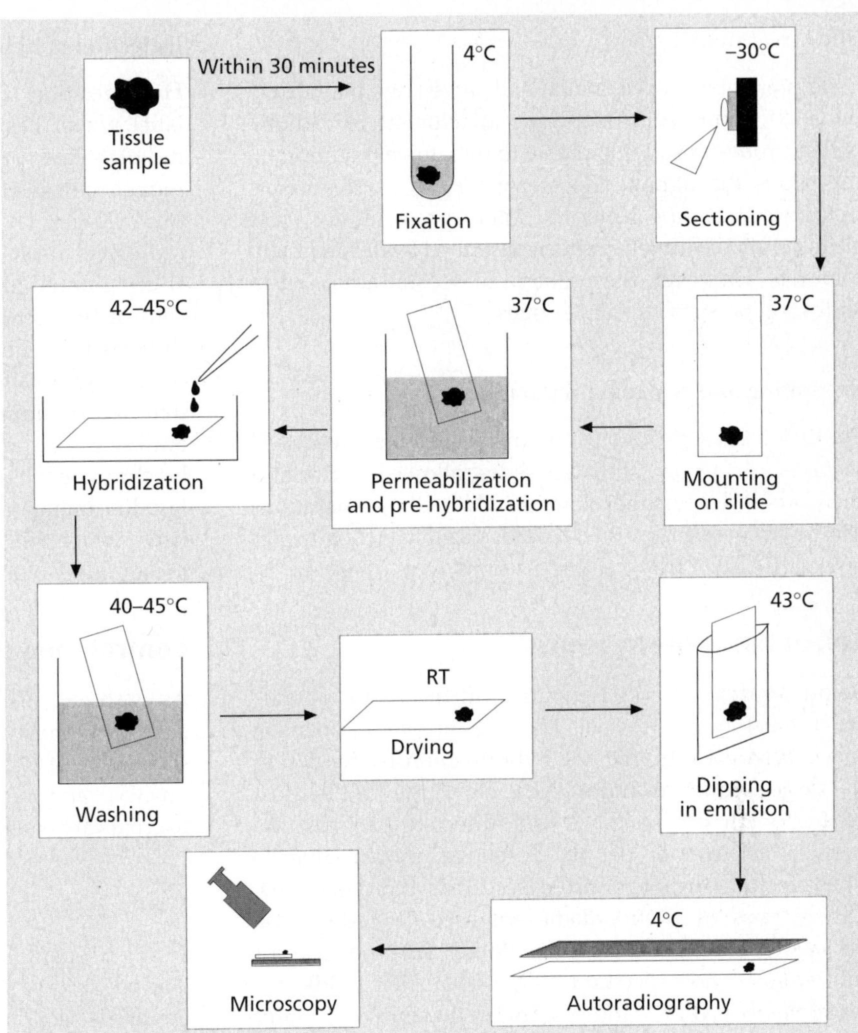

Fig. 44.4 Diagrammatic representation of *in situ* hybridization procedure.

Tissue preparation (Fig. 44.4)

Tissue handling

It is essential to keep the tissue RNase free. Fingertips are rich in RNase, so gloves should always be worn. Sterile knives, containers and solutions should be used whenever possible. Tissue must be collected as fresh as possible, with a maximum delay of 30 minutes.

Fixation for mRNA ISH

Any procedure involving ISH begins with the fixation of the tissue, cytology specimen or cell culture. The fixative must preserve the tissue in a morphologically stable state while retaining the maximal accessible mRNA within the cells, particularly under the rigorous conditions used for hybridization. Several fixatives have been reported to be of use for ISH. These include paraformaldehyde, glutaraldehyde, buffered formalin, Bouin's solution and ethanol/acetic acid. Paraformaldehyde maintains sufficient morphological information while allowing efficient hybridization. Freshly prepared paraformaldehyde should be used before the paraformaldehyde breaks down into several substances, one of which is formic acid, and loses its ability to retain maximum mRNA. The time of fixation differs according to the type of preparation (30 minutes for cytological preparation, 2 hours for endoscopic biopsies and 4 hours for surgical and post-mortem samples). Overfixation decreases the hybridization signal by masking the mRNA. Tissue can be embedded in paraffin or frozen on cryostat chucks. Optimum morphological preservation in paraffin-embedded material may be accompanied by substantial reductions in the density of hybridization in comparison with frozen-section material.

Slide treatment

Slide pretreatment is essential and serves two main functions: to minimize non-specific attachment of radiolabelled probes to slides and also to maximize retention on the slides throughout the various rigorous treatments involved in *in situ* protocols. Many protocols for slide cleaning and coating have been described by different laboratories. However, the problem of section adhesion to slides still persists for some tissues.

Sectioning and cytospin preparations

For ISH, thick sections (10 μm) are usually employed. The sections are cut on precoated slides, allowed to dry and then processed for hybridization. Cytospin preparations can be prepared from body fluids (e.g. bronchoalveolar lavage (BAL)) or from cell suspensions.

Cell or tissue pretreatment

Before starting any ISH experiment, the tissue preparation must be pretreated. The aim of pretreatment is to increase the efficiency of hybridization by rendering the target sequences more accessible to the probe. Most of the methods described are directed towards the permeabilization of the fixed cellular protein matrix. These include the use of proteases, acids and detergents. Other types of pretreatment are used to reduce the background staining. Among these are the use of inhibitors of non-specific binding of nucleic acids, for example prehybridization with acetic anhydride and formamide.

Hybridization

The conditions of hybridization vary to allow probe access, appropriate stringency and tissue preservation. For hybridization, the probe is incubated with the pretreated tissue or cells with an optimal incubation condition, usually overnight, to allow the hybridization between the cRNA probe and the cytoplasmic mRNA equation. However, not all the probes will be hybridized to the mRNA; thus, the preparation needs to be washed with high stringency to remove background signal. Washing conditions determine the stringency of the ISH procedure; they allow diffusion of materials trapped in the section and should select for a 'good fit' between probe and target mRNA. The availability of RNase to digest the unhybridized probe has favoured the use of RNA probes for ISH. This enzyme is a very powerful one and the time and concentration of RNase in the post-hybridization mixture are critical for an optimal signal.

Detection of hybridization

Hybridization signals can be detected according to the label which has been incorporated into the probe. For radiolabelled probes, standard autoradiographic techniques with an emulsion (Ilford K5 or NBT Kodak) can be used (Roger, 1979). The incubation time depends on the radiolabel itself, and the signal will appear as a dark, silver granule overlying the emulsion which covers the cells or the sections. When the morphology of the cell is difficult to identify, dark-field illumination can help. For the non-radiolabelled probes, the RNA hybrid is usually detected by immunocytochemical methods, in which an antibody (e.g. anti-digoxigenin) is used and developed by chromogenes (Ying *et al.*, 1993, 1994). For biotin, streptavidin conjugated to an enzyme fluorescent dye might be used, which will again be developed with an immunocytochemical technique (Giaid *et al.*, 1989).

Controls and specificity of ISH

As with any histochemical method, proper controls are necessary during every ISH experiment to assess the specificity of the reagents and procedures used. Proper positive and negative controls for tissue, probes and reagents are essential.

Tissue

Tissue preparation is critical to selective hybridization. One must have confidence that the nucleic acids within the tissue section have been preserved. Additional tissue slices should be hybridized to probes that hybridize well to the tissue being examined.

The tissue itself should be evaluated for specific mRNA content by Northern blot analysis. This control is critical when studying the absence of specific hybridization or the change in message content under various physiological conditions. Northern blot analysis monitors mRNA levels within a large, often heterogeneous, population of cells. In some cases, ISH reveals mRNA within such a small percentage of cells that a Northern blot analysis of tissue is unable to detect it.

Probes

Northern blotting is the most conclusive analysis of probe specificity. The probe must be able to hybridize to a specific mRNA population containing nucleic acids complementary to the probe. Furthermore, the accurate melting temperature of the probe and mRNA can be determined by Northern blot analysis. These temperatures will reflect the stringency of hybridization required in subsequent experiments on tissue.

Hybridization specificity

Controls for hybridization specificity are required to ensure that the autoradiographic signal is the result of specific nucleic acid interactions. Non-specific interactions include 'edge' artefacts and 'stickiness' of probe to different tissue types. Weak specific interactions include the binding of probe to related sequences and to ribosomal RNA. The use of unrelated probes and 'sense' probes on additional tissue sections addresses the contribution of these interactions.

The specificity of hybridization must be assessed by estimating the melting temperature between probe and signal. A specific signal will withstand increased stringency of hybridization, while non-specific or weak interactions will dissociate at elevated temperatures.

RNase pretreatment is another method of demonstrating that the signals are bound to a digestible RNA species. Loss of signal by RNase pretreatment of slides shows only that the probe was interacting with digestible nucleic acids. For this type of control, treat the preparations with RNase (20 mg/ml) for 30 minutes prior to the prehybridization step and then proceed.

Histological controls

These controls are the least quantitative and the most important controls for ISH. First and foremost, the hybridization signal must conform to known anatomical structures. Signals within a specific cell type should reflect the distribution of that cell type within the tissue. Adjacent histological cell types should be identified by a clear lack of signal if possible.

The combination of ISH with other localization techniques affords the possibility of further control of specificity.

Quantification

Many factors must be carefully considered and controlled if quantitative data are to be collected (Davenport & Nunez, 1990). These include section thickness, nucleic acid retention, consistency of hybridization exposure and development conditions, thickness and uniformity of the emulsion, and availability of proper standards and standard curves. Whatever the case may be, quantification of ISH is at best semiquantitative.

Interpretation of results

Interpretation of ISH results is far from easy. It is essential to be convinced that the hybridization signal is really specific. For example, a number of inflammatory cells, such as eosinophils and macrophages, have the capacity to bind probe non-specifically, especially with ^{35}S-labelled probes. Caution must be exercised in the interpretation of autoradiographic signals at the edge of the section (edge artefact). It is also important to take into consideration other factors, such as the formation of imperfect duplexes with non-homologous nucleic acids, electrostatic interactions among charged groups and physical entrapment of probe in the three-dimensional lattice of the tissue section. A proper microscope with dark-field illumination and phase-contrast facilities is essential for proper interpretation of autoradiographic signals. It is essential to include a positive and negative control in each ISH experiment. Absence of the hybridization signal does not necessarily indicate the absence of a particular mRNA and its translation product. mRNA could be expressed in low copy number which is below the sensitivity of the technique. Moreover, ISH determines the steady-state amount of hybridizable specific mRNA, whereas immunoreactive proteins are localized by immunocytochemistry (ICC). Despite the fact that the expression of the majority of genes is regulated by the amount of specific mRNA, conclusions drawn from 'double-staining' experiments, such as estimation of secretory activity, must be considered carefully. In addition, several other factors at the post-transcriptional and post-translational levels influence the amount and type of detectable gene expression products.

Safety precautions for handling radioisotopes for ISH

Increasing emphasis is being placed today on radiological safety practice. Most of the isotopes used for ISH are β-emitters. In general, there are two major safety precautions that need to be observed: one is to avoid direct interaction with β particles, especially with ^{32}P, and the other is to avoid aerosol-forming operations. Other customary precautions for handling isotopes include allocation of appropriately licensed designated laboratory areas, availability of suitable monitoring equipment and the attendance of training courses.

Examples for mRNA ISH

Preparations which can be processed for mRNA ISH include surgical biopsies, endoscopic biopsies, post-mortem tissue, cytological material (for example, from BAL) and tissue-culture preparations (Fig. 44.5).

Surgical biopsies

Surgically resected specimens are very useful for ISH, as the area of interest can be selected easily. However, the tissue must be collected for fixation from the operating

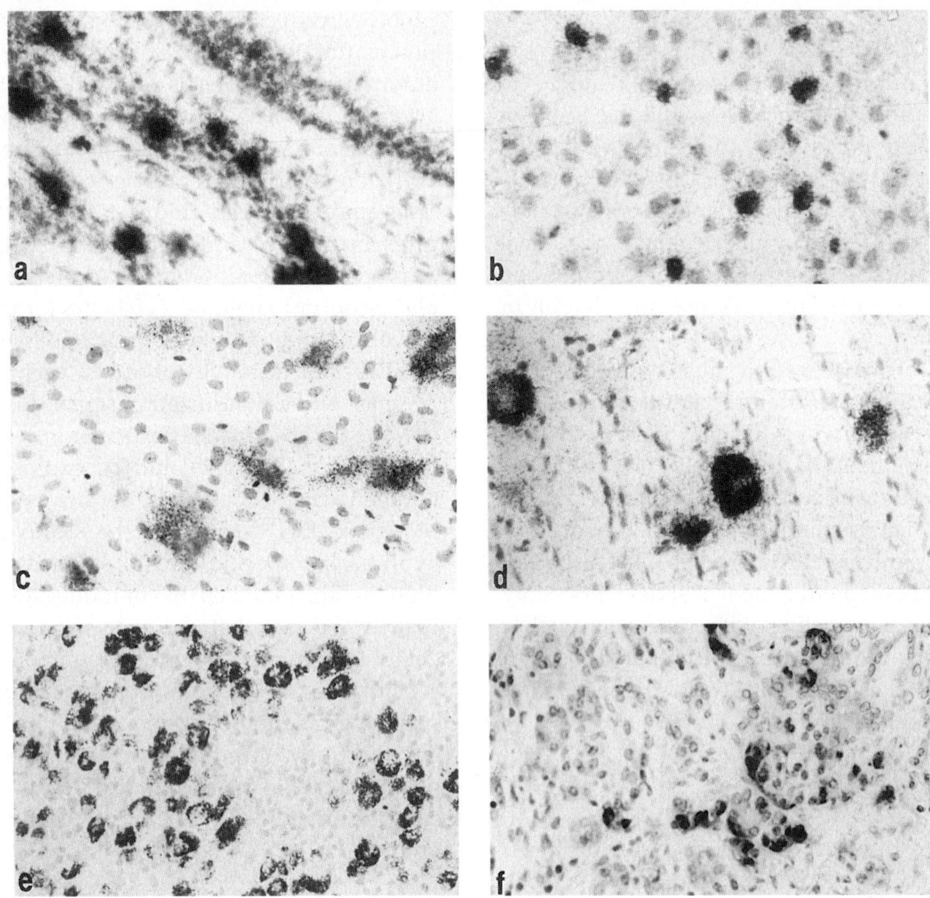

Fig. 44.5 (a) Example of *in situ* hybridization (ISH) using radiolabelled (^{32}P) cRNA probe. Interleukin-5 (IL-5) mRNA localization in endoscopic biopsy of the lung. (b) Example of ISH of bronchoalveolar lavage from a patient with asthma. Granulocyte macrophage colony-stimulating factor (GM-CSF) mRNA localization with ^{35}S-labelled probe. (c) Example of mRNA hybridization in tissue-culture preparation—myocytes hybridized with radiolabelled atrial natriuretic peptide (ANP) probe. (d) Example of mRNA ISH from animal tissue. Preprotachykinin mRNA localization in nodose ganglia of the rat. (e) Example of mRNA ISH in surgically resected lymph node. IL-6 mRNA localization with ^{35}S-labelled probe. (f) Example of non-radiolabelled ISH. Surgically resected bowel, hybridization with digoxigenin-labelled immunoglobulin probe.

theatre within as short a time as possible (less than 30 minutes).

Endoscopic biopsies

mRNA hybridization can be performed easily on small endoscopic biopsies. However, it is essential to take special care in orientating the biopsy to obtain good morphology and avoid edge artefacts, which are very common in crushed endoscopic biopsies (Durham *et al.*, 1992; Bentley *et al.*, 1993).

Cytological preparations

Examples of such preparations are needle aspirates, cervical smears and BAL. Cells can be fixed in solution after adhering to slides. Background and non-specific binding of probes are usually less evident in cytological preparations (Broidie *et al.*, 1992; Robinson *et al.*, 1992; Leung *et al.*, 1995).

Post-mortem tissue

Some human tissues are only accessible for investigation at post mortem. It is inevitable that a large proportion of the mRNA in tissue will be lost after death, especially if the autopsy is performed after more than 24 hours. This has to be considered in the interpretation of the results (Gibson *et al.*, 1988).

Tissue-culture preparations

These are a very good model for mRNA hybridization. The presence of minimal contaminating cells and the absence of endogenous proteins help to a large extent in localization of mRNA to specific types of cell population (Gibson *et al.*, 1988; Cromwell *et al.*, 1992).

Phenotype of cells expressing mRNA

In tissue sections

To identify the cellular source of mRNA in tissue sections the following techniques can be employed.

- Simultaneous ICC and ISH using radiolabelled probes (Hamid *et al.*, 1992).
- Simultaneous ICC and non-radiolabelled ISH (enzymatic methods) (Ying *et al.*, 1994).
- Simultaneous ICC and ISH using immunofluorescence.
- Flip-flop technique (in this technique two sections are cut and mounted in such a way that one represents a mirror image of the other). One section will be treated for ISH and the other for ICC; then they will be visualized and compared.
- Serial-section technique (two thin serial sections can be obtained from cryostat blocks). One section will be treated for ISH and the other for ICC. This technique might be used to phenotype mRNA+ cells that have a diameter greater than 8 μm. It is, for example, not suitable for localizing mRNA in T lymphocytes.
- Combination of ISH and histochemical staining (an example is the use of chromotrope 2R and ISH to colocalize mRNA in eosinophils).

From culture preparations or body fluids (BAL, needle aspiration, nasal and bronchial washes, peripheral blood)

To detect the phenotype of cells expressing specific mRNA, the following techniques can be used.

- Flow-cytometry ISH (FISH) technique. Cells in suspension can be stained with surface markers (using phycoerythrin directly conjugated antibody) and hybridized with biotin-labelled probes, which will be visualized by fluorescent isothiocyanate (FITC)-conjugated streptavidin).
- Hybridization of cells separated by negative or positive selection using magnetic beads. Cells from BAL or peripheral blood can be separated, using immunomagnetic beads that are coupled to specific antibody. The positively or negatively selected cells can then by hybridized in a standard protocol (Robinson *et al.*, 1992).
- Simultaneous ISH and ICC (Ying *et al.*, 1993).

ISH under electron microscopy

This technique can be used under some circumstances, where it is difficult to phenotype the cells by other techniques. The RNA–RNA or DNA–RNA hybrid can be detected using biotin, gold particles or radioactive substances and visualized under transmitted or scanning electromicroscopy.

Colocalization of multiple gene transcript

This technique is usually used to detect more than one mRNA in the same cell, particularly in the case of multiple gene expression and alternative splicing (Broidie *et al.*, 1992). However, it could also be used to identify the phenotype of cells expressing mRNA by combining two probes, one coding for the mRNA in question and the other for an mRNA known to be expressed specifically in one type of cell.

Acknowledgements

I would like to thank Mrs M. Markroyanni and Ms B. Kidd for typing the manuscript and Dr E. Minshall for preparing the diagrams.

References

Bentley, A., Meng, Q., Robinson, D., Hamid, Q., Kay, A.B. & Durham, S. (1993) Increases in activated T lymphocytes, eosinophils and cytokine messenger RNA for IL-5 and GM-CSF in bronchial biopsies after allergen inhalation challenge in atopic asthmatics. *Am. J. Respir. Cell Mol. Biol.*, **8**, 35–42.

Bramwell, N.H. & Burns, B.F. (1988) The effects of fixative type and fixation time on the quantity and quality of extractable DNA for hybridization studies on lymphoid tissue. *Exp. Haematol.*, **16**, 730–2.

Brigati, D.J., Myerson, D., Leary, J.J. *et al.* (1983) Detection of viral genomes in cultured cells and paraffin-embedded tissue sections using biotin-labeled hybridization probes. *Virology*, **126**, 32–50.

Broidie, D. & Firestein, G. (1991) Endobronchial allergen challenge in asthma: demonstration of cellular source of granulocyte macrophage colony-stimulating factor by *in situ* hybridization. *J. Clin. Invest.*, **88**, 1048–53.

Broidie, D., Paine, M.M. & Firestein, G.S. (1992) Eosinophils express interleukin 5 and granulocyte macrophage-colony-stimulating factor mRNA at sites of allergic inflammation in asthmatics. *J. Clin. Invest.*, **90**, 1414–24.

Cox, K.H., DeLeon, D., Angerer, L.M. & Angerer, R.-C. (1984) Detection of mRNA in sea urchin embryos by *in situ* hybridization using RNA probes. *Dev. Biol.*, **101**, 485–502.

Cromwell, O., Hamid, Q.A., Corrigan, C., Barkans, J., Collins, P. & Kay, A.B. (1992) Expression and generation of IL-6, IL-8 and GM-CSF by human bronchial epithelial cells and ehancement by IL-1 beta and TNF-alpha. *Immunology*, **77**, 330–7.

Davenport, A.P. & Nunez, D.J. (1990) Quantification of hybridization signal. In: *In Situ Hybridization: Principles and Practice* (eds J.M. Polak & J. O'D. McGee), pp. 173–281. Oxford University Press, Oxford.

De Block, M. & Debrouwer, D. (1993) RNA–RNA *in situ* hybridization using digoxigenin-labeled probes: the use of high-molecular-weight polyvinyl alcohol in the alkaline phosphatase indoxyl–nitroblue tetrazolium reaction. *Analyt. Biochem.*, **215**, 86.

Denny, P., Hamid, Q.A., Krause, J., Polak, J. & Leagon, S. (1989) Oligoriboprobes, tools for *in situ* hybridization. *Histochemistry*, **89**, 481–3.

Durham, S., Ying, S., Varney, V., Jacobson, M., Kay, A.B. & Hamid, Q.A. (1992) Cytokine messenger mRNA expression for IL-3, IL-4, IL-5 and granulocyte/macrophage-colony-stimulating factor in the nasal mucosa after local allergen provocation: relationship to tissue eosinophilia. *J. Immunol.*, **148**, 2390–4.

Giaid, A., Hamid, Q., Adams, C., Terenghi, G. & Polak, J.M. (1989) Non-isotopic RNA probes: comparison between different labels and detection systems. *Histochemistry*, **93**, 191–6.

Gibson, S.J., Polak, J.M., Giaid, A. *et al.* (1988) Calcitonin gene-related peptide mRNA is expressed in sensory neurones of the dorsal root ganglia and also in spinal motoneurones in man and cat. *Neurosci. Letts.*, **91**, 283–8.

Hamid, Q.A. (1993) Isotopic localization of cellular mRNA in clinical material using RNA probes. In: *Diagnostic Molecular Pathology: a Practical Approach*, Vol. 1 (eds C.S. Herrington & O.D. McGee) pp. 169–85. IRL Press, New York

Hamid, Q., Wharton, J., Terenghi G. *et al.* (1987) Localization of atrial natriuretic peptide mRNA and immunoreactivity in rat heart and human atrial appendage. *Proc. Nat. Acad. Sci. USA*, **84**, 6760–4.

Hamid, Q.A., Corrin, B., Hofler, H., Dewar, A. & Sheppard, M. (1990) Expression of gastrin releasing peptide (human bombesin) gene in large cells undifferentiated carcinoma of the lung. *J. Pathol.*, **161**, 145–51.

Hamid, Q.A., Azzawi, M., Jeffery, P. & Kay, A.B. (1991a) Expression of mRNA for interleukin-5 in mucosal bronchial biopsies from asthma. *J. Clin. Invest.*, **87**, 154–9.

Hamid, Q.A., Corrin, B., Sheppard, M. & Polak, J.M. (1991b) Expression of chromogranin A mRNA in small cell carcinoma of the lung. *J. Pathol.*, **163**, 293–7.

Hamid, Q., Barkans, J., Meng Q., Abrams, J., Kay, A.B. & Moqbel, R. (1992) Human eosinophils synthesize and secrete interleukin-6, *in vitro*. *Blood*, **80**, 1496–501.

Herrington, C.S. & McGee, J. (1990) Non-radiolabelled *in situ* hybridization. In: *In Situ Hybridization: Application to Developmental Biology and Medicine* (eds H. Harris & D. Wilkinson), p. 241. Cambridge University Press, Cambridge.

Herrington, C.S., Burns, J., Graham, A.K. & McGee, J. (1990a) Discrimination of closely homologous HPV types by nonisotopic *in situ* hybridization: definition and derivation of tissue melting temperatures. *Histochem. J.*, **22**, 545–50.

Herrington, C.S., Flannery, D. & McGee, J. (1990b) Non-radiolabelled hybridization. In: *In Situ Hybridization* (eds J. Polak & J. McGee), p. 187. Oxford University Press, Oxford.

Hofler, H., Childer, H., Montminy, M.R., Lachan, R.M., Goodman, R.H. & Wolfe, H.J. (1986) *In situ* hybridization methods for the detection of somatostatin mRNA in tissue sections using antisense RNA probes. *Histochem. J.*, **18**, 597–662.

Hofler, H., Ruhri, C., Putz, B., Wirnsberger, G., Klimplfinger, M. & Smolle, J. (1987) Simultaneous localization of calcitonin mRNA and peptide in a medullary thyroid carcinoma. *Virchows Arch. B*, **53**, 144–51.

Kay, A.B., Ying, S., Varney, V. *et al.* (1991) Messenger RNA expression of the cytokine gene cluster, IL-3, Il-4, Il-5 and GM-CSF in allergen-induced late-phase cutaneous reactions in atopic subjects. *J. Exp. Med.*, **173**, 775–8.

Lawrence, J.B., Villnave, C. & Singer, R.H. (1988) Sensitive, high-resolution chromatic and chromosome mapping *in situ*: presence and orientation of two closely integrated copies of EBV in a lymphoma line. *Cell*, **52**, 51–61.

Leung, D., Martin, R., Szefler, S., Ying, S., Kay, A.B. & Hamid, Q.A. (1995) Dystregulation of interleukin-4, interleukin-5, and interferon-γ gene expression in steroid-resistant asthma. *J. Exp. Med.*, **181**, 33–40.

Morimoto, H., Monden, T., Shimano, T. *et al.* (1987) Use of sulfonated probes for *in situ* detection of amylase mRNA in formalin-fixed paraffin sections of human pancreas and submaxillary gland. *Lab. Invest.*, **57**, 737–41.

Ochman, H., Medhora, M.M., Garza, D. & Hartl, D.L. (1990) Principle of PCR technique. In: *PCR Protocols: a Guide to Methods and Applications* (eds M.A. Innis, D.H. Gelfand, J.J. Sninsky & T. White), pp. 219–27. Academic Press, San Diego.

Pardue, M.L. & Gall, J.G. (1969) Molecular hybridization of radioactive DNA to the DNA of cytological preparations. *Proc. Nat. Acad. Sci. USA*, **64**, 600–4.

Pringle, J.H., Ruprai, A.K., Primrose, L. *et al.* (1990) *In situ* hybridization of immunoglobulin light chain mRNA in paraffin sections using biotinylated or hapten-labelled oligonucleotide. *J. Pathol.*, **162**, 197–207.

Robinson, D., Hamid, Q.A., Ying, S. *et al.* (1992) Predominant Th2-type bronchoalveolar lavage T-lymphocytes population in atopic asthma. *New Engl. J. Med.*, **326**, 298–304.

Roger, A.W. (1979) In: *Techniques in Autoradiography*. Elsevier North-Holland, Amsterdam.

Singer, R.H., Lawrence, J.B. & Villnave, C. (1986) Optimisation of '*in situ*' hybridization using isotopic and non-isotopic detection methods. *Biotechniques*, **4**, 230–3.

Thein, S.L. & Wallace, R.B. (1986) Hybridization histochemistry. In: *Human Genetic Diseases: a Practical Approach* (ed. K.E. Davies), pp. 35–50. IRL Press, Oxford.

Wolfl, S., Quaas, R., Hahn, U. & Wittig, B. (1987) Synthesis of highly radioactive labelled RNA hybridization probes from synthetic single-stranded DNA oligonucleotides. *Nucl. Acids Res.*, **15**, 858.

Yap, E.P., Montero, J. & McGee, J. (1992) Non-radiolabelled RNA probes. In: *Diagnostic Molecular Pathology* (eds C.S. Herrington & J. McGee), pp. 187–205. IRL Press, Oxford.

Ying, S., Durham, S.R., Barkans, J. *et al.* (1993) T cells, mast cells and eosinophils are principal sources of interleukin-5 mRNA in allergen-induced allergic rhinitis. *Am. J. Respir. Cell Mol. Biol.*, 9:356

Ying, S., Durham, S.R., Jacobson, M. *et al.* (1994) T lymphocytes and mast cells express messenger RNA for interleukin-4 in the nasal mucosa in allergen-induced rhinitis. *Immunology*, **82**, 200.

CHAPTER 45

Immunocytochemistry

Q. Hamid

Definition

Immunocytochemistry is the identification of cellular or tissue constituents (antigens) by means of antigen–antibody interaction. The site of interaction is identified by a direct label to the antibody or by the use of a secondary labelling method (Plate 45.1, opposite page 748). It is a tool which allows the precise examination of aspects of cell function and chemical composition and their relationship to our perception of cell and tissue morphology, and as such it has greatly enhanced our understanding of disease processes. The concept of using antibodies raised in the laboratory to localize antigen within tissue has been employed as an important tool in the biological research since the 1940s (Coons *et al.*, 1941). However, since the mid-1970s, with the advent of monoclonal antibodies (Kohler & Milstein, 1975), it has had an increasingly important role.

Light-microscopical immunocytochemistry

Cellular antigen

An antigen is any molecule that has generated an antibody response (antibody generator). The part of the antigen that reacts with a given antibody is the specific antigenic determinant or epitope. A molecule typically has multiple different potential epitopes, although an antibody binds only one specific epitope. Most antigens are proteins, although any type of chemical can be antigenic. For example, the antigen identified in neural tissue by the Leu-7 antibody is a carbohydrate, and some antigens recognized by lupus antibodies are phosphodiesters. Antigenicity is the presence of antibody binding activity. Because antigenicity is dependent on the physicochemical nature of the three-dimensional structure of the antigen, it is influenced by the chemical and physical forces of tissue processing (Pearse, 1985).

Antibodies can be used to a large range of molecular antigens. These include cell structural compounds, cell products (hormones, enzymes, immunoglobulins (Ig)), cell-surface receptors and abnormal proteins produced under pathological conditions. Antibodies can also be raised to the whole cell, as well as to some microorganisms such as bacteria and viruses (Legocki & Verma, 1981; Symington *et al.*, 1981).

Primary antibodies

Antibodies, or Ig, are glycoproteins that bind with high affinity or specificity to antigens. They are classified according to electrophoretic mobility, which depends primarily upon heavy-chain compositions and degree of multimerization. Accordingly, properties of the Ig classes are distinctive — molecular weight, percentage carbohydrates and functional properties in the binding of other substances.

There is a wide range of antibody to human tissue antigen currently available for immunocytochemical investigations. In general, antibodies can be either polyclonal or monoclonal antibodies. Antibodies which are commercially available are usually well characterized. However, for each newly acquired antibody the activity must be assessed and a number of points must be addressed, including the state of specificity of the antibody, establishing appropriate working dilutions for immunodetection systems to be used and tissue fixation and processing, including the use of proteolytic agents. Antibodies are usually stored at either 4°C or –20°C, depending on the nature of the antibody. However, it must be noted that repeated freezing and thawing lead to rapid deterioration of the reagents.

Polyclonal antibodies

The successful immunization of animals produces a variety of antibodies with different specificities and binding affinities (De Mey & Mocremans, 1986). Polyclonal antiserum theoretically maximizes the number of antibodies bound to a moleculae that has little repetitiveness of epitopes. Molecule-specific antibodies of different subclasses may all bind to the desired molecule. Polyclonal antisera are also quicker and simpler to obtain than monoclonal antibodies. A significant disadvantage is the heterogeneous nature of polyclonal antibodies. Because antisera comprise a mixture of antibodies to various epitopes of the antigen and to any other molecules in the immunizing preparation, as well as to Ig already present in animals, and because these various antibodies have different affinities, both specificity and suitability of immunocytochemistry must be assessed. To minimize the development of antibodies to contaminants, the immunogen should be as pure as possible. A further disadvantage of polyclonal sera is that the supply is limited to the serum of one animal. The antibody characteristic of serum from another animal immunized with the identical antigen may be quite different (Vandesande, 1979).

Monoclonal antibodies

Monoclonal antibodies are the secreted Ig of the clonal progeny of a single hybrid plasma cell. Having molecular identity, they have identical antigen specificity and binding affinity. An advantage of great significance for immunocytochemistry was the development of methods to generate immortalized clones that secrete monoclonal antibodies. Such monoclonal antibodies have the following advantages compared with polyclonal antibodies: (i) monospecificity (to a single epitope); (ii) immortality — because they are the progeny of myeloma cells, they can proliferate indefinitely; and (iii) because antibody specificity is generated during selection of a clone to expand, the immunogen does not need to be pure. A potential disadvantage of monoclonal antibodies is that they have a lower sensitivity than polyclonal antibodies. Only single monoclonal antibodies will bind to molecules containing only one copy of the epitope (Galfre & Milstein, 1981). Furthermore, the generation of monoclonal antibodies is more time-consuming and complex than the production of polyclonal antisera (Bastin *et al.*, 1982). Finally, immortality of monoclonal antibody synthesis is not invariable. Monoclonal antibodies may spontaneously lose isotopes or domain. An option is the use of a mix of monoclonal antibodies. By the formation of circular antibody–antigen complexes with a low antibody concentration, such mixes have greater affinity than either antibody alone (Ritter, 1986).

Immunocytochemical methods

Many methods are available for immunocytochemistry, so many that one could easily become confused by the apparent complexity of the situation. The major criteria by which the choice of technique for detecting a particular antigen is made include sensitivity, reliability, cost, versatility and safety. In general, three principal methods are available.

1 *Direct method.* A labelled primary antibody is applied directly to the tissue preparation. This is the simplest immunocytochemical method in which a label is directly conjugated to the antibody (Coons *et al.*, 1955). This conjugate is then applied to tissue sections or preparations in a single step. While simple, this is not particularly sensitive and does not allow the antibody to be used in other methods (Fig. 45.1).

2 *Indirect method.* The primary antibody is unlabelled and is identified by a labelled secondary antibody raised to the Ig of the species providing the primary antibody. Because at least two secondary antibody molecules can bind to each primary antibody molecule, this method is more sensitive than the direct method. An additional advantage is that a labelled secondary antibody to the Ig of one species can be used to identify any number of primary antibodies raised in that species. The sensitivity of this method can be enhanced by applying a third step, a labelled antibody raised against the species in which the second antiserum has been raised (Wick *et al.*, 1982). This is called the three-stage or enhanced indirect technique (Fig. 45.2).

3 *Unlabelled antibody–enzyme methods* (Bullock & Petrusz, 1982). An unconjugated, bridging, secondary antibody is used between the primary antibody and the label detection reagent, which is usually an enzyme–anti-enzyme

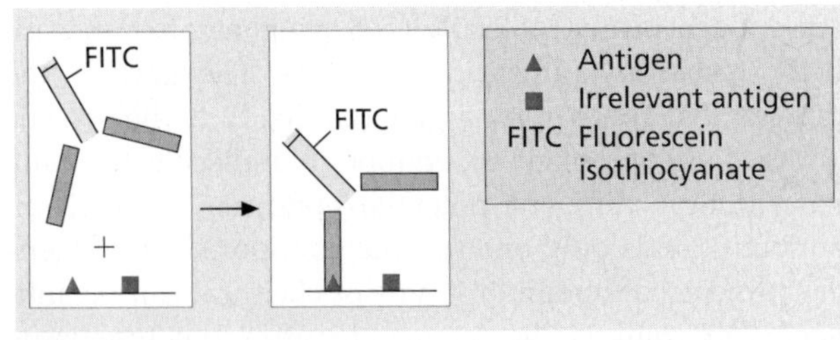

Fig. 45.1 Diagrammatic representation of the principle of the direct immunocytochemistry technique.

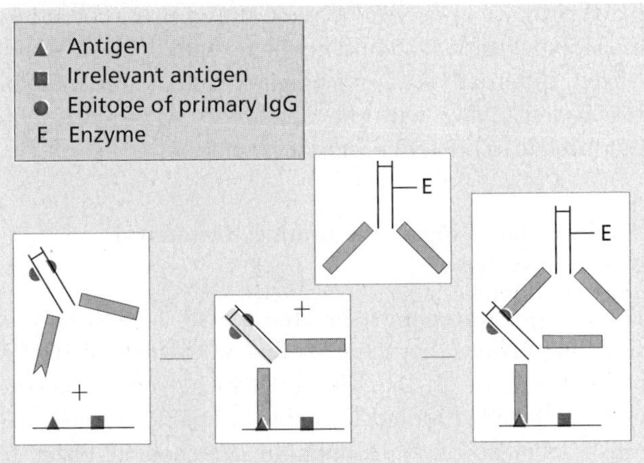

Fig. 45.2 Diagrammatic representation of the indirect immunocytochemistry technique.

complex or an avidin–biotin enzyme complex. Methods utilizing enzyme–anti-enzyme complex approaches include peroxidase–anti-peroxidase (PAP) and alkaline phosphatase–anti-alkaline phosphatase (APAAP) techniques (Cordell *et al.*, 1984).

PAP (Sternberger, 1979)

Sternberger (1979) combined peroxidase with anti-peroxidase to form a stable cyclic complex with three peroxidase molecules to two antibody molecules. The PAP complex is used as a third-layer antigen, the first layer being (rabbit) anti-tissue antigen, the second layer being unconjugated goat anti-rabbit IgG in excess, so that one of the two identical binding sites (Fab protein) is free to combine with the third layer, the rabbit PAP complex. There is thus a high ratio of peroxidase label to primary antigen. The rabbit PAP molecules will react only with the anti-rabbit IgG of the second layer, so that provided there is no unwanted binding to the tissue of the second layer this is a very specific and background-free technique. The increased amount of label allows the primary antibody to be highly diluted, which has the advantage of reducing unwanted background staining. Because the second antibody is unconjugated, it has full activity and, because the peroxidase is bound by an antigen–antibody reaction rather than chemical conjugation, it is fully active. This method is very popular, especially with the use of the polyclonal antibody.

APAAP (Cordell *et al.*, 1984)

This method works on the same principle as the PAP method and can be extremely sensitive. However, to date, only monoclonal mouse anti-alkaline phosphatase has been produced. This method is thus very convenient with the use of monoclonal antibodies and, because it is sensitive, it is extremely valuable for detecting low amounts of antigen in particular receptor antigens.

Avidin–biotin methods (Coggi *et al.*, 1986)

In contrast to other immunocytochemical techniques, avidin–biotin methods were not originally conceived for immunocytochemistry. Indeed, these methods have been routinely used by biochemists in several extraction and chromatographic procedures, based on the same principle (the high affinity between avidin and biotin). All avidin–biotin methods are based generally on four main principles: (i) the extraordinary affinity between avidin and biotin molecules, which link one to the other in a particularly permanent complex; (ii) the possibility of coupling biotin to a large molecule, such as enzymes or antibodies, through a single biochemical reaction; (iii) the possibility of labelling avidin with a variety of markers, such as enzymes, heavy metal and fluorochromes; and (iv) the possibility of using avidin as a bridge between two different biotin-related molecules, such as an antibody and peroxidase. The use of avidin in this system presents some disadvantages, including the reaction with lectin-like endogeneous protein and sticking to other tissue components. These result in the reduction of a specificity-increasing background. In order to overcome these limitations, avidin can be replaced by streptavidin. The reaction between avidin and biotin is due to non-convalent bonds. It has been shown that the reaction is extremely rapid and strong in nature. The two molecules can be separated only by submitting to extreme conditions, such as very low pH.

Immunocytochemical methods employing avidin–biotin do not differ in their essential requirement and in the general outline of the procedure from more traditional methods. This is particularly true for tissue processing, section incubation, washing procedures, controls, etc. The main feature of the immunocytochemical method employing avidin–biotin is that the biotinated antibody used either as the primary in the direct method or as a secondary in the indirect methods can be visualized in three different ways: (i) with label avidin; (ii) with avidin acting as a bridge with biotinated enzymes; and (iii) with the avidin–biotin–peroxidase complex (ABC) method.

Conditions for immunocytochemistry

The necessary conditions for accurate localization of an antigen by a labelled antibody are preservation of the tissue and antigen, production of a specific antibody and efficiency of labelling.

Preservation of tissue and antigen

Conventional formalin fixation in one of its many forms is often quite satisfactory for immunocytochemical detection with the sensitive antibody and detection systems now available. A significant advance in this area was made with the introduction of proteinase digestion to reveal overfixed antigen sites. Alcohol has been used as a fixative, followed by paraffin embedding. Where intracellular Ig are to be detected, the tissue sample has to be washed in saline for 48 hours. This washes out intercellular Ig deposits, giving the Ig-containing cells a better contrast with the background immunofluorescence. However, pretreatment does not do the structure of the tissue much good, and it is thus not suitable for transmitted light-microscopical immunoenzyme methods. If cell-surface antigens (e.g., of lymphoid tissue) are to be studied, the tissue must be fresh-frozen, and well-dried cryostat sections must be used with a short post-fixation in acetone or acetone/methanol mixture. Cryostat sections from lymphoid tissue may be stored at –20°C after drying or freeze-drying. They should be wrapped in foil or cling film and sealed in a bag with some desiccant such as silica gel. Whole-cell preparations, such as smears, imprints, cytospins or cell culture, may need to be made permeable to the antibody, as well as being fixed. One way of achieving permeabilization is to fix the preparation, and then take it through graded alcohol to xyline and back to water, provided that the antigen will survive this treatment. Other fixatives have been used, including Bouin's paraformaldehyde, Zamboni's fixative and benzoquinone.

Tissue fixed in formalin and embedded in paraffin is usually cut on a conventional microtome. Cryostat sections of fresh-frozen tissue are useful for cell-surface and other antigens that are labile to routine fixation and processing methods. Resins are suitable for semithin sections as well as ultrathin sections. Recently, glycol methacrylate methods have also been used for semithin sections. To prevent sections from detaching from the glass slide during immunostaining, particularly when proteinase digestion is used or fragile cryostat sections are involved, it is useful to coat the slide with, for example, poly-L-lysine before mounting the sections.

Preparation of antibodies for immunocytochemistry

Every antiserum must be tested on a non-positive control to find the correct working dilution for the staining method to be used. The dilution will vary according to what the incubation time is to be (1 hour at room temperature or overnight at 4°C). More concentrated antibodies do not necessarily mean better immunostaining. Unconjugated primary antiserum may be stored frozen or at low dilution in buffer. It should not be repeatedly thawed and frozen. Alternatively, unconjugated antiserum may be stored at 4°C neat with the addition of sodium azide or merthiolate to prevent bacterial growth.

Antibody labelling and immunocytochemical detection systems

The label or tracer must be attached to the antibody in such proportions that there are few or no unlabelled antibody molecules in the solution which would compete with the labelled molecules for the variable antigens. As much label as possible must be attached in order to increase the sensitivity of the method, but the antibody must not be so overburdened with label that its reactivity is impaired. However, in the unlabelled antibody–enzyme methods and the PAP method, difficulties arising with labelling antibodies might be avoided. The most common labels used for immunocytochemistry include the following.

Fluorescent

Fluorescent and rhodamine isothiocyanates (FITC or RITC) are well-known fluorescent labels, the former being fluorescent green and the latter fluorescent red. Other fluorescent labels are Texas red and phycoerythrin. The availability of multiple fluorescent labels is very valuable in double-immunostaining (Oi *et al.*, 1982; Titus *et al.*, 1982).

Enzymes

Enzymes are the most popular label, particularly peroxidase and alkaline phosphatese.

- *Peroxidase* can be developed with the diaminobenzidine (DAB)–hydrogen peroxide reaction. This gives an insoluble intensely brown colour. DAB was formerly considered to be potentially carcinogenic but it is now thought to be less dangerous. However, it is probably advisable to treat all reagents with care. Alternatives to DAB for the development of peroxidase are 3-amino-9-ethyl-carbisol, which gives a red product, or 4-chloro-1-naphthol, which gives a blue end-product. These are also useful for double-immunostaining.
- *Alkaline phosphatase* is increasingly popular as a label. It is used in the indirect method, conjugated to a secondary antibody, or in a variant of the end-labelled antibody–enzyme method, using an anti-alkaline phosphatase combined with alkaline phosphatase as either a two-step or a single-step procedure. The alkaline phosphatase is pre-incubated with the antibody to form an APAAP complex. Endogenous alkaline phosphatase

can be inhibited by levimasole, which is very efficient in preventing non-specific binding. Monoclonal APAAP is commercially available and is the recommended method for the localization of receptor antigens in immune regulatory cells. Alkaline phosphatase can be developed to give blue or red products that are alcohol-soluble and must be mounted in an aqueous medium. These multiple detection systems are also useful in double staining.

• *Glucose oxidase*. This label has the advantage of not being present in animal tissue and therefore there are no problems with endogenous enzyme activity in the immunocytochemical preparation. The end-product is an intense navy blue, which provides a good contrast. However, this label is not commonly used in routine immunocytochemistry (Suffin *et al.*, 1979).

• *β-D-Galactosidase*. This is also a popular enzyme label. The endogenous enzyme is not a problem unless there happen to be bacteria in the preparation. The end-product is bright turquoise-blue with the endogenic method of a development, and it can be dehydrated and permanently mounted. It is particularly useful in multiple staining (Bondi *et al.*, 1982).

Haptens

Haptens, such a dinitrophenol, have been used as a label for primary antibodies in the bridging technique. The hapten is localized by an unlabelled anti-hapten, followed by haptenized PAP complex (Cammisuli & Wofsy, 1976).

Colloid metals (Gu *et al.*, 1981; Roth, 1982)

Gold as a label can be seen in the light microscope as deep pink, provided the antibody is used at a high concentration, and has its use in double staining. It can also be seen in dark-field illumination. This has now been replaced by colloidal silver, which gives a yellow colour.

Biotin (Coggi *et al.*, 1986)

This is extremely useful as a bridging label for attachment to avidin and for attaching enzyme or gold to avidin. Details of this have already been discussed.

Radioactive label

A radioactive label can also be used to label a particular antibody; however, this technique is not very popular (Larsson & Schwartz, 1977).

Affinity

Affinity is the binding strength of an antibody to specified antigen. Affinity is characterized as an affinity constant. For immunocytochemistry, the higher the affinity constant, the better the antibody, because the antibody is more likely to remain bound to the antigen sought during the procedure. In contrast, the optimal antibodies for competition immunoasssays, such as radioimmunoassays or enzyme-linked immunosorbent assay (ELISA), have an affinity constant that allows successful competition for a specific labelled antigen. Nonetheless, antibodies used in competition assay have been successfully used in immunocytochemistry.

Sensitivity

The sensitivity of a detection system refers to the minimum concentration of antigen detectable by the assay system. This quality differs from 'antibody efficiency', which refers to the minimum amount of antibodies needed (Bullock & Petrusz, 1983). The sensitivity depends on a number of factors, including the nature of the antigen, distribution of the antigen within the tissue, antigen sequence, antigen sites, functional state of the cell and tissue processing (fixation and embedding).

Antigen accessibility

Location of an antigen may affect sensitivity. In contrast to cell-surface antigens, which are immediately accessible to antibodies, intracellular antigen are shielded by membranes. Because cell membranes are naturally impermeable to Ig, holes must be created to allow antibody access to intracellular antigens. Fixation and sectioning create adequate access for antibodies. This access can be increased by immunoreacting both sides of the tissue (Straus, 1982). However, the other manoeuvres often need to be performed on the intact cell, e.g. freezing, thawing, use of detergents and use of digestion enzymes (Wang & Larsson, 1985).

Specificity

Non-specific immunoreactivity represents the position of reaction products at a site other than the location of this desired antigen. Such false positivity can arise either from antibody binding or from non-antibody-specific binding. In general, non-specificity can be either immunological or non-immunological. Immunological non-specificity refers to the successful immunocytochemical localization of an antigen which provides a false result. Sources of such false positivity include sequence homology, similar antigenicity and contaminating antibodies. Non-immunological non-specificity refers to non-antibody-binding false-positive staining. For example, Fc portions of whole Ig may bind receptors of Fc phagocytes and mast cells. Fc receptors are labile and readily inactivated by fixation.

Complement binding of IgG molecules may localize to complement already present in tissue. Complement is also labile. Certain antibodies and gut endocrine cells have an electrostatically mediated affinity that can mimic antibody–antigen reactivity. Changes in the solution pH and salt concentration of reagents abolish this activity. Free aldehyde groups from incompletely reacted fixatives may non-specifically bind antibodies to tissue.

Endogeneous label activity might present some problems in determining the specificity of any reaction. For example, peroxidase activity is present in epithelial cells, megakaryocytes, mast cells, liver cells, red cells, neutrophils and eosinophils. Alkaline phosphatase activity can also be present in epithelial cells, for example of the bladder, neutrophils and mast cells. Biotin activity can be present in pancreas, liver and kidney and may also cause false localization of avidin–biotin complexes.

Other non-specific reactions including those detected at the edges of the tissue and necrotic tissue. Endogeneous pigment may be confused with labels, particularly lipochromes and melanin. Thus, the determination of the specificity of antibody binding is as important as assessing the result of an immune reaction.

Specificity controls

Positive controls

A positive control preparation known to contain the antigen in question should be carried through with every batch of immunostaining in order to confirm that all the agents are in working order.

Negative controls

The specific antibody should not stain inappropriate tissue and, on appropriate preparation, no reaction should be seen if any of the steps of the reaction are omitted or if an inappropriate antibody or non-immune serum (at the same dilution) is substituted for the primary antibody. If the staining occurs under these circumstances, a cause for the non-specific background should be sought.

Absorption controls

The ultimate test of specificity is to show that the immunoreactivity of the antibody is abolished by prior absorption with an excess of its specific antigen, but not by absorption with similar quantities of related substances. An absorption test should be carried out whenever a new antibody or previously examined tissue is used. A proviso for this absorption test is that the absorbed antibody should not be used to stain tissue that may contain receptors for the antigen.

Multiple-staining techniques

If is often of interest to identify more than one antigen in the same preparation and it is increasingly apparent that several products, even of the same type, may be made by a single cell. Several approaches can be utilized to achieve the goal of identifying multiple antigens.

Serial sections (Pruss *et al.*, 1981)

This method could be used for colocalization by immunostaining serial sections for different antigens and comparing structures that contain them. However, these sections must be very thin (1–2 μm) or there is a risk that the same cell will not be present in both sections. To cut such a thin section, the tissue must be embedded in a special medium, such as resin or methachiolyte, which might affect the antigen of the cell (Holgate *et al.*, 1983). An alternative method is to use mirror-image sections or the flip-flop technique. In this technique, the first section of two is picked up on a slide from the knife in the usual way so that the cut surface will be stained. The second serial section is flipped over on to a cold surface and picked up from that, so that the slide that was originally opposed to the cut surface of the first section is uppermost. Thus, the two surfaces to be stained are those which were separated by the knife. However, this method is not suitable in homogeneous tissue, such as many tumour or lymph tissues, as cell-by-cell comparison can present a problem. If it is desired to see the reaction of one antigen-containing structure with another in the same preparation, other strategies must be adopted.

Double direct method (Brandtzaeg, 1983)

This method is based on using two primary antibodies labelled with different fluorophores, such as fluorescein and rhodamine. Each fluoroscein label is examined with different filters, so that an excess of one antigen does not obscure or confuse localization of the other. Photographs of the two labels on the same frame will show areas of colocalization in a mixed colour.

Double indirect method

In this method, the primary antibodies may be unlabelled and detected by two different, labelled, secondary antibodies. In this case, the primary antibody should be raised in a different species and the detecting antibody should be free of species cross-reactivity. Alternatively, the two primary antibodies could be monoclonal of different Ig subclasses or heavy-chain types, with non-cross-reacting secondary antibodies. In both these methods, enzymes or other markers could be substituted for the fluorescent label.

Double or multiple immunostaining with elution
(Nakane, 1968)

This method is based on the principle that a first antigen can be detected and then the entire Ag/ab complex is eluted from the tissue with glycine–HCl buffer. This will leave, for example, a brown product, and then a second stain is carried out for another antigen. The second antigen–antibody reaction will be developed by another chromogen, for example α-naphthol and pyronine to give a red end-product. However, this method requires a large number of controls to ensure that each entire antigen–antibody complex has been removed before the next sequence is carried out. There is also the problem that high-affinity antibodies are hard to detach from their antigens.

Double staining without elution
(Joseph & Sternberger, 1979)

This method is based on developing two antigen–antibody complexes which will be developed differently. This is suitable when the two antigens to be localized are present in separate cells, because the strong staining of the first reaction may mask any staining for a second antigen on the same side.

Double or multiple immunoenzymatic staining
(Mason & Sammons, 1978)

A double immunoenzymatic staining method which avoids the problems of elution and can allow two antigens to be demonstrated in the same location is described by Mason and Sammons (1978). It consists of the simultaneous application of two primary antibodies, raised in different species, say rabbit and mouse, to two antigens. The second layer consists of two species of Ig-class-specific detecting antibody to Ig (for example, goat and rabbit Ig and goat and mouse Ig). Either these antibodies are conjugated with different enzymes (e.g., perixodase and alkaline phosphatase) or they are unconjugated and the third layer of reagent, say rabbit APAAP and mouse APAAP, is applied. The two enzymes are developed separately to give differently coloured end-products, for example brown for perixodase and blue for alkaline phosphatase. The use of different development methods with different enzymes can result in a variety of single and mixed colours.

Interpretation of immunocytochemistry

Interpretation of an immunocytochemical stain takes into account the sources of false positivity and negativity discussed previously. Good analysis of immunostaining depends upon a final set of considerations, which include the site of synthesis—location of a substance to a given cell usually, but not always, indicates the site of synthesis. Other factors are stable expression, homogeneity of the staining and the significance of the staining.

Quantitative immunostaining

Quantitative immunocytochemistry is the determination of the concentration of an antigen at the light-microscopic level within tissue or cells or at the electron-microscopic level within cell compartments, in either relative or absolute terms. The concentration of an antigen is most easily assessed by estimating relative visual intensity of chromogenic labels. To determine optimal antibody or reagent concentrations in titration studies and to compare antibody efficiencies and sensitivities of different immunostaining protocols, such a semiquantitative method suffices. Several attempts have been made to quantify immunocytochemical reactions by image analysis. However, it has yet to be shown beyond any doubt that these approaches are suitable for quantitative immunocytochemistry. It is possible to quantify the number of cells that are expressing a particular antigen in a specific area, but this does not indicate the amount of antigen which is present in that tissue. Whatever the method to be used for quantitative immunocytochemistry, it should fulfil the following conditions: (i) all antibody–antigen enzyme–substrate reactions must be conducted in conditions where binding is saturated; (ii) the distribution of reagents must be homogeneous; (iii) the matrix and the antigen density should have a predictable effect on immunostaining intensity; and (iv) quantification should be done objectively.

Electron-microscopical immunocytochemistry
(Polak & Varndell, 1984; Varndell & Polak, 1984)

This technique is used to identify antigen at subcellular levels. Among the first electron-microscopical immune labels was peroxidase. This method has now been largely replaced by the use of a colloidal gold labelling reagent, which has several advantages. In particular, the fact that the gold particles can be produced in different sizes means that multiple immunoreactions can be performed on a single tissue section and identified at subcellular levels. As cells often produce more than one protein, multiple immunolabelling has been very useful, as also in the study of the post-translation processing of proteins. In cells which actively secrete their product or have a limited storage ability, immunocytochemistry and electron microscopy give a greater sensitivity than light microscopy. Another advantage of using electron-microscopical immunocytochemistry is that this technique gives precise information about the type of cells that are expressing a particular antigen. Counting gold particles over reactive sites might appear to be an easy method of quantifying an immunoreaction to measure the amount of antigen present in a preparation. However, there are many variables concerned with the fixation, processing, composition of the batch of resin, labelling of the reagent and concentration of the antibodies relative to antigen that affect the amount of labelling on the specimen.

Electron-microscopical immunocytochemistry is not an easy technique to be performed routinely. There are a number of practical aspects to be considered, including fixation, embedding media, adequacy of sectioning, labelling of the antibody and processing of the tissue. Immunolabelling controls are of the same importance in electron-microscopical as in light-microscopic immunocytochemistry. They are of three orders: reagent controls, negative controls and positive controls. High background labelling is a common problem in electron-microscopic immunocytochemistry; it prevents the assessment of a specific labelling and false-negative labelling is not uncommon in this technique.

Conclusion

It is impossible in a short chapter to give a full account of all the immunocytochemical methods that have been and are being used to achieve highly specific localization of cell products and other substances *in situ*. However, a large number of references are available for detailed protocols and more practical applications (Polak & Van Noorden, 1983; Bullock & Petrusz, 1985).

References

Bastin, J., Kirkley, J. & McMichael A.J. (1982) Production of monoclonal antibodies: a practical guide. In: *Monoclonal Antibodies in Clinical Medicine* (eds A.J. McMichael & J.W. Fabre), pp. 503–17. Academic Press, London.

Bondi, A., Chieregatti, G., Eusebi, V., Flucheri, E. & Bussolati, G. (1982) The use of β-galactosidase as a tracer in immunohistochemistry. *Histochemistry*, **76**, 153–8.

Brandtzaeg, P. (1983) Tissue preparation methods for immunocytochemistry. In: *Techniques in Immunocytochemistry*, Vol. 1 (eds G.R. Bullock & P. Petrusz), pp. 1–75. Academic Press, New York.

Bullock, G.R. & Petrusz, P. (eds) (1982) *Techniques in Immunocytochemistry*, Vol. 1. Academic Press, New York.

Bullock, G.R. & Petrusz, P. (eds) (1983) *Techniques in Immunocytochemistry*, Vol. 2. Academic Press, New York.

Bullock, G.R. & Petrusz, P. (eds) (1985) *Techniques in Immunocytochemsitry*, Vol. 3. Academic Press, New York.

Cammisuli, S. & Wofsy, L. (1976) Hapten sandwich labelling. III. Bifunctional reagents for immunospecific labelling of cell surface antigens. *J. Immunol.*, **117**, 1695–704.

Coggi, G., Dell'Orto, P. & Viale, G. (1986) Avidin–biotin methods. In: *Immunocytochemistry*, 2nd edn (eds J. Polak & S. Van Noorden), pp. 54–70. Wright, Bristol.

Coons, A.H., Creech, H.J. & Jones, R.N. (1941) Immunological properties of an antibody containing a fluorescent group. *Proc. Soc. Exp. Biol. Med.*, **47**, 200–2.

Coons, A.H., Leduc, E.H. & Connolly, J.M. (1955) Studies on antibody production. I. A method for the histochemical demonstration of specific antibody and its application to a study of the hyperimmune rabbit. *J. Exp. Med.*, **102**, 49–60.

Cordell, J.L., Falini, B., Erber, W.N. *et al.* (1984) Immunoenzymatic labeling of monoclonal antibodies using immune complexes of alkaline phosphatase and monoclonal anti-alkaline phosphatase (APAAP complexes). *J. Histochem. Cytochem.*, **32**, 219–29.

Cuello, A.C. (ed.) (1983) *Immunohistochemistry*. John Wiley & Sons, Chichester.

De Mey, J. & Mocremans, M. (1986) Raising and testing polyclonal antibodies for immunocytochemistry. In: *Immunocytochemistry*, 2nd edn (eds J. Polak & S. Van Noorden), pp. 3–12. Wright, Bristol.

Galfre, G. & Milstein, C. (1981) Preparation of monoclonal antibodies: strategies and procedures. *Methods Enzymol.*, **73B**, 3–46.

Gu, J., De Mey, J., Moeremans, M. & Polak, J.M. (1981) Sequential use of the PAP and immunogold staining methods for the light microscopical double staining of tissue antigens. *Reg. Peptides*, **1**, 365–74.

Holgate, C.S., Jackson, P., Cowen, P.N. & Bird, C.C. (1983) Immunogold–silver staining — new method of immunostaining with enhanced sensitivity. *J. Histochem. Cytochem.*, **31**, 938–44.

Joseph, F.A. & Sternberger, L.A. (1979) The unlabeled antibody method: contrasting color staining of β-lipotropin and ACTH-associated hypothalamic peptides without antibody removal. *J. Histochem. Cytochem.*, **27**, 1430–7.

Kohler, G. & Milstein, C. (1975) Continuous cultures of fused cells producing antibodies of predefined specificity. *Nature*, **256**, 495–7.

Larsson, L.-I. & Schwartz, T.W. (1977) Radioimmunocytochemistry—a novel immunocytochemical principle. *J. Histochem. Cytochem.*, **25**, 1140–6.

Legocki, R. & Verma D. (1981) Multiple immunoreplica technique: screening for specific proteins with a series of different antibodies using one polyacrylamide gel. *Anal. Biochem.*, **111**, 385–92.

Mason, D.Y. & Sammons, R.E. (1978) Alkaline phosphatase and peroxidase for double immunoenzymatic labelling of cellular constitutents. *J. Clin. Pathol.*, **31**, 454–62.

Nakane, P.K. (1968) Simultaneous localization of multiple tissue antigens using the peroxidase-labeled antibody method: a study in pituitary glands of the rat. *J. Histochem. Cytochem.*, **16**, 557–60.

Oi, V.T., Glazer, A.N. & Stryer, L. (1982) Fluorescent phycobiliprotein conjugates for analyses of cells and molecules. *J. Cell Biol.*, **93**, 981–6.

Pearse, A.G.E. (1985) *Histochemistry, Theoretical and Applied*, Vol. 2. *Analytical Technology*, 4th edn. Churchill Livingstone, Edinburgh.

Polak, J.M. & Van Noorden, S. (eds) (1983) *Immunocytochemistry: Practical Applications in Pathology and Biology*. Wright, Bristol.

Polak, J.M. & Varndell, I.M. (eds) (1984) *Immunolabelling for Electron Microscopy*. Elsevier Science Publishers, Amsterdam.

Pruss, R.M., Mirsky, R., Raff, M.C., Thorpe, R., Dowding, A.J. & Anderton, B.H. (1981) All classes of intermediate filaments share a common antigenic determinant defined by a monoclonal antibody. *Cell*, **27**, 419–28.

Ritter, M. (1986) Raising and testing of monoclonal antibodies for immunocytochemistry. In: *Immunocytochemistry*, 2nd edn (eds J. Polak & S. Van Noorden), pp. 3–12. Wright, Bristol.

Roth, J. (1982) Applications of immunocolloids in light microscopy: preparation of protein A–silver and protein A–gold complexes in their application for the localization of single and multiple antigens in paraffin sections. *J. Histochem. Cytochem.*, **30**, 691–6.

Sternberger, L.A. (1979) *Immunocytochemistry*, 2nd edn. John Wiley & Sons, New York.

Straus, W. (1982) Imidazole increases the sensitivity of the cytochemical reaction for peroxidase with diaminobenzidine at a neutral pH. *J. Histochem. Cytochem.*, **30**, 491–3.

Suffin, S.C., Muck, K.B., Young, J.C., Lewin, K. & Porter, D.D. (1979) Improvement of the glucose oxidase immunoenzyme technic. *Am. J. Clin. Pathol.*, **71**, 492–6.

Symington, J., Green, M. & Brackmann, K. (1981) Immunoautoradiographic detection of proteins after electrophoretic transfer from gels to diazo-paper: analysis of adenovirus encoded proteins. *Proc. Nat. Acad. Sci. USA*, **78**, 177–81.

Titus, J.A., Haugland, R., Sharrow, S.O. & Segal, D.M. (1982) Texas red, a hydrophilic, red-emitting fluorophore for use with fluorescein in dual parameter flow microfluorimetric and fluorescence microscopic studies. *J. Immunol. Methods*, **50**, 193–204.

Vandesande, F. (1979) A critical review of immunocytochemical methods for light microscopy. *J. Neurosci. Methods*, **1**, 3–23.

Varndell, I.M. & Polak, J. (1984) Double immunostaining procedures: techniques and applications. In: *Immunolabelling for Electron Microsocpy* (eds J.M. Polak & I.M. Varndell), pp. 155–77. Elsevier Science Publishers, Amsterdam.

Wang, B.-L. & Larsson, L.-I. (1985) Simultaneous demonstration of multiple antigens by indirect immunofluorescence or immunogold staining. *Histochemistry*, **83**, 47–56.

Wick, G., Traill, K.N. & Schauenstein, K. (eds) (1982) *Immunofluorescence Technology: Selected Theoretical and Clinical Aspects.* Elsevier Biomedical Press, Amsterdam.

CHAPTER 46

Polymerase Chain Reaction

C.J. Corrigan

Basic principles

The polymerase chain reaction (PCR) is a technique for the *in vitro* amplification of specific DNA sequences by the simultaneous primer extension of complementary strands of DNA. The modern PCR technique was devised and named by Mullis and Faloona (1987), although the principle had been described in detail over a decade earlier. The use of PCR was limited until heat-stable DNA polymerase became widely available. The PCR is a major development in the analysis of DNA and RNA, because it allows the amplification of specific sequences from very small amounts of complex mixtures of nuclear acids.

The technique is in essence one of primer extension, utilizing the action of the enzyme DNA polymerase, which catalyses the synthesis of the DNA molecule, whose sequence is directed by the strand being copied, which is known as the template strand. Extension always occurs in a 5′ to 3′ direction and requires the prior annealing of a short oligonucleotide primer. This primer extension reaction forms the principle for a variety of labelling and sequencing techniques using DNA polymerase.

The PCR uses the same principle, but employs two primers, each complementary to the opposite strands of the region of the DNA to be amplified, which have been denatured by heating. The primers are arranged so that each primer extension reaction directs the synthesis of DNA towards the other. Thus, one primer directs the synthesis of a strand of DNA, which can then be primed by the other primer and vice versa. This results in the *de novo* synthesis of the region of DNA flanked by the two primers.

The basic requirements for the reaction are simple: deoxynucleotides (dNT) to provide both the energy and the nucleosides for the synthesis of DNA, DNA polymerase, primer, template and buffer containing magnesium. The dNT and primers are present in large excess, so that the synthesis step can be repeated by heating the newly synthesized DNA to separate the strands and then cooling to allow the primers to anneal to their complementary sequences on the new strands (Fig. 46.1). Initially, synthesis will go beyond the sequence complementary to the other primer, but with each cycle of heating and cooling, the amount of DNA in the region flanked by each primer will increase exponentially, while longer sequences will only accumulate in a linear fashion, provided that the amount of starting DNA is present in limiting quantities. Thus, after several cycles, the predominant reaction product will be that piece of DNA which is flanked by the primers, including the sequences of the primers themselves.

The heating and cooling cycles can be repeated, and DNA will continue to accumulate exponentially until one of the reaction products is exhausted or the enzyme is unable to synthesize new DNA quickly enough. The numbers of cycles required for suitable amplification vary according to the amount of starting material and the efficiency of each amplification step. Generally, 25–35 cycles should be sufficient to amplify up to 1 μg of DNA of a single-copy human sequence from 50 ng of starting DNA. A final incubation step at the extension temperature (usually 72°C; see below) results in fully double-stranded molecules from all nascent products.

The reaction occurs in three steps (Fig. 46.1).

1 *Denaturation*. In this step, the strands of DNA double helix are separated by heating the reaction mixture to

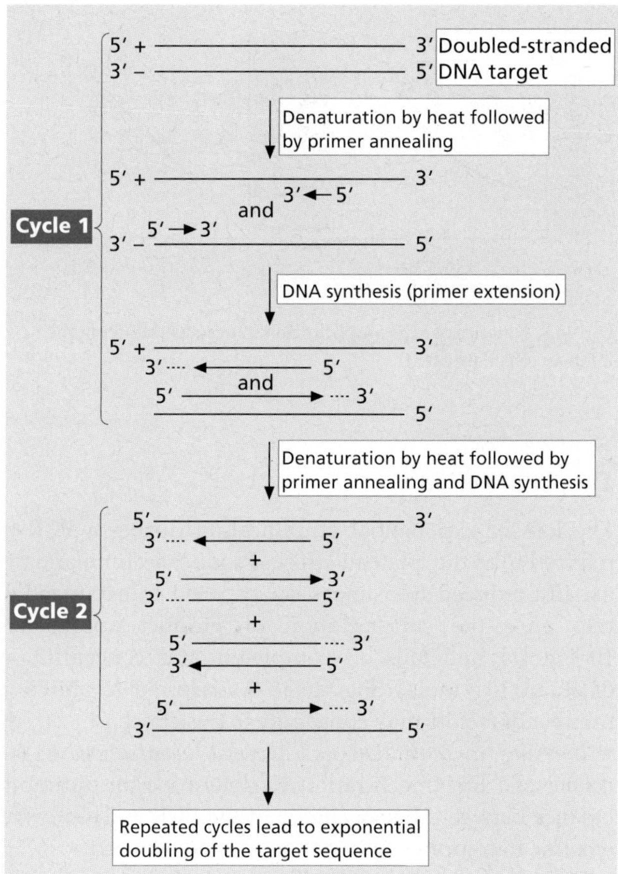

Fig. 46.1 Schematic diagram of the polymerase chain reaction amplification procedure.

94°C. This breaks the hydrogen bonds between bases on complementary strands.

2 *Annealing*. In this step, the temperature is lowered, so that a sequence-specific oligonucleotide primer, as described above, can hybridize to the target DNA, provided that the conditions are suitable.

3 *Extension*. During this step, the annealed primers allow the DNA polymerase enzyme to incorporate nucleotides and extend the nascent DNA molecule, as instructed by the sequence of the target, template DNA. This eventually results in the synthesis of new primer binding sites.

Thus, after one round of amplification there is an effective doubling of the numbers of copies of target sequence. By repeated cycles of denaturation, annealing and extension there is a theoretical exponential increase in the numbers of target sequences until one or other of the reaction components becomes rate-limiting, as described above. Products from previous cycles serve as templates for subsequent cycles.

The widespread use of PCR has depended on the availability of thermostable DNA polymerases (i.e. those whose DNA polymerase activity is retained despite repeated rounds of heating to high temperatures in the denaturation steps). Such enzymes have been isolated from thermophilic viruses and bacteria, notably the organism called *Thermus aquaticus*, from which Taq polymerase is derived. Taq polymerase is optimally active at 72°C, which is the temperature generally chosen for the extension step in the PCR cycle. Although relatively resistant to heat, the enzyme does lose activity at higher temperatures; for example, it has a half-life of 40 minutes at 95°C.

The technique has been automated, with the development of a wide variety of 'thermocyclers'. The design of these machines is essentially similar. Heating in most devices is by a conventional heating element, which is in contact with a metal block that holds the reaction tubes. The metal block is designed to take thin-walled polypropylene reaction tubes of 500 μl capacity. Other blocks can be adapted for larger tubes or microtitre plates. Heating rates are generally about 1 or 2°C/second, and in some machines this ramp rate can be controlled. Methods for cooling the blocks vary between machines. Some machines use a conventional refrigerant, while others use solid-state cooling, which cools slightly faster over the range of 95–50°C. Both of these approaches mean that a reaction product can be stored at 4°C, which facilitates reactions that are set to run overnight. Machines that use water or air as a coolant cannot offer this facility unless connected to a separate refrigeration unit. All machines offer programming facilities in excess of what is really necessary. The minimum that is required is the facility to select three different temperatures for denaturation, annealing and extension in the range of 25–100°C, each with an incubation time in the range of 1 second to 1 hour, and the ability to cycle through these temperatures and times at least up to 40 times. A final extended incubation step at 72°C helps complete the synthesis of all nascent products before analysis, as mentioned above. An initial denaturation period of approximately 5 minutes prior to addition to enzyme is also useful. Some machines offer the opportunity to control more than one heating block independently, which is an advantage for the simultaneous running of PCR cycles requiring differing incubation times and annealing temperatures.

The exponential nature of PCR amplification

Under theoretical conditions the amount of product doubles during each cycle of the PCR (exponential amplification). This may be represented by the equation:

$$N = N_0 2^n$$

where N is the final number of DNA molecules, N_0 is the starting number of molecules and n is the number of cycles of amplification employed (Fig. 46.2). In practice, however, the efficiency of amplification is less than perfect and is more realistically described as:

$$N = N_0(1 + E)^n$$

where E is the efficiency of amplification. Experimentally E has been found to vary from 0.46 to 0.99, depending on the DNA sequence being amplified and the precise reaction conditions. Because of the exponential nature of PCR, a very small change in E can result in dramatic differences in the amount of product, N, even if the initial number of target molecules, N_0, remains the same. Several factors may affect the efficiency of amplification, including the following.

- The sequence being amplified.
- The sequence of the primers.
- The length of the sequence being amplified.
- Impurities in the sample.

The first three of these factors are important because they affect secondary structure formation and the G/C content of the target sequence, both of which may interfere with primer binding, influence the melting-point of the target sequence and reduce the processivity of the polymerase. There is some controversy concerning whether differences in target sequence lengths significantly alter E; in two reports, a weak inverse correlation was observed (Coker *et al.*, 1990; Golde *et al.*, 1990), whereas in a third report E did not vary with target length (Chelly *et al.*, 1988). In addition, variations in E have also been observed when the same DNA molecule is amplified under identical conditions in separate tubes (Gilliland *et al.*, 1990; Kellogg *et al.*, 1990). This phenomenon, called 'the tube effect', is a critical factor to be considered when developing a quantitative PCR protocol (see below).

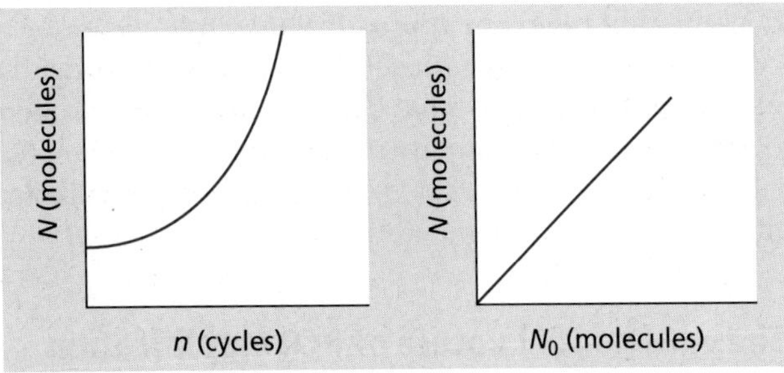

Fig. 46.2 Theoretical kinetics of PCR amplification (see text). Left: the amount of product, N, increases exponentially with the number of cycles (n). Right: for a given number of cycles, the amount of product is linearly related to the starting quantity of template (N_0).

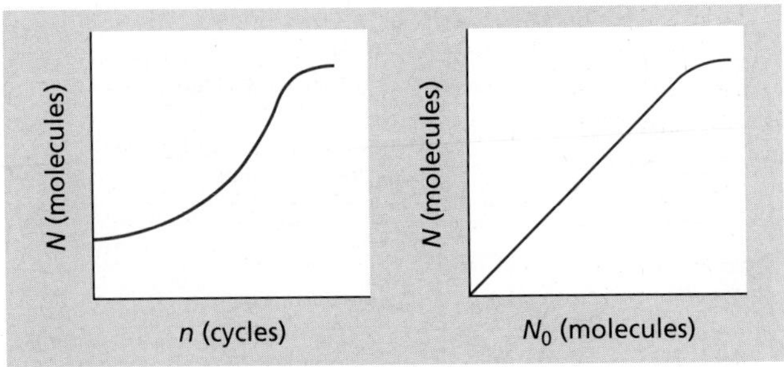

Fig. 46.3 Kinetics of PCR amplification in practice, showing the 'plateau effect' (see text).

The plateau effect

The loss of exponential amplification during a PCR is referred to as the 'plateau effect'. Product accumulation is usually reduced to a linear, as opposed to exponential, rate once the concentration of product approaches 10^{-8} mol/l, and tails off completely at a concentration of about 10^{-7} mol/l (Fig. 46.3). As referred to above, a number of factors may contribute to this effect.

- *Limiting concentration and thermal inactivation of Taq polymerase*. Enzyme titration to determine an optimum balance between the specificity of the PCR and sufficient enzyme to complete the reaction may be required.
- *Reduction in denaturation efficiency*. As the concentration of the target DNA increases, so does its melting temperature. Efficient denaturation at high target DNA concentrations is optimized by the use of thin-walled polypropylene reaction tubes.
- *Accumulation of enzyme inhibitors*. Accumulation of DNA polymerase reaction products, such as pyrophosphates, may inhibit the activity of the DNA polymerase.
- *Inefficiency of primer annealing*. As the concentration of the target DNA increases, the efficiency of annealing between the priming sequences and the target DNA increases, owing to an increased tendency of the target duplex DNA to reanneal to itself (Erlich *et al.*, 1991). If the PCR conditions are suboptimal and mispriming occurs, once the concentration of the major product has reached a plateau, the product resulting from mispriming and originally present at low concentration can then accumulate exponentially. For this reason, it is important to limit the numbers of cycles of the PCR.

PCR components

A PCR mix typically contains the components shown in Table 46.1, with an overlay of mineral oil to prevent evaporation, in a total volume of 30–100 μl.

Table 46.1 Components of a typical PCR reaction mix.

1 × PCR buffer	0.4 µmol/l 5′ (forward) primer
0.2 mmol/l dNTPs	0.4 µmmol/l 3′ (reverse) primer
200 ng BSA	2.5 U Taq polymerase
0.1% Triton X-100	Template DNA

See text for definition of abbreviations.

PCR buffer

Several suitable PCR buffers have been described. A typical buffer contains 50 mmol/l tris-HCl (pH 8.3 at 25°C), 50 mmol/l KCl and 5 mmol/l $MgCl_2$ (final concentrations). For this buffer ΔpK_a is –0.02/°C, so that during the PCR cycle the true pH of the reaction varies between 7.8 and 6.8. Potassium ions participate in primer annealing, although concentrations in excess of 50 mmol/l tend to inhibit Taq polymerase activity, and some buffers dispense with potassium ions completely, replacing these with 16 mmol/l ammonium sulphate. The concentration of magnesium ions in the buffer has the potential to affect many aspects of the PCR, including enzyme activity and fidelity, primer annealing, formation of primer dimers (see below) and the formation of non-specific products. The effects of varying magnesium concentrations with specific primers and templates are very difficult to predict, and it is preferable to establish optimal magnesium concentrations empirically in the range of 1–5 mmol/l. Commercial suppliers of Taq polymerase-like enzymes often provide supplementary solutions of magnesium chloride which can be added to the buffer, so that the final magnesium concentration can be altered within this range. Kits for optimizing magnesium concentrations for a particular set of primers and target DNA are also commercially available. Too little magnesium ion will result in little or no product, while too much may encourage non-specific amplification.

Deoxynucleoside triphosphates

Each of these (deoxyadenosine trychosphate, deoxyguanosine triphosphate, deoxycytidine triphosphate, deoxythymide triphosphate (dATP, dGTP, dCTP, dTTP)) must be present in equal concentrations. If dNTP concentrations are too high, this may contribute to the generation of non-specific PCR products and a reduction of the fidelity of the reaction.

Bovine serum albumin (BSA)

This acts as a carrier protein for the enzyme, which is used in the reaction at very low concentrations. A suitable alternative carrier is 0.01% gelatine.

Ionic and non-ionic detergents

Some detergent is essential in PCR to maximize the processivity of the enzyme: 0.1% Triton X-100, 0.01% NP-40 or 0.01% Tween 20 are all suitable.

Primers

These are included in the reaction at excess, equal concentrations typically in the range 0.1–1 µmol/l. Optimal concentration must be determined empirically. A detailed discussion of optimal primer design is given below under 'Primer design'. If primers are present at too high concentrations, this may result in the generation of non-specific products.

Template DNA

The DNA used for the template in PCR does not need to be highly purified. PCR can be performed directly from bacterial lysates, or from supernatants generated from soil, food and archival material stored in pathological archives and museums. Some substances, however, are known to inhibit the reaction, such as porphyrin, phenol and Ca^{2+}-chelating compounds.

DNA polymerase enzymes used in the PCR

The DNA polymerase isolated from *T. aquaticus*, known as Taq polymerase, is widely used for most PCR. It is a 94 kDa protein. Although it is said to have a relatively low processivity and fidelity of base incorporation, in practice this amounts to approximately only one misincorporation per 50 000 nucleotides. This enzyme exhibits 5′ → 3′ exonuclease activity but lacks 3′ → 5′ exonuclease activity, and therefore has no proofreading facility. The half-life of the enzyme is approximately 130 minutes at 92.5°C, 40 minutes at 95°C and 5 minutes at 97.5°C. The so-called 'Stoffel fragment' of Taq polymerase is also available for PCR. This is a synthetic protein which incorporates the active domain of Taq polymerase but lacks the amino-terminal 289 amino acids. It is more thermostable than Taq polymerase and less sensitive to magnesium ion concentrations in the buffer. A DNA polymerase isolated from the organism *Thermus thermophilus* has higher incorporation fidelity than Taq polymerase and is particularly suitable for gene cloning and sequencing. Other DNA polymerases isolated from *T. thermophilus* exhibit reverse transcriptase activity in the presence of manganese ions, in addition to DNA polymerase activity in the presence of magnesium ions. These enzymes are useful for performing reverse transcription of mRNA prior to PCR amplification without the need for a separate intermediate step.

PCR conditions

The selection of times, temperatures and the numbers of cycles used depends on the particular primer–template set and the initial concentration of the template. In general, for higher-fidelity amplification and the prevention of non-specific products, it is important to keep the number of cycles and the reaction times during each step to a minimum. Typically, 25–40 cycles are required for 10^6-fold amplification of a template DNA.

Denaturation

Generally 94°C for 1 minute is sufficient. Lengthening of this period or raising of the denaturation temperature markedly reduces the lifespan of the Taq polymerase, although an initial denaturation period of 5 minutes is often included at the commencement of the amplification cycle.

Annealing

The optimal annealing temperature depends both on the salt concentration of the buffer and the G + C base content of the primers. If the annealing temperature is too high, the primers will not anneal to the template and the PCR will fail or be very inefficient. Too low a temperature, on the other hand, may allow non-specific priming events and the generation of non-specific products. As a rule of thumb, the approximate melting temperature of an oligonucleotide in °C is given by 4 × (numbers of G + C bases) + 2 × (numbers of A + T bases) – 5. Computer programs are now available to predict annealing temperatures more accurately, although they may also be determined empirically. An annealing time of 30 seconds should be adequate for most primers unless they are particularly long.

Extension

An extension temperature of 72°C is standard. The time allowed for extension should be 1 minute/kb of target DNA. For most short amplified sequences, therefore, an extension time of 1 minute is more than adequate, although this may need to be lengthened if amplification of very long template sequences is attempted.

Primer design

PCR primers are oligonucleotides hybridizing to opposite strands flanking the region of interest in the template DNA. It is useful to bear the following points in mind when designing PCR primers.

- The optimal primer size is 18–30 nucleotides. For a primer composed of 18 nucleotides, the probability that its sequence will occur at random is 4^{18}, or 1 in 7×10^{10}. Since the size of the human genome is 3×10^9 nucleotides, the probability of an oligonucleotide of 18 base pairs cross-reacting randomly with a non-specific DNA sequence in the genome other than the sequence being amplified is extremely remote.
- Avoid complementary bases at the 3′ ends of the primers. This can result in primers binding together during the PCR, resulting in 'primer dimers'.
- The G + C base content of the primers should be at least 50% of the total bases, and both primers should have similar percentages of G + C bases. This will ensure that the annealing temperatures of both primers are similar.
- Avoid palindromes within the primers, which can give rise to secondary structures and inhibit annealing.
- Avoid long runs of single bases.
- Unless it is specifically intended to amplify long regions of target DNA, the distance between the forward and reverse primers should be preferably less than 1 kb.
- For amplification of complementary DNA (cDNA) reverse-transcribed from mRNA (see section on 'Reverse transcription PCR'), it is preferable that the primers span a genomic intron, so that amplification of cDNA and contaminating genomic DNA can be distinguished on the basis of the size of the product. When the cDNA has been primed with oligo(dT) (see under 'Reverse transcription PCR'), the primer location defines the distance that the cDNA must be extended from the 3′ end of the mRNA to provide the 5′ primer template. It is advisable to choose 5′ primer regions no further than 2–3 kb from the 3′ end of the mRNA.
- Primer sequences are synthesized and conventionally written in a 5′ → 3′ direction. Therefore, when specifiying the 3′ primer, this should be designed as the complement and written in the opposite direction to that of the DNA sequence as written.

Non-template, complementary 5′ extensions may be added to primers to allow a variety of useful post-amplification manipulations of the PCR product without significant effect on the amplification itself. These 5′ extensions can be restriction sequences, promoter sequences, etc.

Detection and verification of the amplified PCR product

Several methods are commonly used to detect and quantify amplified PCR products. The simplest approach is to measure the incorporation of labelled nucleotides or primers into PCR products resolved by gel electrophoresis. Other strategies for verification and quantification of PCR products are based on hybridization. The most common of the methods is to probe a Southern blot of the

(a)

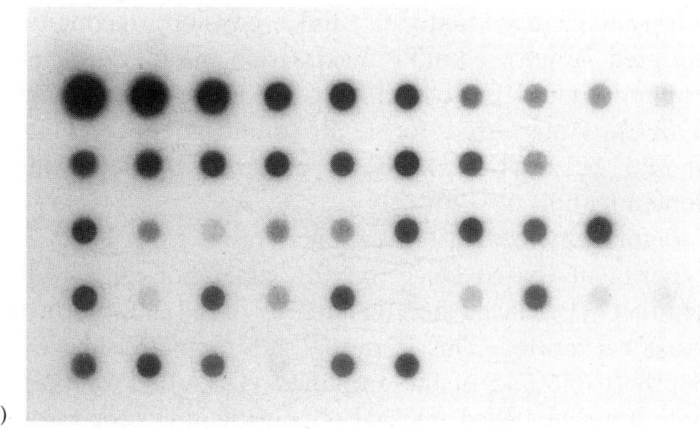

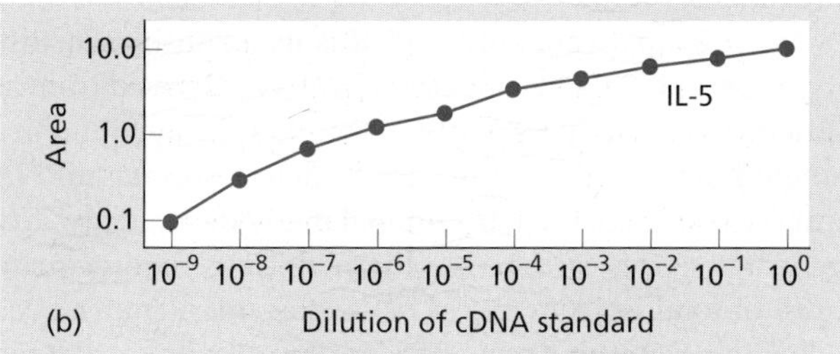

Fig. 46.4 Detection of PCR-amplified DNA template sequences by Southern blotting (in this case interleukin 5 (IL-5)). Top row: amplification of serial 10-fold dilutions (left to right) of standard IL-5 cDNA template demonstrating exponential and non-saturating amplification of the template under the conditions used. Bottom four rows: amplification of reverse-transcribed mRNA encoding IL-5 from clinical specimens. The PCR products have been blotted on to nitrocellulose and probed with an end-labelled, IL-5-specific internal oligonucleotide.

PCR products, using a radiolabelled 'internal' probe designed to hybridize to a unique sequence within the amplified target DNA (Fig. 46.4). To quantitate the amount of probe hybridized, the blot can either be exposed to X-ray film and the resulting autoradiogram densitometrically scanned (Fig. 46.4), or the product can be excised from the blot and its radioactivity measured in a scintillation counter. Because the probe will hybridize only to the amplified product, this method offers the advantage of detecting only the correct product and not non-specific products.

Alternative hybridization methods which avoid Southern blotting have also been utilized (Kellogg *et al.*, 1990; Jalava *et al.*, 1993; Pannetier *et al.*, 1993). One approach uses capture and hybridization of biotinylated PCR products on streptavidin-coated microtitre plates. Another method employs solution hybridization between a radiolabelled probe and denatured PCR products. The hybridized probes are resolved by gel electrophoresis and subsequently quantified by scintillation counting.

Several additional methods exist for quantifying PCR products. They include measurements of the ethidium bromide luminescence of PCR products resolved by gel electrophoresis (Nakayama *et al.*, 1992), use of high-performance liquid chromatography (Katz & Dong, 1990) and assays based on *in vitro* transcription with radiolabelled ribonucleotide substrates (Horikoshi *et al.*, 1992).

Reverse transcription PCR

The process of reverse transcription PCR (RT-PCR) extends the ability of the PCR technique to detect specific mRNA sequences in body fluids or tissues. This can be used for the detection of ongoing gene transcription. Most techniques currently in use employ the properties of reverse transcriptase, an enzyme isolated from retroviruses which has the ability to catalyse the synthesis of a cDNA molecule upon an RNA template. Like all DNA polymerases, reverse transcriptase extends in a $5' \rightarrow 3'$ direction and requires the presence of a previously annealed oligonucleotide primer to initiate synthesis. Total cellular RNA for RT-PCR analysis is typically extracted from body fluids or tissues, or cell pellets or monolayers, by guanidium isothiocyanate solubilization of the cells. The resulting lysate may be layered over a CsCl cushion and ultracentrifuged, when the RNA forms a pellet (Chirgwin *et al.*, 1979). Another technique not requiring ultracentrifugation involves co-extraction with phenol at acid pH to remove protein and DNA (Chomczynski & Sacchi, 1987). This latter technique forms the basis of several commercially available kits for RNA extraction, such as 'TRI reagent' and 'RNAzol'.

When isolating RNA from small amounts of tissue or cells, a carrier nucleic acid such as transfer RNA (tRNA) (Brenner *et al.*, 1989) or polyinosinic acid (Winslow & Henkart, 1991) may be added at the beginning of the extraction to facilitate handling of the RNA and to improve the yield. To ensure optimal RT-PCR, all RNA preparations should be examined by denaturing agarose gel electrophoresis. If the RNA is intact, it will exhibit clear 28S and 18S ribosomal RNA (rRNA) bands, with the 28S band about twice as intense as the 18S band. Isolated RNA is best stored as an ethanol precipitate at –20°C.

There are three ways to prime RNA for cDNA synthesis (Fig. 46.5).

1 Priming with oligo(dT). This method is used most commonly. A 12–18 base oligo(dT) nucleotide anneals to the poly(A) tail of mRNA, thus serving as a primer for reverse transcription of the entire mRNA population in the total cellular RNA. It is rarely necessary to isolate mRNA from the total cellular RNA prior to amplification by RT-PCR.

2 Random priming with short (typically hexamer) oligonucleotides having all possible nucleotides at each position, which anneal to RNA at random sites and thereby prime cDNA synthesis.

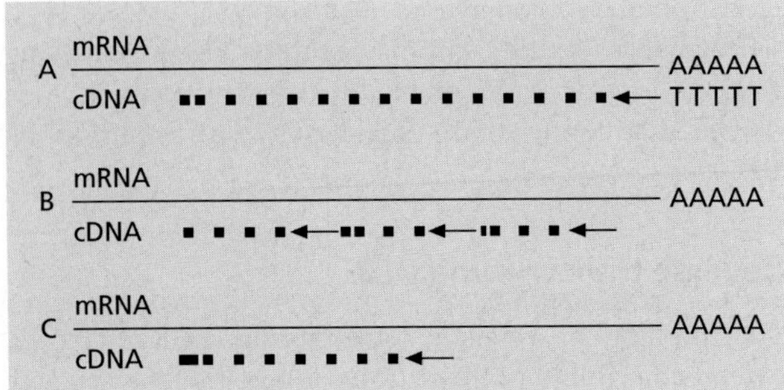

Fig. 46.5 Synthesis of cDNA from mRNA molecules. (a) Oligo(dT)$_{12–18}$ priming, where annealing occurs to the poly(A) tail of mRNA, resulting in reverse transcription of the entire population of mRNA molecules from a cell or tissue. (b) Random priming with short (typically hexamer) random oligonucleotides, which anneal to corresponding sequences in the mRNA molecules and initiate cDNA synthesis. (c) Gene-specific priming, where an antisense gene-specific oligonucleotide is annealed to the mRNA and extended with reverse transcriptase. This same primer (along with a suitable 5′ primer) may be used for subsequent PCR amplification.

Table 46.2 Typical reaction mixture for reverse transcription of total cellular mRNA.

1 × RT buffer	5 μg oligo(dT)$_{12–18}$
0.6 mmol/l dNTPs	20 U placental RNase inhibitor
200 ng BSA	38 U AMV reverse transcriptase
5 mmol/l dithiothreitol	

See text for definition of abbreviations.

3 Specific priming, using a 3′ primer specific for the sequence of the mRNA of interest. This 3′ primer, along with a suitable 5′ primer, can also be used for subsequent PCR amplification.

A typical reaction mixture for reverse transcription of total cellular RNA using oligo(dT) primers is shown in Table 46.2. The buffer used for reverse transcription can be the same as used for the PCR described above. Ribonuclease (RNase) inhibitor is included to inhibit the intrinsic RNase activity of the reverse transcriptase enzyme. The most commonly used reverse transcriptase enzymes are those derived from avian myeloblastosis virus (AMV) and Maloney murine leukaemia virus (MMLV). Before reverse transcription, the RNA solution is heated to 65°C for 5 minutes and then quenched on ice in order to denature the RNA. The reaction components are then incubated at 42°C (MMLV) or 37°C (AMV) for 1 hour. The resulting reverse-transcribed cDNA can be used directly for PCR analysis. Typically, less than one-fortieth of the total reverse transcription mix may be used as a template for subsequent PCR.

In RT-PCR, both nucleic acid and RNase contamination must be controlled. As a general rule, gloves should be worn and changed frequently and a semisterile technique adopted. Water used in RNA extraction and reverse transcription should be treated with diethylypyrocarbonate (DEPC). Water used for PCR amplification reactions should be filter-sterilized to minimize nucleic acid contamination.

Before any conclusion can be drawn from RT-PCR experiments based solely on the generation of a PCR product of predicted size, the identity of the PCR product must be verified. This is most easily accomplished by Southern blotting of the amplified cDNA and probing with a radiolabelled internal oligonucleotide probe (see previous section).

The principal value of RT-PCR is its exquisite sensitivity. Experimental data suggest that cDNA derived from as little as 6 pg of total RNA (the amount typically found in a single human cell) is sufficient to detect specific mRNA transcripts. In contrast, traditional methods for analysis of gene transcripts, such as Northern blotting, require quantities of total RNA in excess of several micrograms, even when the examining gene transcripts are expressed at relatively high concentrations. It is simply not possible to extract such large quantities of RNA from small samples of cells or tissues. In addition, RT-PCR enables rapid, simultaneous detection of multiple mRNA transcripts from a single sample.

Determination of mRNA concentrations in cells and tissues by quantitative PCR

It is useful to be able to compare the concentrations of mRNA encoding specific proteins, either in body tissues *in vivo* following experimental manipulations or therapy, or in cultured cells after experimental manipulations *in vitro*. Since the RT-PCR technique produces a high degree of amplification of the original numbers of reverse-transcribed mRNA sequences originally present in a tissue, and since this amplification is potentially subject to spurious variability, it is clearly critical to ensure, and moreover to demonstrate, that reverse transcription and amplification of different target cDNA sequences are comparable between PCR.

Most commonly, internal standards are used to control for variations in amplification efficiency and to determine absolute concentrations of mRNA. It is possible, however, to perform quantitative PCR without the use of internal standards if two conditions are met. Firstly, tube-to-tube variability in the amplification efficiency (E) must be minimal so that it can be assumed constant (see section on 'The exponential nature of PCR amplification). Secondly, measurements must be made before amplification begins to reach the plateau phase (same section, 'The plateau effect'). Under such conditions, there should be a linear relationship between the logarithm of the concentrations of the PCR products, and the logarithm of the initial concentrations of the target sequence:

$N = N_0(1 + E)^n$

Thus:

$\log N = n[\log(1 + E)] + \log N_0$

For the purpose of relative comparison of quantities of RNA in samples, the variables N and N_0 may be replaced respectively by A, the amount of amplified product (in counts per minute (cpm) or OD_{260} units), and A_0, the starting amount of total RNA (µg) or cDNA (ng). Thus:

$\log A = n[\log(1 + E)] + \log A_0$

which predicts a linear relationship between $\log A$ and $\log A_0$ (Fig. 46.6). Such a relationship has been demonstrated empirically for values of A ranging over two to three orders of magnitude (Abbott *et al*., 1988; Rappolee *et al*., 1988; Singer-Sam *et al*., 1990).

The standard curve generated during exponential product accumulation can be used to compare A_0 between samples (Singer-Sam *et al*., 1990). This analysis has been used to compare relative changes in mRNA levels in single samples, either by plotting $\log A_0$ against log A and comparing values of log A at a given A_0 falling within the linear part of the curve (Fig. 46.7(a)) (Singer-Sam *et al*., 1990), or by plotting A for a number of consecutive amplification cycles (n) for two samples (Fig. 46.7(b)) (Salomon *et al*., 1992). In this case, a value of n is chosen where the two curves are nearly parallel (suggesting equal values of E), and the value of log A for this n is extrapolated from each curve. At this point, the difference between the values of log A is directly proportional to the difference in $\log A_0$ (and hence N_0) between the two samples. This method therefore determines the difference, but not the actual numbers, of starting target molecules between two samples. Analysis of amplification by these techniques is necessary for quantitative PCR to show not only that exponential amplification of products has occurred but also that amplification has not reached a plateau. These methods are still limited, in the sense that they can only compare differences between samples. They do not give an indication of the actual initial concentration of the target cDNA in the samples. Further, they do not control for variability in the amplification efficiency (E) between different samples.

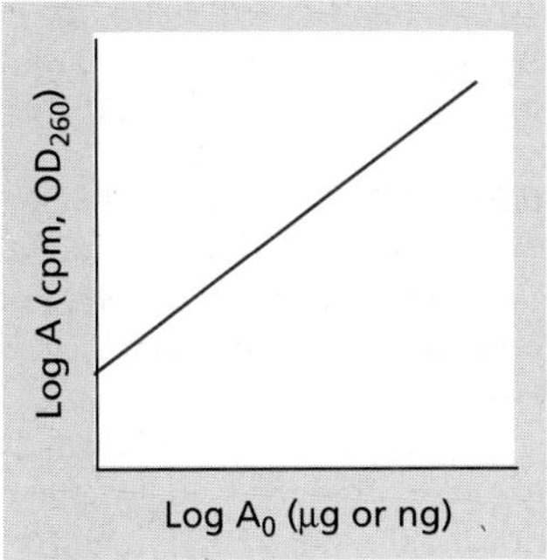

Fig. 46.6 The theoretical relationship between the amount of product, A, and the starting amount of the target sequence, A_0, during polymerase chain amplification (see text).

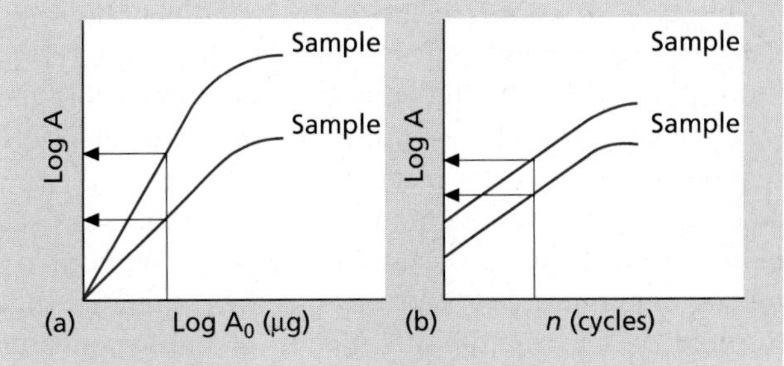

Fig. 46.7 Relative differences in the initial amount of target template cDNA in two samples determined (a) by titration, where serial dilutions of starting cDNA (A_0) are amplified for a given number of cycles, or (b) by kinetic analysis, where similar starting concentrations of template cDNA are amplified for increasing numbers (n) of cycles. In each case the relative concentrations of amplified product (A) can be compared during the exponential phase of amplification (see text).

In order to address the problem of variability in amplification efficiency (E), two types of internal standard, endogenous and exogenous, have been employed, as discussed below.

Endogenous internal standards

In this technique, the amplification of target cDNA is compared with the amplification of cDNA encoding a 'housekeeping gene', such as β-actin or glyceraldehyde-3-phosphate dehydrogenase. It is implicit in this technique that the expression of the 'housekeeping gene' is relatively invariable, an assumption which may not always be justified (Siebert & Fukuda, 1984). The 'housekeeping gene' cDNA is amplified, using a second pair of gene-specific primers, along with the cDNA of the target sequence in contemporaneous reactions in either the same or different reaction tubes. A product ratio between the amplified target and standard cDNA is measured, and data must be obtained before amplification of either the standard or the target cDNA reaches a plateau. The main advantage of this technique is that the standard and target mRNA are isolated and reverse-transcribed together, which acts as a control for variability arising from these two steps. The principal potential flaw with this technique is in the assumption that the concentration of mRNA encoding 'housekeeping genes' does not change following experimental manipulations.

This type of approach has been experimentally validated by performing PCR on mixtures of cDNA (Horikoshi *et al.*, 1992). Although theoretically it is possible and would seem desirable to amplify the target and standard sequences in the same reaction tube, interference may be observed when more than one set of primers is used in the same PCR. For example, addition of both β_2-microglobulin and *mdr-1* primers to the same PCR tube resulted in a premature attenuation of the exponential amplification phase of both PCR products (Murphy *et al.*, 1990). For this reason most researchers use a separate reaction tube for each primer set. The cause of this interference is obscure.

Many examples of the use of endogenous mRNA standards to determine relative concentrations of specific mRNA are to be found in the literature (Chelly *et al.*, 1988; Murphy *et al.*, 1990; Noonan *et al.*, 1990). We have used this technique in our own laboratory to compare relative concentrations of mRNA encoding cytokines in peripheral-blood T lymphocytes from asthmatics and controls (Doi *et al.*, 1994). It is most important when using this technique to obtain measurements of *A* before the amplification reactions reach the plateau phase, especially when the relative degrees of expression of the standard and target sequences differ greatly. For example, in one study (Murphy *et al.*, 1990) amplification of cDNA from β_2-microglobulin mRNA entered the plateau phase before the target, *mdr-1* mRNA, was even detectable.

Exogenous internal standards: competitive PCR

In this technique, an exogenous template is used as an internal standard. The internal standard and target cDNA are designed to have the same primer binding sites, and thus compete with each other for amplification when mixed in the same tube. The exogenous standard template may be a synthetic RNA added to the reverse transcription reaction or a synthetic DNA which would not normally be present in the target sample. The standard, which is of known concentration, is added at serial dilutions to a constant amount of target cDNA and then both are amplified by PCR. The standard and target amplification products can be distinguished, usually on the basis of size, and following amplification the products can be resolved by electrophoresis on an agarose gel. As an alternative to a completely synthetic standard, several reports have described the construction of exogenous RNA and DNA standards that differ from target sequences only by the presence or absence of small introns or restriction sites (Gilliland *et al.*, 1990; Ballagi-Pordany & Funa, 1991). With such standards it seems likely that the amplification efficiencies (*E*) of the standard and target sequences would be very similar. Furthermore, because the ratio of target to standard remains constant during the amplification, it is not necessary to obtain data before the reaction reaches the plateau phase.

If the amplification efficiencies, *E*, of the standard and target are identical, the ratio of standard to target cDNA will remain the same throughout the amplification. This has been confirmed empirically (Bouaboula *et al.*, 1992). Consequently, if the concentration of the standard is known, the concentration of the target can be measured by determination of that concentration of standard which, after amplification, produces an amount of product equal to that of the target (Fig. 46.8). Even this, however, is a minimum estimate, since it assumes that the reverse transcription step is 100% efficient. This problem has been addressed further by using internal RNA standards which are simultaneously reverse-transcribed along with the target mRNA.

In order to generate an RNA standard, an RNA polymerase promoter and a poly(A) tail can be incorporated into the PCR product, using composite primers designed for this purpose. *In vitro* transcription of the PCR product generates synthetic RNAs that contain the target primer sequences and a poly(A) tail. RNA samples can then be titrated with the RNA standard prior to reverse transcription. Transcriptional promoters have been successfully incorporated into PCR products using this technique (Horikoshi *et al.*, 1992) and used to generate competitive RNA fragments (Henvel *et al.*, 1993).

Conclusion

The techniques of PCR and RT-PCR are highly sensitive and specific methods for detecting and quantifying DNA

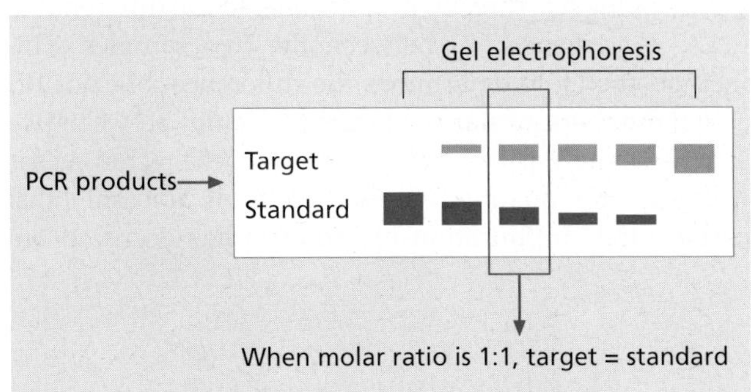

Fig. 46.8 Competitive PCR with exogenous standards. A dilution series of the standard is added to a constant amount of the target cDNA. Following amplification, samples of the amplified products are resolved by gel electrophoresis and their yields quantified by gel scanning. The relative amounts of target and standard product are assumed to be equal in that reaction where the molar ratio of target and standard (competitor) products is equal (after correction for size differences). Because the absolute initial amount of standard is known, the absolute initial amount of target can be inferred. If the competitor standard is a synthetic RNA, a dilution series of this standard is added to a constant amount of sample RNA prior to reverse transcription.

and mRNA from very small samples. The ability to obtain accurate measurements of gene expression in small amounts of tissue or in mixed cell populations will considerably expand our present knowledge of the pathogenesis of many inflammatory processes, not least allergic inflammation and asthma.

A fuller discussion of the entire range of investigations and experimental manipulations which may be performed using PCR lies outside the scope of this volume. The interested reader is encouraged to review new literature in the principal journals mentioned in the references. In addition, several good textbooks are now available on the subject.

References

Abbott, M.A., Poiesz, B.J., Byrne, B.C., Kwok, S., Sninksy, J.J. & Erlich, G.D. (1988) Enzymatic gene amplification: qualitative and quantitative methods for detecting proviral DNA amplified *in vitro*. *J. Infect. Dis.*, **158**, 1158–69.

Ballagi-Pordany, A. & Funa, K. (1991) Quantitative determination of mRNA phenotypes by the polymerase chain reaction. *Analyt. Biochem.*, **196**, 89–94.

Bouaboula, M., Legoux, P., Pessegue, B. *et al.* (1992) Standardisation of mRNA titration using a polymerase chain reaction method involving co-amplification with a multi-specific internal control. *J. Biol. Chem.*, **267**, 21830–8.

Brenner, C.A., Tam, A.W., Nelson, P.A. *et al.* (1989) Message amplification phenotyping (MAPPing): a technique to simultaneously measure multiple mRNAs from small numbers of cells. *Bio Techniques*, **7**, 1096–103.

Chelly, J., Kaplan, J.C., Maire, P., Gautron, S. & Kahn, A. (1988) Transcription of the dystrophin gene in human muscle and non-muscle tissues. *Nature*, **333**, 858–60.

Chirgwin, J.M., Przbyla, A.E., MacDonald, R.J. & Rutter, W.J. (1979) Isolation of biologically-active ribonucleic acid from sources enriched in ribonuclease. *Biochemistry*, **18**, 5294–9.

Chomczynski, P. & Sacchi, N. (1987) Single-step method of RNA isolation by acid guanidium thiocyanate–phenol–chloroform extraction. *Anal. Biochem.*, **162**, 156–9.

Coker, G.T., Studelska, D., Marman, S., Burke, W. & O'Malley, K.L. (1990) Analysis of tyrosine hydroxylase and insulin transcripts in human neuroendocrine tissues. *Mol. Brain Res.*, **8**, 93–8.

Doi, S., Gemou-Engesaeth, V., Kay, A.B. & Corrigan, C.J. (1994) Polymerase chain reaction quantification of cytokine messenger RNA expression in peripheral blood mononuclear cells of patients with acute exucerbations of asthma: effect of glucocorticoid therapy. *Clin. Exp. Allergy*, **24**, 854–67.

Erlich, H.A., Gelfand, D. & Sninsky, J.J. (1991) Recent advances in the polymerase chain reaction. *Science*, **252**, 1643–51.

Gilliland, G., Perrin, S., Blanchard, K. & Bunn, H.F. (1990) Analysis of cytokine mRNA and DNA: detection and quantitation by competitive polymerase chain reaction. *Proc. Nat. Acad Sci. USA*, **87**, 2725–9.

Golde, T.E., Estus, S., Uslak, M., Younkin, L.H. & Younkin, S.G. (1990) Expression of β-amyloid protein precursor mRNAs: recognition of a novel alternatively spliced form and quantitation in Alzheimer's disease using PCR. *Neuron*, **4**, 253–67.

Henvel, J.P.V., Tyson, F.L. & Bell, D.A. (1993) Construction of recombinant RNA templates for use as internal standards in quantitative RT-PCR. *Bio Techniques*, **14**, 395–8.

Horikoshi, T., Danenberg, K.D., Stadlbauer, T.H.W. *et al.* (1992) Quantitation of thymidilate synthase, dihydrofolate reductase and DT-diaphorase gene expression in human tumours using the polymerase chain reaction. *Cancer Res.*, **52**, 108–16.

Jalava, T., Lehtovaara, P., Kallio, A., Ranki, M. & Soderlund, H. (1993) Quantification of hepatitis B virus DNA by competitive amplification and hybridisation on microplates. *Bio Techniques*, **15**, 134–7.

Katz, E.D. & Dong, M.W. (1990) Rapid analysis and purification of polymerase chain reaction products by high performance liquid chromotography. *Bio Techniques*, **8**, 546–54.

Kellogg, D.E., Sninksy, J.J. & Kwok, S. (1990) Quantitation of HIV-1 proviral DNA relative to cellular DNA by the polymerase chain reaction. *Analyt. Biochem.*, **189**, 202–8.

Mullis, K. & Faloona, F. (1987) Specific synthesis of DNA *in vitro* via a polymerase-catalyzed chain reaction. *Methods Enzymol.*, **155**, 335.

Murphy, L.D., Herzog, C.E., Rudick, J.B., Fojo, A.T. & Bates, S.E. (1990) Use of the polymerase chain reaction in the quantitation of *mdr-1* gene expression. *Biochemistry*, **29**, 10351–6.

Nakayama, H., Yokoi, H. & Fujita, J. (1992) Quantification of mRNA by non-radioactive RT-PCR and CCD imaging system. *Nucl. Acids Res.*, **20**, 4939.

Noonan, K.E., Beck, C., Holzmayer, T.A. *et al.* (1990) Quantitative analysis of MDR1 (multidrug resistance) gene expression in human tumors by polymerase chain reaction. *Proc. Nat. Acad. Sci. USA*, **87**, 7160–4.

Pannetier, C., Delassus, S., Darche, S., Saucier, C. & Kourilsky, P. (1993) Quantitative titration of nucleic acids by enzymatic amplification reaction run to saturation. *Nucl. Acids Res.*, **21**, 577–83.

Rappolee, D.A., Mark, D., Banda, M.J. & Werb, Z. (1988) Wound macrophages express TGF-α and other growth factors *in vivo*: analysis by mRNA phenotyping. *Science*, **241**, 708–12.

Salomon, R.N., Underwood, R., Doyle, M.V., Wong, A. & Libby, P. (1992) Increased apoliprotein E and *c-fms* gene expression without elevated interleukin 1 or 6 mRNA levels indicates selective activation of macrophage functions in advanced human atheroma. *Proc. Nat. Acad. Sci. USA*, **89**, 2814–18.

Siebert, P. & Fukuda, M. (1984) Induction of cytoskeletal vimentin and actin gene expression by a tumor-promoting phorbol ester in human leukemic cell line. *J. Biol. Chem.*, **260**, 3868–74.

Singer-Sam, J., Robinson, M.O., Bellve, A.R., Simon, M.I. & Riggs, A.D. (1990) Measurement by quantitative PCR of changes in HPRT, PGK-1, PGK-2, APRT, Mtase and Zfy gene transcripts during mouse spermatogenesis. *Nucl. Acids Res.*, **18**, 1255–9.

Winslow, S.G. & Henkart, P.A. (1991) Polyinosinic acid as a carrier in the microscale purification of total RNA. *Nucl. Acids Res.*, **19**, 3251–3.

APPENDIX

Allergy

Editor's note: The following is a translation of von Pirquet's original article, as it appeared in Gell, P.G.H. & Coombs, R.R.A. (eds) (1963) *Clinical Aspects of Immunology*. Blackwell Scientific Publications, Oxford.

In the course of the last few years a number of facts have been collected which belong to the domain of Immunology but fit poorly into its framework. They are the findings of Supersensitivity in the immunized organism.*

These two terms clash with each other. Do we not regard an organism as immune if it is protected against the disease, is not attacked by it a second time? How can this organism at the same time be supersensitive to the same disease?

Already v. Behring had sensed this contradiction when he described as a 'paradoxical reaction' the death of animals hyperimmunized against tetanus when they were subsequently injected with a small dose of the same toxin.

However, the term 'paradox' can only be accepted in an exceptional case. But the deeper we penetrate into this field, the more closely is it found to obey a definite law. Already a large number of diseases is known in which evidence of supersensitivity has been obtained. Among them are the following:

Tetanus (v. Behring, Kretz), Tuberculosis (Courmont, Strauss and Gamaleia, Babes and Proca, Detre-Deutsch, B. Schick, Löwenstein and Rappaport, Möller, Löwenstein and Ostrowsky), Syphilis (Finger and Landsteiner), Diphtheria (Rigt), Serum sickness (Arthus, v. Pirquet and Schick, Lehndorff, Otto, Rosenau and Anderson), bacteria in general, organ extracts, various proteins, hay fever (A. Wolff-Eisner).

But are Immunity and Supersensitivity really connected with each other, or should one distinguish the processes in which pre-treatment causes immunity, from those in which it leads to supersensitivity?

A. Wolff-Eisner† would insist on such a separation: those processes in which toxins are implicated would lead to the production of antibodies and to immunity; those in which the active agent is an endotoxin to supersensitivity.

Yet from the experience with tetanus it is already evident that in pure antitoxic processes supersensitivity can occur. Wolff-Eisner's objection that it occurs only as an exception, does not seem to me to meet the principle of the problem.

Richet‡ was the first to recognize the significance of supersensitivity, which he called Anaphylaxis. He discovered that his actinia poison produced, at the same time, both immunity and anaphylaxis. If the poison was re-injected after a suitable interval, the animals mostly died acutely; but if they had survived the first shock, they overcame the disease more rapidly than the control animals receiving their first shock injection.

v. Pirquet and Schick§ have come to similar conclusions from their study of Serum sickness: following the re-injec-

* See v. Pirquet und Schick Üeberempfindlichkeit und beschleunigte Reaktion. *Münch. med. Wochenschr.* 1906, 2.

† *Zentralbl. f. Bakteriolog.* 37 (1904); *Münch. med. Wochenschr.* 1906, No. 5; *Das Heufieber*. München: Lehmann (1906).

‡ *Archivio di Fisiologia*, 1904, p. 129. *Soc. de biologie*. 21.1.1905.

§ *Wien. klin. Wochenschr.* 1903, Nos. 26, 45; 1905, No. 17. *'Die Serumkrankheit'*, Wien, Deutike, 1905.

tion of serum the symptoms run a more stormy but a shorter course.

Recently Rosenau and Anderson* have shown that in spite of the very high level of supersensitivity acquired by the guinea-pig after injection of a minute quantity of horse serum, this is nevertheless accompanied by certain processes of immunity. For if instead of giving a single first injection the horse serum is injected for 10 days running, the animal injected ten times will not succumb to the subsequent re-injection of horse serum, whilst the animal pre-injected only once will die.

The relations between immunity and supersensitivity seem to me most clearly exemplified by what is seen in vaccination.† A recently vaccinated individual appears supersensitive as compared with a person receiving his first vaccination, for he reacts far more quickly to the infection; yet at the same time he is protected, for in him the disease process extends only over a small localized area, and he is spared all generalized symptoms. Very similar observations have been made quite recently by Finger and Landsteiner‡ in the case of syphilis. At any stage of the disease re-inoculation has a pronounced effect: this occurs more rapidly than after the primary inoculation (shortened period of incubation). In tertiary syphilis a local erythema may even develop immediately after the re-inoculation; this is equivalent to the 'immediate reaction' seen after repeated serum injection.

'Immunity' and Supersensitivity can therefore be most closely interrelated.

And yet these two terms contradict each other, their union is a forced one. In fact, the concept of immunity has been carried on since a time when supersensitivity was unknown.

As F. Hamburger§ has pointed out, the specific change which an animal undergoes after an experimental disease is almost as often an increase in susceptibility as a raised power of resistance.

What we need is a new generalized term, which prejudices nothing but expresses the change in condition which an animal experiences after contact with any organic poison, be it animate or inanimate.

The vaccinated person behaves towards vaccine lymph, the syphilitic towards the virus of syphilis, the tuberculous patient towards tuberculin, the person injected with serum towards this serum, in a different manner from him who has not previously been in contact with such an agent. Yet he is not insensitive to it. We can only say of him that his power to react has undergone a change.

For this general concept of a *changed reactivity* I propose the term *Allergy*. 'Allos' implies deviation from the original state, from the behaviour of the normal individual, as it is used in the words Allorhythmia, Allotropism.

The vaccinated, the tuberculous, the individual injected with serum becomes *allergic* towards the corresponding foreign substance. A foreign substance which by one or more application stimulates the organism to a change in reaction is an *Allergen*. This term—not quite in accordance with philological usage — traces its origin to the word Antigen (Detre-Deutsch) which implies a substance capable of giving rise to the production of antibody. The term Allergen is more far reaching. The allergens comprise, besides the antigens proper, the many protein substances which lead to no production of antibodies but to supersensitivity. All the agents of infectious diseases which are followed by immunity are allergens. Among the allergens should be included the poisons of mosquitoes and bees in so far as their stings are followed by hypo- or hypersensitivity. For this reason we may also enrol under this term the pollen causing hay fever (Wolff-Eisner), the urticaria-producing substances of strawberries and crabs, and probably too a number of organic substances leading to idiosyncrasy.

The term Immunity must be restricted to those processes in which the introduction of the foreign substance into the organism causes no clinically evident reaction, where, therefore, complete insensitivity exists; may this be due to alexins (natural immunity), antitoxins (active and passive immunity in diphtheria and tetanus), or even to some kind of adaptation to a poison (Wassermann and Citron).

The new names do not conflict with the nomenclature in use up to now. The well-defined concepts of antitoxins, cytolysins, haemolysins, precipitins, agglutinins, coagulins are not affected thereby. Supersensitivity is a new field of research where only in the last few years new concepts have been evolved under laborious adaptation to the old names. From the need to clarify these conceptions I propose the new terms; I hope that by simplifying the outer form I will have made it easier for new research workers to study the interesting phenomena in this field.

C. von Pirquet
Imperial and Royal Paediatric Clinic of the University of Vienna

* 'A study on the cause of sudden death following the injection of horse serum.' *Hyg. Lab. U.S. Pub. Health and Mar. Hosp. Serv., Washington*, 1906, Bull. No. 29.

† v. Pirquet: *Verhandlungen der Gesellschaft deutscher Naturforscher und Aerzte*, Kassel, 1903; *Wien. klin. Wochenschr.* 1906, No. 28. *Klinische Studien über V akzination und vakzinale Allergie*. Wien, Deutike, 1906 (to be published shortly).

‡ Sitzungsbericht der Kais. Akad. d. Wiss. in *Wien. M.-N. Klasse*, April 1906.

§ 'Eine energetische Vererbungstheorie'. 22. *Kongr. f. innere Medizin*, Wiesbaden, 1905.

Editor's note

Clemens von Pirquet had a profound influence on the early development of the field of allergy. In 1906 he coined the term 'allergy'. He also introduced the tuberculin skin test as a diagnostic tool. The skin scarifier for von Pirquet tuberculin testing is shown in the illustration. The instrument was given by von Pirquet to Carl Prausnitz who subsequently gave it to Robin Coombs. Professor Coombs kindly donated it to the editor of this volume.

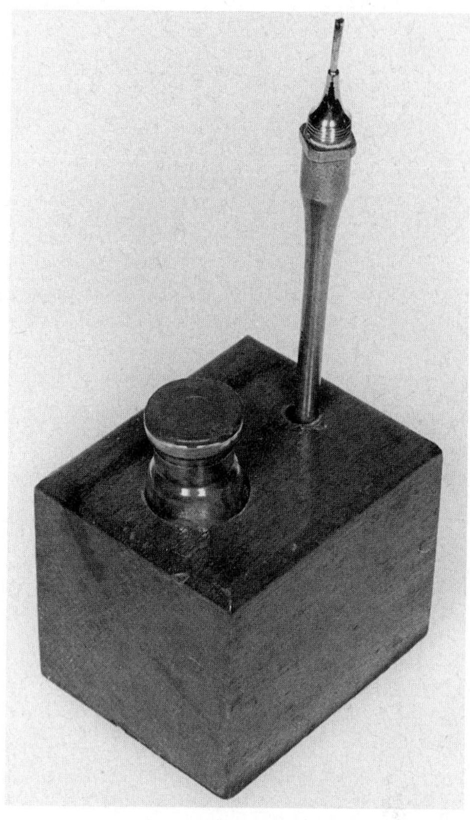

Index

A23187 381–2
A-64077, *see* zileuton
AA-2414, bronchial hyperresponsiveness and effects of 404
abalone 971
abietic acid, *see* colophony
absorption, airway, inflammation affecting 444–6
acaricides, dust mite control 1284, 1711, 1719
accessory cells for culturing T cells 757
  for antigen presentation 755–6
Accuhaler 1444
acetylcholine 488–9
  bronchial responsiveness in rats to 1071, 1072
  enhanced release in asthma 491
  neuropeptide tyrosine and 464
  receptors, *see* muscarinic receptors
  VIP and 459–60, 489
  see also cholinergic nervous system
acetylcysteine and its salts mucolytics 721–2
acetylsalicylic acid, *see* aspirin
achalasia of oesophagus 468
acid aerosols 1395–7
  epidemiology of allergic disease in children related to 1402–3
  laboratory studies 1398
acid anhydrides 916–17
acid particulates 1396
  epidemiology of allergic disease related to
    adults 1400
    children 1402–3
acid phosphatase, honey-bee 930–1
acid protease as allergen 804
acoustic rhinometry 1296, 1303
acrivastine
  in rhinitis 1333
  in urticaria (chronic) 1595
acrylates 921
actin 741
Actinomycetes, thermophilic 880, 880–1
  in hay 869
  pathology
    allergic alveolitis 866
    bagassosis 870
  structure/function 859, 860–1
activator protein-1, *see* AP-1
acupuncture in exercise-induced asthma 701
acute allergic reactions/inflammation
  dendritic cells in 237–8
  primate (monkey) model 252, 292, 1038–40
  rat model 1070
  as type I hypersensitivity 29, 30
  see also specific diseases
addressins 1386
  mucosal, *see* MAdCAM-1
adenoidectomy 1641
adenosine
  airway response in asthmatics 683, 1085
  nucleotides containing, *see* cADP ribose, neutrophil; AMP; ATP
adenylate cyclase activating peptide, pituitary, *see* pituitary adenylate cyclase activating peptide
adhesion (to endothelium), leucocyte (and adhesion molecules/receptors) 244–62, 286–94, 372
  in allergic inflammation (in general) 250–6, 272–4, 287–92, 292–4, 1121
    antagonists of adhesion receptors 252–3
    expression of adhesion receptors 250–2
    in murine model of contact dermatitis 1060
    in primate model 1040, 1042
    in rat model 1073–4
    specificity and selectivity of adhesion processes with each of cell types involved 287–9
  in asthma 272–4, 287–8, 289–90, 292, 293–4, 1372–3
    adhesion-molecule blockers in therapy 1733
    in late response 1121, 1372–3
  chemokines and 372
  migration of leucocytes and role of 253–6, 287–9
    eosinophil migration 42, 173–4, 288–9
  neutrophil adhesion to endothelium 201–3
  in nose
    in late-phase reaction 1150
    in rhinitis 1318, 1319
  soluble adhesion molecules 252
  steroid effects on adhesion molecule expression 620–1
  structure and function of receptors 244–50
  TNF-α and 346
  see also endothelial cells
adjuvant factors in airway sensitization 1370–71, 1717–18
adolapin 931
cADP ribose, neutrophil 206
adrenal cortex, *see* hypothalamic–pituitary–adrenocortical axis
adrenaline, anaphylactic shock treated with 1564–6, 1567–68
  immunotherapy-induced 1255
adrenergic nervous system 482–6, 488
  asthma and 483–6, 504, 568
  cholinergic traffic inhibited by 594
  innervation 482
  neurotransmitters 482–3
adrenoceptors 566–70
  adverse effects 576–8
  agonists 566, 569–78, 578
    mechanism of action 569–70
  alpha, *see* α-adrenoceptors
  beta, *see* β-adrenoceptors
  biology 568–70
  localization 566–8
  nasal 1302–3
  structure 568–9
advice about contact dermatitis 1627
aeroallergens, *see* inhaled allergens
aerosols
  acid, *see* acid aerosols
  hypertonic, *see* hypertonic/hyperosmolar aerosols
  hypotonic, airway response in asthmatics 683
aerosols in asthma treatment 728–39, 1440–50
  advantages 728
  β-adrenoceptor agonists 698–9
    pharmacokinetics 575–6
  calculation of drug delivery 729–31
  delivery systems

children 1460
currently available 731–2
effects with steroids 626
new 731–7
disadvantages 728–9
during inspiratory flow 736–7
in exercise-induced asthma 698–9
see also inhaled agents
affective disorders, *see* mood disorders
afferent pathways
in neuroimmune communication 506–8
nose 1303
vagal, in lungs 595
afferent phase of immune response 119–20
affinity chromatography of allergens 797
African maple 914
Ag (antigen from various species), *see* Antigen (from various species)
age
anaphylaxis severity and 1551
as atopy/atopic disease risk factor 1211–12
as drug allergy risk factor 1672
β-lactams 1684
muscle relaxants 1680
skin changes with 1007
see also elderly
Agostideae 842
agranulocytosis, drug-induced 1675
agriculture, *see* farming
AIDS, drug reactions with 1674, 1685
air
allergens carried in, *see* inhaled allergens
ambient, spore occurrence 862–4
in rats, responses to allergen challenge 1070–4
air-conditioning function, nose 1307–68
air-conditioning systems, microbes in, *see* ventilation pneumonitis
air filters 1719
air-flow, *see* flow
air pollution (pollutant/irritant gases) 1216–17, 1399–11, 1712, 1717–18
airway reactivity in response to 584
allergen interactions with 1397
asthma and 1216–17, 1395–411
occupational 1404, 1467–68
epidemiology of allergic disease and 1399–402, 1467–68, 1712
hayfever/pollen allergens and effects of 845, 1217, 1397
indoor 1403
see also smokers
laboratory studies 1397–9
sensitization and 1370–71, 1402–5, 1717–18
specific gases 1395–7
see also inhaled allergens; irritants
airway/respiratory tract (extrathoracic/upper) 1300–10
air pollutants affecting
adults 1401
children 1402–3
asthma distinguished from obstruction of 1355–6
asthma involving 672–3, 1308–9
nasal 1300–4, 1305–6, 1311–14
anatomy 1300–1, 1311–14
assessment of patency 1298, 1306–7
physiology 1306–8, 1311–14
in rhinitis 1314–18
otitis media and the anatomy of 1634
structure and function 1300–10
airway/respiratory tract (intrathoracic and in general)
absorption, inflammation affecting 444–6
acetylcholine receptor location 596
anaphylaxis 1530, 1561–3
acute management 1567–8
drug-related 1674
anatomy 263–4
antigen-induced response (in animal models)
guinea pig 1095–6
mouse 1061–4
primates 1038–43
rabbit 1081–8
rat 1070–4
sheep 1045–9
in asthma, *see* airway/respiratory tract in asthma
blood flow, *see* blood flow
calibre, *see* calibre
chronic obstructive disease, *see* chronic obstructive pulmonary disease
cytokines produced by various cells of 272
dendritic cells, *see* dendritic cells
drugs adversely affecting 1675
anticholinergic 602, 603
steroid 626
endothelin in 522–3
eosinophils, *see* eosinophil; eosinophilia; eosinophilic lung disease
epithelial cells, *see* epithelial cells
food hypersensitivity reactions 1529–31
function, tests, *see* lung function
heat loss, as stimulus to exercise-induced asthma 702
infection, *see* infection
lumen, *see* lumen
macrophages
distribution/types 228–9
function 230–4, 239–40
in late asthmatic response 1119
population dynamics 230
surface phenotype 229–30
nervous system, *see* nervous system
neuroendocrine regulation 505–6
neutrophilia, E-selectin and 252
occupational disease, *see* occupational disease
particles from aerosols in, *see* particles
plasma exudation, *see* plasma
smooth muscle, *see* smooth muscle
steroid effects on cells in 621–2
tachykinin effects 452–3
vasculature, *see* vasculature
water loss, as stimulus to exercise-induced asthma 699–700, 702, 703
see also reactive airway dysfunction syndrome *and specific regions/components*
airway/respiratory tract in asthma 263–83, 665–73, 1412–28
dimensions, quantitative comparisons 1362
eosinophils, *see* eosinophil; eosinophilia
hyperresponsiveness, *see* bronchial hyperresponsiveness
leukotriene effects 387–90
mucous secretions 389–90
narrowing (of lumen) 665–71
site of (and its determination) 668–71
see also bronchoconstriction; obstruction
pathology (in general) 1412–28
pathophysiology (in general) 161–2, 186, 264, 665–73
structural change/remodelling 298–9, 1364–5
in rabbit model 1087
wall
compliance, *see* compliance
remodelling, *see* structural change/remodelling (*subheading above*)
thickening 666, 1364, 1420
Alaska king crab allergens 913
AlaSTAT inhibition technique 1029
AlaSTAT Microplate 1027–8
AlaTOP 1017
albumin
in BAL fluid in asthmatics 443
bovine serum, in PCR 785
dog serum, as allergen 903–4
human serum, ethylene dioxide-altered 1558
rat serum, as allergen 904
see also conalbumin; ovalbumin; prealbumin
alcuronium anaphylaxis 1558
alder 847
alimentary tract, *see* gastrointestinal tract
alkaline phosphate (AP) in immunocytochemistry 776–7
and anti-AP 775
alkye resin industry 916–17
alkylamines 1330
allelic exclusion, Ig gene rearrangements and 69
allergen(s) 793–993
activity (of extracts)
conservation 826
total (potency) 829
air pollutants and
enhanced allergen responsiveness 1405–7
interactions 1397
in atopic dermatitis
detection 1583
in pathogenesis 1579–80
biochemical properties 795–808
influence on allergenic activity 805
cross-reacting 1017–26
β-lactams 1683, 1684
contact dermatitis and 1613–14, 1619
definition 1013
expected 1017–24
unexpected 1024–5
definition 1013
denaturing sprays 1719
epidemiology of exposure to 1215–16
extract(s)
activity, *see subheading above*
characterization 826–7
cockroach 946
declaration regarding 830
food 962
history 823
for immunotherapy 1244–5, 1286–7
latex 986–7
major allergen molecules in 826–7
preparation 825–6
quantification of allergen molecules 827
regulatory control 830
units 830
extraction/purification/characterization 79 7–8
genes, *see* genes
identification 796–7
by immunoassays, *see* immunoassays
immune response, *see* immune response
major, definition 1013
mixtures, in allergen tests 1017
nomenclature 796, 828
provocation tests, *see* allergen challenge
recombinant 809–22, 829
characterization 826
cloning of genes 809–14
for immunotherapy, number to be cloned 814–15
polymorphisms/variants 814, 816, 828
for standardization purposes 829
synthesis 815–19
see also specific recombinant allergens
reporter, definition 1013

as risk factor in asthma, exposure 1348–9
sensitization, *see* sensitization
sources 823–4
clinical sources 824
common 825
environmental factors affecting 824–5
identification, historical studies 18–19
related 824
standard(s) 828–9
standardization 828–9
for skin tests 1009–10
see also specific (types of) allergens
allergen avoidance 21, 1265, 1283–4, 1720–2
in asthma
children 1456, 1457
in chronic disease 1430
T cell and 1382
in atopic dermatitis 1579–80
in atopic keratoconjunctivitis 1661
bronchial hyperresponsiveness decreased by 685
cockroach 948, 949
extrinsic allergic alveolitis 1497–8
house-dust mite, *see Dermatophagoides pteronyssinus*
latex allergens 988–9
peanuts 1558
pollen 1328
in seasonal allergic conjunctivitis 1651
in rhinitis 1327, 1328
young children 1720–2
see also prevention
allergen challenge/provocation tests 1273
in asthma 186, 1355
drugs modulating effects of 403
cockroach allergens 949
food allergy, *see* food
in immunotherapy 1227–8
in anaphylactic patients 1567
insect venom 1698
plasma exudation response 442–3
urticaria (chronic) 1593
allergen-specific Th2 cells, role in pathogenesis of allergy 104–5, 141
allergen-specific treatment, *see* allergen avoidance; immunotherapy
allergic alveolitis, *see* alveolitis, extrinsic allergic
allergic blepharoconjunctivitis, contact 1661–2
allergic bronchopulmonary mycoses, *see* bronchopulmonary mycoses
allergic conjunctivitis, *see* conjunctivitis
allergic diseases (in general)
causes 49
children, *see* children
contact activation in 333–4
cost 1715
epidemiology, *see* epidemiology
with IgE-driven mechanisms 530
inflammation in, *see* inflammation (allergic)
interleukin-5 in 358–9
models, *see* animal models; human models
neutrophils and 200
pathogenesis of 36–7
allergen-specific Th2 cells in 104–5, 141
phosphodiesterase inhibitor effects 544–9
phosphodiesterases in, *see* phosphodiesterase
prediction 1715–16
prevention, *see* prevention
risk factor, skin test positivity as 1010–11, 1211, 1212
T cell cloning in determining cellular parameters of 760–1
treatment, *see* therapy
allergic encephalomyelitis, experimental, *see* encephalomyelitis
allergic eosinophilic gastroenteritis 1528, 1533
allergic granulomatosis and angiitis 1509–10
allergic persons in history 8
allergic response, *see* anaphylactic reactions
allergic rhinitis, *see* rhinitis, allergic
allergology (and allergological disease)
history/concepts in, diagnostic techniques 20–1
practice 1259–90
as specialty or subspecialty 1261
allergy
children, *see* children
concepts/definitions/terminology 23–35
education, *see* education
milestones in studies of 8–14
in non-specific polysymptomatic illness, role 1268–9, 1283
as otitis media risk factor 1633, 1639, 1640
skin test positivity as risk factor for, evaluation 1010–11
allergy clinic, *see* clinic
allotypes, Ig 61
almond 972
Alnus spp. 847
α-adrenoceptor(s) 483, 567–8
α_1 subtype 567, 568
α_2 subtype 567, 568
asthma and 484, 485–6
localization 567–8
α-adrenoceptor agonists 566, 571, 578
as nasal decongestants 1327–68
α-adrenoceptor antagonists 578–9
α heavy chain, structure 60
see also immunoglobulin A
α-subunits/chains
B cell antigen receptor, structure 73, 74
FcεRI 85–6
as therapeutic target 92
G proteins 742
GM-CSF receptor 354
integrins 247–8
in sheep model of asthma, antibodies to α_4-integrin 1050, 1052
interleukin-3 receptor 354
T cell receptor 1380
Alternaria spp. allergens 875–7
alternata 804, 872
recombinant, synthesis 819
immunotherapy 1237–8
tenuis, neonatal rabbit immunized with 1082–3
alternative therapies, *see* complementary therapies
Altounyan, Roger 22
alveolar macrophages, pulmonary 228–9
in asthma 289–90
depletion, immunological consequences 234
functions 230–4, 239–40
phosphodiesterase inhibitor effects 546–7
in rats challenged with inhaled ovalbumin 1070
surface phenotype 229–30
alveolitis, cryptogenic fibrosing 1496
alveolitis, extrinsic allergic (hypersensitivity pneumonitis) 1269
acute 1493–4, 1496
causes 1489–90
in agriculture, *see* farmer's lung
avian, *see* birds
diisocyanate 1478
fungal spores 866, 869, 1003, 1490
mushroom-workers 869
chronic 1494
clinical features 1493–4
diagnosis 1495–6
differential 1496–7
frequency 1490–1
immunopathogenesis 1492–3
management 1269, 1497–8
natural history/prognosis 1495
pathology 1491
Amaranthaceae 852
Amaranthus spp. 852
Ambrosia spp. (ragweed) pollen 853–4
allergens 801, 1020
canine sensitivity to 1105
cross-reactivity 1020
HLA and 1191
recombinant, synthesis 817–18
American Academy of Allergy and Immunology Aerobiology Committee, pollen/spore 841
Amersham General Hospital, contact allergens
hand and face series 1626
leg-ulcer series 1626
standard series 1622
amiloride in cystic fibrosis 722–3
amines
honey-bee 931
occupational exposure 920, 921
aminophylline in asthma 1285
ammoniated latex 982
sources 987
ammonium compounds, *see* quaternary ammonium compounds; tertiary ammonium compounds
amoxycillin
cephalosporins and, cross-reactivity 1683
reactions
incidence 1682–3
skin tests 1684
AMP, airway response in asthmatics 683
cAMP-responsive element binding (CREB) protein 619
immunosuppressive drugs affecting 644
steroid resistance and 632
cAMP-specific phosphodiesterases 532, 539–40
α-amylase
Aspergillus oryzae 803, 914, 1478, 1480
cereal 914
α-amylase inhibitor protein, wheat/barley 913–14
β-amylase, cereal 914
anaemia
drug-induced 1675
iron-deficiency 1534
anaesthetics, *see* general anaesthetics; local anaesthetics
anaphylactic reactions (immediate/type I/IgE-mediated hypersensitivity) 24, 1161–23
anaphylaxis and 1552–6
chironomid allergens 952–4
genetic aspects 957–8
drugs 1676
muscle relaxants 1680
radiocontrast media 1685
food allergens 1523, 1524
clinical features 1524–7
general principles 1161–23
H_1 receptor in 423–5
antagonists of 431–2
helminthic infection and beneficial effects of 1166–7
insect sting 1693–4
latex 1479
mechanisms 26, 28–9

occupational allergens 1470
anaphylactoid reactions 1558–9
dextran-induced, *see* dextran
anaphylatoxic activity of C3a/C4a/C5a 316
see also C3a; C4a; C5a
anaphylaxis (and anaphylactic shock) 1283, 1550–72
animal models
mouse 1058–9
rabbit 1088
causes (in general) 1550–1, 1551–60
children, immunotherapy-induced 1255
clinical and biochemical features 1561–3
definitions 1550–1, 1551–60
differential diagnosis 1563–4
drug reactions 1551, 1552–4, 1558, 1674
epidemiology 1551
food hypersensitivity reactions 1555–7
gastrointestinal 1525–7
respiratory 1530
historical perspectives 8, 1550–1
immunotherapy-induced, *see* immunotherapy
insect sting allergy 1554–5, 1557, 1567
knowledge of 1268
latex allergens 982, 985, 988, 1551, 1555
skin tests resulting in 987
management 1268, 1283, 1557, 1564–8
of acute attack 1567–8
by immunotherapy 1557, 1566–7
of immunotherapy-induced anaphylaxis 1254, 1255
mechanisms/pathogenesis 1551–60
multifactorial 1559
unknown 1559–60
preventive measures 1564, 1566
prognosis 1568–9
slow-reacting substance of, *see* leukotriene C_4; leukotriene D_4; slow-reacting substance of anaphylaxis
systemic/generalized, *see* systemic reactions/generalized anaphylaxis
Ancylostoma brasiliense 1505–6
androgen therapy, hereditary angioedema 1604
anergy, T cell clonal 38, 131–45
experimental induction 132–3
immunotherapy reversing 50–1
self-reactive peripheral T cells 134–6
angiitis, allergic granulomatosis and 1509–10
angioedema (giant urticaria) 1267–8, 1279, 1586–607
anatomical considerations 1587
angiotensin-converting enzyme inhibitor 1604
aspirin-induced 1687
classification 1588
definition 1586
differential diagnosis 1267, 1592
eosinophilia-associated 1604
food additives and 1593
immunotherapy-induced 1254
children 1255
management 1254, 1255, 1267–8
vibratory 1598–9
angioedema (giant urticaria), hereditary (C1 inhibitor deficiency) 318, 319, 332–3, 1267, 1558–9, 1602–3
anaphylaxis and, differentiation 1563–4
clinical features 1602–3
diagnosis/investigations 1004, 1603
kinin formation in 332–3
screening 1004
treatment 1267–9
acute attacks 1603–4
angiotensin-converting enzyme, tachykinin degradation by 448
angiotensin-converting enzyme inhibitor angioedema 1604
anhydrides 916–17
animal(s) (mainly implying large animals/mammals)
allergens from 803, 889, 900–8, 1023–4, 1275–6, 1711
cross-reactivity 1022–3
immunotherapy 1237, 1239
occupational exposure 910–11, 916, 1276, 1278, 1465, 1478
prevention of exposure 1711
recombinant, synthesis 817
young children exposed to 1718
gastrointestinal anaphylaxis 1525–6
oral tolerance studies 1521
stress-related immune function 508–9
see also pets *and specific animals*
animal models
of asthma (and allergic disease) 1035–110, 1387–8
canine 1103–10
endothelial cells and 292
guinea pig 1093–102
immunosuppressive agents in 654–5
mouse 1063–4
platelets and 218–19
rabbit 1079–92
of autoimmune disease 138, 1060–1
T cell receptor repertoire in 1385
of bronchoconstriction 1045–55
of hyperresponsiveness, *see* bronchial hyperresponsiveness
of ocular allergy 1649
of peripheral T cell tolerance 135
of sensitization involving air pollutants 1404
ant, *see* Formicidae
antihelminthics in helminth-related pulmonary eosinophilia 1504, 1505, 1506
anti-allergy drugs, *see* drugs (allergy-treating)
antibiotics
allergy with 1550–1, 1552–4, 1682–5
topical 1624
in otitis media 1641
see also specific antibiotics
antibody (applied use)
in allergen quantification 827
genetic engineering 63
IgE-specific (to allergens), detection/quantitation, *see* immunoassays
in immunocytochemistry 773–4
affinity 777
for multiple staining 779–80
non-specific immunoreactivity 777, 778
preparation/labelling 776–7
unlabelled 774–5
monoclonal, *see* monoclonal antibodies
antibody (Ig molecule functioning as)
autoimmune, *see* autoantibodies
class-specific differences 61–2
diversity, generation 69–71
membrane-bound forms, *see* membrane-bound Ig
antibody (structure/synthesis/genetics), *see* immunoglobulin
antibody-dependent hypersensitivity reactions, *see* cytotoxic hypersensitivity reactions
anticholinergics, *see* cholinergic antagonists
anticholinesterases reversing atropine toxicity 603
antifibrinolytics, hereditary angioedema 1604
antigen 113–30
binding to/affinity for antibody
affinity maturation 70
binding site 60–1
foreign/exogenous, *see* foreign antigen
in immunocytochemistry 773
accessibility 777
preservation 776
sensitivity depending on 777
internalization 76
presentation to T cells 113–30
accessory cells for (for T cell cultures) 755–6
cellular aspects 119–25
cyclosporin effects 648
molecular aspects 114–19
processing 113–30
cellular aspects 119–25
molecular aspects 14–19
receptor on B cells, *see* membrane-bound Ig
recognition by T cells 37–9, 114–19
molecules for 118–19
self-/endogenous, *see* self-antigen
tolerance to, *see* tolerance
see also Ag
antigen (from various species - Ag)
Alternaria alternata allergens) 872
Aspergillus fumigatus allergens 872, 878
Cavia porcellus allergens (Ag2) 905
Mus musculus allergens (Ag3) 904
rabbit (Ag R1) 905
shrimp (Ag1/2) 970
vespid venom (Ag5) 932, 937
antigen-presenting cells 38, 113
dendritic cells as 234, 238–9, 1069–70
efferent phase of immune response and 124–5
food allergy 1523
macrophages (pulmonary alveolar) as 232
nasal late-phase reaction and 1148
Th1-like vs Th2-like phenotype of, development towards 44
antiglobulin (Coomb's) test 20
antihelminthics in helminth-related pulmonary eosinophilia 1504, 1505, 1506
antihistamines, *see* H_1 receptor antagonists; H_2 receptor; H_3 receptor
anti-inflammatory drugs, *see also specific types*
chronic asthma 1431
phosphodiesterase inhibitors acting as 549–51
rhinitis 1333–7
anti-inflammatory proteins, steroids increasing synthesis of 620
anti-mast cell agents, *see* mast cell inhibitors
anti-myeloperoxidase antibody 1004
antineutrophil cytoplasmic (auto)antibody 1004, 1510
antineutrophil therapeutic strategies 210–11
antinuclear antibodies 1004
antioxidant properties, mucolytics with 722
antiplatelet therapeutic strategies 221–2
antiproteases, *see* protease/proteinase inhibitors
antisense oligonucleotides as immunosuppressants 654
antisense RNA probes, manufacture 765
antithrombin III 331
AP-1 618
steroid-resistant asthma and 631–2, 1387
apamin 930
Apidae (bees) 927
allergens (venom) 929–31, 1278, 1693
immunotherapy 1236
systemic reactions/anaphylaxis 1554, 1694
classification 927, 1693
see also Hymenoptera

Apis mellifera (honey-bee) 927
allergens 804, 929–31
allergenicity 934
nomenclature 936
recombinant, synthesis 819
see also Apidae
aplastic anaemia, drug-induced 1675
apoptosis
eosinophil 356
neutrophil 209–10
apples 973
aquagenic urticaria 1600
Arachia hypogea and Ara h 1 and 2 967–8, 1556
arachidonic acid 380–1
metabolites, *see* lipid mediators
phospholipase A_2 cleavage of, in neutrophils 205
arachin 967, 1556
arrhythmogenic drugs 433–5, 1332, 1333
Artemisia spp. pollen 854
allergens 801
arteries
lower airways, anatomy 1360
nasal 1313–14
ocular tissues 1645, 1646
oxygen tension/partial pressure (Pa_{O_2})
in asthmatics 674
β-adrenoceptor agonist-reduced 577
arterioles, nasal 1305
arteriovenous anastomoses in nose 1305
arthritis (inflammatory joint disease)
food allergens and 1534
rheumatoid, *see* rheumatoid arthritis
tachykinins and 470
arthropod allergens, *see* crustacean; insect; mite
Arthus, Nicholas Maurice 9
Arthus reaction 9, 25, 27
mechanism 27
see immune complex-mediated hypersensitivity
Arundineae 842
Arundinoideae 842
Ascaris spp.
antigen, airway inflammation/hyperresponsiveness
dogs 1105, 1106
primates 252, 292, 1038, 1041
sheep 1045–6
lumbricoides, pulmonary eosinophilia caused by 1505
ascorbate (vitamin C) and asthma occurrence 1218
Aspergillus spp.
cross-reactivity 1021
A. flavus in agricultural environments 869
A. fumigatus allergens 803, 877–8, 1021
crossed immunoelectrophoresis 873, 874
pulmonary eosinophilia caused by, *see* bronchopulmonary mycoses
recombinant, synthesis 819
oryzae allergens 803, 914, 1478, 1480
aspirin 1687–8
allergic reactions 1687–8
anaphylactic 1559
intolerance, nasal polyposis with 1279
in vernal keratoconjunctivitis 1657
aspirin-induced asthma
leukotrienes and 388, 392, 1688
clinical manifestations 1687
diagnosis 1687
therapy 1437
leukotriene antagonists in 394, 1730–1
leukotriene biosynthesis inhibitors in 396–7, 1730–1
nedocromil sodium in 585
assessment of allergic patient 1271–3
see also examination
astemizole
in rhinitis 1331–2
in urticaria (chronic) 1595
asthma, acute, drug therapy of children with 1458
anticholinergics 601–2
asthma, acute severe
anticholinergics in 599–601
combined with β_2-agonists 599–600, 603
emergency management 1266
progression 673–4
steroids in, intravenous 630
asthma, chronic 52, 1379–94, 1429–39
air-flow obstruction, persistent 671–2
initial assessment 1429
leukotriene antagonists in 395
leukotriene biosynthesis inhibitors in 397
stable, in children 602
T cell hypothesis 1379–94
novel approaches to therapy based on 1389–90
therapy 1389–90, 1429–39
aims 1429
anticholinergics 598–9, 602
children 602
choices/options 1435–8
5-lipoxygenase pathway-affecting drugs 1729
self-management 1433
stable disease 598–9, 602
step-down 1432
strategies 1429–30
asthma, exercise-induced, *see* exercise-induced asthma
asthma, extrinsic/atopic/allergic and in general including bronchial asthma 14–17, 36–7, 263–83, 292–4, 298–306, 665–709, 1276–8, 1345–486
airway in, *see* airway
allergen challenge, *see* allergen challenge
in aspergillosis (allergic bronchopulmonary) 1502
treatment 1503
atopic dermatitis and 1578
atopy and, relationship between 1179–81, 1348
basophils in 159–60
β-adrenoceptor agonists, *see* β-adrenoceptor agonists
brittle 1437
causes/aetiology 1366–78
classification by 1347–8
identification 16–17, 49
CD4+ cells in, *see* CD4+ cells
children, *see* children
chronic, *see* asthma, chronic
classification 1347–8
clinical features 1350–1
cockroach allergens and 944, 946–9
cognitive factors 508–10
cough-variant, *see* cough
cytokines, *see* cytokines and *specific cytokines*
death, *see* death
definitions 37, 1347
of phenotype 1197–200, 1209
diagnosis 1276–7, 1351–7
differential 1266, 1355–6
early-phase responses 1372, 1373–4
endothelium and adhesion molecules in, *see* adhesion; endothelial cells
eosinophils in, *see* eosinophil
epidemiological factors 1188, 1208–23
age 1211–12
air pollution 1216–17, 1395–411
exposure to allergens 1215–16
geographical variations 1210–11
infection 1217
prevalence, *see* prevalence
race 1213
fibroblasts and 298–306
genetics, *see* genetics
helminthic infection and, *see* helminthic infection
historical milestones 14–17
immune system and 508–10
immunotherapy-induced 1254, 1255
inflammation in, *see* inflammation (allergic) in asthma
investigations 1266
irreversible air-flow obstruction 623
late-phase reactions (human model of allergic airway inflammation) 1113–30, 1372–3, 1373–4
clinical features 1114
diagnostic uses 1114
methodology 1113–14
pathogenesis (in general) 1121–2
pathophysiology 1117–21
pharmacology 1115–16
predictive factors 1116–17
prevalence 1115
reproducibility 1115
leukotrienes and, *see* leukotrienes
macrophages in 289–90
mast cells in, *see* mast cells
mediators involved in, *see* mediators
mite allergen exposure and 892–3
models
animal, *see* animal models
human, *see* late-phase reactions (*subheading above*)
nasal polyps and 1295
nervous system (autonomic) in 503–4, 508–10, 1423
adrenergic nerves and adrenoceptors 483–6, 504, 568
cholinergic nerves 490–2
higher cortical centres 508–10
non-adrenergic non-cholinergic nerves, *see* non-adrenergic non-cholinergic system
theories of dysfunction 503–4
neuropeptides in 275–6, 468, 469–70, 1085, 1733–4
nitric oxide and 268–71, 525
pathogenesis (in general) 36–7, 1366–76
of late asthmatic response 1121–2
platelets in 217–21
pathology 1360–5, 1412–28
post-mortem, *see* post-mortem
pathophysiology 15–16, 161–2, 263–83, 1117–21
plasma exudation in 161–2, 443
in pregnancy 1437
pre-menstrual 1437
prostanoids in, *see* prostanoids
psychological/psychogenic factors in asthma 490, 509–10
risk factors, *see* risk factors
salivary glands and, minor 287–8
severity of, classification by 1348
severity of exacerbations 1349, 1351
assessment 1349, 1351
classification by 1348
symptoms 1350–1
diagnostic 1351–2, 1357–8
relationship to bronchial hyperresponsiveness 682–4
therapy 358, 394–5, 396–7, 696–72, 1266, 1283–7, 1460–1, 1726–38
alternative 1433
chronic disease, *see* asthma, chronic

difficult asthma 1437
drug, *see* drugs (allergy-treating)
immunotherapy, *see* immunotherapy
novel/future approaches 1389–90, 1460–1, 1726–38
triggers and contributing/exacerbating factors 1276–7, 1349–50, 1354
air pollutants 1400, 1401, 1402, 1403
food 1280–1, 1529–30
at work 1471
upper airway involvement 672–3, 1309
see also specific inducers of asthma
asthma, intrinsic 16, 37
IL-5/GM-CSF and 361
T cells in 1382–3
asthma, nocturnal, *see* nocturnal asthma
asthma, occupational 1277–8
allergens causing/implicated in 37, 909–26, 1277–8, 1464–5, 1477–8
air pollutant/irritants and, *see* air pollution; irritants
cockroach 944
fungal 865, 869, 871
definitions 1464
determinants 1467–71
diagnosis/identification 1471–7
late response in 1114
misdiagnosis (false-positive) 1462, 1477
epidemiology 909–10, 1465–70
investigations 1472–7
management 1266–7, 1437, 1480–1
mechanisms 1470–1
outcome 1469–70
prevention 1481–2
primary 1481–2
secondary 1482
rabbit model 1080
screening for predisposition 1482
T cells in 1382, 1384, 1386
atherosclerosis, nitric oxide and 521–2
atopic diseases/disorders (in general)
food allergy prevalence 1518
organ-specific 1193
see also specific diseases
atopy 32, 36–7
asthma and, relationship between 1179–81, 1344
causes 1187–8
cytokines implicated in 350, 351, 1370
definitions 32, 36–7, 1013, 1208
drug allergy and 1672–3
β-lactams 1683
muscle relaxants 1680
epidemiology, *see* epidemiology
genetics, *see* genetics
helminthic infection and, *see* helminthic infection
historical recognition 11
IgE and, *see* immunoglobulin E
IgG isotype levels in conditions/disorders associated with 1001, 1003
interferon-γ and subsequent, reduced 1722
mononuclear leucocytes and, cAMP phosphodiesterases in 542–3, 553–4
nedocromil sodium and sodium cromoglycate effects on cells/mediators involved in development of 586–7
ocular allergy and 1648, 1650, 1654
prediction 1715–16
pregnancy measures with high-risk infants in prevention of 1722
risk factors, *see* risk factors
Th2-types responses in 108–9
see also sensitization
ATP, mucokinetic properties 723
ATP-sensitive K+ channel, *see* potassium ion channel
atrial natriuretic peptide mRNA *in situ* hybridization 770
atrophic rhinitis 1296
atropine
dose–response 597
pharmacokinetics/dynamics 597
side-effects/toxicity 602
management 603
Austen, K. Frank 12, 13
Austria, allergy training 1264
autoallergic disease, *see* autoimmune disease
autoantibodies
to β-adrenoceptors 485
in systemic vasculitides 1004, 1510
autocrine feedback pathways in asthma 1375
Autohaler 1442–3
autoimmune disease
immunosuppressive drugs 654
immunotherapy 138, 138–9
T cell receptor repertoire and 1385
urticaria (chronic) and 1588–89
autonomic nervous system (airways) 481–504, 503–8, 594–6
asthma and, *see* asthma
cholinergic traffic inhibited by other parts of 594–5
nasal 1302–3, 1313, 1314
neuropeptides involved in 504, 505
neuropeptide tyrosine (NPY) 464, 486–7, 487–8
tachykinins 449–50, 451
VIP 458–60, 486–7, 487–8, 489
nitric oxide in 459, 487
opioid peptides in 465–6
rhinitis and, *see* rhinitis
see also specific components/divisions
autoproteolytic activity of FcεRII 89
autopsy, *see* post-mortem
avian allergens, *see* birds
avidin
as allergen 966
in immunocytochemistry 775, 777
azathioprine 650, 1732
asthma 1732
toxicity 656
azelastine in rhinitis 1331
aztreonam 1554, 1683
skin tests 1684

B cell(s) 36–57
activation
IL-4 in 348, 1371
immunosuppressive drugs affecting 647, 649
T cells and 76
as antigen-presenting cells 124
cytokines produced by, Th cell development and effects of 107
epitopes
chironomid allergens and 955, 956
food allergens and 964
Hymenoptera venoms and 937
Ig/antibodies of
expression/synthesis 59, 73
function 59
IgE synthesis 39–41
membrane-bound forms (antigen receptor), *see* membrane-bound Ig
secreted forms 73
switching 39–40, 71–3, 98–9, 1371
see also secreted immunoglobulins
phosphodiesterase 535
phosphodiesterase inhibitor effects 546
quantitation 1001
T cell cultures requiring EBV-transformed 755–6, 757
T cell interactions with 107
allergy and 125–6
cognate 76
contact-mediated signals, IgE synthesis and 99–101
in efferent phase of immune response 124–5
tolerance in 137–8
B7 32, 1389
T cell activation and 132
T cell antigen recognition 39, 1389
B95.8 line 755–6
Bacillus subtilis proteases 915, 1481
bacteria
exotoxins, *see* exotoxins
infections/sepsis
asthma and 1350
atopic dermatitis and 1575–6, 1582, 1583
chronic, ciliary dysfunction in 713
spores as allergens, *see* Actinomycetes
bagassosis 870
baking industry, allergens and asthma 913–14, 1240, 1278, 1465, 1478–9
balsam of Peru 1623
Bambusoideae 842
banana 973
barbiturates 1681
barrier methods of allergen control 1719
basal airway cells
asthma and 274, 1416
role 445
base pairs, 12/23, Ig joining signals and 63–4
basement membrane, subepithelial 299–1
in asthma, thickening 161, 301, 1417
nose 1302
Basenji greyhounds, airway hyperresponsiveness 1105–6
basidiomycetes 878–9, 1021–2
cross-reactivity 1021–2
basophils 368–71, 1118–19
activation 368–71
in allergic inflammation 162–3, 253–4
in asthma 1422
in asthma, in late-phase response 1118–19
migration of 253–4, 288
in nasal late-phase response 1145, 1146–7
phosphodiesterase and 535
phosphodiesterase inhibitor effects 544, 545
in rhinitis 1317
histamine release assays in food allergy 1538
IgE synthesis and role of 102
mast cells and, common/different features 149–50
mediators (cytokines etc.) 46, 158
allergy and 127–8
BAYK8644 744
BAYu3405 1731
BAYχ1005 396, 1730
beans 968
occupational exposure 915
beclomethasone dipropionate (BDP)
liposomal formulation, deposition 733–5
in rhinitis 1335
systemic effects 626–8
Becotide 735
bedroom in house dust mite control 1328
bee, *see* Apidae; *Apis mellifera*; *Bombus* spp.
Bennich, Hans 12
benzocaine 1625
Bermuda grass, *see Cynodon dactylon*
beryllium disease, chronic 1496

Bet v allergens, *see Betula* spp.
β-adrenoceptor(s) 483
asthma and 483–5, 504, 1108, 1200
atopy and 1193
cholinergic inhibition involving 594
localization 567
β-adrenoceptor agonists 566, 570–8, 571
adverse effects 576–8, 1434
mechanisms 577–8
with regular use 577–8
in asthma 570–8, 686, 1285, 1434–5, 1728–29
bronchial hyperresponsiveness decreased by 686
in chronic asthma 1430–1, 1432, 1434, 1434–5
combined with anticholinergics 599–600, 603
in dog model 1107
in exercise-induced asthma 696, 696–8, 698–9, 1436
late response and effects of 1115
mode of action 1434
oral forms 574–5, 1432, 1434
in rabbit model 1085
regular vs intermittent use 1434–5
as Ca^{2+}-dependent K^+ channel openers 607
children 1459
in cutaneous late-phase reactions 1135
excretion 572
inhaled forms, *see* inhaled agents
long-acting
clinical use 571, 698, 1432
development 1726–7
oral forms, *see* oral route
pharmacokinetics 574–6
parenteral forms, *see* parenteral therapy
physiological effects 573–4
selectivity/affinity/efficacy 572
short-acting
clinical use 571, 698–9
disadvantages 1726
steroid resistance induced by 632
structure/metabolism 570–2
β-adrenoceptor antagonists 578
in anaphylaxis, adverse effects/avoidance 1563, 1566
bronchoconstriction and bronchospasm caused by 684
anticholinergics preventing 598
β-lactam antibiotic reactions 1552–4, 1682–5
clinical manifestations 1683
desensitization 1566
incidence 1682–3
mechanisms 1683–4
risk factors 1683
β-subunits/chains
B cell antigen receptor, structure 73, 74
FcεRI 85
atopy and 49, 1191, 1192, 1203, 1368
G proteins 742
GM-CSF receptor, receptors sharing 343, 354
integrins 247
interleukin-6 receptor, receptors sharing 343
T cell receptor 1380
asthma and 1385
Beta vulgaris 852
Betula spp. 847
verrucosa allergens (Bet v) 799–800, 1019
cross-reactivity 973, 1019, 1024–5
minor 1024–5
recombinant, synthesis 816–17
Betulaceae 1019
Fagaceae and, cross-reaction 850
bimakalim
structure 608
trials in asthma 613
Bioaerosol sampler 840
biopsies
bronchial mucosal, late asthmatic response and 1122
in situ hybridization 769
skin
for deriving T cells for culture 756–7
from eczematous lesions 1135
of tuberculin-induced delayed-type hypersensitivity 1135
biotechnological processes, fungal exposure 871
biotin
in immunocytochemistry 775, 777
RNA probes labelled with 766
birch, *see Betula* spp.
birds
bird (pigeon) fancier's lung 1489
diagnosis 1496
differential diagnosis 1496
epidemiology 1491
management 1498
natural history/prognosis 1495
perennial rhinitis 1276
birth weight, low 1717
Bla g, *see Blatella germanica*
Blackley, Charles 14, 15
Blatella germanica 889
allergens (Bla g) 802–3, 889
exposure 946–7
immunoassays 946–7
immunochemistry 944
immunoreactivity 945–6
molecular biology 944–5
sources 946
in USA 942
bleeding, gastrointestinal, occult 1534
blepharo(kerato)conjunctivitis
atopic dermatitis associated with 1576, 1659–61
contact 1659–2
blood clotting, *see* coagulation
blood flow, airway/bronchial
exercise-induced asthma and 702, 703
in sheep, antigen-induced increases 1049
tachykinins and 452–3
VIP and 460
blood gases, asthmatics 674
blood loss, occult gastrointestinal 1534
blood tests 1273
rhinitis 1297
blood vessels, *see* microvessels; vasculature
Bluescribe vector 765
BN 52021 1729
in rabbit, antigen-induced responses and effects of
airway 1086
skin 1081
BN 52063
in humans 221, 407, 1729
in rabbit, antigen-induced responses and effects of
airway 1084
skin 1081
bombesin 466–7, 495
functional effects 467
localization 466–7, 495
receptors 467
Bombus (bumble bee) spp. 927
venoms 931
see also Apidae
bone metabolism, steroid effects 627
Bos domesticus allergens
milk, *see* milk
occupational exposure 905
Bostock, John 14
Botrytis cinerea 879–80
bovine allergens 905
see also Bos domesticus
bovine serum albumin in PCR 785
bowel (intestine)
diseases 1281–2
food intolerance contributing to 1281–2
inflammatory, *see* inflammatory bowel disease
mast cell, food-allergen induced histamine release 1538
see also gastrointestinal tract
Bra j 1 974
bradykinin
antagonists, in asthma 1731
formation 324–31
functions and control mechanisms 331–2
in hereditary angioedema 333
brain and asthma 508–10
see also central nervous system
Brassica spp.
juncea 974
oleracea 974
brazil nut 972
breast-feeding
rhinitis treatment and 1337
risk for atopy/atopic disease and 1218
food allergy 1541–2, 1720
breath-activated inhalers 736–7
dry powder inhaler 1444
metered dose inhaler 1442–3
breathing
by mouth, aerosols 729
by nose in prevention of exercise-induced asthma 700
brequinar sodium 651
toxicity 656
British Society for Allergy and Clinical Immunology, immunotherapy recommendations 1286
brittle asthma, management 1437
BRL-55834
asthma 613
structure 608
Bromeae 842
bromelin 915, 1480
bronchi
asthmatic, β-adrenoceptors 568
blood flow, *see* blood flow
epithelial cells, *see* epithelial cells
mucosa, *see* mucosa
pressure measurements via catheters in, in asthmatics 670–1
bronchial asthma, *see* asthma
bronchial hyperresponsiveness/hyperreactivity (in general and in diseases other than asthma) 684–5
aetiology 890
mite particles in 890
animal models 1035–110, 1388
dog 1106–7
guinea pig 1096–7
mouse 1056–67, 1388
primate 1040–3
rabbit 1082–7
rat 1071, 1072–3, 1387
sheep 1050–1
defining and measuring of 1209
food allergens and 1529–31
genetics, *see* genetics
ozone-induced 1398
rhinovirus infection resulting in 896, 1712
bronchial hyperresponsiveness/hyperreactivity in asthma 162, 667–8,

680–9, 1412–13
children 1454–68
cholinergic nervous system and 490–1, 492
cytokines and 584
definition 680–1
drugs decreasing/suppressing 685–6
potassium ion channel openers 612
steroids 622, 685–6
genetics 1182
historical background 680
ICAM-1 and 252, 272
leukotriene and 385, 387–8, 388–9, 683
measurement 681–2, 1353–4
delivery of stimulus in 682
diagnostic significance 1353–4
direct stimuli 681, 683, 696
indirect stimuli 681, 683–4
methods 682–3
in occupational asthma 1476–7
origins/mechanisms (in general) 667–8, 682–4
symptoms and their relationship to 682–4
platelets and 217–21
T cells and 1072–3
see also bronchoconstriction; bronchospasm
bronchial tree, nerve number decreasing with descent down 523, 524
bronchitis, chronic
eosinophilic 1351
ipratropium 605–6
bronchoalveolar lavage (BAL) in asthma
albumin 443, 1413–14
eosinophil numbers 186, 187
histopathology 45, 46, 159
T cells 47
bronchoconstriction
in asthma
α-adrenoceptors and 485–6
cholinergic reflex activity and 491
chromone effects 590
leukotriene-associated 385, 387–8, 388–9, 1686
lung parenchyma involved in 673
platelet-activating factor-induced 406–7
platelet and 217–21
prostaglandin-associated 401–4
refractory period 404
tachykinin (substance P/NKA)-induced 451, 494, 495
bombesin-induced 467
CGRP-induced 455
non-adrenergic non-cholinergic 504
paradoxical, with anticholinergics 603
potassium ion channel openers preventing 611
reflex, chromone effects 586, 590
sheep model 1045–55
simulated, anticholinergic effects against 598
sulphur dioxide-induced 1398
see also bronchial hyperresponsiveness; bronchospasm
bronchodilators (drugs)
adrenoceptor agonists, *see* adrenoceptors
aerosol delivery systems, *see* aerosol
anticholinergics, *see* cholinergic antagonists
in chronic asthma 1430–1, 1434–5
additional 1431–2
nebulized 1432–3
leukotriene antagonists as 394–5
leukotriene biosynthesis inhibitors as 397
mucociliary clearance improved by 722
single-dose reversing air-flow limitation, diagnostic significance 1353
steroids combined with 629
theophylline, *see* theophylline
bronchodilators (endogenous), VIP as 458
bronchogram, normal 1360, 1361
bronchopulmonary mycoses, allergic (predominantly aspergillosis) 1500–1
chronic 1497
clinical features 1502
diagnosis/investigations 1502
differential diagnosis 1502–3
pathology 1501–2
treatment and prognosis 1503
bronchoscopy, fibreoptic
in asthma 186, 1367
BAL fluid obtained via, *see* bronchoalveolar lavage
wheezing infant 1453–4
bronchospasm
in asthma
anticholinergics with 598, 603
exercise-induced 392
leukotriene-associated 392
nocturnal, *see* nocturnal asthma
platelets and 217–21
drug-induced 1675
see also bronchial hyperresponsiveness; bronchoconstriction
bronchovascular permeability, *see* vasculature
Brown–Norway rat, allergic response 1068–78
Brugia malayi 1504
budesonide
in rhinitis 1335
systemic effects 626–8
budgerigar-owner's lung 1491
buffers, PCR 785
bumble bee, *see Bombus*
Burkard 7-day volumetric spore trap 839
monitoring programmes in USA 841
BWA4C in inflammatory bowel disease 397
byssinosis 870–1

C gene segment 64
heavy chains (C_H) 39, 65
class switching and 96–7
IgE 83–5
IgM 72–3
rearrangement 71–2
synthesis 72–3
C region/domain of Ig 59
allelic differences (allotypes) 61
genes, *see* C gene segment
structure 59–60
C1 309
activation 309–10, 311
deficiency 318
C1 inhibitor/C1 esterase inhibitor 1602, 1603
deficiency
acquired 1593, 1604
hereditary, *see* angioedema
kallikrein inhibited by 331
C1q 309, 309–10
receptors for 315–16
C1r 309, 310
C1s 309
C2 309, 310
deficiency 318, 319–20
C3 309, 310, 312–13
biological activity 316
deficiency 318, 320
degradation 312
C3 convertase 312, 313
C3a anaphylatoxin
biological activity 316
receptors for 315
C3b (activated C3) 313
receptor for (and for C3b cleavage fragments) 315
C4 310, 311
deficiency 318, 319
measurement 1004
C4 binding protein 311
C4a anaphylatoxin
biological activity 316
receptor for 315
C4b (and its cleavage fragments), receptors for 315
C4bp deficiency 318, 320
C5 310, 313, 314
deficiency 318, 320
C5 convertase 310, 313
C5a anaphylatoxin
biological activity 316
mast cell response 152
receptor for 315
C6 314
deficiency 318, 320
C7 314
deficiency 318, 320
C8 314
deficiency 318, 320
C9 314
deficiency 318, 320
cabbage 974
cachectin, *see* tumour necrosis factor-α
caine mix 1625
Cal c 1 872
calcineurin 643–5
calcitonin gene-related peptide 454–6, 495
asthma and 276
functional effects 455, 495
cutaneous 452
localization 454–5
receptors 455, 495
nasal 1314
calcitriol, pulmonary alveolar macrophage-derived 155
calcium ion(s)
airway smooth muscle tension/contractions and 610, 742–8
birch allergens and 800
chemotaxis of leucocytes and 372
as chromone target 587, 589
in mast cells 587
lectin domain of FcεRII and 88
in neutrophils 206
phospholipase C activation and 204
calcium ion channels
airway smooth muscle cells 743–6
physiological regulation 744–5
receptor-operated 745–6
voltage-dependent, potassium channel openers and 608, 610
antagonists, in asthma 1728
in chronic asthma 1432
calcium ion-dependent K^+ channel openers, β-agonists as 607
calibre, airway
asthma 1364
resting, indomethacin effects 403
calmodulin and airway smooth muscle contraction 746
'calor' as classical sign of inflammation 440
Calvatia cyathiformis 872, 879
calycin 944–5
Can f 1, *see Canis familiaris*
Candida albicans allergens 804, 1022
recombinant, synthesis 819
candidiasis, oropharyngeal, steroid-related 625
Canis familiaris (dog) 803, 902–4, 1024, 1275–6
airway

general characteristics 1103–4
model of asthma and hyperresponsiveness 1103–10
major allergen (Can f 1) 803, 902–3, 1024
allergenic capacity 902
biochemistry 803, 902
cross-reactivity 1024
environmental load/exposure 902–3, 1215
immunotherapy 1237, 1239
other allergens 903–4
prevention of exposure to allergens 1711
CAP system (Pharmacia), venom assay 1796
capillaries
lower airway 1360
nasal 1305, 1313
capsaicin
allergic rabbit and effects of 1086–7
sensory nerves sensitive to
rhinitis and 1303
tachykinin involvement 449–50
Car b allergen, recombinant, synthesis 816–17
carba group of rubber accelerators 1625
carbon dioxide transfer coefficient, asthmatics 675–6
carboxypeptidase, mast cell 155
carcinoid tumour, asthma distinguished from 1356
cardiovascular system
adverse effects/toxicity of drugs
cholinergic antagonists 602, 603
H_1 receptor antagonists 433–5, 1332, 1333
potassium ion channel openers 613
anaphylaxis affecting 1563
drug-related 1673
management 1568
β-adrenoceptors 567
β-adrenoceptor agonist effects 574
adverse 476–7
endothelin localization 520–1
nitric oxide localization 521–2
see also heart
carpeting
in house-dust mite allergen avoidance, treatment 893, 894
as spore reservoir 868
Carpinus betulus allergens (Car b), recombinant, synthesis 816–17
carrier powder in dry-powder inhalers carrier 732
Carrington's (chronic eosinophilic) pneumonia 1507–9, 1510
caseins 965–6
Castanea spp. (chestnut)
nut 972
pollen 849–50
castor beans 915
cat, *see Felis domesticus*
cataracts, steroid-induced 628
catecholamines 483
circulating 486
cathepsin D, mast cell 155
cathepsin G and asthma 275
catheters, endobronchial, pressure measurements in asthmatics 670–1
cationic proteins
eosinophil, *see* eosinophil cationic protein
platelet 215
Cavia porcellus (guinea pig)
allergens from 904–5
laboratory exposure 911
as model of asthma/allergic disease 1093–102
airway response (antigen-induced) 1096–8
antigen challenge conditions 1094–5
immunosuppressive agents in 655
pharmacological relevance 1099
sensitization to antigen 1093–4, 1404
CBP35, *see* ε-binding protein
C-C chemokines 368, 369–71
in allergy/allergic inflammation 369, 374, 374–5
basophil effects 369–71
eosinophil effects 175–6, 369–71
lymphocyte effects 371–2
monocyte effects 371
receptors 372–3
cloned 373–4
structure 367–8
CD markers (in general), expression/function/identification 1001–2
CD3
antigen recognition and subsequent responses and 119
monoclonal antibody to, as immunosuppressant 653
CD4
monoclonal antibodies to, as immunosuppressants 653
T cell antigen recognition and 119
CD4+ eosinophils 178
CD4+ T (helper) cells 755–7
in allergen-specific immunotherapy 50, 1229
antigen-presenting cell interactions with activated 124
in asthma 46–9
in late response 1120, 1122, 1125
clones, antigen/allergen-specific 756–7
studies/uses 761
techniques of manufacture 756–7
cutaneous late-phase reactions and 1134–5
cytokines secreted by 113
dietary allergens and 140
heterogeneity/dichotomy 29–32, 104
in vitro growth 755–6
inhaled allergens and 141
interleukin-13 synthesis by 348
in nasal pathology
in late-phase reaction 1147
rhinitis pathogenesis 46–9, 1318
peptide/antigen recognition and 116
see also Th0 cells; Th1 cells; Th2 cells
CD8
monoclonal antibodies to, as immunosuppressants 653
T cell antigen recognition and 119
CD8+ cells (cytotoxic/suppressor T cells; Tc cells; Ts cells)
in allergen-specific immunotherapy 1230
antigen-presenting cell interactions with activated 124–5
in asthma
in occupational asthma 1384, 1386
theophylline effects 551–2
clones (monoclonal), antigen/allergen-specific 757–60, 761
studies/uses 761
techniques of manufacture 758–60
cyclosporin and FK506 effects 647
deoxyspergualin effects 652
dichotomy 31
dietary allergens and 140
inhaled allergens and 141
lines (oligoclonal) 757–8
peptide/antigen recognition and 116
Tc1 cells 31
Tc2 cells 31
CD11b, *see* Mac-1
CD11c, *see* p150,95
CD16 as eosinophil receptor 176
CD18, CD11's associated with, *see* LFA-1; Mac-1; p150,95
CD19 76
CD21, *see* CR2
CD22 76
CD23, *see* Fcε receptor
CD25 (IL-2 receptor) 344
asthma and 1423
α-subunit/chain of, receptors sharing 343
monoclonal antibody to, immunosuppressant action 653
CD25+ T cells
asthma and 1382
eosinophil function and 188, 1382
CD28 and T cell antigen recognition 38, 1389
CD29, *see* VLA
CD30, grass pollen sensitivity and 105
CD32 as eosinophil receptor 176
CD34, as L-selectin ligand 245
CD34+ eosinophils 173
CD35, *see* CR1
CD40/CD40L and IgE synthesis 41, 100–1
CD43+ lymphocytes in fatal asthma 1414
CD45 76, 1001
isoforms 1001
CD49d, *see* VLA
CD59 315
deficiency 318, 320
CD62, *see* P-selectin
CD64, *see* Fcγ receptors
CD69 on eosinophils 177
CD79a, structure 73, 74
CD79b, structure 73, 74
CD80 (B7-1) 132, 1389
T cell antigen recognition and 39, 1389
CD86 (B7-2) 132, 1389
CDw121a/b 345–6
CDR, *see* complementarity-determining regions
cedar, western red, dust exposure 915
celery 973
cross-reactivity 1025
cell(s) (in general)
culture, *see* cultures
differentiation, drugs interfering with 652
in inflammation, *see* inflammation (allergic), cells involved; inflammatory cells
maturation, drugs interfering with 652
for mRNA detection by *in situ* hybridization
examples 770
pretreatment 768
in mRNA detection by PCR, determination of mRNA concentrations 788–9
in mRNA *in situ*-hybridized tissues/fluids/cells, identifying type 771
phenotype, analysis 1001–2, 1003
cell-mediated hypersensitivity, *see* delayed hypersensitivity
central nervous system
drug toxicity, *see* neurotoxicity
immune system interactions with 503–15
toxicity, H_1 antagonist, second-generation 422–3, 433
vagal output in asthma from, enhanced 490
see also brain
centrifugation, density, lymphocyte preparation via 754–5
cephalopod 971
cephalosporin allergy 1553–4
incidence 1682
skin tests 1684
ceramide metabolism, neutrophil 205–6
cereals 913–14, 972
dust 1278
fungal spores associated with 863, 865, 868–9

proteins, as allergens 913–14, 972
see also baking industry
cetirizine
in nasal late-phase reactions 1151
pharmacokinetics 426–7
in rhinitis 1332
in urticaria (chronic) 1595
CFC propellants 731, 1441
CGRP, *see* calcitonin gene-related peptide
Charcot, Jean Martin 15, 16
Charcot–Leyden crystals 16
protein 91, 181–2
chemical sensitizers in asthma
inhalation challenge 1355
as risk factors 1348–9
chemokines/intecrines 365–79
in allergy 366, 374–5
assays and their value 1000–1
basophil 368–71
endothelial cell-derived 285
eosinophil 175–6, 368–71
in guinea pig model 1098–9
neutrophil 201, 369, 370
receptors 177, 372–4
cloned 373–4
functional characterization 372–3
role/function 368–74
as histamine-releasing factors 374
in modulation of effector cell function (in allergic inflammation) 366
structure 367–8, 374
chemotaxins
C5a as 316
eosinophil 174–6, 368–71, 454
in guinea pig lung 1098
neutrophil 200–1, 369, 454
platelet 214–16
tachykinins as 454
Chenopod(s) 852
Chenopodiaceae 852, 1021
chest deformity, asthmatic children 1457
chest X-rays
allergic bronchopulmonary aspergillosis 1502
eosinophilic pneumonia
acute 1508
chronic 1508
extrinsic allergic alveolitis
acute disease 1493
chronic disease 1494
chestnut 849–50
Chi t allergens, *see* Chironomid non-biting midge
chicken egg, *see* egg allergens
children 1287, 1451–3, 1715–25
aerosols and dose calculation 730–1
air pollutant-related symptoms 1402–3
allergy and allergic disease (in general) 1455–6
prevention 1709–25
stigmata 1457
asthma, *see* children, asthma
atopic dermatitis 1529, 1581–2
bone metabolism, steroid effects 627
diagnosis and management of allergy (in general) 1269, 1287
food/diet-related problems/allergies 1282, 1529, 1581–2, 1710
dietitians 1287
early avoidance of allergens 1370, 1720
food intolerance and hyperkinetic syndrome 1240, 1281
prevalence 1518
severe (anaphylaxis) 1555, 1556–8
growth, steroid effects 627, 628
house-dust mite allergen 1456
exposure in early life 1710–11, 1718–20, 1721
sensitivity 1327
IgE levels 1014
immunotherapy-induced side-effects, treatment 1255
insect sting allergy 1695
otitis media, *see* otitis media
plantar dermatosis 1575
rhinitis (allergic) 1337
skin-test reactivity 1010
smoking (passive) 1214, 1403, 1404–5, 1712, 1717
see also infant; neonate
children, asthma 1451–63
acute, *see* asthma, acute
chronic stable, ipratropium 602
clinical features 1456–7
deaths 1452
diagnostic algorithm 1457
epidemiology 1181–2, 1451–2
exacerbations, epidemiology 1402, 1403
exercise-induced 690
immunotherapy-induced 1255
investigations 1457–8
management 1458–61
delivery of care 1460
drugs 601–562, 623, 1458, 1459–60, 1461
future 1460–1
long term 1458
plan 1458–9
natural history 1452
Chinese restaurant syndrome 1281
chinoform 1624–5
Chironomid non-biting midge (*Chironomus thummi thummi*) allergens (Chi t haemoglobins) 956–64
Chi t 1 804, 954–6
epitopes 955–6
occupational exposure 912
recombinant, synthesis 818–19
three-dimensional structure 954–5
cross-reactivity 954
exposure 952–4
sensitization 952–4
structure, general aspects 954
symptoms 952–3
therapy 958–9
chloride channel
chromone actions 589–90
in cystic fibrosis 714
chlorocresol 1624
chlorofluorocarbon propellants 731, 1441
Chloroideae 842
Chloroidoideae 842
chloromethylisothiazolinone 1624
chocolate 974
cholecystokinin 468
cholinergic (muscarinic) agonists, airway response to
in asthma 683
in dog 1104–5, 1107
cholinergic (muscarinic) antagonists (anticholinergics) 594–606
available 596–7
bronchial hyperresponsiveness decreased by 686
development 1727
dose–response 597–8
pharmacodynamics 597
pharmacokinetics 597
side-effects/toxicity 602–3, 1435
management 603
structure 596
cholinergic (muscarinic) antagonists (anticholinergics), therapeutic use 598–602, 603–4
in asthma 598–600, 603, 686, 698, 1285
in chronic asthma 1432, 1435
mode of action 1435
in chronic obstructive pulmonary disease, *see* chronic obstructive pulmonary disease
in rhinitis 490, 1333
cholinergic nervous system 488–92, 594–606
anatomy/innervation 488, 594–5
in asthma 490–2
cromakalim suppressant effects on 611
nasal 1302–3
in rhinitis 489–90
physiology 595–6
transmission 488–9
neuropeptide tyrosine and 464
opioids and 466
VIP and 459–60
cholinergic urticaria 1599
differentiation from anaphylaxis 1564
from exercise-induced anaphylaxis 1558–60
cholinesterase inhibitors reversing atropine toxicity 603
chromatography of allergens 797, 798
chromium-release cytotoxicity assay 759–60
chromium salts/chromate 918
tests 1622–3
chromones, *see* nedocromil sodium; sodium cromoglycate
chromosomal localization
atopy/allergy/asthma determinants (in general) 1179–80, 1189, 1191–3, 1202–5
atopic dermatitis determinants 1573–4
complement pathway genes 317
cytokine genes 345
chronic allergic reactions/inflammation
dendritic cells in 237–8
primate model 1040–2
in rhinitis 48
as type IV hypersensitivity 29
see also specific disorders
chronic obstructive pulmonary disease/airway disease (COPD/COAD) 600–2
air pollutants and 1400–1
asthma and
differential diagnosis 1356
distinction/overlap between 672, 1356
pathological differences 1412–28
bronchial hyperresponsiveness in 685
smoking-related 672
therapy 1266
anticholinergics in acute exacerbations 601–2
anticholinergics in chronic stable disease 600–1, 603
steroids 623
Churg–Strauss syndrome 1509–10
chymase in mast cells 154–5
asthma and 275
biological properties 154
tryptase and (M_{TC}) 151
chymopapain, adverse reactions
anaphylaxis 1557
atopy and 1673
CI-930
anti-inflammatory effects 549
T cell effects 546
cigarette smokers, *see* smokers
CIIV (compartment for peptide loading) 118
cilia (and ciliated cells) 710–13
dysfunction/dyskinesia 712–13, 1294
primary 712–13, 1294, 1305
in rhinitis 1294
secondary 713
fluid surrounding 713–14

function 711–12
function, measurement/assessment 712, 717–18
in rhinitis 1298
mucus transport 717
nasal, *see* nose
structure 710–11
circadian/diurnal changes in counts
grass pollen 845–6
spores 862, 863
Cladosporium spp. allergens 873–4
cladosporioides 873, 874
herbarum 803–4, 872, 873, 874–5
crossed immunoelectrophoresis 873
immunotherapy 1237–8
clavulanic acid, skin tests 1684
climate and atopic dermatitis 1582–3
see also season; weather
clinic(s), allergy 1264–70, 1287–8
facilities and staff 1287–8
'clinical ecologists' 1289
clinical immunology, links between allergy and 1269–70
clonal anergy, *see* anergy
clonal deletion of T cells, *see* T cell
clonal ignorance 136
Clonorchis sinensis 1506
clotting, *see* coagulation
coagulation 324–39
anaphylactoid reactions and activation of pathways of 1559
disseminated intravascular 334
intrinsic 324–39
cobalt salts 918
Coca, Arthur 11, 21
coccidioidomycosis 1506
cockroaches
allergens 802–3, 889, 942–51
avoidance 947–8, 949
epidemiology 942–4, 949
extracts 946
immunochemistry 944
immunoreactivity 945–6
localization and function *in vivo* 946
molecular biology 944–5, 949
recombinant 819, 945–6
sources 946
treatment 947–8
control 948–9
cod, *see Gadus callarius*
coeliac disease, *see* gluten-sensitive enteropathy
coffee beans/dust 915
cognitive factors in asthma 508–10
cold air hyperventilation in asthmatics, airway response/bronchoconstriction with 683
leukotriene antagonists effects 394
cold urticaria 1596, 1599–600
anaphylaxis and, differentiation 1564
familial essential 1600
reflex 1600
colic, infantile 1526–7
colitis
food-induced 1531–2
ulcerative, *see* ulcerative colitis
collagens 299
basement membrane
in asthma 301
type IV 299
fibrillar 299
non-fibrillar 299
colloid metals in immunocytochemistry 777
colony stimulating factor, granulocyte/macrophage-, *see* granulocyte/macrophage-CSF
colophony (abietic acid; pine-wood resin; solder flux) 920, 1278, 1479–80
asthma and 1479–80
tests 1623
columnar cells
in asthma 273–4
shedding 445
combinatorial diversity with Igs 69–70
community, asthma and atopy studies in 1180
compartment for peptide loading (CPL; CIIV) 118
complement 307–23
alternative pathway 312–13, 318
activation 312–13
components 308, 312
regulation 313
anaphylactoid reactions and 1558–9
assays 1004
biological activities 316–17
classical pathway 309–12, 318
activation 309–11
components 308, 309
regulation 311–12
controlling proteins 308
deficiencies 317–21
drug allergy involving activation 1678
radiocontrast media 1685
nomenclature 307
receptors/receptor proteins 309, 315–16
terminal pathway 314–15
activation 314
components 308, 314
regulation 315
see also specific components/controlling proteins/receptors
complementarity-determining regions (hypervariable regions)
immunoglobulin 61
T cell receptor 1380
complementary (alternative) therapies 1288–9
chronic asthma 1433
compliance, airway wall 665–7
in vivo assessment 667
smooth muscle role in determining 667
Compositae 854, 1021
dermatitis 1625–6
composting, waste 871
computed tomography
allergic alveolitis (extrinsic)
acute disease 1493
chronic disease 1494
allergic bronchopulmonary aspergillosis 1502
eosinophilic pneumonia (chronic) 1508
rhinitis 1297
conalbumin 966
conarachin 967, 1556
concanavalin A-reactive glycoprotein peanut allergen 968
condom, latex
alternatives 989
dermatitis 982, 989
conglycinin 968
conifers 1020
conjunctiva
anatomy 1646, 1648
cytology 1664
histamine provocation test 1649
conjunctivitis
allergic 1651–2, 1658–9, 1662
acute 1662
atopic dermatitis associated with 1576
clinical features 1651, 1653–4, 1662
diagnosis 1269
management 1236–9, 1269, 1651–3, 1654, 1662
pathogenesis 1651, 1653, 1662
pathology/histology 1651, 1653, 1662
perennial, *see* perennial allergic conjunctivitis
seasonal, *see* seasonal allergic conjunctivitis
giant papillary 1658–9
see also blepharo(kerato)conjunctivitis; keratoconjunctivitis; rhinoconjunctivitis
connective tissue
mast cells 150–1
steroid effects 627
constant region of Ig, *see* C region/domain of Ig
contact activation (in blood clotting) 324, 327
in allergic disease 333–4
mechanisms and regulation 328–31
contact blepharoconjunctivitis 1661–2
contact dermatitis 1608–31
common allergens 1621–5
definition 1608
epidemiology 1609
historical perspective 1608–9
investigation/diagnosis 1617–27
management 1626–7
mucosal 1616
predisposing factors 1609–10
prevention 1626
prognosis 1627
protein 1616
contact dermatitis, allergic 1279–80, 1612–17
cellular mechanisms 1612
clinical features/patterns 1614–17
cross-reactions 1612–13
diagnosis/confirmation 1279–81, 1577, 1608–9, 1617–27
patch test, *see* patch test
general features 1615
histopathology 1613–14
immunology 1613–14
latex-containing products 982
management 1268, 1626–7
molecular aspects 1614
murine model 1059–60
specific types 1615–16
tolerance 1613
contact dermatitis, irritant 1610–12
advice/counselling 1627
cumulative insult/chronic injury 1611–12
immunology 1613–14
non-immune 1619
patient history 1614
contact lens wear and conjunctivitis 1658–9
contact reactions, non-eczematous 1617
contact urticaria 1602, 1617
food allergens 1524–5, 1527
immunologically-mediated 1602, 1616
management 1268
non-immunological 1602
contractile proteins 741
contrast media (in radiology), adverse reactions 1566, 1685–7
prevention 1566, 1686–7
risk factors 1673, 1685
Cooke, Robert A. 19, 20
cooling/rewarming hypothesis in exercise-induced asthma 702–3
Coombs, R. Robin A. 20
Coombs' test 20
cord blood IgE and atopy 1709–10, 1715–16
cork factory 870
cornea
anatomy 1646–7
disorders, *see entries under* kerato-
cortical centres in asthma, higher 508–10
corticosteroids, *see* glucocorticosteroids
corticotrophin-releasing factor

cytokine-induced production 506–7
in depressive illness 510
cortisol (hydrocortisone)
in asthma, intravenous 630
IgE synthesis induced by 102
steroid receptor binding 617–18
cost of allergic disease 1715
cot death, food allergy and 1536, 1557–8
cotton mill, byssinosis 870–1
cottonseed 974
cough
asthmatic, chronic (cough-variant) 1350–1, 1356–7
management 1437
non-asthmatic, sodium cromoglycate effects 586
wheeze and, in infants 1452–4
counselling, contact dermatitis 1627
cow, *see Bos domesticus*; milk proteins
CR1 (complement receptor; CD35) 315
on eosinophils 176
CR2 (CD21; complement receptor 2; EBV receptor) 89, 315
CD23 interaction with 41
IgE and 88
FcεRII receptor for 81–2, 88
synthesis of 41
CR3, *see* Mac-1
CR4 (CD11c/CD18) 315
crab allergens, occupational exposure 913
crawfish (crayfish) 971
CREB, *see* cAMP-responsive element binding protein
Crohn's disease 1282
leukotrienes and 393
cromakalim and cromakalim-like drugs, *see* potassium ion channel openers
cromoglycate, sodium/disodium (cromolyn sodium), *see* sodium cromoglycate
crops, fungal spore allergens 863, 865, 868–70
see also farming *and specific crops*
crustacean (seafood) allergens 804–5, 913, 969–71
occupational exposure 913
recombinant, synthesis 819
see also individual genera/species
cryptogenic fibrosing alveolitis 1496
Cryptomera japonica allergens 801
CSF, granulocyte/macrophage-, *see* granulocyte/macrophage-CSF
CTL-A_4/CTLA-4 1389
T cell activation and 132
T cell antigen recognition and 38, 1389
cultural factor in atopy 1187
cultures
lymphocyte 753–5
primary 756–7, 757
tissue, *in situ* hybridization 770–1
Cupressaceae 850–1, 1020
Cupressoidaeae 850
cutaneous lymphocyte-associated antigen (CLA) 287
C-X-C chemokines 175, 368, 369
basophil and eosinophil effects 369
neutrophil effects 201, 369
structure 367
cyclic ADP ribose, neutrophil 206
cyclic AMP, *see* AMP
cyclic GMP, *see* GMP
cyclic nucleotide phosphodiesterase isoenzyme, *see* phosphodiesterase
cyclin D and cyclin-dependent kinases, rapamycin effects on association 648
cyclo-oxygenase 398
gene transcription, steroids affecting 620
inhibitors
in asthma 1731
sheep mediator release and effect of 1048
pathway products, *see* prostanoids
cyclophilin–immunosuppressive drug complexes 642–5
cyclophosphamide 650
toxicity 656
cyclosporin 641–8
in asthma 655–7, 1387, 1732–3
in chronic disease 1387, 1432
in experimental models 655, 1071, 1072
in steroid-resistant asthma 1387
in atopic dermatitis 657, 1584
cellular effects 645–8
gene expression altered by 641–5
liposome-encapsulated 733, 735–6
toxicity 656
in vernal keratoconjunctivitis 1657
Cynodon dactylon (Bermuda grass) allergens 799
cross-reactivity 1018–19
cynomolgus monkey, *see* primate model
cypress 850–1, 1020
cysteinyl leukotrienes, *see* leukotriene C_4; leukotriene D_4; leukotriene E_4
cystic fibrosis
amiloride in 722–3
asthma and 1356
mucous retention 719–20
nasal polyps and 1295
periciliary fluid abnormality 714
cytidine deaminase inhibition 651
cytokines 340–64, 506–7, 1002, 1230–2
activity/action (in general)
immunosuppressive drugs inhibiting 648–9
regulation 341–2
in allergen-specific immunotherapy 1230–2
insect stings and 1702–4
in allergic inflammation (in general) 350, 351, 531–2
guinea pig model 1098–9
assays 1002, 1003
asthma and 46, 47–8, 269–71, 272, 350, 351, 358, 359, 360, 361, 619, 1368, 1373, 1383–4
cytokine antagonists in therapy 1733
epithelial-derived cytokines 1375
guinea pig model 1096, 1097, 1098–9
in late response 1119–20, 1122–3, 1125, 1373
murine model 1064
proliferative and fibrogenic 303
rat model 1074–5
atopy and 350, 351, 1368
basophil 46, 158, 1317
CNS effects 506–7
in contact dermatitis (murine model) 1060
in cutaneous late-phase reactions 1135–6
endothelial cell-derived 285
eosinophil-derived 181, 357
steroid effects 621
eosinophil effects of 158, 173, 174–5, 349, 354–7
in guinea pig model 1097, 1098–9
mast cell-derived cytokines 158
T cell-derived 41–2, 46, 349
eosinophil receptors for 177
epithelial cell release in bronchi, sodium nedocromil effects 584
fibroblast-derived 304
gene transcription 341–2
immunosuppressive drug effects 643, 645
steroid effects 619
in helminthic infection 1171
as histamine-releasing factors 1589
inflammatory cell-derived 46–7
macrophage (pulmonary alveolar)-derived 230–1
T-helper cell selection by 232–3
macrophage (pulmonary alveolar) function in inflammation and the role of 234–5
mast cell, *see* mast cell
monoclonal antibodies to, in studies of allergic disease models 1056–7
in nasal pathology
in late-phase reaction 1149–50, 1153–4
in rhinitis 46, 1316–19
nomenclature 340–1
in plasma exudates 440
precursor processing 342
production/synthesis (in general)
cyclosporin effects 646
regulation 341–2
pro-inflammatory types 345–7
properties of individual 344–50
receptor (haematopoietic receptor) 342–4
antagonists 342
modulation of number 342
superfamily 342–4
sequestration 342
soluble binding proteins 342
steroid resistance caused by, secondary 631–2
structural families 341
Th cell development affected by 106–8, 350
urticaria and 1589
see also specific cytokines
cytokines, T cell-derived 41–2, 42–3, 44, 46, 357
in allergen-specific immunotherapy 1230–2
in allergy (in general) 104–5, 126, 126–7
IgE synthesis and 40–1, 98–9
in immune response 45, 124
in late-phase reactions
in asthma 1119–20, 1122, 1123, 1125
in skin 1135
properties/effects (in general) 348, 349
in rhinitis 1318
cytolytic hypersensitivity reactions, *see* cytotoxic hypersensitivity reactions
cytoplasmic antigens in neutrophils, autoantibodies 1004
cytostatic agent, nitric oxide as 519
cytotoxic hypersensitivity reactions (cytolytic/antibody-dependent/type II reactions) 24–5, 26
drugs 1676
mechanism 26
type IIa 26
type IIb 26
cytotoxic T cell, *see* CD8+ cells; $CTLA_4$
cytotoxicity
eosinophil 183
nitric oxide 519
T cell, assay 759–60

D gene segment
heavy chain 65
immunoglobulin 63
T cell receptor 1380
see also V(D)J region
DAF, *see* decay accelerating factor
Dake, Henry 10
danazol, hereditary angioedema 1604
Dε2 determinant of IgE 1013
death (cell)
immunotherapy-related 1247
programmed, *see* apoptosis
death (individual)
asthmatic

β_2-agonists and 1434
children 1452
depression and 509–10
increases 1210
pathology, *see* post-mortem
steroids reducing 623
sudden infant, food allergy and 1534, 1556–7
decay accelerating factor (DAF) 316
deficiency 318, 320
decongestants, nasal
abuse/overuse 1296, 1329
in allergic rhinitis 1327–9
guidelines for use 1338
in seasonal rhinitis (hayfever) 1284
drug interactions 1329
defence, neutrophils in 198–200
see also immune system
deflazacort 1728
degranulation
eosinophil 172, 183, 1170
mast cell
agents causing 1564
cutaneous late-phase reaction and 1134
food allergy and sudden infant death and 1557
see also mast cell degranulating peptide
dehumidification 1719
dehydration/water loss, airway, in exercise-induced asthma 699–700, 702, 703
delayed hypersensitivity (type IV; T cell/lymphocyte-mediated) 25–8
animal model 1388
drug allergy 1676
food allergy 1523–4
latex allergy 982–3
mechanisms 27
tuberculin-induced, skin biopsy features 1135
type IVa 27
type IVb 27
type IVc 27, 29, 30
delayed pressure urticaria 1598
deletion, T cell, *see* T cell
deletion joining of Igs 64
δ heavy chain, structure 60
δ-opioid receptors 465
denaturing sprays, allergen 1719
dendritic cells 120–4, 235–40
airway/lung 122–3, 235–40
in acute and chronic inflammation 237–8
distribution/density 235–6
origin/ontogeny 237, 239
in rat model of tolerance 1069–70
steady-state kinetics 237
structure/surface phenotype 236–7
allergy and 125, 126
as antigen-presenting cells 234, 238–9, 1069–70
in initiation of immune response 120–4
lymphoid 121–2
migratory pathways 123
non-lymphoid (in general) 122–4
steroid sensitivity 238
T cell interactions with
aeroallergen sensitization and 239
resting 125
Th2 cell development and 106
Denmark, allergy training 1264
density centrifugation, lymphocyte preparation via 754–5
deoxyribonucleic acid, *see* DNA; DNase; nucleotides
deoxyspergualin 652
toxicity 656
depression
in asthma 509–10
immunity and effects of 508–9
Der f and Der p, *see Dermatophagoides farinae; Dermatophagoides pteronyssinus*
dermatitis (eczema) 1573–85, 1608–31
contact, *see* contact dermatitis
inhalant, allergic, canine 1105
seborrhoeic 1577
dermatitis (eczema), atopic 1267, 1279, 1573–85
age and 1212
clinical features 1574–5
major 1574
minor 1574
complications and associated diseases 1575–6, 1659–61
course/prognosis 1577
definition 1209, 1576
differential diagnosis 1577
eosinophilia 187
epidemiology 1210, 1574
food allergens causing 1527–9, 1542, 1581–2, 1583
gender and 1213
genetics 1573–4
investigations/diagnosis 1279, 1577
management 1579–80, 1583–4
H_1 antagonists 432, 1584
immunopharmacological agents 657, 1584
immunotherapy 1239–40
phosphodiesterase inhibitors 552, 553
principles 1267
maternal diet and 1542
murine model 1060
ocular allergy associated with 1576, 1659–60
pathogenesis 1558–83
pathology 1577–9
race and 1213
skin biopsy features 1135
variants 1575
dermatitis herptiformis 1533
dermatographism, *see* dermographism
Dermatophagoides farinae allergens (Der f) 802
recombinant
cloning of gene in manufacture of 811–12
synthesis 815–16
Dermatophagoides pteronyssinus (house-dust mite) allergens (Der p) 802, 888–99, 1023, 1275, 1710–11, 1718
in asthma 1367
children 1456
in late-phase response 1116
atopic eczema and immediate hypersensitivity to 1239–40
avoidance (prevention of exposure/sensitization) 893–4, 1283–4, 1710–11, 1718–20
children 1456, 1710–11, 1718–20, 1721
in rhinitis 1327
biochemical properties 802
allergenic activity and 805
CD23 cleavage by 1167
cross-reactivity 1023
cutaneous reactions induced by, late-phase 1132
epidemiology 891–3
exposure 1215, 1718
measurement 890–1
history 888–9
HLA-D and 50, 1385–6
immunotherapy 894–5, 1236–7, 1239
efficacy 1236–7, 1239
indications 1239
safety 1237, 1239
recombinant
cloning of cDNA 811–12
synthesis 815–16
seasonal perennial conjunctivitis and 1653, 1664
sensitization
prevention, *see* avoidance (*subheading above*)
relationship to exposure 891–2
T cells and 894–5, 1385–6
Th cells 105, 141
treatment 893–5
immunotherapy, *see* immunotherapy
Dermatophytes 1022
dermatosis, juvenile plantar 1575
dermographism (factitious urticaria) 1597–8
pathogenesis 1597
physiological 1597
rarer forms 1598
symptomatic immediate 1597–8
desensitization
to allergen, *see* immunotherapy
β-adrenoceptor 576
desensitization test of chemokine receptor usage 372–93
detergents
allergenic enzymes in 915, 1278, 1480
in PCR 785
Deuteromycotina 860
dextran-induced anaphylactoid reactions 1677–8
prevention 1678
diagnosis
methods, *see* tests
principles and practice 1271–90
dialysis/haemodialysis membranes, adverse reactions 1673
anaphylaxis 1558
diaminobenzidine 776
diarrhoea, adverse food reactions 1536
dichloromethylene diphosphonate 234
dichromate, potassium, testing with 1622–3
diesel particulates 1397
see also traffic fumes
diet
allergens in, *see* food allergens; food allergy
elimination 1536–7
diagnosis via 1536–7
management via 1536, 1540
maternal, in lactation 1541–2, 1720, 1721
food allergy 1541–2, 1720
intervention 1721
maternal, in pregnancy 1721
asthma aetiology and 1368–70
intervention 1721
as risk factor for atopy/atopic disease 1217, 1712
diet diaries 1536
diethylcarbamazine in tropical eosinophilia 1504, 1505
dietitians 1287
dihydrofolate reductase inhibition by methotrexate 650
diisocyanates, *see* isocyanates
dimethylglyoxine test 1621
dipteran allergens 911
Diskhaler 1443–4
Diskus/Accuhaler 1444
disodium cromoglycate, *see* sodium cromoglycate
Disperse dyes 1625
disseminated intravascular coagulation (DIC) 334
diurnal changes, *see* circadian/diurnal changes
DNA
in PCR 785

denaturation 782–3, 786
probes, construction for *in situ* hybridization 764
rearrangement, Ig genes, *see* immunoglobulin, genes
replication/synthesis
activator of 645
Ig genes, class switching and 97–8
immunosuppressive drugs affecting 645, 649–52
subcloned template, complementary/antisense RNA probes made from 765
transcription, *see* transcription
DNA, complementary (cDNA)
allergen gene cloning employing 810–13
screening of cDNA library 811–13
in reverse-transcriptase PCR, synthesis 786, 787–8
DNA polymerases (in PCR) 782, 783, 785–6
inhibitors 784
thermal inactivation 784
DNase treatment, sputum 722
dobutamine in circulatory shock 1568
dog, *see Canis familiaris*
Dolichovespula spp. venom (Dol) 818
maculata (Dol m) 932
Dol m 5 allergen 804, 818
nomenclature 936
recombinant 818
'dolor' as classical sign of inflammation 440
dopamine in circulatory shock 1568
drug(s) (allergy-treating—clinical and experimental) 51, 1284–5
anaphylaxis prevention 1566
asthma 51, 257, 685–6, 1285, 1430–6, 1726–38
aerosols, *see* aerosols
in allergic bronchopulmonary aspergillosis 1503
anticholinergics, *see* cholinergic antagonists
β-agonists, *see* β-adrenoceptor agonists
bronchial hyperresponsiveness decreased by 685–6
children 601–562, 623, 1458, 1459–60, 1461
chromones, *see* nedocromil sodium; sodium cromoglycate
in exercise-induced asthma 696–9, 1436
in guinea pig model 1099
H_1 receptor blockers, *see* H_1 receptor antagonists
immunosuppressive 358, 630, 655–7, 1732–3
in late-phase response 1115–16
leukotriene action-modulating drug 393–8, 699, 1730–1
novel 632, 1726–38
PAF antagonists 221–2, 407–8, 1084, 1116
phosphodiesterase inhibitors, *see* aminophylline; methylxanthines; phosphodiesterase inhibitors; theophylline
potassium ion channel openers, *see* potassium ion channel openers
prostanoid action modulating drug(s) 403–4
in rabbit model 1085–6
routes of delivery 1433–4
in sheep model 1052–3
step-down 1432
steroids, *see* glucocorticosteroids
in chronic obstructive pulmonary disease 600–2
in cutaneous late-phase reaction 1135–6
development 21–2
in food allergy 1285, 1540
interactions
antihistamines 427, 1331, 1333
decongestants 1329
ocular diseases 1663
acute allergic conjunctivitis 1662
atopic keratoconjunctivitis 1660–1
giant papillary conjunctivitis 1659
perennial allergic conjunctivitis 1654
seasonal allergic conjunctivitis 1652–3
vernal keratoconjunctivitis 1656–7
rhinitis (allergic) 1327–38
cholinergic/muscarinic antagonists 490, 1333
leukotriene biosynthesis inhibitors 397
in seasonal allergic rhinitis (hayfever) 1284–5, 1327–38
see also specific (types of) drugs
drug(s) (non-therapeutic aspects)
adverse reactions, *see* drug reactions
in asthma
exacerbation of asthma 1349–50
inhalational challenge with 1355
pulmonary eosinophilia caused by 1506–7
drug reactions
allergic 1278–9, 1671–92
anaphylaxis-inducing drug(s) 1551, 1552–4, 1558, 1674
classification of major mechanisms 1676
clinical classification 1674, 1675
definition 1671
diagnosis 1278–9, 1676–8, 1680–1, 1681, 1682, 1684, 1687
epidemiology, *see* epidemiology
examples 1679–88
extrinsic allergic alveolitis distinguished from disease caused by 1496
foods/drinks 1536
historical studies 19
management 1267, 1678–9, 1682, 1684, 1685, 1686–7, 1688
multidrug allergies 1679
occupational exposure 921, 1465
classification 1671, 1672
idiosyncracy, definition 1671
interactions 1329
definition 1671
intolerance, definition 1671
overdose, definition 1671
pseudoallergic, *see* pseudoallergic drug reactions
side-effects, definition 1671
see also specific drugs
dry air hyperventilation, airway response in asthmatics 683
dry-powder inhalers 731, 1440, 1443–8
drug deposition 1445
ease of use 1445–6
inspiratory flow with 1446–8
steroids in, systemic effects 626
dry-rot fungus 867
dry skin in atopic dermatitis 1574–5, 1578
Durham slide-and-settle plates 881
dust
mixed (inorganic), fibrosis caused by 1497
organic, *see* organic dust
dust mite, *see Dermatophagoides pteronyssinus*; mite allergens
dynein arms of cilia 710
dysphonia, steroid-related 625

E-selectin (ELAM-1) 244, 272, 273
airway neutrophilia and 252
in allergic inflammation (in general) 250–1
antibodies to (treatment with) 1040, 1042
asthma and 294
model of 292, 1040, 1042
leucocyte–endothelial interactions and 292
eosinophil–endothelium 286, 290–1
neutrophil–endothelium 202
ligands 246, 273
EAACI guidelines on immunotherapy 1243, 1247
ear
middle
inflammation, *see* otitis media
structure and function 1634–5
swelling responses in murine model of allergic contact dermatitis 1059
early airway response in asthma (EAR) 1372, 1373–4
ebastine in rhinitis 1332
EBV, *see* Epstein–Barr virus
economic cost of allergic disease 1715
eczema, *see* dermatitis
education in allergy
medical 1262–4
patient 1265
efferent pathways, vagal, in lung 594–5
efferent phase of immune response 120
EG2+ cells and asthma 1420
egg allergens (Gal d)
B cell epitopes 964
occupational exposure 915
Ehrlich, Paul 8, 9
eicosanoids, *see* lipid mediators
eicosapentaenoic acid, asthma and 1218
late response in 1116
ELAM-1, *see* E-selectin
elastase and asthma 275
elasticity of mucus 716
elastin 719
elderly
allergic rhinitis 1337–8
venom immunotherapy 1236
electric blankets 1719
electrical stimulation of tracheal segments in assessment of murine airway function 1061
electron microscopy
immunocytochemistry under 779–80
in situ hybridization under 771
electrophoresis of allergens 796–7
elms 1020
embolism, pulmonary 1356
emergency management, acute severe asthma 1266
emesis (vomiting)
food allergy-related 1536
with phosphodiesterase-4 inhibitors 553
emetics, mucociliary clearance improved by 721
emotional factors causing rhinitis 1296
encapsulated drugs for aerosols, *see* liposome-encapsulated drugs
encephalomyelitis, experimental allergic 138, 1060–1
immunotherapy 139
T cell receptor repertoire and 1385
endobronchial catheters, pressure measurements in asthmatics 670–1
endocardial cells, NO activity 521
endocrine system, *see* hormones; neuroendocrine regulation
endopeptidase, neutral (NEP) 495–6
asthma and 276, 496–7, 1731–2
therapy of 1731–2
neuropeptides degraded by 276, 448, 450, 495–6
endoplasmic reticulum, Ig transport 73

endoscopic biopsies, *in situ* hybridization 770
endoscopy
gastric, in food allergen provocation tests 1538–9
nasal (in rhinitis) 1297, 1306
endosomes 118
endothelial cells (and endothelium) 244–62, 284–97
in allergy/allergic inflammation (in general) 250–6, 272–4, 284–97
mediator production 285–6
phosphodiesterase 535
phosphodiesterase inhibitor effects 545, 548
as target 289–92
in asthma 289–90, 293–4, 1372
contact activation cascade components assembled along surface of 332
leucocyte adhesion to, *see* adhesion and *specific* leucocytes
nitric oxide in 521
in rhinitis 1318, 1319
umbilical vein, *see* umbilical vein endothelial cells
endothelial leucocyte adhesion molecule-1, *see* E-selectin
endothelial nitric oxide synthetase, *see* nitric oxide synthetase
endothelial venule, high (HEV), selectins and 245
endothelin 516–28
biological actions 519
detection 520
localization 520–5
synthesis 516
endothelium, *see* endothelial cells
endotoxic shock
contact activation proteins in 334
nitric oxide and 525–6
enhancer elements, Ig heavy chain gene 71
enteropathy
gluten-sensitive, *see* gluten-sensitive enteropathy
infantile (enterocolitis), food-induced 1282, 1529
environmental factors (aetiological)
asthma, in early life 1368–9
atopy 1187–8, 1213
see also specific factors
environmental measures in prevention of allergy in early life 1718–20
combined with dietary measures 1721
enzyme(s)
as allergens 1167
occupational exposure 914, 915–16, 1278, 1480
gene for, steroids affecting transcription of 620
in immunocytochemistry 774–5, 776–7
for multiple staining 779
see also specific enzymes
enzyme immunoassays (EIA) 1003
cockroach allergens 947
cytokines 1002
eosinophil(s) 171–97, 1117–18, 1229
activation 172, 182–3, 368–71
chemokines in 368–71
priming factors 183
in allergen-specific immunotherapy 1228–9
in allergic inflammation (generally) 185–8, 253–5, 1097–8
phosphodiesterase 536
phosphodiesterase inhibitor effects 545, 547, 548, 550
assays and their value 1000
in asthma 185, 186, 187, 219, 1373, 1382, 1383–4, 1420–1
aspirin/other NSAIDs and 1688
in children 1454
diapedesis 1422
extracellular matrix signals to 303
guinea pig 1096–7, 1097–8
in late response 1117–18, 1122, 1372
post-mortem 185
in primate model 1038, 1039, 1041
in sheep model 1049–50
sodium cromoglycate effects 583–4
T cell interactions with 187–8, 1382, 1383–4
biology 171–85
chemotaxins, *see* chemotaxins
counts, peripheral blood, significance 185–6
cutaneous late-phase reactions and 1134–5
cytokines and, *see* cytokines
cytotoxicity 183
degranulation 172, 183, 1170
density 182
differentiation 173
in disease (in general) 185–8
endothelial cell interactions with 290–1
extracellular matrix adhesion by 254–5
in helminthic infection 1169–70, 1171
maturation 173
mediators produced by 178–82
asthma and 274
secretion/release 183
migration 42, 173–5
adhesion molecules and 42, 173–4, 253–4, 288–9
antibodies inhibiting 252–3
morphology 171–2
in nasal late-phase reaction 1147
receptors on 173–7
adhesion 42, 173–4
in rhinitis 1316–17
role (in health and disease) 185
ultrastructure 171–2
in urticaria 1587
in vernal keratoconjunctivitis 1654–5
eosinophil cationic protein (ECP) 180–1
asthma and 275
helminthic infection and 1169, 1170
infant wheezers and 1454
rhinitis and 1317
eosinophil-derived neurotoxin (EDN) 180, 181
eosinophil peroxidase (EPO) 180, 181, 383
in helminthic infection 1169–70
eosinophilia 185
angioedema associated with 1604
in dermatitis (atopic) 187, 1578
pulmonary/lower airway 1500–16
in asthma 186, 187, 1122
classification and causes 1500, 1501
see also specific causes
clinical approaches to suspected disease 1509
diagnosis and management 1269
ICAM-1 and 252
in rhinitis
in allergic rhinitis 187
in non-allergic rhinitis (NARES) 1295–6
eosinophilia–myalgia syndrome 1507
eosinophilic bronchitis, chronic 1351
eosinophilic gastroenteritis, allergic 1526, 1532
eosinophilic lung disease, diagnosis and management 1269
see also eosinophilia; hypereosinophilic syndrome
eosinophilic pneumonia
acute 1508–9
chronic 1507–8, 1510
eotaxin 371, 1098–9
in guinea pig model 1098–9
ephedrine 578
epidemiology 1208–23, 1715
air pollution/respiratory irritants and allergic disease 1399–400, 1467–8, 1712
anaphylaxis 1551
atopy and atopic disease 1187–8, 1208–23, 1468–9
see also specific atopic diseases
childhood asthma 1181–2, 1451–2
cockroach allergens 942–4, 949
dermatitis
atopic 1210, 1574
contact 1609
drug allergy 1671–4
aspirin/other NSAIDs 1687
β-lactam antibiotics 1682–3
local anaesthetics 1682
muscle relaxants 1679
sulphonamides 1684
extrinsic allergic alveolitis 1490–1
food allergy/intolerance 1518
genetic 1177–9, 1182–3, 1185, 1191, 1191–2
insect sting allergy 1693
mite allergens 891–3
occupational allergic alveolitis 1490–1
occupational asthma 909–10, 1465–70
ocular allergy 1645
otitis media 1633–4
rhinitis (allergic) 1320–41
skin tests in 1010–11, 1208, 1211, 1212, 1609
urticaria 1586–7
physical 1596–7
epidermis, Langerhans cells, *see* Langerhans cells
epinephrine, *see* adrenaline
Epipen autoinjector 1565
epithelial cells, lower airway and airway in general
in asthma 267–70
damage/shedding/inflammatory attack 161–2, 444, 1087, 1374–5, 1414–16
sub-basement membrane thickening 161, 301, 1417
ciliated, *see* cilia
endothelin in 522
nitrogen dioxide effects 1399
phosphodiesterase 535
phosphodiesterase inhibitor effects 545, 549
restitution of denuded 444–6
sodium nedocromil effects on cytokine release from 584
steroid effects 621–2
epithelial cells, upper airway
larynx 1308
nasal
in late-phase reaction 1146
in rhinitis 1314, 1318, 1320
structure 1300–2, 1312
pharynx 1308
epithelial-derived contracting factor, asthma and 267, 268
epithelial-derived relaxing factor, asthma and 267
epithelium, *see* epithelial cells
epitopes
B cell, *see* B cell
chironomid allergens and 955–6
food allergens and 964–5
Hymenoptera venoms and 937
T cell, *see* T cell
epoxy resin industry 916–17, 1278
ε-binding protein (Mac-2; CBP35) 91–2

eosinophils expressing 176
ε heavy chain
production 98–9, 100
structure 60
see also Fcε receptors
Epstein–Barr virus
B cells transformed by, T cell cultures requiring 755–6, 757
IgE synthesis induced by 101–2
receptor, *see* CR2
Equus caballus (horse) allergens 905, 1276
Eragrotideae 842
erythrocytes, sheep, murine model of airway changes using 1063–4
erythro-9-(2-hydroxy-3-nonyl)-adenine 537
ethanolamines 1330
ethnicity and atopy/atopic disease 1213
ethylene dioxide-altered human serum albumin 1558
ethylenediamines 1330, 1624
tests 1624
Europe
pollen in
grass 843–6
tree 847–52
weed 852, 853
training in allergy 1262–3, 1264
European Aeroallergen Network 840–1
birch pollen maps 848
European standard series, contact allergens 1621
European Union on allergen extracts 830
Eurotium spp. 869
Eustachian tube
dysfunction, otitis media due to 1637, 1639
diagnosis 1639–40
obstruction 1635–6
otitis media due to 1635–6
types 1635
structure and function 1634
evidence-based medicine and research 1269
examination, physical 1272
asthma 1351
contact dermatitis 1614–15
rhinitis 1297
exercise-induced anaphylaxis 1559–60
food-dependent 1530–1
exercise-induced asthma 690–709, 1436
epidemiology 692
in general population, identification 692–3
in known/recognized asthmatics 691–2
identification 693–4
in laboratory, identification 693
leukotrienes in 391–2, 394
management 696–702, 1436
leukotriene antagonists 394
phosphodiesterase inhibitors 552
preventive 696–9
prostanoid action modulators in 404
as marker for asthma prevalence 695–6
mechanisms/stimulus/airway response in 683, 702–3
mediators and 703–4
refractory period, use 701
stimulus and mechanism 700–1, 702–3
surrogate challenges to identify 694–5
see also physical training
exercise-induced urticaria, food and 1599
exocytosis, eosinophil 183
exotoxins, bacterial
atopic dermatitis and 1582
ciliary beating slowed by 719
experimental models, *see* animal models; human models
expiration, forced, *see* forced expiration; forced expiratory volume in one second (FEV_1)
expiratory flow in asthmatic 676–7
peak, in classification of disease 1348
peak, in diagnosis 1352–3
of exercise-induced asthma 694
expiratory flow–volume curves, maximum, in asthmatics 668–9
exposure 1467
extracellular matrix 301
in bronchial asthma 301
cellular signals from 303–4
eosinophil adhesion to 254–5
eye 1645–67
allergic diseases (in general) 1645–67
anatomical considerations 1645–8
atopic dermatitis associated with 1576, 1659–60
classification 1648
diagnosis/investigations 1269, 1662–5
differential diagnosis 1662–5
epidemiology 1645
management 1269
models 1649
pathophysiology and mechanisms (overview) 1648–51
see also specific diseases
hayfever-associated symptoms 1284
ipratropium adverse effects 603
steroid adverse effects 628
eyelids, anatomy 1645–6
see also entries under blepharo-

face, allergic contact dermatitis 1615–16
test series 1626
factor B 312–13
deficiency 318, 320
factor D 312–13
deficiency 318, 320
factor H 313
deficiency 318, 320
factor I 312, 313
deficiency 318, 320
factor P deficiency 318, 320
factor XI 326–7
factor XII (Hageman factor) 324, 324–5
activation 324–5
auto- 330
anaphylactoid reactions and 1559
in contact activation 330–1, 332
on endothelial call surface 332
Fagaceae 849–50, 1019
Betulaceae and, cross-reaction 850
Fagales family, allergens 799
familial essential cold urticaria 1600
family (and relatives)
childhood asthma management and 1458
heritability of allergy/asthma and risk to 1200
size of family as risk factor for atopy/atopic disease 1217
family studies (in allergy) 1177–9, 1198–9
asthma 1177–9, 1180, 1198
atopy 1180, 1187, 1188
farmer's lung 1489
diagnosis 1496
differential 1496–7
epidemiology 1490–1
historical observations 18
management 1497–8
natural history/prognosis 1495
farming/agriculture 1465
fungal spore allergens 863, 865, 868–70
fatality, *see* death
Fcα receptors on eosinophils, *see* immunoglobulin A
Fcγ receptors 84–5
FcγRI (CD64)
binding site 84–5
on eosinophils 176
function 62
FcγRII (CD32), on eosinophils 176
FcγRIII (CD16), on eosinophils 176
Fcε receptors 85–92, 176
FcεRI (high-affinity IgE receptor) 62, 81, 83–5, 85–6, 176, 1013
atopy and 49, 1191, 1192, 1202, 1368, 1371
autoantibodies 1004
binding site 83–5
as therapeutic target 92
FcεRII (low-affinity IgE receptor; CD23) 81–2, 87–92, 103–4, 176
allergy and 127
atopy and 1371
binding site 85
CD21 interaction with 41
counter-receptors for 89–92
Dermatophagoides pteronyssinus allergen cleaving 1167
on eosinophils 176
IgE synthesis and 41, 103–4
parasitic proteases cleaving 1167
on platelets 217
soluble fragments 87
FDA, allergen extracts and 830
feed mills 870
feet, atopic winter 1575
Felis domesticus (cat) allergens 803, 900–2, 1023–4, 1275–6
major antigen (Fel d 1) 50, 803, 829, 900–1, 1023
allergenic activity 900–1
biochemistry 803, 901
environmental exposure 902, 1024, 1215
immunotherapy 1237, 1239
recombinant, synthesis 817
standardization 829
other allergens 902
prevention of exposure 1711, 1718
females, *see* breast-feeding; gender differences; pregnancy; pre-menstrual asthma
fetus
in aetiology of allergy 1721–2
asthma 1368–70, 1371
sensitization 1721–2
prevention of allergy 1715–25
FEV_1, *see* forced expiratory volume in one second
fibreoptic bronchoscopy, *see* bronchoscopy, fibreoptic
fibrin deposits in damaged epithelium of asthmatics 1414
fibroblast(s) 298–306
asthma and 298–306
cytokine production 304
transfected murine, as accessory cells for culturing T cells 756
fibroblast growth factor (FGF) in asthma 271
basic type 2 (FGF-2) 304
fibrosing alveolitis, cryptogenic 1496
fibrosis, mixed-dust 1497
filaments, intermediate 741
filaria-associated pulmonary eosinophilia 1504–5
filters, air 1719
filtration of particles in nose 1308, 1312
Finland, occupational asthma 1466
Finn chambers 1617
fire ant, *see Solenopsis*
fish allergens 967
fish oils, asthma and 1218
late response in 1116
fixation, *see* preservation

FK506 (tacrolismus) 641–8
cellular effects 645–8
gene expression altered by 641–5
toxicity 656
FK506-binding protein 642, 645
FLAP, *see* 5-lipoxygenase activating protein
flare, substance P-evoked 451
flare-up reactions, allergic contact dermatitis 1612–13
flour allergens 913–14, 1278, 1478, 1479
immunotherapy 1240
flow (of air)
expiratory, *see* expiratory flow
inspiratory, *see* inspiratory flow; inspiratory peak flow
obstruction, *see* obstruction
resistance in lower airways (pulmonary resistance), in asthmatics 669
resistance in nose
in asthmatics 672, 673
in late-phase reaction 1142
measurement, *see* rhinomanometry
flow-cytometry *in situ* hybridization 771
flow–volume curves in asthmatics 668–9
flower pollen allergens 801
Floyer, John 17
fluids, intravenous, in circulatory shock 1568
flukes, liver 1506
flunisolide, rhinitis 1336
fluorescent antibody labels 776
in multiple staining 778
flurbiprofen, allergen challenge in asthma and effects of 403
fluricasone propionate in rhinitis 1335
flux, solder, *see* colophony
fly allergens 911
follicular variant of atopic dermatitis 1575
food
additives 1281
mimicking allergic reactions 1536
urticaria and angioedema associated with 1593
adverse reactions
definition of term 1517
diagnosis 1534–40
prevalence 1518
aversion 1268, 1280
contaminants/toxins 1517
mimicking allergic reactions 1536
intolerance 1240, 1268, 1280–2
definition 1517
hyperkinetic syndrome and 1240, 1281
management 1268
processing plants 870, 1465
scraps, as spore sources 867
see also diet
food (dietary) allergens 961–80, 1517–49, 1555–7, 1720
atopic dermatitis caused by 1527–9, 1542, 1581–2, 1583
common 965–75
cross-reactivity 962
extracts/preparations 962
IgE antibody tests 1015
immune response to 140–2, 962–3
occupational exposure 911–14, 915, 962
properties 963–5
recombinant 975–6
advantages/disadvantages 975–6
requirements 975
synthesis 819, 975
urticaria and 1524–5, 1527, 1591
food (dietary) allergy/hypersensitivity 804–5, 961–80, 1268, 1280–2, 1517–49, 1555–7, 1720
children, *see* children
clinical features 1524–34
course/prognosis 1540–1
anaphylaxis, *see* anaphylaxis
definitions 962–3, 1517–18
historical studies 18–19
investigations/diagnosis 1280–2, 1288, 1534–40
difficulties 961–2
management 1268, 1540
dietary 1287, 1540
immunotherapy 1240–1, 1540
pharmacological 1285, 1540
otitis media and 1633
pathophysiological mechanisms 1522–4
prevention 1541–2, 1710, 1720
reasons for investigating 961
see also diet
Food and Drug Administration (FDA), allergen extracts and 830
food challenges 1280
chronic urticaria 1593
double-blind placebo-controlled (DBPCFC) 1517, 1518, 1538–40
cutaneous hypersensitivity reactions and 1528
respiratory hypersensitivity reactions and 1529–30
foot, atopic winter 1575
forced expiration, tests of, in asthmatics 669
forced expiratory volume in one second (FEV_1) in asthma 1352
in bronchial hyperresponsiveness studies 682
in diagnosis
exercise-induced asthma 693–4
occupational asthma 1475–6
in experimental allergen challenge in humans 1113–14
leukotrienes and 387, 391, 392
leukotriene antagonists and 394
leukotriene biosynthesis inhibitors and 397
forced oscillation method in assessment of murine airway function 1061
forced residual capacity, asthmatics 676, 677
foreign antigen (non-self/exogenous antigen) 114
IgE responses to 141
recognition/processing mechanisms 116, 117–18, 118
T cell tolerance to 133–7
foreign body-associated conjunctivitis 1658–9
forestry and forest products 870
formaldehyde
occupational exposure 920–1
tests for 1623–4
lutidine 1621
formaldehyde releasers 1624
formalin fixation for immunocytochemistry 776
Formicidae (ants) 928
recombinant allergens 818
formoterol 571
FPL55712 1730
fragrances 1623
France, allergy training 1264
free radicals
asthma and 268–72
atherosclerosis and 522
Freeman, John 21
freezing treatment, mites 1719
fruit allergens 973
cross-reactivity 973, 1019, 1025
fungi (mould) 867–87, 1500–6
entomopathogenic, in cockroach control 949
infection by
atopic dermatitis-associated 1575
pulmonary eosinophilia caused by 1500–6
see also bronchopulmonary mycoses
spores/mycelial fragment allergens 803–4, 871–80, 1020–2
allergenic status 861–2, 1277
in allergic alveolitis 866, 869, 1003, 1492
immunotherapy 1237–8, 1239
indoor occurrence 865–71
mites and 1023
monitoring in USA 841
outdoor occurrence 862–5
recombinant, synthesis 819
young children exposed to 1718
structure/function 858–61
toxins 867
see also yeast infection
Fusarium spp. allergens 804
fyn/$p^{56}{}_{fyn}$ (tyrosine kinase) 85
antigen processing and 119

G proteins 569, 742
eosinophil exocytosis and 183
neutrophil activation and 203–4
receptors coupled to 742
adrenergic 569
Gadus callarius (cod) allergen (Gad c 1; allergen M) 805, 969
B cell epitope 964
Gal d, *see* egg allergens
galactin-1/2 91
β-D-galactosidase 777
galanin 467–8
functional effects 468
localization 467
receptors 467–8
Gallus domesticus allergens, *see* egg allergens
GALT (gut-associated lymphoid tissue) and food allergy 962, 1520–1
γ heavy chain, structure 60
see also Fcγ receptors
γ-subunits/chains
FcεRI 85
G proteins 742
IL-2 receptor, receptors sharing 343
ganglia, peribronchial parasympathetic, β_2-adrenoceptors 573
gases, exchange in lung, asthmatics 674–6
gastric mucosa, food allergen provocation tests under endoscopic control 1538–9
gastrin-releasing peptide 466–7, 495
functional effects 467
localization 466–7, 495
receptors 467
gastroenteritis, allergic eosinophilic 1526, 1533
gastrointestinal tract
blood loss, occult 1534
food allergy and 1281–2, 1519–20, 1524–7, 1531–4
allergen handling and immune system 961–2, 963, 1519–22
clinical features of allergy 1281–2, 1524–7
differential diagnosis of allergy 1538
IgE-mediated 1524–7
non-IgE-mediated 1531–4
pituitary adenylate cyclase activating peptide effects 463
VIP in 456–7
gastro-oesophageal reflux and asthma 1350
gastropods 971–2
GCS 13080 in asthma, allergen challenge and effects of 403
GDP and signal transduction in airway smooth

muscle 742
Gell and Coombs classification of immunopathological reactions with drugs 1676
gender differences/comparisons (in atopy/atopic disease) 1212–13, 1717
in asthma occurrence 1181–2, 1212–13
drug allergy occurrence 1672
barbiturates 1681
muscle relaxants 1679
skin test positivity 1212
gene(s)
allergen 826
cloning/cloned, *see* allergens
for allergy, candidate 1202
for asthma, candidate 1202
chromosomal localization of various, *see* chromosomal localization
complement pathway components, chromosomal localization 317
H_1 receptor 421
HLA, *see* HLA
immunoglobulin, *see* immunoglobulin
immunosuppressive drugs altering expression 641–5
interleukin-4, atopy and 1192–3
phosphodiesterases 533
isoenzyme-1 534
isoenzyme-2 536
isoenzyme-3 537
isoenzyme-4 539
isoenzyme-7 541
steroid-regulated expression 617–21
asthma therapy and 619–21, 633
increasing genomic selectivity 633
tachykinin 447
transcription, *see* transcription
see also specifically named genes
general anaesthetics (allergic reactions) 1279, 1679–81
anaphylaxis 1558
risk factors 1673, 1679–80
genetic counselling, asthmatic parents 1184
genetic linkage/mapping 1202–5
asthma 1183, 1202–5
atopy 1189–90
genetic manipulation/engineering
antibody genes 63
immune and allergic response studies in mouse via 1057–8
genetics (of allergy) 1177–207, 1213, 1716
airway responsiveness/hyperresponsiveness 1182, 1196, 1198, 1201, 1202
in rats 1070
asthma 1177–86, 1196–207, 1213, 1367–8
genetic markers 1182–4
mode of inheritance 1179
occupational disease prevention and 1478
atopy 32, 49, 1179–81, 1187–95, 1213, 1367–8
prediction of atopy 1716
chironomid allergen hypersensitivity 957–8
dermatitis/eczema 1178
atopic dermatitis 1573–4
contact dermatitis 1609–10
drug allergy 1672
urticaria 1587
geographical locations of spore types 863–4
geographical variation of atopy/atopic disease 1210–11
Germany
air pollutant studies in former East and West 1405, 1407
allergy training 1264
giant papillary conjunctivitis 1658–9
giant urticaria, *see* angioedema
glands, submucosal, *see* submucosa
gliadin 972, 1532
glibenclamide as K^+ channel opener antagonists 608, 609
glottis, asthma involving 672–3
gloves, latex 982, 983–4
alternative (non-latex) products 988
diagnosis of allergy 986–7
occupational exposure 985, 1479
routes of exposure 984
glucocorticosteroid(s) (corticosteroids; steroids)
allergic bronchopulmonary aspergillosis 1503
in allergic rabbit 1085, 1086
bronchial hyperresponsiveness decreased by 622, 685–6
conjunctivitis, seasonal allergic 1653
contrast media-related reactions prevented by 1686
dendritic cell sensitivity 238
dermatitis
atopic 1583
contact 1627
eosinophilic pneumonia (chronic) 1508
keratoconjunctivitis
atopic keratoconjunctivitis 1661
vernal keratoconjunctivitis 1657
late response and effects of 1568
asthmatic 1115
cutaneous 1136
nasal 1151–2
leucocyte-derived 507–8
mucociliary clearance improved by 722
neutral endopeptidase and effects of 497
pharmacokinetics 624
receptors 617–18
immunophilin–immunosuppressive drug complexes and 645
resistance in conditions other than asthma 631
reversal of air-flow limitation by course of, diagnostic significance 1354
rhinitis (allergic) including hayfever 1151–2, 1334–6
mode of action 1334
nasal/topical 1284, 1334, 1335–6
systemic 1284–5, 1336
in sheep model of airway inflammation 1049
side-effects 625–9, 1336, 1436
local 625–6, 1336
systemic 626–9, 1336
urticaria (chronic) 1596
glucocorticosteroid(s), in asthma 51, 358, 617–39, 1285, 1768–9
children 623, 1459–60, 1461
chronic asthma 1431, 1434–6
high-dose 1431
maintenance treatment 1432
clinical efficacy 622–3
developments 632, 1460, 1727–8
frequency of administration 624
in allergic bronchopulmonary aspergillosis 1503
guidelines/recommendations 629
hit-and-run 1728
inhaled, *see* inhaled agents/medications; inhalers
intravenous/intramuscular 629
in late response 1115
mechanism of action 617–22, 1436
nasal 1309
oral 617, 629, 1436
resistance to 630–2, 1386–7
alternative means of treatment 358, 1387, 1437
mechanisms 358, 630–1, 1387
secondary 631–2
steroid-sparing strategies 630, 1733
T cells and 1382
glucocorticosteroid response element (GRE) 618
steroid resistance and 631
glucose oxidase 777
glutathione-*S*-transferase as allergen, cockroach 802–3, 946
gluten 972
gluten-sensitive enteropathy (coeliac disease) 972, 1003, 1281–2, 1532–3
course/prognosis 1541
Gly m 30K 968
Glycine max, *see* soybean
glycinin 968
glycoproteins, platelet membrane 216–17
glycosaminoglycans
basement membrane 300
mast cell 153
GM-CSF, *see* granulocyte/macrophage-CSF
GMP, synthesis inhibitors 650–1
cGMP-inhibited phosphodiesterases 532
cGMP-stimulated/specific phosphodiesterases 532
phosphodiesterase isoenzyme-3 537–8
GMP-140, *see* P-selectin
goblet cells
bronchial, in asthma 1418
nasal 1301–2, 1303–4, 1312
gold labels in immunocytochemistry 777
gold salts in asthma 1432, 1732
goosefoot (Chenopodiacae) 852, 1021
Gossypium spp., *see* cotton mill; cottonseed
gout, bradykinin-forming cascade and 334
gp150,95, *see* p150,95
GR 32191 in asthma 402
allergen challenge and effects of 403
bronchial hyperresponsiveness and effects of 404
grafts, *see* transplants
grains, *see* cereals; grass pollen
granules/granular products
asthma and 274, 275
eosinophil, protein in 180
release 183
neutrophil, constituents 198, 199
see also degranulation
granulocyte(s), in antigen-induced airway response in rabbits 1083
see also agranulocytosis; basophil; eosinophil; neutrophil
granulocyte/macrophage-CSF (GM-CSF) 354, 359–60
allergy (in general) and 361
asthma and 47–8, 270, 361
intrinsic 361
biology (in general) 359–61, 1149
eosinophil effects 173, 174–5, 354–7
eosinophil receptors for 177
mRNA *in situ* hybridization 770
receptor 354, 355
β chain, receptors sharing 343, 354
granulomatosis and angiitis, allergic 1509–10
granulomatous vasculitides 1004, 1509–10
grass family, classification 842–3, 1018
grass pollen (grain)
daily/diurnal variation in counts 845–6
seasons 843–5
severity 844–5
timing 843–4
structure 843
grass-pollen allergens 798–9, 842–6

in atopic rhinitis patients, weal diameter induced by 1132
cross-reacting 1018–19
hayfever caused by 105–6
immunotherapy with allergens 51, 105–6, 1236
T cells and 105
recombinant, manufacture 818
see also individual genera/species
Great Britain, *see* United Kingdom
Greece, allergy training 1262–3
Greeks, ancient 4, 5
growth, steroid effects 627, 628
growth factors
in asthma 271
extracellular matrix 304
eosinophil effects 175
monoclonal antibodies to, in studies of allergic disease models 1056–7
GTP and signal transduction in airway smooth muscle 742
GTP-binding proteins, *see* G proteins
guaiphenesin, mucociliary clearance improved by 721
guanine nucleotide(s), *see* GDP; GMP; GTP
guanine nucleotide regulatory proteins, *see* G proteins
guinea pig, *see Cavia porcellus*
gums 914
gustatory rhinorrhoea 1296
gut, *see* gastrointestinal tract
gut-associated lymphoid tissue and food allergy 962, 1520–1

H_1 receptor 421
conjunctiva 1649
function 423
location 423
urticaria and 1588
H_1 receptor antagonists (and antihistamines in general) 421–38
in allergic disorders (in general) 425–6
efficacy 429–32
in asthma 431, 1728–9
chronic asthma 1432
development 1728–9
in conjunctivitis (seasonal allergic) 1652
contrast media-related reactions prevented by 1686
in cutaneous late-phase reactions 1135–6
in dermatitis (atopic) 432, 1583
first-generation 422, 1330–1
adverse effects 432–3, 1330–1
formulation/dosages 428
H_1 receptor blockade by 423–5
in immunotherapy 1253–4
in insect sting allergy 1696
mechanism/mode of action 421–9, 1329–30
in nasal late-phase reactions 1150–1
pharmacodynamics 427–9
pharmacokinetics 426–7, 1331
in pregnancy 425
in rhinitis (seasonal and perennial) 1284, 1329–31, 1338
second-generation 422, 425–6, 1330, 1331–3
adverse effects 422–3, 433–5, 1331, 1332
formulation/dosages 428
relative benefits 427
skin test results influenced by 1009
structure 422
in urticaria
chronic urticaria 431, 1595–6
physical urticaria 1597–8
H_2 receptor
agonists 423
antagonists 423
in anaphylaxis 1568
contrast media-related reactions prevented by 1686
conjunctiva 1649
location and function 423
urticaria and 1588
H-2D 115
H-2I 115
see also I-E molecule
H-2K 115
H_3 receptor
agonists/ antagonists 423
function 423
location 423
nasal 1315
urticaria and 1588
haematological drug reactions
allergic 1675
steroids 628
haematopoietic receptor, *see* cytokines
haemodialysis, *see* dialysis
haemoglobins, chironomid, *see* Chironomid non-biting midge
haemolytic anaemia, immune 1675
Haemophilus influenzae and otitis media 1638
haemosiderosis, food-induced pulmonary 1533–4
Hageman factor, *see* factor XII
hair tint 1625
hands, allergic contact dermatitis 1615
test series 1626
see also MOAHL index
haptens
in allergic contact dermatitis 1614
in drug allergy
inhibition 1678
penicillin 1553, 1678
in immunocytochemistry 777
interaction with host proteins to form neo-antigen 909, 916–21
in models of asthma 1063
harvester ants, *see Pogonomyrmex*
hay, spores associated with 869
hayfever, summer (seasonal allergic rhinitis) 1274–5, 1311–43
causes 1274–5
identification 14
definition 1209
diagnosis 1275
epidemiological factors 1320–1
age 1212
air pollution 845, 1217, 1397
gender 1213
increased prevalence 1210
race 1213
seasonal variation 1216
grass-pollen, *see* grass pollen; grass-pollen allergens
historical background 12–13
management 1265, 1327–43
pharmacological 1284–5, 1327–38
prophylactic 1333–4
otitis media and 1633, 1640
plasma exudation in 444
twin concordance studies 1178
HC14 (MCP-2) 368, 371
headaches
migraine 1534
with potassium ion channel openers 612, 613
health care workers/staff
in allergy clinics 1287
latex allergy 984, 985, 1479
diagnosis 987
prevention 988, 989
other allergies in 1475
heart
arrhythmia-inducing drugs 433–5, 1332, 1333
β-adrenoceptors in 567
β-adrenoceptor agonist effects, adverse 476–7
endothelin in 520–1
transplantation, dendritic cells and 123–4
see also cardiovascular system
heat
loss in airway, as stimulus to exercise-induced asthma 702
mite control using 1719
see also hot air
heat shock proteins, drugs binding to 645, 652
heat urticaria 1596, 1599
localized 1599
heating function, nose 1307–8
heavy (H) chains of Ig/antibody 58
function of different classes of 61–2
genes 65–6
allelic exclusion 69
C region, *see* C gene segment
rearrangement 68–9
transcription 71
structure 58
domain 59
variation between classes 61–2
Heiner's syndrome 1533–4
helium–oxygen mixture, airway response in asthmatics 668–9
helminthic infection 1163–76, 1503–6
allergenicity of helminth allergens 1167
immune response 1169–71
pulmonary eosinophilia caused by 1503–6
relationship to atopy/allergy/asthma 1163–76
allergy/asthmatic state as protective factor (to infection) 1165–6, 1166–9
infection as predisposing factor (to asthma/allergy) 1163–4
infection as preventive or modulating factor (to asthma/allergy) 1164–5
unifying hypothesis 1166
helodermin 461–2
helospectins 461–2
helper T cell, *see* CD4+ T cells; Th
heparan and heparin proteoglycans
basement membrane 300
mast cell 153
heparin, sheep model of bronchoconstriction and effects of 1048
hepatic disorders, *see* liver *and below*
hepatorenal syndrome and leukotrienes 393
hereditary angioedema, *see* angioedema
heredity (in general), *see* family studies; genetics
herpes simplex 1576
5-HETE, asthma and 267
12-HETE, asthma and 267
15-HETE
asthma and 267
eosinophil production 179
Hevea brasiliensis rubber 981–2
known proteins 984
hexahydrophthalic anhydride 917
hexamethylene diisocyanate (HDI) 1476, 1477, 1478
high endothelial venule (HEV), selectins and 245
high-performance liquid chromatography of allergens 798
high-volume pollen samplers 840
himic anhydride 917
Hirschprung's disease 468

Hirst spore trap, pollen trap based on design 839, 840
histamine 999
assays of release 727–8, 999
in drug allergy 1678
in food allergy 1537–8
basophil 1538
biological actions/role 421
canine airway effects of inhalation 1105
conjunctival provocation test 1649
direct release in drug allergy 1680, 1685
IL-6 interactions with 290
IL-8 interactions with 290, 369
mast cell release 153
anaphylaxis and 1559, 1560
food allergy and assays of 1538
urticaria and 1538–9
metabolism, urticaria and 1539
nasal reactivity 1315
antigen-provoked increase 1144
ocular allergy and 1649
platelet 214
receptors and agonists/antagonists, *see* H_1 receptor; H_2 receptor; H_3 receptor
histamine, in asthma/allergic airway disease 275
airway response to 683
in rabbit model 1081
leukotrienes and 388–9
histamine-releasing factors 374
cytokine 1589
food allergy and 1523
rhinitis and 1317
urticaria and 1588–9
histidine–isoleucine, peptide, *see* peptide histidine–isoleucine
histidine–methionine, peptide 486–7
histocompatibility antigens, *see* HLA
history (of allergy/allergological disease) 3–22
allergen extracts 823
anaphylaxis 8, 1550–1
bronchial hyperresponsiveness 680
contact dermatitis 1608–9, 1617
dust mites 888–9
history-taking 1271–2
contact dermatitis, allergic and irritant 1614–15
food allergy 1535–6
muscle relaxant reactions 1680
occupational asthma 1472
rhinitis 1296–7
HIV disease/AIDS, drug reactions with 1674, 1685
hives, *see* urticaria
HLA (human MHC)
allergy and 125
chironomid haemoglobin 957–8
drug 1670
asthma and 1182–3, 1368
occupational 1468
atopic dermatitis and 1574
atopy and 1190–1, 1368
T cells and 1385–6
IgE responsiveness and 32, 108, 1190–1
urticaria and 1587
see also MHC
HLA-D, house-dust mite allergens and 50, 1385–6
HLA-DQA1 and chironomid allergens 958
HLA-DQB1 and chironomid allergens 958
HLA-DR4 alloantigen, IgE synthesis induced by 100
HLA-DRB1 and chironomid allergens 958
Holland, allergy training 1264
homes, nebulizer use 1432–3
see also housing; indoors
homologous restriction factor 315
deficiency 318, 320
honey-bee, *see Apis mellifera*
hookworm 1167
hormones
airway regulation and the role of 505–6
leucocyte-derived 507–8
rhinitis caused by 1296
Th2 cell development and 106
hornbeam (Car b) allergen, recombinant, synthesis 816–17
hornets, *see* vespid
horse allergens 905, 1276
hospital admission studies, air pollutants 1400
hot air in prevention of exercise-induced asthma 702
housing/residential properties
cockroach infestation 946–7
house-dust mite, *see Dermatophagoides pteronyssinus*
spores in 867–8
see also homes; indoors
15-HPETE 179
HRF, *see* homologous restriction factor
human leucocyte antigens, *see* HLA
human models of allergic inflammation 1111–60
airway, *see* asthma
nose 1139–60
skin, *see* skin
humidification function, nose 1307–8
see also dehumidification
humidified air in prevention of exercise-induced asthma 702
humidifier fever 868
actinomycetes 880
diagnosis 1496
hyaluronidases
bee 804, 930
vespid 804, 932
hybridization (cell), T cell 756
hybridization (nucleic acid)
PCR products detected via 787
in situ, *see in situ* hybridization
hydrochloroquine 1732
hydrocortisone, *see* cortisol
hydrogenated soybean phosphatidylcholine liposomes, tolerance/safety 735
15-hydroperoxyeicosatetraenoic acid 179
hydrophilic drugs, liposome-encapsulated 733
hydrophobic drugs, liposome-encapsulated 733
hydroxyeicosatetraenoic acids, *see* HETE
5-hydroxytryptamine, platelet-derived 214
asthma and 220
hygroscopicity of aerosol particles 730
hymenoptera (stinging insects) 927–41
entomology/classification 927–8, 1693
interval from last sting 1698
risk of being stung again 1698
sting morphology 928
hymenoptera allergy 804, 927–41, 1278
allergens (venom)
allergenicity 933–7
cross-reactivity 935–7
recombinant, synthesis 818, 819, 930
sensitization 1693
anaphylaxis 1554–5, 1557, 1567
biochemistry 928–33
clinical features 1694
diagnosis/investigations 1554, 1695–6
drug therapy 1696
epidemiology 1693
immunotherapy 937, 1225–6, 1267, 1278, 1557, 1567, 1694, 1696–703
administration 1699–700
efficacy 1235, 1696
indications 1235–6, 1698–9
mechanism 1701–4
monitoring 1700–2
risk of future reactions 1697–8
safety/side-effects 1235, 1696–7
mechanism 1693–4
natural history 1694–5
principles of management 1267
hyperactivity (hyperkinesis) and food intolerance 1240, 1281
hypereosinophilic syndrome (HES) 182, 1510
hyperimmunoglobulin E syndrome 1575
hyperinflation, asthmatics 676–8
post-mortem 1361–2, 1414
hyperkinetic syndrome and food intolerance 1240, 1281
hypermutation of Ig genes, somatic 70–1
hyperosmolar aerosols and solutions, *see entries under hypertonic*
hyperpolarization, membrane, by K^+ channel openers 607, 609, 609–10
hyperresponsiveness/hyperreactivity, airway, *see* bronchial hyperresponsiveness
hypersensitivity (and hypersensitivity reactions) 24–9
allergen administration reducing, *see* allergen
allergy vs, distinction 23
chironomid allergens 953–5
classification 24–8
cockroach allergens 945–6
food, *see* food allergens; food allergy
Hymenoptera venoms 933–4
type I/immediate/anaphylactic, *see* anaphylactic reactions
type II/cytotoxic/cytolytic/antibody-dependent, *see* cytotoxic hypersensitivity reactions
type III, *see* immune complex-mediated hypersensitivity
type IV/delayed-type/T cell-mediated, *see* delayed hypersensitivity
hypersensitivity pneumonitis, *see* alveolitis, extrinsic allergic
hypertension
bradykinin-forming cascade and 334
pulmonary
asthma distinguished from 1356
neonatal leukotrienes and 392
NO therapy 524
hypertonic/hyperosmolar aerosols (e.g. saline) with asthmatics, airway response 683
in diagnosis of exercise-induced asthma 695
mucociliary clearance improved by 721
hypertonic/hyperosmolar solutions, anaphylaxis induced by infusion 1559
hypervariable regions, *see* complementarity-determining regions
hyperventilation in asthmatics, isocapnic airway response/bronchoconstriction with 683
leukotriene antagonist effects 394
in exercise-induced asthma diagnosis 694–5
hypokalaemia, β-adrenoceptor agonist-induced 577
hypopharynx, physiology 1308
hyposensitization, *see* immunotherapy
hypothalamic–pituitary–adrenocortical (HPAC) axis
cytokine effects 506

depression affecting 510
steroid effects 626–7
hypothalamus, cytokine effects 506, 507
hypotonic aerosols, airway response in asthmatics 683
hypoxaemia, β-adrenoceptor agonist-induced 577

I exon of Ig gene 39–40
ICAM-1 249–50
airway hyperresponsiveness and 252, 272
in allergic inflammation (in general), expression 251, 1121
asthma and 272, 294, 1372, 1373
late response in 1121, 1372, 1373
primate models of 292, 1040, 1042
rat models of 1073
leucocyte–endothelial interactions and 202, 203, 286, 292
eosinophil–endothelium 290–1
neutrophil–endothelium 202, 203
LFA-1 interactions with 249–50
monoclonal antibody to, immunosuppressant action 653
in rhinitis 1318, 1319
ICAM-2 250
leucocyte–endothelial interactions and 273, 286
ICAM-3 250
leucocyte–endothelial interactions and 273
ICI 204,219 (zafirkulast) 1730
in allergen-induced asthma 394
bronchodilator effect 395
in chronic asthma 395, 1730
in exercise-induced asthma 394
idiotypes, Ig 61
I-E molecule, anergy of self-reactive peripheral T cells and 134
ignorance, clonal 136
I-κB 71
ileus with anticholinergics 603
imaging/radiology
allergic alveolitis (extrinsic)
acute disease 1493
chronic disease 1494
allergic bronchopulmonary aspergillosis 1502
contrast media, *see* contrast media
eosinophilic pneumonia
acute 1508
chronic 1508
rhinitis 1297–8
tracheobronchial tree (normal) 1360, 1361
imidazoline derivatives 1329
imipenem 1554, 1683
immediate hypersensitivity, *see* anaphylactic reactions
immune complex(es) 307–23
anaphylaxis associated with formation of 1558
immune complex (antigen–antibody)-mediated hypersensitivity (Arthus reaction) 9, 25, 27
cutaneous late-phase reaction and 1133
drugs 1676
food allergy and 1523, 1524
mechanism 27
immune deficiency syndromes
acquired (AIDS/HIV disease), drug reactions with 1674, 1685
otitis media with 1640–1
immune deviation 136–7
immune haemolytic anaemia 1675
immune responses
afferent phases 119–20
to allergens 997–8
to dietary allergens 140–2, 1520–1
to inhaled allergens 140–2
calcineurin and 643
complement and 317
cyclosporin effects 646
dendritic cells and initiation of 120–4
efferent phases 120
antigen-presenting cells and 124–5
to helminthic infection 1169–71
macrophages (pulmonary alveolar) in 231–5
memory phases 120
peripheral
to self-antigens 133–7
to self-antigens, manipulation 138–9
tolerance and 133–7
to stress 508–9
animal studies 508–9
humans 509
T cells and 45, 49, 119–24
immune system 1–146, 503–15
asthma and 508–10
atopy inheritance and 1190–1
conditioning 510
cutaneous late-phase reactions and 1133–4
dermatitis and
allergic and irritant contact 1613–14
atopic 1578
drugs activating/reacting with
classification of reactions 1676
propensity 1674
extrinsic allergic alveolitis and 1492–3
mouse model for studying 1056–8
nasal late-phase reactions and 1146–50
nervous system and, interactions 503–15
ocular 1647–8
tolerance, *see* tolerance
urticaria and 1591, 1600–1
contact 1602, 1616
see also defence
immunity, historical concepts 4–5
immunization of neonatal rabbit with antigen 1077–8
immunoassays (immunochemical techniques of quantification and detection) with allergen molecules (for allergen-specific IgE antibodies predominantly) 827, 998–9, 1015–29
in asthma (generally) 1355
in cloning of allergens 809, 812
cockroach allergens 946–7
cytokines 1002
drug allergy 1677
β-lactams 1684
food allergens 1537
insect sting allergens 1697–8
latex allergens 983
for mediators of inflammation 999–1001
occupational allergens 921–2, 1477
pollen aeroallergens 840
potential problems 1016–17
predictive value of positive test 1013
rhinitis 1297
routine use 1015
semi-quantification of IgE antibody 1015–17
sensitivity
absolute, definition 1013
clinical, definition 1013
specificity, clinical, definition 1013
spores 882
test kits and procedures 1026–9
testing strategies 1017
see also specific techniques
ImmunoCAP 1026–7
immunocytochemistry, *see* immunostaining
immunodeficiency syndromes, *see* immune deficiency syndromes
immunoelectrophoresis of allergens 797
fungal allergens 873, 874, 875, 876, 877
immunoglobulin (function), *see* antibody
immunoglobulin (genes) 39–40, 63–71
organization 63–71
rearrangement 66–9
cell-type specificity 69
defective 68, 69
genetic analysis of machinery 67–8
order 68–9
regulation 68–9
somatic hypermutation 70–1
immunoglobulin (intravenous) in chronic asthma 1432
immunoglobulin (structure/synthesis/levels) 58–112
allotypes 61
diversity, generation 69–71
eosinophil receptors for 176
idiotypes 61
isotypes/classes, *see* isotype
membrane-bound 72–3
ocular allergy and 1651, 1652
secreted, *see* secreted immunoglobulins
structure 58–63, 73–4
domain 59–60
synthesis 71–4
regulation 71–3
immunoglobulin A
anaphylactoid reactions and 1558
drugs bound by, measurement 1677–8
food antigens bound by 1520–1
multimerization 62
receptors on eosinophils (FcαR) 176
helminthic infection and 1170
secretion 62
see also secreted immunoglobulins
tears 1647–8
immunoglobulin D
IgM co-expressed with 71
membrane-bound (antigen receptor) 73, 74
assembly and surface transport 74
immunoglobulin E 81–112, 1012–34
in allergen-specific immunotherapy, measurement 1228
allergic diseases involving 530
allergic inflammation pathogenesis independent from 530–2
allergic inflammation pathogenesis involving 530–2
phosphodiesterase inhibitors and 549
atopy and 998–9, 1014, 1201, 1371
cord blood IgE 1709–10, 1715–16
in helminthic infection 1168–9
historical studies 12
mast cells and
mast cell mediator release in skin induced by IgE 152
mast cell role in IgE synthesis 102
network 92
components 83
therapy aimed at 92
non-atopic conditions associated with elevated levels of 998
pentapeptide fragment, in seasonal allergic conjunctivitis therapy 1653
quantification 1012–34
as allergen-specific antibodies, *see* immunoassays
total IgE, *see* subheading below
receptors for Fc region of, *see* Fcε receptors
responsiveness to allergens/in allergic disease 36–7

atopy and 1190–2
to extracts of allergens 826–7
HLA and 32, 108, 1190–1
in rat model 1068–70
T cells and 141, 1203
see also anaphylactic reactions
in smokers, levels 1014, 1214
structure 1013
synthesis/production 39–41, 1013
in asthma 162
chromone effects on 586–7
cytokines and 40–1, 98–9
enhancing factors 102–3
inhibitory factors 103
in rat model 1068–70
regulation 96–112
switching to 39–40, 72, 98–9, 1371
T cells and 39–41, 98–101
total (quantification) 998, 1014
in allergic bronchopulmonary aspergillosis 1502
see also hyperimmunoglobulin E syndrome
immunoglobulin G
in allergen-specific immunotherapy 1228
venom-specific 1697–8, 1701–2
drugs bound by, measurement 1677–8
interfering in IgE assays 1016
isotype/subclass levels in atopic disorders 1001, 1003
membrane-bound, assembly and surface transport 74
receptor for Fc region of, *see* Fcγ receptor
immunoglobulin M
drugs bound by, measurement 1677–8
IgD co-expressed with 71
membrane-bound (antigen receptor) 73, 74
multimerization 62
secretion 62
immunoglobulin superfamily (IgSF domain) 59–60, 249–50
cytokine receptor members 344
immunoglobulin superfamily, adhesion receptor members of 249–50
in allergic inflammation (in general)
antagonists/antibodies 252–3
expression 251
integrin interactions with 252–3
in asthma 273
neutrophil–endothelial interactions and 203
immunohistochemistry, *see* immunostaining
immunological tests/techniques 1288
historical development 19–20
occupational asthma 1477
see also immunoassays and specific tests
immunology
clinical, allergy and, links between 1269–70
historical development of science of 4–22
milestones in studies of natural and experimental diseases 7–8
immunophilins 642–6
immunostaining (immunocytochemistry/histochemistry) 773–81
conditions 775–6
definition 773
direct methods 774
double 778
electron-microscopical 779–80
indirect methods 774
double 778–9
interpretation 779
light-microscopical 773–9
endothelin 522
nitric oxide synthase 523
milestones in development 6
multiple-staining techniques 778–9
quantitative 779
sensitivity 777
specificity 777–8
unlabelled antibody–enzyme methods 774–5
immunosuppressive agents 640–61
antisense oligonucleotides as 654
drugs as 640–52
in asthma 358, 630, 655–7, 1732–3
in atopic dermatitis 657, 1584
in experimental models of allergic disease 658–9
future developments 1733
mechanisms of action 640–52
toxicities 656, 657
monoclonal antibodies as, *see* monoclonal antibodies
see also specific (types of) agents
immunotherapy, allergen-specific (desensitization/hyposensitization) 50–1, 1225–57, 1269, 1285–7
anaphylaxis/systemic reactions with 1557, 1566–7
insect venom 1697, 1700
animal proteins 1237, 1239
asthma 50–1, 1236–9, 1688
children 1459
chronic disease 1432
systemic reactions 1246
autoimmune disease 138, 138–9
bronchial hyperresponsiveness decreased by 685
chironomid allergen 958
organization 1243–4
cockroach allergen 949
dermatitis (atopic) 1239–40
dose
dosage and dose modifications 1247–8
increase regimens 1245
top 1245–6
double-blind placebo trials 1234
drug allergies 1678–9
aspirin/other NSAIDs 1688
penicillin 1566, 1679, 1684
radiocontrast media 1686–7
sulphonamides 1685
extracts of allergen for 1244–5, 1286–7
facilities 1244
food allergens 1240, 1540
grass-pollen hayfever 51, 105–6, 1236
guidelines/recommendations 1247, 1248–9, 1286
historical studies 21
house-dust mite, *see Dermatophagoides pteronyssinus*
indications 1234–42
insect venom, *see* Hymenoptera
late-phase reactions and effects of 1230–1
cutaneous 1136, 1227–8, 1230–1
nasal 1152–3, 1228, 1231
mechanisms 1227–33
mixtures of unrelated allergens in 1245
monitoring 1249–51
moulds/fungal spores 1237–8, 1239
peptide, *see* peptide
pregnancy and 1337
provocation tests 1227–8
record form 1250, 1251, 1252
rhinitis 51, 358, 1236–9, 1336–7
guidelines for use 1338
safety/dangers/side-effects/risk factors 1235, 1237, 1239, 1244, 1246–7
prevention of side-effects 1252–4
treatment of mild/moderately severe reactions 1254–5
see also systemic reactions
successful 1243–57
see also peptides
immuno-tyrosine activation motif 85
IMP dehydrogenase, drugs inhibiting 650–1
imputability with drug reactions 1676–7
extrinsic 1676, 1677
intrinsic 1676–7
in situ hybridization to mRNA 764–72
cells for, *see* cells
control and specificity 768–9
detection of hybridization 768
examples 769–70
interpretation of results 769
phenotype of cells expressing 771
principles 764
probe
construction 764–6
labelling 766
size 766
technique (of hybridization) 768
tissues for 768
preparation 767–9, 768
pretreatment 768
sectioning 768
incidence
atopic dermatitis 1574
drug allergy 1671
aspirin/other NSAIDs 1687
β-lactam antibiotics 1682–3
local anaesthetics 1682
muscle relaxants 1679
sulphonamides 1684
occupational asthma in UK, annual 1466
physical urticaria 1596–7
indomethacin, resting airway calibre and effects of 403
indoors
air pollution 1403
see also smokers
allergens 889
fungal spore/mycelial fragment 865–71
see also homes; housing
infants (and young children)
asthma development related to life of 1368–70, 1452–4
atopic dermatitis 1574
food adverse reactions 1534
course/prognosis 1540–1
cow's milk protein 1282, 1532, 1710, 1720
eosinophilic gastroenteritis (allergic) 1524
prevention 1541–2
sudden death related to 1534, 1556–7
newborn and young, *see* neonate
risk factors for allergic disorders 1716–17
T cell sensitization to aeroallergens 239
venom immunotherapy 1236
infection (and sepsis)
asthma and 1457
association 1217, 1454, 1712
exacerbations in 1350
atopic dermatitis and 1575–6, 1582
therapy of 1583
ciliary dysfunction in chronic 713
differentiation
from acute eosinophilic pneumonia 1509
from extrinsic allergic alveolitis 1496
in otitis media, in aetiopathogenesis 1633–4, 1636, 1638–9
rhinitis caused by 1293–4
T cell-derived cytokines in 45
see also specific (types of) pathogen
inflammation (allergic)
acute, *see* acute allergic reactions
adhesion molecules, *see* adhesion
asthmatic, *see* inflammation (allergic) in

asthma
in atopic dermatitis, mechanism 1580–1
chemokines in 366, 374–5
chronic, *see* chronic allergic reactions
cytokines in 350, 351, 531–2
in helminthiases 1167–8
hormones in 506
human models, *see* human models
IgE and, *see* immunoglobulin E
macrophage (pulmonary alveolar) phenotype modified by cytokines during 234–5
mediators, *see* mediators
mucosal, *see* mucosa
neuroimmunomodulatory pathways in, pathophysiological significance 511
opioid peptides in 470–1, 506
picornoviruses and 896
in rhinitis 1314–18
steroid effects 622
inflammation (allergic), cells involved (effector cells/proinflammatory cells) 365
in allergen-specific immunotherapy 1228–30
autonomic networks and 505
basophils as, *see* basophils
dendritic cells as 237–8
endothelial, *see* endothelial cells
eosinophils as, *see* eosinophil
modulation of function 366
monocytes as, *see* monocytes
neutrophils as, *see* neutrophils
phosphodiesterases in, *see* phosphodiesterase
steroid effects 621–2
see also inflammatory cells
inflammation (allergic) in asthma 45–6, 48, 1037, 1371–4
as basis of asthma 1366–7
cell biology and mechanisms 52, 1371–4
children 1454
chromone effects 583–5
tests for biochemical and cellular markers 1355
guinea pig model 1097–8
human model, *see* asthma
primate (monkey) model 252, 292, 1038–43
rabbit model 1082
rat model 1071–2
sheep model 1049–50
T cells and 47–8
inflammation (generally and in normal physiological reaction to injury/infection and disease in general 365
nitric oxide and 525–6
ozone-induced 1398–9
inflammation (neurogenic) 447
inflammatory bowel disease 1282
leukotrienes and 393
leukotriene biosynthesis inhibitors in 397
inflammatory cells 149–306
in asthma 264–76, 1420–1
aspirin/other NSAIDs and 1688
compared with chronic obstructive pulmonary disease 1424
in late phase response 1117–20
tests for 1355
β_2-adrenoceptors on 573–4
CGRP and 456
in cutaneous late-phase reaction 1133–5
cytokine secretion 46–7
in extrinsic allergic alveolitis 1491
immunosuppressive drug effects 645–8
in nasal late-phase reaction 1146–8
nedocromil sodium effects *in vitro* 585
sodium cromoglycate effects *in vitro* 585
steroid effects on 621–2
on survival 620
substance P effects 494
tachykinin effects 453–4
VIP effects 461
see also inflammation (allergic), cells involved and specific cell types
inflammatory model of rhinitis 1318–20
inflation, deep, airway response in asthmatics 669–70
see also hyperinflation
information about contact dermatitis 1627
ingested antigens, *see* food allergens; food allergy
inhaled agents/medications (in asthma) 1433–4
aerosol delivery systems, *see* aerosols
β-adrenoceptor agonists 575–6, 1430–1, 1434–5
development 1726–7
long-acting 1432, 1726–7
mode of action 1434
pharmacokinetics 575–6
regular vs intermittent use 1434–5
side-effects 1434
potassium ion channel openers 613
steroids 617, 622–9, 1285, 1728–9
childhood asthma 623, 1459–60, 1461
in chronic asthma 1431, 1436
clinical efficacy 622–3
comparison between different drugs 623
delivery systems, effects 626
development 1728–9
dose 629
frequency of administration 624
guidelines/recommendations for use 629
increasing selective targeting 633
limiting systemic effects 632–3
liposome-encapsulated formulations 733, 735
pharmacokinetics 624
side-effects 625–9
structures 624
inhaled allergens (respired/aero-allergens) 798–804
atopic dermatitis worsened by skin contact with 1580
common 825
dog model of allergic disease 1105–6
immune response to 140–2
in infancy 239
immunotherapy 1236–9
indications 1238–9
measurement/tests
in extrinsic allergic alveolitis 1496
by IgE antibody tests 1015
in occupational exposure 921–3, 1476–7
preparation 825–6
seasonal, in UK, calendar 1274
sensitization to, *see* sensitization
sheep model of bronchoconstriction 1045–6
skin test positivity with, epidemiology 1010
see also air pollution
inhaled water vapour as mucoactive agent 720–1
inhalers 731–2, 1433–4, 1440–48
children 1460
steroid 731, 1436
systemic effects relating to 626, 1436
inheritance, *see* family studies; genetics
injection immunotherapy, *see* immunotherapy
injury, tissue, neutrophil-mediated 208–9
innervation, *see* nervous system
inosine monophosphate dehydrogenase, drugs
inhibiting 650–1
inositol triphosphate (ins(1,4,5)P_3) metabolism
airway smooth muscle contraction and 746, 747
neutrophils 204
insect allergens 804, 911–12, 927–60
historical studies 19
occupational exposure 911–12
recombinant
immunoreactivity 945–6
synthesis 818–19, 930
stinging insects, *see* Hymenoptera
see also individual genera/species
insecticides, cockroach control 948–9
inspiratory flow, inhalation of aerosols during 736–7
dry powder inhalers and 1446–8
inspiratory peak flow measurements in rhinitis 1298
insulin-like growth factor, asthma and 271
intecrines, *see* chemokines
integrin(s) 246–9
in allergic inflammation (in general) 254
antagonists/antibodies 252–3, 1050, 1052
expression 251
immunoglobulin superfamily interactions with 252–3
in asthma 273
in sheep model 1050, 1052
basophil–endothelial interactions and 254
eosinophil–endothelial interactions and 254, 278, 289
function, regulation 249
neutrophil–endothelial interactions and 202, 202–3
structure 246–8
integrin receptors
eosinophil 42, 174
FcεRII and 82
interdigitating dendritic cells (IDCs) 122
interferon-α, IgE synthesis and 103
interferon-γ 350
asthma and 271
in atopic dermatitis therapy 1584
atopy (subsequent) and reduced 1722
in contact dermatitis, *in vitro* tests 1620
IgE synthesis and 98, 103
properties/effects (in general) 350
interferon receptor superfamily 343, 344
interleukin(s) (in general) 340–53
cyclosporin effects on production 646
interleukin-1 345–6
actions 345, 346
asthma and 269
pulmonary alveolar macrophages and 230–1
interleukin-1 receptor(s) 345–6
steroids inhibiting transcription of 620
interleukin-1 receptor antagonist 345
interleukin-1β, nasal late-phase reaction and 1149
interleukin-2 347
assay 656
asthma/allergic airway disease and 269
rat model 1075
gene transcription 342
immunosuppressive drug affecting 643, 645
IgE synthesis enhanced by 103
properties/effects (in general) 347
receptor, *see* CD25
recombinant 756
T cell cultures requiring 756
interleukin-3 349, 354
allergy (in general) and 361, 1149
asthma and 47–8, 269, 361

basophil 158
eosinophil effects of 173, 174–5, 354–7
eosinophil receptors for 177
receptor 343, 354, 355
interleukin-4 348
asthma and 46, 47–8, 269, 1371, 1421–2
animal model of 1388
chronic 1384
late response in 1118
therapy of 1733
atopic dermatitis and 1578, 1579, 1580, 1581
B cells and 348, 1371
basophil 46, 158
chromone effects on processes involving 586–7
genes, atopy and 1192–3
IgE switching and synthesis involving 72, 98–9, 1371
inflammatory cells secreting 46
mast cell 46, 156–7, 1118, 1316, 1318
biological properties 158
in nasal pathology
in late-phase reaction 1150
in rhinitis 46, 1316, 1318
properties/effects (in general) 348
sensitization to allergen and 1371
Th2 differentiation and effects of 107
vernal keratoconjunctivitis and 1656
interleukin-5 349, 354, 354–9
asthma and 46, 47–8, 269–70, 358, 359, 360, 1421–2
animal model studies 1388
chronic 1384
intrinsic 361
therapy of 1733
basophil 46
effects/actions (in general) 349, 354–7, 1149
eosinophil effects of 41, 158, 173, 174–5, 188, 349, 354–7
in guinea pig 1097, 1098
eosinophil receptors for, in allergic disease 358–9
eosinophil synthesis 181, 357
in helminthic infection 1171
IgE synthesis enhanced by 102
mast cell 46, 157
biological properties 158
mRNA *in situ* hybridization 770
in nasal pathology
in late-phase reaction 1149
in rhinitis 46
T cell-derived 357
interleukin-5 receptor 343, 354, 355, 359
eosinophil 177
interleukin-6 347
asthma and 270
atopic 46
basophil 46
histamine interactions with 290
IgE synthesis enhanced by 102–3
mast cell 46, 157
biological properties 158–9
mRNA *in situ* hybridization 770
properties/effects (in general) 347
receptors 347
β-subunits/chains, receptors sharing 343
rhinitis and, atopic 46
interleukin-8
airway hyperresponsiveness in guinea pig induced by 1097
asthma and 270
as chemokine 368, 369
for neutrophils 201
endothelial cell-derived 285, 290
histamine interactions with 290, 369
IgE synthesis inhibited by 103
mast cell-derived 158
biological properties 159
receptor 368
interleukin-9, properties/effects (in general) 349
interleukin-10 348–9
asthma and 270
IgE synthesis inhibited by 103
interleukin-11, asthma and 270
murine model of 1064
interleukin-12 349–50
in allergen-specific immunotherapy 1231
asthma and 1388, 1389
IgE synthesis inhibited by 103
properties/effects (in general) 349–50
interleukin-13 348
IgE switching involving 99
interleukin-15 347–8
intermediate filaments 741
International Contact Dermatitis Research Group (ICDRG)
patch test reading according to 1618
interstitial macrophages in lung 229
intestine, *see* bowel; gastrointestinal tract
intracellular cell adhesion molecules, *see* ICAM
intradermal tests
drug reactions 1677
muscle relaxants 1680
skin prick tests compared with 1007–8, 1133, 1272–3
intragastric provocation tests under endoscopic control 1538–9
intron enhancer, Ig heavy chain gene 71
invariant chain 118
inversion joining of Igs 64
iodide, mucolytic action 721
ionic composition of mucus 715
see also specific ions
ionic detergents in PCR 785
ionizers 1719–20
ipecacuanha 914
ipratropium
in asthma 598–9, 599–600
in chronic disease 1432, 1435
in exercise-induced asthma 698
mode of action 1435
side-effects 1435
in chronic obstructive pulmonary disease 600, 601
dose–response 597–8
pharmacodynamics 597
pharmacokinetics 597
in rhinitis 490, 1333
side-effects/toxicity 602–3
iron-deficiency anaemia 1534
irritable bowel syndrome 1282
irritant(s) 1610–11
in atopic dermatitis 1583
avoidance 1583
in contact blepharoconjunctivitis 1661
in contact dermatitis, *see* contact dermatitis, irritant
in occupational asthma
adjuvant role 1404, 1467–8
exposure and response 1467
mechanisms 1471
respiratory, *see* air pollution
Ishizaka, Kimshige and Teruko 12, 13
isoallergens/variants/polymorphisms 814, 816, 828
isocyanates/diisocyanates 919–20, 1278, 1477–8
inhalational testing 1476
T cells and asthma induced by 1382, 1384
isoelectric focusing, allergens 796–7
isoprenaline 570
airway smooth muscle effects 609
in allergic rabbits 1085
pharmacokinetics 575
isotope, *see* radionuclide
isotypes/classes of Igs 58–9
IgG, in atopic disorders 1001, 1003
structure/function related to 61–2
switching (by B cells) 39–40, 71–3, 96–8, 1369
molecular mechanisms 97–8
recombinational mechanisms 71–2, 97
Italy, allergy training 1263
ITAM 85

J chain 62
J gene segment
immunoglobulin 63
heavy chain 65
T cell receptor 1380
see also V(D)J region
Jak2 185
Japan, *Trichosporon cutaneum* and allergic alveolitis 1490
Japanese cedar allergens 801
Japanese cedar pollinosis, IL-5 and 359
jet nebulizers 732, 1448
characteristics of liposome aerosols from 733–4
continuous-flow 732
see also nebulizers
Johansson, Gunnar 12
joining with Igs 63–4
imprecision and nucleotide addition at coding joints 67
mechanisms 67
signals 63–4
joint disease, inflammatory, *see* arthritis
junctional diversity with Igs 69–70
Juniperoidaeae 850

kallikrein 324
actions 327–8
inhibitors 331
in disease
in allergic disease 333, 334
in other diseases 334
synthesis 324, 326
κ chain genes 66
κ-opioid receptors 465
Kartagener's syndrome 1294
K^b molecule
anergy of self-reactive peripheral T cells and 135
down-regulation of T cell receptors and 136
KC-128
as anti-asthma drug 613
structure 608
Kellaway, Charles H 11
Kentucky bluegrass allergen, recombinant, synthesis 818
keratinocytes and atopic dermatitis 1578
keratoconjunctivitis 1654–6, 1659–61
atopic (blepharokeratoconjuncitivitis associated with atopic dermatitis) 1576, 1659–61
vernal (spring ophthalmia) 1578, 1654–8
atopic dermatitis associated with 1576
clinical features 1656
histology 1655
pathogenesis 1654–6
prognosis 1658
treatment 1656–8
keratoconus 1576
ketorolac in seasonal allergic conjunctivitis

1653
ketotifen in asthma 1432
kidney, drug reactions 1675
see also hepatorenal syndrome
Kikuyu grass, cross-reactivity with Bermuda grass 1018–19
king crab, Alaska, allergens 913
kinin (human)
formation 324–31
in hereditary angioedema 332–3
rhinitis and 1315
see also bradykinin; cholecystokinin; tachykinin
kinin (wasp) 931
kininogen 324, 327–8
on endothelial call surface 332
high-molecular-weight (HK) 327–8
cleavage/digestion 327–8
in contact activation 330–1, 332
low-molecular-weight (LK) 328
KS-505a 536
Ku80 68
Kunitz soybean trypsin inhibitor 968
Küstner, Heinz 10

L-648051 1730
L cells as accessory cells for culturing T cells 756
L-selectin 244–5, 273
ligands 245–6, 273
neutrophil–endothelial interactions and 202
L-type Ca^{2+} channels in airway smooth muscle cells 743–5
physiological regulation 744–5
laboratory tests/investigations 1288
exercise-induced asthma diagnosis 693
ocular allergy 1664–5
laboratory workers, allergen exposure 1465, 1478
animal 910–11, 1465, 1478
lactation, *see* breast-feeding
β-lactoglobulin 965–6
lactose intolerance 1282
λ chain genes 66
lamina propria, nasal 1305
see also submucosa
lamina reticularis thickening in asthma 161, 301, 1417
laminin 299–300
Langerhans cells
in nose
in late-phase reaction 1148
in rhinitis 1318
in skin/epidermis 122
atopic dermatitis and 1578
skin transplantation and 123
Th2 cell development 106
lanolin 1624
large-volume spacers, *see* spacers
larynx
oedema, food allergens and 1528–30
physiology 1308
late-phase responses/reactions (LPR) 28–9
humans 1111–60, 1230–1
conjunctiva 1651
immunotherapy, *see* immunotherapy
lower airway, *see* asthma
nose, *see* nose
skin, *see* skin
primate model, airways 1042–7
rabbit model, airways 1082–3
rat model, airways 1070–1
sheep model, airways 1046
latex allergens 914, 981–93, 1025, 1479, 1555
anaphylaxis, *see* anaphylaxis
cross-reacting 973, 1025–6
diagnosis of allergy 986–7
extracts 986–7
identification/characterization 983–4
pathophysiology of reactions 982–3
prevention of allergy 988–9
properties/composition 981–0
rabbit immunized with 1080
recommendations 989–90
reduction 988–9
risk groups for allergy 985–6, 1025
routes of exposure 984–5
LECAM, *see* leucocyte–endothelial cell adhesion molecule
lectin(s)
S-type 91
T cells stimulated by 756
lectin domain, soluble FcεRII 87, 88
leflunomide
cytokine actions inhibited by 648–9
toxicity 656
leg-ulcer series 1626
legumes 967–9
lens cataracts, steroid-induced 628
Lepidoglyphus destructor allergens 802, 912–13
occupational exposure 912–13
leucocyte(s)
adhesion (endothelial interactions), *see* adhesion
cytokines, *see* cytokines
as effectors in allergic inflammation, *see* inflammation (allergic)
migration in allergic disease, role of adhesion receptors, *see* adhesion
mononuclear, *see* mononuclear cells/leucocytes
neuroendocrine receptors 506
neutrophil polymorphonuclear, *see* neutrophil
procoagulant activity 1620
steroids synthesized by 507–8
see also specific types
leucocyte adhesion deficiency 321–3
type-1 203
type-2 202
leucocyte antigens, human, *see* HLA
leucocyte function antigen-1, *see* LFA-1
leucocyte–endothelial cell adhesion molecule (LECAM) 202
rhinitis and 1318, 1319
leucocytosis, C3d-K-induced 317
leukotriene(s) (in general) 380, 381–98
actions 384–5
bronchoconstrictive 385, 387–8, 388–9, 1684
pharmacological modulation 393–8, 699, 1726–7
in allergic disease (in general), release 390–2
in sheep model 1048
assays and their value 999
asthma and 266, 390–2, 1084–5
aspirin-induced 388, 392, 1688
bronchial 387–90, 682
biosynthesis 381–2
inhibitors, *see* 5-lipoxygenase inhibitors
PAF and 407
cellular sources 382–3
cysteinyl, *see* leukotriene C_4; leukotriene D_4; leukotriene E_4
metabolism/elimination 383–1
nasal late-phase reaction and 1148
in non-allergic disease, release 392–3
ocular allergy and 1650
platelet 216
receptors 385–7
receptor antagonists 393–5, 699, 1730–1
in allergic rabbit 1086
compared with biosynthesis inhibitors 398
late asthmatic response in 1116
leukotriene A_4 synthesis 381
leukotriene B_4
asthma and 266
biological activity 384–5
cellular sources 382–3
metabolism/elimination 383
neutrophil 179
non-allergic disease and 392–3
receptors 386
synthesis 179, 380
leukotriene C_4 28, 380
asthma and 266
bronchial 387–90
biological activity 385
cellular sources 382–3
eosinophil 179
rhinitis and 1316–17
mast cell 155
metabolism/elimination 383–4
non-allergic disease and 392–3
receptors 386–7
synthesis 179, 381
leukotriene D_4 28, 380
asthma and 266
bronchial 387–90
biological activity 385
metabolism/elimination 384
non-allergic disease and 392–3
receptors 386–7
antagonists 393–5
synthesis 179, 381
leukotriene E_4
asthma and 266, 390–2
bronchial 387–90
biological activity 385
metabolism/elimination 384
non-allergic disease and 393
receptors 386–7
synthesis 179, 381
levocabastine
rhinitis 1332
seasonal allergic conjunctivitis 1652
levocromokalim
airway smooth muscle effects 609
structure 608
trials in asthma 612–13
Leyden, Ernst V. von 16
see also Charcot–Leyden crystals
LFA-1 (CD11a) 247–8
ICAM-1 interactions with 249–50
leucocyte–endothelial interactions and 273
monoclonal antibody to, immunosuppressant action 653
lichenoid eczema, patchy pityriasiform 1575
lifestyle and atopy 1405
light (L) chains of Ig/antibody 58–9
domain structure 60
genes 66
rearrangement 69
light-microscopical immunocytochemistry, *see* immunostaining
lilac allergens 800
limiting-dilution isolation of T cell clones 757
limpet 971
linkage studies, *see* genetic linkage
lipid mediators (arachidonate metabolites/eicosanoids) 380–418
anaphylaxis and 1561
NSAIDs and 1559
assays and their value 999

in asthma 265, 266, 1084–5, 1688
in late response 1117
eosinophil-derived 178–80
eosinophil effects 175
mast cell-derived 155
in nasal late-phase reaction 1148–9
NSAIDs (including aspirin) modulating production of
anaphylaxis and 1559
asthma and rhinosinusitis and 1688
ocular allergy and 1650
platelet-derived 216
steroids affecting gene transcription of enzymes involved in production of 620
see also specific (types of) mediators
lipocalin 944–5
lipocortin 1 expression, steroid effects on 620
liposome-encapsulated drugs 732–7
characteristics of aerosols produced with jet nebulizers 733–4
deposition 733–6
safety/tolerance 735
lipoxins, eosinophil production 179
5-lipoxygenase 179
5-lipoxygenase-activating protein (FLAP) 179, 381
inhibitor 1730
in allergen-induced asthma 396
5-lipoxygenase inhibitors (leukotriene synthesis inhibitors) 395–8, 1729–31
allergic rabbit and airway effects of 1086
late asthmatic response and effects of 1116
15-lipoxygenase 179
lips, contact urticaria confined to 1524–5
liver
drug reactions 1675
leukotrienes and diseases of 393
liver flukes 1506
lobster 971
local anaesthetics 1279, 1681–2
locusts 912
lodoxamide
seasonal allergic conjunctivitis 1653
vernal keratoconjunctivitis 1656–7
Lolium perenne (ryegrass) allergens (Lol p) 798–9
recombinant
cloning of cDNA 812
synthesis 818
lonapalene in psoriasis 397–8
London, 1952 smog 1400
London plane 1019
loratidine
in rhinitis 1332
in urticaria (chronic) 1595
Loveless, Mary 11, 12
low-volume pollen samplers 840
lubricants in metered dose inhalers 1442
lumen, airway
factors determining area 655–8
macrophages 229
narrowing, *see* airway/respiratory tract in asthma; bronchoconstriction; obstruction
lung
β-adrenoceptors 567, 573
capacity
forced residual, asthmatics 676, 677
total, asthmatics 677
chronic obstructive disease, *see* chronic obstructive pulmonary disease
dendritic cells, *see* dendritic cells
embolism 1356
eosinophils in, *see* eosinophilia; eosinophilic lung disease
farmer's, *see* farmer's lung
haemosiderosis, food-induced 1533–4
hyperinflated, *see* hyperinflation
lymphocyte homing/migration in, *see* lymphocyte
mast cells, cytokines 156–7
mucociliary clearance delay in 718
mushroom-workers 869
nitric oxide synthesis 523–5
alterations, physiological consequences 524
parenchyma, asthma involving 673
silo-filler's 1496
vagal afferent pathways 595
vagal efferent pathways 594–5
see also airway
lung function (airway function) tests
in asthma/allergic airway disease 668–72, 1352–3
in bronchial hyperresponsiveness studies 682
in chronic asthma 1430
in guinea pig model 1095
in infant wheezers 1454
mucosal inflammation detected via 671
in murine models 1058, 1061–3
in occupational asthma 1472–3, 1482
post-mortem studies and computer simulations of 1364
in rabbit model 1081–2
see also specific tests,
in extrinsic allergic alveolitis
in acute disease 1493–4
in chronic disease 1494
regular monitoring 1497–8
lupin allergens 969
lutidine test 1621
LY-171,883 394, 1730
Lycopersicon esculentum 973–4
lymphocyte(s)
activation 371–2
in asthma 1420–1
in late asthmatic response 1119–20
cultures, *see* cultures
homing/migration to lung/airway 255
in allergic disease 287–9
homing/migration to lymphoid tissue, autonomic nervous system involvement 504
markers, analysis 1001–2
phosphodiesterase 535
phosphodiesterase inhibitor effects 544–6
re-circulation from blood to lymphoid organs 255–6
in rhinitis 1317–18
sensitization to allergens and 1371
surface marker expression after chironomid allergen stimulation 956–7
transformation tests
contact dermatitis 1620
drug allergy 1678
see also B cell; natural killer cells; T cell
lymphocyte-mediated hypersensitivity, *see* delayed hypersensitivity
lymphocytic choriomeningitis virus antigen, tolerance and 136
lymphoid dendritic cells 121–2
lymphoid system/organs
compartments 255
T cell re-circulation through 255–6
lymphoid tissue
gut-associated, food allergy and 962, 1520
mucosa-associated, conjunctiva 1647
lymphotaxin 368
lyn tyrosine kinase (p53 and p56)
eosinophil 184
T cell 85
antigen processing and 119
lyso-PAF 404–5
lysophospholipase
as Charcot–Leyden crystal protein 91, 181–2
honey-bee 931

M cells 1520
$M_1/M_2/M_3$ receptors, *see* muscarinic receptors
Mac-1 (Mo-1; OKM-1; CR3; CD11b/CD18) 246–8, 315, 369–70
basophil effects 369–70
deficiency 318
on eosinophils 176–7
FcεRII and 82, 91
leucocyte–endothelial interactions and 273
Mac-2, *see* ε-binding protein
Macaca fascicularis, *see* primate models
α_2-macroglobulin, kallikrein inhibited by 331
macrophages 228–35, 289–90
in asthma 289–90
aspirin/other NSAIDs and 1688
in chronic asthma 1383
in late response 1119
cytokines from, Th cell development and effects of 107
distribution in lung 228–9
see also specific types
endothelial cell interactions with 289–90
functions in lung 230–4, 239–40
migration inhibition test 1620
in nasal late-phase reaction 1148
neutrophil removal by 210
phosphodiesterase 535
phosphodiesterase inhibitor effects 545, 546–7
population dynamics 230
surface markers 229–30
tachykinin effects 454
MAdCAM-1 250, 1387
as L-selectin ligand 245–6
Maimonides, Moses 15
major basic protein, eosinophil 180
asthma and 275
murine model of 1064
primate model of 1041
endothelial cells and 290
helminthic infection and 1169
vernal keratoconjunctivitis and 1655
major histocompatibility complex, *see* HLA
males, *see* gender differences
malnutrition as risk factor for atopy/atopic disease 1217, 1712
MALT, conjunctival 1647
maltings 870
mammals, *see* animals
mannan-binding protein 311
manometry, nasal, *see* rhinomanometry
MAP kinase
eosinophils and 184–5
neutrophils and 207
maple, African 914
mass median aerodynamic diameter 729, 730, 731
liposomal formulations and 734
mast cell(s) 149–70, 544, 1118, 1228–9
in allergen-specific immunotherapy 1228–9
anaphylaxis and 1559, 1560, 1561
in asthma 159–62, 274, 1372, 1374, 1422
aspirin/other NSAIDs and 1688
in early response 1372
extracellular matrix signals to 307–8
in late response 1118
basophils and, common/different

features 149–50
cutaneous
atopic dermatitis and 1528
late-phase reactions and 1133–4
urticaria and 1587–8, 1597
cyclosporin and tacrolismus effects 648
cytokines 46, 155–8, 158–9, 1118, 1316
biological properties 158–9
degranulation, *see* degranulation; mast cell degranulating peptide
development 149–50
differential requirement for, in different types 151
endothelial cell interactions with 290
in helminthic infection 1168–9
heterogeneity 150–3
IgE and, *see* immunoglobulin E
intestinal 1538
nasal
in late-phase reaction 1146, 1153
in rhinitis 1314–16, 1318
nedocromil sodium effects 583, 585–6, 587–8
ocular allergy and 1649–50
vernal keratoconjunctivitis 1655
phosphodiesterase 535
phosphodiesterase inhibitor effects 544, 545
protease, *see* protease
sensory nerves and (in airways), association between 453–4
sodium cromoglycate effects 583, 587–8
steroid effects 621
tachykinin effects 152, 453–4, 505
tryptase, *see* tryptase
mast cell degranulating peptide (from *Apis mellifera)* 930
mast cell inhibitors/stabilizers
conjunctivitis
perennial allergic 1654
seasonal allergic 1653
keratoconjunctivitis, vernal 1656
mast cell mediators 152, 153–8, 158–9
allergy and 127–8
anaphylaxis and 1560–1
asthma and 161–2, 274
chymase, *see* chymase
cutaneous
IgE and substance P-induced release 152
urticaria and 1587–8
newly generated 155
ocular allergy and 1649–50
preformed 153–5
mastocytosis, systemic, anaphylaxis and, differentiation 1564
mastoparans 931–2
maternal factors, *see* breast-feeding; diet; pregnancy
maxillary sinusitis, rabbit model 1088
maximum expiratory flow–volume curves in asthmatics 668–9
maximum voluntary ventilation in identification of exercise-induced asthma 694, 695
MBP, *see* major basic protein; mannan-binding protein; myelin basic protein
MCF 316
MCP-1/2/3, *see* monocyte chemotactic protein
meatus, nasal 1300
mechanical stimuli, physical urticaria caused by 1597–9
media, lymphocyte culture 754
mediators, inflammatory 127–8, 307–418, 999–1001
in allergen-specific immunotherapy 1228–30
in asthma 264–76
drugs (other than cromoglycate) affecting 1728–32
in exercise-induced asthma 703–4
late asthmatic response and 1117
in monkey model 1039
in murine model 1064
in rabbit model 1084–5
in sheep model 1046–9
sodium cromoglycate effects, *see* sodium cromoglycate
in atopy, chromone effects 586–7
in cutaneous late-phase reactions 1135
in drug allergy 1678
radiocontrast media 1685
endothelial cell-derived, production 285–6
eosinophil-derived, *see* eosinophil
eosinophil receptors for 178
in helminthic infection 1171
mast cell-derived, *see* mast cell mediators
in nasal late-phase reaction 1148–50, 1153–4
in ocular allergy 1649–50
in seasonal allergic conjunctivitis 1651
in vernal keratoconjunctivitis 1654
platelet-derived 214–16
in urticaria 1588–9, 1590
see also specific (types of) mediators
medical history, *see* history-taking
Medihaler-Epi 1565
megacolon, congenital 468
MEK kinase, eosinophils and 184
mellitin 929–30
melons 973
membrane, plasma
airway smooth muscle cells 741–2, 743–6
macrophage, markers 229–30
platelet, proteins of 216–17
receptors on, *see* receptors and *specific (types of) receptors*
membrane-anchored complement activation regulatory molecules 316
membrane attack complex 314
membrane-bound Ig (B cell antigen receptor) 73–6
accessory molecules associated with 76
assembly/synthesis 72–3, 73–4
function 74–6
ligation 75–6
structure 73–4
surface transport 74
membrane cofactor protein 316
memory T cells 120
men, *see* gender differences
menstrual period, asthma preceding, management 1437
6-mercaptopurine 650
Mercurialis annua 854
metabisulphite, airway response to 684
metabolic burst (respiratory/oxidative burst/phagocytic oxidative killing mechanisms)
eosinophils, phosphodiesterase inhibitor effects 547
neutrophils 208
phosphodiesterase inhibitor effects 548
metabolic disturbances
β-adrenoceptor agonist-induced 577
steroid-induced 628
metals
colloid, in immunocytochemistry 777
salts of, as occupational allergens 917–19, 1277–8, 1465, 1480
Metapenaeus enis 805, 970–1
Metarhizium anisopliae 949
metered dose inhalers, pressurized 731, 1433, 1440–1
for adrenaline administration 1565
breath-activated 1442–3
compared with dry powder inhalers 1445
disadvantages 1441–2
efficient use 1441
for steroids 731
systemic effects 626
methotrexate 650
in asthma 655–7, 1732
in chronic disease 1432
side-effects/toxicity 656, 1732
methoxamine 578
methylene diisocyanate 1477
methylhistamine measurements, drug allergy 1678
methylprednisolone
in allergic rabbit 1085
drug blocking metabolism of 630, 1733
methylxanthines 1727
see also aminophylline; theophylline
MHC 114–19
allergy and 125
antigen/peptide fragment recognition and 37–8, 114–19
atopy and, T cells and 1385–6
class I 114, 115
class II 115, 115–16
human, *see* HLA
mice, *see Mus musculus*
microbes, *see specific types*
microfilaria-associated pulmonary eosinophilia 1504–5
Microplate AlaSTAT 1027–8
microvessels/microvasculature
adhesion molecule expression on 292–4
neutrophil sequestration in 201
neutrophil transmigration of 203
plasma leakage/exudation, *see* plasma
tachykinin effects 451–3
urticaria and 1589–90
midge, non-biting, *see* Chironomid non-biting midge
MIDGET technique 674
migraine headaches 1534
migration inhibition test and migration inhibition factor 1620
milk proteins, cow's 965–6, 1710
B cell epitopes 964
infants
adverse reactions/antigenicity 1282, 1529, 1710, 1720
hydrolysed formulae 1720
intolerance 1282
prevention of allergy 1710
Mini Wright peak-flow meter 1307
Min-I-Jet adrenaline 1565
minor determinant mixture (MDM), β-lactams 1682–3, 1683, 1684
MIP, *see* monocyte inhibitory protein
mite allergens 801–3, 888–99, 912–13, 1022–3
classification 1023
cross-reactivity 1023
epidemiology 88–9
exposure
measurement 890–1, 1023
occupational 912–13, 914
history 888–9
recombinant
cloning of cDNA 811–12, 812
synthesis 815–16
treatment 893–5, 1236–7, 1239
see also individual species
mitochondria 741
mixed-dust fibrosis 1497
mizoribine 651
MK-287 1729
MK-476 (MK-0476) 394

bronchodilator effect 395
MK-571 394
in chronic asthma 395, 1730
MK-0591
in allergen-induced asthma 396
in chronic asthma 397
MK-679 (MK-0679) 394, 1730
in aspirin-induced asthma 394
bronchodilator effect 395
MK-886 396, 1730
Mo-1, *see* Mac-1
MOAHL index (in contact dermatitis) 1609, 1621, 1622
models, experimental, *see* animal models; human models
molecular genetics, atopy studies 1189, 1190–3
molecular immunology, milestones 6–7
mollusc allergens 971
occupational exposure 913
mollusca contagiosa 1576
monkey model, *see* primate model
monoclonal antibodies
in allergen quantification 827
in immunocytochemistry 774
as immunosuppressants 652–3
in experimental models of allergic disease 655
manufacture 63
in mouse model of allergy (as probes) 1056–7
toxicity 656
monocyte(s) 371–2
activation 371–2
in allergic inflammation
adhesion interactions 255
phosphodiesterase 535
phosphodiesterase inhibitor effects 545, 546
in asthma, aspirin and 1688
C5a effects on 316
migration inhibition test 1620
tachykinin effects on 454
monocyte chemotactic protein-1 (MCP-1) 368
in allergic disease 375
receptor 372
monocyte chemotactic protein-2 (MCP-2) 368, 371
monocyte chemotactic protein-3 (MCP-3) 370–1, 371
eosinophils and 175–6
receptor 372–3
monocyte inhibitory proteins (MIP)
MIP-1α 368, 370
receptor 372
MIP-1β 368, 370
mononuclear cells/leucocytes
in atopic individuals, cAMP phosphodiesterases in 542–3, 553–4
peripheral blood
as accessory cells for T cell cultures 755, 756
as sources of T cells for culture 756, 757, 758
in urticaria 1587
see also specific types of mononuclear leucocytes
monosodium glutamate 1281
mood (affective) disorders
in asthma 508–9
immunity and effects of 508–9
Moraxella catarrhalis and otitis media 1638
mortalities, *see* death
mothers, *see* breast-feeding; diet; pregnancy
motifs, sequence
in B cell antigen receptor, transmembrane signalling 75
immuno-tyrosine activation 85
mould allergens, *see* fungi
mouse, *see Mus musculus*
mouth, *see* oral route
μ heavy chain
C gene segment, synthesis 72–3
structure 60
μ-opioid receptors 465
mucins 714–15
Muckle–Wells syndrome 1605
mucociliary system 710–27
clearance 717–23
exercise-induced asthma and 703
measurement 717–18
nasal (normal) 1305
nasal (in rhinitis) 1298
periciliary fluid and 714
in sheep model of asthma 1051–2
clearance, delayed/impaired, pathology 718–19
components 710–17
therapeutic approaches 720–3
see also cilia
mucosa (airway/bronchial and in general)
biopsies, late asthmatic response and 1122
bulk plasma moved to surface of 441
inflammation
in allergic disease (in general) 45–6
in asthma 45–6, 671, 1374
in rhinitis 48, 1314–18
macrophages (airway) 229
mast cells 150–1
middle ear, infection 1637
nasal 1305
autonomic nervous system 487, 489, 489–90, 498
in late-phase reaction 1146, 1154
in rhinitis 48, 489–90
oedema, *see* oedema
mucosa (digestive tract)
in food allergy 963, 1519–20
gastric, provocation tests under endoscopic control 1538–9
oral, contact dermatitis and 1616
mucosal addressin CAM-1, *see* MAdCAM-1
mucosal-associated lymphoid tissue, conjunctiva 1647
mucous, *see* mucus
mucus (mucous), airway 714–17
ciliary transportability 717
composition 714–15
drugs acting on/breaking down 720–3
nasal 1304–15
pathological 715
see also sputum
retention, 'salt' hypothesis 719–20
rheology 715–16, 717, 720
mucus production/secretion 715, 717
in asthma 162
cells involved 1418
leukotriene effects 389–90
bombesin effects 467
gastrin-releasing peptide effects 467
neuropeptide tyrosine effects 464
regulation 715
tachykinin effects 453
VIP effects 460–1
mugwort allergens 801
Muhlenbergia 842
multi-allergen mixtures in allergen tests 1017
multidrug allergies 1679
multiple inert gas elimination technique 674
multiple sclerosis and T cell receptor repertoire 1385
murine species, *see Mus musculus*
Mus musculus (mouse)
allergens from 803, 904
laboratory exposure 911, 1478
major 803, 904
other 904
as allergy/asthma/hyperresponsiveness model 1056–67, 1388
fibroblasts, transfected, as accessory cells for culturing T cells 756
for immune system studies 1056–8
oral tolerance studies 1521
muscarinic (acetylcholine) receptor(s) 489, 595–6, 1727
agonists/antagonists, *see* cholinergic agonists; cholinergic antagonists
location in airways 596
M_1 489, 596, 1727
in asthma 491
M_2 489, 596, 1727
in asthma 491–2
in dog 1104–5, 1108
in rabbit model of asthma 1097
M_3 489, 596, 1727
in asthma 491
in dog 1104–5, 1108
muscle
relaxants 1679–80
smooth, *see* smooth muscle
mushroom farms 869–70
mustard allergens 974
recombinant 975
mycophenolate mofetil (MM) 650–1, 651–2
toxicity 656
mycoses, allergic bronchopulmonary, *see* bronchopulmonary mycoses
mycotoxins 867
myelin basic protein
experimental allergic encephalomyelitis and 138
oral tolerance to 140
myelocyte, eosinophil, morphology 171–2
myeloperoxidase
monocyte 383
neutrophil 383
autoantibody 1004
myocardial infarction and leukotrienes 393
myofibroblasts 301–3
myosin 741
light chain phosphorylation 746–7, 747
Myrmecia spp. 928
allergens (Myr) 933
recombinant, synthesis 818

N regions of Ig coding joints 67
NADPH oxidase, neutrophil 208
naphthalene diisocyanate 1477
narcotic reactions 1681
nasal problems, *see* nose
nasopharynx, physiology 1308
natural killer cells
asthma and 1388
cyclosporin effects 648
identification 1001
nausea with phosphodiesterase-4 inhibitors 553
nebulizers 1440, 1448
children 1460
home 1432–3
jet, *see* jet nebulizers
ultrasonic 1448
Necator americanus 1167
nedocromil sodium 582–93, 1285
adverse effects 1334, 1436
bronchial hyperresponsiveness decreased by 686
in chronic asthma 1436

in exercise-induced asthma 696, 697
late response and effects of
asthmatic 1115
nasal 1151
mechanism/mode of action 587–90, 1334, 1436
pro-inflammatory cells and mediators and
and asthma symptoms 585–6
and asthmatic inflammation 583–5
atopy development 586–7
in rhinitis 1334
guidelines for use 1338
in seasonal allergic conjunctivitis 1653
in sheep model of airway inflammation 1049
structure 583
in vernal keratoconjunctivitis 1656
neomycin 1624
neonates (animals), rabbit, intraperitoneal administration of antigen 1079–80
neonates (human) and young infants
food antigens/allergens
clinical features of disorders caused by 1526–7
course and prognosis of hypersensitivity 1540
gastrointestinal tract handling and immune response 1520, 1522
prematurity and 1541, 1720
prevention of allergy 1709, 1715–25
pulmonary hypertension, leukotrienes and 392
nerve growth factor receptor superfamily 343, 344
nervous system (airways) 481–504
asthma and, *see* asthma
autonomic, *see* autonomic nervous system
central, *see* central nervous system
immune system and, interactions 503–15
nasal 1302–3, 1313–14
late-phase reaction and 1142, 1143–4
neural networks 504
neuropeptides in
neuropeptide tyrosine (NPY) 464, 489
opioid peptides 465–6
tachykinins 449–50, 451
VIP 458–60, 486–7, 487–8, 489
nitric oxide in 459, 487
number of nerves decreasing with descent down bronchial tree 523, 524
rhinitis and, *see* rhinitis
see also neuromodulators; neurotransmission
nervous system (ocular tissues) 1645, 1646, 1647
Netherlands, allergy training 1264
neural mechanisms, *see* nervous system
neural nitric oxide synthetase 517
neuroendocrine receptors, leucocyte 506
neuroendocrine regulation of airways 505–6
neurogenic inflammation 447
neuroimmune communication 503–15
neurokinin A 447, 494–5
in asthma 276, 469
airway response to 684
drugs blocking 1733–4
localization 447–8, 494–5
receptors 448, 449
nasal 1314
smooth muscle effects 451
neurokinin B 447
receptors 448, 449
neuromodulators
neuropeptide tyrosine as 464
opioids as 466
tachykinins as 450
VIP as 459–60
neuronal function and nasal late-phase reaction 1142, 1143–4
neuropeptide(s) 447–80, 493–5, 1085
degradation by neutral endopeptidase 276, 448, 450, 495–6
excitatory 493–7
nasal 1302, 1313, 1314
in neurotransmission, *see* neurotransmission
in pathophysiological conditions 468–71
asthma 275–6, 468, 469–70, 1085, 1733–4
therapy aimed at 471, 1733–4
urticaria 1590–1
receptors 493–5
see also specific peptides
neuropeptide-γ 447
localization 447–8
neuropeptide K 447
localization 447–8
neuropeptide tyrosine (NPY) 463–4
functional effects 464
in cholinergic neurones 464, 489
localization 463–4
nasal 1313
receptors 464
neuropharmacology 510–11
neurotoxicity, drug 1674
H_1 antagonist
first-generation 432, 433
second-generation 422–3, 433
steroids 628
neurotoxin, eosinophil-derived (EDN) 180, 181
neurotransmission (in autonomic nervous system)
adrenergic nerves 482–3
neuropeptides involved in 486–7
neuropeptide tyrosine (NPY) 464
opioid peptides 466
tachykinins 449–50, 451
VIP 458–9, 486–7, 489
nitric oxide in 459, 487
non-adrenergic non-cholinergic nerves 486–7
neutral endopeptidase, *see* endopeptidase, neutral
neutropenia, drug-induced 1675
neutrophil(s) 198–213, 1118
activation 203–8
apoptosis 209–10
in asthma 274
in late response 1118, 1372
in primate model 1039
autoantibodies 1004, 1510
C5a effects on 316
chemotaxins 200–1, 369, 454
chemotaxis and migration into tissues 200–3, 369, 370
defence role 198–200
deformability 201
endothelial cell adhesion 201–3
functional longevity 209–10
in inflammatory/allergic disease (in general) 200
phosphodiesterase 535
phosphodiesterase inhibitor effects 545
leukotriene B_4 179
in microvessels, *see* microvessels
in nasal late-phase reaction 1147
nedocromil sodium effects 585
origin 198
PAF liberation 216
receptors for 201–3
receptors on 203
sodium cromoglycate effects 585
structure 198
therapeutic strategies aimed at 210–11
tissue clearance 209–10
tissue injury mediated by 208–9
in urticaria 1587
neutrophilia, airway, E-selectin and 252
newborn, *see* neonate
NF-AT_c 643–4
NF-κB 71
nickel 918
tests 1621–2
dimethylglyoxine 1621
nicorandil 607
structure 608
nitric oxide (NO) 516–28
asthma and 268–71, 525
in autonomic nervous system/ neurotransmission 459, 487
biological actions 519
damaging effects 519
corticotrophin-releasing factor production and 507
detection 520
inflammation and 525–6
localization 520–5
neutrophil-derived 207
pulmonary alveolar macrophage-derived 155
synthesis 516–19
therapy in pulmonary hypertension 524
nitric oxide synthetases 516–19
endothelial (eNOS) 517–18
atherosclerosis and 521–2
lower airway localization 523, 524
inducible (iNOS) 518–19
atherosclerosis and 522
endotoxic shock and 525–6
gene expression, steroids affecting 620, 622
neural (nNOS) 517
lower airway localization 523, 524
nitrogen dioxide 1216, 1397, 1399
animal studies of sensitization involving 1404
enhanced allergen responsiveness 1406
epidemiological studies of symptoms related to
adults 1401–2
children 1403
indoors 1403
laboratory studies 1399
see also air pollution
nitrogen species, reactive, asthma and 268–71
NK receptors, *see* tachykinin
NO and NO_2, *see* nitric oxide; nitrogen dioxide
nocturnal asthma/bronchospasm
drug therapy 1437
anticholinergics with 598
potassium ion channel openers 612
platelets in 220
non-adrenergic non-cholinergic system/ mechanisms/neurotransmission 449–50, 458–9, 486–8, 492–7, 504
asthma and 487–8, 496–7, 504
occupational 1471
cholinergic transmission inhibited by 594–5
cromakalim suppressing 611
excitatory 492–7
innervation 493
inhibitory 458–9, 486–8
nedocromil sodium effects 586
neuropeptide tyrosine involvement 464
tachykinin involvement 449–50, 451
VIP involvement 458–9
nonarachin 967
non-steroidal anti-inflammatory drugs 1687–8
allergic reactions 1687–8

anaphylaxis 1559
prostanoid action and effects of 403
in seasonal allergic conjunctivitis 1653
in vernal keratoconjunctivitis 1657
Noon, Leonard 21
Northern blot analysis
of mRNA content of tissues 768
of probe specificity 768
nose
absorption and effects of inflammation 444
aerosol deposition in, avoiding 729
airway, *see* airway
anatomy (normal) 1300–5, 1311–16
asthma involving 672
β-adrenoceptors 567
blockage/congestion/obstruction
decongestants, *see* decongestants
H_1 receptor antagonists relieving 430–1
otitis media associated with 1639
breathing through, in prevention of exercise-induced asthma 700
ciliated cells (and cilia) 1300–1
abnormalities 1294, 1305
assessment of function 1298
particle removal by 1308, 1312
congestion, *see subheading above*
hyperreactivity, allergen-provoked 1144–5
IgE, demonstration 1016
inflammation, *see* rhinitis; rhinoconjunctivitis
late-phase reactions 1139–58, 1139–60
clinical presentation 1140–2
definition 1140
immunology 1146–50
mechanism, theoretical considerations and postulates 1153–5
physiology 1142–6
provocation tests following immunotherapy 1228
role, theoretical considerations and postulates 1155–6
therapy 1150–3, 1228, 1231
mucociliary clearance delay in 718
mucosa, *see* mucosa
obstruction, *see subheading above*
physiology 1306–8
pathological 1314–20
pollen protein release on landing in 837
polyposis, *see* polyps
priming effect, allergen-induced 1145–6
NSAIDs, *see* non-steroidal anti-inflammatory drugs
nuclear antigens, autoantibodies 1004
nuclear factor of activated T cells, cytoplasmic component (NF-AT_c) 643–4
nucleic acid, *see* DNA; RNA
nucleoside analogues, DNA synthesis-inhibiting 650
advantages of mycophenolate mofetil over 651
nucleotides (deoxynucleotides)
addition at Ig coding joints 67
in PCR 782, 785
nurses, *see* health care workers
nut(s) 967–8, 972–3
nutrition, *see* diet; food

obeche 914
obstruction/limitation, air-flow
in asthma
assessment 1351, 1352–3
in classifying asthma 1348
increasing severity, response to 673–6
irreversible, distinguished from reversible 1430
irreversible, prevention with steroids 623
in occupational asthma diagnosis 1472–6
persistent, in chronic asthma 671–2
reversibility, diagnostic significance 1353, 1354
reversibility, distinguished from non-reversibility 1430
chronic, *see* chronic obstructive pulmonary disease
in nasal late-phase reaction 1142
upper airway (generally), asthma distinguished from 1355–6
see also bronchoconstriction
occupational allergens 909–26, 1464–86
air pollutants/respiratory agents involved in sensitization to 1404, 1470–1
inhalational testing 921–3, 1476–7
tobacco smoke 1214, 1404
animals 910–11, 916, 1276, 1278
asthma caused by, *see* asthma, occupational
avoidance/prevention of exposure 1283, 1711–12
extrinsic allergic alveolitis caused by 1489
management 1498–9
natural history 1495
food/foodstuffs 911–14, 915, 962
latex 985, 1479
spores
indoor exposure 868–71
outdoor exposure 864–5
occupational disease (predominantly respiratory) 909–26, 1464–86
dermatitis as
contact 1626–7
irritant 1611–12
historical studies 17
rhinitis as 1296
surveillance 909–10
see also specific occupations
oculopathy, *see* eye
odour identification tests in rhinitis 1298
oedema
angioneurotic, *see* angioedema
mucosal airway 440
in asthma 161–2, 1420
food allergens and 1529–30
oesophageal achalasia 468
Oryza sativa 972
OKM-1, *see* Mac-1
OKT3 as immunosuppressant 653
OKY-046 404
Olea europea (olive tree) 851–2
allergens 800–1
Oleaceae 1019, 1020
cross-reactions 851–2
olfactory nerves 1313
olfactory tests in rhinitis 1296
oligonucleotide(s)
allergen genes synthesized from 814
antisense, as immunosuppressants 654
as probes *in situ* hybridization, construction 764–5
oligonucleotide primers in PCR 782, 785
annealing 783, 786
inefficiency 784
design 786
extension 783, 786
in reverse transcriptase-PCR 787–8
olive, *see Olea europea*
Onchocera volvulus, immune response 1170
ONO-1078 (pranlukast) 394
in chronic asthma 395, 1730
oocyte microinjection and murine studies of immunity and allergy 1057–8
ophthalmopathy, *see* eye
opioid analgesics, reactions to 1681
opioid peptides 464–6, 470–1
functional effects 465–6
localization 465
in pathophysiological conditions 470–1, 506
receptors 465
opisthorchiasis 1506
opsonization 316
oral allergy syndrome 1524–5
oral route
aerosols breathed via 729
asthma medications
β-adrenoceptor agonists 574–5, 1432, 1434
steroids 617, 629, 1436
theophyllines 1431
hayfever medications 1284–5
nasal decongestants 1151–2, 1328–9
nasal late-phase reaction medications 1151–2
tolerance to antigens via, induced by feeding antigens 138, 140, 1521–2
organic dust
allergic alveolitis caused by, *see* alveolitis, extrinsic allergic
toxic syndrome (ODTS)
diagnosis 1496–7
epidemiology 1491
Ornithonyssus sylviarium 913
oropharynx
candidiasis, steroid-related 625
contact urticaria confined to 1524–5
physiology 1308
spacers reducing drug deposition in 1442
orthopteran allergens 912
see also cockroach
Oryctolagus cuniculus (rabbit) 1079–92
allergens 905
laboratory exposure 911
as model of allergy/asthma/airway hyperresponsiveness 1079–92
Oryzae 842
osmolarity measurement in exercise-induced asthma 703
see also entries under hypertonic; hypotonic
osmotic shock, pollen grain rupture 838
ostiomeatal complex 1300
otitis media 1632–44
aetiopathogenesis 1633–4, 1636–9
classification 1632, 1633
definition 1632–3
diagnosis 1639–40
differential diagnosis 1640–1
epidemiology 1633–4
pathophysiology 1634–6
risk factors 1633
structural and anatomical considerations 1634–5
treatment 1641
otitis media with effusion (OME)
allergy and 1639
chronic 1639
definition 1632–3
diagnostic techniques 1640
Eustachian tube obstruction resulting in 1635–6
infection and 1638–9
otoscopy, pneumatic 1640
outpatient facilities 1287
ovaflavoprotein 966
ovalbumin 966
immune response to 140, 141
guinea pig 1094
mice 1388
ovalbumin model of asthma/allergic airway disease
mice 1063

rats 1070, 1071
Ovis spp., *see* sheep
ovoinhibitor 966
ovomucin 966
ovomucoid 966
ovotransferrin 966
oxidative burst, *see* metabolic burst
oxitropium
pharmacokinetics 597
side-effects/toxicity 602–3
oxygen species, reactive
asthma and 271–2
atherosclerosis and 522
oxygen tension, arterial, *see* arteries
oxygenation, asthmatics 674–6
oyster allergens, occupational exposure 913
ozone 1396–7, 1398–9
enhanced allergen responsiveness 1405–6
epidemiological studies of symptoms related to
adults 1401–2
children 1403
laboratory studies 1398–9
sensitization studies 1405
animals 1404
see also air pollution

P regions of Ig coding joints 67
P-selectin (CD62; PADGEM; GMP-140) 244, 273
allergic inflammation and 250–1
leucocyte–endothelial interactions and 286
neutrophil–endothelial interactions and 202
ligands 246, 273
p56^{lyn}, *see* lyn
p59^{fyn}, *see* fyn
p150,95 (CD11c) 246–7
FcεRII and 82, 91
leucocyte–endothelial interactions and 273
see also CR4
PADGEM, *see* P-selectin
paediatrics, *see* children
PAF, *see* platelet-activating factor
pancreatitis, bradykinin-forming cascade and 334
Paniceae 842
Panicoideae 842
papain 915, 974–5, 1480
paper wasps, *see Polistes*
papillary conjunctivitis, giant 1658–9
papular urticaria 1601
parabens 1624
paracrine function, leucocyte-derived hormones 507–8
paraformaldehyde fixation for mRNA *in situ* hybridization 767
paranasal sinuses, *see* sinuses
paraphenylenediamine 1625
parasites, helminth, *see* helminthic infection
parasympathetic ganglia, peribronchial, β_2-adrenoceptors 573
parasympathetic nervous system 488–97
nose 1303, 1313
parenteral therapy with β-adrenoceptor agonists in asthma 1434
pharmacokinetics 575
Parietaria spp. pollen 853
allergens 801
Parthenium hysterophorus 854
particles from aerosols (droplets/powders) in airway
deposition 728–9
calculation 729–31
with liposomal formulations 733–6
size 729, 730, 731
with liposomal formulations 734, 735, 736
particles from environment
acid, *see* acid particulates
cockroach allergens carried in, size 947
filtration/clearance in nose 1308, 1312
pollen carried in 838–9
patch tests
allergic contact dermatitis 1268, 1273, 1288, 1608–9, 1617–19
Amersham General Hospital standard series, results 1622
complications 1619
epidemiological studies 1609
false-positives and negatives 1619
reading 1618–19
atopic dermatitis 1580–2
drug allergy 1677
ocular allergy 1664–5
see also photopatch test
pathophysiology of allergy, historical ideas/concepts 5–6, 8–9
see also specific conditions
PDGF 215–16
pea allergens 968–9
peach 973
peak flow measurements
in classification of asthma 1348
in diagnosis of asthma 1352–3
in exercise-induced asthma 694
in occupational asthma 1472–5
nasal (in rhinitis) 1298, 1307
in prevention of occupational asthma 1482
peanut 967–8, 1556
peanut-1 967–8
PECAM-1 273, 287
pellitory, *see Parietaria* spp.
Penaeus spp. allergens
aztecus 805, 970
indicus 804–5, 970
penicillin allergy 1550–1, 1552–3
atopy and 1673
diagnosis 1684
incidence 1682
management 1678
desensitization 1566, 1679, 1684
mechanisms 1683–4
other drug allergies associated with 1679
penicillin polylysine (PPL) skin test 1683, 1684
Penicillium spp. 870
cross-reactivity 1021
notatum 879
peptide(s)/peptide fragments
immunotherapy employing 50–1, 142
in autoimmune disease 139
in house-dust mite allergy 895
in Hymenoptera venom allergy 937
in plasma exudates 440
T cell receptor-antagonizing 139
transporters 117
see also neuropeptide
peptide 401 (of *Apis mellifera*) 930
peptide histidine–isoleucine (PHI) 461
asthma and 276
functional effects 461
localization 461
peptide histidine–methionine 486–7
peptide histidine–valine (PHV-42) 461
peptide–MHC complexes (in T cell antigen recognition) 37–8, 114–19
Pepys, Jack 18
Per a, *see Periplanata americana*
perennial (chronic) allergic conjunctivitis 1649
diagnosis 1265
management 1265
perennial (chronic) allergic rhinitis 1275–6, 1653–4
conditions mimicking 1265, 1276
epidemiology 1321
management 1265–6, 1327–8
pharmacological 1327–8
pathogenesis 1653, 1664
perfumes 1623
periciliary fluid 713–14
peripheral blood
eosinophil counts, significance 185–6
mononuclear cells, density centrifugation 754–5
T cell, following immunotherapy 1231–2
peripheral T cells, *see* T cell
Periplanata americana 889
allergens (Per a) 889
immunoassays 947
molecular biology 945
permeability
airway vasculature, *see* vasculature
gut mucosa, food allergy and 963, 1519–20
peroxidase
eosinophil, *see* eosinophil peroxidase
in immunocytochemistry 776
and anti-peroxidase 775
personality and risk in asthma 510
pesticides
cockroach control 948–9
dust mite 1284, 1711, 1719
pet allergens 1275–6, 1328, 1711, 1718
prevention of exposure 1711, 1718
see also specific animals
petrolatum, allergens tested in 1621–6
Peyer's patches 1520
PF-4 215
PF 5901 in allergic rabbit 1086
PGEM vector 765
Phadiatop 1017
phagocyte oxidative killing, *see* metabolic burst
phagocytosis of foreign antigens 114
pharmaceutical industry, allergen exposure 921, 1465
Pharmacia CAP system, venom assay 1696
pharmacology 419–661
of late response
in asthma 1115–16
in skin 1135–6
see also drugs
pharynx 1308
asthma involving 672–3
physiology 1308
phenothiazines 1330
phenylephrine 578, 1329
phenylpropanolamine 578, 1328–9
Phleum pratense (timothy grass) allergens 799
recombinant, synthesis 818
phosphatidylcholine liposomes
cyclosporin A in 736
hydrogenated soybean, tolerance/safety 735
phosphatidylinositol, metabolism in neutrophils 204
phosphatidylinositol 3-kinase 204–5
phosphodiesterase (PDE)(s), cyclic nucleotide 529–65
in allergic disease/allergic inflammation 542–3, 543–4
distribution 535, 543–4
isoenzyme-1 533, 534–6
tissue distribution 534–6
isoenzyme-2 533, 536–7
tissue distribution 536–7
isoenzyme-3 533

isoenzyme-4 533
characteristics and properties 539
long-term regulation 539–40
short-term regulation 539
tissue distribution 540
isoenzyme-5 533, 540–1
tissue distribution 540–1
isoenzyme-6 533, 541
isoenzyme-7 533, 541
nomenclature 533
pro-inflammatory/immunocompetent cells containing 544–9
effects of PDE inhibitors on 544–9, 549–51
isoenzyme profiles 535
structure/properties/general characteristics 533–4
phosphodiesterase (PDE) inhibitors, isoenzyme-selective 544–52
anti-inflammatory effects *in vivo* 549–51
isoenzyme-1 534–6
therapeutic implications 534–6, 538
isoenzyme-2 536–7, 538
therapeutic implications 536–7
isoenzyme-3 537–8, 538
asthma 530
side-effects/limitations 553
isoenzyme-3/4 (mixed) selective 538
asthma 530
isoenzyme-4 540, 1727
in allergic rabbit 1085, 1086
asthma 530, 1727
side-effects/limitations 553
isoenzyme-5 538, 541
therapeutic implications 541
isoenzyme-6 538
isoenzyme-7 541
therapeutic implications 541
plasma extravasation and effects of 551
pro-inflammatory cells and effects of 544–9, 549–50
rationale for developing 529–30
representative 532
therapeutic uses 530, 552
tissue distribution 538
phosphodiesterase (PDE) inhibitors, non-selective, *see* aminophylline; methylxanthines; theophylline
phospholipase A_1, vespid 932
phospholipase A_2
Apis mellifera (honey-bee) 804, 930
recombinant, synthesis 819, 930
neutrophil 205
phospholipase B, vespid 932
phospholipase C
airway smooth muscle contraction and 747
neutrophil 204
phospholipase D, neutrophil 205
phospholipids of liposomal delivery systems 733
particle size and output of cyclosporin A with various 736
phosphorylation (of proteins)
of contractile proteins in airway smooth muscle 746–7, 747
enzymes responsible for, *see* protein kinase; serine–threonine kinases; tyrosine kinases and tyrosine phosphorylation
of phosphodiesterase isoenzyme-3 537–8
photoallergic reactions, skin 1616
photochemical pollution/smog and allergic disease
adults 1400–1
children 1403
see also nitrogen dioxide; ozone
photopatch test 1619–20
photoreceptors, phosphodiesterase-6 in 541
phototoxic reactions, skin 1616, 1620
physical examination, *see* examination
physical training/activity and exercise-induced asthma 700
phytophotodermatitis 1616
picornavirus infection, airway reactivity following 896
picryl chloride asthma 1063
animal model 1388
pigeon-fancier's lung, *see* birds
pinacidil 607
structure 608
pine-wood resin, *see* colophony
pinocytosis of foreign antigens 114
piperadines 1330
Pirquet, Clemens von 9, 10
pistachio 972–3
pituitary, *see* hypothalamic–pituitary–adrenocortical axis
pituitary adenylate cyclase activating peptide 456, 462–3
functional effects 463
localization 462
receptors 457–8, 462–3
pityriasiform lichenoid eczema, patchy 1575
Pityrosporum spp. 1022, 1575–6
plane, London 1019
plant(s)
cross-reactivity
expected 1018–20
unexpected 1024–5
fungal pathogens, spores from 863
materials
carrying pollen 838
patch testing 1618
occupational exposure to non-pollen allergens from 914–15
pollens, *see* pollens
see also farming; food *and individual species*
plant fibre, fungi growing on 870–1
plantar dermatosis, juvenile 1575
plasma
expansion in circulatory shock 1568
mediators derived from, urticaria and 1590
proteins, in exudates 440
plasma, exudation/extravasation/leakage 439–46, 550–1
as airway end-organ response 440–1
in allergic airway disease/asthma 161–2, 442–3, 550–1
phosphodiesterase inhibitor effects 551
challenge studies 442–3
contents of exudate 440
pathways/mechanisms 441–2
role of exudate 443–4
steroid effects 621
tachykinins and 451, 452
plasma cells, synthesis of membrane-bound vs secreted forms of Ig 73
plasma membrane, *see* membrane
plasmalemmal ATP-sensitive K^+ channel, *see* potassium ion channel
plastics workers 1465
platelet(s) 214–27
activation 217, 217–21
agonists, experiments using 218–19
antagonists 221–2
asthma and 217–21
aspirin and 1688
therapy of 221–2
contact dermatitis (allergic) and role, murine model 1059–60
mediators derived from 214–16
membrane proteins 216–17
phosphodiesterase 535
phosphodiesterase inhibitor effects 545, 548
platelet-activating factor (PAF) 179–80, 404–8
anaphylaxis and 1561
asthma and 217–18, 219, 267, 1084
biological activity 405–7
biosynthesis 404–5
cells releasing 405
eosinophils 179–80
neutrophils 216
platelets 216
cutaneous responses 1081
eosinophil effects 175
in helminthic infection 1171
ocular allergy and 1650–1
rabbit airway responses 1084
platelet-activating factor (PAF) receptor 405
platelet-activating factor (PAF) receptor antagonists
in humans 221–2, 407–8
in asthma 221–2, 407–8, 1084, 1116
in rabbit model, antigen-induced responses and effects of
airway 1084, 1086
skin 1081
platelet-derived growth factor 215–16
asthma and 271
platelet-derived histamine-releasing factor (PDHRF) 214
airway hyperreactivity and 219
platelet-derived hyperreactivity factor (PDHF) 219
platelet endothelial cell adhesion molecule-1 273, 287
platelet factor-4 215
platinum salts 918, 919, 1277–8, 1480
plethysmography in assessment of murine airway function 1061
Pleurotus ostreatus allergens, crossed immunoelectrophoresis 873, 875
plicatic acid 915
neonatal rabbit immunized with 1080
pneumatic otoscopy 1640
pneumonia
differentiation from extrinsic allergic alveolitis 1496
eosinophilic, *see* eosinophilic pneumonia
pneumonitis, hypersensitivity, *see* alveolitis, extrinsic allergic
Poa pratensis (Kentucky bluegrass) allergen, recombinant, synthesis 818
Poaceae, *see* grass family; grass-pollen allergens
Poeae 842
Pogonomyrmex spp. 928
allergens 933
Polistes (paper wasp) spp. 928
nomenclature of allergens 936
Polistinae, classification 928
pollen(s) 798–801, 835–57, 1274–5, 1718
abundance 837–8
air pollutant effects 845, 1217, 1397
avoidance, *see* allergen avoidance
collection devices 838–9, 840
counting (monitoring) 838–41
interpreting count 839–40
monitoring networks 840–1
cross-reacting 1018–20, 1024–5
dispersal 837–8
historical studies 14, 18
immunotherapy 1236, 1239
particles carrying 838–9
seasons, *see* seasons
smokers with increased rates of sensitization 1214
sources of information 838–41
structure/characteristics 835–7
grasses 843

young children exposed to 1718
see also specific (types of) pollens
pollenosis (in general)
air pollution and 845, 1216
symptoms, relation to pollen counts and seasons 840
see also specific pollenoses
pollutant gases, *see* air pollution
polyacrylamide gel electrophoresis of allergens 796
poly(adenosine diphosphate-ribose) synthetase 519
polyadenylation sites on Cμ gene segment 73
polyamine depleting-drugs 652
polyarteritis nodosa (PAN) 1510
trans-polyisoprene 982
polymerase chain reaction 782–91
allergen gene cloning employing 813–14
basic principles 782–3
components 784–6
conditions 786
detection and verification of product 786–7
exponential nature (of amplification) 783–4
loss 784
reverse transcriptase-, *see* reverse transcriptase-PCR
polymorphic/variant allergens 814, 816, 828
polyps/polyposis, nasal 1294–5
with aspirin intolerance 1279
asthma and, association 1350
Pooideae 798, 842
poppy seed 974
Portier, Paul 8, 9
Portugal, allergy training 1263
post-mortem
asthma, pathology 185, 1360–5, 1414, 1424
compared with chronic obstructive pulmonary disease 1414, 1424
indirect measurements 1362–3
in situ hybridization to tissue samples 770
systemic anaphylaxis 1563
potassium dichromate, testing with 1622–3
potassium ion, β-adrenoceptor agonist-induced disturbances 577
potassium ion channel (Ca^{2+}-dependent) openers, β-agonists as 607
potassium ion channel (plasmalemmal ATP-sensitive) openers (cromakalim/cromakalim-like drugs) 607–16
airway smooth muscle effects 607–12
relaxant action 607–8, 610–11
in asthma 607–16, 1728
possible mechanisms of action 611–12
potential 612–13, 1728
trials 612–13
structures 608
unwanted effects 612, 613
potato 973
powder (in dry-powder inhalers), carrier 732
pranlukast, *see* ONO-1078
Prausnitz, Carl 10
Prausnitz–Kustner reactions 1165
prawn allergens 913
prealbumin, mouse 904, 911
precipitins
in allergic bronchopulmonary aspergillosis 1502
in extrinsic allergic alveolitis 1495–6
prednisolone
asthma 358, 360, 629, 630
rhinitis 1335
see also methylprednisolone
pregnancy
asthma (chronic) in 1437
diet in, *see* diet
fetus in, *see* fetus
H_1 receptor antagonists in 425
insect venom immunotherapy 1236, 1567
preventive measures with high risk of infant atopy 1722
rhinitis treatment in 1337
smoking in, *see* smokers
steroid safety 628–9
prekallikrein 324, 326
conversion to kallikrein 324, 326
premature birth and food allergy 1541, 1720
premedication in drug reaction prevention 1678, 1686
pre-menstrual asthma, management 1437
preprotachykinin 447
mRNA *in situ* hybridization 770
preservation/fixation
for immunocytochemistry 776
for mRNA *in situ* hybridization 767
pressure measurements, nasal, *see* rhinomanometry
pressure urticaria, delayed 1598
pressurized metered dose inhalers, *see* metered dose inhalers
preterm neonates and food allergy 1541, 1720
prevalence
air pollution and symptoms
adults 1400–2
children 1402–3
of asthma
evidence for increase 1209–10
exercise-induced asthma as marker of 695–6
gender differences in children 1181–2
in asthma, of late-phase reactions 1115
atopy, evidence for increase 1209
of eczema, evidence for increase 1210
food reactions (adverse) 1518
rhinitis, perennial allergic 1321
rhinitis, seasonal allergic (hayfever) 1320–1
evidence for increase 1210
prevention (of allergic disease) 1709–25
anaphylaxis 1564, 1566
β-adrenoceptor antagonist-induced bronchospasm, anticholinergics in 598
drug reactions 1678
radiocontrast media 1566, 1686
exercise-induced asthma 700, 702
food allergy 1541–2, 1710, 1720
helminthic infection and 1164–5
irreversible air-flow obstruction in asthma 623
latex allergy in health care workers/staff 988, 989
occupational allergens 1711–12
see also asthma, occupational; genetics
primary 1715
seasonal allergic rhinitis 1333–4
secondary 1715
tertiary 1715
see also allergen avoidance
prick tests 1287–9
asthma (chronic) 1430
bronchopulmonary aspergillosis (allergic) 1502
contact dermatitis 1619
drug allergy 1677
muscle relaxants 1680
penicillin 1684
extrinsic allergic alveolitis 1496
food allergens 1537
intradermal methods compared with 1007–8, 1133, 1272–3
ocular allergy 1664
rhinitis 1297
scoring system 1272
primate models of asthma (cynomolgus monkey; *Macaca fascicularis*) 1037–44
endothelial cells and 292
primer oligonucleotides for PCR, *see* oligonucleotide primers
primin 1625
procoagulant activity, leucocyte 1620
profilin 1024–5
propellants for metered dose inhalers 731, 1441–2
prophylaxis, *see* prevention
propranolol 578
airway response to 684
prostacyclin (PGI_2) 402–3
asthma and 266, 402–3, 1731
prostaglandin(s) 380, 398–404
assays and their value 999
biosynthesis 398–400
cellular source 398
receptors 400
prostaglandin D_2
asthma and 266, 400, 401
mast cell 155
nasal
late-phase reaction and 1148
rhinitis and 1315
prostaglandin E_2 402
asthma and 266, 402
therapy of 1731
honey-bee phospholipase A_2 and synthesis of 804
prostaglandin $F_{2\alpha}$ 401
asthma and 266, 400, 401
mast cell 155
prostaglandin G_2, pulmonary alveolar macrophage-derived 155
prostaglandin H synthase, role 398–400
prostaglandin I_2, *see* prostacyclin
prostanoids (cyclo-oxygenase pathway products) 398–404
actions in asthma 401–4
pharmacological modulation 403
biosynthesis 398–400
cellular source 398
eosinophils 179
receptors 400
release 400–1
in asthma 400–1
see also prostaglandin; thromboxane
protamine sulphate 969
atopy and 1673
protease (proteinase)
CD23-cleaving 1167
inhibitors
in contact activation 331
secretory leucocyte, steroid effects on synthesis of 620
mast cell 154, 154–5
neuropeptide actions modulated by 457
occupational exposure 915–16
see also proteolytic activity
proteasomes 116–17
protein(s)
phosphorylation, *see* protein kinase; serine–threonine kinases; tyrosine kinase
plasma, in exudates 440
pollen, first-release 836–7
protein contact dermatitis 1616
protein kinase A, phosphorylation phosphodiesterase isoenzyme-3 537
protein kinase C
airway smooth muscle contraction and 747
as chromone target 588
proteinase, *see* protease
proteoglycan
basement membrane 300
mast cell 153–4

proteolytic activity of FcεRII
auto- 89
see also protease
provocation tests, *see* allergen challenge
pseudoallergic drug reactions, definition 1671, 1676
pseudoephedrine 578, 1328–9
pseudogenes, C region heavy chain 65
PSGL-1 246
psoralens
phototoxic reactions 1620
UV and, in atopic dermatitis therapy 1584
psoriasis
leukotrienes and 392–3
leukotriene biosynthesis inhibitors in 397–8
psychological/psychogenic factors
in asthma 490, 509–10
in atopic dermatitis 1582
in rhinitis 1296
in urticaria (chronic) 1593
Pulmicort 735
pulmonary hypertension, *see* hypertension
pulmonary non-vascular biology/problems, *see* lung
punch biopsy for deriving T cells for culture 756–7
purine biosynthesis inhibitors 650–1
PUVA in atopic dermatitis therapy 1584
pyrimidine biosynthesis inhibitors 651
pyschiatric disturbances, steroids 628
pysyllium 914

Qa 115
Q–T interval, H_1 receptor antagonists affecting 433–5, 1332, 1333
quaternary ammonium compounds
development 597
toxicity/side-effects 602–3
questionnaire, asthma diagnosis 1352, 1356–7
quinoline 1624–5

R68,151 in psoriasis 398
Ra reactive factor 311
rabbit, *see Oryctolagus cuniculus*
Rac1/Rac2 208
race and atopy/atopic disease 1213
Rackemann, Francis 16
radioallergosorbent test (IgE antibody quantification) 1016
drug allergy 1677
β-lactams 1684
food allergy 1537
inhibition technique 1028–9
insect-sting allergy 1696
potential problems 1016–17
rhinitis 1297
radiocontrast media, *see* contrast media
radiology, *see* imaging
radionuclide/radioisotopes
antibodies labelled with 777
monoclonal antibody conjugated to, as immunotoxins 653
RNA probes labelled with 766
safety precautions with radioisotopes 769
scans with, drug–liposome aerosol deposition determined via 734–5
Raf-1 184
RAG-1/RAG-2 67–8
ragweed, *see Ambrosia* spp.
rain, spore release with 862, 863
Ramazzini, Bernadino 17
ramin 914
RANTES 370
endothelial cell-derived 285
eosinophils and 175–6, 370
platelet-derived 215, 216
receptor 372
rapamycin
cytokine actions inhibited by 648–9
in experimental models of allergic disease 655
toxicity 656
RaRF 311
RAST, *see* radioallergosorbent test
rat
allergens 904
laboratory exposure 910–11, 1478
as models of airway responses to allergens 1068–78
reactive airway dysfunction syndrome (RADS) 1464
diagnosis 1472
epidemiology 1467
mechanisms 1471
receptors
Ca^{2+} channels operated by 745–6
as chromone targets 588–9
on endothelial cells 201–3
on eosinophils, *see* eosinophil
for neutrophils 201–3
on neutrophils 203
signalling from, *see* signal transduction
steroids affecting transcription of various 620
see also specific receptors
recombinant allergens, *see* allergen *and specific allergens*
recombination (with Ig genes)
class switch 71–2, 97
RAG genes 67–8
red blood cells, sheep, murine model of airway changes using 1063–4
reflex activity, cholinergic, bronchial hyperreactivity and enhanced 490–1
reflex bronchoconstriction, chromone effects 586, 590
reflex cold urticaria 1600
reflux, gastro-oesophageal, asthma and 1350
relatives, *see* family (and relatives)
remodelling, airway, *see* airway/respiratory tract in asthma
renal tract, *see* kidney
reporter allergen, definition 1013
research
evidence-based 1269
skin tests in 1010–11
residential buildings, *see* housing
resistance to airflow, *see* flow
resistance vessels in nose 1305, 1312–13
respiratory burst, *see* metabolic burst
respiratory distress syndrome, adult, leukotrienes and 392
respiratory syncytial virus infection in early life 1370, 1712
respiratory tract, *see* airway
respired allergens, *see* inhaled allergens
resuscitation in anaphylaxis 1567–78
see also adrenaline
reticular basement membrane (lamina reticularis) thickening in asthma 161, 301, 1417
retina, phosphodiesterase-6 in 541
reverse transcriptase-PCR 787–8
phosphodiesterase-4 subtype identification by 540
rewarming of airways in exercise-induced asthma 702–3
rheology of mucus 715–16, 717, 720
rheumatoid arthritis
bradykinin-forming cascade and 334
leukotrienes and 392
leukotriene biosynthesis inhibitors in 398
tachykinins and 470
Rhi s 1/2 (Rhiz IIIb/VIb) 872, 880
rhinitis (generally and non-allergic forms) 1293–9
asthma and, association 1350
atrophic 1296
capsaicin effects 1303
classification 1293–6
differential diagnosis 1296–8
conditions mimicking 1292, 1294, 1296
definition 1293
infective 1293–4
investigations 1297–8, 1306–7
occupational 1296
pathophysiology 1314–20
structural causes 1294, 1294–5
vasomotor 1295
rhinitis, allergic/atopic 1265–6, 1293–343
adhesion molecules and 293
atopic dermatitis and 1576
autonomic nervous system in
adrenergic nervous system 488
cholinergic nervous system 489–90
children 1337
cutaneous late-phase reactions to allergens in 1132
definitions 1209, 1293
eosinophils 187
epidemiology 1320–1
histopathology 46
historical background 12–13
immunotherapy-induced 1254
children 1255
inflammatory model 1318–20
in lactation 1337
mild intermittent 1338–9
mild persistent 1339
model, nasal late-phase response as 1150, 1155–6
moderate persistent 1339
nature of disease 1311
otitis media and 1633, 1636, 1636–7, 1639, 1640
perennial/chronic, *see* perennial (chronic) allergic rhinitis
in pregnancy 1337
seasonal/summer, *see* hayfever
severe persistent 1339
T cells in pathogenesis of 46–9, 1317–18, 1319
therapy/management 1327–43
guidelines 1338
immunotherapy, *see* immunotherapy
pharmacological, *see* drugs
rhinoconjunctivitis, allergic 1338–9
atopic dermatitis associated with 1576
drug therapy
guidelines 1338–9
H_1 antagonists 431
food-related 1529–30
mild intermittent 1338–9
mild persistent 1339
moderate persistent 1339
severe persistent 1339
rhinomanometry 1298, 1306–7
active anterior 1306
active posterior 1306
passive 1307
rhinometry, acoustic 1298, 1307
rhinorrhoea, gustatory 1296
rhinoscopy, rhinitis 1297, 1306
rhinosinusitis
aspirin/other NSAID-induced 1687, 1688
chronic infective 1293–4

rhinovirus infection, airway reactivity following 896, 1712
Rhizopus stolinifer (*nigricans*) 872, 879–80
crossed immunoelectrophoresis 873, 876
ribonucleic acid, messenger, *in situ* hybridization to, *see in situ* hybridization to mRNA
rice 972
Richet, Charles 8, 9
ricin in rat model 1072
IgE responses to 1068, 1069
Ricinus communis 915
Riley, James F. 11, 12
risk factors
asthma 510, 1348–9
evaluation 1354–5
for atopy/allergy/allergic disease (in general) 1211–18, 1716–17
skin test positivity as 1010–11, 1211, 1212
drug allergy 1672–4
aspirin/other NSAIDs 1687
barbiturates 1681
β-lactams 1683
contrast media 1673, 1685
general anaesthetics 1673, 1679–80
immunotherapy 1246
latex allergy 985–6, 1025
otitis media 1633
RNA
extraction, methods 787
Northern blots, *see* Northern blot analysis
as probe for *in situ* hybridization
construction 765–6
labelling 766
size 766
specificity 768
transfer, as shrimp allergen 970
RNA, messenger (mRNA)
in situ hybridization to, *see in situ* hybridization to mRNA
PCR in detection of 787–90
reverse transcriptase- 787–8
quantitative 788–90
RNases as allergens
fungal 803
grass pollen 799
rodent (and rodent-like animal) allergens 803, 904–5
rodlets of Deuteromycotina 860
rolipram
anti-inflammatory effects 549
inflammatory/immunocompetent cell effects 550
T cells 546
Rotadisk 1443–4
Rotahaler 1443
rotamase activity of FK506-binding protein 645
rotorod system 838–9
RS-61443 (myclophenolate mofetil; MM) 650–1, 651–2
rubber 981–2
biosynthesis 981–2
contact allergens 1625
see also latex
rubber accelerators 1625
rubber elongation factor 973, 982
'rubor' as classical sign of inflammation 440
Rumex spp. 854
rush immunotherapy, insect sting allergy 1699–700
Russian thistle 852
ryegrass, *see Lolium perenne*

S-protein 315
S-type lectins 91
SA-1/II (shrimp allergens) 970
Sac r 1/2/3 872
saccharin test 717
Saccharopolyspora rectivirgula 872, 880–1
salbutamol 570
in exercise-induced asthma 697
pharmacokinetics
inhaled preparations 575
oral preparations 575
parenteral preparations 575
Salicaceae 1019, 1020
saline, hypertonic, *see* hypertonic/hyperosmolar aerosols
salivary glands, minor, of asthmatics 287–8
salmeterol 571–2
Salsola pestifer (*kali*) 852
salt
concentration, effect on regional aerosol particle deposition 730
dietary, asthma and 1218
'salt' hypothesis of mucous retention 719–20
Salter, Henry H. 17
sampling devices
cockroach allergens 946–7
mite allergens 891
pollen 840
spores, *see* spores
Samuelson, Bengt I. 12, 14
sarcoidosis
diagnosis 1497
lymphocytes in 1492
sarcoplasmic reticulum 741
SCA40, airway smooth muscle effects 609, 613
Schistosoma spp.
haematobium, immune response 1170
mansoni, immune response 1169
pulmonary eosinophilia caused by 1506
schools, pet allergens 1710
scintigraphic determination of drug–liposome aerosols 734–5
screening, occupational asthma predisposition 1482
SDS-polyacrylamide gel electrophoresis of allergens 796
SDZ PCO-400
airway hyperreactivity suppressed by 612
structure 608
seafood allergens 804–5, 969–71
occupational exposure 913
recombinant, synthesis 819
see also specific foods
season(s)
pollen 837–8, 1215–16, 1273
grass, *see* grass
severity 837–8, 844–5, 849, 851
tree 847, 847–9, 850, 851
in UK 1273
weed 852, 853
spore 862–3, 864
see also climate; keratoconjunctivitis; weather; winter feet
seasonal aeroallergens (in general) in UK, calendar 1274
seasonal allergic conjunctivitis 1649, 1651–3
diagnosis 1269
management 1269, 1651–3
pathogenesis 1651
pathology 1651
seasonal allergic rhinitis, *see* hayfever
seborrhoeic dermatitis 1577
second messenger systems, *see* signal transduction
secreted immunoglobulins 62
IgA 62
food antigens bound by 1520–1
IgM 62
intracellular transport 73
properties 62
secretion 62
synthesis 72–3
secretions, airway
mucous, *see* mucus
nasal 1303–4
late-phase 1142, 1143
secretory effects
bombesin 467
gastrin-releasing peptide 467
neuropeptide tyrosine 464
pituitary adenylate cyclase activating peptide 463
tachykinins 453
VIP 460–1
secretory functions of pulmonary alveolar macrophages 230–1
secretory leucocyte protease inhibitor, steroid effects on synthesis 620
sectioning of tissue
for immunocytochemistry, serial 778
for *in situ* hybridization to mRNA 768
seeds 974
occupational exposure 915
segregation analysis 1201
asthma and bronchial hyperresponsiveness 1201
atopy 1189, 1201
selectins 244–6, 250–1, 252, 253–4, 273
in allergic inflammation 250–1
antagonists/antibodies to 140, 252, 1040
in primate model 1040, 1041
counter-structures/ligands 245–6, 273
leucocyte–endothelial cell interactions concerning
basophils and 253–4
endothelial cell production 202, 286
eosinophils and 42, 253–4, 289
neutrophils and 202, 253–4
see also E-selectin; L-selectin; P-selectin
self, discrimination from non-self 37–8, 118
self-administered adrenaline in anaphylactic shock 1565
self-antigen (endogenous antigen) 114
recognition of/response to 116, 116–17, 118
elimination 38
tolerance to 133–7
intrathymic 133
seminal plasma proteins, anaphylaxis with 1557–8
sensitization
airway 239, 1370–1
adjuvant factors 1370–1, 1717–18
air pollutants and 1370–1, 1403–5, 1717
cellular biology 1371
chironomid allergens 952–4
guinea pig (in asthma model) 1093–4, 1404
mite allergens, *see Dermatophagoides pteronyssinus*
occupational allergens, *see* occupational allergens
smoking and 1214, 1370, 1404–5, 1717
see also specific factors
eczematous
capacity/susceptibility 1609–10, 1612–13
molecular aspects 1614
fetal/intrauterine 1721–2
hymenoptera allergens (venoms) 1693
prevention 1709–14
see also atopy
sensory nerves
capsaicin-sensitive, tachykinin involvement

449–50
mast cells and (in airways), association between 453–4
nose 1303
opioid peptide effects 465–6
sepsis, *see* infection/sepsis
serine–threonine kinases, neutrophil 206–7
serological tests 1288
seromucous glands in nose 1303, 1312
serotonin, *see* 5-hydroxytryptamine
serous glands in nose 1303
Serpula lacrimans 867
serum sickness and anaphylaxis, differentiation 1564
sesame seed 974
sesquiterpene lactone 1625–6
sex, *see* gender
sheep
as model of bronchoconstriction 1045–55
red blood cells, murine model of airway changes using 1063–4
wool alcohols 1624
shock, *see* anaphylaxis; endotoxic shock
shrimp allergens 804–5, 970
B cell epitopes 964
recombinant, synthesis 819
SI/SI[d] mice, mast cell development 150
signal transduction and second messenger systems
airway smooth muscle 741–2
contraction of 746–8
B cell antigen receptors and 75–6
chromone effects 587–8
eosinophils and 183–5
neutrophils and 204–6
T cells and
activated, immunosuppressive drugs and 644, 649
after antigen recognition 118–19
silo-filler's lung 1496
Sinapsis alba allergens 974
Sin a 1 974
recombinant 975
singulair 1730
sinuses, paranasal
inflammation (sinusitis) 1294
asthma and, association 1350
rabbit model 1088
see also rhinosinusitis
in late-phase reaction 1142
sinusoids/sinuses, venous
lower airway 1361
nasal 1305, 1313
sirolismus, cytokine actions inhibited by 648–9
SI/SI[d] mice, mast cell development 150
SK&F 104,353 1730
in aspirin-induced asthma 394
bronchodilator effect 395
in exercise-induced asthma 394
skin
age-related changes 1007
allergic disease/inflammation 1279–80
diagnosis 1279–80
food allergens causing 1527–9
human models, *see* late-phase reactions (*subheading below*)
management 1267–8
murine models 1057, 1058–61
rabbit models 1080–1
see also specific skin diseases
anaphylaxis affecting 1561, 1562
acute management 1567–8
drug-related 1674
biopsy, *see* biopsies
drug allergy 1675
dry, in atopic dermatitis 1574–5, 1578
Langerhans cells, *see* Langerhans cells
late-phase reactions 1131–8
immunotherapy 1136, 1227–8, 1230–1
steroid therapy 1568
mast cells
cytokines 156
IgE and substance P-induced release of mediators by 152
pituitary adenylate cyclase activating peptide effects on vasculature 463
steroid effects 627
tachykinin effects 152
vasculature 451–2
transplantation 123
skin tests 1007–11, 1287–8
age differences 1211
allergen standardization for 1009–10
asthma allergens/sensitizers 1354–5, 1430
atopy diagnosis 1208
chironomid haemoglobin 958
conditions precluding 1015
drug allergy 1677
barbiturates 1681
β-lactams 1682–3, 1684
local anaesthetics 1682
muscle relaxants 1680
in epidemiology 1010–11, 1208, 1211, 1212, 1609
gender differences 1212
intradermal, *see* intradermal tests
latex allergy 986–7
ocular allergy 1664–5
patch tests, *see* patch tests
prick tests, *see* prick tests
principles/features 998–9, 1007
quantitative, allergen activity assayed by 727–8
in research 1010–11
results
factors influencing 1008–9
interpretation 1010
rhinitis 1297
weal, *see* weal
slide treatment for mRNA *in situ* hybridization 768
slow-reacting substance of anaphylaxis 28
discovery 11, 12
see also leukotriene C_4; leukotriene D_4
small-volume spacers 1442
smell identification tests in rhinitis 1298
smog, *see* photochemical pollution
smokers/smoking 1370, 1717
airway sensitization and 1214, 1370, 1404–5, 1717
chronic obstructive pulmonary disease with 1214–15
asthma distinction from/overlap between 672
IgE levels with 1014, 1214
maternal (in pregnancy)
asthma aetiology 1368, 1370
skin-test reactivity and 1405
passive/environmental 1214, 1403, 1404–5, 1712, 1717
sensitization and, *see* sensitization
smooth muscle (airway) 740–50
β-adrenoceptors in
agonist of, relaxation induced by, mechanism 570
desensitization 576
canine 1103–4
abnormal biochemical pathway 1107–8
pharmacological challenge, effects 1104–5
CGRP effects 455
contraction (and tension) 742–8
in asthma 665–7
Ca^{2+} concentration and 610, 742–8
integrated scheme for 746–8
see also bronchoconstriction
cromakalim-like drug actions on, *see* potassium ion channel openers
hyperresponsiveness, *see* bronchial hyperresponsiveness
mass increase in asthma 1418–20
nerve number decreasing with descent down bronchial tree 523, 524
neuropeptide tyrosine effects 464
pituitary adenylate cyclase activating peptide effects 463
rabbits neonatally immunized with antigen 1087–8
shortening in asthma 1364
structural aspects 740–2
tachykinin effects 451, 494
smooth muscle (non-airway)
CGRP effects 455
neuropeptide tyrosine effects 464
pituitary adenylate cyclase activating peptide effects 463
tachykinin effects 451
snails 971–2
sneezing responsiveness to histamine, antigen-provoked increase 1144
snow-crab allergens 913
sodium, dietary, asthma and 1218
sodium cromoglycate and disodium cromoglycate (cromolyn) 582–93, 1285
adverse effects 1334, 1436
allergic rabbit 1085, 1086
bronchial hyperresponsiveness decreased by 686
in childhood asthma 1459, 1461
in chronic asthma 1436
in conjunctivitis
giant papillary conjunctivitis 1659
seasonal allergic conjunctivitis 1652–3
see also keratoconjunctivitis (*subheading below*)
discovery 22, 582
in exercise-induced asthma 696, 697
in keratoconjunctivitis
atopic keratoconjunctivitis 1661
vernal keratoconjunctivitis 1656
late response and effects of
asthmatic 1115
nasal 1151
mechanism/mode of action 587–90, 1333, 1436
pro-inflammatory cells and mediators and
and asthma symptoms 585–6
and asthmatic inflammation 583–5
and atopy development 586–7
in rhinitis 1333–4
guidelines for use 1338
in seasonal rhinitis (hayfever) 1284
structure 583
sodium ion channel blockers in cystic fibrosis 722–3
solar urticaria 1600
solder flux, *see* colophony
Solenopsis (fire ant) spp. 928
invicta 928
nomenclature of allergens 936
Sol i 5 allergen 818
richteri 928
somatic hypermutation of Ig genes 70–1
somatostatin 468
sorbitan sesquiolate, fragrances tested with addition of 1623
sorrel 854

Southern blots, PCR products detected via 787
soy(a)bean (*G. max*)
allergens 968, 1481
asthma epidemics and 1216
cow's milk substitute made from, intolerance/hypersensitivity 1282, 1531, 1532
phosphatidylcholine liposomes, hydrogenated, tolerance/safety 735
spacers/holding chambers 1442
large-volume 1442
chronic asthma 1434
main uses 1442
small-volume 1442
Spain, allergy training 1262
Spanish toxic oil syndrome 1506–7
specialists 1287
specialty or subspecialty, allergology as 1261
spermine/spermidine metabolism, drugs interfering with 652
sphingomyelin metabolism, neutrophil 205–6
spices 974
spina bifida and latex allergy 985
Spinhaler 1443
spinnability of mucus 716
spiny lobster 971
spirometry in asthma 1352
spores, fungal and bacterial
in air-conditioning systems, *see* ventilation pneumonitis
characteristics for recognition as allergen 861
circadian periodicity 862, 863
geographical locations 863–4
local sources 864
mites and 1023
monitoring in USA 841, 858–87
release mechanisms, weather and 862
seasonality 862–3, 864
structure 860, 860–1
traps and sampling devices 862, 881
Burkard, *see* Burkard 7-day volumetric spore trap
Hirst, pollen trap based on design 839, 840
see also bacteria; fungi
spot tests 1621
sprays, allergen denaturing 1719
spring ophthalmia, *see* keratoconjunctivitis
sputum
asthmatics (compared with chronic obstructive pulmonary disease) 1413–14, 1424
drugs acting on 722–3
general characteristics 715
transportability in disease states 718–19, 719
squid 971
Stachybotrys atra 868
staff, *see* health care workers
Stamper–Woodruff assay
eosinophil recruitment 253, 254
lymphocyte re-circulation in 255–6
stanozolol, hereditary angioedema 1604
Staphylococcus aureus, atopic dermatitis and 1575, 1582
therapy of 1583
stem cell factor, mast cell development and 150
steroids, *see* glucocorticosteroids
stinging insects, *see* Hymenoptera
stocking dermatitis 1625
stomach mucosa, food allergen provocation tests under endoscopic control 1538–9
storage mite allergens 802, 912–13
occupational exposure 912–13, 914
stress, immune response, *see* immune response
Strongyloides stercoralis 1505
submucosa
bronchial, glands, in asthma 1418
nasal
blood supply 1305
glands 1303–4, 1312
sub-specialty or specialty, allergology as 1261
substance P 447, 494
in asthma 276, 469
airway response to 684
localization 447–8
mast cell effects 152, 453, 454, 505
in pathophysiological conditions (other than asthma) 470
receptors 448, 449
nasal 1314
skin and effects of 451–2, 505
smooth muscle effects 451, 494
other effects 494
suction trapping of pollen 839
sugar beet 852
sugar-cane bagasse 870
sulph-hydryl agents as mucolytics 721–2
sulphite sensitivity 1559
sulphonamides 1684–5
sulphur dioxide 1216, 1395–6
airway response to 684
animal studies of sensitization involving 1404
enhanced allergen responsiveness 1406
epidemiology of allergic disease related to
adults 1400
children 1402–3
laboratory studies 1398
see also air pollution
sulphuric acid 1395–6
summer hayfever, *see* hayfever
superoxide anion, atherosclerosis and 522
surfactants
endogenous, mucokinetic properties 723
in metered dose inhalers 1442
surgery
general anaesthetics, *see* general anaesthetics
otitis media 1641
vernal keratoconjunctivitis 1657–8
surgical biopsies, *in situ* hybridization 769–70
Surveillance for Work-related and Occupational Respiratory Diseases 909–10, 1466
suxamethonium 1679, 1680
sweating and atopic dermatitis 1582
Sweden, allergy training 1262
'swelling' ('tumor') as classical sign of inflammation 440
Switzerland, allergy training 1264
SWORD 909–10, 1466
sympathetic nerves, nose 1303, 1313
synovial fluid for deriving T cells for culture 757
Syringa vulgaris allergens 800
syringe for adrenaline self-administration 1565
systemic mastocytosis and anaphylaxis, differentiation 1564
systemic reactions/generalized anaphylaxis 1268, 1550–72
causes 1550–1, 1551–60
food allergens 1530
insect venom 1694, 1695
clinical and biochemical features 1561–3
definitions 1550–1
drugs 1672–3
in immunotherapy 1246, 1246–7
children 1255
for insect stings 1697
management guidelines 1254, 1255
recording 1251, 1252, 1253
mechanisms/pathogenesis 1551–60
murine models 1058–9
need for knowledge of features and management 1268
see also anaphylaxis

T cell(s) 29–32, 36–57, 255–6, 287–8, 291–2, 753–63, 1229–30, 1379–94
activated, *see* T cell(s), activated
activation and proliferation
pulmonary alveolar macrophages in suppression of 232, 233
signals involved in 132–3
aeroallergens recognized by/sensitizing in infancy 239
in rat model 1069, 1072–3
airway hyperresponsiveness and role of 1072–3
in allergen-specific immunotherapy 50, 1229–30, 1230–2
insect stings and 1702–4
peripheral blood 1231–2
antigen and, *see* antigen
antigen-presenting cell interactions with 124–5
asthma and 1379–94, 1421
chronic 1379–94
eosinophil interactions with T cells 187–8, 1382, 1383–4
immunosuppressants and 1733
late response in 1119–20
pathogenesis of 46–9, 287–8, 552
theophylline effects in 552, 553
autoimmune disease and 138
B cell interactions with, *see* B cell
chironomid allergen response 956
clonal anergy, *see* anergy
clonal deletion of 38, 133, 133–4
partial 134
peripheral 133–4
clonal ignorance 136
clones (monoclonal–manufactured)) 753–66
techniques of manufacture 756–7, 758–60
uses 760–1
cutaneous
allergic contact dermatitis and 1612
atopic dermatitis and 1528–9, 1578, 1579, 1580–1, 1582
late-phase reactions and 1134, 1134–5
punch biopsy for deriving, for culture 756–7
cytokines of, *see* cytokines, T cell-derived
cytotoxic/suppressor, *see* CD8+ cells
endothelial cell interactions with 291–2
epitopes
food allergens and 964
Hymenoptera venoms and 937
T cell antigen recognition and 37–8
extrinsic allergic alveolitis and 1492–3
fetal sensitization and 1721–2
GM-CSF synthesis 349
helminthiasis-related responses 1168
helper, *see* CD4+ T cells; Th0; Th1; Th2
heterogeneity/dichotomy 29–32, 104, 113
functional 42–5, 1120
homing receptors 1386
house-dust mite and, *see Dermatophagoides pteronyssinus*
hybridization 756
hypersensitivity mediated by, *see* hypersensitivity

IgE synthesis and role of 39–41, 98–100
immune response and 45, 49, 119–24
interleukin-10 effects 349
lectin-stimulated 756
lines (oligoclonal) 755
established 757
memory 120
migration/movement 291
adhesion molecules controlling 287
re-circulation from blood to lymphoid organs 255–6
monoclonal antibodies to, as immunosuppressant 653
in murine models of allergy 1057, 1059, 1060
in nose
in late-phase reaction 1147–8
in rhinitis 46–9, 1317–18, 1319
phosphodiesterase in 535
phosphodiesterase inhibitor effects 544–6
proliferative assays 755–6
quantitation 1001
resting 119–20
allergy and 125
dendritic cell interactions with 125
immunosuppressive drugs affecting 645
tolerance in
peripheral 133–7
in rat model 1069–70
vernal keratoconjunctivitis and 1656
viral transformation 756
T cell(s), activated 1381–3
allergy and 125–6
asthma and 1381–2, 1421
extrinsic allergic alveolitis and 1492–3
immunosuppressive drugs affecting 643–4, 649, 654–5
nuclear factor of (cytoplasmic component - NF-AT_c) 645–6
T cell receptor 1379–81, 1384–6
agonisms, partial 139–40
antagonists/altered peptide ligands 139
antigen recognition and subsequent responses and 119, 1380
asthma and 1384–6
atopy and 1191
chironomid allergens and 957
down-modulation 136
IgE responses and 141, 1203–5
in murine models of allergy 1057, 1060
repertoire 1385–6
tachykinins 447–54, 468–70
antagonists, therapeutic possibilities 471
in asthma 451, 469–70, 494, 495, 496–7, 1085
airway response to 684
degradation by neutral endopeptidase 448, 450, 496, 496–7
functional effects 449–54
localization 447–8
metabolism 448
in pathophysiological conditions (in general) 468–70
receptors (NK) 448–9, 451, 494
agonists 448, 449
antagonists 448, 449, 510
steroids inhibiting gene transcription 620
types 447
see also specific types
tacrolismus, *see* FK506
TAP1/TAP2 117
Taq polymerase 783, 785
thermal inactivation 784
thermal inhibition 784
tar
atopic dermatitis therapy 1584
phototoxic reactions 1620
target cells for T cell cytotoxicity assay 759–60
tartrazine 1281
Tc cells, *see* CD8+ cells
tea dust 915
tears
IgA in 1647–8
laboratory tests 1666
terbutaline 570
pharmacokinetics
oral preparations 574–5
parenteral preparations 575
terfanadine 1332–3
drugs interacting with 427, 1333
rhinitis 1332–3
urticaria (chronic) 1595
terminal deoxynucleotidyl transferase, Ig gene rearrangement and 67
tertiary ammonium compounds 596–7
toxicity/side-effects 602
tests (in diagnosis and assessment of allergic disease) 995–1034, 1272–3
asthma-associated allergens/sensitizers 1354–5
contact allergens 1621–6
principles and interpretation 997–1006, 1272–3
see also specific (types of) test
Tetranychus urticae 913
TGF-β, *see* transforming growth factor-β
Th0 cells 42–3
atopic dermatitis and 1578, 1581
Th1 cells 29–32, 42–5, 351
in allergen-specific immunotherapy 1229, 1231
insect stings and 1702–4
cytokine secretion 351, 1702–4
development/differentiation 43–4, 350
immunosuppressive drug effects 645
macrophage-derived cytokines and selection of 233
roles 42–5
in allergy (in general) 127
in asthma 1367
in atopic dermatitis 1578, 1581
in fetal sensitization 1721–2
in immune response 45, 49
in late asthmatic response 1120
in tolerance 136–7
Th2 cells 29–32, 42–5, 104–9, 351
in allergen-specific immunotherapy 50, 1229, 1230–1
insect stings and 1702–4
cytokine secretion 351, 1702–4
development/differentiation 43–4
regulatory mechanisms 106–8, 350
immunosuppressive drug effects 645
phosphodiesterase inhibitor effects 546
roles and responses of 42–5
of allergen-specific Th2 cells in pathogenesis of allergy 104–5, 141
in allergy (in general) 127
in asthma 48–9, 1120, 1122, 1125, 1371, 1388–9, 1421, 1733
in atopic dermatitis 1578, 1580–1
in atopy 108–9
in fetal sensitization 1721–2
in immune response 45, 49
in nasal late-phase reaction 1148
in tolerance 136–7
theophylline 543
in allergic rabbit 1085, 1086
in asthma 1285, 1435
in chronic asthma 1431, 1435
in late asthmatic response 1115
clinical use 551–2
inflammatory cell effects
basophils 544
eosinophils 547–8
macrophages 547
mast cells 544
monocytes 547
neutrophils 548
platelets 548
T cells 544
plasma extravasation and effects of 551
side-effects/limitations 552
therapy (of allergic disease) 141–2, 1225–57, 1271–90
alternative methods 1288–9
antineuropeptide strategies 471, 1733–4
antineutrophil strategies 210–11
antiplatelet strategies 221–2
drug, *see* drug
IgE network and 92
milestones 21
new strategies (in general) 50–1, 1726–38
principles and practice 1271–90
see also specific conditions and therapeutic modalities and agents
Thermoactinomyces spp. 881
sacchari 881
bagassosis caused by 870
structure/physiology 859
thalpophilus 881
vulgaris 881
thermophilic actinomycetes, *see* Actinomycetes
Thermus aquaticus DNA polymerase, *see* Taq polymerase
Thermus thermophilus DNA polymerase 785–6
Thiabendazole in parasitic pulmonary eosinophilia 1505, 1506
thiopental 1681
Thistle, Russian 852
thixotropy of mucus 716
thoracic deformity, asthmatic children 1457
thrombocyte, *see* platelet
thrombocytopenia
in asthma, in animal models 218
drug-related 1675
thromboxane (in general) 380
biosynthesis 398–400
inhibitors, *see* thromboxane synthetase inhibitors
cellular source 398
receptor antagonists 404, 1731
thromboxane A_2 401–2
asthma and 266, 400–1, 401–2
platelet 216
receptors 400
thromboxane B_2
asthma and 266, 400–1
eosinophil-derived 179
thromboxane synthetase inhibitors
bronchial hyperresponsiveness and effects of 404
late asthmatic response and effects of 1116
thrush, oropharyngeal, steroid-related 625
Thujoidaeae
pollen 850
Thuja plicata dust exposure 915
thymus
fetal nutrition and, in asthma aetiology 1369–70
self-tolerance and the 133
tidal volume, effect on regional aerosol particle deposition 730
tight dermatitis 1625
timber, *see* wood
timothy grass, *see Phleum pratense*
tissue
for immunocytochemistry, preservation 776

for *in situ* hybridization, *see in situ* hybridization
tissue-culture preparation, *in situ* hybridization 770–1
Tla 115
TNF-α, *see* tumour necrosis factor-α
TNT factory, NO_2 emission 1401
tobacco smokers, *see* smokers
tolerance 131–45
antigen-specific
monoclonal antibodies inducing 652–3
oral, induced by feeding antigens 138, 140, 1521–2
B cell 137–8
contact allergens 1613
in rat model 1069–70
T cell, peripheral 133–7
toluene diisocyanate (TDI) 919–20, 1477, 1478
plasma exudation in response to 443
T cells and asthma induced by 1384
tomato 973–4
topical agents
asthma, *see* inhaled agents
rhinitis
decongestants 1329
steroids 1152, 1334, 1335–6
vernal keratoconjunctivitis, steroids and their side-effects 1657
torsades de point 1332
total lung capacity (TLC), asthmatics 677
toxic oil syndrome 1506–7
toxicity
drugs, *see specific types*
hydrogenated soybean phosphatidylcholine liposomes 735
toxins
fungal 867
monoclonal antibodies conjugated with, as immunotoxins 653
Toxocara canis 1505
immune response 1170–1
trachea
asthma involving 672–3
mucus transport 717, 718, 719
segments, contraction in murine airway functional assessment 1061–2
traffic fumes 1401
see also diesel particulates
training, allergy 1262–4
transcription
cytokine genes, *see* cytokines
Ig genes 71
IL-4-induced 99
immunosuppressive drugs interfering with 641–5
in RNA probe manufacture 765
steroid-regulated 618–21
increasing genomic selectivity 633
transcription factors
steroid receptors as 617–18
interacting with other transcription factors 617, 618–19
steroid resistance and 631–2, 1387
transfer RNA as shrimp allergen 970
transformed cells, *see* virus-transformed cells
transforming growth factor-β
asthma and 271
pulmonary alveolar macrophages 231, 232
transgenic models of peripheral T cell tolerance 135
transmembrane 4 superfamily, platelet 217
transmembrane domain receptors, neutrophil 203
transmembrane signalling by membrane-bound Ig 74–5
transplants/grafts
heart, dendritic cells and 123–4
rejection, monoclonal antibodies in prevention of 653
skin, dendritic cells and 123
transporters associated with antigen processing (TAP) 117
treatment, *see* therapy *and specific conditions*
tree(s), classification 1019, 1020
tree pollen 847–52
allergens 799–801
cross-reactivity 1019–20
recombinant, synthesis 816–17
see also individual genera/species
tremor with β_2-adrenoceptor agonists 576
Trethewie, Everton T. 11
triamcinolone acetonide
asthma 629
rhinitis 1335–6
Trichinella spiralis, immune response 1169, 1170
trichlorophthalic anhydride 917
Trichosporon cutaneum 1490
trigeminal nerves branches in nose 1313
trimellitic anhydride 916–17
trinitrotoluene factory, NO_2 emission 1401
Triticeae 842
troleandomycin 630, 1733
tropical eosinophilia 1504–5
tropomyosin as allergen 804–5, 963
True Test 1617–18
trypsin inhibitor, soybean 968
tryptase
inhibitor, sheep model of bronchoconstriction and effects of 1052
mast cell 154
anaphylaxis and 1560
assays and their value 999
asthma and 275, 1372
biological properties 154
cells containing chymase and (M_{TC}) 151
cells containing only (MC_T) 151
drug allergy and 1678
ocular allergy and 1649–50
L-tryptophan and eosinophilia–myalgia syndrome 1507
tuberculin-induced delayed-type hypersensitivity, skin biopsy features 1135
tuberculosis, pulmonary 1497
'tumor' as classical sign of inflammation 440
tumour, carcinoid, asthma distinguished from 1356
tumour necrosis factor-α (cachectin) 346–7
asthma and 161, 269
atopic 46
late response in 1118
basophil 46
IgE synthesis enhanced by 103
mast cell 46, 157–8, 159, 1118
properties/effects 159, 346
pulmonary alveolar macrophages 231
rhinitis and, atopic 46
Turbuhaler 1444–5, 1446, 1447
systemic effects 626
12/23 base pairs, Ig joining signals and 63–4
twin studies (of allergy) 1178–9, 1200–1
asthma 1178–9, 1181, 1200–1
of bronchial hyperresponsiveness 1182
and its relationship to atopy 1181
atopy 1188
eczema 1178
hayfever 1178
tympanometry 1640
tympanostomy 1641
tyrosine kinases and tyrosine phosphorylation
B cell 85
antigen receptors and 75
eosinophil 184–5
neutrophil 207–8

U-46619 402
ubiquitin system 117
UK, *see* United Kingdom
UK-74,505 221, 407–8, 1729
antigen-induced airway responses in rabbit and effects of 1084
ulcerative colitis 1282
leukotrienes and 393
leukotriene biosynthesis inhibitors in 397
ultrasonic nebulizers 1448
ultraviolet light, *see* UV
umbilical vein endothelial cells, human (HUVEC)
allergic disease/inflammation and 251, 253, 254
selectins and 251
VCAM-1 and 250
United Kingdom/Great Britain
pollen
grass, counts (in 1995) 845
seasons 1273
seasonal aeroallergens (in general), calendar 1274
spore, seasonal periodicity 863, 864
training in allergy 1262
United States of America
cockroach distribution/prevalence 942–3
pollen monitoring 841
training in allergy 1263–4
University of Virginia Allergy Clinic instruction for house-dust mite allergen avoidance 893
uridine triphosphate, mucokinetic properties 723
urine, rat, allergens in 910
urticaria (hives) 1279, 1586–607
acute 1586, 1591–2
allergic 1591
non-allergic 1591–2
anatomical considerations 1587
aquagenic 1600
aspirin-induced 1687, 1688
chronic 1587, 1592–6
autoimmune disease and 1588–9
causes 1592–3
clinical features 1592
pathophysiology 1588
treatment 431, 1595–6
classification 1587, 1588
contact, *see* contact urticaria
definition 1586
diagnosis/investigation 1279, 1593–5
differential diagnosis 1592
epidemiology, *see* epidemiology
factitious, *see* dermographism
food allergen-related 1524–5, 1527, 1591
genetics 1587
giant, *see* angioedema
immune system and, *see* immune system
immunotherapy-induced 1254
children 1255
ordinary/in general 1587–96
histopathology 1587
management 1267–8
pathophysiology 1587–8
papular 1601
physical 1596–9
mechanical stimuli 1597–9
pathogenesis 1597
temperature stimuli, *see* cholinergic urticaria; cold urticaria; heat urticaria

solar 1600
urticaria pigmentosa
anaphylaxis and, differentiation 1564
venom immunotherapy 1236
USA, *see* United States of America
UTP, mucokinetic properties 723
UV (ultraviolet)
atopic dermatitis therapy 1584
photopatch test and effects of 1619–20
urticaria on exposure to 1600

V gene segment
heavy chain 65–6
immunoglobulin 63–4
T cell receptor 1380
in asthma/allergic inflammation 1385
V region/domain of Ig 59
antigen binding site 60–1
genes, *see D* gene; *J* gene; *V* gene
idiotypic differences 61
structure 59, 60
see also V(D)J region
vaccines, desensitizing, *see* immunotherapy
vacuum-cleaners 1719
vagus
afferent pathways in lung 595
in asthma, enhanced output from CNS 490
efferent pathways in lung 594–5
variable region of Ig, *see* V region/domain
vascular addressins 1386
vascular bed of lung, peripheral, macrophages in 229
see also microvessels
vascular cell adhesion molecule-1, *see* VCAM-1
vasculature (airway)
anatomy and physiology (normal)
lower airway 1360–1
nose 1305–6, 1312–13
CGRP effects 455–6
endothelium, *see* endothelial cells
engorgement/congestion
in asthma 1420
in nasal late-phase reaction 1142
exercise-induced asthma mechanisms involving 702–3
neuropeptide tyrosine effects 464
permeability 439–46
CGRP and 455–6
in nasal late-phase reaction 1142, 1143
substance P and 494
pituitary adenylate cyclase activating peptide effects 463
tachykinin effects 451–3
VIP effects 460
see also microvessels
vasculature (general and non-airway)
β-adrenoceptors 567
ocular tissues 1645, 1646
vasculitis
systemic/granulomatous, lung disease 1004, 1509–10
urticarial 1600–1
vasoactive intestinal polypeptide 456–61, 468
analogues, therapeutic possibilities 471, 1733
functional effects 458–61
in autonomic nervous system/neurotransmission 458–9, 486–7, 489
localization 456–7
metabolism 457
in pathophysiological conditions 468
in asthma 276, 468, 1733–4
receptors 457–8, 462–3, 487
vasoactive intestinal polypeptide-related peptides 461–3
vasoconstriction
leukotriene-induced 385
neuropeptide tyrosine-induced 464
in seasonal allergic conjunctivitis therapy 1651
vasodilation
CGRP-induced 455
tachykinin-induced 451
VIP-induced 455
vasomotor rhinitis 1295
vasovagal attack vs anaphylaxis 1563–4
VCAM-1 250, 286–7
in allergic inflammation (in general) 291–2
antibodies to, effects 253
expression 251, 1121
in asthma 273, 292, 294, 1373
late response in 1121, 1373
eosinophils and 42, 290–1
in nose
in late-phase reaction 1150
in rhinitis 1318
T cells and 291
VLA-4 interactions with 250, 292
V(D)J region of immunoglobulin 39, 64
rearrangement 69
defective 68
V(D)J region of T cell receptor 1380
asthma/allergic inflammation and 1385
vectors for *in situ* hybridization 765
vecuronium 1679, 1680
vegetable allergens 973, 974
veins, *see* venous system
venoms, stinging insect, *see* Hymenoptera
venous system
airway 1361
nasal 1305, 1313, 1313–14
ocular tissues 1645, 1646
ventilation, maximum voluntary, in identification of exercise-induced asthma 694, 695
ventilation–perfusion ratios, asthmatics 674–6
ventilation pneumonitis (caused by microbial spores in ventilation systems) 867, 868, 1490
humidifier fever distinguished from 1497
venule
high endothelial (HEV), selectins and 245
nasal post-capillary 1305
vernal keratoconjunctivitis, *see* keratoconjunctivitis
very late antigens, *see* VLA
vesarininone 538
vespid (wasp/hornet) 927–8, 931–3
allergens 804, 931–3, 1278, 1693
allergenicity 934–5
anaphylaxis 1554
nomenclature 936
recombinant, synthesis 818
classification 927–8, 1693
see also Hymenoptera
vibratory angioedema 1598–9
vioform 1624–5
VIP, *see* vasoactive intestinal polypeptide
virus infections
atopic dermatitis and 1576
lower respiratory tract
asthma and 1350, 1454–5, 1457, 1712
in early life 1371–2
upper respiratory tract, otitis media and 1633–4, 1636–7, 1638–9
virus-transformed cells
B-cells, as accessory cells for T cell cultures 755–6
T cells, growth 756
viscosity of mucus 715–16, 716
vitamin C and asthma occurrence 1218
vitronectin 315
VLA 248
structure 248
VLA-4 (CD49d/CD29)
animal models of asthma and 292, 1073
eosinophils and 42
late asthmatic response and 1121
leucocyte–endothelial interactions and 273
VCAM-1 interactions with 250, 292
V·m/V·p ratios, asthmatics 670
in tests of mucosal inflammation 671
voice, steroid-related hoarseness 625
voltage-dependent calcium ion channels in airway smooth muscle cells 743–5
physiological regulation 744–5
potassium channel openers and 608, 610
volume (plasma) expansion in circulatory shock 1568
volumetric pollen traps 839
in European Aeroallergen Network 840
vomiting, *see* emesis; emetics
von Leyden, Ernst V. 16
see also Charcot–Leyden crystals
von Pirquet, Clemens 9, 10
V·/Q· rations, asthmatics 674–6

W/W^v mice, mast cell development 150
walls
airway, *see* airway
buildings, spores isolated from 867
warm-up, severity of exercise-induced asthma and effects of 701–2
washing powders (detergents), allergenic enzymes in 915, 1278, 1480
wasp, *see* vespid
waste composting 871
water
inhaled vapour, as mucoactive agent 720–1
loss in airway, as stimulus to exercise-induced asthma 699–700, 702, 703
urticaria on contact with 1600
watermelons 973
wattles 1020
weal(s)
substance P-evoked 451
urticaria
chronic 1592
physical 1597
weal in skin test 1008, 1132
diameter 1008, 1132
in cutaneous late-phase reactions 1132, 1134–5
weather
pollen and 838
grass 846
spore release and 862
see also climate; season
WEB 2086 221–2, 407, 1729
antigen-induced airway responses in rabbit and effects of 1084
late asthmatic response and effects of 1116
weed pollen 882–4, 1020
allergens 801, 1020
cross-reactivity 1020
recombinant, synthesis 817–18
weight at birth, low 1717
West, Geoffrey B. 11, 12
western red cedar, dust exposure 915
wheat allergens 972
occupational exposure 913–14, 1478
wheeze, occurrence
age-related 1211–12
in infants 1452–4

maternal smoking-related 1215
white-faced hornet, *see Dolichovespula maculata*
WHO, allergen standards 829
Willis, Thomas 15, 16
wine 1281
winter feet, atopic 1575
Wiskott–Aldrich syndrome 1577
women, *see* breast-feeding; gender differences; pregnancy; pre-menstrual asthma
wood/timber
dusts, occupational exposure 914–15, 1465
spores associated with
occupational exposure 870
residential places 867, 868
wool alcohols 1624
workplace, allergens and disease in, *see* asthma, occupational; occupational allergens; occupational disease
World Health Organization, allergen standards 829
Wucheria bancrofti 1504
W/Wv mice, mast cell development 150

X-ray radiograph
allergic bronchopulmonary aspergillosis 1502
eosinophilic pneumonia
acute 1508
chronic 1508
extrinsic allergic alveolitis
acute disease 1493
chronic disease 1494
rhinitis 1297
xanthines, *see aminophylline; methylxanthines;* theophylline
xerosis in atopic dermatitis 1574–5, 1578

yeast infections 1022, 1575–6
yellow jackets 927–8
allergen
nomenclature 936
recombinant 818
YM-934, structure 608
Young's syndrome 714, 1294

zafirkulast, *see* ICI 204,219
zaprinast 541
basophil effects 544
clinical use 554
in exercise-induced asthma 552
ZD2138
in allergen-induced asthma 396
in aspirin-induced asthma 397
bronchodilator effect 397
zileuton (A-64077) 1730
allergen-induced asthma 396
aspirin-induced asthma 397
bronchodilator effect 397
chronic asthma 397, 1730
exercise-induced asthma 396
rheumatoid arthritis 398
rhinitis (allergic) 397
zinc, allergy to salts 918–19
zinc fingers of steroid receptors 617
Zoysieaeae 842